D0069987

A

Inhalation route (nebulizer)
- Use Lamira Nebulizer System
- May pretreat with short-acting beta 2 agonists
- Allow to warm to room temperature
- Shake well, pour medication into reservoir
- Press and hold on/off button, mist will flow
- Insert mouthpiece, take slow deep breaths, when done a beep will be heard
- Clean after each use

Intermittent IV INF route
- **Dilute** 500 mg of product/100-200 ml of **IV** D₅W, 0.9% NaCl and **give** over ½-1 hr; dilute D₅W, 0.9% NaCl and **give** over ½-1 hr; dilute insufficient volume to allow inf over 1-2 hr (infants); **flush** after administration with D₅W or 0.9% NaCl; solution is clear or pale yellow; discard if precipitate or dark color develops
- In children, amount of fluid depends on ordered dose; in infants infuse over 1-2 hr
- Give in evenly spaced doses to maintain blood level

Y-site compatibilities: Acyclovir, alatrofloxacin, aldesleukin, alemtuzumab, alfentanil, amifostine, aminophylline, amiodarone, amsacrine, anidulafungin, argatroban, ascorbic acid, atracurium, atropine, aztreonam, benztropine, bivalirudin, bumetanide, buprenorphine, butorphanol, calcium chloride/gluconate, CARBOplatin, caspofungin, ceFAZolin, cefepime, cefonicid, cefotaxime, cefoTEtan, cefOXitin, cefTAZidime, ceftizoxime, cefTRIAXone, cefuroxime, chloramphenicol, chlorproMAZINE, cimetidine, cisatracurium, CISplatin, clindamycin, codeine, cyanocobalamin, cyclophosphamide, cycloSPORINE, cytarabine, DACTINomycin, DAPTOmycin, dexamethasone, dexmedetomidine, digoxin, diltiazem, diphenhydrAMINE, DOBUTamine, DOCEtaxel, DOPamine, doripenem, doxacurium, DOXOrubicin, doxycycline, enalaprilat, ePHEDrine, EPINEPHrine, epirubicin, epoetin alfa, eptifibatide, ertapenem, erythromycin, esmolol, etoposide, famotidine, fentaNYL, filgrastim, fluconazole, fludarabine, fluorouracil, foscarnet, furosemide, gemcitabine, gentamicin, glycopyrrolate, granisetron, hydrocortisone, HYDROmorphone, IDArubicin, ifosfamide, IL-2, imipenem-cilastatin, isoproterenol, ketorolac, labetalol, levofloxacin, lidocaine, linezolid, LORazepam, magnesium sulfate, mannitol, mechlorethamine, melphalan, meperidine, metaraminol, methotrexate, methoxamine, methyldopate, methylPREDNISolone, metoclopramide, metoprolol, metroNIDAZOLE, midazolam, milrinone, mitoXANtrone, morphine, multivitamins, nafcillin, nalbuphine, naloxone, niCARdipine, nitroglycerin, nitroprusside, norepinephrine, octreotide, ondansetron, oxaliplatin, oxytocin, PACLitaxel, palonosetron, pantoprazole, papaverine, PEMEtrexed, penicillin G, pentazocine, perphenazine, PHENobarbital, phenylephrine, phytonadione, piperacillin-tazobactam, potassium chloride, procainamide, prochlorperazine, promethazine, propranolol, protamine, pyridoxine, quinupristin-dalfopristin, ranitidine, remifentanil, riTUXimab, rocuronium, sargramostim, sodium acetate, sodium bicarbonate, succinylcholine, SUFentanil, tacrolimus, teniposide, theophylline, thiamine, thiotepa, ticarcillin/clavulanate, tigecycline, tirofiban, tobramycin, tolazoline, trimetaphan, urokinase, vancomycin, vasopressin, vecuronium, verapamil, vinCRIStine, vinorelbine, voriconazole, warfarin, zidovudine, zoledronic acid

Patient/family education
- Advise patient to contact prescriber if vaginal itching, loose foul-smelling stools, furry tongue occur; may indicate superinfection
- Advise patient to report hypersensitivity: rash, itching, trouble breathing, facial edema and notify prescriber

> **BLACK BOX WARNING:** Monitor for hyper-**kalemia:** *MS:* fatigue, muscle weakness; *NEURO; CARDIAC:* dysrhythmias, hypotension; *NEURO:* paresthesias, confusion; *RESP:* dyspnea, monitor potassium level baseline and each dosage change, hyperkalemia is more common in renal disease, geriatrics, diabetes, if potassium ≥ 5.5 mEq/L immediately notify prescriber

Evaluation
Positive therapeutic outcome
- Absence of signs/symptoms of infection: WBC <10,000/mm³, temp WNL; absence of red draining wounds; absence of earache
- Reported improvement in symptoms of infection

TREATMENT OF OVERDOSE: Withdraw product; administer EPINEPHrine, hemodialysis, exchange transfusion in the newborn; monitor serum levels of product; may give ticarcillin or carbenicillin

---

aMILoride (Rx)
(a-mill'oh-ride)
Midamor
Func. class.: Potassium-sparing diuretic
Chem. class.: Pyrazine

Do not confuse: aMILoride/amLODIPine/amiodarone

ACTION: Inhibits sodium, potassium ATPase ion exchange in the distal tubule, cortical collecting duct resulting in inhibition of sodium reabsorption

High Alert header highlights drugs that pose the greatest risk if administered improperly

⚠ HIGH ALERT

metoprolol (Rx)
(met-oh-proe'lole)
BEtaloc ✦, Lopressor ✦, Lopressor
SR ✦, Nu-Metop ✦, Toprol-XL
Func. class.: Antihypertensive, antianginal
Chem. class.: β₁-Adrenergic blocker

Do not confuse: Lopressor/Lyrica
Toprol-XL/Topamax

Canadian drugs identified with maple-leaf icon

ACTION: Lowers B/P by β-blocking effects; reduces elevated renin plasma levels; blocks β₂-adrenergic receptors in bronchial, vascular smooth muscle only at high doses, negative chronotropic effect

Therapeutic outcome: Decreased B/P, heart rate, AV conduction

Genetic warning icon highlights drugs with genetic contraindications

USES: Mild to moderate hypertension, acute MI to reduce cardiovascular mortality, angina pectoris, New York Heart Association class II, III heart failure, cardiomyopathy

Pharmacokinetics

Absorption	Well absorbed (PO); completely absorbed (IV)
Distribution	Crosses blood-brain barrier, placenta
Metabolism	Liver, extensively ✦ by CYP2D6, some may be poor metabolizers
Excretion	Kidneys, breast milk
Half-life	3-7 hr

Pharmacodynamics

	PO	IV
Onset	15 min	Immediate
Peak	2-4 hr	20 min
Duration	6-19 hr	5-8 hr

CONTRAINDICATIONS

Hypersensitivity to β-blockers, cardiogenic shock, heart block (2nd and 3rd degree), sinus bradycardia, pheochromocytoma, sick sinus syndrome

Precautions: Pregnancy, breastfeeding, geriatric, major surgery, diabetes mellitus, thyroid/renal/hepatic disease, COPD, CAD, nonallergic bronchospasm, HF, bronchial asthma, CVA, children, depression, vasospastic angina

BLACK BOX WARNING: Abrupt discontinuation

DOSAGE AND ROUTES
Hypertension
Adult: PO 50 mg bid, or 100 mg/day; may give 100-450 mg in divided doses; ext rel 25-100 mg qday, titrate at weekly intervals, max 400 mg/day
Child/adolescent 6-16 yr: PO ext rel 1 mg/kg up to 50 mg qday
Geriatric: PO 25 mg/day initially, increase weekly as needed

Myocardial infarction
Adult: IV BOL (early treatment) 5 mg q2min × 3 doses, then 50 mg PO 15 min after last dose and q6hr × 48 hr (late treatment); PO maintenance 50-100 mg bid for 1-3 yr

Heart failure (NYHA class II/III)
Adult: PO ext rel 25 mg qd × 2 wk (class 12.5 mg qd (class III)

Angina
Adult: PO 100 mg/day as a single dose or 2 divided doses, increase qwk as needed, 100 mg ext rel tab daily, max 400 mg/day ext

Migraine prevention (unlabeled)
Adult: PO 25-100 mg bid-qid; 50-200 mg daily (XL)

Available forms: Tabs 25, 50, 100 mg; inj 1 mg/ml; ext rel tabs (tartrate) 100 mg; ext rel tabs (succinate) (XL) 25, 50, 100, 200 mg

Pediatric, geriatric, and other special dosages included throughout

ADVERSE EFFECTS
CNS: *Insomnia, dizziness,* mental changes, hallucinations, depression, anxiety, headaches, nightmares, confusion, fatigue, weakness
CV: HF, *palpitations,* dysrhythmias, cardiac arrest, *hypotension,* bradycardia, pulmonary/peripheral edema, chest pain
EENT: Blurred vision
GI: *Nausea, vomiting,* colitis, cramps, *diarrhea,* constipation, flatulence, dry mouth, *hiccups*
GU: Impotence, urinary frequency
HEMA: Agranulocytosis, eosinophilia, thrombocytopenic purpura
INTEG: Rash, purpura, alopecia, dry skin, urticaria, pruritus
RESP: Bronchospasm, dyspnea, wheezing
ENDO: Hyper/hypoglycemia

Common and life-threatening adverse effects grouped by body system

INTERACTIONS
Individual drugs
Cimetidine: increased metoprolol level
Digoxin, diltiazem, EPINEPHrine, hydrALAZINE, methyldopa prazosin, verapamil: increased hypotension, bradycardia
Insulin: increased hypoglycemia
Dopamine, theophylline: Decreased effect of each

MOSBY'S
DRUG GUIDE
for NURSING
STUDENTS

FOURTEENTH EDITION

Linda Skidmore-Roth, RN, MSN, NP
Consultant
Littleton, Colorado

Formerly, Nursing Faculty
New Mexico State University
Las Cruces, New Mexico
El Paso Community College
El Paso, Texas

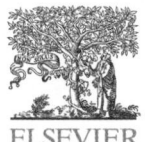

ELSEVIER

Elsevier
3251 Riverport Lane
St. Louis, Missouri 63043

MOSBY'S DRUG GUIDE FOR NURSING STUDENTS,   ISBN: 978-0-323-87489-2
FOURTEENTH EDITION   ISSN: 2213-4409

Notices

Knowledge and best practice in this field are constantly changing. As new research and experience broaden our understanding, changes in research methods, professional practices, or medical treatment may become necessary.

Practitioners and researchers must always rely on their own experience and knowledge in evaluating and using any information, methods, compounds, or experiments described herein. In using such information or methods they should be mindful of their own safety and the safety of others, including parties for whom they have a professional responsibility.

With respect to any drug or pharmaceutical products identified, readers are advised to check the most current information provided (i) on procedures featured or (ii) by the manufacturer of each product to be administered, to verify the recommended dose or formula, the method and duration of administration, and contraindications. It is the responsibility of practitioners, relying on their own experience and knowledge of their patients, to make diagnoses, to determine dosages and the best treatment for each individual patient, and to take all appropriate safety precautions.

To the fullest extent of the law, neither the Publisher nor the authors, contributors, or editors, assume any liability for any injury and/or damage to persons or property as a matter of products liability, negligence or otherwise, or from any use or operation of any methods, products, instructions, or ideas contained in the material herein.

Previous editions copyrighted 2021, 2019, 2017, 2015, 2013, 2011, 2009, 2007, 2005, 2003, 2001, 1999, 1997, 1996.

Library of Congress Control Number: 2021933795

Executive Content Strategist: Sonya Seigafuse
Senior Content Development Manager: Luke Held
Senior Content Development Specialist: Sarah Vora
Publishing Services Manager: Julie Eddy
Senior Project Manager: Jodi M. Willard
Design Direction: Ryan Cook; Bridget Hoette

Printed in the United States of America

Last digit is the print number: 9   8   7   6   5   4   3   2   1

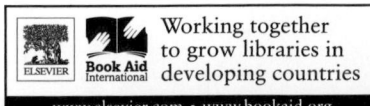

Working together
to grow libraries in
developing countries

www.elsevier.com • www.bookaid.org

Consultants

James Graves, Pharm D
Clinical Pharmacist
Inpatient Pharmacy
University of Missouri Health Center
Columbia, Missouri

Kathleen S. Jordan, DNP, MS, FNP-BC, ENP-BC, ENP-C, SANE-P
Nurse Practitioner
Mid-Atlantic Emergency Medicine Associates
Clinical Assistant Professor
School of Nursing
The University of North Carolina
Charlotte, North Carolina

Janis McMillan, MSN, RN, CNE
Associate Clinical Professor
School of Nursing
Northern Arizona University
Flagstaff, Arizona

Meera K. Shah, PharmD, AAHIVP
Clinical Pharmacist
Saint Louis, Missouri

Travis E. Sonnett, PharmD
Inpatient Pharmacy Supervisor
Mann-Grandstaff VA Medical Center
Spokane, Washington
Residency Program Director
Pharmacy
Washington State University
College of Pharmacy
Spokane, Washington

Wm. Kendall Wyatt, MD, RN, EMT-P
Chief resident Physician
West Virginia University
Charleston Area Medical Center
Charleston, West Virginia

Preface

Mosby's Drug Guide for Nursing Students, fourteenth edition, is the most in-depth handbook available for nursing students! Since its first publication in 1996, more than 100 U.S. and Canadian pharmacists and consultants have reviewed the book's content closely. Today, *Mosby's Drug Guide for Nursing Students* is more up-to-date than ever—with features that make it easy to find critical information fast!

NEW FEATURES
• Over 50 recent FDA-approved drugs for 2021 are located throughout the book and in Appendix A.
• A new appendix with commonly used herbs and natural supplements delivers easy-to-reference information about these commonly mentioned products.
• New Patient Problems subheading under Nursing Considerations provides International Classification for Nursing Practice (ICNP) classifications that are applicable to individual drugs..

NEW FACTS
This edition features thousands of new drug facts, including:
• New drugs and new dosage information
• Newly researched adverse effects
• Updated Black Box Warnings
• The latest precautions, interactions, and contraindications
• IV therapy updates
• Revised nursing considerations
• Updated patient/family education guidelines
• Updates on key new drug research

ORGANIZATION
This handbook is organized into four main sections:
• Individual drug monographs (in alphabetical order by generic name)
• Drug Categories
• Appendixes
• Illustrated mechanisms and sites of action
The guiding principle behind this book is to provide fast, easy access to drug information and nursing considerations. Every detail—from the cover, binding, and paper to the typeface, four-color design, and appendixes—has been carefully chosen with the user in mind. Here's what you'll find in each section of the handbook:

Individual Drug Monographs
This book includes monographs for more than 4000 generic and trade medications—those most commonly administered by students. Common trade names are given for all drugs

regularly used in the United States and Canada, with drugs available only in Canada identified by a maple leaf icon (🍁). Select monographs, important to learn and know for the NCLEX examination, have been identified by a ▓. You'll see drug-specific information within monographs identified with a >>. A special icon highlights drugs that may have genetic contraindications ▧.

Each monograph provides the following information, whenever possible, for safe, effective administration of each drug:

High-alert status: Identifies drugs with the most potential to cause harm to patients if administered incorrectly.

"Tall Man" lettering: Uses the capitalization of distinguishing letters to avoid medication errors and is required by the FDA for drug manufacturers.

Pronunciation: Helps the nurse master complex generic names.

Rx, OTC: Identifies prescription or over-the-counter drugs.

Functional and chemical classifications: Helps the nurse recognize similarities and differences among drugs in the same functional but different chemical classes.

Do not confuse: Presents drug names that might easily be confused within each appropriate monograph.

Action: Describes pharmacologic properties concisely.

Therapeutic outcome: Details all possible results of medication use.

Uses: Lists the conditions the drug is used to treat.

Unlabeled uses: Describes drug uses that may be encountered in practice but are not yet FDA approved.

Dosages and routes: Lists all available and approved dosages and routes for adult, pediatric, and geriatric patients.

Available forms: Includes tablets, capsules, extended release, injectables (IV, IM, SUBCUT), solutions, creams, ointments, lotions, gels, shampoos, elixirs, suspensions, suppositories, sprays, aerosols, and lozenges.

Adverse effects: Groups these reactions by alphabetical body system, with common side effects *italicized* and life-threatening reactions in red type for emphasis.

Contraindications: Lists conditions under which the drug absolutely should not be given.

Precautions: Lists conditions that require special consideration when the drug is prescribed.

Black Box Warnings: Identifies FDA warnings that highlight serious and life-threatening adverse effects.

Pharmacokinetics/pharmacodynamics: Features a quick-reference chart of concise facts of pharmacokinetics (absorption, distribution, metabolism, excretion, half-life) and pharmacodynamics (onset, peak, duration).

Interactions: Lists confirmed drug, food, herb, and lab test interactions.

Nursing considerations: Identifies key nursing considerations for each step of the nursing process: Assessment, Patient Problem, Implementation, Patient/Family Education, and Evaluation, including positive therapeutic outcomes. Instructions for giving drugs by various routes (e.g., IV, PO, IM, SUBCUT, topically, rectally) appear under Implementation, with route subheadings in bold.

Compatibilities: Lists syringe, Y-site, and additive compatibilities and incompatibilities. If no compatibilities are listed for a drug, the necessary compatibility testing has not been done and that compatibility information is unknown. To ensure safety, assume that the drug may not be mixed with other drugs unless specifically stated.

Treatment of overdose: Lists drugs and treatments for overdoses where appropriate.

Drug Categories

The Drug Categories section, following the individual drug monographs, provides general information about the various functional classes to promote learning about the similarities and differences among drugs in the same functional class. It summarizes action, uses, adverse effects, contraindications, precautions, pharmacokinetics, interactions, and nursing considerations for each functional class.

Appendixes

Selected new drugs: Includes comprehensive information on 20+ key drugs approved by the FDA during the last 12 months.

Ophthalmic, nasal, topical, and otic products: Provides essential information for 140 ophthalmic, nasal, topical, and otic products commonly used today, grouped by chemical drug class.

Vaccines and toxoids: Features an easy-to-use table with generic and trade names, uses, dosages and routes, and contraindications for 39 key vaccines and toxoids.

Abbreviations: Lists abbreviations alphabetically with their meanings and explains the five FDA pregnancy categories.

Immunization schedules: Recommended childhood and adolescent immunization schedules.

Standard Precautions: Used in the care of all patients regardless of their diagnosis or disease.

Illustrated mechanisms and sites of action: These 13 detailed, full-color illustrations are added to help enhance the understanding of the mechanism or site of action for the following drugs and drug classes:
- Anticholinergic bronchodilators
- Antidepressants
- Antidiabetic agents
- Antifungal agents
- Antiinfective agents
- Antiretroviral agents
- Benzodiazepines
- Diuretics
- Laxatives
- Narcotic agonist-antagonist analgesics
- Narcotic analgesics
- Phenytoin
- Sympatholytics

Photo atlas of drug administration: This practical resource for students and practitioners lists standard precautions and provides more than 20 full-color illustrations depicting the physical landmarks and administration techniques used for IV, IM, SUBCUT, and ID drug delivery.

Common Herbs

This appendix, new to the fourteenth edition, provides easy-to-reference information for the most commonly used herbs and natural supplements.

The following sources were consulted in the preparation of this edition:

Blumenthal M: *The Complete German Commission E Monographs: Therapeutic Guide to Herbal Medicines,* Austin, 1998, American Botanical Council.

Brunton L, Lazo J, Parker K: *Goodman and Gilman's The Pharmacological Basis of Therapeutics,* ed 13, New York, 2018, McGraw-Hill.

Clinical Pharmacology powered by ClinicalKey [database online], Tampa, Florida, 2016, Elsevier. https://www.clinicalkey.com/pharmacology/. Updated March 2018.

Gahart BL, Nazareno AR: *Intravenous Medications,* ed 36, St. Louis, 2020, Mosby.

Acknowledgments

I am indebted to the nursing and pharmacology consultants who reviewed the manuscript and pages and thank them for their criticism and encouragement. I would also like to thank Sarah Vora, my editor, whose active encouragement and enthusiasm have made this book better than it might otherwise have been. I am likewise grateful to Jodi Willard at Elsevier, and Cassie Carey at Graphic World Inc., for the coordination of the production process and assistance with the development of the new edition, and to Craig Roth for his editorial assistance.

Linda Skidmore-Roth

Contents

INDIVIDUAL DRUG MONOGRAPHS, 1

DRUG CATEGORIES, 1042

APPENDIXES

INDEX, 1173

NEW DRUGS FOR 2022, 1205

EVOLVE WEBSITE CONTENTS

Canadian Resources
- Canadian Controlled Substance Chart
- Canadian Recommended Immunization Schedules for Infants and Children
- High Alert Canadian Medications

Content Changes

Drug Monographs—Additional Monographs

Drug Monographs—Recently Approved

A HIGH ALERT

abacavir (Rx)

(a-ba-ka'veer)

Ziagen

Func. class.: Antiretroviral

Chem. class.: Nucleoside reverse transcriptase inhibitor (NRTI)

ACTION: Inhibitory action against HIV; inhibits replication of HIV by incorporating into cellular DNA by viral reverse transcriptase, thereby terminating the cellular DNA chain

Therapeutic outcome: Decreased symptoms, progression of HIV, increased CD4 counts, decreased viral load

USES: In combination with other antiretroviral agents for HIV-1 infection

Pharmacokinetics

Absorption	Rapid/extensive
Distribution	50% protein binding, extravascular space, then erythrocytes
Metabolism	Extensively, to inactive metabolite by liver
Excretion	Kidneys, feces
Half-life	1½-2 hr

Pharmacodynamics

Unknown

CONTRAINDICATIONS

BLACK BOX WARNING: Hypersensitivity, moderate to severe hepatic disease, lactic acidosis

Precautions: Pregnancy, breastfeeding, child <3 mo, granulocyte count <1000/mm³ or Hgb <9.5 g/dl, severe renal disease, impaired hepatic function, ✋ HLA B5701 (Black, Caucasian, Asian patients), abrupt discontinuation; Guillain-Barré syndrome, immune reconstitution syndrome, MI, obesity, polymyositis

DOSAGE AND ROUTES

Adult/adolescent ≥16 yr: PO 300 mg bid or 600 mg daily with other antiretrovirals

Adolescent <16 yr/child ≥3 mo: PO 8 (oral solution) mg/kg bid or 16mg/kg q day, max 300 mg bid with other antiretrovirals; tablets 14-19 kg: 150 mg BID or 300 mg q day; 20-24 kg: 150 mg AM and 300 mg PM or 450 mg q day; ≥ 25 kg: 300 mg BID or 600 mg q day

Hepatic dose

Adult: (Child-Pugh A 5-6) PO oral/sol 200 mg bid; moderate to severe hepatic disease, do not use

Available forms: Tabs 300 mg; oral sol 20 mg/ml

ADVERSE EFFECTS

CNS: *Fever, headache, insomnia*

GI: *Nausea, vomiting, diarrhea, anorexia,* hepatotoxicity, hepatomegaly with steatosis

INTEG: *Rash*, urticaria

META: Lactic acidosis

MISC: Fatal hypersensitivity reactions, fat redistribution, immune reconstitution

INTERACTIONS

Individual drugs

Do not coadminister with abacavir-containing products, ribavirin, interferon

Alcohol: increased abacavir levels; do not use with alcohol

Ribavirin: possible lactic acidosis

Methadone: decreased levels of methadone, may require higher dose of methadone

Tipranavir: decreased abacavir levels

Drug/lab test

Increased: serum glucose, triglycerides, AST, ALT, amylase, CK

NURSING CONSIDERATIONS

Assessment

• Assess for symptoms of HIV and possible infection, increased temp baseline and throughout treatment

BLACK BOX WARNING: Assess for lactic acidosis (elevated lactate levels, increased liver function tests) and severe hepatomegaly with steatosis; discontinue treatment and do not restart; women and the obese are at greater risk for lactic acidosis; monitor serum lactate, liver function studies that may be increased, palpate liver for enlargement

BLACK BOX WARNING: Assess for fatal hypersensitivity reactions: fever, rash, nausea, vomiting, fatigue, cough, dyspnea, diarrhea, abdominal discomfort; those with ✋ HLA-B 5701 are at greater risk, obtain genetic testing for HLA-B 5701 before beginning treatment; treatment should be discontinued and not restarted; register at the Abacavir Hypersensitivity Registry (800-270-0425)

• Fat redistribution: May occur during treatment, buffalo hump, breast growth, moon face, trunk obesity

BLACK BOX WARNING: Assess for pancreatitis: abdominal pain, nausea, vomiting, elevated liver enzymes; product should be discontinued because condition can be fatal

• Monitor CBC, differential, platelet count qmo; withhold product if WBC is <4000/mm³ or platelet count is <75,000/mm³; notify prescriber of results; monitor viral load and CD4 counts during treatment, perform hepatitis B virus (HBr) screening to confirm correct treatment

> **BLACK BOX WARNING: Hepatotoxicity:**
> Monitor liver function tests before, during therapy (bilirubin, AST, ALT, amylase, alkaline phosphatase, creatine phosphokinase, creatinine prn or qmo)

• **Immune reconstitution syndrome:** may occur anytime during treatment; response to CMV, mycobacterium avium infection

Implementation
PO route
• Reduce dose in hepatic disease, use oral solution
• May give without regard to food q12hr around the clock
• Give in combination with other antiretrovirals with or without food
• Store in cool environment; protect from light, oral solution stored at room temperature; do not freeze

Patient problem
Infection (uses)

Patient/family education
• **Advise patient to report signs of infection:** increased temp, sore throat, flulike symptoms; to avoid crowds and those with known infections; to carry emergency ID with condition, products taken; do not take other products that contain abacavir
• Instruct patient to report signs of anemia: fatigue, headache, faintness, shortness of breath, irritability
• Advise patient to report bleeding; avoid use of razors or commercial mouthwash
• Inform patient that product is not a cure but will control symptoms
• Inform patient that major toxicities may necessitate discontinuing product
• **Pregnancy/breastfeeding:** Register pregnant patients with the Antiretroviral Pregnancy Registry 1-800-258-4263, use only if benefits outweigh fetal risk, identify if pregnancy is planned or suspected, avoid breastfeeding; consider the use of contraception during treatment
• Caution patient to avoid OTC products or other medications without approval of prescriber, that other products may be necessary to prevent infections, and that product is taken with other products for HIV
• That body fat redistribution may occur, not to share product
• Caution patient not to have any sexual contact without use of a condom; needles should not be shared; blood from infected individual should not come in contact with another's mucous membranes
• Give Medication Guide and Warning Card; discuss points on guide
• Advise patient to notify prescriber if skin rash, fever, cough, shortness of breath, GI symptoms occur; advise all health care providers that allergic reactions have occurred with this product
• To use exactly as prescribed, not to drink alcohol, not to stop or change dose, not to use with other products unless approved by prescriber

Evaluation
Positive therapeutic outcome
• Increased CD4 count
• Decreased viral load
• Decreased symptoms, progression of HIV

> **⚠ HIGH ALERT**
>
> ## abacavir/dolutegravir/lamivudine
> Ah-back′ ah-veer/doe-loo-teg′ ra-vir/la-mi-vyoo-deen
> **Triumeq**
> *Func. class.:* Antiretroviral
> *Chem. class.:* Nucleoside reverse transcriptase inhibitor (NRTI)

ACTION: Inhibitory action against HIV; inhibits replication of HIV by incorporating into cellular DNA by viral reverse transcriptase, thereby terminating the cellular DNA chain

Therapeutic use: Decreased symptoms, progression of HIV

USES: HIV

Pharmacokinetics

Abacavir

Absorption	83%
Distribution	Extravascular space, erythrocytes
Metabolism	Liver
Excretion	1% unchanged urine
Half-life	1.5 hr

A

Dolutegravir

Absorption	Unknown
Distribution	CSF, protein binding 99%
Metabolism	Liver by UGT1A1, CYP3A4
Excretion	Unchanged feces, metabolites urine; ⚥ poor metabolizers, increased levels
Half-life	14 hr

Lamivudine

Absorption	86% adult, 66% child
Distribution	Extravascular space, CSF
Metabolism	Liver minimal
Excretion	Unchanged urine

Pharmacodynamics

Onset	Unknown
Peak	Unknown
Duration	Up to 24 hr

CONTRAINDICATIONS

BLACK BOX WARNING: Hypersensitivity, moderate-to-severe hepatic disease, lactic acidosis

Precautions:
Pregnancy, breastfeeding, child <3 mo, impaired hepatic function, ⚥ HLA B5701 (Black, Caucasian, Asian patients), abrupt discontinuation; immune reconstitution syndrome, MI, obesity, polymyositis

DOSAGE AND ROUTES
Adult: PO 1 tablet (600 mg abacavir, 50 mg dolutegravir, 300 mg lamivudine) q day; if given with efavirenz, fosamprenavir/ritonavir, tipranavir/ritonavir, carbamazepine, or rifampin, administer an additional 50 mg dolutegravir separate by 12 hr

Available forms: Tablets 600 mg abacavir, 50 mg dolutegravir, 300 mg lamivudine

ADVERSE REACTIONS
CNS: Fever, headache, malaise, insomnia, paresthesia, peripheral neuropathy
CV: MI
GI: *Nausea, vomiting, diarrhea,* anorexia, cramps, abdominal pain, *increased AST, ALT,* hepatotoxicity, hepatomegaly with steatosis
INTEG: *Rash,* urticaria
META: Lactic acidosis
MISC.: Fatal hypersensitivity reactions, fat redistribution, immune reconstitution syndrome

INTERACTIONS:
Abacavir
Individual drugs
Do not coadminister with abacavir-containing products: ribavirin, interferon
Alcohol: increased abacavir levels; do not use with alcohol
Ribavirin: possible lactic acidosis
Methadone: decreased levels of methadone

Dolutegravir
Individual drugs
Efavirenz, RifAMPin tenofovir, tipranavir/ritonavir: decreased levels of each product

Drug classifications
Antacids, buffered products, laxatives/sucralfate, oral iron products, oral calcium products, buffered products: decreased effect of dolutegravir

Drug/herb
St. John's wort: avoid concurrent use

Lamivudine
Individual drugs
AMILoride, dofetilide, entecavir, metFORMIN, memantine, procainamide, trospium, trimethoprim/sulfamethoxazole: increased level of lamiVUDine
Emtricitabine: do not combine, duplication
Other products that cause pancreatitis or increase pancreatitis
Sulfamethoxazole/trimethoprim: increase: lamotrigine level

Drug/lab test
Increased: glucose, triglycerides, AST, ALT, amylase, CK

NURSING CONSIDERATIONS
Assessment
• Assess for symptoms of HIV and possible infection, increased temperature, flulike symptoms

BLACK BOX WARNING: Assess for lactic acidosis (elevated lactate levels, increased liver function tests) and severe hepatomegaly with steatosis; discontinue treatment and do not restart; women and the obese are at greater risk for lactic acidosis

• **Fat distribution:** May occur during treatment, buffalo hump, breast growth, moon face, trunk

BLACK BOX WARNING: Assess for fatal hypersensitivity reactions: fever, rash, nausea, vomiting, fatigue, cough, dyspnea, diarrhea, abdominal discomfort; those with HLA-B 5701 are at greater risk, obtain genetic testing for HLA-B 5701 before beginning treatment; treatment should be discontinued and not restarted; register at the Abacavir Hypersensitivity Registry (800-270-0425)

> **BLACK BOX WARNING: Assess for pan-creatitis:** abdominal pain, nausea, vomiting, elevated liver enzymes; product should be discontinued because condition can be fatal

• Monitor viral load and CD4 counts during treatment; perform hepatitis B virus (HBr) screening to confirm correct treatment

> **BLACK BOX WARNING: Hepatotoxicity:** Monitor liver function tests before and during therapy (bilirubin, AST, ALT, amylase, alkaline phosphatase, creatine phosphokinase, creatinine prn or qmo)

• **Immune reconstitution syndrome:** may occur anytime during treatment; response to CMV, mycobacterium avium infection
• **Peripheral neuropathy:** Assess for burning, tingling in extremities; if severe, product may need to be discontinued

Patient problem
Infection (uses)
Risk for injury (adverse reactions)

Implementation
PO route
• Use 2 hrs prior to or 6 hrs after drugs that reduce absorption like antacids
• May give without regard to food

Patient/family education
• **Infection:** Advise patient to report increased temperature, sore throat, flulike symptoms; to avoid crowds and those with known infections; to carry emergency ID with condition, products taken; do not take other products that contain abacavir

> **BLACK BOX WARNING: Lactic acidosis:** Teach patient to notify health care professional immediately of fatigue, muscle weakness, trouble breathing, fever, rash, nausea, vomiting, cough, diarrhea, abdominal discomfort

> **BLACK BOX WARNING: Hepatotoxicity:** Teach patient to report dark urine, clay-colored stools, yellow eyes and skin, no appetite, abdominal pain

• Inform patient that product is not a cure but will control symptoms
• Inform patient that major toxicities may necessitate discontinuing product
• Teach patient that body fat redistribution may occur
• Advise patient not to share product
• Caution patient to avoid OTC products or other medications without approval of prescriber, that other products may be necessary to prevent infections, and that product is taken with other products for HIV
• Caution patient not to have any sexual contact without use of a condom; needles should not be shared; blood from infected individual should not come into contact with another's mucous membranes
• Give Medication Guide and Warning Card; discuss points on guide
• **Immune reconstitution syndrome and hypersensitivity reactions:** Advise patient to immediately report skin rash, fever, cough, shortness of breath, GI symptoms; advise all health care providers that allergic reactions have occurred with this product
• Teach patient to use exactly as prescribed, not to drink alcohol, not to stop or change dose
• Advise patient that regular followup exams and blood-work will be needed
• **Pregnancy/breastfeeding:** Pregnant patients should be registered with the Antiretroviral Pregnancy, registry (1-800-258-4263), identify if pregnancy is planned or suspected, avoid breastfeeding; consider the use of contraception during treatment

Evaluation
Positive therapeutic outcome
• Increased CD4 count
• Decreased viral load
• Decreased symptoms, progression of HIV

> **⚠ HIGH ALERT**
>
> ## abemaciclib
> (uh-beh′muh-sy′klib)
> **Verzenio**
> *Func. class.:* Antineoplastic
> *Chem. class.:* Protein kinase inhibitor

ACTION: Inhibits cyclin-dependent kinases 4, 6, a protein kinase inhibitor needed for cancer cell growth

Therapeutic use: Decreased spread of cancer

USES: HER 2-negative advanced or metastatic breast cancer after endocrine therapy and prior chemotherapy as monotherapy or in combination with fulvestrant

Pharmacokinetics

Absorption	45%
Distribution	Extensively to tissues, protein binding 96.3%
Metabolism	Liver by CYP3A4 to active metabolites
Excretion	Feces (80%), urine (3%)
Half-life	18.3 hr

A

Pharmacodynamics

Onset	Unknown
Peak	8 hr
Duration	Up to 24 hr

CONTRAINDICATIONS
Hypersensitivity

Precautions: Breastfeeding, contraception requirement, pregnancy, pregnancy testing, breastfeeding, hepatic disease, hepatotoxicity, infertility, reproductive risk, thromboembolic disease

DOSAGE AND ROUTES
Adult: PO (Monotherapy) 200 mg bid until disease progression or unacceptable toxicity; **(with fulvestrant)** 150 mg bid continue until disease progression or unacceptable risk; **(with CYP3A4 strong inhibitors)** 100 mg bid, adverse reactions are present and dose at 100 mg lower to 50 mg bid

Hepatic dose
Adult PO (Child–Pugh C) reduce dose to 150 mg q day (with fulvestrant), 200 mg q day (monotherapy); CYP3A4 inhibitors 100 mg q dat (with fulvestrant or monotherapy)

Available forms: Tablets 50, 100, 150, 200 mg

ADVERSE EFFECTS:
CNS: Dizziness, drowsiness, fatigue, fever
CV: Venous thromboembolism
GI: Nausea, vomiting, diarrhea, anorexia, stomatitis, abdominal pain, weight loss, hepatotoxicity
GU: Infertility
INTEG: *Rash, alopecia*
MS: Arthralgia
HEMA: Anemia, leukopenia, neutropenia, thrombocytopenia
Misc.: Infection, cough

INTERACTIONS
Drug classifications
CYP3A4 inhibitors, strong or moderate (itraconazole, ketoconazole): increase—abemaciclib effect, avoid using together
CYP3A4 inducers, strong or moderate (rifampin): decrease—abemaciclib effect, avoid using together

NURSING CONSIDERATIONS
Assessment
• **Diarrhea:** at first sign of loose stools, start antidiarrheal therapy, increase oral fluids; **grade 1** no dosage modification; **grade 2** suspend therapy until resolves to grade 1, if persists hold dose until resolves to grade 1 or lower, resume at lower dose, **grade 3 or**

4 with hospitalization, suspend until resolves to grade 1 or lower, resume at another lower dose
• **Neutropenia:** CBC baseline then q 2 wk for the first 2 mo, then monthly for the next 2 mo and as needed
• **Venous thromboembolism:** monitor for signs and symptoms of thrombosis, pulmonary embolism
• **Pulmonary embolism:** monitor for chest pain that is worse when breathing deeply or coughing, coughing up blood, dizziness, fainting, tachypnea, rapid or irregular heartbeat, shortness of breath
• **Hepatotoxicity:** monitor liver function tests before, during therapy (bilirubin, AST, ALT) q 2 wk X first 2 mo, then monthly for next 2 mo; if **grade 1** (ULN X 3), **grade 2** (3.1-5 X ULN) without increase in bilirubin above 2 X ULN no change; if **grade 2** persists hold; after resolution to grade 1 or less, resume at next lower dose; **grade 2 or 3** (3.1-20 X ULN) with bilirubin greater than 2 X ULN, discontinue

Patient problem
Infection (uses)
Risk for injury (adverse reactions)

Implementation
PO route
• May give without regard to food
• Swallow tablets whole, do not crush, chew, break; do not use if cracked or broken
• If dose is missed, do not replace missed dose, resume with next scheduled daily dose

Patient/family education
• **Infection:** Advise patient to report increased temp, sore throat, flulike symptoms; to avoid crowds and those with known infections; to carry emergency ID with condition and products taken
• **Hepatotoxicity:** Teach patient to report dark urine, clay-colored stools, yellow eyes and skin, no appetite, abdominal pain
• **Diarrhea:** Teach patient to start antidiarrheal therapy at first sign of loose stools, increase fluids, notify health care provider
• Inform patient that major toxicities may necessitate discontinuing product
• **Venous thromboembolism:** Teach patient to report immediately chest pain, worse when breathing or coughing, coughing up blood, dizziness, fainting, tachypnea, rapid or irregular heartbeat, shortness of breath, pain, swelling of extremity with redness and warmth, discoloration including a bluish color
• Caution patient to avoid OTC products or other medications without approval of prescriber

and that other products may be necessary to prevent infections

- Give "Patient information" to read
- Teach patient to use exactly as prescribed, not to stop or change dose
- Advise patient that regular follow-up exams and blood-work will be needed
- **Pregnancy/breastfeeding:** Identify if pregnancy is planned or suspected, or if breastfeeding, not to be used in pregnancy or breastfeeding, to use contraception during and for at least 3 wk after last dose

Evaluation
Positive therapeutic outcome

- Decrease in size, spread of cancer cells

> ⚠ **HIGH ALERT**
>
> ## abiraterone
> **Zytiga**
> (a-bir-a′ter-one)
> *Func Class.:* Antineoplastic
> *Chem Class.:* Androgen inhibitor

ACTION: Converted to abiraterone, which inhibits CYP17, the enzyme required for androgen biosynthesis; androgen-sensitive prostate cancer responds to treatment that decreases androgens

Therapeutic outcome: Decreases spread of malignancy

USES: Metastatic castration-resistant prostate cancer in combination with prednisone

Pharmacokinetics

Absorption	Food increases effect; give on empty stomach; increased effect in hepatic disease
Distribution	99% protein binding
Metabolism	Converted to abiraterone (active metabolite)
Excretion	88% (feces), 5% (urine)
Half-life	Mean terminal half-life 12 hr

Pharmacodynamics

Onset	Unknown
Peak	Unknown
Duration	Unknown

CONTRAINDICATIONS
Pregnancy, women, children, breastfeeding

Precautions
Adrenal insufficiency, cardiac disease, MI, heart failure, hepatic disease, hypertension, hypokalemia, infection, surgery, ventricular dysrhythmia, stress, trauma

DOSAGE AND ROUTES
Adult Males: PO 1000 mg q day with predniSONE 5 mg bid; **with strong CYP3A4 inducers** 1000 mg BID

Hepatic dose
Adult Males: (Child-Pugh B) PO 250 mg qday with predniSONE

Available forms: Tab 250, 500 mg

ADVERSE EFFECTS
CV: Angina, dysrhythmia exacerbation, chest pain, edema, hypertension
ENDO: Adrenocortical insufficiency
GI: Diarrhea, dyspepsia, hepatotoxicity
GU: Increased urinary frequency, nocturia
META: Adrenocortical insufficiency, hyperbilirubinemia, hypertriglyceridemia, hypokalemia, hypophosphatemia
MS: Arthralgia, myalgia, fracture
RESP: Cough, upper respiratory infection
SYST: Infection

INTERACTIONS
Drug classifications
CYP3A4 inducers (carBAMazepine, phenytoin, rifampin, rifabutin, rifapentine, PHENobarbital): decreased abiraterone effect
CYP2D6 substrates (dextromethorphan, pioglitazone, thioridazine): increased action, dose of these products should be reduced, avoid concurrent use if possible

Drug/Lab
Increase: ALT, AST, bilirubin, triglycerides
Decrease: Potassium, phosphate, testosterone, lymphocytes

Drug/Food
Must be taken on an empty stomach, increased product effect if taken with food

NURSING CONSIDERATIONS
Assessment

- Prostate cancer: Monitor prostate-specific antigen (PSA), serum potassium, serum bilirubin
- **Hepatotoxicity:** Monitor liver function tests (AST/ALT) baseline and every 2 wk for 3 mo and monthly thereafter in those with no known hepatic disease; interrupt treatment in patients without known hepatic disease at baseline who develop ALT/AST >5 times ULN or total bilirubin >3 times ULN; in baseline moderate hepatic disease, measure ALT, AST, and bilirubin before the start of treatment, every week for the first month, every 2 weeks for the following 8 wk, and monthly thereafter; if elevations in ALT and/ or AST >5 times ULN or total bilirubin >3 times ULN occur in patients with baseline

moderate hepatic impairment, discontinue and do NOT restart. Measure serum total bilirubin, AST, and ALT if hepatotoxicity is suspected. Elevations of AST, ALT, bilirubin from baseline should prompt more frequent monitoring.

• Monitor B/P, pulse, edema, if hypertensive, control symptoms

• **Monitor musculoskeletal pain, joint swelling, discomfort:** Assess for arthritis, arthralgia, joint swelling, and joint stiffness, some severe. Muscle discomfort that includes muscle spasms, musculoskeletal pain, myalgia, musculoskeletal discomfort, and musculoskeletal stiffness may be relieved with analgesics.

• Assess for signs and symptoms of adrenocorticoid insufficiency (anorexia, nausea, vomiting, fatigue, weight loss), corticosteroids may be needed during times of stress, surgery, trauma; monthly for hypertension, hypokalemia, and fluid retention

• **Pregnancy/breastfeeding:** Do not use in pregnancy, breastfeeding

Patient problem
Lack of knowledge (teaching)

Implementation
PO route

• Give whole, on empty stomach 2 hrs before or 1 hr after meals with full glass of water; do not crush, break, chew

• Women who are pregnant or may become pregnant should not touch tabs without gloves

• Storage of tabs at room temperature

Patient/family education

• Teach patient that women must not come in contact with tabs, wear gloves if product needs to be handled, males need to wear condoms and use of another form of contraception if partner is pregnant, not to be used in pregnancy, breastfeeding

• Instruct patient to report chest pain, swelling of joints, burning/pain when urinating

• Teach patient to take 2 hr before or 1 hr after meals, swallow whole, take with water, to use with predniSONE, if dose is missed contact health care professional

• Advise patient not to stop abruptly without prescriber's consent

• Teach patient not to use with other medications, herbs, supplements without prescriber approval

• Teach patient: Some formulations may vary and are not interchangeable

Evaluation
Positive therapeutic outcome

• Decreasing spread, progression of prostate cancer

RARELY USED

⚠ HIGH ALERT

acalabrutinib
Calquence
Func. class.: Antineoplastic

USES: For the treatment of mantle cell lymphoma

Dosage and routes
For the treatment of mantle cell lymphoma (MCL) in patients who have received at least 1 prior therapy
Adult: PO 100 mg bid (approximately 12 hr apart) until disease progression.

acetaminophen (PO/rectal) (OTC)/IV (Rx) (Paracetamol)
(a-seat-a-mee'noe-fen)
222AF ✤, Abenol ✤, ACET ✤, Aceta, Acetab ✤, Aminofen, Apacet, APAP, Apra, Atasol ✤, Children's Feverall, Acephen, Infant Feverall, Exdol ✤, Fortolin ✤, Genapap, Mapap, Maranox, Meda, Neopap, Novo-Gesic ✤, Oraphen-PD, Pediaphen ✤, Pediatrix ✤, Q-Pap, Q-Pap Children's, Rapid Action Relief ✤, Redutemp, Ridenol, Robigesic ✤, Rounox ✤, Silapap, Taminol ✤, Tapanol, Tempra ✤, T-Painol, Tylenol, Uni-Ace ✤, XS Pain Reliever

Acetaminophen (IV)
Ofirmue ✤
Func. class.: Nonopioid analgesic, antipyretic
Chem. class.: Nonsalicylate, paraaminophenol derivative

Do not confuse: Anacin/Aspirin 3/Anacin-3

ACTION: May block pain impulses peripherally that occur in response to inhibition of prostaglandin synthesis; does not possess antiinflammatory properties; antipyretic action results from inhibition of prostaglandins in the CNS (hypothalamic heat-regulating center)

Therapeutic outcome: Decreased pain, fever

USES: Mild to moderate pain or fever; arthralgia, dental pain, dysmenorrhea, headache, myalgia, osteoarthritis

Pharmacokinetics

Absorption	Well absorbed (PO), variable (RECT), complete (IV)
Distribution	Widely distributed; crosses placenta in low concentrations
Metabolism	Liver 85%-95%; metabolites are toxic at high levels
Excretion	Kidneys—metabolites, breast milk
Half-life	3-4 hr

Pharmacodynamics

	PO	RECT	IV
Onset	½-1 hr	½-1 hr	Rapid
Peak	1-3 hr	1-3 hr	30-120 min
Duration	3-4 hr	3-4 hr	3-4 hr

CONTRAINDICATIONS

Hypersensitivity to this product, aspartame, saccharin, tartrazine, phenacetin

Precautions: Pregnancy, breast-feeding, geriatric, anemia, renal/hepatic disease, chronic alcoholism

> **BLACK BOX WARNING:** Hepatotoxicity

DOSAGE AND ROUTES

Adult and child >12 yr: PO/RECT 325-650 mg q4-6hr prn, max 4 g/day; **weight ≥50 kg IV** 1000 mg q6hr or 650 mg q4hr prn, max single dose 1000 mg, minimum dosing interval 4 hr; **weight <50 kg IV** 15 mg/kg/dose q6hr or 12.5 mg/kg/dose q4hr, max single dose 15 mg/kg minimum dosing interval 4 hr, max 75 mg/kg/day from all sources, **ext rel** 650-1300 mg q8hr as needed, max 4 g/day
Child ≥2 yr and <50 kg: IV 15 mg/kg/dose q6hr or 12.5 mg/kg/dose q4hr, max single dose 15 mg/kg, minimum dosing interval 4 hr, max 75 mg/kg/day from all sources

Renal dose

Adult: IV CCr <30 ml/min reduce dose and prolong interval; CCr <10 ml/min PO/IM/IV minimal interval q8h

Available forms: Rectal supp 120, 325, 650 mg; chewable tabs 80, 160 mg; caps 500 mg; elix 120, 160, 325 mg/5 ml; tabs 160, 325, 500, 650 mg; sol for injection 1000 mg/100 ml; disintegrating tab 80, 160 mg; oral drops 80 mg/10.8 ml; liquid 500 mg/5 ml, 160 mg/5 ml, 1000 mg/30 ml, 80 mg/ml; ext rel tabs 650 mg

ADVERSE EFFECTS

GI: Nausea, vomiting, abdominal pain; hepatotoxicity, hepatic seizure (overdose)
GU: Renal failure (high, prolonged doses)
NS: Agitation (child) (IV); headache, fatigue, anxiety (IV)
Resp: dyspnea (IV), atelectasis (IV, child)
CV: Hyper-hypotension (IV)
HEMA: neutropenia, hemolytic anemia (long-term use), pancytopenia
INTEG: Rash, urticaria, injection site pain
SYST: Stevens-Johnson syndrome
TOXICITY: Cyanosis, anemia, neutropenia, jaundice, pancytopenia, CNS stimulation, delirium followed by vascular collapse, seizures, coma, death

INTERACTIONS

Individual drugs

Alcohol, carBAMazepine, dasatinib mipomersen, diflunisal, imatinib, isoniazid, lamoTRIgine, rifabutin, rifampin, zidovudine: increased hepatotoxicity
Colestipol, cholestyramine: decreased absorption of acetaminophen
Lomitapide: increase effect of lomitapide, consider a lower dose
Nitric oxide, pilocarpine: increased methoglobinemia, avoid concurrent use
Decrease: zidovudine, lamoTRIgine effect
Avoid use with salicylates
Warfarin: hypoprothrombinemia; long-term use, high doses of acetaminophen

Drug classifications

Barbiturates, hydantoins: decreased effect; increased hepatotoxicity, monitor for hepatotoxicity
NSAIDs, salicylates: increased renal adverse reactions

Drug/herb

St. John's wort: increased hepatotoxicity due to acetaminophen metabolism

Drug/lab test

Increased: LFTs, potassium, bilirubin, LDH, pro-time
Decreased: Hgb/Hct, WBC, RBC, platelets; albumin, magnesium, phosphate (pediatrics)

NURSING CONSIDERATIONS

Assessment

• **Pain/fever:** Assess for location, duration, type, aggravating/alleviating factors, intensity; assess for diaphoresis, fever; baseline and periodically
• **Monitor liver function studies:** AST, ALT, bilirubin, creatinine before therapy if long-term therapy is anticipated; may cause hepatic toxicity at doses >4 g/day with chronic use

---

• Monitor renal function studies: BUN, urine creatinine, occult blood; albumin indicates nephritis, check I&O ratio; decreasing output may indicate renal failure (long-term therapy)

• Monitor blood studies: CBC, PT if patient is on long-term therapy

• **Assess for chronic poisoning:** rapid, weak pulse; dyspnea; cold, clammy extremities; report immediately to prescriber

> **BLACK BOX WARNING: Assess hepatotoxicity:** dark urine, clay-colored stools, yellowing of skin and sclera; itching, abdominal pain, fever, diarrhea if patient is on long-term therapy; doses > 4 gm/day, may require liver transplant, patients malnourished or use alcohol chronically are at higher chance of hepatotoxicity

• **Potentially fatal hypersensitivity/allergic reactions:** rash, urticaria; Stevens-Johnson syndrome, may occur when beginning treatment or any other dose

• **Pregnancy/breastfeeding:** Use cautiously in pregnancy, breastfeeding (PO), use only if clearly needed (IV)

Patient problems
Pain (uses)
Risk for impaired thermoregulation (uses)

Implementation
PO route
• **Do not confuse:** 2 × 325 (650 mg), with 650 mg ER tab

• Administer to patient crushed or whole; chewable tabs may be chewed; do not crush or chew EXT REL product

• Give with food or milk to decrease gastric symptoms; give 30 min before or 2 hr after meals; absorption may be slowed

• Shake susp well; check all product concentrations carefully; check elixir, liquid, suspension concentration carefully; susp and caps are bioequivalent

Intermittent IV infusion route
• No further dilution needed, do not add other medications to vial or infusion device

• For doses equal to single vial, a vented IV set may be used to deliver directly from vial; for doses less than a single vial, withdraw dose and place in an empty sterile syringe, plastic IV container, or glass bottle, infuse over 15 mins

• Discard unused portion, once seal is broken or vial penetrated or transferred to another container, give within 6 hr

• Check IV dose carefully to prevent dosing errors

Y-site incompatibilities: acyclovir, chlorpromazine, diazepam, metronidazole

Additive incompatability: Do not admix

Rectal route
• Store suppositories <80° F (27° C)

Patient/family education

> **BLACK BOX WARNING:** Teach patient not to exceed recommended dosage; the elixir, liquid, and suspension come in several concentrations, read label carefully; acute poisoning with liver damage may result; acute toxicity includes symptoms of nausea, vomiting, and abdominal pain; prescriber should be notified immediately

• Inform patient that toxicity may occur when used with other combination products

• Advise patient not to use with alcohol, OTC products, or herbals without prescriber approval

• **Teach patient to recognize signs of chronic overdose:** bleeding, bruising, malaise, fever, sore throat

• Inform patient that urine may become dark brown as a result of phenacetin (metabolite of acetaminophen)

• Tell patient to notify prescriber for pain or fever lasting more than 3 days, not to be used in <2 yr unless approved by prescriber

• **Hypersensitivity:** Teach patient to stop product, notify provider if rash occurs

• **Pregnancy/breastfeeding:** May be used when breastfeeding short-term

Evaluation
Positive therapeutic outcome
• Decreased pain, use pain scoring
• Decreased fever

TREATMENT OF OVERDOSE:
Product level, gastric lavage; administer oral acetylcysteine to prevent hepatic damage (*see acetylcysteine monograph*)

---

acetylcholine ophthalmic
See Appendix B

---

acetylcysteine (Rx)
(a-se-teel-sis'tay-een)
Acetadote, Cetylev
Func. class.: Mucolytic; antidote—acetaminophen
Chem. class.: Amino acid L-cysteine

ACTION: Decreases viscosity of secretions in respiratory tract by breaking disulfide links of mucoproteins; serves as a substrate of glutathione, which is necessary to inactivate toxic metabolites in acetaminophen overdose

Therapeutic outcome: Decreased hepatotoxicity from acetaminophen overdose (PO); decreased viscosity of mucus in respiratory disorders (inh)

USES: Acetaminophen toxicity, bronchitis, cystic fibrosis, COPD, atelectasis, meconium ileus

Unlabeled Uses: PO: Prevention of radio-contrast renal reactions

Pharmacokinetics

Absorption	Extensive (PO), locally (inh)
Distribution	Protein binding 83%
	Peak ½-1 hr
Metabolism	Liver
Excretion	Kidneys
Half-life	5.6 hr (adult), 11 hr (newborn)

Pharmacodynamics

	PO	IV	INH
Onset	unknown	unknown	1 min
Peak	up to 60 mins	unknown	5-10 mins
Duration	4 hr	unknown	unknown

CONTRAINDICATIONS
Hypersensitivity

Precautions: Pregnancy, breastfeeding, hypothyroidism, Addison's disease, CNS depression, brain tumor, asthma, renal/hepatic disease, COPD, psychosis, alcoholism, seizure disorders, bronchospasms, asthma, anaphylactoid reactions, fluid restriction, weight <40 kg, increased intracranial pressure, status asthmaticus

DOSAGE AND ROUTES
Mucolytic
Adult and child 1-12 yr: Instill 1-2 ml (10%-20% sol) q2-8hr prn, or 3-5 ml (20% sol) or 6-10 ml (10% sol) tid or qid; **nebulization (face, mask, mouthpiece, tracheostomy)** 1-10 ml of a 20% sol or 2-20 ml of a 10% sol q2-6hr; **nebulization (tent, croupette)** may require large dose, up to 300 ml

Diagnostic bronchial lab studies
Adult/child: Nebulizer 2-3 uses of 1-2 ml or a 20% solution or 2-4 ml of a 10% solution

Tracheostomy care
Adult/child: Instill 1-2 ml of a 10% or 20% solution directly into the tracheostomy q1-4hr

Acetaminophen toxicity
Adult and child: PO 140 mg/kg, then 70 mg/kg q4hr × 17 doses to total 1330 mg/kg; loading dose 150 mg/kg over 60 min, then 50 mg/kg over 4 hr, then 100 mg/kg over 16 hr

Prevention of radio contrast-induced renal reactions
Adult PO 600 mg BID x 2 days, starting day before radiocontrast

Available forms: Oral sol 10%, 20%; inj 20% (200 mg/ml); effervescent tab for solution 500, 2500 mg

ADVERSE EFFECTS
CNS: Chills, *dizziness, drowsiness,* fever, headache
CV: Flushing, hypotension, tachycardia
EENT: *Rhinorrhea,* tooth damage
GI: Anorexia, constipation, diarrhea, hepatotoxicity, *nausea,* stomatitis, vomiting
INTEG: Clamminess, fever, pruritus, rash, urticaria
MISC: Anaphylaxis, angioedema, unpleasant odor
RESP: Bronchospasm, burning, chest tightness, cough, hemoptysis, dyspnea

INTERACTIONS
Individual drugs
Activated charcoal: Do not use with acetylcysteine

NURSING CONSIDERATIONS
Assessment
Mucolytic use
• **Assess cough:** type, frequency, character, including sputum; bronchospasm
• **Assess characteristics, rate, rhythm of respirations,** increased dyspnea, sputum; discontinue if bronchospasm occurs; ABGs for increased CO_2 retention in asthma patients
• Monitor VS, cardiac status including checking for dysrhythmias, increased rate, palpitations
Antidotal use
• Use within 8 hr for best result, 24 hr of acetaminophen toxicity, give within 10 hr of acetaminophen to minimize hepatotoxicity
• Assess liver function tests, acetaminophen levels, PT, glucose, electrolytes, BUN, creatinine; inform prescriber if dose is vomited or vomiting is persistent; 150 mg/kg may be toxic, check acetaminophen level q4hr; provide adequate hydration; decrease dosage in hepatic encephalopathy
• Assess for nausea, vomiting, rash; notify prescriber if these occur
• **Hypersensitivity:** Anaphylaxis may occur with IV dose; if present, stop infusion, treat, restart; assess for dyspnea, swelling of face, lips, tongue; rash; itching

---

⚠ Nurse Alert   ✴ Key NCLEX® Drug   >> Drug Specifics

• **Pregnancy/breastfeeding:** Use only if clearly needed, cautious use in breastfeeding, excretion unknown

Patient problems
Impaired airway clearance (uses)
Lack of knowledge of medication (teaching)

Implementation
• Give decreased dosage to geriatric patients; their metabolism may be slowed; give gum, hard candy, frequent rinsing of mouth for dryness of oral cavity
• Use only if suction machine is available

PO route (Antidotal use)
• Give within 24 hr; dilute 10% or 20% sol to a 5% sol with diet soda; may use water if giving via gastric tube; dilution of 10% sol 1:1, 20% sol 1:3; use within 1 hr, store open undiluted solution refrigerated ≤96 hr, repeat dose if vomited within 1 hr

PO route and effervescent tablets
• Dissolve in 100 ml of water for 50 mg/ml (1-19 kg weight), in 150 mL (20-59 kg weight) or 300 mg/ml (≥ 60 kg weight)

Direct intratracheal INSTILL
• Use ½-1 hr before meals for better absorption to decrease nausea; only after patient clears airway by deep breathing, coughing
• Give by syringe 2-3 doses of 1-2 ml of 10%-20% sol up to q1hr
• Store in refrigerator: use within 96 hr of opening
• Provide assistance with inhaled dose: bronchodilator if bronchospasm occurs; wash face and rinse mouth after use to remove sticky feeling
• Use decreased dose in geriatric, metabolism may be slowed
• Use mechanical suction if cough insufficient to remove excess bronchial secretions
• Store in refrigerator; use within 96 hr of opening

IV route
21-hr regimen:
• **Loading dose: dilute** 150 mg/kg in 200 ml D_5W; maintenance dose no. 1 **dilute** 50 mg/kg in 500 ml D_5W; maintenance dose no. 2 **dilute** 100 mg/kg in 1000 ml D_5W
• **Give** loading over 15 min; **give** maintenance dose no. 1 over 4 hr; **give** maintenance dose no. 2 over 16 hr; **give** sequentially without time between doses

Incompatibilities: Rubber, metals, stability with other products unknown

Patient/family education
Mucolytic use
• Inform patient that foul odor and smell may be unpleasant
• Instruct patient to clear airway for inhalation

• Teach patient to report vomiting, as dose may need to be repeated
Acetaminophen toxicity
• Explain reason for product, expected result

Evaluation
Positive therapeutic outcome
• Absence of purulent secretions when coughing (mucolytic use)
• Clear lung sounds bilaterally (mucolytic use)
• Absence of hepatic damage (acetaminophen toxicity)
• Decreasing blood toxicology (acetaminophen toxicity)

---

aclidinium
(a'kli-din'ee-um)
Tudorza Genuair ✦, Tudorza Pressair
Func. class.: Anticholinergic, bronchodilator
Chem. class.: Synthetic quaternary ammonium compound

ACTION: Anticholinergic action, inhibits the M3 receptor in bronchials

Therapeutic use: Bronchodilation and ease of breathing

USES: Long-term maintenance treatment of bronchospasm in COPD, emphysema, chronic bronchitis, not indicated for initial treatment of acute episodes

Pharmacokinetics
Absorption	6%
Distribution	Unknown
Metabolism	Hydrolyzed to inactive metabolites
Excretion	Feces (20-30%), urine (55-65%)
Half-life	5-8 hr

Pharmacodynamics
Onset	Up to 1 hr
Peak	2-4hr
Duration	Up to 12 hr

CONTRAINDICATIONS
Hypersensitivity to this product or milk protein

Precautions: Narrow angle glaucoma, bladder neck obstruction, hypersensitivity to atropine, breastfeeding, pregnancy

DOSAGE AND ROUTES
Adult: Inhalation 400 mcg (1 inhalation) bid

Available forms: Dry powder metered dose inhaler 400 mcg/actuation

ADVERSE REACTIONS
CNS: Headache
EENT: Narrow angle glaucoma increased
RESP: Paradoxical bronchospasm
GU: Urinary retention
MISC: Hypersensitivity, angioedema, anaphylaxis, rash, itching, pruritus

INTERACTIONS
Drug classifications
Anticholinergics: Increased effect

NURSING CONSIDERATIONS
Assessment
• **Respiratory status:** Assess breathing patterns, breath sounds, b/p, pulse, respiratory rate, baseline and 1-2 hr after use, avoid use in bronchospasm, hold if dyspnea, wheezing occurs after dose
• **Hypersensitivity:** Angioedema; anaphylaxis; assess for rash, itching, swelling of face, lips, which may be more severe if there was a past reaction to milk proteins, or atropine; discontinue immediately; notify provider

Patient problems
Impaired breathing (uses)
Impaired airway clearance (uses)

Implementation
Inhalation route
• Use q 12 hr
• Give adrenergics first if prescribed, then this product, then corticosteroids, wait 5 mins between each

Patient/family education
• Caution patient to avoid OTC, Rx, herbals, supplements without discussing with provider
• Discuss how to use the product, that the product should be used every 12 hr, and to avoid smoking and getting powder in eyes
• Teach patient to use exactly as prescribed, not to stop or change dose
• Advise patient that regular follow-up exams will be needed as well as pulmonary function tests
• **Pregnancy/breastfeeding:** Identify if pregnancy is planned or suspected, or if breastfeeding

Evaluation
Positive therapeutic outcome
• Improved ease of breathing

acyclovir (Rx)
(ay-sye′kloe-veer)
Avirax ✦, Sitavig, Xerese ✦, Zovirax
Func. class.: Antiviral
Chem. class.: Purine nucleoside analog

Do not confuse: Zovirax/Zyvox/Valtrex/Zostrix

ACTION: Converted to acyclovir monophosphate by virus-specific thymidine kinase, then further converted to acyclovir triphosphate by other cellular enzymes

Therapeutic outcome: Decreased amount and time of healing of lesions

USES: Mucocutaneous herpes simplex virus, herpes genitalis (HSV-1, HSV-2), varicella infections, herpes zoster, herpes simplex encephalitis

Pharmacokinetics

Absorption	Minimal (PO)
Distribution	Widely distributed, crosses placenta; CSF concentration 50% plasma; protein binding 9%-33%
Metabolism	Liver, minimal
Excretion	Kidneys, 95% unchanged
Half-life	2.0-3.5 hr, increased in renal disease; child 2-3 hr; neonates up to 4 hr

Pharmacodynamics

	PO	IV	Buccal
Onset	Unknown	Rapid	unknown
Peak	2.5-3.3 hr	Infusion's end	8 hr
Duration	Unknown	8 hr	unknown

CONTRAINDICATIONS
Hypersensitivity to this product or valacyclovir, milk protein (buccal)

Precautions: Pregnancy, breastfeeding, renal/hepatic disease, electrolyte imbalance, dehydration, neurologic disease; hypersensitivity to famciclovir, ganciclovir, penciclovir, valganciclovir, obesity

DOSAGE AND ROUTES
Base dose in obese patients on ideal body weight, not actual weight

Herpes simplex (recurrent)
Adult: PO 400 mg 3 ×/day for 5 days or 200 mg 5 ×/day × 5 days

---

Adult and child >12 yr (use ideal weight in obesity): IV INF 5 mg/kg over 1 hr q8hr × 5 days
Infant >3 mo/child <12 yr: IV INF 10 mg/kg q8hr × 7 days; if HIV infected 5-10 mg/kg q8hr (moderate to severe)

Neonate: IV infusion 10mg/kg q8hr × 10 days, may use higher dose

Genital herpes initial episode

Adult: PO 400 mg tid or 200 mg 5 times per day × 7-10 days, may extend treatment if healing is not complete after 10 days; topical 5 times per day; IV 5 mg/kg q 8 h or 750 mg/m2/day divided q 8 h × 5-7 days

Genital herpes, episodic treatment

Adult: PO 400 mg tid or 800 bid × 5 days or 800 mg × 2 days, initiate within 1 day of lesion onset

Genital herpes, suppression therapy

Adult: PO 400 mg bid for up to 12 mo

Genital herpes, initial limited, mucocutaneous HSV in immunocompromised patients, non-life-threatening

Adult and child ≥12 yr: TOP cover lesions q3hr 6 times/day

Herpes simplex encephalitis

Adult: IV 10 mg/kg over 1 hr q8hr × 10 days
Child 3 mo-12 yr: IV 20 mg/kg q8hr × 10 days
Child birth-3 mo: IV 10–15 mg/kg q 8 h × 14–21 days
Neonates, premature: IV 10 mg/kg q 12 h × 14–21 days

Herpes labialis

Adult and child ≥12 yr: TOP apply cream 5 times a day × 4 days, start as soon as symptoms appear; buccal 50 mg as a single dose in upper gum region within 1 hr after prodromal symptoms and before cold sore formation

Herpes zoster (shingles): immuno-compromised patients

Adult and adolescent: PO 800 mg q4hr 5 times/day × 7–10 days; IV 10–15 mg/kg q 8 h × 10–14 days
Infant and child <12 yr: IV 10 mg/kg q8hr × 7-10 days

Herpes zoster (shingles): immuno-competent patient

Adult: PO 800 mg q4hr 5 times/day × 7-10 days; start within 48-72 hr of rash onset; IV 10 mg/kg q8hr × 7 days

Varicella (chickenpox):

Adult/Child ≥2 yr: PO 20 mg/kg (max 800 mg) PO 4 times per day × 5 days, start within 24 hr of rash onset

Mucosal/cutaneous herpes simplex infections in immunosuppressed patients

Adult and child >12 yr: IV 5 mg/kg q8hr × 7 days
Infant >3 mo/child <12 yr: IV 10 mg/kg q8hr × 7 days
Adult: Top 0.5 in ribbon of 5% ointment for every 4 square in q 3 hr (6 times/day) × 7 days

Renal dose

Adult and child: PO/IV CCr >50 ml/min 100% dose q8hr; CCr 25-50 ml/min 100% dose q12hr; CCr 10-24 ml/min 100% dose q24hr; CCr 0-10 ml/min 50% of dose q24hr
Base dose in obese patients on ideal body weight, not actual body weight

Available forms: Caps 200 mg; tabs 400, 800 mg; powder for inj 500, 1000 mg; sol for inj 50 mg/ml; oral susp 200 mg/5 ml; ointment/cream 5%; buccal tab 50 mg

ADVERSE EFFECTS

CNS: Tremors, confusion, hallucinations, seizures, *dizziness, headache*
EENT: Gingival hyperplasia
GI: *Nausea, vomiting, diarrhea,* increased ALT, AST, abdominal pain
GU: Crystalluria, vaginitis, moniliasis, acute renal failure, purpura, hemolytic uremic syndrome (immunocompromised patient)
INTEG: Rash, urticaria, pruritus, pain or phlebitis at **IV** site, unusual sweating, alopecia, Stevens-Johnson syndrome, acne, hives
MS: Joint pain, leg pain, muscle cramps

INTERACTIONS
Individual drugs

Aminoglycosides: increased nephrotoxicity
Entecavir, PEMEtrexed, tenofovir, theophylline: increased concentration of each product
Probenecid: increased neurotoxicity, nephrotoxicity
Phenytoin, Valproic acid: decreased action of valproic acid, monitor drug level
Zidovudine, IT methotrexate: increased CNS side effects

NURSING CONSIDERATIONS
Assessment

• **Monitor for signs of infection,** type of lesions, area of body covered, purulent drainage frequency
• Check I&O ratio; report hematuria, oliguria, fatigue, weakness; may indicate nephrotoxicity; check for protein in urine during treatment
• Monitor liver studies: AST, ALT
• **Monitor renal studies:** urinalysis, protein, BUN, creatinine, CCr; increased BUN, creatinine indicates renal failure and nephrotoxicity

• Assess allergies before treatment, reaction of each medication; place allergies on chart in bright red letters; allergic reaction: burning, stinging, swelling, redness, rash, vulvitis, pruritus
• **Pregnancy/breastfeeding:** Identify if pregnancy is planned or suspected, use cautiously in pregnancy, avoid breastfeeding if lesions are around breasts

Patient problems
Infection (uses)
Impaired skin integrity (uses)

Implementation
PO route
• May be taken orally before infection occurs or when itching or pain occurs, usually before eruptions
• Do not break, crush, or chew caps
• Give with food to lessen GI symptoms; may give without regard to meals with 8 oz of water
• Store at room temperature in dry place
• Must be taken at equal intervals around the clock
• Shake susp before use
• **Buccal:** use on the same side at the herpes labialis lesion, after removing tab from blister, place rounded side of tab to the upper gum above incisor tooth, hold in place for 30 sec, once adhered, the tab will dissolve, if tab fell off within 6 hr, reposition the same tab

IV route
• Provide increased fluids to 3 L/day to decrease crystalluria, most critical during first 2 hr after IV infusion
Intermittent IV infusion route
• Reconstitute with 10 ml sterile water for injection/500 mg of product (50 mg/ml) or 1 g/20 mL of product; shake; **further dilute** in 50-125 ml compatible sol, shake well use within 12 hr; **give** over at least 1 hr (constant rate) by infusion pump to prevent nephrotoxicity; do not reconstitute with sol containing benzyl alcohol or parabens; check infusion site for redness, pain, induration; rotate sites
• Lower dosage in acute or chronic renal failure
• Store at room temp for up to 12 hr after reconstitution; if refrigerated, sol may show a precipitate that clears at room temperature; yellow discoloration does not affect potency

Y-site compatibilities: Alemtuzumab, allopurinol, amikacin, aminophylline, amphotericin B cholesteryl, amphotericin B liposome, ampicillin, anidulafungin, argatroban, atracurium, bivalirudin, buprenorphine, busulfan, butorphanol, calcium chloride/gluconate, CARBOplatin, ceFAZolin, cefonicid, cefotaxime, cefOXitin, cefTAZidime, ceftizoxime, cefTRIAXone, cefuroxime, chloramphenicol, cholesteryl sulfate complex, cimetidine, clindamycin, dexamethasone sodium phosphate, dimenhyDRINATE, DOXOrubicin, doxycycline, erythromycin, famotidine, filgrastim, fluconazole, gentamicin, granisetron, heparin, hydrocortisone sodium succinate, HYDROmorphone, imipenem-cilastatin, LORazepam, magnesium sulfate, melphalan, methylPREDNISolone sodium succinate, metoclopramide, metroNIDAZOLE, multivitamin, nafcillin, oxacillin, PACLitaxel, penicillin G potassium, PENTobarbital, perphenazine, piperacillin, potassium chloride, propofol, ranitidine, remifentanil, sodium bicarbonate, teniposide, theophylline, thiotepa, ticarcillin, tobramycin, trimethoprim-sulfamethoxazole, vancomycin, vasopressin, voriconazole, zidovudine

Topical route
• Use finger cot or glove to cover all lesions completely, do not get in eyes, wash hands after use

Patient/family education
• Teach patient that product may be taken orally before infection occurs or when itching or pain occur, usually before eruptions; that partners need to be told that patient is infected; they can become infected, so condoms must be worn to prevent reinfections
• Tell patient to report sore throat, fever, fatigue; may indicate superinfection; that product must be taken at equal intervals around the clock to maintain blood levels for duration of therapy
• Teach patient not to use topical products on lesions, spreading may occur
• Adequate intake of fluids (2 L) to prevent deposits in kidneys, more likely to occur with rapid administration or in dehydration
• Teach female patients with genital herpes to have regular Pap smears to prevent undetected cervical cancer
• **Pregnancy/breastfeeding:** Teach patient to advise prescriber if pregnancy is planned or suspected or if breastfeeding
• **Topical:** Not to use on or around eyes, to use enough ointment to cover lesions q 3 h, 6 x/day × 7 days, use finger cot or gloves to apply

Evaluation
Positive therapeutic outcome
• Absence of itching, painful lesions
• Crusting and healed lesions
• Decreased pain with herpes zoster
• Decreased symptoms of chicken pox

TREATMENT OF OVERDOSE:
Discontinue product, hemodialysis

adalimumab (Rx)
(add-a-lim'yu-mab)
Amjevita, Humira, Humira Pen
Func. class.: Antirheumatic agent
Chem. class.: immunomodulator, anti-TNF

Do not confuse: Humira/Humalin/
Humalog/Humira Pen/Humapen Memoir

ACTION: A form of human IgG1 monoclonal antibody specific for human tumor necrosis factor (TNFα); elevated levels of TNFα are found in patients with rheumatoid arthritis

Therapeutic outcome: Decreased pain, inflammation in joints, better ROM

USES: Moderate to severe active rheumatoid arthritis in patients ≥18 years of age who have not responded to other disease-modifying agents, JRA, psoriatic arthritis, Crohn's disease, moderate-severe plaque psoriasis, ankylosing spondylitis, noninfectious uveitis

Pharmacokinetics

Absorption	65% (subcut)
Distribution	synovial fluid
Metabolism	Unknown
Excretion	Unknown
Half-life	2 wk

Pharmacodynamics (inflammation decreased)

Onset	Up to 24 wk
Peak	Unknown
Duration	2 wk

CONTRAINDICATIONS
Hypersensitivity, breastfeeding, use of anakinra, abatacept

Precautions: Pregnancy, children, geriatric, CNS demyelinating disease, lymphoma, latent TB, HF, hepatitis B carriers, mannitol hypersensitivity, latex allergy, neoplastic disease, TB

> **BLACK BOX WARNING:** Active infections, risk of lymphomas/leukemias

DOSAGE AND ROUTES
Rheumatoid arthritis, ankylosing spondylitis, psoriatic arthritis
Adult: SUBCUT 40 mg every other wk or every week if not combined with methotrexate

Juvenile rheumatoid arthritis (JRA) Ⓐ
Child ≥2 yr/adolescent ≥30 kg: SUBCUT 40 mg every other wk
Child ≥2 yr/adolescent ≥15 kg to <30 kg: SUBCUT 20 mg every other wk
Child ≥2 yr/adolescent 10 kg to <15 kg: SUBCUT 10 mg every other wk

Crohn's disease
Adult: SUBCUT 160 mg given as 4 inj on day 1, or 2 inj on days 1 and 2, then 80 mg at wk 2 and 40 mg every other wk, starting at wk 4
Child > 6 yr and ≥40 kg (88 lb) SUBCUT 160 mg day 1 (as 4 injections 40 mg or 40 mg as 2 injections) × 2 days then 80 mg after 2 wk (day 15 then 40 mg q other wk, day 29
Child > 6 yr and 17-40 kg (37-88 lb) SUBCUT 80 mg day 1 (as 2 injections then 40 mg after 2 wk (day 15) then 20 mg q other week (day 29)

Plaque psoriasis/noninfectious uveitis
Adult: SUBCUT 80 mg baseline as 2 inj, then 40 mg every other week starting 1 wk after initial dose (plaque psoriasis)

Available forms: Inj 40 mg/0.8 ml; 20 mg/0.4 ml (pediatric)

ADVERSE EFFECTS
CNS: Headache, Guillain-Barré syndrome multiple sclerosis
CV: Hypertension, HF
EENT: Sinusitis, optic neuritis
GI: Abdominal pain, nausea, hepatic damage, GI bleeding
HEMA: Leukopenia, thrombocytopenia, neutropenia
INTEG: Rash, *inj site reaction*
MISC: Flulike symptoms, risk of cancer, risk of infection (TB, invasive fungal infections, other opportunistic infections); may be fatal, Stevens-Johnson syndrome, anaphylaxis, hyperlipidemia
RESP: URI, pulmonary fibrosis, bronchitis

INTERACTIONS
Individual drugs
Anakinra, abatacept: do not use together, serious infections may occur
Azathioprine, methotrexate: Increased HSTCL
Rilonacept: increase serious infections

Drug classifications
Live-virus vaccines: do not give concurrently; immunization should be brought up to date before treatment

> **BLACK BOX WARNING:** Other TNF blockers: increased serious infections

Drug/lab test
Increased: ALT, cholesterol, lipids

NURSING CONSIDERATIONS
Assessment
• **Rheumatoid arthritis:** assess for pain, stiffness, ROM, swelling of joints during treatment
• Check for inj site pain, swelling, redness; usually occur after 2 inj (4-5 days) use cold compress to relieve pain/swelling
• **Crohn's disease/ulcerative colitis:** assess bowel pattern, cramping, abdominal pain, bleeding

> **BLACK BOX WARNING:** Assess for infections, fever, flulike symptoms, dyspnea, change in urination, redness/swelling around wounds, stop treatment if present, some serious infections, including sepsis, may occur; patients with active infections should not be started on this product

• May reactivate hepatitis B in chronic carriers, may be fatal

> **BLACK BOX WARNING:** Assess for latent TB prior to therapy; treat before starting this product

• Assess for anaphylaxis, latex allergy; stop therapy if lupuslike syndrome develops
• Assess for blood dyscrasias: CBC, differential periodically

> **BLACK BOX WARNING:** Assess for neoplastic disease (lymphomas/leukemia); in children, adolescents, hepatosplenic T-cell lymphoma is more likely in adolescent males with Crohn's disease or ulcerative colitis

• **Pregnancy/breastfeeding:** Use only if clearly needed, no well-controlled studies, cautious use in breastfeeding, excreted in breast milk

Patient problems
Pain (uses)
Impaired mobility (uses)
Infection (adverse reactions)

Implementation
SUBCUT route
• Do not admix with other sol or medications, do not use filter, protect from light
• Don't inject in bruised, red, tender areas

Patient/family education
• Teach patient about self-administration if appropriate: inj should be made in thigh, abdomen, upper arm; rotate sites at least 1 inch from old site; do not inject in areas that are bruised, red, hard, review provided medication guide with patient
• Advise patient that if medication is not taken when due, inject next dose as soon as remembered and inject next dose as scheduled

• Advise patient not to take any live-virus vaccines during treatment
• Instruct patient to report signs of infection, allergic reactions, immediately
• Teach patient to do regular skin assessments and report any changes in the skin to provider since skin cancers do occur
• Teach patient to refrigerate the product, to dispose of needles and equipment as instructed
• Teach patient to advise health care professionals of OTC, Rx, herbals, supplements taken
• Advise health care professional if pregnancy is planned or suspected or if breastfeeding; to register if pregnant at 1-877-311-8972
Prefilled pen use:
• Using alcohol swab, clean area (do not use if solution is discolored or contains particulate), the pen is activated by removing gray cap, pinch skin and place at 90-degree angle and press button, hold until solution is inserted, remove, use cotton ball for a few seconds, dispose of properly

Evaluation
Positive therapeutic outcome
• Decreased inflammation, pain in joints, decreased joint destruction

---

⚠ HIGH ALERT

adenosine (Rx)
(ah-den'oh-seen)
Adenocard, Adenoscan ✤
Func. class.: Antidysrhythmic—miscellaneous
Chem. class.: Endogenous nucleoside

ACTION: Slows conduction through AV node, can interrupt reentry pathways through AV node, and can restore normal sinus rhythm in patients with paroxysmal supraventricular tachycardia (PSVT), decreases cardiac oxygen demand decreasing hypoxia

Therapeutic outcome: Normal sinus rhythm in patients diagnosed with SVT or diagnosis of perfusion defect

USES: PSVT, as a diagnostic aid to assess myocardial perfusion defects in CAD; Wolff-Parkinson-White (WPW) syndrome

Pharmacokinetics

Absorption	Complete bioavailability
Distribution	Erythrocytes, cardiovascular endothelium
Metabolism	Liver, converted to inosine and adenosine monophosphate
Excretion	Kidneys
Half-life	10 sec

Pharmacodynamics	
Onset	Rapid
Peak	Unknown
Duration	1-2 min

CONTRAINDICATIONS
Hypersensitivity, 2nd- or 3rd-degree heart block, AV block, sick sinus syndrome, bradycardia

Precautions: Pregnancy, breastfeeding, children, geriatric, asthma, atrial flutter, atrial fibrillation, ventricular tachycardia, bronchospastic lung disease, symptomatic bradycardia, bundle branch block, heart transplant, unstable angina, COPD, hypotension, hypovolemia, vascular heart disease, CV disease

DOSAGE AND ROUTES
Converting paroxysmal supraventricular tachycardia to sinus rhythm (Adenocard)
Adult and child >50 kg: IV BOL 6 mg; if conversion to normal sinus rhythm does not occur within 1-2 min, give 12 mg by rapid IV BOL; may repeat 12 mg dose again in 1-2 min
Infant and child <50 kg: IV BOL 0.05 mg/kg; if not effective, increase dose by 0.05-0.1 mg/kg q2min to a max of 0.3 mg/kg/dose

(Adenoscan) Diagnostic Use
Adult and Child >50 kg: 140 mcg/kg/min × 6 min (0.84 mg/kg total)

Available forms: 3 mg/ml solution for injection

ADVERSE EFFECTS
CNS: Light-headedness, dizziness, arm tingling, numbness, headache; seizures, stroke (adenoscan)
CV: Chest pain/pressure, atrial tachydysrhythmias, sweating, palpitations, hypotension, *facial flushing*, AV block, cardiac arrest, ventricular dysrhythmias, atrial fibrillation
GI: *Nausea*, metallic taste
RESP: *Dyspnea, chest pressure*, hyperventilation, bronchospasm (asthmatics)
EENT: Blurred vision
MS: Back pain

INTERACTIONS
Individual drugs
Caffeine, theophylline: decreased effects of adenosine, dose may need to be increased
CarBAMazepine: increased heart block
Digoxin, verapamil: increased ventricular fibrillation, monitor ECG
Dipyridamole: increased effects of adenosine, dose may need to be reduced
Smoking: increased tachycardia

Drug/herb
Ginger: increased effect
Green tea, guarana: decreased effect

NURSING CONSIDERATIONS
Assessment
• **Assess cardiopulmonary status:** pulse, respiration, ECG intervals (PR, QRS, QT); check for transient dysrhythmias (PVCs, PACs, sinus tachycardia, AV block)
• Assess respiratory status: rate, rhythm, lung fields for crackles, watch for respiratory depression; bilateral crackles may occur in HF patient; if increased respiration, increased pulse occurs, product should be discontinued
• Assess CNS effects: dizziness, confusion, paresthesias; product should be discontinued
• **Pregnancy/breastfeeding:** Identify if pregnancy is planned or suspected or if breastfeeding, do not breastfeed

Patient problems
Impaired cardiac function (uses)

Implementation
IV, direct (bolus) route
• Give IV BOL undiluted; give 6 mg or less by rapid inj; if using an IV line, use port near insertion site, flush with 0.9% NaCl (20 ml), then elevate arm, reduce dose if given via central line
• Store at room temperature; sol should be clear; discard unused product
Intermittant infusion (diagnostic)
• Uses 30 ml vial undiluted (3 mg/ml), give at 140 mcg/kg/min over 6 min (total 0.84 mg/kg), thallium-201 should be given after 3 min of infusion

Patient/family education
• Tell patient to report facial flushing, dizziness, sweating, palpitations, chest pain, IV discomfort
• Advise to change positions slowly to prevent orthostatic hypertension
• Teach patient to avoid products that are xanthines before image study
• **Pregnancy/breastfeeding:** Teach patient to advise prescriber if pregnancy is planned or suspected or if breastfeeding, do not breastfeed

Evaluation
Positive therapeutic outcome
• Normal sinus rhythm
• Diagnosis of perfusion defect

⚠ HIGH ALERT

ado-trastuzumab (Rx)

(a'doe-tras-tooz'ue-mab)

Kadcyla

Func. class.: Antineoplastic-biologic response modifier

Chem. class.: Signal transduction inhibitor (STI), humanized anti-HER2 antibody

Do not confuse: ado-trastuzumab/ trastuzumab

ACTION: Humanized ❦ anti-HER2 monoclonal antibody that is linked to DM1, a small molecule microtubular inhibitor. Once the antibody is bound to the ❦ HER2 receptor, the complex is internalized and the DM1 is released to bind with tubulin to lead to apoptosis

Therapeutic outcome: Decrease in size of tumors

USES: Breast cancer, metastatic with overexpression of HER2, in patients who previously received trastuzumab and a taxane separately or in combination

Pharmacokinetics

Absorption	Unknown
Distribution	93% protein binding
Metabolism	Liver by CYP3A4
Excretion	
Half-life	4 days

Pharmacodynamics

Onset	unknown
Peak	unknown
Duration	unknown

CONTRAINDICATIONS

Hypersensitivity to this product, Chinese hamster ovary cell protein, pregnancy

> **BLACK BOX WARNING:** Pregnancy

Precautions: Breastfeeding, children, acute bronchospasm, anticoagulants, ❦ Asian patients, asthma, cardiomyopathy/HF, COPD, extravasation, fever, hepatitis, human anti-human antibody, hypotension, neuropathy, hepatotoxicity, interstitial lung disease/pneumonitis; pulmonary disease, thrombocytopenia

> **BLACK BOX WARNING:** Heart failure, hepatotoxicity

DOSAGE AND ROUTES

Adult: IV 3.6 mg/kg over 30-90 min q3wk; give first infusion over 90 min; if tolerated, give over 30 min for 14 cycles

• Permanently discontinue treatment in patients diagnosed with nodular regenerative hyperplasia (NRH)

Available forms: Lyophilized powder 100 mg/vial, 160 mg/vial

ADVERSE EFFECTS

CNS: Dizziness, insomnia, neuropathy, chills, fatigue, fever, flushing, headache

CV: Hypertension, peripheral edema, left ventricular dysfunction

EENT: stomatitis

GI: Diarrhea, nausea, vomiting, constipation, dyspepsia, hepatotoxicity

HEMA: Anemia, bleeding, thrombocytopenia

INTEG: Rash, infusion-related reactions

MISC: Elevated LFTs, hand-foot syndrome

MS: Arthralgia, pain

SYST: Anaphylaxis

INTERACTIONS
Drug classifications

Anticoagulants, 5% dextrose, platelets: avoid concurrent use

CYP3A4 inhibitors (clarithromycin, ketoconazole, ritonavir, saquinavir, atazanavir): Increased: ado-trastuzumab effect, avoid concurrent use

Do not give with other IV products

NURSING CONSIDERATIONS
Assessment

• Monitor liver function tests; CBC

• **Pregnancy/breastfeeding:** Identify if pregnancy is planned or suspected or if breastfeeding, this product is contraindicated in pregnancy, do not breastfeed; enroll pregnant patient in MotherHER Pregnancy Registry 800-690-6720

> **BLACK BOX WARNING:** Heart failure, other cardiac symptoms: assess for dyspnea, coughing; gallop; obtain full cardiac workup including ECG, echo, MUGA, LVEF baseline and q 3 min

• Monitor for symptoms of infection; may be masked by product

• CNS reaction: monitor LOC, mental status, dizziness, confusion

> **BLACK BOX WARNING:** Monitor hypersensitive reactions, anaphylaxis

• **Infusion reactions that may be fatal:** monitor fever, chills, nausea, vomiting, pain, headache, dizziness, hypotension; discontinue product, monitor for infusion reactions

---

⚠ Nurse Alert   ✳ Key NCLEX® Drug   ≫ Drug Specifics

during and for 1-1/2 hr after conclusion of infusion, slowing of infusion may be needed
- **Pulmonary toxicity:** monitor dyspnea, interstitial pneumonitis, pulmonary hypertension, ARDs: can occur after infusion reaction; those with lung disease may have more severe toxicity in those with pneumonitis, interstitial lung disease
- **Bleeding:** Monitor for bleeding, grade 3 or 4 blooding with fatalities has occurred, check platelets baseline and before each dose
- **Hepatotoxicity:** Monitor LFTs baseline and before each dose, fatal liver damage may occur, reduced dose or discontinuing treatment may be required; AST/ALT >5 to ≤20× ULN: withhold, resume at a reduced dose when AST/ALT is ≤5× ULN
- **First dose reduction:** reduce the dose to 3 mg/kg
- **Second dose reduction:** reduce the dose to 2.4 mg/kg
- **Requirement for further dose reduction:** discontinue
AST/ALT >20× ULN: discontinue
Total bilirubin >3 to ≤10× ULN: withhold; resume treatment at a reduced dose when total bilirubin recovers to ≤1.5
- **First dose reduction:** reduce the dose to 3 mg/kg
- **Second dose reduction:** reduce the dose to 2.4 mg/kg
- **Requirement for further dose reduction:** discontinue treatment
Total bilirubin >10× ULN: permanently discontinue
- Permanently discontinue treatment in patients with AST/ALT > 3× ULN and total bilirubin > 2× ULN
- **Left ventricular ejection fraction (LVEF) 40%-45% and decrease is <10% points from baseline:** continue treatment; repeat LVEF assessment within 3 wk
- **LVEF 40%-45% and decrease is ≥10% points from baseline:** withhold; repeat LVEF assessment within 3 wk; if LVEF remains ≥10% points from baseline, discontinue
- **LVEF < 40%:** withhold; repeat LVEF assessment within 3 wk; if LVEF remains <40%, discontinue
- **Thrombocytopenia**
Platelet count 25,000/mm³ to <50,000/mm³: withhold; resume treatment at same dose when platelet count recovers to ≥75,000/mm³
Platelet count <25,000/mm³: withhold; resume treatment at a reduced dose when platelet count recovers to ≥75,000/mm³

- **First dose reduction:** reduce the dose to 3 mg/kg
- **Second dose reduction:** reduce the dose to 2.4 mg/kg
- **Requirement for further dose reduction:** discontinue

Patient problem
Lack of knowledge of medication (teaching)

Implementation

IV route
- Visually inspect for particulate matter and discoloration prior to use
- Give as IV infusion with a 0.22-micron in-line filter; do not administer as an IV push or bolus
- Use cytotoxic handling procedures; do not mix with, or administer as an infusion with, other IV products

Reconstitution
- Slowly inject 5 ml of sterile water for injection into each 100 mg vial, or 8 ml of sterile water for injection into each 160 mg vial, to yield a single-use solution of 20 mg/ml
- Direct the stream of sterile water toward the wall of the vial and not directly at the cake or powder
- Gently swirl the vial to aid in dissolution; do not shake
- After reconstitution, withdraw desired amount from the vial and dilute immediately in 250 ml of 0.9% sodium chloride; do not use dextrose 5% solution; gently invert the bag to mix the solution in order to avoid foaming
- The reconstituted single-use product does not contain a preservative. Use the diluted solution immediately or store at 2-8 °C (36-46 °F) for up to 24 hr after reconstitution; discard any unused drug after 24 hr. Do not freeze.

IV infusion
- Closely monitor for possible subcutaneous infiltration during drug administration
- First infusion: Give over 90 min. The infusion rate should be slowed or interrupted if the patient develops an infusion-related reaction. Patients should be observed for at least 90 min following the initial dose for fever, chills, or other infusion-related reactions. Permanently discontinue for life-threatening infusion-related reactions.
- Subsequent infusions: Administer over 30 min if prior infusions were well tolerated. The infusion rate should be slowed or interrupted if the patient develops an infusion-related reaction. Patients should be observed for at least 30 min after the infusion. Permanently discontinue for life-threatening infusion-related reactions

Patient/family education

- Advise patient of reasons for product, expected result
- Teach patient to take acetaminophen for fever
- Teach patient to avoid hazardous tasks because confusion, dizziness may occur
- Teach patient to report signs of infection: sore throat, fever, diarrhea, vomiting, bleeding, decreased heart function/SOB with exertion, neuropathy, liver toxicity, to report weight gain, swelling of extremities, fatigue, coughing, bleeding
- Teach patient to use effective contraception while taking this product and for additional 7 months after discontinuing this drug; to avoid breastfeeding
- Teach patient to report pain at infusion site

Evaluation

Positive therapeutic outcome
- Decrease in size, spread of breast cancer

RARELY USED

afatinib (Rx)

(a-fat′i-nib)
Gilotrif ✦, Giotrif
Func. class.: Antineoplastic
Chem. class.: Signal transduction inhibitors (STIs), epidermal growth factor receptor tyrosine kinase inhibitor

USES: Treatment of non-small cell lung cancer whose tumors have epidermal growth factor receptor Exon 19 deletions or 21 substitution mutations

CONTRAINDICATIONS

Pregnancy, hypersensitivity

DOSAGE AND ROUTES

Adult: PO 40 mg/day until disease progresssion or unacceptable toxicity

---

albuterol (Rx)

(al-byoo′ter-ole)
AccuNeb, Salbutamol ✦, Airomir, ProAir HFA, ProAir RespiClick, Proventil HFA, Ventolin HFA, Ventolin Diskus ✦, Ventolin Nebules ✦, Vospire ER
Func. class.: Bronchodilator
Chem. class.: Adrenergic β_2-agonist, sympathomimetic, bronchodilator

Do not confuse: albuterol/atenolol/Albutein, **Proventil**/Prinivil, **Ventolin**/Vantin

---

ACTION: Causes bronchodilation by action on β_2 (pulmonary) receptors by increasing levels of cyclic AMP, which relaxes smooth muscle; produces bronchodilatation; CNS, cardiac stimulation, increased diuresis, and increased gastric acid secretion; longer acting than isoproterenol

Therapeutic outcome: Increased ability to breathe because of bronchodilation

USES: Prevention of exercise-induced asthma, acute bronchospasm, bronchitis, emphysema, bronchiectasis, reversible airway obstruction

Pharmacokinetics

Absorption	Well absorbed (PO)
Distribution	Unknown
Metabolism	Liver extensively, tissues
Excretion	Unknown, breast milk
Half-life	3-4 hr

Pharmacodynamics (bronchodilation)

	PO	PO–ext rel	INH
Onset	½ hr	½ hr	5-15 min
Peak	2½ hr	2-3 hr	1½-2hr
Duration	4-6 hr	12 hr	4-6 hr

CONTRAINDICATIONS

Hypersensitivity to sympathomimetics

Precautions: Pregnancy, breastfeeding, exercise-induced bronchospasm (aerosol) in children <12 yr, cardiac/renal disease, hyperthyroidism, diabetes mellitus, hypertension, prostatic hypertrophy, closed-angle glaucoma, seizures, hypoglycemia, tachydysrhythmias, severe cardiac disease, heart block

DOSAGE AND ROUTES

Bronchospasm, prophylaxis/treatment
Adult and child ≥4 yr: INH (metered dose inhaler) 2 puffs (180 mcg) q4-6hr prn; **Powdered inhaler** (ProAir RespiClick) >12 yrs 180 mcg (2 INH) q4-6hr as needed
Adult/child ≥ 13 yr: PO-EXT REL 4-8 mg q12h, max 32 mg/day; PO 2-4 mg tid, max 32 mg/day
Child 6-13 yr: PO- EXT REL 4 mg q12h, max 24 mg/day; PO 2 mg tid-qid, max 24 mg/day
Child 2-5 yr: PO 0.1 mg/kg tid, max 23 mg/day
Adult/child ≥ 15 yr: PO- Syrup 2-4 mg (1-2 tsp) tid-qid, max 32 mg/day
Child 6-14 yr: PO-Syrup 2 mg (1 tsp) tid-qid, max 24 mg /day
Child 2-5 yr: PO-Syrup 0.1 mg/kg tid, max 12 mg/day

To prevent exercise-induced bronchospasm (not ProAir RespiClick)
Adult/child ≥ 4 yr: INH 2 inhalations before exercise, max 12 INH/24 hr; **ProAir RespiClick** INH 2 inhalations 15-30 min before exercise

Other respiratory conditions
Adult and child ≥12 yr: INH (metered dose inhaler) 1 puff q4-6hr; PO 2-4 mg tid-qid, max 32 mg/day, depending on formulation, NEB/IPPB 2.5 mg tid-qid
Geriatric: PO 2 mg tid-qid, may increase gradually to 8 mg tid-qid
Child 2-12 yr: INH (metered dose inhaler) 0.1 mg/kg tid (max 2.5 mg tid-qid); NEB/IPPB 0.1-0.15 mg/kg/dose tid-qid or 1.25 mg tid-qid for child 10-15 kg or 2.5 mg tid-qid >15 kg

Available forms: INH aerosol 108 mcg/actuation; tabs 2, 4 mg; oral syr 2 mg/5 ml; ext rel 4, 8 mg; inh sol 0.083, 0.5, 0.042%, 0.02%; metered dose aerosol 90 mcg/actuation

ADVERSE EFFECTS
CNS: *Tremors, anxiety,* insomnia, headache, stimulation, *restlessness*
CV: *Tachycardia, hypertension,* angina, dysrhythmias, chest pain
EENT: Dry nose, irritation of nose and throat
GI: *nausea, vomiting*
MISC: Hypokalemia, hyperglycemia
RESP: paradoxical bronchospasm

INTERACTIONS
Individual drugs
Digoxin: increased digoxin level

Drug classifications
Adrenergics: increased action of albuterol; do not use together
β-Adrenergic blockers: block therapeutic effect
Bronchodilators (aerosol): increased action of bronchodilator
CNS stimulants: increased CNS stimulation
Diuretics (potassium-losing): increased ECG changes/hypokalemia
MAOIs, tricyclics: increased chance of hypertensive crisis; do not use together
Oxytocics: severe hypotension; do not use together
Theophylline: toxicity

Drug/herb
Black tea, green tea, kola nut, guarana, yerba maté: increased stimulation

Drug/food
Caffeine products, chocolate: increased stimulation

Drug/lab test
Decreased: potassium

NURSING CONSIDERATIONS
Assessment
• Assess respiratory function: vital capacity, pulse oximetry, forced expiratory volume, ABGs, lung sounds; heart rate, rhythm; B/P, sputum (baseline and during therapy)
• Determine that patient has not received theophylline therapy before giving dose, to prevent additive effect, client's ability to self-medicate
• Assess for paradoxical bronchospasm, trouble breathing with wheezing, notify health care professional immediately

Patient problem
Impaired airway clearance (uses)

Implementation
PO route
• Do not break, crush, or chew ext rel tabs
• Give PO with meals to decrease gastric irritation; oral sol for children (no alcohol, sugar)
• In geriatric patients, a spacing device is advised
Aerosol route
• Give after shaking inhaler; have patient exhale and place mouthpiece in mouth, inhale slowly while depressing inhaler, hold breath, remove inhaler, exhale slowly; allow at least 1 min between inhalations; avoid using near flames or source of heat
• Track number of inhalations used and discard when labeled inhalations have been used
• Store in light-resistant container; do not expose to temperatures >86° F (30° C)
• **ProAir RespiClick:** Dose counter window should show number 200. The dose counter only displays even numbers; hold the inhaler upright while opening the cap fully; make sure a "click" is heard; do not open the cap unless ready to give dose; the patient should breathe out through the mouth; be careful that the patient does not breathe out into the inhaler mouthpiece; put the mouthpiece in the mouth and have patient close lips around it; the patient should breathe in deeply through the mouth; hold breath for about 10 sec; remove the inhaler; check dose counter to make sure the dose was received; do not wash or put any part of the inhaler in water; if the mouthpiece needs cleaning, wipe with a dry cloth or tissue; when there are 20 doses left, the counter will change to red; refill
Nebulizer/IPPB route
• **Dilute** 5 mg/ml sol/2.5 ml 0.9% NaCl for inhalation; other solutions do not require dilution for nebulizer O_2 flow or compressed air 6-10 L/min, once treatment lasts 10 min; IPPB lasts 5-20 min

Patient/family education
• Tell patient not to use OTC medications before consulting prescriber; excess stimulation may occur; instruct patient to use this medication before other medications and allow at least 5 min between each to prevent overstimulation; to limit caffeine products such as chocolate, coffee, tea, and cola, to avoid smoking, smoke-filled rooms, or other noxious odors or irritants
• Teach patient to use inhaler; to prime with 4 sprays; review package insert with patient; to avoid getting aerosol in eyes or blurring may result; to wash inhaler in warm water and dry daily; to rinse mouth after using; to avoid smoking, smoke-filled rooms, persons with respiratory infections; about when to empty and when to renew, bad taste may occur
• Teach patient that if paradoxic broncho-spasm occurs to stop product immediately and notify prescriber, usually from first dose of new inhaler
• Instruct patient on administration of dose, not to use more than prescribed; serious side effects may occur; if taking PO regularly and dose is missed, take when remembered; space other doses on new time schedule; do not double doses, notify health care professional immediately if product does not relieve symptoms, corticosteroids may be needed
• In geriatric patients, a spacing device is advised
• **Pregnancy/breastfeeding:** teach patient to notify provider if pregnancy is planned or suspected, or if breastfeeding

Evaluation
Positive therapeutic outcome
• Absence of dyspnea and wheezing after 1 hr
• Improved airway exchange
• Improved ABGs

TREATMENT OF OVERDOSE:
Administer a β_1-adrenergic blocker, **IV** fluids

---

alclometasone
(al-kloe-met′a sone)
Aclovate
Func. class.: Corticosteroid, topical

ACTION: Anti-inflammatory, decreases immune responses

Therapeutic use: Decreased inflammation

USES: Skin inflammation in various dermatological conditions

Absorption	Minimal
Distribution	Skin
Metabolism	Skin
Excretion	None
Half-life	None

Onset	Mins
Peak	Hours
Duration	Hours

CONTRAINDICATIONS
Hypersensitivity, untreated skin infections

Precautions: Preexisting skin infections

DOSAGE AND ROUTES
Adult/child: **Topical** apply 1-4 times per day to affected skin

Available forms: Cream 0.05%, ointment 0.05%

ADVERSE REACTIONS
INTEG: Dermatitis, burning, hypersensitivity, irritation

INTERACTIONS
None significant

NURSING CONSIDERATIONS
Assessment
• **Skin area:** Assess area that is being treated for cuts, scrapes, maceration, burns, infections. Do not use on these areas
Hypersensitivity: Assess for rash, itching

Patient problems
Impaired skin integrity (uses)

Implementation
Topical route
• Apply a thin film to area, use gloves when applying

Patient/family education
• Teach patient how to apply product and not to use on broken, cut, scraped skin, or skin with an active infection

Evaluation
Positive therapeutic outcome
• Improved skin integrity

⚠ HIGH ALERT
RARELY USED

alectinib
(al-ek'ti-nib)
Alecensa
Func. class.: Antineoplastics

USES: Anaplastic lymphoma kinase (ALK)–positive metastatic non-small cell lung cancer that has progressed or is intolerant to crizotinib

CONTRAINDICATIONS
Hypersensitivity

DOSAGE AND ROUTES
Adult: PO 600 mg bid, with food, until disease progression or unacceptable toxicity

alendronate (Rx)
(al-en'droe-nate)
Binosto, Fosamax, Fosamax plus D
Func. class.: Bone-resorption inhibitor
Chem. class.: Bisphosphonate

Do not confuse: Fosamax/Flomax

ACTION: Decreases rate of bone resorption and may directly block dissolution of hydroxyapatite crystals of bone; inhibits osteoclast activity

Therapeutic outcome: Prevention, decrease in progression of osteoporosis in women; treatment of Paget's disease; treatment of osteoporosis in men

USES: Treatment and prevention of osteoporosis in postmenopausal women, treatment of osteoporosis in men, Paget's disease, treatment of corticosteroid-induced osteoporosis in postmenopausal women not receiving estrogen, or in men who are continuing corticosteroid treatment with low bone mass

Pharmacokinetics

Absorption	Minimal absorption
Distribution	Mainly to bones; protein binding 78%
Metabolism	Unknown
Excretion	Via kidneys after bound to bone
Half-life	>10 yrs

Pharmacodynamics (bone resorption inhibition)

Onset	30 days
Peak	3-6 mo
Duration	1-7 mo

CONTRAINDICATIONS
Hypersensitivity to bisphosphonates, delayed esophageal emptying, inability to sit or stand for 30 min, hypocalcemia

Precautions: Pregnancy, breastfeeding, children, CCr <35 ml/min, esophageal disease, increased esophageal cancer risk, ulcers, gastritis, poor dental health

DOSAGE AND ROUTES
Osteoporosis
Adult and geriatric: PO 10 mg daily or 70 mg qwk

Paget's disease
Adult and geriatric: PO 40 mg daily × 6 mo, consider retreatment for relapse

Prevention of osteoporosis in postmenopausal women (excluding Binosto and oral solution)
Adult (postmenopausal females): PO 5 mg daily or 35 mg qwk

Glucocorticoid-induced osteoporosis in those receiving glucocorticoids (daily dose >7.5 mg or predniSONE) and low bone density (excluding Binosto and oral solution)
Adult: PO 5 mg qday, those not receiving estrogen 10 mg qday

Renal dose
Adult: PO CCr ≤35 ml/min, not recommended

Available forms: Tabs 5, 10, 35, 40, 70 mg, tabs 70 mg with 2800 IU Vit D_3, 70 mg with 5600 IU Vit D_3; oral sol 70 mg/75 ml, effervescent tab 70 mg

ADVERSE EFFECTS
CNS: Headache
GI: Abdominal pain, constipation, nausea, vomiting, esophageal ulceration, acid reflux, dyspepsia, esophageal perforation, diarrhea, esophageal cancer
CV: Atrial fibrillation
Integ: Rash, photosensitivity
Resp: Asthma exacerbation
META: Hypophosphatemia, hypocalcemia
MS: Bone pain, osteonecrosis of the jaw, bone fractures

INTERACTIONS
Drug classifications
Antacids, calcium supplements: decreased absorption, give alendronate at least 30-60 min before other products
H_2 blockers, proton pump inhibitors (PPIs), gastric mucosal agents, NSAIDs, salicylates: adverse GI reactions, monitor for GI reactions

Drug/food
Caffeine, food, orange juice: decreased product absorption, take food at least 30 min after this product

Drug/lab test
Decreased: calcium, phosphate

NURSING CONSIDERATIONS
Assessment
• Assess dental status, regular dental exams should be done; dental extractions (cover with antiinfectives) prior to procedure
• Hormonal status of women, prior to treatment
• **Osteoporosis:** assess for bone density testing baseline and during treatment, history of fractures
• **Paget's disease:** assess for increased skull size, bone pain, headache, monitor alkaline phosphatase; level of 2 × upper limit of normal is indicated for Paget's disease
• Monitor renal studies and electrolytes (calcium, potassium, magnesium, phosphorous) BUN/creatinine
• **Hypercalcemia:** assess for paresthesia, twitching, laryngospasm, Chvostek's, Trousseau's signs; monitor calcium, Vitamin D baseline and during treatment, correct before use
• MS or bone pain: may occur in a few days after start of treatment to years later, usually pain resolves after stopping treatment

Patient problem
Risk for injury (uses)

Implementation
• Give PO for 6 mo to be effective in Paget's disease; take with 8 oz of water 30 min before 1st food, beverage, or medication of the day
• Patient to remain upright for 30 min after dose to prevent esophageal irritation
• Store in cool environment out of direct sunlight
Tablet:
• Do not lie down for ≥30 min after dose, do not take at bedtime
Effervescent tablet:
• Dissolve in 4 oz of water, after 5 min stir, drink
Liquid:
• Use oral syringe or calibrated device; give in AM with ≥2 oz of water ≥30 min before food, beverage, or medication

Patient/family education
• Teach patient to remain upright for 30 min after dose to prevent esophageal irritation; if dose is missed, skip dose, do not double doses or take later in day
• Teach patient to take in AM, only before food, other meds, to take with 6-8 oz of water (not mineral water)
• Teach patient to take calcium, vit D if instructed by provider

• Advise patient to use sunscreen, protective clothing to prevent photosensitivity
• Teach patient to avoid smoking, alcohol intake that increase osteoporosis
• Teach patient to use weight-bearing exercise to increase bone density
• Teach patient to let provider know if pregnancy is planned or suspected or if nursing
• Advise to maintain good oral hygiene, to use antiinfectives before dental procedures as directed by prescriber

Evaluation
Positive therapeutic outcome
• Increased bone mass, absence of fractures

---

alfuzosin (Rx)
(al-fyoo′zoe-sin)
Uroxatral, Xatral ✤
Func. class.: Urinary tract, antispasmodic, α_1-agonist
Chem. class.: Quinazolone

ACTION: Binds preferentially to α_{1A}-adrenoceptor subtype located mainly in the prostate, relaxing smooth muscles

Therapeutic outcome: Resolution of symptoms of benign prostatic hyperplasia

USES: Symptoms of benign prostatic hyperplasia

Pharmacokinetics	
Absorption	50%
Distribution	Protein bound (82%-90%)
Metabolism	Liver (by CYP3A4 enzyme)
Excretion	Urine 11%
Half-life	10 hr

Pharmacodynamics	
Onset	Up to 1 hr
Peak	8 hr
Duration	Up to 24 hr

CONTRAINDICATIONS
Hypersensitivity, moderate to severe hepatic impairment, not indicated for use in women or children, breastfeeding (but not used in women)

Precautions: Pregnancy, geriatric, coronary artery disease, coronary insufficiency, mild hepatic disease, mild/moderate/severe renal disease, history of QT prolongation or coadministration with medications known to prolong QT interval, torsades de pointes, syncope, surgery, prostate cancer, orthostatic hypotension, ocular surgery, CAD, dysrhythmias, angina

---

DOSAGE AND ROUTES
Adult: PO EXT REL 10 mg daily

Available forms: EXT REL tabs 10 mg

ADVERSE EFFECTS
CNS: *Dizziness, headache,* fatigue, flushing
CV: Postural hypotension (dizziness, light-headedness, fainting) within a few hours of administration
GI: Nausea, abdominal pain, dyspepsia, constipation, diarrhea, liver injury, jaundice
GU: Impotence, priapism
HEMA: Thrombocytopenia
INTEG: Rash, toxic epidermal necrolysis
MISC: Floppy iris syndrome
RESP: Upper respiratory tract infection, pharyngitis, bronchitis, sinusitis

INTERACTIONS
Individual drugs
Alcohol: increased hypotension
Atenolol, cimetidine, diltiazem: Increased effects of these individual drugs

Drug classifications
β-Blockers, nitrates, antihypertensives, phosphodiesterase 5 inhibitors: increased hypotension
CYP3A4 inhibitors, cimetidine (ketoconazole, itraconazole, ritonavir): do not take concurrently

NURSING CONSIDERATIONS
Assessment
• **Prostatic hyperplasia:** change in urinary patterns, baseline and throughout treatment
• **Orthostatic hypotension:** Take BP lying and standing, pulse baseline and frequently, usually occurs within 2-4 hr after beginning dose
• Monitor BUN, uric acid, urodynamic studies (urinary flow rates, residual volume)
• **Serious skin reactions:** Assess for toxic epidermal necrolysis, notify prescriber immediately, stop product

Patient problem
Risk for injury (adverse reactions)

Implementation
• Swallow tabs whole; do not break, crush, or chew tabs, give with food at same time of day
• Store in tight container in cool environment

Patient/family education
• Advise not to drive or operate machinery until reaction is known; dizziness, drowsiness may occur
• Teach patient to take at the same time of the day with food; do not double doses, take missed dose when remembered
• Advise patient about orthostatic hypotension, to rise slowly from sitting or lying

• Inform patient to avoid all OTC, herbal unless approved by prescriber
• Advise patient to inform prescriber of rash, dizziness, chest pain
• Teach patient follow-up exams and lab work may be necessary
• Teach patient to inform health care professionals of use before surgery

Evaluation
Positive therapeutic outcome
• Decreased symptoms of benign prostatic hyperplasia

alirocumab (Rx)
(al′-i- rok′-ue-mab)
Praluent
Func. class.: Antilipemic
Chem. class.: Proprotein convertase subtilism kexin type q inhibitor

ACTION: Binds to low-density lipoproteins, a human monoclonal antibody (IgG1)

Therapeutic outcome: Decreased LDL

USES: Heterozygous, familial hypercholesterolemia, atherosclerotic disease

Pharmacokinetics
Absorption	Well
Distribution	Circulation, crosses placenta
Metabolism	Unknown
Excretion	Binds to PCSK9
Half-life	17-20 days

Pharmacodynamics
Onset	Unknown
Peak	Up to 8 h
Duration	Up to 14 days

CONTRAINDICATIONS
Hypersensitivity

Precautions: Pregnancy, breastfeeding

DOSAGE AND ROUTES
Adult: SUBCUT 75 mg q2wk, may increase to 150 mg q2wk if needed or 300 mg q 4 wk

Available forms: Prefilled pen or prefilled syringe 75 mg/1 ml, 150 mg/1 ml

ADVERSE EFFECTS
CNS: Memory impairment, confusion
INTEG: Pruritus, injection-site reaction, vasculitis

INTERACTIONS
None known

NURSING CONSIDERATIONS
Assessment
• **Hypercholesterolemia:** Obtain diet history: fat content, lipid levels (triglycerides, LDL, LDL-C 4-8 wk after start of titration, HDL, cholesterol); LFTs at baseline, periodically during treatment
Hypersensitivity: Monitor for rash, pruritus, vasculitis; if severe, product may need to be discontinued

Implementation
• If dose is missed give within 7 days of next dose; if over 7 days, wait until next scheduled dose
• Visually inspect for particulate matter and discoloration; solution is clear, colorless to pale yellow
• Warm to room temperature for 30-40 min before use. Use as soon as possible after warming
• Do NOT use the pre-filled pen or syringe if it has been at room temperature for ≥24 hr
• Give by SUBCUT inj into the thigh, abdomen, or upper arm. Rotate inj site with each inj.
• Do NOT inject into areas of active skin disease or injury (sunburn, rash, inflammation, skin infection)
• Do NOT administer with other injectable drugs at the same inj site

Patient/family education
• Teach patient that compliance is needed
• Teach patient how to correctly self-inject, provide patient information sheet
• Advise that risk factors should be decreased: high-fat diet, smoking, alcohol consumption, absence of exercise
• Advise patient to notify prescriber if pregnancy suspected, planned, or if breastfeeding
• Inform patient to report confusion, injection-site reactions

Evaluation
• Therapeutic response: decreased LDL-C

---

allopurinol (Rx)
(al-oh-pure′i-nole)
Alloprin ✦, **Aloprim, Zyloprim**
Func. class.: Antigout drug, antihyperuricemic
Chem. class.: Xanthine enzyme inhibitor

Do not confuse: Zyloprim/Zovirax/ZORprin/zolpidem

ACTION: Inhibits the enzyme xanthine oxidase, reducing uric acid synthesis

Therapeutic outcome: Decreasing serum uric acid levels, decreasing joint pain

USES: Chronic gout, hyperuricemia associated with malignancies, recurrent calcium oxalate calculi, uric acid calculi

Pharmacokinetics

Absorption	80% (PO), complete (IV)
Distribution	Widely distributed, protein binding minimal
Metabolism	Liver to oxypurinol
Excretion	Kidneys
Half-life	1-2 hr

Pharmacodynamics

	PO	IV
Onset	Unknown	Unknown
Peak	1½ hr	Up to 30 min
Duration	Unknown	Unknown

CONTRAINDICATIONS
Hypersensitivity

Precautions: Pregnancy, breastfeeding, children, renal/hepatic disease

DOSAGE AND ROUTES
Increased uric acid levels in malignancies
Adult: PO 600-800 mg/day in divided doses, for 2-3 days; start up to 1-2 days prior to chemotherapy; **IV** INF 200-400 mg/m²/day, max 600 mg/day 24-48 hr prior to chemotherapy, may be divided at 6-, 8-, 12-hr intervals
Child 6-10 yr: PO 300 mg/day, adjust dose after 48 hr
Child <6 yr: PO 150 mg/day, adjust dose after 48 hr
Child: IV INF 200 mg/m²/day, initially as a single dose or divided q6-12hr

Gout
Adult: PO 100 mg/day, titrating upward; maintenance 100-200 mg BID-TID

Renal dose
Adult: PO/IV CCr 81-100 ml/min 300 mg/day; CCr 61-80 ml/min 250 mg/day; CCr 41-60 ml/min 200 mg/day; CCr 21-40 ml/min 150 mg/day; CCr 10-20 ml/min 100-200 mg/day; CCr 3-9 ml/min 100 mg/day or 100 mg every other day; CCr <3 ml/min 100 mg q24hr or longer or 100 mg every third day

Available forms: Tabs, scored, 100, 300 mg; powder for inj 500 mg/vial

---

ADVERSE EFFECTS
CNS: Drowsiness
CV: Hypo-hypertension; HF (IV)
GI: *Nausea, vomiting, malaise,* diarrhea, hepatitis
GU: Renal failure
INTEG: rash
Misc: Hypersensitivity, bone marrow depression

INTERACTIONS
Individual drugs
Ampicillin, amoxicillin: increased risk of rash, avoid concurrent use
AzaTHIOprine; mercaptopurine: increased bone marrow depression
Rasburicase: increased xanthine nephropathy, calculi
Theophylline: increased theophylline toxicity

Drug classifications
ACE inhibitors: increased hypersensitivity, toxicity
Anticoagulants (oral): increased action of oral anticoagulants
Diuretics (thiazide): increased hypersensitivity

NURSING CONSIDERATIONS
Assessment
• Assess for **pain** including location, characteristics, onset/duration, frequency, quality, intensity or severity of pain, precipitating factors; **gout:** joint pain, swelling, do not initiate any new therapy during acute gout flare
• Check I&O ratio, increase fluids to 2 L/day to prevent stone formation, toxicity
• Monitor CBC, AST, BUN, creatinine, ALT before starting treatment, monthly; check blood glucose in diabetic patients receiving oral antidiabetic agents
• Assess for rash, hypersensitivity reactions, if present discontinue this product immediately; after rash is resolved, treatment may continue at a lower dose

Patient problem
Pain (uses)

Implementation
PO route
• Give with meals to prevent GI symptoms; crush and mix with food or fluids for patients with swallowing difficulties
• Increase fluid intake to 2 L/day
• Begin 1-2 days before antineoplastic therapy if using for hyperuricemia associated with malignancy

Intermittent IV infusion route
• Use in tumor lysis before starting chemotherapy (24-48 hr)
• Reconstitute 30-ml vial with 25 ml of sterile water for inj; dilute to desired conc (≤6 mg/ml) with 0.9% NaCl for inj or D_5 for inj, begin inf within 10 hr

IV compatibilities: Acyclovir, aminophylline, amphotericin B lipid complex, anidulafungin, argatroban, atenolol, aztreonam, bivalirudin, bleomycin, bumetanide, buprenorphine, butorphanol, calcium gluconate, CARBOplatin, caspofungin, ceFAZolin, cefoTEtan, cefTAZidime, ceftizoxime, cefTRIAXone, cefuroxime, CISplatin, cyclophosphamide, DACTINomycin, DAUNOrubicin liposome, dexamethasone, dexmedetomidine, DOCEtaxel, DOXOrubicin liposomal, enalaprilat, etoposide, famotidine, fenoldopam, filgrastim, fluconazole, fludarabine, fluorouracil, furosemide, gallium, ganciclovir, gatifloxacin, gemcitabine, gemtuzumab, granisetron, heparin, hydrocortisone phosphate, hydrocortisone succinate, HYDROmorphone, ifosfamide, linezolid, LORazepam, mannitol, mesna, methotrexate, metroNIDAZOLE, milrinone, mitoXANtrone, morphine, nesiritide, octreotide, oxytocin, PACLitaxel, pamidronate, pantoprazole, PEMEtrexed, piperacillin, piperacillin-tazobactam, plicamycin, potassium chloride, ranitidine, sodium, sulfamethoxazole-trimethoprim, teniposide, thiotepa, ticarcillin, ticarcillin clavulanate, tigecycline, tirofiban, vancomycin, vasopressin, vinBLAStine, vinCRIStine, voriconazole, zidovudine, zoledronic acid

Patient/family education
• Tell patient to increase fluid intake to 2 L/day; to avoid taking large doses of vit C; kidney stone formation may occur; to maintain a diet enhancing urine alkalinity (e.g., milk, other dairy products); if taking for calcium oxalate stones, reduce dairy products, refined sugar, sodium, meat
• Tell patient to report skin rash, stomatitis, malaise, fever, aching; product should be discontinued
• Advise patient to avoid hazardous activities if drowsiness or dizziness occurs; response may take several days to determine
• Tell patient to avoid alcohol, caffeine, foods high in purines, meats, processed foods; these substances increase uric acid levels and decrease allopurinol levels
• Teach patient to report side effects and adverse reactions to prescriber, including rash, itching, nausea, vomiting
• Teach patient an alkaline diet may be required
• Inform patient that follow-up exams and blood-work will be necessary
• Teach patient to identify triggers and avoid

Evaluation
Positive therapeutic outcome
- Decreased pain in joints
- Decreased stone formation in kidney
- Decreased uric acid level to 6 mg/dl

---

almotriptan (Rx)
(al-moh-trip′tan)
Axert
Func. class.: Antimigraine agent
Chem. class.: 5-HT$_1$ receptor agonist, triptan

Do not confuse: Axert/Antivert

ACTION: Binds selectively to the vascular 5-HT$_{1B/1D/1F}$ receptor subtype, exerts antimigraine effect; causes vasoconstriction in cranial arteries

Therapeutic outcome: Absence of migraines

USES: Acute treatment of migraine with or without aura (Adults/adolescents/children ≥12 yr)

Pharmacokinetics

Absorption	Well absorbed (~70%)
Distribution	35% protein bound
Metabolism	Liver (metabolite); metabolized by MAO-A, CYP2D6, CYP3A4
Excretion	Urine 40%, feces 13%
Half-life	3-4 hr

Pharmacodynamics

Onset	Unknown
Peak	1-3 hr
Duration	3-4 hr

CONTRAINDICATIONS
Hypersensitivity, acute MI, angina, CV disease, CAD, stroke, vasospastic angina, ischemic heart disease or risk for, peripheral vascular syndrome; uncontrolled hypertension, basilar or hemiplegic migraine

Precautions: Pregnancy, breastfeeding, children <18 yr, geriatric, postmenopausal women, men >40 yr, risk factors for coronary artery disease, MI, hypercholesterolemia, obesity, diabetes, impaired renal/hepatic function, sulfonamide hypersensitivity, cardiac dysrhythmias, Raynaud's disease, tobacco smoking, Wolff-Parkinson-White syndrome

DOSAGE AND ROUTES
Adult/adolescent/child ≥12 yr: PO 6.25-12.5 mg, may repeat dose after 2 hr; max 2 doses/ 24 hr, 25 mg/day, or 4 treatment cycles within any 30-day period

Renal/hepatic dose (CCr 10-30 ml/hr)
Adult: PO 6.25 mg initially, max 12.5 mg

Available forms: Tabs 6.25 or 12.5 mg

ADVERSE EFFECTS
CNS: *Dizziness,* headache, paresthesias
CV: *Flushing,* palpitations, tachycardia, coronary artery vasospasm, MI, ventricular fibrillation, ventricular tachycardia
GI: Nausea, xerostomia

INTERACTIONS
Individual drugs
Ergot: increased vasospastic effects, avoid concurrent use
Erythromycin, itraconazole, ketoconazole, ritonavir: increased effects of almotriptan, avoid concurrent use in renal/hepatic disease

Drug classifications
5-HT$_1$ agonists, ergot derivatives: increased vasospastic effects, avoid concurrent use
MAOIs: increased almotriptan effect; do not use together
SSRIs, SNRIs, serotonin-receptor agonists, sibutramine: increased serotonin syndrome

Drug/herb
Feverfew: avoid use
St. John's wort: increased serotonin syndrome

NURSING CONSIDERATIONS
Assessment
- **Migraine:** Assess for pain, location, aura, duration, intensity, nausea, vomiting, before using product and after use
- Assess B/P, signs/symptoms of coronary vasospasms
- Assess for tingling, hot sensation, burning, feeling of pressure, numbness, flushing
- Assess for stress level, activity, recreation, coping mechanisms
- Assess neurologic status: LOC, blurring vision, nausea, vomiting, tingling in extremities preceding headache
- **Serotonin syndrome:** Assess for serotonin syndrome that occurs in those taking SSRIs, SNRIs; agitation, confusion, hallucinations, diaphoresis, hypertension, diarrhea, fever, tremor, usually occurs when dose is increased
- **Pregnancy/breastfeeding:** Identify if pregnancy is planned or suspected, use only if benefits outweigh fetal risk, use cautiously in breastfeeding

Patient problems
Pain (uses)

Implementation
- Swallow tabs whole; do not break, crush, or chew tabs, without regard to food 2 times/24 hr
- Provide quiet, calm environment with decreased stimulation from noise, bright light, excessive talking

Patient/family education
- Instruct patient to use contraception while taking product, notify prescriber if pregnancy is planned or suspected, avoid breastfeeding
- Advise patient to have dark, quiet environment available
- Inform patient that product does not prevent or reduce number of migraine attacks, max 4 doses/30 days, do not take MAOIs for ≥ 24 hr
- Advise patient to report chest pain, drowsiness, dizziness, tingling, flushing
- **Serotonin syndrome:** Teach patient to report immediately signs of serotonin syndrome
- Advise patient to report immediately chest tightness or pain
- Advise patient not to drive or operate machines until reaction is known; drowsiness, dizziness may occur
- Advise patient to inform all health care professionals of all OTC, Rx, herbs, supplements taken

Evaluation
Positive therapeutic outcome
- Decrease in severity of migraine

TREATMENT OF OVERDOSE:
Gastric lavage; clinical and ECG monitoring for ≥20 hr after overdose

---

⚠ HIGH ALERT

alogliptin
(al'oh glip'tin)
Nesina
Func. class.: Antidiabetic
Chem. class.: Dipeptidyl peptidase-4 (DPP-4) inhibitor

ACTION: A dipeptidyl peptidase-4 (DPP-4) inhibitor for the treatment of type 2 diabetes mellitus (monotherapy or in combination with other antidiabetic agents), potentiates the effects of the incretin hormones by inhibiting their breakdown by DPP-4

Therapeutic outcome: Decrease in polyuria, polydipsia, polyphagia; clear sensorium, absence of dizziness; improvement in A1c, daily blood glucose monitoring

USES: Type 2 diabetes mellitus

Pharmacokinetics
Absorption	100%
Distribution	Well
Metabolism	Not metabolized
Excretion	Unchanged (urine)
Half-life	2 hr

Pharmacodynamics
Onset	Unknown
Peak	1-2 hr
Duration	Up to 24 hr

CONTRAINDICATIONS
Hypersensitivity, ketoacidosis, type 1 diabetes

Precautions: Pregnancy, breastfeeding, hepatic disease, burns, diarrhea, fever, GI obstruction, hyper/hypoglycemia, hyper/hypothyroidism, hypercortisolism, children, ileus, malnutrition, pancreatitis, surgery, trauma, vomiting, kidney disease, adrenal insufficiency, angioedema

DOSAGE AND ROUTES
Adult: PO 25 mg/day

Renal dose
Adult: PO CCr 30-59 ml/min: 12.5 mg/day; CCr 30 ml/min: 6.25 mg/day; intermittent hemodialysis: 6.25 mg/day; give without regard to the timing of hemodialysis

Available forms: Tab 6.25, 12.5, 25 mg

ADVERSE EFFECTS
CNS: Headache
CV: Heart failure
GI: Pancreatitis, hepatotoxicity
SYST: Rash, hypersensitivity, angioedema, Stevens–Johnson syndrome, anaphylaxis

INTERACTIONS
Hypoglycemia-insulin, sulfonylureas, androgens: increased effect, dose adjustment may be needed
Thiazides: decrease; hypoglycemia, adjust dose if needed

Drug/lab test
Increased: LFTs
Decrease: Glucose

NURSING CONSIDERATIONS
Assessment
- **Diabetes:** monitor blood glucose, glycosylated hemoglobin (A1c), LFTs, serum creatinine/BUN baseline and throughout treatment
- **Pancreatitis:** can occur anytime during use, assess for severe abdominal pain with or without vomiting
- **Hypersensitivity reactions:** angioedema
- Assess for Stevens-Johnson syndrome

• **Pregnancy/breastfeeding:** Use only if clearly needed, cautious use in breastfeeding

Patient problem
Excess food intake (uses)

Implementation
Give without regard to food

Patient/family education
• Advise patient to notify all health care professionals of OTC, Rx, herbs, supplements used
• **Hypersensitivity: Inform patient to notify health care professional and stop taking product if hypersensitivity occurs (rash, trouble breathing, swelling of face)**
• **Hepatotoxicity: Advise patient to report immediately yellowing of skin and urine, clay-colored stools, nausea, vomiting**
• Inform patient that diabetes is a life-long condition; product does not cure disease
• Advise patient to consume all food on diet plan, to continue other medical and lifestyle regimens
• Teach patient to carry emergency ID with prescriber, medications, and condition listed

Evaluation
Positive therapeutic outcome
• Decrease in polyuria, polydipsia, polyphagia, clear sensorium, absence of dizziness, improvement in A1c

---

ALPRAZolam (Rx)
(al-pray′zoe-lam)
Xanax, Xanax XR
Func. class.: Antianxiety
Chem. class.: Benzodiazepine, short/intermediate acting
Controlled substance schedule IV

Do not confuse: ALPRAZolam/LORazepam, **Xanax**/Zantac

ACTION: Depresses subcortical levels of CNS, including limbic system, reticular formation

Therapeutic outcome: Decreased anxiety

USES: Anxiety, panic disorders with or without agoraphobia, anxiety with depressive symptoms

Unlabeled uses: Premenstrual dysphoric disorder, insomnia, PMS, alcohol withdrawal syndrome

Pharmacokinetics

Absorption	Slow, complete
Distribution	Widely distributed; crosses placenta; crosses blood-brain barrier, protein binding 80%
Metabolism	Liver, to active metabolites
Excretion	Kidneys, breast milk
Half-life	12-15 hr immediate release 11-16 hr extended release

Pharmacodynamics

	PO	Oral Disintegrating
Onset	1 hr	Unknown
Peak	1-2 hr	1.5-2 hr
Duration	4-6 hr, therapeutic response 2-3 days	Unknown

CONTRAINDICATIONS
Pregnancy, breastfeeding, hypersensitivity to benzodiazepines, closed-angle glaucoma, psychosis, addiction

Precautions: Geriatric, debilitated, hepatic disease, obesity, severe pulmonary disease

DOSAGE AND ROUTES
Anxiety disorder
Adult: PO 0.25-0.5 mg tid, may increase q3-4days if needed, max 4 mg/day in divided doses
Geriatric: PO 0.125-0.25 mg bid; increase by 0.125 mg prn

Panic disorder
Adult: PO 0.5 mg tid, may increase up to 1 mg/day q3-4days, max 10 mg/day; **EXT REL TABS** (Xanax XR) give daily in AM 0.5-1 mg initially, maintenance 3-6 mg daily

Premenstrual dysphoric disorder (unlabeled)
Adult: PO 0.25 mg tid-qid, starting on day 16-18 of menses cycle, taper over 2-3 days when menses occurs, max 4 mg/day

Hepatic dose
Reduce dose by 50%

Available forms: Tabs 0.25, 0.5, 1, 2 mg; ext rel tabs (Xanax XR) 0.5, 1, 2, 3 mg; orally disintegrating tabs 0.25, 0.5, 1, 2 mg; oral sol, 1 mg/ml

ADVERSE EFFECTS
CNS: *Dizziness, drowsiness,* confusion, headache, anxiety, tremors, stimulation, poor coordination

---

EENT: *Blurred vision*
GI: Constipation, dry mouth, nausea, vomiting, anorexia, diarrhea, weight gain/loss
INTEG: Rash, dermatitis

INTERACTIONS
Individual drugs
Alcohol: increased CNS depression
Carbamazepine, rifampin: decreased action of ALPRAZolam

Drug classifications
Anticonvulsants, antihistamines, opioids, sedatives/hypnotics: increased CNS depression
CYP3A4 inducers (barbiturates): decreased action of ALPRAZolam
CYP3A4 inhibitors (cimetidine, disulfiram, erythromycin, fluoxetine, isoniazid, itraconazole, ketoconazole, metoprolol, propranolol, valproic acid): increased action of ALPRA-Zolam, adjust if needed

Drug/herb
Chamomile, kava, melatonin, St. John's wort, valerian: increased CNS depression

Drug/food
Grapefruit juice: increased product level, avoid concurrent use

Drug/lab test
Increased: ALT, AST, alkaline phosphatase

NURSING CONSIDERATIONS
Assessment
• Assess mental status: mood, sensorium, anxiety, affect, sleeping pattern, drowsiness, dizziness, especially geriatric; physical dependency, withdrawal symptoms: anxiety, panic attacks, agitation, headache, nausea, vomiting, muscle pain, weakness; suicidal tendencies; withdrawal seizures may occur after rapid decrease in dose or abrupt discontinuation; short duration of action makes it the product of choice in the geriatric; suicidal thoughts, behaviors
• Monitor blood studies: CBC during long-term therapy; blood dyscrasias have occurred rarely; decreased hematocrit, neutropenia may occur
• Monitor hepatic studies: AST, ALT, bilirubin, creatinine LDH, alkaline phosphatase, renal studies if on long-term treatment
• Monitor I&O; indicate renal dysfunction if on long-term treatment
• **Pregnancy:** Assess if planned or suspected, not to use in pregnancy, to avoid breastfeeding
• **Beers:** Avoid in older adults, increased risk of cognitive impairment

Patient problems
Anxiety (uses)
Nonadherence (teaching)

Implementation
• Give with food or milk for GI symptoms; high-fat meal decreases absorption; tab may be crushed, if patient is unable to swallow medication whole, and mixed with foods or fluids; may divide total daily dose into more times/day, if anxiety occurs between doses, conversion from regular release tab to extended release is at same dose, do not crush, chew, break extended release tablets
• Give sugarless gum, hard candy, frequent sips of water for dry mouth
• Taper by 0.5 mg q3days
• **Orally disintegrating tabs:** Place orally disintegrating tabs on tongue to dissolve and swallow, protect from moisture, discard unused portion of tab if split
• Give ext rel tab in AM
• **Oral solution:** mix with water, applesauce, or other soft foods, use calibrated dropper supplied

Patient/family education
• Tell patient that product may be taken with food or fluids and tabs may be crushed or swallowed whole
• Tell patient not to use for everyday stress or longer than 4 mo unless directed by prescriber; not to take more than prescribed amount; may be habit forming; not to double doses or skip doses; memory impairment is a sign of long-term use
• Tell patient to avoid OTC preparations unless approved by prescriber; alcohol and CNS depressants increase CNS depression; not to use with grapefruit juice
• **Pregnancy/breastfeeding:** Teach patient not to use during pregnancy, avoid breastfeeding
• Tell patient to avoid driving, activities that require alertness, since drowsiness may occur; to avoid alcohol ingestion or other psychotropic medications; to rise slowly, or fainting may occur, especially geriatric; that drowsiness may worsen at beginning of treatment
• Tell patient not to discontinue medication abruptly after long-term use; withdrawal symptoms include vomiting, cramping, tremors, seizures

> **BLACK BOX WARNING:** Caution patient not to use with opioids, increased respiratory depression

• **Oral disintegrating:** Place on tongue and allow to dissolve, swallow; if only half of the tab is required, discard the other half
• **Oral solution:** Mix with water, soft food, juice, use measuring device supplied

Evaluation
Positive therapeutic outcome
- Decreased anxiety, restlessness, sleeplessness (short-term treatment only)
- Decreased panic attacks

TREATMENT OF OVERDOSE:
Lavage, VS, supportive care, flumazenil

⚠ HIGH ALERT

alteplase (Rx)
(al-ti-plaze')
Activase, Activase rt-PA ✸, Cathflo
Func. class.: Thrombolytic enzyme
Chem. class.: Tissue plasminogen activator (TPA)

Do not confuse: alteplase/Altace, Activase/Cathflo Activase/TNKase

ACTION: Produces fibrin conversion of plasminogen to plasmin; able to bind to fibrin, convert plasminogen in thrombus to plasmin, which leads to local fibrinolysis, limited systemic proteolysis

Therapeutic outcome: Lysis of thrombi in MI, pulmonary emboli (life threatening)

USES: Lysis of obstructing thrombi associated with acute MI; conditions requiring thrombolysis (e.g., PE, unclotting arteriovenous shunts, acute ischemic CVA); central venous catheter occlusion (Cathflo)

Pharmacokinetics

Absorption	Complete
Distribution	Unknown
Metabolism	>80% liver
Excretion	Kidneys
Half-life	35 min

Pharmacodynamics

Onset	Immediate
Peak	1 hr
Duration	unknown

CONTRAINDICATIONS
Active internal bleeding, recent CVA, severe uncontrolled hypertension, intracranial/intraspinal surgery/trauma (within 3 mo), aneurysm, brain tumor, platelets <100,000 mm^3, bleeding diathesis including INR >1.7 or PT >15 sec, arteriovenous malformation, subarachnoid hemorrhage, intracranial hemorrhage, uncontrolled hypertension, seizure at onset of stroke

Precautions: Pregnancy, breastfeeding, children, geriatric, neurologic deficits, mitral stenosis, recent GI/GU bleeding, diabetic retinopathy, subacute bacterial endocarditis, arrhythmias, diabetic hemorrhage retinopathy, CVA, recent major surgery, hypertension, acute pericarditis, hemostatic defects, significant hepatic disease, septic thrombophlebitis, occluded AV cannula at seriously infected site

DOSAGE AND ROUTES
Pulmonary embolism (Activase)
Adult: IV 100 mg over 2 hr, then heparin

Acute ischemic stroke (Activase)
Adult: IV 0.9 mg/kg, max 90 mg; give as INF over 1 hr, give 10% of dose IV BOL over 1st min

Myocardial infarction (standard infusion)
Adult >65 kg: IV a total of 100 mg, given over 3 hr; 6-10 mg given IV BOL over 1-2 min, then the remaining 50-54 mg over the remainder of the hr, during 2nd, 3rd hr 20 mg is given by cont IV INF (20 mg/hr)
Adult <65 kg: IV 1.25 mg/kg over 3 hr; 60% in first 1 hr (10% as a bolus), remaining 40% over next 2 hr

Myocardial infarction (accelerated infusion) (Activase)
Adult >67 kg: 100 mg total dose: give 15 mg IV BOL, then 50 mg over 30 min, then 35 mg over 60 min
Adult <67 kg: 15 mg IV BOL: then 0.75 mg/kg over 30 min (max 50 mg); 0.5 mg/kg over the next 60 min (max 35 mg)

Occlusion prophylaxis (unlabeled) (Cathflo, Activase)
Adult/child ≥30 kg: IV Max 2 mg in 2 ml; may use up to 2 doses (120 min apart)
Adult/child <30 kg: IV 110% of lumen volume (max 2 mg/2 ml) in occluded catheter may repeat after 2 hr

Available forms: Powder for inj 50 mg (29 million international units/vial), 100 mg (58 million international units/vial); Cathflo Activase: lyophilized powder for injection 2 mg

ADVERSE EFFECTS
CV: recurrent ischemic stroke
INTEG: Urticaria, rash
SYST: GI, GU, intracranial, retroperitoneal bleeding, anaphylaxis, fever

INTERACTIONS
Individual drugs
Abciximab, clopidogrel, dipyridamole, eptifibatide, plicamycin, ticlopidine, tirofiban, valproic acid: increased bleeding

---

⚠ Nurse Alert   ✸ Key NCLEX® Drug   >> Drug Specifics

Drug classifications
Anticoagulants (oral), cephalosporins (some), NSAIDs, salicylates: increased bleeding

Drug/herb
Feverfew, garlic, ginger, ginkgo, ginseng, green tea: increased risk of bleeding

Drug/lab test
Increased: PT, APTT, TT

NURSING CONSIDERATIONS
Assessment
• Perform noncontrast CT of brain or MRI to rule out intracranial hemorrhage prior to systemic administration

• Monitor VS q15min, B/P, pulse, respirations (including peripheral), neurologic signs, temp at least q4hr; temp >104° F (40° C) indicates internal bleeding; monitor rhythm closely; ventricular dysrhythmias may occur with hyperperfusion; monitor heart, breath sounds, neurologic status, and peripheral pulses, those with severe neurologic deficit

• Start treatment as soon as possible when symptoms occur

• **Assess for bleeding during first hr of treatment and 24 hr after procedure:** hematuria, hematemesis, bleeding from mucous membranes, epistaxis, ecchymosis, puncture sites; guaiac all body fluids and stools; obtain blood studies (Hct, platelets, PTT, PT, TT, APTT) before starting therapy; PT or APTT must be <2 times control before starting therapy; PTT or PT q3-4hr during treatment

• **Assess hypersensitivity:** fever, rash, facial swelling, dyspnea, itching, chills; mild reaction may be treated with antihistamines; report to prescriber

• **Occlusion:** have patient exhale then hold breath when connecting/disconnecting syringe to prevent air embolism

• **Myocardial infarction:** monitor ECG; watch for dysrhythmias, monitor cardiac enzymes, radionuclide myocardial scanning/coronary angiography

• **Pulmonary embolism:** monitor pulse, B/P, ABGs, rate/rhythm of respirations; symptoms include dyspnea, tachypnea, chest pain, cough, hemoptysis

• **Pregnancy/breastfeeding:** Usually considered contraindicated in pregnancy except in serious conditions, use cautiously in breastfeeding

Patient problem
Ineffective tissue perfusion (uses)

Implementation
Intermittent IV infusion route
• Errors can be fatal, confirm all doses give after reconstituting with provided diluent; add appropriate amount of sterile water for inj (no preservatives); 20-mg vial/20 ml or 50-mg vial/50 ml (1 mg/ml); mix by slow inversion or dilute with 0.9% NaCl, D₅W to a concentration of 0.5 mg/ml further dilution; 1.5 to <0.5 mg/ml may result in precipitation of product; use 18-G needle; flush line with 0.9% NaCl after administration; use reconstituted IV sol within 8 hr or discard, within 6 hr of coronary occlusion for best results

• Store powder at room temperature or refrigerate; protect from excessive light

• Avoidance of invasive procedures, inj, rectal temp

• Pressure for 30 sec to minor bleeding sites; 30 min to sites of atrial puncture followed by pressure dressing; inform prescriber if this does not attain hemostasis; apply pressure dressing

• Do not use 150 mg or more total dose; intracranial bleeding may occur

• Give heparin therapy after thrombolytic therapy is discontinued and when thrombin time, ACT, and APTT <2 times control (about 3-4 hr), treatment can be initiated before coagulation study results, infusion should be discontinued if pretreatment is INR >1.7, PT >15 sec, or an elevated APPT is identified

• Avoid invasive procedures, inj, rect temp; apply pressure for 30 sec to minor bleeding sites; 30 min to sites of arterial puncture, followed by pressure dressing; inform prescriber if this does not attain hemostasis; apply pressure dressing

• **Cathflo Activase:** Use this product after other options used for declotting a line; reconstitute by using 2.2 ml of sterile water provided and injecting into vial, direct flow into powder (1 mg/ml), foam will disappear after standing, swirl, do not shake, sol will be pale yellow or clear, use sol within 8 hr, instill 2 ml of reconstituted sol into occluded catheter, try to aspirate after ½ hr, if unable to remove allow 2 hrs; a second dose may be used; aspirate 5 ml of blood to remove clot and product; irrigate with normal saline

Y-site compatibilities: Eptifibatide, lidocaine, metoprolol, propranolol

Y-site incompatibilities: Bivalirudin, DOBUTamine, DOPamine, heparin, nitroglycerin

Patient/family education
• Teach patient reason for alteplase, signs and symptoms of bleeding, allergic reactions, when to notify prescriber

---

Evaluation
Positive therapeutic outcome
- Lysis of thrombi
- Adequate hemodynamic state
- Absence of heart failure
- Cannula/catheter leak by occlusion

---

aluminum hydroxide (OTC)
AlternaGEL, Alu-Cap, Alugel ✹,
Alu-Tab ✹, Amphojel ✹, Basaljel ✹
Func. class.: Antacid, hypophosphatemic, antiulcer
Chem. class.: Aluminum product, phosphate binder

ACTION: Neutralizes gastric acidity, binds phosphates in GI tract; these phosphates are excreted

Therapeutic outcome: Decreased acidity, healing of ulcers; decreased phosphate levels in chronic renal failure

USES: Antacid, adjunct in peptic, gastric, duodenal ulcers; hyperphosphatemia in chronic renal failure; reflux esophagitis, hyperacidity, heartburn, stress ulcer prevention in critically ill, GERD

Pharmacokinetics

Absorption	Not usually absorbed
Distribution	Widely distributed if absorbed; crosses placenta
Metabolism	Unknown
Excretion	Feces; kidneys (small amounts), breast milk
Half-life	Unknown

Pharmacodynamics

Onset	20-40 min
Peak	½ hr
Duration	1-3 hr

CONTRAINDICATIONS
Hypersensitivity to this product or aluminum products

Precautions: Pregnancy, breastfeeding, geriatric, fluid restriction, decreased GI motility, GI obstruction, dehydration, renal disease, sodium-restricted diets, GI bleeding, hypokalemia

DOSAGE AND ROUTES
Antacid
Adult: SUSP PO 500-1500 mg 3-6 times/day; max 6 times/day

Hyperphosphatemia
Adult: PO susp 30-40 mL (regular) or 15-20 mL (concentrated) TID-QID
Child: PO 50-150 mg/kg/day in 4-6 divided doses

Available forms: Capsules 475, 500 mg; tablets 300, 500, 600 mg; SUSP 320 mg/5 ml, 450 mg/5 mL, 600 mg/5 ml, 675 mg/5mL

ADVERSE EFFECTS
GI: *Constipation,* anorexia
META: *Hypophosphatemia*

INTERACTIONS
Individual drugs
Allopurinol, amprenavir, delavirdine, digoxin, gabapentin, gatifloxacin, isoniazid, ketoconazole, penicillamine, phenytoin, quiNIDine, ticlopidine: decreased effect of each of these drugs

Drug classifications
Anticholinergics, cephalosporins, corticosteroids, H_2 antagonists, iron salts, phenothiazines, quinolones, tetracyclines, thyroid hormones: decreased effect of each of these drug classifications

Drug/food
High-protein meal: decreased product effect

Drug/lab test
Decreased: Phosphate

NURSING CONSIDERATIONS
Assessment
- Assess GI pain symptoms: location, duration, intensity, alleviating/precipitating factors; monitor for blood in stools, emesis, in ulcer disease
- Monitor phosphate levels, since product is bound in GI system; urinary pH, calcium, electrolytes; hypophosphatemia
- Monitor constipation; increase bulk in diet if needed, may use stool softeners or laxatives; record amount and consistency of stools
- **Monitor aluminum toxicity:** severe renal disease; may also be used for hyperphosphatemia
- **Pregnancy/breastfeeding:** Usually considered safe if used occasionally at recommended dose in pregnancy, breastfeeding

Patient problem
Pain (uses)
Constipation (adverse reactions)
Nonadherence (teaching)

Implementation
- 2 tsp (10 ml) neutralizes 20 mEq of acid
PO route
- Give laxatives or stool softeners if constipation occurs, especially geriatric
- Give after shaking suspension; follow with water to facilitate passage

---

A

- Tab may be chewed if patient is unable to swallow, drink 8 oz of water after chewing; or by nasogastric tube if patient unable to swallow
- Give with 8 oz of water for hyperphosphatemia unless contraindicated
- Give 1 hr before or after other medications to prevent poor absorption
- Give 15 ml 30 min after meals and at bedtime (esophagitis)

NG tube route

- May be given as prescribed q1-2hr and given by gastric tube after diluting with water (peptic ulcer)

Patient/family education

- **Hyperphosphatemia:** Instruct patient to avoid phosphate-containing foods (most dairy products, eggs, fruits, carbonated beverages) during product therapy; to add cheese, corn, pasta, plums, prunes, lentils after product (hypophosphatemia)
- Instruct patient not to use for prolonged periods if serum phosphate is low or if on a low-sodium diet, shake liquid well; HF patients should check for sodium content and use sodium-reduced products
- Instruct patient that stools may appear white or speckled; constipation may result; to report black tarry stools, which indicate gastric bleeding
- Instruct patient to check with prescriber after 2 wk of self-prescribed antacid use; may be used for 4-6 wk after symptoms subside or as prescribed
- Instruct patient to separate other medications by 2 hr
- Teach patient to notify prescriber of black tarry stools, which may indicate bleeding

Evaluation

Positive therapeutic outcome

- Absence of GI pain, decreased acidity
- Increased pH of gastric secretions
- Decreased phosphate levels

---

amikacin (Rx)

(am-i-kay'sin)

Amikan ✦, Arikayce

Func. class.: Antibiotic
Chem. class.: Aminoglycoside

Do not confuse: amikacin/Kineret

ACTION: Interferes with protein synthesis in bacterial cell by binding to ribosomal subunit, which causes misreading of genetic code; inaccurate peptide sequence forms in protein chain, causing bacterial death

Therapeutic outcome: Bactericidal effects for the following organisms: *Staphylococcus aureus (MSSA), Pseudomonas aeruginosa, Escherichia coli, Enterobacter, Acinetobacter, Providencia, Citrobacter, Serratia, Proteus, Klebsiella pneumoniae*

USES: Severe systemic infections of CNS, respiratory, GI, urinary tract, bone, skin, soft tissues caused by susceptible organisms

Unlabeled uses: *Mycobacterium avium* complex (intrathecal or intraventricular) in combination; actinomycotic mycetoma, cystic fibrosis

Pharmacokinetics

Absorption	Well absorbed (IM), completely absorbed (**IV**)
Distribution	Widely distributed in extracellular fluids, poor in CSF; crosses placenta
Metabolism	Minimal; liver
Excretion	Mostly unchanged (79%) in kidneys, removed by hemodialysis
Half-life	2-3 hr, prolonged up to 7 hr in infants; increased in renal disease

Pharmacodynamics

	IM	IV	INH
Onset	Rapid	Rapid	Unknown
Peak	15-30 min	1-2 hr	Unknown
Duration	Unknown	Unknown	Unknown

CONTRAINDICATIONS

Pregnancy, hypersensitivity to aminoglycosides, sulfites

Precautions: Neonates, breastfeeding, geriatric, myasthenia gravis, Parkinson's disease, dehydration, mild to moderate infections

> **BLACK BOX WARNING:** Hearing impairment, renal/neuromuscular disease

DOSAGE AND ROUTES

Adult and child: IV INF 10-15 mg/kg/day in 2-3 divided doses q8-12hr in 100-200 ml D$_5$W over 30-60 min, not to exceed 1.5 g/day; **pulse dosing** (once-daily dosing) may be used with some infections; **IM** 10-15 mg/kg/day in divided doses q8-12hr; or extended internal dosing as an alternative dosing regimen

Neonate: IM/IV 10 mg/kg initially, then 7.5 mg/kg q12hr

Mycobacterium avian complex
Adult and adolescent: IV 7.5-15 mg/kg divided q12-24hr as part of a multiple-drug regimen; **Neb (Arikayce)** 590 mg q day in combination
Child: IV 15-30 mg/kg/day divided q12-24hr as part of a multiple-drug regimen, max 1.5 g/day

Renal dose (extended interval dosing)
Adult: IV/IM CCr 40-59 ml/min 15 mg/kg IV q36hr; CCr 20-39 ml/min 15 mg/kg IV q48hr; <20 ml/min adjust based on serum concentrations and MIC (use traditional dosing)

Available forms: Injection 50, 250 mg/ml; suspension for oral inhalation 590 mg/8.4 mL

ADVERSE EFFECTS
CNS: Dizziness, vertigo, tinnitus, neuromuscular blockade with respiratory paralysis
EENT: Ototoxicity, deafness
HEMA: Eosinophilia, anemia
INTEG: *Rash*, burning, urticaria, dermatitis, alopecia
RESP: Apnea
SYST: Hypersensitivity

INTERACTIONS
Individual drugs

> **BLACK BOX WARNING:** Acyclovir, amphotericin B, cidofovir, cycloSPORINE, vancomycin: increased nephrotoxicity

> **BLACK BOX WARNING:** DimenhyDRINATE, ethacrynic acid: increased masking of ototoxicity

Drug classifications

> **BLACK BOX WARNING:** Anesthetics, nondepolarizing neuromuscular blockers: increased neuromuscular blockade, respiratory depression

> **BLACK BOX WARNING:** Increased: Ototoxicity-IV loop diuretics

Penicillins, cephalosporins: decreased effect of amikacin in renal disease
NSAIDs: neurotoxicity

Drug/lab test
Increased: BUN, creatinine, urea levels (urine), increased AST/ALT, alkaline phosphatase, bilirubin, LDH

NURSING CONSIDERATIONS
Assessment
- Assess patient for previous sensitivity reaction
- Assess patient for signs and symptoms of infection, including characteristics of wounds, sputum, urine, stool, WBC >10,000/mm^3, earache, temp; obtain baseline information before and during treatment
- Assess for allergic reactions: rash, urticaria, pruritus

> **BLACK BOX WARNING: Nephrotoxicity:** Assess renal impairment; obtain urine for CCr, BUN, serum creatinine; lower dosage should be given in renal impairment; nephrotoxicity may be reversible if product is stopped at first sign. Notify prescriber of increased BUN and creatinine, urine CCr <80 ml/min; urinalysis daily for protein, cells, casts

- Monitor blood studies: AST, ALT, CBC, Hct, bilirubin, LDH, alkaline phosphatase
- Assess for **overgrowth of infection:** perineal itching, fever, malaise, redness, pain, swelling, drainage, rash, diarrhea, change in cough, sputum
- Obtain weight before treatment; calculation of dosage is usually based on ideal body weight but may be calculated on actual body weight; in those underweight and nonobese, use total body weight (TBW) instead of ideal body weight
- Assess **IV** site for thrombophlebitis including pain, redness, swelling; change site if needed; apply warm compresses to discontinued site

> **BLACK BOX WARNING: Ototoxicity:** Deafness by audiometric testing, ringing, roaring in ears, vertigo; assess hearing before, during, after treatment

- **Dehydration:** high specific gravity, decrease in skin turgor, dry mucous membranes, dark urine, keep well hydrated 2000 mL/day
- **Vestibular dysfunction:** nausea, vomiting, dizziness, headache; product should be discontinued if severe
- **Pregnancy/breastfeeding:** Identify if pregnancy is planned or suspected or if breastfeeding; do not use in pregnancy or breastfeeding

Patient problem
Infection (uses)
Impaired hearing (adverse reactions)

Implementation
- Obtain C&S before administration, begin treatment before results if received
IM route
- Give deeply in large muscle mass, rotate inj sites
- Obtain peak 1 hr after IM, trough before next dose

Inhalation route (nebulizer)
- Use Lamira Nebulizer System
- May pretreat with short-acting beta 2 agonists
- Allow to warm to room temperature
- Shake well, pour medication into reservoir
- Press and hold on/off button, mist will flow
- Insert mouthpiece, take slow deep breaths, when done a beep will be heard
- Clean after each use

Intermittent IV INF route
- **Dilute** 500 mg of product/100-200 ml of **IV** D₅W, 0.9% NaCl and **give** over ½-1 hr; dilute insufficient volume to allow inf over 1-2 hr (infants); **flush** after administration with D₅W or 0.9% NaCl; solution is clear or pale yellow; discard if precipitate or dark color develops
- In children, amount of fluid depends on ordered dose; in infants infuse over 1-2 hr
- Give in evenly spaced doses to maintain blood level

Y-site compatibilities: Acyclovir, alatrofloxacin, aldesleukin, alemtuzumab, alfentanil, amifostine, aminophylline, amiodarone, amsacrine, anidulafungin, argatroban, ascorbic acid, atracurium, atropine, aztreonam, benztropine, bivalirudin, bumetanide, buprenorphine, butorphanol, calcium chloride/gluconate, CARBOplatin, caspofungin, ceFAZolin, cefepime, cefonicid, cefotaxime, cefOTEtan, cefOXitin, cefTAZidime, ceftizoxime, cefTRIAXone, cefuroxime, chloramphenicol, chlorproMAZINE, cimetidine, cisatracurium, CISplatin, clindamycin, codeine, cyanocobalamin, cyclophosphamide, cycloSPORINE, cytarabine, DACTINomycin, DAPTOmycin, dexamethasone, dexmedetomidine, digoxin, diltiazem, diphenhydrAMINE, DOBUTamine, DOCEtaxel, DOPamine, doripenem, doxacurium, DOXOrubicin, doxycycline, enalaprilat, ePHEDrine, EPINEPHrine, epirubicin, epoetin alfa, eptifibatide, ertapenem, erythromycin, esmolol, etoposide, famotidine, fentaNYL, filgrastim, fluconazole, fludarabine, fluorouracil, foscarnet, furosemide, gemcitabine, gentamicin, glycopyrrolate, granisetron, hydrocortisone, HYDROmorphone, IDArubicin, ifosfamide, IL-2, imipenem-cilastatin, isoproterenol, ketorolac, labetalol, levofloxacin, lidocaine, linezolid, LORazepam, magnesium sulfate, mannitol, mechlorethamine, melphalan, meperidine, metaraminol, methotrexate, methoxamine, methyldopate, methylPREDNISolone, metoclopramide, metoprolol, metroNIDAZOLE, midazolam, milrinone, mitoXANtrone, morphine, multivitamins, nafcillin, nalbuphine, naloxone, niCARdipine, nitroglycerin, nitroprusside, norepinephrine, octreotide, ondansetron, oxaliplatin, oxytocin, PACLitaxel, palonosetron, pantoprazole, papaverine, PEMEtrexed, penicillin G, pentazocine, perphenazine, PHENobarbital, phenylephrine, phytonadione, piperacillin-tazobactam, potassium chloride, procainamide, prochlorperazine, promethazine, propranolol, protamine, pyridoxine, quinupristin-dalfopristin, ranitidine, remifentanil, riTUXimab, rocuronium, sargramostim, sodium acetate, sodium bicarbonate, succinylcholine, SUFentanil, tacrolimus, teniposide, theophylline, thiamine, thiotepa, ticarcillin/clavulanate, tigecycline, tirofiban, tobramycin, tolazoline, trimetaphan, urokinase, vancomycin, vasopressin, vecuronium, verapamil, vinCRIStine, vinorelbine, voriconazole, warfarin, zidovudine, zoledronic acid

Patient/family education
- Advise patient to contact prescriber if vaginal itching, loose foul-smelling stools, furry tongue occur; may indicate superinfection
- Advise patient to report hypersensitivity: rash, itching, trouble breathing, facial edema and notify prescriber

Evaluation
Positive therapeutic outcome
- Absence of signs/symptoms of infection: WBC <10,000/mm³, temp WNL; absence of red draining wounds; absence of earache
- Reported improvement in symptoms of infection

TREATMENT OF OVERDOSE:
Withdraw product; administer EPINEPHrine, O₂, hemodialysis, exchange transfusion in the newborn; monitor serum levels of product; may give ticarcillin or carbenicillin

aMILoride (Rx)
(a-mill′oh-ride)
Midamor
Func. class.: Potassium-sparing diuretic
Chem. class.: Pyrazine

Do not confuse: aMILoride/amLODIPine/amiodarone

ACTION: Inhibits sodium, potassium ATPase ion exchange in the distal tubule, cortical collecting duct resulting in inhibition of sodium reabsorption and decreasing potassium secretion

Therapeutic outcome: Diuretic and antihypertensive effect while retaining potassium

USES: Edema in HF in combination with other diuretics; for hypertension, adjunct with other diuretics to maintain potassium

Pharmacokinetics

Absorption	Variable (20%-90%)
Distribution	Widely distributed, crosses placenta
Metabolism	Unchanged in urine (50%), in feces (40%)
Excretion	Renal; breast milk
Half-life	6-9 hr

Pharmacodynamics

Onset	2 hr
Peak	6-10 hr
Duration	24 hr

CONTRAINDICATIONS

Anuria, hypersensitivity, diabetic neuropathy, renal failure

> **BLACK BOX WARNING:** Hyperkalemia

Precautions: Pregnancy, breastfeeding, children, geriatric, dehydration, diabetes, acidosis, respiratory hyponatremia, impaired renal function

DOSAGE AND ROUTES

Adult: PO 5-10 mg daily in 1-2 divided doses; may be increased to 10-20 mg daily if needed
Infant/child (6-20 kg): PO 0.4-0.625 mg/kg/dose q day, max 20 mg/day

Renal dose

Adult: PO CCr 10-50 ml/min reduce dose by 50%; CCr <10 ml/min contraindicated

Available forms: Tabs 5 mg

ADVERSE EFFECTS

CNS: Dizziness, weakness, paresthesias, tremor, depression, anxiety, encephalopathy
CV: Orthostatic hypotension, dysrhythmias, angina
ELECT: Hyperkalemia, dehydration, hyponatremia
GI: *Nausea, diarrhea,* dry mouth, *vomiting, anorexia,* constipation, abdominal pain, jaundice
INTEG: *Rash, pruritus,* Stevens-Johnson syndrome, toxic epidermal necrolysis
MS: *Muscle cramps*

INTERACTIONS

Individual drugs

> **BLACK BOX WARNING:** CycloSPORINE, tacrolimus: increased hyperkalemia

Lithium: increased lithium toxicity, monitor lithium levels

Drug classifications

> **BLACK BOX WARNING:** ACE inhibitors, diuretics (potassium-sparing), potassium products, salt substitutes: increased hyperkalemia. Avoid concurrent use; if using together, monitor K level

Antihypertensives: increased action
NSAIDs: decreased effectiveness of aMILoride, avoid concurrent use

Drug/herb

Hawthorn, horse chestnut: increased aMILoride effect

Drug/food

Potassium foods: increased hyperkalemia, potassium-based salt substitutes

Drug/lab test

Interference: GTT
Increased: LFTs, BUN, potassium, sodium, bilirubin, calcium, cholesterol
Decrease: potassium, magnesium, sodium

NURSING CONSIDERATIONS
Assessment

> **BLACK BOX WARNING:** Monitor for **hyperkalemia:** *MS:* fatigue, muscle weakness; *CARDIAC:* dysrhythmias, hypotension; *NEURO:* paresthesias, confusion; *RESP:* dyspnea, monitor potassium level baseline and each dosage change, hyperkalemia is more common in renal disease, geriatrics, diabetes, if potassium ≥ 5.5 mEq/L immediately notify prescriber

• Assess fluid volume status: distended red veins, crackles in lung, color, quality, and specific gravity of urine, skin turgor, adequacy of pulses, moist mucous membranes, bilateral lung sounds, peripheral pitting edema; dehydration symptoms of decreasing output, thirst, hypotension, dry mouth and mucous membranes should be reported
• Monitor electrolytes: potassium, sodium, calcium, magnesium; also include BUN, ABGs, uric acid, CBC, blood glucose
• Assess B/P before, during therapy
• **Beers:** Avoid in older adults, may decrease sodium, increase potassium, decrease creatinine clearance; use with caution, may exacerbate or cause inappropriate antidiuretic hormone secretion/hyponatremia, monitor sodium levels often

• **Pregnancy/breastfeeding:** Identify if pregnancy is planned or suspected or if breastfeeding, use only if clearly needed.

Patient problem
Fluid imbalance (uses)

Implementation
• Give in AM to avoid interference with sleep
• With food; if nausea occurs, absorption may be increased

Patient/family education
• Teach patient to take medication early in the day to prevent nocturia, to avoid alcohol
• Instruct patient to take with food or milk if GI symptoms of nausea and anorexia occur
• Teach patient to maintain a weekly record of weight and notify prescriber of weight loss >5 lb
• Caution patient that this product causes an increase in potassium levels, so foods high in potassium and potassium supplements or potassium salt substitutes should be avoided; refer to dietitian for assistance, planning
• Caution patient not to exercise in hot weather or stand for prolonged periods since orthostatic hypotension is enhanced
• Teach patient not to use alcohol or any OTC medications without prescriber's approval; serious product reactions may occur
• Emphasize the need to contact prescriber immediately if muscle cramps, weakness, nausea, dizziness, or numbness occurs
• Teach patient to take own B/P and pulse and record
• Advise patient that dizziness and confusion may occur; avoid driving or other hazardous activities if alertness is decreased
• Teach patient to continue taking medication even if feeling better; this product controls symptoms but does not cure the condition, to use as directed, not to double or skip doses
• Advise patient with hypertension to continue other medical treatment (exercise, weight loss, relaxation techniques, cessation of smoking)
• Teach patient to avoid hazardous activities if dizziness occurs

Evaluation
Positive therapeutic outcome
• Prevention of hypokalemia (diuretic use)
• Decreased edema
• Decreased B/P
• Increased diuresis

TREATMENT OF OVERDOSE:
Lavage if taken orally; monitor electrolytes; administer **IV** fluids; monitor hydration, CV, renal status

> ### ⚠ HIGH ALERT
> ## amiodarone (Rx)
> (a-mee-oh′da-rone)
> **Nexterone, Pacerone**
> *Func. class.:* Antidysrhythmic (Class III)
> *Chem. class.:* Iodinated benzofuran derivative

Do not confuse: amiodarone/amantadine

ACTION: Prolongs action potential duration and effective refractory period, noncompetitive α- and β-adrenergic inhibition; increases PR and QT intervals, decreases sinus rate, decreases peripheral vascular resistance

Therapeutic outcome: Decreased amount and severity of ventricular dysrhythmias

USES: Hemodynamically unstable ventricular tachycardia, supraventricular tachycardia, ventricular fibrillation not controlled by 1st-line agents

Unlabeled uses: Supraventricular tachyarrhythmias, ventricular fibrillation, pulseless ventricular tachycardia after CPR and defibrillation failure (ACLS/PALS guidelines)

Pharmacokinetics

Absorption	Slow, variable (PO) up to 65%
Distribution	Body tissues; crosses placenta
Metabolism	Liver, an inhibitor of CYP1A2, CYP3A4, CYP2C8, CYP2C9, CYP2C19, CYP2A6, CYP2B6, CYP2D6, P-glycoprotein, organic cation transporter
Excretion	Bile, kidney (minimal)
Half-life	15-100 days, increased in geriatrics

Pharmacodynamics

	PO	IV
Onset	1-3 wk	2 hr
Peak	3-7 hr	3-7 hr
Duration	Up to several months	Unknown

CONTRAINDICATIONS
Pregnancy, breastfeeding, neonates, infants, severe sinus node dysfunction, hypersensitivity to this product/iodine/benzyl alcohol, cardiogenic shock, 2nd- and 3rd-degree AV block

Precautions: Goiter, Hashimoto's thyroiditis, electrolyte imbalances, HF, severe respiratory disease, children, torsades de pointes

> **BLACK BOX WARNING:** Cardiac arrhythmias, pneumonitis, pulmonary fibrosis, severe hepatic disease, requires a specialized setting

DOSAGE AND ROUTES
Ventricular dysrhythmias
Adult: PO loading dose 800-1600 mg/day for 1-3 wk; then 600-800 mg/day × 1 mo; maintenance 400 mg/day; **IV** loading dose (first rapid) 150 mg over the first 10 min then slow 360 mg over the next 6 hr; maintenance 540 mg given over the remaining 18 hr

Supraventricular tachycardia
Adult PO 600-800 mg/day × 1 wk until desired response, then decrease to 400 mg/day × 3 wk, then 200-400 mg/day (maintenance)
Child PO 10 mg/kg/day × 10 days or until desired response, then decrease to 5 mg/kg/day for several weeks, then decrease to 2.5 mg/kg/day or lower (maintenance)

Available forms: Tabs 100, 200, 400 mg; inj 50 mg/ml

ADVERSE EFFECTS
CNS: *Headache, dizziness,* involuntary movement, tremors, peripheral neuropathy, malaise, fatigue, ataxia, paresthesias, insomnia, confusion, hallucinations
CV: *Hypotension,* bradycardia, HF, dysrhythmias
EENT: Photophobia, *corneal microdeposits,* dry eyes
ENDO: Hyper/hypothyroidism
GI: Nausea, vomiting, diarrhea, abdominal pain, anorexia, constipation, hepatotoxicity pancreatitis
GU: Epididymitis, ED
INTEG: Rash, photosensitivity, blue-gray skin discoloration, alopecia, spontaneous ecchymosis, toxic epidermal necrolysis, urticaria, phlebitis (IV)
MISC: Flushing, abnormal taste or smell, edema, abnormal salivation, coagulation abnormalities
RESP: Pulmonary fibrosis/toxicity, ARDS, gasping syndrome in neonates

INTERACTIONS
Individual drugs
CycloSPORINE, dextromethorphan, digoxin, disopyramide, flecainide, methotrexate, phenytoin, procainamide, quiNIDine, theophylline: increased blood levels, increased toxicity
Loratadine, trazodone: Increased QT prolongation
Warfarin: increased bleeding, dabigatran

Drug classifications
Azoles, fluoroquinolones, macrolides: increased QT prolongation
β-Adrenergic blockers, calcium channel blockers: increased bradycardia, sinus arrest, AV block
Class I antidysrhythmics: increased levels
HMG-CoA reductase inhibitors: increased myopathy
Protease inhibitors: increased amiodarone concentrations, possible serious dysrhythmias, reduce dose

Drug/herb
St. John's wort: decreased amiodarone effect

Drug/food
Grapefruit juice: toxicity

Drug/lab test
Increased: T_4, ALT, AST, GGT, alk phos, cholesterol, lipids, PT, INR
Decrease: T_3

NURSING CONSIDERATIONS
Assessment

> **BLACK BOX WARNING:** Assess for **pulmonary toxicity** including ARDS, pulmonary fibrosis: dyspnea, fatigue, cough, fever, chest pain; product should be discontinued if these occur, increased at higher doses (400 mg/day), toxicity is common

- Monitor electrolytes: potassium, sodium, chloride
- Monitor chest x-ray, PFTs with diffusion capacity, thyroid function tests
- Monitor liver function studies: AST, ALT, bilirubin, alkaline phosphatase

> **BLACK BOX WARNING: Cardiac dysrhythmias:** Monitor ECG continuously to determine product effectiveness; measure PR, QRS, QT intervals; check for PVCs, other dysrhythmias; monitor B/P continuously for hypo/hypertension; check for rebound hypertension after 1-2 hr

- Monitor for dehydration or hypovolemia, monitor PT, INR if using warfarin
- Assess for **CNS symptoms**: confusion, psychosis, numbness, depression, involuntary movements; if these occur, product should be discontinued
- Assess for **hypothyroidism**: lethargy, dizziness, constipation, enlarged thyroid gland, edema of extremities, cool, pale skin
- Monitor **hyperthyroidism**: restlessness, tachycardia, eyelid puffiness, weight loss, frequent urination, menstrual irregularities, dyspnea, warm, moist skin, may cause fatal thyrotoxicosis, cardiac dysrhythmias, product may need to be reduced or discontinued

• Monitor cardiac rate, respiration: rate, rhythm, character, chest pain, ventricular tachycardia, supraventricular tachycardia or fibrillation
• Assess sight and vision before treatment and throughout therapy; microdeposits on the cornea may cause blurred vision, halos, and photophobia, to prevent corneal deposits use methylcellulose
• **Beers:** Avoid as first-line therapy for atrial fibrillation in older adults unless heart failure
• **Stevens-Johnson syndrome, toxic epidermal necrolysis;** monitor for rash, blistering, discontinue immediately, notify prescriber

Patient problem

Impaired cardiac output (uses)
Impaired gas exchange (uses)

Implementation

Start with patient hospitalized and monitored
PO route
• Give reduced dosage slowly with ECG monitoring only
• Loading dose with food to decrease nausea

IV, direct route
• **Peripheral:** max 2 mg/ml for longer than 1 hr; preferred through central venous line with in-line filter; concentration >2 mg/ml should be given by central line
• **Cardiac arrest:** give 300 mg IV bol diluted to a total volume of 20 ml D₅W; may repeat 150 mg after 3-5 min
Intermittent IV INF route
• **Rapid loading:** add 3 ml (150 mg), 100 ml D₅W (1.5 mg/ml), give over 10 min
• **Slow loading:** add 18 ml (900 mg), 500 ml D₅W (1.8 mg/ml), give over next 6 hr

Continuous IV infusion route

• After 24 hr, dilute 50 ml to 1-6 mg/ml, give 1-6 mg/ml at 1 mg/ml for the first 6 hr, then 0.5 mg/min

Y-site compatibilities: Amikacin, bretylium, clindamycin, DOBUTamine, DOPamine, doxycycline, erythromycin, esmolol, gentamicin, insulin (regular), isoproterenol, labetalol, lidocaine, metaraminol, metroNIDAZOLE, midazolam, morphine, nitroglycerin, norepinephrine, penicillin G potassium, phentolamine, phenylephrine, potassium chloride, procainamide, tobramycin, vancomycin

Patient/family education

• Instruct patient to report side effects immediately to prescriber; more common at high dose
• Instruct patient that skin discoloration is usually reversible, but skin may turn bluish on neck, face, arms when used for long periods
• Advise patient that dark glasses may be needed for photophobia
• Instruct patient to use sunscreen and protective clothing to prevent burning associated with photosensitivity
• Instruct patient to take medication as prescribed, not to double doses, do not discontinue abruptly, not to use other drugs, herbs without prescriber approval, many interactions
• Instruct patient to complete follow-up appointment with health care provider, including pulmonary function studies, chest x-ray, ophthalmic examinations
• Teach patient to report vision changes, weight change, rash, blistering, numbness, temperature intolerance
• **Pregnancy/breastfeeding:** Teach patient product is not to be used during pregnancy or breastfeeding

Evaluation

Positive therapeutic outcome
• Decreased ventricular tachycardia
• Decreased supraventricular tachycardia or fibrillation

TREATMENT OF OVERDOSE:

Administer O₂, artificial ventilation, ECG, DOPamine for circulatory depression, diazepam or seizures; isoproterenol

amitriptyline (Rx)

(a-mee-trip′ti-leen)
Elavil ✦, Levate ✦
Func. class.: Antidepressant—tricyclic
Chem. class.: Tertiary amine

Do not confuse: amitriptyline/ nortriptyline/aminophylline

ACTION: Blocks reuptake of norepinephrine, serotonin into nerve endings that increase action of norepinephrine, serotonin in nerve cells

Therapeutic outcome: Decreased symptoms of depression after 2-3 wk

USES: Major depression

Unlabeled uses: Neuropathic pain, fibromyalgia, anxiety, insomnia

Pharmacokinetics

Absorption	Well absorbed
Distribution	Widely distributed; crosses placenta, protein binding >95%
Metabolism	Liver, extensively
Excretion	Kidneys, breast milk
Half-life	10-46 hr

Pharmacodynamics (antidepressant action)

Onset	up to 30 days
Peak	2-6 wk
Duration	up to several weeks

CONTRAINDICATIONS

Hypersensitivity to tricyclics, recovery phase of MI

Precautions: Pregnancy, breastfeeding, geriatric, seizure disorders, prostatic hypertrophy, schizophrenia, psychosis, severe depression, increased intraocular pressure, closed-angle glaucoma, urinary retention, cardiac disease, renal/hepatic disease, hyperthyroidism, electroshock therapy, elective surgery

> **BLACK BOX WARNING:** Child <12 yr, suicidal patients

DOSAGE AND ROUTES

Adults: PO Initially, 75 mg/day in divided doses or 50-100 mg qday at bedtime may increase max 300 mg/day

• **Geriatric:** PO 10-25 mg at bedtime may increase by 10-25 mg q wk, max 150 mg/ day

Available forms: Tabs 10, 25, 50, 75, 100, 150 mg

ADVERSE EFFECTS

CNS: *Dizziness, drowsiness, insomnia,* EPS (geriatric), increased psychiatric symptoms, suicidal thoughts
CV: *Orthostatic hypotension,* ECG changes, palpitations, dysrhythmias, QT prolongation, torsade de pointes
EENT: Amblyopia
GI: *Constipation, dry mouth,* weight gain, paralytic ileus, increased appetite, cramps, epigastric distress, jaundice, hepatitis, stomatitis
GU: *Urinary retention,* sexual dysfunction
HEMA: Agranulocytosis, thrombocytopenia, eosinophilia, leukopenia, aplastic anemia
INTEG: Rash

INTERACTIONS
Individual drugs

Alcohol: increased CNS depression
Amiodarone, procainamide, quiNIDine: increased QT prolongation
CarBAMazepine, cimetidine, fluoxetine, ritonavir: increased levels, increased toxicity, may need dosage reduction
CloNIDine: Increase: hypertensive crisis, avoid use
Linezolid, methylene blue, tramadol, trazodone: increased serotonin syndrome, use cautiously

Drug classifications

Antidepressants, antidysrhythmics (class IC), phenothiazines, SSRIs, SNRI: increased amitriptyline levels, toxicity
Antidysrhythmics (class IA, III), tricyclic antidepressants: increased QT prolongation
Barbiturates, benzodiazepines, CNS depressants, opioids, sedative/hypnotics, sympathomimetics (direct acting): increased CNS effects
MAOIs: hypertensive crisis, seizures, hyperpyretic crisis, do not use within 14 days of MAOIs
Oral contraceptives: increased effects, toxicity

Drug/herb

Chamomile, hops, kava, lavender, valerian: increased CNS depression
SAM-e, St. John's wort, yohimbe: increased serotonin syndrome, avoid concurrent use

Drug/lab test

Increased: blood glucose, LFTs
Decreased: WBCs, platelets, granulocytes, blood glucose

NURSING CONSIDERATIONS
Assessment

• Monitor B/P (with patient lying, standing), pulse; if systolic B/P drops 20 mm Hg, hold product, notify prescriber; take VS more frequently in patients with cardiovascular disease
• Monitor blood studies: CBC, leukocytes, differential, cardiac enzymes if patient is receiving long-term therapy, thyroid function tests
• Monitor hepatic studies: AST, ALT, bilirubin
• Check weight weekly; appetite may increase with product
• Assess ECG baseline, periodically in those with cardiac disease, avoid use immediately after MI
• Assess for EPS primarily in geriatric: rigidity, dystonia, akathisia

> **BLACK BOX WARNING:** Assess mental status: mood, sensorium, affect, suicidal tendencies; increase in psychiatric symptoms: depression, panic; suicidal tendencies are higher in those ≤ 24 yr, restrict amount of product available, not to use in child <12 yr

• Monitor urinary retention, constipation; constipation is more likely to occur in children or geriatric
• Assess for paralytic ileus, glaucoma exacerbation
• Assess for **withdrawal symptoms:** headache, nausea, vomiting, muscle pain, weakness; do not usually occur unless product was discontinued abruptly
• Identify alcohol consumption; if alcohol is consumed, hold dose until morning

---

- Assess for sexual dysfunction: erectile dysfunction, decreased libido; usually resolves after discontinuing product
- **Pain syndromes:** monitor for location, intensity, alleviating/aggravating factors baseline and periodically
- **Beers:** Avoid in older adults, highly anticholinergic, sedating, causes orthostatic hypotension
- **Pregnancy/breastfeeding:** Teach patient to notify health care professional if pregnancy is planned or suspected, or if breastfeeding

Patient problem
Risk for injury (uses, adverse reactions)
Pain (uses)

Implementation
- Give with food or milk for GI symptoms
- Crush if patient is unable to swallow medication whole and given with fluids, foods
- Give dose at bedtime if oversedation occurs during day; may take entire dose at bedtime; geriatric may not tolerate once/day dosing; use tapering when withdrawing product
- Store at room temperature; do not freeze

Patient/family education
- Teach patient that therapeutic effects may take 2-3 wk, to take as directed, usually at bedtime, not to discontinue quickly after long-term use, usually used for at least 3-4 mo
- Advise patient follow-up exams will be needed
- Pregnancy/breastfeeding: Teach patient to notify health care professional if pregnancy is planned or suspected, or if breastfeeding
- Instruct patient to use caution in driving or other activities requiring alertness because of drowsiness, dizziness, blurred vision; to avoid rising quickly from sitting to standing, especially geriatric; management of anticholinergic effects
- Advise patient to avoid alcohol ingestion, other CNS depressants; overheating
- Advise patient to wear sunscreen or large hat, since photosensitivity occurs; hyperthermia can occur
- Teach patient to increase fluids, bulk in diet if constipation, urinary retention occur, especially geriatric
- Teach patient to use gum, hard sugarless candy, or frequent sips of water for dry mouth

> **BLACK BOX WARNING:** Teach patient, caregivers to watch for suicidal ideation, thoughts of dying, making a plan or attempts, panic attacks, changes in mood

Evaluation
Positive therapeutic outcome
- Decreased depression
- Absence of suicidal thoughts

TREATMENT OF OVERDOSE: A
ECG monitoring, lavage, administer anticonvulsant, sodium bicarbonate

amLODIPine (Rx)
(am-loe′di-peen)
Norvasc
Func. class.: Antianginal, calcium channel blocker, antihypertensive
Chem. class.: Dihydropyridine

Do not confuse: amLODIPine/aMILoride

ACTION: Inhibits calcium ion influx across cell membrane during cardiac depolarization; produces relaxation of coronary vascular smooth muscle and peripheral vascular smooth muscle; dilates coronary vascular arteries; increases myocardial oxygen delivery in patients with vasospastic angina

Therapeutic outcome: Decreased angina pectoris, dysrhythmias, B/P

USES: Chronic stable angina pectoris, hypertension, variant angina (Prinzmetal's angina)

Pharmacokinetics
Absorption	Well absorbed up to 90%
Distribution	Crosses placenta, protein binding 93%
Metabolism	Liver, extensively by CYP3A4
Excretion	Kidneys to metabolites (90%)
Half-life	30-50 hr; increased in geriatric, hepatic disease

Pharmacodynamics (CV action)
Onset	Unknown
Peak	6-10 hr
Duration	24 hr

CONTRAINDICATIONS
Hypersensitivity to this product, severe aortic stenosis, severe obstructive CAD

Precautions: Pregnancy, breastfeeding, children, geriatric, HF, hypotension, hepatic injury, GERD

DOSAGE AND ROUTES
Hypertension
Adult: PO 5 mg daily initially, max 10 mg/day
Adolescents/child 6-17 yr
PO 2.5-5 mg q day max 5 mg/day
Geriatric: PO 2.5 mg/day; may increase to 5 mg/day, max 10 mg/day

Hepatic dose
Adult: PO 2.5 mg/day, may increase to 10 mg/day (antihypertensive); 5 mg/day, may increase to 10 mg/day (antianginal)

Available forms: Tabs 2.5, 5, 10 mg

ADVERSE EFFECTS

CNS: Headache, fatigue, dizziness, asthenia, anxiety, depression, insomnia, paresthesia, somnolence

CV: Angina, peripheral edema, bradycardia, hypotension, palpitations

GI: Nausea, anorexia, gingival hyperplasia, dyspepsia

INTEG: Rash, flushing, photosensitivity

INTERACTIONS
Drug classifications
Cyclosporine: Increased level
Simvastatin: Increased myopathy
Strong CYP3A4 inhibitors (clarithromycin, ketoconazole, itraconazole, ritonavir): Increased levels

NURSING CONSIDERATIONS
Assessment
• Assess fluid volume status: distended red neck veins, crackles in lung; color, quality, and specific gravity of urine, skin turgor, adequacy of pulses, moist mucous membranes, bilateral lung sounds, peripheral pitting edema; dehydration symptoms of decreasing output, thirst, hypotension, dry mouth and mucous membranes should be reported
• **Angina:** Assess for angina: intensity, location, duration of pain
• Monitor B/P and pulse; if B/P drops, notify health care professional; monitor ECG during treatment
• **Pregnancy/breastfeeding:** Identify if pregnancy is planned or suspected or if breastfeeding, data are limited on pregnancy or breastfeeding

Patient problem
Ineffective tissue perfusion (uses)
Pain (uses)

Implementation
• Give once a day, without regard to meals

Patient/family education
• Advise patient to avoid hazardous activities until stabilized on product, dizziness is no longer a problem
• Instruct patient to avoid alcohol and OTC, Rx, herbs, supplements products unless directed by prescriber
• Advise patient to comply in all areas of medical regimen: diet, exercise, stress reduction, smoking cessation, product therapy; to notify prescriber of irregular heartbeat, shortness of breath, swelling of feet, face, and hands, severe dizziness, constipation, nausea, hypotension; use nitroglycerin when angina is severe
• Teach patient to use as directed even if feeling better; may be taken with other cardiovascular products (nitrates, β-blockers), not to double or skip doses
• Teach patient how to take pulse correctly, to hold dose if <50 bpm and notify health care professional
• Advise patient to wear sunscreen, protective clothing to prevent photosensitivity
• Inform patient to keep regular dental exam and good dental hygiene to prevent gingival hyperplasia
• Teach patient to change positions for lying, sitting, standing slowly to minimize orthostatic hypertension

Evaluation
Positive therapeutic outcome
• Decreased anginal pain
• Decreased B/P
• Increased exercise tolerance

TREATMENT OF OVERDOSE:
Defibrillation, β-agonists, **IV** calcium inotropic agents, diuretics, atropine for AV block, vasopressor for hypotension

amoxicillin (Rx)
(a-mox-i-sill′in)
Moxatag, Novamoxin ✦
Func. class.: Antiinfective, antiulcer
Chem. class.: Aminopenicillin

ACTION: Interferes with cell wall replication of susceptible organisms by binding to the bacterial cell wall; the cell wall; bactericidal, lysis mediated by bacterial cell wall autolysis

Therapeutic outcome: Bactericidal effects for the following organisms: effective for gram-positive cocci *(Staphylococcus aureus, Streptococcus pyogenes, Streptococcus faecalis, Streptococcus pneumoniae)*, gram-negative cocci *(Neisseria gonorrhoeae, Neisseria meningitidis)*, gram-negative bacilli *(Haemophilus influenzae, Proteus mirabilis, Escherichia coli, Salmonella)*, in combination for *Helicobacter pylori*, gram-positive bacilli *(Corynebacterium diphtheriae, Listeria monocytogenes)*; gastric ulcer, β-lactamase-negative organisms

USES: Infections of respiratory tract, skin, GI tract, GU tract, otitis media, meningitis, septicemia, sinusitis, anthrax treatment and prophylaxis, and bacterial endocarditis prophylaxis, ulcers due to Helicobacter pylori

---

⚠ Nurse Alert   ✴ Key NCLEX® Drug   ≫ Drug Specifics

Unlabeled uses: Lyme disease

Pharmacokinetics

Absorption	Well absorbed (90%)
Distribution	Readily in body tissues, fluids, CSF; crosses placenta
Metabolism	Liver (30%)
Excretion	Breast milk, kidney, unchanged (70%)
Half-life	1-1.3 hr, extended in renal disease

Pharmacodynamics

Onset	½ hr
Peak	1-2 hr
Duration	8-12 hr

CONTRAINDICATIONS
Hypersensitivity to penicillins

Precautions: Pregnancy, breastfeeding, neonates, hypersensitivity to cephalosporins, carbapenems; severe renal disease, mononucleosis, phenylketonuria, diabetes, geriatrics, asthma, child, colitis, dialysis, eczema, pseudomembranous colitis, syphilis

DOSAGE AND ROUTES
Most respiratory infections
Adults: PO (immediate-release) 500 mg q12hr or 250 mg q8hr for mild/moderate infections and 875 mg q12hr or 500 mg q8hr for severe infections

Infants >3 mo, children, and adolescents: PO (immediate release) 20 mg/kg/day in divided doses every 8 hr (max: 250 mg/dose) or 25 mg/kg/day PO in divided doses every 12 hr (max: 500 mg/dose) for mild to moderate infections and 40 mg/kg/day PO in divided doses every 8 hr (max: 500 mg/dose) or 45 mg/kg/day PO in divided doses every 12 hr (max: 875 mg/dose) for severe infections
Neonates and infants 3 mo and younger: 30 mg/kg/day PO given in divided doses every 12 hr

Tonsillitis and/or pharyngitis (rheumatic fever prophylaxis) secondary to *Streptococcus pyogenes*
• Adults, adolescents, and children 12 yr and older PO (Moxatag 775 mg extended-release tablets) 775 mg qday, given within 1 hr of completing a meal, for 10 days
Adults: PO (immediate-release) 1 g qday or 500 mg bid for 10 days
• Infants, children, and adolescents PO (immediate-release) 25 mg/kg/dose (max: 500 mg/dose) bid for 10 days

Sinusitis
Children and adolescents 2 yr and older (standard-dose therapy): PO (immediate-release) 45 mg/kg/day divided q12hr
Children and adolescents 2 yr and older (high-dose therapy): PO (immediate-release) 80 to 90 mg/kg/day divided q12hr (max: 2 g/dose)
Children younger than 2 yr: PO Children younger than 2 yr should be treated with amoxicillin plus clavulanic acid, not amoxicillin alone

Acute otitis media
Adults: PO (immediate-release) 500 mg q12hr or 250 mg q8hr for mild/moderate infections and 875 mg q12hr or 500 mg q8hr for severe infections
• **Infants ≥ 6 mo, children, and adolescents** PO (immediate-release) 80 to 90 mg/kg/day divided q12hr
• **Infants 4 to 5 mo PO (immediate-release)** 80 to 90 mg/kg/day divided q12hr for 10 days
• **Infants ≤ 3 mo PO (immediate-release)** 30 mg/kg/day divided q12hr

H. Pylori
Adult PO 1000 mg bid with lansoprazole 30 mg bid with clarithromycin 500 mg bid × 14 days or 1000 mg bid with omeprazole 20 mg bid, with clarithromycin 500 mg bid × 14 days or 1000 mg
BID with esomeprazole 40 mg daily with clarithromycin 500 mg bid × 10 day; 1000 mg tid with lansoprazole 30 mg tid × 14 days

Gonorrhea
Adult and child ≥ 40 kg: PO 3 g single dose
Child >2 yr and <40 kg: 50 mg/kg with probenecid 25 mg/kg single dose

Prevention of endocarditis
Adult PO 2 g 60 min prior to procedure
Child PO 50 mg/kg 60 min prior to procedure, max adult dose

Renal disease
Adult: PO CCr 10-30 ml/min 250-500 mg q12hr; CCr <10 ml/min 250-500 mg q24hr; do not use 775, 875 mg strength if CCr <30 ml/min

Available forms: Caps 250, 500 mg; chewable tabs 125, 200, 250, 400 mg; tabs 250, 500, 875 mg; ext rel tab (Moxatag) 775 mg; powder for susp 125, 200, 250, 400 mg/5 ml; suspension 50 mg/mL

ADVERSE EFFECTS
CNS: Headache, seizures
GI: *Nausea, vomiting, diarrhea*, increased AST, ALT, CDAD

HEMA: Anemia, bone marrow depression, granulocytopenia, hemolytic anemia, eosinophilia, thrombocytopenia, agranulocytosis
INTEG: *Urticaria, rash*
SYST: Anaphylaxis, serum sickness, overgrowth of infection

INTERACTIONS
Individual drugs
Allopurinol: increased risk of rash
Methotrexate: increased methotrexate levels, monitor for toxicity
Probenecid: increased amoxicillin levels, decreased renal excretion, used for this reason
Warfarin: increased anticoagulant effects

Drug classifications
Contraceptives (hormonal): may decrease contraceptive effectiveness

Drug/lab test
Decreased: Hgb, WBC, platelets
Increase: AST/ALT, alk phos, LDH, eosinophils

NURSING CONSIDERATIONS
Assessment
• Assess patient for previous sensitivity reaction to penicillins or other cephalosporins; cross-sensitivity between penicillin products and cephalosporins is common
• Assess patient for signs and symptoms of **infection**, including characteristics of wounds, sputum, urine, stool, WBC >10,000/mm^3, earache, fever; obtain baseline information and monitor symptoms during treatment
• Obtain C&S before beginning product therapy to identify if correct treatment has been initiated
• **Assess for allergic reactions during treatment:** rash, urticaria, pruritus, chills, fever, joint pain; angioedema may occur a few days after therapy begins; EPINEPHrine and resuscitation equipment should be available for anaphylactic reactions, rash is more common if allopurinol is taken concurrently
• Assess bowel pattern daily; diarrhea, cramping, blood in stools; if severe diarrhea occurs, notify prescriber; product should be discontinued; CDAD may occur even weeks after discontinuing product
• Assess for overgrowth of infection: perineal itching, fever, malaise, redness, pain, swelling, drainage, rash, diarrhea, change in cough, sputum

Patient problem
Infection (uses)
Nonadherence (teaching)

Implementation
PO route
• Identify allergies before use
• Give in even doses around the clock without regard to food; if GI upset occurs, give with food; product must be given for 10-14 days to ensure organism death and prevent superinfection; store in tight container
• The caps may be opened and contents taken with fluids
• **Suspension:** shake well before each dose, may be used alone or mixed in drinks, use immediately; susp may be stored in refrigerator for 14 days
• **Extended release:** do not crush, chew, or break; take with food

Patient/family education
• Advise patient to contact prescriber if vaginal itching, loose foul-smelling stools, diarrhea, sore throat, fever, fatigue, furry tongue occur; may indicate superinfection or agranulocytopenia
• Instruct patient to take all medication prescribed for the length of time ordered; not to double dose; chew form is available to use equally around the clock
• Advise patient to notify prescriber of diarrhea with blood or pus, abdominal pain, which may indicate pseudomembranous colitis
• **Pregnancy/breastfeeding:** Identify if pregnancy is planned or suspected, or if breastfeeding, usually considered safe in pregnancy, use cautiously in breastfeeding; advise those taking oral contraceptives to use an alternate contraceptive, since oral contraceptive effect may be decreased

Evaluation
Positive therapeutic outcome
• Absence of signs/symptoms of infection (WBC <10,000/mm^3, temp WNL, absence of red draining wounds or earache)
• Prevention of endocarditis
• Resolution of ulcer symptoms

TREATMENT OF ANAPHYLAXIS:
Withdraw product, maintain airway, administer EPINEPHrine, aminophylline, O$_2$, **IV** corticosteroids

---

amoxicillin/clavulanate (Rx)
(a-mox-i-sill'in)
Augmentin, Augmentin ES, Augmentin XR, Clavulin ✿
Func. class.: Broad-spectrum antiinfective (extended spectrum)
Chem. class.: Aminopenicillin-β lactamase inhibitor

ACTION: Interferes with cell wall replication of susceptible organisms; lysis mediated by bacterial cell wall autolytic enzymes, combination increases spectrum of activity against β-lactamase resistance organisms

Therapeutic outcome: Bactericidal effects for *Actinomyces, Bacillus anthracis, Bacteroides, Bordetella pertussis, Borrelia burgdorferi, Brucella, Burkholderia pseudomallei, Clostridium perfringens, Clostridium tetani, Corynebacterium diphtheriae, Eikenella corrodens, Enterobacter, Enterococcus faecalis, Erysipelothrix rhusiopathiae, Escherichia coli, Eubacterium, Fusobacterium, Haemophilus ducreyi, Haemophilus parainfluenzae* (positive/negative beta-lactamase), *Helicobacter pylori, Klebsiella, Lactobacillus, Listeria monocytogenes, Moraxella catarrhalis, Neisseria gonorrhoeae, Neisseria meningitis, Nocardia brasiliensis, Peptococcus, Peptostreptococcus, Prevotella melaninogenica, Propionibacterium, Salmonella, Shigella, Staphylococcus aureus* (MSSA), *Staphylococcus epidermidis, Staphylococcus saprophyticus, Streptococcus agalactiae* (group B Streptococci), *Streptococcus dysgalactiae, Streptococcus pneumoniae, Streptococcus pyogenes* (group A Streptococci), *Treponema pallidum, Vibrio cholerae,* viridans streptococci

USES: Infections of lower respiratory tract, skin, GU tract; impetigo; otitis media, sinusitis, pneumonia, and endocarditis prophylaxis

Pharmacokinetics

Absorption	Well absorbed (90%)
Distribution	Readily in body tissues, fluids, CSF; crosses placenta
Metabolism	Liver (30%)
Excretion	Breast milk; kidney, unchanged (70%), removed by hemodialysis
Half-life	1-1.3 hr

Pharmacodynamics

Onset	½ hr
Peak	1-2.5 hr
Duration	8-12 hr

CONTRAINDICATIONS
Hypersensitivity to penicillins, severe renal disease, dialysis, jaundice

Precautions: Pregnancy, breastfeeding, neonates, children, hypersensitivity to cephalosporins, GI/renal disease, asthma, colitis, diabetes, eczema, leukemia, mononucleosis, viral infections, phenylketonuria

DOSAGE AND ROUTES
Most infections
Adult/child >40 kg: PO 250 mg q 8 hr or 500 mg q 12 hr

Recurrent/persistent otitis media (*Streptococcus pneumoniae, Haemophilus influenzaem, Moreaxella catarrhalis)* in those exposed to antiinfectives within the past 3 mo (≤ 2 yr or in daycare)
Child >3 mo PO 90 mg/kg/day (600 mg amoxicillin/42.9mg clavulanate) q12hr × 10 days

Lower respiratory infections, otitis media, sinusitis, skin/skin structure infections; UTIs
Adult: PO 250-500 mg q8hr or 500-875 mg q12hr depending on severity of infection
Child ≤40 kg: PO 20-90 mg/kg/day in divided doses q8-12hr

Community-acquired pneumonia or acute bacterial sinusitis
Adult: PO 2000 mg/125 mg (Augmentin XR) q12hr x 7-10 days (pneumonia), 10 days (sinusitis)

Renal dose
Adult: PO CCr 10-30 ml/min dose q12hr; CCr <10 ml/min dose q24hr; do not use 875 mg strength if CCr <30 ml/min; Augmentin XR is contraindicated in renal disease

Available forms: Tabs 250, 500, 875 mg amoxicillin/125 mg clavulanate; chewable tabs 200 amoxicillin/28.5 mg clavulanate, 400 mg amoxicillin/57 mg clavulanate; powder for oral susp 125 amoxicillin mg/31.25 mg clavulanate, 250/28.5, 200/28.5, 400/57 mg clavulanate, 600/42.9 mg clavulanate mg/5 ml; (XR) ext rel tabs 1000 mg amoxicillin/62.5 mg clavulanate; (ES) powder for oral susp 600 mg amoxicillin; 42.9 mg clavulanate/5 ml

ADVERSE EFFECTS
CNS: Headache, seizures
GI: *Nausea, diarrhea, vomiting,* increased AST, ALT, CDAD

GU: *Vaginitis*

HEMA: Anemia, bone marrow depression, granulocytopenia, leukopenia, eosinophilia, thrombocytopenic purpura

INTEG: Rash, urticaria

SYST: Anaphylaxis, serum sickness, superinfection

INTERACTIONS
Individual drugs
Probenecid: increased amoxicillin levels, used for this reason

Warfarin: increased anticoagulant effect, monitor closely: dose adjustment may be needed

Oral contraceptives: decreased contraceptive effect

Drug/food
High-fat meal: decreased absorption

Drug/lab test
Increased: AST/ALT, alk phos, LDH

False-positive: Direct Coombs test

NURSING CONSIDERATIONS
Assessment
• Assess patient for previous sensitivity reaction to penicillins or other cephalosporins; cross-sensitivity between penicillins and cephalosporins is common

• Assess patient for signs and symptoms of **infection**, including characteristics of wounds, sputum, urine, stool, WBC >10,000/mm^3, earache, fever; obtain baseline information and during treatment

• Complete C&S before beginning product therapy to identify if correct treatment has been initiated

• **Assess for anaphylaxis:** rash, urticaria, pruritus, chills, dyspnea, laryngeal edema, fever, joint pain; angioedema may occur a few days after therapy begins; EPINEPHrine and resuscitation equipment should be available for anaphylactic reaction

• Monitor blood studies: AST, ALT, CBC, Hct, bilirubin, LDH, alkaline phosphatase, Coombs' test baseline and monthly if patient is on long-term therapy

• Assess bowel pattern daily; diarrhea, cramping, blood in stools, report to prescriber; if severe diarrhea occurs, product should be discontinued; may indicate CDAD

• Assess for **overgrowth of infection:** perineal itching, fever, malaise, redness, pain, swelling, drainage, rash, diarrhea, change in cough, sputum

Patient problem
Infection (uses)

Nonadherence (teaching)

Implementation
PO route
• Give in even doses around the clock; if GI upset occurs, give with food; product must be taken for 10-14 days to ensure organism death and prevent superinfection; store in tight container; cap can be opened and mixed with food or liquid; chewable tabs should be chewed

• Administer only as directed; two 250-mg tabs not equivalent to one 500-mg tab due to strength of clavulanate

• Shake susp well before each dose; may be used alone or mixed in drinks, use immediately; susp may be stored in refrigerator for 10 days

Patient/family education
• Advise patient to contact prescriber if vaginal itching, loose foul-smelling stools occur; may indicate superinfection

• Instruct patient to take all medication prescribed for the length of time prescribed, not to double or skip doses

• Advise patient to notify prescriber of diarrhea with blood or pus, which may indicate CDAD

• **Pregnancy/breastfeeding:** Teach patient to notify all health care professionals if pregnancy is planned or suspected or if breastfeeding, to use another form of contraception if taking oral contraception, as effect may be decreased

Evaluation
Positive therapeutic outcome
• Absence of signs/symptoms of infection (WBC <10,000/mm^3, temp WNL)

• Reported improvement in symptoms of infection

TREATMENT OF ANAPHYLAXIS:
Withdraw product, maintain airway, administer EPINEPHrine, aminophylline, O$_2$, **IV** corticosteroids

---

⚠ HIGH ALERT

amphotericin B lipid complex (ABLC)
(am-foe-ter'i-sin)

Abelcet

Func. class.: Antifungal

Chem. class.: Amphoteric polyene

Do not confuse: Abelcet/amphotericin B

ACTION: Increases cell membrane permeability in susceptible fungi by binding sterols;

---

alters cell membrane, thereby causing leakage of cell components, cell death

Therapeutic outcome: Decreased fever, malaise, rash; negative C&S for infecting organism

USES: Indicated for the treatment of invasive fungal infections in patients who cannot tolerate or have failed conventional amphotericin B therapy; broad-spectrum activity against many fungal, yeast and mold pathogen infections, including *Aspergillus, Zygomycetes, Fusarium, Cryptococcus,* and many hard-to-treat *Candida* species; *Aspergillus fumigatus, Aspergillus, Blastomyces dermatitidis, Candida albicans, Candida guilliermondii, Candida stellatoidea, Candida tropicalis, Coccidioides immitis, Cryptococcus, Histoplasma, Sporotrichosis*

Precautions: Hypersensitivity, anemia, breastfeeding, cardiac disease, children, electrolyte imbalance, geriatric, hematological/hepatic/ renal disease, hypotension, pregnancy

Pharmacokinetics

Absorption	Complete bioavailability (IV)
Distribution	Body tissues
Metabolism	Liver
Excretion	Kidneys, detectable for several weeks
Half-life	7 days

Pharmacodynamics

Onset	Immediate
Peak	2 hr
Duration	Unknown

DOSAGE AND ROUTES
Adult: IV 5 mg/kg/day

Renal dose
Adult: IV CCr <10 ml/min; give 5 mg/kg q24-36hr

Available forms: Susp for inj 5 mg/mL

ADVERSE EFFECTS
CNS: *Headache, fever, chills,* confusion, anxiety, insomnia
CV: Hypotension, tachycardia edema, chest pain, hypertension
EENT: Tinnitus, deafness, diplopia, blurred vision
GI: *Nausea, vomiting, anorexia,* diarrhea, cramps, bilirubinemia
GU: Nephrotoxicity
HEMA: Anemia, thrombocytopenia, agranulocytosis, leukopenia
INTEG: *Burning, irritation,* pain, necrosis at inj site with extravasation, dermatitis, rash, pruritus

META: Hyponatremia, hypomagnesemia, hypokalemia
MS: Arthralgia, myalgia
RESP: Dyspnea, wheezing
SYST: Toxic epidermal neurolysis, exfoliative dermatitis, anaphylaxis

INTERACTIONS
Digoxin: increased hypokalemia

Drug classifications
Other nephrotoxic antibiotics (aminoglycosides, CISplatin, vancomycin, cycloSPORINE, polymyxin B), antineoplastics, salicylates): increased nephrotoxicity
Azole antifungals: decreased amphotericin B lipid complex effect; antifungals may still be used concurrently in serious resistant infections
Corticosteroids, skeletal muscle relaxants, thiazides, loop diuretics: increased hypokalemia, monitor electrolytes

Drug/lab test
Increased: AST/ALT, alk phos, BUN, creatinine, LDH, bilirubin
Decreased: magnesium, potassium, Hgb, WBC, platelets

NURSING CONSIDERATIONS
Assessment
• Monitor vital signs every 15-30 min during first inf; note changes in pulse, B/P
• I&O ratio; watch for decreasing urinary output, change in specific gravity; discontinue product to prevent permanent damage to renal tubules
• Blood studies: monitor CBC, potassium, sodium, calcium, magnesium every 2 wk; BUN, creatinine 2-3 ×/wk
• Weight weekly; if weight increases by more than 2 lb/wk, edema is present; renal damage should be considered
• **For renal toxicity:** Assess for increasing BUN, serum creatinine; if BUN is >40 mg/dl or if serum creatinine is >3 mg/dl, product may be discontinued, dosage reduced
• **Assess for hepatotoxicity:** Assess for increasing AST, ALT, alk phos, bilirubin
• **For allergic reaction:** dermatitis, rash; product should be discontinued, antihistamines (mild reaction) or EPINEPHrine (severe reaction) should be administered
• **For hypokalemia:** anorexia, drowsiness, weakness, decreased reflexes, dizziness, increased urinary output, increased thirst, paresthesias
• **Infusion reactions:** fever, chills, pain, swelling at site

Patient problem
Infection (uses)

Implementation

- Do not confuse the four different types; these are not interchangeable: conventional amphotericin B, amphotericin B cholesteryl, amphotericin B lipid complex, amphotericin B liposome
- May premedicate with acetaminophen, diphenhydrAMINE

IV route

- Give product only after C&S confirms organism, product needed to treat condition; make sure product is used for life-threatening infections
- Handle with aseptic technique because amphotericin B lipid complex (ABLC) has no preservatives; visually inspect parenteral products for particulate matter and discoloration before use

Filtration and dilution

- Prior to dilution, store at 36°-46° F (2°-8° C), protected from moisture and light; do not freeze; the diluted, ready-for-use admixture is stable for up to 48 hours at 36°-46° F (2°-8° C) and an additional 6 hr at room temperature; do not freeze
- Prepare the admixture for infusion by first shaking the vial until there is no remaining yellow sediment on the bottom of the vial
- Transfer the appropriate amount of drug from the required number of vials into one or more sterile syringes using an 18-gauge needle
- Attach the provided 5-micron filter needle to the syringe; inject the syringe contents through the filter needle, into an IV bag containing the appropriate amount of D₅W injection; each filter needle may be used on the contents of no more than four 100-mg vials
- The suspension must be diluted with D₅W injection to a final concentration of 1 mg/ml; for pediatric patients and patients with cardiovascular disease, the final concentration may be 2 mg/ml; DO NOT USE SALINE SOLUTIONS OR MIX WITH OTHER DRUGS OR ELECTROLYTES
- The diluted ready-for-use admixture is stable for up to 48 hr at 36°-46° F (2°-8° C) and an additional 6 hr at room temperature; do not freeze

IV INF

- Flush IV line with D₅W injection before use or use a separate IV line; DO NOT USE AN IN-LINE FILTER
- Before infusion, shake the bag until the contents are thoroughly mixed; max rate 2.5 mg/kg/hr; if the infusion time exceeds 2 hr, mix the contents by shaking the infusion bag every 2 hr

Y-site compatibilities: Acyclovir, allopurinol, aminocaproic acid, aminophylline, amiodarone, anidulafungin, argatroban, arsenic trioxide, atracurium, azithromycin, aztreonam, bumetanide, buprenorphine, busulfan, butorphanol, CARBOplatin, carmustine, ceFAZolin, cefepime, cefotaxime, cefoTEtan, cefOXitin, cefTAZidime, ceftizoxime, cefTRIAXone, cefuroxime, chloramphenicol, chlorproMAZINE, cimetidine, cisatracurium, clindamycin, cyclophosphamide, cycloSPORINE, cytarabine, DACTINomycin dexamethasone, digoxin, diphenhydrAMINE, DOCEtaxel, doxacurium, DOXOrubicin liposomal, enalaprilat, EPINEPHrine, eptifibatide, ertapenem, etoposide, famotidine, fentaNYL, fludarabine, fluorouracil, fosphenytoin, furosemide, ganciclovir, granisetron, heparin, hydrocortisone, HYDROmorphone, ifosfamide, insulin, regular ketorolac, lepirudin, lidocaine, linezolid, LORazepam, mannitol, melphalan, meperidine, methotrexate, methylPREDNISolone, metoclopramide, mitoMYcin, mivacurium, nafcillin, nesiritide, nitroglycerin, nitroprusside, octreotide, oxaliplatin, PACLitaxel, pamidronate, pantoprazole, PEMEtrexed, pentazocine, PENTobarbital, PHENobarbital, phentolamine, piperacillin-tazobactam, procainamide, ranitidine, succinylcholine, SUFentanil, tacrolimus, telavancin, teniposide, theophylline, thiopental, thiotepa, ticarcillin, ticarcillin-clavulanate, trimethobenzamide, verapamil, vinBLAStine, vinCRIStine, zidovudine, zoledronic acid

Patient/family education

- Teach patient that long-term therapy may be needed to clear infection (2 wk-3 mo, depending on type of infection), that frequent blood draws will be required
- Instruct patient to notify prescriber of bleeding, bruising, or soft-tissue swelling, neurologic, renal symptoms
- **Pregnancy/breastfeeding:** Advise patient to notify provider if pregnancy is planned or suspected, not to breastfeed

Evaluation

Positive therapeutic outcome

- Resolution of infection; negative C&S for infecting organism

---

⚠ HIGH ALERT

amphotericin B liposomal (LAmB)

(am-foe-ter'i-sin)

AmBisome

Func. class.: Antifungal
Chem. class.: Amphoteric polyene

Do not confuse: AmBisome/amphotericin B

ACTION: Increases cell membrane permeability in susceptible fungi by binding to membrane sterols; alters cell membrane, thereby causing leakage of cell components, cell death

---

Therapeutic outcome: Resolution of infection

USES: Empirical therapy for presumed fungal infection in febrile neutropenic patients; treatment of *Cryptococcal* Meningitis in HIV-infected patients; treatment of *Aspergillus, Candida,* and/or *Cryptococcus* infections refractory to amphotericin B deoxycholate, or in patients where renal impairment or unacceptable toxicity precludes the use of amphotericin B deoxycholate *(Aspergillus flavus, Aspergillus fumigatus, Blastomyces dermatitidis, Candida albicans, Candida krusei, Candida lusitaniae, Candida parapsilosis, Candida tropicalis, Cryptococcus neoformans)*; treatment of visceral leishmaniasis

Pharmacokinetics

Absorption	Complete bioavailability (IV)
Distribution	Body tissues
Metabolism	Liver
Excretion	Kidneys, detectable for several weeks
Half-life	4-6 days

Pharmacodynamics

Onset	Immediate
Duration	Unknown

CONTRAINDICATIONS
Hypersensitivity

Precautions: Anemia, breastfeeding, cardiac disease, children, electrolyte imbalance, geriatric, hematological/hepatic/renal disease, hypotension, pregnancy, severe bone marrow depression

DOSAGE AND ROUTES
Systemic fungal infections
Adults and children: IV 3-6 mg/kg/dose q 24 hr

Cryptococcal meningitis in HIV patients
Adults/adolescents/children/infants: IV 6 mg/kg/dose q24hr

Visceral leishmaniasis
Adult IV 3 mg/kg q 24 hr on days 1-5, then 3 mg/kg q 24 hr on days 14 and 21 (immunocompetent); 4 mg/kg q 24 hr on days 1-5, then 4 mg/kg q 24 hr on days 10, 17, 24, 31, 38 (immunosuppressed)

Renal dose
Adult: IV CCr <10 ml/min; use 3 mg/kg q24hr

Available forms: Powder for inj 50-mg vial

ADVERSE EFFECTS
CNS: *Headache, fever, chills,* insomnia, tachycardia edema

CV: Hypotension, tachycardia, edema
GI: *Nausea, vomiting, anorexia,* diarrhea, cramps, bilirubinemia
GU: Nephrotoxicity
HEMA: Anemia, thrombocytopenia, agranulocytosis, leukopenia, hypomagnesemia
INTEG: *Burning, irritation,* pain, necrosis at inj site with extravasation, flushing; dermatitis, skin rash (topical route)
MS: Arthralgia, myalgia
RESP: Dyspnea, wheezing
SYST: Stevens–Johnson syndrome, toxic epidermal neurolysis, exfoliative dermatitis, anaphylaxis

INTERACTIONS
Drug classifications
Other nephrotoxic antibiotics (aminoglycosides, CISplatin, vancomycin, cycloSPORINE, polymyxin B): increased nephrotoxicity
Azole antifungals: decreased amphotericin B liposomial; antifungals may still be used concurrently in serious resistant infections
Corticosteroids, skeletal muscle relaxants, thiazides/loop diuretics: increased hypokalemia

NURSING CONSIDERATIONS
Assessment
• Monitor vital signs every 15-30 min during first inf; note changes in pulse, B/P
• I&O ratio; watch for decreasing urinary output, change in specific gravity; discontinue product to prevent permanent damage to renal tubules
• Blood studies: CBC, potassium, sodium, calcium, magnesium every 2 wk, BUN, creatinine 2-3 ×/wk
• Weight weekly; if weight increases by more than 2 lb/wk, edema is present; renal damage should be considered
• **For renal toxicity:** Assess for increasing BUN, serum creatinine; if BUN is >40 mg/dl or if serum creatinine is >3 mg/dl, product may be discontinued, dosage reduced
• **For hepatotoxicity:** Assess for increasing AST, ALT, alk phos, bilirubin, monitor LFTs
• **For allergic reaction:** Assess for dermatitis, rash; product should be discontinued, antihistamines (mild reaction) or EPINEPHrine (severe reaction) administered
• **For hypokalemia:** Assess for anorexia, drowsiness, weakness, decreased reflexes, dizziness, increased urinary output, increased thirst, paresthesias
• **Infusion reaction:** chills, fever, pain, swelling at site

Patient problem
Infection (uses)

Implementation
• Do not confuse four different types; these are not interchangeable: conventional amphotericin B, amphotericin B cholesteryl, amphotericin B lipid complex, amphotericin B liposome
• May premedicate with acetaminophen, diphenhydrAMINE

IV route
• Give product only after C&S confirms organism, product needed to treat condition
• Make sure product is used for life-threatening infections
• Administer by IV infusion only; handle with aseptic technique as LAmB does not contain any preservatives
• Visually inspect products for particulate matter and discoloration

Reconstitution
• LAmB *must* be reconstituted using sterile water for injection (without a bacteriostatic agent); do not reconstitute with saline or add saline to the reconstituted suspension, do not mix with other drugs; doing so can cause a precipitate to form
• Reconstitute vials containing 50 mg of LAmB/12 ml of sterile water (4 mg/ml)
• Immediately after the addition of water, SHAKE THE VIAL VIGOROUSLY for 30 sec; the suspension should be yellow and translucent; visually inspect vial for particulate matter and continue shaking until product is completely dispersed
• Store suspension for up to 24 hours refrigerated if using sterile water for injection; do not freeze

Filtration and dilution
• Calculate the amount of reconstituted (4 mg/ml) suspension to be further diluted and withdraw this amount into a sterile syringe
• Attach the provided 5-micron filter to the syringe; inject the syringe contents through the filter, into the appropriate amount of D₅W injection; use only one filter per vial
• The suspension must be diluted with D₅W injection to a final concentration of 1-2 mg/ml before administration; for infants and small children, lower concentrations (0.2-0.5 mg/ml) may be appropriate to provide sufficient volume for infusion
• Use injection of LAmB within 6 hr of dilution with D₅W

IV INF
• Flush intravenous line with D₅W injection before infusion; if this cannot be done, then a separate IV line must be used

• An inline membrane filter may be used provided the mean pore diameter of the filter is not less than 1 micron
• Administer by IV infusion using a controlled infusion device over a period of approximately 120 min; infusion time may be reduced to approximately 60 min in patients who tolerate the infusion; if discomfort occurs during infusion, the duration of infusion may be increased

Acetaminophen and diphenhydrAMINE
• 30 min before inf to reduce fever, chills, headache
• Store protected from moisture and light; diluted solution is stable for 24 hr at room temp

Y-site compatibilities: Acyclovir, amifostine, aminophylline, anidulafungin, atropine, azithromycin, bivalirudin, bumetanide, buprenorphine, busulfan, butorphanol, CARBOplatin, carmustine, ceFAZolin, ceFOXitin, ceftizoxime, cefTRIAXone, cefuroxime, cimetidine, clindamycin, cyclophosphamide, cytarabine, DACTINomycin, DAPTOmycin, dexamethasone, dexmedetomidine, diphenhydrAMINE, doxacurium, enalaprilat, ePHEDrine, EPINEPHrine, eptifibatide, ertapenem, esmolol, etoposide, famotidine, fenoldopam, fentaNYL, fludarabine, fluorouracil, fosphenytoin, furosemide, granisetron, haloperidol, heparin, hydrocortisone, HYDROmorphone, ifosfamide, isoproterenol, ketorolac, levorphanol, lidocaine, linezolid, mesna, methotrexate, methylPREDNISolone, metoprolol, milrinone, mitoMYcin, nesiritide, nitroglycerin, nitroprusside, octreotide, oxaliplatin, oxytocin, palonosetron, pancuronium, pantoprazole, PEMEtrexed, PENTobarbital, PHENobarbital, phenylephrine, piperacillin/tazobactam, potassium chloride, procainamide, ranitidine, SUFentanil, tacrolimus, theophylline, thiopental, thiotepa, ticarcillin/clavulanate, tigecycline, trimethoprim-sulfamethoxazole, vasopressin, vinCRIStine, voriconazole, zidovudine

Patient/family education
• Teach patient that long-term therapy may be needed to clear infection (2 wk-3 mo, depending on type of infection)
• Instruct patient to notify prescriber of bleeding, bruising, or soft-tissue swelling, renal, neurological side effects

Pregnancy/breastfeeding:
• Advise patient to notify provider if pregnancy is planned or suspected, not to breastfeed
• Advise patient that frequent blood draws will be required with long-term therapy to monitor for side effects

---

⚠ Nurse Alert   ✴ Key NCLEX® Drug   ≫ Drug Specifics

Evaluation
Positive therapeutic outcome
• Resolution of infection

ampicillin (Rx)
(am-pi-sill'in)
Func. class.: Broad-spectrum antiinfective
Chem. class.: Aminopenicillin

ACTION: Interferes with cell wall replication of susceptible organisms; the cell wall, rendered osmotically unstable, swells and bursts from osmotic pressure, lysis mediated by cell wall autolysis

Therapeutic outcome: Bactericidal effects for the following organisms: effective for gram-positive cocci *(Streptococcus aureus, Streptococcus pyogenes, Streptococcus faecalis, Streptococcus pneumoniae),* gram-negative cocci *(Neisseria meningitidis),* gram-negative bacilli *(Haemophilus influenzae, Proteus mirabilis, Salmonella, Shigella, Listeria monocytogenes),* gram-positive bacilli

USES: Infections of respiratory tract, skin, skin structures, GI/GU tract; otitis media, meningitis, septicemia, sinusitis, and endocarditis prophylaxis, bacterial endocarditis

Pharmacokinetics

Absorption	Moderate, in duodenum (35%-50%)
Distribution	Readily in body tissues, fluids, CSF; crosses placenta
Excretion	Breast milk; kidney unchanged (70%), removed by dialysis
Half-life	50-110 min

Pharmacodynamics

	PO	IM	IV
Onset	Rapid	Rapid	Rapid
Peak	2 hr	1 hr	Infusion end
Duration	4-6 hr	4-6 hr	4-6 hr

CONTRAINDICATIONS
Hypersensitivity to penicillins, antimicrobial resistance, skin infection

Precautions: Pregnancy, breastfeeding, neonates, hypersensitivity to cephalosporins, renal disease, mononucleosis

DOSAGE AND ROUTES
Systemic infections
Adult and child ≥40 kg (88 lb): PO 250-500 mg q6hr; **IV/IM** 2-8 g daily in divided doses q4-6hr

Child <40 kg: PO 50-100 mg/kg/day in divided doses q6-8hr; **IV/IM** 100-150 mg/kg/day divided q 6 hr

Bacterial meningitis
Adult/adolescent: IM/**IV** 150-200 mg/kg/day in divided doses, q3-4hr; IDSA IV 2 g q 4 hr
Infant/child: IM/**IV** 150-200 mg/kg/day in divided doses q3-4hr; IDSA dose IV 200-400 mg/kg/day divided q6hr
Neonate >7 days and >2000 g: IM/**IV** 200 mg/kg/day divided q6hr; IDSA dose IV 200 mg/kg/day divided q6-8hr

Prevention of bacterial endocarditis
Adult: IM/**IV** 2 g 30 min before procedure
Child: IM/**IV** 50 mg/kg 30 min before procedure, max 2 g

GI/GU infections other than caused by *N. gonorrhoeae*
Adult and child >40 kg: PO 250-500 mg q6hr, may use larger dose for more serious infections
Child <40 kg: PO 50 mg/kg/day in divided doses q6-8hr

Renal dose
Adult and child: CCr 10-50 ml/min extend to q6-12hr; CCr <10 ml/min dose q12-16hr

Available forms: Powder for inj 125, 250, 500 mg, 1, 2, 10 g/vial; caps 250, 500 mg; powder for oral susp, 125, 250, 500 mg/5 mg

ADVERSE EFFECTS
CNS: Seizures (high doses)
GI: *Nausea, vomiting, diarrhea,* CDAD, stomatitis
HEMA: Anemia, increased bleeding time, bone marrow depression, granulocytopenia, leukopenia, eosinophilia
INTEG: *Rash,* urticaria
SYST: Anaphylaxis, serum sickness

INTERACTIONS
Individual drugs
Allopurinol: increased ampicillin-induced skin rash, monitor for rash
Probenecid: increased ampicillin levels, decreased renal excretion

Drug classifications
Contraceptives (oral): may decrease contraceptive effectiveness; use reliable contraception, use alternative contraception
H2 antagonists, proton pump inhibitors: decreased ampicillin level
Oral anticoagulants: increased bleeding, monitor INR/PT

Drug/lab test
Increased: eosinophil, ALT, AST
Decreased: conjugated estrogens in pregnancy, conjugated estriol, Hgb, WBC, platelets
False positive: urine glucose
Interfere: urine glucose (Clinitest, Benedict's reagent, cupric SO_4)

NURSING CONSIDERATIONS
Assessment
• Assess patient for previous sensitivity reaction to penicillins or other cephalosporins; cross-sensitivity between penicillins and cephalosporins is common
• Assess patient for signs and symptoms of **infection**, including characteristics of wounds, sputum, urine, stool, WBC $>10,000/mm^3$, earache, fever; obtain baseline information and during treatment
• Obtain C&S before beginning product therapy to identify if correct treatment has been initiated, product can be started before results are received
• **Assess for allergic reactions:** rash, urticaria, pruritus, chills, fever, joint pain; angioedema may occur a few days after therapy begins; EPINEPHrine and resuscitation equipment should be on unit for anaphylactic reaction; also, check for ampicillin rash: pruritic, red, raised; identify allergies before using
• Monitor blood studies: AST, ALT, CBC, Hct, bilirubin, LDH, alkaline phosphatase, Coombs' test monthly if patient is on long-term therapy
• **CDAD:** Assess bowel pattern daily; if severe diarrhea occurs, product should be discontinued
• Assess for **overgrowth of infection:** perineal itching, fever, malaise, redness, pain, swelling, drainage, rash, diarrhea, change in cough, sputum

Patient problem
Infection (uses)

Implementation
• Check allergies before using; obtain C&S before using, begin before results are received
PO route
• Give in even doses around the clock; store caps in tight container; store after reconstituting in refrigerator up to 2 wk, 1 wk room temperature
• Tabs may be crushed or caps opened and mixed with water
• Shake susp well before each dose; store for 2 wk in refrigerator or 1 wk at room temperature
IM route
• **Reconstitute** with 125 mg/0.9-1.2 ml; 250 mg/0.9-1.9 ml; 500 mg/1.2-1.8 ml; 1 g/2.4-7.4 ml; 2 g/6.8 ml
• **Give** deep in large muscle mass

IV route
• **Reconstitute** with 125 mg/0.9-1.2 ml; 250 mg/0.9-1.9 ml; 500 mg/1.2-1.8 ml; 1 g/2.4-7.4 ml; 2 g/6.8 ml
Direct IV route
• **Give** over 3-5 min in lower dosages (125-500 mg) or over 15 min in higher dosages (1-2 g)
Intermittent IV infusion route
• **Give** after diluting with 0.9% NaCl, LR, D_5W, $D_5/0.45\%$ NaCl; use 50 ml of sol and dilute to concentration of <30 mg/ml

Y-site compatibilities: Acyclovir, alemtuzumab, amifostine, allopurinol, argatroban, azithromycin, aztreonam, carmustine, cyclophosphamide, cytarabine, DAUNOrubicin, dexrazoxane, doxapram, DOXOrubicin liposome, enalaprilat, esmolol, etoposide phosphate, famotidine, filgrastim, fludarabine, foscarnet, gallium, gemtuzumab, granisetron, heparin, regular insulin, labetalol, lepirudin, leucovorin, liposome, magnesium sulfate, mannitol, melphalan, meperidine, milrinone, morphine, multivitamins, ofloxacin, penicillin G potassium, perphenazine, phytonadione, potassium acetate, potassium chloride, propofol, remifentanil, thiotepa, tolazoline, vecuronium, vinBLAStine, vit B with C, zoledronic acid

Patient/family education
• Teach patient to report sore throat, bruising, bleeding, joint pain; may indicate blood dyscrasias (rare)
• Advise patient to contact prescriber if vaginal itching, loose foul-smelling stools, furry tongue occur; may indicate superinfection
• Instruct patient to take all medication prescribed for the length of time ordered
• Advise patient to notify prescriber of diarrhea with blood or pus, which may indicate pseudomembranous colitis
• Tab may be crushed; cap may be opened and mixed with water
• **Pregnancy/breastfeeding:** Advise patient to notify health care professional if pregnancy is planned or suspected, or if breastfeeding, to use additional contraception if using oral contraception, as effect may be decreased

Evaluation
Positive therapeutic outcome
• Absence of signs/symptoms of infection (WBC $<10,000$, temp WNL)
• Reported improvement in symptoms of infection

TREATMENT OF ANAPHYLAXIS:
Withdraw product, maintain airway, administer EPINEPHrine, aminophylline, O_2, **IV** corticosteroids

---

ampicillin/sulbactam (Rx)

(am-pi-sill'in/sul-bak'tam)

Unasyn

Func. class.: Broad-spectrum antiinfective

Chem. class.: Aminopenicillin, lactase inhibitor

ACTION: Interferes with cell wall replication of susceptible organisms; the cell wall, rendered osmotically unstable, swells and bursts from osmotic pressure; lysis due to cell wall autolytic enzymes; this combination extends the spectrum of activity and inhibits β-lactamase that may inactivate ampicillin

Therapeutic outcome: Bactericidal against *Actinobacter, Actinomyces, Bacillus anthracis, Bacteroides, Bifidobacterium, Bordetella pertussis, Borrelia burgdorferi, Brucella, Clostridium, Corynebacterium diptheriae/xerosis, Eikenella corrodens, Enterococcus faecalis, Eubacterium, Erysipelothrix rhusiopathiae, Escherichia coli, Eubacterium, Fusobacterium, Gardnerella vaginalis, Haemophilus influenzae* (beta-lactamase negative/positive), *Helicobacter pylori, Klebsiella, Lactobacillus, Leptospira, Listeria monocytogenes, Moraxella catarrhalis, Morganella morganii, Neisseria gonorrhoeae, Pasteurella multocida, Peptococcus, Peptostreptococcus, Porphyromonas, Prevotella, Propionibacterium, Proteus mirabilis, Proteus vulgaris, Providencia rettgeri, Providencia stuartii, Salmonella, Shigella, Staphylococcus aureus* (MSSA)/*epidermidis/saprophyticus, Streptococcus agalactiae/dysgalactiae/pneumoniae/pyrogenes, Treponema pallidum,* viridans streptococci

USES: Skin infections, intraabdominal infections, gynecological infections, asthma, cellulitis, diabetes mellitus, diabetic foot ulcer, dialysis, diarrhea, eczema, IBS, leukemia, meningitis, nosocomial pneumonia, ulcerative colitis

Pharmacokinetics

Absorption	Well absorbed (IM)
Distribution	Readily in body tissues, fluids, CSF; crosses placenta
Metabolism	Liver (10%-50%)
Excretion	Breast milk; kidney unchanged (75%)
Half-life	50-110 min (ampicillin), sulbactam 1-1.4 hr

Pharmacodynamics

	IM	IV
Onset	Rapid	Immediate
Peak	1 hr	Infusion's end
Duration	up to 8 hr	up to 8 hr

CONTRAINDICATIONS

Hypersensitivity to ampicillin, or sulbactam

Precautions: Pregnancy, breastfeeding, neonates, hypersensitivity to cephalosporins, renal disease, mononucleosis, viral infections, syphilis

DOSAGE AND ROUTES

Adult and child >40 kg: IM/IV 1 g ampicillin and 0.5 g sulbactam to 2 g ampicillin, and 1 g sulbactam q6hr, max 4 g/day sulbactam

Child <40 kg: IV 100-200 mg/kg/day (ampicillin component) divided q6hr, max 4 g/day

Renal dose

Adult ≥40 kg: IM/IV CCr 15-29 ml/min dose q12hr; CCr 5-14 ml/min dose q24hr

Available forms: Powder for inj 1.5 g (1 g ampicillin, 0.5 g sulbactam), 3 g (2 g ampicillin, 1 g sulbactam), 15 g (10 g ampicillin, 5 g sulbactam)

ADVERSE EFFECTS

CNS: Seizures (high doses)

GI: *Nausea, vomiting, diarrhea,* increased AST, ALT, abdominal pain, glossitis, colitis, CDAD, hepatotoxicity

HEMA: Anemia, bone marrow depression, granulocytopenia, leukopenia, eosinophilia

INTEG: Injection site reactions, rash, edema, urticaria

SYST: Anaphylaxis, serum sickness, Stevens-Johnson syndrome, hypoalbuminemia

INTERACTIONS

Individual drugs

Allopurinol: ampicillin-induced skin rash, check for rash

Probenecid: increased ampicillin levels, decreased renal excretion

Drug classifications

Oral anticoagulants: increased bleeding risk, check INR, PT

Drug/lab test

False positive: urine glucose, urine protein

NURSING CONSIDERATIONS

Assessment

• Assess patient for previous sensitivity reaction to penicillins or cephalosporins; cross-sensitivity between penicillins and cephalosporins is common

• Assess patient for signs and symptoms of **infection,** including characteristics of wounds, sputum, urine, stool, WBC >10,000/mm³, earache, fever; obtain baseline information and during treatment; complete C&S before beginning product therapy to identify if correct treatment has been initiated

• **Assess for allergic reactions:** rash, urticaria, pruritus, chills, fever, joint pain; angioedema may occur a few days after therapy begins; EPINEPHrine and resuscitation equipment should be on unit for anaphylactic reaction

• Monitor blood studies: AST, ALT, CBC, Hct, bilirubin, LDH, alkaline phosphatase, Coombs' test monthly if patient is on long-term therapy

• Assess bowel pattern daily; if severe diarrhea occurs, product should be discontinued; may indicate pseudomembranous colitis

• **Assess for superinfection:** perineal itching, fever, malaise, redness, pain, swelling, drainage, rash, diarrhea, change in cough, sputum

Patient problem
Infection (uses)

Implementation
• Scratch test to assess allergy after securing order from prescriber; usually done when penicillin is only product choice

IM route
• Reconstitute by adding 3.2 ml/1.5 g or 6.4 ml/3 g; use sterile water, 0.5% or 2% lidocaine; give within 1 hr of preparation; give deep in large muscle mass, aspirate
• Do not use IM in child
• Give after C&S completed; on empty stomach

IV direct route
• Give **IV** after diluting 1.5 g/3.2 ml sterile water for inj; or 3 g/6.4 ml (250 mg ampicillin/125 mg sulbactam); allow to stand until foaming stops; give directly over 10-15 min, inject slowly

Intermittent IV infusion route
• Dilute further in 50 ml or more of D₅W, D₅/10.45% NaCl, 10% invert sugar in water, LR, 6% sodium lactate, isotonic NaCl; administer within 1 hr after reconstitution; give as an intermittent inf over 15-30 min

Y-site compatibilities: Alemtuzumab, amifostine, aminocaproic acid, anidulafungin, argatroban, atenolol, bivalirudin, bleomycin, CARBOplatin, carmustine, cefepime, CISplatin, codeine, cyclophosphamide, cytarabine, DAPTOmycin, DAUNOrubicin liposome, dexmedetomidine, DOCEtaxel, doxacurium, DOXOrubicin liposomal, eptifibatide, etoposide, fenoldopam, filgrastim, fludarabine, fluorouracil, foscarnet, gallium, gatifloxacin, gemcitabine, granisetron, irinotecan, levofloxacin,

linezolid, methotrexate, metroNIDAZOLE, octreotide, oxaliplatin, PACLitaxel, palonosetron, pamidronate, pancuronium, pantoprazole, PEMEtrexed, remifentanil, riTUXimab, rocuronium, tacrolimus, teniposide, thiotepa, tigecycline, tirofiban, TNA, TPN, trastuzumab, vecuronium, vinCRIStine, voriconazole, zoledronic acid

Patient/family education
• Teach patient to report sore throat, bruising, bleeding, joint pain, persistent diarrhea; may indicate blood dyscrasias (rare)
• Advise patient to contact prescriber if vaginal itching, loose foul-smelling stools, furry tongue occur
• Instruct patient to use another form of contraception other than oral contraceptives
• **Instruct patient to report immediately CDAD:** fever, diarrhea with pus, blood, or mucus; may occur up to 4 wk after treatment
• Instruct patient to wear or carry emergency ID if allergic to penicillin products
• **Pregnancy/breastfeeding:** Advise patient to report if pregnancy is planned or suspected, or if breastfeeding, and to use additional contraception if using oral contraceptives, as effect may be decreased

Evaluation
Positive therapeutic outcome
• Absence of signs/symptoms of infection (WBC <10,000/mm³, temp WNL, absence of red draining wounds)
• Reported improvement in symptoms of infection
• Resolution of infection
• Negative C&S

TREATMENT OF OVERDOSE:
Withdraw product, maintain airway, administer EPINEPHrine, aminophylline, O₂, **IV** corticosteroids for anaphylaxis

---

⚠ HIGH ALERT

anastrozole (Rx)
(an-ass-stroh′zole)

Arimidex

Func. class.: Antineoplastic
Chem. class.: Aromatase inhibitor

ACTION: Highly selective nonsteroidal aromatase inhibitor that lowers serum estradiol concentrations; many breast cancers have strong estrogen receptors

Therapeutic outcome: Prevention of rapidly growing malignant cells

USES: Advanced breast carcinoma in estrogen-receptor-positive patients (usually postmenopausal); patients with advanced disease on tamoxifen, adjunct therapy, endometriosis

Pharmacokinetics

Absorption	85%
Distribution	Unknown
Metabolism	Liver 83%
Excretion	Feces, urine
Half-life	50 hr

Pharmacodynamics

Onset	Unknown
Peak	4-7 hr
Duration	Unknown

CONTRAINDICATIONS
Pregnancy, hypersensitivity, breastfeeding

Precautions: Children, geriatric, cardiac/hepatic disease, premenopausal females, osteoporosis

DOSAGE AND ROUTES
Adult: PO 1 mg daily; continue for 5 yr in ERT early breast cancer who have already received 2-3 yr of tamoxifen and are switched to anastrozole, max 5 yr; may also combine with tamoxifen for up to 10 yr

Available forms: Tabs 1 mg

ADVERSE EFFECTS
CNS: Hot flashes, headache, light-headedness, depression, dizziness, confusion, insomnia, anxiety, fatigue, mood changes, weakness
CV: Chest pain, edema, MI, angina
GI: Nausea, vomiting, altered taste leading to anorexia, diarrhea, constipation, abdominal pain, dry mouth
GU: Vaginal bleeding, vaginal dryness, pelvic pain
INTEG: *Rash,* Stevens-Johnson syndrome, anaphylaxis, angioedema
MISC: Hypercholesterolemia
MS: Bone pain, myalgia, arthralgia, fractures, back pain
RESP: Cough, sinusitis, dyspnea
EENT: Pharyngitis

INTERACTIONS
Drug/drug
• None known

Drug/lab test
Increased: GGT, AST, ALT, alkaline phosphatase, cholesterol, LDL

NURSING CONSIDERATIONS
Assessment
• Monitor bone mineral density, cholesterol, lipid panel periodically
• **Assess serious skin reactions:** Stevens-Johnson syndrome
• Assess for tumor flare—increase in size of tumor, increased bone pain—may occur and will subside rapidly; may take analgesics for pain

Patient problem
Pain (adverse reactions)

Implementation
• Do not break, crush, or chew enteric products
• Give with food or fluids for GI upset; repeat dose may be needed if vomiting occurs
• Store in light-resistant container at room temperature

Patient/family education
• Instruct patient to report any complaints, side effects to health care prescriber; if dose is missed, do not double next dose
• Advise patient that vaginal bleeding, pruritus, hot flashes, can occur and are reversible after discontinuing treatment
• Teach patient to take adequate calcium, vitamin D; risk of bone loss/fractures
• Inform patient that rash or lesions are temporary and may become large during beginning therapy
• **Tumor flare:** Teach patient that the increase in size of tumor, increased bone pain may occur and will subside rapidly, may take analgesics for the pain
• **Pregnancy/breastfeeding:** Identify if pregnancy is planned or suspected or if breastfeeding, do not use in pregnancy or breastfeeding during therapy, 15 days after last dose

Evaluation
Positive therapeutic outcome
• Decreased spread of malignant cells in breast cancer

anidulafungin (Rx)
(a-nid-yoo-luh-fun′jin)
Eraxis
Func. class.: Antifungal, systemic
Chem. class.: Echinocandin

ACTION: Inhibits fungal enzyme synthesis; causes direct damage to fungal cell wall

Therapeutic outcome: Decreased symptoms of candida infection, negative culture

USES: Esophageal candidiasis, *Aspergillosis,*
Candida albicans, Candida glabrata, Candida
parapsilosis, Candida tropicalis

Pharmacokinetics

Absorption	complete
Distribution	crosses placenta, protein binding 84%
Metabolism	no metabolism
Excretion	minimal
Half-life	40-50 hr

Pharmacodynamics

Onset	A few mins
Peak	Infusion end
Duration	24 hr

CONTRAINDICATIONS

Hypersensitivity to this product or other echinocandins

Precautions: Pregnancy, breastfeeding, children, severe hepatic disease

DOSAGE AND ROUTES
Candidemia and other candidal in-
fections

Adult: **IV** loading dose 200 mg on day 1, then
100 mg/day until 14 days or more since last
positive culture

Esophageal candidiasis

Adult: **IV** loading dose 100 mg on day 1, then
50 mg/day for at least 14 days and for at least
7 days after symptoms are resolved

Available forms: Powder for injection,
lyophilized 50 mg/vial for IV use

ADVERSE EFFECTS

CNS: Dizziness, *headache*
CV: Hypotension
GI: *Nausea; anorexia; vomiting; diarrhea;
increased AST, ALT*
META: Hypokalemia
Misc: Anaphylaxis, infusion site reactions
INTEG: *Rash,* urticaria, itching, flushing

INTERACTIONS
Drug/drug
None known

Drug/lab test
Increased: amylase, bilirubin, CPK, creatinine,
ECG, lipase, PT, alk phos
Decreased: platelets, magnesium, potassium,
transferase, urea

NURSING CONSIDERATIONS
Assessment

• Assess for **infection**, clearing of cultures
during treatment; obtain culture at baseline and
throughout; product may be started as soon
as culture is taken, those with HIV pharyngeal
candidiasis may need antifungals
• **Anaphylaxis: Asess for rash, dyspnea,
low B/P, flushing, itching, bronchospasm;
an emergency; max rate of infusion 1.1 mg/
min; crash cart should be nearby**
• Assess for GI symptoms: frequency of stools,
cramping, if severe diarrhea occurs, electrolytes
may need to be given

Patient problem
Infection (uses)

Implementation
IV route

• Visually inspect prepared infusions for
particulate matter and discoloration—do not
use if present; give by IV infusion only, after
dilution
• **Reconstitution:** Reconstitute each 50 mg or
100 mg vial/15 ml or 30 ml of sterile water for
injection, respectively (3.33 mg/ml)
• **Storage:** Reconstituted solutions are stable
for ≤24 hr at room temperature
• **Dilution:** Do not use any other diluents
besides dextrose 5% in water (D_5W) or sodium
chloride 0.9% (NS)
• *Preparation of the 200-mg loading
dose infusion:* Withdraw the contents of
either four 50-mg reconstituted vials OR two
100-mg reconstituted vials and add to an IV
infusion bag or bottle containing 200 ml
of D_5W or NS to give a total infusion volume
of 260 ml
• *Preparation of the 100-mg daily infusion:* Withdraw the contents of one 100-mg
reconstituted vial OR two 50-mg reconstituted
vials and add to an IV infusion bag or bottle
containing 100 ml of D_5W or NS to give a total
infusion volume of 130 ml
• *Preparation of a 50-mg daily infusion:* Withdraw the contents of one 50-mg
reconstituted vial and add to an IV infusion bag
or bottle containing 50 ml of D_5W or NS to give
a total infusion volume of 65 ml
Intermittent IV INF route
• Do not mix or co-infuse with other medications
• Administer as a slow IV infusion at a rate of
1.4 ml/min or 84 ml/hr; minimum duration of
infusion is 180 min for the 200-mg dose, 90 min
for the 100-mg dose, and 45 min for the 50-mg
dose

- Store reconstituted vials at 59°-86° F (15°-30° C) for up to 24 hr; do not freeze (dehydrated alcohol); store reconstituted vials at 36°-46° F (2°-7° C) (sterile water) for up to 24 hr; do not freeze

Y-site compatibilities: Acyclovir, alemtuzumab, alfentanil, allopurinol, amifostine, amikacin, aminocaproic acid, aminophylline, amiodarone hydrochloride, amphotericin B lipid complex, amphotericin B liposome, ampicillin, ampicillin sulbactam, argatroban, arsenic trioxide, atenolol, atracurium, azithromycin, aztreonam, bivalirudin, bleomycin, bumetanide, buprenorphine, busulfan, butorphanol, calcium chloride/gluconate, CARBOplatin, carmustine, caspofungin, ceFAZolin, cefepime, cefotaxime, cefoTEtan, cefOXitin, cefTAZidime, ceftizoxime, cefTRIAXone, cefuroxime, chloramphenicol, chlorproMAZINE, cimetidine, ciprofloxacin, cisatracurium, CISplatin, clindamycin, cyclophosphamide, cycloSPORINE, cytarabine, dacarbazine, DACTINomycin, DAUNOrubicin, DAUNOrubicin liposome, dexamethasone, dexmedetomidine, dexrazoxane, diazepam, digoxin, diltiazem, diphenhydrAMINE, DOBUTamine, DOCEtaxel, dolasetron, DOPamine, doripenem, doxacurium, DOXOrubicin, DOXOrubicin liposomal, doxycycline, droperidol, enalaprilat, ePHEDrine, EPINEPHrine, epirubicin, eptifibatide, erythromycin, esmolol, etoposide, etoposide phosphate, famotidine, fenoldopam, fentaNYL, fluconazole, fludarabine, fluorouracil, foscarnet, fosphenytoin, furosemide, gallium, ganciclovir, gatifloxacin, gemcitabine, gentamicin, glycopyrrolate, granisetron, haloperidol, heparin, hydrALAZINE, hydrocortisone, HYDROmorphone, hydrOXYzine, IDArubicin, ifosfamide, imipenem-cilastatin, inamrinone, insulin (regular), irinotecan, isoproterenol, ketorolac, labetalol, leucovorin, levofloxacin, lidocaine, linezolid injection, LORazepam, mannitol, mechlorethamine, melphalan, meperidine, meropenem, mesna, metaraminol, methotrexate, methyldopate, methylPREDNISolone, metoclopramide, metoprolol, metroNIDAZOLE, midazolam, milrinone, mitoMYcin, mitoXANtrone, mivacurium, morphine, moxifloxacin, mycophenolate mofetil, nafcillin, naloxone, nesiritide, niCARdipine, nitroglycerin, nitroprusside, norepinephrine, octreotide, ondansetron, oxaliplatin, oxytocin, PACLitaxel, palonosetron, pamidronate, pancuronium, pantoprazole, pentamidine, pentazocine, PENTobarbital, PHENobarbital, phentolamine, phenylephrine, piperacillin-tazobactam, polymyxin B, potassium acetate/chloride, procainamide, prochlorperazine, promethazine, propranolol, quiNIDine, quinupristin-dalfopristin, ranitidine, remifentanil, rocuronium, sodium acetate, streptozocin, succinylcholine, SUFentanil citrate, sulfamethoxazole-trimethoprim, tacrolimus, teniposide, theophylline, thiopental, thiotepa, ticarcillin, ticarcillin-clavulanate, tirofiban, tobramycin, topotecan, trimethobenzamide, vancomycin, vasopressin, vecuronium, verapamil, vinBLAStine, vinCRIStine, vinorelbine, voriconazole, zidovudine, zoledronic acid

Patient/family education
- Advise patient to notify prescriber if pregnancy is suspected or planned; use nonhormonal form of contraception while taking this product; avoid breastfeeding
- **Anaphylaxis: Teach patient to report anaphylaxis symptoms**
- **Advise patient of reason for product, expected result**

Evaluation
Positive therapeutic outcome
- Decreased symptoms of candidal infection, negative culture

apixaban
(a-pix′a-ban)
Eliquis
Func. class.: Anticoagulant
Chem. class.: Factor Xa inhibitor

ACTION: Inhibits factor Xa and thereby decreases thrombin and clot formation

Therapeutic use: Prevention/treatment of DVT, adequate anticoagulation

USES: Deep vein thrombosis (DVT) after hip or knee replacement, to prevent stroke and embolism in atrial fibrillation (nonvalvular)

Pharmacokinetics

Absorption	50%
Distribution	Unknown
Metabolism	By CYP3A4 25%
Excretion	Urine, feces
Half-life	12 hr

Pharmacodynamics

Onset	Unknown
Peak	3-4 hr
Duration	Up to 24 hr

CONTRAINDICATIONS
Hypersensitivity, active bleeding

Precautions: Breastfeeding, dialysis, hepatic/renal disease, labor, pregnancy, surgery, prosthetic heart valves

---

BLACK BOX WARNING: Abrupt discontinuation, epidural, spinal anesthesia, lumbar puncture

DOSAGE AND ROUTES
Stroke, systemic embolism prophylaxis
Adult: PO 5 mg bid; in those with any 2 of the following—age ≥80 yr, body weight ≤60 kg or serum creatinine ≥1.5 mg/dl, reduce dose to 2.5 mg bid; strong CYP3A4 and P-glycoprotein 2.5 mg bid

Prevention of deep vein thrombosis (knee/hip replacement)
Adult: PO 2.5 mg bid started 12-24 hr after surgery continuing for 35 days or more (hip), 12 days (knee)

Treatment of DVT or PE
Adult: PO 10 mg bid × 7 days, then 5 mg bid

Reduction in risk of recurrent DVT or PE after acute DVT or PE
Adult: PO 2.5 mg bid after at least 6 mo of treatment

Renal dose
Adult PO serum CCr ≥1.5 mg/dl, <60 kg, and/or ≥80 yr; if two of these three are present then dose should be 2.5 mg bid

Available forms: Tablets 2.5, 5 mg

ADVERSE REACTIONS
CNS: Syncope, intracranial bleeding
HEMA: Bleeding
INTEG: Rash
MISC: Hypersensitivity

INTERACTIONS
Drug classifications
Anticoagulants, salicylates, thrombolytics, NSAIDs, SNRIs, SSRIs: Increased bleeding, dosage should be reduced
CYP3A4 inhibitors, P-gp (clarithromycin, ritonavir): Increase: apixaban effect, use 2.5 mg of apixaban
CYP3A4 inducers (carbamazepine, ketoconazole, itraconazole, phenytoin, rifampin): Decrease: apixaban effect, avoid using together

Drug/herb
St. John's wort: Decrease: apixaban effect

Drug/lab test
Increase: PT, PTT, INR, coagulation studies

NURSING CONSIDERATIONS
Assessment
• **Bleeding:** Assess for bleeding that may occur in any body system; may be fatal

BLACK BOX WARNING: Neurologic status: Monitor for impairment, including numbness, paresthesia, weakness, confusion, back pain, bowel/bladder impairment; notify prescriber immediately

BLACK BOX WARNING: Abrupt discontinuation: Do not discontinue abruptly; if bleeding occurs, consider using another anticoagulant to prevent thromboembolic events

BLACK BOX WARNING: Epidural, spinal anesthesia, lumbar puncture: Avoid use in these conditions, risk of hematoma, and permanent paralysis; may be increased with use of other anticoagulants, thrombolytics, antiplatelets

• **Hypersensitivity:** Assess for rash, itching, chills, fever, report to provider
• **Beers:** Avoid in older adults; may cause increased risk of bleeding, decreased creatinine clearance

Patient problems
Ineffective tissue perfusion (uses)

Implementation
PO route
• May take without regard to food
• If unable to swallow whole, may crush and suspend the tablet in 60 ml 5% dextrose solution, give immediately via NG
• If dose is missed take as soon as remembered if possible on the same day; twice daily dosing should be resumed. Do not double the dose to make up for a missed dose

Patient/family education

BLACK BOX WARNING: Teach patient not to discontinue without prescriber approval; stroke, clots may occur

• **Bleeding:** Advise patient to report bleeding, bruising, weakness, numbness of limbs
• Teach patient to discuss all OTC, Rx, herbals, supplements taken with provider; serious product interactions may occur
• Advise patient to carry emergency ID with product taken; to inform all health providers of product use
• Advise patient to report hypersensitivity reactions: rash, chills, fever, itching

Evaluation
Positive therapeutic outcome
• Prevention of DVT, stroke, adequate anticoagulation

apraclonidine ophthalmic
See Appendix B

aprepitant (Rx) (PO)
(ap-re'pi-tant)
Emend
fosaprepitant (IV)
(fos-a-prep'i-tant)
Emend
Func. class.: Antiemetic
Chem. class.: Neurokinin antagonist

Do not confuse: aprepitant/fosaprepitant

ACTION: Selective antagonist of human substance P/neurokinin 1 (NK₁) receptors, decreasing emetic reflex

Therapeutic outcome: Decreased nausea, vomiting during chemotherapy

USES: Prevention of nausea, vomiting associated with cancer chemotherapy (highly emetogenic/moderately emetogenic) including high-dose cisplatin; used in combination with other antiemetics; postop nausea, vomiting

Pharmacokinetics

Absorption	Complete (IV)
Distribution	95% protein bound, crosses blood/brain barrier
Metabolism	Liver (CYP3A4 enzymes to an active metabolite)
Excretion	Not in kidneys
Half-life	10-12 hr

Pharmacodynamics

	PO	IV
Onset	1 hr	immediate
Peak	4 hr	infusion end
Duration	up to 24 hr	up to 24 hr

CONTRAINDICATIONS
Hypersensitivity to this product, polysorbate 80, pimozide

Precautions: Pregnancy, breastfeeding, children, geriatric, hepatic disease

DOSAGE AND ROUTES
Prevention of nausea/vomiting after chemotherapy antineoplastics
Adult: **PO** day 1 (1 hr prior to chemotherapy) aprepitant 125 mg with 12 mg 1st dose of aprepitant on day 1 of regimen; **IV:** 150 mg give 30 min prior to chemotherapy

Child ≥ 12 yr: PO capsules 125 mg 1 hr prior to chemotherapy: suspension 3 mg/kg 1 hr prior to chemotherapy, max 125 mg

Prevention of postop nausea/vomiting
Adult: **PO** 40 mg within 3 hr of induction of anesthesia

Available forms: Caps 40, 80, 125 mg; lyophilized powder for inj, 150 mg; powder for oral suspension 125 mg/pouch

ADVERSE EFFECTS
CNS: *Headache, dizziness,* weakness
INTEG: Injection reaction
MISC: Hiccups
SYST: Stevens-Johnson syndrome

INTERACTIONS
Individual drugs
ALPRAZolam, midazolam, triazolam: increased level of each product, decrease dose of each product
Paroxetine: decreased action of both products

Drug classifications
CYP2C9 substrates (phenytoin, TOLBUTamide, warfarin), hormonal contraceptives: decreased action
CYP3A4 inhibitors (clarithromycin, diltiazem, itraconazole, ketoconazole, nefazodone, nelfinavir, ritonavir, troleandomycin): increased aprepitant action of each, use alternate contraception if taking with hormonal contraceptives
CYP3A4 inducers (carBAMazepine, phenytoin, rifampin): decreased aprepitant action
CYP3A4 substrates (ALPRAZolam, dexamethasone, DOCEtaxel, etoposide, ifosfamide, imatinib, irinotecan, methylPREDNISolone, midazolam, PACLitaxel, pimozide, triazolam, vinBLAStine, vinCRIStine, vinorelbine): increased action, avoid concurrent use

Drug/food
Grapefruit juice: decreased effect

Drug/lab
Increase: AST/ALT, alkaline phosphatase
Decrease: Hgb, WBC

NURSING CONSIDERATIONS
Assessment
• Assess for hypersensitivity reactions: pruritus, rash, urticaria, anaphylaxis
• Assess for absence of nausea, vomiting during chemotherapy
• CBC, LFTs, creatinine baseline and periodically

Patient problems
Nausea (uses)

Do not open, break, crush capsules; day 1 use 1 hr prior to chemotherapy; day 2 and 3 give in AM, may use with or without food

Implementation
• Given with dexamethasone and a 5-HT3 antagonist

PO route
• Give PO on 3-day schedule, given with other antiemetics

Suspension: Use for children unable to swallow capsules, give slowly, store for 3 hr at room temperature

IV route
• Reconstitution: use aseptic technique; inject 5 ml 0.9% NaCl into the vial, directing stream to wall of vial to prevent foam; swirl; do not shake
• Prepare inf bag with 145 ml/150 mg do not dilute or reconstitute with any divalent cations such as calcium, magnesium, including LR, Hartmann's sol
• Withdraw the entire volume from vial and transfer to inf bag; total volume 115 ml (1 mg/1 ml)
• Gently invert bag 2-3 times; reconstituted sol is stable for 24 hr at lower room temperature or <25° C
• Visually inspect for particulates and discoloration
• Infuse over 20-30 min, stable for 24 hr at room temperature

Patient/family education
• Advise to take only as prescribed; to take (PO) first dose 1 hr before chemotherapy or within 3 hr of surgery to prevent nausea/vomiting
• Advise to report all medication to prescriber prior to taking this medication
• Instruct to use nonhormonal form of contraception while taking this agent, to avoid breastfeeding
• Advise those on warfarin to have clotting monitored closely during 2-wk period following administration of aprepitant

Evaluation
Positive therapeutic outcome
• Absence of nausea, vomiting during cancer chemotherapy or post op

---

⚠ HIGH ALERT

argatroban (Rx)
(are-ga-troe′ban)
Func. class.: Anticoagulant
Chem. class.: Direct thrombin inhibitor

Do not confuse: argatroban/Aggrastat/L

ACTION: Direct inhibitor of thrombin that is derived from L-arginine; it reversibly binds to the thrombin active site

Therapeutic outcome: Prevention of or decrease of thrombosis

USES: Thrombosis prophylaxis or treatment; anticoagulation prevention/treatment of thrombosis in heparin-induced thrombocytopenia (HIT); percutaneous coronary intervention (PCI) in those with a history of HIT, deep vein thrombosis, pulmonary embolism

Pharmacokinetics

Absorption	complete (IV)
Distribution	To extracellular fluid, 54% plasma protein binding
Metabolism	Liver
Excretion	Feces
Half-life	39-51 min

Pharmacodynamics (anticoagulant action)

Onset	Rapid
Peak	1-2 hr
Duration	2-4 hr

CONTRAINDICATIONS
Hypersensitivity, overt major bleeding

Precautions: Pregnancy, breastfeeding, children, intracranial bleeding, impaired renal function, hepatic disease, severe hypertension, after lumbar puncture, spinal anesthesia, major surgery/trauma, congenital or acquired bleeding, GI ulcers, abrupt discontinuation

DOSAGE AND ROUTES
Prevention/treatment of thrombosis (heparin-induced thrombocytopenia)
Adult: CONT IV inf 2 mcg/kg/min; adjust dose until steady-state aPPT is 1.5-3 × initial baseline, not to exceed 100 sec, max dose 10 mcg/kg/min

Percutaneous coronary intervention (PCI) in HIT
Adult: IV inf 25 mcg/kg/min and a bol of 350 mcg/kg given over 3-5 min, check ACT 5-10 min after bol is completed, proceed if ACT

>300 sec; if ACT <300 sec, give another 150 mcg/kg bol and increase infusion rate to 30 mcg/kg/min; recheck ACT in 5-10 min; if ACT >450 sec, decrease infusion rate to 15 mcg/kg/min; recheck ACT in 5-10 min; once ACT is therapeutic, continue for duration of procedure

Hepatic dose
Adult: Cont inf 0.5 mcg/kg/min, adjust rate based on APTT

Available forms: Inj 100 mg/ml (2.5 ml) (must dilute 100-fold), 50 mg/50 ml, 125 mg/125 ml

ADVERSE EFFECTS
CNS: Headache
CV: Hypotension
GI: Nausea, vomiting, abdominal pain, diarrhea
HEMA: bleeding
SYST: Anaphylaxis

INTERACTIONS
Individual drugs
Clopidogrel, dipyridamole, heparin, ticlopidine, warfarin: increased bleeding risk, avoid using concurrently

Drug classifications
Antiplatelets, glycoprotein IIb/IIIa antagonists (abciximab, eptifibatide, tirofiban), NSAIDs, other anticoagulants, salicylates, thrombolytics (alteplase, reteplase, tenecteplase, urokinase): increased risk of bleeding, avoid using concurrently

Drug/herb
Garlic, ginger, ginkgo, horse chestnut: increased bleeding risk

Drug/lab
Decrease: Hgb/HcT

NURSING CONSIDERATIONS
Assessment
• Obtain baseline aPTT before treatment; do not start treatment if aPTT ratio ≥2.5, then aPTT 4 hr after initiation of treatment and at least daily thereafter; if aPTT above target, stop inf for 2 hr, then restart at 50%, take aPTT in 4 hr; if below target, increase inf rate by 20%, take aPTT in 4 hr, do not exceed inf rate of 0.21 mg/kg/hr without checking for coagulation abnormalities
• **Bleeding:** Assess for bleeding gums, petechiae, ecchymosis, black tarry stools, hematuria/epistaxis, decreased B/P, HCT, vaginal bleeding, and possible hemorrhage
• Fever, skin rash, urticaria
• **Anaphylaxis:** assess for dyspnea, rash during treatment

Patient problem
Impaired tissue perfusion (uses)

Implementation
• Avoid all IM inj that may cause bleeding

IV, direct route
• For PCL: 350 mg/kg bol, and continuous inf of 25 mcg/kg/min, check ACT 5-10 min after bolus

Intermittent IV INF route
• **Dilute** in 0.9% NaCl, D₅W, LR to a final conc 1 mg/ml; **dilute** each 2.5-ml vial 100-fold by mixing with 250 ml of diluent, mix by repeated inversion of the diluent bag for 1 min; may be slightly hazy briefly
• Dosage adjustment may be made after review of aPTT, not to exceed 10 mcg/kg/min

Patient/family education
• Teach patient reason for product, expected result
• Advise patient to use soft-bristle toothbrush to avoid bleeding gums, avoid contact sports, use electric razor, avoid IM inj
• Instruct patient to report any signs of bleeding: gums, under skin, urine, stools; trouble breathing, wheezing, skin rash
• Pregnancy/breastfeeding: Teach patient to notify provider if planning to become pregnant, breastfeeding
• Advise patient to notify provider of hepatic/GI disease, recent surgery, injury

Evaluation
Positive therapeutic outcome
• Prevention or decrease of thrombosis

ARIPiprazole (Rx)
(a-rip-ip-pra′zol)
Abilify, Abilify Discmelt, Abilify Maintena, Aristada
Func. class.: Antipsychotic/neuroleptic

Do not confuse: ARIPiprazole/RABEprazole

ACTION: Exact mechanism unknown; may be mediated through both dopamine type 2 (D₂) and serotonin type 2 (5-HT₂) antagonism, dopamine system stabilizer

Therapeutic outcome: Decreased excitement, hallucinations, delusions, paranoia, reorganization of patterns of thought, speech

USES: Schizophrenia and bipolar disorder (adults and adolescents), agitation, mania, major depressive disorder, short-term mania or mixed episodes of bipolar disorder, irritability in autism

Pharmacokinetics

Absorption	well
Distribution	Protein binding, 90% extravascular
Metabolism	Liver, extensively to major active metabolism by CYP3A4/CYP2D6
Excretion	Unknown
Half-life	Unknown 75 hr

Pharmacodynamics

	PO	Ex Rel
Onset	Unknown	Unknown
Peak	Up to 2 wk	Unknown
Duration	Unknown	Unknown

CONTRAINDICATIONS

Hypersensitivity, breastfeeding, seizure disorders

Precautions: Pregnancy, geriatric, renal/cardiac/hepatic disease, neutropenia

> **BLACK BOX WARNING:** Children with depression, dementia, suicidal ideation

DOSAGE AND ROUTES
Schizophrenia
Adult: PO 10-15 mg/day; if needed, dosage may be increased to 30 mg daily after 2 wk; maintenance 15 mg/day, periodically reassess; IM/EXT REL (monthly inj susp) 400 mg qmo
Adolescent 13-17 yr: 2 mg/day, may increase to 5 mg after 2 days, then 10 mg after 2 more days, max 30 mg/day

Major depressive disorder
Adult: PO 2-5 mg/day as an adjunct to other antidepressant treatment; adjust by 5 mg at ≥1 wk (range, 2-15 mg/day)

Agitation in bipolar disorder/schizophrenia
Adult: IM 9.75 mg as a single dose; may start with a lower dose, max 30 mg/day

Bipolar disorder
Adult: 15 mg/day, may increase to 30 mg/day if needed (monotherapy): adjunctive to lithium or valproate PO 10-15 mg qd, may increase to 30 mg as needed
Child ≥10 yr/adolescent: PO 2 mg, titrate to 5 mg/day after 2 days to a target of 10 mg/day after another 2 days

Irritability associated with autism
Child ≥6 yr/adolescent: PO 2 mg/day, increase to 5 mg/day after 1 wk, may increase to 10-15 mg/day if needed, dose changes should not occur more frequently than q1wk

Tourette's disorder
Child 6-18 yr and ≥ 50 kg: PO 2 mg/day × 2 days, then increase to 5 mg/day, target 10 mg/day on day 8
Child 6-18 yr and <50 kg: PO 2 mg/day × 2 days, then increase to 5 mg/day then gradually increase in weekly intervals, max 10 mg/day

Potential CYP2D6 inhibitor, strong CYP3A4 inhibitors
Adult: PO reduce to 50% of usual dose, increase dose when CYP2D6, CYP3A4 inhibitor is withdrawn

Combination of strong CYP3A4/CYP2D6 inhibitors
Adult: PO reduce to 25% of usual dose
Available forms: Tabs 2, 5, 10, 15, 20, 30 mg; inj 9.75 mg/1.3 ml; orally disintegrating tab 10, 15 mg; oral sol 1 mg/ml; susp for injection 441 mg/1.6 ml, 662 mg/2.4 ml, 882 mg/3.2 ml; susp EXT REL 300, 400 mg

ADVERSE EFFECTS
CNS: *Drowsiness, insomnia, agitation, anxiety, headache,* seizures, neuroleptic malignant syndrome, *lightheadedness, akathisia,* tardive dyskinesia, tremor, suicidal ideation
CV: Orthostatic hypotension, tachycardia, chest pain, hypertension, peripheral edema
EENT: Blurred vision, rhinitis
GI: Constipation, *nausea,* vomiting, weight gain, anorexia
INTEG: *Rash,* dry skin, sweating
META: Hyperglycemia, dyslipidemia
MS: Myalgia
RESP: *Cough*
HEMA: Agranulocytosis, anemia, leukopenia
SYST: Death in geriatric patients with dementia, hypersensitivity

INTERACTIONS
Individual drugs
Alcohol: increased sedation
CarBAMazepine: decreased effects of ARIPiprazole

Drug classifications
CNS depressants: increased sedation
CYP3A4/CYP2D6 inhibitors Clarithromycin, ketoconazole, fluoxetine, paroxetine, quinidine) increased effects of ARIPiprazole, reduce dose
CYPA34 inducers: decreased effects of ARIPiprazole; increase dose as needed

Drug/herb
St. John's wort: decreased ARIPiprazole effect

Drug/Lab
False positive: amphetamine drug screen

NURSING CONSIDERATIONS
Assessment

> **BLACK BOX WARNING:** Assess mental status before initial administration, children/young adults may exhibit suicidal thoughts/behaviors, the smallest amount of product should be given; elderly patients with dementia-related psychosis are at increased risk of death

• Check for swallowing of PO medication; check for hoarding or giving of medication to other patients
• Assess affect, orientation, LOC, reflexes, gait, coordination, sleep pattern disturbances
• Monitor B/P standing and lying; also pulse, respirations; take q4hr during initial treatment; establish baseline before starting treatment; report drops of 30 mm Hg; watch for ECG changes
• Assess for dizziness, faintness, palpitations, tachycardia on rising
• Assess for EPS, including akathisia (inability to sit still, no pattern to movements), tardive dyskinesia (bizarre movements of the jaw, mouth, tongue, extremities), pseudoparkinsonism (rigidity, tremors, pill rolling, shuffling gait)
• **Assess for neuroleptic malignant syndrome:** hyperthermia, increased CPK, altered mental status, muscle rigidity
• Monitor weight, lipid profile, fasting blood glucose
• **Beers:** Avoid in older adults, high risk of CVA, delirium, may use in schizophrenia, bipolar, or short-term use as an antiemetic in chemotherapy
• **Pregnancy/breastfeeding:** Identify if pregnancy is planned or suspected, pregnant patient should be enrolled in the National Pregnancy Registry for Atypical Antipsychotics (866-961-2388), avoid breastfeeding, use only if benefits outweigh fetal risk

Patient problem
Distorted thinking process (uses)

Implementation
• Administer reduced dose in geriatric
• Supervise ambulation until patient is stabilized on medication; do not involve in strenuous exercise program because fainting is possible; patient should not stand still for a long time
• Store in tight, light-resistant container
• **PO route:** Give without regard to meals
• Oral sol can be substituted for tablet mg per mg up to 25-mg dose; patients receiving 30-mg tablets should receive 25 mg of sol
• IM (Ext Rel) route monthly (Abilify Maintena)
• Do not give IV or subcut

Patient/family education
• Advise patient that orthostatic hypotension may occur and to rise from sitting or lying position gradually
• Advise patient to avoid hot tubs, hot showers, tub baths; hypotension may occur
• Instruct patient to avoid abrupt withdrawal of this product; EPS may result; product should be withdrawn slowly
• Teach patient to avoid OTC preparations (cough, hayfever, cold) unless approved by prescriber, because serious product interactions may occur; avoid use with alcohol, CNS depressants; increased drowsiness may occur
• Advise patient to avoid hazardous activities if drowsy or dizzy
• Explain importance of compliance with product regimen
• Advise patient, family to report impaired vision, tremors, muscle twitching
• Instruct patient to take extra precautions to stay cool in hot weather, that heat stroke may occur

> **BLACK BOX WARNING:** Teach patient to report suicidal thoughts/behaviors, dementia immediately

• Inform patient that blood work will be needed during treatment
• Teach patient that weight gain may occur and to notify health care professional of large weight gain

Evaluation
Positive therapeutic outcome
• Decreased emotional excitement, hallucinations, delusions, paranoia; reorganization of patterns of thought, speech

TREATMENT OF OVERDOSE:
Lavage if orally ingested; provide airway; *do not induce vomiting*

asenapine (Rx)
(a-sen'a-peen)
Saphris
Func. class.: Antipsychotic, atypical; DOPamine/serotonin antagonist
Chem. class.: Dibenzazepine

ACTION: Unknown; may be mediated through both dopamine type 2 (D_2) and serotonin type 2 (5-HT_{2A}) antagonism

Therapeutic outcome: Decrease in delusions, hallucinations

USES: Bipolar 1 disorder, schizophrenia

Pharmacokinetics

Absorption	35%
Distribution	Protein binding 95% rapidly
Metabolism	Liver by CYP1A2/UGTA14
Excretion	Urine 50%, feces 40% (metabolites)
Half-life	24 hr

Pharmacodynamics

Onset	Unknown
Peak	½-1½ hr
Duration	up to 24 hr

CONTRAINDICATIONS
Breastfeeding, hypersensitivity

Precautions: Pregnancy, children, geriatric patients, cardiac/renal/hepatic disease, breast cancer, Parkinson's disease, dementia, seizure disorder, CNS depression, agranulocytosis, QT prolongation, torsades de pointes, suicidal ideation, substance abuse, diabetes mellitus

> **BLACK BOX WARNING:** Increased mortality in elderly patients with dementia-related psychosis

DOSAGE AND ROUTES
Schizophrenia
Adult: SL 5 mg bid, may increase to 10 mg bid after 1 wk, max 20 mg/day

Acute mania, mixed episodes (bipolar 1 disorder monotherapy)
Adult: SL 10 mg bid, may decrease to 5 mg bid as needed, max 20 mg/day; with lithium or valproate 5 mg bid, may increase to 10 mg bid
Child: 10-17 SL 2.5 mg bid, may increase after 3 days to 5 mg bid, then after 3 more days, increase to 10 mg bid as tolerated

Available forms: SL tab 2.5 mg, 5 mg, 10 mg

ADVERSE EFFECTS
CNS: *EPS, pseudoparkinsonism, akathisia, dystonia, tardive dyskinesia, drowsiness, insomnia, agitation, anxiety, headache,* seizures, neuroleptic malignant syndrome, dizziness, suicidal ideation
CV: Orthostatic hypotension, tachycardia, heart failure, QT prolongation
ENDO: Hyperglycemia
GI: *Nausea,* vomiting; oral hypoesthesia/paresthesia (SL)
HEMA: Agranulocytosis, anemia, leukopenia
INTEG: Serious allergic reaction (anaphylaxis, angioedema)

INTERACTIONS
Individual drugs
Alcohol: increased sedation
Chloroquine, clarithromycin, droperidol, erythromycin, haloperidol, methadone, pentamidine: increased QT prolongation
CarBAMazepine: increased asenapine excretion

Drug classifications
Other CNS depressants: increased sedation
CYP2D6 inhibitors/substrates (SSRIs), other antipsychotics: increased EPS
Class IA/III antidysrhythmics, some phenothiazines, β-agonists, local anesthetics, tricyclics: increased QT prolongation
CYP2D6 inducers (carBAMazepine, barbiturates, phenytoin, rifampin): decreased asenapine action
SSRIs: increased serotonin syndrome

Drug/herb
Kava: increased CNS depression, increased EPS
Betel palm: increased EPS

Drug/lab test
Increased: cholesterol, glucose, LFTs, lipids, prolactin levels, triglycerides
Decreased: sodium

NURSING CONSIDERATIONS
Assessment

> **BLACK BOX WARNING:** Assess mental status before initial administration; watch for suicidal thoughts and behaviors; dementia and death may occur in the elderly

• Assess for affect, orientation, LOC, reflexes, gait, coordination, sleep pattern disturbances
• Monitor B/P standing and lying, pulse, respirations; take these during initial treatment; establish baseline before starting treatment; report drops of 30 mm Hg; watch for ECG changes; QT prolongation may occur
• Monitor for dizziness, faintness, palpitations, tachycardia on rising
• Assess for **EPS,** including akathisia, tardive dyskinesia (bizarre movements of the jaw, mouth, tongue, extremities), pseudoparkinsonism (rigidity, tremors, pill rolling, shuffling gait)
• **Assess for neuroleptic malignant syndrome:** hyperthermia, increased CPK, altered mental status, muscle rigidity, dyspnea, hypo-hypertension, discontinue immediately, notify professional health care provider
• Assess for constipation daily; increase bulk and water in diet if needed
• Assess for weight gain, hyperglycemia, metabolic changes in diabetes

Beers: avoid use in older adults; high risk of delirium, CVA, worsening Parkinsonian symptoms; increased CNS effects, may use in schizophrenia, bipolar disorder, or as antiemetic in chemotherapy

Patient problem
Distorted thinking process (uses)

Implementation
PO route
- Give anticholinergic agent for EPS
- Avoid use with CNS depressants
- **SL tab:** remove tab, place tab under tongue; after it dissolves, swallow; advise not to chew, crush or swallow tabs, not to eat or drink for 10 min
- Supervise ambulation until patient is stabilized on medication; do not involve in strenuous exercise program because fainting is possible; patient should not stand still for a long time
- Store in tight, light-resistant container

Patient/family education
- Caution patient that orthostatic hypotension may occur and to rise from sitting or lying position gradually
- Teach patient to avoid hot tubs, hot showers, tub baths; hypotension may occur, to take as directed, not to double or skip doses
- Advise patient to avoid abrupt withdrawal of this product; EPS may result; product should be withdrawn slowly
- Advise patient to avoid OTC preparations (cough, hay fever, cold) unless approved by prescriber, serious product interactions may occur; avoid use of alcohol, increased drowsiness may occur
- Advise patient to avoid hazardous activities if drowsy or dizzy
- Advise patient about compliance with product regimen
- Advise patient that heat stroke may occur in hot weather; take extra precautions to stay cool
- Advise patient to report suicidal thoughts/ behaviors immediately
- Advise patient that follow-up exams will be needed
- Pregnancy/breastfeeding: Identify if pregnancy is planned or suspected, if pregnant register at the National Pregnancy Registry for Atypical Antipsychotics (866-961-2388) do not breastfeed, use only if benefits outweigh fetal risk

Evaluation
Positive therapeutic outcome
- Therapeutic response: decrease in emotional excitement, hallucinations, delusions, paranoia; reorganization of patterns of thought, speech

TREATMENT OF OVERDOSE:
Lavage if orally ingested; provide airway; *do not induce vomiting*

⚠ HIGH ALERT
RARELY USED
asparaginase erwinia chrysanthemi (Rx)
Erwinaze
Func. class.: Antineoplastic

USES: Treatment of acute lymphocytic leukemia (ALL) in combination with other chemotherapeutic agents in patients who have developed hypersensitivity to *Escherichia coli*–derived asparaginase

CONTRAINDICATIONS
Hypersensitivity, breastfeeding, history of serious pancreatitis, bleeding, or serious thrombosis with prior L-asparaginase therapy

DOSAGE AND ROUTES
Adult, adolescent, child ≥2 yr (substitute for pegaspargase): IM 25,000 IU/m2 3 times per week (Monday, Wednesday, Friday) × 6 doses for each planned dose of pegaspargase within a treatment
Adult (substitute for L-asparaginase *E. Coli*): IM 25,000 IU/m2 for each scheduled dose of native *E. coli* asparaginase within a treatment

⚠ HIGH ALERT
asparaginase (Erwina chrysanthemi)
Erwinase ✦, Erwinaze
Func. class.: Antineoplastic
Chem class.: Plant alkaloid

ACTION: The enzyme L-asparaginase catalyzes asparagine to aspartic acid and ammonia, which causes reduced circulating concentrations of asparagine

Therapeutic use: Decreased progression of leukemia

USES: Treatment of acute lymphocytic leukemia (ALL) in combination with other chemotherapeutic agents in patients who have developed hypersensitivity to *E. coli*–derived asparaginase

Pharmacokinetics	
Absorption	Complete (IV)
Distribution	Intravascular space
Metabolism	unknown
Excretion	unknown
Half-life	8-30 hr (IV), 40-49 hr (IM)

Pharmacodynamics

Onset	Unknown
Peak	Unknown
Duration	Unknown

CONTRAINDICATIONS

Hypersensitivity, history of pancreatitis, thrombosis

Precautions: Pregnancy, breastfeeding

DOSAGE AND ROUTES

Adult: IM/IV To substitute for pegaspargase: 25,000 IU/m^2 IV/IM 3 × a week (Monday/Wednesday/Friday) × 6 doses for each planned dose of pegaspargase within a treatment; to substitute for L-asparaginase *Escherichia coli*: 25,000 IU/m^2 for each scheduled dose of native *E. coli* asparaginase within a treatment

Available forms: Powder for injection 10,000 IU/vial

ADVERSE REACTIONS

GI: Pancreatitis, nausea, vomiting, anorexia, increased AST, ALT

INTEG: Rash, urticaria

ENDO: Hyperglycemia

HEMA: Thrombosis, bleeding

MISC: Hypersensitivity, anaphylaxis

Interactions

None known

NURSING CONSIDERATIONS

Assessment

• **Hypersensitivity reactions:** fever, rash, dyspnea
• **Assess for pancreatitis:** abdominal pain, nausea, vomiting, elevated liver enzymes; product should be discontinued because condition can be fatal
• **Hepatotoxicity:** Monitor liver function tests before, during therapy (bilirubin, AST, ALT, amylase, alkaline phosphatase, creatine phosphokinase, creatinine prn or qmo)
• Monitor CBC and coagulation studies baseline and periodically; after a 2 wk course fibrinogen, protein C, protein S, and antithrombin III were decreased; bleeding may occur; may require discontinuing or holding dose
• Monitor nadir (predose) serum asparaginase activity (NSAA) concentrations when administering asparaginase Erwinia chrysanthemi IV and switching to IM administration if desired NSAA concentrations are not achieved

Patient problem

Risk for injury (adverse reactions)

Implementation

• Use cytotoxic handling precautions
• Visually inspect parenteral products for particulate matter and discoloration prior to use

Reconstitution:
• Slowly inject 1 or 2 mL of preservative-free sterile 0.9% sodium chloride injection against the inner vial wall, gently mix, do not shake
• The reconstituted solution should be clear and colorless; discard if any visible particles or protein aggregates are present
• Calculate the dose needed and the volume needed to obtain the calculated dose. Withdraw the volume containing the calculated dose from the vial into a polypropylene syringe within 15 min
• Do not freeze or refrigerate the reconstituted solution; discard any unused portions

IV intermittent infusion:
• Slowly inject the calculated volume of reconstituted solution into an IV infusion bag containing 100 mL of 0.9% sodium chloride at room temperature; do not shake or squeeze the bag
• Infuse over 1 to 2 hours within 4 hours of reconstitution; do not infuse other IV drugs through the same line

IM route:
• Use within 4 hrs of reconstitution; limit the volume to 2 mL per injection site; multiple injection sites may be needed

Patient/family education

• Infection: Advise patient to report increased temperature, sore throat, flulike symptoms and to avoid crowds and those with known infections
• Hepatotoxicity: Teach patient to report dark urine, clay-colored stools, yellow eyes and skin, no appetite, abdominal pain
• Caution patient to avoid OTC products or other medications without approval of prescriber
• Advise patient that regular follow-up exams and blood work will be needed
• Pregnancy/breastfeeding: Identify if pregnancy is planned or suspected, or if breastfeeding

Evaluation

Positive therapeutic outcome
• Decreased symptoms, progression of leukemia

⚠ HIGH ALERT

aspirin (acetylsalicylic acid, ASA) (OTC)

(as'pir-in)

Acuprin, A.S.A., Asaphen ♥, Asatab ♥, Ascriptin Enteric, Aspergum, Aopir Low, Aspirtrin, Bayer Aspirin, Easprin, Ecotrin, Entrophen ♥, Halfprin, Lowprin ♥, Novasen ♥, Rivasa ♥, Sloprin, St. Joseph's Adult, Zorprin

Func. class.: Nonopioid analgesic
Chem. class.: Salicylate

ACTION: Blocks pain impulses by blocking COX-1 in CNS, reduces inflammation by inhibition of prostaglandin synthesis; antipyretic action results from vasodilatation of peripheral vessels; decreases platelet aggregation

Therapeutic outcome: Decreased pain, inflammation, fever; absence of MI, transient ischemic attacks, thrombosis

USES: Mild to moderate pain or fever including rheumatoid arthritis, osteoarthritis, thromboembolic disorders, transient ischemic attacks, rheumatic fever, post-MI, prophylaxis of MI, ischemic stroke, angina; acute MI, Kawasaki disease

Pharmacokinetics

Absorption	Well absorbed, small intestine (PO); erratic (enteric); slow (RECT)
Distribution	Rapidly, widely distributed; crosses placenta, protein binding 90%
Metabolism	Liver, extensively
Excretion	Inactive metabolites, kidney; breast milk
Half-life	2-3 hr (low doses); 9-30 hr (high doses)

Pharmacodynamics

	PO	RECT
Onset	15-30 min	Slow
Peak	1-2 hr	4-5 hr
Duration	4-6 hr	6-7 hr

CONTRAINDICATIONS

Pregnancy, breastfeeding, children <12 yr, children with flulike symptoms, hypersensitivity to salicylates, tartrazine (FDC yellow dye #5), GI bleeding, bleeding disorders, vit K deficiency, peptic ulcer, acute bronchospasm, agranulocytosis, increased intracranial pressure, intracranial bleeding, nasal polyps, urticaria

Precautions: Abrupt discontinuation, acetaminophen/NSAIDs hypersensitivity, acid/base imbalance, alcoholism, ascites, asthma, bone marrow suppression, geriatric patients, dehydration, G6PD deficiency, gout, heart failure, anemia, renal/hepatic disease, pre/postoperatively, gastritis, pregnancy C 1st trimester

DOSAGE AND ROUTES
Pain/fever

Adult: PO/RECT 325-1000 mg q4hr prn, max 4 g/day

Child 2-11 yr: PO 10-15 mg/kg/dose q4hr, max 4 g/day

Inflammatory conditions

Adult: PO 2.4 g/day in divided doses q4-6hr, maintenance 3.6-5.4 g/day; extended release 650 mg q 8 hr or 800 mg q 12 hr, target salicylate level 150-300 mcg/ml

Juvenile rheumatoid arthritis

Child: PO or RECT 90-130 mg/kg/day in divided doses, target salicylate level 150-300 mcg/ml

MI, stroke prophylaxis

Adult: PO 50-325 mg/day

Thromboembolic disorders

Adult: PO 325-650 mg/day or bid

Transient ischemic attacks

Adult: PO 50-325 mg/day (grade 1A)

Prevention of recurrent MI/Antiplatelet

Adult: PO 80-325 mg/day

Kawasaki disease

Child PO 80-100 mg/kg/day in 4 divided doses until fever resolves, if maintenance is needed 3-5 mg/kg/day as a single dose up to 8 wk
Child PO 3-10 mg/kg/day q day

Available forms: Tabs 81, 162.5 325, 500, 650, 975 mg ♥; chewable tabs 81 mg; supp 60, 120, 125, 130, 150 ♥, 160 ♥, 195, 200, 300, 320 ♥, 325 ♥, 600, 640, 650, 1.2 g mg; chewing gum 227 mg; enteric coated tabs 81, 325, 500, 600 ♥, 650, 975 mg; del rel tabs 325, 500 mg;

ADVERSE EFFECTS

EENT: Tinnitus, hearing loss
GI: *Nausea, vomiting,* GI bleeding, heartburn, anorexia, hepatotoxicity
HEMA: Hemolytic anemia, increased PT, PTT, bleeding time
INTEG: *Rash,* urticaria, bruising

SYST: Reye's syndrome (children), anaphylaxis, laryngeal edema, angioedema

INTERACTIONS
Individual drugs
Alcohol, cefamandole, clopidogrel, eptifibatide, heparin, plicamycin, ticlopidine, tirofiban: increased risk of bleeding, monitor for bleeding

Ammonium chloride, nizatidine: increased salicylate level

Insulin, methotrexate, phenytoin, valproic acid, increased effects of each specific product, monitor for increased effects of each product

Nitroglycerin: increased hypotension

Probenecid: decreased effects of probenecid

Spironolactone, sulfinpyrazone: decreased effects

Drug classifications
ACE inhibitors: decreased antihypertensive effect, monitor BP

Antacids (high doses), corticosteroids, urinary alkalizers: decreased effects of aspirin, monitor for decreased aspirin effects

Anticoagulants, thrombolytics: increased risk of bleeding

Diuretics (loop), sulfonylamides, NSAIDs, β-blockers: decreased effect of each specific product

NSAIDs, antiinflammatories, steroids: increased gastric ulcers

Penicillins, oral hypoglycemics, sulfonamides, thrombolytic agents: increased effects of each specific product

Salicylates: decreased blood glucose levels

Urinary acidifiers: increased salicylate levels

Drug/herb
Feverfew, garlic, ginger, ginkgo, ginseng *(Panax)*, horse chestnut: increased risk of bleeding

Drug/food
Foods acidifying urine may increase aspirin levels

Fish oil (omega-3-fatty acids): increased risk of bleeding

Drug/lab test
Increased: coagulation studies, liver function studies, serum uric acid, amylase, CO_2, urinary protein

Decreased: serum potassium, cholesterol

Interference: VMA, 5-HIAA, xylose tolerance test, TSH, pregnancy test

NURSING CONSIDERATIONS
Assessment
• Assess for **pain:** character, location, intensity, ROM before and 1 hr after administration

• Assess for fever: temperature before and 1 hr after administration

• Monitor liver function studies: AST, ALT, bilirubin, creatinine if patient is on long-term therapy

• Monitor renal function studies: BUN, urine creatinine if patient is on long-term therapy

• Monitor blood studies: CBC, Hct, Hgb, PT if patient is on long-term therapy

• Check I&O ratio; decreasing output may indicate renal failure (long-term therapy)

• **Assess for hepatotoxicity:** dark urine, clay-colored stools, yellowing of the skin and sclera, itching, abdominal pain, fever, diarrhea if patient is on long-term therapy

• **Assess for allergic reactions:** rash, urticaria; if these occur, product may have to be discontinued; in patients with asthma, nasal polyps, allergies, severe allergic reactions may occur

• Assess for **ototoxicity:** tinnitus, ringing, roaring in ears; audiometric testing needed before, after long-term therapy

• Monitor **salicylate level:** therapeutic level 150-300 mcg/ml for chronic inflammation

• Identify prior product history; there are many product interactions

• **Beers:** Avoid chronic use in older adults, GI bleeding may occur

Patient problem
Pain (uses)

Impaired mobility (uses)

Implementation
PO route
• Do not break, crush, or chew enteric product

• Administer to patient crushed or whole (regular PO product); chewable tab should be chewed

• Give with food or milk to decrease gastric symptoms; separate by 2 hr of enteric product; absorption may be slowed

• Give antacids 1-2 hr after enteric products

• Give with 8 oz of water and have patient sit upright for 30 min after dose; discard tabs if vinegar-like smell is present; avoid if allergic to tartrazine

Rectal route
• Place suppository in refrigerator for at least 30 min before removing wrapper

Patient/family education
• Teach patient to report any symptoms of renal/hepatic toxicity, visual changes, ototoxicity, allergic reactions, bleeding (long-term therapy)

• Instruct patient to take with 8 oz of water and sit upright for 30 min after dose to facilitate product passing into the stomach; to discard tabs if vinegar-like smell is present; to avoid if allergic to tartrazine

• Instruct patient not to exceed recommended dosage; acute poisoning may result

• Advise patient to read label on other OTC products; many contain aspirin

---

• Inform patient that the therapeutic response takes 2 wk (arthritis)
• Teach patient to report tinnitus, confusion, diarrhea, sweating, hyperventilation
• Advise patient to avoid alcohol ingestion; GI bleeding may occur
• Advise patient with allergies, nasal polyps, asthma, that allergic reactions may develop
• Teach patient not to use in children with flulike symptoms or chicken pox, risk of Reye's syndrome
• Instruct patient to read labels on other OTC products: may contain salicylates
• Teach patient not to give to children or teens with flulike symptoms or chicken pox; Reye's syndrome may develop
• Instruct patient not to use during 3rd trimester of pregnancy
• Teach patient to take with a full glass of water

Evaluation
Positive therapeutic outcome
• Decreased pain
• Decreased inflammation
• Decreased fever
• Absence of MI
• Absence of transient ischemic attacks, thrombosis

TREATMENT OF OVERDOSE:
Lavage, monitor electrolytes, VS

---

atazanavir (Rx)
(at-a-za-na′veer)
Reyataz
Func. class.: Antiretroviral
Chem. class.: Protease inhibitor

ACTION: Inhibits human immunodeficiency virus (HIV-1) protease, which prevents maturation of the infectious virus

Therapeutic outcome: Decreasing symptoms of HIV

USES: HIV-1 infection in combination with other antiretroviral agents

Pharmacokinetics

Absorption	Rapid, increased with food
Distribution	86% protein bound
Metabolism	Liver extensively by CYP3A4
Excretion	27% excreted unchanged in urine/feces (minimal)
Half-life	7 hr

Pharmacodynamics

Onset	Unknown
Peak	2 hr
Duration	up to 24 hr

CONTRAINDICATIONS
Hypersensitivity, hepatic disease moderate to severe

Precautions: Pregnancy, breastfeeding, children, geriatric, liver disease, alcoholism, antimicrobial resistance, AV block, diabetes, dialysis, elderly, women, hemophilia, hypercholesterolemia, immune reconstitution syndrome, lactic acidosis, pancreatitis, cholelithiasis, serious rash

DOSAGE AND ROUTES
Antiretroviral-naive patients
Adult: PO 400 mg daily
Child ≥6 yr/adolescent ≤40 kg: PO 300 mg with ritonavir 100 mg qd
Child ≥6 yr/adolescent 20 to <40 kg: PO 200 mg with ritonavir 100 mg qd
Child ≥6 yr/adolescent 15 to <20 kg: PO 150 mg with ritonavir 80 mg qd

Antiretroviral-experienced patients
Adult: PO 300 mg daily and ritonavir 100 mg daily
Pregnant adult/adolescent (2nd/3rd trimester) with H$_2$ blocker or tenofovir: PO 400 mg with ritonavir 100 mg qd
Child ≥6 yr/adolescent ≥40 kg: PO 300 mg with ritonavir 100 mg qd
Child ≥6 yr/adolescent 20 to <40 kg: PO 200 mg with ritonavir 100 mg qd
Infants ≥ 3 months and children 10 to <25 kg: Oral powder 15 to <25 kg 250 mg/dose q24hr with ritonavir 80 mg/dose q24hr; 10 to <15 kg 200 mg/dose q24hr with ritonavir 80 mg/dose q24hr

Hepatic dose
Adult: PO (Child-Pugh B) 300 mg daily; (Child-Pugh C) do not use

Renal dose
Adult: PO Therapy-naïve and HD 300 mg q day with ritonavir 100 mg q day; therapy experienced and HD: do not use

Available forms: Caps 100, 150, 200, 300 mg, oral powder 50 mg/packet

ADVERSE EFFECTS
CNS: Headache, depression, dizziness, insomnia, peripheral neuropathy
CV: Increased PR interval
GI: *Diarrhea, abdominal pain, nausea,* vomiting, hepatotoxicity, cholelithiasis
INTEG: *Rash,* Stevens-Johnson syndrome, *photosensitivity,* DRESS
MISC: Fatigue, fever, arthralgia, back pain, cough, lipodystrophy, nephrolithiasis, immune reconstitution syndrome

---

INTERACTIONS
Individual drugs
Alfuzisun, ariprazole, brentuximab, cabazitaxel, carBAMazepine, cilostazol, colchine, eletriptan, eplerenone, crizotinib, DOCEtaxel, ixabepilone, iloperidine, lurasidone, maraviroc, nilotinib, vilazodone, vemurafenib, dasatinib, lapatinib, SORAfenib, trazodone, risperiDONE, raltegravir, QUEtiapine
Clarithromycin, romiDEPsin, ranolazine, salmeterol: increased QT prolongation
Chlorazepate, clarithromycin, cycloSPORINE, diazepam, irinotecan, midazolam, pimozide, sildenafil, sirolimus, tacrolimus, triazolam, warfarin: increased levels resulting in toxicity, monitor for toxicity
Didanosine, efavirenz, rifampin: decreased atazanavir levels
Indinavir: increased hyperbilirubinemia
Ritonavir, telaprevir: decreased telaprevir levels when used with atazanavir and ritonavir

Drug classifications
Antacids, H$_2$-receptor antagonists, proton pump inhibitors, CYP3A4 inducers: decreased atazanavir levels, give atazanavir 2 hr before or 1 hr after these products
Antidepressants (tricyclics), antidysrhythmics, antifungals (itraconazole, ketoconazole, voriconazole) ergots, calcium channel blockers, HMG-CoA reductase inhibitors, immunosuppressants, other protease inhibitors (amprenavir, darunavir, fosamprenavir, indinavir, nelfivanavir, ritonavir, saquinavir): increased levels resulting in increased toxicity, monitor for toxicity
Contraceptives (oral), estrogens: increased effects (unboosted), decreased (boosted with ritonavir)
CYP3A4 substrates, CYP3A4 inhibitors: increased atazanavir levels

Drug/herb
St. John's wort: decreased atazanavir levels, avoid concurrent use

Drug/lab test
Increased: AST, ALT, total bilirubin, amylase, lipase, CK
Decreased: Hgb, neutrophils, platelets

Drug/food
Increased: drug bioavailability (to be taken with food)

NURSING CONSIDERATIONS
Assessment
• **Immune reconstitution syndrome:** when given with combination antiretroviral therapy
• Assess for hepatic failure; ALT, AST, bilirubin, do not use in Child-Pugh C
• Assess for signs of infection, anemia
• Monitor liver function studies: ALT, AST, bilirubin
• Monitor bowel pattern before, during treatment; if severe abdominal pain with bleeding occurs, product should be discontinued; monitor hydration
• If pregnant, call Antiretroviral Pregnancy Registry (800-258-4263), do not breastfeed, use additional contraception when boosted with ritonivir
• PR interval in those taking calcium channel blockers, digoxin
• Monitor viral load, CD4 count throughout treatment
• **Serious rash (Stevens-Johnson syndrome, DRESS):** most rashes last 1-4 wk; if serious, discontinue product

Patient problem
Infection (uses)
Nonadherence (teaching)

Implementation
• Administer with food; take 2 hr before or 1 hr after antacid or didanosine; swallow cap whole, do not open
• Oral powder: Use with food or beverage, mix 1 tablespoon of food with powder, then add another tablespoon of food to container, mix and feed; mix with 30 ml of liquid, give and mix another 15 ml to cup to remove residual and give, use within 1 hr of mixing

Patient/family education
• Advise to take as prescribed with other antiretrovirals as prescribed; if dose is missed, take as soon as remembered up to 1 hr before next dose; do not double dose; do not share with others
• Teach that product must be taken daily to maintain blood levels for duration of therapy
• To report yellowing of skin, sclera
• Instruct to notify prescriber if diarrhea, nausea, vomiting, rash occur; dizziness, lightheadedness; ECG may be altered
• Inform that product interacts with many products and St. John's wort; advise prescriber of all products, herbal products used
• Advise that redistribution of body fat may occur; the effect is not known
• Teach that product does not cure HIV-1 infection or prevent transmission to others, only controls symptoms
• Advise that if taking sildenafil with atazanavir, there may be an increased risk of phosphodiesterase type 5 inhibitor–associated

adverse events, including hypotension and prolonged penile erection; notify physician promptly of these symptoms

• **Pregnancy/breastfeeding:** Encourage patient to register with the Antiretroviral Pregnancy Registry if pregnant, to notify provider if pregnancy is planned or suspected, not to breastfeed

Evaluation

Positive therapeutic outcome

• Increasing CD4 counts; decreased viral load, resolution of symptoms of HIV-1 infection

---

⚠ HIGH ALERT

atenolol (Rx)

(a-ten′oh-lole)

Tenormin ✦

Func. class.: Antihypertensive

Chem. class.: β-Blocker

Do not confuse: atenolol/albuterol/Altenol, **Tenormin**/thiamine/Imuran

ACTION: Competitively blocks stimulation of β-adrenergic receptor within vascular smooth muscle; produces negative chronotropic activity (decreases rate of SA node discharge, increases recovery time), slows conduction of AV node, decreases heart rate, negative inotropic activity, decreases O_2 consumption in myocardium; also decreases renin-aldosterone-angiotensin system at high doses, inhibits $β_2$-receptors in bronchial system at higher doses

Therapeutic outcome: Decreased B/P, heart rate, prevention of angina pectoris, MI

USES: Hypertension; angina pectoris; suspected or known MI (**IV** use), MI prophylaxis

Pharmacokinetics

Absorption	50%-60% (PO)
Distribution	Crosses placenta; protein binding (5%-15%)
Metabolism	Not metabolized
Excretion	Breast milk, kidneys (50%), feces
Half-life	7 hr

Pharmacodynamics

	PO
Onset	1 hr
Peak	2-4 hr
Duration	24 hr

CONTRAINDICATIONS

Pregnancy, hypersensitivity to β-blockers, cardiogenic shock, 2nd- or 3rd-degree heart block, bradycardia, cardiac failure

Precautions: Major surgery, breastfeeding, diabetes mellitus, renal disease, thyroid disease, HF, COPD, asthma, well-compensated heart failure, dialysis, myasthenia gravis, Raynaud's disease, pulmonary edema

> **BLACK BOX WARNING:** Abrupt discontinuation, may precipitate angina, MI

DOSAGE AND ROUTES

Hypertension

Adult: PO 25-50 mg daily, increasing q1-2wk to 100 mg daily; may increase to 200 mg daily for angina or up to 100 mg for hypertension

Child: PO 0.8-1 mg/kg/dose initially, range 0.8-1.5 mg/kg/day, max 2 mg/kg/day

Geriatric: PO 25 mg/day initially

Angina

Adult: PO 50 mg q day, then 100 mg/day prn after 7 days, max 200 mg/day

MI

Adult: PO 100 mg/day, in 1-2 divided doses, may need for 1-3 yr post MI

Renal dose

Adult: PO CCr 15-35 ml/min, max 50 mg/day; CCr <15 ml/min max 25 mg/day; hemodialysis 25-50 mg after dialysis

Available forms: Tabs 25, 50, 100 mg

ADVERSE EFFECTS

CNS: *Insomnia, fatigue, dizziness, mental changes,* memory loss, hallucinations, depression, lethargy, drowsiness, strange dreams, catatonia

CV: Profound hypotension, bradycardia

ENDO: Hyper-hypoglycemia

GI: *Nausea, diarrhea,* vomiting, constipation

GU: Impotence, decreased libido, urinary frequency

INTEG: Rash

RESP: Bronchospasm, dyspnea, wheezing, pulmonary edema

INTERACTIONS

Individual drugs

Digoxin, diltiazem, hydrALAZINE, methyldopa, prazosin, reserpine, verapamil: increased hypotension, bradycardia

Amphetamine, epinephrine, norepinephrine, pseudoephedrine: increased hypertension

DOPamine, insulin, theophylline: decreased effect of each of these drugs

---

Drug classifications

Aluminum antacids, NSAIDs, penicillins, salicylates: decreased atenolol effect

Anticholinergics, antihypertensives: cardiac glycosides, calcium channel blockers: increased hypotension, bradycardia, monitor and adjust dose if needed

Antidiabetic agents (oral): decreased effect of each of these drugs

MAOIs: Increase hypertension, avoid use within 2 wks

Sympathomimetics (cough, cold preparations): mutual inhibition

Drug/herb

Hawthorn: increased atenolol effect

Ephedra (ma huang): decreased atenolol effect

Drug/lab test

Increased: uric acid, potassium, triglyceride, blood, BUN, ANA titer, platelets, alkaline phosphatase, creatinine, LDH, AST/ALT

Decreased: glucose

NURSING CONSIDERATIONS

Assessment

• Monitor **hypertension,** B/P during beginning treatment, periodically thereafter; pulse q4hr; note rate, rhythm, quality: apical/radial pulse before administration; notify prescriber of any significant changes (pulse <50 bpm); ECG baseline and throughout treatment

• Hypoglycemia: monitor for tachycardia, weakness, may be masked in diabetes mellitus

• Assess for edema in feet, legs daily; monitor I&O, daily weight; check for jugular vein distention, crackles bilaterally, dyspnea (HF)

Patient problem

Impaired cardiac output (uses)

Nonadherence (teaching)

Implementation

PO route

• Given before meals, at bedtime; tablet may be crushed or swallowed whole; give with food, same time of day to prevent GI upset; reduced dosage in renal dysfunction; take at same time each day

• Store protected from light, moisture; place in cool environment

Patient/family education

> **BLACK BOX WARNING:** Teach patient not to discontinue product abruptly; taper over 2 wk (angina) as directed, **may precipitate angina, MI,** if stopped abruptly; take at same time each day

• Teach patient not to use OTC products containing α-adrenergic stimulants (such as nasal decongestants, OTC cold preparations); to limit alcohol, smoking; to limit sodium intake as prescribed

• Teach patient how to take pulse and B/P at home; advise when to notify prescriber (<50 bpm)

• Instruct patient to comply with weight control, dietary adjustments, modified exercise program

• Advise patient to carry/wear emergency ID for products, allergies, conditions being treated; tell patient product controls symptoms but does not cure

• Caution patient to avoid hazardous activities if dizziness, drowsiness is present

• Teach patient to report symptoms of HF: difficult breathing, especially on exertion or when lying down, night cough, swelling of extremities or bradycardia, dizziness, confusion, depression, fever

• Teach patient to take product as prescribed, not to double doses, skip doses; take any missed doses as remembered if at least 6 hr until next dose

• Advise to change position slowly to limit orthostatic hypotension

• Advise patient that product may mask symptoms of hypoglycemia in diabetic patients

• **Pregnancy/breastfeeding:** Advise patient to use contraception while taking this product, do not use in pregnancy, breastfeeding

Evaluation

Positive therapeutic outcome

• Decreased B/P in hypertension (after 1-2 wk)

• Absence of dysrhythmias

• Absence of MI

• Decreased angina/pain

• Increased activity tolerance

TREATMENT OF OVERDOSE:

Lavage, **IV** atropine for bradycardia, **IV** theophylline for bronchospasm, digoxin, O₂, diuretic for cardiac failure, hemodialysis, **IV** glucose for hyperglycemia, **IV** diazepam (or phenytoin) for seizures

> **⚠ HIGH ALERT**
> **RARELY USED**
>
> ## atezolizumab
> (a-te-zoe-liz′ue-mab)
> **Tecentriq**
> *Func. class.:* Antineoplastic

USES: Treatment of locally advanced or metastatic urothelial carcinoma, including bladder cancer and other urinary system cancers, in patients who progress during or after platinum-containing chemotherapy for advanced disease, or within 12 months of neoadjuvant or adjuvant platinum-containing chemotherapy

CONTRAINDICATIONS
Hypersensitivity

DOSAGE AND ROUTES
Adult: IV INF 1200 mg over 60 min q3wk until disease progression or unacceptable toxicity.

atomoxetine (Rx)
(at-o-mox′eh-teen)
Strattera
Func. class.: Psychotherapeutic—miscellaneous
Chem. class.: Selective norepinephrine reuptake inhibitors (SNRIs)

Do not confuse: atomoxetine/atorvastatin

ACTION: May inhibit the presynaptic norepinephrine transporter

Therapeutic outcome: Decreased hyperactivity, impulsivity; increased attention, organization, ability to complete tasks

USES: Attention deficit hyperactivity disorder

Pharmacokinetics
Absorption	Unknown
Distribution	Protein binding, 98%
Metabolism	Liver 🖎 some are poor metabolizers
Excretion	Kidneys
Half-life	5 hr

Pharmacodynamics
Onset	Unknown
Peak	1-2 hr
Duration	Up to 24 hr

CONTRAINDICATIONS
Hypersensitivity, closed-angle glaucoma, MAOI therapy, history of pheochromocytoma

Precautions: Pregnancy, breastfeeding, hypertension, hepatic disease, angioedema, bipolar disorder, dysrhythmias, CAD, hypo/hypertension, arteriosclerosis, cardiac disease, cardiomyopathy, heart failure, jaundice

> **BLACK BOX WARNING:** Children <6 yr, suicidal ideation

DOSAGE AND ROUTES
Child ≤70 kg, and <6 yr: PO 0.5 mg/kg/day, increase after 3 days to a target daily dose of 1.2 mg/kg in AM or evenly divided doses AM, late afternoon; max 1.4 mg/kg/day or 100 mg daily, whichever is less
Adult and child >6 yr and >70 kg: PO 40 mg daily, increase after 3 days to a target daily dose of 80 mg in AM or evenly divided doses AM, late afternoon; max 100 mg daily

Initial dosage titration with strong CYP2D6 inhibitors
Adult and child >6 yr weighing >70 kg: PO 40 mg/day each AM or 2 evenly divided doses, titrate to target of 80 mg/day if symptoms do not improve after 4 wk and dose is well tolerated

Hepatic dose
Adult/child PO: Child-Pugh B: reduce dose by 50%
Child-Pugh C: reduce dose by 75%

Available forms: Caps 10, 18, 25, 40, 60, 80, 100 mg

ADVERSE EFFECTS
CNS: *Insomnia,* dizziness, irritability, crying, mood swings, fatigue, suicidal ideation
CV: *Palpitations,* tachycardia, increased B/P, orthostatic hypotension, QT prolongation
ENDO: Growth retardation
GI: Dyspepsia, nausea, anorexia, dry mouth, weight loss, vomiting, diarrhea, constipation, hepatotoxicity
GU: Urinary hesitancy, retention, dysmenorrhea, erectile disturbance, ejaculation failure, impotence, priapism, prostatitis, abnormal orgasm, male pelvic pain
INTEG: Sweating, rash
MISC: Ear infection, rhabdomyolysis, angioneurotic edema, anaphylaxis

INTERACTIONS
Individual drug
Albuterol: increased cardiovascular effects

Drug classifications
CYP2D6 inhibitors (amiodarone, cimetidine [weak], citalopram, clomiPRAMINE, delavirdine, escitalopram, FLUoxetine, gefitinib, imatinib, PARoxetine, propafenone, quiNIDine [potent], ritonavir, sertraline, thioridazine, venlafaxine): increased effects of atomoxetine, dose decrease may be needed
MAOIs or within 14 days of MAOIs, vasopressors: increased risk of hypertensive crisis, avoid use within 2 wk of this product

Increase: QT prolongation, torsade de pointes, dofetilide, grepafloxacin, mesoridazine, pimozide, probucol, sparfloxacin, ziprasidone
Pressor agents: increased cardiovascular effects

NURSING CONSIDERATIONS
Assessment
• Monitor VS, B/P; check patients with cardiac disease more often for increased B/P
• **Hepatic injury:** may cause liver failure: monitor LFT; assess for jaundice, pruritus, flu-like symptoms, upper right quadrant pain; if these occur product should be discontinued permanently

> **BLACK BOX WARNING:** Assess mental status: mood, sensorium, affect, stimulation, insomnia, aggressiveness, suicidal ideation in children/young adults

• Assess appetite, sleep, speech patterns
• **ADHD:** Assess for attention span, decreased hyperactivity, growth rate, weight; therapy may need to be discontinued
• **Priapism:** Monitor for urinary function (hesitancy, retention, sexual changes)
• **Pregnancy/breastfeeding:** Identify if pregnancy is planned or suspected, or if breastfeeding, use only if benefits outweigh fetal risk

Patient problem
Distorted thinking process (uses)
Impaired interactive behavior (uses)

Implementation
• Swallow whole; do not break, crush, or chew
• Give without regard to food
• Provide gum, hard candy, frequent sips of water for dry mouth

Patient/family education
• Advise patient to avoid OTC preparations, other medications, herbs, supplements unless approved by prescriber, no tapering needed when discontinuing product
• Advise patient to avoid hazardous activities until stabilized on medication
• Advise patient to get needed rest; patients will feel more tired at end of day; do not take dose late in day, insomnia may occur

> **BLACK BOX WARNING: Suicidal ideation**

• Teach patient to notify prescriber immediately if erection >4 hr
• To report immediately: Fatigue, chest pain, difficulty breathing
• **Pregnancy/breastfeeding:** Teach patient to notify provider if pregnancy is planned or suspected, avoid use in pregnancy, breastfeeding

Evaluation
Positive therapeutic outcome
• Decreased hyperactivity (ADHD) in school, work, or social situations

atorvastatin (Rx)
(a-tore′va-stat-in)
Lipitor
Func. class.: Antilipidemic
Chem. class.: HMG-CoA reductase inhibitor

Do not confuse: atorvastatin/atomoxetine, Lipitor/ZyrTEC

ACTION: Inhibits HMG-CoA reductase enzyme, which reduces cholesterol synthesis, high doses lead to plaque regression

Therapeutic outcome: Decreased cholesterol levels and LDLs, increased HDLs

USES: As an adjunct in primary hypercholesterolemia (types Ia, Ib), dysbetalipoproteinemia, elevated triglyceride levels; prevention of cardiovascular disease by reduction of heart risk in those with mildly elevated cholesterol

Pharmacokinetics
Absorption	Rapid
Distribution	Protein binding >98%
Metabolism	Liver
Excretion	Bile, feces, kidneys
Half-life	14 hr

Pharmacodynamics
Onset	Unknown
Peak	Unknown
Duration	Up to 30 hr

CONTRAINDICATIONS
Pregnancy, breastfeeding, hypersensitivity, active liver disease

Precautions: Past liver disease, alcoholism, severe acute infections, trauma, severe metabolic disorders, electrolyte imbalance

DOSAGE AND ROUTES
Adult: PO 10-20 mg daily, usual range 10-80 mg, dosage adjustments may be made in 2-4 wk intervals, max 80 mg/day; patients requiring >45% reduction in LDL may be started at 40 mg daily
Child 10-17 yr: PO 10 mg q day, adjust q4 wk, max 20 mg/day; concurrent use with clarithromycin, itraconazole, saquinavir/ritonavir, darunavir/ fosamprenivir, fosaamprenavir/ritonavir, max 20 mg/day

Available forms: Tabs 10, 20, 40, 80 mg

ADVERSE EFFECTS
CNS: Headache, insomnia
EENT: Lens opacities
GI: *Abdominal cramps, constipation, diarrhea, heartburn,* nausea, dyspepsia, *flatus,* liver dysfunction, pancreatitis, increased serum transaminase
GU: Impotence
INTEG: Rash, pruritus
MISC: Hypersensitivity
MS: Myalgia, rhabdomyolysis, arthralgia
RESP: Pharyngitis, sinusitis

INTERACTIONS
Individual drugs
Colchicine, erythromycin, nelfinavir, cyclo-SPORINE, gemfibrozil, niacin: increased risk of rhabdomyolysis, use lower dose
Digoxin: increased action of digoxin, monitor digoxin levels often
Warfarin: increased action of warfarin

Drug classifications
Antifungals (azole): possible rhabdomyolysis
Contraceptives (oral): increased levels
CYP3A4 inhibitors (erythromycin, ketoconazole, itraconazole, posaconazole, voriconazole, protease inhibitors): Do not use concurrently

Drug/food
Grapefruit juice (large amounts): possible toxicity

Drug/lab test
Increased: ALT, AST, CK
Interference: thyroid function tests

NURSING CONSIDERATIONS
Assessment
• **Hypercholesterolemia:** assess nutrition: fat, protein, carbohydrates; nutritional analysis should be completed by dietitian before treatment; assess for muscle pain, tenderness; obtain CK if these occur, product may need to be discontinued; monitor triglycerides, cholesterol at baseline and throughout treatment
• Monitor bowel pattern daily; diarrhea may be a problem
• Monitor liver function studies q1-2mo during the first 1½ yr of treatment; AST, ALT, liver function tests may be increased
• **Rhabdomyolysis:** Assess for muscle pain, tenderness, obtain CPK baseline, if markedly increased, product may need to be discontinued, many drug interactions make the possibility of rhabdomyolysis greater
• **Pregnancy/breastfeeding:** Identify if pregnancy is planned or suspected, do not breastfeed or use in pregnancy

Patient problem
Nonadherence (teaching)

Implementation
• Administer total daily dose at any time of day
• Store in cool environment in airtight, light-resistant container

Patient/family education
• Inform patient that compliance is needed for positive results to occur, not to double or skip doses
• Teach patient that risk factors should be decreased: high-fat diet, smoking, avoid alcohol consumption, absence of exercise
• Advise patient to notify prescriber if the GI symptoms of diarrhea, abdominal or epigastric pain, nausea, vomiting; chills, fever, sore throat; muscle pain, weakness occur
• Advise patient that blood work will be necessary during treatment
• Advise not to take if pregnant or breastfeeding

Evaluation
Positive therapeutic outcome
• Decreased cholesterol levels, serum triglyceride
• Improved HDL:LDL ratio

atovaquone (Rx)
(a-toe′va-kwon)
Mepron
Func. class.: Antiprotozoal
Chem. class.: Analog of ubiquinone

ACTION: Interferes with DNA/RNA synthesis in protozoa

Therapeutic outcome: Antiprotozoal for *Pneumocystis jiroveci* only

USES: *P. jiroveci* infections in patients intolerant of trimethoprim/sulfamethoxazole (cotrimoxazole)

Pharmacokinetics
Absorption	Poor; increased when taken with fatty foods
Distribution	CSF (minimal), protein binding >99%
Metabolism	Hepatic recycling
Excretion	Feces, unchanged (94%)
Half-life	2-3 days

Onset	Unknown
Peak	1-8 hr
Duration	up to 12 hr

CONTRAINDICATIONS
Hypersensitivity or history of developing life-threatening allergic reactions to any component of the formulation, benzyl alcohol sensitivity

Precautions: Pregnancy, breastfeeding, GI/hepatic disease, neonates, respiratory insufficiency

DOSAGE AND ROUTES
Adult and adolescent 13-16 yr: PO 750 mg bid for 21 days
Child: **PO** (unlabeled) 40 mg/kg/day

Pneumocystis jiroveci pneumonia prophylaxis
Adult and adolescent: PO 1500 mg daily with meal

Available forms: Susp 750 mg/5 ml

ADVERSE EFFECTS
CNS: *Headache,* insomnia, fever
CV: Hypotension
GI: *Nausea, vomiting, diarrhea,* anorexia
HEMA: Anemia, neutropenia
INTEG: Pruritus, urticaria, *rash*
META: Hypoglycemia, hyponatremia
OTHER: Cough, dyspnea

INTERACTIONS
Individual drugs
Metoclopramide, rifampin, rifabutin, tetracycline: decreased effectiveness of atovaquone, avoid concurrent use
Zidovudine: increased level of zidovudine, monitor for toxicity

Drug/food
• Increased absorption

Drug/lab test
Increase: AST, ALT, alk phos
Decrease: glucose, neutrophils, Hgb, sodium

NURSING CONSIDERATIONS
Assessment
• Assess for *Pneumocystis jiroveci:* monitor WBC, bilateral lung sounds, sputum for C&S; these should be checked before, periodically during, after treatment; after collection of 1st sputum, therapy may begin
• Monitor for signs of **infection;** anemia; monitor bowel pattern before, during treatment
• Assess for dizziness, confusion, hallucination
• Assess for allergies before treatment, reaction of each medication; place allergies on chart; notify all people giving products

• **Pregnancy/breastfeeding:** Identify if pregnancy is planned or suspected, use only if benefits outweigh fetal risk, cautious use in breastfeeding

Patient problem
Infection (uses)

Implementation
• Give with food (preferably fatty) to increase absorption of the product and higher plasma concentrations; give tid × 3 wk
• Give oral suspension after shaking

Patient/family education
• Instruct patient to take with food, preferably fatty foods, to increase plasma concentrations, to take as prescribed, not to skip or double dose
• Advise patient to take product exactly as prescribed
• Teach patient to shake suspension gently; if vomiting occurs after ingestion, notify prescriber for further instructions

Evaluation
Positive therapeutic outcome
• C&S negative
• Decreased infection signs/symptoms

---

atropine (Rx)
(a'troe-peen)
Atro-Pen
Func. class.: Antidysrhythmic, anticholinergic parasympatholytic, antimuscarinic
Chem. class.: Belladonna alkaloid

ACTION: Blocks acetylcholine at parasympathetic neuroeffector sites; increases cardiac output, heart rate by blocking vagal stimulation in heart; dries secretions by blocking vagus

Therapeutic outcome: Drying of secretions, increased heart rate, cycloplegia, mydriasis

USES: Bradycardia <40-50 bpm, bradydysrhythmia, reversal of anticholinesterase agents, insecticide poisoning, blocking cardiac vagal reflexes, decreasing secretions before surgery, antispasmodic with GU and biliary surgery, bronchodilator, AV heart block, irinotecan-induced diarrhea, rapid-sequence intubation

Absorption	Well absorbed (SUBCUT, IM)
Distribution	Crosses blood-brain barrier, placenta
Metabolism	Liver
Excretion	Kidneys, unchanged (50%); breast milk
Half-life	4-5 hr

Pharmacodynamics

	IM/ SUBCUT	IV	Ophth
Onset	rapid	Immediate	½ hr
Peak	30 min	2-4 min	30-60 min
Duration	4-6 hr	4-6 hr	1-2 wk

CONTRAINDICATIONS

Hypersensitivity to belladonna alkaloids, closed-angle glaucoma, GI obstructions, myasthenia gravis, thyrotoxicosis, ulcerative colitis, prostatic hypertrophy, tachycardia/tachydysrhythmias, asthma, acute hemorrhage, severe hepatic disease, myocardial ischemia, paralytic ileus

Precautions: Pregnancy, breastfeeding, child <6 yr, geriatric, renal disease, HF, hyperthyroidism, COPD, hypertension, intraabdominal infections, Down syndrome, spastic paralysis, gastric ulcer

DOSAGE AND ROUTES
Bradycardia/bradydysrhythmias

Adult: IV bol 0.5-1 mg given q3-5min, not to exceed 2 mg

Child: IV 0.02 mg/kg, may repeat X 1, minimum dose 0.1 mg to avoid paradoxical reaction, max single dose 0.5 mg, max total dose 1 mg; **endotracheal:** IV dose, dilute before use

Organophosphate poisoning

Adult and child: IM (AtroPen)/**IV** 1-2 mg q 20-30 min until muscarinic symptoms disappear; may need 6 mg qhr

Adult and child ≥90 lb, usually >10 yr: 2 mg IM (AtroPen)

Child 40-90 lb, usually 4-10 yr: 1 mg IM (AtroPen)

Child 15-40 lb, 6 mo-4 yr: 0.5 mg IM (AtroPen)

Infant <15 lb: IM/IV 0.05 mg/kg q5-20min

Presurgery

Adult and child >20 kg: SUBCUT/IM/ **IV** 0.4-0.6 mg 30-60 min before anesthesia

Child <20 kg: IM/SUBCUT 0.01 mg/kg up to 0.4 mg ½-1 hr preop, max 0.6 mg/dose

Available forms: Inj 0.05, 0.1, 0.4, 0.8, 1 mg/ml; inj prefilled autoinjectors (AtroPen) 0.25, 0.5, 1, 2 mg/0.7 mL

ADVERSE EFFECTS

CNS: Confusion, *coma*, flushing, drowsiness, decreased sweating

CV: Paradoxical bradycardia, angina, PVCs, *tachycardia*, palpitations

EENT: Blurred vision, photophobia

GI: Dry mouth, constipation

GU: Retention, hesitancy, impotence, dysuria

INTERACTIONS
Individual drugs

Potassium chloride (oral): increased mucosal lesions, avoid concurrent use

Drug classifications

Antacids: decreased absorption of atropine
Antidepressants (tricyclic), antiparkinson agents, phenothiazines, antidysrhythmics: increased anticholinergic effect
Beta blockers: Increased altered response

NURSING CONSIDERATIONS
Assessment

• Monitor I&O ratio; check for urinary retention and daily output in geriatric or postoperative patients

• Monitor vital signs, ECG during treatment for ectopic ventricular beats, PVC, tachycardia in cardiac patients

• Monitor for bowel sounds; check for constipation; abdominal distention and constipation may occur

• **Beers:** Avoid in older adults, highly anticholinergic, high risk of delirium, in men decreases urinary flow

• **Pregnancy/breastfeeding:** Identify if pregnancy is planned or suspected, use only if benefits outweigh fetal risk

Patient problem

Impaired cardiac output (uses)
Constipation (adverse reactions)

Implementation
IM route

• Expect atropine flush 15-20 min after inj; it may occur in children and is not harmful

AtroPen

• Use no more than 3 AtroPen injections unless under the supervision of trained provider

• Use as soon as symptoms appear (tearing, wheezing, muscle fasciculations, excessive oral secretions), may use through clothing

IV route

• Give **IV** undiluted or diluted with 10 ml sterile water; give at a rate of 0.6 mg/min; give through Y-tube or 3-way stopcock; do not add to **IV** sol; may cause paradoxical bradycardia lasting 2 min

Y-site compatibilities: Amrinone, etomidate, famotidine, heparin, hydrocortisone sodium succinate, meropenem, nafcillin, potassium chloride, SUFentanil, vit B/C

Endotracheal route

• Dilate with 5-10 mL of 0.9% NaCl, inject into endotracheal tube, then positive pressure ventilations

Patient/family education

- Advise patient not to perform strenuous activity in high temperatures; heat stroke may result
- Instruct patient to take as prescribed; not to skip doses
- Instruct patient to report change in vision; blurring or loss of sight; sweating; flushing, constipation, urinary retention
- Caution patient not to operate machinery if drowsiness occurs
- Advise patient not to take OTC products, herbals, supplements without approval of prescriber
- Teach patient not to freeze or expose to light (Astropen)

Evaluation

Positive therapeutic outcome
- Decreased dysrhythmias
- Increased heart rate
- Decreased secretions, GI, GU spasms
- Bronchodilatation

TREATMENT OF OVERDOSE:

O_2, artificial ventilation, ECG; administer DOPamine for circulatory depression; administer diazepam or thiopental for seizure; assess need for antidysrhythmics

---

atropine ophthalmic

See Appendix B

avanafil (Rx)

(a-van´a-fil)
Stendra
Func. class: Impotence agent
Uses: Erectile dysfunction

CONTRAINDICATIONS

Hypersensitivity, severe renal/hepatic disease, current nitrates/nitrites, patients <18 yr, potent CYP3A4 inhibitors

DOSAGE AND ROUTES

Adult: 100 mg, 30 mins before sexual activity, dose may be reduced to 50 mg or increased to 200 mg; usual dose 1 time/day

---

⚠ HIGH ALERT

avelumab

a-vel´ue-mab)
Bavencio
Func. class.: Antineoplastic monoclonal antibody
Chem. class.: Human IgG1 monoclonal antibody

ACTION: A human IgG1 monoclonal antibody that binds to the programmed death ligand found on T cells and blocks the interaction on receptors on the tumor cell

USES: For the treatment of Merkel cell carcinoma

Half-life	6.1 days, steady state 4-6 wk

CONTRAINDICATIONS

Pregnancy, hypersensitivity

Precautions: Adrenal insufficiency, autoimmune disease, breastfeeding, colitis, Crohn's disease, contraception requirements, diabetes mellitus, diarrhea, hepatic disease, hepatitis, hyperglycemia, infertility, infection, infusion-related reactions, organ transplant, pulmonary disease, pneumonitis, reproductive risk, thyroid disease

DOSAGE AND ROUTES

Merkel cell carcinoma

Adult, Adolescent, and Child > 12 yr of age: IV 10 mg/kg IV over 60 min q2wk until disease progression. Give antihistamine (diphenhydramine) and acetaminophen 30 to 60 min before the first 4 infusions

Urothelial carcinoma

Adult: IV 10 mg/kg IV over 60 min q2wk until disease progression or unacceptable toxicity. Give antihistamine (diphenhydramine) and acetaminophen 30 to 60 min before the first 4 infusions

Management of treatment-related toxicity
Immune-mediated reactions

Colitis: *Grade 2 or 3 toxicity:* Hold and give corticosteroids (predniSONE 1 to 2 mg/kg/day or equivalent, then taper); resume therapy when the adverse event recovers to grade 1 or less after the corticosteroid taper; permanently discontinue if grade 3 toxicity occurs or recurs. *Grade 4 toxicity:* Permanently discontinue, give corticosteroids (predniSONE 1 to 2 mg/kg/day or equivalent, then taper)

Endocrinopathies (including hyperglycemia, hypothyroidism, hyperthyroidism, adrenal insufficiency): *Grade 3 or 4 toxicity:* Hold, give corticosteroids and manage the endocrinopathy with the following: insulin or antihyperglycemics for hyperglycemia, hormone replacement therapy for hypothyroidism; resume when the adverse event recovers to grade 1 or less after the corticosteroid taper

Hepatitis: *Grade 2 toxicity (AST or ALT level of 3 to 5 times the upper limit of normal [ULN] or a total bilirubin level of 1.5 to 3 times the ULN):* Hold, give corticosteroids (predniSONE 1 to 2 mg/kg/day equivalent initially, then taper); resume when the adverse event recovers to grade 1 or less after the corticosteroid taper. *Grade 3 or 4 toxicity (AST or ALT level greater than 5 times the ULN or a total bilirubin level greater than 3 times the ULN):* Permanently discontinue, give corticosteroids (predniSONE 1 to 2 mg/kg/day or equivalent initially, then taper).

Nephritis: *Grade 2 or 3 toxicity (serum creatinine [SCr] level of 1.5- to 6-times the ULN):* Hold, give corticosteroids predniSONE 1 to 2 mg/kg/day or equivalent initially, then taper); resume therapy when the adverse event recovers to grade 1 or less after the corticosteroid taper. *Grade 4 toxicity (SCr level greater than 6-times the ULN):* Permanently discontinue, give corticosteroids (predniSONE 1 to 2 mg/kg/day or equivalent initially then taper).

Pneumonitis: *Grade 2 toxicity:* Hold, give corticosteroids (predniSONE 1 to 2 mg/kg/day or equivalent initially, then taper); resume when the adverse event recovers to grade 1 or less after the corticosteroid taper; permanently discontinue if grade 2 toxicity occurs or recurs. *Grade 3 or 4 toxicity:* Permanently discontinue, give corticosteroids (predniSONE 1 to 2 mg/kg/day or equivalent initially, then taper).

Infusion-related reactions: *Grade 1 or 2 toxicity:* Temporarily hold or slow the infusion. *Grade 3 or 4 toxicity:* Permanently discontinue. Available forms: Solution for injection 200 mg/10 ml

ADVERSE EFFECTS
CNS: Fatigue, chills, fever, dizziness, headache, flushing
GI: Nausea, vomiting, diarrhea, constipation, abdominal pain, anorexia
HEMA: Anemia, thrombocytopenia, lymphopenia
INTEG: Urticaria
MS: Back pain, arthralgia, myalgia

INTERACTIONS
None known

NURSING CONSIDERATIONS
Assessment
• **Serious infection:** Some may be fatal. Monitor patients for signs and symptoms of infection; hold therapy for grade 3 or higher infection. Serious *Pneumocystis jiroveci* pneumonia (PJP) has occurred; consider PJP prophylaxis in at-risk patients before starting treatment, hold if PJP is suspected. If PJP diagnosis is confirmed, treat the infection until resolution and then resume at the previous dose and give PJP prophylaxis for the duration of therapy

• **Myelosuppression:** Assess for anemia, thrombocytopenia, neutropenia; obtain a CBC at least weekly during treatment
• **Pregnancy/breastfeeding:** Product can cause fetal harm; females of reproductive potential should avoid becoming pregnant while taking this product; do not breastfeed during and for at least 1 mo after the last dose

Patient problems
Risk for injury (adverse reactions)

Implementation
IV route
• Visually inspect for particulate matter and discoloration before use

Dilution
• Add the required amount/volume of drug to a 250-ml bag of 0.9% sodium chloride injection or 0.45% sodium chloride injection; mix by gentle inversion
• Discard any unused drug left in the vial
• *Storage after dilution:* Store at room temperature (up to 25° C or 77° F) for up to 4 hr or refrigerated (2 to 8° C; 36 to 46° F) for up to 24 hr from the time of dilution. Do not freeze or shake; protect from light. If refrigerated, allow the diluted solution to warm to room temperature before use

Intermittent IV infusion
• Administer the diluted solution IV over 60 min
• Use a sterile, nonpyrogenic, low-protein-binding, 0.2-micron inline filter
• Do not administer other drugs through the same infusion line
• Follow cytotoxic handling procedures

Patient/family education
• Teach patient to report adverse reactions immediately, report diarrhea, flu-like symptoms
• Teach patient about reason for treatment, expected results
• **Pregnancy/breastfeeding:** Advise patient to notify provider if pregnancy is planned or suspected, to use effective contraception during treatment and up to 30 days after discontinuing treatment, not to use during pregnancy, breastfeeding, and for at least 1 mo after last dose

Evaluation
Positive therapeutic outcome
Improving blood counts

axicabtagene ciloleucel
(ax-i-cab'tay-jeen-sye-lo'loo-sel)
Yescarta
Func. class.: Antineoplastic, cellular immunotherapies
Chem. class.: Chimeric antigen receptor (CAR) T-cell therapy

ACTION: A chimeric antigen receptor (CAR) T-cell therapy that works by redirecting T cells to target an antigen on B cells in patients with hematologic malignancies.

USES: For the treatment of non-Hodgkin's lymphoma (NHL)

Pharmacokinetics

Absorption, distribution, metabolism, excretion	Unknown

Pharmacodynamics

Onset, duration	Unknown
Peak	7-14 days

CONTRAINDICATIONS
Hypersensitivity

Precautions: Neurotoxicity, allergic reactions, anemia, neutropenia, thrombocytopenia, secondary malignancy, hypogammaglobulinemia, B-cell aplasia, pregnancy, breastfeeding, hepatitis B, vaccinations, infection

> **BLACK BOX WARNING:** Cytokine release syndrome

DOSAGE AND ROUTES
Relapsed or refractory large B-cell lymphoma
Adult: IV 2×10^6 CAR-positive viable T cells per kg of body weight (max dose of 2×10^8 CAR-positive viable T-cells) as a single IV dose

Therapeutic drug monitoring
Management of treatment-related toxicity

Cytokine release syndrome (CRS) (without concurrent neurologic toxicity): For ≥ grade 2 toxicity, give tocilizumab 8 mg/kg IV over 1 hr (max 800 mg); repeat tocilizumab 8 mg/kg IV q8hr as needed if IV fluids or supplemental oxygen is not effective. Max 3 doses/24 hr, or max 4 doses. *Grade 2 toxicity (oxygen requirement <40% FiO₂, hypotension responsive to fluids or a low dose of 1 vasopressor agent, or grade 2 organ toxicity):* No improvement within 24 hr after starting tocilizumab, start methylprednisolone 1 mg/kg IV bid or dexamethasone 10 mg IV q6hr, continue corticosteroids until the toxicity resolves to ≤ grade 1, then taper over 3 days. *Grade 3 toxicity (oxygen requirement of ≥ 40% FiO2, hypotension requiring high-dose or multiple vasopressor agents, grade 3 organ toxicity, or grade 4 transaminitis):* Start methylprednisolone 1 mg/kg IV bid or dexamethasone 10 mg IV q6hr; continue corticosteroids until the toxicity resolves to ≤ grade 1, then taper over 3 days. *Grade 4 toxicity (i.e., requirements for ventilator support, continuous venovenous hemodialysis [CVVHD], or grade 4 organ toxicity (excluding transaminitis):* Give methylprednisolone 1000 mg IV/day for 3 days. If the condition improves, begin methylprednisolone 1 mg/kg IV bid or dexamethasone 10 mg IV q6hr. Continue corticosteroids until the toxicity resolves to ≤ grade 1, then taper over 3 days

Neurologic toxicity (without concurrent CRS): Nonsedating antiseizure medication. *Grade 2 toxicity:* Start dexamethasone 10 mg IV q6hr until the toxicity resolves to ≤ grade 1, then taper over 3 days. *Grade 3 toxicity:* Start dexamethasone 10 mg IV q6hr until the toxicity resolves to ≤ grade 1, then taper over 3 days. *Grade 4 toxicity:* Give methylprednisolone 1000 mg IV daily for 3 days. If condition improves, begin dexamethasone 10 mg IV q6hr. Continue corticosteroids until the toxicity resolves to ≤ grade 1, then taper over 3 days.

ADVERSE EFFECTS
CNS: Confusion, chills, delirium, dizziness, drowsiness, fatigue, fever, hallucinations, irritability, malaise, neurotoxicity, paranoia, tremor, weakness
CV: Atrial fibrillation/flutter, AV block, bundle branch block, orthostatic hypotension, QT prolongation, sinus tachycardia, supraventricular tachycardia, ventricular tachycardia, hypotension
GI: Abdominal pain, nausea, vomiting, anorexia, constipation, diarrhea, weight loss
HEMA: Anemia, leukopenia, lymphopenia, neutropenia, thrombocytopenia, thromboembolism, thrombosis
META: Hypokalemia, hyponatremia, hypophosphatemia, hyperuricemia

INTERACTIONS
None known

NURSING CONSIDERATIONS
Assessment
• **Allergic reactions, anaphylaxis:** Premedicate acetaminophen and diphenhydramine before use. Use with caution in those with DMSO, aminoglycoside hypersensitivity

• **Cytopenias (anemia, neutropenia, and thrombocytopenia):** Monitor complete blood counts regularly until recovery

• **Secondary malignancy:** Lifelong monitoring for the development of secondary malignancies is recommended. Report cases of secondary malignancy to Kite at 844-454-5483; instructions will be provided regarding patient sample collection for testing

• **Hypogammaglobulinemia and B-cell aplasia:** Monitor immunoglobulin levels after therapy; provide infection precautions, antibiotic therapy, and immunoglobulin replacement as required

• **Hepatitis B virus (HBV) reactivation:** May cause hepatitis B exacerbation, fulminant hepatitis, hepatic failure, and death; may occur with drugs directed against B cells. Screen all patients for HBV, hepatitis C virus, and HIV before cell collection (leukapheresis)

• **Serious infections (bacterial, fungal, viral):** Some may be life-threatening or fatal. Monitor for infection before and after use; antiinfective therapy should be used as needed. Febrile neutropenia has also been reported; it may occur concurrently with cytokine release syndrome, assess for infection and give broad-spectrum antibiotics, fluids as needed

• Patients should avoid cell, organ, tissue, and blood donation

• **Pregnancy/breastfeeding:** Should be avoided; there are not any studies available; pregnancy testing is needed before starting treatment, contraception should be used during treatment, but length of time after treatment concludes is unknown; avoid breastfeeding, excretion is unknown

BLACK BOX WARNING: Cytokine release syndrome (CRS) may be fatal or life-threatening. Do not use in active infection or inflammatory disorders. Confirm that 2 tocilizumab doses are available before infusion. Observe for CRS qday for ≥ 7 days in a certified facility after the infusion, continue monitoring for ≥ 4 wk after the infusion. Assess for fever, hypoxia, and hypotension. Treat severe or life-threatening CRS with tocilizumab or tocilizumab and corticosteroids. Those with mild symptoms (fever, nausea, fatigue, headache, myalgia, and malaise) may require symptomatic treatment only. Monitor patients with grade 2 or higher CRS (hypotension, not responsive to fluids, or hypoxia requiring supplemental oxygenation) with continuous cardiac telemetry and pulse oximetry. Possible ECG to assess cardiac function. Available only through a restricted program under a Risk Evaluation and Mitigation Strategy (REMS) called the YESCARTA REMS.

• **Severe neurotoxicity** (encephalopathy, seizures, cerebral edema) some fatal, usually occurs within 8 wk. Assess for neurotoxicity daily ≥ 7 days in a certified healthcare facility after infusion and for ≥ 4 wk after the infusion. Monitor those with grade 2 or higher neurotoxicity with continuous cardiac telemetry and pulse oximetry. Nonsedating, antiseizure medicines (levetiracetam) may be required for seizure prophylaxis

Patient problems
• Give as an IV infusion within 30 min via gravity or a peristaltic pump until the infusion bag is empty

• Gently agitate during the infusion to prevent cell clumping

• Rinse the tubing with normal saline at the same infusion rate to ensure all product is given

Implementation
IV route
• Premedicate patients with acetaminophen 650 mg and diphenhydramine 12.5 mg IV or PO 1 hr before use

• Confirm that tocilizumab is available at the facility before the infusion

• Visually inspect the infusion bag for any breaks or cracks before thawing. Do not infuse if the bag is compromised; follow local guidelines or call Kite Pharma at 844-454-5483

• For autologous and IV use

• Each dose contains a max of 2×10^8 CAR-positive viable T cells suspended in a single patient-specific infusion bag; the total infusion bag volume is about 68 ml

• Ensure tocilizumab and emergency equipment are available before use

• Coordinate the timing of the product's thaw and infusion; confirm the infusion time in advance, and adjust the start time for thaw so that the patient will be ready

• Premedicate with acetaminophen and diphenhydramine approximately 1 hr before the infusion; avoid corticosteroid use except in the case of a life-threatening emergency

Preparation

• Match the patient's identity with the patient identifiers on the cassette; do not remove the product bag from the cassette if the patient-specific label does not match the intended recipient

• Remove the product bag from the cassette; verify that the patient information on the cassette label matches the bag label

• Put the infusion bag inside a second, sterile bag to protect against leaks and port contamination

• Thaw the infusion bag at 37° Celsius (C) using a water bath or dry thaw method; once there is no visible ice, gently mix the contents of the bag

• If visible cell clumps remain, continue to gently mix; small clumps should disperse

• Do not wash, spin down, and/or resuspend in new media before use

• *Storage*: After thawing, may store at room temperature (20 to 25° C) ≤ 3 hr

Intravenous (IV) infusion

• Confirm the patient's identity with the patient identifiers on the infusion bag

• Prime the tubing with normal saline before use; do not use a leukocyte-depleting filter

Patient/family education

• Advise patient to avoid driving, operating machinery, or performing other dangerous duties for 8 wk after treatment; mental status changes, seizures may occur or change in consciousness or coordination

• Do not donate blood, organs, tissues

• Teach patient to report fever, fast heartbeat, confusion, inability to speak to healthcare provider

• Advise patient to avoid vaccinations (live virus) during and for 6 wk after treatment

Evaluation

Positive therapeutic outcome

• Prevention of spread of cancer

azaTHIOprine (Rx)
(ay-za-thye′oh-preen)
Azasan, Imuran
Func. class.: Immunosuppressant
Chem. class.: Purine antagonist

Do not confuse: azaTHIOprine/azaCITIDine

ACTION: Produces immunosuppression by inhibiting purine synthesis in cells

Therapeutic outcome: Absence of graft rejection, slowing of rheumatoid arthritis

USES: Renal transplants to prevent graft rejection, refractory rheumatoid arthritis

Unlabeled uses: Chronic ulcerative colitis, Crohn's disease

Pharmacokinetics

Absorption	Readily (PO)
Distribution	Crosses placenta
Metabolism	Liver to mercaptopurine
Excretion	Kidney, minimal
Half-life	3 hr

Pharmacodynamics

	PO	IV
Onset	Unknown	Unknown
Peak	4 hr	Unknown
Duration	Unknown	Unknown

CONTRAINDICATIONS
Pregnancy, breastfeeding, hypersensitivity

Precautions: Severe renal/hepatic disease, geriatric, ⚫ thiopurine methyltransferase deficiency, infection, bone marrow suppression, must be used by an experienced clinician

> **BLACK BOX WARNING:** neoplastic disease

DOSAGE AND ROUTES
Immunosuppression in kidney transplantation
Adult and child: PO/IV 3-5 mg/kg/day, then maintenance (PO) of at least 1-3 mg/kg/day,

Renal dose
Adult: PO; give lower dose in tubular necrosis in immediate postcadaveric transplant period, CCr 10-50 ml/min 75% of dose; CCr <10 ml/min 50% of dose

Refractory rheumatoid arthritis
Adult: PO 1 mg/kg/day; may increase dosage after 2 mo by 0.5 mg/kg/day and then q4wk; not to exceed 2.5 mg/kg/day

---

Crohn's disease or ulcerative colitis (unlabeled)

Adult/child: PO 50 mg/day, may increase by 25 mg/day q 1-2 wk up to 2-3 mg/kg/day if tolerated

Available forms: Tabs 50, 75, 100 mg; inj Powder for injection 50 mg ✤, 100 mg/vial

ADVERSE EFFECTS

CNS: Progressive multifocal leukoencephalopathy

GI: Nausea, vomiting, pancreatitis, hepatotoxicity, hepatic

EENT: Retinopathy

RESP: Pulmonary edema

HEMA: Leukopenia, thrombocytopenia, anemia, pancytopenia

INTEG: Rash, alopecia

MISC: Raynaud's symptoms, serum sickness, secondary malignancy, infection

MS: Arthralgia, chills, fever

INTERACTIONS
Individual drugs

Do not admix with other products

Allopurinol: increased action of azaTHIOprine, use decreased dose of azaTHIOprine or avoid using

CycloSPORINE: increased myelosuppression

Drug classifications

Antineoplastics: increased myelosuppression, monitor for increased myelosupression

Toxoids, vaccines: decreased immune response

Drug/herb

• Echinacea, melatonin: Decreased immunosuppression, avoid concurrent use

Drug/lab test

Increased: liver function tests

Decreased: uric acid

Interference: CBC, diff count

NURSING CONSIDERATIONS
Assessment

• Assess symptoms of **rheumatoid arthritis:** pain in joints, stiffness, poor range of motion, mobility, inflammation before and during treatment

• Monitor **blood studies:** CBC, Hgb, WBC, platelets during treatment monthly; if leukocytes are <3000/mm³ or platelets <100,000/mm³, product should be discontinued or reduced; decreased Hgb level may indicate bone marrow suppression

• **Bone marrow suppression:** severe leukopenia, pancytopenia, thrombocytopenia

• **Hepatotoxicity:** alkaline phosphatase, AST, ALT, amylase, bilirubin: Assess for dark urine, jaundice, itching, light-colored stools; product should be discontinued

• Monitor I&O, weight daily, report decreasing urine output, toxicity may occur

• Assess for **infection:** increased temp, WBC; sputum, urine, vital signs baseline and during treatment

Patient problem

Risk for infection (uses)

Implementation
PO route

• Give with meals to reduce GI upset; nausea is common

IV route

• Prepare in biological cabinet using gown, gloves, mask

Direct, IV route

• **Dilute** to 10 mg/ml with 0.9% NaCl, 0.45% NaCl, D_5W, **give** over 5 min

Intermittent IV INF route

• **Reconstitute** 100 mg/10 ml of sterile water for inj; rotate to dissolve; **further dilute** with 50 ml or more saline or glucose in saline, **give** over ½-1 hr

Y-site compatibilities: Alfentanil, atracurium, atropine, benztropine, calcium gluconate, cycloSPORINE, enalaprilat, epoetin alfa, erythromycin, fentaNYL, fluconazole, folic acid, furosemide, glycopyrrolate, heparin, insulin, mannitol, mechlorethamine, metoprolol, naloxone, nitroglycerin, oxytocin, penicillin G, potassium chloride, propranolol, protamine, SUFentanil, trimethaphan, vasopressin

Patient/family education

• Teach patient to take as prescribed, do not miss doses; if dose is missed on daily regimen, skip dose; if on multiple dosing/day, take as soon as remembered

• Teach patient that therapeutic response may take 3-4 mo in rheumatoid arthritis, to continue with prescribed exercise, rest, other medications; that product is needed for life in renal transplant

• Instruct patient to report fever, rash, severe diarrhea, chills, sore throat, fatigue, since serious infections may occur; or clay-colored stools and cramping (hepatotoxicity)

• Advise patient to use contraceptive measures during treatment for 16 wk after ending therapy; product is teratogenic

• Advise patient to avoid live vaccinations, bring vaccinations up-to-date prior to starting therapy

• Tell patient to avoid crowds and persons with known infections to reduce risk of infection

• Advise patient to avoid OTC, herbals, supplements unless approved by health care professional

- **RA:** Advise patient to continue with other prescribed treatment, other medications, physical therapy

Evaluation
Positive therapeutic outcome
- Absence of graft rejection
- Immunosuppression in autoimmune disorders
- Increased joint mobility without pain in rheumatoid arthritis

azelaic acid topical
See Appendix B

azelastine nasal agent
See Appendix B

azelastine ophthalmic
See Appendix B

azilsartan
(ay-zil-sar'tan)
Edarbi
Func. class.: Antihypertensive
Chem class.: Angiotensin II receptor antagonist

ACTION: Antagonizes angiotensin II at the AT$_1$ receptor in tissues like vascular smooth muscle and the adrenal gland.

Therapeutic outcome: Decreased B/P

USES: Hypertension, alone or in combination with other antihypertensives

Pharmacokinetics
Absorption	60%
Distribution	Protein binding, >99%, to serum albumin
Metabolism	Metabolized by CYP2C9
Excretion	55% eliminated (feces), 42% (urine)
Half-life	Elimination half-life 11 hr

Pharmacodynamics
Onset	Unknown
Peak	1.5-3 hr
Duration	Unknown

CONTRAINDICATIONS

> **BLACK BOX WARNING:** Pregnancy

Precautions: Angioedema, ◆♦ African descent, renal disease, renal artery stenosis, children, geriatrics, heart failure, hypovolemia, breastfeeding, pregnancy 1st trimester

DOSAGE AND ROUTES
Adult: PO 80 mg/day, may give an initial dose of 40 mg/day in patients receiving high-dose diuretic therapy

Available forms: Tabs 40, 80 mg

ADVERSE EFFECTS
CNS: Dizziness, fatigue, insomnia, headache, depression
CV: Hypotension, orthostatic hypotension
GI: Nausea, diarrhea, vomiting, abdominal pain
HEMA: Anemia
INTEG: Angioedema, rash, pruritus
MS: Muscle cramps, arthralgia, myalgia
META: Hyperkalemia

INTERACTIONS
Individual drugs
CycloSPORINE: in those with poor renal function, increased renal failure risk: monitor closely
Digoxin: Increased digoxin level
Lithium: increased lithium toxicity

Drug classifications
Antidiabetics: increased hypoglycemia
NSAIDs in those with poor renal function: monitor closely: increased renal failure risk
Diuretics, potassium-sparing, potassium salt substitute, potassium products: Increased hyperkalemia, monitor potassium levels
Other antihypertensives, other angiotensin receptor antagonists, MAOIs: increased hypotensive effect

Drug/herb
Black licorice, ephedra: decreased antihypertensive effect
Garlic, hawthorn: increased antihypertensive effect

NURSING CONSIDERATIONS
Assessment
- **Angioedema:** Assess for facial swelling, difficulty breathing; stop product, notify health care professional immediately

> **BLACK BOX WARNING:** Pregnancy, can cause fetal death, avoid breastfeeding

- **HF:** B/P, pulse during beginning therapy and periodically thereafter; note rhythm, rate, quality; obtain electrolytes before beginning therapy; monitor daily weight for fluid overload (dyspnea, jugular venous distention, edema, crackles)

• Monitor renal function studies: BUN, creatinine; electrolytes (potassium)

Patient problems
Nonadherence (teaching)

Implementation
• May administer without regard to food
• Use original package to protect from light, moisture, and heat

Patient/family education
• Instruct patient to comply with dosage schedule even if feeling better
• Advise patient that diarrhea, dehydration, excessive perspiration, vomiting; may lead to fall in B/P, to consult prescriber if these occur
• Instruct patient to rise slowly from lying or sitting to minimize orthostatic hypotension; that product may cause dizziness
• Instruct patient to avoid OTC medications unless approved by prescriber; to inform all health care providers of product use
• Instruct patient to use proper technique for obtaining B/P

Evaluation
Positive therapeutic outcome
• Decreased B/P

---

azithromycin (Rx)

(ay-zi-thro-my′sin)
AzaSite, Zithromax, Zmax
Func. class.: Antiinfective
Chem. class.: Macrolide

Do not confuse: azithromycin/
erythromycin, **Zithromax**/Zinacef

ACTION: Binds to 50S ribosomal subunits of susceptible bacteria and suppresses protein synthesis; much greater spectrum of activity than erythromycin; more effective against gram-negative organisms

Therapeutic outcome: Bacteriostatic against the following susceptible organisms: PO, acute pharyngitis/tonsillitis (group A streptococcal); acute skin/soft tissue infections; community-acquired pneumonia

USES: Mild to moderate infections of the upper respiratory tract, in children: acute otitis media, lower respiratory tract; uncomplicated skin and skin structure infections, nongonococcal urethritis, or cervicitis; prophylaxis of disseminated *Mycobacterium avium* complex (MAC); *Bacillus anthracis, Bacteroides bivius, Bordetella pertussis, Borrelia burgdorferi, Campylobacter jejuni,* CDC coryneform group G, *Chlamydia trachomatis, Chlamydophila pneumoniae, Clostridium perfringens, Gardnerella vaginalis, Haemophilus ducreyi/influenzae* (beta-lactamase negative/positive), *Helicobacter pylori, Klebsiella granulomatis, Legionella pneumoniae/moraxella/catarrhalis, Mycobacterium avium/intracellulare, Mycoplasma genitalium/hominis/pneumoniae, Neisseria gonorrhoeae, Peptostreptococcus, Prevotella bivia, Rickettsia tsutsugamushi, Salmonella typhi, Staphylococcus aureus* (MSSA)*/epidermidis, Streptococcus, Toxoplasma gondii, Treponema pallidum, Ureaplasma urealyticum, Vibrio cholerae,* viridans streptococci; **opthalmic:** bacterial conjunctivitis

Pharmacokinetics

Absorption	Rapid (PO) up to 50%
Distribution	Widely distributed
Metabolism	Minimal
Excretion	Unchanged (bile); kidneys, minimal
Half-life	11-70 hr

Pharmacodynamics

	PO	IV
Onset	Rapid	Rapid
Peak	2-4 hr	End of infusion
Duration	24 hr	24 hr

CONTRAINDICATIONS

Hypersensitivity to azithromycin, erythromycin, or any macrolide; hepatitis, jaundice

Precautions: Pregnancy, breastfeeding, child <6 mo for otitis media, child <2 yr for pharyngitis, geriatric, renal/hepatic/cardiac disease, tonsillitis, QT prolongation, ulcerative colitis, torsades de pointes, sunlight exposure, sodium restriction, myasthenia gravis, pseudomembranous colitis, contact lenses, hypokalemia, hypomagnesemia

DOSAGE AND ROUTES
Most infections
Adult: PO 500 mg on day 1, then 250 mg daily on days 2-5 for a total dose of 1.5 g or 500 mg a day × 3 days
Child 2-15 yr: PO 10 mg/kg on day 1, then 5 mg/kg × 4 days

Pelvic inflammatory disease
Adult: PO/**IV** 500 mg **IV** q24hr × 2 doses, then 250 mg PO q24hr × 7-10 days

Cervicitis, chlamydia, chancroid, nongonococcal urethritis, syphilis
Adult: PO 1 g single dose

Gonorrhea
Adult: PO 1 g single dose with ceftriaxine 250 mg IM

Endocarditis prophylaxis
Adult: PO 500 mg 1 hr prior to procedure
Child: PO 15 mg/kg 1 hr prior to procedure

Community acquired pneumonia
Adult: PO/IV 500 mg q 24 hr (IV, severe) $\times$ 2 doses, then 500 mg q 24 hr $\times$ 7-10 days; 500 mg (PO), then 250 mg/day $\times$ 4 more days or 2 g single dose (Zmax)
Child: >6 mg PO 10 mg/kg on day 1, then 5 mg/kg q day $\times$ 4 more days

Disseminated MAC infections
Adult: PO 600 mg/day in combination with ethambutol 15 mg/kg/day; **MAC in HIV** PO 1.2 g qwk, alone or with rifabutin

Lower respiratory tract infections
Adult: PO 500 mg day 1, then 250 mg $\times$ 4 days
Child: PO 5-12 mg/kg/day $\times$ 5 days

Acute otitis media
Child >6 mo: PO 30 mg/kg as a single dose or 10 mg/kg daily $\times$ 3 days or 10 mg/kg as a single dose on day 1, max 500 mg/day, then 5 mg/kg on days 2-5, max 250 mg/day

Bacterial conjunctivitis
Adult/child ≥ 1 yr: opthalmic instill 1 drop in affected eye bid $\times$ 2 days then 1 drop in eye q day $\times$ 5 days

Available forms: Tabs 250, 500, 600 mg; powder for inj 500 mg; powder for oral susp 1 g/packet; susp 100, 200 mg/5 ml; extended release oral suspension (Zmax) 2 g single dose bottle; ophthalmic drops 1% sol

ADVERSE EFFECTS
CNS: Dizziness, headache, vertigo, somnolence, fatigue, seizures
CV: Palpitations, chest pain, QT prolongation, torsades de pointes (rare)
GI: *Nausea, diarrhea,* hepatotoxicity, abdominal pain, stomatitis, heartburn, dyspepsia, flatulence, melena, cholestatic jaundice, CDAD
GU: Vaginitis, nephritis
HEMA: Anemia leukopenia, thrombocytopenia
INTEG: Rash, photosensitivity, pain at injection site
SYST: Angioedema, Stevens-Johnson syndrome, toxic epidermal necrolysis

INTERACTIONS
Individual drugs
Bromocriptine, carBAMazepine, cycloSPORINE, digoxin, disopyramide, methylPREDNISolone, nelfinavir, phenytoin, tacrolimus, theophylline, triazolam: increased effects of specific products
Ergotamine: ergot toxicity
Amiodarone, droperidol, methadone, nilotinib, propafenone, quiNIDine: increased QT prolongation
Pimozide: increased dysrhythmias; fatal reaction; do not use concurrently
Triazolam: decreased clearance of triazolam

Drug classifications
Aluminum, magnesium antacids: decreased levels of azithromycin, separate by ≥2 hr
Anticoagulants (orals): increased effect of oral anticoagulants

Drug/food
Decreased: absorption—food (suspension)

Drug/lab test
Increased: bilirubin, alkaline phosphatase, CPK, BUN, creatinine, AST, ALT, potassium, blood glucose
Decreased: blood glucose, potassium, sodium

NURSING CONSIDERATIONS
Assessment
• **QT prolongation, torsades de pointes:** assess for patients with serious bradycardia, ongoing pro-arrhythmic conditions, or elderly; more common in these patients
• Assess for signs and symptoms of **infection:** drainage, fever, increased WBC >10,000/mm³, urine culture positive, sore throat, sputum culture positive
• Monitor respiratory status: rate, character, wheezing, tightness in chest; discontinue product if these occur
• Monitor allergies before treatment, reaction of each medication; place allergies on chart, notify all people giving products; skin eruptions, itching
• Monitor I&O ratio, renal studies; report hematuria, oliguria in renal disease; check urinalysis, protein, blood
• Monitor liver studies: AST, ALT, bilirubin, LDH, alkaline phosphatase; CBC with diff
• Monitor C&S before product therapy; product may be taken as soon as culture is taken; C&S may be repeated after treatment
• **Assess for serious skin reactions:** Stevens-Johnson syndrome, toxic epidermal necrolysis, angioedema, discontinue if rash occurs

- **Assess for CDAD:** blood or pus in diarrhea stool, abdominal pain, fever, fatigue, anorexia; obtain CBC, serum albumin
- Assess for **superinfection:** sore throat, mouth, tongue; fever, fatigue, diarrhea, anogenital pruritus
- Pregnancy/breastfeeding: Use only if clearly needed, cautious use in breastfeeding, excreted in breast milk

Patient problem
Infection (uses)

Implementation
Opthalmic route
- Store in refrigerator
- Do not touch dropper to eye

PO route
- Provide adequate intake of fluids (2 L) during diarrhea episodes
- Give with a full glass of water; give susp 1 hr before or 2 hr after meals; tabs may be taken without regard to food; do not give with fruit juices
- Store at room temperature
- Reconstitute 1 g packet for susp with 60 ml water, mix, rinse glass with more water and have patient drink to consume all medication; packets not for pediatric use
- Do not take aluminum/magnesium-containing antacids or food simultaneously with this product

Intermittent IV infusion route
- **Reconstitute** 500 mg product/4.8 ml sterile water for inj (100 mg/ml), shake, **dilute** with ≥ 250 ml 0.9% NaCl, 0.45% NaCl, or LR to 1-2 mg/ml; diluted solution is stable for 24 hr or 7 days if refrigerated
- **Give** 1 mg/ml sol over 3 hr or 2 mg/ml sol over 1 hr, never give IM or as a bolus

Y-site compatibilities: Acyclovir, alatrofloxacin, alemtuzumab, alfentanil, aminocaproic acid, aminophylline, amphotericin B liposome/complex, ampicillin, ampicillin-sulbactam, anidulafungin, atenolol, bivalirudin, bleomycin, bumetanide, buprenorphine, butorphanol, calcium chloride/gluconate, CARBOplatin, carmustine, ceFAZolin, cefepime, cefoTEtan, cefOXitin, ceftaroline, cefTAZidime, ceftizoxime, cimetidine, cisatracurium, CISplatin, cyclophosphamide, cycloSPORINE, cytarabine, DAPTOmycin, DAUNOrubicin liposome, dexamethasone, dexmedetomidine, dexrazoxane, digoxin, dilTIAZem, diphenhydrAMINE, DOBUTamine, DOCEtaxel, dolasetron, doripenem, doxacurium, DOXOrubicin liposomal, doxycycline, droperidol, enalaprilat, EPINEPHrine, epiRUBicin, eptifibatide, ertapenem, esmolol, etoposide, etoposide phosphate, fenoldopam, fluconazole, fluorouracil, foscarnet, fosphenytoin, gallium, ganciclovir, gatifloxacin, gemcitabine, granisetron, haloperidol, heparin, hydrocortisone phosphate/succinate, HYDROmorphone, hydrOXYzine, IDArubicin, ifosfamide, inamrinone, irinotecan, isoproterenol, labetalol, lepirudin, magnesium sulfate, mannitol, meperidine, meropenem, mesna, mechlorethamine, methohexital, methotrexate, methylPREDNISolone, metoclopramide, metroNIDAZOLE, milrinone, minocycline, mivacurium, nalbuphine, naloxone, nesiritide, nitroglycerin, nitroprusside, octreotide, ofloxacin, ondansetron, oxaliplatin, oxytocin, PACLitaxel, palonosetron, pamidronate, pantoprazole, PEMEtrexed, PENTobarbital, phenylephrine, piperacillin, potassium acetate/phosphates, procainamide, prochlorperazine, promethazine, propranolol, raNITIdine, remifentanil, rocuronium, sodium acetate, succinylcholine, SUFentanil, sulfamethoxazole-trimethoprim, tacrolimus, telavancin, teniposide, thiotepa, ticarcillin, tigecycline, tirofiban, TPN, trimethobenzamide, vancomycin, vasopressin, vecuronium, verapamil, vinCRIStine, voriconazole, zidovudine, zoledronic acid

Patient/family education
- Instruct patient to report sore throat, black furry tongue, fever, loose foul-smelling stool, vaginal itching, discharge, fatigue; may indicate **superinfection**
- Caution patient not to take aluminum/magnesium-containing antacids or food simultaneously with this product; blood levels of azithromycin will be decreased
- Instruct patient to notify prescriber of diarrhea stools, dark urine, pale stools, yellow discoloration of eyes or skin, severe abdominal pain; cholestatic jaundice is a severe adverse reaction
- Teach patient to take Zmax 1 hr prior to or 2 hr after a meal; shake well before use
- Teach patient to complete dosage regimen; to notify prescriber if symptoms continue
- Teach patient to use protective clothing or stay out of the sun: photosensitivity may occur
- Teach patient to notify prescriber if pregnancy is suspected

Evaluation
Positive therapeutic outcome
- C&S negative for infection
- WBC within 5000-10,000/mm^3

azithromycin ophthalmic
See Appendix B

aztreonam
(az tree'oh-nam)
Azactam, Cayston
Func. class.: Antibiotic, misc.
Chem. class.: Monobactam

ACTION: Binds to bacterial cell wall, causing cell death

Therapeutic use: Treatment of susceptible bacteria

USES: Urinary tract infection; septicemia; skin, muscle, bone infection; lower respiratory tract, intraabdominal infections; other infections caused by gram-negative organisms; used for *E. coli, Serratia, Klebsiella oxytoca, K. pneumoniae, Citrobacter, Proteus mirabilis, Pseudomonas aeruginosa, Enterobacter, Haemophilis influenza*

Pharmacokinetics

Absorption	Well IM, poor inhalation
Distribution	Widely, crosses placenta, enters breast milk (minimal), inhalation high in sputum, protein binding 56%
Metabolism	Liver minimal
Excretion	70% (urine, unchanged)
Half-life	1.5-2 hrs (adult), 1.7 hr (child), extended in renal disease

Pharmacodynamics

	IM	IV	Inhal
Onset	Unknown	Rapid	Rapid
Peak	1 hr	Infusion end	Unknown
Duration	Up to 8 hr	Up to 8 hr	Unknown

CONTRAINDICATIONS
Hypersensitivity, severe renal disease

Precautions: Breastfeeding, hepatic/renal disease, pregnancy

DOSAGE AND ROUTES
Urinary tract infections
Adult: IM/IV 500 mg-1 g q 8-12 hr

Systemic infections
Adult: IM/IV 1-2 g q 8-12 hr
Child: IM/IV 90-120 mg/kg/day in divided doses q 6-8 hr, max 8 g/day IV

Severe systemic infections
Adult: IM/IV 2 g q6-8 hr; max 8 g/day continue treatment for 48 hr after negative culture or until patient is asymptomatic

Cystic fibrosis with *Pseudomonas aeruginosa*
Adult, adolescent, child ≥7 yr: NEB 75 mg tid x 28 days, then 28 days off; give q 4 hr or more, give bronchodilator before aztreonam

Renal dose
Adult: (IV) CCr 10-30 mL/min 1-2 g, may give 50% of usual dose thereafter; **CCr <10 mL/min** 500 mg-2 g, then 25% of usual dose thereafter

Available forms: Solution for injection 500 mg, 1 g, 2 g/vial; premixed 1 g, 2 g/50 ml; lyophilized powder for use in nebulizer system 75/mg/1 vial

ADVERSE REACTIONS
CNS: Seizures
GI: CDAD
CV: Chest pressure (inhal)
EENT: Nasal congestion (inhal)
RESP: Cough, wheezing (inhal)
INTEG: Rash, pain at injection site (IV/IM)
MISC: Hypersensitivity, anaphylaxis, superinfection; fever (inhal)

INTERACTIONS
Individual drugs
Furosemide, probenecid: Increased levels

Drug/Lab
Increase: LFTs, LDH, BUN, creatinine, PTT, pro-time

NURSING CONSIDERATIONS
Assessment
• **Infection:** Assess for characteristics of sputum, wounds, urine, stools; monitor vital signs often
• **Culture and sensitivity:** Obtain specimens before use or first dose; may use before results are received
• **Hypersensitivity/anaphylaxis:** Assess for rash, itching, wheezing, trouble breathing, chills, fever, report to provider immediately
• **CDAD:** Assess for diarrhea with mucus or blood, abdominal pain, fever, report to provider immediately; may occur several days to weeks after last dose

Patient problems
Infection (uses)
Impaired airway clearance (uses, inhal)

Implementation
• Add diluent provided to vial, shake

IM route
• Dilute each 1 g/3 mL or more 0.9% NaCl, sterile, bacteriostatic water for injection, give deeply in muscle mass
• Stable at room temperature 48 hr or refrigerated for 1 wk

IV direct route
• Reconstitute 15 mL vial/6-10 mL of sterile water for injection, give over 3-5 min into turbine of running IV of compatible solution; do not use rapidly

Intermittent IV infusion route
• Reconstitute 15 mL vial/3 mL of sterile water for injection; further dilute with 0.9% NaCl, Ringer's or LR, D5W; infuse over 20-60 min

Inhalation route
• Open vial, twist top of diluent ampule, place contents in vial, replace top and swirl, give immediately by using the Alterna Nebulizer System, do not use IM/IV

• Give bronchodilator 15 min-4 hr prior to use with this system

Patient/family education
• Superinfection: Advise patient to notify provider of vaginal itching; loose, foul-smelling stools; black, furry tongue
• **Hypersensitivity/anaphylaxis:** Advise patient to report immediately rash, itching, wheezing, trouble breathing, chills, fever
• **CDAD:** Advise patient to report immediately diarrhea with mucus or blood, abdominal pain, fever; may occur several days to weeks after last dose

Evaluation
• Resolution of infection
• Negative culture and sensitivities

baclofen (Rx)
(bak'loe-fen)
Gablofen, Lioresal Intrathecal
Func. class.: Skeletal muscle relaxant, central acting
Chem. class.: GABA, chlorophenyl derivative

Do not confuse: Lioresal/Lotensin, baclofen/Bactroban/bacitracin

ACTION: Inhibits synaptic responses in CNS by stimulating GABA$_B$ receptor subtype, which decreases neurotransmitter function, decreasing frequency, severity of muscle spasms

Therapeutic outcome: Decreased spasticity of muscles

USES: Spasticity in spinal cord injury, multiple sclerosis

Unlabeled use: Trigeminal neuralgia pain

Pharmacokinetics

Absorption	Well (PO)
Distribution	Widely, crosses placenta, protein binding 30%
Metabolism	Liver, partially
Excretion	Kidney, unchanged 70%-80%
Half-life	2½-4 hr

Pharmacodynamics

	IT	PO
Onset	0.5-1 hr	Unknown
Peak	2-3 hr	Unknown
Duration	>8 hr	Unknown

CONTRAINDICATIONS
Hypersensitivity; epidural, IM, IV, subcut use

Precautions: Pregnancy, breastfeeding, geriatric, peptic ulcer, renal/hepatic disease, stroke, seizure disorder, diabetes mellitus, psychosis. Abrupt discontinuation (Intrathecal); CNS depressants, especially opiates

DOSAGE AND ROUTES
Adult, child ≥12 yr: PO 5 mg tid × 3 days, then 10 mg tid × 3 days, then 15 mg tid × 3 days, then 20 mg tid × 3 days, then titrated to response, max 80 mg/day (20 mg qid); **IT** use implantable **IT** inf pump; use screening trial of 3 separate bol doses if needed 24 hr apart (50 mcg/ml, 75 mcg/1.5 ml, 100 mcg/2 ml)
Child ≥8 yr: As above, max 60 mg/day

Child 2-7 yr: PO 10-15 mg/day divided q8hr; titrate every 3 days by 5-15 mg/day, max 40 mg/day
Child: IT initial test dose same as adult; for small children, initial dose of 25 mcg/dose; 25-1200 mcg/day inf, titrated to response in screening phase

Available forms: Tabs 5, 10, 20 mg; **IT inj** 10,000 mcg/20 ml, 20,000 mcg/20 ml, 40,000 mcg/20 ml; 50 mcg/ml, 0.05 mcg/ml, 10 mg/20 ml, 10 mg/5 ml, 50 mg/20 ml

ADVERSE EFFECTS
CNS: *Dizziness, weakness, fatigue, drowsiness,* headache, disorientation, seizures (IT); insomnia
CV: Hypotension, bradycardia, edema
EENT: Nasal congestion, blurred vision, tinnitus
GI: *Nausea,* constipation, anorexia
GU: Urinary frequency
INTEG: Rash, pruritus
MISC: Hypersensitivity, sweating, hyperglycemia

INTERACTIONS
Individual drugs
Alcohol: Increased CNS depression

Drug classifications
Antidepressants (tricyclics), antihistamines, barbiturates, MAOIs, opioids, sedative/hypnotics: increased CNS depression, avoid concurrent use
Antihypertensives: increased hypotension

Drug/herb
Kava, valerian, chamomile: increased CNS depression

Drug/lab test
Increased: AST, ALT, alkaline phosphatase, blood glucose, CK

NURSING CONSIDERATIONS
Assessment
• **Multiple sclerosis/spinal cord lesions:** Assess for spasms, spasticity, ataxia; mobility, improvement should occur
• Monitor B/P, weight, blood glucose, and hepatic function periodically
• **Withdrawal symptoms:** Agitation, tachycardia, insomnia, hyperpyrexia
• Check for increased seizure activity in patients with epilepsy; this product decreases seizure threshold, monitor EEG
• Check for urinary retention, frequency, hesitancy

- **Allergic reactions:** rash, fever, respiratory distress; severe weakness, numbness in extremities
- Assess CNS depression: dizziness, drowsiness, psychiatric symptoms
- **Intrathecal:** Have emergency equipment nearby; assess test dose and titration, if there is no response, check pump and catheter for proper functioning
- **Pregnancy/breastfeeding:** Use in pregnancy only if benefits outweigh fetal risk, avoid breastfeeding, excretion unknown

Patient problems
Impaired mobility (uses)

Implementation
PO route
- Give with meals for GI symptoms; gum, frequent sips of water for dry mouth
- Store in airtight container at room temperature
IT route
- **For screening,** dilute to a concentration of 50 mcg/ml with NaCl for inj (preservative-free); give test over 1 min; watch for decreasing muscle tone, frequency of spasm; if inadequate, use two more test doses q24hr, those with inadequate response should not receive chronic IT therapy; **maintenance inf** via implantable pump of 500-2000 mcg/ml dosage because individual titration is required
- Do not give IT dose by inj, **IV,** IM, SUBCUT, epidural

BLACK BOX WARNING: Don't discontinue abruptly, may be fatal (intrathecal)

Patient/family education

BLACK BOX WARNING: IT: Advise patient not to discontinue medication quickly; hallucinations, spasticity, tachycardia will occur; product should be tapered off over 1-2 wk, especially intrathecal form

- Advise patient not to take with alcohol, other CNS depressants
- Teach patient to avoid hazardous activities if drowsiness, dizziness occurs; to rise slowly to prevent orthostatic hypotension
- Teach patient to avoid using OTC medications: cough preparations, antihistamines, unless directed by prescriber; to take with food or milk
- Teach patient to notify prescriber if nausea, headache, tinnitus, insomnia, confusion, constipation, or inadequate, painful urination continues
- **Pregnancy/breastfeeding:** To notify if pregnancy is planned or suspected, avoid breastfeeding
- May require 1-2 mo for full response

Evaluation
Positive therapeutic outcome
- Decreased pain, spasticity, ability to perform ADLs

TREATMENT OF OVERDOSE:
Induce emesis of conscious patient, dialysis, physostigmine to reduce life-threatening CNS side effects

⚠ HIGH ALERT

basiliximab (Rx)
(bas-ih-liks′ih-mab)
Simulect
Func. class.: Immunosuppressant
Chem. class.: Murine/human monoclonal antibody (interleukin-2) receptor antagonist

ACTION: Binds to and blocks the IL-2 receptor, which is selectively expressed on the surface of activated T lymphocytes; impairs the immune system to antigenic challenges

Therapeutic outcome: Prevention of graft rejection

USES: Acute allograft rejection in renal transplant patients when used with cycloSPORINE and corticosteroids

Pharmacokinetics

Absorption	Complete IV
Distribution	Unknown
Metabolism	Unknown
Excretion	Unknown
Half-life	7 days (adult), 9½ days (child)

Pharmacodynamics

Onset	2 hr
Peak	Unknown
Duration	30-40 days

CONTRAINDICATIONS
Mannitol, murine protein hypersensitivity

Precautions: Pregnancy, children, geriatric, infections, breastfeeding, neoplastic disease, vaccination

BLACK BOX WARNING: Requires a specialized care setting and experienced clinician

DOSAGE AND ROUTES
Adult/child ≥35 kg: **IV** 20 mg × 2 doses; first dose within 2 hr before transplant surgery; second dose given 4 days after transplantation

Child <35 kg: IV 10 mg × 2 doses; first dose within 2 hr before transplant surgery; second dose given 4 days after transplantation

Available forms: Powder for inj 10, 20 mg/vial

ADVERSE EFFECTS

CNS: *Pyrexia, chills, tremors, headache, insomnia, weakness,* dizziness; psychiatric/behavioral changes (child)

CV: *Chest pain,* angina, cardiac failure, hypo/hypertension, edema

GI: *Vomiting, nausea, diarrhea,* constipation, abdominal pain, GI bleeding, gingival hyperplasia, stomatitis

GU: Weight gain

INTEG: *Acne,* pruritus, impaired wound healing

META: Hypercholesterolemia, hyperuricemia, hypo/hyperkalemia, hypocalcemia, hypophosphatemia

MISC: Infection, moniliasis, anaphylaxis, anemia, allergic reaction, dysuria

MS: Arthralgia, myalgia

RESP: *Cough*

INTERACTIONS
Drug classifications
Immunosuppressants: increased immunosuppression

Drug/herb
Echinacea, melatonin: St. John's wort, turmeric: Decreased immunosuppression

Drug/lab test
Increased: BUN, cholesterol, uric acid, creatinine, calcium, blood glucose, Hgb, Hct
Decreased: Hgb, Hct, platelets, magnesium, phosphate, glucose, potassium

NURSING CONSIDERATIONS
Assessment
• Assess for infection, increased temp, WBC, sputum, urine, may be fatal (bacterial, protozoal, fungal)
• Monitor blood studies: Hgb, WBC, platelets baseline and during treatment
• Monitor liver function studies: alkaline phosphatase, AST, ALT, bilirubin baseline
• **Assess for anaphylaxis, hypersensitivity:** dyspnea, wheezing, rash, pruritus, hypotension, tachycardia; if severe hypersensitivity reactions occur, product should not be used again

Patient problems
Infection (adverse reaction)

Implementation
IV direct route
• May give undiluted by bolus at 4 mg/mL given over 30 min by central or peripheral IV line
Intermittent IV INF route
• **Reconstitute** 10 mg vial/2.5 ml or 20 mg vial in 5 ml sterile water for inj; shake gently to dissolve, **dilute** reconstituted sol in 25 ml (10 mg vial) or 50 ml (20 mg vial) with 0.9% NaCl or D₅W, gently invert bag, do not shake, **give** over ½ hr, do not admix, usually given with corticosteroids and other immunosuppressants
• Storage of reconstituted sol refrigerated for up to 24 hr or at room temp for 4 hr

Patient/family education
• Instruct patient to report fever, chills, sore throat, fatigue, since serious infection may occur; avoid crowds, persons with known upper respiratory infections; use contraception during treatment
• Teach patient reason for product, expected result
• Advise patient not to drive or engage in hazardous activities, dizziness
• Bring vaccinations up to date 2 wk prior to therapy
• **Pregnancy/breastfeeding:** Advise patient to report if pregnancy is planned or suspected, or if breastfeeding

Evaluation
Positive therapeutic outcome
• Absence of graft rejection

becaplermin
(be-kap′ler-min)
Regranex
Func. class.: Decubiti agent
Chem. class.: Growth factor

ACTION: Repairs wounds and decubiti by promoting cell regeneration and granulation

Therapeutic use: Healing of tissues

USES: Decubiti ulcers in the lower extremity of diabetic patients with adequate blood supply to area

Pharmacokinetics

Absorption	Poor
Distribution	Local area
Metabolism	Unknown
Excretion	Unknown
Half-life	Unknown

Pharmacodynamics

Onset	Unknown
Peak	Unknown
Duration	Unknown

CONTRAINDICATIONS

Hypersensitivity to this product or parabens, neoplastic disease

Precautions: Malignancy, pregnancy

DOSAGE AND ROUTES

Adults and adolescents ≥16: One application left in place for 12 hr q day. The amount of gel to be used is determined by ulcer size; measure the greatest length by the greatest width. If the ulcer width and length are measured in centimeters, use ulcer length × ulcer width divided by 4 for a 15 g tube. If the ulcer width and length are measured in inches, use ulcer length × ulcer width × 0.6 for a 15 g tube. If the ulcer does not decrease in size by approximately 30% after 10 wk of treatment or if complete healing does not occur in 20 wk, reassess

Available forms: Gel 100 mcg in 2, 7.5, 15 g tubes

ADVERSE REACTIONS:

INTEG: Malignancy, rash at application site

NURSING CONSIDERATIONS
Assessment

• **Wound/decubiti:** Assess area, color, drainage, and surrounding tissue at least weekly. Each week the amount of gel needed will be recalculated on size of area

• **Malignancy:** Assess for a new primary malignancy distant from the site being treated; patients prescribed this product 3 or more times are at greater risk

Patient problems

Impaired skin integrity (uses)

Implementation
Topical route (gel)

• Apply to affected area and cover with saline dressing for 12 hr

• The amount to be applied will vary depending on the size of the ulcer area (see Dosage). The physician or wound-care giver needs to recalculate the needed amount of gel at weekly or biweekly intervals depending on the rate of change in ulcer area

• Thoroughly wash your hands before applying the gel. Squeeze the calculated length of gel on to a clean, firm, nonabsorbable surface such as wax paper. Do not touch the tip of the tube to the ulcer or to any other surface. Tightly recap the tube after each use.

• Use a clean cotton swab, tongue depressor, or similar application aid to evenly spread the measured amount of gel over the ulcer surface. A thin, continuous layer of gel that is approximately 1/16 of an inch in thickness is needed. Cover the ulcer with a saline moistened gauze dressing

• After approximately 12 hr, gently rinse the ulcer with saline or water to remove residual gel. Cover the ulcer with a saline-moistened gauze dressing for the remaining 12 hr

Patient/family education

• Teach patient/family member or caregiver method of use and not to touch the tube to affected area

Evaluation

• Decreased size of wound
• Improved healing

beclomethasone (Rx, inhalation)
(be-kloe-meth′a-sone)
QVAR Redi Haler

beclomethasone (Rx, nasal)
Beconase AQ, QNASL, Rivanase AQ ✦

Func. class.: antiasthmatic/antiinflammatory
Chem. class.: corticosteroid

Do not confuse: beclomethasone/betamethasone

ACTION: Prevents inflammation by suppression of migration of polymorphonuclear leukocytes, fibroblasts, reversal of increased capillary permeability and lysosomal stabilization; does not suppress hypothalamus and pituitary function

Therapeutic outcome: Decreased inflammation and normal immunity

USES: Seasonal, perennial allergic/vasomotor rhinitis, nasal polyps, chronic steroid-dependent asthma

Pharmacokinetics

Absorption	Locally only
Distribution	Not distributed
Metabolism	Lungs, liver (by CYP3A)
Excretion	Feces, urine
Half-life	2.8 hr (INH/nasal)

Pharmacodynamics

	Inh	Nasal
Onset	1-4 wk	10 min
Peak	Unknown	Unknown
Duration	Unknown	Unknown

CONTRAINDICATIONS

Hypersensitivity, status asthmaticus (primary treatment)

Precautions: Pregnancy, breastfeeding, child <12, nasal disease/surgery, nonasthmatic bronchial disease, bacterial, fungal, viral infections of mouth, throat, lungs, HPA suppression, osteoporosis, Cushing's syndrome, diabetes mellitus, measles, cataracts, corticosteroid hypersensitivity, glaucoma, herpes infection

DOSAGE AND ROUTES

Adult and child >12 yr: INH 48-80 mcg bid (alone) or 40-160 mcg bid (with inhaled corticosteroids), max 320 bid; **nasal** 1-2 sprays in each nostril bid

Child 5-12 yr: INH 40 mcg bid, max 80 mcg bid, **nasal** 1-2 sprays in each nostril bid

Available forms: Oral inh 40, 80, 250 ✚ mcg/metered spray; nasal 42 mcg/metered spray, 80 mcg/metered spray; 50 mcg/metered spray ✚

ADVERSE EFFECTS

Inhalation

CNS: *Headache;* psychiatric/behavioral changes (child)

EENT: *Candidal infection of oral cavity, hoarseness,* sore throat, dysgeusia, loss of taste/smell, pharyngitis, rhinitis, sinusitis, cataracts, fungal infections, epistaxis

ENDO: Hypothalamic-pituitary (HPA) suppression

GI: Dry mouth, dyspepsia

MISC: Angioedema, adrenal insufficiency, facial edema, Churg-Strauss syndrome (rare)

RESP: Bronchospasm, wheezing, cough

Nasal

CNS: Headache, dizziness

EENT: Nasal burning/irritation, sneezing

GI: Dry mouth, esophageal candidiasis

RESP: Cough

NURSING CONSIDERATIONS

Assessment

• Assess adrenal suppression: 17-KS, plasma cortisol for decreased levels, adrenal function periodically for HPA axis suppression during prolonged therapy; if indicated, monitor growth and development

• Check nasal passages during long-term treatment for changes in mucus; check for burning, stinging; assess for glucocorticoid withdrawal

• Assess for fungal infections in mucous membranes

• **Bronchospasm:** Use short-acting bronchodilator

• **Beers:** Avoid use in older adults, high risk of delirium

• **Pregnancy/breastfeeding:** Inhaled product: fetal harm appears remote, acceptable to use in breastfeeding

Patient problems

Impaired airway clearance (uses)
Infection (side effects)
Lack of knowledge of medication (teaching)
Nonadherence (teaching)

Implementation

Oral route

• Give PO, spacer device, priming or shaking is not needed

• Use after cleaning aerosol top daily with warm water; dry thoroughly

• Store in cool environment; do not puncture or incinerate container

Nasal route

• Shake inhaler, invert, tilt head backward, insert nozzle into nostril, away from septum; hold other nostril closed and depress activator, inhale through nose, exhale through mouth

Patient/family education

• Teach patient to gargle/rinse mouth after each use to prevent oral fungal infections

• Teach patient to continue using product even if mild nasal bleeding occurs; is usually transient

• Teach patient method of administration after providing written instructions from manufacturer

• Teach patient to notify prescriber if pregnancy is planned or suspected, do not breastfeed

• Teach patient to check growth in child on long-term therapy

• Teach patient to taper PO products before starting inhalation products

• Teach patient to carry medical alert ID with corticosteroid user listed

• Teach patient how to use nasal and inhalation products; clean inhaler by wiping with dry cloth

• **Allergic reactions: Teach patient to inform healthcare professional immediately of rash, itching, swelling of face, lips, trouble breathing**

• Advise patient to take as prescribed, not to double or skip doses

• Teach patient the symptoms of **adrenal insufficiency:** nausea, anorexia, fatigue, dizziness, dyspnea, weakness, joint pain, depression

Evaluate

Positive therapeutic outcome

• Decrease in runny nose, improved symptoms of bronchial asthma

• Nasal polyps are reduced

belatacept (Rx) REMS
(bel-a-ta'sept)
Nulojix
Func. class.: Immunosuppressant
Chem. class.: Fusion protein

ACTION: Activated T lymphocytes are the mediators of immunologic rejection, and this product is a selective T-cell costimulation blocker; blocks the CD28-mediated co-stimulation of T lymphocytes by binding to CD80 and CD86 on antigen-presenting cells; inhibits T-lymphocyte proliferation and the production of the cytokines

Therapeutic outcome: Absence of kidney transplant rejection

USES: Kidney transplant rejection prophylaxis given with basiliximab induction, mycophenolate mofetil, corticosteroids

Pharmacokinetics

Absorption	Complete (IV)
Distribution	Steady state by week 8 after transplantation and by month 6 during the maintenance phase
Metabolism	Unknown
Excretion	Unknown
Half-life	Half-life range 6.1-15.1 days

Pharmacodynamics

Onset	Unknown
Peak	Infusion end
Duration	Up to 1 month

CONTRAINDICATIONS

Hypersensitivity, Epstein-Barr Virus (EPV) seronegative, and specialized setting, EBV status unknown

> **BLACK BOX WARNING:** Infection, organ transplant, requires an experienced clinician, secondary malignancy, posttransplant lymphoproliferation disorder (PTLD)

Precautions: Breastfeeding, immunosuppression, child/infant/neonate, pregnancy, diabetes mellitus, progressive multifocal leukoencephalopathy, immunosuppression, sunlight exposure, TB

DOSAGE AND ROUTES

Adult: **IV** *initial:* 10 mg/kg rounded to nearest 12.5 mg increment give over 30 min the day of transplantation (day 1) but before transplantation, on day 5 approximately 96 hours after the day 1 dose 1, at the end of wk 2, at the end of wk 4, at the end of wk 8, and at the end of wk 12; *maintenance* 5 mg/kg rounded to nearest 12.5 mg increment given over 30 min at the end of wk 16 and q4wk ± 3 days thereafter; doses should be calculated on actual body weight on the transplantation day unless the patient's weight varies by >10%

Available forms:
Powder for inj 250 mg

ADVERSE EFFECTS

CNS: Progressive multifocal leukoencephalopathy (PML), headache, fever
GI: Abdominal pain, constipation, diarrhea, nausea, vomiting
GU: Proteinuria
HEMA: Anemia, leukopenia
INTEG: Infusion reaction
META: Hyperglycemia, hyper/hypokalemia
RESP: *Cough*
SYST: Secondary malignancy, posttransplant lymphoproliferation disorder (PTLD), wound dehiscence

INTERACTIONS
Individual drugs
• Mycophenolic acid: Increased effect, toxicity
• Live virus vaccines: Do not use 30 days before or with this product

Drug classifications
• Corticosteroids: increased belatacept effect
• Vaccines: avoid concurrent use
• Immunosuppressives: avoid increased dose

NURSING CONSIDERATIONS
Assessment
• Progressive multifocal leukoencephalopathy (PML): Assess for apathy, confusion, ataxia may occur during treatment, may occur up to 3 yr after transplant

> **BLACK BOX WARNING: Transplant rejection:** Assess for flulike symptoms, decreasing urinary output, malaise; some may experience pain in area (rare; monitor BUN/creatinine)

> **BLACK BOX WARNING: Infection:** Monitor for fever, immunosuppression occurs, chills, increased WBC, wound dehiscences

> **BLACK BOX WARNING: Posttransplant lymphoproliferation disorder (PTLD):** May lead to secondary malignancy (lymphoma) or infectious mononucleosislike lesions (assess for mood change, confusion, memory loss, change in gait, talking); may be treated with antivirals or immunosuppressant; may need to be discontinued

• **Pregnancy/breastfeeding:** Use in pregnancy if benefits outweigh fetal risk, pregnant patients should enroll in the pregnancy registry 1-877-681-6296, use adequate contraception during and for 4 months after last dose, discontinue breastfeeding or product, excretion in breast milk unknown

Evaluation
Positive therapeutic outcome
• Absence of renal transplant rejection

Patient problems
Risk for infection (adverse reactions)
Risk for injury (adverse reactions)

Implementation

> **BLACK BOX WARNING:** Only providers skilled in the use of immunosuppressant and management of transplant should use these products

IV route
• Visually inspect for particulate matter, discoloration, discard if present
• Calculate the number of vials required
• **Reconstitute** each vial/10.5 ml of sterile water for injection, 0.9% sodium chloride, D$_5$W using the silicone-free disposable syringe provided with each vial and an 18G to 21G needle. If using a silicone-free disposable syringe, use a new silicone-free disposable syringe. If you need additional silicone-free disposable syringes, call 888-685-6549. If the powder is accidentally reconstituted using a different syringe than the one provided, the solution may develop a few translucent particles. Discard any solutions prepared using siliconized syringes.
• Using aseptic technique, inject the diluent into the vial and direct the stream of diluent to the glass wall of the vial. To minimize foaming, rotate and invert with gentle swirling until the contents are dissolved. Do not shake; when reconstituted (25 mg/mL), product should be clear to slightly opalescent and colorless to pale yellow. Do not use if opaque particles, discoloration, or other foreign particles are present.
• Calculate the total volume of the reconstituted 25 mg/ml sol required to provide the prescribed dose. **Further dilute** this volume with a volume of infusion fluid equal to the volume of the reconstituted drug solution required. Use either NS or D$_5$W if drug was reconstituted with SWFI; use NS if drug was reconstituted with NS; use D$_5$W if drug was reconstituted with D$_5$W. With the same silicone-free disposable syringe used for reconstitution, withdraw the required amount, inject it into the infusion container, gently rotate; final concentration in infusion container should range 2-10 mg/ml. Volume of 100 ml will be appropriate for most doses, but total inf volumes ranging from 50-250 ml

may be used. Discard any unused drug solution; after reconstitution, immediately transfer the reconstituted sol from the vial to the inf bag or bottle; complete within 24 hr.

IV INF route
• **Give** over 30 min, use an infusion set and a sterile, nonpyrogenic low-protein-binding filter (0.2-1.2 mm), use a separate line
• **Storage:** refrigerate, protect from light ≤24 hr; max 4 hr of the total 24 hr can be at room temp and room light

Patient/family education
• Teach reason for product and expected result, use REMS guidelines
• Teach to avoid exposure to sunlight, tanning beds, risk of secondary malignancy, including skin cancer
• Teach to avoid crowds, persons with known infections
• Advise that repeated lab test will be needed, to inform providers of all OTC, Rx medications, herbs, supplements
• Advise to avoid with vaccines
• Advise that immunosuppressants will be needed for life to prevent rejection/infection; teach symptoms of rejection and to call provider immediately

belimumab (Rx)
(be-lim'ue-mab)
Benlysta
Func. class.: Immunosuppressant, monoclonal antibody
Chem. class.: Disease-modifying antirheumatic drugs (DMARDs)

ACTION: Inhibits B-lymphocyte stimulator (BLyS), which is needed for B-cell survival; normally, soluble BLyS binds to its receptors on B cells and allows B-cell survival; binds BLyS and prevents binding to its receptors on B cells

Therapeutic outcome: Decreasing symptoms of systemic lupus erythematosus (SLE): decreased fever, malaise, joint pains, myalgias, fatigue

USES: Active, autoantibody-positive, SLE in combination with standard therapy

Pharmacokinetics

Absorption	Complete
Distribution	Unknown
Metabolism	Unknown
Excretion	Unknown
Half-life	19.4 days

Pharmacodynamics

Onset	Unknown
Peak	Unknown
Duration	Unknown

CONTRAINDICATIONS
Hypersensitivity

Precautions: African descent patients, depression, children/infants, ✺ immunosuppression, infection, pregnancy, breastfeeding, suicidal ideation, vaccination, geriatrics, secondary malignancy, cardiac disease, requires experienced clinician

DOSAGE AND ROUTES
Adult/child/adolescents 5-17 yr: 10 mg/kg **IV** over 1 hr q2wk for the first 3 doses, then q4wk; **subcut** 200 mg q wk

Available forms: Powder for injection 120, 400 mg; auto injection 200 mg/mL; prefilled syringe solution 200 mg/mL

ADVERSE EFFECTS
CNS: *Depression,* dizziness, fever, *insomnia, migraine,* suicidal ideation, progressive multifocal leukoencephalopathy
CV: Bradycardia
GU: UTI
GI: Diarrhea, nausea
MISC: Allergic reactions, myalgia, rash
SYST: Anaphylaxis, infection, infusion reactions, secondary malignancy

INTERACTIONS
Individual drugs
IV cyclophosphamide, biologic therapies (riTUXimab, ofatumumab): avoid concurrent use

Drug classifications
Vaccines: within 30 days of belimumab, response to vaccine will be decreased

Drug/Herb
Echinacea: decreases product effect, avoid using together

Drug/lab test
Decrease: leukocytes

NURSING CONSIDERATIONS
Assessment
• **SLE:** Monitor for improvement including decreasing fever, malaise, fatigue, joint pain, myalgias
• **Progressive multifocal leukoencephalopathy:** Apathy, confusion, ataxia, cognitive problems
• **Suicidal ideation:** More common in those with preexisting depression
• **Infection:** Determine if a chronic or acute infection is present, may be fatal; do not begin therapy if any products are being used for a chronic infection; leukopenia may occur and susceptibility to infections increased
• **Anaphylaxis, infusion site reactions:** If these occur, stop infusion (angioedema, rash, pruritus, wheezing)
• **African descent patients:** Use cautiously in these patients, may not respond to this product
• **Pregnancy/breastfeeding:** Determine if pregnant or if pregnancy is planned or suspected, if pregnant call Belimumab Pregnancy Registry (877-681-6269) to enroll in registry; do not breastfeed; contraception is required during and for 4 mo after conclusion of therapy

Patient problems
Risk for infection (adverse reactions)
Risk for injury (adverse reactions)

Implementation
• Only health care providers prepared to manage anaphylaxis should administer this product, may give premedication for prophylaxis against infusion and hypersensitivity reactions (antihistamine/antipyretic)

Subcut Route
Use of the prefilled syringe or auto-injector:
• Remove from refrigerator and allow 30 minutes to reach room temperature. Do not warm in any other way.
• Inspect syringe or autoinjector for particulate matter and discoloration prior to use; product should be clear to opalescent and colorless to pale yellow. It is normal to see 1 or more air bubbles in the solution.
• Do not use the autoinjector or prefilled syringe if dropped on a hard surface.
• *Storage of unopened prefilled syringes or autoinjectors:* Protect from light and store refrigerated at 2° to 8° C (36° to 46° F) until time of use. Do not freeze and do not use if the injection has been frozen. Do not shake. Avoid exposure to heat Administration:
• Subcutaneous administration sites include the abdomen and thigh. Do not inject within 2 inches of the umbilicus. Do not administer where skin is tender, bruised, erythematous, or hard.
• For the pre-filled syringe, insert the entire needle into the pinched area of the skin at a slight 45-degree angle using a dart-like motion. Push the plunger all the way down until all of the solution is injected. While keeping your hold on the syringe, slowly move your thumb back, allowing the plunger to rise up. The needle will automatically rise up into the needle guard.
• For the auto-injector, position the auto-injector straight over the injection site at a 90-degree

angle. Make sure the gold needle guard is flat on the skin. To start the injection, firmly press the auto-injector all the way down onto the injection site and hold in place. A "click" will be heard at the start of the injection. Continue to hold the auto-injector down until you see that the purple indicator has stopped moving. A second "click" may be heard. The injection may take up to 15 seconds to complete. When the injection is complete, lift the injector from the injection site.

• Dispose of any used pre-filled syringes or auto-injectors immediately after use.

• Rotate sites of injection with each dose.

• *Missed dose:* If a dose is missed, administer as soon as possible. Thereafter, the patient can resume dosing on their usual day of administration or start a new weekly schedule from the day that the missed dose was administered. Do not give 2 doses on the same day.

Intermittent IV infusion route

• Visually inspect particulate matter and discoloration whenever solution and container permit

• **Give** as IV infusion only, do not give IV bolus or push, give over 1 hr and slow or stop if infusion reactions occur

• Do not give with any other agents in the same IV line

• Allow to stand at room temperature for 10-15 min before using

• **Reconstitute** with the appropriate amount of sterile water for injection (80 mg/ml); add 1.5 ml of sterile water (120 mg/vial) or 4.8 ml of sterile water (400 mg/vial)

• Direct the stream of sterile water toward the side of the vial to minimize foaming; gently swirl for 60 sec and allow to sit during reconstitution, gently swirling for 60 secs q5min until the powder is dissolved; do not shake; reconstitution is complete in 10 to 30 min

• If a mechanical reconstitution device (swirler) is used, max 500 rpm swirled for ≤30 min

• The solution should be opalescent, colorless to pale yellow, and without particles; small air bubbles are expected; protect from sunlight

• **Dilution:** Only dilute in NS, 0.45% NaCl, LR for injection; dilute reconstituted solution with enough compatible solution to 250 ml. From a 250-ml infusion bag or bottle of normal saline, withdraw and discard a volume equal to the volume of the reconstituted solution required for dose; add the required volume of the reconstituted solution to the infusion bag/bottle; gently invert to mix

• Discard any unused solution

• Storage in refrigerator or at room temp; total time from reconstitution to completion of inf max 8 hr

Patient/family education

• Advise patient to seek treatment immediately for serious hypersensitive reactions

• Advise patient not to receive live vaccinations during treatment

• Teach patient/caregiver in correct subcut injection technique; must give at same time of day q wk

• Advise patient to take as prescribed, not to double or skip doses; if dose is missed take as soon as remembered then resume correct schedule; provide Medication Guide and review with patient

• Advise patient to bring vaccinations up-to-date before starting therapy

• **Infection:** Report for fever, shortness of breath, diarrhea, urinary frequency/burning, sweating, chills;

• Teach patient that compliance is required

• Teach patient to avoid others with known infections

• Teach patient to report history of cancer in patient or family

Evaluation

• Decreasing symptoms of SLE: decreasing fatigue, fever, malaise

benazepril (Rx)

(ben-a′za-pril)

Lotensin

Func. class.: Antihypertensive

Chem. class.: ACE inhibitor

Do not confuse: benazepril/Benadryl

ACTION: Selectively suppresses renin-angiotensin-aldosterone system; inhibits ACE, preventing conversion of angiotensin I to angiotensin II

Therapeutic outcome: Decreased B/P in hypertension

USES: Hypertension, alone or in combination with thiazide diuretics

Pharmacokinetics

Absorption	<40%
Distribution	Unknown; crosses placenta; protein binding 97%
Metabolism	Liver metabolites
Excretion	Kidney, breast milk (minimal)
Half-life	10-11 hr (metabolite); increased in renal disease

Pharmacodynamics (B/P action)	
Onset	30-60 min
Peak	2-4 hr
Duration	Up to 24 hr

CONTRAINDICATIONS

Breastfeeding, children, hypersensitivity to ACE inhibitors, hereditary angioedema

> **BLACK BOX WARNING:** Pregnancy

Precautions: Impaired renal/liver function, dialysis patients, hypovolemia, blood dyscrasias, HF, COPD, asthma, geriatric, bilateral renal artery stenosis

DOSAGE AND ROUTES

Adult: PO 10 mg daily initially, then 20-40 mg/day divided bid or daily (without a diuretic); 5 mg PO daily (with a diuretic); max 80 mg daily
Child ≥6 yr: PO 0.2 mg/kg q day, may increase to 0.6 mg/kg/day

Renal dose

Adult: PO 5 mg daily with CCr <30 ml/min or CCr >3 mg/d/use; increase as needed to max of 40 mg/day
Child ≥6 yr: PO CCr < 30 ml/min do not use

Available forms: Tabs 5, 10, 20, 40 mg

ADVERSE EFFECTS

CNS: Insomnia, headache, dizziness, fatigue, drowsiness, fever
CV: Hypotension, postural hypotension
GI: Nausea, constipation, vomiting, gastritis, diarrhea
GU: Increased BUN, creatinine, decreased libido, impotence, renal insufficiency
HEMA: Agranulocytosis
INTEG: Rash, flushing, sweating, pruritus
META: Hyperkalemia
MISC: Angioedema, Stevens-Johnson syndrome, hypersensitivity, dry cough

INTERACTIONS

Individual drugs

AzaTHIOprine: increased myelosuppression
Digoxin, lithium: increased serum levels, may cause toxicity, monitor lithium or digoxin levels
Aliskiren: Increase 1 Hypotension, hyperkalemia in diabetes, renal disease; aliskiren, do not use in diabetes, avoid use in GFR<60 ml/min

Drug classifications

Antihypertensives, diuretics, nitrates, phenothiazines: increased hypotension
Diuretics (potassium-sparing), potassium supplements: increased hyperkalemia, monitor potassium, BUN, creatinine
Cox-2 inhibitors, NSAIDs: decreased hypotensive effects, may need to reduce dose, monitor B/P

Drug/herb

Black licorice, Ephedra (Ma huang): avoid concurrent use; decreased antihypertensive effect
Garlic, hawthorn: increased antihypertensive effect

Drug/lab test

Increased: AST, ALT, alkaline phosphatase, bilirubin, uric acid, blood glucose, potassium, BUN, creatinine

NURSING CONSIDERATIONS
Assessment

• **Hypertension:** Monitor B/P, pulse baseline and periodically; monitor compliance, check for orthostatic hypotension, syncope; if changes occur, dosage change may be required; notify prescriber of changes; monitor compliance
• Monitor renal studies: protein, BUN, creatinine; watch for increased levels that may indicate and renal failure; monitor urine for protein; monitor renal symptoms: polyuria, oliguria, frequency, dysuria
• Check potassium levels throughout treatment, although hyperkalemia rarely occurs; diuretic should be discontinued 3 days prior to initiation with benazepril; if hypertension is not controlled, a diuretic can be added; measure B/P at peak 2-4 hr and trough (before next dose); this product is less effective in African-American descendants
• Monitor CBC, AST/ALT, alkaline phosphatase during treatment
• **Assess for allergic reactions:** Rash, fever, pruritus, urticaria; swelling of lips, tongue, face; dyspnea; product should be discontinued if antihistamines fail to help; angioedema, Stevens-Johnson syndrome is more common in African-American descendants

Patient problems

Impaired cardiac output (uses)
Nonadherence (teaching)

Implementation

• Severe hypotension may occur after 1st dose of this medication; decreased hypotension may be prevented by reducing or discontinuing diuretic therapy 3 days before beginning benazepril therapy
• Storage in tight container at 86° F (30° C) or less

Patient/family education

• Instruct patient not to discontinue product abruptly; advise patient to tell all persons associated with care that product is being used
• Teach patient not to use OTC products (cough, cold, allergy) unless directed by prescriber; serious side effects can occur; xanthines such as coffee, tea, chocolate, cola can prevent action of product

• Emphasize the importance of complying with dosage schedule, even if feeling better; to continue with medical regimen to decrease B/P: exercise, cessation of smoking, decreasing stress, diet modifications

• Emphasize the need to rise slowly to sitting or standing position to minimize orthostatic hypotension, not to exercise in hot weather because increased hypotension can occur

• Teach patient to notify prescriber of mouth sores, sore throat, fever, swelling of hands or feet, irregular heartbeat, chest pain, coughing, shortness of breath, bruising, bleeding, swelling of face, tongue, lips, difficulty breathing, signs of infection, cough

• Caution patient to report excessive perspiration, dehydration, vomiting, diarrhea; strenuous exercise may lead to fall in B/P; to consume adequate fluids

• To use caution in hot weather

• Caution patient that product may cause dizziness, fainting, light-headedness; may occur during first few days of therapy; to avoid activities that may be hazardous

• **Hypertension:** Teach patient how to take B/P; teach normal readings for age group; ensure patient takes own B/P

> **BLACK BOX WARNING:** Advise patient to notify prescriber of pregnancy, product will need to be discontinued

Evaluation
Positive therapeutic outcome
• Decreased B/P in hypertension

TREATMENT OF OVERDOSE:
0.9% NaCl **IV** inf, hemodialysis

benzocaine topical
See Appendix B

benztropine (Rx)
(benz′troe-peen)
Cogentin
Func. class.: Anticholinergic, antiparkinson agent
Chem. class.: Tertiary amine

Do not confuse: benztropine/bromocriptine

ACTION: Blockade of central acetylcholine receptors in the CNS; neurotransmitters are balanced, balances cholinergic activity

Therapeutic outcome: Decreased involuntary movements

USES: Parkinsonian symptoms, EPS associated with neuroleptic products, acute dystonia

Pharmacokinetics

Absorption	Good (PO, IM), complete (**IV**)
Distribution	Unknown
Metabolism	Unknown
Excretion	Unknown
Half-life	Unknown

Pharmacodynamics

	IM/IV	PO
Onset	15 min	1 hr
Peak	7 hr	Unknown
Duration	6-10 hr	6-24 hr

CONTRAINDICATIONS
Hypersensitivity, closed-angle glaucoma, dementia, tardive dyskinesia

Precautions: Pregnancy, breastfeeding, children, geriatric, tachycardia, renal/hepatic disease, product abuse history, dysrhythmias, hypo/hypertension, psychosis; myasthenia gravis, GI/GU obstruction, child ≤3 yr, peptic ulcer, megacolon, prostate hypertrophy

DOSAGE AND ROUTES
Drug-induced extrapyramidal symptoms
Adult: IM/IV 1-4 mg daily/bid; give PO dose as soon as possible; PO 1-2 mg bid/tid; increase by 0.5 mg q5-6days
Child >3 yr: IM/IV 0.02-0.05 mg/kg/dose 1-2 ×/day
Geriatric: PO 0.5 mg daily-bid, increase by 0.5 mg q5-6days; max 4 mg/day

Parkinsonian symptoms
Adult: PO 1-2 mg daily, in 1-2 divided doses; increased 0.5 mg q5-6days titrated to patient response; max 6 mg daily

Postencephalitic parkinsonism
Adult: PO/IM/IV 2 mg qday in one dose or divided, max 6 mg qday

Acute dystonic reactions
Adult: IM/IV 1-2 mg, may increase to 1-2 mg bid (PO)

Available forms: Tabs 0.5, 1, 2 mg; inj 1 mg/ml (2-mg ampules)

ADVERSE EFFECTS

CNS: Confusion; hallucinations, headache, sedation, depression, incoherence, dizziness, memory loss; delirium (geriatric)
CV: Palpitations, tachycardia, hypotension, bradycardia
EENT: Blurred vision, photophobia, dry eyes, mydriasis
GI: *Dryness of mouth, constipation,* nausea
GU: Hesitancy, retention
INTEG: Rash
MISC: Decreased sweating

INTERACTIONS
Individual drugs
Bethanechol: decreased cholinergic effects
Disopyramide, quiNIDine: increased anticholinergic 5 effects, reduce dose, monitor response

Drug classifications
Antidepressants (tricyclic), antihistamines, phenothiazines: increased anticholinergic effects
Antidiarrheals, antacids: decreased absorption

NURSING CONSIDERATIONS
Assessment
• Assess for **parkinsonism**, EPS: shuffling gait, muscle rigidity, involuntary movements, loss of balance, pill rolling, muscle spasms, drooling before and during treatment, tardive dyskinesia (TD), exacerbation of symptoms may occur
• Monitor I&O ratio; retention commonly causes decreased urinary output, distention, frequency
• Palpate bladder if retention occurs
• Monitor for constipation, cramping, pain in abdomen, abdominal distention; increase fluids, bulk, exercise if this occurs
• Assess for tolerance over long-term therapy; dosage may have to be increased or changed
• Assess for mental status: affect, mood, CNS depression, worsening of mental symptoms during early therapy
• Assess for benztropine "buzz" or "high," patients may imitate EPS
• Do not discontinue abruptly, taper
• **Beers:** Avoid in older adults, high risk of delirium, CNS effects, decreased urinary flow

Patient problems
Risk for injury (uses)
Impaired mobility (uses)

Implementation
PO route
• Give with or after meals to prevent GI upset; may give with fluids other than water; hard candy, frequent drinks, gum to relieve dry mouth
• Give at bedtime to avoid daytime drowsiness in patient with parkinsonism

• May be crushed and mixed with food
• Store at room temperature
IM route
• Inject deeply in muscle; use filtered needle to remove solution from ampule
• Give in large muscle mass for dystonic symptoms

IV direct route
• Use in emergencies, not used often; **Rate:/** 1 mg/min

Y-site compatibilities: Alfentanil, amikacin, aminophylline, ascorbic acid injection, atracurium, atropine, azaTHIOprine, aztreonam, bumetanide, buprenorphine, butorphanol, calcium chloride, gluconate, ceFAZolin, cefotaxime, cefoTEtan, cefOXitin, cefTAZidime, ceftizoxime, cefTRIAXone, cefuroxime, chlorproMAZINE, cimetidine, clindamycin, cyanocobalamin, cycloSPORINE, dexamethasone, digoxin, diphenhydrAMINE, DOBUTamine, DOPamine, Doxycycline, enalaprilat, ePHEDrine, EPINEPHrine, epoetin alfa, erythromycin lactobionate, esmolol, famotidine, fentaNYL, fluconazole, folic acid (as sodium salt), gentamicin, glycopyrrolate, heparin, hydrocortisone sodium succinate, hydrOXYzine, imipenem-cilastatin, inamrinone, insulin, regular, isoproterenol, ketorolac, labetalol, lactated Ringer's, lidocaine, magnesium sulfate, mannitol, meperidine, metaraminol, methyldopate, methylPREDNISolone, metoclopramide, metoprolol, midazolam, minocycline, morphine, multiple vitamins injection, nafcillin, nalbuphine, naloxone, netilmicin, nitroglycerin, nitroprusside, norepinephrine, ondansetron, oxacillin, oxytocin, papaverine, penicillin G potassium, sodium, pentamidine, pentazocine, PHENobarbital, phentolamine, phenylephrine, phytonadione, piperacillin, polymyxin B, potassium chloride, procainamide, prochlorperazine, promethazine, propranolol, protamine, pyridoxine, quiNIDine, raNITIdine, Ringer's injection, sodium bicarbonate, succinylcholine, SUFentanil, tacrolimus

Patient/family education
• Teach patient to report urinary hesitancy/retention, dysuria
• Teach patient to use caution in hot weather; product may increase susceptibility to stroke since perspiration is decreased; patient should remain indoors
• Teach patient to avoid strenuous exercise or activities in hot weather, overheating may occur
• Advise patient not to discontinue this product abruptly; to taper off over 1 wk to prevent withdrawal symptoms (insomnia, involuntary movements, anxiety, tachycardias), to take as directed, not to double doses
• Advise patient that tabs may be crushed, mixed with food; may take whole dose at bedtime if approved by prescriber

- Caution patient to avoid driving or other hazardous activities; drowsiness, dizziness may occur
- Teach patient to avoid OTC medication: cough, cold preparations with alcohol, antihistamines, antacids, or antidiarrheals within 2 hr unless directed by prescriber; increased CNS depression may occur
- Advise patient to rise from sitting or recumbent position slowly to minimize orthostatic hypotension
- Teach patient to use good oral hygiene; to use sugarless gum, hard candy, frequent sips of water to decrease dry mouth; if dry mouth continues, saliva substitutes may be prescribed
- Instruct patient that doses should not be doubled, but missed dose may be taken up to 2 hr before next dose
- Advise patient routine exams will be needed
- Inform patient to separate antacids by 2 hr of taking this product

Evaluation
Positive therapeutic outcome
- Absence of involuntary movements (pill rolling, tremors, muscle spasms) after 2 days of treatment

betamethasone topical
See Appendix B

betamethasone (augmented) topical
See Appendix B

betaxolol ophthalmic
See Appendix B

⚠ HIGH ALERT
betrixaban (Rx)
(be-trix'-a-ban)
Bevyxxa
Func. class.: Antithrombotic agent
Chem. class.: Synthetic, selective factor Xa inhibitor

ACTION: Inhibits factor Xa; neutralization of factor Xa interrupts blood coagulation and thrombin formation

USES: Prevention/treatment of deep venous thrombosis, PE at-risk, acutely ill, hospitalized medical patients

Pharmacokinetics

Absorption	Unknown
Distribution	Protein binding 60%
Metabolism	Affected cytochrome P450 isoenzymes and drug transporters: P-gp, betrixaban is a substrate of P-glycoprotein (P-gp)
Excretion	85% of the dose is recovered in the feces and 11% in the urine
Half-life	19 to 27 hr

CONTRAINDICATIONS
Hypersensitivity, active major bleeding

Precautions: Pregnancy, breastfeeding, children, geriatric patients, hepatic disease, renal disease

> **BLACK BOX WARNING:** Spinal/epidural anesthesia, lumbar puncture

DOSAGE AND ROUTES
For venous thromboembolism prophylaxis
Adult: PO 160 mg once, followed by 80 mg qday for 35 to 42 days

ADVERSE EFFECTS
CNS: Headache
GI: Nausea, constipation, diarrhea
HEMA: Bleeding, major bleeding (intracranial, cerebral, retroperitoneal hemorrhage)
META: Hypokalemia
EENT: Ocular hemorrhage

INTERACTIONS
Drug classifications
Salicylates, NSAIDs: Increased bleeding risk

Individual drugs
Abciximab, eptifibatide, tirofiban, clopidogrel, dipyridamole, quiNIDine, valproic acid: Increased bleeding risk

Drug/herb
Feverfew, garlic, ginger, ginkgo, ginseng, green tea, horse chestnut, kava: Increased bleeding risk

NURSING CONSIDERATIONS
Assessment

> **BLACK BOX WARNING:** Monitor patients who have received epidural/spinal anesthesia or lumbar puncture for neurologic impairment, including spinal hematoma; may lead to permanent disability or paralysis

---

- Assess for bleeding: Gums, petechiae, ecchymosis, black tarry stools, hematuria; decreased Hct, notify prescriber
- Assess for risk of hemorrhage if coadministering with other products that may cause bleeding
- Assess for hypersensitivity: Rash, fever, chills; notify prescriber
- **Beers:** Avoid in older adults; increased risk of bleeding, lower creatinine clearance

Patient problems
Risk for injury (uses, adverse reactions)

Implementation
- Give capsules with food
- If a dose is not taken at the scheduled time, the dose should be taken as soon as possible on the same day. Do not take a double dose

Patient/family education
- Teach patient to use soft-bristle toothbrush to avoid bleeding gums; to use electric razor
- Advise patient to report any signs of bleeding: Gums, under skin, urine, stools
- Advise patient to avoid OTC products containing aspirin, NSAIDs
- Prgnancy/breastfeeding: Teach patient to notify healthcare provider if pregnancy is planned or suspected, or if breasfeeding

Evaluation
Positive therapeutic outcome
- Prevention of DVT

> ### ⚠ HIGH ALERT
>
> ## bevacizumab (Rx)
> (beh-va-kiz'you-mab)
> **Avastin**
> *Func. class.:* Antineoplastic—miscellaneous
> *Chem. class.:* Monoclonal antibody

ACTION: Monoclonal antibody selectively binds to and inhibits activity of human vascular endothelial growth factor to reduce microvascular growth and inhibition of metastatic disease progression

Therapeutic outcome: Decreased tumor size, growth

USES: Metastatic carcinoma of the colon or rectum in combination, renal cell carcinoma, glioblastoma, non–small cell lung cancer

Pharmacokinetics

Absorption	Complete
Distribution	Unknown
Metabolism	Unknown
Excretion	Unknown
Half-life	20 days

Pharmacodynamics

Onset	Unknown
Peak	Infusion end
Duration	2 wk

CONTRAINDICATIONS
Hypersensitivity, serious bleeding, hypertensive crisis, recent surgery

Precautions: Pregnancy, breastfeeding, children, geriatric, HF, blood dyscrasias, CV disease, hypertension, surgery, thromboembolic disease, hamster protein/murine hypersensitivity

> **BLACK BOX WARNING:** GI perforation, wound dehiscence, bleeding

DOSAGE AND ROUTES
Epithelial, ovarian, fallopian tube, or primary peritoneal cancer
Adult: IV 15 mg/kg with PACLitaxel (175 mg/m2 IV over 3 hr) and CARBOplatin (AUC 5 IV on day 1 and q3wk × 6-8 cycles), then bevacizumab 15 mg/kg IV q3wk as a single agent until disease progression or unacceptable toxicity

Colorectal cancer
Adult: IV INF in combination with 5-fluorouracil 5 mg/kg q14 days given over 90 min; if well tolerated, the next infusion may be given over 60 min; if 60 min infusions are well tolerated, subsequent infusions may be given over 30 min; (second-line) 5 mg/kg q2wk or 7.5 mg/kg q3wk with fluoropyrimidine and irinotecan or fluoropyrimidine and oxaliplatin-based agent

Lung cancer
Adult: IV 15 mg/kg

Glioblastoma
Adult: IV 10 mg/kg q 14 days

Cervical cancer
Adult: IV 15 mg/kg q3wk

Renal cell carcinoma
Adult: IV 10 mg/kg q2wk

Available forms: Solution for injection 25 mg/ml

ADVERSE EFFECTS
CNS: *Asthenia, dizziness,* headache, fatigue, confusion, weakness, reversible posterior leukoencephalopathy syndrome (RPLS)
CV: Deep vein thrombosis, hypo/hypertension, hypertensive crisis, heart failure
GI: Nausea, vomiting, anorexia, GI hemorrhage/perforation
GU: Proteinuria, nephrotic syndrome, ovarian failure
HEMA: Leukopenia, bleeding
META: Bilirubinemia, hypokalemia, hyponatremia

MISC: Wound dehiscence, *impaired wound healing,* osteonecrosis of the jaw
RESP: Dyspnea, upper respiratory infection
INTEG: Necrotizing fasciitis, infusion reactions

INTERACTIONS
Individual drugs
SUNItinib: avoid concurrent use; microangiopathic hemolytic anemia may occur

NURSING CONSIDERATIONS
Assessment
• Monitor B/P; if hypertension is severe or uncontrolled, discontinue, as hypertensive crisis has occurred
• Assess for symptoms of infection; may be masked by product
• Monitor **CNS reaction:** dizziness, confusion
• Assess for **HF:** crackles, jugular vein distention, dyspnea during treatment
• Assess **GU status** (proteinuria); nephrotic syndrome may occur; monitor urinalysis for increasing protein level; products should be held if protein ≥2 g/24 hr

> **BLACK BOX WARNING: Wound dehiscence:** discontinue 28 days before elective surgery, hold for ≥28 days until incision is healed

> **BLACK BOX WARNING:** Assess for GI perforation, serious bleeding, nephrotic syndrome, hypertensive crisis; GI perforation (constipation, fever, abdominal pain, nausea, vomiting)

• **Serious bleeding:** Assess for bleeding from any orifice, stroke, deep vein thrombosis, product should be discontinued permanently; for surgery, product should be discontinued temporarily
• **Reversible posterior leukoencephalopathy syndrome (RPLS):** discontinue if this disorder develops (headache, vision changes, seizures, altered mental status); MRI may be ordered, occurs 16 hr-1 yr after beginning treatment
• Thromboembolic events: Assess for stroke, TIA, MI, usually occurs in geriatric patients who used this product previously
• **Fistulas:** May occur within 6 mo of beginning treatment, may be fatal

Patient problems
Risk for injury (adverse reactions)
Ineffective tissue perfusion (adverse reactions)
Risk for infection (adverse reactions)

Implementation
IV intermittent infusion route
• Do not give by **IV** bolus or **IV** push, do not admix
• Give as **IV** inf over 90 min for first dose and 60 min thereafter, if well tolerated

> **BLACK BOX WARNING: Wound dehiscence:** do not give for ≥28 days after surgery, make sure wounds are healed prior to use

Patient/family education
• Instruct patient to avoid hazardous tasks, since confusion, dizziness may occur
• Instruct patient to report signs of infection: sore throat, fever, diarrhea, vomiting
• Advise patient to notify prescriber if pregnant or planning a pregnancy, discuss possible infertility with patient, to use adequate contraception and for ≥6 mo after last dose
• Advise patient about the need to discontinue a month before surgery and not restart until wound is healed

> **BLACK BOX WARNING:** Teach patient to report bleeding, changes in urinary patterns, edema, abdominal pain

Evaluation
Positive therapeutic outcome
• Decrease in size of tumors

bezlotoxumab
(bez′loe-tox′ue-mab)
Zinplava
Func. class.: Antidiarrheal
Chem. class.: Monoclonal antibody

ACTION: Binds to *Clostridium difficile* toxin B, and neutralizing its effects

Therapeutic outcome: No recurrence of CDI when used with antibiotic therapy

USES: For *C. difficile* infection (CDI) in patients who are receiving antibacterial treatment of CDI and are at a high risk for CDI recurrence

Pharmacokinetics
Absorption	Complete
Distribution	Minimal
Metabolism	Unknown
Excretion	Catabolism
Half-life	19 days

Pharmacodynamics
Unknown

CONTRAINDICATIONS
Hypersensitivity

Precautions: Breastfeeding, pregnancy, heart failure

DOSAGE AND ROUTES:
Adult: IV 10 mg/kg as a single dose

Available forms: Solution for injection 25 mg/mL

ADVERSE EFFECTS
CNS: Fever, headache
CV. Heart failure, hypertension
Misc: *Infusion-related reactions*

INTERACTIONS
None known

NURSING CONSIDERATIONS
Assessment
• **CDAD:** Assess for diarrhea that is watery or bloody, fever, abdominal cramping/pain, pus or mucus in the stools, dehydration
• **Heart failure:** Monitor for heart failure during administration, death has occurred from heart failure; causes of death included infections, cardiac failure, and respiratory failure, in those with existing heart failure
• **Pregnancy/breastfeeding:** Identify if the patient is pregnant or breastfeeding

Patient problems
Diarrhea (uses)
Infection (uses)

Implementation
Intermittent IV infusion:
• **Give by** IV infusion, visually inspect parenteral products for particulate matter and discoloration prior to use
• **Dilution of the vials:** Do not shake, withdraw the required volume from the vial based on the patient's weight and transfer into an IV bag of either 0.9% NaCl or D5 injection to 1-10 mg/ml. Mix the diluted solution by gentle inversion, do not shake
• Infuse the diluted solution IV over 60 min using a sterile, nonpyrogenic, low-protein–binding 0.2-0.5 micron inline or add-on filter, give via a central line or a peripheral catheter, do not give IV push or bolus, do not coadminister other drugs simultaneously through the same infusion line
• **Storage:** The diluted solution may be stored at room temperature for 16 hr or refrigerated 2-8° C (36-46° F) up to 24 hr; if refrigerated, allow the solution to come to room temperature before use, do not freeze

Y-site incompatibility: Do not give other products through same infusion line, concurrently

Patient/family education
• Advise on the reason for product and expected result

• **CDAD:** Teach patient to report immediately diarrhea that is watery or bloody, fever, abdominal cramping/pain, pus or mucus in the stools, dehydration
• **Infusion-related reactions:** Teach patient to report immediately infusion-related reactions, redness, swelling; if these occur, infusion should be discontinued

Evaluation
Positive therapeutic outcome
No recurrence when used with antibiotic therapy

---

bicalutamide (Rx)
(bye-ka-loot'a-mide)
Casodex
Func. class.: Antineoplastic hormone
Chem. class.: Nonsteroidal antiandrogen

ACTION: Competitively inhibits the action of androgens by binding to cytosol androgen receptors in target tissue

Therapeutic outcome: Prevention of growth of malignant cells

USES: Stage D-2 metastatic prostate cancer in combination with luteinizing hormone–releasing hormone (LHRH) analog

Pharmacokinetics

Absorption	Well absorbed
Distribution	Unknown
Metabolism	Liver
Excretion	Urine, feces
Half-life	5.2 days

Pharmacodynamics

Onset	Unknown
Peak	31.5 hr
Duration	Unknown

CONTRAINDICATIONS
Pregnancy, women, hypersensitivity

Precautions: Breastfeeding, geriatric, renal/hepatic disease, diabetes mellitus

DOSAGE AND ROUTES
Adult: PO 50 mg daily with LHRH

Available forms: Tabs 50 mg

ADVERSE EFFECTS
CNS: Dizziness, paresthesia, insomnia, anxiety, neuropathy, headache
CV: Hot flashes, hypertension, chest pain, HF, edema
GI: *Diarrhea, constipation, nausea,* vomiting, increased liver enzyme test, anorexia, dry mouth, melena, abdominal pain, hepatitis, hepatotoxicity

---

GU: Nocturia, hematuria, UTI, impotence, gynecomastia, urinary incontinence, frequency, dysuria, retention, urgency, breast tenderness, decreased libido
INTEG: Rash, sweating, dry skin, pruritus, alopecia
MISC: Infection, anemia, dyspnea, bone pain, headache, asthenia, *back pain*, flulike symptoms

INTERACTIONS
Individual drugs
Warfarin: Increase warfarin effects

Drug/herb
St. John's wort: may require dosage change

Drug/food
Grapefruit juice: do not use together

Drug/lab test
Increased: AST, ALT, bilirubin, BUN, creatinine
Decreased: Hgb, WBC

NURSING CONSIDERATIONS
Assessment
• Assess for diarrhea, constipation, nausea, vomiting
• Assess for hot flashes, gynecomastia; assure patient that these are common side effects
• Monitor prostate-specific antigen (PSA) liver function tests
• **Hepatotoxicity:** Monitor serum transaminase levels should be measured baseline and at regular intervals × 4 months and then periodically; if nausea, vomiting, abdominal pain, anorexia, dark urine, jaundice, or right upper quadrant tenderness, the serum transaminases, in particular the ALT, should be measured immediately. If jaundice or their ALT rises above 2-times the upper limit of normal, discontinue and assess liver function.

Patient problems
• Risk for injury (uses, adverse reactions)
• Lack of knowledge of medication (teaching)
• Diarrhea (adverse reactions)

Implementation
• Give at same time each day (for both products) either AM or PM with or without food
• Give only with LHRH treatment

Patient/family education
• Teach patient to recognize and report signs of anemia, renal/hepatic toxicity
• Advise patient that hair may be lost, but loss is reversible after therapy is discontinued
• Advise patient not to use other products unless approved by prescriber
• Advise patient to use contraception during and for130 days last dose

Evaluation
Positive therapeutic outcome
• Decreased tumor size, spread of malignancy

bimatoprost ophthalmic
See Appendix B

bisacodyl (Rx, OTC)
(bis-a-koe′dill)
Bisac-Evac, Bisacolax ✹**, Bisacolax, Correctol, Carter's Little Pills** ✹**, Codulax** ✹**, Dacodyl, Doxidan, Dulcolax, Ex-Lax Ultra Tab, Femilax, Fleet, Soflax-Ex** ✹
Func. class.: Laxative, stimulant
Chem. class.: Diphenylmethane

Do not confuse: Dulcolax (bisacodyl), Dulcolax (docusate)

ACTION: Acts directly on intestine by increasing peristalsis; thought to irritate colonic intramural plexus; increases water in the colon

Therapeutic outcome: Decreased constipation, removal of stool from colon

USES: Short-term treatment of constipation, bowel or rectal preparation for surgery, examination

Pharmacokinetics
Absorption	Poor
Distribution	Unknown
Metabolism	Liver, minimally
Excretion	Kidneys
Half-life	Unknown

Pharmacodynamics
	PO	Rect
Onset	6-10 hr	15-60 min
Peak	Unknown	Unknown
Duration	Unknown	Unknown

CONTRAINDICATIONS
Hypersensitivity, abdominal pain, nausea, vomiting, appendicitis, acute surgical abdomen, ulcerated hemorrhoids, acute hepatitis, fecal impaction, intestinal/biliary tract obstruction

Precautions: Pregnancy, breastfeeding, rectal fissures, severe CV disease

DOSAGE AND ROUTES
Adult/child ≥12 yr: PO 5-15 mg in PM or AM; may use up to 30 mg for bowel or rectal preparation; **RECT** 10 mg (single dose), 30 ml enema
Child 6-11 yr: PO 5-10 mg as a single dose; **RECT** 5 mg as a single dose

Available forms: Tabs del rel 5, 10 mg; enteric-coated tabs 5 mg; supp 5, 10 mg; rectal solution 10 mg/30 ml

ADVERSE EFFECTS
CNS: MS, Muscle weakness (extended use)
GI: *Nausea, vomiting, anorexia, cramps,* diarrhea, rectal burning (supp)
META: Protein-losing enteropathy (extended use), alkalosis, hypokalemia, tetany

INTERACTIONS
Drug classifications
Antacids, gastric acid pump inhibitors, H_2-blockers: increased gastric irritation

Drug/food
Increased irritation—dairy products: separate by 2 hr

Drug/lab test
Increased: sodium phosphate
Decreased: calcium, magnesium

Drug/herb
Flax, lily of the valley, pheasant's eye, senna, squill: increased laxative action

NURSING CONSIDERATIONS
Assessment
• Monitor blood, urine electrolytes if used often by patient; check I&O ratio to identify fluid loss
• Assess **GI symptoms:** cramping, rectal bleeding, nausea, if these symptoms occur, product should be discontinued; identify cause of constipation; identify whether fluids, bulk, or exercise are missing from lifestyle
• Multiple products/routes may be used for bowel prep

Patient problems
Constipation (uses)

Implementation
Oral route
• Swallow tabs whole; do not break, crush, or chew
• Give alone with water only for better absorption; do not take within 1 hr of antacids, milk
• Administer in AM or PM (oral dose)
Rectal route
• Lubricate before insertion, patient should retain for ½ hr
• Insert high in rectum

Patient/family education
• Discuss with the patient that adequate fluid and bulk consumption is necessary
• Advise patient that normal bowel movements do not always occur daily
• Teach patient not to use in presence of abdominal pain, nausea, vomiting; tell patient to notify prescriber if constipation is unrelieved or if symptoms of electrolyte imbalance occur: muscle cramps, pain, weakness, dizziness, excessive thirst

• Teach patient to take with a full glass of water; if using with dairy products, separate by 2 hr; separate from other foods by 1 hr
• Teach patient to identify bulk, water, constipating products, exercise in patient's life
• Instruct patient not to use laxatives for long-term therapy because bowel tone will be lost; 1 wk use is usually sufficient

Evaluation
Positive therapeutic outcome
• Decreased constipation within 3 days
• Evacuation of colon before surgery or other procedures
• Evacuation of colon in spinal cord injury

⚠ HIGH ALERT

bisoprolol (Rx)
(bis-oh′pro-lole)
Func. class.: Antihypertensive
Chem. class.: β_1-Blocker (selective)

ACTION: Blocks stimulation of β_1-adrenergic receptor within cardiac muscle (decreases rate of SA node discharge, increases recovery time), slows conduction of AV node, decreases heart rate, which decreases O_2 consumption in myocardium; decreases renin-aldosterone-angiotensin system

Therapeutic outcome: Decreased B/P, heart rate

USES: Mild to moderate hypertension

Pharmacokinetics
Absorption	Well
Distribution	Unknown; protein binding (30%)
Metabolism	Liver, inactive metabolites
Excretion	Urine, unchanged (50%)
Half-life	9-12 hr

Pharmacodynamics
Onset	Unknown
Peak	2-4 hr
Duration	24 hr

CONTRAINDICATIONS
Hypersensitivity to β-blockers, cardiogenic shock, heart block (2nd or 3rd degree), sinus bradycardia, acute cardiac failure

Precautions: Pregnancy, breastfeeding, children, major surgery, diabetes mellitus, HF, renal/hepatic/thyroid/peripheral vascular/aortic/mitral valve disease, COPD, asthma, well-compensated heart failure, myasthenia gravis, abrupt discontinuation

DOSAGE AND ROUTES
Adult: PO 2.5-5 mg/day, may increase if necessary to 20 mg once daily, max 20 mg/day

Renal/hepatic dose
Adult: PO CCr <40 ml/min 2.5 mg, titrate upward

Available forms: Tabs 5, 10 mg

ADVERSE EFFECTS
CNS: Insomnia, fatigue, dizziness, mental changes, memory loss, depression, lethargy, drowsiness
CV: Pulmonary edema, bradycardia, HF, cold extremities, postural hypotension
EENT: Sore throat, dry burning eyes, dry mouth, blurred vision
GI: Nausea, diarrhea, vomiting, constipation
INTEG: Rash
ENDO: Hypo-hyperglycemia
MISC: Lupus-like syndrome
RESP: Dyspnea, cough
GU: Erectile dysfunction, decreased libido, urinary frequency

INTERACTIONS
Individual drugs
Amiodarone, clonidine, diltiazem, veramil, digoxin: increased bradycardia
Phenytoin (IV), verapamil: increased myocardial depression

Drug classifications
ACE inhibitors, α-blockers, calcium channel blockers, diuretics, nitrates: increased antihypertensive effect
Antidiabetics: increased antidiabetic effect

Drug/herb
Hawthorn: increased β-blocking effect
Ephedra: decreased β-blocking effect

Drug/lab test
Increased: AST, ALT, blood glucose, BUN, uric acid, potassium

NURSING CONSIDERATIONS
Assessment
• **Hypertension:** Monitor B/P, pulse during beginning treatment, periodically thereafter; pulse: note rate, rhythm, quality; apical/radial pulse before administration; notify prescriber of any significant changes (pulse <50 bpm), monitor ECG baseline and periodically
• Check for baselines in renal, liver function tests before therapy begins
• **HF:** assess for edema in feet, legs daily, monitor I&O, daily weight; check for jugular vein distention, crackles, bilaterally, dyspnea

• Monitor skin turgor, dryness of mucous membranes for hydration status, especially geriatric

Patient problems
Implementation
• Take apical pulse before each dose, if <50 bpm withhold, notify health care professional
• Give daily; give with food to prevent GI upset; may be crushed
• Store protected from light, moisture; place in cool environment

Patient/family education
• Teach patient not to discontinue product abruptly, taper over 1 wk; may cause precipitate angina if stopped abruptly; evaluate noncompliance
• Teach patient not to use OTC products containing α-adrenergic stimulants (such as nasal decongestants, cold preparations) unless approved by prescriber; to avoid alcohol, smoking; to limit sodium intake as prescribed
• Teach patient how to take pulse and B/P at home; advise when to notify prescriber
• Instruct patient to comply with weight control, dietary adjustments, modified exercise program
• Tell patient to carry/wear emergency ID to identify product being taken, allergies; tell patient product controls symptoms but does not cure
• Caution patient to avoid hazardous activities if dizziness, drowsiness present
• Teach patient to take product as prescribed, not to double doses, skip doses; take any missed doses as soon as remembered if at least 8 hr until next dose
• Advise patient to avoid alcohol and smoking and limit sodium
• Advise patient to report slow heart rate, dizziness, confusion, depression, fever, cold extremities
• Teach diabetic patient drug may mask signs of hypoglycemia or alter blood glucose levels
• **Pregnancy/breastfeeding:** Teach patient to notify health care professional if pregnancy is planned or suspected or if breastfeeding

Evaluation
Positive therapeutic outcome
• Decreased B/P (after 1-2 wk)

TREATMENT OF OVERDOSE:
Lavage, **IV** atropine for bradycardia, digoxin, O_2, diuretic for cardiac failure, hemodialysis, **IV** glucose for hypoglycemia, **IV** diazePAM (or phenytoin) for seizures

⚠ HIGH ALERT

bivalirudin (Rx)
(bye-val-i-rue'din)
Angiomax
Func. class.: Anticoagulant
Chem. class.: Thrombin inhibitor

ACTION: Direct inhibitor of thrombin that is highly specific; able to inhibit free and clot-bound thrombin

Therapeutic outcome: Anticoagulation in percutaneous transluminal coronary angioplasty (PTCA), used with aspirin; heparin-induced thrombocytopenia with thrombosis syndrome

USES: Unstable angina in patients undergoing PTCA, used with aspirin; heparin-induced thrombocytopenia; heparin-induced thrombocytopenia with thrombosis syndrome, PCI with IIb/IIIa

Pharmacokinetics

Absorption	Unknown
Distribution	No protein binding
Metabolism	Unknown
Excretion	Kidneys
Half-life	25 min

Pharmacodynamics

Onset	Unknown
Peak	Unknown
Duration	1 hr

CONTRAINDICATIONS
Hypersensitivity, active bleeding, cerebral aneurysm, intracranial hemorrhage, recent surgery, CVA

Precautions: Pregnancy, breastfeeding, children, geriatric, renal function impairment, hepatic disease, asthma, blood dyscrasias, thrombocytopenia, GI ulcers, hypertension, inflammatory bowel disease, vitamin K deficiency

DOSAGE AND ROUTES
PCI/PTCA
Adult: **IV** bol 0.75 mg/kg, then **IV** infusion 1.75 mg/kg/hr for 4 hr; another **IV** infusion may be used at 0.2 mg/kg/hr for ≤20 hr; this product is intended to be used with aspirin (325 mg daily) adjusted to body weight

HIT/HITTS
Adult: **IV** bolus 0.75 mg/kg, then continuous INF 1.75 mg/kg/hr for duration of procedure

DVT prophylaxis (major hip or knee surgery)
Adult: Subcut 1 mg/kg q 8 hr up to 14 days

Renal dose
Adult: IV CCr ≥ 30 ml/min no change; CCr 10-29 ml/min consider reduction to 1 ml/kg/hr

Available forms: Inj, lyophilized 250 mg vial

ADVERSE EFFECTS
CNS: *Headache, insomnia, anxiety, nervousness*
CV: *Hypo/hypertension, bradycardia,* ventricular fibrillation
GI: *Nausea, vomiting, abdominal pain, dyspepsia*
HEMA: Hemorrhage, thrombocytopenia
MISC: Pain at inj site, pelvic pain, urinary retention, fever, anaphylaxis, infection
MS: *Back pain*
GU: Urinary retention, renal failure, oliguria

INTERACTIONS
Individual drugs
Abciximab, aspirin: increased risk of bleeding, use together cautiously

Drug classifications
Anticoagulants, low molecular weight heparins, thrombolytics: increased risk of bleeding

Drug/herb
Angelica, chamomile, devil's claw, dong quai, garlic, ginger, ginkgo, ginseng, horse chestnut, saw palmetto, avoid concurrent use

NURSING CONSIDERATIONS
Assessment
• Assess for fall in B/P or Hct that may indicate hemorrhage; hematoma, hemorrhage at puncture site are more common in the elderly; baseline and periodic ACT, aPTT, PT, INR, TT, platelets, Hct, Hgb
• Assess for fever, skin rash, urticaria
• Assess **bleeding:** check arterial and venous sites, IM inj sites, catheters; all punctures should be minimized
• **PCI use:** assess for possible thrombosis, stenosis, unplanned stent, prolonged ischemia, decreased reflow

Patient problems
Impaired tissue perfusion (uses)
Risk for injury (adverse reactions)

Implementation
• Prior to PTCA, give with aspirin, 325 mg **IV** direct 1 mg/kg as a bolus; then intermittent infusion

Intermittent IV infusion route
• To each 250-mg vial add 5 ml of sterile water for inj, swirl until dissolved, further dilute reconstituted vial with 50 ml of D₅W or 0.9% NaCl (5 mg/ml); the dose is adjusted to body weight, run at 2.5 mg/kg/hr, do not admix before or during administration
• Give reduced dose in renal impairment

Y-site compatibilities: Abciximab, acyclovir, alfentanil, allopurinol, amifostine, amikacin, aminocaproic acid, aminophylline, amphotericin B liposome, ampicillin, ampicillin-sulbactam, anidulafungin, argatroban, arsenic trioxide, atenolol, atracurium, atropine, azithromycin, aztreonam, bleomycin, bumetanide, buprenorphine, busulfan, butorphanol, calcium chloride/gluconate, capreomycin, CARBOplatin, carmustine, ceFAZolin, cefepime, cefotaxime, cefoTEtan, cefOXitin, cefTAZidime, ceftizoxime, cefTRIAXone, cefuroxime, chloramphenicol, cimetidine hydrochloride, ciprofloxacin, cisatracurium, CISplatin, clindamycin, cyclophosphamide, cycloSPORINE, cytarabine, dacarbazine, DACTINomycin, DAPTOmycin, DAUNOrubicin, DAUNOrubicin liposome, dexamethasone, dexmedetomidine, dexrazoxane, digoxin, dilTIAZem, diphenhydrAMINE, DOCEtaxel, dolasetron, DOPamine, DOXOrubicin, DOXOrubicin liposomal, doxycycline, droperidol, enalaprilat, ePHEDrine, EPINEPHrine, epiRUBicin, epoprostenol, eptifibatide, ertapenem, erythromycin, esmolol, etoposide, etoposide phosphate, famotidine, fenoldopam, fentaNYL, fluconazole, fludarabine, fluorouracil, foscarnet, fosphenytoin, furosemide, gallium, ganciclovir, gatifloxacin, gemcitabine, gentamicin, glycopyrrolate, granisetron, haloperidol, heparin, hydrALAZINE, hydrocortisone, HYDROmorphone, hydrOXYzine, IDArubicin, ifosfamide, imipenem-cilastatin, inamrinone, insulin, irinotecan, isoproterenol, ketorolac, labetalol, leucovorin, levofloxacin, lidocaine, linezolid, LORazepam, magnesium, mannitol, mechlorethamine, melphalan, meperidine, meropenem, mesna, methohexital, methotrexate, methyldopate, methylPREDNISolone, metoclopramide, metoprolol, metroNIDAZOLE, midazolam, milrinone, mitoMYcin, mitoXANtrone, mivacurium, morphine, moxifloxacin, mycophenolate, nafcillin, nalbuphine, naloxone, nesiritide, niCARdipine, nitroglycerin, nitroprusside, norepinephrine, octreotide, ofloxacin, ondansetron, oxaliplatin, oxytocin, PACLitaxel, palonosetron, pamidronate, pancuronium, PEMEtrexed, PENTobarbital, PHENobarbital, phenylephrine, piperacillin, piperacillin-tazobactam, polymyxin B, potassium acetate/chloride/phosphates, procainamide, promethazine, propranolol, raNITIdine, remifentanil, rocuronium, sodium acetate/bicarbonate/phosphates, streptozocin, succinylcholine, SUFentanil, sulfamethoxazole-trimethoprim, tacrolimus, teniposide, theophylline, thiopental, thiotepa, ticarcillin, ticarcillin-clavulanate, tigecycline, tirofiban, tobramycin, topotecan, vasopressin, vecuronium, verapamil, vinBLAStine, vinCRIStine, vinorelbine, voriconazole, warfarin, zidovudine, zoledronic acid

Patient/family education

• Explain reason for product and expected results
• Teach patient not to use other OTC products unless approved by prescriber
• Teach patient not to use hard-bristle toothbrush, regular razor to avoid any injury: hemorrhage may result, notify health care professional of bleeding

Evaluation
Positive therapeutic outcome
• Anticoagulation in PTCA

⚠ HIGH ALERT

bleomycin (Rx)

(blee-oh-mye′sin)

Blenoxane ✦

Func. class.: Antineoplastic, antibiotic
Chem. class.: Glycopeptide

ACTION: Inhibits synthesis of DNA, RNA, protein; derived from *Streptomyces verticillus;* phase specific in the G_2 and M phases; a nonvesicant, sclerosing agent

Therapeutic outcome: Prevention of rapidly growing malignant cells

USES: Cancer of head, neck, penis, cervix, vulva of squamous cell origin, Hodgkin's/non-Hodgkin's disease, testicular carcinoma, as a sclerosing agent for malignant pleural effusion

Pharmacokinetics

Absorption	Well absorbed (IM, SUBCUT, intrapleural, intraperitoneal)
Distribution	Widely distributed
Metabolism	Liver, 30%
Excretion	Kidneys, unchanged (70%)
Half-life	2-4 hr; increased in renal disease

Pharmacodynamics

IV, IM SUBCUT	Peak 30-60 min

CONTRAINDICATIONS
Pregnancy, breastfeeding, hypersensitivity

Precautions: Renal/hepatic/respiratory disease, patients >70 yr old

---

BLACK BOX WARNING: Idiosyncratic reaction, pulmonary fibrosis, requires specialized care setting, experienced clinician

---

DOSAGE AND ROUTES
Non-Hodgkin's lymphoma, testicular cancer, squamous cell carcinoma
Adult and child: IM/SUBCUT/**IV** 0.25-0.5 units/kg q1-2wk or 10-20 units/m^2; then 1 unit/day or 5 units/wk; max total dose, 400 units in lifetime

Hodgkin's disease (test dose)
Adult and child (unlabeled): IM/IV/SUBCUT <2 units for first 2 doses followed by 24 hr observation

Hodgkin's lymphoma
Adult/adolescent/child: IV, IM, SUBCUT 5-20 units/m2 may give in combination

Malignant pleural effusion
Adult: 60 units diluted in 100 ml of 0.9% NaCl intrapleural inj given through a thoracotomy tube following drainage of excess pleural fluid and complete lung expansion, remove after 4 hr

Testicular cancer
Adult: IV 10-20 units/m^2 1-2 × per wk, may be given in combination

Renal Dose
Adult/child: CCr 40-50 ml/min reduce dose by 30%; CCr 30-39 ml/min reduce dose by 40%; CCr 20-29 ml/min reduce dose by 45%; CCr 10-19 ml/min reduce dose by 55%; CCr 5-10 ml/min reduce dose by 60%

Available forms: Injection 15, 30 units/vial

ADVERSE EFFECTS
CNS: Pain at tumor site, headache, confusion, fever, chills, malaise
CV: Hypotension, peripheral vasoconstriction
GI: *Nausea, vomiting, anorexia, stomatitis, weight loss,* weight loss
INTEG: *Rash, alopecia,* hyperpigmentation, mucocutaneous toxicity
HEMA: Anemia, leukopenia, thrombocytopenia
RESP: Fibrosis, pneumonitis, pulmonary toxicity
SYST: Anaphylaxis

INTERACTIONS
Individual drugs
Cisplatin: increased bleomycin toxicity
Radiation: increased toxicity, bone marrow suppression

Drug classifications
Anesthetics (general), antineoplastics: increased toxicity, use together cautiously
Live virus vaccines: avoid concurrent use, adverse reactions may occur

Drug/lab test
Increase: uric acid
Decrease: Pulmonary function tests

NURSING CONSIDERATIONS
Assessment
• Assess buccal cavity q8hr for dryness, sores or ulceration, white patches, oral pain, bleeding, dysphagia; obtain prescription for viscous lidocaine (Xylocaine)
• **Assess symptoms indicating anaphylaxis:** rash, pruritus, urticaria, purpuric skin lesions, itching, flushing, wheezing, hypotension; have emergency equipment available

> **BLACK BOX WARNING: Pulmonary toxicity/fibrosis:** Risk increases >70 yr, assess pulmonary function tests; chest x-ray before, during therapy; monitor q2wk during treatment; pulmonary diffusion capacity for carbon monoxide (DL$_{CO}$) monthly; if <40% of pretreatment value, stop treatment; assess for dyspnea, crackles, unproductive cough, chest pain, tachypnea, fatigue, increased pulse, pallor, lethargy, more common in the elderly, radiation therapy, pulmonary disease; usually occurs with cumulative doses >400 units

• Monitor vital signs baseline and often during treatment
• Monitor CBC, differential, may cause leukopenia and thrombocytopenia (nadir 12 days)

> **BLACK BOX WARNING: Idiosyncratic reaction:** Severe reaction in those with lymphoma; assess hypotension, mental confusion, fever, chills, wheezing in lymphoma

> **BLACK BOX WARNING:** Requires a specialized care setting and experienced clinician due to severe reactions

• Monitor temp (may indicate beginning of infection)
• Monitor liver function tests before, during therapy (bilirubin, AST, ALT, LDH) as needed or monthly
• Assess for bleeding: hematuria, stool guaiac, bruising or petechiae, mucosa or orifices q8hr; inflammation of mucosa, breaks in skin
• Treat pulmonary infection prior to treatment; identify dyspnea, crackles, unproductive cough, chest pain, tachypnea
• Identify effects of alopecia on body image; discuss feelings about body changes; if edema in feet, joint pain, stomach pain, shaking present, prescriber should be notified; identify inflammation of mucosa, breaks in skin

Patient problems
Risk of injury (adverse reactions)

Implementation
• Avoid contact with skin; very irritating; wash completely to remove

- Give fluids **IV** or PO before chemotherapy to hydrate patient
- Give antacid before oral agent; give antiemetic 30-60 min before giving product and prn to prevent vomiting; give antibiotics for prophylaxis of infection
- Provide liquid diet: carbonated beverages, gelatin may be added if patient is not nauseated or vomiting
- Rinse mouth tid-qid with water, club soda; brush teeth bid-qid with soft brush or cotton-tipped applicators for stomatitis; use unwaxed dental floss

IM/SUBCUT route
- IM test dose in lymphoma
- Reconstitute with 1-5 ml sterile water for inj; max conc 5 units/ml, D_5W, 0.9% NaCl, rotate inj sites

IV route
- Product should be prepared by experienced personnel using proper precautions
- Two test doses 2-5 units before initial dose in lymphoma; monitor for anaphylaxis
- Give by direct **IV** after reconstituting 15- or 30-unit vial with 5 or 10 ml of 0.9% NaCl; give 15 units or less/10 min through Y-tube or 3-way stopcock initial dose; monitor for anaphylaxis

Intermittent IV infusion route
- Administer after diluting 50-100 ml 0.9% NaCl, D_5W and giving at prescribed rate

Y-site compatibilities: Acyclovir, alfentanil, allopurinol, amifostine, amikacin, aminocaproic acid, aminophylline, amiodarone, ampicillin, ampicillin-sulbactam, anidulafungin, atenolol, atracurium, azithromycin, aztreonam, bivalirudin, bumetanide, buprenorphine, busulfan, butorphanol, calcium chloride/gluconate, CARBOplatin, carmustine, caspofungin, ceFAZolin, cefepime, cefotaxime, cefoTEtan, cefOXitin, cefTAZidime, ceftizoxime, cefTRIAXone, cefuroxime, chloramphenicol, chlorproMAZINE, cimetidine, ciprofloxacin, cisatracurium, CISplatin, clindamycin, codeine, cyclophosphamide, cycloSPORINE, cytarabine, dacarbazine, DACTINomycin, DAPTOmycin, DAUNOrubicin, dexamethasone, dexmedetomidine, dexrazoxane, digoxin, dilTIAZem, diphenhydrAMINE, DOBUTamine, DOCEtaxel, DOPamine, doxacurium, DOXOrubicin, DOXOrubicin liposomal, doxycycline, droperidol, enalaprilat, ePHEDrine, EPINEPHrine, epiRUBicin, ertapenem, erythromycin, esmolol, etoposide, famotidine, fenoldopam, fentaNYL, filgrastim, fluconazole, fludarabine, fluorouracil, foscarnet, fosphenytoin, furosemide, ganciclovir, gatifloxacin, gemcitabine, gentamicin, glycopyrrolate, granisetron, haloperidol, heparin, hydrALAZINE, hydrocortisone sodium succinate, HYDROmorphone, hydrOXYzine, IDArubicin, ifosfamide, imipenem-cilastatin, inamrinone, insulin (regular), irinotecan, isoproterenol, ketorolac, labetalol, leucovorin, levofloxacin, levorphanol, lidocaine, linezolid, LORazepam, magnesium sulfate, mannitol, mechlorethamine, melphalan, meperidine, meropenem, mesna, metaraminol, methohexital, methotrexate, methyldopa, methylPREDNISolone, metoclopramide, metoprolol, metroNIDAZOLE, midazolam, milrinone, minocycline, mitoMYcin, mitoXANtrone, mivacurium, morphine, nafcillin, nalbuphine, naloxone, nesiritide, niCARdipine, nitroglycerin, nitroprusside, norepinephrine, octreotide, ondansetron, oxaliplatin, palonosetron, pamidronate, pancuronium, pantoprazole, PEMEtrexed, pentamidine, pentazocine, PENTobarbital, PHENobarbital, phenylephrine, piperacillin, piperacillin-tazobactam, polymyxin B, potassium chloride, potassium phosphates, procainamide, prochlorperazine, promethazine, propranolol, quiNIDine, raNITIdine, remifentanil, riTUXimab, rocuronium, sargramostim, sodium acetate, sodium bicarbonate, sodium phosphates, succinylcholine, SUFentanil, sulfamethoxazole-trimethoprim, tacrolimus, teniposide, theophylline, thiopental, thiotepa, ticarcillin, ticarcillin-clavulanate, tirofiban, tobramycin, tolazoline, trastuzumab, trimethobenzamide, vancomycin, vasopressin, vecuronium, verapamil, vinBLAStine, vinCRIStine, vinorelbine, voriconazole, zidovudine

Patient/family education
- Instruct patient to report any changes in breathing or coughing even several months after treatment; to avoid crowds and persons with respiratory tract or other infections, to avoid smoking and smoke-filled rooms
- Inform patient that hair may be lost during treatment; a wig or hairpiece may make patient feel better; new hair may be different in color, texture
- Caution patient not to have any vaccinations without the advice of the prescriber; serious reactions can occur
- Advise patient that continuing exams and lab tests will be needed
- **Skin toxicity:** Teach patient to report rash, color changes, sensitivity, irritation
- **Stomatitis:** Teach patient that mouth ulcerations, redness may occur and to use soft toothbrush
- **Pregnancy/breastfeeding:** Advise patient contraception is needed during treatment and for several months after completion of therapy

Evaluation
Positive therapeutic outcome
- Prevention of rapid division of malignant cells

> **⚠ HIGH ALERT**
>
> ## bortezomib (Rx)
> (bor-tez′oh-mib)
> **Velcade**
> *Func. class.:* Antineoplastic—miscellaneous
> *Chem. class.:* Proteasome inhibitor

ACTION: Reversible inhibitor of chymotrypsin-like activity; causes a delay in tumor growth by disrupting normal homeostatic mechanisms

Therapeutic outcome: Decreased growth and spread of malignant cells

USES: Multiple myeloma previously untreated or when at least two other treatments have failed; mantle cell lymphoma

Pharmacokinetics

Absorption	Complete (IV)
Distribution	Protein binding 83%
Metabolism	P450 enzymes (3A4, 2D6, 2C19, 2C9, 1A2)
Excretion	Unknown
Half-life	9-15 hr

Pharmacodynamics

Unknown

CONTRAINDICATIONS

Pregnancy, breastfeeding, hypersensitivity to this product, boron, or mannitol

Precautions: Peripheral neuropathy, children, geriatric, cardiac/hepatic disease, hypotension, tumor lysis syndrome, thrombocytopenia, infection, diabetes mellitus, bone marrow suppression, intracranial bleeding, injection-site irritation

DOSAGE AND ROUTES
Multiple myeloma (previously untreated)

Adult: IV bol/subcut Give for 9 6-wk cycles; cycle 1-4, 1.3 mg/m²/dose given on days 1, 4, 8, 11, then a 10-day rest period (days 12-21) and again on days 22, 25, 29, 32, then a 10-day rest period (days 33-42) given with melphalan (9 mg/m²/day on days 1-4) and predniSONE (60 mg/m²/day on days 1-4); this 6-wk cycle is considered one course; in cycles 5-9, give bortezomib 1.3 mg/m²/dose on days 1, 8, 22, 29 with melphalan (9 mg/m²/day on days 1-4) and predniSONE (60 mg/m²/day on days 1-4); this 6-wk cycle is considered one course; at least 72 hr should elapse between consecutive doses

Mantle cell lymphoma in combination

Adult: IV bol/subcut 1.3 mg/m²/dose (days 1, 4, 8, 11) followed by 10-day rest period (days 12 to 21); × 6 (3wk) cycles with riTUXimab 375 mg/m2, cyclophosphamide 750 mg/m2, DOXOrubicin 50mg/m2 all on day 1, and predniSONE 100mg/m2 q day on day 1-5, give bortezomib before riTUXimab

Neuropathic pain

Grade 1 with pain or grade 2, reduce to 1 mg/m²; grade 2 with pain or grade 3, hold product until toxicity resolves, then start at 0.7 mg/m² qwk; grade 4 hematologic toxicities, withhold use

Relapsed multiple myeloma or mantle cell lymphoma

Adult: IV BOL/SUBCUT 1.3 mg/m²/2 × per wk followed by a 10-day rest period

Hepatic dose

Adult: IV bilirubin >1.5 × ULN reduce to 0.7 mg/m² in cycle 1, consider dose escalation to 1 mg/m² or further reduction to 0.5 mg/m² in next cycles based on tolerability

Available forms: Lyophilized powder for inj 3.5 mg (must reconstitute)

ADVERSE EFFECTS

CNS: Reversible posterior encephalopathy syndrome (PRESS), progressive multifocal leukoencephalopathy (PML), dizziness, headache, *peripheral neuropathy,* fever
CV: Hypotension, edema, HF
GI: Abdominal pain, *constipation,* diarrhea, *nausea, vomiting,* anorexia, hepatotoxicity
HEMA: Anemia, neutropenia, thrombocytopenia
MISC: Dehydration, weight loss, herpes zoster, *rash,* pruritus, blurred vision
MS: *Fatigue, malaise, weakness,* tumor lysis syndrome
RESP: Cough, pneumonia, dyspnea

INTERACTIONS
Individual drugs

Amiodarone, amprenavir, chloramphenicol, CISplatin, colchicine, cycloSPORINE, dapsone, didanosine, disulfiram, DOCEtaxel, gold salts, INH, iodoquinol, isoniazid, lamiVUDine, metroNIDAZOLE, nitrofurantoin, oxaliplatin, PACLitaxel, penicillAMINE, phenytoin, ritonavir, stavudine, sulfaSALAzine, thalidomide, vinBLAStine, vinCRIStine, zacatabine, zidovudine, and others: increased peripheral neuropathy

---

Drug classifications
Anticoagulants, NSAIDs, platelet inhibitors, salicylates, thrombolytics: increased bleeding risk

Antivirals, statins, HMG-CoA reductase inhibitors: increased peripheral neuropathy

Decreased: effect of norethindrone, estradiol, combination oral contraceptives, another nonhormonal contraceptive should be used

Drug/herb
St. John's wort: toxicity or decreased efficacy

Drug/lab tests
Increase: LFTs, glucose, platelets, Hb

NURSING CONSIDERATIONS
Assessment
• Assess hematologic status: platelets, CBC throughout treatment
• PRES: Assess for headache, malaise, confusion, seizures, blindness, hypertension, usually occurs within a few hr to up to 1 yr after beginning treatment; most symptoms do not need treatment; test by MRI to confirm diagnosis
• Fatal pulmonary toxicity: assess for risk factors, or new worsening pulmonary symptoms
• Tumor lysis syndrome: usually with those with a high tumor burden, assess for hypotension, tachycardia, pulmonary edema
• Monitor vital signs baseline and frequently; hypotension may occur; patients that are dehydrated are at greater risk
• GI toxicity: Assess for nausea, vomiting, diarrhea, constipation; may require antiemetics, antidiarrheals
• **Thrombocytopenia/neutropenia:** Monitor CBC baseline and periodically; monitor platelets before each dose; dose adjustments may be required (nadir day 11 platelets)

Patient problems
Risk for injury (adverse reactions)
Risk for infection (adverse reactions)

Implementation
SUBCUT route
• Only Velcade can be given subcut
• Reconstitute with 1.4 ml NS (2.5 mg/ml) or 3.5 ml NS (1 mg/ml); the 1 mg/ml may be used for local inj site reaction with the 2.5 mg/ml solution; if injection-site reaction occurs, use 1 mg/ml; the final product should be a clear, colorless solution; if any discoloration or particulate matter is observed, do not use
• Store reconstituted at room temperature, give within 8 hr of reconstitution, store ≤8 hr in a syringe; total storage time must be ≤8 hr when exposed to normal light

• Determine the volume of reconstituted bortezomib to be administered by multiplying the desired dose in mg/m^2 by the patient's BSA and dividing the result by the concentration (1 mg/ml or 2.5 mg/ml); discard unused drug, as no preservative is present
• Place a sticker that indicates subcut use on the syringe

SUBCUT inj
• Inject subcutaneously in the thigh or abdomen; do not inject into a site that is tender, bruised, erythematous, or indurated; rotate injection sites; new sites should be at least 1 inch from an old site
• Use of gloves and protective clothing are recommended to prevent skin contact

IV direct
• **Reconstitute** each vial with 3.5 ml 0.9% NaCl (1 mg/ml), sol should be clear/colorless; **inject** bol over 3-5 sec
• Store unopened product at room temperature, protect from light
• Use protective clothing during handling, preparation; avoid contact with skin
• Monitor for extravasation at inj site

Patient/family education
• **Pregnancy/breastfeeding:** Teach to use contraception while on this product, do not breastfeed
• Advise diabetic to monitor blood glucose levels
• Instruct to contact prescriber if new or worsening peripheral neuropathy, severe vomiting, diarrhea, easy bruising, bleeding, infection
• Advise to avoid driving, operating machinery until effect is known
• Advise to avoid using other medications unless approved by prescriber
• Bleeding risk (report bruising, bleeding)
• Provide fluids and electrolytes as needed
• Teach patient to report immediately, headache, confusion, lethargy (PRES)
• **Pregnancy/breastfeeding:** do not use in pregnancy, breastfeeding and advise to use contraception

Evaluation
Positive therapeutic outcome
• Improvement of multiple myeloma symptoms

> **⚠ HIGH ALERT**

brentuximab vedotin (Rx)

(bren-tak'see-mab)

Adcetris

Func. class.: antineoplastic
Chem. class.: monoclonal antibody

ACTION: The anticancer activity is due to the binding of the ᴼⁱᵍ⁴ ADC to CD30-expressing cells, followed by the internalization and transportation of the ADC-CD30 complex to lysosomes, and the release of MMAE via selective proteolytic cleavage. MMAE binds to tubulin and disrupts the microtubule network within the cell, inducing cell cycle arrest and apoptotic death of the cells

Therapeutic outcome: Decreasing symptoms of Hodgkin's disease (increased lymph nodes, night sweats, weight loss, splenomegaly, hepatomegaly)

USES: Hodgkin's lymphoma after failure of autologous stem cell transplant (ASCT) or after failure of at least 2 prior multiagent chemotherapy regimens in patients who are not ASCT candidates; non-Hodgkin's lymphoma (NHL): systemic anaplastic large cell lymphoma (sALCL) after failure of at least one prior multiagent chemotherapy regimen

Pharmacokinetics

Absorption	Complete
Distribution	Protein binding, 68%-82%
Metabolism	Small amount, potent inhibitors or inducers of CYP3A4, may alter action
Excretion	Minimal
Half-life	Terminal 4-6 days; three components are released

Pharmacodynamics

Onset	Unknown
Peak	Unknown
Duration	Unknown

CONTRAINDICATIONS

Hypersensitivity, pregnancy

> **BLACK BOX WARNING:** Progressive multifocal leukoencephalopathy (PML)

Precautions: Breastfeeding, children, infants, neonates, neutropenia, peripheral neuropathy, tumor lysis syndrome (TLS)

DOSAGE AND ROUTES

Adult: IV 1.8 mg/kg IV every 3 weeks until disease progression or unacceptable toxicity.

Renal dose
Adult IV: CCr <30 mL/min avoid use

Hepatic dose
Adult IV: (Child-Pugh A) 1.2 mg/kg q 3 wk; (child-Pugh B or C) avoid use

Available forms: Powder for IV injection 50 mg/vial

ADVERSE EFFECTS

CNS: Headache, dizziness, *fever,* peripheral neuropathy, anxiety, chills, *fatigue,* paresthesias, insomnia, night sweats, progressive multifocal leukoencephalopathy (PML)
CV: Peripheral edema
GI: *Abdominal pain, nausea, vomiting,* constipation, *diarrhea,* weight loss, GI hemorrhage, perforation/obstruction, hepatotoxicity, pancreatitis, ileus
HEMA: Anemia, neutropenia, thrombocytopenia
INTEG: *Rash,* pruritus, toxic epidermal necrolysis
RESP: Pneumothorax, pneumonitis, pulmonary embolism, dyspnea, *cough*
SYST: Anaphylaxis, tumor lysis syndrome, Stevens-Johnson syndrome, infusion reactions

INTERACTIONS
Individual drugs
Boceprevir, dalfopristin; delavirdine, isoniazid, indinavir, itraconazole, ketoconazole, quinupristin, rifAMPin, ritonavir; telithromycin, tipranavir: increased brentuximab component action
Bleomycin: increased noninfectious pulmonary toxicity; do not use together

Drug classifications
CYP3A4 inhibitors: increase brentuximab action
Decrease: brentuximab action-CYP3A4 inducers

Drug/herb
St. John's wort: increased brentuximab action

NURSING CONSIDERATIONS
Assessment
• **Tumor lysis syndrome (TLS):** Assess for hyperkalemia, hyperphosphatemia, hypocalcemia; may develop renal failure; may use allopurinol or rasburicase to prevent TLS; monitor serum BUN/creatinine
• **Progressive multifocal leukoencephalopathy (PML):** Assess for weakness, or paralysis, vision loss, impaired speech, and cognitive deterioration; often fatal
• **Pancreatitis:** Assess for severe abdominal pain, nausea, and vomiting

• **Anaphylaxis, Stevens-Johnson syndrome:** Assess for rash; swelling of face, lips, throat; dyspnea; pruritus; stop immediately
• **Infusion-related reactions:** Check site frequently, if reactions occur (redness, swelling at site), stop infusion; may give antihistamines
• **Pulmonary toxicity:** Assess for dyspnea, cough; if these occur product may need to be discontinued
• **Hepatotoxicity:** Monitor AST/ALT, bilirubin baseline and periodically; if elevated, product may need to be discontinued or decreased
• Monitor CBC and differential, LFTs, serum bilirubin (direct and indirect), electrolytes, uric acid, neurologic function

Patient problems
Risk fior infection (adverse reactions)
Risk for injury (adverse reactions)

Implementation:
Intermittent IV infusion route
• Visually inspect for particulate matter and discoloration whenever solution and container permit
• Give only as an IV infusion, do not give as an IV push or bolus
• Use cytoxic handling procedures
• Do not mix with, or administer as an infusion with, other IV products
• Calculate the dose (mg) and the number of vials required. For patients weighing >100 kg, use 100 kg to calculate the dose; reconstitute each 50 mg vial/10.5 ml of sterile water for injection (5 mg/ml)
• Direct the stream of sterile water toward the wall of the vial and not directly at the cake or powder; gently swirl the vial to aid in dissolution, do not shake
• Discard any unused portion left in the vial
• After reconstitution, dilute immediately with ≥100 ml of 0.9% sodium chloride, 5% dextrose, or lactated Ringer's solution to a final concentration (0.4 mg/ml-1.8 mg/ml)
• Use the diluted solution immediately or store in refrigerator for ≤24 hrs after reconstitution; do not freeze
• Infuse over 30 min

Patient/family education
• **Pulmonary toxicity:** Teach patient cough, trouble breathing, report immediately
• **Infection:** Teach patient to report immediately fever, chills
• **PML:** Teach patient to report immediately confusion, mood changes, vision/speech changes, weakness
• Advise patient to use reliable contraception, do not use in breastfeeding

• Use the diluted sol immediately or store in refrigerator for ≤24 hr after reconstitution; do not freeze

Evaluation
Positive therapeutic outcome
• Decreasing symptoms of Hodgkin's disease (decreased lymph nodes, night sweats, splenomegaly, hepatomegaly)

brimonidine ophthalmic
See Appendix B

brinzolamide ophthalmic
See Appendix B

bromfenac ophthalmic
See Appendix B

brexpiprazole
(brex-pip′-ra-zole)
Rexulti
Func. class.: Antipsychotic, atypical

ACTION: Although the exact mechanism of action is unknown, may exert its effects through a combination of partial agonist activity at dopaminergic D-2 receptors and serotonergic 5-HT1A receptors and antagonist activity at serotonergic 5-HT2A receptors

USES: Adjunctive treatment of major depressive disorder, schizophrenia

Pharmacokinetics	
Half-life	91 hr

Pharmacodynamics	
Onset	Unknown
Peak	4 hr
Duration	Unknown

CONTRAINDICATIONS
Hypersensitivity

DOSAGE AND ROUTES
Schizophrenia
Adult: PO Initially, 1 mg qday, on Day 5, increase to 2 mg qday, on Day 8, may increase to 4 mg qday based on response and tolerability. The recommended dose range is 2 to 4 mg/day (max: 4 mg/day)

Major depression
Adult: PO initially, 0.5 to 1 mg qday, after titration to 1 mg/day, increase to the target dose of 2 mg qday, titrate dosage at weekly intervals based on response and tolerability

Hepatic dose
Adult: PO Mild hepatic impairment: No change, moderate to severe hepatic impairment (Child-Pugh score 7 or more): Max 2 mg qday for major depression and 3 mg qday for schizophrenia

Renal dose
Adult: PO CCr $\geq$ 60 ml/min: No change; CCr <60 ml/min, including end stage renal disease (ESRD): Max is 2 mg qday for major depression and 3 mg qday for schizophrenia

Available forms: Tablet: 0.25, 0.50, 1, 2, 3, 4 mg

ADVERSE EFFECTS
CNS: Akathisia, fatigue, drowsiness, dizziness, tremor, sedation, insomnia, EPS, neuroleptic malignant syndrome
EENT: Blurred vision, dry mouth, nasopharyngitis
GI: Constipation, diarrhea, nausea, flatulence, abdominal cramping/pain
GU: UTI
MISC: Weight gain, myalgia, anaphylaxis

INTERACTIONS
Drug classifications
Anticholinergics: Increased temperature
Other CNS depressants: Increased CNS depression
Strong CYP2D6 inhibitors, strong CYP3A4 inhibitors: Increased brexiprazole effect

Drug/herb
Decrease: Brexiprazole effect: St. John's wort, may need to increase product dose

Drug/food
Increase: Brexiprazole effect: Grapefruit juice, avoiding using together

NURSING CONSIDERATIONS
Assessment
• **Hypersensitivity:** Do not use in hypersensitivity, rash, facial swelling, urticaria, and anaphylaxis have been observed; discontinue immediately

> **BLACK BOX WARNING: Suicidal ideation:**
> Provide close supervision and control, patient should receive the smallest quantity to reduce the risk of overdose. In those who exhibit changes in symptoms, worsening of depression, suicidality, or other unusual changes in mood or behaviors, a decision should be made to change or discontinue treatment. If discontinuing, the medication should be tapered as rapidly as possible, but with recognition that abrupt discontinuation of the drug can also cause adverse symptoms. Children and young adults < 24 yr are at increased risk

• **Tardive dyskinesia:** Assess for movement disorders (AIMS). If tardive dyskinesia appear, discontinuation may be needed
• **Seizure disorder:** Assess for seizures. Conditions that lower the seizure threshold may be more prevalent in elderly patients who are 65 yr or older
• **Orthostatic hypotension:** Monitor for dizziness, lightheadedness, and tachycardia at the beginning of treatment and during dose escalation. May be at increased risk include those with dehydration, hypovolemia, treatment with antihypertensive medications, history of cardiac disease (heart failure, myocardial infarction, coronary artery disease, ischemia, or conduction abnormalities), history of cerebrovascular disease, and those patients who are antipsychotic-naïve. Elderly patients may be at higher risk for syncope and cardiovascular and cerebrovascular events. A fall risk assessment should be completed recurrently in at-risk patients on long-term antipsychotic therapy
• **Hematological disease:** Those with a history of clinically significant low WBC count or drug-induced leukopenia/neutropenia should have frequent complete blood count (CBC) during the first few months of treatment. Discontinuation may be needed if a decline in WBC occurs in the absence of an identifiable cause. Patients with clinically significant neutropenia should be closely monitored for fever and infection. Discontinue in patients with severe neutropenia (ANC < 1000/mm^3)
• **Pregnancy/breastfeeding:** Neonates exposed to antipsychotics during the third trimester of pregnancy are at risk for extrapyramidal and/or withdrawal symptoms after delivery. Enroll patient at The National Pregnancy Registry for Psychiatric Medications at https://womensmentalhealth.org/clinical-and-research-programs/pregnancyregistry or by phone 866-961-2388.

Patient problems
Distorted thinking processes (uses)
Excess food intake (adverse reactions)

Implementation
• Initiate treatment at the low end of the dosage range in geriatric adults
• Coadministration of certain drugs may need to be avoided or dosage adjustments may be necessary; review drug interactions. In those who are poor metabolizers (PMs) of CYP2D6 (CYP2D6 PMs), give one–half of the usual dose. In those who are CYP2D6 PMs and receiving a moderate

or strong CYP3A4 inhibitor, give one–quarter of the usual. If the coadministered drug is discontinued, adjust the dose accordingly for those who are CYP2D6 PMs. Periodically reassess for need of continued maintenance therapy
• Without regard to food

Patient/family education
• Advise patient to use caution when driving or operating machinery or performing other tasks that require mental alertness until they know how the drug affects them. Patients should also be advised to avoid ethanol ingestion during treatment. Somnolence from antipsychotic use could lead to falls with the potential for fractures and other injuries
• Teach patient that on-going lab work and exams will be needed
• Advise patient that weight may increase
• Advise patient and caregiver to report immediately thought/behavior of suicide
• Inform patient to rise slowly to minimize orthostatic hypotension

Evaluation
Positive therapeutic outcome:
• Decreased depression
• Increased organized thought

RARELY USED

⚠ HIGH ALERT

brigatinib
(bri-ga'-ti-nib)
Alunbrig
Func. class.: Antineoplastic

USES: For the treatment of advanced ALK-positive metastatic non small cell lung cancer that has progressed on or is intolerant to crizotinib

DOSAGES AND ROUTES
Adult: PO 90 mg qday × 7 days, if tolerated during the first 7 days, increase to 180 mg qday. Continue until disease progression or unacceptable toxicity

---

⚠ HIGH ALERT

brivaracetam
(briv-a-ra'se-tam)
Briviact
Func. class.: Anticonvulsant

ACTION: The exact mechanism not known, may occur in modulation of synaptic vesicle proteins, additional anticonvulsant activity may be related to the modulation of voltage-dependent sodium channels

USES: For the adjunctive treatment of partial seizures

Pharmacokinetics

Absorption	Unknown
Distribution	Protein binding 20%
Metabolism	By hydrolysis to form a hydroxy metabolite metabolized by CYP2C19
Excretion	Urine, feces <1%
Half-life	9 hr

Pharmacodynamics

Onset	Unknown
Peak	1 hr without food; high-fat meal slows absorption

CONTRAINDICATIONS
Hypersensitivity renal failure

Precautions: Abrupt discontinuation, breastfeeding, depression, driving or operating machinery, geriatric, hepatic disease, pregnancy, suicidal ideation, children < 16 yr

DOSAGE AND ROUTES
Adult and adolescent 16 yr and older: PO/IV 50 mg bid. Adjust dose to 25 mg bid IV or 100 mg bid based on clinical response; max 100 mg bid. Use IV when PO is temporarily not feasible

Available forms: Tabs 10, 25, 50, 75, 100; oral solution 10 mg/ml; solution for injection 50 mg/5 ml (10 mg/ml)

ADVERSE EFFECTS
CNS: *Dizziness, drowsiness,* ataxia, euphoria, fatigue, irritability, depression, emotional lability, hallucinations, psychosis, suicidal ideation
GI: Constipation, nausea, vomiting
HEMA: Leukopenia
INTEG: Angioedema
RESP: Bronchospasm

INTERACTIONS
Drug classifications
CYP2C19 inducers (rifampin): Decreased product effect
Tricyclic antidepressants, antihistamines, benzodiazepines, other CNS depressants: Increased sedation

Individual drugs
Carbamazepine: Increased toxicity possible
Phenytoin: Increased phenytoin levels
Sevelamer: Decreased brivaracetam absorption

Drug/lab test
Increase: LFTs
Decrease: Hct/Hgb, WBC, RBC

NURSING CONSIDERATIONS
Assessment
• **Seizures:** Assess for type, location, duration, character; provide seizure precautions
• Renal studies: Monitor urinalysis, BUN, urine creatinine q3mo
• **Bronchospasm:** Assess for dyspnea, wheezing
• Blood studies: Monitor CBC, LFTs
• Mental status: Assess mood, sensorium, affect, behavioral changes, suicidal thoughts/ behaviors; if mental status changes, notify prescriber
• Provide assistance with ambulation during early part of treatment, dizziness, drowsiness occurs

Patient problems
Risk for injury (adverse reactions)
Suicide (adverse reactions)

Implementation
• May be administered without regard to meals
• To discontinue, gradually reduce the dose to minimize the risk for increased seizure frequency and status epilepticus

Tablets: Swallow tablets whole; do not crush or chew
Oral solution:
• No dilution is necessary
• Measure and administer the oral solution using a calibrated measuring device
• A nasogastric tube or gastrostomy tube may be used for administration
• **Storage:** Discard any unused solution after 5 mo of first opening the bottle
IV Infusion
• Visually inspect parenteral products for particulate matter and discoloration before use; do not use if discoloration or particulate matter is present; injection is a clear, colorless solution
• May be given IV without further dilution or may be mixed with a diluent, including 0.9% NaCl Injection, LR injection, or D5 injection
• Infuse over 2 to 15 min
• **Storage:** After dilution, the solution may be stored ≤ 4 hr at room temperature and may be stored in polyvinyl chloride (PVC) bags. Discard any unused injection vial contents, for single dose only

Patient/family education
• Teach patient to carry emergency ID stating patient's name, medications taken, condition, prescriber's name, and phone number
• Teach patient how to use oral solution, use calibrated device to measure
• Advise the patient to notify prescriber if pregnancy is planned or suspected
• Advise the patient to avoid driving, other activities requiring alertness until response is known, drowsiness occurs during beginning therapy
• Teach patient not to discontinue quickly after long-term use, withdrawal seizure may occur
• Teach patient not to breastfeed
• Teach patient to report suicidal thoughts/ behaviors immediately

Evaluation
Positive therapeutic outcome
• Decreased seizure activity

brodalumab (Rx)
(broe-dal´-ue-mab)
Siliq
Func. class.: Immunosuppressive
Chem. class.: Recombinant human IgG1 monoclonal antibody

ACTION: Human IgG2 monoclonal antibody that binds to interleukin-17 receptor A (IL-17RA) and prevents IL-17 cytokines from activating the receptor

USES: For the treatment of moderate to severe plaque psoriasis in those who are candidates for phototherapy or systemic therapy and have failed to respond or have lost response to other systemic therapies

Pharmacokinetics
Absorption	55%
Distribution	Unknown
Metabolism	Unknown
Excretion	Unknown
Half-life	Unknown

Pharmacodynamics
Onset	Unknown
Peak	3 days
Duration	Unknown

CONTRAINDICATIONS
Hypersensitivity, Crohn's disease, TB

Precautions: Pregnancy, breastfeeding, children, depression, geriatric patients, immunosuppression, infection, suicidal ideation, vaccination

DOSAGE AND ROUTES

Adult: SUBCUT 210 mg at weeks 0, 1, and 2 then 210 mg q2wk. Discontinue if inadequate response after 12 to 16 wk

Available form: Prefilled syringe 210 mg/ 1.5 ml

ADVERSE EFFECTS

CNS: Headache, fatigue, suicidal ideation
EENT: Sinusitis
GI: Nausea, diarrhea
MS: Arthralgia
INTEG: Erythema, pruritus
HEMA: Bleeding, **neutropenia**
MISC: Infection, injection site reactions, antibody formation, pharyngitis, TB

INTERACTIONS

Drug classifications

CYP 450 enzymes (carbamazepine, cyclosporine, ethosuximide, fosphenytoin, phenytoin, tacrolimus, theophylline, aminophylline, warfarin). Increased altered effect of each product, monitor if products are initiated or discontinued, dose adjustments may be needed

Do not give concurrently with live virus vaccines; immunizations should be brought up to date before treatment

NURSING CONSIDERATIONS

Assessment

• Assess for injection site pain, swelling, redness—use cold compress to relieve pain/ swelling; give at 45-degree angle using abdomen, thighs; rotate injection sites; discard unused portions

• **Infection:** Assess for infections (fever, flulike symptoms, dyspnea, change in urination, redness/swelling around any wounds), stop treatment if present; some serious infections including sepsis may occur, may be fatal; patients with active infections should not be started on this product

• **TB:** Obtain a TB test before starting this product, do not use in active TB; for latent TB, give antituberculosis therapy before use of this product, monitor closely for signs and symptoms of active tuberculosis infection during and after treatment

• **Suicidal ideation:** Assess for suicidal thought/behaviors, worsening depression, panic attacks, anxiety

Patient problems

Risk for injury (adverse reactions)
Suicide (adverse reactions)

Implementation

SUBCUT route

• Due to the product's association with suicidal ideation/behavior, this product is only available through a restricted program (SILIQ Risk Evaluation and Mitigation Strategy (REMS) Program). Those prescribing this product must be certified in the SILIQ REMS Program. Patients must sign a Patient-Prescriber Agreement Form. For information, visit the SILIQ REMS website or telephone 855-511-6135

• Remove prefilled syringe from refrigerator and allow to reach room temperature (about 30 min) without removing the needle cap; once brought to room temperature, do not place back into the refrigerator. If needed, the prefilled syringe may be stored at room temperature for up to 14 days. Any prefilled syringe that has been stored at room temperature for more than 14 days MUST be discarded.

• Do not shake the prefilled syringe. DO NOT use the prefilled syringe if it has been dropped on a hard surface. Use a new syringe and call 800-321-4576.

• Visually inspect for particulate matter and discoloration; the solution should be clear to slightly opalescent, colorless to slightly yellow, and may contain a few small translucent particles. Do not use if discolored, cloudy, or foreign particulate matter is present

• Only an individual trained in subcutaneous drug delivery should administer the injection. A patient who is properly trained in injection technique may self-inject using the prefilled syringe or vial, if his or her prescriber deems the action appropriate. However, the first injection needs to be under the supervision of a qualified health care professional

• Use front part of the middle thigh, the gluteal or abdominal region, and the outer area of the upper arm. For injection sites, rotate injection sites. Do not use where skin is tender, bruised, red, hard, thick, scaly, or affected by psoriasis

• Gently pinch the skin and insert the needle at a 45-degree angle subcutaneously. Push the plunger slowly and evenly to deliver the dose, remove the needle, and release the pinched skin. Do not rub the injection site; slight bleeding may occur

• No preservatives are present; discard any unused portion

• Protect from light, do not freeze

Patient/family education
• Teach patient about self-administration if appropriate: Injection should be made in thigh, abdomen, upper arm; rotate sites at least 1 inch from old site; do not inject in areas that are bruised, red, hard
• Teach patient that if medication is not taken when due, inject next dose as soon as remembered and inject next dose as scheduled
• Teach patient not to take any live virus vaccines during treatment
• Teach patient to report signs of infection (fever, sweats, or chills; muscle aches; weight loss; cough; warm, red, or painful skin or sores on body different from psoriasis; diarrhea or stomach pain; shortness of breath; blood in phlegm (mucus); burning when urinate or urinating more often than normal); allergic reactions (itching, rash)
• Advise patient to tell provider of all prescription, OTC, herbals, and supplements currently taken
• **Suicidal ideation:** Advise patients and caregivers to seek medical attention for suicidal ideation, new-onset or worsening depression, anxiety, or other mood changes

Evaluation
Positive therapeutic outcome
• Decreased in lesions

---

budesonide (Rx)
(byoo-des'oh-nide)
Inhalation
Pulmicort Respules, Pulmicort Flexhaler
Nasal
Rhinocort Allergy, Rhinocort Aqua
Systemic
Entocort EC, Uceris
Func. class.: Glucocorticoid

ACTION: Prevents inflammation by depression of migration of polymorphonuclear leukocytes, fibroblasts, reversal of increased capillary permeability and lysosomal stabilization; does not suppress hypothalamus and pituitary function

USES: Rhinitis; prophylaxis for asthma; Crohn's disease, ulcerative colitis, nasal polyps

Pharmacokinetics
Absorption	39%
Distribution	In airways, protein binding 85%-90%
Metabolism	Liver
Excretion	In urine (60%), small amounts in feces, enters breast milk
Half-life	2-3.6 hr

Pharmacodynamics
Onset	Respules 2-8 days, Rhinocort Aqua 10 hr
Peak	Respules 4-6 wk, Rhinocort Aqua 2 wk
Duration	Unknown

CONTRAINDICATIONS
Hypersensitivity, status asthmaticus, acute bronchospasm

Precautions: Pregnancy; breastfeeding, children, TB, fungal, bacterial, systemic viral infections, ocular herpes simplex, nasal septal ulcers; hepatic disease, diabetes, GI disease, increased intraoccular pressure

DOSAGE AND ROUTES
Rhinitis
Adult and child >6 yr: Nasal Spray/inh 2 sprays in each nostril AM, PM, or 4 sprays in each nostril AM

Asthma
Adult and child >6 yr: INH 400-1200 mcg/day
Child 1-8 yrs previously taking bronchodilator alone: Plumicort (Respules) 0.5 mg q day or 0.25 mg bid susp via jet nebulizer, max 0.5 mg q day; previously using inhaled corticosteroid 0.5 mg q day or 0.25 mg bid susp via jet nebulizer, max 0.5 mg bid

Crohn's disease, ulcerative colitis (Uceris)
Adult: PO 9 mg daily AM × 8 wk

Laryngotracheobronchitis (croup) (unlabeled)
Infant ≥3 months-child ≤5 yr: (Pulmicort Respules INH susp) 2 mg inhaled as a single dose

Available forms: Dry powder for INH 90, 100 ❧ 180, 200 ❧, 400 ❧ 32 mcg/actuation (Rhinocort Aqua) nasal spray; susp for inh 0.5 mg/2 ml, 0.25 mg/2 ml; ext rel tab (Uceris) 9 mg; cap 3 mg, rectal foam 2 mg/actuation

ADVERSE EFFECTS
CNS: *Headache,* insomnia, hypertonia, syncope, dizziness, drowsiness
CV: Chest pain, hypertension, sinus tachycardia, palpitation, syncope
EENT: *Sinusitis, pharyngitis,* rhinitis, oral candidiasis
ENDO: Adrenal insufficiency, growth suppression in children
GI: Dry mouth, dyspepsia, nausea, vomiting, abdominal pain; diarrhea (inhalation)
MISC: Ecchymosis, fever, *hypersensitivity,* flu-like symptoms, epistaxis, dysuria
MS: Back pain, myalgias, fractures

❧ Canada only   ⚠ Genetic Warning   Adverse effects: *italics* = common; red = life-threatening

RESP: Nasal irritation, cough, nasal bleeding, *respiratory infections,* bronchospasm

INTERACTIONS
Individual drugs
Varicella live vaccine: avoid concurrent use in pediatric patients

Drug classifications
CYP3A inhibitors: increased budesonide effect; dose adjustment may be required

NURSING CONSIDERATIONS
Assessment
• **Crohn's disease/ulcerative colitis:** Assess for improvement: decreased stools, abdominal cramps, urgency
• **HPA axis suppression:** may occur if stopped abruptly, taper
• Assess respiratory status: rate, rhythm, increase in bronchial secretions, wheezing, chest tightness; provide fluids to 2 L/day to decrease thickness of secretions; check for oral candidiasis
• For bronchospasm, stop treatment and give bronchodilator
• With viral infections, corticosteroid use can mask infections
• For increased intraocular pressure, discontinue use if increase occurs
• **Pregnancy/breastfeeding:** Fetal harm appears remote, excreted in breast milk, consider risk factors
• **Beers:** Avoid in older adults, high risk of delirium

Patient problems
Impaired airway clearnace (uses)
Risk for infection (adverse reactions)

Implementation
PO route (Crohn's disease)
• Swallow caps whole; do not break, crush, or chew, take in AM
• May repeat 8-wk course if needed; may taper to 6 mg/day for 2 wk before cessation
Oral inh route (dry powder for inh) (Pulmicort Turbuhaler)
• A new Turbuhaler should be primed before use; to load the dose on a primed inhaler, twist the brown grip fully to the right as far as it will go, then twist it back fully to the left; there will be the sound of a "click"
• When inhaling, the Turbuhaler may be held upright or horizontally; turn head away from the inhaler and breathe out; place the mouthpiece between the lips and inhale deeply and forcefully; exhale normally
• After the last dose, rinse the mouth with water; do not swallow the water; keep inhaler clean and dry

Inh susp route for nebulization (Pulmicort Respules)
• Use via jet nebulizer connected to an air compressor with adequate airflow and equipped with a mouthpiece or suitable face mask; do not use ultrasonic nebulizers
• See manufacturer's direction on use of nebulizer and preparation of the solution
• Gently shake the ampule in a circular motion before opening it and placing the suspension in the nebulizer reservoir; using the "blow by" technique (i.e., holding the face mask or open tube near the patient's nose and mouth) is not recommended; use inh susp separately in the nebulizer
• Store inhal susp upright at controlled room temperature and protected from light; after opening the envelope, the shelf life of the unused respules is 2 wk; return unused respules to the aluminum foil envelope to protect from light; opened respule should be used promptly
Intranasal inhalation route
• Shake inhaler well; prior to initial use, the Rhinocort Aqua container must be shaken gently and the pump must be primed by actuating 8 times; if used daily, the pump does not need to be reprimed; if not used for 2 consecutive days, reprime with 1 spray or until a fine spray appears; if not used for more than 14 days, rinse the applicator and reprime with 2 sprays or until a fine spray appears; blow nose gently, without squeezing; with head upright, spray into each nostril; sniff while squeezing the bottle quickly and firmly; after use, rinse the tip of the bottle with hot water, taking care not to suck water into the bottle, and dry with a clean tissue; replace the cap
• To avoid the spread of infection, do not use the container for more than one person
• Store at 59°-86° F (15°-30° C); keep away from heat, open flame
Rectal Foam Route
• Product is flammable, may use prior to bedtime, applicators are single use only

Patient/family education
• Teach patient to notify prescriber of pharyngitis, nasal bleeding, oral candidiasis
• Instruct patient not to exceed recommended dosage; adrenal suppression may occur
• Teach patient to carry/wear emergency ID identifying steroid use
• Instruct patient to read and follow package directions
• Instruct patient to prevent exposure to infections, especially viral
• Advise to use good oral hygiene if using by nebulizer or inhaler

- Teach patient to avoid breastfeeding
- Teach patient that product is not a bronchodilator and is not to be used for asthma; to use regularly
- Teach how to use as described in "administer"
- Advise to notify prescriber if symptoms persist after 3 wk, that results usually take 2 wk
- Advise to notify prescriber if exposure to measles, chickenpox occurs

Evaluation
Positive therapeutic outcome
- Absence of asthma, rhinitis

budesonide nasal agent
See Appendix B

bumetanide (Rx)
(byoo-met′a-nide)
Burinex ✦
Func. class.: Loop diuretic, antihypertensive
Chem. class.: Sulfonamide derivative

ACTION: Acts on the ascending loop of Henle in the kidney to inhibit the reabsorption of the electrolytes sodium and chloride

Therapeutic outcome: Decreased edema in lung tissue and peripherally; decreased B/P

USES: Edema in heart failure, ascites, renal disease

Pharmacokinetics

	PO/IM
Absorption	Rapidly, (IV), well (PO/IM)
Distribution	Crosses placenta, protein binding >72%
Metabolism	Liver (30%-40%)
Excretion	Breast milk, urine (50% unchanged), feces (20%)
Half-life	1-1½ hr

Pharmacodynamics

	PO	IM	IV
Onset	½-1 hr	½-1 hr	5 min
Peak	1-2 hr	1-2 hr	½ hr
Duration	4-6 hr	4-6 hr	2-3 hr

CONTRAINDICATIONS
Hypersensitivity to this product, sulfonamides, anuria, hepatic coma

BLACK BOX WARNING: Fluid and electrolyte depletion

Precautions: Pregnancy, breastfeeding, neonates, severe renal disease, ascites, hepatic cirrhosis, blood dyscrasias, ototoxicity, hyperuricemia, hypokalemia, hyperglycemia, oliguria, hypomagnesemia, hypovolemia

BLACK BOX WARNING: Dehydration

DOSAGE AND ROUTES
Adult/adolescent: PO 0.5-2 mg daily max 10 mg/day; IM/IV 0.5-1 mg; may give 2nd or 3rd dose at 2-3 hr intervals; max 10 mg/day
Child (unlabeled): PO/IM/IV 0.015-0.1 mg/kg/dose, max 10 mg/day
Neonates: PO/IM/IV 0.01-0.05 mg/kg dose q 12-24 hr

Available forms: Tabs 0.5, 1, 2, 5 mg ✦; inj 0.25 mg/ml

ADVERSE EFFECTS
CNS: Headache, fatigue, weakness, dizziness, encephalopathy
CV: *Hypotension*
EENT: Loss of hearing
ELECT: *Hypokalemia, hypochloremic alkalosis, hypomagnesemia, hyperuricemia, hypocalcemia, hyponatremia*
ENDO: *Hyperglycemia*
GI: Dry mouth, vomiting, anorexia, diarrhea, nausea upset stomach
GU: *Polyuria*
INTEG: *Rash, pruritus*
MS: Myalgia, arthralgia

INTERACTIONS
Individual drugs
Digoxin: increased toxicity if potassium is low
Lithium: decreased renal clearance causing increased toxicity

Drug classifications
Aminoglycosides: increased ototoxicity, avoid concurrent use
Antihypertensives, nitrates: Increased hypotension
Antidiabetics: decreased antidiabetic effects
NSAIDs: decreased diuretic effect
Corticosteroids, diuretics, laxatives (stimulant): increased hypokalemia, monitor closely

Drug/herb
Hawthorn, horse chestnut: increased diuretic effect

Drug/Lab
Increase: Glucose
Decrease: Chloride, potassium, sodium, calcium, phosphorus

NURSING CONSIDERATIONS
Assessment
• Assess patient for tinnitus, hearing loss, ear pain; periodic testing of hearing is needed when high doses of this product are given by **IV** route

> **BLACK BOX WARNING: Dehydration:** Assess fluid volume status: I&O ratio and record, distended red veins, crackles in lung, color, quality and specific gravity of urine, skin turgor, adequacy of pulses, moist mucous membranes, bilateral lung sounds, peripheral pitting edema; dehydration symptoms of decreasing output, thirst, hypotension, dry mouth and mucous membranes should be reported

> **BLACK BOX WARNING:** Monitor for fluid and electrolyte depletion: potassium, sodium, calcium, magnesium; also include BUN, blood pH, ABGs, uric acid, CBC, blood glucose; severe electrolyte imbalances should be corrected before starting treatment

• Assess B/P, pulse before and during therapy with patient lying, standing, and sitting as appropriate; orthostatic hypotension can occur rapidly
• Monitor for digoxin toxicity (anorexia, nausea, vomiting, confusion, paresthesia, muscle cramps) in patients taking digoxin; lithium toxicity in those taking lithium
Stevens-Johnson Syndrome/toxic epidermal necrolysis:
• Assess for rash during treatment, discontinue if rash occurs
• **Beers:** Use cautiously in older adults, may cause or exacerbate syndrome of inappropriate antidiuretic hormone secretion, falls

Patient problems
Fluid imbalance (uses)

Implementation
PO route
• Give in AM to avoid interference with sleep
IV route
• Do not use solution that is yellow or has a precipitate or crystals
IV, direct route
• Give undiluted through Y-tube or 3-way stopcock; give 20 mg or less/min
Intermittent IV infusion route
• May be added to 0.9% NaCl, D₅W, use within 24 hr to ensure compatibility; give through Y-tube or 3-way stopcock; give at 4 mg/min or less; use infusion pump

Y-site compatibilities: Acyclovir, alfentanil, allopurinol, amifostine, amikacin, aminocaproic acid, aminophylline, amiodarone, amoxicillin, amphotericin B lipid complex (Abelcet), amphotericin B liposome (AmBisome), anidulafungin, ascorbic acid injection, atenolol, atracurium, atropine, aztreonam, benztropine, bivalirudin, bleomycin, buprenorphine, butorphanol, calcium chloride/gluconate, CARBOplatin, caspofungin, cefamandole, ceFAZolin, cefepime, cefmetazole, cefonicid, cefotaxime, cefoTEtan, cefOXitin, cefTAZidime, ceftizoxime, ceftobiprole, cefTRIAXone, cefuroxime, cephapirin, chloramphenicol, cimetidine, cisatracurium, CISplatin, cladribine, clarithromycin, clindamycin, codeine, cyanocobalamin, cyclophosphamide, cycloSPORINE, cytarabine, DACTINomycin, DAPTOmycin, dexamethasone, dexmedetomidine, digoxin, dilTIAZem, diphenhydrAMINE, DOBUTamine, DOCEtaxel, DOPamine, doripenem, doxacurium, DOXOrubicin, doxycycline, enalaprilat, ePHEDrine, EPINEPHrine, epiRUBicin, epoetin alfa, eptifibatide, ertapenem, erythromycin, esmolol, etoposide, famotidine, fentaNYL, filgrastim, fluconazole, fludarabine, fluorouracil, folic acid, furosemide, gatifloxacin, gemcitabine, gentamicin, glycopyrrolate, granisetron, heparin, hydrocortisone sodium succinate, HYDROmorphone, hydrOXYzine, IDArubicin, ifosfamide, imipenemcilastatin, indomethacin, insulin (regular), irinotecan, isoproterenol, ketorolac, labetalol, levofloxacin, lidocaine, linezolid, LORazepam, magnesium sulfate, mannitol, mechlorethamine, melphalan, meperidine, metaraminol, methotrexate, methoxamine, methyldopate, methylPREDNISolone, metoclopramide, metoprolol, metroNIDAZOLE, mezlocillin, micafungin, miconazole, milrinone, mitoXANtrone, morphine, moxalactam, multiple vitamins injection, mycophenolate, nafcillin, nalbuphine, naloxone, netilmicin, nitroglycerin, nitroprusside, norepinephrine, octreotide, ondansetron, oxacillin, oxaliplatin, oxytocin, palonosetron, pamidronate, pancuronium, pantoprazole, PEMEtrexed, penicillin G potassium/sodium, pentazocine, PENTobarbital, PHENobarbital, phenylephrine, phytonadione, piperacillin, piperacillin-tazobactam, polymyxin B, potassium chloride, procainamide, promethazine, propofol, propranolol, protamine, pyridoxine, quiNIDine, raNITIdine, remifentanil, rifAMPin, ritodrine, riTUXimab, rocuronium, sodium acetate, sodium bicarbonate, succinylcholine, SUFentanil, tacrolimus, teniposide, theophylline, thiamine, thiotepa, ticarcillin, ticarcillin-clavulanate, tigecycline, tirofiban, TNA, tobramycin, tolazoline, TPN, traMADol, trastuzumab, trimetaphan, urokinase, vancomycin, vasopressin, vecuronium, verapamil, vinCRIStine, vinorelbine, voriconazole

Patient/family education

• Teach patient to take the medication early in the day to prevent nocturia; if another dose is needed, take after noon, not to double or miss doses

• Instruct the patient to take with food or milk if GI symptoms of nausea and anorexia occur

• Teach patient to maintain weekly record of weight and notify prescriber of weight loss of >5 lb

• Caution the patient that this product causes a loss of potassium, so food rich in potassium should be added to the diet; refer to a dietitian for assistance in planning

• Caution the patient not to exercise in hot weather or stand for prolonged periods since orthostatic hypotension will be enhanced

• Teach patient not to use alcohol or any OTC medications without prescriber's approval; serious product reactions may occur

• Emphasize the need to contact prescriber immediately if muscle cramps, weakness, nausea, dizziness, or numbness occur

• Teach patient to take own B/P and pulse and record

• Teach patient to weigh daily

• Caution the patient that orthostatic hypotension may occur; patient should rise slowly from sitting or reclining positions and lie down if dizziness occurs

• Teach patient to continue taking medication even if feeling better; this product controls symptoms but does not cure the condition

• Advise the patient with hypertension to continue other medical treatment (exercise, weight loss, relaxation techniques, cessation of smoking); edema, weight gain

• Advise patient that continuing exams and blood work will be needed

• Inform patient to notify other health care providers of condition being treated, medication taken

• Advise patient to report if pregnancy is planned or suspected or if breastfeeding

Evaluation

Positive therapeutic outcome

• Decreased edema
• Decreased B/P
• Increased diuresis

⚠ HIGH ALERT

buprenorphine (Rx) (REMS)
(byoo-pre-nor'feen)

Belbuca, Buprenex, Butrans, Probuphine, Sublocade

Func. class.: Opioid analgesic, partial agonist

Chem. class.: Thebaine derivative

Controlled substance schedule III

ACTION: Depresses pain impulse transmission at the spinal cord level by interacting with opioid receptors, partial agonist at MU-opioid receptor

Therapeutic outcome: Relief of pain

USES: Moderate to severe pain, opiate agonist withdrawal/dependence

Pharmacokinetics

Absorption	Well absorbed IM, SL
Distribution	Crosses placenta, protein binding 96%
Metabolism	Liver, extensively by CYP3A4
Excretion	Kidneys, feces, breast milk
Half-life	2.2 hr (**IV**); 26 hr (transdermal); 37 hr (SL)

Pharmacodynamics

	IM	IV
Onset	15 min	Immediate
Peak	1 hr	5 min
Duration	6-10 hr	6 hr

SL	TD	Buccal
Unknown	Unknown	Unknown
Unknown	Unknown	Unknown
Unknown	Unknown	Unknown

CONTRAINDICATIONS

Hypersensitivity, ileus, status asthmaticus

BLACK BOX WARNING: Respiratory depression

Precautions: Pregnancy, breastfeeding, substance abuse/alcoholism, increased intracranial pressure, MI (acute), severe heart disease, respiratory depression, renal/hepatic/pulmonary disease, hypothyroidism, Addison's disease

BLACK BOX WARNING: QT prolongation, use of heating pad, accidental exposure, potential for overdose/poisoning, substance abuse, IM, neonatal opioid withdrawal syndrome, coadministration with other CNS depressants, implant insertion and removal

---

DOSAGE AND ROUTES

Adult: IM/IV 0.3 mg q 4-6 hr as needed may repeat after 30-60 min; TD: each patch is worn for 7 days (moderate-severe pain); **opioid-naïve patients** (those taking <30 mg oral morphine or equivalent prior to beginning treatment with q 4-6 hr as needed buprenorphine), 5 mcg/hr q7days, overestimating dose can be fatal; **conversion from other opiate agonist therapy,** titrate from other opioids for up to 7 days to no more than 30 mg oral morphine or equivalent prior to beginning q 4-6 hr as needed therapy, begin with 5 mcg/hr q7days; for those with daily dose of 30-80 mg oral morphine or equivalent, start with 10 mcg/hr q7days; for those >80 mg oral morphine or equivalent start with 20 mcg/hr q7days; geriatric/debilitated: IM/IV 0.15 mg slowly

Child 2-12 yr: IM/IV 2-6 mcg/kg q4-8hr

Opiate dependence

Adult/adolescent ≥16 yr: SL 8 mg day 1, 16 mg days 2-4; subdermal: 4 implants inserted in the inner side of the upper arm

Hepatic Dose

Adult SL (severe hepatic disease): decrease dose by 50% initially

Available forms: **Inj** 0.3 mg/ml (1-ml vials); SL tab 2, 8 mg as base, **TD** system 5, 7.5, 10, 15, 20 mcg/hr (weekly); **oral dissolving film** (buccal); solution for injection extended release 100 mg/ 0.5 mL, 300 mg/1.5 mL; subdermal implant 74.2 mg/implant 75, 150, ✷ 300, 450, 600, 750, 900 mcg

ADVERSE EFFECTS

CNS: *Drowsiness, dizziness, confusion, headache, sedation, euphoria, hallucinations, strange dreams*
CV: Palpitations, QT prolongation, hypo/hypertension
EENT: blurred vision, *miosis,* diplopia
GI: *Nausea,* vomiting, anorexia, constipation, cramps, dry mouth, abdominal pain, hepatotoxicity
GU: urinary retention
INTEG: *Rash,* diaphoresis, pruritus
RESP: Respiratory depression, bronchospasm
MISC: Anaphylaxis, angioedema, dependency

INTERACTIONS

Individual drugs

Alcohol: increased respiratory depression, hypotension, sedation
Linezolid, methylene blue: Increased serotonin syndrome
Tramadol, trazadone: Increased seizure risk

Drug classifications

5-HT3 receptor antagonists, MAOIs, SSRIs, SNRIs, tricyclic antidepressants: Increased serotonin syndrome
Antidysrhythmics (class IA, III): increased QT prolongation
Antihistamines, antipsychotics, CNS depressants, Opioids, sedatives/hypnotics, skeletal muscle relaxants: increased respiratory depression, hypotension
Benzodiazepines: Increased chance of coma, death; do not use together
CYP3A4 inducers (carBAMazepine, PHENobarbital, phenytoin, rifAMPin): decreased buprenorphine effect
CYP3A4 inhibitors (erythromycin, indinavir, ketoconazole, ritonavir, saquinavir): increased buprenorphine effect

Drug/herb

Chamomile, kava, St. John's wort: increased CNS depression

NURSING CONSIDERATIONS

Assessment

• Assess **pain characteristics:** location, intensity, type, severity before medication administration and after treatment 5, 15, 30 min (IV)

> **BLACK BOX WARNING: Overdose:** Potential for overdose may occur from chewing, swallowing, snorting, or injecting extracted product from TD formulation

• **QT prolongation:** Assess often in those taking class Ia, III antidysrhythmics; patients with hypokalemia or cardiac instability (TD), max TD 20 mcg/hr q7 days

> **BLACK BOX WARNING: Respiratory depression:** Assess respiratory rate during treatment, do not combine with benzodiazepines

• Monitor VS after parenteral route; note muscle rigidity, product history, liver, kidney function tests, respiratory dysfunction: respiratory depression, character, rate, rhythm; notify prescriber if respirations are <10/min
• Monitor CNS changes: dizziness, drowsiness, hallucinations, euphoria, LOC, pupil reaction; withdrawal in opioid-dependent persons
• Monitor allergic reactions: rash, urticaria
• Monitor bowel pattern; severe constipation can occur

> **BLACK BOX WARNING: Accidental exposure:** Keep away from children and pets, may be fatal

---

• **Beers:** Avoid in older adults unless safer alternatives are available, may cause impaired psychomotor function, syncope
• **Pregnancy/breastfeeding:** Avoid use in pregnancy and breastfeeding, watch infant for decreased respiration, lethargy, decreased heart rate

Patient problems
Pain (uses)
Risk for injury (adverse reactions)

Implementation
• Give by inj (**IM**, **IV**), only with resuscitative equipment available; give slowly to prevent rigidity

SL route
• Do not chew, dissolve under tongue or take 2 or more at same time

Transdermal route (REMS)
• Apply to clean, dry, intact skin; each patch should be worn for 7 days, do not exceed dose, QTc prolongation may occur, may use first aid tape if edge of patch is not adhering

> **BLACK BOX WARNING:** Do not apply direct heat source to patch

• Apply to upper outer arm, upper chest/back, or side of chest

IM route
• Give deep in large muscle mass; rotate sites of inj

Subdermal route
• Inserted in inner side of upper arm
• Patient must be on a maintenance dose of 8 mg/day or less
• Follow manufacturer guidelines
• Available through the REMS program (844-859-6341); health care professional must complete training program
• Inserts are removed after 6 mo; if other inserts are not used after 6 mo, use transmucosal route

Subcut route (extended-release injection-Sublocade)
• Only inject in abdominal region. DO NOT use IM/IV
• Visually inspect for particulate matter, discoloration before use; product is clear, colorless to yellow to amber solution
• Give monthly with a minimum of 26 days between doses
• Only use the syringe and safety needle included. Do not attach the needle until the time of use

• Choose an injection site in the abdominal region. Do not inject into an area where the skin is irritated, reddened, bruised, infected, or scarred in any way
• Do not rub area after the injection. If bleeding occurs, use a gauze pad or bandage but only use minimal pressure
• Advise patient that there may be a lump for several weeks that decreases in size over time
• To avoid irritation, rotate the injection site with each injection
• The injection site should be examined for infection, evidence of tampering, or attempts to remove the depot
• *Storage:* Store unopened prefilled syringes in the refrigerator in the original packaging; do not freeze. Once outside the refrigerator this product may be stored in its original packaging at room temperature, 15° to 30° C (59° to 86° F), for up to 7 days prior to administration. Discard the injection if left at room temperature for longer than 7 days.

IV route
• **Give IV** direct undiluted over ≥3-5 min (0.3 mg/2 min); give slowly
• With antiemetic if nausea, vomiting occur
• When pain is beginning to return; determine dosage interval by patient response; rapid injection will increase side effects

Y-site compatibilities: Acyclovir, alfentanil, allopurinol, amifostine, amikacin, aminocaproic acid, amphotericin B liposome (AmBisome), anidulafungin, ascorbic acid injection, atenolol, atracurium, atropine, aztreonam, benztropine, bivalirudin, bleomycin, bumetanide, butorphanol, calcium chloride/gluconate, CARBOplatin, cefamandole, ceFAZolin, cefepime, cefotaxime, cefoTEtan, cefOXitin, cefTAZidime, ceftizoxime, cefTRIAXone, cefuroxime, chloramphenicol, chlorproMAZINE, cimetidine, cisatracurium, CISplatin, cladribine, clindamycin, cyanocobalamin, cyclophosphamide, cycloSPORINE, cytarabine, D₅W-dextrose 5%, DACTINomycin, DAPTOmycin, dexamethasone, dexmedetomidine, digoxin, dilTIAZem, diphenhydrAMINE, DOBUTamine, DOCEtaxel, DOPamine, doxacurium, DOXOrubicin HCl, doxycycline, enalaprilat, ePHEDrine, EPINEPHrine, epiRUBicin, epoetin alfa, eptifibatide, ertapenem, erythromycin, esmolol, etoposide, famotidine, fenoldopam, fentaNYL, filgrastim, fluconazole, fludarabine, gatifloxacin, gemcitabine, gentamicin, glycopyrrolate, granisetron, heparin, hydrocortisone, hydrOXYzine, IDArubicin, ifosfamide, imipenem-cilastatin, inamrinone, insulin (regular), irinotecan, isoproterenol, ketorolac, labetalol, lactated Ringer's injection, levofloxacin, lidocaine, linezolid, LORazepam, magnesium sulfate, mannitol, mechlorethamine, melphalan, meperidine, metaraminol, methicillin, methotrexate, methoxamine, methyldopate, methylPREDNISolone, metoclopramide, metoprolol, metroNIDAZOLE, mezlocillin, miconazole, midazolam, milrinone, minocycline, mitoXANtrone, morphine, moxalactam, multiple vitamins injection, mycophenolate mofetil, nafcillin, nalbuphine, naloxone, nesiritide, netilmicin, nitroglycerin, nitroprusside, norepinephrine, octreotide, ondansetron, oxacillin, oxaliplatin, oxytocin, palonosetron, pamidronate, pancuronium, papaverine, PEMEtrexed, penicillin G potassium/sodium, pentamidine, pentazocine, phenylephrine, phytonadione, piperacillin, piperacillin-tazobactam, polymyxin B, potassium chloride, procainamide, prochlorperazine promethazine, propofol, propranolol, protamine, pyridoxine, quiNIDine, raNITIdine, remifentanil, Ringer's injection, riTUXimab, rocuronium, sodium acetate, succinylcholine, SUFentanil, tacrolimus, teniposide, theophylline, thiamine, thiotepa, ticarcillin, ticarcillin-clavulanate, tigecycline, tirofiban, TNA (3-in-1), tobramycin, tolazoline, TPN, trastuzumab, trimetaphan, urokinase, vancomycin, vasopressin, vecuronium, verapamil, vinCRIStine, vinorelbine, voriconazole

Patient/family education
• Instruct patient to report any symptoms of CNS changes, allergic reactions
• Caution patients to avoid CNS depressants: alcohol, sedative/hypnotics for at least 24 hr after taking this product
• Teach patient to notify provider immediately if feeling faint, dizzy, or breathing is much slower than normal

> **BLACK BOX WARNING:** Advise that psychologic dependence leading to substance abuse may result when used for extended periods; long-term use is not recommended

SL route:
• Teach patient to place under tongue and allow to dissolve; do not double, skip doses

Transdermal route
• Teach patient how to apply and dispose of patch
• Teach patient not to use a heating pad or other heat source; do not cut, remove liner from adhesive layer, press firmly with hand for 30 sec, make sure edges are adhering to skin; when removing, fold, flush down toilet, use different site each time
• Advise to avoid driving, other hazardous activities until reaction is known

• Discuss with patient that dizziness, drowsiness, and confusion are common; to avoid getting up without assistance; to avoid hazardous activities
• Discuss in detail all aspects of the product
• Do not start new meds/herbs without prescriber approval
• Start stool softener/ laxatives to lessen constipation

Evaluation
Positive therapeutic outcome
• Relief of pain
• Decreased withdrawl symptoms when detoxifying

TREATMENT OF OVERDOSE:
Naloxone 0.4 mg ampule diluted in 10 ml 0.9% NaCl, give by direct **IV** push 0.02 mg q2min (adult)

---

buPROPion (Rx)
(byoo-proe'pee-on)
Aplenzin, Forfivo XL, Wellbutrin SR, Wellbutrin XL, Zyban
Func. class.: Antidepressant—miscellaneous, smoking deterrent
Chem. class.: Aminoketone

Do not confuse: buPROPion/busPIRone

ACTION: Inhibits reuptake of DOPamine, norepinephrine, serotonin

Therapeutic outcome: Decreased symptoms of depression after 2-3 wk

USES: Depression (Wellbutrin), smoking cessation (Zyban); seasonal affective disorder, substance abuse, glaucoma, smoking, cardiac disease, heart failure

Unlabeled uses: Attention-deficit/hyperactivity disorder (ADHD) (SR); increases libido in women

Pharmacokinetics
Absorption	Well absorbed; bioavailability poor
Distribution	Unknown
Metabolism	Liver extensively
Excretion	Kidneys
Half-life	14 hr, (antidepressant action)

Pharmacodynamics
Onset	Up to 4 wk
Peak	Unknown
Duration	Unknown

CONTRAINDICATIONS

Hypersensitivity, eating disorders, seizure disorder

Precautions: Pregnancy, breastfeeding, geriatric, renal/hepatic disease, recent MI, cranial, head trauma, stroke, intracranial mass, trauma, seizure disorders, substance abuse, glaucoma, smoking, cardiac disease, heart failure, Tourette's syndrome, tics, tobacco smoking, abrupt discontinuation

BLACK BOX WARNING: Children <18 yr, suicidal thinking/behavior (young adults)

DOSAGE AND ROUTES
Depression

Adult: PO 100 mg bid initially, then increase after 3 days to 100 mg tid if needed, max 150 mg single dose; **ER/SR**, initially 150 mg AM, increase to 300 mg/day if initial dose is tolerated, after no less than 4 days; after several wk, titrate to 200 mg bid; **Aplenzin** 174 mg qAM; may increase to 348 mg qAM on day 4; may increase to 522 mg after several weeks if needed; **Forfivo XL** (not for initial treatment) 450 mg q day after titration with another product (300mg/day × ≥ 2 wks)
Geriatric: PO 50-100 mg/day, may increase by 50-100 mg q3-4days

Hepatic Dose

Adult PO (moderate to severe hepatic disease): Aplenzin max 174 mg every other day

Smoking cessation (Zyban)

Adult: SR 150 mg q day × 3 days, then 150 mg bid for remainder of treatment, (7-12 wk)

Seasonal affective disorder

Adult: PO (Wellbutrin XL) 150 mg as a single dose in the AM, after 1 wk may be increased to 300 mg/day; (Aplenzin) 174 mg/day in AM, after 7 days may increase to 348 mg/day

Hepatic Dose

Adult PO (moderate-severe hepatic disease): Aplenzin max dose 174 mg every other day

Available forms: Tabs 75, 100 mg; sus rel tabs (**SR**), 100, 150, 200 mg; ext rel tab (XL) 100, 150, 300, 450 mg (SR-12 hr, XL-24 hr); ext rel tab (Aplenzin) 174, 348, 522 mg

ADVERSE EFFECTS

CNS: *Headache, agitation, confusion,* seizures, delusions, *insomnia, tremors,* dizziness, suicidal ideation, homicidal ideation, mania, hot flashes, myoclonia, chest pain, flushing
CV: Dysrhythmias, *hypertension,* chest pain
GI: *Nausea, vomiting, dry mouth,* anorexia, diarrhea, increased appetite, *constipation,* altered taste
INTEG: Photosensitivity
ENDO: Hypo-hyperglycemia, SIADH secretion

INTERACTIONS
Individual drugs

Alcohol, amantadine, haloperidol, levodopa, theophylline: increased risk of seizures
CarBAMazepine, cimetidine, PHENobarbital, phenytoin: decreased buPROPion effect
Citalopram: increased citalopram action

Drug classifications

Antidepressants, (SSRIs, tricyclics), benzodiazepines, beta blockers, corticosteroids, phenothiazines, steroids (systemic): increased risk of toxicity
MAOIs: increased risk of serious hypertension

Drug/herb

Kava, valerian: increased CNS depression

Drug/lab test

Positive urine drug screen for amphetamine possible

NURSING CONSIDERATIONS
Assessment

• Assess for increased risk of seizures; if patient has used CNS depressant or CNS stimulants, dosage of buPROPion should not be exceeded
• Monitor hepatic studies: AST, ALT, bilirubin if on long-term treatment
• Check weight weekly; appetite may increase with product

BLACK BOX WARNING: Assess mental status: mood, sensorium, affect, suicidal tendencies; increase in psychiatric symptoms: depression, panic

• Identify alcohol consumption; if alcohol was consumed, hold dose
• **Beers:** Avoid in older adults, lowers seizure threshold, may be acceptable in those with well-controlled seizures, where other treatment hasn't been effective

Patient problems

Nonadherence (teaching)

Implementation

• Give with food or milk for GI symptoms
• Give sugarless gum, hard candy, or frequent sips of water for dry mouth, do not crush, chew ext rel product
• When switching to Aplenzin from Wellbutrin, Wellbutrin SR, or XL use these equivalents: 174 buPROPion HBr = 150 mg buPROPion HCl; 348 mg buPROPion HBr = 300 mg buPROPion HCl; 522 mg buPROPion HBr = 450 mg buPROPion HCl
• **Wellbutrin immediate rel,** separate by ≥6 hr, give in 3 divided doses; **Wellbutrin SR,** if multiple doses are used, separate by ≥8 hr;

Wellbutrin XL, give q day in AM; **Zyban SR,** give in 2 divided doses ≥8 hr apart; **Aplenzin ER,** give q day in AM, a larger dose of Aplenzin is needed because these products are not equivalent

• Store at room temperature; do not freeze

Patient/family education

• Advise patients to notify all health care professionals of all Rx, OTC, herbals, supplements taken, not to start new products unless discussed with health care professional

• **Photosensitivity:** Use sunscreen, protective clothing to prevent burns

• Inform patient that extended release shell may be seen in stools

• Advise patient that lab work and continuing exams will be needed

• Teach patient that therapeutic effects may take 2-3 wk; not to increase dose without prescriber's approval; that treatment for smoking cessation lasts 7-12 wk

• Teach patient to use caution in driving or other activities requiring alertness because of drowsiness, dizziness, blurred vision; to avoid rising quickly from sitting to standing, especially geriatric

• Teach patient to avoid alcohol ingestion; alcohol may increase risk of seizures, obtain approval for other products

• Teach patient to take gum, hard sugarless candy, or frequent sips of water for dry mouth

• Advise patient not to use with nicotine patches unless directed by prescriber, may increase B/P

> **BLACK BOX WARNING:** Teach patient that risk of seizures increases when dose is exceeded or if patient has seizure disorder; suicidal ideas, behavior, hostility, depression may occur in children or young adults

• **Pregnancy/breastfeeding:** Teach patient to notify prescriber if pregnancy is suspected or planned or if breastfeeding

• Report hearing, visual, CNS changes

• May need to use stool softener/laxative

Evaluation
Positive therapeutic outcome

• Decrease in depression

• Absence of suicidal thoughts

• Smoking cessation

TREATMENT OF OVERDOSE:

ECG monitoring, induce emesis, lavage, administer anticonvulsant

---

bupropion/naltrexone (Rx)
(byoo-proe′ pee-on′nal-trex′one)
Contrave
Func. class.: Weight control product
Chem. class.: Aminoketone, opioid antagonist

ACTION: Bupropion/naltrexone consists of naltrexone, an opioid antagonist, and bupropion, a relatively weak inhibitor of the neuronal reuptake of dopamine and norepinephrine. Naltrexone and bupropion have effects on two separate areas of the brain involved in the regulation of food intake: the hypothalamus (appetite regulatory center) and the mesolimbic dopamine circuit (reward system)

Therapeutic outcome: Weight loss

USES: For the treatment of obesity as an adjunct to a reduced-calorie diet and increased physical activity

Pharmacokinetics

Bupropion	
Absorption	Well absorbed; bioavailability poor; high-fat meal enhances absorption
Distribution	Unknown
Metabolism	Liver extensively
Excretion	Kidneys
Half-life	21 hr
Naltrexone	
Absorption	Well absorbed; high-fat meal enhances absorption
Distribution	Enters breast milk
Metabolism	Liver extensively to active metabolites and parent drug
Excretion	Kidneys
Half-life	5-13 hr

Pharmacodynamics

Onset	Up to 4 wk
Peak	Unknown
Duration	Unknown

CONTRAINDICATIONS

Hypersensitivity, eating disorders, seizure disorder, uncontrolled hypertension, severe renal disease, MAOIs within 14 days, withdrawal of alcohol, benzodiazepines, barbiturates, anticonvulsants, pregnancy, lactation, children

Precautions: geriatric, renal/hepatic disease, recent MI, cranial, head trauma, stroke, intracranial mass, trauma, seizure disorders,

---

substance abuse, glaucoma, smoking, cardiac disease, heart failure, Tourette's syndrome, tics, tobacco smoking, abrupt discontinuation

> **BLACK BOX WARNING:** Children <18 yr, suicidal thinking/behavior (young adults), psychiatric events, suicidal ideation

DOSAGE AND ROUTES
Adults: PO Ext Rel Titrate to target dose during the first 4 wk of treatment, as follows: (week 1) 1 tablet (8 mg naltrexone/90 mg bupropion) qd in the morning, no evening dose; (week 2) 1 tablet bid in the morning and evening; (week 3) 2 tablets in the morning, 1 tablet in the evening; (week 4 and onward) 2 tablets bid in the morning and evening. Max daily dose: 32 mg/360 mg per day (2 tablets bid). Evaluate response after 12 wk at the maintenance dosage. If the patient has not lost at least 5% of baseline body weight, discontinue; **CYP2B6 inhibitors:** max 1 tab bid

Hepatic Dose
Adult: PO Max 1 tablet (8 mg naltrexone with 90 mg bupropion) qday each morning, do not use in severe hepatic disease (Child-Pugh class C)

Renal Dose
Mild renal impairment (CrCL 50 to 79 mL/minute): No change; *moderate to severe renal impairment (CrCl 30 to 49 mL/minute):* max 1 tablet (8 mg naltrexone with 90 mg bupropion) each morning and evening (max: 2 tablets/day); *severe renal impairment, end-stage renal disease (ESRD), or on dialysis (estimated GFR less than 30 mL/minute):* Do not use

Available forms: Tabs, ext rel 90 mg bupropion/8 mg naltrexone

ADVERSE EFFECTS
CNS: Headache, agitation, confusion, seizures, delusions, *insomnia, sedation, tremors,* tremor dizziness, akinesia, suicidal ideation, homicidal thoughts, mania
CV: *Hypertension, tachycardia*
EENT: Angle-closure glaucoma, tinnitus
GI: *Nausea, vomiting, dry mouth,* anorexia, diarrhea, increased appetite, *constipation,* altered taste, dry mouth
INTEG: Rash, pruritus, sweating, Stevens-Johnson syndrome, anaphylaxis
MISC: *Weight loss*

INTERACTIONS
Individual drugs
Alcohol, levodopa, theophylline: increased risk of seizures

CarBAMazepine, cimetidine, PHENobarbital, phenytoin: decreased buPROPion effect
Cimetidine: increased buPROPion levels
Ritonavir: increased buPROPion toxicity
Tamoxifen: decreased effect of tamoxifen

Drug classifications
Antidepressants, benzodiazepines, MAOIs, phenothiazines, steroids (systemic): increased risk of seizures, do not use together
CYP2D6/CYP2B6 inhibitors: increased buPROPion effect
CYP450, CYP2D6 products: decreased buPROPion effects
CYP2D6, CYP2B6 inducers: decreased buPROPion effect
MAOIs: acute toxicity, do not use within 14 days

Drug/lab test
Positive urine drug screen for amphetamine possible

NURSING CONSIDERATIONS
Assessment
• **Weight loss:** check weight baseline and periodically, weight loss should be significant within 12 wk or consider discontinuation
• Monitor B/P (with patient lying, standing), pulse q4hr; if systolic B/P drops 20 mm Hg hold product, notify prescriber; take vital signs more often in patients with CV disease
• Assess for increased risk of seizures if patient has used CNS depressant or CNS stimulants

> **BLACK BOX WARNING:** Assess mental status: mood, sensorium, affect, suicidal tendencies; increase in psychiatric symptoms: depression, panic, suicidal/homicidal ideation; notify provider of changes in mood with depression, panic immediately

• **Allergic reactions/anaphylaxis:** Monitor for allergic reactions during treatment (rash, hives, trouble breathing), discontinue and provide antihistamines if mild, or more aggressive treatment if severe

Patient problems
Excess food intake (uses)
Nonadherence (teaching)

Implementation
• Do not cut, chew, or crush
• May be given with or without food; avoid administering with high-fat meals because of significant increases in bupropion and naltrexone systemic exposure

Patient/family education

• Teach patient that therapeutic effects may take 2-3 wk; not to increase dose without prescriber's approval; that treatment for smoking cessation lasts 7-12 wk

• Teach patient to use caution in driving or other activities requiring alertness because of drowsiness, dizziness, blurred vision; to avoid rising quickly from sitting to standing, especially geriatric

• Teach patient to avoid alcohol ingestion; alcohol may increase risk of seizures, obtain approval for other products

• Teach patient to chew gum, eat hard sugarless candy, or take frequent sips of water for dry mouth

> **BLACK BOX WARNING:**
> • Teach patient that risk of seizures increases when dose is exceeded or if patient has seizure disorder; suicidal ideas, behavior, hostility, depression may occur in children or young adults

• Report hearing, visual, CNS changes

• Teach patient to notify prescriber if pregnancy is suspected or planned

Evaluation
Positive therapeutic outcome
• Weight loss

⚠ HIGH ALERT

busPIRone (Rx)
(byoo-spye′rone)
Buspirex ✖, **Bustab** ✖
Func. class.: Antianxiety, sedative
Chem. class.: Azaspirodecanedione

Do not confuse: busPIRone/buPROPion

ACTION: Acts by inhibiting the action of serotonin (5-HT) by binding to serotonin and DOPamine receptors; also increases norepinephrine metabolism

Therapeutic outcome: Decreased anxiety

USES: Generalized anxiety disorders

Pharmacokinetics

Absorption	Rapid
Distribution	Protein binding 86%
Metabolism	Liver, extensively (CYP3A4)
Excretion	Feces (30-40%)
Half-life	2-4 hr

Pharmacodynamics

Onset	Unknown
Peak	40-90 min
Duration	Unknown

CONTRAINDICATIONS
Hypersensitivity, child <18 yr, MAOIs

Precautions: Pregnancy, breastfeeding, geriatric, impaired renal/hepatic function

DOSAGE AND ROUTES
Adult: PO 7.5 mg bid; may increase by 5 mg/day q2-3days; max 60 mg/day

Renal/hepatic dose
Adult: PO reduce by 25%-50% in mild to moderate hepatic disease, do not use in severe hepatic disease; CCr 11-70 ml/min reduce dose by 25%-50%, CCr <10 ml/min do not use

Available forms: Tabs 5, 7.5, 10, 15, 30 mg

ADVERSE EFFECTS
CNS: *Dizziness, headache, stimulation, insomnia, nervousness, light-headedness, numbness, paresthesia, incoordination, tremors,* excitement
CV: *Tachycardia, palpitations,* hypo/hypertension, chest pain
EENT: *Sore throat, tinnitus, blurred vision, nasal congestion,* change in taste, smell
GI: *Nausea, dry mouth, diarrhea, constipation,* flatulence, increased appetite, rectal bleeding
GU: Frequency, hesitancy, change in libido
INTEG: *Rash,* edema, pruritus, alopecia, dry skin
MISC: *Sweating,* fatigue, fever, serotonin syndrome
MS: *Pain, weakness,* muscle cramps, myalgia
RESP: Hyperventilation, chest congestion, shortness of breath

INTERACTIONS
Individual drugs
Alcohol: increased CNS depression; avoid use

Drug classifications
CYP3A4 (erythromycin, itraconazole, nefazodone, ketoconazole, ritonavir, verapamil, dilTIAZem, several other protease inhibitors): increased busPIRone levels
MAOIs, procarbazine: increased B/P, do not use together
Products induced by CYP3A4 inducers (rifAMPin, phenytoin, PHENobarbital, carBAMazepine, dexamethasone): decreased busPIRone action
Psychotropics: increased CNS depression, avoid use
CYP3A4 inhibitors (erythromycin, ketoconazole, itraconazole, ritonavir): increased buspirone action
Selective serotonin reuptake inhibitors (SNRIs, serotonin receptor agonists): increase serotonin syndrome

---

Drug/herb

Chamomile, kava, valarian: increased CNS depression

Drug/food

Grapefruit juice: increased peak concentration of busPIRone

NURSING CONSIDERATIONS

Assessment

• Assess anxiety reaction: inability to sleep, apprehension, dread, foreboding, or uneasiness related to unidentified source of danger

• Assess for previous product dependence or tolerance; if patient is product dependent or tolerant, amount of medication should be restricted

• Monitor B/P (lying, standing), pulse; if systolic B/P drops 20 mm Hg, hold product, notify prescriber; check I&O; may indicate renal dysfunction

• Monitor mental status: mood, sensorium, affect, sleeping patterns, drowsiness, dizziness, suicidal tendencies; withdrawal symptoms when dose is reduced or product discontinued

• Assess for CNS reaction, some reactions may be unpredictable

• **Pregnancy/breastfeeding:** Avoid in pregnancy/breastfeeding

• **Beers:** Avoid in older adults with delirium or a high risk of delirium

Patient problems
Implementation

• Give with food or milk for GI symptoms (avoid grapefruit juice); sugarless gum, hard candy, frequent sips of water for dry mouth

• May be crushed

Patient/family education

• Teach patient that product may be taken consistently with or without food; if dose is missed take as soon as remembered; do not double doses

• Caution patient to avoid OTC medications unless approved by the prescriber; to avoid alcohol ingestion and other psychotropic medications unless prescribed; that 2 wk of therapy may be required before therapeutic effects occur; to avoid large amounts of grapefruit juice; max effect 3-6 wk

• Caution patient to avoid driving and activities requiring alertness since drowsiness may occur; until medication response is known, tell patient that drowsiness may worsen at beginning of treatment

• Instruct patient not to discontinue medication abruptly after long-term use; if dose is missed, do not double

• Advise patient to rise slowly or fainting may occur, especially in geriatric

• **Serotonin syndrome:** Teach patient to report immediately (fever, tremor, sweating, diarrhea, delirium)

Evaluation
Positive therapeutic outcome

• Increased well-being

• Decreased anxiety, restlessness, sleeplessness, dread

busulfan (Rx)

(byoo-sul′fan)

Busulfex, Myleran

Func. class.: Antineoplastic alkylating agent

Chem. class.: Bifunctional alkylating agent

Do not confuse: Alkeran/Myleran

ACTION: Changes essential cellular ions to covalent bonding with resultant alkylation; this interferes with normal biological function DNA; activity is not phase specific; action is due to myelosuppression

Therapeutic outcome: Prevention of rapid growth of malignant cells in chronic myelocytic leukemia

USES: Chronic myelocytic leukemia, bone marrow ablation, stem cell transplant preparation in CML

Pharmacokinetics

Absorption	Rapidly absorbed
Distribution	Unknown; crosses placenta
Metabolism	Live, extensively
Excretion	Kidneys, breast milk
Half-life	2.5 hr

Pharmacodynamics

Unknown

CONTRAINDICATIONS

Pregnancy (3rd trimester), breastfeeding, radiation, chemotherapy, blastic phase of chronic myelocytic leukemia, hypersensitivity

Precautions: Child-bearing age men and women, leukopenia, thrombocytopenia, anemia, hepatotoxicity, renal toxicity, seizures, tumor lysis syndrome, hyperkalemia, hyperphosphatemia, hypocalcemia, hyperuricemia

BLACK BOX WARNING: Neutropenia, secondary malignancy, thrombocytopenia

DOSAGE AND ROUTES
Chronic myelocytic leukemia

Adult: PO 4-8 mg/day or 1.8-4 mg/m²/day initially; reduce dosage if WBC levels reach 30,000-40,000/mm³; stop if WBC ≤20,000/mm³; maintenance 1-3 mg/day

Child: PO 0.06-0.12 mg/kg/day or 1.8-4.6 mg/m²/day, reduce if WBC is 30,000-40,000/mm³; discontinue if WBC ≤20,000/mm³

Allogenic hemopoietic stem cell transplantation

Adult: **IV** 0.8 mg/kg over 2 hr, q6hr × 4 days (total 16 doses); give cyclophosphamide **IV** 60 mg/kg over 1 hr/day for 2 days, starting after 16th dose of busulfan

Available forms: Tabs 2 mg; sol for inj 6 mg/ml

ADVERSE EFFECTS

CV: *Hypotension*, thrombosis, *chest pain*, tachycardia, atrial fibrillation, heart block, pericardial effusion, cardiac tamponade (high dose with cyclophosphamide)
GI: Anorexia, constipation, dry mouth, nausea, vomiting, *diarrhea*
RESP: Alveolar hemorrhage, atelectasis, cough, hemoptysis, hypoxia, pleural effusion, pneumonia, sinusitis, pulmonary fibrosis
CNS: *Depression, dizziness, insomnia, headache*
EENT: *Blurred vision*
GU: Impotence, sterility, amenorrhea, gynecomastia, renal toxicity, hyperuremia, adrenal insufficiency–like syndrome
HEMA: Thrombocytopenia, leukopenia, pancytopenia, severe bone marrow depression
INTEG: Dermatitis, hyperpigmentation, alopecia
MISC: Chromosomal aberrations
RESP: Irreversible pulmonary fibrosis, pneumonitis
• Advise patient that contraception is needed during treatment and for ≥3 months after the completion of therapy (pregnancy); avoid breastfeeding; may cause infertility; discuss family planning before initiating therapy

INTERACTIONS
Individual drugs
Acetaminophen, itraconazole, decreased busulfan clearance
Cyclophosphamide: cardiac tamponade
Phenytoin: decreased busulfan level
Radiation: increased toxicity, bone marrow suppression
Thioguanine: hepatotoxicity

Drug classifications
Anticoagulants, salicylates: increased risk of bleeding
Antineoplastics: increased toxicity, bone marrow suppression
Live virus vaccines: decreased antibody reaction

Drug/lab test
False positive: breast, bladder, cervix, lung cytology tests

NURSING CONSIDERATIONS
Assessment
• Monitor CBC, differential, platelet count weekly; withhold product for WBC <15,000/mm³; notify prescriber of results; institute thrombocytopenia precautions, levels to withhold product are different in children

> **BLACK BOX WARNING:** Assess bone marrow status prior to chemotherapy; bone marrow suppression may be prolonged (up to 2 mo); seizure history

• **Pulmonary fibrosis:** Monitor pulmonary function tests, chest x-ray films before, during therapy; chest film should be obtained q2wk during treatment; check for dyspnea, crackles, nonproductive cough, chest pain, tachypnea; pulmonary fibrosis may occur up to 10 yr after treatment with busulfan
• Assess for increased uric acid levels, swelling, joint pain primarily in extremities; patient should be well hydrated to prevent urate deposits
• Monitor renal function studies: BUN, serum uric acid, urine CCR before, during therapy; I&O ratio; report fall in urine output of 30 ml/hr; check for hyperuricemia
• Monitor for cold, fever, sore throat (may indicate beginning infection); identify edema in feet, joint, or stomach pain, shaking; prescriber should be notified
• Assess for bleeding: hematuria, guaiac, bruising or petechiae, mucosa or orifices q 8 hr; no rectal temps

> **BLACK BOX WARNING:** Assess for secondary malignancy within 5-8 yr of chronic oral therapy, long-term follow-up may be required

Patient problems
Risk for injury (adverse reactions)

Implementation
• Give 1 hr before or 2 hr after meals to lessen nausea and vomiting; give at same time daily
• Increased fluid intake to 2-3 L/day to prevent grain deposits, calcium formations
• Administer antibiotics for prophylaxis of infection; may be prescribed since infection potential is high

Intermittant IV infusion route
• Prepared in biologic cabinet using gloves, gown, mask; dilute with 10 times the volume of product with D5W or 0.9% NaCl (0.5 mg/ml), when withdrawing product, use needle with

5 micron filter provided, remove amount needed, remove filter and inject product into diluent; always add product to diluent, not vice versa; stable for 8 hr at room temperature (using D5W) or 12 hr refrigerated; give by central venous catheter over 2 hr q6hr x 4 days, use infusion pump, do not admix
• Give antiemetics before IV route, on schedule; in those with history of seizures, give phenytoin before IV route, to prevent seizures using 0.9% NaCl)

Y-site compatibilities: Acyclovir, amphotericin B lipid complex, amphoteracin B liposome, anidulafungin, atenolol, bivalirudin, bleomycin, caspofungin, codeine, daptomycin, dexmedetomidine, diltizem, docetaxel, ertapenem, gatifloxacin, granisetron, hydromorphone, nesiritide, ocetreotide acetate, ondesetron, palsonosetron, pancuronium, piperacillin tazobactam, ritTUXimab, sodium acetate, tacrolimus, tigecycline, tirofiban, trastuzumab, vasopressin

Patient/family education
• Teach patient to avoid use of products containing aspirin or ibuprofen, razors, commercial mouthwash since bleeding may occur; to report symptoms of bleeding (hematuria, tarry stools)

• Instruct patient to report signs of anemia (fatigue, headache, irritability, faintness, shortness of breath), jaundice, congestion, skin pigmentation, darkening of skin, sudden weakness, weight loss (may resemble adrenal insufficiency)
• Instruct patient to report any changes in breathing or coughing, even several months after treatment; to avoid crowds and persons with respiratory tract or other infections
• Teach patient that hair loss may occur; discuss the use of wigs or hair pieces
• Advise patient that contraception is needed during treatment and for ≥3 months after completion of therapy (pregnancy D); avoid breastfeeding; may cause infertility; discuss family planning before initial therapy

Evaluation
Positive therapeutic outcome
• Decreased leukocytes to normal limits
• Absence of sweating at night
• Increased appetite, increased weight

butoconazole vaginal antifungal
See Appendix B

RARELY USED

C1 esterase inhibitor subcutaneous, human
Haegarda

USES: For the routine prophylaxis to prevent hereditary angioedema attacks

DOSAGE AND ROUTES
For the treatment of acute attacks of hereditary angioedema (HAE)
Adult and adolescent: ≥ 84 kg IV Inject 4200 International Units (2 vials) as a slow intravenous injection over approximately 5 min; may give a second dose

Adult and adolescent: < 84 kg IV Inject 50 International Units per kg body weight up to 4200 International Units as a slow intravenous injection over approximately 5 min; may give second dose

For routine angioedema prophylaxis in patients with hereditary angioedema
Adult/adolescent: SUBCUT 60 International Units/kg twice weekly (every 3 or 4 days)

CONTRAINDICATIONS
Leporine protein hypersensitivity

cabazitaxel (Rx)
(ka-baz_i-tax_el)
Jevtana
Func. class.: Antineoplastic
Chem. class.: Taxane

ACTION: A taxane that binds to tubulin and inhibits microtubule depolymerization, cell division, cell cycle arrest (G2/M) phase, cell proliferation; unlike other taxanes, this product may be useful for treating multidrug-resistant tumors

Therapeutic outcome: Decreased tumor size, spread of malignancy

USES: Hormone-refractory prostate cancer in combination with prednisone in patients that have been previously treated with a docetaxel-containing regimen

Pharmacokinetics

Absorption	89%-92% protein binding, primarily bound to albumin and lipoproteins
Distribution	Equally distributed between blood and plasma
Metabolism	Extensively metabolized by CYP3A4/5 in the liver and CYP2C8 to a lesser extent
Excretion	80% eliminated within 2 wk mainly in feces
Half-life	Half-life alpha, beta, gamma of 4 min, 2 hr, 95 hr respectively

Pharmacodynamics

Onset	Unknown
Peak	Infusion's end
Duration	Unknown

CONTRAINDICATIONS
Hypersensitivity to this product, pregnancy

BLACK BOX WARNING: Hypersensitivity to polysorbate 80, neutropenia (ANC 1500/mm^3)

Precautions: Breastfeeding, children, diarrhea, elderly, hepatic disease, renal disease, sepsis, vomiting

DOSAGE AND ROUTES
Adult: IV INF 25 mg/m^2 over 1 hr on day 1 with predniSONE 10 mg/day continuously; give q3wk cycles for up to 10 cycles

Hepatic dose
Adult: IV INF do not use if total bilirubin ULN or AST and/or ALT _1.5 times ULN

Available forms: Solution for injection 60 mg/1.5 ml

ADVERSE EFFECTS
CNS: *Peripheral neuropathy, dysgeusia, dizziness, headache, fatigue, fever*
CV: Dysrhythmia, peripheral edema, hypotension
GI: *Diarrhea, nausea, vomiting, constipation, abdominal pain, dyspepsia, anorexia*
GU: Renal failure, dehydration, hematuria, urinary tract infection, dysuria, obstructive uropathy, infertility
HEMA: Neutropenia, febrile neutropenia, anemia, leukopenia, thrombocytopenia
MS: Back pain, arthralgia, muscle spasms
RESP: Cough, dyspnea
SYST: Fatal infections, sepsis, anaphylaxis

INTERACTIONS
Individual drugs
Radiation: increased bone marrow depression

Drug classifications
Other antineoplastics: increased bone marrow depression
Strong CYP3A4 inhibitors (conivaptan, chloramphenicol, danazol, dalfopristin, delavirdine, ethinyl estradiol, fluvoxamine, imatinib, isoniazid, tipranavir, troleandomycin, zafirlukast, ketoconazole, itraconazole, clarithromycin,

atazanavir, indinavir, nefazodone, nelfinavir, ritonavir, saquinavir, telithromycin, voriconazole); mild or moderate CYP3A4 inhibitors (basiliximab, fluoxetine, niCARdipine, ranolazine, amiodarone, darunavir, diltiazem, miconazole, mifepristone [RU-486], posaconazole, propoxyphene, tamoxifen, erythromycin, verapamil, fluconazole): increased cabazitaxel concentrations

CYP3A4 inducers (rifampin, phenytoin, carBAMazepine, rifabutin, rifapentine): decreased cabazitaxel concentrations

Vaccines: decreased immune response

NURSING CONSIDERATIONS
Assessment
• **Assess for symptoms of anaphylaxis:** hypotension, dyspnea, generalized urticaria, bronchospasm, discontinue immediately; keep emergency equipment near; usually occurs during the first or second infusion, do not use this product again after severe hypersensitivity reactions
• Check infusion site for reactions: if given by regular **IV**, not port (redness, inflammation, warmth)
• **Assess for bone marrow depression:** monitor CBC with differential, prior to and after 1 wk, withhold if WBC <1500/mm³ or platelets <100,000/mm³. May not be a concern if an erythropoietin agent is given
• Assess for neurological side effects: peripheral neuropathy, dizziness, headache. During infusion of product, ice extremities periodically, may prevent peripheral neuropathy
• Assess for musculoskeletal reactions: back pain, arthralgia, muscle spasms
• **Monitor for renal failure:** monitor BUN, creatinine, and serum electrolytes; usually associated with sepsis, dehydration, or obstructive uropathy; renal failure has been fatal
• **Assess for bleeding:** bruising, petechiae, hematuria, blood in emesis or stools; check mucosa orifices for stomatitis, obtain order for vicious Xylocaine if needed
• Monitor temp periodically, increased temperature may indicate beginning infection
• Monitor hepatic studies: AST, ALT, bilirubin, LDH, prior to and periodically; jaundice of skin, eyes, clay-colored stools, dark urine, itching skin, abdominal pain, fever, diarrhea
• Identify effects of alopecia on body image, discuss feelings about body changes

Patient problems
• Risk for infection (adverse reactions)
• Risk for injury (adverse reactions)
• Lack of knowledge of medication (teaching)

Implementation
• Use cytotoxic handling procedures
• Obtain neutrophil counts prior to administration, count should be _1500/mm³
• Do not use PVC infusion containers or polyurethane infusion sets for preparation or administration
• Premedicate with diphenhydramine 25 mg IV or equivalent, dexamethasone 8 mg or equivalent and ranitidine 50 mg or equivalent and antiemetics
• Do not use solution if it is discolored or if particulate is present; solution should be clear, yellow to brownish; discard if first or second dilution is not clear; remove immediately if solution comes in contact with skin

Intermittent IV infusion
• Two dilutions are required, both product and dilution are overfilled; first dilution: mix each vial of product (60 mg/1.5 ml) with the entire contents of supplied diluent (10 mg/ml); when transferring diluent, direct needle on side of vial and inject slowly to limit foaming; remove syringe and needle and gently mix by several inversions, do not shake; let stand for a few min; second dilution: withdraw the required dose, further dilute the withdrawn product with 0.9% NaCL or D5 in a PVC-free container; remove syringe and needle; mix by gently inverting the bag/bottle (final concentration 0.1-0.26 mg/ml); if a dose of 65 mg use a larger volume of infusion solution, so the concentration is max 0.26 mg/ml; do not mix with other drugs; solution may crystallize over time, discard if this occurs; use solution within 8 hr (room temperature), 24 hr (refrigerated); give over 1 hr, use 0.22 micrometer in-line filter

Patient/family education
• **Instruct patient to use a nonhormonal form of contraception** and to notify prescriber if pregnancy is planned or suspected, pregnancy category (D); not to breastfeed
• Advise patient that hair may be lost during treatment; a wig or hairpiece may make the patient feel better; new hair will be different in color, texture
• Instruct patient to avoid receiving vaccinations while using this product
• **Teach patient to report signs of infection:** fever, sore throat, flulike symptoms; avoid persons with known respiratory infections

Evaluation
Positive therapeutic outcome
• Decreased size, spread of malignancy

cabergoline
(ka-ber'goe-leen)
Func. class.: Hyperprolactinemic
Chem. class.: Dopamine agonists

ACTION: Acts as a dopamine agonist to reduce prolactin secretion

USES: Hyperprolactinemia, pituitary adenoma

Pharmacokinetics

Absorption	Well
Distribution	Widely to pituitary, protein binding 40%
Metabolism	Liver extensively via hydrolysis
Excretion	Minimal urine, unchanged
Half-life	65-69 hr

Pharmacodynamics

Onset	Unknown
Peak	1-3 hr
Duration	Unknown

CONTRAINDICATIONS

Hypersensitivity to this product or ergots; severe hypertension; pulmonary, pericardial, cardiac valvular, or retroperitoneal fibrotic disorders

Precautions: Pregnancy, breastfeeding

DOSAGE AND ROUTES

Adult: PO 0.25 twice weekly, may be increased after 4 wk, max 1 mg twice weekly

Available forms: Tablet 0.5 mg

SIDE EFFECTS

CNS: *Dizziness,* fatigue, *headache,* poor impulse control (sex, food, gambling), paresthesia, depression
CV: Postural hypotension, hot flashes, CV fibrosis
EENT: Blurred vision
RESP: Pleural effusion, pulmonary fibrosis
GI: Constipation, nausea, retroperitoneal fibrosis
GU: Dysmenorrhea, breast soreness
INTEG: Rash

INTERACTIONS
Individual drugs
Haloperidol, metoclopramide: Decrease: effect of cabergoline, avoid using together

Drug classifications
Antihypertensives: Increase: hypotension
Phenothiazines, thioxanthenes: Decrease: effect of cabergoline, avoid using together
SSRIs, SNRIs: Increase: serotonin syndrome

NURSING CONSIDERATIONS
Assessment:
• Monitor serum prolactin levels baseline and monthly, chest x-ray, echocardiogram, LFTs
• **Orthostatic hypotension:** Monitor B/P baseline and periodically, as hypotension may occur and may be worse if taking antihypertensives
• **Pulmonary fibrosis:** Assess for dry cough, dyspnea, inability to lie down to sleep, edema in extremities; use chest X-ray and/or CT scan baseline and periodically to confirm
• **CV effects:** Monitor ECG baseline and q 6-12 months, assess for coughing, dyspnea, murmurs that may indicate valvular heart disease, if these occur, product should be discontinued
• Pregnancy: Identify if pregnancy is planned or suspected or if breastfeeding; do not use in pregnancy or breastfeeding

Patient problems
Risk for injury (uses)

Implementation:
• Give without regard to food

Patient/family education:
• **Pituitary adenoma:** Teach patient to immediately report blurred vision, severe headaches, nausea, vomiting
• Advise patient to rise slowly to minimize orthostatic hypotension
• Inform patient to avoid use of alcohol or tobacco products while taking this product
• Advise patient to notify provider of impulse control disorders (sexual, eating, gambling)
• Inform the patient dizziness, drowsiness may occur and not to drive or engage in other hazardous activities until response is known
• Teach patient that follow-up exam and blood work will be needed
• Teach patient to take as prescribed; if dose is missed, take when remembered if within 2 days
• Pregnancy: Advise patient to notify prescriber if pregnancy is planned or suspected, not to breastfeed, and to use nonhormonal contraception while taking this product

Evaluation:
• Positive therapeutic outlook: decreasing prolactin secretion, decrease galactorrhea

calcitonin (salmon) (Rx)
Calcimar ✦, Miacalcin
Func. class.: Parathyroid agents (calcium regulator)
Chem. class.: Polypeptide hormone

Do not confuse: Fortical/Foradil

ACTION: Decreases bone resorption, blood calcium levels; increases deposits of calcium in bones; opposes parathyroid hormone

Therapeutic outcome: Lowered calcium level, decreasing symptoms of Paget's disease

USES: Paget's disease, postmenopausal osteoporosis, hypercalcemia

Pharmacokinetics

Absorption	Completely absorbed (IM/subcut)
Distribution	Unknown
Metabolism	Rapid; kidneys, tissue, blood
Excretion	Kidneys, inactive metabolite
Half-life	1 hr

Pharmacodynamics

	SUBCUT/IM	Nasal
Onset	15 min	Rapid
Peak	4 hr	30 min
Duration	8-24 hr	Unknown

CONTRAINDICATIONS
Hypersensitivity to this product or fish

Precautions: Pregnancy, breastfeeding, children, hypotension, hypocalcemia, secondary malignancy

DOSAGE AND ROUTES
Postmenopausal osteoporosis
Adult: SUBCUT/IM 100 units/day; **nasal** 200 units (1 spray) alternating nostrils daily

Paget's disease
Adult: SUBCUT/IM 100 units daily, maintenance 50-100 units daily or every other day

Hypercalcemia
Adult: SUBCUT/IM 4 units/kg q12hr, increase to 8 units/kg q12hr if response is unsatisfactory, may increase to 8 units/kg q 6 hr if needed after 2 more days

Available forms: Inj 200 units/ml; nasal spray 200 units/actuation

ADVERSE EFFECTS
CNS: Headache (nasal), tetany, chills, weakness, dizziness, fever, tremors
CV: Chest pressure, hypertension
EENT: Nasal congestion
GI: Nausea, diarrhea, vomiting, anorexia (IM/SUBCUT)
GU: Diuresis, nocturia, urine sediment, frequency (IM/subcut)
INTEG: Rash, flushing, inj site reaction
MS: Backache, myalgia, arthralgia (nasal)
RESP: Dyspnea, flulike symptoms
SYST: Anaphylaxis

INTERACTIONS
Individual drugs
Lithium: decreased lithium effect, monitor lithium level

Drug classifications
Disphosphonates (Paget's disease): decreased effect of nasal spray, monitor for adequate effect

NURSING CONSIDERATIONS
Assessment
• **Anaphylaxis, hypersensitivity:** Assess for inability to breathe, rash, fever; have emergency equipment nearby
• Assess for GI symptoms, polyuria, flushing, head swelling, tingling, headache; may indicate **hypercalcemia**; nervousness, irritability, twitching, seizures, spasm, paresthesia indicate **hypocalcemia** during beginning of treatment
• Identify nutritional status; check diet for sources of vit D (milk, some seafood), calcium (dairy products, dark green vegetables), phosphates
• **Postmenopausal osteoporosis:** Monitor BUN, creatinine, uric acid, chloride, electrolytes, urine pH, urinary calcium, magnesium, phosphate, urinalysis; vit D 50-135 international units/dl), alkaline phosphatase baseline and q3-6mo; check urine sediment for casts throughout treatment; monitor urine hydroxyproline in Paget's disease, biochemical markers of bone formation/absorption, radiologic evidence of fracture; bone density (osteoporosis)
• **Toxicity (can occur rapidly):** Assess for increased product level, since toxic reactions occur rapidly; have parenteral calcium or gluconate on hand if calcium level drops too low; check for tetany (irritability, paresthesia, nervousness, muscle twitching, seizure, tetanic spasm)

Patient problem
Pain (uses)

Implementation
Test dose
• Dilute 10 units/mL, withdraw 0.5 mL and add to 1 mL 0.9% NaCl for injection give intradermally (0.1 mL) on forearm, check after 15 min, if reaction is more than mild, do not use
SUBCUT route
• Rotate inj sites, check for injection site reaction
IM route
• **Give** after test dose of 10 international units/ml, 0.1 ml intradermally; watch 15 min; **give** only with EPINEPHrine and emergency meds available

• IM inj in deep muscle mass slowly; rotate sites; preferred route if volume is >2 ml, use within 2 hr of reconstitution

Nasal route
• Use alternating nostrils for nasal spray; store in refrigerator, allow to warm to room temperature, prime to get full spray
• Discard after 30 days

Patient/family education
• Advise patients to report difficulty swallowing or change in side effects to prescriber immediately
• **Pregnancy/breastfeeding:** Advise prescriber if pregnancy is planned or suspected, avoid breastfeeding

SUBCUT route/ IM route
• Teach method of inj if patient will be responsible for self-medication
• Instruct patient to notify prescriber for hypercalcemic relapse: renal calculi, nausea, vomiting, thirst, lethargy, deep bone or flank pain
• Teach patient that warmth and flushing occur and last 1 hr
• Provide a low-calcium diet as prescribed (Paget's disease, hypercalcemia)

Postmenopausal osteoporosis
• Teach patient to take vitamin D and calcium as directed
• Teach patient that nausea, vomiting, and facial flushing occur often

Nasal route
• Teach patient to use alternating nostrils for nasal spray; use after warming to room temperature, prime to get full spray, discard after 30 days, report serious symptoms of rhinitis
• Advise patients with osteoporosis to increase calcium and vit D in diet and to continue with moderate exercise to prevent continued bone loss

Evaluation
Positive therapeutic outcome
• Calcium levels 9-10 mg/dl
• Decreasing symptoms of Paget's disease, including pain
• Decreased bone loss in osteoporosis

calcitriol (Rx)
(kal-si-tree′ole)
Calcijex ✦, Rocaltrol, Silkis ✦
Func. class.: Parathyroid agent (calcium regulator)
Chem. class.: Vitamin D hormone

Do not confuse: calcitriol/Calciferol

ACTION: Increases intestinal absorption, renal reabsorption of calcium, provides calcium for bones, increases renal tubular resorption of phosphate

Therapeutic outcome: Calcium at normal level

USES: Hypocalcemia in chronic renal disease, hyperparathyroidism, pseudohypoparathyroidism, psoriasis, renal osteodystrophy

Pharmacokinetics

Absorption	Well absorbed (PO), complete (IV)
Distribution	To liver, crosses placenta, protein binding >99%
Metabolism	Liver, undergoes hepatic recycling
Excretion	Bile
Half-life	4-8 hr

Pharmacodynamics

	PO	IV
Onset	2-6 hr	Unknown
Peak	10-12 hr	Unknown
Duration	Up to 5 days	Unknown

CONTRAINDICATIONS
Hypersensitivity, hyperphosphatemia, hypercalcemia, vit D toxicity

Precautions: Pregnancy, breastfeeding, renal calculi, CV disease

DOSAGE AND ROUTES
Hypocalcemia, on dialysis
Adult and child ≥6 yr: PO 0.25 mcg/day; **IV** 0.5 mcg (0.01 mcg/kg)[33] × per wk, may increase by 0.25-0.5 mcg/dose q 2-4 wk
Child 1-5 yr: PO 0.25-2 mcg/day; **IV** 0.01-0.05 mcg/kg[33] × per wk

Hypoparathyroidism
Adult and child ≥6 yr: PO 0.25 mcg/day, may increase q2-4wk, maintenance 0.5-2 mcg/day
Child 1-5 yr: PO 0.25-0.75 mcg daily
Child <1 yr: PO 0.04-0.08 mcg/kg/day

Available forms: Caps 0.25, 0.5 mcg; inj 1 mcg/ml, 2 mcg/ml; oral sol 1 mcg/ml; top 3 mcg/g

ADVERSE EFFECTS
CNS: Drowsiness, headache, vertigo
CV: Palpitations, edema, hypertension, dysrhythmias
ENDO: Hypercalcemia
EENT: Blurred vision, photophobia, rhinorrhea
GI: Nausea, vomiting, jaundice, anorexia, dry mouth, constipation, cramps, pancreatitis metallic taste
GU: Polyuria, hematuria, thirst, azotemia, albuminuria
MS: Myalgia, arthralgia, weakness

SYST: Anaphylaxis
INTEG: Pain at injection site, rash, pruritus

INTERACTIONS
Individual drugs
Cholestyramine, mineral oil: decreased absorption of calcitriol, avoid concurrent use
Phenytoin: increased vit D metabolism
Verapamil: increased dysrhythmias use cautiously

Drug classifications
Antacids (magnesium): increased hypermagnesemia
Calcium supplements, diuretics (thiazide): increased hypercalcemia
Cardiac glycosides: increased dysrhythmias
Vitamin D products: increased toxicity
Vitamins (fat-soluble): decreased calcitriol absorption

Drug/food
Large amounts of high-calcium foods may cause hypercalcemia

Drug/lab test
Increase: AST/ALT, BUN, creatinine
False: increase cholesterol
Interference: alkaline phosphatase, electrolytes

NURSING CONSIDERATIONS
Assessment
• **Vitamin D deficiency:** Assess baseline and periodically
• Assess GI symptoms, polyuria, flushing, head swelling, tingling, headache; may indicate hypercalcemia
• **Hypercalcemia:** dry mouth, metallic taste, polyuria, bone pain, muscle weakness, headache, fatigue, change in LOC, anorexia, nausea, vomiting, cramps, diarrhea, twitching
• **Hypocalcemia:** Assess for dysrhythmias, constipation, confusion, paresthenia, twitching
• Identify nutritional status; check diet for sources of vit D (milk, some seafood), calcium (dairy products, dark green vegetables), phosphates
• Monitor calcium phosphate 2 × per wk at beginning treatment; serum calcium, PTH, alkaline phosphatase q mo (calcium should be kept at 9-10 mg/dl; vit D 50-135 units/dl)

Patient problem
Impaired nutritional intake (uses)

Implementation
PO route
• Do not break, crush, or chew caps
• Give with meals for GI symptoms
• Store protected from light, heat, moisture

Topical route
• Rub into skin

IV route
• **Hypocalcemia** Give by direct **IV** over 1 min through catheter at hemodialysis conclusion

Patient/family education
• Teach patient the symptoms of hypercalcemia (renal stones, nausea, vomiting, anorexia, lethargy, thirst, bone or flank pain) and about foods rich in calcium
• Advise patient to follow prescribed diet, to avoid products with high levels of sodium: cured meats, dairy products, cold cuts, olives, beets, pickles, soups, meat tenderizers in chronic renal failure, usually to avoid potassium: oranges, bananas, dried fruit, peas, dark green leafy vegetables, milk, melons, beans in chronic renal failure
• Advise patient to avoid OTC products containing calcium, potassium, or sodium in chronic renal failure; to take as prescribed, not to double or skip doses
• Advise patient to avoid large doses of vitamins or supplements
• Instruct patient to monitor weight weekly; maintain fluid intake

Evaluation
Positive therapeutic outcome
• Calcium levels 9-10 mg/dl
Treatment of overdose:
• Discontinue treatment, IV hydration, diuretics, hemodialysis

calcium acetate (OTC)
(kal′see-um ass′e-tate)
Calphron, Eliphos, PhosLo, Phoslyra

calcium carbonate (PO-OTC, Rx)
Alka-Mints, Amitone, Apo-Cal ✿, BioCal, Calcarb, Calci-Chew, Calciday, Calci-Mix, Calcite ✿, Calglycine ✿, Cal-Plus, Calsan ✿, Caltrate, Chooz, Dicarbosil Equilet, Gencalc, Liqui-cal, Maalox Antacid, Os-Cal, Rolaids Extra Strength Soft-chew, Tums, Tums E-X
Func. class.: Antacid, calcium supplement
Chem. class.: Calcium product

Do not confuse: Os-Cal/Asacol

ACTION: Neutralizes gastric acidity

Therapeutic outcome: Neutralized gastric acidity; calcium at normal levels

USES: Antacid, calcium supplement

✿ Canada only   ⚠ Genetic Warning   Adverse effects: *italics* = common; red = life-threatening

Pharmacokinetics

Absorption	⅓ absorbed by small intestines, must have adequate vit D for absorption
Distribution	Extracellular fluid
Metabolism	Unknown
Excretion	Feces, crosses placenta, excreted in breast milk
Half-life	Unknown

Pharmacodynamics

Onset	Unknown
Peak	Unknown
Duration	Unknown

CONTRAINDICATIONS
Hypersensitivity, hypercalcemia

Precautions: Pregnancy, breastfeeding, geriatric, fluid restriction, decreased GI motility, GI obstruction, dehydration, renal disease, hyperparathyroidism, bone tumors

DOSAGE AND ROUTES
Hypocalcemia prevention, osteoporosis
Adult: PO 1-2 g

Chronic hypocalcemia
Adult: PO 2-4 g/day elemental calcium (5-10 g calcium carbonate) in 3-4 divided doses
Child: PO 45-65 mg/kg/day elemental calcium (112.5-162.5 mg/kg calcium carbonate) in 4 divided doses
Neonate: PO 50-150 mg/kg/day elemental calcium (125-375 mg/kg/day in 4-6 divided doses, max 1 g/day)

Supplementation
Child: PO 45-65 mg/kg/day

Hyperphosphatemia
Adult: PO (acetate) 1334 mg with meals

Heartburn, dyspepsia, hyperacidity (OTC)
Adult: PO 1-2 tabs q2hr, max 9 tabs/24 hr (Alka-mints); chew 2-4 tab q1hr prn, max 16 tabs (Tums regular strength); chew 2-4 tab q1hr prn, max 10 tabs (Tums E-X); chew 2-3 tabs q1hr prn, max 10 tabs/24 hr (Tums Ultra)

Available forms: Calcium carbonate: chewable tabs 350, 420, 450, 500, 750, 1000, 1250 mg; **tabs** 500, 600, 650, 667, 1000, 1250, 1500 mg; **gum** 300, 450 500 mg; **susp** 1250 mg/5 ml; **caps** 1250 mg; **powder** 6.5 g/packet; **calcium acetate: tabs** 667 mg (169 mg Ca), **caps** 500 mg (125 mg Ca); **gelcaps:** 667 mg (169 mg elemental Ca)

ADVERSE EFFECTS
GI: *Constipation,* anorexia, nausea, vomiting, diarrhea
GU: Calculi, hypercalciuria

INTERACTIONS
Individual drugs
Atenolol, etidronate, phenytoin, risedronate, ketoconazole: decreased levels of each drug
Digoxin: increased toxicity from hypercalcemia
QuiNIDine: increased quiNIDine levels

Drug classifications
Amphetamines: increased levels of amphetamines
Calcium channel blockers, calcium supplements, fluoroquinolones, iron products, salicylates, tetracyclines: PO decreased levels of each specific product
Thiazide diuretics: increased hypercalcemia

Drug/food
Cereal, spinach, decreased calcium supplement effect

Drug/lab test
Decrease: phosphates
False increase: chloride
False decrease: magnesium, oxalate, lipase
False positive: benzodiazepines

NURSING CONSIDERATIONS
Assessment
• Monitor Ca^+ (serum, urine); Ca^+ should be 8.5-10.5 mg/dl, urine Ca^+ should be 150 mg/day
• **Assess for milk-alkali syndrome:** nausea, vomiting, disorientation, headache
• Assess for constipation; increase bulk in the diet if needed
• Assess for **hypercalcemia:** headache, nausea, vomiting, confusion; **hypocalcemia:** paresthesia, twitching, colic, dysrhythmias, Chvostek's/Trousseau's sign
• Assess those taking digoxin for toxicity
• Assess those taking for abdominal pain, heartburn, indigestion before, after administration
• **Pregnancy/breastfeeding:** Considered compatible with breastfeeding

Patient problem
Impaired nutritional intake (uses)

Implementation
PO route
• Administer as antacid 1 hr after meals and at bedtime
• Administer as supplement 1½ hr after meals and at bedtime
• Administer only with regular tablets or capsules; do not give with enteric-coated tablets
• Administer laxatives or stool softeners if constipation occurs

Patient/family education
- **Pregnancy/breastfeeding:** Considered to be compatible with breastfeeding
- Advise patient not to switch antacids unless directed by prescriber, not to use as antacid for >2 wk without approval by prescriber
- Teach patient that therapeutic dose recommendations are figured as elemental calcium
- Advise to avoid excessive use of alcohol, caffeine, tobacco
- Teach to avoid spinach, cereals, dairy products in large amounts
- **Hypocalcemia:** Advise patient to report confusion, memory loss, muscle spasms
- **Hypercalcemia:** Advise patient to report nausea, vomiting, constipation, confusion
- Teach patient to avoid other products with calcium (supplements, antacids)

Evaluation
Positive therapeutic outcome
- Absence of pain, decreased acidity
- Decreased hyperphosphatemia in renal failure (Acetate)

CALCIUM SALTS
calcium acetate
calcium chloride (Rx)
calcium citrate (OTC)
Cal-Citrate
Citracal
calcium glubionate
Kalcinate
calcium gluceptate (Rx)
calcium gluconate (Rx)
calcium phosphate (OTC)
calcium lactate
Cac-Lac
tricalcium phosphate
Posture
Func. class.: Electrolyte replacement—calcium product

ACTION: Calcium needed for maintenance of nervous, muscular, skeletal systems, enzyme reactions, normal cardiac contractility, coagulation of blood; affects secretory activity of endocrine, exocrine glands

Therapeutic outcome: Calcium at normal level, absence of increased magnesium, potassium

USES: Prevention and treatment of hypocalcemia, hypermagnesemia, hypoparathyroidism, neonatal tetany, cardiac toxicity caused by hyperkalemia, lead colic, hyperphosphatemia, vit D deficiency, osteoporosis prophylaxis, calcium antagonist toxicity (calcium channel blocker toxicity)

Pharmacokinetics
Absorption	Complete (**IV**)
Distribution	Readily extracellular fluid; crosses placenta, protein binding 40%-50%
Metabolism	Liver
Excretion	Feces (80%), kidney (20%), breast milk
Half-life	Unknown

Pharmacodynamics
	PO	IV
Onset	Unknown	Immediate
Peak	Unknown	Rapid
Duration	Unknown	½-1½ hr

CONTRAINDICATIONS
Hypercalcemia, digoxin toxicity, ventricular fibrillation, renal calculi

Precautions: Pregnancy, breastfeeding, children, renal disease, respiratory disease, cor pulmonale, digitalized patient, respiratory failure, diarrhea, dehydration

DOSAGE AND ROUTES
>> **Acute hypocalcemia:**
Adults: IV 7-14 mEq; **for tetany**, 4.5-16 mEq.
Child/infant: 1-7 mEq. **For tetany**, 0.5-0.7 mEq/kg tid-qid.

>> **For nutritional supplementation:**
PO (any oral calcium salt; dosage expressed as elemental calcium):
Adults: PO 1-2 g
Child: PO 45-65 mg/day

Available forms:
Calcium chloride: Injection 10% (1.36 mEq); calcium glubionate: syrup 1.8 g/5 mL; calcium gluconate: Tabs 500, 650, 975 mg, 1.2 g; Calcium citrate: tabs 250 mg; Calcium lactate: tabs 325, 500, 650 mg; tricalcium phosphase 600 mg

ADVERSE EFFECTS
CV: Bradycardia, dysrhythmias; cardiac arrest (**IV**)
GI: Vomiting, nausea, constipation
GU: Hypercalcemia, renal calculi
META: Hypercalcemia
INTEG: Pain, burning at **IV** site, extravasation

INTERACTIONS
Individual drugs
Atenolol: decreased effect
Phenytoin, tetracyclines, thyroid: decreased absorption when calcium is taken PO

DilTIAZem, verapamil: decreased effects, increased toxicity

Drug classifications
Antacids: milk-alkali syndrome (renal disease)
Digoxin glycosides: increased dysrhythmias
Diuretics (thiazide): increased hypercalcemia
Fluoroquinolones: decreased absorption of fluoroquinolones when calcium is taken PO
Iron salts: decreased absorption of iron when calcium is taken PO

Drug/herb
Lily of the valley, pheasant's eye, shark cartilage, squill: increased side effects, action

Drug/food
Cereal, spinach: Decreased calcium absorption

Drug/lab test
Increased: calcium

NURSING CONSIDERATIONS
Assessment
• **Monitor ECG for decreased QT interval and T-wave inversion during rapid administration:** in hypercalcemia, product should be reduced or discontinued
• Monitor calcium levels during treatment (9-10 mg/dl is normal level), urine calcium if hypercalciuria occurs
• Assess cardiac status: rate, rhythm, CVP (PWP, PAWP if being monitored directly)
• Assess digitalized patients closely, an increase in calcium increases digoxin toxicity risk
• **Hypocalcemia:** Assess for muscle twitching, paresthesia, dysrhythmias, laryngospasm

Patient problems
Impaired nutritional intake (uses)

Implementation
PO route
• Give PO with or following meals to enhance absorption
• Store at room temperature
IM route
• Can cause severe tissue necrosis, do not use IM
• Do not give chloride, or gluconate IM
IV route
• Warm to room temperature, administer **IV** undiluted or diluted with equal amounts of 0.9% NaCl for inj to a 5% sol; give 0.5-1 ml/min, give slowly, rapid administration may cause cardiac arrest
• Give through small-bore needle into large vein; do not use scalp vein if extravasation occurs, necrosis will result (**IV**); IM inj may cause severe burning, necrosis, and tissue sloughing; warm sol to body temp before administering (only gluconate/glucceptate)

• Provide seizure precautions: padded side rails, decreased stimuli (noise, light); place airway suction equipment, padded mouth gag if calcium levels are low
• Patient should remain recumbent 30 min after IV dose, drop in B/P may result

>> Calcium chloride

Y-site compatibility: Acyclovir, alemtuzumab, alfentanil, amikacin, aminocaproic acid, aminophylline, amiodarone, anidulafungin, argatroban, arsenic trioxide, ascorbic acid injection, asparaginase, atenolol, atracurium, atropine, azithromycin, aztreonam, benztropine, bivalirudin, bleomycin, bumetanide, buprenorphine, butorphanol, calcium gluconate, CARBOplatin, carmustine, caspofungin acetate, cefotaxime, cefoTEtan, cefOXitin, ceftaroline, ceftizoxime, chloramphenicol, chlorothiazide, chlorpheniramine, chlorproMAZINE, cimetidine, CISplatin, clindamycin, cloxacillin, colistimethate, cyanocobalamin, cyclophosphamide, cycloSPORINE, cytarabine, DACTINomycin, DAPTOmycin, DAUNOrubicin, dexmedetomidine, dexrazoxane, digoxin, dilTIAZem, diphenhydrAMINE, DOBUTamine, DOCEtaxel, dolasetron, DOPamine, doxacurium, doxapram, DOXOrubicin, doxycycline, edetate calcium disodium, enalaprilat, ePHEDrine, EPINEPHrine, epiRUBicin, epoetin alfa, eptifibatide, ergonovine, ertapenem, erythromycin, esmolol, etoposide, etoposide phosphate, famotidine, fenoldopam, fentaNYL, fluconazole, fludarabine, furosemide, gallamine, gallium, ganciclovir, gatifloxacin, gemcitabine, gentamicin, glycopyrrolate, granisetron, heparin sodium, HYDROmorphone, hydrOXYzine, IDArubicin, ifosfamide, inamrinone, insulin, regular, irinotecan, isoproterenol, kanamycin, labetalol, lactated Ringer's, lepirudin, leucovorin, lidocaine, lincomycin, linezolid, LORazepam, mannitol, mechlorethamine, meperidine, mephentermine, mesna, metaraminol, methohexital, methotrexate, methyldopate, metoclopramide, metoprolol, metroNIDAZOLE, micafungin, midazolam, milrinone, minocycline, mitoMYcin, mitoXANtrone, mivacurium, morphine, moxifloxacin, multiple vitamins injection, mycophenolate mofetil, nafcillin, nalbuphine, nalorphine, naloxone, nesiritide, niCARdipine, nitroglycerin, nitroprusside, norepinephrine, octreotide, ondansetron, oxytocin, PACLitaxel (solvent/surfactant), pancuronium, papaverine, penicillin G potassium/sodium, pentazocine, PENTobarbital, PHENobarbital, phentolamine, phenylephrine, phytonadione, piperacillin-tazobactam, polymyxin B, potassium, potassium chloride, procainamide, prochlorperazine, promazine, promethazine, propranolol, protamine,

C

pyridoxine, quinupristin-dalfopristin, raNITI-dine, Ringer's injection, rocuronium, streptomycin, succinylcholine, SUFentanil, tacrolimus, teniposide, theophylline, thiamine, thiotepa, ticarcillin-clavulanate, tigecycline, tirofiban, TNA (3-in-1), tobramycin, tolazoline, topotecan, trimetaphan, tubocurarine, urokinase, vancomycin, vasopressin, vecuronium, verapamil, vinBLAStine, vinCRIStine, vinorelbine, voriconazole

Calcium gluconate Y-site compatibilities: Acyclovir, aldesleukin, alemtuzumab, alfentanil, allopurinol, amifostine, amikacin, aminocaproic acid, aminophylline, amiodarone, anidulafungin, argatroban, arsenic trioxide, ascorbic acid injection, asparaginase, atenolol, atracurium, atropine, azaTHIOprine, azithromycin, aztreonam, benztropine, bivalirudin, bleomycin, bumetanide, buprenorphine, butorphanol, calcium chloride, CARBOplatin, carmustine, caspofungin, cefamandole, ceFAZolin, cefepime, cefoperazone, cefotaxime, cefoTEtan, cefOXitin, ceftaroline, cefTAZidime, ceftizoxime, cefuroxime, chloramphenicol sodium succinate, chlorothiazide, chlorpheniramine, chlorproMAZINE, cimetidine, ciprofloxacin, cisatracurium, CISplatin, cladribine, clindamycin, cloxacillin, codeine, colistimethate, cyanocobalamin, cyclophosphamide, cycloSPORINE, cytarabine, DACTINomycin, DAPTOmycin, DAUNOrubicin, DAUNOrubicin liposome, dexmedetomidine, dexrazoxane, digoxin, dilTIAZem, dimenhyDRINATE, diphenhydrAMINE, DOBUTamine, DOCEtaxel, dolasetron, DOPamine, doripenem, doxacurium, doxapram, DOXOrubicin, DOXOrubicin liposomal, doxycycline, edetate calcium disodium, enalaprilat, ePHEDrine, EPINEPHrine, epiRUBicin, epoetin alfa, eptifibatide, ergonovine, ertapenem, erythromycin, esmolol, etoposide, etoposide phosphate, famotidine, fenoldopam, fentaNYL, filgrastim, fludarabine, fluorouracil, folic acid (as sodium salt), furosemide, gallamine, gallium, ganciclovir, gatifloxacin, gemcitabine, gentamicin, glycopyrrolate, granisetron, heparin sodium, HYDROmorphone, hydrOXYzine, IDArubicin, ifosfamide, insulin, regular, irinotecan, isoproterenol, kanamycin, ketamine, labetalol, lactated Ringer's injection, lepirudin, leucovorin, levofloxacin, lidocaine, lincomycin, linezolid, LORazepam, magnesium sulfate, mannitol, mechlorethamine, melphalan, meperidine, mephentermine, mesna, metaraminol, methohexital, methotrexate, methyldopate, metoclopramide, metoprolol, metroNIDAZOLE, micafungin, midazolam, milrinone, mitoMYcin, mitoXANtrone, mivacurium, morphine, moxifloxacin, multiple vitamins injection, nafcillin, nalbuphine, nalorphine, naloxone, nesiritide, netilmicin, niCARdipine, nitroglycerin, nitroprusside, norepinephrine, octreotide, ondansetron, oritavancin, oxaliplatin, oxytocin, PACLitaxel (solvent/surfactant), palonosetron, pancuronium, papaverine, penicillin G potassium/sodium, pentamidine, pentazocine, PENTobarbital, PHENobarbital, phentolamine, phenylephrine, phytonadione, polymyxin B, potassium acetate/chloride, procainamide, prochlorperazine, promazine, promethazine, propofol, propranolol, protamine, pyridoxine, quiNIDine, raNITIdine, remifentanil, Ringer's, riTUXimab, rocuronium, sargramostim, sodium acetate, streptomycin, succinylcholine, SUFentanil, tacrolimus, telavancin, teniposide, theophylline, thiamine, thiotepa, ticarcillin, ticarcillin-clavulanate, tigecycline, tirofiban, TNA (3-in-1), tobramycin, tolazoline, TPN (2-in-1), trastuzumab, trimethaphan, tubocurarine, urokinase, vancomycin, vasopressin, vecuronium, verapamil, vinBLAStine, vinCRIStine, vinorelbine, vitamin B complex with C, voriconazole

Patient/family education

• **Pregnancy/breastfeeding:** Considered to be compatible with breastfeeding
• Advise patient not to switch antacids unless directed by prescriber, not to use as antacid for >2 wk without approval by prescriber
• Teach patient that therapeutic dose recommendations are figured as elemental calcium
• Advise to avoid excessive use of alcohol, caffeine, tobacco
• Teach to avoid spinach, cereals, dairy products in large amounts
• **Hypocalcemia:** Advise patient to report confusion, memory loss, muscle spasms
• **Hypercalcemia:** Advise patient to report nausea, vomiting, constipation, confusion
• Teach patient to avoid other products with calcium (supplements, antacids)

Evaluation
Positive therapeutic outcome
• Decreased twitching, paresthesias, muscle spasms
• Absence of tremors, seizures, dysrhythmias, dyspnea, laryngospasm, negative Chvostek's sign, negative Trousseau's sign

canagliflozin
(kan'a-gli-floe'zin)
Invokana
Func. class.: Oral antidiabetic
Chem. class.: Sodium glucose cotransporter 2, SGLT-2 inhibitor

ACTION: Blocks reabsorption by the kidney, increases glucose excretion, lowers blood glucose concentrations by inhibiting proximal renal tubular sodium glucose transporter 2 (SGLT2)

Therapeutic outcome: Improved signs/symptoms of diabetes mellitus (decreased polyuria, polydipsia, polyphagia; clear sensorium; absence of dizziness; stable gait

USES: Type 2 diabetes mellitus, with diet and exercise, may use in combination

Pharmacokinetics

Absorption	Well PO
Distribution	99% protein binding, extensive to all tissues
Metabolism	By UGT1A9, UGT2B4
Excretion	33% in urine
Half-life	10 hr

Pharmacodynamics

Onset	Unknown
Peak	Unknown
Duration	Up to 24 hr

CONTRAINDICATIONS

Dialysis, renal failure, hypersensitivity, breastfeeding, diabetic ketoacidosis

Precautions: Pregnancy, children, renal/hepatic disease, hypothyroidism, hyperglycemia, hypotension, pituitary insufficiency, type 1 diabetes mellitus, malnutrition, fever, dehydration, adrenal insufficiency, geriatrics

> **BLACK BOX WARNING:** Lower limb amputation

DOSAGE AND ROUTES

Adult: PO eGFR ≥60 mL/min/1.73 m² 100 mg/day, may increase to 300 mg/day
Renal dose
Adult: PO eGFR 45-59 ml/min/1.73 m², max 100 mg/day; <45 ml/min/1.73 m², do not use

Available forms: Tabs 100, 300 mg

ADVERSE EFFECTS

GU: Candidiasis, urinary frequency, polydipsia, polyuria, renal impairment
INTEG: Photosensitivity, rash, pruritus
META: Hypercholesterolemia, lipidemia, hypoglycemia, hyperkalemia, hypermagnesemia, hyperphosphatemia, hypersensitivity, ketoacidosis
MISC: Bone fractures
CV: Hypotension, orthostatic hypotension

INTERACTIONS
Individual drugs
Baclofen, cycloSPORINE, estrogen, isoniazid, tacrolimus: decreased effect, hyperglycemia
Gatifloxacin: do not use concurrently
Lithium: increased or decreased glycemic control
Increase: Hyperkalemia, potassium-sparing diuretics

Drug classifications
ACE inhibitors, angiotensin II receptor antagonists, β-blockers, bile acid sequestrants, fibric acid derivatives, insulin, MAOIs, salicylates, sulfonylureas: increased hypoglycemia, monitor for hypoglycemia
Atypical antipsychotics, carbonic anhydrase inhibitors, corticosteroids, digestive enzymes, intestinal absorbents, loop diuretics, oral contraceptives, phenothiazines, progestins, protease inhibitors, sympathomimetics, thiazide diuretics: decreased effect, hyperglycemia

Drug/lab tests
Increase: Magnesium, phosphate, uric acid, serum creatinine
Decrease: Serum glucose, eGFR
UGT inducers PHENobarbital, ritonavir; dose may need to be increased

NURSING CONSIDERATIONS
Assessment
• Assess for hypoglycemia (weakness, hunger, dizziness, tremors, anxiety, tachycardia, sweating), hyperglycemia; even though product does not cause hypoglycemia, if patient is on sulfonylureas or insulin, hypoglycemia may be additive; if hypoglycemia occurs, treat with dextrose, or, if severe, with IV glucagon

> **BLACK BOX WARNING:** Lower limb amputation: monitor frequently for wound complications; inspect feet, wounds for new ulcerations

• Monitor for stress, surgery, or other trauma that may require a change in dose
• Monitor A1c q3mo, serum glucose; 1 hr PP throughout treatment; serum cholesterol, serum creatinine/BUN, serum electrolytes
• **Bone fractures:** Monitor bone density, other conditions that may lead to bone fractures, fractures may occur within 3 mo of starting therapy
• **Renal impairment:** Monitor those with renal disease more frequently, increased creatinine, BUN may occur, monitor for increased creatinine, eGFR may be decreased

Patient problem
Impaired nutritional intake (uses)

Implementation
PO route
• Once daily with first meal of the day
• Adjust dose in times of stress, surgery, trauma
• Store at room temperature

Patient/family education
• Teach patient the symptoms of hypoglycemia/hyperglycemia, what to do about each
• Instruct patient that medication must be taken as prescribed; explain consequences of discontinuing

medication abruptly; that insulin may need to be used for stress, including trauma, fever, surgery, to take as soon as remembered if dose is missed unless close to next dose, then skip and take at next dose, do not take double dose

• Instruct patient to avoid OTC medications and herbal supplements unless discussed with health care professional

• Instruct patient that diabetes is a lifelong illness; that the diet and exercise regimen must be followed; that this product is not a cure

• Instruct patient to carry emergency ID and glucose source

• Teach patient that blood glucose monitoring is required to assess product effect

> **BLACK BOX WARNING:** Instruct patient to notify prescriber of new ulcerations, inspect feet daily

• **Yeast infections (women/men):** Advise women that yeast infections can occur with this product, women (vaginal), men (penile), to report discharge, itching, swelling

• **Pregnancy/breastfeeding:** To advise prescriber if pregnancy is planned or suspected or if breastfeeding

• **Ketoacidosis:** Advise patient to notify prescriber immediately of nausea, vomiting, lack of appetite, sleepiness, difficulty breathing

Evaluation

Therapeutic response: improved signs/symptoms of diabetes mellitus (decreased polyuria, polydipsia, polyphagia; clear sensorium, absence of dizziness, stable gait)

candesartan (Rx)

(can-deh-sar′tan)

Atacand

Func. class.: Antihypertensive

Chem. class.: Angiotensin II receptor (type AT₁)

Do not confuse: Atacand/antacid

ACTION: Blocks the vasoconstrictor and aldosterone-secreting effects of angiotensin II; selectively blocks the binding of angiotensin II to the AT₁ receptor found in tissues

Therapeutic outcome: Decreased B/P, decreased heart failure–related complications or death

USES: Hypertension, alone or in combination; heart failure NYHA Class II-IV and ejection fraction ≤40%, diabetic nephropathy in hypertension and diabetes (type 2)

Pharmacokinetics

Absorption	Well absorbed
Distribution	Protein binding >90%
Metabolism	Minimal
Excretion	Feces, urine, breast milk
Half-life	9 hr

Pharmacodynamics (antihypertensive action)

Onset	2-4 hr
Peak	4 wk
Duration	24 hr

CONTRAINDICATIONS

Hypersensitivity

> **BLACK BOX WARNING:** Pregnancy

Precautions: Breastfeeding, children, geriatric, hypersensitivity to ACE inhibitors, volume depletion, renal/hepatic impairment, renal artery stenosis, hypotension, electrolyte abnormalities

DOSAGE AND ROUTES

Hypertension

Adult: PO (single agent) 16 mg daily initially in patients who are not volume depleted, range 8-32 mg/day; with diuretic or volume depletion, 8-32 mg/day as a single dose or divided bid

Adult and child ≥6 yr and weight >50 kg: PO 8-16 mg/day or divided bid, adjust to B/P, usual range 4-32 mg/day max 32 mg/day

Child ≥6 yr and weight <50 kg: PO 4-8 mg/day or divided bid, adjust to B/P

Child ≥1 yr and <6 yr: PO 0.2 mg/kg/day in 1 dose or divided in 2 doses/day, adjust B/P, max 0.4 mg/kg/day, max 16 mg/day

Heart failure

Adult: PO 4 mg/day, may be doubled ≥2 wk, target dose 32 mg/day

Renal/hepatic dose

Adult: PO ≤8 mg/day in severe renal disease/moderate hepatic disease, adjust dose as needed

Available forms: Tabs 4, 8, 16, 32 mg

ADVERSE EFFECTS

CNS: *Dizziness,* fatigue, headache, syncope, insomnia

CV: Chest pain, peripheral edema, hypotension, palpitations

EENT: Sinusitis, rhinitis, pharyngitis

GI: *Diarrhea,* nausea, abdominal pain, vomiting

GU: Renal dysfunction

MS: Arthralgia, back pain, myalgia

SYST: Angioedema, hypersensitivity reactions

INTERACTIONS
Individual drugs
Lithium: increased lithium level

Drug classifications
ACE inhibitors, β-blockers, calcium channel blockers, diuretics, MAOIs: increased hypotension

Diuretics (potassium sparing): increased hypokalemia

Cox 2 inhibitors, NSAIDs, salicylates: decreased hypotensive effect

Potassium-sparing diuretics, potassium salt substitutes, potassium supplements: Increased hyperkalemia, check potassium levels

Drug/herb
Astragalus, cola tree: increased or decreased antihypertensive effect

Black licorice, Ephedra: decreased antihypertensive effect

Hawthorn: increased antihypertensive effect

Drug/Lab
Increase: albumin, ALT/AST, potassium

NURSING CONSIDERATIONS
Assessment
Hypertension: Assess B/P, pulse q4hr; note rate, rhythm, quality, notify prescriber of significant changes

• **Serious hypersensitivity reactions:**
Assess for angioedema, anaphylaxis; facial swelling, difficulty breathing (rare)

• **Heart failure:** Monitor for jugular vein distention, weight, peripheral edema, dyspnea, crackles

• Monitor electrolytes: potassium, sodium, chloride; hyperkalemia is more common with other diuretics

• Assess blood studies: BUN, creatinine, liver function tests before treatment, liver function studies, BUN, creatinine may be increased

• Assess for skin turgor, dryness of mucous membranes for hydration status; correct volume depletion

> **BLACK BOX WARNING:** Assess for pregnancy; pregnancy/breastfeeding: this product can cause fetal death when given in pregnancy, breastfeeding

Patient problem
Nonadherance (teaching)

Implementation
• Administer without regard to meals
• Oral liquid (compounded) shake well, do not freeze

Patient/family education
• If a dose is missed, instruct patient to take as soon as possible, unless it is within 1 hour before next dose

> **BLACK BOX WARNING: Pregnancy/breastfeeding:** Advise patient to inform prescriber if pregnancy is planned or suspected, or if breastfeeding

• **Hypersensitivity:** Advise patient to report immediately difficulty breathing, hives, swelling of face, lips

• Teach patient to notify prescriber of fever, swelling of hands and feet, irregular heartbeat, chest pain

• Advise patient that excessive perspiration, dehydration, diarrhea may lead to fall in blood pressure—consult prescriber if these occur

• Inform patient that product may cause dizziness, fainting; light-headedness may occur, not to drive or operate machinery until effect is known

• Advise patient that continuing blood work and follow-up exams will be needed

• Inform patient to limit potassium foods or salt substitutes containing potassium or supplements with potassium unless approved by health care professional

• Advise patient to avoid all OTC medications unless approved by prescriber; to inform all health care providers of medication use, full effect 4 wk, onset 2 wk, that product may be taken with or without meals, to store at room temperature

• Caution patient to rise slowly to sitting or standing position to minimize orthostatic hypotension

• **Hypertension:** Teach proper technique for obtaining B/P and acceptable parameters; to continue to follow other requirements (no smoking, weight loss/exercise)

Evaluation
Positive therapeutic outcome
• Decreased B/P, decreased heart failure–related complications, death

> **⚠ HIGH ALERT**
>
> ## capecitabine (Rx)
> (cap-eh-sit'ah-bean)
> **Xeloda**
> *Func. class.:* Antineoplastic, antimetabolite
> *Chem. class.:* Fluoropyrimidine carbamate

Do not confuse: Xeloda/Xenical

ACTION: Competes with substrate of DNA synthesis, thus interfering with cell replication in the S phase of cell cycle (before mitosis); also interferes with RNA and protein synthesis; product is converted to 5-fluorouracil (5-FU)

Therapeutic outcome: Decreasing spread of cancer cells

USES: Metastatic breast cancer, after failure with PACLitaxel and anthracycline colorectal cancer when 5-FU monotherapy is preferred; treatment of patients with colorectal cancer who have undergone complete resection of their primary tumor

Pharmacokinetics

Absorption	Readily absorbed, decreased with food
Distribution	Unknown
Metabolism	Liver, extensively
Excretion	Kidneys
Half-life	45 min

Pharmacodynamics

Onset	Unknown
Peak	1½ hr
Duration	Unknown

CONTRAINDICATIONS
Pregnancy, infants, hypersensitivity to 5-FU, severe renal impairment (CCr <30 ml/min), ⁂ DPD deficiency

Precautions: Renal/hepatic/cardiac disease, breastfeeding, children, geriatric patients, radiation therapy, DPD deficiency ⁂

> **BLACK BOX WARNING:** Anticoagulant therapy

DOSAGE AND ROUTES
Adult: PO 1250 mg/m² bid × 14 days, then 7 day rest period, use in 3 wk cycles

Renal dose
Adult: PO CCr 30-50 ml/min; decrease initial dose to 75% of usual dose; CCr < 30 ml/min contraindicated

Available forms: Tabs 150, 500 mg

ADVERSE EFFECTS
CNS: Dizziness, headache, *paresthesia, fatigue,* insomnia
CV: Edema, chest pain
GI: *Nausea, vomiting, anorexia, diarrhea, stomatitis, abdominal pain, constipation, dyspepsia,* intestinal obstruction, necrotizing enterocolitis, hyperbilirubinemia, hepatic failure
HEMA: Neutropenia, lymphopenia, thrombocytopenia, anemia
INTEG: *Hand and foot syndrome,* dermatitis, nail disorder, alopecia, rash
MISC: Eye irritation, edema, myalgia, limb pain, *pyrexia,* dehydration, renal impairment, Stevens Johnson syndrome
RESP: *Cough, dyspnea,* pulmonary embolism

INTERACTIONS
Individual drugs
Leucovorin: increased toxicity, monitor for toxicity
Phenytoin: increased phenytoin level, monitor phenytoin level

Drug classifications
Antacids (aluminum, magnesium): increased capecitabine absorption

> **BLACK BOX WARNING:** Anticoagulants: NSAIDs, salicylates, platelet inhibitors, thrombolytics; increased risk of bleeding, monitor PT and INR

Food/drug
Increased absorption; give within 30 min of a meal

Drug/lab test
Increased: bilirubin
Decreased: Hgb/Hct/RBC, neutrophils, platelets, WBC

NURSING CONSIDERATIONS
Assessment
• **Bone marrow suppression:** Monitor CBC, differential, platelet count weekly; withhold product if WBC <1000/mm³ or platelet count is <50,000/mm³ or RBC, Hct, Hgb is low; notify prescriber of results; frequently monitor INR in those receiving warfarin
• Assess buccal cavity q8hr for dryness, sores or ulceration, white patches, pain, bleeding, dysphagia; obtain prescription for viscous lidocaine (Xylocaine)
• Assess symptoms indicating severe allergic reaction: rash, pruritus, urticaria, purpuric skin lesions, itching, flushing; product should be discontinued
• **Assess for hand/foot syndrome, Stevens Johnson syndrome:** paresthesia, tingling, painful/painless swelling, blistering, erythema with severe pain of hands/feet; toxicity divided into grade 1, 2, 3; if grade 2 or 3, product should be discontinued until grade 1
• **Assess for GI toxicity:** severe diarrhea (multiple times/day or at night), nausea, vomiting, stomatitis, adjust dose, stop treatment if severe
• Monitor liver function tests before and during therapy (bilirubin, AST, ALT, LDH) as needed or monthly; note jaundice of skin or sclera, dark urine, clay-colored stools, itchy skin, abdominal pain, fever, diarrhea

> **BLACK BOX WARNING: Assess for bleeding:** hematuria, stool guaiac, bruising or petechiae, mucosa or orifices q8hr; inflammation of mucosa, breaks in skin, monitor INR and PT in those taking coumarin-derivative anticoagulants, adjustment of dose may be needed

---

Patient problem
Risk for infection (adverse reactions)
Impaired nutritional intake (adverse reactions)

Implementation
• Give q 12 h × 2 wk, then 1 7 day rest period, do not crush, break, or chew, use with water

Patient/family education
• Advise patient to avoid use of products containing aspirin or ibuprofen, razors, commercial mouthwash, since bleeding may occur; to report symptoms of bleeding (hematuria, tarry stools)
• Teach patient that continuing blood work and exams will be needed
• Instruct patient to report signs of **anemia** (fatigue, headache, irritability, faintness, shortness of breath); **infection:** increased temp, sore throat, flulike symptoms to avoid crowds, persons with known infections
• Advise patient to notify prescriber if pregnancy is planned or suspected or if breast-feeding, use adequate contraception during and for 6 mo after last dose; males should use contraception during and for 3 mo after last dose, if partner is of child-bearing potential
• Advise patient not to double dose, if dose is missed, how to take (on for 14 days then 7 days off) then start new cycle; do not crush, cut, to take with water
• Advise patient to report immediately severe diarrhea, vomiting, stomatitis, fever ≥100° F, hand/foot syndrome, anorexia, stop taking this product
• Advise patient to avoid foods with citric acid, hot or rough texture if stomatitis is present; take with water within 30 min at end of meal

Evaluation
Positive therapeutic outcome
• Prevention of rapid division of malignant cells

---

captopril (Rx)
(kap'toe-pril)
Func. class.: Antihypertensive
Chem. class.: Angiotensin-converting enzyme (ACE) inhibitor

Do not confuse: captopril/carvedilol

ACTION: Selectively suppresses renin-angiotensin-aldosterone system; inhibits ACE; prevents conversion of angiotensin I to angiotensin II

Therapeutic outcome: Decreased B/P in hypertension; decreased preload, afterload in HF

USES: Hypertension, HF, left ventricular dysfunction (LVD) after MI, diabetic nephropathy, proteinuria

Absorption	Well absorbed
Distribution	Widely distributed; crosses placenta, excreted in breast milk (small amounts)
Metabolism	Liver (50%)
Excretion	Kidneys, unchanged (50%)
Half-life	2 hr increased in renal disease

Pharmacodynamics

Onset	¼-1 hr
Peak	1 hr
Duration	6-12 hr

CONTRAINDICATIONS
Breastfeeding, children, hypersensitivity, heart block, potassium-sparing diuretics, bilateral renal artery stenosis, ACE inhibitors, ACE inhibitor–induced angioedema

BLACK BOX WARNING: Pregnancy

Precautions: Dialysis patients, hypovolemia, leukemia, scleroderma, LE, blood dyscrasias, HF, diabetes mellitus, renal/hepatic disease, thyroid disease, ⬥ African descent, pregnancy 1st trimester, collagen-vascular disease, hyperkalemia, hyponatremia

DOSAGE AND ROUTES
Hypertension
Adult: Initial dose: PO 12.5-25 mg bid-tid; may increase to 50 mg bid-tid at 1-2 wk intervals; usual range 25-150 mg bid-tid; max 450 mg/day
Unlabeled child: PO 0.3-0.5 mg/kg/dose, may titrate up to 6 mg/kg/day in 2-4 divided doses

Unlabeled neonate: PO 0.01-0.1 mg/kg bid-tid, may increase as needed

HF
Adult: PO 25 mg tid; may increase to 50 mg bid-tid; after 14 days may increase to 150 mg tid if needed

Post MI
Adult: PO 6.25 mg test dose, then 12.5 mg TID, may increase to 50 mg TID

Diabetic nephropathy
Adult: PO 25 mg tid

Renal dose
Adult: PO; CCr 10-50 ml/min, decrease dose by 25%; CCr <10 ml/min, decrease dose by 50%

Available forms: Tabs 12.5, 25, 50, 100 mg

ADVERSE EFFECTS

CNS: Fever, chills, dizziness, drowsiness, fatigue, headache, insomnia, weakness

CV: *Hypotension,* postural hypotension, *tachycardia,* angina

GI: Loss of taste, increased liver function tests

GU: Impotence, dysuria, nocturia, proteinuria, nephrotic syndrome, acute reversible renal failure, polyuria, oliguria, frequency

HEMA: Neutropenia, agranulocytosis, pancytopenia, thrombocytopenia, anemia

INTEG: Rash, pruritus

MISC: Angioedema, hyperkalemia

RESP: Bronchospasm, *dyspnea, cough*

INTERACTIONS
Individual drugs
Alcohol (acute ingestion): increased hypotension Aliskren: increased hyperkalemia (large amounts)

Digoxin, lithium: increased serum levels, toxicity, monitor blood glucose

Insulin: increased hypoglycemia, monitor individual drug levels

Drug classifications
Antacids, NSAIDs, Cox-2 inhibitors, salicylates: decreased captopril effect

Antidiabetics (oral): increased hypoglycemia

Antihypertensives, diuretics: increased hypotension

Diuretics (potassium-sparing), potassium supplements: increased toxicity, hyperkalemia

Sympathomimetics: do not use

Drug/herb
Black licorice, Ephedra: decreased antihypertensive effect

Garlic, Hawthorn: increased antihypertensive effect

Drug/food
Food: decreased absorption of captopril

Drug/lab test
Increased: AST, ALT, alkaline phosphatase, bilirubin, uric acid, potassium

Decreased: platelets, WBC, RBC, Hgb/Hct

Positive: ANA titer

False positive: urine acetone, ANA titer

NURSING CONSIDERATIONS
Assessment
• **Blood dyscrasias:** Monitor blood studies: decreased platelets; CBC with diff baseline q2wk × 3 mo and periodically during 1 yr, periodically, if neutrophils are <1000/mm³, discontinue treatment

• **Hypertension:** Monitor B/P, pulse, check for orthostatic hypotension, syncope; if changes occur, dosage change may be required; notify prescriber of significant changes

• **Heart failure:** Monitor for dyspnea, jugular venous distention, weight gain, edema, rales/crackles in lungs

• Monitor renal studies: protein, BUN, creatinine, electrolytes; watch for increased levels, if increased dose may need to be reduced

• **Cough:** Monitor for development of dry cough unexplained by other illness, notify health care professional

• Monitor AST, ALT, alkaline phosphatase, glucose, urine protein, bilirubin, uric acid baseline and periodically

• **Angioedema:** Assess for allergic reactions: rash, fever, pruritus, urticaria; product should be discontinued if antihistamines fail to help; swelling of lips, mouth, face, difficulty breathing/swallowing (angioedema), provide supportive care, discontinue product

Patient problem
Impaired cardiac output (uses)

Nonadherence (teaching)

Implementation
• Store in air-tight container at 86° F (30° C) or less

• Severe hypotension may occur after first dose of this medication; decreasing hypotension may be prevented by reducing or discontinuing diuretic therapy 3 days before beginning captopril therapy

• Correct volume depletion before starting treatment

• Administer 1 hr before or 2 hr after meals

• **Oral sol:** May crush tab and dissolve in water, give within ½ hr, make sure tab is completely dissolved

Patient/family education
• Caution patient not to discontinue product abruptly; advise patient to tell all persons associated with care that product is being used

• Teach patient not to use OTC products (cough, cold, allergy) unless directed by prescriber; serious side effects can occur

• Teach patient importance of complying with dosage schedule, even if feeling better; to continue with medical regimen to decrease B/P: exercise, smoking cessation, decreasing stress, diet modifications

• Emphasize the need to rise slowly to sitting or standing position to minimize orthostatic hypotension; not to exercise in hot weather or increased hypotension can occur

• Teach patient to notify prescriber of mouth sores, sore throat, fever, swelling of hands or feet, irregular heartbeat, chest pain, coughing, shortness of breath

• Caution patient to report excessive perspiration, dehydration, vomiting, diarrhea; may lead to fall in B/P

• Caution patient that product may cause dizziness, fainting, light-headedness; may occur during first few days of therapy; to avoid activities that may be hazardous, avoid activities that require concentration
• Teach patient how to take B/P, and teach normal readings for age-group; ensure patient takes regularly
Diabetes: Teach diabetic patients to monitor blood glucose often, hypoglycemia may occur with this product

> **BLACK BOX WARNING:** Advise patient to tell prescriber if pregnancy is suspected or planned, or if breastfeeding; do not breastfeed; contraception should be used, if pregnancy occurs discontinue medication

Evaluation
Positive therapeutic outcome
• Decreased B/P in hypertension
• Decreased diabetic nephropathy symptoms
• Decreased HF after MI

TREATMENT OF OVERDOSE:
0.9% NaCl **IV** infusion, hemodialysis

carbachol ophthalmic
See Appendix B

carBAMazepine (Rx)
(kar-ba-maz′e-peen)
Carbatrol, Carnexiv, Epitol, Equetro, Mazepine ✤, TEGretol ✤, TEGretol-XR
Func. class.: Anticonvulsant
Chem. class.: Iminostilbene derivative

Do not confuse: carBAMazepine/OXcarbazepine/**TEGretol**/Tegrotol XR/Tequin/TRENtal

ACTION: Exact mechanism unknown; appears to decrease polysynaptic responses and block posttetanic potentiation

Therapeutic outcome: Absence of seizures; decreased trigeminal neuralgia pain

USES: Tonic-clonic, complex-partial, mixed seizures; trigeminal neuralgia; bipolar disorder (Equetro only); diabetic neuropathy

Unlabeled uses: Neurogenic pain

Pharmacokinetics

Absorption	Slow; completely absorbed
Distribution	Widely distributed; protein binding 76%
Metabolism	Extensively, liver, metabolized by CYP3A4

Excretion	Urine, feces, breast milk
Half-life	18-65 hr, then 8-29 hr after first month

Pharmacodynamics

	PO	IV
Onset	Slow	Unknown
Peak	4-5 hr (PO), 1.5 hr (susp)	Unknown
Duration	Unknown	Unknown

CONTRAINDICATIONS
Pregnancy, hypersensitivity to carBAMazepine or tricyclics, bone marrow suppression

Precautions: Glaucoma, renal/hepatic/cardiac disease, psychosis, breastfeeding, child <6 yr, alcoholism, hepatic porphyria, AV or bundle branch block

> **BLACK BOX WARNING:** Hematologic disease, agranulocytosis, leukopenia, neutropenia, thrombocytopenia, ✖⊶ Asian patients or those with positive HLA-B 1502, serious rash

DOSAGE AND ROUTES/NTI
Seizures
Adult and child >12 yr: **PO** 200 mg bid; may be increased by 200 mg/day in weekly intervals, give in divided doses q6-8hr; maintenance 800-1200 mg/day; max 1600 mg/day (adult); max child 12-15 yr 1000 mg/day; max child >15 yr 1200 mg/day; EXT REL give bid; **oral SUSP** 200 mg/10 ml or 6 mg/kg as a single dose
Child 6-12 yr: PO tabs 100 mg bid or **SUSP** 50 mg qid; may increase by <100 mg qwk, max 1000 mg/day, usual dose 15-30 mg/kg/day
Child <6 yr: PO 10-20 mg/kg/day in 2-3 divided doses or 4 divided doses (susp), may increase qwk, don't use ext rel, max 35 mg/kg/day

Trigeminal neuralgia
Adult: PO 100 mg/bid; may increase 100 mg q12hr until pain subsides; max 1200 mg/day; maintenance is 200-400 mg bid

Bipolar disorder
Adult: PO (Equetro only) 200 mg bid, increase by 200 mg/day until response max 1600 mg/day

Available forms: Chewable tabs 100, 200 ✤ mg; oral susp 100 mg/5 ml; ext rel tabs 100, 200, 400 mg; ext rel caps (Equetro, Carbatrol) 100, 200, 300 mg

ADVERSE EFFECTS
CNS: *Drowsiness,* dizziness, fatigue, paralysis, headache, suicidal ideation
CV: Hypertension, HF, hypotension, aggravation of CAD, dysrhythmias, AV block

EENT: Dry mouth, blurred vision, diplopia, nystagmus, conjunctivitis

ENDO: Syndrome of inappropriate antidiuretic hormone (SIADH) (geriatric)

GI: *Nausea*, anorexia, hepatotoxicity, increased liver enzymes, hepatitis, weight gain

GU: Retention, glycosuria, impotence, increased BUN, renal failure

HEMA: Thrombocytopenia, leukopenia, agranulocytosis, leukocytosis, aplastic anemia, eosinophilia, lymphadenopathy

INTEG: *Rash*, Stevens-Johnson syndrome, urticaria, photosensitivity, toxic epidermal necrolysis, DRESS, alopecia, pruritus

MS: Osteoporosis

RESP: Pulmonary hypersensitivity (fever, dyspnea, pneumonitis)

INTERACTIONS
Individual drugs

Cimetidine, clarithromycin, danazol, dilTIAZem, erythromycin, FLUoxetine, fluvoxaMINE, isoniazid, propoxyphene, valproic acid, verapamil, voriconazole, may increase toxicity, increased carBAMazepine levels

Darunavir, delavirdine, DOXOrubicin, felbamate, nefazodone, OXcarbazepine, PHENobarbital, phenytoin, primidone, rifAMPin, theophylline: decreased carBAMazepine levels

Delavirdine, doxycycline, felbamate, haloperidol, nefazodone, OXcarbazepine, PHENobarbital, phenytoin, primidone: decreased effect of these products

Desmopressin, lithium, hypressin, vasopressin: increased effects of each specific product

Lithium: increased CNS toxicity, avoid concurrent use

Phenytoin: increased and decreased plasma levels; decreased carBAMazepine plasma levels

Thyroid: decreased effect of thyroid hormones

Warfarin: decreased effect of warfarin, adjust dose as needed

Drug classifications

CYP3A4 inducers, benzodiazepines: decreased carBAMazepine levels

CYP3A4 inhibitors: increased carBAMazepine levels, monitor carBAMazepine effectiveness

Contraceptives (oral): decreased effect of oral contraceptives

• **MAOIs:** fatal reaction; do not use together, do not use within 14 days of beginning carBAMazepine

• **Do not use with:** NNRTIs (non-nucleoside reverse-transcriptase inhibitors), nefazodone

Drug/herb

Echinacea: decreased carBAMazepine metabolism, increased levels

St. John's wort: decreased anticonvulsant action

Drug/food

Grapefruit juice: increased peak concentration of carBAMazepine, avoid use

Drug/lab test

Decreased: serum calcium, sodium

Increased: cholesterol

NURSING CONSIDERATIONS
Assessment

> **BLACK BOX WARNING:** Serious skin reactions: Asian patient, obtain genetic test prior to administration, these patients may develop toxic epidermal necrolysis, Stevens Johnson syndrome, DRESS may be fatal, avoid using

• **Assess for seizures:** assess character, location, duration, intensity, frequency, presence of aura

• Assess for **trigeminal neuralgia:** facial pain including location, duration, intensity, character, activity that stimulates pain

• Monitor liver function tests (AST, ALT) and urine function tests, BUN, urine protein periodically during treatments; serum calcium may be decreased and lead to osteoporosis; cholesterol periodically

• **DRESS:** Assess for fever, lymphadenopathy with multiorgan development, including liver, kidney, cardiac, discontinue carBAMazepine

• **Bone marrow supression:** Assess blood studies: RBC, Hct, Hgb, reticulocyte counts qwk for 4 wk then q3-6mo if on long-term therapy; if myelosuppression occurs, product should be discontinued

• **Beers:** Avoid use in older adults unless safer alternative is not available, ataxia, impaired psychomotor function may occur

• Check blood levels during treatment or when changing dose; therapeutic level 4-12 mcg/ml

• Assess for **blood dyscrasias:** fever, sore throat, bruising, rash, jaundice, epistaxis (long-term treatment only)

• **Assess mental status:** mood, sensorium, affect, behavioral changes, suicidal thoughts/ behaviors

• **Toxicity:** Assess for bone marrow suppression, nausea, vomiting, ataxia, diplopia, CV collapse, Stevens-Johnson syndrome

Patient problem

Risk for injury (uses, adverse reactions)

Pain (uses)

Distorted thinking process (uses)

Implementation

- Do not break, crush, or chew ext rel tabs and caps: ext rel caps may be opened and beads mixed with food; chewable tabs should be chewed, not swallowed whole
- When converting from tabs to oral susp give same amount/day, or regular release to extended release same amount
- Give with food for GI symptoms
- Shake oral susp before use
- **Suspension:** Turn off N/G, internal feeding 15 min before and hold for 15 min after; mix an equal amount of water, D₅W, 0.9% NaCl when giving by NG tube, flush tube with 15-30 ml of above sol
- Store at room temperature

Patient/family education

- Teach patient to carry/wear emergency ID stating patient's name, products taken, condition, prescriber's name, phone number
- Caution patient to avoid driving, other activities that require alertness until stabilized on medication, dizziness, drowsiness occurs
- Advise patient not to use with grapefruit juice
- Teach patient not to discontinue medication quickly after long-term use
- Advise patient to use sunscreen to prevent burns
- Teach patient to take exactly as prescribed; do not double or omit doses, overdose symptoms can occur rapidly
- Teach patient to report immediately chills, rash, light-colored stools, dark urine, yellowing of skin/eyes, abdominal pain, sore throat, mouth ulcers, bruising, blurred vision, dizziness, skin rash, fever
- **Pregnancy/breastfeeding:** Teach patient to notify if pregnancy is planned or suspected, avoid breastfeeding, if pregnant, patient should register with American Antiepileptic Drug Pregnancy Registry 888-233-2334, to use nonhormonal contraceptive
- That ophthalmic exams will be needed, to report changes in vision

Evaluation

Positive therapeutic outcome
- Decreased seizure activity

TREATMENT OF OVERDOSE:
Lavage, VS

⚠ HIGH ALERT

CARBOplatin (Rx)
(kar′boe′pla-tin)
Func. class.: Antineoplastic alkylating agent
Chem. class.: Platinum coordination compound

Do not confuse: CARBOplatin/CISplatin

ACTION: Produces interstrand DNA cross-links and to a lesser extent DNA-protein cross-links; activity is not cell cycle phase specific

Therapeutic outcome: Prevention of rapidly growing malignant cells

USES: Advanced ovarian cancer in combination with other agents; palliative treatment of recurrent ovarian carcinoma after treatment with other antineoplastic agents

Pharmacokinetics

Absorption	Complete (IV)
Distribution	Unknown
Metabolism	Liver
Excretion	Kidneys
Half-life	2-6 hr; increased in renal disease

Pharmacodynamics

Onset	½ hr
Peak	Unknown
Duration	4-6 hr

CONTRAINDICATIONS

Pregnancy, hypersensitivity to this product, breast-feeding, significant bleeding, aluminum products used to prepare or administer CARBOplatin

> **BLACK BOX WARNING:** Severe bone marrow depression, platinum compound hypersensitivity

Precautions: Geriatric patients, radiation therapy within 1 mo, other cancer, chemotherapy within 1 mo, renal disease, liver disease, hearing impairment, infection

> **BLACK BOX WARNING:** Anemia, chemotherapy-induced nausea/vomiting, requires a specialized care setting and experienced clinician

DOSAGE AND ROUTES

Adult: **IV** INF 300 mg/m² on day 1 with cyclophosphamide, 600 mg/m² **IV** on day 1, repeat q4wk × 6 cycles; refractory tumors 360 mg/m² single dose, may repeat q4wk as needed

Renal dose

Adult: IV INF CCr 41-59 ml/min 250 mg/m², CCr 16-40 ml/min 200 mg/m²; do not use in CCr <15 ml/min

Available forms: Solution for injection 10 mg/ml

ADVERSE EFFECTS

CNS: Seizures, central neurotoxicity, peripheral neuropathy, dizziness, confusion, weakness
EENT: Tinnitus, hearing loss

GI: Severe nausea, vomiting, diarrhea, weight loss, mucositis, anorexia, constipation, taste change
GU: Nephrotoxicity
HEMA: Thrombocytopenia, leukopenia, pancytopenia, neutropenia, anemia, bleeding
INTEG: Alopecia, dermatitis, rash, erythema, pruritus, urticaria
META: Hypomagnesemia, hypocalcemia, hypokalemia, hyponatremia, hyperuricemia
SYST: Anaphylaxis, hypersensitivity

INTERACTIONS
Individual drugs
Amphotericin B: increased nephrotoxicity or ototoxicity
Aspirin, anticoagulants, platelet inhibitors: increased risk of bleeding
Phenytoin: decreased levels, monitor levels
Radiation: increased toxicity, bone marrow suppression

Drug classifications
Aminoglycosides: ototoxicity, increased nephrotoxicity
Antineoplastics, bone marrow–suppressing products: increased bone marrow suppression, monitor blood counts often
Myelosuppressives: increased myelosuppression
Live virus vaccines: Do not use this product within 3 mo of these vaccines

Drug/lab test
Increased: AST, BUN, alkaline phosphatase, bilirubin, creatinine
Decreased: platelets, neutrophils, WBC, RBC, Hgb/Hct, calcium, potassium, magnesium, phosphate

NURSING CONSIDERATIONS
Assessment

> **BLACK BOX WARNING: Nausea/vomiting:** May occur a few hr after administration, antiemetics are used, give fluids and food as tolerated

> **BLACK BOX WARNING:** To be used only by person experienced in the use of chemotherapeutic products, in a specialized care setting

> **BLACK BOX WARNING: Bone marrow depression:** Monitor CBC, differential, platelet count weekly; withhold product if neutrophil count is <2000/mm³ or platelet count is <100,000/mm³; notify prescriber of results, calcium, magnesium, phosphate, potassium, sodium, uric acid, CCR, bilirubin; creatinine clearance < 60 ml/min may be responsible for increased bone marrow suppression; assess frequently for infection

> **BLACK BOX WARNING: Assess for anaphylaxis:** pruritus, wheezing, tachycardia; may occur within a few minutes of use; notify physician after discontinuing products; resuscitation equipment should be available

• **Peripheral neuropathy:** may be increased in geriatrics
• Monitor renal function studies: BUN, creatinine, serum uric acid, urine CCr before, during therapy; I&O ratio; report fall in urine output to <30 ml/hr
• **Ototoxicity:** Hearing test baseline and before each dose; may occur more frequently in children
• Monitor liver function tests before, during therapy (bilirubin, AST, ALT, LDH) as needed or monthly; note jaundice of skin or sclera, dark urine, clay-colored stools, itchy skin, abdominal pain, fever, diarrhea

Patient problem
Risk of infection (adverse reactions)
Risk for injury (adverse reactions)

Implementation

> **BLACK BOX WARNING:** Give antiemetic 30-60 min before giving product to prevent vomiting, and prn

IV route
• Do not use needles or IV administration sets containing aluminum; may cause precipitate or loss of potency
• Use cytotoxic handling procedures
• **Reconstitute** CARBOplatin 50, 150, or 450 mg with 5, 15, or 45 ml, respectively, of sterile water for inj, D₅W, or NaCl (10 mg/ml); then further **dilute** with the same sol to 0.5-4 mg/ml; **give** over 15 min - 1hr **(intermittent INF)**
• **Continuous IV INF** over 24 hr; max dose based on (GFR = 125 mg/ml)
• Store protected from light at room temperature; reconstituted sol is stable for 8 hr at room temperature

Y-site compatibilities: Acyclovir, alfentanil, allopurinol, amifostine, amikacin, aminocaproic acid, aminophylline, amiodarone, amphotericin B lipid complex, amphotericin B liposome, ampicillin, ampicillin sulbactam, anidulafungin, atenolol, atracurium, azithromycin, aztreonam, bivalirudin, bleomycin, bumetanide, buprenorphine, butorphanol, calcium chloride/gluconate, caspofungin, ceFAZolin, cefepime, cefoperazone, cefotaxime, cefoTEtan, cefOXitin, cefTAZidime, ceftizoxime, cefTRIAXone, cefuroxime, cimetidine, ciprofloxacin, cisatracurium, CISplatin, cladribine, clindamycin, codeine, cyclophosphamide, cycloSPORINE, cytarabine, DAPTOmycin, DAUNOrubicin, dexamethasone, dexmedetomidine, dexrazoxane, digoxin, dilTIA-Zem, diphenhydrAMINE, DOBUTamine, DOCEtaxel, DOPamine, doripenem, doxacurium, DOXOrubicin, DOXOrubicin liposomal, doxycycline, droperidol, enalaprilat, ePHEDrine, EPINEPHrine, epiRUBicin, ertapenem, erythromycin, esmolol, etoposide, famotidine, fenoldopam, fentaNYL, filgrastim, fluconazole, fludarabine, fluorouracil, foscarnet, fosphenytoin, furosemide, ganciclovir, gatifloxacin, gemcitabine, gentamicin, granisetron, haloperidol, heparin, hydrocortisone, HYDROmorphone, hydrOXYzine, IDArubicin, ifosfamide, imipenem-cilastatin, inamrinone, insulin (regular), irinotecan, isoproterenol, ketorolac, labetalol, levofloxacin, levorphanol, lidocaine, linezolid injection, LORazepam, magnesium sulfate, mannitol, melphalan, meperidine, meropenem, mesna, methohexital, methotrexate, methylPREDNISolone, metoclopramide, metoprolol, metroNIDAZOLE, micafungin, midazolam, milrinone, minocycline, mitoXANtrone, mivacurium, morphine, nafcillin, nalbuphine, naloxone, nesiritide, niCARdipine, nitroglycerin, nitroprusside, norepinephrine, octreotide, ofloxacin, ondansetron, oxaliplatin, PACLitaxel, palonosetron, pamidronate, pancuronium, pantoprazole, PEMEtrexed, pentamidine, PENTobarbital, PHENobarbital, phentolamine, piperacillin, piperacillin-tazobactam, potassium chloride, potassium phosphates, prochlorperazine, promethazine, propofol, propranolol, raNITIdine, remifentanil, riTUXimab, rocuronium, sargramostim, sodium acetate, sodium bicarbonate, sodium phosphates, succinylcholine, SUFentanil, sulfamethoxazole-trimethoprim, tacrolimus, teniposide, theophylline, thiotepa, ticarcillin, ticarcillin-clavulanate, tigecycline, tirofiban, TNA, tobramycin, topotecan, TPN, trastuzumab, trimethobenzamide, vancomycin, vasopressin, vecuronium, verapamil, vinBLAStine, vinCRIStine, vinorelbine, voriconazole, zidovudine

Patient/family education

• Advise patient to report ringing/roaring in the ears, numbness, tingling in face, extremities, weight gain
• Instruct patient to report signs of **anemia** (fatigue, headache, irritability, faintness, shortness of breath); sore throat, bleeding, bruising, chills, back pain, blood in stools, dyspnea
• Instruct patient to report any changes in breathing or coughing even several months after treatment; to avoid crowds and persons with respiratory tract or other infections
• Advise patient that hair may be lost during treatment; a wig or hairpiece may make patient feel better; new hair may be different in color, texture

• Caution patient not to have any vaccinations without the advice of the prescriber; serious reactions can occur
• **Pregnancy/breastfeeding:** Teach patient that impotence or amenorrhea can occur; that this is reversible after treatment is discontinued; to notify prescriber if pregnancy is planned or suspected; that contraception should be used if patient is fertile; not to breastfeed
• Teach patient to notify prescriber immediately of fever, fatigue, sore throat, bleeding, bruising, chills, back pain, blood in stools, urine, emesis, dyspnea, tingling in extremities

Evaluation

Positive therapeutic outcome

• Prevention of rapid division of malignant cells

cariprazine

(kar-ip′ra-zeen)
Vraylar
Func. class.: Antipsychotic
Chem. class.: Partial dopamine receptor agonist

Do not confuse: Vraylar/Valchlor

ACTION: Partial agonist activity at central dopamine D-2 and serotonin 5-HT1A receptors, and antagonist activity at serotonin 5-HT2A

USES: Schizophrenia, mania, or mixed episodes associated with bipolar disorder (bipolar I disorder)

Pharmacokinetics

Absorption	Well
Distribution	Unknown, protein binding 91%-97%
Metabolism	Liver extensively by CYP3A4, and to a lesser extent CYP2D6 to DCAR, DDCAR
Excretion	Feces, 30% (urine, unchanged)
Half-life	2-4 days, metabolite 1-3 wk

Pharmacodynamics

Onset	Unknown
Peak	3-6 hr
Duration	Up to 2 wk

CONTRAINDICATIONS

Hypersensitivity, strong CYP3A4 inhibitors or inducers, history of angioedema

Precautions: CV disease, renal/hepatic disease, antihypertensive, diuretics, leukopenia,

---

neutropenia, acute MI, breast cancer, breastfeeding, pregnancy, agranulocytosis, suicidal ideation, seizure disorder

---

BLACK BOX WARNING: Dementia-related psychosis

DOSAGE AND ROUTES
Adults: PO Initially, 1.5 mg q day, increasing to 3 mg q day on day 2. Further dose adjustments can be made in 1.5 mg to 3 mg increments based upon response and tolerability, range: 1.5 mg to 6 mg q day, max: 6 mg/day
Concurrent CYP3A4 inhibitors: Reduce dose by 50%

Available forms: Capsules 1.5, 3, 4.5, 6 mg

SIDE EFFECTS
CNS: Dizziness, fatigue, headache, insomnia, drowsiness, restlessness, EPS
CV: Orthostatic hypotension, tachycardia, hypertension
GI: Diarrhea, constipation, nausea, vomiting, dry mouth, diarrhea, anorexia
INTEG: Rash
EENT: Blurred vision
RESP: Cough
HEMA: Leukopenia, neutropenia, agranulocytosis
MS: Arthralgia, back pain
META: Hyperglycemia, increased lipids
SYST: Neuroleptic malignant syndrome

INTERACTIONS
Drug classifications
Antihypertensives, diuretics: Increase-orthostatic hypotension
CYP3A4 inhibitors (ketoconazole, itraconazole): Increase toxicity, avoid using together
CYP3A4 inducers (carbamazepine, rifampin): Decrease effect, avoid using together

Drug/lab test
Increase: CK, LFTs
Decrease: WBC

NURSING CONSIDERATIONS
Assessment:
• Monitor HbA1c, lipids, B/P prior to initiation and 3-6 mo after; monitor CBC at baseline and periodically in those with leukopenia. Product may cause low WBCs, agranulocytosis, neutropenia; avoid use if WBC $<1,000$ mm^3
• Monitor for EPS (tardive dyskinesia, dystonic reactions); report immediately if they occur
• **Neuroleptic malignant syndrome:** Dyspnea, seizures, fever, hyper/hypotension,

change in mental status; notify provider immediately
• **Beers:** May use in mania and schizophrenia; there is increased risk of cerebrovascular accident (stroke) and greater rate of cognitive decline and mortality in persons with dementia
• **Pregnancy:** Identify if pregnancy is planned or suspected or if breastfeeding; do not use in pregnancy or breastfeeding

Patient problems
Distorted thinking process (uses)
Impaired nutritional intake (adverse reactions)

Implementation:
• Take capsules with or without food
• Make sure product is swallowed and not saved
• Store at room temperature

Patient/family education:
• Advise patient to take as directed, not to double or skip doses; if a dose is missed, take when remembered unless close to time for next dose; if not taken, then take at next regularly scheduled time
• Teach patient to advise all providers of product use before surgery or other medical regimens
• **Orthostatic hypotension:** Advise patient to make position changes slowly
• Advise patient to avoid ambient temperature increases like hot tubs, as patient's temperature may increase
• Advise to discuss all OTC, Rx, herbs, supplements taken with health care professional
• **Suicidal ideation:** Teach patient, family caregiver to report immediately suicidal thoughts, behaviors, deepening depression, hostility, panic
• Inform patient that drowsiness, dizziness may occur and not to drive or engage in other hazardous activities until response is known
• **EPS:** Review with the patient and caregiver the symptoms of EPS and when to notify the provider
• **Neuroleptic malignant syndrome:** Have patient report immediately dyspnea, seizures, fever, hyper/hypotension, change in mental status
• **Pregnancy/breastfeeding:** Advise patient to notify prescriber if pregnancy is planned or suspected and not to breastfeed; pregnant patients should enroll in the national pregnancy registry for atypical antipsychotics (1-866-961-2388)
Evaluation:
• Positive therapeutic outlook:
  • Decreasing episodes of mania

• Decreasing disorganized thought processes, delusions, and hallucinations

carisoprodol (Rx)
(kar-i-soe-proe′dole)
Soma
Func. class.: Skeletal muscle relaxant, central acting
Chem. class.: Meprobamate congener
Controlled substance schedule IV

Do not confuse: Soma/Soma compound

ACTION: Depresses CNS by blocking interneuronal activity in descending reticular formation of spinal cord, producing sedation and possibly altering pain perception

Therapeutic outcome: Relaxation of skeletal muscles

USES: Relieving pain, stiffness in musculoskeletal disorders

Pharmacokinetics

Absorption	Well absorbed
Distribution	Crosses placenta
Metabolism	Liver, extensively, substrate of CYP2C19 ✸☞ some Asians, Blacks, and Caucasians are poor metabolizers
Excretion	Kidney, unchanged; breast milk
Half-life	8 hr

Pharmacodynamics

Onset	½ hr
Peak	4 hr
Duration	4-6 hr

CONTRAINDICATIONS
Hypersensitivity to these products or carbamates, intermittent porphyria

Precautions: Pregnancy, breastfeeding, geriatric, renal/hepatic disease, substance abuse, seizure disorder, CNS depression, abrupt discontinuation, ✸☞ Asian patients

DOSAGE AND ROUTES
Adult and child ≥16 yr: PO 250-350 mg qid

Available forms: Tabs 250, 350 mg

ADVERSE EFFECTS
CNS: *Dizziness, weakness, drowsiness,* headache, insomnia, irritability
CV: Postural hypotension, tachycardia
GI: Nausea, vomiting, hiccups, epigastric discomfort

HEMA: Eosinophilia
INTEG: Rash, pruritus, fever, facial flushing
RESP: Asthmatic attack
SYST: Angioedema, anaphylaxis

INTERACTIONS
Individual drugs
Alcohol: increased CNS depression

Drug classifications
Antidepressants (tricyclic), barbiturates, opioids, sedative/hypnotics: avoid concurrent use, increased CNS depression
CYP2C19 inhibitors (FLUoxetine, fluvoxaMINE, isoniazid, modafinil): increased carisoprodol effect
CYP2C19 inducers (rifAMPin): decreased carisoprodol metabolite, decreasing carisoprodol effect

Drug/herb
Kava, valerian: increased CNS depression
St. John's wort: increased metabolism of carisoprodol

Drug/lab test
Increased: eosinophils
Decreased: RBC, WBC, platelets

NURSING CONSIDERATIONS
Assessment
• **Pain:** Monitor ROM, atrophy, stiffness, and pain in muscles; assess baseline throughout treatment
• **Beers:** Avoid in older adults, may decrease urinary flow, cause retention (men), sedation, anticholinergic effects
• Assess for idiosyncratic reaction within a few min or 1 hr of administration (disorientation, restlessness, weakness, euphoria, blurred vision); patient should be reassured that reaction is temporary, withhold and notify prescriber, usually seen in poor CYP2C19 metabolizers
• **Check for allergic reactions:** rash, fever
• **CNS depression:** Assess for dizziness, drowsiness, psychiatric symptoms, abuse potential
• **Abrupt discontinuation:** withdrawal reactions do occur but may be mild; dependence may occur
• **Pregnancy/breastfeeding:** Advise prescriber if pregnancy is planned or suspected or if breastfeeding

Patient problem
Pain (uses)
Impaired mobility (uses)

Implementation
• Give with meals for GI symptoms
• Have patient use gum, frequent sips of water for dry mouth

- Store in tight container at room temperature
- Use for short term (2-3 wk), potential for habituation

Patient/family education
- Caution patient not to take with alcohol, other CNS depressants
- Advise patient to avoid rapid position changes, postural hypotension occurs, not to use for >2-3 wk
- Caution patient to avoid hazardous activities if drowsiness or dizziness occurs
- Caution patient to avoid using OTC medication such as cough preparations, antihistamines, unless directed by prescriber
- **Teach patient to report allergic reactions immediately:** rash, swelling of tongue/lips, hives, dyspnea
- Advise patient to take with food for GI symptoms

Evaluation
Positive therapeutic outcome
- Decreased pain, spasticity

TREATMENT OF OVERDOSE:
Lavage, dialysis

carteolol ophthalmic
See Appendix B

⚠ HIGH ALERT
carvedilol (Rx)
(kar-veh′dee-lol)
Coreg, Coreg CR
Func. class.: Antihypertensive α/β-blocker

Do not confuse: carvedilol/Captopril

ACTION: A mixture of nonselective β-blocking and α-blocking activity; decreases cardiac output, exercise-induced tachycardia, reflex orthostatic tachycardia; causes reduction in peripheral vascular resistance and vasodilatation

Therapeutic outcome: Decreased B/P in hypertension

USES: Hypertension alone or in combination with other antihypertensives, HF, left ventricular dysfunction following MI, cardiomyopathy

Pharmacokinetics
Absorption	Readily and extensively absorbed
Distribution	>98% protein binding
Metabolism	Extensively liver, by CYP2D6, CYP2C9 some patients may be poor metabolizers
Excretion	Via bile into feces

Half-life	Half-life 7-10 hr, increased in the geriatric, hepatic disease

Pharmacodynamics
	PO	Ext rel
Onset	45 min	Unknown
Peak	1-2 hr	5 hr
Duration	12 hr	24 hr

CONTRAINDICATIONS
Hypersensitivity, asthma, class IV decompensated cardiac failure, 2nd- or 3rd-degree heart block, cardiogenic shock, severe bradycardia, pulmonary edema, severe hepatic disease

Precautions: Pregnancy, breastfeeding, children, geriatric, cardiac failure, hepatic injury, peripheral vascular disease, anesthesia, major surgery, diabetes mellitus, thyrotoxicosis, emphysema, chronic bronchitis, renal disease, abrupt discontinuation

DOSAGE AND ROUTES
Hypertension
Adult: PO 6.25 mg bid × 7-14 days may increase if needed to 25 mg bid, max 50 mg daily; ext rel cap 20 mg/day, double after 7-14 days to 40 mg/day, max 80 mg/day

Heart failure
Adult: PO 3.125 mg bid × 2 wk; may increase to 6.25 mg bid × 2 wk, then double q2wk to max dose 25 mg bid <85 kg or 50 mg bid >85 kg; ext rel cap (Coreg CR) 10 mg/day × 2 wk, increase to 20, 40, 80 mg/day over successive intervals of 2 wk

Post MI
Adult: PO 6.25 mg bid ×3-10 days, may increase to 12.5 mg bid, then titrate to 25 mg bid; **ext rel** 20 mg/day, 10 mg/day may be used and titrate upwards after 3-10 days, increase to 80 mg/day as required

Available forms: Tabs 3.125, 6.25, 12.5, 25 mg; ext rel cap 10, 20, 40, 80 mg

ADVERSE EFFECTS
CNS: *Dizziness,* somnolence, insomnia, drowsiness, memory loss, paresthesia, vertigo, depression, *fatigue, weakness,* headache
CV: *Bradycardia, postural hypotension,* HF, pulmonary edema
GI: *Diarrhea,* abdominal pain, constipation, nausea, vomiting
GU: Decreased libido, *impotence,* UTI
INTEG: Rash, Stevens-Johnson syndrome, toxic epidermal necrolysis, pruritus
MISC: Injury, back pain, viral infection, hypertriglyceridemia, thrombocytopenia, *hyperglycemia,* abnormal weight gain, **anaphylaxis, angioedema**

RESP: Dyspnea, bronchospasm, lupus-like syndrome
EENT: Blurred vision, floppy iris syndrome, dry eyes

INTERACTIONS
Individual drugs
CYP2D6 inhibitors FLUoxetine, quiNIDine, increase: Carvediol level
Alcohol (acute ingestion), cimetidine: increased toxicity, monitor for toxicity, hypotension
CloNIDine: decreased heart rate, B/P, monitor B/P, pulse frequently
Digoxin: increased concentrations of digoxin, bradycardia
Reserpine, levodopa: increased hypotension, bradycardia
RifAMPin: decreased levels of carvedilol

Drug classifications
Antihypertensives, nitrates: increased hypotension
Antidiabetic agents: increased hypoglycemia, insulin; monitor blood glucose level, dose of antidiabetics may need to be decreased
Calcium channel blockers: increased conduction disturbance
CYP2D6 inhibitors (FLUoxetine, quiNIDine): increased digoxin
MAOIs: increased bradycardia, hypotension
NSAIDs, thyroid hormones: decreased levels of carvedilol

Drug/herb
Black licorice, Ephedra: decreased antihypertensive effect
Garlic, Hawthorn: increased antihypertensive effect

Drug/lab test
Increased: alk phos, serum creatinine blood glucose, potassium, triglycerides, uric acid, bilirubin, cholesterol, creatinine
Decreased: sodium, HDL

NURSING CONSIDERATIONS
Assessment
• **HF:** Assess for edema in feet and legs daily, fluid overload: dyspnea, weight gain, jugular vein distention, fatigue, crackles monitor I&O, worsening of heart failure may occur during beginning of treatment, check for compliance
• Monitor I&O, weight daily
• **Hypertension:** Monitor B/P during beginning treatment and periodically thereafter; pulse q4hr, note rate, rhythm, quality
• Monitor apical/radial pulse before administration; in those with lower heart rate (<55 bpm) dose may need to be lowered, notify prescriber of significant changes, identify orthostatic hypotension when patient rises pulse <50 bpm hold product, notify prescriber

Patient problem
Impaired cardiac output (uses)
Nonadherence (teaching)

Implementation
• Take apical pulse before use, notify prescriber if <50 bpm and hold dose
• Tablets may be crushed or swallowed whole, give with food to decrease orthostatic hypotension; do not break, crush, or chew ext rel cap; decreased anginal pain
• Administer reduced dosage in renal dysfunction
• Do not discontinue prior to surgery
• Conversion from immediate release to extended release 3.125 mg bid is 10 mg qday; 6.25 mg bid is 20 mg qday; 12.5 mg bid is 40 mg; 25 mg bid is 8 mg

Patient/family education
• **Hypertension:** Teach patient that other treatment regimens should continue; exercise, no smoking, weight control
• Teach patient not to break, crush, or chew ext rel cap
• Instruct patient to comply with dosage schedule even if feeling better, that improvement may take several weeks, not to crush, chew caps
• Teach patient to rise slowly to sitting or standing position to minimize orthostatic hypotension

> **BLACK BOX WARNING:** Encourage patient to report bradycardia, dizziness, confusion, depression, fever, weight gain, shortness of breath, cold extremities, rash, sore throat, bleeding, bruising

• Teach patient to take pulse at home; advise when to notify prescriber
• Encourage patient not to discontinue product abruptly, taper over 1-2 wk, life-threatening dysrhythmias may occur
• Advise patient to avoid hazardous activities until stabilized on medication; dizziness may occur
• Teach patient that product may mask hypoglycemia, thyroid symptoms
• Advise patient to carry/wear emergency ID with product name, prescriber at all times
• Advise patient to inform all health care providers of products, supplements taken; advise patient to avoid all OTC medications unless approved by prescriber
• **Pregnancy/breastfeeding:** Teach patient to report if pregnancy is planned or suspected, pregnancy, or if breastfeeding

Evaluation
Positive therapeutic outcome
• Decreased B/P
• Decreased symptoms of HF or angina

caspofungin (Rx)
(cas-po-fun'gin)
Cancidas
Func. class.: Antifungal, systemic
Chem. class.: Echinocandin

ACTION: Inhibits an essential component in fungal cell walls; causes direct damage to fungal cell wall

USES: Treatment of invasive aspergillosis and candidemia that has not responded to other treatment, including peritonitis and intraabdominal abscesses; susceptible species: *Aspergillus flavus, A. fumigatus, A. terreus, Candida albicans, C. glabrata, C. krusei, C. lusitaniae, C. parapsilosis, C. tropicalis*, esophageal candidiasis; empirical therapy for presumed fungal infection in febrile, neutropenic patients

Pharmacokinetics

Absorption	Complete (IV)
Distribution	Widely to tissues, protein binding 97%
Metabolized	Liver extensively
Excretion	Urine minimal unchanged
Half-life	Biphasic 9-11 hr, 40-50 hr

Pharmacodynamics

Onset	Unknown
Peak	Infusion's end
Duration	Up to 24 hr

CONTRAINDICATIONS
Hypersensitivity

Precautions: Pregnancy, breastfeeding, children, geriatric patients, severe hepatic disease

DOSAGE AND ROUTES
Adult: IV loading dose 70 mg on day 1, then 50 mg/day maintenance dose, depending on condition; max 70 mg/day
Adolescent/child/infant ≥3 mo: IV INFUSION 70 mg/m² loading dose, then 50 mg/m²/day; max 70 mg/day
Neonate and infant <3 mo (unlabeled): IV 25 mg/m²/day

Esophageal candidiasis
Adult: IV 50 mg × 7-14 days over 1 hr

Hepatic dose
• **Adult:** IV (Child-Pugh 7-9, class B) loading dose 70 mg, then 35 mg/day
• **Child 3 mo-17 yr:** IV 70 mg/m² loading dose, then 50 mg/m² daily; max 70 mg/m²

Available forms: Powder for inj 50, 70 mg

ADVERSE EFFECTS
CNS: Dizziness, *headache*, fever, chills
CV: Sinus tachycardia, hypertension
GI: Abdominal pain, *nausea, anorexia, vomiting, diarrhea, increased AST/ALT, alk phos*
GU: Renal failure
HEMA: Thrombophlebitis, vasculitis, anemia
INTEG: *Rash, pruritus, inj site pain*
META: Hypokalemia
MS: Myalgia
RESP: Acute respiratory distress syndrome (ARDS), pleural effusions
SYST: Anaphylaxis, histamine-related reactions, Stevens-Johnson syndrome

INTERACTIONS
Individual Drugs
Carbamazepine, dexamethasone, efavirenz, nelfinavir, nevirapine, phenytoin, rifAMPin: decrease: caspofungin levels; caspofungin dose may need to be increased
Cyclosporine: Increase: caspofungin levels, hepatic toxicity, avoid concurrent use
Sirolimus, tacrolimus: Decrease: levels of tacrolimus, sirolimus

Drug/lab test
Increase: AST, ALT, RBC, eosinophils, glucose, bilirubin, alk phos, serum creatinine
Decrease: Hct/Hgb, WBC, potassium, magnesium

NURSING CONSIDERATIONS
Assessment:
• **Infection:** Assess for clearing of cultures during treatment; obtain culture at baseline, throughout treatment; product may be started as soon as culture is taken (esophageal candidiasis); monitor cultures during hematopoietic stem cell transplantation (HSCT) for prevention of *Candida* infections
• Blood studies before and during treatment: monitor bilirubin, AST, ALT, alk phos, as needed; obtain baseline renal studies; CBC with differential, serum potassium
• Hypersensitivity: Assess for rash, pruritus, facial swelling; also for phlebitis, anaphylaxis (rare)
• GI symptoms: Assess for frequency of stools, cramping; if severe diarrhea occurs, electrolytes may need to be given

Patient Problems
Infection (uses)
Risk for injury (uses, adverse reactions)

Implementation:
• Do not mix or confuse with other medications; do not use dextrose-containing products to dilute; do not give as bolus

• Store at room temperature for up to 24 hr or refrigerated for 48 hr; store reconstituted sol at room temperature for 1 hr before preparation of sol for administration

Intermittent IV INFUSION route
• Allow to warm to room temperature
• May administer loading dose on day 1
• **Reconstitute** 50 mg vial or 70 mg vial with 10.8 mL 0.9% NaCl, sterile water for inj or bacteriostatic water for inj (5 mg/mL or 7 mg/mL, respectively); **swirl** to dissolve; withdraw 10 mL reconstituted sol and **further dilute** with 250 mL 0.9% NaCl, 0.45% NaCl, 0.225% NaCl, RL; **run** over 1 hr or more

Teach patient/family:
• **Pregnancy/breastfeeding:** Teach patient to notify prescriber if pregnancy is suspected or planned; to use cautiously in breastfeeding
• Advise patient to inform prescriber of renal/hepatic disease
• Teach patient to report bleeding, facial swelling, wheezing, difficulty breathing, itching, rash, hives, increasing warmth, flushing; anaphylaxis can occur

Evaluation:
• Positive therapeutic outcome: decreased symptoms of *Candida* and *Aspergillus* infections

cefaclor
See cephalosporins—2nd generation

cefadroxil
ceFAZolin
See cephalosporins—1st generation

cefdinir
cefditoren
cefepime
cefotaxime
See cephalosporins—3rd generation

cefoTEtan
cefOXitin
See cephalosporins—2nd generation

cefpodoxime
See cephalosporins—3rd generation

cefprozil
See cephalosporins—2nd generation

ceftaroline (Rx)
(sef-tar'oh-leen)
Teflaro
Func. class.: Anti-infective, Cephalosporin derivative (fifth generation)

ACTION: Inhibits cell wall synthesis through binding to essential penicillin-binding protein (PBP)

Therapeutic outcome: Negative C&S, resolution of symptoms of infection

USES: Acute bacterial skin/skin structure infections, bacterial community acquired pneumonia

Pharmacokinetics

Absorption	Complete (IV)
Distribution	Unknown
Metabolism	Not hepatically metabolized
Excretion	Urine 88%, feces 6%
Half-life	1.6 hr

Pharmacodynamics

Onset	Immediately
Peak	Unknown
Duration	Up to 12 hr

CONTRAINDICATIONS
Cephalosporin hypersensitivity

Precautions: Antimicrobial resistance, breastfeeding, carbapenem/penicillin hypersensitivity, child/infant/neonate, coagulopathy, colitis, dialysis, diarrhea, geriatrics, GI disease, hypoprothrombinemia, IBS, pregnancy, pseudomembranous colitis, renal disease, ulcerative colitis, viral infection, vitamin K deficiency

DOSAGE AND ROUTES
Adult: IV 600 mg q12hr × 5-14 days (skin/skin structure infections), × 5-7 days (bacterial community acquired pneumonia)
Child: IV 2-17 yr and >33 kg: 400 mg q 8 h or 600 mg q 12 h; 2-17 yr and <33kg: 12 mg/kg q 8 h
Child 2 mo-<2 yr: **IV 8 mg/kg q 8 h**

Renal dose
Adult: IV CCr >30-≤50 ml/min 400 mg q12hr; CCr ≥15-≤30 ml/min 300 mg q12hr, CCr <15 ml/min 200 mg q12hr (includes hemodialysis)

Available forms: Powder for injection 400 mg, 600 mg/vial

ADVERSE EFFECTS
CNS: Dizziness, seizures
GI: Diarrhea, nausea, vomiting, *Clostridium difficile*-associated diarrhea (CDAD)
HEMA: Hemolytic anemia

INTEG: Rash, anaphylaxis
MISC: Injection-site reactions

INTERACTIONS
Drug classifications
Anticoagulants: increased prothrombin time risk

Drug/lab test
Increased: LFTs
Decreased: potassium, eosinophils, platelets

NURSING CONSIDERATIONS
Assessment
• **Assess for infection:** vital signs, sputum, WBC prior to and during therapy; culture and sensitivity should be done before starting treatment, may start medications before results are received
• **Assess for hypersensitivity:** prior to use, obtain a history of hypersensitivity reactions to cephalosporins, carbapenems, penicillins; cross sensitivity may occur
• **Assess for anaphylaxis (rare):** rash, pruritus, laryngeal edema, dyspnea, wheezing; discontinue and notify health care provider immediately, keep emergency equipment nearby
• **Monitor for *Clostridium difficile*-associated diarrhea (CDAD):** diarrhea, abdominal pain, fever, bloody stools; report immediately if these occur, may occur several weeks after terminating therapy
• Hemolytic anemia (rare): discontinue product, obtain direct Coomb's test, result will be positive

Patient problem
Infection (uses)
Diarrhea (adverse reactions)

Implementation
• Obtain C&S before use, first dose may be given before results are received
• Visually inspect for particulate matter or discoloration if solution or container permit
• Identify allergies before use
Intermittent IV infusion route
• **Reconstitute:** add 20 mg of sterile water to 400 or 600 mg vial (20 ml/ml for 400 mg), (30 mg/ml for 600 mg), mix gently until dissolved: **Dilute:** in 250 ml of 0.9% NaCl, 0.45% NaCl, LR, D5, D2.5, give over 1 hr, do not admix, use within 6 hrs at room temperature or 24 hr refrigerated
• Store reconstituted solution in the refrigerator

Patient/family education
• Explain reason for treatment and expected result
• Instruct patient to report immediately rash, itching, difficulty breathing, bloody diarrhea, fever, abdominal pain

Pregnancy/breastfeeding: Advise patient to tell health care professional if pregnancy is planned or suspected or if breastfeeding

Evaluation
Positive therapeutic outcome
• Negative C&S, resolution of symptoms of infection

---

cefTAZidime
ceftibuten
ceftizoxime
cefTRIAXone
See cephalosporins—3rd generation

cefuroxime
See cephalosporins—2nd generation

ceftazidime/avibactam (Rx)
(sef-tay′ zi-deem av-i-bak′ tam)
Avycaz
Func. class.: Broad-spectrum antiinfective
Chem. class.: Cephalosporin (3rd generation)

ACTION: **Ceftazidime:** Inhibits bacterial cell wall synthesis, rendering cell wall osmotically unstable, leading to cell death; **avibactam:** Inhibits beta-lactamase

Therapeutic outcome: Bactericidal effects for the following: *Citrobacter freundii, Citrobacter koseri, Enterobacter cloacae, Escherichia coli, Haemophilus influenzae* (beta-lactamase negative), *Haemophilus influenzae* (beta-lactamase positive), *Klebsiella aerogenes, Klebsiella oxytoca, Klebsiella pneumoniae, Morganella morganii, Proteus mirabilis, Providencia rettgeri, Providencia stuartii, Pseudomonas aeruginosa, Serratia marcescens*

USES: Complicated urinary tract infection (UTI), including pyelonephritis; complicated intraabdominal infections in combination with metronidazole; nosocomial pneumonia, including hospital-acquired pneumonia (HAP) and ventilator associated pneumonia (VAP)

Pharmacokinetics

Absorption	Complete
Distribution	Widely distributed; enters breast milk
Metabolism	Minimal
Excretion	Kidneys, unchanged
Half-life	Ceftazidime: 2.8-3.2 hr; avibactam: 2.2-2.7 hr

Pharmacodynamics

Onset	Immediate
Peak	Infusion's end
Duration	8 hr or longer

CONTRAINDICATIONS

Hypersensitivity to cephalosporins, infants <6 mo

Precautions: Pregnancy, breastfeeding, children, hypersensitivity to penicillins, renal/GI disease, geriatrics, CDAD, viral infection

DOSAGE AND ROUTES

Adults: IV 2.5 g (2 g ceftazidime and 0.5 g avibactam) q 8 hr for 7 to 14 days.

Children and adolescents: 2 to 17 years IV 62.5 mg/kg/dose (50 mg/kg/dose ceftazidime and 12.5 mg/kg/dose avibactam) q 8 hrs (max: 2.5 g [2 g ceftazidime and 0.5 g avibactam]) for 7 to 14 days

Infants and children 6 mo to 1 year: IV 62.5 mg/kg/dose (50 mg/kg/dose ceftazidime and 12.5 mg/kg/dose avibactam) q 8 hr for 7 to 14 days

Infants 3 to 5 months: IV 50 mg/kg/dose (40 mg/kg/dose ceftazidime and 10 mg/kg/dose avibactam) q 8 hr for 7 to 14 days

Renal dose

Adults: IV CCr >50 mL/min: no change; CCr 31 to 50 mL/min: 1.25 g (1 g ceftazidime and 0.25 g avibactam) q 8 hr; CCr 16 to 30 mL/min: 0.94 g (0.75 g ceftazidime and 0.19 g avibactam) q 12 hr; CCr 6 to 15 mL/min: 0.94 g (0.75 g ceftazidime and 0.19 g avibactam) q 24 hr; CCr ≤5 mL/min: 0.94 g (0.75 g ceftazidime and 0.19 g avibactam) q 48 hr

Child 2 to 17 yrs: CCr >50 mL/min: no change; CCr 31 to 50 mL/min: 31.25 mg/kg/dose (25 mg/kg/dose ceftazidime and 6.25 mg/kg/dose avibactam) q 8 hr (max: 1.25 g [1 g ceftazidime and 0.25 g avibactam]); CCr 16 to 30 mL/min: 23.75 mg/kg/dose (19 mg/kg/dose ceftazidime and 4.75 mg/kg/dose avibactam) q 12 hr (max: 0.94 g [0.75 g ceftazidime and 0.19 g avibactam]); CCr 6 to 15 mL/min: 23.75 mg/kg/dose (19 mg/kg/dose ceftazidime and 4.75 mg/kg/dose avibactam) q 24 hr (max: 0.94 g [0.75 g ceftazidime and 0.19 g avibactam]); CCr ≤5 mL/min: 23.75 mg/kg/dose (19 mg/kg/dose ceftazidime and 4.75 mg/kg/dose avibactam) q 48 hr (max: 0.94 g [0.75 g ceftazidime and 0.19 g avibactam])

Available forms: Powder for injection 2.5 g

ADVERSE EFFECTS

CNS: Headache, dizziness, seizures, dyskinesia, encephalopathy

GI: Nausea, vomiting, diarrhea, anorexia, CDAD

HEMA: Thrombocytopenia, eosinophilia

INTEG: Rash, urticarial

SYST: Anaphylaxis, Stevens-Johnson syndrome, toxic epidermal necrolysis

INTERACTIONS

Individual drugs

Probenecid: decreased avibactam excretion, avoid using together

Drug/lab test

Increased: ALT, AST, alkaline phosphatase, LDH, bilirubin, BUN, creatinine

False positive: urinary protein, direct Coombs' test, urine glucose

NURSING CONSIDERATIONS

Assessment

• Assess patient for previous sensitivity reaction to penicillins or other cephalosporins; cross-sensitivity between penicillins and cephalosporins is common

• Assess patient for signs and symptoms of **infection,** including characteristics of wounds, sputum, urine, stool, WBC 10,000/mm³, fever; obtain information baseline and during treatment

• Obtain C&S before beginning product therapy to identify if correct treatment has been initiated

• **Assess for anaphylaxis:** rash, urticaria, pruritus, chills, fever, joint pain; angioedema may occur a few days after therapy begins; EPINEPHrine and resuscitation equipment should be available for anaphylactic reaction

• Monitor blood studies: AST, ALT, CBC, Hct, bilirubin, LDH, alkaline phosphatase, Coombs' monthly if patient is on long-term therapy

• Assess bowel pattern daily; if severe diarrhea occurs, product should be discontinued; may indicate CDAD

• Assess for **overgrowth of infection:** perineal itching, fever, malaise, redness, pain, swelling, drainage, rash, diarrhea, change in cough, sputum

• **Encephalopathy:** Assess for confusion, seizures during treatment; report to provider immediately

Patient problems

Infection (uses)

Risk for injury (adverse reactions)

Implementation

Intermittent IV Infusion route

• Give for 7-14 days to ensure organism death, prevent superinfection

• Visually inspect parenteral products for particulate matter and discoloration. The diluted solution ranges from clear to light yellow

Reconstitution:

• Using aseptic technique, reconstitute the dry powder with 10 mL of 1 of the following solutions: Sterile Water for Injection, Lactated Ringer's Injection, 0.9% sodium chloride injection, 5% dextrose injection, or any combination of dextrose and sodium chloride that contains up to 2.5% dextrose injection and 0.45% sodium chloride injection; concentration (167 mg/mL/42 mg/mL/12 mL)

• Ensure the dry powder is dissolved by mixing
• Do not give by direct injection; must be diluted before IV infusion
• *Storage:* the solution should be further diluted within 30 min of reconstitution

Dilution: Withdraw the needed volume from the reconstituted vial

• Adults and pediatric patients weighing 40 kg or more
  • *For a 2.5 g dose (2 g ceftazidime and 0.5 g avibactam)*, withdraw 12 mL (entire contents) of the reconstituted solution for further dilution
  • *For a 1.25 g dose (1 g ceftazidime and 0.25 g avibactam)*, withdraw 6 mL of the reconstituted solution for further dilution
  • *For a 0.94 g dose (0.75 g ceftazidime and 0.19 g avibactam)*, withdraw 4.5 mL of the reconstituted solution for further dilution
• Pediatric patients weighing less than 40 kg
  • Withdraw needed dose of the reconstituted solution based on a final concentration of 209 mg/mL (167 mg/mL ceftazidime and 42 mg/mL avibactam)
• *Adults and pediatric patients weighing 40 kg or more*: using the same solution that was selected for reconstitution, dilute to a total volume of 50 to 250 mL (8 to 40 mg/mL ceftazidime and 2 to 10 mg/mL avibactam). Dilution to 250 mL should only be used for the 2.5 g dose. If Sterile Water for Injection was used for reconstitution, use any other appropriate diluent for dilution
• *Pediatric patients weighing less than 40 kg*: using the same solution that was selected for reconstitution, dilute to a total volume of 8 to 40 mg/mL ceftazidime and 2 to 10 mg/mL avibactam. If Sterile Water for Injection was used for reconstitution, use any other appropriate diluent for dilution. *Gently mix.*
• *Storage: Administer diluted solution* within 12 hr if stored at room temperature of 25° C (77° F). Diluted solution may be stored for up to 24 hr under refrigeration at 2 to 8° C (36 to 46° F), with subsequent storage for up to 12 hr at room temperature
• Give over 2 hr

Patient/family education

• Advise patient to contact prescriber if vaginal itch, loose foul-smelling stools, furry tongue occur; may indicate superinfection

Advise patient to notify prescriber of diarrhea with blood or pus, may indicate CDAD
• Teach patient to report if pregnancy is planned or suspected or if breastfeeding

Evaluation
Positive therapeutic outcome
• Absence of signs/symptoms of infection (WBC 10,000/mm³, temp WNL, absence of red draining wounds, earache)
• Reported improvement in symptoms of infection
• Negative C&S

TREATMENT OF ANAPHY-LAXIS: EPINEPHrine, antihistamines, resuscitate if needed

---

ceftolozone/tazobactam (Rx)
(sef-tol' o-zane taz-oh-bak' tam)
Zerbaxa
Func. class.: Broad-spectrum antiinfective
Chem. class.: Cephalosporin derivative (beta-lactamase inhibitor)

ACTION: Ceftolozone: Inhibits bacterial cell wall synthesis, rendering cell wall osmotically unstable, leading to cell death; **tazobactam:** inhibits beta-lactamase

Therapeutic outcome: Bactericidal effects for the following: *Bacteroides fragilis, Citrobacter koseri, Enterobacter cloacae, Escherichia coli, Haemophilus influenzae (beta-lactamase negative), Haemophilus influenzae (beta-lactamase positive), Klebsiella aerogenes, Klebsiella oxytoca, Klebsiella pneumoniae, Morganella morganii, Proteus mirabilis, Proteus vulgaris, Providencia rettgeri, Providencia stuartii, Pseudomonas aeruginosa, Serratia liquefaciens, Serratia marcescens, Streptococcus agalactiae (group B streptococci), Streptococcus anginosus, Streptococcus constellatus, Streptococcus intermedius, Streptococcus salivarius*

USES: Complicated urinary tract infection (UTI), including pyelonephritis; complicated intraabdominal infections in combination with metronidazole

Pharmacokinetics

Absorption	Complete
Distribution	Unknown
Metabolism	Minimal
Excretion	Kidneys, unchanged
Half-life	Ceftolozone: 2.8 hr; tazobactam: 1 hr

Pharmacodynamics

Onset	Immediate
Peak	Infusion's end
Duration	8 hr or longer

CONTRAINDICATIONS

Hypersensitivity to beta lactams

Precautions: Pregnancy, breastfeeding, children, hypersensitivity to penicillins, renal/GI disease, geriatrics, CDAD, viral infection

DOSAGE AND ROUTES

Adults IV 1.5 g (1 g ceftolozane and 0.5 g tazobactam) q 8 hr x 4-14 days (intraabdominal infections), 7 days UTIs

Available forms: Powder for injection 1.5 g

ADVERSE EFFECTS

CNS: Headache, dizziness, seizures, dyskinesia, encephalopathy
GI: Nausea, vomiting, diarrhea, anorexia, CDAD
HEMA: Thrombocytopenia, eosinophilia
INTEG: Rash, urticarial
SYST: Anaphylaxis, Stevens-Johnson syndrome, toxic epidermal necrolysis

INTERACTIONS

None significant

Drug/lab test

Increased: creatinine clearance

NURSING CONSIDERATIONS
Assessment

• Assess patient for previous sensitivity reaction to penicillins, cephalosporins, or beta lactam inhibitors; cross-sensitivity between penicillins, cephalosporins, and beta lactam inhibitors may occur
• Assess patient for signs and symptoms of **infection,** including characteristics of wounds, sputum, urine, stool, WBC 10,000/mm^3, fever; obtain information at baseline and during treatment
• Obtain C&S before beginning product therapy to identify if correct treatment has been initiated
• **Assess for anaphylaxis:** rash, urticaria, pruritus, chills, fever, joint pain; angioedema may occur a few days after therapy begins; EPINEPHrine and resuscitation equipment should be available for anaphylactic reaction
• Monitor creatinine clearance daily in renal disease
• Assess bowel pattern daily; if severe diarrhea occurs, product should be discontinued; may indicate CDAD
• Assess for **overgrowth of infection:** perineal itching, fever, malaise, redness, pain, swelling, drainage, rash, diarrhea, change in cough, sputum

Patient problems

Infection (uses)
Risk for injury (adverse reactions)

Implementation
Intermittent IV Infusion route:

• Visually inspect parenteral products for particulate matter and discoloration
• Do not mix with other drugs or physically add to solutions containing other drugs
Reconstitution:

• Reconstitute each vial with 10 mL of Sterile Water for Injection or 0.9% sodium chloride injection
• Gently shake to dissolve
• The final volume after reconstitution is approximately 11.4 mL
• Further dilution is required
• For doses above 1.5 g (1 g ceftolozane and 0.5 g tazobactam), reconstitute a second vial and add the appropriate volume to the same IV infusion bag
• *Storage:* the reconstituted solution may be held for 1 hr before further dilution. Do not freeze
Dilution:

• To prepare the required dose, withdraw the appropriate volume from the reconstituted vial(s) and aseptically add to an IV infusion bag containing 100 mL of 0.9% sodium chloride injection or 5% dextrose injection.
• To prepare a dose of 3 g (2 g ceftolozane and 1 g tazobactam), withdraw 11.4 mL (entire contents) from two reconstituted vials
• To prepare a dose of 2.25 g (1.5 g ceftolozane and 0.75 g tazobactam), withdraw 11.4 mL (entire contents) from one reconstituted vial and 5.7 mL from a second reconstituted vial
• To prepare a dose of 1.5 g (1 g ceftolozane and 0.5 g tazobactam), withdraw 11.4 mL (entire contents) of one reconstituted vial
• To prepare a dose of 750 mg (500 mg ceftolozane and 250 mg tazobactam), withdraw 5.7 mL of one reconstituted vial
• To prepare a dose of 450 mg (300 mg ceftolozane and 150 mg tazobactam), withdraw 3.5 mL of one reconstituted vial
• To prepare a dose of 375 mg (250 mg ceftolozane and 125 mg tazobactam), withdraw 2.9 mL of one reconstituted vial
• To prepare a dose of 150 mg (100 mg ceftolozane and 50 mg tazobactam), withdraw 1.2 mL of one reconstituted vial
• *Storage:* the diluted solution may be stored for 24 hr at room temperature or for 7 days

when refrigerated (2 to 8° C or 36 to 46° F). Do not freeze
• Infuse over 1 hr

Patient/family education
• Advise patient to contact prescriber if vaginal itching, loose foul-smelling stools, furry tongue occur; may indicate superinfection
• Advise patient to notify prescriber of diarrhea with blood or pus, may indicate CDAD
• Teach patient to report if pregnancy is planned or suspected or if breastfeeding

Evaluation
Positive therapeutic outcome
• Absence of signs/symptoms of infection (WBC 10,000/mm³, temp WNL, absence of red draining wounds, earache)
• Reported improvement in symptoms of infection
• Negative C&S

TREATMENT OF ANAPHYLAXIS: EPINEPHrine, antihistamines, resuscitate if needed

▲ HIGH ALERT

celecoxib (Rx)
(cel-eh-cox'ib)
CeleBREX
Func. class.: Nonsteroidal antiinflammatory, antirheumatic
Chem. class.: COX-2 inhibitor

Do not confuse: CeleBREX/CeleXA/Cerebyx

ACTION: Inhibits prostaglandin synthesis by selectively inhibiting cyclooxygenase 2 (COX-2), an enzyme needed for biosynthesis

Therapeutic outcome: Decreased pain, inflammation

USES: Acute, chronic rheumatoid arthritis, osteoarthritis, acute pain, primary dysmenorrhea, ankylosing spondylitis, juvenile rheumatoid arthritis (JRA)

Pharmacokinetics

Absorption	Well absorbed (PO)
Distribution	Crosses placenta, protein binding ~97%
Metabolism	Liver by CYP2C9, ✎ some patients may be poor metabolizers
Excretion	Feces/kidneys, small amount
Half-life	11 hr

Pharmacodynamics

Onset	Unknown
Peak	3 hr
Duration	Unknown

CONTRAINDICATIONS
Pregnancy, hypersensitivity to salicylates, iodides, other NSAIDs, sulfonamides, CABG

Precautions: breastfeeding, children <18 yr, geriatric, renal/hepatic disease, hypertension, severe dehydration, bleeding, GI, cardiac disorders, PVD, asthma, peptic ulcer disease, stroke, MI

> **BLACK BOX WARNING:** GI bleeding/perforation, thromboembolism

DOSAGE AND ROUTES
Acute pain/primary dysmenorrhea
Adult: PO 400 mg initially, then 200 mg if needed on first day, then 200 mg bid as needed on subsequent days, if needed; start with ½ dose in poor CYP2C9 metabolizers
Geriatric: PO use lowest possible dose

Osteoarthritis
Adult: PO 200 mg/day as a single dose or 100 mg bid; start with ½ dose in poor CYP2C9 metabolizers

Rheumatoid arthritis
Adult: PO 100-200 mg bid; start with ½ dose in poor CYP2C9 metabolizers

Ankylosing spondylitis
Adult: PO 200 mg daily or in divided dose (bid); start with ½ dose in poor CYP2C9 metabolizers

Juvenile rheumatoid arthritis (JRA)
Adolescent and child ≥2 yr (>25 kg): PO 100 mg bid; start with ½ dose in poor CYP2C9 metabolizers
Child ≥2 yr (10-25 kg): PO 50 mg bid; start with ½ dose in poor CYP2C9 metabolizers

Hepatic dose
Adult: PO (Child-Pugh B) reduce dose by 50%; (Child-Pugh C) do not use

Available forms: Caps 50, 100, 200, 400 mg

ADVERSE EFFECTS
CNS: *Fatigue, nervousness, paresthesia,* dizziness, insomnia, headache
CV: Stroke, MI, tachycardia, HF, angina, palpitations, dysrhythmias, hypertension, fluid retention
GI: *Nausea, anorexia, dry mouth,* diarrhea, GI bleeding/ulceration

---

INTEG: Purpura, Stevens-Johnson syndrome, toxic epidermal necrolysis, exfoliative dermatitis

INTERACTIONS
Individual drugs
Aspirin: decreased effectiveness; increased adverse reactions

Fluconazole: increased celecoxib level

Furosemide, cidofovir: decreased effect of each drug

Lithium: increased toxicity

Drug classifications
ACE inhibitors, diuretics: may decrease effects of ACE inhibitors

Anticoagulants, antiplatelets, SNRIs, SSRIs, salicylates, thrombolytics: increased risk of bleeding

CYP2C inhibitors: increase celecoxib levels, dose may need to be reduced

Drug/lab test
Increased: ALT, AST, BUN, cholesterol, glucose, potassium, sodium

Decreased: glucose, sodium, WBC, platelets

NURSING CONSIDERATIONS
Assessment
• Assess for **pain** of rheumatoid arthritis, osteoarthritis; check ROM, inflammation of joints, characteristics of pain baseline and periodically

> **BLACK BOX WARNING:** Assess for cardiac disease that may be worse after taking this product; do not use in coronary artery bypass graft (CABG)

> **BLACK BOX WARNING:** Assess for thromboembolism including MI, stroke

• **Assess for GI bleeding/perforation:** black, tarry stools; abdominal pain, monitor stool guaiac
• **Assess for serious skin disorders:** Stevens-Johnson syndrome, toxic epidermal necrolysis; may be fatal, treat symptomatically, may recur after therapy is discontinued, if severe may require discontinuing
• **Beers:** Avoid use in older adults, may increase risk of kidney injury, exacerbate heart failure, increase fluid retention

Patient problem
Pain (uses)

Impaired mobility (uses)

Implementation
• Do not break, crush, chew, or dissolve caps; caps may be opened and mixed with applesauce, ingest immediately with water
• Administer with food or milk to decrease gastric symptoms

Patient/family education

> **BLACK BOX WARNING:** Do not exceed recommended dose; notify prescriber, immediately of chest pain, skin eruptions, stop product; hepatotoxicity: nausea, pruritus, yellowing skin, eyes; lethargy, itching, upper abdominal pain

• Teach patient that product must be continued for prescribed time to be effective; to avoid other NSAIDs, sulfonamides, salicylates; if allergic, do not use this product

> **BLACK BOX WARNING: GI bleeding/perforation:** Caution patient to report bleeding, bruising, fatigue, malaise, since blood abnormalities do occur; to report GI symptoms: black tarry stools, cramping

• Teach patient to take with a full glass of water to enhance absorption
• Teach patient to check with prescriber to determine when product should be discontinued before surgery
• **Pregnancy/breastfeeding:** Teach patient to report if pregnancy is planned or suspected, do not use in breastfeeding or pregnancy, those who are pregnant and taking this product should register with the Teratology Information Specialists of Autoimmune Disease in Pregnancy Study 877-311-8972, discontinue breastfeeding or product

Evaluation
Positive therapeutic outcome
• Decreased pain in arthritic conditions
• Decreased inflammation in arthritic conditions
• Decreased number of polyps (FAP)

cemiplimab
(seh-mip′lih-mab)

Libtayo

Func. class.: Antineoplastic-monoclonal antibody

Chem. class.: Death receptor-1 (PD-1)/PD-L1

ACTION: Binds to the programmed death receptor-1 (PD-1) found on T-cells. Blocking the PD-1/PD-L1 pathway improves the antitumor immune response by reducing immunosuppressive signals between immune cells and tumor cells and causes inhibition of T-cell proliferation and cytokine production

Therapeutic outcome: Decreased spread of skin cancer

USES: Treatment of squamous cell skin carcinoma in patients who are not candidates for curative surgery/radiation

Pharmacokinetics

Absorption	Unknown
Distribution	Unknown
Metabolism	Unknown
Excretion	Unknown
Half-life	19 days

Pharmacodynamics

Onset	Unknown
Peak	Unknown
Duration	Unknown

CONTRAINDICATIONS: Hypersensitivity, pregnancy, breastfeeding

PRECAUTIONS: Adrenal insufficiency, autoimmune disease, colitis, contraception requirements, Crohn's disease, hepatitis, hyperthyroidism, immune-mediated reactions, infusion-related reactions, organ transplant, pneumonitis, pregnancy testing, renal impairment, reproductive risk, serious rash, type 1 diabetes mellitus, ulcerative colitis

DOSAGE AND ROUTES
Adults: IV 350 mg over 30 min q3 wk until disease progression; visually inspect parenteral products for particulate matter and discoloration prior to administration whenever solution and container permit

Available forms: Solution for injection 350 mg/7 ml

ADVERSE EFFECTS
CNS: Fatigue, asthenia
EENT: Immune-mediated optic nephritis
Endo: Immune-mediated hypophysitis, immune-mediated hypothyroidism/hyperthyroidism, immune-mediated type 1 diabetes mellitus
GI: *Anorexia, nausea, vomiting, abdominal pain, constipation, diarrhea,* immune-mediated colitis, immune-mediate hepatitis
GU: Immune-mediated nephritis
Hema: Anemia
Integ: *Rash, pruritus,* infusion-related reactions
MS: Immune-mediated rhabdomyolysis, back pain, myalgia, MS pain
Resp: Immune-mediated pneumonitis

INTERACTIONS
None known

NURSING CONSIDERATIONS
Assessment
• **Immune-mediated pneumonitis:** Assess for shortness of breath, chest pain, new or worsening cough periodically; if present obtain X-ray; withhold product until grade ≤1; usually treated with corticosteroids

• **Immune-mediated colitis:** Monitor for severe diarrhea or abdominal pain, blood or mucus in stool; if present, therapy may need to be interrupted or discontinued based on the severity; corticosteroids may be used; permanently discontinue if grade 4 toxicity

• **Immune-mediated hepatitis:** Assess for jaundice of skin/eyes, severe nausea/vomiting; obtain liver function tests prior to starting and periodically during therapy; if hepatitis occurs, therapy may need to be interrupted or discontinued based on the severity of the toxicity; corticosteroids may be given

• **Infusion-related reactions:** Assess for fever, pruritus, wheezing, rigors; if severe grade 3 or 4 discontinue permanently

• **Immune-mediated dermatologic reactions:** monitor for erythema multiform, Stevens-Johnson syndrome; toxic epidermal necrolysis has occurred with other similar products; interrupt or discontinue therapy in patients who develop severe skin toxicity; provide corticosteroids followed by a 1-month taper starting when the toxicity resolves to grade 1 or less

• **Immune-mediated hypophysitis: Immune-mediated pneumonitis:** shortness of breath, chest pain, new or worsening cough periodically; if present obtain X-ray; withhold product until grade ≤1; usually treated with corticosteroids

• **Immune-mediated colitis:** Severe diarrhea or abdominal pain, blood or mucus in stool; if present, therapy may need to be interrupted or discontinued based on the severity; corticosteroids may be used; permanently discontinue if grade 4 toxicity

• **Immune-mediated hepatitis:** Jaundice of skin/eyes, severe nausea/vomiting; obtain liver function tests prior to starting and periodically during therapy; if hepatitis occurs, therapy may need to be interrupted or discontinued based on the severity of the toxicity; corticosteroids may be given

• **Infusion-related reactions:** Fever, pruritus, wheezing, rigors; if severe grade 3 or 4, discontinue permanently

• **Immune-mediated dermatologic reactions:** erythema multiform, Stevens-Johnson syndrome; toxic epidermal necrolysis has occurred with other similar products; interrupt or discontinue therapy in patients who develop severe skin toxicity; provide corticosteroids followed by a 1-month taper starting when the toxicity resolves to grade 1 or less

• **Immune-mediated hypophysitis:** Continual headache, weakness, fatigue, blurred vision, dizziness; provide corticosteroids for grade 2; if severe (grade 3), withhold or discontinue product until toxicity resolves to grade 1 or less; permanently discontinue for grade 4

• **Immune-mediated nephritis:** Monitor serum creatinine and BUN baseline and periodically; corticosteroids may be used for ≥ grade 2 nephritis; withhold for grade 2, resume when recovery is grade ≤1; discontinue for grade 4

• **Pregnancy/breastfeeding:** Product should not be used in pregnancy or breastfeeding; a pregnancy test should be performed in all women of childbearing potential

• Monitor blood glucose at baseline and periodically; may cause hyperglycemia

• Monitor thyroid function test at baseline and periodically; may cause hypo/hyperthyroidism; corticosteroids may be used for grade 3 hypothyroidism; withhold product for severe grade 3; permanently discontinue for grade 4

• Monitor for headache, weakness, fatigue, blurred vision, dizziness; provide corticosteroids for grade 2; if severe (grade 3), withhold or discontinue product until toxicity resolves to grade 1 or less; permanently discontinue for grade 4

• **Immune-mediated nephritis:** Monitor serum creatinine and BUN at baseline and periodically; corticosteroids may be used for ≥ grade 2 nephritis; withhold for grade 2, resume when recovery is grade ≤1; discontinue for grade 4

• Blood glucose at baseline and periodically; may cause hyperglycemia

• Thyroid function test at baseline and periodically, may cause hypo/hyperthyroidism; corticosteroids may be used for grade 3 hypothyroidism; withhold product for severe grade 3; permanently discontinue for grade 4

Patient problems
Risk for injury (adverse reactions)

Implementation
IV Infusion Route
• Visually inspect for particulate matter and discoloration prior to use; product is clear to slightly opalescent, colorless to pale yellow and may contain trace amounts of translucent to white particles

• Do not shake the vial
Dilution:
• Withdraw the required amount/volume, dilute in 0.9% sodium chloride injection or 5% dextrose injection to a final concentration between 1 and 20 mg/ml; mix by gentle inversion; do not shake
• Discard any unused portion
• **Storage following dilution:** Store at room temperature (up to 25° C or 77° F) for up to 8 hr or refrigerated (2 to 8° C; 36 to 46° F) for up to 24 hr from the time of dilution; do not freeze

Administration:
• If refrigerated, allow to warm to room temperature
• Give the diluted solution over 30 min through a sterile, in-line, or add-on 0.2-to-0.5 micron filter

Patient/family education
• Teach patient that product treats a type of skin cancer by working with your immune system
• Notify prescriber immediately of new or worsening cough; shortness of breath; chest pain; diarrhea; stools that are black, tarry, sticky, or have blood or mucus; abdominal pain; yellowing of skin/eyes; severe nausea/vomiting; bleeding or bruising more easily; unusual headaches; rapid heartbeat; increased sweating; extreme tiredness; weight gain/weight loss; dizziness/fainting; feeling more hungry or thirsty than usual; hair loss; feeling cold; constipation; skin rash with blisters
• **Pregnancy/breastfeeding:** Inform healthcare provider if pregnancy is planned or suspected. This product should not be used in pregnancy and breastfeeding. A pregnancy test will be required before treatment begins. A nonhormonal form of contraception will be needed to prevent pregnancy during and for 4 months after treatment is concluded. Do not breastfeed during or for 4 months after last dose
• Advise patients to tell their healthcare provider about all Rx, OTC, vitamins, and herbals taken, and not to take others without prescriber's approval
• Teach patient that blood work and regular exams will be needed throughout treatment

Evaluation
• Decreased spread of skin cancer

cephalexin
See cephalosporins—1st generation

CEPHALOSPORINS— 1ST GENERATION

cefadroxil (Rx)
(sef-a-drox'ill)
Duricef ✦
ceFAZolin (Rx)
(sef-a'zoe-lin)
Ancef ✦, Kefzol ✦
cephalexin (Rx)
(sef-a-lex'in)
Keflex ✦
Func. class.: Antiinfective-cephalosporin

ACTION: Inhibits bacterial cell wall synthesis, rendering cell wall osmotically unstable, leading to cell death

>> cefadroxil

Therapeutic outcome: Bactericidal effects for the following: gram-negative bacilli *Escherichia coli, Proteus mirabilis, Klebsiella pneumoniae* (UTI only); gram-positive organisms *Streptococcus pneumoniae, Streptococcus pyogenes, Staphylococcus aureus/epidermidis*

USES: Upper, lower respiratory tract, urinary tract, skin infections; otitis media; tonsillitis, UTI

>> cefadroxil
Pharmacokinetics

Absorption	Well absorbed
Distribution	Widely distributed; crosses placenta
Metabolism	Not metabolized
Excretion	Unchanged by kidneys; enters breast milk
Half-life	1½-2 hr

Pharmacodynamics

	PO
Onset	Rapid
Peak	1½-2 hr
Duration	12-24 hr

>> ceFAZolin

Therapeutic outcome: Bactericidal effects for the following: gram-negative organisms *Haemophilus influenzae, Escherichia coli, Proteus mirabilis, Klebsiella;* gram-positive organisms *Staphylococcus aureus*

USES: Upper, lower respiratory tract, urinary tract, skin infections; bone, joint, biliary, genital infections; endocarditis; surgical prophylaxis; septicemia; *Streptococcus*

>> ceFAZolin
Pharmacokinetics

Absorption	Well absorbed
Distribution	Widely distributed; crosses placenta
Metabolism	Not metabolized
Excretion	Unchanged by kidneys; enters breast milk
Half-life	1½-2½ hr

Pharmacodynamics

	IM	IV
Onset	Rapid	10 min
Peak	1-2 hr	Infusion's end
Duration	6-12 hr	Unknown

>> cephalexin

Therapeutic outcome: Bactericidal effects for the following: gram-negative organisms *Haemophilus influenzae, Escherichia coli, Proteus mirabilis, Klebsiella pneumoniae;* gram-positive organisms *Streptococcus pneumoniae, Streptococcus pyogenes, Streptococcus agalactiae, Staphylococcus aureus*

USES: Upper, lower respiratory tract, urinary tract, skin, bone infections; otitis media

>> cephalexin
Pharmacokinetics

Absorption	Well absorbed
Distribution	Widely distributed; crosses placenta
Metabolism	Not metabolized
Excretion	Kidneys, unchanged; enters breast milk
Half-life	½-1 hr; increased in renal disease

Pharmacodynamics

Onset	15-30 min
Peak	1 hr
Duration	6-12 hr

CONTRAINDICATIONS
Hypersensitivity to cephalosporins, infants <1 mo

Precautions: Pregnancy, breastfeeding, hypersensitivity to penicillins, renal disease

DOSAGE AND ROUTES
>> cefadroxil
Adult: PO 1-2 g daily or divided q12hr, give a loading dose of 1 g initially
Child: PO 30 mg/kg/day in divided doses bid, max 2 g/day

✦ Canada only   ✤☞ Genetic Warning   Adverse effects: *italics* = common; red = life-threatening

Catheter-related bloodstream infections
Adults: IV 2 g q8hr

Renal dose
Adult: PO CCr 25-50 ml/min, 1 g, then 500 mg q12hr; CCr 10-24 ml/min, 1 g, then 500 mg q24hr; CCr < 10 ml/min, 1 g, then 500 mg q36hr

Available forms: Caps 500 mg; tabs 1 g; oral susp 250, 500 mg/5 ml

>> ceFAZolin
Life-threatening infections
Adult: IM/**IV** 1-2 g q6-8hr, max 12 g/day
Child >1 mo: IM/**IV** 75-100 mg/kg/day in 3-4 divided doses, max 6 g/day

Mild/moderate infections
Adult: IM/**IV** 250 mg-1 g q8hr, max 12 g/day
Child >1 mo: IM/**IV** 25-50 mg/kg in 3-4 equal doses, max 6 g/day or 2 g as a single dose

Renal dose
Adult: IM/IV following loading dose CCr 35-54 ml/min dose q8hr; CCr 10-34 ml/min 50% of dose q12hr; CCr <10 ml/min 50% of dose q18-24hr
Child: IM/IV CCr >70 ml/min, no dosage adjustment; CCr 40-70 ml/min following loading dose, reduce dose to 7.5-30 mg/kg q12hr; CCr 20-39 ml/min, give 3.125-12.5 mg/kg after loading dose q12hr; CCr 5-19 ml/min, 2.5-10 mg/kg after loading dose q24hr

Available forms: Powder for injection 500 mg/vial, 1 g/vial, 10 g/vial, 20 g/vial; Premixed 1 g/50mL D5W, 2g/50 mL D$_5$W

>> cephalexin
Moderate infections
Adult: PO 250-500 mg q6hr, max 4 g/day
Child: PO 25-100 mg/kg/day in 4 equal doses, max 4 g/day

Moderate skin infections
Adult: PO 500 mg q12hr

Endocarditis prophylaxis
2 g 1 hr before procedure

Severe infections
Adult: PO 500 mg-1 g q6hr, max 4 g
Child: PO 50-100 mg/kg/day in 4 equal doses, max 4 g/day
Otitis media
Child: PO 18.75-25 mg/kg q 6 hr, max 4 g/day

Renal dose
Adult: PO CCr 30-59 ml/min max 1000 mg/day; CCr 15-29 ml/min 250 mg q 8-12 hr; CCr 5-14 ml/min 250 mg q 24 hr; CCr 1-4 ml/min 250 mg q 48-60 hrs

Available forms: Caps 250, 500, 750 mg; tabs 250, 500 mg, 1 g; oral susp 125, 250 mg/5 ml

ADVERSE EFFECTS
CNS: Headache, dizziness, seizures
GI: Nausea, vomiting, *diarrhea, anorexia,* abdominal pain, *Clostridium difficile*-associated diarrhea (CDAD)
HEMA: Leukopenia, thrombocytopenia, agranulocytosis, neutropenia, hemolytic anemia
INTEG: Rash, urticaria, dermatitis, injection site reactions
SYST: Anaphylaxis, serum sickness, superinfection, Stevens-Johnson syndrome, toxic epidermal necrolysis

INTERACTIONS
Individual drugs
Probenecid: increased toxicity

Drug classifications
Aminoglycosides, diuretics (loop): increased toxicity

Drug/lab test
Increased: AST, ALT, alkaline phosphatase, LDH, BUN, creatinine, bilirubin
False positive: urinary protein, direct Coombs' test, urine glucose
Interference: cross-matching

NURSING CONSIDERATIONS
Assessment
• Assess patient for signs and symptoms of **infection** including characteristics of wounds, sputum, urine, stool, WBC >10,000/mm^3, earache, fever; obtain baseline information and during treatment
• Assess patient for previous sensitivity reaction to penicillins or other cephalosporins; cross-sensitivity between penicillins and cephalosporins is common
• Obtain C&S before beginning product therapy to identify if correct treatment has been initiated, may start treatment before receiving results
• **Assess for anaphylaxis:** rash, urticaria, pruritus, chills, fever, joint pain; angioedema may occur a few days after therapy begins; EPINEPHrine and resuscitation equipment should be available for anaphylactic reaction
• Monitor blood studies: AST, ALT, CBC, Hct, bilirubin, LDH, alkaline phosphatase, Coombs' test if patient is on long-term therapy
• **Assess for Stevens-Johnson syndrome, toxic epidermal necrolysis:** monitor for painful rash, flu-like symptoms, discontinue product and do not restart
• CDAD: Assess bowel pattern daily, if severe diarrhea occurs, product should be discontinued, may indicate CDAD

⚠ Nurse Alert   ✶ Key NCLEX® Drug   >> Drug Specifics

C

• **Assess for superinfection:** perineal itching, fever, malaise, redness, pain, swelling, drainage, rash, diarrhea, change in cough, sputum

Patient problem
Infection (uses)
Diarrhea (adverse reactions)

>> cefadroxil
Implementation
• Give in even doses around the clock; if GI upset occurs, give with food; product must be given for prescribed time to ensure organism death and prevent superinfection
• Shake susp, refrigerate, discard after 2 wk

>> ceFAZolin
Implementation
IM route
• Reconstitute 250-500 mg of product with 2 ml sterile or bacteriostatic water for inj, or 0.9% NaCl; reconstitute 1 g of product with 2.5 ml; give deep in large muscle mass, massage

IV route
• Check for irritation, extravasation, phlebitis daily, change site q72hr
• For **direct IV** dilute in 2 ml/500 mg or 2.5 ml/ 1 g of sterile water for inj; give over 5 min
• For **intermittent inf** dilute reconstituted sol (500 mg or 1 g) in 50-100 ml D$_5$W, D$_{10}$W, D$_5$/0.25% NaCl, D$_5$/0.45% NaCl, D$_5$/0.9% NaCl, D$_5$/LR, or LR, 0.9% NaCl; give over 10-60 min; may be refrigerated up to 96 hr or stored 24 hr at room temperature

Y-site compatibilities: Acyclovir, alfentanil, allopurinol, alprostadil, amifostine, amikacin, aminocaproic acid, aminophylline, amphotericin B liposome, anidulafungin, ascorbic acid injection, atenolol, atracurium, atropine, aztreonam, benztropine, bivalirudin, bleomycin, bumetanide, buprenorphine, butorphanol, calcium gluconate, CARBOplatin, cefamandole, cefmetazole, cefonicid, cefoperazone, cefoTEtan, cefOXitin, cefpirome, cefTAZidime, ceftizoxime, cefTRIAXone, cefuroxime, cephalothin, cephapirin, chloramphenicol, cimetidine, CISplatin, clindamycin, codeine, cyanocobalamin, cyclophosphamide, cycloSPORINE, cytarabine, DACTINomycin, DAPTOmycin, dexamethasone, dexmedetomidine, digoxin, dilTIAZem, DOCEtaxel, doxacurium, doxapram, DOXOrubicin liposomal, enalaprilat, ePHEDrine, EPINEPHrine, epiRUBicin, epoetin alfa, eptifibatide, esmolol, etoposide, fenoldopam, fentaNYL, filgrastim, fluconazole, fludarabine, fluorouracil, folic acid (as sodium salt), foscarnet, furosemide, gallium, gatifloxacin, gemcitabine, gentamicin, glycopyrrolate, granisetron, heparin, hydrocortisone, hydrOXYzine, IDArubicin, ifosfamide, imipenem-cilastatin, indomethacin, insulin (regular), irinotecan, isoproterenol, ketorolac, lidocaine, linezolid, LORazepam, LR's injection, mannitol, mechlorethamine, melphalan, meperidine, metaraminol, methicillin, methotrexate, methoxamine, methyldopate, methylPREDNISolone, metoclopramide, metoprolol, metroNIDAZOLE, mezlocillin, miconazole, midazolam, milrinone, morphine, moxalactam, multiple vitamins injection, nafcillin, nalbuphine, naloxone, nesiritide, niCARdipine, nitroglycerin, nitroprusside, norepinephrine, octreotide, ondansetron, oxacillin, oxaliplatin, oxytocin, PACLitaxel, palonosetron, pamidronate, pancuronium, pantoprazole, penicillin G potassium/sodium, peritoneal dialysis solution, perphenazine, PHENobarbital, phenylephrine, phytonadione, piperacillin, Plasma-Lyte M in dextrose 5%, polymyxin B, potassium chloride, procainamide, propofol, propranolol, raNITIdine, remifentanil, Ringer's injection, ritodrine, riTUXimab, sargramostim, sodium acetate, sodium bicarbonate, succinylcholine, SUFentanil, tacrolimus, teniposide, tenoxicam, theophylline, thiamine, thiotepa, ticarcillin, ticarcillin-clavulanate, tigecycline, tirofiban, TNA, tolazoline, trastuzumab, trimetaphan, urokinase, vasopressin, vecuronium, verapamil, vinCRIStine, vitamin B complex with C, voriconazole, warfarin, zoledronic acid

>> cephalexin
Implementation
• Do not break, crush, or chew caps
• Give in even doses around the clock; if GI upset occurs, give with food; product must be taken for 10-14 days to ensure organism death and prevent superinfection
• Shake susp, refrigerate, discard after 2 wk, use calibrated oral syringe, spoon or measuring cup

Patient/family education
• Advise patient to contact prescriber if vaginal itching, loose foul-smelling stools, furry tongue occur; may indicate superinfection
• Instruct patient to take all medication prescribed for the length of time ordered, take missed dose as soon as remembered, unless close to next dose, do not take a double dose, use calibrated device for suspension
• Advise patient to notify prescriber of diarrhea with blood, pus, mucus, which may indicate *Clostridium difficile*-associated diarrhea (CDAD)
• Teach patient to report immediately rash, flu-like symptoms, blisters, stop product

Evaluation
Positive therapeutic outcome
• Absence of signs/symptoms of infection (WBC <10,000/mm³, temp WNL, absence of red draining wounds, earache)
• Reported improvement in symptoms of infection
• Negative C&S

TREATMENT OF ANAPHY-LAXIS: EPINEPHrine, antihistamines, resuscitate if needed

CEPHALOSPORINS— 2ND GENERATION

cefaclor (Rx)
(sef′a-klor)
Ceclor ✦
cefoTEtan (Rx)
(sef′oh-tee-tan)
Cefotan
cefOXitin (Rx)
(se-fox′i-tin)
Mefoxin
cefprozil (Rx)
(sef-proe′zill)
Cefzil
cefuroxime (Rx)
(sef-yoor-ox′eem)
Ceftin, Kefurox ✦, Zinacef
Func. class.: Antiinfective
Chem. class.: Cephalosporin (2nd generation)

Do not confuse: cefaclor/cephalexin, **Cefotan**/Ceftin, **cefprozil**/ceFAZolin/cefuroxime, **Cefzil**/Ceftin

ACTION: Inhibits bacterial cell wall synthesis, rendering cell wall osmotically unstable, leading to cell death by binding to cell wall membrane

>> cefaclor
Therapeutic outcome: Bactericidal effects for the following: gram-negative bacilli *Haemophilus influenzae, Escherichia coli, Proteus mirabilis, Klebsiella;* gram-positive organisms *Streptococcus pneumoniae, Streptococcus pyogenes, Staphylococcus aureus*

USES: Lower respiratory tract, urinary tract, skin infections; otitis media; infections

>> cefaclor
Pharmacokinetics

Absorption	Well absorbed
Distribution	Widely distributed; crosses placenta
Metabolism	Not metabolized
Excretion	Unchanged by kidneys (60%-80%); enters breast milk
Half-life	36-54 min; increased in renal disease

Pharmacodynamics

Onset	15 min
Peak	½-1 hr
Duration	Up to 12 hr

>> cefoTEtan
Therapeutic outcome: Bactericidal effects for the following: gram-negative organisms *Citrobacter, Haemophilus influenzae, Escherichia coli, Enterobacter aerogenes, Proteus mirabilis, Klebsiella, Salmonella, Shigella, Acinetobacter, Bacteroides fragilis, Neisseria, Serratia;* gram-positive organisms *Streptococcus pneumoniae, Streptococcus pyogenes, Staphylococcus aureus*

USES: Serious upper or lower respiratory tract, urinary tract, gynecologic, skin, bone, joint, gonococcal, intraabdominal infections

>> cefoTEtan
Pharmacokinetics

Absorption	Well absorbed (IM)
Distribution	Widely distributed; crosses placenta
Metabolism	Not metabolized
Excretion	Kidneys, unchanged; enters breast milk
Half-life	5 hr; increased in renal disease

Pharmacodynamics

	IM	IV
Onset	Rapid	Immediate
Peak	1-3 hr	Infusion's end
Duration	Up to 12 hr	Up to 12 hr

>> cefOXitin
Therapeutic outcome: Bactericidal effects for the following: gram-negative bacilli *Bacteroides fragilis, Haemophilus influenzae, Escherichia coli, Proteus, Klebsiella, Neisseria gonorrhoeae;* gram-positive organisms *Streptococcus pneumoniae, Streptococcus pyogenes, Staphylococcus aureus;* anaerobes including *Clostridium*

USES: Lower respiratory tract, urinary tract, skin, bone, gynecologic, gonococcal infections; septicemia, peritonitis

>> cefOXitin
Pharmacokinetics

Absorption	Well absorbed (IM)
Distribution	Widely distributed; crosses placenta
Metabolism	Not metabolized
Excretion	Kidneys, unchanged; enters breast milk
Half-life	½-1 hr; increased in renal disease

Pharmacodynamics

	IM	IV
Onset	Rapid	Immediate
Peak	½ hr	Infusion's end
Duration	6-8 hr	6-8 hr

>> cefprozil
Therapeutic outcome: Bactericidal effects for the following: gram-negative bacilli *Haemophilus influenzae, Escherichia coli;* gram-positive organisms *Streptococcus pneumoniae, Streptococcus pyogenes, Staphylococcus aureus*

USES: Pharyngitis/tonsillitis, otitis media, secondary bacterial infection of acute bronchitis, and acute bacterial exacerbation of chronic bronchitis and uncomplicated skin and skin structure infections; acute sinusitis

>> cefprozil
Pharmacokinetics

Absorption	Well absorbed
Distribution	Widely distributed; crosses placenta
Metabolism	Not metabolized
Excretion	Kidneys (60%), unchanged; enters breast milk
Half-life	1.3 hr (normal renal function); 2 hr (hepatic disease); 5¼-6 hr (end-stage renal disease)

Pharmacodynamics

Onset	Unknown
Peak	1-2 hr
Duration	Up to 24 hr

>> cefuroxime
Therapeutic outcome: Bactericidal effects for the following: gram-negative bacilli *Haemophilus influenzae, Escherichia coli, Neisseria, Proteus mirabilis, Klebsiella;* gram-positive organisms: *Streptococcus pneumoniae, Streptococcus pyogenes, Staphylococcus aureus*

USES: Serious lower respiratory tract, urinary tract, skin, bone, joint, gonococcal infections; septicemia, meningitis, surgery prophylaxis

>> cefuroxime
Pharmacokinetics

Absorption	Well absorbed
Distribution	Widely distributed
Metabolism	Crosses placenta
Excretion	Kidneys, unchanged, enters breast milk
Half life	60-120 min

Pharmacodynamics

	PO	IM	IV
Onset	Unknown	Rapid	Rapid
Peak	2-4 hr	Infusions	6-12 hr
Duration	8-12 hr	6-12 hr	6-12 hr

CONTRAINDICATIONS
Hypersensitivity to cephalosporins or related antibiotics, seizures

Precautions: Pregnancy, breastfeeding, children, renal/GI disease, diabetes mellitus, coagulopathy, pseudomembranous colitis

DOSAGE AND ROUTES
>> cefaclor
Adult: PO 250-500 mg q8hr; EXT REL 375-500 mg q12hr; max 1.5 g/day (cap, oral susp); 1 g/day (EXT REL)
Child >1 mo: PO 20-40 mg/kg daily in divided doses q8hr, or total daily dose may be divided and given q12hr, max 1 g/day

Available forms: Caps 250, 500 mg; oral susp 125, 187, 250, 375 mg/5 ml; EXT REL tab 375, 500 mg

>> cefoTEtan
Adult: IV/IM 1-3 g q12hr × 5-10 days

Perioperative prophylaxis
Adult: IV 1-2 g ½-1 hr before surgery

Renal dose
Adult: IM/IV CCr 30-50 ml/min 1-2 g, then 1-2 g q8-12hr; CCr 10-29 ml/min 1-2 g, then 1-2 g q12-24hr; CCr 5-9 ml/min 1-2 g, then 0.5-1 g q12-24hr; CCr <5 ml/min 1-2 g, then 0.5-1 g q24-48hr

Available forms: Inj 1, 2, 10 g

>> cefOXitin
Adult: IM/IV 1-2 g q6-8hr
Child/infant >3 mo: IM/IV most infections 13.3-26.7 mg/kg q 4 h or 20-40 mg/kg q 6 hr

Severe infections
Adult: IM/IV 2 g q4hr
Child ≥3 mo: IM/IV 80-160 mg/kg/day divided q4-6hr; max 12 g/day

Available forms: Powder for inj 1, 2, 10 g; premixed 1 g/50 mL D_5W, 2 g/50 mL D_5W

>> cefprozil
Upper respiratory infections
Adult: PO 500 mg q24hr × 10 days

Lower respiratory infections
Adult: PO 500 mg q12hr × 10 days

Skin/skin structure infections
Adult: PO 250-500 mg q12hr × 10 days

C

Otitis media
Child 6 mo-12 yr: PO 15 mg/kg q12hr × 10 days

Renal dose
CCr <30 ml/min 50% of dose

Available forms: Tabs 250, 500 mg; susp 125, 250 mg/5 ml

>> **cefuroxime**
Oral tablets and suspension are not bio-equivalent

Lower respiratory tract infections (mild-moderate)/uncomplicated skin/skin structure infections
Adult/adolescent: PO 250-500 mg q12hr × 5-10 days; IV/IM 750 mg q8hr
Child (unlabeled): PO 125 mg q12hr; 750 mg IV or IM q8hr
Adolescent/child/infant ≥3 mo: IV/IM 50-100 mg/kg/day divided q6-8hr (not to exceed adult dose)

Serious lower respiratory tract infections/serious skin/skin structure infections
Adult: IV/IM 0.75-1.5 g q8hr; life-threatening infections or infections caused by less-susceptible organisms, IV 1.5 g q6hr
Adolescent/child/infant ≥3 mo: IV/IM 50-150 mg/kg/day divided q6-8hr; max 6 g/day

Impetigo
Child: PO (tab unlabeled) 250 mg PO q12hr
Child/infant ≥3 mo: (PO-Susp) 30 mg/kg/day divided into two doses; max 1000 mg/day

Urinary tract infection (UTI)
Adult/adolescent: PO 250 mg q12hr × 7-10 days; IV/IM 0.75-1.5 g q8hr (general) or 0.75 g q8hr (uncomplicated)
Adolescent/child/infant ≥3 mo: IV/IM 50-100 mg/kg/day in divided doses q6-8hr (max adult dose)

Bone and joint infections
Adult: IV/IM 1.5 g q8hr; for life-threatening infections or infections caused by less-susceptible organisms, 1.5 g IV q6hr
Adolescent/child/infant ≥3 mo: IV/IM 150 mg/kg/day in divided doses q8hr; max 6 g/day

Upper respiratory tract infections (e.g., pharyngitis, tonsillitis)
Adult/adolescent: PO (tabs) 250 mg q12hr × 10 days
Child/infant ≥3 mo: PO (susp) 20 mg/kg/day divided into 2 doses × 10 days, max 500 mg/day

Acute bacterial maxillary sinusitis
Adult/adolescent: PO (tabs) 250 mg bid × 10 days
Child (who can swallow tablets whole): PO (tabs) 250 mg bid × 10 days
Child/infant ≥3 mo: PO (susp) 15 mg/kg bid × 10 days, max 1000 mg/day

Early Lyme disease
Adult/adolescent: PO (tabs) 500 mg q12hr × 20 days
Child (unlabeled): PO (susp) 30 mg/kg/day in 2 divided doses (max 1000 mg/day) or 1000 mg/day × 14-21 days

Acute otitis media
Child (who can swallow whole tablets): PO (tabs) 250 mg bid × 10 days
Child/infant ≥3 mo: PO (susp) 30 mg/kg/day divided into 2 doses × 10 day, max 1000 mg/day

Septicemia
Adult: IV/IM 1.5-3 g q8hr, max 9 g/day
Adolescent/child/infant ≥3 mo: IV/IM 200-240 mg/kg/day divided doses q6-8hr, max 9 g/day

Renal dose
Adult: CCr 10-20 ml/min: IV/IM 0.75-1.5 g, then 750 mg q12hr; CrCl <10 ml/min: IV/IM 0.75-1.5 g, then 750 mg q24hr
Child: The frequency of dosing should be modified consistent with the recommendations for adults

Available forms: Tabs 125, 250, 500 mg; inj 150, 750 mg, 1.5, 7.5 g; inj 750 mg; 1.5 g powder, susp 125, 250 mg/5 ml

ADVERSE EFFECTS
CNS: Dizziness, headache, fatigue, paresthesia, fever, chills, confusion, seizures
GI: *Diarrhea*, nausea, vomiting, anorexia, Clostidium difficile-associated diarrhea (CDAD)
HEMA: Leukopenia, thrombocytopenia, agranulocytosis, neutropenia, lymphocytosis, eosinophilia, pancytopenia, hemolytic anemia, leukocytosis, granulocytopenia
INTEG: Rash, urticaria, dermatitis, Stevens-Johnson syndrome, IV site reactions
RESP: Dyspnea
SYST: Anaphylaxis, serum sickness, super-infection

INTERACTIONS
Individual drugs
Antacids: decreased absorption of cephalosporins
Probenecid: decreased excretion of product and increased blood levels/toxicity

---

Drug classifications

Aminoglycosides: increased effect/toxicity

Anticoagulants, antiplatelets, NSAIDs, thrombolytics: increased bleeding (cefoTEtan)

Drug/lab test

False: increased creatinine (serum urine), urinary 17-KS

False positive: urinary protein, direct Coombs' test, urine glucose (Clinitest)

Interference: cross-matching

NURSING CONSIDERATIONS

Assessment

• Assess patient for signs and symptoms of **infection** including characteristics of wounds, sputum, urine, stool, WBC >10,000/mm³, earache, fever; obtain baseline information and during treatment

• Assess patient for previous sensitivity reaction to penicillins or other cephalosporins; cross-sensitivity between penicillins and cephalosporins is common

• Obtain C&S before beginning product therapy to identify if correct treatment has been initiated, may begin treatment before results are received

• **Assess for anaphylaxis:** rash, urticaria, pruritus, dyspnea, chills, fever, joint pain; angioedema may occur a few days after therapy begins; EPINEPHrine and resuscitation equipment should be available for anaphylactic reaction

• Identify urine output; if decreasing, notify prescriber (may indicate nephrotoxicity); also check for increased BUN, creatinine, urine output; if decreasing notify prescriber

• Monitor blood studies: AST, ALT, CBC, Hct, bilirubin, LDH, alkaline phosphatase, Coombs' test monthly if patient is on long-term therapy

• Monitor electrolytes: potassium, sodium, chloride monthly if patient is on long-term therapy

• *Clostridium difficile*–associated diarrhea **CDAD):** Assess bowel pattern daily; if severe diarrhea occurs, product should be discontinued

• Monitor for bleeding: ecchymosis, bleeding gums, hematuria, stool guaiac daily if on long-term therapy

• Assess for **overgrowth of infection:** perineal itching, fever, malaise, redness, pain, swelling, drainage, rash, diarrhea, change in cough, sputum

Patient problem

Infection (uses)

Diarrhea (adverse reactions)

Implementation

>> cefaclor

• Do not break, crush, chew, or cut EXT REL tabs

• Give in even doses around the clock; if GI upset occurs, give with food; product must be given for 10-14 days to ensure organism death and prevent superinfection

• Shake susp, refrigerate, discard after 2 wk

>> cefoTEtan

IM route

• Reconstitute 1 g/2 ml or 2 g/3 ml of sterile or bacteriostatic water for inj; may be diluted with 0.5% of 1% lidocaine to prevent pain; give deep in large muscle mass, massage

IV route

• May be stored 96 hr refrigerated or 24 hr at room temperature

• Check for irritation, extravasation, phlebitis daily; change site q72hr

• Direct IV route dilute in 1 g/10 ml or more and give over 5 min

• Intermittant IV infusion further dilute in 50-100 ml of 0.9% NaCl or D₅W; give over 3-5 min; discontinue primary line while running intermittent inf

Y-site compatibilities: Allopurinol, amifostine, aztreonam, dilTIAZem, famotidine, filgrastim, fluconazole, fludarabine, heparin, regular insulin, melphalan, meperidine, morphine, PACLitaxel, sargramostim, tacrolimus, teniposide, theophylline, thiotepa

>> cefOXitin

IV route

• Check for irritation, extravasation, phlebitis daily; change site q72hr

• Direct IV route, dilute 1 g/10 ml or 2 g/20 ml of sterile water for inj; shake, let stand until clear; give over 3-5 min

• Intermittent IV infusion route, further dilute with 50-100 ml of D₅W, D₁₀W, D₅/0.25% NaCl, D₅/0.45% NaCl, D₅/0.9% NaCl, 0.9% NaCl D₅/LR, D₅/0.02%, sodium bicarbonate, Ringer's, or LR; give over 15-30 min; may store 96 hr refrigerated or 24 hr room temperature

• Continuous infusion route, dilute in 500-1000 ml; give over prescribed rate

Y-site compatibilities: Acyclovir, amifostine, aztreonam, cyclophosphamide, dilTIAZem, famotidine, fluconazole, foscarnet, HYDROmorphone, magnesium sulfate, meperidine, morphine, ondansetron, perphenazine, teniposide, thiotepa

>> cefprozil
PO route
- May be given without regard to meals
- Shake oral suspension well before use

>> cefuroxime
PO route
- Give for 10-14 days to ensure organism death, prevent superinfection, discard after 14 days
- Give with food if needed for GI symptoms
- Five after C&S obtained

Intermittant IV infusion route
- Solution for infusion may be further diluted in 50-100 mL (10-40 mg/mL) of 0.9% NaCl, D5W, stable refrigerated 48 hr, 24 hr room temperature give over 15-60 min

Continuous IV infusion route
- Dilute solution for infusion in 500-100 mL

Patient/family education
- Advise patient to contact prescriber if vaginal itching, loose foul-smelling stools, furry tongue occur; may indicate **superinfection**
- Instruct patient to take all medication prescribed for the length of time ordered; take missed dose as soon as remembered unless close to next dose, do not take double dose, use calibrated device for syrup, liquid, suspension
- Advise patient to notify prescriber of diarrhea with blood or pus, which may indicate *Clostridium difficile*-associated diarrhea

Evaluation
Positive therapeutic outcome
- Absence of signs/symptoms of infection (WBC <10,000/mm^3, temp WNL, absence of red draining wounds, earache)
- Reported improvement in symptoms of infection
- Negative C&S

TREATMENT OF ANAPHYLAXIS: EPINEPHrine, antihistamines, resuscitate if needed

---

CEPHALOSPORINS—3RD/4TH GENERATION

cefdinir (Rx)
(sef'dih-ner)
cefditoren pivoxil (Rx)
(sef-dit'oh-ren pih-vox'il)
Spectracef
(4th generation) cefepime (Rx)
(sef'e-peem)
Maxipime

---

cefixime (Rx)
(sef-iks'ime)
Suprax
cefotaxime (Rx)
(sef-oh-taks'eem)
Claforan
cefpodoxime (Rx)
(sef-poe-docks'eem)
cefTAZidime (Rx)
(sef'tay-zi-deem)
Fortaz, Tazicef
ceftibuten (Rx)
(sef-ti-byoo'tin)
Cedax
cefTRIAXone (Rx)
(sef-try-ax'one)
Func. class.: Antiinfective
Chem. class.: Cephalosporin (3rd generation)

Do not confuse: cefTAZidime/ceftizoxime

ACTION: Inhibits bacterial cell wall synthesis, rendering cell wall osmotically unstable, leading to cell death

>> cefdinir
Therapeutic outcome: Bactericidal effects for the following: *Citrobacter diversus, Escherichia coli, Haemophilus influenzae, Haemophilus parainfluenzae, Klebsiella pneumoniae, Moraxella catarrhalis, Proteus mirabilis, Staphylococcus aureus, Staphylococcus epidermidis, Streptococcus agalactiae* (group B), *Streptococcus pneumoniae, Streptococcus pyogenes,* viridans streptococci alpha

USES: Uncomplicated skin and skin structure infections, community-acquired pneumonia, acute exacerbations of chronic bronchitis, acute maxillary sinusitis, pharyngitis, tonsillitis, otitis media

>> cefdinir
Pharmacokinetics

Absorption	Well absorbed
Distribution	Widely distributed; crosses placenta
Metabolism	Not metabolized
Excretion	Kidneys, unchanged; enters breast milk
Half-life	1.7 hr

Pharmacodynamics

Unknown

>> cefditoren pivoxil
Therapeutic outcome: Bactericidal effects for the following organisms: *Haemophilus influenzae, Haemophilus parainfluenzae, Streptococcus pneumoniae, Moraxella catarrhalis, Streptococcus pyogenes, Staphylococcus aureus*

USES: Acute bacterial exacerbation of chronic bronchitis, pharyngitis/tonsillitis; uncomplicated skin, skin structure infections, community-acquired pneumonia, viridans streptococci

>> cefditoren pivoxil
Pharmacokinetics

Absorption	Well absorbed after it is broken down (prodrug)
Distribution	Widely
Metabolism	Unknown
Excretion	Unknown
Half-life	100 mins

Pharmacodynamics

Onset	Rapid
Peak	1.5-3 hr
Duration	12 hrs

>> cefixime
Therapeutic outcome: Bactericidal effects for the following organisms: *Escherichia coli, Proteus mirabilis, Streptococcus pyogenes, Haemophilus influenzae, Moraxella catarrhalis, Streptococcus pneumoniae*

USES: Uncomplicated UTI, pharyngitis/tonsillitis, otitis media, acute bronchitis, exacerbations of chronic bronchitis, uncomplicated gonorrhea

>> cefixime
Pharmacokinetics

Absorption	Unknown
Distribution	Protein binding 65%-70%
Metabolism	Unknown
Excretion	Urine, bile
Half-life	3-4 hr

Pharmacodynamics

Onset	Unknown
Peak	2-6 hr
Duration	Unknown

>> cefotaxime
Therapeutic outcome: Bactericidal effects for the following: *Haemophilus influenzae, Haemophilus parainfluenzae, Escherichia coli, Enterococcus faecalis, Neisseria gonorrhoeae, Neisseria meningitidis, Proteus mirabilis, Klebsiella, Citrobacter, Serratia, Salmonella, Shigella Pseudomonas;* gram-positive organisms *Streptococcus pneumoniae, Streptococcus pyogenes, Staphylococcus aureus*

USES: Lower serious respiratory tract, urinary tract, skin, bone, gonococcal infections; bacteremia, septicemia, meningitis, skin, skin structure infections, CNS infections, perioperative prophylaxis, intraabdominal infections, PID, UTI, ventriculitis

>> cefotaxime
Pharmacokinetics

Absorption	Widely distributed
Distribution	Breast milk, small amounts
Metabolism	Liver, active metabolites
Excretion	40%-65% unchanged, kidney
Half-life	1 hr

Pharmacodynamics

	IV	IM
Onset	5 min	30 min
Peak	Unknown	Unknown
Duration	Unknown	Unknown

>> cefpodoxime
Therapeutic outcome: Bactericidal effects for the following: *Neisseria gonorrhoeae, Haemophilus influenzae, Escherichia coli, Proteus mirabilis, Klebsiella;* gram-positive organisms *Streptococcus pneumoniae, Streptococcus pyogenes, Staphylococcus aureus*

USES: Upper and lower respiratory tract, urinary tract, skin infections; otitis media, STDs

>> cefpodoxime
Pharmacokinetics

Absorption	Well absorbed
Distribution	Widely distributed; crosses placenta, protein binding 13%-38%
Metabolism	Not metabolized
Excretion	Kidneys, unchanged; enters breast milk
Half-life	1-1.5 hr, increased in renal disease

Pharmacodynamics

Unknown

>> cefTAZidime
Therapeutic outcome: Bactericidal effects for the following: *Haemophilus influenzae, Escherichia coli, Enterobacter aerogenes, Proteus mirabilis, Klebsiella, Citrobacter, Enterobacter, Salmonella, Serratia, Pseudomonas aeruginosa, Shigella, Acinetobacter, Bacteroides fragilis, Neisseria; Streptococcus pneumoniae, Streptococcus pyogenes, Staphylococcus aureus*

USES: Serious upper or lower respiratory tract, urinary tract, skin, gynecologic, bone, joint, intraabdominal infections; septicemia, meningitis, febrile neutropenia

>> cefTAZidime
Pharmacokinetics

Absorption	Well absorbed (IM)
Distribution	Widely distributed; crosses placenta
Metabolism	Not metabolized
Excretion	Kidneys, unchanged; enters breast milk
Half-life	1-2 hr; increased in renal disease

Pharmacodynamics

	IM	IV
Onset	Rapid	Immediate
Peak	1.5-2 hr	Infusion's end

>> ceftibuten
Therapeutic outcome: Bactericidal effects for the following: *Haemophilus influenzae, Escherichia coli; Streptococcus pneumoniae, Streptococcus pyogenes, Staphylococcus aureus*

USES: Pharyngitis, tonsillitis, otitis media, secondary bacterial infection of acute bronchitis

>> ceftibuten
Pharmacokinetics

Absorption	Well absorbed
Distribution	Widely distributed; crosses placenta
Metabolism	Not metabolized
Excretion	Kidneys, unchanged; enters breast milk
Half-life	1-1½ hr; increased in renal disease

Pharmacodynamics

Unknown

>> cefTRIAXone
Therapeutic outcome: Bactericidal effects on the following: gram-negative organisms *Haemophilus influenzae, Escherichia coli, Enterobacter aerogenes, Proteus mirabilis, Klebsiella, Citrobacter, Enterobacter, Salmonella, Shigella, Acinetobacter, Bacteroides fragilis, Neisseria, Serratia;* gram-positive organisms *Streptococcus pneumoniae, Streptococcus pyogenes, Staphylococcus aureus*

USES: Serious lower respiratory tract, urinary tract, skin, gonococcal, intraabdominal infections; septicemia, meningitis; bone, joint infections, otitis media, PID

>> cefTRIAXone
Pharmacokinetics

Absorption	Well absorbed
Distribution	Widely distributed; crosses placenta; enters CSF, protein binding 58%-96%
Metabolism	Liver
Excretion	Kidneys, partly
Half-life	6-9 hr

Pharmacodynamics

	IM	IV
Onset	Rapid	Immediate
Peak	1.5-4 hr	30 min

CONTRAINDICATIONS
Hypersensitivity to cephalosporins, infants <1 mo

Precautions: Pregnancy, breastfeeding, children, hypersensitivity to penicillins, renal/GI disease, geriatrics, pseudomembranous colitis, viral infection, vit K deficiencies, diabetes

DOSAGE AND ROUTES
>> cefdinir
Uncomplicated skin and skin structure infections/community-acquired pneumonia
Adult and child ≥13 yr: PO 300 mg q12hr × 10 days or 600 mg q 24 hr
Child 6 mo-12 yr: PO 7 mg/kg q12hr or 14 mg/kg q24hr × 10 days

Acute exacerbations of chronic bronchitis/acute maxillary sinusitis
Adult and child ≥13 yr: PO 300 mg q12hr or 600 mg q24hr × 10 days

---

Pharyngitis/tonsillitis
Adult and child ≥13 yr: PO 300 mg q12hr or 600 mg q24hr × 5-10 days
Child 6 mo-12 yr: PO 7 mg/kg q12hr × 5-10 days or 14 mg/kg q24hr × 5-10 days

Renal dose
Adult/child ≥13 yr: PO CCr <30 mL/min 300 mg q 24 hr
Child 6 mo-12 yr: PO CCr 30 mL/min 7 mg/kg q 24 hr

Available forms: Caps 300 mg, oral susp 125 mg/5 ml, 250 mg/5 ml

>> cefditoren pivoxil
Adult: PO 200-400 mg bid × 10-14 days

Renal dose
Adult: PO CCr 30-49 ml/min, max 200 mg bid; CCr <30 ml/min, max 200, 400 mg daily

Available forms: Tabs 200, 400 mg

>> cefepime
Febrile neutropenia
Adult/adolescent >16 yr/child ≥40 kg: IV 2 g q8hr × 7 days or until neutropenia resolves
Infant ≥2 mo/child/adolescent ≤16 yr and weighing up to 40 kg: IV 50 mg/kg/dose q8hr × 7-10 days or until resolution

Urinary tract infections (mild to moderate)
Adult: IV/IM 0.5-1 g q12hr × 7-10 days

Urinary tract infections (severe)
Adult/adolescent >16 yr/child ≥40 kg: IV 2 g q12hr × 10 days

Pneumonia (moderate to severe)
Adult: IV 1-2 g q12hr × 10 days

Available forms: Powder for inj 500 mg, 1, 2 g; 1 g/50 ml, 2 g/100 ml

>> cefixime
Adult/adolescent/child >12 yr or >45 kg: PO 400 mg/day divided q12-24hr
Child: PO 8 mg/kg/day divided q12-24hr

Renal dose
CCr 21-59 ml/min give 65% of dose; CCr <20 ml/min give 50% of dose

Available forms: Powder for oral susp 100 mg/5 ml, 200 mg/5mL, 500 mg/5mL; chew tabs 100, 150, 200 mg; cap 400 mg

>> cefotaxime
Adult/adolescent/child ≥50 kg: IV/IM (uncomplicated infections) 1 g q12hr, (moderate-severe infections) 1-2 g q8hr, (severe infections)

2 g q6-8hr, (life-threatening infections) 2 g q4hr, max 12 g/day
Adolescent/child <50 kg and infant: IV/IM 50-180 mg/kg/day divided q6-8hr, max 2 g/dose, (severe infections 200-225 mg/kg/day divided q4-6hr max 12 g)
Neonate >7 days: IV/IM 50 mg/kg/dose q8-12hr

Renal dose
Adult: IM CCr <20 ml/min 50% dose reduction

Available forms: Powder for inj 500 mg, 1, 2, 10 g

>> cefpodoxime
Pneumonia
Adult >13 yr: PO 200 mg q12hr for 14 days

Skin and skin structure
Adult >13 yr: PO 400 mg q12hr for 7-14 days

Pharyngitis and tonsillitis
Adult >13 yr: PO 100 mg q12hr for 5-10 days
Child 5 mo-12 yr: PO 5 mg/kg q12hr (max 100 mg/dose or 200 mg/day) × 5-10 days

Uncomplicated UTI
Adult >13 yr: PO 100 mg q12hr for 7 days; dosing interval increased in presence of severe renal impairment

Acute otitis media
Child 5 mo-12 yr: PO 5 mg/kg q12hr for 5 days

Available forms: Tabs 100, 200 mg; granules for susp 50, 100 mg/5 ml

>> cefTAZidime
Adult: IV/IM 1-2 g q8-12hr × 5-10 days
Child: IV/IM 30-50 mg/kg q8hr, max 6 g/day
Neonate: IV/IM 30-50 mg/kg q8-12hr

Renal dose
Adult: IV CCr 31-50 ml/min 1 g q12hr; CCr 16-30 ml/min 1 g q24hr; CCr 6-15 ml/min 1 g loading dose, then 0.5 g q24hr; CCr <5 ml/min 1 g loading dose, then 0.5 g q48hr

Available forms: Inj 500 mg, 1, 2, 6 g/vial

>> ceftibuten
Adult: PO 400 mg daily × 10 days
Child 6 mo-12 yr: PO 9 mg/kg daily × 10 days

Renal dose
Adult: PO CCr 30-49 ml/min 200 mg q24hr; CCr 5-29 ml/min 100 mg q24hr

Available forms: Caps 400 mg; susp 90, 180 mg/5 ml

>> cefTRIAXone
Adult: IM/IV 1-2 g daily, max 4 g q24hr
Child: IM/IV 50-75 mg/kg/day in equal doses q12-24hr

Uncomplicated gonorrhea
Adult: 250 mg IM as single dose
Reduce dosage in severe renal impairment (CCr <10 ml/min)

Available forms: Inj 250, 500 mg, 1, 2, 10 g

ADVERSE EFFECTS
CNS: Headache, dizziness, seizures
GI: *Nausea, vomiting, diarrhea, anorexia,* abdominal pain, *Clostridium difficile*-associated diarrhea (CDAD), cholestasis (cefotaxime)
GU: Pruritus, *candidiasis,* increased BUN, nephrotoxicity, renal failure
HEMA: Leukopenia, thrombocytopenia, agranulocytosis, neutropenia, lymphocytosis, eosinophilia, hemolytic anemia
INTEG: Rash, urticaria, dermatitis, injection site reaction
MS: Arthralgia (cefditoren)
SYST: Anaphylaxis, serum sickness, Stevens-Johnson syndrome, toxic epidermal necrolysis

>> cefepime
Pharmacokinetics

Absorption	Well absorbed (IM)
Distribution	Widely distributed; crosses placenta
Metabolism	Not metabolized
Excretion	Kidneys, unchanged; enters breast milk
Half-life	2 hr; increased in renal disease

Pharmacodynamics

	IM	IV
Onset	Rapid	Immediate
Peak	79 min	Infusion's end
Duration	Unknown	Unknown

INTERACTIONS
Individual drugs
Many products should not be used with calcium salts (mixed or administered) or H_2 blockers antacids (PO)
Probenecid: increased levels of each product

Drug classifications
Aminoglycosides, diuretics (loop), NSAIDs: increased toxicity

Anticoagulants, NSAIDs, thrombolytics: increased bleeding (ceftriaxone)

Drug/food
Iron-rich cereal, infants' formula: decreased absorption

Drug/lab test
Increased: ALT, AST, alkaline phosphatase, LDH, bilirubin, BUN, creatinine
False increase: creatinine (serum urine), urinary 17-KS
False positive: urinary protein, direct Coombs' test, urine glucose
Interference: cross-matching

NURSING CONSIDERATIONS
Assessment
• Assess patient for previous sensitivity reaction to penicillins or other cephalosporins; cross-sensitivity between penicillins and cephalosporins is common
• Assess patient for signs and symptoms of **infection** including characteristics of wounds, sputum, urine, stool, WBC >10,000/mm^3, fever; obtain baseline information and during treatment
• Obtain C&S before beginning product therapy to identify if correct treatment has been initiated, may start treatment before results are received
• **Assess for anaphylaxis:** rash, urticaria, pruritus, chills, fever, joint pain; angioedema may occur a few days after therapy begins; EPINEPHrine and resuscitation equipment should be available for anaphylactic reaction
• Monitor blood studies: AST, ALT, CBC, Hct, bilirubin, LDH, alkaline phosphatase, Coombs' test monthly if patient is on long-term therapy
• Monitor electrolytes: potassium, sodium, chloride monthly if patient is on long-term therapy
• *Clostridium difficile*-associated diarrhea: Assess bowel pattern daily; if severe diarrhea occurs, product should be discontinued; may indicate pseudomembranous colitis
• **Serious skin disorders:** Assess for beginning rash, toxic epidermal necrolysis, Stevens Johnson syndrome may occur
• Assess for **overgrowth of infection:** perineal itching, fever, malaise, redness, pain, swelling, drainage, rash, diarrhea, change in cough, sputum

Patient problem
Infection (uses)
Diarrhea (adverse reactions)

Implementation

>> cefdinir
PO route
• Give oral susp after adding 39 ml water to the 60 ml bottle; 65 ml water to the 12.0 ml bottle; discard unused portion after 10 days, give without regard to food, do not give within 2 hr of antacids, iron supplements

>> cefditoren pivoxil
• Give for 10 days to ensure organism death, prevent superinfection
• Give with food if needed, do not give with antacids
• Give after C&S is completed

>> cefepime
IV route
• Check for irritation, extravasation, phlebitis daily; change site q72hr
• For **intermittent inf** dilute with 50-100 ml of D_5W, give over 30 min

Solution compatibilities: 0.9% NaCl, D_5, 0.5, 1.0% lidocaine, bacteriostatic water for inj with parabens/benzyl alcohol

>> cefixime
• Give for 10-14 days to ensure organism death, prevent superinfection

>> cefotaxime
IV route
• **Dilute** 1 g/10 ml D_5W, NS, sterile water for inj and **give** over 3-5 min by Y-tube or 3-way stopcock; may be **diluted further** with 50-100 ml of 0.9% NaCl or D_5W; **run** over ½-1 hr; discontinue primary inf during administration; or may be diluted in larger volume of sol and given as a cont inf
• Give for 10-14 days to ensure organism death, prevent superinfection
• Thaw frozen container at room temperature or refrigeration, do not force thaw by immersion or microwave; visually inspect container for leaks

Y-site compatibilities: Acyclovir, alfentanil, alprostadil, amifostine, amikacin, aminocaproic acid, aminophylline, anidulafungin, ascorbic acid injection, atenolol, atracurium, atropine, aztreonam, benztropine, bivalirudin, bleomycin, bumetanide, buprenorphine, butorphanol, caffeine, calcium chloride/gluconate, CARBOplatin, cefamandole, cefmetazole, cefonicid, cefoperazone, cefoTEtan, cefOXitin, cefTAZidime (L-arginine), cefTRIAXone sodium, cefuroxime, cimetidine, CISplatin, clindamycin, codeine, cyanocobalamin, cyclophosphamide, cycloSPORINE, cytarabine, DACTINomycin, DAPTOmycin, dexamethasone, dexmedetomidine, digoxin, dilTIAZem, DOCEtaxel, DOPamine, doxacurium, doxycycline, enalaprilat, ePHEDrine, EPINEPHrine, epiRUBicin, epoetin alfa, eptifibatide, erythromycin, esmolol, etoposide, famotidine, fenoldopam, fentaNYL, fludarabine, fluorouracil, folic acid, furosemide, gatifloxacin, gentamicin, glycopyrrolate, granisetron, heparin, hydrocortisone, HYDROmorphone, ifosfamide, imipenem-cilastatin, insulin (regular), isoproterenol, ketorolac, lidocaine, linezolid, LORazepam, LR, magnesium sulfate, mannitol, mechlorethamine, melphalan, meperidine, metaraminol, methicillin, methotrexate, methoxamine, methyldopate, metoclopramide, metoprolol, metroNIDAZOLE, mezlocillin, miconazole, midazolam, milrinone, minocycline, mitoXANtrone, morphine, moxalactam, multiple vitamins, mycophenolate, nafcillin, nalbuphine, naloxone, nesiritide, netilmicin, nitroglycerin, nitroprusside, norepinephrine, normal saline, octreotide, ofloxacin, ondansetron, ornidazole, oxacillin, oxaliplatin, oxytocin, PACLitaxel, palonosetron, pamidronate, pancuronium, pantoprazole, papaverine, pefloxacin, PEMEtrexed, penicillin G potassium/sodium, pentamidine, pentazocine, PENTobarbital, peritoneal dialysis solution, perphenazine, PHENobarbital, phenylephrine, phenytoin, phytonadione, piperacillin, polymyxin B, potassium chloride, procainamide, prochlorperazine, promethazine, propofol, propranolol, protamine, quiNIDine, quinupristin, raNITIdine, remifentanil, Ringer's injection, ritodrine, riTUXimab, rocuronium, sargramostim, sodium acetate/bicarbonate, sodium fusidate, sodium lactate, succinylcholine, SUFentanil, sulfamethoxazole-trimethoprim, tacrolimus, teniposide, theophylline, thiamine, thiotepa, ticarcillin, ticarcillin-clavulanate, tigecycline, tirofiban, TNA, tobramycin, tolazoline, TPN, trastuzumab, trimetaphan, urokinase, vancomycin, vasopressin, vecuronium, verapamil, vinorelbine, voriconazole

>> cefpodoxime
PO route
• Do not break, crush, or chew tabs due to taste
• Give for 10-14 days to ensure organism death, prevent superinfection
• With food for better absorption, do not give within 2 hr of antacids, H_2 receptor antagonists
• Shake susp well, refrigerate, discard after 2 wk

>> cefTAZidime
IM route
• **Fortaz, Tazidime vials:** Reconstitute 500 mg or 1 g with 1.5 or 3 ml, respectively, of sterile or bacteriostatic water for injection, or 0.5%-1% lidocaine (approx. 280 mg/ml)
• **Tazicef vials:** Reconstitute 1 g/3 ml sterile water for injection (approx. 280 mg/ml)
• **Ceptaz vials:** Reconstitute 1 g/3 ml sterile or bacteriostatic water for injection or 0.5%-1% lidocaine (approx. 250 mg/ml)

• Withdraw the dose, making sure the needle remains in the vial; ensure that no CO_2 bubbles are present; inject deeply in large muscle mass; aspirate prior to injection

IV route
• If possible, visually inspect for particulate matter and discoloration
• **Fortaz, Tazicef, Tazidime packs:** Reconstitute 1 or 2 g/100 ml sterile water for injection or other compatible **IV** sol (10 or 20 mg/ml, respectively). Reconstitution is done in two stages. First, inject 10 ml of the diluents into the pack and shake well to dissolve and become clear; CO_2 pressure inside the container will occur; insert a vent needle to release the pressure; add remaining diluents and remove vent needle
• **Fortaz, Tazicef, Tazidime vials:** Reconstitute 500 mg, 1 g, 2 g with 5, 10, 10 ml, respectively, of sterile water for injection or other compatible **IV** sol (100, 95-100, or 170-180 mg/ml, respectively; shake well to dissolve
• **Fortaz, Tazidime-ADD-Vantage vials** (for **IV** only): Reconstitute 1 or 2 g with NS, ½ NS, D_5W in either 50 or 100 ml flexible diluents container; to release CO_2 pressure, insert a vent needle after dissolving; remove vent before using
• **Ceptaz packs:** Reconstitute 1 or 2 g/100 ml sterile water for injection or compatible **IV** sol (10 or 20 mg/ml, respectively). Reconstitution is done in two stages. First, inject 10 ml of the diluent into the pack and shake well to dissolve; add the remaining diluents; insert as vent needle before giving
• **Ceptaz vials:** Reconstitute 1 or 2 g/10 ml of sterile water for injection or compatible **IV** sol (90-95, or 170-180 mg/ml, respectively)
• **Ceptaz ADD-Vantage vials** (for **IV** infusion only): Reconstitute 1 or 2 g with NS, ½ NS, or D_5W in either 50 or 100 ml diluent container as appropriate
Direct intermittent IV infusion route
• **Vials:** Withdraw the correct dose, making sure the needle opening remains in the solution; make sure there are no CO_2 bubbles in the syringe before injection; inject directly over 3-5 min or slowly into the tubing of a free-flowing compatible IV solution
Intermittent IV infusion route
• **Vials:** Withdraw the correct dose, making sure the needle opening remains in the solution; make sure there are no CO_2 bubbles in the syringe before injection; infusion packs and ADD-Vantage systems are ready for infusion after reconstitution; infuse over 15-30 min

>> ceftibuten
• Administer for 10 days to ensure organism death, prevent superinfection
• Administer after C&S
• Administer on empty stomach

>> cefTRIAXone
• Give IM inj deep in large muscle mass
• Give for 10-14 days to ensure organism death, prevent superinfection

IV route
• Give **IV** after reconstituting 250 mg/2.4 ml of 500 mg/4.8 ml, 1 g/9.6 ml, 2 g/19.2 ml D_5W, water for inj, 0.9% NaCl; further diluted with 50-100 ml (40 mg/mL) of 0.9% NaCl, D_5W, $D_{10}W$, shake; run over ½ hr
• Do not mix with calcium salts

Y-site compatibilities: Acyclovir, allopurinol, aztreonam, cisatracurium, dilTIAZem, DOXOrubicin liposome, fludarabine, foscarnet, heparin, melphalan, meperidine, methotrexate, morphine, PACLitaxel, remifentanil, sargramostim, tacrolimus, teniposide, theophylline, vinorelbine, warfarin, zidovudine

Patient/family education
• Teach patient to report sore throat, bruising, bleeding, joint pain; may indicate blood dyscrasias (rare)
• Advise patient to contact prescriber if vaginal itching, loose foul-smelling stools, furry tongue occur; may indicate superinfection
• Advise patient to notify prescriber of diarrhea with blood or pus, may indicate *Clostridium difficile*-associated diarrhea
• To complete full course of treatment, take missed dose as soon as remembered unless close to next dose, do not take a double dose, use calibrated device for suspension

Evaluation
Positive therapeutic outcome
• Absence of signs/symptoms of infection (WBC <10,000/mm³, temp WNL, absence of red draining wounds, earache)
• Reported improvement in symptoms of infection
• Negative C&S

TREATMENT OF ANAPHYLAXIS: EPINEPHrine, antihistamines, resuscitate if needed

cephradine
See cephalosporins—1st generation

⚠ HIGH ALERT

ceritinib
(cerr-ah-tin'ib)
Zykadia
Func. class.: Antineoplastic—Miscellaneous
Chem. class.: Protein-tyrosine kinase inhibitor

ACTION: A tyrosine kinase inhibitor targeting anaplastic lymphoma kinase (ALK); also targets insulinlike growth factors

Therapeutic outcome: Decreased progression of tumor

USES: 🔎 Anaplastic lymphoma kinase (ALK)-positive metastatic non-small cell lung cancer (NSCLC)

Pharmacokinetics

Absorption	Unknown
Distribution	Protein 97%
Metabolism	CYP3A4
Excretion	68% (feces)
Half-life	41 hr

Pharmacodynamics

Onset	Unknown
Peak	4-6 hr
Duration	Unknown

CONTRAINDICATIONS
Pregnancy, hypersensitivity, breastfeeding, QT prolongation

Precautions: Children, geriatric patients, cardiac/hepatic disease, GI bleeding, bone marrow suppression, infection, diarrhea, hyperglycemia, diabetes mellitus, nausea/vomiting, pancreatitis, pneumonitis, torsade de pointes, bradycardia, cardiac arrhythmias, electrolyte imbalances, corticosteroid therapy

DOSAGE AND ROUTES
Adults: PO 450 mg qday on an empty stomach until disease progression or unacceptable toxicity; decrease dose by 1/3 round to nearest 150 mg strong 3A4 inhibitors

Hepatic dose
Adult: PO ALT or AST >5 times above ULN and total bilirubin ≤ 2 times ULN: Hold product. When ALT/AST return to baseline or ≤ 3 times ULN, resume with a 150-mg dose reduction. Do not resume those unable to tolerate 300 mg qday

Available forms: Cap 150 mg

ADVERSE EFFECTS
CNS: Weakness, fatigue, paresthesias
CV: QT prolongation, torsade de pointes, bradycardia
GI: *Nausea,* hepatotoxicity, vomiting, *anorexia,* pancreatitis, GERD, *abdominal pain,* diarrhea, constipation
INTEG: *Rash*
META: Hyperglycemia, hyperphosphatemia, hyperamylasemia
MISC: Renal failure
RESP: Cough, dyspnea, pneumonitis

INTERACTIONS
Individual drugs
Warfarin: increased plasma concentration of warfarin; avoid use with warfarin; use low molecular weight anticoagulants instead
Beta blockers: increased bradycardia, avoid using concurrently

Drug classifications
CYP3A4 inhibitors (ketoconazole, itraconazole, erythromycin, clarithromycin): increased ceritinib concentrations, avoid using together
CYP3A4 inducers (dexamethasone, phenytoin, carBAMazepine, rifampin, PHENobarbital): decreased ceritinib concentrations
CYP3A4/CYP2C9 substrates: increased toxicity of each of these products

Drug/food
Grapefruit and its juice: increase effect, toxicity of ceritinib

Drug/herb
Decreased: ceritinib concentration—St. John's wort

Drug/lab test
Increased: bilirubin, amylase, LFTs

NURSING CONSIDERATIONS
Assessment
• **Bradycardia:** Symptomatic, but not life-threatening: Hold and evaluate other medications that may cause bradycardia. When asymptomatic or heart rate ≥60 bpm, resume with an adjusted dose, do not resume in those unable to tolerate 300 mg qday; life-threatening: discontinue product
• **Severe or intolerable nausea, vomiting, or diarrhea:** Hold dose; when improved, resume with a 150-mg dose reduction. Do not resume in those unable to tolerate 300 mg qday
• **QT prolongation:** Assess for a history of cardiac arrhythmias, congestive heart failure, bradycardia, electrolyte imbalance, or congenital long QT syndrome. Correct electrolyte abnormalities before starting product; monitor ECG

• Dosage adjustments due to treatment-related toxicity QTc prolongation: QTc >500 msec on at least 2 separate ECGs: Hold. When QTc returns to <481 msec (or baseline if >481 msec), resume with a 150-mg dose reduction. Do not resume in those unable to tolerate 300 mg qday.
• Any occurrence, QTc prolongation in combination with torsade de pointes or polymorphic ventricular tachycardia or signs/symptoms of serious arrhythmia: Permanently discontinue
• **Hyperglycemia:** Monitor for hyperglycemia, may be 6-8-fold in diabetic patients
• **Persistent hyperglycemia >250 mg/dL despite optimal antihyperglycemic therapy:** Do not resume in those unable to tolerate 300 mg qday. If blood sugars cannot be controlled medically, discontinue
• **Pancreatitis:** Monitor for nausea, vomiting, severe abdominal pain
• **Lipase or amylase >2 times the upper limit of normal (ULN):** Hold product and monitor serum lipase/amylase. When improved to <1.5 x ULN, resume with a 150-mg dose reduction. Do not resume in those unable to tolerate 300 mg qday

Patient problem
Risk for injury (adverse reactions)
Lack of knowledge of medication (teaching)

Implementation
• **Any grade interstitial lung disease (ILD) or pneumonitis:** Permanently discontinue
• **Strong CYP3A4 inhibitors:** Close monitoring of the QT interval is recommended. If the strong CYP3A4 inhibitor is discontinued, resume the previous dosage
• Take on an empty stomach. Do not give within 2 hr of a meal; swallow tablets whole; do not crush or dissolve; if a dose is missed, take as soon as remembered unless the next dose is due within 12 hr. Do not take 2 doses at the same time if missed; if vomiting occurs, do not give an additional dose. Take the next dose at the next scheduled time
• Store at 77°F (25°C).

Patient/family education
• **Pregnancy:** Teach patient to notify their provider immediately if pregnancy is suspected; effective contraception is needed during and for ≥ 2wk after treatment; if product is used during pregnancy or if the patient becomes pregnant during use, the woman should be apprised of the potential hazard to the fetus
• Teach patient about reason for treatment, expected results, to avoid grapefruit juice

• Teach patient to report adverse reactions immediately: abdominal pain, nausea, vomiting, increased blood glucose in diabetics
• Advise patient to avoid OTC products unless approved by prescriber, to take as directed, not to double or miss doses

Evaluation
Positive therapeutic outcome
• Decreased spread of tumor

RARELY USED

cerliponase alfa
Brineura
Func. class.: Alimentary tract and metabolism agents; lysosomal storage disorder agents

USES: For the treatment of late infantile neuronal ceroid lipofuscinosis type 2

DOSAGE/ROUTES
Late-infantile neuronal ceroid lipofuscinosis type 2 (CLN2) disease, a form of Batten disease
Child and adolescent 3 to 17 yr: IV 300 mg every other wk. Give first at an infusion rate of 2.5 ml/hr, then with the required infusion of intraventricular electrolytes at the same infusion rate of 2.5 ml/hr (complete infusion time is 4.5 hr). Pretreatment with antihistamines with or without antipyretics or corticosteroids is recommended 30 to 60 min before the start of the infusion

---

certolizumab (Rx)
(ser'tue-liz'oo-mab)
Cimzia
Func. class.: GI antiinflammatory, antirheumatic
Chem. class.: Anti-TNF (tissue necrosis factor) agent

ACTION: Monoclonal antibody that neutralizes the activity of tumor necrosis factor-α (TNF-α) found in Crohn's disease; decreased infiltration of inflammatory cells

Therapeutic outcome: Absence of fever, mucus in stools, decreased abdominal cramping or other symptoms of Crohn's disease; ability to move without pain

USES: Crohn's disease (moderate-severe) that has not responded to conventional therapy, rheumatoid arthritis (moderate-severe), psoriatic arthritis, ankylosing spondylitis

---

Pharmacokinetics

Absorption	Unknown
Distribution	Unknown
Metabolism	Unknown
Excretion	Unknown
Half-life	Terminal 14 days

Pharmacodynamics

Onset	Unknown
Peak	54-171 hr
Duration	Unknown

CONTRAINDICATIONS
Influenza, **IV** administration, sepsis, hypersensitivity

Precautions: Pregnancy, breastfeeding, children, geriatric patients, AIDS, coagulopathy, diabetes, fungal infection, heart failure, hepatitis, human anti-chimertic antibody, immunosuppression, leukopenia, MS, cancer, neurologic disease, surgery, thrombocytopenia, TB, vaccinations, renal disease

> **BLACK BOX WARNING:** Infection, neoplastic disease in children

DOSAGE AND ROUTES
Crohn's disease (moderate-severe)
Adult: SUBCUT 400 mg given as 2 inj at wk 0, 2, 4; if clinical response occurs, give 400 mg q4wk

Rheumatoid arthritis (moderate-severe), Ankylosing spondolytis, Psoriatic Arthritis
Adult: SUBCUT 400 mg (as two injections of 200 mg) once, then repeat at wk 2 and 4; maintenance, 200 mg q2wk or 400 mg q4wk

Available forms: Solution for inj 200 mg/mL; Subcut injection (prefilled syringe) 400 mg kit

ADVERSE EFFECTS
CNS: Anxiety, bipolar disorder, suicidal ideation
CV: Heart failure, MI, cardiac dysrhythmia
GI: Abdominal pain
HEMA: Anemia, pancytopenia
INTEG: *Rash, urticaria,* angioedema
MISC: *Infection*
SYST: Anaphylaxis, malignancies, serum sickness, arthralgia

INTERACTIONS
Individual drugs
Abatacept, adalimumab, anakinra, etanercept, infliximab, rilonacept, do not use concurrently, increased possible infections

Drug classifications
Immunosuppressive agents: increased possible infections, do not use concurrently

Live vaccines, toxoids: do not administer concurrently

NURSING CONSIDERATIONS
Assessment
• Monitor antibody test (ANA), hepatitis B serology, CBC with differential
• **Assess rheumatoid arthritis/ankylosing spondylitis** pain, range of motion baseline and during treatment
• Assess GI symptoms: nausea, vomiting, abdominal pain, hepatitis, increased LFTs
• **Assess for allergic reaction, anaphylaxis:** rash, dermatitis, urticaria, dyspnea, hypotension, fever, chills; discontinue if severe, administer EPINEPHrine, corticosteroids, antihistamines; assess for allergies to murine proteins before starting therapy
• **Hepatitis B virus:** Carriers of HBV should be monitored, those at risk for HBV should be evaluated before use

> **BLACK BOX WARNING: Fungal infection:** Fever, weight loss, diaphoresis, fatigue, dyspnea; assess infections: discontinue if infection occurs; do not administer to patients with active infections

> **BLACK BOX WARNING:** Identify TB, risk for HBV before beginning treatment; a TB test should be obtained; if present, TB should be treated prior to receiving inFLIXimab

> **BLACK BOX WARNING:** Do not use in children, lymphoma may occur

Patient problem
Risk for infection (adverse reactions)
Risk for injury (adverse reactions)

Implementation
SUBCUT route
• TB testing: TB testing is required before use, TB testing should be done baseline and periodically, use in TB or active infections is contraindicated
• Give by SUBCUT only
• Allow reconstitution to warm to room temp; add 1 ml sterile water for inj to each vial; two vials will be needed for Crohn's disease
• Gently swirl; do not shake; full reconstitution may take up to 30 min; reconstituted product may remain at room temp for up to 2 hr or refrigerated up to 24 hr
• Warm to room temperature if reconstituted product has been refrigerated
• Use 2 syringes and 2 20-G needles

- Withdraw reconstituted sol from each vial into separate syringes; each will contain 200 mg; switch 20-G to 23-G needle; inject into 2 separate sites in abdomen or thigh
- Store in refrigerator; do not freeze

Patient/family education
- Inform patient to discuss with provider all OTC, Rx, herbals, supplements taken
- **Anaphylaxis, angioedema, hypersensitivity:**
- Inform patient to report immediately rash, itching, swollen lips, tongue, face
- Discuss with patient the possibility of secondary malignancies
- Teach patient not to receive live virus vaccines while taking this product
- Teach patient how to inject medication if given prefilled syringes for same use
- Advise patient to notify prescriber of GI symptoms, infections, redness, pain, swelling at injection site
- Caution patient not to operate machinery, drive if dizziness, vertigo occur
- **Pregnancy/breastfeeding:** Advise patient to report if pregnancy is planned or suspected, or if breastfeeding; women who are pregnant should enroll in the mother to baby study by OTIS at 1-877-311-8972

Evaluation
Positive therapeutic outcome
- Absence of fever, mucus in stools; decreased inflammation in joints, improved ROM, pain

---

cetirizine (Rx)
(se-tear′i-zeen)
Reactine ✽, **AllerRelief** ✽, **Rhinaris Relief** ✽, **ZyrTEC**
Func. class.: Antihistamine, peripherally selective (2nd generation)
Chem. class.: Piperazine, H_1 histamine antagonist

Do not confuse: Cetirizine/sertraline/ stavudine, **ZyrTEC**/Xanax/Zantac/Zocor/ ZyPREXA/Zerit

ACTION: Acts on blood vessels, GI, respiratory system by competing with histamine for H_1-receptor site; decreases allergic response by blocking pharmacologic effects of histamine; minimal anticholinergic/sedative action

Therapeutic outcome: Absence of allergy symptoms, rhinitis, and chronic idiopathic urticaria

USES: Rhinitis, allergy symptoms, and chronic idiopathic urticaria

Absorption	Well absorbed
Distribution	Protein binding 93%
Metabolism	Not metabolized
Excretion	Kidneys
Half-life	8.3 hr, decreased in children, increased in renal/ hepatic disease

Onset	½ hr
Peak	1-2 hr
Duration	24 hr

CONTRAINDICATIONS
Hypersensitivity to this product or hydrOXYzine, breastfeeding, newborn or premature infants, severe hepatic disease

Precautions: Pregnancy, children, geriatric, respiratory disease, closed-angle glaucoma, prostatic hypertrophy, bladder neck obstruction, asthma

DOSAGE AND ROUTES
Adult and child ≥6 yr: PO 5-10 mg daily
Child 2-5 yr: PO 2.5 mg daily, may increase to 5 mg daily or 2.5 mg bid
Child 1-2 yr: PO 2.5 mg daily, may increase to 2.5 mg q12hr
Child 6-11 mo: PO 2.5 mg daily
Geriatric: PO 5 mg daily, may increase to 10 mg/day

Renal dose
Adult: PO CCr 11-31 ml/min 5 mg daily

Hepatic dose/hemodialysis
Adult: PO 5 mg daily
Child 6-11 yr: PO <2.5 mg/day initially

Available forms: Tabs 5, 10 mg; syr 5 mg/ 5 ml; chew tab 5, 10 mg; orally disintegrating tab 10 mg

ADVERSE EFFECTS
CNS: *Headache, drowsiness,* sedation, *fatigue*
GI: *Dry mouth*
EENT: Pharyngitis
INTEG: Rash, eczema

INTERACTIONS
Individual drugs
Alcohol: increased CNS depression

Drug classifications
CNS depressants, opioids, sedative/hypnotics: increased CNS depression
MAOIs: increased anticholinergic effect

Drug/food
Prolongs absorption by 1.7 hr

Drug/lab test
False negative: skin allergy tests (discontinue antihistamine 3 days before testing)

NURSING CONSIDERATIONS
Assessment
- Assess respiratory status: rate, rhythm; increase in bronchial secretions, wheezing, chest tightness; provide fluids to 2 L/day to decrease secretion thickness
- Assess for **allergy symptoms:** pruritus, urticaria, watering eyes, baseline, during treatment

Patient problem
Impaired airway clearance (uses)

Implementation
- Give without regard to meals
- Store in tight, light-resistant container
- **Chew tabs:** chew before swallowing, may use without or with water
- **Syrup:** use calibrated measuring device

Patient/family education
- Teach all aspects of product uses; to notify prescriber if confusion, sedation, hypotension occur; to avoid driving or other hazardous activity if drowsiness occurs; to avoid alcohol or other CNS depressants that may potentiate effect
- Instruct patient to take without regard to meals
- Advise patient to use sugarless gum, candy, frequent sips of water to minimize dry mouth
- Teach patient to take at night as drowsiness may occur, especially in children

Evaluation
Positive therapeutic outcome
- Absence of runny or congested nose, rashes

TREATMENT OF OVERDOSE:
Lavage, diazePAM, vasopressors, phenytoin IV

---

cetuximab (Rx)
(se-tux'i-mab)
Erbitux
Func. class.: Antineoplastic—miscellaneous, monoclonal antibody
Chem. class.: Epidermal growth factor receptor inhibitor

ACTION: Not fully understood; binds to ⚠ K-RAS wild type epidermal growth factor receptors (EGFRs); inhibits phosphorylation and activation of receptor-associated kinase resulting in inhibition of cell growth

Therapeutic outcome: Decrease in tumor size

USES: Alone or in combination with irinotecan for K-RAS wild type EGFR expressing metastatic colorectal carcinoma, head/neck cancer

Pharmacokinetics

Absorption	Complete
Distribution	Unknown
Metabolism	Unknown
Excretion	Unknown
Half-life	114 hrs

Pharmacodynamics

Onset	Unknown
Peak	Unknown
Duration	Unknown

CONTRAINDICATIONS
Hypersensitivity to this product or murine proteins, ⚠ RAS-mutant metastatic colorectal cancer or unknown RAS mutation

Precautions: Pregnancy, breastfeeding, child, geriatric, CV/renal/hepatic disease, ocular, pulmonary disorders, arrhythmias, CAD, platinum-based therapy infusion-related reactions, radiation, cardiac, respiratory arrest

> **BLACK BOX WARNING:** Cardiac arrest

DOSAGE AND ROUTES
Adult: IV INF 400 mg/m^2 loading dose given over 120 min, max INF rate 5 ml/min, weekly maintenance dose (all other infusions) is 250 mg/m^2 given over 60 min, max INF rate 5 ml/min (10 mg/min); premedicate with an H$_1$ antagonist (diphenhydrAMINE 50 mg **IV**); dosage adjustments are made for INF reactions or dermatologic toxicity; other protocols are used

Available forms: Sol for inj 2 mg/mL

ADVERSE EFFECTS
CNS: *Headache, insomnia, depression,* aseptic meningitis
CV: Cardiac arrest
GI: *Nausea, diarrhea, vomiting, anorexia, mouth ulceration, dehydration, constipation, abdominal pain*
HEMA: Leukopenia, anemia, neutropenia
INTEG: Rash, pruritus, acne, dry skin, toxic epidermal necrolysis, angioedema, *cheilitis, cellulitis, cysts, alopecia, skin/nail disorder,* acute infusion reactions, other skin toxicities
MISC: *Conjunctivitis,* photosensitivity, hypomagnesemia

MS: *Back pain*
RESP: Interstitial lung disease, *cough, dyspnea,* pulmonary embolus, *peripheral edema,* respiratory arrest
SYST: Anaphylaxis, sepsis, infection, Stevens-Johnson syndrome, toxic epidermal necrolysis

INTERACTIONS
Drug/lab test
Increase: LFTs

NURSING CONSIDERATIONS
Assessment
• Monitor pulmonary changes: lung sounds, cough, dyspnea; interstitial lung disease may occur, may be fatal; discontinue therapy if confirmed

> **BLACK BOX WARNING: Cardiac arrest:** monitor electrolytes; in those undergoing radiation therapy, electrolytes may be decreased

• Assess for toxic epidermal necrosis, angioedema, anaphylaxis, Stevens-Johnson syndrome
• Assess GI symptoms: frequency of stools, dehydration, abdominal pain, stomatitis
• Obtain ⚕ **K-RAS mutation test** in metastatic colorectal carcinoma; if K-RAS mutation in codon 12 or 13 is detected, then patient should not receive anti-EGFR antibody therapy

Patient problem
Risk for injury (adverse reactions)
Impaired skin integrity (adverse reactions)

Implementation
Intermittent infusion route
• Administer by **IV** infusion only, do not give by **IV** push or bolus
• Do not shake or dilute
• Do not dilute with other products
• **Infusion pump:** draw up volume of a vial using appropriate syringe/needle (a vented spike or other appropriate transfer device); fill Erbitux into sterile evacuated container/bag, repeat until calculated volume has been put into the container. Use a new needle for each vial; give through in-line filter (low protein binding 0.22-micrometer); affix inf line and prime before starting inf, max rate 5 ml/min; flush line at end of inf with 0.9% NaCl
• **Syringe pump:** Draw up volume of a vial using appropriate syringe/needle (a vented spike); place syringe into syringe driver of a syringe pump and set rate; use an in-line filter 0.22 micrometer (low protein binding); connect inf line and start inf after priming; repeat until calculated volume has been given

• Use a new needle and filter for each vial, max 5 ml/min rate; use 0.9% NaCl to flush line after inf
• Do not piggyback to patient inf line
• Observe patient for adverse reactions for 1hr after inf

> **BLACK BOX WARNING:** Inf reactions (bronchospasm, stridor, urticaria, hypotension, MI): if mild (grade 1 or 2) reduce all doses by 50%; if severe (grade 3 or 4) permanently discontinue, monitor for at least 1 hr after completion of therapy, reactions usually occur during first dose, have emergency equipment nearby

• Store refrigerated 36°-46° F, discard unused portions

Patient/family education
• Instruct patient to report adverse reactions immediately: SOB, severe abdominal pain, skin eruptions
• Explain reason for treatment, expected results

> **BLACK BOX WARNING: Pregnancy/breastfeeding:** Instruct patient to use contraception during treatment and for 6 mo after treatment, both female and male, not to breastfeed during and for 6 mo after treatment

• Advise patient to wear sunscreen and hat to limit sun exposure; sun exposure can exacerbate any skin reactions

Evaluation
Positive therapeutic outcome
• Decrease growth, spread of cancer

chlorothiazide (Rx)
(klor-oh-thye_a-zide)
Diuril
Func. class.: Diuretic, antihypertensive
Chem. class.: Thiazide; sulfonamide derivative

Do not confuse: chlorothiazide/chlorproMAZINE/chlorproPAMIDE/chlorthalidone

ACTION: Acts on the distal tubule and thick ascending limb of the loop of Henle in the kidney, increasing excretion of sodium, water, chloride, magnesium, and potassium

Therapeutic outcome: Decreased B/P, decreased edema in tissues peripherally, diuresis

USES: Hypertension, diuresis, CHF, edema, nephrotic syndrome

Pharmacokinetics

	PO
Absorption	GI tract (10%-20%)
Distribution	Extracellular spaces; crosses placenta
Metabolism	Liver
Excretion	Urine, unchanged; breast milk
Half-life	1-2 hr

Pharmacodynamics

	PO	IV
Onset	2 hr	15 min
Peak	4 hr	1/2 hr
Duration	6-12 hr	2 hr

CONTRAINDICATIONS: Hypersensitivity to thiazides or sulfonamides, anuria, renal decompensation, breastfeeding, hepatic coma

Precautions: Pregnancy, geriatric, hypokalemia, renal/hepatic disease, gout, COPD, LE, diabetes mellitus, hyperlipidemia

DOSAGE AND ROUTES
Hypertension
Adult: PO/IV 500 mg-1 g daily; may divide bid, max 2 g/day in divided doses

Edema
Adult: IV 250 mg q6-12 hr
Child, Infant 6 month and older: PO 10-20 mg/kg/day may divide bid

Renal dose
Adult: PO/IV CCr _30 ml/min; do not use

Available forms: Tabs 250, 500 mg; oral susp 250 mg/5 ml; powder for inj 500 mg chlorothiazide

ADVERSE EFFECTS
CNS: Paresthesia, headache, *dizziness, fatigue*
CV: Irregular pulse, orthostatic hypotension, volume depletion
EENT: Blurred vision
ELECT: *Hypokalemia*, hypercalcemia, hyponatremia, hypochloremia, hypomagnesemia, hyperuricemia
GI: Nausea, vomiting, anorexia, constipation, diarrhea, pancreatitis, GI irritation, **hepatitis**
GU: *Frequency*, polyuria, incontinence, ED
HEMA: Aplastic anemia, hemolytic anemia, leukopenia, agranulocytosis, thrombocytopenia, neutropenia
INTEG: Rash, urticaria, purpura, photosensitivity, alopecia, fever, **exfoliative dermatitis**

META: Hyperglycemia, *hyperuricemia*, increased creatinine, BUN
SYST: Anaphylaxis

INTERACTIONS
Individual drugs
Alcohol: increased hypotension
Allopurinol, digoxin, lithium: increased toxicity
Amphotericin, mezlocillin, piperacillin, ticarcillin: increased hypokalemia
Cholestyramine, colestipol: decreased absorption of thiazides

Drug classifications
Antihypertensives: increased antihypertensive effect
Glucocorticoids: increased hypokalemia
Nitrates: increased hypotension
NSAIDs: decreased diuretic action
Nondepolarizing skeletal muscle relaxants: increased toxicity

Drug/herb
Ephedra: decreased antihypertensive
Hawthorn, horse chestnut: increased antihypertensive effect

Drug/lab test
Increased: calcium, amylase, parathyroid test, CPK
Decreased: PBI
False negative: tyramine tests
Interference: urine steroid tests

NURSING CONSIDERATIONS
Assessment
• Monitor improvement in CVP q8hr
• Check for rashes, temp elevation daily
• Assess for confusion, especially in geriatric; take safety precautions if needed
• Monitor electrolytes: potassium, sodium, calcium, magnesium; also include BUN, blood pH, ABGs, uric acid, CBC, blood glucose
• Assess B/P before, during therapy with patient lying, standing, and sitting as appropriate; orthostatic hypotension can occur rapidly

Patient problems
• Fluid imbalance (uses)
• Lack of knowledge of medication, deficient (teaching)
• Impaired urination (adverse reactions)

Implementation
• Give in AM to avoid interference with sleep
• Potassium replacement if potassium level is 3.0 mg/dl
• Give whole or use oral solution; product may be crushed if patient is unable to swallow

PO route
• Give with food; if nausea occurs, absorption may be increased
IV route
• Do not use solution that is yellow or has a precipitate or crystals
IV direct/IV infusion route
• May be given undiluted over 5 min or as an infusion
• Reconstitute: add 18 ml of sterile water for injection to the vial (28 mg/ml)

Patient/family education
• Teach patient to take medication early in the day to prevent nocturia
• Instruct patient to take with food or milk if GI symptoms of nausea and anorexia occur
• Teach patient to maintain a weekly record of weight and notify prescriber of weight loss >5 lb
• Caution patient that this product causes a loss of potassium, so food rich in potassium should be added to the diet; refer to a dietitian for assistance in planning
• Caution patient not to exercise in hot weather or stand for prolonged periods, since orthostatic hypotension will be enhanced, and to use sunscreen to prevent burning
• Teach patient not to use alcohol or any OTC medications without prescriber's approval; serious product reactions may occur
• Emphasize the need to contact prescriber immediately if muscle cramps, weakness, nausea, dizziness, or numbness occur
• Teach patient to take own B/P and pulse and record

---

chlorthalidone (Rx)
(klor-thal' doan)
Func. class.: Diuretic, antihypertensive
Chem. class.: Thiazide-like phthalimidine derivative

ACTION: Acts on the distal tubule and thick ascending limb of the loop of Henle in the kidney, increasing excretion of sodium, water, chloride, magnesium, potassium, and bicarbonate; possible arteriolar dilatation

Therapeutic outcome: Decreased B/P, decreased edema in lung tissues and peripherally, diuresis

USES: Edema, hypertension, edema in congestive heart failure

Absorption	Well absorbed
Distribution	Extracellular spaces; crosses placenta
Metabolism	Liver
Excretion	Urine, unchanged (30%-60%)
Half-life	40 hr

Pharmacodynamics

Onset	2 hr
Peak	6 hr
Duration	24-72 hr

CONTRAINDICATIONS: Hypersensitivity to thiazides or sulfonamides, anuria, renal decompensation, breastfeeding

Precautions: Pregnancy, geriatric, hypokalemia, renal/hepatic disease, gout, diabetes mellitus, hyperlipidemia, SLE, hypotension, CCr <25 ml/min

DOSAGE AND ROUTES
Adult: PO 12.5-100 mg q day

Available forms: Tabs 25, 50, 100 mg

ADVERSE EFFECTS
CNS: Paresthesia, headache, dizziness, fatigue, weakness, fever
CV: Hypertension, orthostatic hypotension, palpitations, volume depletion
EENT: Blurred vision
ELECT: *Hypokalemia*, hypercalcemia, hyponatremia, hypochloremia, hypomagnesemia
GI: *Nausea, vomiting, anorexia*, constipation, diarrhea, pancreatitis, GI irritation, jaundice
GU: *Frequency*, polyuria, uremia, glucosuria, impotence
HEMA: Aplastic anemia, hemolytic anemia, leukopenia, agranulocytosis, thrombocytopenia, neutropenia
INTEG: Rash, urticaria, purpura, photosensitivity
META: *Hyperglycemia, hyperuricemia*, increased creatinine, BUN, gout

INTERACTIONS
Individual drugs
Alcohol: increased hypotensive effect
Allopurinol, lithium: increased toxicity
Amphotericin B: increased hypokalemia
Cholestyramine, colestipol: decreased absorption of thiazides
Diazoxide: increased hyperglycemia, hypotension

Drug classifications
Glucocorticoids: increased hypokalemia
Nondepolarizing skeletal muscle relaxants: increased toxicity

---

Drug/herb
Ephedra: decreased antihypertensive effect
Hawthorn, horse chestnut: increased
hypotension

Drug/lab test
Increased: triglycerides, calcium, amylase,
cholesterol, bilirubin, creatinine, low-density
lipoproteins, serum/urine glucose (diabetics),
uric acid
Decreased: PBI, parathyroid test, magnesium,
potassium, sodium, urinary calcium

NURSING CONSIDERATIONS
Assessment
• Monitor for **hypokalemia;** *CV:* hypotension,
broad T wave, U wave, ectopy, tachycardia, weak
pulse; *GI:* anorexia, nausea, cramps, constipation, distention, paralytic ileus; *NEURO:* muscle
weakness, altered LOC, drowsiness, apathy,
lethargy, confusion, depression; *RENAL:* acidic
urine, reduced urine, osmolality, nocturia;
RESP: hypoventilation, respiratory muscle
weakness
• Assess fluid volume status: I&O ratios and
record; weight; distended red veins; crackles in
lung, color, quality, and specific gravity of urine;
skin turgor; adequacy of pulses; moist mucous
membranes; bilateral lung sounds; peripheral
pitting edema; dehydration symptoms of decreasing output, thirst, hypotension, dry mouth,
and mucous membranes should be reported
• Monitor electrolytes: potassium, sodium,
calcium, magnesium; also include BUN, blood
pH, ABGs, uric acid, CBC, blood glucose
• **Hypertension:** Assess B/P before and during
therapy with patient lying, standing, and sitting
as appropriate; orthostatic hypotension can
occur rapidly
• Assess for signs of **metabolic alkalosis:**
drowsiness, restlessness

Patient problems
• Fluid imbalance (uses, adverse reactions)
• Lack of knowledge of medication (teaching)
• Impaired urination (adverse reactions)

Implementation
• Give in AM to avoid interference with sleep
• Provide potassium replacement if potassium
level is 3.0 mg/dl; give whole or use oral solutions lightly; product may be crushed if patient is
unable to swallow
• Give with food if nausea occurs; may crush tab
and mix with fluids or applesauce for swallowing

Patient/family education
• Teach patient to take the medication early in
the day to prevent nocturia
• Instruct patient to take with food or milk if GI
symptoms of nausea and anorexia occur
• Teach patient to maintain weekly record of
weight and notify prescriber of weight loss >5 lb
• Caution patient that this product causes a loss
of potassium, so foods rich in potassium should
be added to the diet; refer to a dietitian for assistance in planning
• Caution the patient not to exercise in hot
weather or stand for prolonged periods, since
orthostatic hypotension will be enhanced, and to
use sunscreen to prevent burns
• Teach patient not to use alcohol or any OTC
medications without prescriber's approval;
serious product reactions may occur
• Emphasize the need to contact prescriber
immediately if muscle cramps, weakness, nausea,
dizziness, or numbness occur
• Teach patient to take own B/P and pulse and
record
• Caution patient that orthostatic hypotension
may occur; patient should rise slowly from
sitting or reclining positions and lie down if
dizziness occurs
• Teach patient to continue taking medication
even if feeling better; this product controls
symptoms but does not cure the condition
• Advise patient with hypertension to continue
other medical treatment (exercise, weight loss,
relaxation techniques, cessation of smoking)

Evaluation
Positive therapeutic outcome
• Decreased edema
• Decreased B/P
• Increased diuresis

TREATMENT OF OVERDOSE:
Lavage if taken orally, monitor electrolytes; ad-
minister dextrose in saline; monitor hydration,
CV, renal status

ciclesonide
(sye-kles'oh-nide)
Alvesco, Drymira 🍁, Omnaris, Zetonna
Func. class.: Corticosteroid, nasal

ACTION: Reduces inflammation in nasal
passages

USES: Allergic rhinitis, nasal polyps

Pharmacokinetics

Absorption	Minimal
Distribution	Cross placenta, enter breast milk
Metabolism	Liver
Excretion	Unknown
Half-life	Unknown

Pharmacodynamics

Onset	1-2 days
Peak	2-4 wk
Duration	Unknown

CONTRAINDICATIONS

Hypersensitivity to this product, child <6 yr

Precautions: Breastfeeding, acute broncho-spasm, corticosteroid hypersensitivity, pregnancy, infections, cataracts, HPA suppression, geriatrics, osteoporosis, Cushing's syndrome, increased intracranial pressure, increased intraocular pressure, nasal surgery/trauma

DOSAGE AND ROUTES

Adult and child > 12 yr nasal (Omnaris): 2 sprays in each nostril q day, max 2 sprays in each nostril per day

Adult and child > 12 yr nasal (Zetonna): 1 spray in each nostril q day, max 1 spray in each nostril per day

Available forms: Nasal spray (Omnaris) 50 mcg/metered spray (12.5 g bottle); (Zetonna) 37 mcg/actuation in 6.1 g bottle

ADVERSE EFFECTS

CNS: Headache
EENT: Pharyngitis, epistaxis, nasal congestion
GI: Nausea, vomiting, dry mouth, esophageal candidiasis
INTEG: Rash
ENDO: Adrenal suppression (high dose)
RESP: Bronchospasm, cough
SYST: Anaphylaxis, Angioedema

INTERACTIONS

None significant

NURSING CONSIDERATIONS

Assessment:
• **Nasal condition:** Assess nasal congestion, dryness, discharge, sneezing, cough
• Anaphylaxis, angioedema (assess for rash, trouble breathing): discontinue treatment and notify provider immediately
• **HPA suppression:** Monitor children for growth suppression in long-term therapy

Patient problems

Impaired airway clearance (uses)
Risk for infection (adverse reactions)
Nonadherence (teaching)

Implementation

• Prime the inhaler prior to the initial use by releasing 3 sprays into the air away from the face and other people.

• If the inhaler is not used for more than 10 consecutive days, it should be primed by releasing 3 sprays into the air.
• The canister contains a dose counter. The inhaler should be discarded after the counter reads zero; although the canister is still operational and may contain medication, the accuracy of medication delivery cannot be assured.
• When the dose indicator shows a red zone, approximately 20 inhalations are left, and a refill is required.
• Instruct patient on proper inhalation technique.
• To avoid the spread of infection, do not use the inhaler for more than one person.

Intranasal inhalation administration Omnaris:
• For intranasal use only.
• Prior to first use, shake the inhaler gently and prime the pump by actuating eight times.
• If not used in 4 consecutive days, shake gently and prime with one spray or until fine mist appears.
• Product should be discarded after 120 sprays following initial priming, or 4 months after removal from pouch.
• Blow nose gently if needed. Insert spray tip into nostril, and close the other nostril with finger. With head slightly tilted forward and bottle upright, press pump quickly and firmly while inhaling through nose. Avoid spraying into eyes and directly onto the nasal septum. After administration, wipe the applicator tip with a clean tissue and replace dust cap. If applicator is clogged or needs further cleaning, remove nasal applicator and rinse with warm water. Dry and replace applicator and prime the unit with one spray or until a fine mist appears, then replace cap. To avoid the spread of infection, do not use the container for more than one person.

Zetonna:
• For intranasal use only.
• Prior to first use or if not used in 10 consecutive days, shake the inhaler gently and prime the pump by actuating three times.
• Product should be discarded after 60 sprays following initial priming, or when the dose indicator reads zero.
• Clean the nose piece weekly by wiping with a clean, dry tissue or cloth; do not wash or put any part of the canister or applicator in water.
• Blow nose gently if needed. Insert spray tip into nostril, and close the other nostril with finger. With head slightly tilted back and bottle upright, press pump quickly and firmly while inhaling through nose. Avoid spraying into eyes and directly onto the nasal septum. To avoid the spread of infection, do not use the container for more than one person.

Patient/family education
• Teach patient to take as prescribed, not to skip or double doses
• Teach patient and caregiver how to use
• Advise patient to discuss with provider all OTC, Rx, herbs, supplements taken
• Advise patient to notify provider if pregnancy is planned or suspected, or if breastfeeding
• Inform patient that continuing follow-up exams may be needed

ciclopirox (Rx)
(sye-kloe-peer′ ox)
Loprox, Pentac, Stieprox ✿
Func. class.: Antifungal, topical

ACTION: Inhibits RNA, DNA synthesis in fungus

Therapeutic outcome: Decreased fungal infections including *Candida albicans, Epidermophyton floccosum, Malassezia furfur, Microsporum canis, Trichophyton mentagrophytes, Trichophyton rubrum*

USES: Topical treatment of mild to moderate onychomycosis of fingernails and toenails without lunula involvement, due to *Trichophyton rubrum* in immunocompetent patients; topical treatment of seborrheic dermatitis of the scalp; topical treatment of tinea corporis, tinea cruris, or tinea pedis (*Epidermophyton floccosum; Microsporum canis; Trichophyton mentagrophytes; Trichophyton rubrum*); tinea versicolor (*Malassezia furfur*); or cutaneous candidiasis due to *Candida albicans*

Pharmacokinetics
Absorption	Minimal
Distribution	Local
Metabolism	Unknown
Excretion	Unknown
Half-life	Unknown

Pharmacodynamics
Onset	Unknown
Peak	Unknown
Duration	Unknown

CONTRAINDICATIONS
Hypersensitivity

Precautions: infections (nails, scalp), pregnancy, breastfeeding, children

DOSAGE AND ROUTES
Mild to moderate onychomycosis of fingernails and toenails

Adults, Adolescents, and Children ≥12 years: Topical, nail lacquer, apply q day (bedtime or 8 hr before washing nails) to affected nails with the applicator brush provided; cream/lotion/gel apply bid for up to 4 wk; shampoo 5-10 mL applied to scalp and lather and leave for 3 min, rinse, repeat, twice weekly for 4 wk

Available forms: Topical cream, gel, lotion 0.77%; nail lacquer 8%; shampoo 1%; 1.5% (✿)

ADVERSE EFFECTS
INTEG: Rash, burning, redness, stinging

INTERACTIONS
None significant

NURSING CONSIDERATIONS
Assessment
• Assess area involved—skin, nails, scalp—baseline and during treatment; do not use with occlusive dressings (topical); avoid skin (nail lacquer)
• **Assess** rash, burning, itching, redness

Patient problems
Infection (uses)

Implementation
• **Topical: Gel, lotion, cream** apply to affected area twice a day
• **Nail lacquer:** Apply to nails using brush supplied

Patient/family education
• Advise patient to use as directed, not to double or skip doses
• Teach patient to report if pregnancy is planned or suspected or if breastfeeding

Evaluation
Positive therapeutic outcome
• Reported improvement in symptoms of fungal infection

cholecalciferol
See vitamin D

cilastatin
See imipenem/cilastatin

⚠ HIGH ALERT
cilostazol (Rx)
(sih-los′ tah-zol)
Func. class.: Antiplatelet, Platelet aggregation inhibitor
Chem. class.: Quinolinone derivative

ACTION: Multifactorial effects (antithrombotic, antiplatelet vasodilation)

Therapeutic outcome: Increased walking distance

USES: Intermittent claudication associated with PVD

Pharmacokinetics

Absorption	Unknown
Distribution	95%-98% protein binding
Metabolism	Hepatic extensively by CYP3A41, CYP2C19 enzymes (active metabolite)
Excretion	Urine (74%), feces (20%)
Half-life	11-13 hr

Pharmacodynamics (antiplatelet effect)

Onset	Up to 4 wk
Peak	Up to 12 wk
Duration	Unknown

CONTRAINDICATIONS
Hypersensitivity, acute MI, active bleeding conditions, hemostatic conditions

> **BLACK BOX WARNING:** HF

Precautions: Pregnancy, breastfeeding, children, geriatric, past liver disease, renal/cardiac disease, increased bleeding risk, low platelet count, platelet dysfunction, smoking

DOSAGE AND ROUTES
Adult: PO 100 mg bid or 50 mg bid, if using products that inhibit CYP3A4 and CYP2C19

Available forms: Tabs 50, 100 mg

ADVERSE EFFECTS
CNS: *Dizziness, headache*
CV: *Palpitations, tachycardia,* nodal dysrhythmia, postural hypotension, chest pain
GI: *Diarrhea, flatulence*
INTEG: *Rash*
RESP: *Cough, pharyngitis, rhinitis,* asthma, pneumonia

INTERACTIONS
Individual drugs
Abciximab, eptifibatide, ticlopidine, tirofiban: increased bleeding tendencies
Clarithromycin, dilTIAZem, erythromycin, omeprazole, verapamil: increased cilostazol levels
Fluconazole, FLUoxetine, fluvoxaMINE, gemfibrozil, isoniazid, itraconazole, ketoconazole, omeprazole, voriconazole: may increase cilostazol levels; exercise caution when coadministering and reduce dose to 50 mg bid

Drug classifications
Anticoagulants, NSAIDs, thrombolytics: may increase bleeding tendencies
CYP3A4 inducers: decreased cilostazol
Protease inhibitors, CYP3A4 inhibitors, CYP2C19 inhibitors: increased cilostazol levels

Drug/food
Grapefruit juice: do not use; toxicity may occur
High-fat meals: increased cilostazol action; avoid giving with food

Drug/herb
Feverfew, garlic, ginger, ginkgo biloba: decreased cilostazol action

NURSING CONSIDERATIONS
Assessment

> **BLACK BOX WARNING:** Assess for underlying CV disease since CV risk is great; for CV lesions with repeated oral use; do not use in heart failure of any severity

- Assess for CV lesions with repeated oral administration
- Assess for HF
- Monitor blood studies: CBC, Hct, Hgb, pro-time if patient is on long-term therapy; thrombocytopenia, neutropenia may occur
- **Beers:** Avoid in older adults, may promote fluid retention and/or exacerbate heart failure

Patient problem
Risk for injury (uses)
Activity intolerance (uses)

Implementation
- Give bid ≥1 hr before or 2 hr after meals with a full glass of water; do not give with grapefruit juice

Patient/family education
- Teach patient to avoid hazardous activities until effect is known
- Advise patient to report any unusual bleeding to prescriber
- Caution patient to report side effects such as diarrhea, skin rashes, subcutaneous bleeding
- Teach patient that effects may take 2-4 wk, treatment of up to 12 wk may be required for necessary effect
- Teach patients with HF about potential risks
- Advise patient to take ≥1 hr before or 2 hr after meals
- Advise patient that reading patient information is necessary
- Advise patient to discontinue tobacco use, not to drink grapefruit juice
- Advise that there are many drug and herb interactions; obtain approval by prescriber before use

---

Evaluation
Positive therapeutic outcome
- Increased walking distance and duration
- Decreased pain

cimetidine (OTC, Rx)
(sye-met′i-deen)
Tagamet, Tagamet HB
Func. class.: H$_2$-receptor antagonist
Chem. class.: Imidazole derivative

ACTION: Inhibits histamine at H$_2$-receptor site in the gastric parietal cells, which inhibits gastric acid secretion

Therapeutic outcome: Healing of duodenal or gastric ulcers; prevention of duodenal ulcers; decreases symptoms of gastroesophageal reflux disease (GERD) and Zollinger-Ellison syndrome

USES: Short-term treatment of duodenal and gastric ulcers and maintenance; management of GERD, Zollinger-Ellison syndrome; prevention of upper GI bleeding; prevent, relieve heartburn, acid indigestion

Pharmacokinetics

Absorption	Well absorbed (PO)
Distribution	Widely distributed; crosses placenta
Metabolism	Liver (30%)
Excretion	Kidneys, unchanged (70%); breast milk
Half-life	1½-2 hr; increased in renal disease

Pharmacodynamics

	PO
Onset	½ hr
Peak	45-90 min
Duration	4-5 hr

CONTRAINDICATIONS
Hypersensitivity to this product, H$_2$ blockers, benzyl alcohol

Precautions: Pregnancy, breastfeeding, child <16 yr, geriatric, organic brain syndrome, renal/hepatic disease

DOSAGE AND ROUTES
Treatment of active ulcers
Adult/adolescent ≥16 yr: PO 300 mg qid 800 mg at bedtime or 400-600 mg bid, max 2.4 g/day × 8 wk
Child: PO 5-10 mg/kg q 6 hr

Prophylaxis of duodenal ulcer
Adult and child >16 yr: PO 400 mg at bedtime or 300 mg bid

GERD
Adult: PO 800-1600 mg/day in divided doses × ≤12 wk

Gastric hypersecretory conditions
Adult: PO 300-600 q 6h, max 2400 mg/day

OTC use
Adult: PO up to 200 mg bid, max 2 wk

Heartburn
Adult/child ≥12 yr: PO 200 mg up to bid, may use prior to eating, max 400 mg/day, max daily use up to 2 wk

Renal dose
Adult: PO/IV CCr <30 ml/min 300 mg q12hr

Available forms: Tabs 200, 300, 400, 800 mg; liquid 300 mg/5 ml

ADVERSE EFFECTS
CNS: *Confusion, headache,* depression, dizziness, psychosis, tremors, seizures
CV: Bradycardia, tachycardia, dysrhythmias
GI: *Diarrhea,* abdominal cramps, constipation
GU: Gynecomastia, impotence
INTEG: Urticaria, rash

INTERACTIONS
Individual drugs
CarBAMazepine, chloroquine, lidocaine, metroNIDAZOLE, moricizine, phenytoin, quiNIDine, quiNINE, valproic acid, warfarin: increased toxicity
Carmustine: increased bone marrow suppression
Itraconazole: decreased absorption of itraconazole
Ketoconazole: decreased absorption of ketoconazole
Sucralfate: decreased cimetidine absorption

Drug classifications
Antacids: decreased absorption of cimetidine
Antidepressants (tricyclic), benzodiazepines, β-adrenergic blockers, calcium channel blockers, phenytoin, sulfonylureas, theophyllines: increased toxicity (CYP450 pathway)

Drug/lab test
Increased: alkaline phosphatase, AST, creatinine, prolactin
False positive: Hemoccult, Gastroccult tests
False negative: TB skin tests

NURSING CONSIDERATIONS
Assessment
- **Ulcer symptoms:** Assess patient with ulcers or suspected ulcers: epigastric or abdominal pain, hematemesis, occult blood in stools, blood

in gastric aspirate before and/or throughout treatment

• **Beers:** Avoid in older adults with or at high risk of delirium, adverse CNS effects

Patient problem
Pain (uses)

Implementation
PO route
• Give with meals for lengthened product effect; antacids 1 hr before or 1 hr after cimetidine

Patient/family education
• Advise patient that any gynecomastia or impotence that develops is reversible after treatment is discontinued
• Caution patient to avoid driving, other hazardous activities until stabilized on this medication; drowsiness or dizziness may occur
• Advise patient to avoid black pepper, caffeine, alcohol, harsh spices, extremes in temperature of food; tell patient to avoid OTC preparations: aspirin, cough, cold preparations; condition may worsen, OTC therapy is used for short term (2 wk)
• Advise patient that smoking decreases the effectiveness of the product; smoking cessation should be considered
• Teach patient to use increased fluids, bulk in diet to decrease constipation
• Teach patient that product must be continued for prescribed time to be effective and taken exactly as prescribed; doses are not to be doubled; to take missed dose when remembered up to 1 hr before next dose; if taking OTC, not to use maximum dose >2 wk, unless directed by prescriber
• Have patient report to prescriber immediately any diarrhea, black tarry stools, sore throat, dizziness, confusion, or delirium
• **Pregnancy/breastfeeding:** Advise patient to report if pregnancy is planned or suspected or if breastfeeding

Evaluation
Positive therapeutic outcome
• Decreased pain in abdomen
• Healing of ulcers
• Absence of gastroesophageal reflux
• Gastric pH of ≥5

cinacalcet (Rx)
(sin-a-kal'set)
Sensipar
Func. class.: Calcium receptor agonist
Chem. class.: Polypeptide hormone

ACTION: Directly lowers PTH levels by increasing sensitivity of calcium sensing receptors to extracellular calcium

Therapeutic outcome: Decreased symptoms of hypercalcemia

USES: Hypercalcemia in parathyroid carcinoma, secondary hyperparathyroidism in chronic kidney disease on dialysis, primary hyperparathyroidism

Pharmacokinetics

Absorption	Protein binding
Distribution	93%–97%
Metabolism	Proteins metabolized by CYP3A4, CYP2D6, CYP1A2
Excretion	Renal (80% renal, 15% feces)
Half-life	30-40 hr

Pharmacodynamics (PTH effect)

Onset	Unknown
Peak	4–6 hr
Duration	6–12 hr

CONTRAINDICATIONS
Hypersensitivity, hypocalcemia

Precautions: Pregnancy, breastfeeding, children, seizure disorders, hepatic disease

DOSAGE AND ROUTES
Parathyroid carcinoma
Adult: PO 30 mg bid, titrate q2-4wk, with sequential doses of 30 mg bid, 60 mg bid, 90 mg bid, 90 mg tid-qid to normalize calcium levels

Secondary hyperparathyroidism
Adult: PO 30 mg daily, titrate no more frequently than 2-4 wks with sequential doses of 30, 60, 90, 120, 180 mg daily

Available forms: Tabs 30, 60, 90 mg

ADVERSE EFFECTS
CNS: Dizziness, asthenia, seizures, paresthesias, fatigue, depression, headache
CV: Dysrhythmia exacerbation, hypotension
GI: Nausea, diarrhea, vomiting, anorexia, constipation
MISC: Infection, noncardiac chest pain, hypocalcemia dehydration, arthralgia, hypercalcemia, anemia
MS: Myalgia, bone fractures

INTERACTIONS
Individual drugs
Flecainide, thioridazine, vinBLAStine: increased levels of CYP2D6 inhibitors; adjustments may be necessary

Drug classifications
CYP3A4 inhibitors (erythromycin, itraconazole, ketoconazole): increased cinacalcet levels, dose may need to be decreased
Tricyclics: increased levels of CYP2D6 inhibitors)

⚠ Nurse Alert   ✴ Key NCLEX® Drug   ≫ Drug Specifics

Drug/food
High-fat meal: increased action

NURSING CONSIDERATIONS
Assessment
• Assess for **hypocalcemia:** cramping, seizures, tetany, myalgia, paresthesia
• Monitor calcium, phosphorous within 1 wk and iPTH 1-4 wk after initiation or dosage adjustment when maintenance is established; measure calcium, phosphorus monthly; iPTH q1-3mo, target range 150-300 pg/ml for iPTH level; biochemical markers of bone formation/resorption, radiologic evidence of fracture; if calcium <8.4 mg/dl, do not start therapy, if calcium is 7.5-8.4 mg/dl give calcium-containing phosphate binders, vitamin D sterols to increase calcium, if calcium <7.5 mg/day or if symptoms of hypocalcemia continue and vitamin D cannot be increased, withhold product until calcium reaches 8.0 mg/dl, symptoms resolve, start product at next lowest dose
• **Renal disease (without dialysis):** These patients should not receive treatment with this product, high risk of hypocalcemia
• **Pregnancy/breastfeeding:** advice to patient report if pregnancy is planned or suspected or if breastfeeding, pregnant patients should enroll in Amgen's Pregnancy Surveillance Program 800-772-6436

Patient problem
Lack of knowledge of medication (teaching)

Implementation
• Swallow tabs whole; do not break, crush, chew, or divide tabs
• Can be used alone or in combination with vit D sterols and/or phosphate binders
• Take with food or shortly after meal
Secondary hyperthyroidism
• **Chronic kidney disease:** if iPTH drops below 150-300 pg/ml, reduce dose of cinacalcet and/or vit D sterols or discontinue treatment
• Store at <77° F (25° C)

Patient/family education
• Instruct patient to take with food or shortly after a meal, to take tabs whole, not to take any other meds, supplements without prescriber approval
• Instruct patient to immediately report cramping, seizures, muscle pain, tingling, tetany, sign of GI bleeding
• Teach patient continuing exams and lab work will be needed

Evaluation
Positive therapeutic outcome
• Calcium levels 9-10 mg/dl, decreasing symptoms of hypercalcemia

ciprofloxacin (Rx)
(sip-ro-floks'a-sin)
Cipro, Cipro XR
Func. class.: Antiinfectives, broad-spectrum
Chem. class.: Fluoroquinolone

Do not confuse: ciprofloxacin/cephalexin

ACTION: Interferes with conversion of intermediate DNA fragments into high-molecular-weight DNA in bacteria; DNA gyrase inhibitor

Therapeutic outcome: Bactericidal action against the following: gram-positive organisms *Staphylococcus epidermidis,* methicillin-resistant strains of *Staphylococcus aureus;* gram-negative organisms *Escherichia coli, Klebsiella* species, *Enterobacter, Salmonella, Proteus vulgaris, Pseudomonas aeruginosa, Serratia, Campylobacter jejuni, Streptococcus pyogenes, Bacillus anthracis*

USES: Adult urinary tract infections (including complicated); chronic bacterial prostatitis; acute sinusitis; infectious diarrhea; typhoid fever; plague, complicated intraabdominal infections; nosocomial pneumonia; exposure to inhalation anthrax

Pharmacokinetics
Absorption	Well absorbed (75%) (PO)
Distribution	Widely distributed
Metabolism	Liver (15%)
Excretion	Kidneys (40%-50%)
Half-life	4 hr; increased in renal disease

Pharmacodynamics
	PO	PO ER	IV
Onset	Rapid	Rapid	Immediate
Peak	4 hr	1–4 hr	Infusion's end
Duration	12 hr	Up to 24 hr	

CONTRAINDICATIONS
Hypersensitivity to quinolones

Precautions: Pregnancy, breastfeeding, children, geriatric, renal disease, seizure disorder, stroke, CV disease, hepatic disease, QT prolongation, hypokalemia, colitis

BLACK BOX WARNING: Tendon pain/rupture, tendonitis, myasthenia gravis, neurotoxicity

DOSAGE AND ROUTES
Uncomplicated urinary tract infections
Adult: PO 250 mg q12hr × 3 days or XL 500 mg q24hr × 3 days

Complicated/severe urinary tract infections
Adult: PO 500 mg q12hr or XL 1000 mg q24hr × 7-14 days; **IV** 400 mg q12hr

Respiratory, bone, skin, joint infections (mild-moderate)
Adult: PO 500-750 mg q12hr × 7-14 days; **IV** 400 mg q12hr

Nosocomial pneumonia
Adult: IV 400 mg q8hr × 10-14 days

Intraabdominal infections, complicated
Adult: PO 500 mg q12hr × 7-14 days, **IV** 400 mg q12hr × 7-14 days, usually given with metroNIDAZOLE

Acute sinusitis, mild/moderate
Adult: PO 500 mg q12hr × 10 days; **IV** 400 mg q12hr × 10 days

Inhalational anthrax (postexposure)
Adult: PO 500 mg q12hr × 60 days; **IV** 400 mg q12hr × 60 days
Child: PO 15 mg/kg/dose q12hr × 60 days, max 500 mg/dose; **IV,** 10 mg/kg q12hr, max 400 mg/dose

Infectious diarrhea
Adult: PO 500-750 mg q12hr × 5-7 days

Chronic bacterial prostatitis
Adult: PO 500 mg q12hr × 28 days; **IV** 400 mg q12hr × 28 days

Renal dose
Adult: PO CCr 30-50 ml/min PO 250-500 mg q12hr; CCr 5-29 ml/min PO 250-500 mg q18hr; CCr 5-29 mL/min IV 200-400 mg q18-24hr

Available forms: Tabs 100, 250, 500, 750 mg; ext rel tabs (XR) 500, 1000 mg; inj 200 mg/ 20 ml, 400 mg/40 ml, 200 mg/100 ml D$_5$, 400 mg/200 ml D$_5$W; oral susp 250, 500 mg/5 ml

ADVERSE EFFECTS
CNS: *Headache,* dizziness, fatigue, insomnia, depression, *restlessness,* seizures, confusion, hallucinations, suicidal ideation, pseudotumor cerebri
GI: *Nausea,* increased ALT, AST, flatulence, *vomiting, diarrhea,* abdominal pain, pancreatitis, *Clostridium difficile*-associated diarrhea (CDAD)
GU: Vaginitis
META: Hypo-hyperglycemia

INTEG: *Rash,* pruritus, urticaria, photosensitivity, toxic epidermal necrolysis, injection site reactions
MISC: Anaphylaxis, Stevens-Johnson syndrome, QT prolongation, pseudotumor cerebri
MS: Arthralgia, tendon rupture

INTERACTIONS
Individual drugs
Alfuzosin, arsenic trioxide, astemizole, chloroquine, cloZAPine, cyclobenzaprine, dasatinib, dolasetron, droperidol, flecainide, haloperidol, lapatinib, levomethadyl, methadone, octreotide, ondansetron, paliperidone, palonosetron, pentamidine, probucol, propafenone, ranolazine, risperiDONE, sertindole, SUNItinib, tacrolimus, terfenadine, vardenafil, vorinostat, ziprasidone: increased QT prolongation; less likely than other quinolones
Calcium, enteral feeding, iron, sucralfate, sevelamer, zinc sulfate: decreased ciprofloxacin absorption
CycloSPORINE: increased nephrotoxicity
Probenecid: increased blood levels of ciprofloxacin, increased toxicity
Theophylline: increased theophylline levels, monitor blood levels, reduce dose, if needed
Warfarin: increased warfarin effect, monitor blood levels

Drug classifications
Antacids (containing magnesium, aluminum), iron salts: decreased absorption of ciprofloxacin
Antidiabetics: increased hypoglycemia risk
β-agonists, class IA/III antidysrhythmics, halogenated anesthetics, local anesthetics, macrolides, phenothiazines, tetracyclines, tricyclics: increased QT prolongation

> **BLACK BOX WARNING:** Corticosteroids: increased tendonitis, tendon rupture

Drug/food
Dairy products, food: decreased absorption

Drug/lab test
Increased: AST, ALT, bilirubin, BUN, creatinine, alkaline phosphatase, LDH, glucose, proteinuria, albuminuria
Decreased: WBC, glucose

NURSING CONSIDERATIONS
Assessment
• Assess patient for previous sensitivity reaction
• Assess patient for signs and symptoms of **infection** including characteristics of wounds, sputum, urine, stool, WBC >10,000/mm^3, fever; obtain baseline information before, during treatment

---

• Assess for **Stevens Johnson syndrome, anaphylaxis:** rash, urticaria, dyspnea, pruritus, chills, fever, joint pain; discontinue immediately, have emergency equipment nearby may occur a few days after therapy begins; EPINEPHrine and resuscitation equipment should be available for anaphylactic reaction

• Monitor blood studies: AST, ALT, CBC, Hct, bilirubin, LDH, alkaline phosphatase, Coombs' test monthly if patient is on long-term therapy

> **BLACK BOX WARNING: Myasthenia gravis:** avoid use in these patients, increases muscle weakness

• **QT prolongation:** monitor for changes in QTc if taking other products that increase QT
• Assess for **CNS symptoms:** headache, dizziness, fatigue, insomnia, depression, seizures
• Assess for **overgrowth of infection:** perineal itching, fever, malaise, redness, pain, swelling, drainage, rash, diarrhea, change in cough, sputum

> **BLACK BOX WARNING: Tendonitis, tendon rupture:** discontinue at first sign of tendon pain, inflammation; increased in those >60 yr, those taking corticosteroids, organ transplant recipients; assess for tendon pain, especially in children

• **Pseudomotor cerebri:** may occur at excessive doses
• ***Clostridium difficile*–associated diarrhea (CDAD):** monitor for diarrhea, abdominal pain, cramps, fever, bloody stools, usually occurs several weeks after completion of therapy, report to prescriber immediately

Patient problem
Infection (uses)

Implementation
Obtain C&S before use, may give first dose before results are received
PO route
• Give around the clock to maintain proper blood levels
• Administer 6 hr before or 2 hr after antacids, zinc, iron, calcium; use adequate fluids to prevent crystalluria
• Do not give oral sup by GI tube
• Limit intake of alkaline soda, products with milk, dairy products, alkaline antacids, sodium bicarbonate
• Ext rel and regular release are not interchangeable
• Use calibrated measuring device for suspension

IV route
• Check for irritation, extravasation, phlebitis daily
• For **intermittent inf,** dilute to 1-2 mg/ml of D₅W, 0.9% NaCl; give over 60 min; it will remain stable for 2 wk, diluted vials can be stored for 14 days at room temperature or in refrigerator, do not freeze

Y-site compatibilities: Amifostine, anakinra, anidulafungin, argatroban, arsenic, atenolol, aztreonam, bivalirudin, bleomycin, calcium gluconate, CARBOplatin, caspofungin, cefTAZidime, cisatracurium, CISplatin, clarithromycin, codeine, cytarabine, DACTINomycin, DAPTOmycin, dexmedetomidine, digoxin, diltiaZEM, diphenhydrAMINE, DOBUTamine, DOCEtaxel, doripenem, DOPamine, doxacurium, DOXOrubicin, epiRUBicin, eptifibatide, ertapenem, etoposide, fenoldopam, fludarabine, gallium, gemcitabine, gentamicin, granisetron, HYDROmorphone, hydrOXYzine, IDArubicin, ifosfamide, irinotecan, lidocaine, linezolid, LORazepam, LR, mechlorethamine, meperidine, methotrexate, metoclopramide, metroNIDAZOLE, midazolam, midodrine, milrinone, mitoXANTRONE, mycophenolate, nesiritide, octreotide, ondansetron, oxaliplatin, oxytocin, PACLitaxel, palonosetron, pamidronate, pancuronium, piperacillin, potassium acetate/chloride, promethazine, raNITIdine, remifentanil, rocuronium, sodium chloride, tacrolimus, teniposide, thiotepa, tigecycline, tirofiban, TNA, tobramycin, trastuzumab, vasopressin, vecuronium, verapamil, vinCRIStine, vinorelbine, voriconazole

Patient/family education
• Teach patient to contact prescriber if adverse reaction occurs or if inflammation or pain in tendon occurs before, 6 hr after
• Teach patient not to crush or chew the extended-release product
• Instruct patient to take all medication prescribed for the length of time ordered; product must be taken around the clock to maintain blood levels; do not give medication to others

> **BLACK BOX WARNING:** Teach patient to report tendon pain, chest pain, palpitations

• **Suicidal thoughts/behaviors:** Advise patient, family to report immediately suicidal thoughts, behaviors
• Teach patient to notify prescriber if rash occurs, discontinue product
• Teach patient to notify prescriber if pregnancy is planned or suspected, do not breastfeed
• Teach patient to contact prescriber if taking theophylline, warfarin

Evaluation
Positive therapeutic outcome
- Absence of signs/symptoms of infection
- Reported improvement in symptoms of infection

ciprofloxacin ophthalmic
See Appendix B

⚠ HIGH ALERT

CISplatin (Rx)
(sis′pla-tin)
Func. class.: Antineoplastic alkylating agent
Chem. class.: Inorganic heavy metal

Do not confuse: CISplatin/CARBOplatin

ACTION: Alkylates DNA, RNA; inhibits enzymes that allow synthesis of amino acids in proteins; activity is not cell cycle phase specific

Therapeutic outcome: Prevention of rapidly growing malignant cells

USES: Advanced bladder cancer; adjunctive in metastatic testicular cancer and metastatic ovarian cancer, head, neck, lung cancer

Pharmacokinetics

Absorption	Complete
Distribution	Widely distributed, accumulates in body tissues for several months
Metabolism	Liver
Excretion	Kidneys, breast milk
Half-life	30-90 hr

Pharmacodynamics (blood counts)

Onset	Unknown
Peak	20 days
Duration	40 days

CONTRAINDICATIONS
Pregnancy, breastfeeding

> **BLACK BOX WARNING:** Bone marrow suppression, platinum compound hypersensitivity

Precautions: Geriatric patients, vaccination, infections, extravasation, peripheral neuropathy, radiation therapy

> **BLACK BOX WARNING:** Chemotherapy-induced nausea/vomiting; in children, nephrotoxicity, ototoxicity; requires a specialized care setting and an experienced clinician

DOSAGE AND ROUTES
Dosage protocols may vary

Metastatic testicular cancer
Adult: IV 20 mg/m^2 daily × 5 days, repeat q3wk for 2 cycles or more, depending on response

Advanced bladder cancer
Adult: IV 50-70 mg/m^2 q3-4wk

Metastatic ovarian cancer
Adult: IV 100 mg/m^2 q4wk or 75-100 mg/m^2 q3wk with cyclophosphamide therapy

Available forms: Inj 0.5 mg/ml ✲, 1 mg/ml

ADVERSE EFFECTS
CNS: Seizures, *peripheral neuropathy*, reversible posterior leukoencephalopathy syndrome (RPLS)
EENT: *Tinnitus, hearing loss, vestibular toxicity,* blurred vision, altered color perception
GI: *Severe nausea, vomiting, diarrhea, weight loss, hepatotoxicity*
GU: Renal tubular damage, *renal insufficiency,* sterility
HEMA: Thrombocytopenia, leukopenia, pancytopenia, *anemia*
INTEG: *Alopecia,* dermatitis
META: *Hypomagnesemia, hypocalcemia, hypokalemia*
SYST: Anaphylaxis

INTERACTIONS
Individual drugs
Alcohol, aspirin: increased risk of bleeding
Bumetanide, ethacrynic acid, furosemide: ototoxicity
Phenytoin: decreased phenytoin effect

Drug classifications
Aminoglycosides, diuretics (loop), salicylates: increased nephrotoxicity
Diuretics loop: decreased potassium, magnesium levels
Myelosuppressive agents, radiation: increased myelosuppression
NSAIDs: increased risk of bleeding
Vaccines, live virus: decreased antibody response

Drug/lab test
Increased: uric acid, BUN, creatinine
Decreased: CCr, calcium, phosphate, potassium, magnesium
Positive: Coombs' test

NURSING CONSIDERATIONS
Assessment

> **BLACK BOX WARNING:** Monitor for **bone marrow depression:** CBC, differential, platelet count weekly; withhold product if WBC count is <4000/mm^3 or platelet count is <100,000/mm^3; notify prescriber of results if WBC <20,000/mm^3, platelets <150,000/mm^3

> **BLACK BOX WARNING:** Monitor for **renal toxicity:** BUN, creatinine, serum uric acid, urine CCr before, during therapy; I&O ratio; report fall in urine output to <30 ml/hr; dose should not be given if BUN <25 mg/dl; creatinine <1.5 mg/dl, toxicity is cumulative, withhold until renal function returns to normal

> **BLACK BOX WARNING:** Assess for anaphylaxis: wheezing, tachycardia, facial swelling, fainting; discontinue product and report to prescriber; resuscitation equipment should be nearby, may occur within minutes; often EPINEPHrine, corticosteroids, antihistamines may alleviate symptoms

• **Hepatotoxicity:** Monitor liver function tests before, during therapy (bilirubin, AST, ALT, LDH) as needed or monthly; note yellowing of skin or sclera, dark urine, clay-colored stools, itchy skin, abdominal pain, fever, diarrhea

• **RPLS:** Assess for headache, change in eyesight, confusion, seizures, increased B/P, usually occurs a few hrs up to 1 year after treatment starts, discontinue treatment

• Assess for increased uric acid levels, swelling, joint pain primarily in extremities; patient should be well hydrated to prevent urate deposits, may use products to lower uric acid levels

• Assess for **bleeding:** hematuria, stool guaiac, bruising or petechiae, mucosa or orifices q8hr; note inflammation of mucosa, breaks in skin

> **BLACK BOX WARNING: Ototoxicity:** more common in genetic variants TPMT 3B and 3C in children; use audiometric testing baseline and before each dose, usually tinnitus or loss of high-frequency sounds are first indication of ototoxicity

Patient problem
Risk for infection (adverse reactions)
Risk for injury (adverse reactions)

Implementation

IV route
• Prepare in biological cabinet using gown, gloves, mask; do not allow product to come in contact with skin; use soap and water if contact occurs, use cytotoxic handling procedures
• Hydrate patient with 1-2 L 0.9% NaCl over 8-12 hr before treatment
• Give all medications PO, if possible; avoid IM inj when platelets <100,000/mm³

• Give EPINEPHrine, antihistamines, corticosteroids for hypersensitivity reaction; antiemetic 30-60 min before giving product to prevent vomiting, and prn; allopurinol or sodium bicarbonate to maintain uric acid level, alkalinization of urine; antibiotics for prophylaxis of infection; diuretic (furosemide 40 mg **IV**) or mannitol after infusion
• Do not use aluminum equipment during any preparation or administration, will form precipitate; do not refrigerate unopened powder or solution; protect from sunlight

Intermittent IV infusion route
• Check solution for particulate and color, do not use if particulate is present or product is colored
• Give after **diluting** 10 mg/10 ml or 50 mg/50 ml sterile water for inj; **withdraw** prescribed dose, **dilute** ½ dose with 1000 ml D₅ 0.2 NaCl or D₅ 0.45 NaCl with 37.5 g mannitol; **IV** inf is **given** over 3-4 hr; use a 0.45 μm filter; total dose 2000 ml over 6-8 hr; check site for irritation, phlebitis; do not use equipment containing aluminum

Continuous IV infusion route
• Give over 24 hr × 5 days

Y-site compatibilities: Acyclovir, alfentanil, allopurinol, amikacin, aminophylline, amiodarone, ampicillin, ampicillin-sulbactam, anidulafungin, atenolol, atracurium, azithromycin, aztreonam, bivalirudin, bleomycin, bumetanide, buprenorphine, butorphanol, calcium chloride/gluconate, carmustine, caspofungin, ceFAZolin, cefoperazone, cefotaxime, cefoTEtan, cefOXitin, cefTAZidime, ceftizoxime, cefTRIAXone, cefuroxime, chlorproMAZINE, cimetidine, ciprofloxacin, cisatracurium, cladribine, clindamycin, codeine, cyclophosphamide, cycloSPORINE, cytarabine, DACTINomycin, DAPTOmycin, DAUNOrubicin, dexamethasone, dexmedetomidine, dexrazoxane, digoxin, dilTIAZem, diphenhydrAMINE, DOBUTamine, DOCEtaxel, DOPamine, doripenem, doxacurium, DOXOrubicin, DOXOrubicin liposomal, doxycycline, droperidol, enalaprilat, ePHEDrine, EPINEPHrine, epiRUBicin, ertapenem, erythromycin, esmolol, etoposide, famotidine, fenoldopam, fentaNYL, filgrastim, fluconazole, fludarabine, fluorouracil, foscarnet, fosphenytoin, furosemide, ganciclovir, gatifloxacin, gemcitabine, gentamicin, glycopyrrolate, granisetron, haloperidol, heparin, hydrocortisone, HYDROmorphone, IDArubicin, ifosfamide, imipenem-cilastatin, inamrinone, indomethacin, irinotecan, isoproterenol, ketorolac, labetalol, leucovorin, levofloxacin, levorphanol, lidocaine, linezolid, LORazepam, magnesium sulfate, mannitol, melphalan, meperidine, meropenem, methohexital, methotrexate, methylPREDNISolone, metoclopramide, metoprolol, metroNIDAZOLE, midazolam, milrinone, minocycline, mitoMYcin, mitoXANtrone, mivacurium, nafcillin, naloxone, nesiritide, niCARdipine, nitroglycerin, nitroprusside, norepinephrine, octreotide, ofloxacin, ondansetron, oxaliplatin, PACLitaxel, palonosetron, pamidronate, pancuronium, PEMEtrexed, pentamidine, pentazocine, PENTobarbital, PHENobarbital, phenylephrine, phenytoin, piperacillin, polymyxin B, potassium chloride/phosphates, procainamide, prochlorperazine, promethazine, propofol, propranolol, quiNIDine, quinupristindalfopristin, raNITIdine, remifentanil, riTUXimab, sargramostim, sodium acetate/bicarbonate/phosphates, succinylcholine, SUFentanil, sulfamethoxazole-trimethoprim, tacrolimus, teniposide, theophylline, thiopental, ticarcillin, ticarcillin-clavulanate, tigecycline, tirofiban, TNA, tobramycin, topotecan, trastuzumab, vancomycin, vasopressin, vecuronium, verapamil, vinBLAStine, vinCRIStine, vinorelbine, voriconazole, zidovudine, zoledronic acid

Patient/family education
• Advise patient to report numbness, tingling in face or extremities, poor hearing or joint pain, swelling
• Instruct patient to report signs of anemia (fatigue, headache, irritability, faintness, shortness of breath)
• **Infection:** to avoid crowds and persons with respiratory tract or other infections, to report signs of infection, cough, fever, sore throat
• Advise patient that hair may be lost during treatment; a wig or hairpiece may make patient feel better; new hair may be different in color, texture
• Tell patient not to have any vaccinations without the advice of the prescriber; serious reactions can occur

> **BLACK BOX WARNING: Ototoxicity:** teach patient to report loss of hearing, ringing or roaring in the ears

• **Pregnancy/breastfeeding:** caution patient contraception is needed during treatment and for 4 months after the completion of therapy, pregnancy

Evaluation
Positive therapeutic outcome
• Prevention of rapid division of malignant cells

citalopram (Rx)
(sigh-tal′oh-pram)
CeleXA
Func. class.: Antidepressant
Chem. class.: Selective serotonin reuptake inhibitor (SSRI)

Do not confuse: CeleXA/CeleBREX/Cerebyx/ZyPREXA

ACTION: Inhibits CNS neuron uptake of serotonin but not of norepinephrine; weak inhibitor of CYP450 enzyme system, making it more appealing than other products

Therapeutic outcome: Decreased symptoms of depression after 2-3 wk

USES: Major depressive disorder

Unlabeled uses: Compulsive disorder in adolescents

Pharmacokinetics
Absorption	Well absorbed
Distribution	Unknown
Metabolism	Liver, by ⚕ CYP1A2, CYP2D6 several patients are poor metabolizers
Excretion	Kidneys, steady state 28-35 days
Half-life	35 hr

Pharmacodynamics (antidepressant action)
Onset	Up to 4 wk
Peak	Unknown
Duration	Unknown

CONTRAINDICATIONS
Hypersensitivity

Precautions: Pregnancy, breastfeeding, geriatric, renal/hepatic disease, seizure disorder, hypersensitivity to escitalopram, bradycardia, recent MI, abrupt discontinuation, QT prolongation

> **BLACK BOX WARNING:** Children, suicidal ideation

DOSAGE AND ROUTES
Depression
Adult: PO 20 mg daily AM or PM, may increase if needed to 40 mg/day after 1 wk; maintenance: after 6-8 wk of initial treatment, continue for 24 wk (32 wk total); ⚕ **poor metabolizers**

---

of **CYP2C19, or CYP2C19 inhibitors** max 20 mg/day

Hepatic dose/geriatric
Adult: PO 20 mg/day

Available forms: Tabs 10, 20, 40 mg; oral SOL 10 mg/5 ml

ADVERSE EFFECTS
CNS: *Headache, insomnia, drowsiness, anxiety, tremor, dizziness, fatigue, sedation, poor concentration,* seizures, suicidal attempts, malignant neuroleptic-like syndrome reactions
CV: Tachycardia, QT prolongation, orthostatic hypotension, torsades de pointes
EENT: Vision changes
GI: Nausea, diarrhea, dry mouth, anorexia, dyspepsia, vomiting, taste changes, flatulence, decreased appetite
GU: Dysmenorrhea, decreased libido, urinary frequency, urinary tract infection, amenorrhea, impotence
INTEG: *Sweating, rash, pruritus,* acne, alopecia, urticaria, photosensitivity
MS: *Pain,* arthritis, twitching myalgia
RESP: *Infection, cough, dyspnea*
SYST: Serotonin syndrome

INTERACTIONS
Individual drugs
Alcohol: increased CNS depression
CarBAMazepine, cloNIDine: decreased citalopram levels
Lithium, linezolid, methylene blue, tricyclics, fentaNYL, busPIRone, triptans, traMADol, traZODone: increased serotonin syndrome
Pimoside, ziprasidone: increased QTc interval; do not use together

Drug classifications
Anticoagulants, antiplatelets, NSAIDs, salicylates, thrombolytics: increased risk of bleeding
Antidepressants (tricyclics): increased effect, use cautiously
Antifungals (azole), macrolides: increased citalopram levels
β-Adrenergic blockers: increased plasma levels of β-blockers
Barbiturates, benzodiazepines, CNS depressants, sedatives/hypnotics: increased CNS depression
MAOIs: hypertensive crisis, seizures, fatal reactions; do not use together within 14 days
Quinolones: increased QTc interval; do not use together
Serotonin receptor agonists, SNRIs, SSRIs: increased serotonin syndrome

Drug/herb
SAM-e, St. John's wort: serotonin syndrome; do not use with citalopram; fatal reaction may occur
Yohimbe: increased CNS stimulation

Drug/lab test
Increased: serum bilirubin, blood glucose, alkaline phosphatase
Decreased: VMA, 5 HIAA
False increase: increased urinary catecholamines

NURSING CONSIDERATIONS
Assessment
• Monitor B/P (lying, standing), pulse q4hr; if systolic B/P drops 20 mm Hg, hold product and notify prescriber; take vital signs q4hr in patients with cardiovascular disease
• Check weight qwk; appetite may increase with product
• **QT prolongation:** Assess ECG for flattening of T wave, bundle branch block, AV block, dysrhythmias in cardiac patients, torsades de pointes, QT prolongation

> **BLACK BOX WARNING:** Assess suicidal: mood, sensorium, affect, suicidal tendencies; increase in psychiatric symptoms: depression, panic, risk for suicide is greater in children and those ≤ 24 yr, these patients should be evaluated q4wk and q3wk × 4 wk, only small amounts of product should be given, continue with exams at least weekly for a month

• Monitor urinary retention, constipation; constipation is more likely to occur in children or geriatric
• **Assess for serotonin syndrome:** increased heart rate, sweating, dilated pupils, tremors, twitching, hyperthermia, agitation, hyperreflexia, nausea, vomiting, diarrhea, coma, hallucinations; may be worse in those taking (SSRIs, SNRIs, triptans)
• Identify patient's alcohol consumption; if alcohol is consumed, hold dose until AM
• **Beers:** Avoid in older adults unless safer alternative is not available, may cause ataxia, impaired psychomotor function

Patient problem
Depression (uses)
Risk for injury (adverse reactions)
Impaired sexual functioning (adverse reactions)

Implementation
• Give with food or milk for GI symptoms
• Give dosage at bedtime if oversedation occurs during day
• Store at room temperature; do not freeze
• Do not give within 14 days of MAOIs

Patient/family education
• Teach patient that therapeutic effects may take 4-6 wk, not to discontinue abruptly
• Instruct patient to use caution in driving or other activities requiring alertness because of drowsiness, dizziness, blurred vision; to avoid rising quickly from sitting to standing, especially geriatric patients

> **BLACK BOX WARNING:** Advise that **suicidal ideas,** behavior may occur in children or young adults, to watch closely for suicidal thoughts, behaviors, notify prescriber immediately

• Caution patient to avoid alcohol ingestion, other CNS depressants
• To use sunscreen, protective clothing to prevent photosensitivity
• Teach patient to notify prescriber if planned or suspected pregnancy, not to breastfeed
• Instruct patient to increase fluids, bulk in diet if constipation, urinary retention occur, especially geriatric
• Advise patient to take gum, hard sugarless candy, or frequent sips of water for dry mouth
• Teach patient how to use orally disintegrating tabs
• **Teach patient to report serotonin syndrome:** sweating, dilated pupils, tremors, twitching, extreme heat, agitation
• **Pregnancy/breastfeeding:** Advise patient to report if pregnancy is planned or suspected or if breastfeeding and to use contraception
• Advise patient that lab work and continuing exams will be needed
• Inform patient to report immediately, swelling, redness, pain at injection site

Evaluation
Positive therapeutic outcome
• Decrease in depression
• Absence of suicidal thoughts

clarithromycin (Rx)
(clare-i-thro-mye′sin)
Biaxin, Biaxin XL
Func. class.: Antiinfective
Chem. class.: Macrolide

ACTION: Binds to 50S ribosomal subunits of susceptible bacteria and suppresses protein synthesis

Therapeutic outcome: Bactericidal action against the following: *Streptococcus pneumoniae, Streptococcus pyogenes, Mycoplasma pneumoniae, Corynebacterium diphtheriae, Bordetella pertussis, Listeria monocytogenes, Haemophilus influenzae, Staphylococcus aureus, Mycobacterium avium (MAC), Legionella pneumophila, Moraxella catarrhalis, Neisseria gonorrhoeae,* complex infections in AIDS patients, *Helicobacter pylori* in combination with omeprazole, *Helicobacter parainfluenzae*

USES: Mild to moderate infections of the upper respiratory tract, lower respiratory tract; uncomplicated skin and skin structure infections

Pharmacokinetics
Absorption	50%
Distribution	Widely distributed, protein binding 70%
Metabolism	Liver
Excretion	Kidneys, unchanged (20%-30%)
Half-life	5-7 hr

Pharmacodynamics
Onset	Unknown
Peak	2 hr; Ext release: 4 hr;
Duration	12 hr; 24 hr (ext rel)

CONTRAINDICATIONS
Hypersensitivity to this product or other macrolides, torsades de pointes, QT prolongation

Precautions: Pregnancy, breastfeeding, geriatric, renal/hepatic disease, heart disease

DOSAGE AND ROUTES
Acute exacerbation of chronic bronchitis
Adult: PO 250-500 mg q12hr × 14 days or 1000 mg/day × 7 days (XL)

Pharyngitis/tonsillitis
Adult: PO 250 mg q12hr × 14 days

Community-acquired pneumonia
Adult: PO 250 mg q12hr × 7-14 days or 1000 mg/day × 7 days (XL)

Endocarditis prophylaxis
Adult: PO 500 mg 1 hr before procedure
Child: PO 15 mg/kg 1 hr prior to procedure

MAC prophylaxis/treatment
Adult: PO 500 mg bid, will require an additional antiinfective for active infection

H. pylori infection
Adult: PO 500 mg with 30 mg lansoprazole and 1 g amoxicillin together q12hr × 10-14 days or 500 mg with omeprazole 20 mg and 1 g amoxicillin together q12hr × 10 days or 500 mg q8hr and omeprazole 40 mg q d × 14 days, continue omeprazole for 14 more days

Acute maxillary sinusitis
Adult: PO 500 mg q12hr × 14 days

Most infections
Child: PO 7.5 mg/kg q12hr × 10 days, max 500 mg/dose for MAC

Renal dose
Adult: PO CCr 30-60 ml/min; decrease dose by 50% if using with ritonavir; CCr < 30 ml/min reduce dose by 50%, if used with ritonavir, reduce by 75%

Available forms. Tabs 250, 500 mg; oral susp 125, 250 mg/5 ml; ext rel tab (XL) 500 mg

ADVERSE EFFECTS
CV: Ventricular dysrhythmias, QT prolongation, torsades de pointes
GI: Nausea, diarrhea, hepatotoxicity, abdominal pain, anorexia, abnormal taste, *Clostridium difficile*-associated diarrhea (CDAD), pancreatitis
INTEG: Rash, urticaria, pruritus, Stevens-Johnson syndrome, toxic epidermal necrolysis, angioedema
MISC: Headache, hearing loss

INTERACTIONS
Individual drugs
ALPRAZolam, busPIRone, carBAMazepine, cycloSPORINE, digoxin, disopyramide, felodipine, fluconazole, omeprazole, tacrolimus, theophylline: increased levels, increased toxicity
CarBAMazepine: increased toxicity, from increased levels of carBAMazepine
Increase: Myopathy risk: atorvastatin, pravastatin, use lowest effective dose
Increase: Rhabdomyolysis risk: lovastatin, simvastatin, do not use concurrently
Increase: Bleeding risk, monitor INR
Increase: Levels of each sildenafil, tadalafil, vardenafil, avoid concurrent use

Drug classifications
All products metabolized by CYP3A enzyme system: increased action, risk of toxicity
Antidiabetics: increased toxicity
Digoxin: increased blood levels of digoxin, increased digoxin effects
Calcium channel blockers, benzodiazepines: increased effects
Class IA, III antidysrhythmics, quiNIDine, procainamide, dofetilide, sotalol, amiodarone or other products that prolong QT: increased QT prolongation
Benzodiazepines, Ergots: increased levels, increased toxicity

Drug/herb
Decrease: Clarithromycin effect: St. John's wort

Drug/lab test
Increased: AST, ALT, BUN, creatinine, LDH, total bilirubin, INR, PT

NURSING CONSIDERATIONS
Assessment
• Assess patient for signs and symptoms of **infection** including characteristics of wounds, sputum, urine, stool, WBC > 10,000/mm³, earache, fever; obtain baseline information before, during treatment; obtain C&S before beginning product therapy to identify if correct treatment has been initiated, product may be given as soon as culture is taken, repeat after treatment
• Bleeding: check INR if anticoagulants are taken
• Monitor blood studies: AST, ALT, bilirubin, LDH, alkaline phosphatase, Coombs' test monthly if patient is on long-term therapy
• **Assess for QT prolongation, ventricular dysrhythmias:** monitor ECG, cardiac status in those with cardiac abnormalities
• **Assess for serious skin reaction:** Stevens-Johnson syndrome, toxic epidermal necrolysis, assess for rash, product should be discontinued immediately, may occur after therapy is concluded
• *Clostridium difficile*–associated diarrhea **(CDAD):** Monitor for diarrhea, cramping, blood in stools, fever, report immediately to prescriber, may start up to several weeks after conclusion of treatment

Patient problem
Infection (uses)
Diarrhea (adverse reactions)

Implementation
• Do not break, crush, or chew ext rel tab
• Ensure adequate fluid intake (2 L) during diarrhea episodes
• Give q12hr to maintain serum level
• Store at room temperature
• **Susp:** Shake well, store at room temperature, discard after 2 wk
• **Ext Rel:** Give with food

Patient/family education
• **Superinfection:** Advise patient to contact physician if vaginal itching, loose foul-smelling stools, furry tongue occur
• Instruct patient to take all medication prescribed for the length of time ordered, ext rel with food
• **Pregnancy/breastfeeding:** Advise prescriber if pregnancy is planned or suspected, or if breastfeeding
• *Clostridium difficile*-associated diarrhea **(CDAD):** Teach patient to notify prescriber of diarrhea, severe abdominal pain, fever, blood in stools

Evaluation
Positive therapeutic outcome
- Absence of signs/symptoms of infection
- Reported improvement in symptoms of infection
- Prevention of endocarditis

clavulanate
See amoxicillin/clavulanate, ticarcillin/clavulanate

clindamycin HCl (Rx)
(klin-dah-my′sin)
Cleocin T, Clinda-Derm, Clinda-T ✤, Clindagel, Clindesse, Clindets, Dalacin T ✤, Evoclin
Func. class.: Antiinfective—miscellaneous
Chem. class.: Lincomycin derivative

ACTION: Binds to 50S subunit of bacterial ribosomes; suppresses protein synthesis

Therapeutic outcome: Absence of infection

USES: Skin/skin structures, respiratory tract infections, septicemia, intra-abdominal infections, endocarditis prophylaxis caused by staphylococci, streptococci, *Rickettsia, Fusobacterium, Actinomyces, Peptococcus, Bacteroides*

Unlabeled uses: *P. jiroveci* pneumonia

Pharmacokinetics

Absorption	Well absorbed (PO, IM), minimal (TOP)
Distribution	Widely distributed; crosses placenta, protein binding 94%
Metabolism	Liver, extensively by CYP3A4
Excretion	Kidneys, breast milk
Half-life	2½ hr

Pharmacodynamics

	PO	IM	IV
Onset	Rapid	Rapid	Rapid
Peak	1 hr	1-3 hr	Infusion's end

CONTRAINDICATIONS
Hypersensitivity to this product or lincomycin, tartrazine dye, ulcerative colitis/enteritis

> **BLACK BOX WARNING:** Pseudomembranous colitis

Precautions: Pregnancy, breastfeeding, geriatric, renal/liver/GI disease, asthma, allergy, diarrhea

DOSAGE AND ROUTES
Most infections
Adult: PO 150-450 mg q6hr, max 2.7 g/day; IM/IV 1.2-2.7 g/day in 2-4 divided doses q6-12hr, max 4.8 g/day (IV)
Child >1 mo: PO 8-25 mg/kg/day in divided doses q6-8hr; IM/IV 20-40 mg/kg/day in divided doses q6-8hr in 3-4 equal doses
Neonate: 15-20 mg/kg/day divided q6-8hr

PID
Adult: IV 900 mg q8hr plus gentamicin

Bacterial endocarditis prophylaxis
Adult: PO/IV 600 mg 1 hr before procedure; 30 min (IV)

P. jiroveci pneumonia
Adult: PO 1200-1800 mg/day in divided doses with 15-30 mg primaquine/day × 21 days

Bacterial vaginosis
Adult/Adolescent: Vag (Cleocin, CLindamax) 1 applicator (5 g at bedtime × 3-7 day; (clindesse) 1 applicator (5 g) single, or 1 suppository (100 mg) at bedtime × 3 nights

Available forms: Phosphate: inj 150 mg/mL base/6 ml; inj inf in D₅ 300, 600, 900 mg; **HCl:** caps 75, 150, 300 mg; **palmitate:** oral sol 75 mg/5 ml

ADVERSE EFFECTS
CV: Dysrhythmias, hypotension
GI: *Nausea, vomiting, abdominal pain, diarrhea,* pseudomembranous colitis, *anorexia*
INTEG: Rash, urticaria, pruritus, abscess at inj site
SYST: Stevens-Johnson syndrome, exfoliative dermatitis
MISC: Candidiasis

INTERACTIONS
Individual drugs
Erythromycin, decreased action of clindamycin, avoid using together
Kaolin/pectin: decreased absorption

Drug/lab test
Increased: alkaline phosphatase, bilirubin, CPK, AST, ALT

NURSING CONSIDERATIONS
Assessment
- Assess patient for signs and symptoms of infection: characteristics of wounds, sputum, urine, stool, WBC >10,000/mm³, fever; obtain baseline information before, during treatment; complete C&S testing before beginning product therapy; this will identify if correct treatment has

been initiated, give product as soon as culture is taken, monitor appearance of wounds, sputum, stools, urine baseline and periodically
• Assess for **allergic reactions:** rash, urticaria, pruritus, chills, fever, joint pain; may occur a few days after therapy begins; EPINEPHrine and resuscitation equipment should be available in case of an anaphylactic reaction
• Monitor blood studies: CBC

> **BLACK BOX WARNING:** Assess bowel pattern daily; if severe diarrhea occurs, product should be discontinued; may indicate **CDAD**, may occur several weeks after therapy is terminated

• Assess for overgrowth of infection: perineal itching, fever, malaise, redness, pain, swelling, drainage, rash, diarrhea, change in cough, sputum
• **Assess for serious skin infections:** Stevens-Johnson syndrome, exfoliative dermatitis (monitor for rash), discontinue at first appearance of rash, may occur after conclusion of therapy

Patient problems
Infection (uses)
Diarrhea (adverse reactions)

Implementation
• Obtain C&S before use; may start treatment before results are labeled
PO route
• Do not break, crush, or chew caps
• Give with 8 oz of water; give with meals for GI symptoms
• Shake liquids well
• Do not refrigerate oral preparations; stable at room temperature for 2 wk
Oral sol
• Do not refrigerate reconstituted product, store at room temperature ≤2 wk
• Reconstitute granules with most of 75 ml of water, shake well, add remaining water, shake well (75 mg/5 ml)
Vaginal route
• Use applicator supplied
• Partner is not treated
Topical route
• Do not get in eyes, cuts
IM route
• If more than 600 mg must be given, divide into 2 inj
• Give deeply in large muscle mass; rotate sites

IV route
• Visually inspect parenteral products for particulate matter and discoloration prior to use
• **Vials:** Dilute 300 and 600 mg doses with 50 ml of a compatible diluent. Dilute 900 mg doses with 50-100 ml of a compatible diluent. Dilute 1200 mg doses with 100 ml of a compatible diluent, final concentration max 18 mg/ml
• **ADD-Vantage vials:** Dilute 300 and 600 mg ADD-Vantage containers with 50 or 100 mg, respectively, of NS or D_5W
• **Storage:** When diluted in D_5W, NS, or LR, solutions with concentrations of 6, 9, or 12 mg/ml are stable for 16 days at room temperature or 32 days under refrigeration when stored in glass bottles or minibags. When diluted in D_5W, solutions with a concentration of 18 mg/ml are stable for 16 days at room temperature
Intermittent IV infusion
• Infuse over at least 10-60 min, infusion rates max 30 mg/min and ≤1.2 g should be infused in a 1 hr period
• Infuse 300 mg doses over 10 min; 600 mg doses over 20 min, 900 mg doses over 30 min, and 1200 mg doses over 40 min
Continuous IV infusion
• Give first dose rapidly, and then follow with continuous infusion; rate is based on desired serum clindamycin levels
• To maintain serum concentrations above 4 mcg/ml, use a rapid infusion rate of 10 mg/min for 30 min and a maintenance rate of 0.75 mg/min; to maintain serum concentrations above 5 mcg/ml, use a rapid infusion rate of 15 mg/min for 30 min and a maintenance rate of 1 mg/min; to maintain serum concentrations above 5 mcg/ml, use a rapid infusion rate of 20 mg/min for 30 min and a maintenance rate of 1.25 mg/min

Y-site compatibilities: Acyclovir, alfentanil, amifostine, amikacin, aminocaproic acid, aminophylline, amiodarone, amphotericin B cholesteryl, amphotericin B lipid complex, amsacrine, anakinra, anidulafungin, ascorbic acid injection, atenolol, atracurium, atropine, aztreonam, benztropine, bivalirudin, bleomycin, bumetanide, buprenorphine, butorphanol, calcium chloride/gluconate, CARBOplatin, cefamandole, ceFAZolin, cefmetazole, cefonicid, cefoperazone, cefotaxime, cefoTEtan, cefOXitin, cefpirome, cefTAZidime, ceftizoxime, ceftobiprole, cefuroxime, cephalothin, cephapirin, chloramphenicol, cimetidine, cisatracurium, CISplatin, codeine, cyanocobalamin, cyclophosphamide, cycloSPORINE, cytarabine, DACTINomycin, DAPTOmycin, dexamethasone, dexmedetomidine, digoxin, dilTIAZem, diphenhydrAMINE, DOCEtaxel, DOPamine, doxacurium, DOXOrubicin, DOXOrubicin liposomal, doxycycline, enalaprilat, ePHEDrine, EPINEPHrine, epiRUBicin, epoetin alfa, eptifibatide, esmolol, etoposide, famotidine, fenoldopam, fentaNYL, fludarabine, fluorouracil, folic acid, foscarnet, furosemide, gatifloxacin, gemcitabine, gemtuzumab, gentamicin, glycopyrrolate, granisetron, heparin, hydrocortisone, HYDROmorphone, ifosfamide, imipenem-cilastatin, indomethacin, insulin (regular), irinotecan, isoproterenol, ketorolac, levofloxacin, lidocaine, linezolid, LORazepam, LR, magnesium sulfate, mannitol, mechlorethamine, melphalan, meperidine, metaraminol, methicillin, methotrexate, methoxamine, methyldopate, methylPREDNISolone, metoclopramide, metoprolol, metroNIDAZOLE, mezlocillin, miconazole, milrinone, morphine, moxalactam, multiple vitamins injection, nafcillin, nalbuphine, naloxone, nesiritide, netilmicin, niCARdipine, nitroglycerin, nitroprusside, norepinephrine, octreotide, ondansetron, oxacillin, oxaliplatin, oxytocin, PACLitaxel, palonosetron, pamidronate, pancuronium, pantoprazole, PEMEtrexed, penicillin G potassium/sodium, pentazocine, perphenazine, PHENobarbital, phenylephrine, phytonadione, piperacillin, piperacillin-tazobactam, potassium chloride, procainamide, propofol, propranolol, protamine, pyridoxine, raNITIdine, remifentanil, Ringer's, ritodrine, riTUXimab, rocuronium, sargramostim, sodium acetate/bicarbonate, succinylcholine, SUFentanil, tacrolimus, teniposide, theophylline, thiamine, thiotepa, ticarcillin, ticarcillin-clavulanate, tigecycline, tirofiban, TNA, tobramycin, tolazoline, TPN, trimetaphan, urokinase, vancomycin, vasopressin, vecuronium, verapamil, vinCRIStine, vinorelbine, vitamin B complex/C, voriconazole, zidovudine, zoledronic acid

Patient/family education
• Tell patient to take oral product with full glass of water; may take with food if GI symptoms occur; antiperistaltic products may worsen diarrhea
• Teach patient aspects of product therapy: need to complete entire course of medication to ensure organism death (10-14 days); culture may be taken after medication course has been completed
• **Superinfections:** Advise patient to report sore throat, fever, fatigue; may indicate superinfection
• Advise patient that product must be taken at equal intervals around clock to maintain blood levels

> **BLACK BOX WARNING:** Teach patient to report diarrhea with pus, mucus, rash

Pregnancy/breastfeeding: Advise patient to report if pregnancy is planned or suspected or if breastfeeding

Evaluation
Positive therapeutic outcome
• Negative C&S
• Prevention of endocarditis
• Absence of signs/symptoms of infection

TREATMENT OF HYPERSENSITIVITY: Withdraw product; maintain airway; administer EPINEPHrine, O_2, **IV** corticosteroids

clindamycin topical
See Appendix B

clobetasol topical
See Appendix B

clocortolone (Rx)
(kloe-kore′toe-lone)
Cloderm
Func. class.: Antiinflammatory, topical
Chem. class.: Corticosteroid

ACTION: Inhibits inflammation

Therapeutic outcome: Decreased inflammation

USES: Topical treatment of mild to moderate inflammation of skin disorders

Pharmacokinetics

Absorption	Minimal
Distribution	Local
Metabolism	Unknown
Excretion	Unknown
Half-life	Unknown

Pharmacodynamics

Onset	Unknown
Peak	Unknown
Duration	Unknown

CONTRAINDICATIONS
Hypersensitivity

Precautions: infections, pregnancy, breastfeeding, children, cataracts, glaucoma

DOSAGE AND ROUTES
Adult: Topical, apply 1-4 times per day

Available forms: Topical cream 0.1%

ADVERSE EFFECTS
INTEG: Rash, burning, redness, stinging

INTERACTIONS
None significant

NURSING CONSIDERATIONS
Assessment
• Assess area involved baseline and during treatment; use occlusive dressings if directed
• **Assess** rash, burning, itching, redness

Patient problems
Impaired skin integrity (uses)

Implementation
• **Topical:** apply cream to affected area once to four times per day; wear gloves when applying

Patient/family education
• Advise patient to use as directed, not to double or skip doses
• Teach patient to report if pregnancy is planned or suspected or if breastfeeding

Evaluation
Positive therapeutic outcome
• Reported improvement in skin integrity, absence of itching

⚠ HIGH ALERT

clonazePAM (Rx)
(kloe-na′zi-pam)
KlonoPIN, Rivotril ♦
Func. class.: Anticonvulsant
Chem. class.: Benzodiazepine derivative
Controlled substance schedule IV

Do not confuse: clonazePAM/LORazepam/ cloNIDine, **KlonoPIN**/cloNIDine

ACTION: Inhibits spike, wave formation in absence seizures (petit mal), decreases amplitude, frequency, duration, spread of discharge in minor motor seizures

Therapeutic outcome: Decreased frequency, severity of seizures

USES: Absence, atypical absence, akinetic, myoclonic seizures, Lennox-Gastaut syndrome, panic disorder

Unlabeled uses: Restless leg syndrome, acute mania, psychosis, insomnia, neuralgia

Pharmacokinetics

Absorption	Well absorbed
Distribution	Crosses blood-brain barrier, placenta, protein binding 85%
Metabolism	Liver
Excretion	Kidneys
Half-life	18-50 hr

Pharmacodynamics

Onset	½-1 hr
Peak	1-2 hr
Duration	6-12 hr

CONTRAINDICATIONS
Pregnancy, hypersensitivity to benzodiazepines, acute closed-angle glaucoma, psychosis, severe liver disease

Precautions: Open-angle glaucoma, chronic respiratory disease, renal/hepatic disease, breastfeeding, geriatric

> **BLACK BOX WARNING:** Coadministration with other CNS depressants, especially opiates

DOSAGE AND ROUTES
Lennox-Gastaut syndrome/ atypical absence seizures/akinetic and myoclonic seizures
Adult: PO 1.5 mg/day in 3 divided doses; may be increased 0.5-1 mg q3day until desired response; max 20 mg/day
Child <10 yr or <30 kg: PO 0.01-0.03 mg/kg/ day in divided doses q8hr, max 0.05 mg/kg/day; may be increased 0.25-0.5 mg q3day until desired response; max 0.1-0.2 mg/kg/day
Geriatric: PO 0.25 daily-bid initially, increase by 0.25 daily q7-14day as needed

Panic disorder
Adult: PO 0.25 mg bid, increase to 1 mg/day after 3 days, max 4 mg/day

Available forms: Tabs 0.5, 1, 2 mg; **orally disintegrating tabs** 0.125, 0.25, 0.5, 1, 2 mg

ADVERSE EFFECTS
CNS: *Drowsiness,* dizziness, confusion, behavioral changes, tremors, insomnia, headache, suicidal tendencies, slurred speech, fatigue
CV: Palpitations, bradycardia
EENT: *Nystagmus, diplopia*
GI: *Nausea, constipation,* anorexia, diarrhea
GU: Dysuria, nocturia, retention, libido changes
HEMA: Thrombocytopenia, leukopenia, anemia, eosinophilia
INTEG: Rash
RESP: Respiratory depression, congestion

INTERACTIONS
Individual drugs

> **BLACK BOX WARNING:** Alcohol: increased CNS depression

CarBAMazepine: decreased clonazePAM effect
Cimetidine, clarithromycin, dilTIAZem, erythromycin, FLUoxetine: increased clonazePAM effect
PHENobarbital: decreased clonazePAM effect
Phenytoin: decreased clonazePAM levels, monitor effect

Drug classifications

Anticonvulsants, antidepressants, barbiturates, general anesthetics, opiates, sedative/hypnotics: increased CNS depression

Azoles, oral contraceptives: increased clonazePAM effect, adjust dosages

CYP3A4 inducers: decreased clonazePAM effect

Drug/herb

Ginkgo, melatonin: increased clonazePAM effect

Ginseng, St. John's wort: decreased clonazePAM effect

Kava, chamomile, valerian: increased sedative effect

Drug/lab test

Increased: AST, alkaline phosphatase

Decreased: platelets, WBC

NURSING CONSIDERATIONS

Assessment

• Assess **seizures:** Monitor duration, type, intensity, with or without aura

• **Assess mental status:** mood, sensorium, affect, memory (long, short), especially geriatric; behavioral changes, suicidal thoughts/behaviors

• Monitor blood studies: RBCs, Hct, Hgb, reticulocyte counts periodically

• Monitor hepatic studies: ALT, AST, bilirubin, creatinine periodically

• **Abrupt discontinuation:** do not discontinue abruptly, seizures may increase; assess for signs of physical withdrawal if medication suddenly discontinued

• Assess allergic reaction: red raised rash; if this occurs, product should be discontinued

• **Monitor for toxicity:** bone marrow depression, nausea, vomiting, ataxia, diplopia; monitor drug levels during initial treatment (therapeutic 20-80 ng/ml)

• **Beers:** May be appropriate in older adults for seizure disorders, rapid eye movement sleep disorders, benzodiazepine/ethanol withdrawal; avoid in those with or at high risk of delirium

> **BLACK BOX WARNING:** Assess for concomitant use of benzodiazepines and opioids, which may result in profound sedation, respiratory depression, coma, death

Patient problem

Risk for injury (uses)

Implementation

PO route

• Give on empty stomach for best absorption, or with food for GI upset

Orally disintegrating tablets: Remove from blister package when ready to use, place on tongue, allow to dissolve

Rectal route

• **IV** sol may be used rectally, 1 ml syringe inserted 3 cm into rectum

• Oral susp may be used rectally (1 mg/ml of product with 1 ml of water), use plastic tube (volume 2.2-3.3 ml)

• Store at room temperature

Patient/family education

• Teach patient to notify prescriber of yellowing skin/eyes, pale stools, bleeding, fever, extreme fatigue, sore throat, suicidal thoughts/behaviors

• **Pregnancy/breastfeeding:** Teach patient to notify prescriber if pregnancy is planned or suspected or if breastfeeding to register with North American Antiepileptic Drug Pregnancy Registry 888-233-2334, do not use in pregnancy/breastfeeding

• Teach patient to carry/wear emergency ID card stating patient's name, products taken, condition, physician's name, phone number, discuss tolerance, withdrawal, to continue with follow-up exams, lab work

• Caution patient to avoid driving, other activities that require alertness

• Advise patient to take as prescribed, not to double or skip doses; provide Medication Guide

• Advise patient to inform all health care professionals of all OTC, Rx, herbs, supplements taken

• Caution patient to avoid alcohol ingestion or CNS depressants; increased sedation may occur

• Teach patient not to discontinue medication quickly after long-term use; taper off over several weeks

Evaluation

Positive therapeutic outcome

• Decreased seizure activity

• Decreased restless legs

• Decreased panic attacks

TREATMENT OF OVERDOSE:

Lavage, VS, flumazenil, monitor electrolytes, sodium bicarbonate

cloNIDine (Rx)

(klon'i-deen)

**Catapres, Catapres-TTS, Dixarit ❧,
Duraclon, Kapvay**

Func. class.: Antihypertensive, centrally acting analgesic

Chem. class.: Centrally acting α-adrenergic agonist

Do not confuse: cloNIDine/KlonoPIN/clonazePAM

ACTION: Inhibits sympathetic vasomotor center in CNS, which reduces impulses in sympathetic nervous system; B/P, pulse rate, cardiac output decreased; prevents pain signal transmission in CNS by α-adrenergic receptor stimulation of the spinal cord

Therapeutic outcome: Decreased B/P in hypertension

USES: Mild to moderate hypertension, used alone or in combination; severe pain in cancer patients (epidural), attention-deficit/hyperactivity disorder (ADHD)

Unlabeled uses: Opioid withdrawal

Pharmacokinetics

Absorption	Well absorbed (PO, TD)
Distribution	Widely distributed; crosses blood-brain barrier
Metabolism	Liver, extensively
Excretion	Kidneys, unchanged (45%)
Half-life	12-21 hr

Pharmacodynamics

	PO	TD	Epidural
Onset	½-1 hr	3 days	Unknown
Peak	2-4 hr	Unknown	Unknown
Duration	8-12 hr	8 hr	Unknown

CONTRAINDICATIONS

Hypersensitivity; (epidural) bleeding disorders, anticoagulants

Precautions: Pregnancy, breastfeeding, child <12 yr (transdermal), geriatric, MI (recent), diabetes mellitus, chronic renal failure, Raynaud's disease, thyroid disease, depression, COPD, asthma, noncompliant patients

BLACK BOX WARNING: Labor (transdermal)

DOSAGE AND ROUTES
Hypertension

Adult: PO 0.1 mg bid, then increase by 0.1-0.2 mg/day at weekly intervals, until desired response; range 0.2-0.6 mg/day in divided doses or transdermal q7 days, start 0.1 mg and adjust q1-2wk
Geriatric: PO 0.1 mg at bedtime, may increase gradually
Child: PO 5-10 mcg/kg/day in divided doses q8-12hr, max 0.9 mg/day

Severe pain

Adult: CONT EPIDURAL INF 30 mcg/hr
Child: CONT EPIDURAL INF 0.5 mcg/kg/hr, then titrate to response

Opioid withdrawal (unlabeled)

Adult: PO 0.3-1.2 mg/day; may decrease by 50% × 3 days, then decrease by 0.1-0.2 mg/day or discontinue

Available forms: **Tabs** 0.025 ❧, 0.1, 0.2, 0.3 mg; **transdermal** 2.5, 5, 7.5 mg delivering 0.1, 0.2, 0.3 mg/24 hr, respectively; **inj** 100, 500 mcg/ml, **ext rel tab** 0.1 mg (Kapvay)

ADVERSE EFFECTS

CNS: *Drowsiness,* nightmares, insomnia, mental changes, anxiety, depression, hallucinations, delirium, syncope, dizziness, paresthesia
CV: *Orthostatic hypotension, palpitations,* HF, ECG abnormalities
EENT: Taste change, dry eyes
ENDO: Hyperglycemia
GI: *Nausea, vomiting, malaise,* constipation, *dry mouth*
GU: Impotence
INTEG: *Rash,* pruritus, hives, (TD patches)
MISC: *Withdrawal symptoms*

INTERACTIONS
Individual drugs

Alcohol: increased CNS depression
Levodopa: decreased levodopa effect
Prazosin: decreased hypotensive effects
Verapamil, dilTIAZem: Increased bradycardia

Drug classifications

Amphetamines, appetite suppressants, MAOIs, tricyclics: decreased hypotensive effects
Increase: Bradycardia, amphetamines, beta blockers, digoxin, dilTIAZem, MAOI inhibitors, verapamil, Increased: Bradycardia
Anesthetics, opiates, sedatives/hypnotics: increased CNS depression
Antidepressants (tricyclic), β-adrenergic blockers: life-threatening increase in B/P
Diuretics, nitrates: increased hypotensive effects

Drug/herb
Ephedra, ginseng: decreased antihypertensive effect

Hawthorn: increased antihypertensive effect

Drug/lab test
Increased: blood glucose

Decreased: VMA, urinary catecholamines, aldosterone

Positive: Coomb's test

NURSING CONSIDERATIONS
Assessment
• Monitor B/P, pulse if the product is being used for **hypertension;** notify prescriber of changes

• Assess **pain:** location, intensity, character, alleviating, aggravation factors, baseline and frequency

• Monitor baselines for renal/liver function tests before therapy begins; check potassium levels, although hyperkalemia rarely occurs

• Assess for **opiate withdrawal** (unlabeled) in patients receiving the product for opioid withdrawal, including fever, diarrhea, nausea, vomiting, cramps, insomnia, shivering, dilated pupils, weakness

• Assess **allergic reaction:** rash, fever, pruritus, urticaria; product should be discontinued if antihistamines fail to help

• ADHD: monitor B/P, pulse, palpitations, syncope, mental status

> **BLACK BOX WARNING: Pregnancy/ breastfeeding:** Do not use for labor (epidural), excreted in breast milk, discontinue breastfeeding or product

• **Beers:** Avoid as first line in older adults, high risk of CNS effects, bradycardia, orthostatic hypotension

Patient problems
Risk for injury (uses)

Implementation
PO route
• Give last dose at bedtime

• Do not crush, cut, chew, or break ER tabs; Kapvay is not interchangeable with other products

Transdermal route
• Apply patch weekly; remove old patch and wash off residue; apply to site without hair; best absorption over chest or upper arm; rotate sites with each application; clean site before application; apply firmly, especially around edges, may secure with adhesive tape if loose; fold sticky sides together and discard

• Should be removed before MRI

• Store patches in cool environment

Epidermal route
• Dilute 500 mcg/mL with 0.9% NaCl (100 mcg/mL)

> **BLACK BOX WARNING:** Do not use for labor

Patient/family education
• **Heart failure:** Advise patient to continue with regimen including weight, no smoking, exercise, sodium-restricted diet

• **Instruct patient not to discontinue product abruptly, or withdrawal symptoms may occur:** anxiety, increased B/P, headache, insomnia, increased pulse, tremors, nausea, sweating

• Caution patient not to use OTC (cough, cold, or allergy), alcohol or CNS depressant products unless directed by prescriber

• Teach patient to comply with dosage schedule even if feeling better; product controls symptoms, does not cure

• Caution patient to change position slowly, to rise slowly to sitting or standing position to minimize orthostatic hypotension, especially geriatric

• Teach patient about excessive perspiration, dehydration, vomiting; diarrhea may lead to fall in B/P; consult prescriber if these occur

• Tell patient that product may cause dizziness, fainting; light-headedness may occur during first few days of therapy; use hard candy, saliva product, or frequent rinsing of mouth for dry mouth

• **Transdermal:** teach patient how to use patch; that patch comes in two parts: product patch and overlay to keep patch in place; not to trim or cut patch; remove for MRI; can use during bathing, swimming

• Advise patient that compliance is necessary; not to skip or stop product unless directed by prescriber

• Teach patient that product may cause skin rash or impaired perspiration

• Teach patient that response may take 2-3 days if product is given TD; instruct on administration of patch; return demonstration

• Teach patient to avoid hazardous activities, since product may cause drowsiness, dizziness

• Teach patient to administer 1 hr before meals

Evaluation
Positive therapeutic outcome
• Decrease in B/P in hypertension
• Decrease in withdrawal symptoms
• Decrease in pain
• Decrease in vascular headaches
• Decrease in dysmenorrhea
• Decrease in menopausal symptoms

TREATMENT OF OVERDOSE:
Supportive treatment; administer atropine, DOPamine prn

> ⚠ **HIGH ALERT**
>
> ## clopidogrel (Rx)
> (klo-pid'oh-grel)
> **Plavix**
> *Func. class.:* Platelet aggregation inhibitor
> *Chem. class.:* Thienopyridine derivative

Do not confuse: Plavix/Paxil/Elavil

ACTION: Inhibits first and second phases of ADP-induced effects in platelet aggregation

Therapeutic outcome: Decreased possibility of stroke, MI by decreasing platelet aggregation

USES: Reducing the risk of stroke, MI, vascular death, peripheral arterial disease in high-risk patients, acute coronary syndrome, transient ischemic attack (TIA), unstable angina

Pharmacokinetics

Absorption	Rapidly absorbed
Distribution	Unknown
Metabolism	Liver, extensively, by protein binding 95%, CYP2B6, CYP1A2, CYP2C8
Excretion	Kidneys, unchanged product
Half-life	6 hr

Pharmacodynamics

Onset	Unknown
Peak	Unknown
Duration	Unknown

CONTRAINDICATIONS
Hypersensitivity, active bleeding

Precautions: Pregnancy, breastfeeding, children, past liver disease, increased bleeding risk, neutropenia, agranulocytosis, renal disease, ⚠ Asian/Black/Caucasian patients

> **BLACK BOX WARNING:** ⚠ CYP2C19 allele (poor metabolizers)

DOSAGE AND ROUTES
Recent MI, stroke, peripheral arterial disease, TIA
Adult: PO 75 mg daily with aspirin

Acute coronary syndrome
Adult: PO loading dose 300 mg then 75 mg daily with aspirin

Available forms: Tabs 75, 300 mg

ADVERSE EFFECTS
CNS: Headache, dizziness, depression, fatal intracranial bleeding
CV: Edema, hypertension, chest pain
GI: Diarrhea, GI discomfort
HEMA: Bleeding (major/minor from any site), neutropenia, aplastic anemia, agranulocytosis, thrombotic thrombocytopenic purpura
INTEG: Rash, pruritus
MISC: UTI, hypercholesterolemia, chest pain, fatigue, toxic epidermal necrolysis, Stevens-Johnson syndrome, flu-like syndrome, anaphylaxis
MS: Arthralgia, back pain
RESP: Upper respiratory tract infection, dyspnea, rhinitis, bronchitis, cough, bronchospasm

INTERACTIONS
Individual drugs
Abciximab, aspirin, eptifibatide, rifAMPin, ticlopidine, tirofiban, treprostinil, SNRIs, prasugrel: increased bleeding tendencies
Fluvastatin, phenytoin, tamoxifen, TOLBUTamide, torsemide, warfarin: increased action of each specific product

Drug classifications
Anticoagulants, NSAIDs, SSRIs, thrombolytics: increased bleeding tendencies
CYP3A4 inhibitors/substrates (atorvastatin, cerivastatin, esomeprazole, omeprazole, simvastatin): decreased effects

> **BLACK BOX WARNING:** ⚠ CYP2C19 inhibitors (omeprazole, esomeprazole): avoid use

NSAIDs: increased action of some NSAIDs
Proton pump inhibitors (PPIs): decreased clopidogrel effect

Drug/herb
Bilberry, saw palmetto: decreased clopidogrel effect
Feverfew, fish oil, garlic, ginger, ginkgo biloba, green tea, horse chestnut, omega-3 fatty acids: increased clopidogrel effect

Drug/lab test
Increased: AST, ALT, bilirubin, uric acid, total cholesterol, nonprotein nitrogen (NPN)

C

NURSING CONSIDERATIONS
Assessment

> **BLACK BOX WARNING:** ✏️⚠ CYP2C19 allele (poor metabolizers): Consider using another antiplatelet product, higher CV reaction occurs after acute coronary syndrome or PCI, tests are available to determine CYP2C19 allele

- Assess for thrombotic/thrombocytic purpura: fever, thrombocytopenia, neurolytic anemia, treat immediately
- Monitor liver function tests: AST, ALT, bilirubin, creatinine if patient is on long-term therapy (4 mo or more)
- Monitor blood studies: CBC, Hct, Hgb, bleeding time if patient is on long-term therapy; thrombocytopenia, hemolytic anemia, neurologic changes occur (rare)

Patient problem
Pain (uses)
Risk for injury (adverse reactions)

Implementation
- Without regard to food, give with food to decrease gastric symptoms
- Product should be discontinued 5 days before elective surgery if an antiplatelet action is not desired

Patient/family education
- **Pregnancy/breastfeeding:** Use only if clearly needed
- Advise patient that blood work will be necessary during treatment
- Advise patient to report any unusual bleeding to prescriber, that it may take longer to stop bleeding
- Teach patient to take without regard to food
- Caution patient to report diarrhea, skin rashes, subcutaneous bleeding, chills, fever, sore throat, yellowing of skin, eyes, weakness
- Teach patient to tell all health care providers that clopidogrel is being used; may be held for 5 days before surgery, restart as soon as remembered
- **Hypersensitivity:** Rash, pruritus may occur, notify health care professional immediately
- **Pregnancy/breastfeeding:** If pregnancy is planned or do not breastfeed

Evaluation
Positive therapeutic outcome
- Absence of stroke

---

clotrimazole topical
See Appendix B

clotrimazole vaginal antifungal
See Appendix B

---

cloZAPine (Rx)
(kloz′a-peen)
Clozaril, Fazaclo, Versacloz
Func. class.: Antipsychotic
Chem. class.: Tricyclic dibenzodiazepine derivative

Do not confuse: Clozaril/Colazal/cloZAPine/cloNIDine/clofazimine/clonazePAM/KlonoPIN

ACTION: Interferes with DOPamine receptor binding with lack of EPS and tardive dyskinesia; also acts as an adrenergic, cholinergic, histaminergic, serotoninergic antagonist

Therapeutic outcome: Decreased psychotic behavior

USES: Management of psychotic symptoms in schizophrenic patients for whom other antipsychotics have failed, recurrent suicidal behavior; orally disintegrating tabs are not used for recurrent suicidal behavior

Pharmacokinetics

Absorption	Well absorbed
Distribution	Widely distributed; crosses blood-brain barrier, placenta; 95% protein binding
Metabolism	✏️⚠ Liver, by CYP1A2, 2D6, 3A4
Excretion	Kidneys (50%), feces (30%) (metabolites)
Half-life	8-12 hr

Pharmacodynamics

Onset	Unknown
Peak	Unknown
Duration	8-12 hr

CONTRAINDICATIONS
Hypersensitivity, severe granulocytopenia (WBC <3500/mm^3 before therapy)

Precautions: Pregnancy, breastfeeding, children <16 yr, geriatric, renal/hepatic/cardiac/CV/pulmonary disease, seizures, prostatic enlargement, closed-angle glaucoma, stroke

> **BLACK BOX WARNING:** Bone marrow suppression, hypotension, myocarditis, orthostatic hypotension, elderly patients with dementia-related psychosis, seizures, syncope

DOSAGE AND ROUTES
Adult: PO 12.5 mg daily or bid; may increase by 25-50 mg/day over 2 wk, dose > 500 mg requires 3 divided doses; max 900 mg/day; if dose is to be discontinued, taper over 1-2 wk

---

Available forms: Tabs 25, 50, 100, 200 mg; orally disintegrating tabs 12.5, 25, 100 150, 200 mg; oral suspension 50 mg/ml

ADVERSE EFFECTS

CNS: *Sedation, dizziness, headache,* seizures, *confusion, insomnia, EPS, anxiety,* neuroleptic malignant syndrome, agitation, dystonia, obsessive-compulsive symptoms
CV: *Tachycardia, hypo/hypertension,* HF, DVT, torsade de pointes, orthostatic hypotension
EENT: Blurred vision
GI: *Drooling or excessive salivation, constipation, nausea, abdominal discomfort, vomiting, diarrhea,* anorexia, weight gain, dry mouth, dyspepsia, hepatotoxicity
GU: *Urinary abnormalities,* incontinence
HEMA: Leukopenia, neutropenia, agranulocytosis, eosinophilia
RESP: Dyspnea, pulmonary embolism
OTHER: Diaphoresis
SYST: Death in geriatric patients with dementia, aggravation of diabetes mellitus

INTERACTIONS
Individual drugs
Alcohol: increased CNS depression
Caffeine, citalopram, erythromycin, FLUoxetine, fluvoxaMINE, ketoconazole, risperiDONE, ritonavir, sertraline: increased cloZAPine levels
CarBAMazepine, omeprazole, PHENobarbital, rifAMPin: decreased cloZAPine level
Digoxin: increased plasma concentration of digoxin
Warfarin: increased plasma concentrations

Drug classifications
Benzodiazepines: increased hypotension, respiratory, cardiac arrest, collapse
Increase: Bone marrow suppression: antineoplastic radiation therapy
Increase: Seizures: lithium
β-blockers, class IA/III antidysrhythmics, and other drugs that increase QT: increased QT prolongation
CNS depressants, psychoactives, antihistamines, opioids, sedatives/hypnotics: increased CNS depression
CYP1A2 inducers CYP3A4 inducers: decreased cloZAPine levels
CYP1A2 inhibitors, CYP2D6 inhibitors, CYP3A4 inhibitors: increased cloZAPine level
Highly protein-bound products: increased plasma concentrations

Drug/herb
St. John's wort: Decreased clozepine action

Drug/lab test
Increased: Triglycerides, cholesterol, blood glucose
Decreased: WBC, ANC

NURSING CONSIDERATIONS
Assessment
• Assess for **myocarditis**: dyspnea, fever, palpitations, ECG changes, if suspected, discontinue; myocarditis usually occurs during first month of treatment
• Obtain AIMS assessment, blood glucose, CBC differential, glycosylated hemoglobin A1C, LFTs, neurologic function, pregnancy test, serum creatinine, electrolytes, lipid profile, prolactin, thyroid function tests, weight

> **BLACK BOX WARNING:** Assess for **seizures;** usually occurs with higher doses (>600 mg/day) or dosage change >100 mg/day; do not use in uncontrolled seizure disorder; use cautiously in those with a predisposition to seizures

• Assess mental status: orientation, mood, behavior, presence of hallucinations, and type before initial administration and monthly; this product should significantly reduce psychotic behavior
• Assess affect, orientation, LOC, reflexes, gait, coordination, sleep pattern disturbances
• Check for swallowing of PO medication; check for hoarding or giving of medication to other patients

> **BLACK BOX WARNING: Bone marrow depression:** Monitor bilirubin, CBC, liver function test monthly; discontinue treatment if WBC <3000-3500/mm³ or if ANC <1500/mm³; test qwk; may resume when normal; if WBC <2000/mm³ or ANC <1000/mm³, discontinue; if agranulocytosis develops, never restart product

> **BLACK BOX WARNING: Hypotension, bradycardia, syncope:** Monitor B/P with patient sitting, standing, and lying; take pulse and respirations q4hr during initial treatment; establish baseline before starting treatment; report drops of 30 mm Hg check for dizziness, faintness, palpitations, tachycardia on rising

• **Assess for neuroleptic malignant syndrome:** hyperpyrexia, muscle rigidity, increased CPK, altered mental status; product should be discontinued
• Assess for **EPS** including akathisia (inability to sit still, no pattern to movements), tardive dyskinesia (bizarre movements of the jaw,

mouth, tongue, extremities), pseudoparkinsonism (rigidity, tremors, pill rolling, shuffling gate)
• **Beers:** Avoid in older adults except for schizophrenia, bipolar disorder, increased risk of stroke and cognitive decline

Patient problems
Risk for Injury (adverse reactions)
Disturbed thought process (uses)

Implementation
• Decrease dosage in geriatric since metabolism is slowed
• Give tablets with full glass of water, milk; or give with food to decrease GI upset
• Store in tight, light-resistant container; oral sol in amber bottle
• Patient-specific registration is required before administration (clozapine REMS program); if WBC <3500 cells/mm³ or ANC <2000 cells/mm², therapy should not be started, pharmacist may only dispense the 7, 14, 28 day supply upon receipt of lab report that is appropriate
• **Orally disintegrating tab:** do not push through foil, leave in foil blister until ready to take, peel back foil, place tab in mouth, allow to dissolve, swallow; water is not needed
• **Oral suspension:** Shake before using, use oral syringe and syringe adapter

Patient/family education
• Teach patient to use good oral hygiene; frequent rinsing of mouth, sugarless gum for dry mouth
• Caution patient to avoid hazardous activities until product response is determined
• Inform patient that orthostatic hypotension occurs often and to rise from sitting or lying position gradually
• Caution patient to avoid hot tubs, hot showers, tub baths, since hypotension may occur
• Advise patient to notify all health care professionals of product use
• Inform patient that continued labs and follow up will be needed
• Explain reason for product, expected result, procedure for REMS program
• Advise patient to take product as directed, not to double or skip doses; product should be withdrawn gradually if on long-term treatment
• Teach patient to avoid OTC preparations (cough, hay fever, cold) unless approved by prescriber, since serious product interactions may occur; avoid use with alcohol, CNS depressants; increased drowsiness may occur
• Teach patient about EPS, to report immediately
• Teach patient to report sore throat, malaise, fever, bleeding, mouth sores; if these occur, CBC should be performed and product discontinued

BLACK BOX WARNING: Teach patient symptoms of agranulocytosis and need for blood test qwk for 6 mo, then q2wk; report flulike symptoms

• **Pregnancy/breastfeeding:** a pregnancy test is recommended before starting treatment, advise patient to notify health care professional if pregnancy is planned or suspected, or if breastfeeding

Evaluation
Positive therapeutic outcome
• Decrease in emotional excitement, hallucinations, delusions, paranoia
• Reorganization of patterns of thought, speech

TREATMENT OF ANAPHYLAXIS: Withdraw product, maintain airway; if diabetic, check blood glucose levels

---

⚠ HIGH ALERT
RARELY USED

cobimetinib
(koe-bi-me'ti-nib)
Cotellic
Func. class.: Antineoplastic

USES: Orphan drug. For the treatment of unresectable or metastatic melanoma in patients with a BRAF V600E or V600K mutation, in combination with vemurafenib

CONTRAINDICATIONS
Hypersensitivity

DOSAGE AND ROUTES
Adult: PO 60 mg (three 20-mg tablets) qday × 21 days, in combination with vemurafenib 960 mg bid × 28 days; repeat cycle q28days until disease progression or unacceptable toxicity

---

⚠ HIGH ALERT

codeine (Rx)
(koe'deen)
Func. class.: Opiate, phenanthrene derivative
Controlled substance schedule II, III, IV, V (depends on content)

Do not confuse: codeine/Lodine/Iodine

ACTION: Depresses pain impulse transmission at the spinal cord level by interacting with opioid receptors; decreases cough reflex, GI motility

---

Therapeutic outcome: Pain relief, decreased cough, decreased diarrhea depending on route

USES: Mild to moderate to severe pain, cough

Unlabeled uses: Diarrhea

Pharmacokinetics

Absorption	Bioavailability 60%-90%
Distribution	Widely distributed, crosses placenta, protein binding 🐟 7%
Metabolism	Liver, extensively by CYP3A4 to morphine; 🐟 altered in ethnic groups
Excretion	Kidneys (up to 15%), breast milk
Half-life	3-4 hr

Pharmacodynamics

	PO
Onset	30-60 min
Peak	1-2 hr
Duration	4 hr

CONTRAINDICATIONS

Hypersensitivity to opiates, respiratory depression, increased intracranial pressure, seizure disorders, severe respiratory disorders, breast-feeding

> **BLACK BOX WARNING:** Children (tonsillectomy/adenoidectomy), ultra-rapid metabolizers

Precautions: Pregnancy, geriatric, cardiac dysrhythmias, prostatic hypertrophy, bowel impaction

DOSAGE AND ROUTES
Pain
Adult: PO 15-60 mg q4hr
Child: PO 6-17 yr 3 mg/kg/day in divided doses q4hr prn

Renal dose
Adult: PO CCr 10-50 ml/min 75% of dose; CCr <10 ml/min 50% of dose

Cough
Adult: PO 10-20 mg q4-6hr, max 120 mg/day

Diarrhea (unlabeled)
Adult: PO 30 mg; may repeat qid

Available forms: Tabs 15, 30, 60 mg; oral sol 10 mg/5 mL ✤, 25 mg/5 mL ✤

ADVERSE EFFECTS
CNS: *Drowsiness, sedation,* dizziness, hallucinations, headache, confusion

CV: Bradycardia, palpitations, orthostatic hypotension
GI: *Nausea, vomiting, anorexia, constipation,* dry mouth
GU: Urinary retention
INTEG: Flushing, rash, sweating
RESP: Respiratory depression

INTERACTIONS
Individual drugs
Alcohol: increased CNS depression

Drug classifications
Antipsychotics, 🐟; CYP3A4 inhibitors (clarithromycin, erythromycin, ketoconazole, protease inhibitors; antihistamine, antidepressants, sedative, hypnotics, opiates, skeletal muscle relaxants: increased CNS depression
MAOIs: increased toxicity; use cautiously

Drug/herb
Chamomile, kava, valerian: Increased CNS depression

Drug/lab test
Increased: amylase, lipase
Decrease: Opioid effect: opioid antagonists

NURSING CONSIDERATIONS
Assessment
• Assess **pain:** intensity, type, alleviating factors, type, location, need for pain medication, tolerance, use pain scoring, evaluate baseline and after 1 hr
• Assess GI function: nausea, vomiting, constipation
• Monitor B/P, pulse respirations baseline and periodically
• Assess **cough:** type, duration, ability to raise secretion for productive cough; do not use to suppress a productive cough
• Monitor CNS changes: dizziness, drowsiness, hallucinations, euphoria, LOC, pupil reaction

> **BLACK BOX WARNING:** Child (tonsillectomy/adenoidectomy) and are ultra-rapid metabolizers: deaths have occurred, use is contraindicated

• Monitor allergic reactions: rash, urticaria
• **Assess for Respiratory dysfunction:** respiratory depression, character, rate, rhythm, especially in the first 24-72 hr after dosage increase; notify prescriber if respirations are <10/min, shallow
• **Beers:** Avoid in older adults unless safer alternative is not available, may cause ataxia, impaired psychomotor function

Patient problem
Risk for Injury (adverse reactions)

Implementation

- Give with antiemetic if nausea, vomiting occur
- Administer when pain is beginning to return, determine dosage interval by patient response; continuous dosing of medication is more effective given prn; explain analgesic effect
- Medication should be slowly withdrawn after long-term use to prevent withdrawal symptoms, use stool softener, laxative for constipation
- Store in light-resistant container at room temp

PO route
- May be given with food or milk to lessen GI upset

Patient/family education

- Teach patient to report any symptoms of CNS changes, allergic reactions; to avoid CNS depressants: alcohol, sedative/hypnotics for at least 24 hr after taking this product
- Discuss with patient that dizziness, drowsiness, and confusion are common, to change positions slowly to minimize orthostatic hypotension
- Advise patient to avoid getting up without assistance
- Discuss in detail with patient all aspects of the product
- Teach patient to use increased fiber in diet, water for constipation
- Teach patient that physical dependency may result after extended periods
- Advise patient to use frequent mouth rinses, gum, frequent oral hygiene to prevent dry mouth
- **Cough:** Have patient use turn, coupling, and deep breath if unable to walk frequently with assistance
- **Pregnancy/breastfeeding:** Identify if pregnancy is planned or suspected, infants born to those using opioids are at risk of neonatal opiate withdrawal, do not breastfeed

Evaluation
Positive therapeutic outcome
- Decreased pain
- Decreased cough
- Decreased diarrhea

TREATMENT OF OVERDOSE:
Naloxone 0.4 ampule diluted in 10 ml 0.9% NaCl and given by direct **IV** push 0.02 mg q2min (adult)

colchicine (Rx)
(kol′chih-seen)
Colcrys, ColciGel, Mitigare
Func. class.: Antigout agent
Chem. class.: Colchicum autumnale alkaloid

Do not confuse colchicine/Cortrosym

ACTION: Inhibits microtubule formation of lactic acid in leukocytes, which decreases phagocytosis and inflammation in joints

Therapeutic outcome: Decreased pain, inflammation of joints

USES: Gout, gouty arthritis (prevention, treatment); to arrest progression of neurologic disability in multiple sclerosis

Pharmacokinetics

Absorption	45%
Distribution	WBCs
Metabolism	Deacetylates in liver
Excretion	Feces (metabolites/active product)
Half-life	30 (Gout effect) hr

Pharmacodynamics

	PO
Onset	12 hr
Peak	Up to 72 hr
Duration	Unknown

CONTRAINDICATIONS
Hypersensitivity; serious GI disorders, severe renal/hepatic/cardiac disorders

Precautions: Pregnancy, breastfeeding, children, geriatric, blood dyscrasias, hepatic disease

DOSAGE AND ROUTES
Gout prevention
Adult: PO 0.6-1.8 mg in 1-2 divided doses daily depending on severity

Gout treatment
Adult: PO 1.2 mg initially, then 0.6 mg 1 hr later (1.8 mg); those on strong CYP3A4 inhibitor (past 14 days) 0.6 mg initially, then 0.3 mg 1 hr later

P-glycoprotein inhibitors or with strong CYP3A4 inhibitors
Adult PO 0.6 mg for 1 dose, then 0.3 mg 1 hr later

With moderate CYP3A4 inhibitors
Adult PO 1.2 mg for 1 dose

Renal dose
Adult: PO CCr <30 ml/min for acute gout, do not repeat course for 2 wk; familial Mediterranean fever 0.3 mg daily, increase cautiously

Available forms: Tabs 0.6 mg; caps 0.6 mg; topical gel $4\times$

ADVERSE EFFECTS
GI: *Nausea, vomiting, anorexia,* cramps, diarrhea
HEMA: Agranulocytosis, thrombocytopenia, aplastic anemia, leukopenia
MISC: Alopecia, peripheral neuritis

INTERACTIONS
Individual drugs
CycloSPORINE, radiation: increased bone marrow depression
Ethanol: increased GI effects
Vitamin B_{12}: decreased action of vit B_{12}; may cause reversible malabsorption

Drug classifications
Bone marrow depressants: increased bone marrow depression
HMG-COA reductase inhibitors Increase: rhabdomyolysis
Moderate/strong CYP3A4 inhibitors, (atazanavir, clarithromycin, indinavir, itraconazole, ketoconazole, ritonavir, saquinavir, telithromycin); P-glycoprotein inhibitors reduce dose: increased colchicine level/toxicity
NSAIDs: increased GI effects

Drug/food
Grapefruit juice: increased colchicine level

Drug/lab test
Increased: alkaline phosphatase, AST
Decreased: platelets, WBC, granulocytes
False positive: urine Hgb
Interference: urinary 17-hydroxycorticosteroids

NURSING CONSIDERATIONS
Assessment
• **Gout:** Assess pain and mobility of joints, uric acid levels returning to normal, monitor response to treatment q1hr
• **Familial Mediterranean fever:** Chest pain, fever, joint pain, lesions, baseline and periodically monitor I&O ratio; observe for decrease in urinary output; CBC, platelets, reticulocytes before, during therapy (q3mo); may cause aplastic anemia, agranulocytosis, decreased platelets
• Monitor I&O, increase to 2,000 mL/day unless contraindicated
• **Assess for toxicity:** weakness, abdominal pain, nausea, vomiting, diarrhea, product should be discontinued, report symptoms immediately

• **Beers:** Reduce dose in older adults, monitor for adverse reactions

Patient problem
Pain (uses)

Implementation
PO route
• Give without regard to food
• Cumulative doses ≤4 mg, renal patients ≤2 mg, when reached, administer only for 3 wks

Patient/family education
• Caution patient to avoid alcohol, OTC preparations that contain alcohol
• Instruct patient to report any pain, redness, or hard area, usually in legs; rash, sore throat, fever, bleeding, bruising, weakness, numbness, tingling, nausea, vomiting, abdominal pain, muscle pain, weakness
• Advise patient to take as prescribed, not to double or skip doses; during acute attacks other products may be needed
• Teach patient to avoid grapefruit and juice, may increase colchicine level
• Teach patient importance of complying with medical regimen (diet, weight loss, product therapy); bone marrow depression may occur
• Advise patient to tell all providers of product use, surgery may increase possibility of acute gout symptoms
• **Pregnancy/breastfeeding:** Identify if pregnancy is planned or suspected

Evaluation
Positive therapeutic outcome
• Decreased stone formation on x-ray
• Decreased pain in kidney region
• Absence of hematuria
• Decreased pain in joints, reduced familial Mediterranean fever episodes

TREATMENT OF OVERDOSE:
Discontinue medication, may need opioids to treat diarrhea

colesevelam (Rx)
(coal-see-vel'am)
Lodalis ✤, **Welchol**
Func. class.: Antilipemic
Chem. class.: Bile acid sequestrant

ACTION: Adsorbs, combines with bile acids to form insoluble complex that is excreted through feces; loss of bile acids lowers cholesterol levels

Therapeutic outcome: Decreasing LDL cholesterol

USES: Elevated LDL cholesterol, alone or in combination with HMG-CoA reductase inhibitor; type 2 diabetes (adjunct)

Pharmacokinetics

Absorption	Not absorbed
Distribution	Unknown
Metabolism	Unknown
Excretion	Feces
Half-life	Unknown

Pharmacodynamics (cholesterol effect)

Onset	1-2 days
Peak	Up to 14 days
Duration	Unknown

CONTRAINDICATIONS
Hypersensitivity, bowel disease, primary biliary cirrhosis, triglycerides >300 mg/dl, bowel obstruction, pancreatitis, biliary obstruction; dysphagia, fat-soluble vitamin deficiency

Precautions: Pregnancy, breastfeeding, children

DOSAGE AND ROUTES
Hyperlipidemia
Adult: PO 3 625 mg tabs bid with meals or 6 tabs daily with a meal; may increase to 7 tabs if needed (monotherapy)
Adult: PO 3 tabs bid with meals or 6 tabs daily with a meal given with an HMG-CoA reductase inhibitor, combination therapy

Type 2 diabetes
Adult and geriatric: PO approx 3.8 g (6 tabs)/day or approx 1.9 g (3 tabs) bid

Heterozygous familial hypercholesterolemia
Females (postmenarchal and >10 yr) and males ≥10 yr: PO 1.875 g packet bid or 3.75 g packet q day dissolved in 4-8 oz of water with a meal

Available forms: Tabs 625 mg, granules for oral susp 3.75 g/packet

ADVERSE EFFECTS
GI: *Constipation, nausea,* flatulence

INTERACTIONS
Individual drugs
Digoxin, dilTIAZem, gemfibrozil, glyBURide, iron, mycophenolate, penicillin G, phenytoin, propanolol, warfarin: decreased absorption of each specific product
Thyroid hormones: decreased absorption of thyroid

Drug classifications
Corticosteroids/fluoroquinolones: decreased corticosteroid action
Oral contraceptives: decreased action of oral contraceptives, give ≥ 4 hr before colesevelam
Tetracyclines: decreased absorption of tetracyclines
Thiazides: decreased absorption of thiazides
Vitamins (fat-soluble): decreased absorption of fat-soluble vitamins

Drug/lab test
Increased: liver function tests

NURSING CONSIDERATIONS
Assessment
• Assess cardiac glycoside level if use with a HMG-CoA
• Assess for signs of vit A, D, K deficiency
• **Hypercholesterolemia:** monitor fasting LDL, HDL, total cholesterol, triglyceride levels baseline and q4wk after initiation of treatment and periodically, electrolytes if on extended therapy; monitor blood glucose, A1c
• Monitor bowel pattern daily; increase bulk, water in diet for constipation
• **Diabetes:** Assess for hypoglycemia (weakness, hunger, dizziness, diaphoresis), can result from use of this product

Patient problem
Constipation (adverse reactions)
Nonadherence (teaching)

Implementation
• Give product daily, bid with meals; give all other medications 4 hr before colesevelam to avoid poor absorption; take with liquid
• Give supplemental doses of vit A, D, K if levels are low
Granules for oral susp
• Empty contents of packet into a cup/glass; add ½-1 cup (4-8 oz) of water, fruit juice, or diet soda; stir well before drinking

Patient/family education
• To take with meal and fluids
• Teach the importance of compliance; toxicity may result if doses missed, timing of dose 4 hr after other meds
• **Hypercholesterolemia:** Teach that risk factors should be decreased: high-fat diet, smoking, alcohol consumption, absence of exercise
• **Diabetes:** Advise patient to continue to monitor glucose, that this product does not cure diabetes but helps control symptoms, to use emergency ID and sugar source
• Advise patient to discuss all Rx, OTC, herbs, supplements with health care professional, to

use oral contraceptives at least 4 hr before this product
• **Pregnancy/breastfeeding:** Identify if pregnancy is planned or suspected or if breastfeeding, insulin may be used in diabetes during pregnancy; to use another form of contraception other than oral contraceptives

Evaluation
Positive therapeutic outcome
• Decreased cholesterol level (hyperlipidemia); diarrhea, pruritus (excess bile acids)

conivaptan (Rx)
(kon-ih-vap′tan)
Vaprisol
Func. class.: Vasopressin receptor antagonist

ACTION: Dual arginine vasopressin (AVP) antagonist with affinity for V_{1A}, V_2 receptors; level of AVP in circulating blood is critical for regulation of water, electrolyte balance and is usually elevated in euvolemic/hypervolemic hyponatremia

Therapeutic outcome: Correct serum sodium levels

USES: Euvolemia hyponatremia in those hospitalized, not indicated for HF, hypervolemia, hyponatremia

Pharmacokinetics
Absorption	Complete
Distribution	Protein binding 99%
Metabolism	By CYP3A4
Excretion	Feces (85%)
Half-life	5 hr

Pharmacodynamics
Onset	Unknown
Peak	½ hr
Duration	Infusion's end

CONTRAINDICATIONS
Hypersensitivity, hypovolemia

Precautions: Pregnancy, breastfeeding, orthostatic/renal disease, heart failure, rapid correction of serum sodium

DOSAGE AND ROUTES
Adult: IV INF loading dose 20 mg given over 30 min, then CONT **IV** over 24 hr; after 1 day, give for an additional 1-3 days as a CONT INF of 20 mg/day total, can be titrated up to 40 mg/day if serum sodium is not rising at the desired rate; max time 4 days

Hepatic/renal dose
Adult: IV Child-Pugh A-C or CCr 30-60 ml/min: Give IV loading dose over 10 min, then cont IV INF 10 mg over 24 hr × 2-4 days

Available forms: Injection (premixed) 0.2 mg/ml in 100 ml D_5W

ADVERSE EFFECTS
CNS: Headache, confusion, insomnia
CV: Hypo/hypertension, orthostatic hypotension, phlebitis
GI: Nausea, vomiting, constipation, dry mouth, diarrhea
GU: Polyuria, infertility (women)
INTEG: Erythema, inj site reaction
META: Dehydration, hypomagnesia, hyponatremia
MISC: Oral candidiasis

INTERACTIONS
Drug classifications
CYP3A4 substrates (alfuzosin, ARIPiprazole, bexarotene, bortezomib, bosentan, bupivacaine, buprenorphine, carBAMazepine, cevimeline, cilostazol, cinacalcet, clopidogrel, colchicine, cyclobenzaprine, dapsone, darifenacin, disopyramide, DOCEtaxel, donepezil, DOXOrubicin, dutasteride, eletriptan, eplerenone, ergots, erlotinib, eszopiclone, ethinyl estradiol, ethosuximide, etoposide, fentaNYL, galantamine, gefitinib, halofantrine, ifosfamide, irinotecan, levobupivacaine, levomethadyl, lidocaine, loperamide, loratadine, mefloquine, methadone, modafinil, PACLitaxel, pimozide, praziquantel, quiNIDine, quiNINE, ramelteon, reboxetine, repaglinide, rifabutin, sibutramine, sildenafil, sirolimus, SUFentanil, SUNItinib, tacrolimus, tamoxifen, teniposide, testosterone, tiaGABine, tinidazole, trimetrexate, vardenafil, vinca alkaloids, ziprasidone, zolpidem, zonisamide): increased effects, do not use concurrently

NURSING CONSIDERATIONS
Assessment
• Monitor renal/hepatic function
• Assess neurologic status: confusion, headache; monitor serum sodium levels of 2-3 hr until stable
• Assess CV status: hyper/hypotension, orthostatic hypotension; monitor B/P, pulse baseline and often if severe decrease in B/P, pulse product should be discontinued
• Monitor other electrolytes (magnesium and potassium)

• Assess for injection site reactions: redness, inflammation, pain; if these occur product may need to be discontinued

Patient problem
Risk for injury (uses)
Lack of knowledge of medication (teaching)

Implementation

Intermittent IV infusion
• Premixed do not need dilution (0.2 mg/mL) give over 30 min; in large vein, change site q24hr to minimize vascular irritation
Continuous IV infusion route
• Premixed do not need dilution (0.2 mg/mL) give over 24 hr; 20 mg or 40 mg over 24 hr

Patient/family education
• Advise patient to report neurologic changes: headache, insomnia, confusion
• Teach patient administration procedure and expected result
• Advise patient to report inj site pain, redness, swelling

Evaluation
Positive therapeutic outcome
• Correction of serum sodium levels

CONTRACEPTIVES, HORMONAL

MONOPHASIC, ORAL
ethinyl estradiol/ desogestrel (Rx)
Apri-28, Desogen, Emoquette, Enkyce, Isibroom, Kalliga, Reclipsen, Solia
ethinyl estradiol/ drospirenone (Rx)
Beyaz, Gianvil Loryna, Nikki, Ocella, Yasmin, Safyral, Syeda, Vestura, Yaz 28, Yaela, Zarah
ethinyl estradiol/ ethynodiol (Rx)
Kelnor, Zovia 1/35, Zovia 1/50
ethinyl estradiol/ levonorgestrel (Rx)
Aviane-28, Altavera, Aubra Chateal, Falmina, Kuruelo, Lessina, Levora, Lutera, Marlissa, Sronyx, Vienva

ethinyl estradiol/ norethindrone (Rx)
Alyacen 1/35, Brevicon, Briellin, Cyclafem 1/35, Dasetta 1/35, Femcon Fe, Femhrt, Generess Fe, Junel 1/20, Junel 21 1.5/20, Larin 1/20, Larin Fe 1.5/30, Loestrin 21 1.5/30, Loestrin 21 1/20, 1/35E, Norinyl 1+35, Norlestrin 1/50, Norlestrin 2.5/50, Nortrel 1/35, Nortrel 7/7/7
ethinyl estradiol/ norgestimate (Rx)
Estrayella, Mono-Linyah, MonoNessa, Ortho-Cyclen, Previfem, Sprintec
ethinyl estradiol/norgestrel (Rx)
Cryselle, Elinest, Lo/Ovral, Low-Ogestrel, Ogestrel
mestranol/norethindrone (Rx)
Genora 1/50, Nelova 1/50m, Norethin 1/50m, Necon 1/50, Norinyl 1+50, Ortho-Novum 1/50

BIPHASIC, ORAL
ethinyl estradiol/ norethindrone (Rx)
Nelova 10/11, Ortho-Novum 10/11

TRIPHASIC, ORAL
ethinyl estradiol/ desogestrel (Rx)
Azurette, Bekyree, Kariva, Kimidess, Pimtrea, Viorele
ethinyl estradiol/ norethindrone (Rx)
Necor 7/7/7, Nortrel 7/7/7, Ortho-Novum 7/7/7, Tri-Norinyl
ethinyl estradiol/ norgestimate (Rx)
Ortho Tri-Cyclen, Tri-E Starylla, Tri-Linyah, Ortho Tri-Cyclen Lo
ethinyl estradiol/ levonorgestrel (Rx)
Enpresse, Levonest, Myzilra, Tri-Levlen, Triphasil
fourphasic, oral estradiol valerate/dienogest
Natazia

FOURPHASIC, ORAL
estradiol valorate/dienoget
Natazia

EXTENDED CYCLE, ORAL
ethinyl estradiol/
levonorgestrel (Rx)
Seasonale

PROGESTIN, ORAL
norethindrone (Rx)
Errin, Jencycla, Ortho Micronor,
Camila, Jolivette, Nor-Q D, Nora-BE

PROGRESSIVE ESTROGEN, ORAL
ethinyl estradiol/
norethindrone acetate (Rx)
Estrostep, Estrostep Fe

EMERGENCY
levonorgestrel (Rx)
Plan B, Fallback Solo
ulipristal
Ella, Logilia
medroxyPROGESTERone
(Rx)
Depo-Provera, Depo-Subq Provera 104

INTRAUTERINE
levonorgestrel (Rx)
Mirena, Skyla

IMPLANT
etonogestrel (Rx)
Implanon, Nexplanon

VAGINAL RING
ethinyl estradiol/
etonogestrel (Rx)
Nuva Ring

TRANSDERMAL
ethinyl estradiol/
norelgestromin (Rx)
Yulane

ACTION: Prevents ovulation by contraceptives suppressing FSH, LH; *monophasic:* estrogen/progestin (fixed dose) used during a 21-day cycle; ovulation is inhibited by suppression of FSH and LH; thickness of cervical mucus and endometrial lining prevents pregnancy; *biphasic:* ovulation is inhibited by suppression of FSH and LH; alteration of cervical mucus, endometrial lining prevents pregnancy; *triphasic:* ovulation is inhibited by suppression of FSH and LH; change of cervical mucus, endometrial lining prevents pregnancy; variable doses of estrogen/progestin combinations may be similar to natural hormonal fluctuations; *extended cycle:* estrogen/progestin continuous for 84 days, off for 7 days, result 4 menstrual periods/yr; *progressive estrogen:* constant progestin with 3 progressive doses of estrogen; *progestin-only pill, implant, intrauterine:* change of cervical mucus and endometrial lining prevents pregnancy; ovulation may be suppressed

Therapeutic outcome: Prevention of pregnancy, decreased severity of endometriosis, hypermenorrhea

USES: To prevent pregnancy, regulation of menstrual cycle, treatment of acne in women >14 yr that other treatment has failed, emergency contraception; *injection:* inhibits gonadotropin secretion, ovulation, follicular maturation; *emergency:* inhibits ovulation and fertilization, decreases transport of sperm and egg from fallopian tube to uterus; *vaginal ring, transdermal:* inhibits ovulation, prevents sperm entry into uterus; *antiacne:* may decrease sex hormone binding globulin, results in decreased testosterone

Pharmacokinetics

Absorption	Unknown
Distribution	Unknown
Metabolism	Unknown
Excretion	Breast milk
Half-life	Unknown

Pharmacodynamics

Onset	1 mo
Peak	1 mo
Duration	Varies

CONTRAINDICATIONS
Pregnancy, breastfeeding, women 40 yr and over, reproductive cancer, thrombophlebitis, MI, hepatic tumors, hepatic disease, CAD, CVA, breast cancer, jaundice, stroke, vaginal bleeding

Precautions: Depression, hypertension, renal disease, seizure disorders, lupus erythematosus, rheumatic disease, migraine headache, amenorrhea, irregular menses, gallbladder disease, diabetes mellitus, heavy smoking, acute mononucleosis, sickle cell disease

BLACK BOX WARNING: Tobacco smoking

DOSAGE AND ROUTES
Monophasic
Adult: PO take first tab on Sunday after start of menses × 21 days; skip 7 days; then repeat cycle; start on 1st day of menses × 21 days; skip

7 days, then repeat cycle; may contain 7 placebo tabs, where 1 tab is taken daily

Biphasic
Adult: PO Take 10 days of small progestin, then large progestin; estrogen is the same during cycle; skip 7 days, then repeat cycle; may contain 7 placebo tabs, where 1 tab is taken daily

Triphasic
Adult: PO estrogen dose remains constant, progestin changes throughout 21 day cycle, some products contain 28 tabs per month

Extended cycle
Adult: PO start taking on first day of menses; continue for 84 days of active tab, then 7 days of placebo; repeat cycle

Progestin
Adult: PO start on 1st day of menses, then daily and continuously

Progressive estrogen
Adult: PO progestin dose remains constant, estrogen increases q7days throughout 21-day cycle, may include 7 placebo tabs for 28-day cycle

Emergency
Adult and adolescent: Give within 72 hr of intercourse, repeat 12 hr later; Plan B 1 tab, then 1 tab 12 hr later; Preven 2 tab, then 2 tab 12 hr later; Ovral 2 white tabs; Lo/Ovral 4 white tabs; Levlen, Nordette 4 orange tabs; Triphasil, Tri-Levlen 4 yellow tabs; ulipristal 1 tab as soon as possible within 120 hr

Injectable
Adult: IM (Depo-Provera) 150 mg within 5 days of start of menses, or within 5 days postpartum (must not be breastfeeding); if breastfeeding, give 6 wk postpartum, repeat q3mo

Intrauterine
Adult: To be inserted using the levonorgestrel-releasing intrauterine system (LRIS) by those trained in procedure; inserted into uterine cavity within 7 days of the onset of menstruation; use should not exceed 5 years per implant

Vaginal ring
Adult: VAG insert 1 ring on or prior to day 5 of cycle, leave in place 3 wk; remove for 1 wk, then repeat

Transdermal
Adult: Transdermal apply patch within 7 days of menses, change weekly × 3 wk; no patch wk 4, repeat cycle

Implant
Adult: Subdermal in inner side of upper arm on days 1-5 of menses, replace q3yr

Acne
Adult: PO (Ortho Tri-Cyclen) take daily × 21 days, off 7 days

ADVERSE EFFECTS
CNS: Depression, fatigue, dizziness, nervousness, anxiety, headache
CV: Increased B/P, cerebral hemorrhage, thrombosis, pulmonary embolism, fluid retention, edema, MI
EENT: Optic neuritis, retinal thrombosis, cataracts
ENDO: Decreased glucose tolerance, increased TBG, PBI, T_4, T_3, temporary infertility
GI: *Nausea,* vomiting, cramps, diarrhea, bloating, constipation, change in appetite, cholestatic jaundice, weight change
GU: Breakthrough bleeding, amenorrhea, spotting, dysmenorrhea, galactorrhea, endocervical hyperplasia, vaginitis, cystitis-like syndrome, breast change
HEMA: Increased fibrinogen, clotting factor
INTEG: *Chloasma, melasma,* acne, rash, urticaria, erythema, pruritus, hirsutism, alopecia, photosensitivity

INTERACTIONS
Individual drugs
Griseofulvin, rifAMPin: decreased effectiveness of oral contraceptive

Drug classifications
Analgesics, antibiotics, anticonvulsants, antihistamines: decreased action of oral contraceptives
Anticoagulants (oral): decreased action of oral anticoagulants

Drug/herb
Black cohosh: altered action
Saw palmetto, St. John's wort: decreased oral contraceptive effect

Drug/food
Grapefruit juice: increased peak level

Drug/lab test
Increased: pro-time; clotting factors VII, VIII, IX, X; TBG, PBI, T_4, platelet aggregation, BSP, triglycerides, bilirubin, AST, ALT
Decreased: T_3, antithrombin III, folate, metyraPONE test, GTT, 17-OHCS

NURSING CONSIDERATIONS
Assessment
• Assess for reproductive changes: change in breasts, tumors, positive Pap smear; product should be discontinued if changes occur
• Monitor glucose, thyroid function, liver function tests, B/P
• **Pregnancy/breastfeeding:** Do not use in pregnancy, breastfeeding

Patient problems
Risk for injury (adverse reactions)
Nonadherence (teaching)

Implementation
PO route
• If GI symptoms occur, medication may be taken with food; take at same time each day
Implant route
• Inject 6 cap subdermally
• Implant is effective for 5 yr, should be removed after that
IM route
• Administer inj deep in large muscle mass after shaking susp well; ensure pregnancy has not occurred if inj are 2 wk or more apart

Patient/family education
• Teach patient about detection of venous thrombosis; teach monitoring technique for heat, redness, pain, swelling
• Teach patient to use sunscreen or to avoid sunlight; photosensitivity can occur
• Teach patient to take at same time each day to ensure equal product level; to take another tab as soon as possible if one is missed
• Teach patient that after product is discontinued, pregnancy may not occur for several mo
• Instruct patient to report GI symptoms that occur after 4 mo
• Advise patient to use another birth control method during first 3 wk of oral contraceptive use, many antibiotics interfere with oral contraceptive effect
• Teach patient to report abdominal pain, change in vision, shortness of breath, change in menstrual flow, spotting, breakthrough bleeding, breast lumps, swelling, headache, severe leg pain, mental changes; that continuing medical care is needed: Pap smear and gynecologic exam q6mo

BLACK BOX WARNING: Teach patient not to smoke, increased risk of CV side effects

• Teach patient to notify physicians and dentist of oral contraceptive use

Evaluation
Positive therapeutic outcome
• Absence of pregnancy
• Decreased severity of endometriosis
• Decreased severity of hypermenorrhea

⚠ HIGH ALERT

copanlisib
(koh-pan′-lih-sib)
Aliqopa
Func. class.: Antineoplastic biologic response modifiers
Chem. class.: Tyrosine kinase inhibitor

ACTION: Inhibits tyrosine kinase created in patients with non-Hodgkin's lymphoma, induces tumor cell death by apoptosis and by inhibiting the proliferation of primary malignant B-cell lines

USES: For the treatment of non-Hodgkin's lymphoma (NHL)

Pharmacokinetics

Distribution	Protein binding 84.2%
Metabolism	Avoid use with strong CYP3A inhibitors or inducers, this product is a substrate of the P-glycoprotein (P-gp) and breast cancer resistance protein (BCRP) transporters and a multidrug and toxin extrusion member 2 (MATE2)-K inhibitor

CONTRAINDICATIONS
Pregnancy, hypersensitivity

Precautions: Breastfeeding, contraception requirements, children, diabetes mellitus, diarrhea, geriatric patients, hepatic/pulmonary disease, hyperglycemia, hypertension, infertility, male-mediated teratogenicity, neutropenia, pneumonitis, bone marrow suppression, infection, reproductive risk, serious rash, thrombocytopenia

DOSAGE AND ROUTES
Follicular lymphoma
Adult: **IV** 60 mg over 1 hr on days 1, 8, and 15 repeated q28days until disease progression

Dosage adjustment for related toxicities
Infection:
Grade 3 or higher toxicity: Hold until the infection resolves; *suspected* **Pneumocystis jiroveci** *pneumonia (PJP) infection (any grade):* Hold, if PJP diagnosis is confirmed, treat the infection until resolution and then resume product at the previous dose. PJP prophylaxis is recommended for the duration of therapy
Hyperglycemia:
Predose fasting blood glucose of 160 mg/dl or higher or a random/nonfasting blood glucose of 200 mg/dl or higher: Hold until the fasting glucose is 160 mg/dl or less or a random/nonfasting blood glucose is 200 mg/dl or less; *pre- or postdose blood glucose of 500 mg/dl or higher (first occurrence):* Hold until fasting glucose is 160 mg/dl or less or a random/nonfasting blood glucose is 200 mg/dl or less; resume product at 45 mg; *pre- or postdose blood glucose of 500 mg/dl or higher (subsequent occurrences):* Hold product until fasting glucose is 160 mg/dl or less or a random/nonfasting blood glucose is 200 mg/dl or

less; resume at 30 mg. Discontinue if hyperglycemia persists at the 30-mg dose

Hypertension:

Predose systolic B/P of 150 mm Hg or higher or predose diastolic B/P of 90 mm Hg or higher: Hold until B/P is less than 150/90 mm Hg based on two consecutive measurements (taken at least 15 min apart); *postdose B/P of 150/90 mm Hg or higher (nonlife threatening):* Continue product at the previous dose if antihypertensive treatment is not required. Consider a dose reduction (from 60 mg to 45 mg or from 45 mg to 30 mg) if antihypertensive treatment is required. Discontinue if hypertension persists despite antihypertensive treatment; *post-dose B/P (life threatening):* Discontinue

Noninfectious pneumonitis;

grade 2 toxicity: Hold and treat with systemic corticosteroids. Resume at 45 mg when the toxicity recovers to grade 1 or less. Discontinue if grade 2 toxicity recurs; *grade 3 or higher toxicity:* Discontinue

Neutropenia:

Absolute neutrophil count (ANC) of 0.5 to 1 × 10³ cells/mm³: Continue at the previous dose and monitor the ANC at least weekly; *ANC of less than 0.5 × 10³ cells/mm³:* Hold, monitor the ANC at least weekly until the ANC is 0.5 × 10³ cells/mm³ or greater; resume at the previous dose. Reduce to 45 mg if an ANC of 0.5 × 10³ cells/mm³ or less recurs

Thrombocytopenia:

Platelet count less than 25 × 10⁹ cells/L: Hold, resume at a reduced dose (from 60 mg to 45 mg or from 45 mg to 30 mg) if the platelet count recovers to 75 × 10⁹ cells/L or greater within 21 days. Discontinue if the platelet count does not recover to 75 × 10⁹ cells/L within 21 days

Severe cutaneous reactions:

Grade 3 toxicity: Hold until the toxicity resolves. Resume at a reduced dose (from 60 mg to 45 mg or from 45 mg to 30 mg); *life-threatening (grade 4) toxicity:* Discontinue

Other severe and non-life-threatening toxicities:

Grade 3 toxicity: Hold until the toxicity resolves, resume at a reduced dose (from 60 mg to 45 mg or from 45 mg to 30 mg); *grade 4 or life-threatening toxicity:* Discontinue

Available forms: Powder for injection 60 mg

ADVERSE EFFECTS

CNS: Fatigue

GI: Nausea, vomiting, diarrhea, stomatitis

HEMA: *Anemia,* neutropenia, thrombocytopenia, bleeding, lymphopenia

INTEG: Rash, exfoliative dermatitis

ENDO: Hyperglycemia, hypophosphatemia

MISC: Hypertriglyceridemia, hyperuricemia

INTERACTIONS

CYP3A4 inhibitors (ketoconazole, itraconazole, erythromycin, clarithromycin), P-gp inhibitors: Increased copanlisib concentrations

Increased plasma concentrations of simvastatin, calcium channel blockers, ergots

CYP3A4 inducers (dexamethasone, phenytoin, carBAMazepine, rifampin, PHENobarbital), antacids, proton pump inhibitors: Decreased copanlisib concentrations

Drug/food

Increased copanlisib effect—grapefruit juice; avoid use while taking product

Drug/herb

Decreased copanlisib concentration—St. John's wort

Drug/lab test

Increased uric acid, blood glucose, triglycerides

Decreased phosphate

NURSING CONSIDERATIONS

Assessment

• **Serious infection:** Some may be fatal. Monitor patient for signs and symptoms of infection; hold therapy for grade 3 or higher infection. Serious *Pneumocystis jiroveci* pneumonia (PJP) has occurred; consider PJP prophylaxis in at-risk patients before starting treatment, hold if PJP is suspected. If PJP diagnosis is confirmed, treat the infection until resolution and then resume at the previous dose and give PJP prophylaxis for the duration of therapy

• **Myelosuppression:** Anemia, thrombocytopenia, neutropenia; obtain a CBC at least weekly during treatment

• **Pregnancy/breastfeeding:** Product can cause fetal harm, females of reproductive potential should avoid becoming pregnant while taking this product; malformations may occur; do not breastfeed during and for at least 1 mo after the last dose; men with female partners of reproductive potential should avoid fathering a child and use effective contraception during and for at least 1 mo after therapy

• **Severe hyperglycemia:** Elevated HbA1c and infusion-related hyperglycemia have occurred; monitor blood glucose levels before and after the infusion, product interruption, dose reduction, or discontinuation may be needed for hyperglycemia. Blood glucose levels typically peak at 5 to 8 hr postinfusion and then decline to baseline levels in most patients. Use with caution in diabetes mellitus. Initiate product

---

⚠ Nurse Alert   ✷ Key NCLEX® Drug   ≫ Drug Specifics

after these patients have achieved optimal blood glucose control; monitor blood glucose levels in these patients closely
• **Severe hypertension and infusion-related hypertension:** Use with caution in those with preexisting hypertension; monitor B/P before and after the infusion; optimal B/P control should be achieved before each dose. Therapy interruption, dose reduction, or therapy discontinuation may be necessary in patients who develop hypertension. A mean increase in systolic (+16.8 mm Hg) and diastolic (+7.8 mm Hg) B/P was observed at 2 hr postinfusion on day 1 of cycle 1; B/P may remain elevated for 6-8 hr after the start of the infusion

Evaluation
Positive therapeutic outcome
• Improving blood counts

Patient problems
Risk for injury (adverse reactions)

Implementation
IV route
• Visually inspect for particulate matter and discoloration before use
Reconstitution:
• Add 4.4 ml of sterile 0.9% NaCl injection to the 60-mg lyophilized powder vial (15/ml)
• Gently shake and then allow to stand for 1 min letting the bubbles rise to the surface; repeat if needed, solution will be colorless to slightly yellowish
• Storage of reconstituted vial: If not diluted immediately, store refrigerated at 2 to 8° C (36 to 46° F) for up to 24 hr before use; protect from direct sunlight
Dilution
• Into an infusion bag containing 100 ml of sterile 0.9% sodium chloride injection, add the appropriate volume (based on the desired dose) from the reconstituted vial as follows: **60-mg dose:** 4 ml; **45-mg dose:** 3 ml; **30-mg dose:** 2 ml
• Invert the infusion bag to mix
• Discard any unused contents from the reconstituted vial
• *Storage of diluted admixture:* If not used immediately, store refrigerated at 2 to 8° degrees C (36 to 46° F) for up to 24 hr (from vial reconstitution) before use; protect from direct sunlight

Intermittent IV Infusion
• Allow the diluted admixture in the infusion bag to warm to room temperature (if stored in refrigerator) before use
• Give over 1 hr
• Do not mix or inject product with other drugs or diluents
• Follow cytotoxic handling procedures

Patient/family education
• Teach patient to report adverse reactions immediately, bleeding; report diarrhea, hepatic, hematologic symptoms/toxicity, flulike symptoms
• Teach patient about reason for treatment, expected results
• **Pregnancy/breastfeeding:** Teach patient to notify provider if pregnancy is planned or suspected, to use effective contraception during treatment and up to 30 days after discontinuing treatment, not to use during pregnancy, breastfeeding; men with female partners of reproductive potential should be cautioned to avoid fathering a child and use effective contraception during and for at least 1 mo after therapy

cotrimoxazole
See trimethoprim/sulfamethoxazole

crisaborole
(kris' a-bor-ole)
Eucrisa
Func. class.: Dermatologic agent
Chem. class.: Phosphodiesterase 4 inhibitor

ACTION: Increases intracellular cAMP levels in the skin

Therapeutic outcome: Decreasing redness, itching, inflammation

USES: Mild to moderate atopic dermatitis

Pharmacokinetics
Absorption	Unknown
Distribution	Unknown
Metabolism	Unknown
Excretion	Unknown
Half-life	Unknown

Pharmacodynamics
Onset	Unknown
Peak	Unknown
Duration	Unknown

CONTRAINDICATIONS: Hypersensitivity

PRECAUTIONS: Children, pregnancy, breastfeeding

DOSAGE AND ROUTES
Adult/child ≥2 yr: Apply ointment in a thin film to cover area bid

Available forms: Topical ointment 2%
ADVERSE EFFECTS
Integ: Burning, stinging

INTERACTIONS
None known

NURSING CONSIDERATIONS
Assessment
- **Contact dermatitis**: For redness, itching, inflammation; assess if these symptoms are relieved after application
- **Hypersensitivity**: For pruritus, inflammation, rash; if present, product should be discontinued
- **Pregnancy/breastfeeding**: No adverse reactions in animal studies, no human studies are available; consider benefits to mother and infant if breastfeeding, product is systemically absorbed

Patient problems
Impaired skin integrity (uses)

Implementation
Topical route:
- For external use only, store at room temperature
- Tube should be tightly closed
- Apply only to affected areas

Patient/family education
- **Contact dermatitis**: Identify if the symptoms are relieved after application; apply a thin film and wash hands after use; use externally only
- **Hypersensitivity**: Report immediately itching, inflammation, rash; if present, product should be discontinued
- **Pregnancy/breastfeeding**: If pregnant or planning to get pregnant, or if breastfeeding, advise prescriber; effects are unknown

Evaluation
Therapeutic response
- Decreasing redness, itching, inflammation

⚠ HIGH ALERT

crizotinib
(kriz-oh′ti-nib)
XALKORI
Func. class.: Antineoplastic
Chem. class.: Kinase inhibitors

ACTION: An inhibitor of ⟡ receptor tyrosine kinases (anaplastic lymphoma kinase (ALK), hepatocyte growth factor receptor (HGFR, c-Met), recepteur d'origine nantais (RON).

Therapeutic outcome: Decreased spread of malignancy

USES: ⟡ Locally advanced or metastatic non–small-cell lung cancer (NSCLC) that is anaplastic lymphoma kinase (ALK)-positive as detected by an FDA-approved test

Pharmacokinetics
Absorption	43%
Distribution	Steady state 15 days, protein binding 91%, distribution tissue, plasma
Metabolism	By 3YPA4/5, oxidation to metabolites
Excretion	63% feces, unchanged 53%; 22% urine, unchanged 2, 3%
Half-life	42 hr

Pharmacodynamics
Onset	Unknown
Peak	4-6 hr
Duration	Unknown

CONTRAINDICATIONS
Pregnancy, breastfeeding, hypersensitivity, concurrent use of strong CYP3A4 inducers/inhibitors

Precautions: Pneumonitis, severe hepatic disease, congenital long QT syndrome, neonates, infants, children, adolescents, severe renal impairment, end-stage renal disease, vision disorders ⟡, Asian patients

DOSAGE AND ROUTES
Adult: PO 250 mg bid; continue as long as is beneficial

Available forms: Caps 200, 250 mg

ADVERSE EFFECTS
CNS: Dizziness, peripheral neuropathy headache, insomnia
CV: QT prolongation, disseminated intravascular coagulation (DIC), septic shock, bradycardia, chest pain
EENT: *Diplopia, blurred vision, reduced visual acuity*
GI: *Nausea, diarrhea, vomiting, constipation,* decreased appetite, dysgeusia, abdominal pain, abdominal discomfort/pain, stomatitis, hepatotoxicity
HEMA: Grade 3/4 neutropenia, thrombocytopenia, lymphopenia
MISC: Fever, *edema*, chest pain
RESP: Severe, life-threatening pneumonitis, dyspnea, cough

INTERACTIONS
Individual drugs
Abarelix, alfuzosin, amoxapine, apomorphine, arsenic trioxide, asenapine, chloroquine, ciprofloxacin, citalopram, clarithromycin,

---

cloZAPine, cyclobenzaprine, dasatinib, dolasetron, dronedarone, droperidol, eriBULin, erythromycin, ezogabine, flecainide, fluconazole, gatifloxacin, gemifloxacin, grepafloxacin, halofantrine, haloperidol, iloperidone, indacaterol, lapatinib, levofloxacin, levomethadyl, lopinavir/ritonavir, magnesium sulfate, maprotiline, mefloquine, methadone, moxifloxacin, nilotinib, norfloxacin, octreotide, ofloxacin, OLANZapine, ondansetron, paliperidone, palonosetron, pentamidine, certain phenothiazines (chlorproMAZINE, mesoridazine, thioridazine, fluPHENAZine, perphenazine, prochlorperazine, trifluoperazine), pimozide, posaconazole, potassium sulfate, probucol, propafenone, QUEtiapine, quiNIDine, ranolazine, rilpivirine, risperiDONE, saquinavir, sodium, sparfloxacin, SUNItinib, tacrolimus, telavancin, **telithromycin**, tetrabenazine, troleandomycin, vardenafil, **vemurafenib**, venlafaxine, vorinostat, ziprasidone: increased QT prolongation, torsades de pointes, avoid using together

Midazolam: increased midazolam action

Drug classifications

CYP2B6 substrates (prasugrel, selegiline, cyclophosphamide): increased action of these products

β-agonists, Class IA antiarrhythmics (disopyramide, procainamide, quiNIDine), Class III antiarrhythmics (amiodarone, dofetilide, ibutilide, sotalol), halogenated anesthetics, local anesthetics, tricyclic antidepressants: increased QT prolongation, torsades de pointes, avoid using together

CYP3A4 inhibitors (ketoconazole, atazanavir, indinavir, itraconazole, nefazodone, nelfinavir, ritonavir, voriconazole, boceprevir, delavirdine, isoniazid, dalfopristin-quinupristin, tipranavir): increased crizotinib, avoid using together

CYP3A4 inducers (rifAMPin, carBAMazepine, PHENobarbital, phenytoin, rifabutin); antacids, H2-blockers, proton pump inhibitors (PPIs): decreased crizotinib, avoid using together

CYP3A4 substrates (alfentanil, cycloSPORINE, ergotamine, dihydroergotamine fentaNYL, sirolimus, colchicine): avoid concurrent use

Drug/herb

Do not use with St. John's wort

Drug/food

Do not use with grapefruit juice, or grapefruit

NURSING CONSIDERATIONS
Assessment

• **Severe, life-threatening, or fatal treatment-related pneumonitis:** All cases occurred within 2 months of treatment

initiation; assess for dyspnea, cough, fever permanently discontinue in pneumonitis

• **Hepatic disease:** Monitor liver function test (LFT) abnormalities, altered bilirubin levels, may occur during treatment; monitor LFTs and bilirubin levels prior to treatment, then monthly; more frequent testing is needed in those presenting with grade 2 or greater toxicities; Laboratory alterations should be managed with dose reduction, treatment interruption, or discontinuation

• **QT prolongation:** Monitor ECG and electrolytes in those with HF, bradycardia, electrolyte imbalance (hypokalemia, hypomagnesemia), or in those who are taking concomitant medications known to prolong the QT interval; treatment interruption, dosage adjustment, or treatment discontinuation may be needed in those who develop QT prolongation

For Grade 3 QTc prolongation: Interrupt treatment until toxicity resolves to grade ≤1; when resuming treatment, reduce dosage to 200 mg PO bid; in case of recurrence, interrupt treatment until toxicity resolves to grade ≤1 and when resuming treatment, reduce dosage to 250 mg PO daily; permanently discontinue in case of further recurrence

For Grade 4 QTc prolongation: Permanently discontinue

• **Vision disorders:** Generally started within 2 weeks of the start of therapy; ophthalmologic evaluation should be considered, particularly if patients experience photopsia or new/ increased vitreous floaters; caution should be used when driving or operating machinery by patients who experience vision disorders

• CBC with differential; Baseline and monthly, hematologic toxicity

Patient problem

Impaired gas exchange (uses)
Risk for injury (adverse reactions)

Implementation

• May be taken orally with or without food
• Have the patient swallow capsule whole; do not crush or chew
• If a dose is missed, it can be taken up to 6 hr before the next dose is due to maintain the twice daily regimen. Do not take both doses at the same time
• Store capsules at room temperature

Patient/family education

• Advise patient to discuss with health care professional use of OTC, Rx, herbs, supplements
• Missed doses can be taken up to 6 hr before the next dose is due to maintain the twice daily

regimen, to take as prescribed not to double or skip doses
• **Pregnancy/breastfeeding:** Identify if pregnancy is planned or suspected, do not use in pregnancy, avoid breastfeeding
• Teach patient to use reliable contraception; both women and men of childbearing age should use adequate contraceptive methods during therapy and for at least 90 days after completing treatment; pregnancy
• Teach patient to report immediately shortness of breath, cough, fatigue, visual changes
• Teach patient not to take with grapefruit juice
• Teach patient to avoid activities requiring mental alertness until effects are known, blurred vision and other vision problems occur
• Teach patient to report signs of QT prolongation (abnormal heartbeats, dizziness, syncope)
• Teach patient to report immediately nausea; vomiting; abdominal pain; yellowing of skin, eyes; dark urine; itching
• Teach patient to swallow caps whole and avoid contact with broken cap; not to use with grapefruit/grapefruit juice; avoid St. John's wort

Evaluation
Positive therapeutic outcome
• Decreased spread of malignancy

cyclobenzaprine (Rx)
(sye-kloe-ben′za-preen)
Amrix
Func. class.: Skeletal muscle relaxant, central acting
Chem. class.: Tricyclic amine salt

ACTION: Reduction of tonic muscle activity at the brain stem; may be related to antidepressant effects

Therapeutic outcome: Relaxation of skeletal muscle

USES: Adjunct for relief of muscle spasm and pain in musculoskeletal conditions

Unlabeled uses: Fibromyalgia

Pharmacokinetics

Distribution	Widely
Metabolism	Liver, partially
Excretion	Kidney (unchanged)
Half-life	1-3 days, 32 hr ext rel

Pharmacodynamics

Onset	1 hr
Peak	3-8 hr
Duration	12-24 hr

CONTRAINDICATIONS
Acute recovery phase of MI, dysrhythmias, heart block, HF, hypersensitivity, intermittent porphyria, thyroid disease, within 14 days of MAOIs

Precautions: Pregnancy, breastfeeding, geriatric, renal/hepatic disease, addictive personality, CV disease, child <15 yr

DOSAGE AND ROUTES
Musculoskeletal disorders
Adult/adolescent ≥15 yr: PO 5 mg tid × 1 wk, max 30 mg/day × 3 wk
Adult: EXT REL 15 mg q day, max 30 mg q day × 3 wk
Geriatric: PO 5 mg tid

Hepatic dose
Adult (mild hepatic disease): PO 5 mg, titrate slowly

Fibromyalgia (unlabeled)
Adult: PO 10 mg at bedtime, titrated up

Available forms: Tabs 5, 7.5, 10 mg; ext rel tab 15, 30 mg

ADVERSE EFFECTS
CNS: *Dizziness, weakness, drowsiness,* headache, insomnia, confusion, nervousness, fatigue
CV: Postural hypotension, dysrhythmias
EENT: Diplopia, dry mouth, blurred vision
GI: *Nausea,* dry mouth, constipation
GU: Urinary retention
INTEG: Rash

INTERACTIONS
Individual drugs
Alcohol: increased CNS depression
Bupropion, TraMADol: increased serotonin syndrome

Drug classifications
Antidepressants (tricyclic), barbiturates, opiates, sedative/hypnotics: increased CNS depression
MAOIs: do not use within 14 days
SSRIs, SNRIs, tricyclics, triptans, increased serotonin syndrome

Drug/herb
Kava, chamomile, hops, valerian: increased CNS depression

NURSING CONSIDERATIONS
Assessment
- **Serotonin syndrome:** if using with SSRIs, SNRIs, monitor closely; if syndrome occurs, discontinue both products immediately assess for hallucinations, nausea, vomiting, diarrhea, tachycardia, hyperthermia
- Assess pain periodically: location, duration, mobility, stiffness, baseline
- **Beers:** Avoid use in older adults, anticholinergic effects

Patient problems
Pain (uses)
Impaired mobility (uses)

Implementation
- Give without regard to meals, give with food for GI symptoms
- Store in airtight container at room temperature
- Extended release capsules should be swallowed whole; do not break, chew, crush; may open and sprinkle on food

Patient/family education
- Teach patient not to discontinue medication quickly; insomnia, nausea, headache, spasticity, tachycardia will occur; product should be tapered off over 1-2 wk
- Caution patient not to take with alcohol, other CNS depressants or MAOIs
- Advise to avoid altering activities while taking this product
- Caution patient to avoid hazardous activities if drowsiness/dizziness occurs
- Caution patient to avoid using OTC medication: cough preparations, antihistamines, unless directed by prescriber
- Inform patient to report feeling of fullness of bladder, inability to void adequate amounts
- Teach patient to use fluids, bulk in diet to prevent constipation
- Teach patient to use gum, frequent sips of water for dry mouth
- Teach patient to notify prescriber of serotonin syndrome

Evaluation
Positive therapeutic outcome
- Decreased pain, spasticity; muscle spasms of acute, painful musculoskeletal conditions are generally short term; long-term therapy is seldom warranted

TREATMENT OF OVERDOSE:
Gastric lavage, then use anticonvulsants if indicated; monitor cardiac function

cyclopentolate ophthalmic
See Appendix B

⚠ HIGH ALERT

cyclophosphamide (Rx)
(sye-kloe-foss'fa-mide)
Procytox ✦
Func. class.: Antineoplastic alkylating agent
Chem. class.: Nitrogen mustard

Do not confuse: cyclophosphamide/cycloSPORINE

ACTION: Alkylates DNA; responsible for cross-linking DNA strands; activity is not cell cycle phase specific

Therapeutic outcome: Prevention of rapidly growing malignant cells

USES: Hodgkin's disease, lymphomas, leukemia, multiple myeloma, neuroblastoma, retinoblastoma, Ewing's sarcoma, cancer of female reproductive tract, breast, nephrotic syndrome

Pharmacokinetics

Absorption	Well absorbed
Distribution	Widely distributed; crosses placenta, blood-brain barrier (50%)
Metabolism	Liver to active product
Excretion	Kidneys, unchanged (30%)
Half-life	4-6½ hr

Pharmacodynamics (blood count action)

Onset	1 wk
Peak	1-2 wk
Duration	3 wk

CONTRAINDICATIONS
Pregnancy, hypersensitivity, prostatic hypertrophy, bladder neck obstruction

Precautions: Radiation therapy, cardiac disease, anemia, dysrhythmias, child, dental disease/work, dialysis, geriatrics, heart failure, hematuria, infections, leukopenia QT prolongation, secondary malignancy surgery, tumor lysis syndrome, vaccinations, breastfeeding, severely depressed bone marrow function

DOSAGE AND ROUTES
Acute lymphocytic leukemia (ALL)
Adult/adolescent/child: IV 300-1500 mg/m² have been used with induction, intensification, and consolidation regimens that may include prediSONE, vinCRIStine and others; PO 1-5 mg/kg/day adjusted to response

---

Neuroblastoma
Adult/child: **IV** For induction, 40-50 mg/kg in divided doses over 2-5 days or 10-15 mg/kg q7-10 days, 3-5 mg/kg 2 times/wk or 1-5 mg/kg daily
Child and infant: PO 150 mg/m^2/day, days 1-7 with DOXOrubicin (**IV** 35 mg/m^2 on day 5) q21days × 5 cycles
Child: **IV** 70 mg/kg/day with hydration on days 1 and 2 with DOXOrubicin and vinCRIStine q21days for courses 1, 2, 4, 6, alternating with CISplatin and etoposide q21days for courses 3, 5, 7

Breast cancer
Adult: PO 100-200 mg/m^2/day or 2 mg/kg/day × 4-14 days; **IV** 500-1000 mg/m^2 on day 1 in combination with fluorouracil and methotrexate or DOXOrubicin, or DOXOrubicin alone; also cyclophosphamide 600 mg/m^2, may be given dose-dense on day 1 of q14day with DOXOrubicin (60 mg/m^2) with growth factor support

Operable node-positive breast cancer
IV (TAC regimen) Adult: 500 mg/m^2 with DOXOrubicin (50 mg/m^2 **IV**) then DOCEtaxel (75 mg/m^2) **IV** given 1 hr later × 6 cycles q3wk

Available forms: Powder for Inj **IV** ❦, 500 mg, 1, 2 g/vials; capsules 25, 50 mg

ADVERSE EFFECTS
CV: Cardiotoxicity (high doses), myocardial fibrosis, hypotension
ENDO: Syndrome of inappropriate antidiuretic hormone (SIADH), gonadal suppression
GI: *Nausea, weight loss,* anorexia
GU: Hemorrhagic cystitis, hematuria
HEMA: Thrombocytopenia, leukopenia, myelosuppression
INTEG: *Alopecia,* dermatitis
META: Hyperuricemia
MISC: Secondary neoplasms
RESP: Pulmonary fibrosis, interstitial pneumonia

INTERACTIONS
Individual drugs
Allopurinol: increased bone marrow suppression
Digoxin: decreased digoxin levels
Succinylcholine: increased neuromuscular blockade
Warfarin: increased warfarin action

Drug classifications
Other antineoplastics, radiation diuretics (thiazides): increased bone marrow suppression
Live virus vaccines: decreased antibody reaction

Drug/herb
St. John's wort: increased toxicity
Drug/lab test
Increased: uric acid
False positive: Pap smear
False negative: PPD, mumps trichophytin, *Candida, Trichophyton,* Pap smear

NURSING CONSIDERATIONS
Assessment
• **Bone marrow suppression:** Monitor CBC, differential, platelet count baseline and weekly; withhold product if WBC count is <2500/mm^3 or platelet count is <75,000/mm^3; notify prescriber of results avoid vein punctures, rectal temperatures
• Infection: Monitor temperature, flu-like symptms
• **Assess for hemorrhagic cystitis:** renal function studies including BUN, creatinine, serum uric acid, urine CCr before, during therapy; I&O ratio; report fall in urine output to <30 ml/hr, monitor
• **Hepatotoxicity:** Monitor liver function tests before, during therapy (bilirubin, AST, ALT, LDH) as needed or monthly; note jaundice of skin or sclera, dark urine, clay-colored stools, itchy skin, abdominal pain, fever, diarrhea
• **Beers:** Avoid in older adults, delirium, dementia may occur; avoid in men due to decreased urine flow, retention
• **Assess for bleeding:** hematuria, stool guaiac, bruising or petechiae, mucosa or orifices q8hr
• **Pulmonary fibrosis/interstitial pneumonia:** Identify dyspnea, crackles, unproductive cough, chest pain, tachypnea
• Identify effects of alopecia on body image; discuss feelings about body changes

Patient problems
Risk for infection (adverse reactions)
Risk for injury (adverse reactions)

Implementation
• Give fluids **IV** or PO before chemotherapy to hydrate patient
• Give antacid before oral agent, after PM meals, before bedtime; antiemetic 30-60 min before giving product to prevent vomiting and prn; antibiotics for prophylaxis of infection
• Give top or syst analgesics for pain; give in AM so product can be eliminated before bedtime
• Use cytotoxic handling procedures
PO route
• To be taken on empty stomach; do not crush, break, chew capsule, wash hands immediately if in contact with capsule
• Take in AM

Direct IV
- Reconstitute with NS only, 100 mg/5 mL, swirl, inject slowly
- Store in tight container at room temperature

Intermittent IV infusion route
- Use cytotoxic handling procedures
- Give **IV** after diluting 100 mg/5 ml of 0.9% NaCl or sterile or water, shake, let stand until clear; may be further diluted in up to 250 ml D$_5$ 0.9% NaCl, 0.45% NaCl, (2 mg/mL) give 100 mg or less/min
- Use 21-, 23-, or 25-G needle; check site for irritation, phlebitis

Y-site compatibilities: Amifostine, amikacin, ampicillin, azlocillin, aztreonam, bleomycin, cefamandole, ceFAZolin, cefepime, cefoperazone, cefotaxime, cefOXitin, cefuroxime, cephalothin, cephapirin, chloramphenicol, chlorproMAZINE, cimetidine, CISplatin, cladribine, clindamycin, dexamethasone, diphenhydrAMINE, DOXOrubicin, doxycycline, droperidol, erythromycin, famotidine, filgrastim, fludarabine, fluorouracil, furosemide, gallium, ganciclovir, gentamicin, granisetron, heparin, HYDROmorphone, IDArubicin, kanamycin, leucovorin, LORazepam, melphalan, methotrexate, methylPREDNISolone, metoclopramide, metroNIDAZOLE, mezlocillin, minocycline, mitoMYcin, moxalactam, nafcillin, ondansetron, oxacillin, PACLitaxel, penicillin G potassium, piperacillin, piperacillin/tazobactam, prochlorperazine, promethazine, propofol, raNITIdine, sargramostim, sodium bicarbonate, teniposide, tetracycline, thiotepa, ticarcillin, ticarcillin-clavulanate, tobramycin, trimethoprim-sulfamethoxazole, vancomycin, vinBLAStine, vinCRIStine, vinorelbine

Patient/family education
- Teach patient to avoid use of products containing aspirin or ibuprofen, razors, commercial mouthwash, since bleeding may occur; to report symptoms of bleeding (hematuria, tarry stools, bruising)
- Instruct patient to report signs of anemia (fatigue, headache, irritability, faintness, shortness of breath)
- Teach patient to report any changes in breathing or coughing even several months after treatment
- Advise patient that hair may be lost during treatment; a wig or hairpiece may make patient feel better; new hair may be different in color, texture, skin, fingernails may become darker
- Advise patient on proper handling and disposal of chemotherapy drugs

- Teach patient not to have any vaccinations without the advice of the prescriber; serious reactions can occur
- **Pregnancy/breastfeeding:** Advise patient contraception is needed during treatment and for several months (men use condoms); 1 yr (women) after the completion of therapy
- Teach patient to take adequate fluids to eliminate product

Evaluation
Positive therapeutic outcome
- Prevention of rapid division of malignant cells
- Increased appetite, increased weight

cycloSPORINE (Rx)
(sye-kloe-spor'een)
SandIMMUNE, Gengraf, Neoral
Func. class.: Immunosuppressant (antirheumatic, DMARD)
Chem. class.: Fungus-derived peptide

Do not confuse: cycloSPORINE/CycloSERINE/cyclophosphamide, **SandIMMUNE**/SandoSTATIN

ACTION: Produces immunosuppression by inhibiting T lymphocytes

Therapeutic outcome: Absence of transplant rejection

USES: Organ transplants (liver, kidney, heart, GVHD) to prevent rejection, rheumatoid arthritis, psoriasis

Unlabeled uses: Recalcitrant ulcerative colitis, aplastic anemia, Crohn's disease, thrombocytopenia purpura, lupus, nephritis, myasthenia gravis, psoriatic arthritis

Pharmacokinetics

Absorption	Poorly absorbed (PO)
Distribution	Crosses placenta, enters breast milk, protein binding 98%
Metabolism	Liver extensively to mercaptopurine by CYP3A4
Excretion	Kidney, minimal
Half-life	25 hr

Pharmacodynamics

	PO	IV
Onset	Unknown	Unknown
Peak	2-6 hr	Infusion's end
Duration	Unknown	

CONTRAINDICATIONS

Hypersensitivity to polyoxyethylated castor oil (inj only), psoriasis or rheumatoid arthritis in renal disease (Neoral/Gengraf), Gengraf/Neoral used with PUVA/UVB; methotrexate, coal tar, breastfeeding, ocular infections

> **BLACK BOX WARNING:** Neoplastic disease, sunlight (UV) exposure, renal disease/failure, uncontrolled, malignant hypertension; radiation in psoriasis

Precautions: Pregnancy, geriatric, severe renal/hepatic disease

> **BLACK BOX WARNING:** Immunosuppression, requires a specialized care setting and experienced clinician, nephrotoxicity, infection, new primary malignancy (lymphoma, skin cancer)

DOSAGE AND ROUTES/NTI

Prevention of transplant rejection (unmodified) (Sandimmune)

Adult and child: PO 15 mg/kg 4-12 hr before surgery, daily for 2 wk, reduce dosage by 2.5 mg/kg/wk to 5-10 mg/kg/day; **IV** 5-6 mg/kg 4-12 hr before surgery, daily, switch to PO form as soon as possible

Prevention of transplant rejection (modified) (Neoral)

Adult and child: PO 4-12 mg/kg/day divided q12hr, depends on organ transplanted

Rheumatoid arthritis (Neoral/Gengraf)

Adult: PO 2.5 mg/kg/day divided bid, may increase 0.5-0.75 mg/kg/day after 8-12 wk, max 4 mg/kg/day

Psoriasis (Neoral/Gengraf)

Adult: PO 2.5 mg/kg/day divided bid × 4 wk, then increase by 0.5 mg/kg/day q2wk, max 4 mg/kg/day

Autoimmune diseases (Neoral)

Adult/child: PO 1-3 mg/kg/day

Available forms: Oral sol (Gendraf, Neoral) 100 mg/ml; soft gel cap 25, 50, 100 mg; inj 50 mg/ml

ADVERSE EFFECTS

CNS: *Tremors, headache,* seizures, paresthesia, confusion, progressive multifocal leukoencephalopathy, encephalopathy

GI: Nausea, vomiting, diarrhea, *oral candida, gum hyperplasia,* hepatotoxicity, pancreatitis

GU: Nephrotoxicity

INTEG: Rash, acne, *hirsutism,* pruritus

META: Hyperkalemia, hypomagnesemia, hyperlipidemia, hyperuricemia

MISC: *Infection,* gingival hyperphasia, hypersensitivity, malignancy

INTERACTIONS

Individual drugs

Allopurinol, amiodarone, amphotericin B, bromocriptine, carvedilol, cimetidine, colchicine, foscarnet, imipenem-cilastatin, melphalan, metoclopramide: increased action, cycloSPORINE toxicity

Aminoglycosides, ciprofloxacin, NSAIDs, fibric acid derivatives, vancomycin, melphalan, ketoconazole; increased renal impairment

Digoxin: increased digoxin level

Etoposide: increased etoposide level

Methotrexate: increased methotrexate level

Nafcillin, orlistat, PHENobarbital, phenytoin, terbinafine, ticlopidine, trimethoprim/sulfamethoxazole: decreased cycloSPORINE action

Sirolimus: increased sirolimus level, toxicity

Tacrolimus: increased tacrolimus level, toxicity

Drug classifications:

Androgens, antifungals (azole), β-blockers, calcium channel blockers, contraceptives (oral), corticosteroids, fluoroquinolones, macrolides, NSAIDs, selective serotonin reuptake inhibitors: increased cycloSPORINE levels, toxicity

Anticonvulsants, rifamycins: decreased cycloSPORINE levels

HMG-CoA reductase inhibitors, diuretics (potassium-sparing): increased effects of each product, toxicity

Live virus vaccines: decreased antibody reaction

Potassium-sparing diuretics, potassium supplements, ACE inhibitors: increase renal dysfunction

Drug/food

Grapefruit juice, food: increased slowed metabolism of product

Drug/herb

• Possible decreased effect of cyclosporine: St. John's wort

• Decreased immunosuppression: echinacea, melatonin

NURSING CONSIDERATIONS

Assessment

• **Posterior reversible, encephalopathy:** Assess for impaired cognition, seizures, vision changes including blindness, loss of motor function, movement disorders, psychiatric changes; dosage reduction or discontinuation may be needed in severe cases

• **Progressive multifocal leukoencephalopathy (PML):** Assess for apathy, confusion, cognitive changes, may be fatal, withhold dose, notify prescriber immediately

- **Nephrotoxicity:** monitor renal studies: BUN, creatinine at least monthly during treatment, 3 mo after treatment, nephrotoxicity increases with increasing doses and duration of treatment
- Monitor liver function studies: alkaline phosphatase, AST, ALT, bilirubin
- Monitor product blood levels during treatment (Therapeutic range: 100-400 mg/ml)

> **BLACK BOX WARNING: Assess for hepatotoxicity:** dark urine, jaundice, itching, light-colored stools; product should be discontinued

Psoriasis: Assess lesions baseline and during treatment
RA: Assess pain, ROM, ADLs baseline and during treatment

Patient problems
Risk for infection (adverse reactions)
Immunologic impairment (uses)

Implementation
PO route
- Some brands are not interchangeable
- Do not break, crush, or chew caps
- Use pipette provided to draw up oral sol; may mix with milk or juice, wipe pipette, do not wash (Neoral)
- Give for several days before transplant surgery with corticosteroids
- Microemulsion products (Neoral) and other products are not interchangeable
- Give with meals for GI upset or place product in chocolate milk (SandIMMUNE)

Intermittent IV infusion route
- Give **IV** after diluting each 50 mg/20-100 ml of 0.9% NaCl or D_5W (2.5 mg/mL); run over 2-6 hr; use an inf pump

Continuous IV infusion route
- May run over 24 hr
- **For SandIMMUNE parenteral:** give 1/3 of PO dose, initial dose 4-12 hr prior to transplantation as a single **IV** dose 5-6 mg/kg/day, continue the single daily dose until PO can be used

Y-site compatibilities: Abciximab, alatrofloxacin, alfentanil, amikacin, aminocaproic acid, aminophylline, amphotericin B lipid complex, anidulafungin, argatroban, ascorbic acid injection, atenolol, atracurium, atropine, azaTHIOprine, aztreonam, benztropine, bivalirudin, bleomycin, bretylium, bumetanide, buprenorphine, butorphanol, calcium chloride/gluconate, CARBOplatin, carmustine, caspofungin, ceFAZolin, cefmetazole, cefonicid, cefotaxime, cefoTEtan, cefOXitin, cefTAZidime, ceftizoxime, cefTRIAXone, cefuroxime, chloramphenicol,

chlorproMAZINE, cimetidine, ciprofloxacin, CISplatin, clindamycin, codeine, cyanocobalamin, cyclophosphamide, cytarabine, DACTINomycin, DAPTOmycin, DAUNOrubicin, dexamethasone, dexmedetomidine, digoxin, dilTIAZem, diphenhydrAMINE, DOBUTamine, DOCEtaxel, DOPamine, doripenem, doxacurium, DOXOrubicin, doxycycline, enalaprilat, ePHEDrine, EPINEPHrine, epiRUBicin, epoetin alfa, eptifibatide, ertapenem, erythromycin, esmolol, etoposide, famotidine, fenoldopam, fentaNYL, fluconazole, fludarabine, fluorouracil, folic acid, furosemide, gallium, ganciclovir, gatifloxacin, gemcitabine, gentamicin, glycopyrrolate, granisetron, heparin, hydrocortisone, HYDROmorphone, hydrOXYzine, ifosfamide, imipenem-cilastatin, indomethacin, irinotecan, isoproterenol, ketorolac, labetalol, lansoprazole, levofloxacin, lidocaine, linezolid, LORazepam, mannitol, mechlorethamine, meperidine, meropenem, methotrexate, methyldopa, methylPREDNISolone, metoclopramide, metoprolol, metroNIDAZOLE, micafungin, miconazole, midazolam, milrinone, minocycline, mitoXANtrone, morphine, multiple vitamins injection, nafcillin, naloxone, nesiritide, netilmicin, nitroglycerin, nitroprusside, norepinephrine, octreotide, ondansetron, oxacillin, oxaliplatin, oxytocin, PACLitaxel, palonosetron, pamidronate, pancuronium, pantoprazole, papaverine, PEMEtrexed, penicillin G potassium/sodium, pentamidine, pentazocine, phentolamine, phenylephrine, phytonadione, piperacillin, piperacillin-tazobactam, polymyxin B, potassium acetate/chloride, procainamide, prochlorperazine, promethazine, propofol, propranolol, protamine, pyridoxine, quiNIDine, quinupristin-dalfopristin, raNITIdine, ritodrine, sargramostim, sodium acetate/bicarbonate, succinylcholine, SUFentanil, tacrolimus, teniposide, theophylline, thiamine, thiotepa, ticarcillin, ticarcillin-clavulanate, tigecycline, tirofiban, tobramycin, trimetaphan, urokinase, vancomycin, vasopressin, vecuronium, verapamil, vinCRIStine, vinorelbine, zoledronic acid

Patient/family education
- Advise patient to report fever, rash, severe diarrhea, chills, sore throat, fatigue, since serious infections may occur; also to report clay-colored stools, cramping (may indicate hepatotoxicity); tremors, bleeding gums, increased B/P

> **BLACK BOX WARNING:** Advise patient to limit UV exposure

- Caution patient to avoid crowds and persons with known infections to reduce risk of infection

• Teach patient to take at the same time of day, every day; do not skip or double a missed dose; not to use with grapefruit juice or receive vaccines; there are many drug interactions, do not add or discontinue products without prescriber approval
• Teach patient that treatment is lifelong to prevent rejection; to identify signs of rejection
• Advise patient to report severe diarrhea as drug loss may result in rejection

> **BLACK BOX WARNING:** Nephrotoxicity: Teach patient to notify prescriber of increased B/P, tremors of the hands, change in gums, increased hair on body/face

• Advise patient to continue with lab work and follow-up appointment
• Teach patient types of products are not interchangeable
• Teach patient not to wash syringe/container with water; a variation in dose may result
• Teach patient to notify prescriber of all medications, herbal, supplements that are taken
• **Pregnancy/breastfeeding:** Caution patient to use contraceptive measures during treatment and for 12 wk after ending therapy; product is teratogenic, to notify prescriber if pregnancy is planned or suspected

Evaluation
Positive therapeutic outcome
• Absence of graft rejection, decreased pain in rheumatoid arthritis, decreased lesions in psoriasis

---

⚠ HIGH ALERT

cytarabine (Rx)
(sye-tare′a-been)
Cytosar ✚
cytarabine liposomal (Rx)
Depo Cyt
Func. class.: Antineoplastic, antimetabolite
Chem. class.: Pyrimidine nucleoside

Do not confuse: Cytosar ✚/Cytovene/Cytoxan

ACTION: Competes with physiologic substrate of DNA synthesis, thus interfering with cell replication in the S phase of the cell cycle (before mitosis)

Therapeutic outcome: Prevention of rapidly growing malignant cells

USES: Acute myelocytic leukemia, acute lymphocytic leukemia, chronic myelocytic leukemia, lymphomatous meningitis (IT/intraventricular)

Absorption	Complete (IV)
Distribution	Widely distributed; crosses blood-brain barrier, placenta
Metabolism	Liver, extensively
Excretion	Kidneys (<10%)
Half-life	IV/subcut 1-3 hr; IT 100-236 hr

Pharmacodynamics

	IV/Subcut	IT
Onset	24 hr	Unknown
Peak	7-10 days	5 hr
Duration	12 days	2-4 wk

CONTRAINDICATIONS
Pregnancy, hypersensitivity

Precautions: Renal/hepatic disease, breastfeeding, children, tumor lysis syndrome, infection, hyperkalemia, hyperphosphatemia, hyperuricemia, hypocalcemia

> **BLACK BOX WARNING: Bone marrow suppression,** arachnoiditis, abdominal pain, chemotherapy-induced nausea/vomiting, diarrhea, hepatotoxicity, stomatitis, requires a specialized care setting and experienced clinician

DOSAGE AND ROUTES
Acute myelogenous leukemia (AML)
Regimens vary
Adult: cont IV infusion 100 mg/m²/day × 7 days q2wk as a single agent or 2-3 divided doses × 5-10 days until remission used in combination; maintenance 70-200 mg/m²/day × 2-5 days qmo; **SUBCUT** maintenance 100 mg/m²/day × 5 days q28days
Adult/child: IV For induction, 40-50 mg/kg in divided doses over 2-5 days or 10-15 mg/kg q7-10 days, 3-5 mg/kg 2 times/wk or 1-5 mg/kg daily

Meningeal leukemia
Adult and child: Intrathecal For induction 50 mg (liposomal) q14 days × 2 doses (wk 1, 3); consolidation 50 mg (liposomal) q14 days × 3 doses (wk 5, 7, 9) then another dose at wk 13; maintenance 50 mg (liposomal) q28 days (wks 17, 21, 25, 29)

Carcinomatous meningitis (liposoma)
Adult: Intrathecal 50 mg over 1-5 min q14days, during induction and consolidation wk 1, 3, 5, 7, 9, give another 50 mg wk 13; maintenance 50 mg q28days on wk 17, 21, 25, 29 use with dexamethasone 4 mg PO/IV × 5 days on each day of cytarabine

---

Renal dose
Adult CCr ≤60 ml/min, serum creatinine 1.5-1.9 mg/dl or increase of 0.5-1.2 mg/dl from baseline: during treatment reduce to 1 g/m^2/dose; serum creatinine ≥2 mg/dl or change from baseline serum creatinine was 1.2 mg/dl reduce to 100 mg/m^2/day

Available forms: Solution for injection 20 mg/mL, 100 mg/mL; liposomal intrathecal injection 10 mg/mL

ADVERSE EFFECTS
CNS: Neuritis, dizziness, headache, confusion, drowsiness, cerebellar syndrome, personality changes, ataxia, mechanical dysphasia, coma; chemical arachnoiditis (IT), fever
CV: Chest pain, cardiopathy, edema
EENT: Sore throat, conjunctivitis, visual changes
GI: *Nausea, vomiting, anorexia, diarrhea, stomatitis,* hepatotoxicity, abdominal pain, GI ulceration (high doses)
GU: Urinary retention, renal failure, hyperuricemia
HEMA: Thrombophlebitis, bleeding, thrombocytopenia, leukopenia, myelosuppression, anemia
INTEG: *Rash*
META: Hyperuricemia
MISC: Cytarabine syndrome—fever, myalgia, bone pain, chest pain, rash, conjunctivitis, malaise (6-12 hr after administration)
RESP: Dyspnea, pulmonary edema **(high doses)**
SYST: Anaphylaxis, tumor lysis syndrome

INTERACTIONS
Individual drugs
Cyclophosphamide: increase cardiomyopathy (high doses)
Digoxin oral: decreased digoxin effects
Filgrastim, G-CSF, GM-CSF, sargramostim: do not use within 24 hr
Gentamicin: decreased effects
Radiation: increased toxicity, bone marrow suppression

Drug classifications
Anticoagulants, NSAIDs, platelet inhibitors, salicylates, thrombolytics: increased bleeding risk
Immunosuppressants, antineoplastics: increased toxicity, bone marrow suppression
Live virus vaccines: do not use together

NURSING CONSIDERATIONS
Assessment

> **BLACK BOX WARNING: Stomatitis:** Assess buccal cavity q8hr for dryness, sores or ulceration, white patches, pain, bleeding, dysphagia; obtain prescription for viscous lidocaine (Xylocaine)

• **Assess symptoms indicating anaphylaxis:** rash, pruritus, urticaria, purpuric skin lesions, itching, flushing; resuscitation equipment should be nearby

> **BLACK BOX WARNING: Assess for chemical arachnoiditis (IT):** headache, nausea, vomiting, fever; neck rigidity/pain, meningism, CSF pleocytosis; may be decreased by dexamethasone

• Assess tachypnea, dyspnea, edema, fatigue; identify dyspnea, crackles, unproductive cough, chest pain, tachypnea; pulmonary edema may be fatal (rare)
• **Assess for cytarabine syndrome 6-12 hr after infusion:** fever, myalgia, bone pain, chest pain, rash, conjunctivitis, malaise; corticosteroid may be ordered

> **BLACK BOX WARNING: Bone marrow suppression:** Monitor CBC (RBC, Hct, Hgb), differential, platelet count weekly; withhold product if WBC count is <1000/mm^3 or platelet count is <50,000/mm^3 or if RBC, Hct, Hgb are low; notify prescriber of results

• Assess for increased uric acid levels, swelling, joint pain primarily in extremities; patient should be well hydrated to prevent urate deposits
• Monitor renal function studies: BUN, creatinine, serum uric acid, urine CCr before and during therapy; I&O ratio; report fall in urine output to <30 ml/hr

> **BLACK BOX WARNING: Hepatotoxicity:** Monitor liver function tests before and during therapy (bilirubin, AST, ALT, LDH) as needed or monthly; note yellowing of skin or sclera, dark urine, clay-colored stools, pruritus, abdominal pain, fever, diarrhea; an antispasmodic may be used for GI symptoms

• **Assess for bleeding:** hematuria, stool guaiac, bruising or petechiae, mucosa or orifices q8hr; identify inflammation of mucosa, breaks in skin

Patient problems
Risk for infection (adverse reactions)
Risk for injury (adverse reactions)

Implementation

- Avoid contact with skin; very irritating; wash completely to remove
- Give fluids **IV** or PO before chemotherapy to hydrate patient
- Give antiemetic 30-60 min before giving product to prevent vomiting, and prn; antibiotics for prophylaxis of infection
- Increase fluids to 3 L/day
- Give in AM so product can be eliminated before bedtime
- Use cytotoxic handling precautions

Intrathecal route

- **Liposomal: withdraw** product immediately before use; **use** within 4 hr, do not save unused portions or use in-line filter; **give** directly into CSF by intraventricular reservoir or by direct inj into lumbar site
- **Give** slowly over 1-5 min; follow with lumbar puncture; instruct patient to lie flat; **give** dexamethasone 4 mg bid PO or **IV** × 5 days beginning on day of liposomal inj

Direct IV route

- Give undiluted (100 mg/mL) **give** over 1-3 min through a free-flowing IV

Intermittent IV infusion route

- May be diluted in 50-100 ml NS or D$_5$W and **give** over 30 min-24 hr, depending on dose

Continuous IV infusion route

- May be given as continuous IV infusion

Y-site compatibilities: Acyclovir, alfentanil, amifostine, amikacin, aminocaproic acid, aminophylline, amphotericin B lipid complex, amphotericin B liposome, ampicillin, ampicillin-sulbactam, amsacrine, anidulafungin, atenolol, atracurium, azithromycin, aztreonam, bivalirudin, bleomycin, bumetanide, buprenorphine, butorphanol, calcium chloride/gluconate, CARBOplatin, ceFAZolin, cefepime, cefotaxime, cefoTEtan, cefOXitin, cefTAZidime, ceftizoxime, cefTRIAXone, cefuroxime, chlorproMAZINE, cimetidine, ciprofloxacin, cisatracurium, CISplatin, cladribine, clindamycin, codeine, cyclophosphamide, cycloSPORINE, DAUNOrubicin, dexamethasone, dexmedetomidine, dexrazoxane, digoxin, dilTIAZem, diphenhydrAMINE, DOBUTamine, DOCEtaxel, dolasetron, DOPamine, doxacurium, DOXOrubicin, DOXOrubicin liposomal, doxycycline, droperidol, enalaprilat, ePHEDrine, EPINEPHrine, ertapenem, erythromycin, esmolol, etoposide, famotidine, fenoldopam, fentaNYL, filgrastim, fluconazole, fludarabine, foscarnet, fosphenytoin, furosemide, gatifloxacin, gemcitabine, gemtuzumab, gentamicin, granisetron, haloperidol, heparin, hydrocortisone, HYDROmorphone, hydrOXYzine, IDArubicin, ifosfamide, imipenem-cilastatin, inamrinone, insulin (regular), irinotecan, isoproterenol, ketorolac, labetalol, leucovorin, levofloxacin, levorphanol, lidocaine, linezolid, LORazepam, magnesium sulfate, mannitol, melphalan, meperidine, meropenem, mesna, methohexital, methotrexate, methylPREDNISolone, metoclopramide, metoprolol, metroNIDAZOLE, midazolam, milrinone, minocycline, mitoXANtrone, mivacurium, morphine, nalbuphine, naloxone, nesiritide, niCARdipine, nitroglycerin, nitroprusside, norepinephrine, octreotide, ofloxacin, ondansetron, oxaliplatin, PACLitaxel, palonosetron, pamidronate, pancuronium, pantoprazole, PEMEtrexed, pentamidine, PENTobarbital, PHENobarbital, phenylephrine, piperacillin, piperacillin-tazobactam, potassium chloride/phosphates, procainamide, prochlorperazine, promethazine, propofol, propranolol, quinupristin-dalfopristin, raNITIdine, rapacuronium, remifentanil, riTUXimab, rocuronium, sargramostim, sodium acetate/bicarbonate/phosphates, succinylcholine, SUFentanil, sulfamethoxazole-trimethoprim, tacrolimus, teniposide, theophylline, thiopental, thiotepa, ticarcillin, ticarcillin-clavulanate, tigecycline, tirofiban, TNA, tobramycin, trastuzumab, trimethobenzamide, vancomycin, vasopressin, vecuronium, verapamil, vinCRIStine, vinorelbine, voriconazole, zidovudine, zoledronic acid

Patient/family education

- Teach patient to avoid use of products containing aspirin or ibuprofen, NSAIDs, razors, commercial mouthwash, since bleeding may occur; to report symptoms of bleeding (hematuria, tarry stools)
- Advise that fever, headache, nausea, vomiting are likely to occur but to continue using dexamethasone with IT administration
- Provide liquid diet: carbonated beverages; gelatin may be added if patient is not nauseated or vomiting
- Provide rinsing of mouth tid-qid with water, club soda; brushing of teeth bid-qid with soft brush or cotton-tipped applicators for stomatitis; use unwaxed dental floss
- Advise patient to report signs of anemia (fatigue, headache, irritability, faintness, shortness of breath)
- **Stomatitis:** Advise patient to avoid foods with citric acid, hot flavor, or rough texture if stomatitis is present, to use sponge brush and rinse with water after each meal; to report stomatitis: any bleeding, white spots, ulcerations in mouth; tell patient to examine mouth daily, report any symptoms

• Instruct patient to report any changes in breathing or coughing even several months after treatment; to avoid crowds and persons with respiratory tract or other infections
• Caution patient not to have any vaccinations without the advice of the prescriber; serious reactions can occur
• Advise patient to take 3 L/day fluids to prevent renal damage

• **Pregnancy/breastfeeding:** Advise patient that contraceptive measures are recommended during and 4 mo after therapy, do not use in pregnancy, breastfeeding

Evaluation
Positive therapeutic outcome
• Decrease in size, spread of tumor
• Improvement in CBC with differential, platelets, leukocytes

dabigatran (Rx)
(da-bye-gat'ran)
Pradaxa
Func. class.: Anticoagulant
Chem. Class.: Thrombin inhibitor

ACTION: Direct thrombin inhibitor that inhibits both free and clot-bound thrombin, prevents thrombin-induced platelet aggregation and thrombus formation by preventing conversion of fibrinogen to fibrin

Therapeutic outcome: Decreased thrombus formation/extension, absence of emboli, postthrombotic effects

USES: Stroke/systemic embolism prophylaxis with nonvalvular atrial fibrillation, DVT, pulmonary embolism in hip replacement

Pharmacokinetics

Absorption	7%
Distribution	Unknown
Metabolism	Unknown
Excretion	Feces 86%
Half-life	12-17 hr (extended in renal disease)

Pharmacodynamics

Onset	Unknown
Peak	1 hr; high-fat meal delays peak
Duration	Unknown

CONTRAINDICATIONS
Hypersensitivity, active bleeding, use with P-gp inducers

Precautions: Abrupt discontinuation, anticoagulant therapy, breastfeeding, pregnancy, children, geriatrics, labor, obstetric delivery, renal disease, surgery

> **BLACK BOX WARNING:** Abrupt discontinuation, epidural/spinal anesthesia, lumbar puncture

DOSAGE AND ROUTES
Stroke prophylaxis/Systemic embolism (nonvalvular atrial fibrillation)
Adult: PO 150 mg bid

Renal dose
Adult PO CCr more than 30 ml/min: No dosage adjustment; CCr 15 to 30 ml/min: 75 mg bid;

Deep vein thrombosis/pulmonary embolism
Adult: PO 150 mg bid

Renal dose
Adult PO CCr >30 ml/min: No change; CCr 30 ml/min or less: avoid use

Prevention of DVT/PE after hip replacement surgery
Adult PO 110 mg 1-4 hr after surgery, then 220 mg q d ×28-35 days

With concomitant use of P-glycoprotein (P-gp) inhibitors: CCr <50 ml/min: Avoid use

Available forms: Cap 75, 110, 150 mg

ADVERSE EFFECTS
GI: Abdominal pain, dyspepsia, peptic ulcer, esophagitis, gastritis, diarrhea
HEMA: Bleeding (any site)
SYST: Anaphylaxis (rare), angioedema

INTERACTIONS
Individual drugs
Amiodarone, clopidogrel, ketoconazole, quiNIDine, verapamil: increased bleeding risk, avoid use in those with renal disease (CCr 15-30 ml/min)
RifAMPin: decreased dabigatran effect, avoid use

Drug classifications
Anticoagulants, antiplatelets, antifibrinolytics; NSAIDs (chronic use), solicylates, thrombolytics: increased bleeding risk,
P-gp inhibitors: Dose should be reduced to 150 mg/day (75 mg bid) in those with CCr 30-50 ml/min

Drug/herb
Garlic, ginger, Ginkgo biloba: Increased bleeding risk, avoid use
St. John's wort: decreased dabigatran effect, avoid use

NURSING CONSIDERATIONS
Assessment
• **Stroke:** Assess for facial palsy, weakness, headache, blurred vision, speaking difficulty
• **DVT/PE:** Assess for pain in calf swelling or behind knee, trouble breathing, chest pain, light headedness
• **Assess for bleeding:** blood in urine or emesis, dark tarry stools, lower back pain. Caution with arterial/venous punctures, catheters, NG tubes. Monitor vital signs frequently, aPTT or ECT if needed. The elderly are more prone to serious bleeding
• **Assess for thrombosis emboli:** swelling, pain, redness, difficulty breathing, chest

pain, tachypnea, cough, coughing up blood, cyanosis

> **BLACK BOX WARNING:** Epidural/spinal anesthesia, lumbar puncture

• Teach patient risk of hematoma that may cause paralysis, indwelling epidural catheters and products that cause coagulation may increase the risk of paralysis
• **Assess for postthrombotic syndrome:** pain, heaviness, itching/tingling, swelling, varicose veins, brownish/reddish skin discoloration, ulcers; ambulation, compression stockings and adequate anticoagulation can prevent this syndrome
• Monitor renal studies baseline and during treatment

> **BLACK BOX WARNING:** Do not discontinue abruptly

Patient problem
Risk for injury (uses)

Implementation
• Before surgery, discontinue product, restart after surgery is completed
• Do not crush, break, chew, or empty contents of capsule
• Take without regard to food
• Store in original package until time of use at room temperature, discard after 30 days, protect from moisture

Patient/family education
• Explain the purpose and expected results of this product, store in original container, protect from moisture

> **BLACK BOX WARNING: Neurologic changes:** To report bladder or bowel changes, numbness in lower extremities, back pain; notify prescriber immediately

• If dose is missed take as soon as remembered if on the same day, do not administer if <6 hr before next dose, do not stop taking without discussing with prescriber; increases risk of clotting stroke
• Instruct patient to report if bleeding or bruising is present, check with prescriber about when to discontinue
• Advise patient not to use any other OTC products, herbs, supplements without prescriber approval
• Inform patient that lab tests will be required during treatment
• **Pregnancy/breastfeeding:** Advise patient to notify health care professional

if pregnancy is planned or suspected or if breastfeeding

Evaluation
Positive therapeutic outcome
• Decreased thrombus formation/extension, absence of emboli

D

dabrafenib
(da braf'e-nib)
Tafinlar
Func. class.: Antineoplastic
Chem. class.: Signal transduction inhibitor, kinase inhibitor

ACTION: Inhibits kinase, inhibitor against mutated forms of ⚠ BRAF kinases in melanoma cells

Therapeutic outcome: Decrease in melanoma progression

USES: ⚠ Unresectable or metastatic BRAD V600E-mutated malignant melanoma, or *V600K*-mutated melanoma in combination with trametinib

Pharmacokinetics

Absorption	Well
Distribution	Protein binding 99.7%
Metabolism	By CYP2C8, CYP344
Excretion	71% (feces), 23% (urine)
Half-life	8 hr (dabrafenib); 10 hr, 21-22 hr metabolites

Pharmacodynamics

Onset	Unknown
Peak	Unknown
Duration	Unknown

CONTRAINDICATIONS
Pregnancy, hypersensitivity

Precautions: Breastfeeding, children, infection, dehydration, diabetes mellitus, fever, G6PD deficiency, hemolytic anemia, hyperglycemia, hypotension, infertility, iritis, renal failure, secondary malignancy

DOSAGE AND ROUTES
Adult: PO 150 mg q12hr until disease progression, avoid strong CYP3A4/CYP2C8 inhibitors or inducers

Available forms: Caps 50, 75 mg

ADVERSE EFFECTS
EENT: Uveitis, retinal detachment
CNS: Headache, fever, fatigue
GI: Pancreatitis, constipation
CV: Cardiomyopathy, HF, thromboembolism

INTEG: Rash, alopecia
MISC: hand-foot syndrome, hyperglycemia, hypophosphatemia, hyponatremia, secondary malignancy
MS: Myalgia, arthralgia, back pain

INTERACTIONS
Drug classifications
Antacids, CYP3A4 inducers (dexamethasone, phenytoin, carBAMazepine, rifAMPin, PHENobarbital), proton-pump inhibitors: decreased dabrafenib concentrations

CYP3A4, CYP2C9 substrates: decreased effect of these products

CYP3A4 inhibitors (ketoconazole, itraconazole, erythromycin, clarithromycin): altered dabrafenib concentrations, toxicity

Drug/food
Grapefruit juice: increased dabrafenib effect; avoid use while taking product

Drug/herb
St. John's wort: decreased dabrafenib concentrations

NURSING CONSIDERATIONS
Assessment
• **Secondary malignancy:** Perform a dermatologic evaluation before therapy, q2mo while on therapy, and for up to 6 mo after discontinuing therapy
• **Serious fever and febrile reaction:** Assess for hypotension, rigors/chills, dehydration, renal failure may occur; the incidence and severity of fever are higher when given with trametinib. Interruption of therapy, a dose reduction, or permanent therapy discontinuation may be needed. Monitor for signs and symptoms of infection. If a severe fever or febrile reaction occurs, monitor renal function (BUN/serum creatinine) during and after the event and give antipyretic agents when therapy is resumed. In those who develop a febrile reaction that does not resolve within 3 days of onset, give corticosteroids (prednisone 10 mg/day PO) for at least 5 days; ensure there is no evidence of active infection before starting corticosteroids
• **Hyperglycemia:** Monitor serum glucose levels at baseline and as indicated
• **Uveitis, iritis, and iridocyclitis:** Steroid and mydriatic ophthalmic drops may provide symptomatic relief for these conditions. Monitor for visual signs and symptoms of uveitis (blurred vision, photophobia, and eye pain). Continue

at the same dose in iritis. Hold for mild or moderate uveitis that does not respond to ocular therapy, severe uveitis, or iridocyclitis; initiate treatment as indicated. Permanently discontinue in those who develop persistent grade 2 or higher uveitis that lasts longer than 6 wk
• **Bleeding:** Major intracranial bleeding/GI bleeding can occur when used in combination with trametinib. Monitor for signs of bleeding; (frank blood, blood in stools, urine, vomit) evaluate any unexplained fall in hematocrit, hypotension, grade 3 hold product, grade 4 discontinue
• **Cardiomyopathy:** A decrease in left ventricular ejection fraction (LVEF) of 10% or greater from baseline and below the lower limit of normal (LLN) may occur and was higher when given in combination with trametinib. Obtain an echocardiogram or multigated acquisition (MUGA) scan before starting combination therapy, 1 month after starting dabrafenib, and then q2-3mo during treatment. Hold dabrafenib for symptomatic congestive heart failure or LVEF below the LLN with an absolute decrease of greater than 20% from baseline. Resume dabrafenib at the same dose if LVEF improves to the institutional LLN and an absolute decrease of 10% or less from baseline
• **Palmar-plantar erythrodysesthesia syndrome (hand and foot syndrome):** May occur when given in combination with trametinib, usually within 37 days; hospitalization may be required due to a secondary infection of the skin. Interruption of therapy, a dose reduction, or permanent therapy discontinuation may be needed in those who develop severe skin toxicity

Patient problem
Risk for injury (adverse reactions)
Impaired skin integrity (adverse reactions)

Implementation
PO route
• Obtain testing for genetic evidence of BRAF V600E or K
• Swallow whole, do not open, crush, chew caps
• If dose is missed, take within 6 hr of missed dose, if >6 hr have passed, skip dose
• Space doses q12hr
• Take at least 1 hr before or 2 hr after a meal

Patient/family education
• Advise patient to notify prescriber of new lesions
• Teach patient to notify all providers of all OTC, Rx, herbal products taken

- Teach patient to take as prescribed 1 hr before or 2 hr after meals, take a missed dose within 6 hr of next dose
- Instruct patient to report adverse reactions immediately
- Teach patient about reason for treatment, expected results
- Advise patients to report symptoms of severe hyperglycemia (excessive thirst, increased urinary frequency)
- Advise patient that other malignancies are possible
- **Pregnancy:** Identify if pregnancy is planned or suspected, if breastfeeding, instruct patient to use effective nonhormonal contraception during treatment, after discontinuing treatment, do not breastfeed

Evaluation
Positive therapeutic outcome
- Decrease in melanoma progression

⚠ HIGH ALERT

dacarbazine (Rx)
(da-kar′ba-zeen)
miscellaneous agent
Chem. class.: Triazine

ACTION: Alkylates DNA, RNA; inhibits RNA, DNA synthesis; also responsible for breakage, cross-linking DNA strands; activity is not cell cycle phase specific

Therapeutic outcome: Prevention of rapidly growing malignant cells

USES: Hodgkin's disease, malignant melanoma

Pharmacokinetics

Absorption	Complete bioavailability (**IV**)
Distribution	Widely distributed; concentrates in liver
Metabolism	Liver (50%, 5% protein bound)
Excretion	Kidneys, unchanged (50%)
Half-life	5 hr

Pharmacodynamics

Unknown

CONTRAINDICATIONS
Hypersensitivity, breastfeeding

Precautions: Renal disease, infection

BLACK BOX WARNING: Pregnancy (1st trimester), radiation therapy, hepatic disease, bone marrow suppression, secondary malignancy, requires an experienced clinician

DOSAGE AND ROUTES
Metastatic malignant melanoma
Adult· IV 2 4.5 mg/kg daily × 10 days or 100-250 mg/m² daily × 5 days; repeat q3wk depending on response

Hodgkin's disease
Adult: IV 150 mg/m² daily × 5 days with other agents, repeat q4wk or 375 mg/m² on days 1 and 15 when given in combination, repeat q28day

Available forms: Powder for injection 100, 200, 500 mg vials

ADVERSE EFFECTS
GI: *Nausea, anorexia, vomiting,* hepatotoxicity
HEMA: Thrombocytopenia, leukopenia, anemia
INTEG: *Alopecia,* dermatitis, pain at inj site, photosensitivity, severe sun reactions (high doses)
MISC: Flulike symptoms, malaise, fever, myalgia, hypotension
SYST: Anaphylaxis

INTERACTIONS
Individual drugs
Carbamazepine, PHENobarbital, phenytoin: increased metabolism; decreased dacarbazine effect

Drug classifications
Antineoplastics, bone marrow–suppressing products: increased toxicity, bone marrow suppression
Live virus vaccines: increased adverse reactions; decreased antibody reaction

Drug/Lab
Increase: BUN, AST, ALT
Decrease: Platelets, WBC, RBC

NURSING CONSIDERATIONS
Assessment
- **Assess symptoms indicating severe allergic reaction:** rash, pruritus, urticaria, purpuric skin lesions, itching, flushing; product should be discontinued

BLACK BOX WARNING: Assess for bone marrow suppression: Monitor CBC, differential, platelet count weekly; withhold product if WBC is <4000/mm³ or platelet count is <75,000/mm³

- Monitor renal function tests: BUN, creatinine, urine CCr before, during therapy; I&O ratio; report fall in urine output to <30 ml/hr

• Monitor temp (may indicate beginning of infection), I&O, for nausea, appetite

BLACK BOX WARNING: Hepatotoxicity: Monitor liver function tests before, during therapy (bilirubin, AST, ALT, LDH) as needed or monthly; note jaundice of skin or sclera, dark urine, clay-colored stools, itchy skin, abdominal pain, fever, diarrhea; hepatotoxicity can be serious and fatal

• Assess for **bleeding:** hematuria, stool guaiac, bruising or petechiae, mucosa or orifices q8hr; check for inflammation of mucosa, breaks in skin

BLACK BOX WARNING: Product must be administered by those experienced in the use of cancer chemotherapy

• Assess IV site for irritation, redness, pain; if infiltration occurs use hot packs at site
• Identify effects of alopecia on body image; discuss feelings about body changes

BLACK BOX WARNING: Secondary malignancy: Assess for secondary malignancy that may occur with this product

Patient problem
Risk for infection (adverse reactions)
Risk for injury (adverse reactions)

Implementation
• Give fluids **IV** or PO before chemotherapy to hydrate patient
• Nausea/vomiting may be severe and last several hours
• Give antiemetic 30-60 min before giving product to prevent vomiting, and prn; antibiotics for prophylaxis of infection
• Clarify all orders, double-check original order, may be fatal if wrong dose is given
• Use cytotoxic handling procedures

Direct IV route
• After diluting 100 mg/9.9 ml or 200 mg/19.7 ml of sterile water for inj (10 mg/ml), give by direct **IV** over 2-3 min through Y-tube or 3-way stopcock

Intermittent IV infusion route
• May be further diluted in 50-250 ml of D₅W or normal saline for inj and given over 30-60 min
• Watch for extravasation; stop infusion, apply ice to area
• Store in light-resistant container in a dry area

Y-site compatibilities: Amifostine, aztreonam, filgrastim, fludarabine, granisetron, melphalan, ondansetron, PACLitaxel, sargramostim, teniposide, thiotepa, vinorelbine

Patient/family education
• Teach patient to avoid use of products containing aspirin or ibuprofen, razors, commercial mouthwash, since bleeding may occur; to report symptoms of bleeding (hematuria, tarry stools)
• Advise patient that hair may be lost during treatment; a wig or hairpiece may make patient feel better; new hair may be different in color, texture
• Teach patient to use sunscreen or protective clothing to prevent burns
• Caution patient not to have any vaccinations without the advice of prescriber; serious reactions can occur

BLACK BOX WARNING: Pregnancy: to notify prescriber if pregnancy is planned or suspected. Advise patient contraception is needed during treatment and for several months after the completion of therapy; product has teratogenic properties

• **Teach patient to report signs of infection:** fever, sore throat, flulike symptoms

Evaluation
Positive therapeutic outcome
• Prevention of rapid division of malignant cells

daclatasvir
(dak-lat'-as-vir)
Daklinza
Func. class.: Antiviral, antihepatitis agent
Chem. class.: NS5A inhibitor

ACTION: Active against chronic infections caused by ⋙ genotype 3 hepatitis C virus (HCV); prevents viral RNA replication by impairing protein function

Therapeutic outcome: Decreased symptoms of chronic hepatitis C

USES: Chronic hepatitis C, genotype 3 with complicated liver disease

Pharmacokinetics

Absorption	Unknown
Distribution	99% protein binding
Metabolism	Liver, by CYP3A4, affected by P-glycoprotein (P-gp), organic anion transporting polypeptides (OATP1B1 and OATP1B3), breast cancer resistance protein (BCRP)
Excretion	Feces 88%
Half-life	Half-life 12-15 hr

Pharmacodynamics

Onset	Unknown
Peak	2 hr
Duration	Unknown

CONTRAINDICATIONS
Hypersensitivity

Precautions: Pregnancy, antimicrobial resistance, hepatic disease, hepatitis C with HIV coinfection, liver transplant

DOSAGE AND ROUTES
HCV genotype 1 or 3
Adult: PO 60 mg q day × 12 wk in combination with sofosbuvir

Adults without cirrhosis or who have compensated (Child-Pugh A): PO 60 mg once daily in combination with sofosbuvir 400 mg PO once daily for 12 wk.

Adults receiving strong CYP3A inhibitors who do not have cirrhosis or who have compensated (Child-Pugh A) cirrhosis: PO 30 mg once daily in combination with sofosbuvir 400 mg PO once daily for 12 wk.

Adults receiving moderate CYP3A inducers who do not have cirrhosis or who have compensated (Child-Pugh A) cirrhosis: PO 90 mg once daily in combination with sofosbuvir 400 mg PO once daily for 12 wk.

Available forms: Tabs 30, 60, 90 mg

ADVERSE EFFECTS
CNS: Headache, fatigue
GI: Diarrhea, nausea
MISC: HBV reactivation

INTERACTIONS
Drug classifications
Do not use with potent CYP3A4 inducers

Individual drugs
Amiodarone: Increased bradycardia; use cardiac monitoring if used together
Dabigatra: Increased dabigatran level
Digoxin: Increased digoxin level
P-glycoprotein (P-gp) substrates: increase of each product
Potent CYP3A4 inhibitors: Increased daclatasvir effect, reduce dose of daclatasvir
Moderate CYP3A4 inducers. Decreased daclatasvir effect, increase dose of daclatasvir

NURSING CONSIDERATIONS
Assessment
• **Liver transplant/cirrhosis:** May have lower sustained virologic response rates in cirrhosis and use in prior liver transplant is unknown

• **HIV/ hepatitis C coinfection:** All patients with HIV infection should be tested for hepatitis C, with continued annual screening for persons considered high risk for acquiring hepatitis C. If hepatitis C and HIV coinfection is identified, treating both viral infections concurrently is used.
• **Bradycardia:** Monitor for bpm ,60, dizziness, confusion, memory problems, notify health care professional immediately
• **Strong CYP3A4 inducers:** Do not use concurrently, may lead to treatment failure, review patient's medication profile for potential drug interactions before starting treatment
• **Hepatitis C:** Monitor plasma hepatitis C RNA and plasma HIV RNA baseline and during treatment, HBsAg, and anti-HBC NS5A resistance testing in Type 1a with cirrohsis

Patient problem
Infections (uses)

Implementation
• Give by mouth without regard to food
• Do not use as monotherapy, must be given with sofosbuvir

Patient/family education
• Teach patient that optimal duration of treatment is 12 wk; that product is not a cure; that transmission may still occur and must be taken with sofosbuvir, not to skip or double doses
• Inform patient to avoid use with other medications, herbs, supplements unless approved by prescriber
• Teach patient not to stop abruptly unless directed; worsening of hepatitis may occur
• **Pregnancy/breastfeeding: Advise patient to notify prescriber if pregnancy is planned or suspected or if breastfeeding**

Evaluation
Positive therapeutic outcome
• Therapeutic response: decreased symptoms of chronic hepatitis C

dalbavancin
(dal-ba-van'sin)
Dalvance
Func. class.: Antiinfective-glycopeptide

ACTION: Binds to the bacterial cell walls, inhibiting their synthesis

USES: Treatment of acute bacterial skin and skin structure infections due to gram-positive organisms (cellulitis, major abscess, wound infections); *Staphylococcus aureaus, Streptococcus agalactiae, S. anginosus, S.pyogenes*

Pharmacokinetics

Absorption	Complete (IV)
Distribution	Protein binding 93%, primarily to albumin, tissues
Metabolism	Unknown
Excretion	Feces (13%) and urine (33%), decreased in renal disease
Half-life	8 days

Pharmacodynamics

Onset	Unknown
Peak	Infusion's end
Duration	Unknown

CONTRAINDICATIONS
Hypersensitivity

Precautions: Antimicrobial resistance, breast-feeding, colitis, diarrhea, GI disease, inflammatory bowel disease, infusion-related reactions, pregnancy, CDAD, ulcerative colitis, vancomycin hypersensitivity, viral infection

DOSAGE AND ROUTES
Adult: IV 1500 mg once or 1000 mg once, then 500 mg **IV** 1 wk later

Renal dose
Adult: IV CCr ,30 mL/min 1125 mg as a single dose or 750 mg once then 375 mg 1 week later

Available forms: Powder for injection 500 mg/vial

SIDE EFFECTS
CNS: Dizziness, headache, flushing
GI: Nausea, vomiting, CDAD, GI bleeding, abdominal pain, diarrhea
SYST: Red man syndrome, hypersensitivity reactions
INTEG: Rash, urticaria, infusion-related reactions, pruritus

INTERACTIONS
Drug classifications
None significant

Drug/lab test
Increase: LFTs, INR, alkaline phosphatase
Decrease: platelets, WBC

NURSING CONSIDERATIONS
Assessment:
• Monitor BUN/creatinine; lower dose may be required in severe renal disease
• Infection: Monitor B/P, pulse, temperature, characteristics of urine, stools, sputum, baseline and periodically

• **CDAD:** Monitor bowel pattern daily; if severe diarrhea occurs, product should be discontinued
• Assess IV site for infusion-site reactions
• Anaphylaxis: Monitor for rash, urticaria, pruritus, wheezing; may occur a few days after administration
• Red man–like syndrome: Assess for flushing, rash over upper torso and neck; may occur after a few minutes of infusion; may be treated with antihistamines and a slower infusion

Patient problems
Infection (uses)

Implementation:
IV infusion route
• Visually inspect parenteral products for particulate matter and discoloration
• Reconstitute each 500 mg/25 mL sterile water for injection; to avoid foaming, alternate between gentle swirling and inversion until completely dissolved, do not shake; further dilution is required
• **Storage:** Refrigerate or store at room temperature. Do not freeze. The total time from reconstitution to dilution to use should not exceed 48 hr
• **Dilution:** Transfer the dose of reconstituted solution from the vial(s) to an IV bag or bottle containing D5W (1-5 mg/mL) discard unused product
Intermittent IV infusion
• Give over 30 min, do not infuse with other medications or electrolytes, saline-based infusion solutions may cause precipitation and should not be used; if a common IV line is being used to administer other drugs, the line should be flushed before and after each dose

Teach patient/family:
• Teach patient to report sore throat, bruising, bleeding, joint pain (blood dyscrasias); diarrhea with mucus, blood (pseudomembranous colitis); rash, pruritus, wheezing (hypersensitivity reactions)
• **Pregnancy/breastfeeding:** Identify if pregnancy is planned or suspected, or if breastfeeding; advise patient to use nonhormonal contraceptive if on long-term therapy
• Teach patient to notify prescriber of all OTC, prescription medications, and herbals used

Evaluation: Positive therapeutic outcome: decreased symptoms of infection, negative C&S

---

dalfampridine (Rx)
(dal-fam'pri-deen)
Ampyra, Fampyra ✤
Func. class.: Neurological agent—MS
Chem. class.: Broad-spectrum potassium channel blocker

ACTION. Mechanism of action is not fully understood, a broad-spectrum potassium channel blocker inhibits potassium channels and increased action potential conduction in demyelinated axons

Therapeutic outcome: Ability to walk at improved speed in MS

USES: For improved walking in patients with multiple sclerosis

Pharmacokinetics
Absorption	Bioavailability 96%
Distribution	Largely unbound to plasma proteins
Metabolism	Unknown
Excretion	96% is recovered in the urine
Half-life	5-6 hr

Pharmacodynamics
Onset	Unknown
Peak	3-4 hr (fasting), longer if taken with food
Duration	Unknown

CONTRAINDICATIONS
Renal failure (CCr <50 ml/min), seizures

Precautions: Pregnancy, breastfeeding, renal disease, elderly

DOSAGE AND ROUTES
Adult: PO 10 mg q12hr

Renal dose
Adult: PO CCr 51-80 ml/min no dosage adjustment needed, but seizure risk is unknown; CCr ≤50 ml/min, do not use

Available forms: Ext rel tab 10 mg

ADVERSE EFFECTS
CNS: Seizures, paresthesias, headache, dizziness, asthenia, insomnia
GI: Nausea, constipation, dyspepsia
GU: Urinary tract infection
MS: Back pain
SYST: Anaphylaxis

INTERACTIONS
None known

NURSING CONSIDERATIONS
Assessment
• **Multiple sclerosis:** assess walking, including speed baseline and during treatment
• **Assess for seizures:** more common in those with previous seizure disorder, risk increases with higher doses, discontinue if seizures occurred
• **Anaphylaxis:** Assess for wheezing, rash, urticaria, pruritus, angioedema

Patient problem
Impaired walking (uses)
Impaired balance (adverse reaction)

Implementation
• Do not break, crush, or chew; give without regard to meals
• Do not give closer together than q12hr, seizures may occur
• Do not double doses, if a dose is missed, skip it

Patient/family education
• Teach patient about expected results, side effects including seizures
• Teach patient to notify prescriber of all OTC/Rx/herbals, supplements taken
• **Anaphylaxis:** Teach patient to notify prescriber immediately of wheezing, throat tightening, rash, swelling of face, lips
• **Seizures:** Teach patient to notify prescriber immediately
• Advise patient to take as directed, not to double or skip doses, to take 12 hr apart; provide "Medication Guide" and ask patient to read
• Teach patient to notify prescriber if pregnancy is planned or suspected or if breastfeeding

Evaluation

Positive therapeutic outcome
• Ability to walk at improved speed in MS

⚠ HIGH ALERT

dalteparin (Rx)
(dahl'ta-pear-in)
Fragmin
Func. class.: Anticoagulant
Chem. class.: Low-molecular-weight heparin

ACTION: Inhibits factor Xa/IIa (thrombin), resulting in anticoagulation

Therapeutic outcome: Absence of deep vein thrombosis

USES: Unstable angina/non-Q-wave MI; prevention/treatment of deep vein thrombosis in abdominal surgery, hip replacement patients or those with restricted mobility during acute illness; pulmonary embolism

Pharmacokinetics

Absorption	87%
Distribution	Unknown
Metabolism	Unknown
Excretion	Unknown
Half-life	2-2.3 hr

Pharmacodynamics

Onset	Rapid
Peak	4 hr
Duration	Up to 24 hr

CONTRAINDICATIONS

Hypersensitivity to this product, heparin, pork products; active major bleeding, hemophilia, leukemia with bleeding, thrombocytopenic purpura, cerebrovascular hemorrhage, cerebral aneurysm, those undergoing regional anesthesia for unstable angina, non–Q-wave MI, dalteparin-induced thrombocytopenia

Precautions: Hypersensitivity to benzyl alcohol, pregnancy, recent childbirth, breastfeeding, child, geriatric, hepatic disease, severe renal/cardiac disease, blood dyscrasias, bacterial endocarditis, acute nephritis, peptic ulcer disease, pericarditis, pericardial effusion, recent lumbar puncture, vasculitis, other diseases where bleeding is possible, uncontrolled hypertension; recent brain, spine, eye surgery; congenital or acquired disorders, hemorrhagic stroke, history of HIT

> **BLACK BOX WARNING:** Epidural/spinal anesthesia, lumbar puncture

DOSAGE AND ROUTES
Deep vein thrombosis/pulmonary embolism

Adult: SUBCUT 200 units/kg/day during 1st month (max single dose 18,000 units), then 150 IU/kg/day in month 2-6 (max single dose 18,000 units), use prefilled syringe that is closest to calculated dose; if platelets are 50,000-100,000/mm^3 reduce dose by 2500 units until platelets ≥100,000/mm^3; if platelets <50,000/mm^3 discontinue until >50,000/mm^3

Hip replacement surgery/DVT prophylaxis

Adult: SUBCUT 2500 units 2 hr before surgery and 2nd dose in the evening the day of surgery (4-8 hr postop), then 5000 units SUBCUT 1st postop day and daily 5-10 days

Unstable angina/non-Q-wave MI

Adult: SUBCUT 120 units/kg q12hr × 5-8 days; max 10,000 units q12hr × 5-8 days with concurrent aspirin, continue until stable

Deep vein thrombosis, prophylaxis for abdominal surgery

Adult: SUBCUT 2500 units 1-2 hr prior to abdominal surgery and repeat daily × 5-10 days; in high-risk patients >3400 international units should be used

Renal dose

Adult: SUBCUT cancer patient with CCr <30 ml/min, monitor and adjust based on antifactor Xa

Available forms: Prefilled syringes, 2500, 5000 units/0.2 ml; 7500 units/0.3 ml, 10,000, 12,500, 15,000, 18,000 units/ml, solution for injection 95,000 units/3.8 mL (25,000 units/mL)

ADVERSE EFFECTS

CNS: Intracranial bleeding
HEMA: Thrombocytopenia, DIC
INTEG: Alopecia, skin necrosis, injection site reaction
SYST: Hypersensitivity, anaphylaxis, hemorrhage

INTERACTIONS
Drug classifications

Anticoagulants, NSAIDs, platelet inhibitors, some cephalosporins, salicylates, thrombolytics: increased risk of bleeding

Drug/herb

Angelica, capsicum, chamomile, dandelion, danshen, feverfew, garlic, ginger, ginkgo, horse chestnut: increased bleeding risk

Drug/lab test

Increase: AST/ALT
Decrease: Platelets

NURSING CONSIDERATIONS
Assessment

• Assess for bleeding (Hct, occult blood in stools) during treatment since bleeding can occur
• Assess for bleeding gums, petechiae, ecchymosis, black tarry stools, hematuria, epistaxis, decrease in Hct, B/P; may indicate bleeding, possible hemorrhage; notify prescriber immediately; product should be discontinued
• **Assess for hypersensitivity:** fever, skin rash, urticaria; notify prescriber immediately
• Assess for needed dosage change q1-2wk; dosage may need to be decreased if bleeding occurs

Patient problem
Ineffective tissue perfusion (uses)
Risk for injury (adverse reactions, uses)

Implementation
SUBCUT route
- **Cannot be used interchangeably unit for unit with unfractionated heparin or other LMWHs**
- Do not give IM or **IV** product route; approved in SUBCUT only; do not mix with other inj or sol, solution should be clear
- Give by SUBCUT only; have patient sit or lie down; SUBCUT inj may be 2 in from umbilicus in a U-shape, upper outer side of thigh, around navel, or upper outer quadrangle of the buttocks; rotate inj sites
- Change inj site daily, use at same time of day

Patient/family education
- Advise patient to avoid OTC preparations that contain aspirin, other anticoagulants; serious product interactions may occur
- Advise patient to use soft-bristle toothbrush to avoid bleeding gums, avoid contact sports, use electric razor, avoid IM inj
- **Bleeding; Instruct patient to report any signs of bleeding:** gums, under skin, urine, stools; unusual bruising

Evaluation
Positive therapeutic outcome
- Absence of deep vein thrombosis/PE
- Prevention complications (unstable angina, non-Q-wave MI)

TREATMENT OF OVERDOSE:
Protamine sulfate 1% given IV; 1 mg protamine/100 anti-Xa international units of dalteparin given

---

▲ HIGH ALERT
dantrolene (Rx)
(dan′troe-leen)
Dantrium, Revonto, Ryanodex
Func. class.: Skeletal muscle relaxant, direct acting
Chem. class.: Hydantoin

Do not confuse: Dantrium/danazol

ACTION: Interferes with intracellular release from the sarcoplasmic reticulum of calcium necessary to initiate contraction; slows catabolism in malignant hyperthermia

Therapeutic outcome: Decreased muscle spasticity; absence of malignant hyperthermia

USES: Spasticity in multiple sclerosis, stroke, spinal cord injury, cerebral palsy, prevention and treatment of malignant hyperthermia

Unlabeled uses: Neuroleptic malignant syndrome

Pharmacokinetics
Absorption	PO (30%-35%), poor
Distribution	Unknown
Metabolism	Liver, extensively
Excretion	Kidney
Half-life	9 hr

Pharmacodynamics
	PO	IV
Onset	Unknown	Immediate
Peak	5 hr	Unknown
Duration	Dose related	Dose related

CONTRAINDICATIONS
Hypersensitivity, hepatic disease, hepatitis

Precautions: Pregnancy, breastfeeding, geriatric, peptic ulcer disease, renal/cardiac/hepatic, stroke, seizure disorder, diabetes mellitus, ALS, COPD, MS, mannitol/gelatin hypersensitivity, labor, lactase deficiency, extravasation

BLACK BOX WARNING: Hepatotoxicity

DOSAGE AND ROUTES
Spasticity
Adult: PO 25 mg/day × 7 days; may increase to 25-100 mg bid-qid, max 400 mg/day, may be increased q7days as needed
Child: PO 0.5 mg/kg/day given in divided doses bid; may be increased q7days as needed; max 400 mg daily

---

Malignant hyperthermia
Adult and child: **IV** 1 mg/kg × 7 days; may repeat to total dose of 10 mg/kg; PO 4-8 mg/kg/day in 4 divided doses × 1-3 days to prevent further hyperthermia; postcrisis follow-up 4-8 mg/kg/day for 1-3 days

Prevention of malignant hyperthermia
Adult and child: PO 4-8 mg/kg/day in 3-4 divided doses × 1-2 days before procedures; give last dose 4 hr preoperatively; **IV** 2.5 mg/kg 1.25 hr prior to anesthesia

Neuroleptic malignant syndrome (unlabeled)
Adult: PO 100-300 mg/day in divided doses, **IV** 1.25-1.5 mg/kg

Available forms: Caps 25, 50, 100 mg; powder for inj 20 mg/vial, 250 mg/vial

ADVERSE EFFECTS
CNS: *Dizziness, weakness, drowsiness,* headache, insomnia, seizures, flushing
CV: Hypotension, tachycardia
EENT: blurred vision, excessive lacrimation
GI: Hepatic injury, *nausea,* constipation, vomiting, increased AST and alkaline phosphatase, abdominal pain, dry mouth, anorexia, hepatitis, dyspepsia, hepatotoxicity
GU: Urinary frequency, nocturia, impotence, crystalluria
HEMA: Eosinophilia, aplastic anemia, leukopenia, thrombocytopenia/lymphoma
INTEG: Rash, pruritus, photosensitivity, extravasation (tissue necrosis), phlebitis
RESP: Pleural effusion, pulmonary edema, respiratory depression, dyspnea
SYST: Anaphylaxis

INTERACTIONS
• Considered incompatible in sol or syringe; compatibility unknown

Individual drugs
Alcohol: increased CNS depression
Verapamil: increased dysrhythmias

Drug classifications
Antidepressants (tricyclic), antihistamines, barbiturates, opiates, sedative/hypnotics: increased CNS depression
Estrogens, hepatotoxic agents: increased hepatotoxicity

NURSING CONSIDERATIONS
Assessment
• **Spasticity:** Assess muscle, nervous system status baseline and during treatment, identify improvement

• **Malignant hyperthermia:** Assess for patient, family reactions if malignant hyperthermia has been a problem in the past, monitor ECG, B/P, pulse, I&O
• **Seizures:** Monitor ECG in epileptic patients; poor seizure control has occurred with patients taking this product; assess for increased seizure activity in epilepsy patient

> **BLACK BOX WARNING: Active hepatic disease:** Monitor hepatic function by frequent determination of AST, ALT, bilirubin, alkaline phosphatase, GGTP; renal function studies; CBC; use lowest dose possible; check for jaundice, dark urine, diarrhea, weakness; product should be discontinued, occurs with oral form

• **Assess for allergic reactions:** rash, fever, respiratory distress
• Monitor for severe weakness, numbness in extremities; prescriber should be notified, product discontinued
• **Respiratory status:** Assess for dyspnea, trouble swallowing

Patient problem
Pain (uses)
Impaired mobility (uses)

Implementation
PO route
• Do not crush or chew caps; caps may be opened and mixed with juice and swallowed; drink immediately after mixing
• Give with meals for GI symptoms
• Store in airtight container at room temperature

IV route
• **Dantrium:** Administer **IV** after reconstituting each 20 mg/60 ml sterile water for inj without bacteriostatic agent (333 mcg/ml); shake until clear; give by rapid **IV** push through Y-tube or 3-way stopcock; follow by prescribed doses immediately; may also give by intermittent inf over 1 hr before anesthesia; assess site for extravasation, phlebitis
• Protect diluted sol from light; use reconstituted sol within 6 hr
• Considered incompatible in sol or syringe
• **Ryanodex:** Add 5 mL sterile water for injection

Patient/family education
• Caution patient not to discontinue product quickly, hallucinations, spasticity, tachycardia will occur; product should be tapered over 1-2 wk; notify prescriber of abdominal pain, jaundiced sclera, clay-colored stools, change in color of urine, rash, itching
• Caution patient not to take with alcohol, other CNS depressants; severe CNS depression can occur; avoid using OTC medication (cough

preparations, antihistamines, alcohol, other CNS depressants), unless directed by prescriber, to take with meals
• Tell patient that if improvement does not occur within 6 wk, prescriber may discontinue
• Caution patient to avoid hazardous activities if drowsiness, dizziness, blurred vision occurs; wait several days to identify patient response to medication
• Advise patient to report severe weakness, seizures, signs of liver insufficiency
• Instruct patient to take medication as prescribed; do not double doses; take missed dose within 1 hr of scheduled time
• **Malignant hyperthermia:** These patients should use a medical ID stating condition, products used

Evaluation

Positive therapeutic outcome
• Decreased pain, spasticity
• Absence or decreased symptoms of malignant hyperthermia

DAPTOmycin (Rx)
(dap′toe-mye-sin)
Cubicin, Cubicin RF
Func. class.: Antiinfective—miscellaneous
Chem. class.: Lipopeptides

ACTION: New class of antiinfective; binds to the bacterial membrane and results in a rapid depolarization of the membrane potential, leading to inhibition of DNA, RNA, and protein synthesis

Therapeutic outcome: Absence of infections

USES: Complicated skin, skin structure infections caused by *Staphylococcus aureus,* (MRSA, MSSA) including methicillin-resistant strains, *Streptococcus pyogenes, S. agalactiae, S. dysgalactiae* (vancomycin-susceptible strains only), *Streptococcus pyogenes* (group A beta hemolytic), *Staphylococcus aureus, Staphylococcus epidermidis,* bone, joint infection, infectious arthritis, orthopedic device-related infection, osteomyelitis

Absorption	Complete
Distribution	Protein binding 92%
Metabolism	Unknown
Excretion	Breast milk, kidneys
Half-life	8.1 hr

Pharmacodynamics

Onset	Rapid
Peak	Infusion End
Duration	24 hr

CONTRAINDICATIONS
Hypersensitivity

Precautions: Pregnancy, breastfeeding, children, geriatrics, GI/renal disease, myopathy, ulcerative/pseudomembranous colitis, rhabdomyolysis, eosinophilic pneumonia

DOSAGE AND ROUTES
Complicated skin or skin structure infection
Adult: IV INF 4-6 mg/kg over ½ hr diluted in 0.9% NaCl, give q24hr × 7-14 days
Adolescent/child/infant ≥5 mo (unlabeled): IV 4-6 mg/kg/day

Staphylococcus aureus bacteremia, right-sided infective endocarditis
Adult: IV INF 6 mg/kg/day × 2-6 wk, up to 8-10 mg/kg/day, treatment failures should use another agent

Renal dose
Adult: IV CCr <30 ml/min; hemodialysis, CAPD 4 mg/kg q48hr, 6 mg/kg q48hr (bacteremia)

Available forms: Lyophilized powder for inj 500 mg/vial

ADVERSE EFFECTS
CNS: Headache, insomnia, dizziness
CV: Hypo/hypertension
GI: Nausea, constipation, diarrhea, vomiting, dyspepsia, *Clostridium difficile*–associated diarrhea abdominal pain
GU: Nephrotoxicity: increased BUN
HEMA: anemia
INTEG: Rash, pruritus
MS: Rhabdomyolysis, injection site reactions
RESP: Cough, eosinophilic pneumonia, dyspnea
SYST: Anaphylaxis, DRESS, Stevens-Johnson syndrome, angioedema

INTERACTIONS
Drug classifications
Individual drugs: Warfarin, monitor PT, INR, or discontinue, may alter anticoagulant levels
Increase: DAPTOmycin action-tobramycin
Increase: tobramycin levels
HMG-CoA reductase inhibitors: myopathy

Drug/lab test
Increased: CPK, AST, ALT, BUN, creatinine, albumin, LDH

Increased/decreased: glucose
Decreased: alk phos, magnesium, phosphate, bicarbonate

NURSING CONSIDERATIONS
Assessment
• Assess signs of infection, C&S, product may be given as soon as culture is taken
• **Rhabdomyolysis:** check for myopathy CPK >1000 U/L (5×ULN), discontinue product, muscle pain, weakness
• **DRESS:** Assess for swelling, rash, fever; may lead to organ involvement, discontinue product
• **Nephrotoxicity:** Monitor any patient with compromised renal system: BUN, creatinine; toxicity may occur
• **Bowel function:** Assess for diarrhea, fever, abdominal pain; report to prescriber; *Clostridium difficile*–associated diarrhea (CDAD) occur
• **Monitor I&O ratio:** report hematuria, oliguria; nephrotoxicity may occur
• **Eosinophilic pneumonia:** Assess for dyspnea, fever, cough, shortness of breath, if left untreated can lead to respiratory failure and death, product should be discontinued
• Monitor B/P during administration; hypo/ hypertension may occur
• Identify allergies before treatment, reaction of each medication
• **Pregnancy/breastfeeding:** Identify if pregnancy is planned or suspected, or if breastfeeding

Patient problem
Infection (uses)

Implementation
• Obtain culture and sensitivity, can begin treatment before results

Intermittent IV infusion route-Cubicin
• Give after reconstitution with 10 ml 0.9% NaCl (500 mg/10 ml), further dilution is needed with 0.9% NaCl; infuse over 30 min
Direct IV route (push)
• Give reconstituted sol (50 mg/ml) by direct **IV** inj over 2 min
• Refrigerate vials, for single use only, discard unused portion; prepared solutions are stable for 12 hr at room temperature or 48 hr refrigerated
Cubicin RF
Direct IV route (push)
• Reconstitute 500 mg/10 mL (50 mg/mL), sterile water for injection, use ≤21 G needle, swirl, give over 2 min
Intermittent IV infusion route
• Further dilute in 50 mL 0.9% NaCl, give over 30 min; child ≥7 yr give over 30 min at 1.67 mL/min

Y-site compatibilities: Alfentanil, amifostine, amikacin, aminocaproic acid, aminophylline, amiodarone, amphotericin B liposome, ampicillin, ampicillin-sulbactam, argatroban, arsenic trioxide, atenolol, atracurium, azithromycin, aztreonam, bivalirudin, bleomycin, bumetanide, buprenorphine, busulfan, butorphanol, calcium chloride/ gluconate, CARBOplatin, carmustine, caspofungin, ceFAZolin, cefepime, cefotaxime, cefoTEtan, cefOXitin, cefTAZidime, ceftizoxime, cefTRIAXone, cefuroxime, chloramphenicol, chlorproMAZINE, cimetidine, ciprofloxacin, cisatracurium, CISplatin, clindamycin, cyclophosphamide, cycloSPORINE, dacarbazine, DACTINomycin, DAUNOrubicin, dexamethasone, dexmedetomidine, dexrazoxane, diazePAM, digoxin, dilTIAZem, diphenhydrAMINE, DOBUTamine, DOCEtaxel, DOPamine, doripenem, doxacurium, DOXOrubicin, DOXOrubicin liposomal, doxycycline, droperidol, enalaprilat, ePHEDrine, EPINEPHrine, epiRUBicin, eptifibatide, ertapenem, erythromycin, esmolol, etoposide, famotidine, fenoldopam, fentaNYL, fluconazole, fludarabine, fluorouracil, foscarnet, fosphenytoin, furosemide, ganciclovir, gentamicin, glycopyrrolate, granisetron, haloperidol, heparin, hydrALAZINE, hydrocortisone, HYDROmorphone, hydrOXYzine, IDArubicin, ifosfamide, inamrinone, insulin (regular), irinotecan, isoproterenol, ketorolac, labetalol, lepirudin, leucovorin, levofloxacin, lidocaine, linezolid, LORazepam, magnesium sulfate, mannitol, mechlorethamine, melphalan, meperidine, meropenem, mesna, metaraminol, methyldopate, methylPREDNISolone, metoclopramide, metoprolol, midazolam, milrinone, mitoXANtrone, mivacurium, morphine, moxifloxacin, mycophenolate mofetil, nafcillin, nalbuphine, naloxone, niCARdipine, nitroprusside, norepinephrine, octreotide, ondansetron, oxaliplatin, oxytocin, PACLitaxel, palonosetron, pamidronate, pancuronium, PEMEtrexed, pentamidine, PHENobarbital, phenylephrine, piperacillin-tazobactam, polymyxin B, potassium acetate/chloride/phosphates, procainamide, prochlorperazine, promethazine, propranolol, quinupristin-dalfopristin, raNITIdine, rocuronium, sodium acetate/bicarbonate/citrate/phosphates, succinylcholine, sulfamethoxazole-trimethoprim, tacrolimus, teniposide, theophylline, thiotepa, ticarcillin, ticarcillin-clavulanate, tigecycline, tirofiban, tobramycin, topotecan, trimethobenzamide, vasopressin, vecuronium, verapamil, vinBLAStine, vinCRIStine, vinorelbine, voriconazole, zidovudine, zoledronic acid

Patient/family education
• Teach all aspects of product therapy
• Advise patient to report sore throat, fever, fatigue; could indicate superinfection; shortness of breath; diarrhea; muscle weakness, pain

- Teach patient may cause dizziness, to avoid driving, hazardous activities until response is known
- Advise patient to report darkening urine, muscle pain (rhambdomyolysis)

Evaluation

Positive therapeutic outcome
- Negative culture, resolution of infection

⚠ HIGH ALERT

darbepoetin (Rx)
(dar′bee-poh′-eh-tin)
Aranesp
Func. class.: Hematopoietic agent
Chem. class.: Recombinant human erythropoietin

ACTION: Stimulates erythropoiesis by the same mechanism as endogenous erythropoietin; in response to hypoxia, erythropoietin is produced in the kidney and released into the bloodstream, where it interacts with progenitor stem cells to increase red cell production

Therapeutic outcome: Decreased anemia with increased RBCs

USES: Anemia associated with chronic renal failure in patients on and not on dialysis and anemic in nonmyeloid malignancies receiving coadministered chemotherapy

Pharmacokinetics

Absorption	Slow, rate-limiting (SUBCUT)
Distribution	Vascular space
Metabolism	Metabolized in body (**IV**), extent unknown
Excretion	Unknown
Half-life	49 hr (subcut), 12 hr (IV)

Pharmacodynamics

Onset	Onset of increased reticulocyte count 1-6 wk
Peak	Unknown
Duration	Unknown

CONTRAINDICATIONS

Hypersensitivity to hamster proteins, human albumin, polysorbate 80; uncontrolled hypertension, red cell aplasia

Precautions: Pregnancy, breastfeeding, children, seizure disorder, porphyria, hypertension, sickle cell disease, vit B_{12}, folate deficiency, chronic renal failure, dialysis, latex hypersensitivity, CABG, angina, anemia

BLACK BOX WARNING: Hgb >11 g/dl, neoplastic disease, MI, stroke, thrombolic disease

DOSAGE AND ROUTES
Correction of anemia in chronic renal failure
Adult: SUBCUT/IV 0.45 mcg/kg as a single inj, titrate max target Hgb of 11 g/dl

Anemia due to Chemotherapy
Adult: SUBCUT 2.5 mcg/kg/wk or 500 mcg q3wk

Epoetin alfa to darbepoetin conversion
Adult: SUBCUT/IV (epoetin alfa <2500 units/wk) 6.25 mcg/wk; (epoetin alfa 2500-4999 units/wk) 12.5 mcg/wk; (epoetin alfa 5000-10,999 units/wk) 25 mcg/wk; (epoetin alfa 11,000-17,999 units/wk) 40 mcg/wk; (epoetin alfa 18,000-33,999 units/wk) 60 mcg/wk; (epoetin alfa 34,000-89,999 units/wk) 100 mcg/wk; (epoetin alfa >90,000 units/wk) 200 mcg/wk

Available forms: Sol for inj 25, 40, 60, 100, 150, 200, 300, 500 mcg/ml; solution for injection, prefilled syringes

ADVERSE EFFECTS
CNS: Seizures, headache, dizziness, stroke
CV: *Hypo/hypertension,* cardiac arrest, *angina pectoris,* thrombosis, HF, acute MI, dysrhythmias, chest pain, transient ischemic attacks, edema
GI: *Diarrhea, vomiting, nausea, abdominal pain, constipation*
HEMA: Red cell aplasia
MISC: *Infection, fatigue, fever*
MS: *Bone pain, myalgia, limb pain, back pain*
RESP: *Upper respiratory infection, dyspnea, cough, bronchitis,* pulmonary embolism
SYST: Allergic reactions, anaphylaxis

INTERACTIONS
Drug classifications
Androgens: increased darbepoetin alfa effect

Drug/lab test
Increased: WBC, platelets, Hgb
Decreased: bleeding time

NURSING CONSIDERATIONS
Assessment
- **Assess for serious allergic reactions:** rash, urticaria; if anaphylaxis occurs, stop product, administer emergency treatment (rare)

BLACK BOX WARNING: Hemoglobin >11 g/dl: monitor Hgb before and weekly × 4 wk or after change in dose and then often after target range has been reached, a rise >1 g/dl over 2 wk may increase risks, reduce dose

BLACK BOX WARNING: Assess blood studies: ferritin, transferrin monthly; transferrin sat ≥20%, ferritin ≥100 ng/ml; Hgb 2 ×/wk until stabilized in target range (30%-33%), then at regular intervals; those with endogenous erythropoietin levels of <500 units/L respond to this agent, if there is lack of response, obtain folic acid, iron, B_{12} levels

BLACK BOX WARNING: Assess renal studies: urinalysis, protein, blood, BUN, creatinine, and electrolytes, those with renal dysfunction may be at greater risk of death, keep Hgb <10 g/dl in chronic kidney disease

• Assess B/P, Hct; check for rising B/P as Hct rises; antihypertensives may be needed

BLACK BOX WARNING: Assess CV status: hypertension may occur rapidly, leading to hypertensive encephalopathy; Hgb >11 g/dl may lead to, stroke, MI, death

• Assess I&O ratio; report drop in output to <50 ml/hr
• Assess for **seizures** if Hgb is increased within 2 wk by 4 points, institute seizure precautions
• Assess CNS symptoms: cold sensation, sweating, pain in long bones

BLACK BOX WARNING: Assess **dialysis patients** for thrill, bruit of shunts; monitor for circulation impairment

BLACK BOX WARNING: Neoplastic disease: breast, non-small cell lung, head and neck, lymphoid or cervical cancers, increased tumor progression, use lowest dose to avoid RBC transfusion. Facility must be enrolled in the ESA APPRISE oncology program (866-284-8089) to use this product in cancer treatment

Patient problems
Fatigue (uses)

Implementation
• Transfusions may still be required for anemia, use iron supplements with this product

Subcut route
• May be used without diluting, give into vein or venous return line of dialysis tubing after dialysis

IV/SUBCUT route
• Do not shake, do not dilute, do not mix with other products or solutions
• Check for discoloration, particulate matter; do not use if present; discard unused portion; do not pool unused portion

• Give over 1-3 min by direct injection or after dialysis
• Store refrigerated, do not freeze, protect from light

Patient/family education
• Caution patient to avoid driving or hazardous activity during beginning of treatment
• Advise patient to monitor B/P, max Hgb 11 g/dl
• Advise patient to take iron supplements, vit B_{12}, folic acid as directed

BLACK BOX WARNING: Advise patient to report chest pain, shortness of breath, swelling/pain in legs, confusion, inability to speak to prescriber, to comply with treatment regimen

• Teach patient that menses may return, use contraception
• Teach home administration and review information for patients and caregivers if home administration is deemed appropriate
• **Chronic renal failure:** Teach patient that product does not cure condition, that other treatment regimens should be followed
• **Seizures:** Teach patient that seizures may occur if Hgb is increased too rapidly, how to protect patient from injury, to report immediately if seizures occur
• **Pregnancy/breastfeeding:** Teach patient to notify health care professional if pregnancy is planned or suspected or if breastfeeding, those who become pregnant should register with Amgen's Pregnancy Surveillance program 800-772-6436

Evaluation
Positive therapeutic outcome
• Increased reticulocyte count, Hgb/Hct
• Increased appetite
• Enhanced sense of well-being

TREATMENT OF OVERDOSE: If polycythemia occurs, discontinue product temporarily

darifenacin
(da-ree-fen'ah-sin)
Enablex
Func. class.: Antispasmodic/GU anticholinergic

Do not confuse: Enablex/Effexor XR

ACTION: Bladder smooth muscle relaxation by decreasing the action of muscarinic receptors, thereby relieving overactive bladder

Therapeutic outcome: Decreasing urgency, frequency of urination

USES: Urge incontinence, frequency, urgency in overactive bladder

Pharmacokinetics

Absorption	15%
Distribution	Protein binding 98%
Excretion	Unknown
Metabolism	Extensively metabolized by CYP2D ⍾⍾, less metabolism in poor metabolizers; some metabolism by CYP3A4
Half-life	12-19 hr

Pharmacodynamics

Onset	Unknown
Peak	7 hr
Duration	24 hr

CONTRAINDICATIONS

Hypersensitivity, urinary retention, narrow-angle glaucoma (uncontrolled)

Precautions: Severe hepatic disease (Child-Pugh), GI/GU obstruction, controlled narrow-angle glaucoma, ulcerative colitis, myasthenia gravis, moderate hepatic disease (Child-Pugh B), elderly patients

DOSAGE AND ROUTES

Adult: PO 7.5 mg/day, initially, may increase to 15 mg/day after 14 days if needed

With taking a potent CYP3A4 inhibitor

Adult: PO Max 7.5 mg/day

Hepatic dose

Adult: PO (Child-Pugh B) max 7.5 mg, do not use in severe hepatic disease

Available forms: Tabs, EXT REL 7.5, 15 mg

ADVERSE EFFECTS

CNS: Dizziness, headache, confusion
EENT: Blurred vision, hallucinations, drowsiness
GI: Constipation, dry mouth, abdominal pain, nausea, vomiting, dyspepsia
INTEG: Rash, pruritus, skin drying
MISC: angioedema
META: Heat intolerance

INTERACTIONS

Drug classifications

Anticholinergics: increased anticholinergic effect
CYP3A4 and CYP2D6 inhibitors: (ketoconazole, itraconazole, ritonavir) increased darifenacin levels
Drugs metabolized by CYP2D6 (fluoxetine, tricyclics): increased levels of these products

NURSING CONSIDERATIONS

Assessment

• **Urinary function:** Assess for urgency, frequency, retention in bladder outflow obstruction
• Bowel pattern: Assess for constipation, abdominal pain, increase fluids in bulk in diet if constipation occurs

Patient problem

Impaired urination (uses)

Implementation

PO route

• Give without regard to meals
• Do not crush, break, chew EXT REL tabs
• Store at room temperature

Patient/family education

• **Angioedema:** Teach patient to report facial swelling or large tongue
• Instruct patient to advise prescriber if pregnancy is planned or suspected; breastfeeding
• Teach patient about anticholinergic symptoms (dry mouth, constipation, dry eyes, heat prostration), not to become overheated, not to use other products unless approved by prescriber
• Teach patient to avoid hazardous activities until reaction is known, dizziness, blurred vision may occur
• Advise patient not to double or skip doses, provide patient information and instruct to read
• Advise patient to discuss with health care professional all OTC, Rx, herbals, supplements used

Evaluation

Positive therapeutic outcome

• Decreasing urgency, frequency of urination

⚠ HIGH ALERT

DAUNOrubicin (Rx)

(daw-noe-roo'bi-sin)
Cerubidine
Func. class.: Antineoplastic, antibiotic
Chem. class.: Anthracycline glycoside

Do not confuse: DAUNOrubicin/ DOXOrubicin

ACTION: Inhibits DNA synthesis, primarily; derived from *Streptomyces coeruleorubidus;* replication is decreased by binding to DNA, binds DNA causing confirmational changes; a vesicant

Therapeutic outcome: Prevention of rapidly growing malignant cells; immunosuppression

USES: Acute lymphocytic leukemia (ALL), acute myelogenous leukemia (AML)

Pharmacokinetics

Absorption	Complete
Distribution	Widely distributed; crosses placenta
Metabolism	Liver, extensively
Excretion	Biliary (40%-50%)
Half-life	18½ hr

Pharmacodynamics

Onset	7-10 days
Peak	14 days
Duration	21 days

CONTRAINDICATIONS

Pregnancy, breastfeeding, hypersensitivity, systemic infections, cardiac disease, bone marrow depression

BLACK BOX WARNING: IM/Subcut use

Precautions: Renal/hepatic disease, gout, tumor lysis syndrome, MI, infection, thrombocytopenia

BLACK BOX WARNING: Bone marrow suppression, cardiac disease, extravasation, renal failure, hepatic disease, requires a specialized care setting and an experienced clinician

DOSAGE AND ROUTES

Adult < 60 yr: IV 45 mg/day × 3 days, 1st cycle, then 2 days, 2nd cycle
Adult ≥ 60 yr: IV 30 mg/m^2/day × 3 days, then 2 days of subsequent courses in combination, max 400-600 mg/m^2 total cumulative dose
Child ≥ 2 yr: IV 25 mg/m^2 depending on cycle weekly in combination, <2 yr or BSA <0.5 m^2 determine on mg/kg basis

Available forms: Inj 20 mg powder/vial

ADVERSE EFFECTS

CNS: Fever, chills
CV: HF, cardiotoxicity, peripheral edema, tachycardia
GI: *Nausea, vomiting, anorexia, mucositis,* hepatotoxicity
GU: Impotence, sterility, orange urine
HEMA: Thrombocytopenia, leukopenia, anemia
INTEG: *Rash, extravasation,* dermatitis, alopecia, thrombophlebitis at inj site
MISC: Anaphylaxis, tumor lysis syndrome, secondary malignancies

INTERACTIONS
Individual drugs
Cyclophosphamide, radiation: increased toxicity

Arsenic trioxide, chloroquine, clarithromycin, dasatinib, dolasetron, droperidol, erythromycin, flecainide, halofantrine, haloperidol, levomethadyl, methadone, ondansetron, palonosetron, pentamide, propafenone, risperiDONE, sparfloxacin, vorinstat, ziprasidone: increase QT prolongation, torsades de pointes

Drug classifications
Antineoplastics: increased toxicity
Class IA/III antidysrhythmics, some phenothiazines, tricyclic antidepressants (high doses): increased QT prolongation, torsades de pointes
Live virus vaccines: decreased antibody reaction

Drug/lab test
Increased: uric acid

NURSING CONSIDERATIONS
Assessment
• Assess buccal cavity for dryness, sores or ulceration, white patches, pain, bleeding, dysphagia; obtain prescription for viscous lidocaine (Xylocaine)
• **Assess symptoms indicating severe allergic reaction:** rash, pruritus, urticaria, purpuric skin lesions, itching, flushing; product should be discontinued

BLACK BOX WARNING: Cardiac toxicity: assess chest x-ray, echocardiography, radionuclide angiography, MUGA, ECG; watch for ST-T wave changes, low QRS and T, QT prolongation possible, dysrhythmias (sinus tachycardia, heart block, PVCs); watch for HF (jugular vein distention, weight gain, edema, crackles), may occur after 2-6 mo of treatment, cumulative dose (400-550 mg/m^2), 450 mg/m^2 if used in combination with radiation, cyclophosphamide

BLACK BOX WARNING: Bone marrow suppression, monitor CBC, differential, platelet count weekly, leukocyte nadir within 2 wk after administration, recovery within 3 wk; do not administer if absolute granulocyte count is <750/mm^3 (liposome)

• Assess for increased uric acid levels, swelling, joint pain primarily in extremities; patient should be well hydrated to prevent urate deposits
• **Acute renal failure, uric acid nephropathy:** Monitor renal function tests: BUN, creatinine, serum uric acid, urine CCr baseline and before each dose; I&O ratio; report fall in urine output to <30 ml/hr, provide aggressive alkalinization of the urine as use of allopurinol can prevent urate nephropathy
• **Hepatotoxicity:** Monitor liver function tests baseline and before each dose (bilirubin,

AST, ALT, LDH) as needed or monthly; note jaundice of skin or sclera, dark urine, clay-colored stools, itchy skin, abdominal pain, fever, diarrhea; hepatotoxicity can be severe
• Assess for bleeding: hematuria, stool guaiac, bruising or petechiae, mucosa or orifices q8hr; check for inflammation of mucosa, breaks in skin
• Identify effects of alopecia on body image; discuss feelings about body changes
• **Tumor lysis syndrome.** Assess for hyperkalemia, hyperphosphatemia, hyperuricemia, hypocalcemia

---

BLACK BOX WARNING: Extravasation: swelling, pain, decreased blood return, if extravasation occurs stop infusion, remove tubing, attempt to aspirate the drug prior to removing the needle, elevate area, treat with ice

---

Patient problem
• Risk for infection (uses)
• Impaired cardiac output (adverse reactions)
• Risk for injury (adverse reactions)

Implementation
• Avoid contact with skin; very irritating; wash completely to remove
• Give fluids **IV** or **PO** before chemotherapy to hydrate patient; give antiemetic 30-60 min before giving product to prevent vomiting, and prn; antibiotics for prophylaxis of infection
• Provide liquid diet: carbonated beverages; gelatin may be added if patient is not nauseated or vomiting

---

BLACK BOX WARNING: To be used in a care setting with emergency equipment available; to be used by a clinician knowledgeable in cytotoxic therapy, do not give by IM/SUBCUT route

---

• Help patient rinse mouth tid-qid with water, club soda, brush teeth bid-qid with soft brush or cotton-tipped applicators for stomatitis, use unwaxed dental floss
• Product should be prepared by experienced personnel using proper precautions
• Do not give by IM/SUBCUT inj

IV route
• Give after diluting 20 mg/4 ml sterile water for inj (5 mg/ml); rotate; further dilute in 10-15 ml 0.9% NaCl; give over 3-5 min by direct **IV** through **Y**-tube or 3-way stopcock of inf of D₅W or 0.9% NaCl, may use premix vial 5 mg/ml
Intermittent IV infusion route
• Dilute further in 50-100 ml 0.9% NaCl, LR, D₅W; give over 15 min (50 ml), 30 min (100 ml) for extravasation

Y-site compatibilities: Amifostine, anidulafungin, atenolol, bivalirudin, bleomycin, CARBOplatin, caspofungin, CISplatin, codeine, cyclophosphamide, cytarabine, DACTINomycin, DAPTOmycin, dexmedetomidine, etoposide, fenoldopam, filgrastim, gemcitabine, gemtuzumab, granisetron, melphalan, meperidine, methotrexate, nesiritide, octreotide, ondansetron, oxaliplatin, PACLitaxel, palonosetron, quinupristin-dalfopristin, riTUXimab, sodium acetate/bicarbonate, teniposide, thiotepa, tigecycline, trastuzumab, vinCRIStine, vinorelbine, voriconazole, zoledronic acid

Patient/family education
• Teach patient to avoid use of products containing aspirin or ibuprofen, razors, commercial mouthwash, since bleeding may occur; to report symptoms of bleeding (hematuria, tarry stools)
• Instruct patient to report signs of **anemia** (fatigue, headache, irritability, faintness, shortness of breath); signs of **infection;** bleeding, bruising, shortness of breath, swelling, change in heart rate; to avoid crowds, those with known infections
• Advise patient that hair may be lost during treatment; a wig or hairpiece may make patient feel better; new hair may be different in color, texture
• Caution patient not to have any vaccinations without the advice of the prescriber; serious reactions can occur
• **Pregnancy/breastfeeding:** Do not use in pregnancy, breastfeeding
• Advise patient that contraception is needed during treatment and for 4 mo after the completion of therapy
• Inform patient that urine and other body fluids may be red-orange for 48 hr
• Teach patient to avoid crowds, those with known infections
• Advise patient continued exams and lab work will be needed

Evaluation

Positive therapeutic outcome
• Prevention of rapid division of malignant cells

⚠ HIGH ALERT

RARELY USED

daunorubicin/cytarabine
(daw-noe-roo'bi-sin sye-tare'a-been)
Vyxeos
Func. class.: Antineoplastic

USES: For the treatment of newly diagnosed therapy-related AML or AML with myelodysplasia-related changes

---

DOSAGES AND ROUTES

Adult: IV First induction, 44 mg/m^2 daunorubicin liposomal and 100 mg/m^2 cytarabine liposomal over 90 min on days 1, 3, and 5; patients who do not achieve a response may receive a second induction. Second induction (given 2 to 5 wk after the first induction cycle), 44 mg/m^2 daunorubicin liposomal and 100 mg/m^2 cytarabine liposomal on days 1 and 3. Consolidation therapy (given 5 to 8 wk after the start of the last induction), 29 mg/m^2 daunorubicin liposomal and 65 mg/m^2 cytarabine liposomal on days 1 and 3. Patients without disease progression or unacceptable toxicity should receive a second cycle of consolidation therapy given 5 to 8 wk after the start of the previous consolidation

---

RARELY USED

delafloxacin

(dela-flox′-a-sin)

Baxdela

Func. class.: Antiinfective

USES: For the treatment of acute bacterial skin and skin structure infections

DOSAGE AND ROUTES

Adult: PO 450 mg q12hr × 5 to 14 days; **IV** 300 mg q12hr × 5 to 14 days

---

deferoxamine (Rx)

(de-fer-ox′a-meen)

Desferal

Func. class.: Antidote, heavy metal

ACTION: Ferric ions bind to deferoxamine, creating ferrioxamine, a stable, water-soluble complex that is then readily excreted by the kidneys

Therapeutic outcome: Removes iron and aluminum

USES:

Pharmacokinetics

Absorption	Minimal
Distribution	Widely
Metabolism	Tissues
Excretion	Kidneys
Half-life	1 hr

Pharmacodynamics

Onset	Unknown
Peak	Unknown
Duration	Unknown

CONTRAINDICATIONS

Hypersensitivity, severe renal disease, anuria

Precautions: pregnancy, breastfeeding, children, heart failure, infection

DOSAGE AND ROUTES

Acute iron overload

Adult/Child ≥3 yr: IM/IV Initially 1 g then 500 mg q 4 hr × 2 doses, then 500 mg q 4 to 12 hr if needed

Chronic iron overload

Adult/Child ≥3 yr: IV/IM 500mg-1 g q day IM, may give additional 2 g IV for each unit of blood, max 1g/day no transfusions, 6g/day with transfusions

SUBCUT: 1-2 g/day over 8-24 hr; use continuous infusion pump

Available forms: Powder for injection 500, 2 g/vial

ADVERSE EFFECTS

CV: Tachycardia, hypotension

EENT: Hearing loss, blurred vision, cataracts

GI: Diarrhea, abdominal pain, vomiting

GU: Pink or red urine

MS: Muscle cramps

INTEG: Rash, flushing, pain at injection site, allergic reactions, anaphylaxis, angioedema

INTERACTIONS

Individual drugs

Ascorbic acid (vitamin C): increase effect, avoid use until prescribed

NURSING CONSIDERATIONS

Assessment

• **Iron poisoning:** Assess type, amount time ingested, reason for ingesting; monitor for bloody vomiting and diarrhea, abdominal pain, nausea; metabolic acidosis, shock, death may occur

• Monitor I&O, notify provider of significant changes

• Monitor hearing, serum iron, total iron-binding capacity, ferritin levels LFTs, serum creatinine, BUN baseline and periodically

• Monitor vital signs during IV administration. Epinephrine, an antihistamine, and resuscitation equipment should be readily available in case of an anaphylactic reaction

Patient problems

Risk for injury (uses)

Implementation

• Give IM, IV, SUBCUT, use by IM unless patient is in shock

• Visually inspect parenteral products for particulate matter and discoloration prior to use. Do not use turbid solutions.

• Once reconstructed, use within 3 hr; the solution may be stored at room temperature for up to 24 hr. Do not refrigerate.

IV infusion route:
• Reconstituted with sterile water for injection is for single use only. Discard any unused portion.
• Reconstitute each vial of deferoxamine 500 mg with 5 mL of sterile water for injection, for a total volume of 5.3 mL, to give a final concentration of 95 mg/mL. For each vial of 2000 mg, reconstitute with 20 mL of sterile water for injection, for a total volume of 21.1 mL, to give a concentration of 95 mg/mL. The drug must be completely dissolved before withdrawing into the syringe to further dilute.
• Dilute the reconstituted IV solution in 5% dextrose for injection, 0.45% sodium chloride for injection, 0.9% sodium chloride for injection, or lactated Ringer's solution.
• Infuse IV at a rate of max 15 mg/kg per hr. Rapid infusion may cause hypotension, erythema, urticaria, wheezing, convulsions, tachycardia, or shock.
• If the patient is also receiving blood, deferoxamine should be administered in a line that is separate from the blood.
• Switch to IM as soon as possible.

IM route
• Reconstitute with sterile water for injection, for single use only. Discard any unused portion.
• Reconstitute each vial of deferoxamine 500 mg with 2 mL of sterile water for injection for a total volume of 2.35 mL, to give a final concentration of 213 mg/mL. For each vial of 2000 mg, reconstitute with 8 ml of sterile water for injection, for a total volume of 9.4 mL, to give a final concentration of 213 mg/mL. The drug must be completely dissolved before withdrawing into the syringe.
• Inject deeply into a large muscle mass. Aspirate prior to injection to avoid injecting into a blood vessel. Massage area following administration. Transient severe pain may occur following injection. Rotate sites of injection.

SUBCUT infusion route:
• Reconstitute with sterile water for injection; is for single use only. Discard any unused portion.
• Reconstitute each vial of deferoxamine 500 mg with 5 mL of sterile water for injection, for a total volume of 5.3 mL, to give a final concentration of 95 mg/mL. For each vial of 2000 mg, reconstitute with 20 mL of sterile water for injection, for a total volume of 21.1 mL, to give a final concentration of 95 mg/mL. The drug must be completely dissolved before withdrawing into the syringe.

• Give in the abdominal subcutaneous tissue using an infusion pump. Infuse over 8–24 hr per treatment, preferably overnight. Infusion duration must be individualized for each patient, because in some patients as much iron will be excreted after a short infusion of 8–12 hr as with the same dose given over 24 hr.

Patient/family education
• Advise patient to avoid driving or other hazardous activities if dizziness or change in vision occurs
• Teach patient that follow-up exams and blood work will be needed in chronic iron overload
• Teach patient to report if pregnancy is planned or suspected or if breastfeeding

Evaluation
Positive therapeutic outcome
• Serum iron WNL

degarelix
(day-gah-rel′iks)
Firmagon
Func. class.: Antineoplastic
Chem. class.: GnRH-receptor antagonist

ACTION: Reduces release of gonadotropins and testicular steroidogenesis by reversibly binding to GnRH receptors

USES: Advanced prostate cancer

Pharmacokinetics	
Absorption	Well
Distribution	Unknown
Metabolism	Liver 80%
Excretion	Feces, 30% (urine, unchanged)
Half-life	53 days

Pharmacodynamics	
Onset	unknown
Peak	2 days
Duration	50 days

CONTRAINDICATIONS
Hypersensitivity, QT prolongation, osteoporosis, severe hepatic/renal disease, pregnancy, breastfeeding

Precautions: CV disease, electrolyte abnormalities, geriatric patients

DOSAGE AND ROUTES
Adult (male): SUBCUT 240 mg given as two 120 mg injections (40 mg/mL concentrations); maintenance 80 mg (20 mg/mL concentration) every 28 days, starting 28 days after first dose

Available forms: Injection 80, 120 mg vial

SIDE EFFECTS
CNS: Chills, dizziness, fatigue, fever, headache, insomnia
CV: Increased QT prolongation, hypotension, hot flashes, hypertension
GI: Diarrhea, constipation, nausea
GU: ED, UTI, gynecomastia, testicular atrophy
INTEG: Injection site reactions, pain at site, redness, swelling
MS: Back pain, decreased bone density
SYST: Hypersensitivity, anaphylaxis, angioedema

INTERACTIONS
Individual drugs
Methyldopa, metoclopramide, reserpine: Increase QT prolongation

Drug classifications
Class IA/III antidysrhythmics: Increase QT prolongation

Drug/lab test
Increase: PSA, LFTs
Decrease: bone density test

NURSING CONSIDERATIONS
Assessment:
• Monitor HbA1c, lipids, B/P prior to initiation and 3-6 mo after
  QT prolongation: more common in those taking Class IA/III antidysrhythmics, heart failure, congenital long QT syndrome; monitor cardiac status at baseline and often thereafter, include ECG periodically
  Anaphylaxis, angioedema (assess for rash, trouble breathing): discontinue treatment and do not restart in serious reactions; assess for rash, dyspnea, wheezing, facial swelling
• Monitor liver function studies, PSA, GGT that may be elevated; bone density that may be decreased; electrolytes; if PSA is elevated, monitor testosterone levels

Patient problems
Impaired sexual functioning (uses)

Implementation:
• Do not give IV, subcut only
General reconstitution information:
• Use double gloves, gown, aseptic technique during preparation and administration
• Keep vials vertical at all times; do *not* shake the vials; give reconstituted drug within 1 hr after addition of sterile water for injection
Reconstitution of 120 mg vial (240 mg dose *only*):
• For a 240 mg dose, use two 120 mg vials; repeat for each 120 mg vial: draw up 3 mL of sterile water for injection with a 2 inch, 21 G needle; do not use bacteriostatic water for injection; inject the sterile

water slowly into vial containing 120 mg; to maintain sterility, do not remove the syringe or the needle from the vial; keep the vial in an upright position and swirl gently; avoid shaking; reconstitution can take up to 15 min; tilt the vial slightly and withdraw 3 mL (40 mg/mL); avoid turning the vial upside down; repeat with a new vial, needle, and syringe for the second 120 mg dose (total dose = 240 mg)
Reconstitution of 80 mg vial:
• Draw up 4.2 mL of sterile water for injection with a 2 inch, 21 G needle; do not use bacteriostatic water for injection; inject the sterile water slowly into vial containing 80 mg; do not remove the syringe or the needle from the vial; swirl gently; avoid shaking; reconstitution can take up to 15 min; withdraw 4 mL (20 mg/mL); avoid turning upside down during withdrawal
Subcut injection:
• Exchange the reconstitution needle with a 1.25 inch, 27G needle; remove air bubbles; give in the abdominal region; rotate injection site periodically; use area not exposed to pressure; grasp the skin of abdomen, elevate the subcutaneous tissue, and insert the needle deeply at an angle $\geq$45 degrees; aspirate before injection; inject the dose subcut; when giving the loading dose of two 120 mg doses, the second dose should be injected at a different site

Patient/family education:
• Advise to notify all prescribers of cardiac disease or use of all cardiac products, irregular pulse, heartbeat
• Advise on injection technique if patient/family will be giving product (provide patient information)

Evaluation:
• Positive therapeutic outlook: decreasing spread, size of cancer

---

denosumab (Rx)
(den-oh′sue-mab)
Prolia, Xgeva
Func. class.: Bone resorption inhibitor
Chem. class.: Monoclonal antibody, bone resorption

ACTION: Neutralizes activity of receptor activator nuclear factor kappa-B ligand (RANKL) by binding to it and blocking its interaction with cell surface receptors, use of a RANKL inhibitor may reduce bone turnover and decrease tumor burden

Therapeutic outcome: Increased/maintained bone density

USES: Prolia: Osteoporosis in postmenopausal women or men at high risk for fractures,

---

who are receiving androgen deprivation therapy for prostate cancer, and women receiving aromatase inhibitor therapy for breast cancer; **Xgeva:** prevention of skeletal-related events in bone metastases from solid tumors; giant cell tumor of bone

Pharmacokinetics

Absorption	Bioavailability 62%
Distribution	Unknown
Metabolism	Unknown
Excretion	Unknown
Half-life	25.4 days

Pharmacodynamics (bone resorption effect)

Onset	1 mo
Peak	Serum concentration 3-21 days
Duration	12 mo after treatment conclusion

CONTRAINDICATIONS

Hypersensitivity, hypocalcemia, pregnancy

Precautions: Anemia, breastfeeding, child/infant/neonate, coagulopathy, diabetes mellitus, dialysis, eczema, hypoparathyroidism, immunosuppression, latex hypersensitivity, malabsorption syndrome, neonates, neoplastic disease, pancreatitis, parathyroid disease, pregnancy, dental/renal/thyroid disease, TB, vitamin D deficiency

DOSAGE AND ROUTES

Postmenopausal osteoporosis (Prolia)
Adult female: SUBCUT 60 mg q6mo

Bone metastases from solid tumors (Xgeva)
Adult: SUBCUT 120 mg q4wk

Giant cell tumor of bone (Xgeva)
Adult: SUBCUT 120 mg on days 1, 8, 15, then 120 mg q4wk

Hypercalcemia of malignancy (Xgeva)
Adult: Subcut 120 mg q 4 wk, another dose of 120 mg given on day 8 and 15 of first month of treatment

Available forms: Solution for injection 60 mg/ml (Prolia); 120 mg/1.7 ml (Xgeva)

ADVERSE EFFECTS

CNS: Headache, vertigo, insomnia, fatigue
CV: Angina, atrial fibrillation
GI: Abdominal pain, constipation, *diarrhea*, flatulence, GERD, *vomiting, nausea*, pancreatitis
GU: Cystitis
HEMA: Anemia, neutropenia
INTEG: Atopic dermatitis, pruritus
META: Hypercholesterolemia, hypocalcemia, hypophosphatemia
MS: Back/bone pain, MS pain, myalgia, osteonecrosis of the jaw
RESP: Cough, *dyspnea*
SYST: Infection, secondary malignancy, anaphylaxis

INTERACTIONS
Drug classifications
Immunosuppressives (except cytarabine liposomal), corticosteroids: possible increased infection
Antineoplastics, corticosteroids: possible increased osteonecrosis of the jaw

Drug/lab test
Increase: cholesterol

NURSING CONSIDERATIONS
Assessment
• **Assess for acute acute-phase reaction:** fever, myalgia, headache, flulike symptoms, for 72 hr after injection, usually resolves after 72 hr
• Monitor blood tests: serum calcium/creatinine/BUN/magnesium/phosphate; provide adequate calcium D, magnesium
• **Assess for hypocalcemia (may be fatal):** paresthesia, twitching, laryngospasm, Chvostek's/Trousseau's signs; preexisting hypocalcemia prior to treatment; patient with vitamin D deficiency may require higher doses of vitamin D
• **Assess for hypercalcemia:** nausea, vomiting, anorexia, weakness, thirst, constipation, dysrhythmias
• **Monitor dental status:** correct dental complications prior to product use, good oral hygiene should be maintained; if dental work is to be performed, antiinfectives should be given to prevent osteonecrosis of the jaw
• **Assess for infection:** Do not start treatment in those with active infections, infections should be resolved first

Patient problem
Risk for injury (uses)

Implementation
SUBCUT route
• Give acetaminophen before and for 72 hr after to decrease pain
• Do not use if particulate matter or discoloration is present; solution is clear and colorless

to slightly yellow with small white/opalescent particles, remove from refrigerator and allow to warm to room temperature (15-30 min)
• **Use of prefilled syringe with needle safety guard:** Leave green guard in original position until after administration, remove and discard needle cap immediately before injection, give by SUBCUT injection in upper arm, thigh, or abdomen; after injection, point needle away from people and slide green guard over needle
• **Use of single-use vials:** Use 27G needle, give in upper arm/thigh, or abdomen, do not re-insert needle in vial, discard supplies as appropriate
• Avoid direct sunlight/heat, do not freeze, use within 14 days after removal from refrigerator, store unopened containers in refrigerator

Patient/family education
• Teach patient reason for treatment, expected result
• Advise patient to report hypercalcemic relapse: nausea, vomiting, bone pain, thirst
• Teach patient to notify prescriber immediately of rash, infection, cramps, twitching
• Teach patient to continue with dietary recommendations including additional calcium 1000 mg/day and vitamin D ≥ 400 units (Prolia product labeling)
• **Pregnancy/breastfeeding:** Women who become pregnant should enroll in Amgen's Pregnancy Surveillance Program (800-772-6436), do not use in pregnancy, breastfeeding, notify prescriber if pregnancy is planned or suspected, Xgeva: to use contraception during and for 5 mo after completion of therapy, males should use contraception if partner is pregnant
• Instruct patient to use acetaminophen prior to and for 72 hrs after injection to lessen bone pain
• Explain the purpose of this product and expected results
• Advise patient to avoid OTC, Rx, or herbs and supplements unless approved by prescriber
• Teach patient to use regular exercise, stop smoking, and avoid alcohol to maintain bone health
• Teach patient that product must be continued or fractures may occur
• Advise patient to inform all health care providers of product use, avoid dental procedures/surgery if possible, practice good oral hygiene
• Teach patient that lab tests and follow-up exams will be required

Evaluation
Positive therapeutic outcome
• Increased/maintained bone density

desipramine (Rx)
(dess-ip'ra-meen)
Norpramin
Func. class.: Antidepressant, tricyclic
Chem. class.: Dibenzazepine, secondary amine

Do not confuse desipramine/
disopyramide

ACTION: Blocks reuptake of norepinephrine, serotonin into nerve endings, increasing action of norepinephrine, serotonin in nerve cells

Therapeutic outcome: Decreased depression

USES: Depression

Unlabeled uses: Chronic pain, insomnia, anxiety

Pharmacokinetics

Absorption	Well
Distribution	Widely, protein binding 92%
Metabolism	Extensively, liver by CYP2D6, 7% of population may be poor metabolizers
Excretion	Unknown
Half-life	15-24 hr

Pharmacodynamics (antidepressant)

Onset	2-3 wk
Peak	2-6 wk
Duration	Unknown

CONTRAINDICATIONS
Hypersensitivity to tricyclics, carBAMazepine; closed-angle glaucoma, acute MI, MAOIs

Precautions: Pregnancy, breastfeeding, geriatric, severe depression, increased intraocular pressure, seizure disorder, CV disease, urinary retention, cardiac dysrhythmias, cardiac conduction disturbances, family history of sudden death, prostatic hypertrophy, thyroid disease

> **BLACK BOX WARNING:** Suicidal patients, children <18 yr

DOSAGE AND ROUTES
Major depression
Adult: PO 50-75 mg/day in 1-4 divided doses; titrate by 25-50 mg qwk up to 300 mg/day in

single or divided doses (inpatient), 200 mg/day (outpatient)

Geriatric: PO 25 mg/day at bedtime, titrate qwk; may increase to 150 mg/day

Child >12 yr: PO 25-50 mg/day in divided doses, max 100 mg/day

Child 6-12 yr: PO 1-3 mg/kg/day in divided doses, max 5 mg/kg/day

Available forms: Tabs 10, 25, 30, 75, 100, 150 mg

ADVERSE EFFECTS

CNS: *Dizziness, drowsiness,* fatigue, confusion, headache, anxiety, tremors, stimulation, insomnia, nightmares, EPS (geriatric), increased psychiatric symptoms, paresthesia, suicidal ideation, impaired memory, seizures, serotonin syndrome

CV: *Orthostatic hypo/hypertension,* ECG changes, *tachycardia, palpitations*

EENT: *Blurred vision,* mydriasis

GI: *Dry mouth,* paralytic ileus, increased appetite, hepatitis, stomatitis, constipation, weight gain

GU: *Retention,* decreased libido, ED

HEMA: Agranulocytosis, thrombocytopenia, eosinophilia, leukopenia

INTEG: Rash, urticaria, sweating, pruritus, photosensitivity

INTERACTIONS
Individual drugs

Alcohol: increased CNS depression

Cimetidine, dilTIAZem, fluvoxaMINE, FLUoxetine, PARoxetine, sertraline, verapamil: increased desipramine level, monitoring drug levels

CloNIDine: increased life-threatening B/P elevations, do not use concurrently

EPINEPHrine, norepinephrine: increased hypertension

Bupropion, cylcobenazaprine, gatifloxacin, levofloxacin, linezolid, methylene blue, moxifloxacin, sparfloxacin, SUNItinib, tramadol, trazodone, vorinostat, ziprasidone: increased serotonin syndrome, neuroleptic malignant syndrome

Drug classifications

Antihistamines: Increased anticholinergic effect

Barbiturates, opioids, CNS depressants: increased CNS depression, skeletal muscle relaxants

MAOIs: increased hyperpyrexia, seizures, excitation; do not use within 14 days of MAOIs

SSRIs, SNRIs, serotonin-receptor agonists, other tricyclic antidepressants: increased serotonin syndrome, neuroleptic malignant syndrome

Class IA/III dysrhythmics, tricyclic antidepressants: increased QT interval

Drug/herb

Kava, valerian: increased CNS depression

St. John's wort, SAM-e, yohimba: may increase serotonin syndrome; avoid concurrent use

Drug/lab test

Increase: serum bilirubin, blood glucose, alkaline phosphatase, LFTs

NURSING CONSIDERATIONS
Assessment

• **Pain:** Assess characteristics including location, intensity, alleviating and aggravating factors before and periodically

• Monitor B/P (lying, standing), pulse q4hr; if systolic B/P drops 20 mm Hg, hold product, notify prescriber; take vital signs

• Monitor ECG in cardiac patients

• Monitor blood studies: CBC, leukocytes, differential, cardiac enzymes if patient is receiving long-term therapy

• Monitor hepatic studies: AST, ALT, bilirubin, monitor blood glucose and cholesterol in those who are overweight

• Check weight qwk, BMI initially and periodically; appetite may increase with this product

• Assess for **EPS** primarily in geriatric: rigidity, dystonia, akathisia

• Assess for **seizure activity** in those with a history of seizures, may be before cardiac events

> **BLACK BOX WARNING: Depression:** assess mental status: mood, sensorium, affect, **suicidal tendencies,** increase in psychiatric symptoms: depression, panic; this product is not indicated for children, monitor mental status baseline and during first few months of treatment

• Assess for urinary retention, constipation; constipation most likely in children

• Assess for **withdrawal symptoms:** headache, nausea, vomiting, muscle pain, weakness; not usual unless product is discontinued abruptly

• **Beers:** avoid in older adults with delirium or high risk for delirium, assess for confusion

Patient problem

Depression (uses)
Pain (uses)

Implementation

• Increase fluids, bulk in diet for constipation, especially in geriatric

• Take with food or milk for GI symptoms

• Crush if patient is unable to swallow medication whole, without regard to food

---

• Give dosage at bedtime if oversedation occurs during day; may take entire dose at bedtime; geriatric may not tolerate once a day dosing
• Store at room temperature
• Provide assistance with ambulation during beginning of therapy for drowsiness/dizziness
• Provide safety measures, primarily in the geriatric
• Check to see that PO medication is swallowed

Patient/family education
• Advise patient that therapeutic effects may take 2-3 wk
• **Pregnancy/breastfeeding:** Teach patient to notify health care professional if pregnancy is planned or suspected or if breastfeeding

> **BLACK BOX WARNING:** Teach patient that suicidal thoughts and behavior may occur, notify prescriber immediately

• Advise patient to use caution in driving, other activities requiring alertness because of drowsiness, dizziness, blurred vision
• Teach patient to avoid alcohol ingestion, other CNS depressants
• Teach patient not to discontinue medication quickly after long-term use; may cause nausea, headache, malaise
• Teach patient to wear sunscreen or large hat, since photosensitivity occurs

Evaluation
Positive therapeutic outcome
• Decreased depression

TREATMENT OF OVERDOSE:
ECG monitoring; induce emesis; lavage, administer anticonvulsant

---

desmopressin (Rx)
(des-moe-press′in)
DDAVP, DDAVP Melt ❋, DDAVP Rhinal Tube ❋, DDAVP Rhinyle Nocdurma ❋, Noctiva, Stimate
Func. class.: Pituitary hormone
Chem. class.: Synthetic antidiuretic hormone

ACTION: Promotes reabsorption of water by action on renal tubular epithelium in the kidney; causes smooth muscle constriction and increase in plasma factor VIII levels, which increases platelet aggregation resulting in vasopressor effect; similar to vasopressin

Therapeutic outcome: Prevention of nocturnal enuresis, decreased bleeding in hemophilia A, von Willebrand's disease type 1, control and stabilization of water in diabetes insipidus

USES: Hemophilia A, von Willebrand's disease type 1, nonnephrogenic diabetes insipidus, symptoms of polyuria/polydipsia caused by pituitary dysfunction, nocturnal enuresis

Pharmacokinetics

Absorption	Nasal (up to 20%), poor PO, SL
Distribution	Breast milk
Metabolism	Unknown
Excretion	Urine

Pharmacodynamics

	PO	Intranasal	SUBCUT/ IV
Onset	1 hr	1 hr	Rapid
Peak	4-7 hr	1-4 hr	15-30 min
Duration	Unknown	8-20 hr	3 hr

CONTRAINDICATIONS
Hypersensitivity, nephrogenic diabetes insipidus, severe renal disease

> **BLACK BOX WARNING:** Hyponatremia

Precautions: Pregnancy, breastfeeding, CAD, hypertension, cystic fibrosis, thrombus, electrolyte imbalances, male infertility

DOSAGE AND ROUTES
Primary nocturnal enuresis
Adult and child ≥6 yr: INTRANASAL 20 mcg (half in each nostril) at bedtime, may increase to 40 mcg; **PO** 0.2 mg at bedtime, may be increased to max 0.6 mg at bedtime

Diabetes insipidus
Adult: INTRANASAL 10-40 mcg in divided doses (1-4 sprays with pump); SUBCUT/IV 2-4 mcg/day or SUBCUT in 2 divided daily in divided doses
Child 3 mo-12 yr: INTRANASAL 5-30 mcg in divided doses

Hemophilia/von Willebrand's disease
Adult and child >3 mo: IV 0.3 mcg/kg in NaCl over 15-30 min; may repeat if needed
Adult/child >11 mo: Nasal spray: 33 mcg (1 spray in each nostril), give 2 hr before surgery

Antihemorrhagic
Adult and child >3 mo: IV 0.3 mcg/kg
Adult and child <50 kg: INTRANASAL 1 spray in one nostril
Adult and child >50 kg: 1 spray each nostril
Adult: SUBCUT/IV 0.2-0.4 mcg/kg dose

Nocturia
Adults: 50-64 yr, Noctiva nasal spray 1 spray in each nostril 30 min before going to bed (use in those not at increased risk for hyponatremia)

Available forms: Inj 4, 15 mcg/ml, Rhinal Tube delivery 2.5 mg/vial (0.1 mg/ml); tabs 0.1, 0.2 mg; nasal spray pump (DDAVP) 10 mcg/spray (0.1 mg/ml); nasal spray (Stimate) 1.5 mg/ml (150 mcg/dose)

ADVERSE EFFECTS
CNS: Drowsiness, headache, lethargy, flushing, seizures
CV: Increased B/P, palpitations, tachycardia
EENT: Nasal irritation, congestion, rhinitis
GI: Nausea, heartburn, cramps
GU: *Vulval pain*
META: Hyponatremia, hyponatremia-induced seizures
SYST: Anaphylaxis (IV)

INTERACTIONS
Individual drugs
Alcohol, demeclocycline, EPHINEPHrine (large doses), heparin, lithium: decreased antidiuretic action
CarBAMazepine, chlorproPAMIDE, clofibrate: increased antidiuretic action, SSRIs, lamoTRIgine

Drug classifications
Pressor products: increased pressor effect

NURSING CONSIDERATIONS
Assessment
• Monitor I&O ratio, urine osmolality, specific gravity, weight daily; check for edema in extremities; if water retention is severe, diuretic may be prescribed; check pulse, B/P when giving product **IV** or SUBCUT
• **Assess for water intoxication:** lethargy, behavioral changes, disorientation, neuromuscular excitability, dehydration, poor skin turgor, severe thirst, dry skin, tachycardia
• Assess intranasal use: nausea, congestion, cramps, headache; usually decreased with decreased dosage
• Assess for allergic reaction, including anaphylaxis **(IV route)**, notify prescriber, discontinue use
• Assess for nasal mucosa changes: congestion, edema, discharge, scarring (nasal route)
• **Diabetes insipidus:** Monitor urine volume osmolality and plasma osmolality, monitor for dry skin, poor turgor, thirst (dehydration)
• Nocturia enuresis: Identify how often enuresis is occurring, avoid use in those prone to water intoxication or sodium depletion

• **Hemophilia/Von Willebrand's disease:** Monitor factor VIII coagulant activity before using for hemostasis, assess for bleeding frank and occult
• **Pregnancy/breastfeeding:** No well-controlled studies, use only if benefit outweighs fetal risk, cautious use in breastfeeding, excretion is unknown

Patient problem
Fluid imbalance (uses)

Implementation
PO route
• Store at room temperature
• Draw medication into tube, insert tube into nostril to instill product and blow on other end to deliver sol into nasal cavity; rinse after use
• Store in refrigerator or cool environment
Nasal route
• DDAVP and Stimate are not interchangeable
• Prime prior to first dose (press down 4 times), pump stays primed for 1 wk; to reprime, press down 1 time
• Noctiva: Do not shake bottle, prime by pumping 5 times into the air, away from the face, if not used >3 days, reprime with 2 actuations, have patient blow nose, tilt head back slightly, close then open nostril, inhale while pumping 1 time, wipe applicator, and replace cap

IV, direct route
• Give undiluted over 1 min in diabetes insipidus

Intermittent IV infusion route
• Give single dose diluted in 50 ml of 0.9% NaCl (adult and child >10 kg) as a single dose/10 ml as an **IV** inf over 15-30 min in von Willebrand's disease or hemophilia A
• Store in refrigerator

Patient/family education
• Use demonstration, return demonstration to teach technique for nasal instillation, clear nasal passage before use
• Teach patient to notify prescriber of dyspnea, vomiting, cramping, drowsiness, headache, nasal congestion
• Caution patient to avoid OTC products (cough, hay fever), since these preparations may contain EPINEPHrine and decrease product response; do not use with alcohol
• Advise patient to carry/wear emergency ID or other identification specifying disease and medication used
• Advise patient if dose is missed, take when remembered, up to 1 hr before next dose; do not double doses; avoid fluids from 1 hr to up to 8 hr after PO dose

---

- Teach patient to report upper respiratory infection, nasal congestion
- How to use subcut, rotate sites

Evaluation

Positive therapeutic outcome

- Absence of severe thirst
- Decreased urine output, osmolality
- Absence of bleeding (hemophilia)

---

desonide topical
See Appendix B

desoximetasone topical
See Appendix B

desvenlafaxine (Rx)
Khedezla, Pristiq
Func. class.: Antidepressant
Chem. class.: Serotonin receptor norepinephrine reuptake inhibitor (SNRI)

Do not confuse: Pristiq/PriLOSEC

ACTION: May work by blocking the central presynaptic reuptake of 5-HT and NE, resulting in an increased sustained level of these neurotransmitters.

Therapeutic outcome: Decreased depression, increased sense of well-being and renewed interest in activities

USES: Major depressive disorder

Unlabeled uses: Vasomotor symptoms (hot flashes) associated with menopause

Pharmacokinetics

Absorption	Unknown
Distribution	Protein binding 30%; enters breast milk
Metabolism	Liver, 55%
Excretion	Urine, unchanged, 45%
Half-life	Elimination 11 hr, increased in hepatic/renal disease

Pharmacodynamics

Onset	Unknown
Peak	7.5 hr
Duration	24 hr

CONTRAINDICATIONS

Hypersensitivity to this product or venlafaxine, MAOI therapy

Precautions: CNS depression, abrupt discontinuation, hypertension, hepatic/renal disease, hyponatremia, geriatric patients, pregnancy, labor and delivery, breastfeeding, angina, bleeding, cardiac dysrhythmias, MI, stroke, mania, hypovolemia, dehydration, increased intraocular pressure

> **BLACK BOX WARNING:** Children, suicidal ideation

DOSAGE AND ROUTES
Adult: PO Initially, 50 mg daily; max 400 mg/day with adjustments as needed

Renal/hepatic dose
Adult: PO CCr 30-50 ml/min 50 mg daily; CCr <30 ml/min or end-stage renal disease 50 mg every other day; moderate to severe hepatic disease, max 100 mg/day

Available forms: Ext rel tabs 25, 50, 100 mg

ADVERSE EFFECTS
CNS: *Dizziness,* drowsiness, *headache,* tremor, paresthesias, asthenia, suicidal thoughts and behaviors, seizures, chills, yawning, hot flashes, flushing, *irritability, insomnia, anxiety, abnormal dreams, fatigue*
CV: Palpitations, sinus tachycardia, increased blood pressure, orthostatic hypotension
EENT: Blurred vision, mydriasis, tinnitus, bruxism
GI: *Nausea,* xerostomia, *diarrhea,* constipation, vomiting, anorexia, weight loss, dysgeusia, hypercholesterolemia, hypertriglyceridemia
GU: Urinary retention/hesitancy, orgasm dysfunction, decreased libido, impotence, proteinuria
HEMA: Impaired platelet aggregation
INTEG: Photosensitivity, hyperhidrosis, diaphoresis, rash
SYST: Serotonin syndrome, neuroleptic malignant syndrome-like symptoms, toxic epidermal necrolysis, Stevens-Johnson syndrome, erythema multiforme, angioedema; neonatal abstinence syndrome (fetal exposure)

INTERACTIONS
Individual drugs
Dexfenfluramine, dexmethylphenidate, dextromethorphan, fenfluramine, linezolid, lithium, nefazodone, meperidine, methylphenidate, mirtazapine, pentazocine, phentermine, promethazine, sibutramine, SUMAtriptan, traZODone, tryptophan: do not administer concurrently; increased serotonin syndrome, neuroleptic malignant syndrome-like reactions
Zolpidem: increased hallucinations, delusions, disorientation

Drug classifications
Anticoagulants, NSAIDs, platelet inhibitors, salicylates, thrombolytics: increased bleeding risk

---

Alcohol, antihistamines, opioids, sedatives/
hypnotics: increased CNS depression
Ergots, MAOIs, serotonin receptor agonists
(almotriptan, eletriptan, frovatriptan,
methylene blue IV, naratriptan, rizatriptan,
SUMAtriptan, ZOLMitriptan), SSRIs, other
SNRIs, TCAs, tricyclics: do not administer
concurrently; increased serotonin
syndrome, neuroleptic malignant syndrome-like reactions

Drug/herb
Kava, valerian: increased desvenlafaxine action

Drug/lab test
Increased: sodium, cholesterol, triglycerides
False positive: amphetamine, phencyclidine

NURSING CONSIDERATIONS
Assessment

> **BLACK BOX WARNING: Suicidal thoughts/
> behaviors:** Assess mental status and mood,
> identify suicidal ideation

• **Serotonin syndrome, neuroleptic malignant syndrome-like symptoms:** Assess
for nausea/vomiting, sedation, dizziness,
diaphoresis (sweating), facial flush, hallucinations, mental status changes, myoclonia, restlessness, shivering, elevated blood pressure,
hyperthermia, muscle rigidity, autonomic instability, and mental status changes; if serotonin
syndrome occurs discontinue desvenlafaxine,
and any other serotonergic agents
• **Serious skin reactions:** assess during
treatment and after, discontinue product
immediately if rash develops
• Monitor B/P baseline and periodically during
treatment, lipid levels, signs of glaucoma
• Assess appetite and nutritional intake, weight loss
is common, change diet as need to support weight

Patient problem
Depression (uses)
Risk for injury (adverse reaction)

Patient/family education
• Teach patient to take as directed, not to
double or skip doses; if a dose is missed, take as
soon as remembered unless close to next dose,
do not discontinue abruptly, decreased gradually

> **BLACK BOX WARNING:** Advise patient to
> report immediately suicidal thoughts or behav-
> iors, have family members look for symptoms
> of suicidal ideation

• Inform patient not to operate machinery or
engage in hazardous activities until reaction is
known, may cause dizziness, drowsiness

• Teach patient to avoid all others products
unless approval by prescriber
• Teach patient to report if pregnancy is planned
or suspected, pregnancy, or if breastfeeding
• **Serious skin reactions:** Teach patient
to report immediately allergic reactions
including, rash, hives, difficulty breathing, or
swelling of face, lips
• Advise patient that continuing follow-up
exams will be needed
• **Serotonin syndrome, neuroleptic malignant syndrome:** Teach patient to report
immediately nausea, vomiting, sedation,
dizziness, sweating, facial flush
• **Pregnancy/breastfeeding:** Identify if pregnancy is planned or suspected or if breastfeeding

Evaluation
Positive therapeutic outcome
• Decreased depression, increased sense of
well-being and renewed interest in activities

> **RARELY USED**
> # deutetrabenazine
> Austedo

USES: For the treatment of chorea associated
with Huntington's disease or tardive dyskinesia

DOSAGE AND ROUTES
(Huntington's chorea) or tardive dyskinesia
Adult: PO in treatment-naive patients (patients
not switching from tetrabenazine) initially, 6 mg
qday, increase at weekly intervals by increments
of 6 mg/day to a max of 48 mg/day; in patients
switching from tetrabenazine: Discontinue tetrabenazine and start deutetrabenazine the next day.
Current tetrabenazine dosage of 12.5 mg/day,
initiate deutetrabenazine 6 mg once daily; tetrabenazine 25 mg/day, initiate deutetrabenazine
6 mg twice daily; tetrabenazine 37.5 mg/day,
initiate deutetrabenazine 9 mg twice daily; tetrabenazine 50 mg/day, initiate deutetrabenazine
12 mg twice daily; tetrabenazine 62.5 mg/day,
initiate deutetrabenazine 15 mg twice daily; tetrabenazine 75 mg/day, initiate deutetrabenazine
18 mg twice daily; tetrabenazine 87.5 mg/day,
initiate deutetrabenazine 21 mg twice daily; tetrabenazine 100 mg/day, initiate deutetrabenazine
24 mg twice daily

Contraindications
Hypersensitivity, hepatic disease, MAOIs

> **BLACK BOX WARNING:** Suicidal ideation

dexamethasone (Rx)

(dex-ah-meth′ah-sone)

Decadron, Dexasone ✱, DoubleDex, DexPak, Dxevo

Func. class.: Corticosteroid, synthetic

Chem. class.: Glucocorticoid, long-acting

Do not confuse: **Decadron**/Percodan

ACTION: Decreases inflammation by suppressing migration of polymorphonuclear leukocytes, fibroblasts, reversing increased capillary permeability and lysosomal stabilization, suppresses normal immune response, no mineralocorticoid effects

USES: Inflammation, allergies, neoplasms, cerebral edema, septic shock, collagen disorders, dexamethasone suppression test for Cushing syndrome, adrenocortical insufficiency, TB, meningitis, acute exacerbations of MS

Pharmacokinetics

Absorption	Unknown
Distribution	Unknown
Metabolism	Liver
Excretion	Kidneys
Half-life	1-2 days

Pharmacodynamics

	PO	IM	IV
Onset	1 hr	1 hr	1 hr
Peak	1-2 hr	1 hr	1 hr
Duration	2½ days	6 days-3 wk	Varies

CONTRAINDICATIONS

Psychosis, hypersensitivity to corticosteroids, sulfites, or benzyl alcohol, idiopathic thrombocytopenia, acute glomerulonephritis, amebiasis, fungal infections, nonasthmatic bronchial disease, child <2 yr, AIDS, TB, glaucoma, ocular infection

Precautions: Pregnancy, breastfeeding, diabetes mellitus, osteoporosis, seizure disorders, ulcerative colitis, HF, myasthenia gravis, renal disease, peptic ulcer, esophagitis, recent MI, hypertension, TB, active hepatitis, psychosis, sulfite hypersensitivity, thromboembolic disorders, abrupt discontinuation, coagulopathy, ulcerative colitis, seizure disorders

DOSAGE AND ROUTES

Inflammatory condition

Adult: PO 0.75-9 mg/day, in divided doses q6-12hr; or phosphate IM 0.5-9 mg/day divided q6-12hr

Child: PO 0.024-0.34 mg/kg/day in divided doses q6-12hr

Shock

Adult: **IV** (phosphate) single dose 1-6 mg/kg or **IV** 40 mg q2-6hr as needed up to 72 hr

Airway edema/extubation

Adult: PO/IM/IV 0.5-2 mg/kg/day divided q6hr, use 24 hr before extubation

Chemotherapy-induced vomiting

Adult: PO/IV 10-28 mg 15-30 min before chemotherapy or 10 mg q12hr on each treatment day

Child: IV 5-20 mg 15-30 min before chemotherapy

Cerebral edema

Adult: **IV** (phosphate) 10 mg, then 4-6 mg IM q6hr × 2-4 days, then taper over 1 wk

Child: PO/IM/**IV** loading dose 1-2 mg/kg, then 1-1.5 mg/kg/day, max 16 mg/day divided q4-6hr for 2-4 days, then taper down qwk

Palliative management of recurrent or inoperable brain tumors

Adult: IM/IV 2 mg bid-tid maintenance

Adrenocortical insufficiency

Adult: PO 0.75-9 mg/day in divided doses

Child: PO 0.03-0.3 mg/kg/day divided in 2-4 doses

Suppression test for Cushing's syndrome

Adult: PO 1 mg at 11 PM or 0.5 mg q6hr × 48 hr

Available forms: Tabs 0.5, 0.75, 1, 1.5, 2, 4, 6 mg; oral sol 0.5 mg/5 ml, 1 mg/ml; injection 4 mg/mL, 10 mg/mL

ADVERSE EFFECTS

CNS: *Depression,* headache, mood changes, euphoria, psychosis, seizures

CV: *Hypertension*

EENT: Increased intraocular pressure, blurred vision, cataracts

ENDO: Phenochromocytoma, adrenal suppression, hyperglycemia

GI: *Nausea,* peptic ulceration, vomiting

INTEG: Acne, poor wound healing, ecchymosis, petechiae, hirsutism

META: Hypokalemia, fluid retention, hypokalemic alkalosis

MS: Fractures, osteoporosis, weakness, arthralgia, myopathy

MISC: Cushingoid symptoms

INTERACTIONS

Individual drugs

Alcohol, amphotericin B, cycloSPORINE, digoxin, indomethacin: increased side effects

Ambemonium, isoniazid, neostigmine, sometrem: decreased effects of each specific product

Bosentan, carBAMazepine, cholestyramine, colestipol, ePHEDrine, ethotoin, phenytoin, rifAMPin, theophylline: decreased action of dexamethasone

CycloSPORINE, tacrolimus: increased effect of each drug

Ketoconazole, NSAIDs: increased action of dexamethasone

Drug classifications

Antacids, barbiturates: decreased action of dexamethasone

Antibiotics (macrolide), contraceptives (hormonal), estrogens, salicylates: increased action of dexamethasone

Anticholinesterases, anticoagulants, anticonvulsants, antidiabetics, salicylates, toxoids/vaccines: decreased effects of each specific product

Antidiabetics: decreased effect of these products

Diuretics, NSAIDs, salicylates: increased side effects

Quinolones: decreased risk of tendinitis, tendon rupture

Thiazide diuretics: decreased potassium levels/ loop, amphotericin B

Drug/lab test

Increased: cholesterol, Na, blood glucose

Decreased: Ca, potassium, T_4, T_3, thyroid ^{131}I uptake test

False negative: skin allergy tests

NURSING CONSIDERATIONS
Assessment

• Monitor blood, urine glucose, potassium while on long-term therapy; hypokalemia and hyperglycemia, may occur

• Monitor weight daily; notify prescriber of weekly gain >5 lb

• Monitor B/P, pulse; notify of significant changes

• Monitor I&O ratio; be alert for decreasing urinary output, increasing edema

• **Cerebral edema:** LOC and headache, baseline and periodically

• **Adrenal insufficiency:** weight loss, nausea, vomiting, anorexia, confusion, decreased B/P, baseline and periodically

• **Epidural injections (unlabeled):** may cause rare events (vision loss, paralysis, stroke, death)

• Monitor plasma cortisol levels during long-term therapy (normal: 138-635 nmol/L when assessed at 8 AM), prolonged use can cause **cushingoid symptoms** (buffalo hump, moon face, increased B/P)

• **Assess infection:** fever, WBC even after withdrawal of medication; product masks infection

• **Assess potassium depletion:** paresthesias, fatigue, nausea, vomiting, depression, polyuria, dysrhythmias, weakness

• Assess edema, hypertension, cardiac symptoms

• Assess mental status: affect, mood, behavioral changes, aggression

• **Abrupt withdrawal:** acute adrenal insufficiency and death may occur following abrupt discontinuation of systemic therapy; withdraw gradually

• **Pregnancy/breastfeeding:** No well-controlled studies, use only if benefits outweigh fetal risk, discontinue breastfeeding or product

Patient problem

Risk for infection (adverse reaction)

Risk for injury (adverse reactions)

Implementation
PO route

• Give with food or milk to decrease GI symptoms

• Provide assistance with ambulation in patient with bone tissue disease to prevent fractures, give once a day in AM for less toxicity, less adverse reactions

IM route

• IM inj deep in large muscle mass; rotate sites; avoid deltoid; use 21-G needle

• In one dose in AM to prevent adrenal suppression; avoid SUBCUT administration, may damage tissue

Intraarticular/intralesion

• Use rarely as injections may damage joints

Direct IV route (sodium phosphate)

• **IV** undiluted direct over 1 min or less

• Titrated dose; use lowest effective dose

Intermittent IV infusion route

• Diluted with 0.9% NaCl or D_5W and give as an **IV** inf at prescribed rate

Continuous IV infusion

Change solution q 24 h

Y-site compatibilities: Acetaminophen, acyclovir, alfentanil, allopurinol, amifostine, amikacin, aminocaproic acid, aminophylline, amphotericin B cholesteryl, amphotericin B lipid complex, amphotericin B liposome, amsacrine, anidulafungin, argatroban, ascorbic acid injection, atenolol, atracurium, atropine, aztreonam, benztropine, bivalirudin, bleomycin, bumetanide, buprenorphine, butorphanol, CARBOplatin, carmustine, ceFAZolin, cefepime, cefonicid, cefoTEtan, cefOXitin, cefpirome, ceftaroline, cefTAZidime, ceftizoxime, cefTRIAXone, chloramphenicol, cimetidine, cisatracurium, CISplatin, cladribine, clindamycin, codeine, cyanocobalamin, cyclophosphamide, cycloSPORINE, cytarabine, DACTINomycin, DAPTOmycin, DAUNOrubicin liposome, dexmedetomidine, digoxin, dilTIAZem, DOCEtaxel, DOPamine, doripenem, doxacurium, DOXOrubicin, DOXOrubicin liposomal, enalaprilat, ePHEDrine, EPINEPHrine, epoetin alfa, eptifibatide, ertapenem, etoposide, etoposide phosphate, famotidine, fentaNYL, filgrastim, fluconazole, fludarabine, fluorouracil, folic acid, fosaprepitant, foscarnet, furosemide, ganciclovir, gatifloxacin, gemcitabine, glycopyrrolate, granisetron, heparin, hydrocortisone, HYDROmorphone, ifosfamide, imipenem-cilastatin, indomethacin, insulin (regular), irinotecan, isoproterenol, ketorolac, lansoprazole, leucovorin, levofloxacin, lidocaine, linezolid, liposome, LORazepam, LR, mannitol, mechlorethamine, melphalan, meropenem, metaraminol, methadone, methyldopate, methylPREDNISolone, metoclopramide, metoprolol, metroNIDAZOLE, mezlocillin, milrinone, morphine, multiple vitamins injection, nafcillin, nalbuphine, naloxone, nitroglycerin, nitroprusside, norepinephrine, octreotide, ondansetron, oxacillin, oxaliplatin, oxyCODONE, oxytocin, PACLitaxel, palonosetron, pamidronate, pancuronium, PEMEtrexed, penicillin G potassium/sodium, PENTobarbital, PHENobarbital, phenylephrine, phytonadione, piperacillin, piperacillin-tazobactam, potassium chloride, procainamide, propofol, propranolol, pyridoxine, raNITIdine, remifentanil, Ringer's, ritodrine, riTUXimab, sargramostim, sodium acetate/bicarbonate, succinylcholine, SUFentanil, tacrolimus, telavancin, teniposide, theophylline, thiamine, thiotepa, ticarcillin, ticarcillin-clavulanate, tigecycline, tirofiban, TNA, tolazoline, topotecan, trastuzumab, urokinase, vancomycin, vasopressin, vecuronium, verapamil, vinCRIStine, vinorelbine, vitamin B complex/C, voriconazole, zidovudine, zoledronic acid

Patient/family education
• Advise that emergency ID as corticosteroid user should be carried or worn
• Teach to notify prescriber if therapeutic response decreases; dosage adjustment may be needed
• Teach not to discontinue abruptly or adrenal crisis can result
• Teach to avoid OTC products: salicylates, alcohol in cough products, cold preparations unless directed by prescriber
• Instruct patient to contact prescriber if surgery, trauma, stress occurs, dosage may need to be adjusted
• Teach patient all aspects of product use, including cushingoid symptoms
• Instruct patient to notify prescriber of infection
• Teach patient to take with food or milk
• Teach patient that bruising may occur easily

• Teach patient that if on long-term therapy, a high-protein diet may be needed
• Teach symptoms of adrenal insufficiency: nausea, anorexia, fatigue, dizziness, dyspnea, weakness, joint pain
• Advise patient to avoid exposure to chickenpox or measles, persons with infections

Evaluation
Positive therapeutic outcome
Decreased inflammation

dexamethasone ophthalmic
See Appendix B

dexlansoprazole (Rx)
(dex-lan-so-prey′zole)
Dexilant
Func. class.: Anti-ulcer–proton pump inhibitor
Chem. class.: Benzimidazole

ACTION: Suppresses gastric secretion by inhibiting hydrogen/potassium ATPase enzyme system in gastric parietal cell; characterized as gastric acid pump inhibitor, since it blocks final step of acid production

Therapeutic outcome: Reduction in gastric pain, swelling, fullness

USES: Gastroesophageal reflux disease (GERD), severe erosive esophagitis, heartburn

Pharmacokinetics

Absorption	57%-64%
Distribution	Protein binding 97%
Metabolism	Liver extensively 🐾 by CYP2C19/CYP3A4; 15%-20% of Asian patients, 3%%-5% of Black and Caucasian patients are poor metabolizers
Excretion	Urine, feces; clearance decreased in geriatric, renal/hepatic disease
Half-life	Plasma 1-2 hr, 4-5 hr

Pharmacodynamics
Unknown

CONTRAINDICATIONS
Hypersensitivity

Precautions: Pregnancy, breastfeeding, children, proton-pump hypersensitivity, gastric cancer, hepatic disease, vit B_{12} deficiency, colitis

DOSAGE AND ROUTES
Erosive esophagitis
Adult/child >12 yr: PO 60 mg qd for up to 8 wk; maintenance: PO 30 mg qd for up to 6 mo
GERD
Adult/child >12 yr: PO: 30 mg qd × 4 wk
Hepatic disease
Adult: PO (Child-Pugh D). max 30 mg/day

Available forms: Del rel caps 30, 60 mg

ADVERSE EFFECTS
CNS: Headache, dizziness, confusion, agitation, amnesia, depression, anxiety, seizures, insomnia
CV: Chest pain, angina, bradycardia, palpitations, CVA, hypertension, MI
EENT: Tinnitus
GI: Diarrhea, abdominal pain, vomiting, nausea, constipation, flatulence, colitis, dysgeusia, pseudomembranous colitis
HEMA: Anemia, neutropenia, thrombocytopenia, pernicious anemia, thrombosis
INTEG: Rash, urticaria, pruritus
META: Gout
MS: Arthralgia, myalgia
RESP: Upper respiratory infections, cough, epistaxis, dyspnea
SYST: Anaphylaxis, Stevens-Johnson syndrome, toxic epidermal necrolysis, exfoliative dermatitis, pneumonia

INTERACTIONS
Individual drugs
Ampicillin, calcium carbonate, delavirdine, iron, itraconazole, ketoconazole: decreased absorption of each specific product
Drug classifications
CYP2C19, CYP3A4 (fluvoxamine, voriconazole): increased dexlansoprazole effect
Sucralfate: delayed absorption of dexlansoprazole
Drug/herb
Decrease: dexlansoprazole effect, St. John's wort
Drug/lab test
Increased: LFTs, bilirubin, creatinine, glucose, lipids
Decreased: platelets, magnesium

NURSING CONSIDERATIONS
Assessment
• **CDAD:** diarrhea, abdominal cramps, fever, report to prescriber promptly (rare)
• Anaphylaxis, serious skin disorders requiring emergency intervention (rare)
• **Hepatotoxicity:** Hepatitis, jaundice, monitor liver enzymes (AST, ALT, alkaline phosphatase) during treatment if hepatic adverse reactions occur (rare)

• **Hypomagnesemia:** Usually 3 months to 1 yr after beginning therapy; monitor magnesium level, assess for irregular heart beats, muscle spasms; in children fatigue, upset stomach, dizziness; magnesium supplement may be used
• **Pregnancy/breastfeeding:** use only if clearly needed, no well-controlled studies, discontinue breastfeeding or product, excretion unknown
• **Beers:** Avoid scheduled use >8 wk in older adults who are at high risk for erosive esophagitis, pathological hypersecretory conditions

Patient problem
Pain (uses)
Implementation
• Swallow del rel cap whole; do not break, crush, chew; caps may be opened and contents sprinkled on food, use immediately; do not chew contents of caps, give without regard to food
Patient/family education
• **CDAD:** report to prescriber at once abdominal cramps, bloody diarrhea, fever
• Inform diabetic patient that hypoglycemia may occur
• Encourage patient to avoid hazardous activities; dizziness may occur
• Tell patient to avoid alcohol, salicylates, ibuprofen; may cause GI irritation
• Teach patient to report allergic reactions, symptoms of low magnesium levels
• Teach patient to notify prescriber if pregnancy is planned or suspected, not to breastfeed
• Advise patient to swallow cap whole, not to chew, crush, to report all products being used to prescriber
Evaluation
Positive therapeutic outcome
• Absence of gastric pain, swelling, fullness; healing of erosive esophagitis

dexmedetomidine (Rx)
(deks-med-ee-tome_a-dine)
Precedex
Func. class.: Sedative/hypnotic

ACTION: Produces alpha-agonist activity as seen at low and moderate doses

USES: Sedation in mechanically ventilated, intubated patients in ICU

Pharmacokinetics

Absorption	Rapid
Distribution	Protein binding 94%
Metabolism	Liver
Excretion	Urine
Half-life	2 hr

Pharmacodynamics

Onset	Unknown
Peak	Unknown
Duration	Unknown

CONTRAINDICATIONS
Hypersensitivity, chronic hypertension

Precautions
Pregnancy, breastfeeding, children, geriatric, respiratory depression, severe respiratory disorders, cardiac dysrhythmias, hypovolemia, diabetes, CV/renal/hepatic disease

DOSAGE AND ROUTES
Adult IV loading dose of 1 mcg/kg over 10 min, then 0.2-0.7 mcg/kg/hr; do not use for more than 24 hr

Available forms
Inj 100 mcg/ml

ADVERSE EFFECTS
CV: *Bradycardia, hypo/hypertension,* atrial fibrillation, infarction, cardiac arrest
GI: Nausea, thirst
GU: Oliguria
HEMA: Leukocytosis, anemia
MISC: Hyperkalemia
RESP: Pulmonary edema, pleural effusion, hypoxia, respiratory acidosis

INTERACTIONS
Individual drugs
Alcohol: increased CNS depression

Drug classifications
Anesthetics (inhalational), antipsychotics, opiates, sedative/hypnotics, skeletal muscle relaxants: increased CNS depression
Antihypertensives: increased hypotension

NURSING CONSIDERATIONS
Assessment
• Assess inj site: phlebitis, burning, stinging
• Monitor ECG for changes: atrial fibrillation; monitor geriatric more closely
• Assess CNS changes: movement, jerking, tremors, dizziness, LOC, pupil reaction
• Assess respiratory dysfunction: respiratory depression, character, rate, rhythm; notify prescriber if respirations are <10/min
• Assess cardiac status: B/P, heart rate

Patient problems
Risk for injury (uses)

Implementation
Continuous IV infusion route
• Give after diluting with 0.9% NaCl; withdraw 2 ml of product and add to 48 ml of 0.9% NaCl to a total of 50 ml (4 mcg/ml); shake gently to mix well; use controlled infusion device
• Give only with resuscitative equipment available
• Give loading dose over 10 min by continuous IV infusion, do not give by bol or rapid IV inj, use for 24 hr
• Give only by qualified persons trained in management of ICU sedation

Solution compatibilities: LR, D5W, 0.9% NaCl, 20% mannitol

Y-site compatibilities: Acyclovir, alfentanil, allopurinol, amifostine, amikacin, aminocaproic acid, aminophylline, amiodarone, amphotericin B liposome, ampicillin, ampicillin/sulbactam, anidulafungin, atenolol, atracurium, atropine, azithromycin, aztreonam, bivalirudin, bleomycin, bumetanide, buprenorphine, busulfan, butorphanol, calcium chloride/gluconate, CARBOplatin, carmustine, caspofungin, ceFAZolin, cefepime, cefoperazone, cefotaxime, cefotetan, cefoxitin, ceftazidime, ceftizoxime, cefTRIAXone, cefuroxime, chlorproMAZINE, cimetidine, ciprofloxacin, cisatracurium, CISplatin, clindamycin, cyclophosphamide, cycloSPORINE, cytarabine, dacarbazine, DACTINomycin, DAPTOmycin, DAUNOrubicin, dexamethasone, dexrazoxane, digoxin, diltiazem, diphenhydrAMINE, DOBUTamine, docetaxel, dolasetron, DOPamine, doxacurium, DOXOrubicin, doxycycline, droperidol, enalaprilat, ePHEDrine, EPINEPHrine, ertapenem, erythromycin, esmolol, etomidate, etoposide, famotidine, fenoldopam, fentaNYL, fluconazole, fludarabine, fluorouracil, foscarnet, fosphenytoin, furosemide, ganciclovir, gatifloxacin, gemcitabine, gentamicin, glycopyrrolate, granisetron, haloperidol, heparin, hydrocortisone, HYDROmorphone, hydrOXYzine, IDArubicin, ifosfamide, imipenem-cilastatin, inamrinone, insulin (regular), isoproterenol, ketorolac, labetalol, leucovorin, levofloxacin, levorphanol, lidocaine, linezolid, LORazepam, magnesium sulfate, mannitol, mechlorethamine, meperidine, meropenem, mesna, methohexital, methotrexate, methylPREDNISolone, metoclopramide, metoprolol, metroNIDAZOLE, midazolam, milrinone, minocycline, mitomycin, mitoxantrone, mivacurium, morphine, mycophenolate mofetil, nalbuphine, naloxone, nesiritide, niCARdipine, nitroglycerin, nitroprusside, norepinephrine, octreotide, oflaxacin, ondansetron, oxaliplatin, oxytocin, paclitaxel, palonosetron, pamidronate, pancuronium, pemetrexed, pentamidine, PENTobarbital, PHENobarbital, phenylephrine, piperacillin, piperacillin-tazobactam, potassium chloride/phosphates, procainamide, prochlorperazine, promethazine, propofol, propranolol, quinupristin-dalfopristin, ranitidine, rapacuronium, remifentanil, rocuronium, sodium acetate/bicarbonate/phosphates, succinylcholine, SUFentanil, sulfamethoxazole-trimethoprim, tacrolimus, teniposide, theophylline, thiopental, thiotepa, ticarcillin, ticarcillin-clavulanate, tigecycline, tirofiban, tobramycin, topotecan, vancomycin, vasopressin, vecuronium, verapamil, vinBLAStine, vinCRIStine, vinorelbine, voriconazole, zidovudine, zoledronic acid

Patient/family education
• Explain reason for treatment, expected results

Evaluation
Positive therapeutic outcome
• Induction of sedation

dexrazoxane (Rx)
(dex-ra-zox'ane)
Totect
Func. class.: Cardioprotective

ACTION: Acts as an intracellular heavy metal chelator and protects against anthracycline-induced free radical damage to the myocardium

Therapeutic outcome: Removes iron and aluminum

USES: Anthracycline-induced cardiomyopathy prophylaxis; treatment of extravasation resulting from IV anthracycline chemotherapy

Pharmacokinetics
Absorption	Complete
Distribution	Unknown
Metabolism	Liver
Excretion	Kidneys (42%)
Half-life	2-2.5 hr

Pharmacodynamics
Onset	Immediate
Peak	Unknown
Duration	Unknown

CONTRAINDICATIONS
Hypersensitivity, pregnancy

Precautions: Renal disease, breastfeeding, children

DOSAGE AND ROUTES
Anthracycline-induced cardiomyopathy prophylaxis
Adults: IV Give in a 10:1 ratio to doxorubicin (e.g., 500 mg/m^2 dexrazoxane to 50 mg/m^2 doxorubicin); give prior to doxorubicin

Treatment of extravasation resulting from IV anthracycline chemotherapy
Adults: IV (Totect) 1,000 mg/m^2 IV (max 2,000 mg) on days 1 and 2 and then dexrazoxane 500 mg/m^2 IV (max 1,000 mg) on day 3; give over 1 to 2 hr via a large caliber vein in an extremity/area other than the one affected by the extravasation. Begin the first infusion as soon as possible and within the 6 hr after extravasation. Infusions on days 2 and 3 should start at the same hour (or within 3 hrs) as on the first day. Regularly monitor the extravasation site after treatment and until resolution

Available forms: Injection (Totect) 500 mg/vial

ADVERSE EFFECTS
INTEG: Pain at injection site
HEMA: Thrombocytopenia, neutropenia, leukopenia
SYST: Secondary malignancy

INTERACTIONS
Individual drugs
Cyclophosphamide, fluorouracil: Decreased chemotherapy effect

Drug classifications
Antineoplastics, radiation: Increase bone marrow suppression

NURSING CONSIDERATIONS
Assessment
• **Cardiac effects:** Assess for dyspnea, rales, left ventricular ejection fraction (LVEF) decline; if LVEF declines may need to discontinue
• Monitor CBC, LFTs (in those with liver disorders), BUN/creatinine (in those with renal disease) baseline and periodically
• **Iron Poisoning:** Assess type, amount time ingested, reason for ingesting; monitor for bloody vomiting and diarrhea, abdominal pain, nausea; metabolic acidosis, shock, death may occur late
• Monitor I&O, notify provider of significant changes
• Monitor vital signs during IV administration. Epinephrine, an antihistamine, and resuscitation equipment should be readily available in case of an anaphylactic reaction

Patient problems
Risk for injury (uses)

Implementation
IV route
- Visually inspect parenteral products for particulate matter and discoloration prior to use
- Use cytototoxic handling procedures
- **Cardioprotectate agent use:** Give doxorubicin within 30 min after the completion of dexrazoxane use
- Totect may be prepared in two different ways to produce the final solution for use
- The prepared solution is slightly yellow

Reconstitution:
- Add 50 mL of Sterile Water for Injection to the dexrazoxane 500 mg vial for a final vial concentration of 10 mg/mL
- *Storage after reconstitution:* Further dilute immediately or within 30 min; discard the unused portion of the vial

Dilution:
- Dilute 1,000 mL of Lactated Ringer's Injection.
- *Storage after dilution:* Use the diluted solution immediately or within 4 hr (from preparation time) when stored at room temperature (up to 25° C or 77° F) or within 12 hr when refrigerated (2 to 8° C or 36 to 46° F).

Reconstitution:
- Compound the diluent by adding 1.67 mL of 5 mEq/mL sodium lactate injection to 50 mL of Sterile Water for Injection to make 50 mL of a 0.167 molar sodium lactate injection solution.
- Add 50 mL of the 0.167 molar sodium lactate injection solution to the dexrazoxane 500 mg vial for a final vial concentration of 10 mg/mL
- *Storage after reconstitution:* Further dilute immediately or within 30 min; discard the unused portion of the vial

Dilution:
- Dilute the dose in 1000 mL of 0.9% sodium chloride injection
- *Storage after dilution:* Use the diluted solution immediately or within 4 hr (from preparation time) when stored at room temperature (up to 25° C or 77° F) or within 12 hr when refrigerated (2 to 8° C or 36 to 46° F).

IV infusion
- Give over 1 to 2 hr in a large caliber vein in an extremity/area other than the one affected by the extravasation; do NOT administer as an IV push
- Remove cooling devices (ice packs) from the extravasation area at least 15 min before use

Patient/family education
- Teach patient reason for medication and expected results

- Teach patient to report if pregnancy is planned or suspected or if breastfeeding

Evaluation
Positive therapeutic outcome
- Prevention of cardiac toxicity
- Prevention of necrosis, nerve damage from extravasation

---

dextromethorphan (OTC)
(dex-troe-meth-or′fan)
Balminil DM ✶, Benylin DM ✶, Bronchophan Forte DM ✶, Buckley's Mixture, Delsym 12-Hour, ElixSure Cough, Koffex ✶, Robafen Cough Gels, Robitussin, Robitussin Cough with Honey, Robitussin Long-Acting Cough, Scot-Tussin Diabetes CF, Triaminic Long-Acting Cough, Vicks Formula 44 Cough Relief, Cough Syrup DM ✶, Creo-Terpin, Wal-Tussin
Func. class.: Antitussive, nonopioid
Chem. class.: Levorphanol derivative

ACTION: Depresses cough center in medulla by direct effect related to levorphanol

Therapeutic outcome: Absence of cough

USES: Nonproductive cough carried by minor respiratory tract infections or irritants that might be inhaled

Pharmacokinetics

Absorption	Rapid (PO); slow (SUS REL)
Distribution	Unknown
Metabolism	Liver
Excretion	Kidneys
Half-life	Terminal 11 hr

Pharmacodynamics

	PO	PO-sus
Onset	15-30 min	Unknown
Peak	Unknown	Unknown
Duration	3-6 hr	12 hr

CONTRAINDICATIONS
Hypersensitivity, MAOIs, SSRIs

Precautions: Pregnancy, fever, hepatic disease, asthma/emphysema, chronic cough, child <4 yr, breastfeeding

DOSAGE AND ROUTES
Adult and child ≥12 yr: PO 10-20 mg q4hr, or 30 mg q6-8hr, max 120 mg/day; SUS REL LIQUID 60 mg q12hr, max 120 mg/day

---

Child 6-12 yr: PO 5-10 mg q4hr; SUS REL LIQUID 30 mg bid, max 60 mg/day; LOZENGE 5-10 mg q1-4hr, max 60 mg/day

Child 4-6 yr: PO 2.5-5 mg q 4 hr or 7.5 mg q 6-8 hr or 15 mg (Ext Rel) q 12 hr, max 30 mg/day

Available forms: Liquid, 3.5, 7.5, 15 mg/5 ml; syr 7.5 mg/5 mL, 15 mg/15 ml, 10 mg/5 ml; 15 mg/5 ml, 30 mg/15 ml; caps 15 mg; gel caps 30 mg; EXT REL SUSP 30 mg/5 ml; drops 7.5 mg/0.8 mL, 7.5 mg/1mL; orally disintegrating strips 7.5 mg, 15 mg

ADVERSE EFFECTS
CNS: *Dizziness*, sedation, confusion, ataxia, fatigue
GI: *Nausea*

INTERACTIONS
Individual drugs
Alcohol: increased CNS depression
Amiodarone, quiNIDine, sibutramine: increased adverse reactions

Drug classifications
Antihistamines, antidepressants, opiates, sedative-hypnotics: increased CNS depression
MAOIs: increased hypotension, hyperpy-rexia, do not give within 2 wk of MAOIs

NURSING CONSIDERATIONS
Assessment
• Assess **cough**: type, frequency, character, lung sounds including sputum; provide adequate hydration to 2 L/day to decrease viscosity of secretions unless contraindicated
• **Pregnancy/breastfeeding:** No well-controlled studies, use only if benefits out-weigh fetal risk, avoid use in breastfeeding

Patient problem
Impaired airway clearance (uses)

Implementation
• Give **chew tabs:** chew well; **syrup:** use cali-brated measuring device; **ext rel susp:** shake well, use calibrated measuring device
• Administer decreased dosage to geriatric patients; their metabolism may be slowed; do not provide water within 30 min of administra-tion because it dilutes product
• Shake susp before administration

Patient/family education
• Caution patient to avoid driving or other hazardous activities until stabilized on this medication; may cause drowsiness, dizziness in some individuals
• Advise patient to avoid smoking, smoke-filled rooms, perfumes, dust, environmental pollutants, cleaners, which increase cough; may use gum, hard candy to prevent dry mouth

• Advise patient to avoid alcohol or other CNS depressants while taking this medication; drowsiness will be increased
• Caution patient that any cough lasting over a few days should be assessed by prescriber
• Teach patient not to use if breastfeeding, or in child <4 yr

Evaluation
Positive therapeutic outcome
• Absence of dry, irritating cough

⚠ HIGH ALERT

diazePAM (Rx)
(dye-az'e-pam)
Diastat, Valium
Func. class.: Antianxiety, anticonvulsant, skeletal muscle relaxant, central acting
Chem. class.: Benzodiazepine, long-acting
Controlled substance schedule IV

Do not confuse: diazePAM/Ditropan/LORazepam

ACTION: Potentiates the actions of GABA, especially in limbic system, reticular formation; enhances presympathetic inhibition, inhibits spi-nal polysynaptic afferent paths

Therapeutic outcome: Decreased anxi-ety, restlessness, insomnia

USES: Anxiety, acute alcohol withdrawal, ad-junct in seizure disorders; preoperative skeletal muscle relaxation; rectally for acute repetitive seizures

Pharmacokinetics

Absorption	Rapid (PO); erratic (IM)
Distribution	Widely distributed; crosses blood-brain barrier, pla-centa; protein binding 99%
Metabolism	Liver, extensively, CYP2C19, CYP3A4 15%-20% of 🧬 Asian patients and up to 5% of Caucasians and Black pa-tients are poor metabolizers
Excretion	Kidneys, breast milk
Half-life	1-12 days

Pharmacodynamics

	PO	IM	IV
Onset	½ hr	15 min	Immediate
Peak	Peak 2 hr	½-1½ hr	15 min
Duration	Up to 24 hr	1-1½ hr	15 min-1 hr

CONTRAINDICATIONS

Pregnancy, hypersensitivity to benzodiazepines, closed angle glaucoma, coma, myasthenia gravis, ethanol intoxication, hepatic disease, sleep apnea

Precautions: Breastfeeding, geriatric, debilitated, addiction, child <6 mo, asthma, renal disease, bipolar disorder, COPD, CNS depression, labor, Parkinson's disease, neutropenia, psychosis, seizures, substance abuse, smoking

> **BLACK BOX WARNING:** Coadministration with other CNS depressants, respiratory depression

DOSAGE AND ROUTES
Anxiety/convulsive disorders

Adult: PO 2-10 mg bid-qid; IM/IV 2-10 mg q3-4hr
Geriatric: PO 2-2.5 mg daily-bid, increase slowly as needed
Child >6 mo: IM/IV 0.04-0.3 mg/kg/dose q2-4hr, max 0.6 mg/kg in an 8-hr period

Precardioversion

Adult: IV 5-15 mg 5-10 min precardioversion

Preendoscopy

Adult: IV 2.5-20 mg, IM 5-10 mg ½ hr preendoscopy

Muscle relaxation

Adult: PO 2-10 mg tid-qid or EXT REL 15-30 mg daily; IM/IV 5-10 mg repeat in 2-4 hr

Tetanic muscle spasms

Child >5 yr: IM/IV 5-10 mg q3-4hr prn
Infant >30 days: IM/IV 1-2 mg q3-4hr prn

Status epilepticus

Adult: IM/IV 5-10 mg, 2 mg/min, may repeat q10-15min; max 30 mg; may repeat in 2-4 hr if seizures reappear
Child >5 yr: IV 1 mg slowly; IM 1 mg q2-5min
Child 1 mo-5 yr: IV 0.2-0.5 mg slowly; IM 0.2-0.5 mg slowly q2-5min up to 5 mg; may repeat in 2-4 hr prn

Seizures other than status epilepticus

Adult: RECT 0.2 mg/kg, may repeat 4-12 hr later

Child 6-11 yr: RECT 0.3 mg/kg, may repeat 4-12 hr later
Child 2-5 yr: RECT 0.5 mg/kg, may repeat 4-12 hr later

Alcohol withdrawal

Adult: IV 10 mg initially, then 5-10 mg q3-4hr prn

Psychoneurotic reactions

Adult IM/IV 2-10 mg, may repeat in 3-4 hr

Available forms: Tabs 2, 5, 10 mg; inj 5 mg/ml; oral sol 5 mg/5 ml; rectal 2.5 (pediatric), 10, 20 mg, twin packs; ext rel cap 15 mg; rectal gel

ADVERSE EFFECTS

CNS: *Dizziness, drowsiness,* headache, depression, hangover, slurred speech, paradoxical excitation
CV: Hypotension
EENT: *Blurred vision*
GI: Constipation, dry mouth, nausea, vomiting, diarrhea, weight gain
HEMA: Neutropenia
INTEG: Rash, dermatitis, itching, phlebitis (IV), venous thrombosis
RESP: Respiratory depression
MISC: Psychological/physical dependency, tolerance

INTERACTIONS
Individual drugs

Alcohol: increased CNS depression
Amiodarone, cimetidine, clarithromycin, dalfopristin, delavirdine, dilTIAZem, disulfiram, efavirenz, erythromycin, fluconazole, fluvoxaMINE, imatinib, itraconazole, ketoconazole, IV miconazole, nefazodone, niCARdipine, quinupristin, ranolazine, troleandomycin, valproic acid, verapamil, voriconazole, zafirlukast, zileuton: increased diazePAM effect
Cimetidine, valproic acid: increased toxicity
CYP3A4 inducers (carBAMazepine, ethotoin, fosphenytoin, phenytoins, rifAMPin), smoking: decreased diazePAM effect, monitor for increased sedation
Disulfiram, isoniazid, propranolol, valproic acid: decreased metabolism of diazePAM

Drug classifications

Barbiturates, CNS depressants, CYP3A4 inhibitors, SSRIs: increased toxicity
CNS depressants: increased CNS depression
CYP3A4 inducers (barbiturates): decreased diazePAM effect
Oral contraceptives: decreased metabolism of diazePAM

Drug/herb

Increase: CNS depression, kava, chamomile, valerian

Drug/lab test
Increased: AST/ALT, alk phos

NURSING CONSIDERATIONS
Assessment
• **Assess for anxiety;** what precipitates anxiety and whether product controls symptoms; other signs of anxiety: dilated pupils, inability to sleep, restlessness, inability to focus
• **Assess for alcohol withdrawal symptoms,** including hallucinations (visual, auditory), delirium, irritability, agitation, fine to coarse tremors
• **IV site:** assess frequently, watch for phlebitis
• Monitor B/P (with patient lying, standing), pulse; if systolic B/P drops 20 mm Hg, hold product, notify prescriber
• Monitor blood studies: CBC during long-term therapy; blood dyscrasias have occurred (rarely); hepatic studies: ALT, AST

> **BLACK BOX WARNING:** Avoid coadministration with other CNS depressants, do not use with opioids

• **Respiratory depression:** Monitor for respiratory depression, respirations 5-15 min if given IV
• **Monitor for seizure control:** type, duration, and intensity of seizures; what precipitates seizures
• Monitor hepatic studies: AST, ALT, bilirubin, creatinine, LDH, alkaline phosphatase
• **Assess mental status:** mood, sensorium, affect, sleeping pattern, drowsiness, dizziness, suicidal tendencies, and ability of product to control these symptoms; check for tolerance, withdrawal symptoms: headache, nausea, vomiting, muscle pain, weakness after long-term use, high dose
• Assess for muscle spasms, pain relief
• **Pregnancy/breastfeeding:** Use in pregnancy not recommended, do not breastfeed, excreted in breast milk
• **Beers:** Avoid use in older adults, may be appropriate for seizures, sleep disorders, benzodiazepine/ethanol withdrawal, severe anxiety disorders

Patient problem
Anxiety (uses)
Risk for Injury (adverse reactions)

Implementation
PO route
• Crush tab if patient is unable to swallow medication whole, use with water, food
• Reduce opioid dosage by one third if given concomitantly with diazePAM

• Check to see if PO medication has been swallowed
• **Oral solution:** Use calibrated dropper only; mix with water, juice, pudding, applesauce; consume immediately
Rectal route
• Do not use more than 5 ×/mo or for an episode q5day (Diastat)

IM route
• Painful, use deltoid if IM is necessary

Direct IV route
• Have emergency equipment nearby
• Administer **IV** into large vein; do not dilute or mix with any other product; give **IV** 5 mg or less/min or total dose over 3 min or more (children, infants); cont inf is not recommended; inject closest vein insertion as possible; do not dilute or mix with other products
• Check **IV** site for thrombosis or phlebitis, which may occur rapidly
• Observe for several hours after IV, if used in combination with opioids, decrease opioid dose

Sterile emulsion for injection route
• Use **IV** only, within 6 hr, flush line after use and after 6 hr

Patient/family education
• Advise patient that product may be taken with food; that product is not to be used for everyday stress or used longer than 4 mo unless directed by prescriber; take no more than prescribed amount; may be habit forming, review package insert with patient, take exactly as prescribed
• Caution patient to avoid OTC preparations unless approved by a prescriber; to avoid alcohol, other psychotropic medications unless prescribed; that smoking may decrease diazePAM effect by increasing diazePAM metabolism; not to discontinue medication abruptly after long-term use, gradually taper
• Inform patient to avoid driving, activities that require alertness; drowsiness may occur; to rise slowly or fainting may occur, especially in geriatric
• Inform patient that drowsiness may worsen at beginning of treatment
• Teach patient to notify prescriber if pregnancy is planned or suspected, avoid breastfeeding

Evaluation
Positive therapeutic outcome
• Decreased anxiety, restlessness, insomnia

TREATMENT OF OVERDOSE:
Lavage, VS, supportive care, flumazenil

dibucaine topical
See Appendix B

diclofenac ophthalmic
See Appendix B

diclofenac (Rx)
Zorvorex
diclofenac epolamine (Rx)
(dye-kloe′fen-ak)
Flector
diclofenac potassium (Rx)
Cambia, Zipsor
diclofenac sodium
Voltaren Gel, Voltaren, Voltaren SR, Pennsaid, Solaraze
Func. class.: Nonsteroidal antiinflammatory drug (NSAID), nonopioid analgesic
Chem. class.: Phenylacetic acid

Do not confuse: Cataflam/Catapres

ACTION: Inhibits COX-1, COX-2 by blocking arachidonate, resulting in analgesic, antiinflammatory, antipyretic effects

Therapeutic outcome: Decreased pain, inflammation

USES: Acute, chronic rheumatoid arthritis, osteoarthritis, ankylosing spondylitis, analgesia, primary dysmenorrhea; patch: mild to moderate pain

Pharmacokinetics

Absorption	Well absorbed (PO, ophth)
Distribution	Crosses placenta; 99% bound to plasma proteins
Metabolism	Liver (50%)
Excretion	Breast milk
Half-life	1-2 hr, patch 12 hr

Pharmacodynamics

	PO	Ophth	TOP (Patch)
Onset	Unknown	Unknown	Unknown
Peak	2-3 hr	Unknown	12 hr
Duration	Unknown	Unknown	Unknown

CONTRAINDICATIONS
Hypersensitivity to aspirin, iodides, other NSAIDs, bovine protein; asthma, serious CV disease; eczema, exfoliative dermatitis, skin abrasions (gel patch); treatment of perioperative pain in CABG surgery

Precautions: Breastfeeding, children, bleeding disorders, GI/cardiac disorders, hypersensitivity to other antiinflammatory agents, CCr <30 ml/min, accidental exposure, acute bronchospasm, hypersensitivity to benzyl alcohol; pregnancy patch, top sol, cap, powder for oral solution (pregnancy <30 wk, D >30 wk)

> **BLACK BOX WARNING:** GI bleeding/perforation, MI, stroke

DOSAGE AND ROUTES
Osteoarthritis
Adult: PO (Cataflam) 50 mg bid-tid, max 150 mg/day; DEL REL (Voltaren) 50 mg bid-tid or 75 mg bid, max 150 mg/day; EXT REL (Voltaren-XR) 100 mg daily, max 150 mg/day; TOP gel 1% (Voltaren gel) 4 g for each lower extremity qid, max 16 g/day; 2 g for each upper extremity qid, max 8 g/day; TOP SOL (Pennsaid) apply 40 drops to each affected knee qid, apply 10 drops at a time, spread over entire knee

Rheumatoid arthritis
Adult: PO (Cataflam) 50 mg tid-qid, max 200 mg/day; DEL REL (Voltaren) 50 mg tid-qid or 75 mg bid, max 200 mg/day; EXT REL (Voltaren-XR) 100 mg qd, may increase to 200 mg/day, max 200 mg/day

Ankylosing spondylitis
Adult: PO DEL REL (Voltaren) 25 mg qid and 25 mg at bedtime, max 125 mg/day

Acute migraine with/without aura
Adult: PO (powder for oral SOL) (Cambia) 50 mg as a single dose; mix contents of packet in 1-2 oz water

Mild to moderate pain
Adult: PO (Zipsor) 25 mg qid

Dysmenorrhea or nonrheumatic inflammatory conditions
Adult: PO (Cataflam) 50 mg tid or 100 mg initially, then 50 mg tid, max 200 mg 1st day, then 150 mg/day, immediate release only

Pain of strains/sprains
Adult: TOP patch (Flector) apply patch to area bid

Actinic keratosis
Adult: TOP gel (Solaraze) apply to area bid

Hepatic dose
Adult: PO max 18 mg tid

Renal dose
Avoid use of top gel, patch, sol, potassium oral tab in advanced renal disease

Available forms: Epolamine: topical patch 1.3%; **potassium:** tabs 50 mg tabs, liquid filled 25 mg; **sodium:** del rel tabs (enteric-coated)

25, 50, 75, 100 mg; oral powder for sol 50 mg; topical gel 1%, 3%

ADVERSE EFFECTS
CNS: *Dizziness, headache*
CV: HF, hypertension, MI, stroke, edema
EENT: Tinnitus, hearing loss, blurred vision, laryngeal edema
GI: Nausea, anorexia, vomiting, diarrhea, constipation, flatulence, GI bleeding, hepatotoxicity,
GU: Nephrotoxicity: dysuria, hematuria, oliguria, azotemia, cystitis, UTI
HEMA: Anemia
INTEG: Rash, pruritus, photosensitivity, alopecia
SYST: Anaphylaxis, Stevens-Johnson syndrome, exfoliative dermatitis, toxic epidermal necrolysis

INTERACTIONS
Individual drugs
Aspirin: increased GI side effects
Cidofovir, cycloSPORINE, digoxin, lithium, methotrexate, phenytoin: increased toxicity

Drug classifications
ACE inhibitors, β-blockers, diuretics: decreased antihypertensive effect
Anticoagulants, NSAIDs, platelet inhibitors, salicylates, SSRIs, thrombolytics: increased risk of bleeding
Antidiabetic agents: increased need for dosage adjustment
Diuretics: decreased effect of these products
Diuretics (potassium-sparing): hyperkalemia
NSAIDs, bisphosphonates, corticosteroids: increased GI side effects

Drug/herb
Garlic, ginger, ginkgo: monitor for bleeding; increased bleeding risk

NURSING CONSIDERATIONS
Assessment
• **CABG:** do not use oral, top, gel, patch in perioperative pain in CABG surgery for 10-14 days

> **BLACK BOX WARNING: Stroke/MI:** may increase HF and hypertension, increased CV thrombotic events that may be fatal; those with CV disease may be at greater risk

• Assess for pain of rheumatoid arthritis, osteoarthritis, ankylosing spondylitis; check ROM, inflammation of joints, characteristics of pain
• Assess for asthma, aspirin hypersensitivity, nasal polyps; may develop hypersensitivity
• Actinic keratosis: Check lesions prior to use and periodically

• Monitor liver function tests (may be elevated) and uric acid (may be decreased in serum, increased in urine) periodically; also BUN, creatinine, electrolytes (may be elevated)
• **Serious skin disorders/anaphylaxis:** Assess for rash, if rash develops discontinue immediately, may be fatal
• **Stroke/MI:** Teach patient to notify prescriber immediately, seek medical attention if chest pain, slurred speech, weakness, shortness of breath occur
• **Beers:** Avoid chronic use in older adults unless other alternatives are not effective, increased risk of GI bleeding

Patient problem
Pain (uses)
Impaired mobility (uses)

Implementation
PO route
• Do not break, crush, chew, or dissolve enteric-coated or ext rel tabs
• Administer with food or milk to decrease gastric symptoms
• Remain upright for ½ hr
• Store at room temperature
Powder:
• Mix powder in 30-60 ml water only, mix solution, have patient drink immediately
• Powder (Cambia and Zorvolex) may be less effective if taken with food
• Zorvolex capsules aren't interchangeable with other formulations or oral product
Topical route (patch) (Flector)
• Wash hands before handling patch
• Remove and release liner before administering
• Use only on normal, intact skin
• Remove before bath, shower, swimming, do not use heat or occlusive dressings
• Discard removed patch in trash away from children, pets
• Store at room temperature
Topical route (gel)
• Apply to intact skin, do not use heat or occlusive dressings
• Use only for osteoarthritis: mild-moderate pain
• Store at room temperature, avoid heat, do not freeze
Ophthalmic route
• Administer with patient recumbent or tilting head back; pull down on lower lid; when conjunctival sac is exposed, instill 1 drop; wait a few minutes before instilling other drops

Patient/family education

• Teach patient that product must be continued for prescribed time to be effective; to avoid aspirin, NSAIDs, acetaminophen, or other OTC medications unless approved by prescriber, alcoholic beverages; to contact prescriber before surgery regarding when to discontinue this product

• Teach patient to notify prescriber immediately, stop product if rash occurs

• **Advise patient to report hepatotoxicity:** flulike symptoms, nausea, vomiting, jaundice, pruritus, lethargy

• Instruct patient to use sunscreen to prevent photosensitivity

• Instruct patient to use caution when driving; drowsiness, dizziness may occur

• Teach patient to take with a full glass of water to enhance absorption; remain upright for ½ hr; if dose is missed, take as soon as remembered within 2 hr if taking 1-2 ×/day; do not double doses

• **Gel:** Use dosing card to measure, do not apply where cosmetics, sunscreen have been applied

• **Transdermal:** Not to use in water (swimming/bathing), only use on intact skin, do not cover with occlusive dressing, if peeling occurs, apply adhesive tape or mesh sleeve

• Advise to notify all providers that product is being used

• Teach patient to notify prescriber if pregnancy is planned or suspected

Evaluation

Positive therapeutic outcome

• Decreased pain in arthritic conditions

• Decreased inflammation in arthritic conditions

• Decreased ocular irritation

dicloxacillin (Rx)

(dye-klox-a-sill′in)

Nallpen

Func. class.: Broad-spectrum antiinfective

Chem. class.: Penicillinase resistant penicillin, beta lactam

ACTION: Inhibits bacterial cell wall synthesis, rendering cell wall osmotically unstable, leading to cell death; action on penicillin binding protein

Therapeutic outcome: Bactericidal effects for the following: *Staphylococcus sp.*

USES: Treatment of infections due to penicillinase-producing *Staphylococcus sp.*, including bacteremia, skin and skin structure infections (including impetigo), bone and joint infections (osteomyelitis or infectious arthritis), pneumonia, or endocarditis; mastitis

Pharmacokinetics

Absorption	Up to 75%
Distribution	Widely distributed; enters breast milk, crosses placenta
Metabolism	Liver 10%
Excretion	Kidneys, 60%
Half-life	0.1-1 hr

Pharmacodynamics

Onset	30 min
Peak	30-120 min
Duration	6 hr

CONTRAINDICATIONS

Hypersensitivity to penicillins

Precautions: Pregnancy, breastfeeding, children, hypersensitivity to cephalosporins, renal/GI disease, geriatrics, CDAD, viral infection

DOSAGE AND ROUTES

Treatment of infections due to penicillinase-producing *Staphylococcus sp.*, including bacteremia, skin and skin structure infections (including impetigo), bone and joint infections (osteomyelitis or infectious arthritis), pneumonia, or endocarditis

Adults, adolescents, and children weighing ≥40 kg PO 125- 250 mg q 6 hr for mild to moderate infections and 250-500 mg q 6 hr for severe infections, max 4 g/day

Infants, children, and adolescents weighing <40 kg PO 12.5 to 25 mg/kg/day q 6 hr for mild to moderate infections and 25 to 50 mg/kg/day q 6 hr for severe infections

Mastitis

Adults PO 125 to 500 mg q 6 hr × 10 to 14 days

Available forms: Capsules 250, 500 mg; oral suspension 62.5 mg/mL

ADVERSE EFFECTS

CNS: Headache, dizziness, seizures

GI: Nausea, vomiting, diarrhea, anorexia, CDAD, *hepatitis*

HEMA: Eosinophilia, leukopenia

INTEG: Rash, urticarial

GU: Interstitial neuritis

SYST: Anaphylaxis, Stevens-Johnson syndrome, toxic epidermal necrolysis, serum sickness

---

INTERACTIONS
Individual drugs
Methotrexate: decreased excretion, increased toxicity

Probenecid: decreased excretion, avoid using together

Drug classifications
Hormonal contraceptives: decreased contraceptive effect possible, use another form of contraception

Drug/lab test
Increased: ALT, AST, alkaline phosphatase, LDH, Alkaline phosphatase, bilirubin, BUN, creatinine
False positive: direct Coombs' test

NURSING CONSIDERATIONS
Assessment
• Assess patient for previous sensitivity reaction to penicillins or other cephalosporins; cross-sensitivity between penicillins and cephalosporins is common

• Assess patient for signs and symptoms of infection, including characteristics of wounds, sputum, urine, stool, WBC $>10,000/mm^3$, fever; obtain baseline information and during treatment

• Obtain C&S before beginning product therapy to identify if correct treatment has been initiated

• **Assess for anaphylaxis:** rash, urticaria, pruritus, chills, fever, joint pain; angioedema may occur a few days after therapy begins; EPINEPHrine and resuscitation equipment should be available for anaphylactic reaction

• Monitor blood studies: AST, ALT, CBC, Hct, bilirubin, LDH, alkaline phosphatase, Coombs' monthly if patient is on long-term therapy

• Assess bowel pattern daily; if severe diarrhea occurs, product should be discontinued; may indicate CDAD

• Assess for **overgrowth of infection:** perineal itching, fever, malaise, redness, pain, swelling, drainage, rash, diarrhea, change in cough, sputum

Patient problems
Infection (uses)
Risk for injury (adverse reactions)

Implementation
PO route
• Food decreases bioavailability, take on an empty stomach (at least 1 hr prior to or 2 hr after a meal)

Patient/family education
• Advise patient to contact prescriber if vaginal itching, loose foul-smelling stools, furry tongue occur; may indicate superinfection

• Advise patient to notify prescriber of diarrhea with blood or pus; may indicate CDAD

• Teach patient to report if pregnancy is planned or suspected or if breastfeeding

Evaluation
Positive therapeutic outcome
• Absence of signs/symptoms of infection (WBC $<10,000/mm^3$, temp WNL, absence of red draining wounds, earache)

• Reported improvement in symptoms of infection

• Negative C&S

TREATMENT OF ANAPHYLAXIS
EPINEPHrine, antihistamines, resuscitate if needed

diflorasone (Rx)
(dye-flor'a-sone)
Func. class.: Antiinflammatory, topical
Chem. class.: Corticosteroid

ACTION: Inhibits inflammation

Therapeutic outcome: Decreased inflammation

USES: Topical treatment of mild to moderate inflammation of skin disorders

Pharmacokinetics
Absorption	Minimal
Distribution	Local
Metabolism	Unknown
Excretion	Unknown
Half-life	Unknown

Pharmacodynamics
Onset	Unknown
Peak	Unknown
Duration	Unknown

CONTRAINDICATIONS
Hypersensitivity

Precautions: Infections, pregnancy, breastfeeding, children, cataracts, glaucoma

DOSAGE AND ROUTES
Adult: Topical apply 1-4 times per day

Available forms: Topical cream, ointment 0.5%

ADVERSE EFFECTS
INTEG: Rash, burning, redness, stinging

INTERACTIONS
None significant

NURSING CONSIDERATIONS
Assessment
- Assess area involved baseline and during treatment, use occlusive dressings if directed
- **Assess** rash, burning, itching, redness

Patient problems
Impaired skin integrity (uses)

Implementation
- **Topical:** apply cream to affected area once to four times per day, wear gloves when applying

Patient/family education
- Advise patient to use as directed, not to double or skip doses
- Teach patient to report if pregnancy is planned or suspected or if breastfeeding

Evaluation
Positive therapeutic outcome
- Reported improvement in skin integrity, absence of itching

didanosine (Rx)
(dye-dan'oh-seen)
ddI, Pediatric Videx, Videx EC
Func. class.: Antiretroviral
Chem. class.: Synthetic purine nucleoside reverse transcriptase inhibitor (NRTI)

ACTION: Nucleoside analog incorporating into cellular DNA by viral reverse transcriptase, thereby terminating the cellular DNA chain and preventing viral replication

Therapeutic outcome: Antiviral against the retroviruses, primarily HIV-1

USES: HIV-1 infection in combination with at least 2 other antiretrovirals

Pharmacokinetics

Absorption	Rapidly absorbed (up to 40%)
Distribution	Unknown
Metabolism	Not metabolized
Excretion	Kidneys (55%), feces
Half-life	48 min, shorter in children

Pharmacodynamics

Onset	Unknown
Peak	Up to 1 hr, del rel 2 hr
Duration	Unknown

CONTRAINDICATIONS
Hypersensitivity, lactic acidosis, pancreatitis, phenylketonuria

Precautions: Pregnancy, breastfeeding, children, renal disease, sodium-restricted diets, elevated amylase, preexistent peripheral neuropathy, hyperuricemia, gout, HF, noncirrhotic portal hypertension

> **BLACK BOX WARNING:** Hepatic disease, lactic acidosis, pancreatitis

DOSAGE AND ROUTES
Ext rel cap
Adult/adolescent/child ≥6 yr and ≥60 kg: PO ext rel cap 400 mg daily; if used with tenofovir, reduce to 250 mg daily
Adult/adolescent/child ≥6 yr and 25 kg to <60 kg: PO ext rel cap 250 mg daily; if used with tenofovir, reduce to 200 mg daily
Adolescent 20 kg to <25 kg: PO ext rel cap 200 mg daily

Oral dosage (powder for oral solution)
Adult ≥60 kg: PO 200 mg bid or 400 mg daily; if used with tenofovir, reduce to 250 mg daily
Adult <60 kg: PO 125 mg bid or 250 mg daily; if used with tenofovir, reduce to 200 mg daily
Adolescent/child/infant >8 mo: PO 120 mg/m² q12hr, max adult dosing
Infant ≤8 mo/neonate ≥2 wk: PO 100 mg/m² q12hr for up to 3 months

Renal dose
Adult: PO CrCl ≥60 ml/min: no change
Adult/adolescent ≥60 kg: PO CCr 30-59 ml/min: reduce oral solution to 100 mg q12hr or 200 mg q24hr, reduce ext rel capsules to 200 mg daily; CCr 10-29 ml/min: reduce oral solution to 150 mg q24hr, reduce ext rel capsules to 125 mg q24hr; CCr <10 ml/min: reduce oral solution to 100 mg q24hr, reduce ext rel capsules to 125 mg q24hr
Adult/adolescent <60 kg: PO CCr 30-59 ml/min: reduce oral solution to 75 mg q12hr or to 150 mg q24hr, reduce ext rel capsules to 125 mg daily; CCr 10-29 ml/min: reduce oral solution to 100 mg q24hr, reduce ext rel capsules to 125 mg daily; CCr <10 ml/min: reduce oral solution to 75 mg q24hr, ext rel capsules are not recommended

Intermittent hemodialysis/continuous ambulatory peritoneal dialysis
≥60 kg, give 100 mg oral solution or 125 mg ext rel capsules q24hr; <60 kg, give 75 mg oral solution q24hr, ext rel capsules are not recommended

Available forms: Powder for oral sol 10 mg/ml; del rel caps 125, 200, 250, 400 mg

---

⚠ Nurse Alert ✴ Key NCLEX® Drug >> Drug Specifics

ADVERSE EFFECTS

CNS: Peripheral neuropathy, seizures, confusion, *anxiety,* hypertonia, abnormal thinking, asthenia, *insomnia, CNS depression,* pain, dizziness, chills, fever

CV: Hypertension, vasodilatation, dysrhythmia, syncope, HF, palpitations

EENT: Ear pain, otitis, photophobia, visual impairment, retinal depigmentation, optic neuritis

GI: Pancreatitis, *diarrhea, nausea,* vomiting, *abdominal pain,* constipation, stomatitis, dyspepsia, liver abnormalities, flatulence, taste perversion, dry mouth, oral thrush, melena, increased ALT, AST, alkaline phosphatase, amylase, hepatic failure, noncirrhotic portal hypertension

GU: Increased bilirubin, uric acid

HEMA: Leukopenia, granulocytopenia, thrombocytopenia, anemia

INTEG: *Rash, pruritus,* alopecia, ecchymosis, hemorrhage, petechiae, sweating

MS: Myalgia, arthritis, myopathy, muscular atrophy

RESP: Cough, pneumonia, dyspnea, asthma, epistaxis, hypoventilation, sinusitis

SYST: Lactic acidosis, anaphylaxis

INTERACTIONS
Individual drugs
Allopurinol, tenofovir

> **BLACK BOX WARNING:** Increase: fatal lactic acidosis: stavudine, tenofovir, other antiretrovirals, do not use together

Dapsone, ketoconazole: decreased absorption of each specific product

Gatifloxacin, gemifloxacin, grepafloxacin, levofloxacin, lomefloxacin, moxifloxacin, norfloxacin, sparfloxacin, trovafloxacin: Do not use didanosine with these products (PO)

Itraconazole: decreased concentrations

Methadone: decreased didanosine level

Stavudine: increased pancreatitis risk

Drug classifications
Aluminum, antacids, magnesium: increased side effects

Antiretrovirals, other: decreased concentration

Fluoroquinolones, tetracyclines: decreased concentrations of each specific product

Drug/food
Do not use with acidic juices

Decreased: absorption 50%, do not use with food

NURSING CONSIDERATIONS
Assessment

> **BLACK BOX WARNING: Pancreatitis:** do not use in those with symptoms of pancreatitis (may be dose-related) or advanced HIV, alcoholism, history of pancreatitis

• **Assess for peripheral neuropathy:** tingling or pain in hands and feet, distal numbness; onset usually occurs 2-6 mo after beginning treatment; if these occur during therapy, product may be decreased or discontinued

> **BLACK BOX WARNING: Assess for pancreatitis:** abdominal pain, nausea, vomiting, elevated liver enzymes; product should be discontinued since condition can be fatal

• Assess children by dilated retinal examination q6mo to rule out retinal depigmentation

• Monitor CBC, differential, platelet count monthly, viral load, $CD4^+$ count; notify prescriber of results

• Monitor renal function studies: BUN, serum uric acid, urine CCr before, during therapy; these may be elevated throughout treatment

> **BLACK BOX WARNING: Lactic acidosis, severe hepatomegaly, pancreatitis:** assess for abdominal pain, nausea, vomiting, elevated hepatic enzymes; product should be discontinued because condition can be fatal

• Monitor temp; may indicate beginning of infection

• Monitor liver function tests before, during therapy (bilirubin, AST, ALT, amylase, alkaline phosphatase) as needed or monthly

• **Pregnancy/breastfeeding:** Identify if pregnancy is planned or suspected, product is not recommended in initial treatment due to toxicity, do not breastfeed, enroll in the Antiretroviral Pregnancy Registry 800-258-4263

Patient problems
Infection (uses)

Implementation
• Give on empty stomach 1 hr before or 2 hr after meals q12hr; food decreases effectiveness of product; adjust dose in renal impairment

• Pediatric powder for oral sol should be prepared in the pharmacy; shake before using

• Packets for oral sol must be mixed with ½ glass of water, not fruit juice; stir until dissolved; drink immediately

• Store caps, tabs in tightly closed bottle at room temperature; store oral sol after dissolving at room temperature ≤4 hr

• Do not take dapsone at same time as ddI

Patient/family education
• Advise patient to take on empty stomach, 30 min before or 2 hr after eating; not to mix powder with fruit juice; to drink powder immediately after mixing; to use exactly as prescribed
• Instruct patient to report signs of **infection:** increased temp, sore throat, flulike symptoms; to avoid crowds and those with known infections
• Instruct patient to report signs of **anemia:** fatigue, headache, faintness, shortness of breath, irritability
• Advise patient to report numbness/tingling in extremities
• Instruct patient to report **bleeding;** avoid use of razors and commercial mouthwash
• Advise patient that hair may be lost during therapy; a wig or hairpiece may make patient feel better
• Caution patient to avoid OTC products and other medications without approval of prescriber; to avoid alcohol

> **BLACK BOX WARNING: Pancreatitis:** Teach patient to report immediately abdominal pain, diarrhea, nausea, vomiting

• That product does not cure symptoms, only controls them, that infection of others may occur via sex or blood
• Teach patient not to have any sexual contact without use of a condom; needles should not be shared; blood from infected individual should not come in contact with another's mucous membranes
• **Pregnancy/breastfeeding:** Identify if pregnancy is planned or suspected, product is not recommended in initial treatment due to toxicity, do not breastfeed, enroll if pregnant in the Antiretroviral Pregnancy Registry (800-258-4263)

Evaluation
Positive therapeutic outcome
• Absence of opportunistic infection, symptoms of HIV

> **⚠ HIGH ALERT**
> ## digoxin (Rx) NTI
> (di-jox′in)
> **Lanoxin ✲, Digitek, Toloxin ✲**
> *Func. class.:* Inotropic antidysrhythmic, cardiac glycoside
> *Chem. class.:* Digitalis preparation

Do not confuse: Lanoxin/Lasix/Lonox/Lomotil/Xanax/Levoxine

ACTION: Inhibits sodium-potassium ATPase, which makes more calcium available for contractile proteins, resulting in increased cardiac output; increases force of contraction (positive inotropic effect); decreases heart rate (negative chronotropic effect); decreases AV conduction speed

Therapeutic outcome: Decreased edema, pulse, respiration, crackles

USES: Atrial fibrillation/flutter, heart failure

Pharmacokinetics

Absorption	Unknown
Distribution	Widely distributed; 20%-25% protein bound
Metabolism	Liver, small amount; also intestinal bacteria
Excretion	Urine
Half-life	30-40 hr

Pharmacodynamics

	PO	IV
Onset	½-1½ hr	5-30 min
Peak	2-6 hr	1-4 hr
Duration	After steady state	2-6 days

CONTRAINDICATIONS
Hypersensitivity to digoxin, ventricular fibrillation, ventricular tachycardia, carotid sinus syndrome, 2nd- or 3rd-degree heart block

Precautions: Pregnancy, breastfeeding, geriatric, renal disease, acute MI, AV block, severe respiratory disease, hypothyroidism, sinus nodal disease, hypokalemia, electrolyte disturbances, hypertension, cor pulmonale, Wolff-Parkinson-White syndrome

DOSAGE AND ROUTES
Loading dose: IV
Adult: IV 400-600 mcg as a single dose, effect in 5-30 min, max effect 1-4 hr, give subsequent doses of 100-300 mcg q6-8hr
Adolescent/child >10 yr: IV 8-12 mcg/kg, divided into 3 or more doses, with the first dose equaling approximately half of the total, give subsequent doses q4-8hr
Child 5-10 yr: IV 15-30 mcg/kg divided into 3 or more doses, with the first dose equaling approximately half of the total, give subsequent doses q4-8hr
Child 2-4 yr: IV 25-35 mcg/kg, divided into 3 or more doses, with the first dose equaling approximately half of the total, give subsequent doses q4-8hr
Child <2 yr/infant: IV 30-50 mcg/kg, divided into 3 or more doses, with the first dose equaling approximately half of the total, give subsequent doses q4-8hr

---

Full-term neonate: IV 20-30 mcg/kg, divided into 3 or more doses, with the first dose equaling approximately half of the total, give subsequent doses q4-8hr

Premature neonate: IV 15-25 mcg/kg, divided into 3 or more doses, with the first dose equaling approximately half of the total, give subsequent doses q4-8hr

Loading dose: oral dosage (tablets)
Tablets are 60%-80% bioavailable; oral elixir should be used to obtain the appropriate dose in infants, young pediatric patients, or patients with very low body weight

Adult/adolescent/child >10 yr: PO Total dose of 10-15 mcg/kg, in 3 divided doses, give half of the total loading dose initially, then one-fourth the loading dose q4-8hr × 2 doses

Child 5-10 yr: PO Total dose of 20-45 mcg/kg, in 3 divided doses, give half of the total loading dose initially, then one fourth of the loading dose q4-8hr × 2 doses

Loading dose: oral dosage (elixir)
Adult/adolescent/child >10 yr: PO Total dose of 10-15 mcg/kg, give half of the total loading dose initially, then additional fractions of the planned total dose at 4-8 hr

Child 5-10 yr: PO Total dose of 20-35 mcg/kg, give half of the total loading dose initially, then additional fractions of the planned total dose at 4-8 hr

Child 2-4 yr: PO Total dose of 30-45 mcg/kg, give half of the total loading dose initially, then additional fractions of the planned total dose at 4-8 hr

Infant/child <2 yr: PO Total dose of 35-60 mcg/kg, give half of the total loading dose initially then additional fractions of the planned total dose at 4-8 hr

Full-term neonate: PO Total dose of 25-35 mcg/kg, give half of the total loading dose initially, then additional fractions of the planned total dose at 4-8 hr

Premature neonate: PO Total dose of 20-30 mcg/kg, give half of the total loading dose initially, then additional fractions of the planned total dose at 4-8 hr

Available forms: Elix 0.05 mg/ml; tabs 0.125, 0.25, 0.5, 0.0625, 0.1875 mg, 0.25 mg; inj 0.5 ✸, 0.25 mg/ml; pediatric inj 0.1 mg/ml

ADVERSE EFFECTS

CNS: *Headache,* drowsiness, apathy, confusion, disorientation, fatigue, depression, hallucinations

CV: Dysrhythmias, hypotension, bradycardia, AV block

EENT: Blurred vision, yellow-green halos, photophobia, diplopia

GI: Nausea, vomiting, anorexia, abdominal pain, diarrhea

INTERACTIONS
Individual drugs
AMILoride, cholestyramine, colestipol, metoclopramide, thyroid hormones: decreased digoxin levels

Amiodarone, dilTIAZem, indomethacin, NIFEdipine, propantheline, quiNIDine, verapamil: increased digoxin levels

Amphotericin B, carbenicillin, ticarcillin: increased hypokalemia, increased toxicity

Calcium IV: increased hypercalcemia, hypomagnesemia, digoxin toxicity, monitor electrolytes

Kaolin/pectin: decreased absorption

Drug classifications
Antacids: decreased digoxin absorption

Anticholinergics: increased digoxin blood levels

Antidysrhythmics, β-adrenergic blockers: increased bradycardia

Azole antifungals, macrolides, tetracyclines: increased toxicity, monitor for toxicity

Diuretics (thiazide) corticosteroids: increased hypokalemia, hypercalcemia, hypomagnesemia, digoxin toxicity

Sympathomimetics: increased cardiac dysrhythmia risk

Drug/herb
Increase: Cardiac effects: foxglove, golden seal, hawthorn, rue

St. John's wort: decreased product effect

Drug/food
Flaxseed, psyllium: decreased digoxin effect: food, separate by ≥1 hr absorption

Drug/lab test
Increased: CPK

NURSING CONSIDERATIONS
Assessment
• Assess and document apical pulse for 1 min before giving product; if pulse <60 in adult or <90 in an infant or is significantly different, take again in 1 hr; if <60 in adult, call prescriber; note rate, rhythm, character, monitor I&O, daily weight, check for edema

• Monitor electrolytes: potassium, sodium, chloride, magnesium, calcium; renal function studies: BUN, creatinine; other blood studies: ALT, AST, bilirubin, Hct, Hgb, product levels (therapeutic level 0.5-2 ng/ml) before initiating treatment and periodically thereafter, draw ≥ 6-8 hr after last dose, optimally 12-24 hr after a dose, monitor for decreased potassium, or increased potassium

• Monitor resolution of atrial dysrhythmias by ECG; if tachydysrhythmia develops, hold product; delay cardioversion while product levels are determined

- Monitor ECG continuously during parenteral loading doses and for patients with suspected toxicity; provide hemodynamic monitoring for patients with heart failure or administer multiple cardiac products
- **Beers:** Avoid dosage >0.125 mg/dl in atrial fibrillation, heart failure in older adults; decreased renal clearance may lead to toxicity

Patient problem
Impaired cardiac output (uses)
Lack of Knowledge of medication (teaching)
Nonadherence (teaching)

Implementation
- Do not give at same time as antacids or other products that decrease absorption

PO route
- Bioavailability varies between different oral dosage forms of digoxin and between different brands of the same dosage form. Changing from one preparation to another may require dosage adjustments.
- All dosage forms may be administered without regard to meals.
- Tab may be crushed and administered with food or fluids
- Pediatric elixir should be administered using a calibrated measuring device

Injectable routes
- When changing from PO to IM/IV use 20%-25% less
- IV is preferred over IM, as it is less painful
- PO should replace parenteral therapy as soon as possible
- Visually inspect parenteral products for particulate matter and discoloration prior to use

IV route
- Monitor ECG during and for 6 hr after IV use, watch for dysrhythmias, or bradycardia, notify prescriber
- May be given undiluted or each 1 ml may be diluted in 4 ml of sterile water for injection, NS, D₅W, or LR; diluent volumes less than 4 ml will cause precipitation; use diluted solutions immediately
- Inject over at least 5 min via Y-site or 3-way stopcock; in patients with pulmonary edema, administer over 10-15 min to avoid inadvertent overdosage, do not flush the syringe following administration
- Check for potency and site for redness, inflammation, infiltration, tissue sloughing can occur

IM route
- Do not administer more than 2 ml at any one IM injection site
- Inject deeply into gluteal muscle, then massage area

Y-site compatibilities: Acyclovir, alfentanil, amikacin, aminocaproic acid, aminophylline, amphotericin B lipid complex, amrinone, anidulafungin, ascorbic acid injection, atenolol, atracurium, atropine, aztreonam, benztropine, bivalirudin, bleomycin, bumetanide, buprenorphine, butorphanol, calcium chloride/gluconate, CARBOplatin, ceFAZolin, cefonicid, cefotaxime, cefoTEtan, cefOXitin, cefTAZidime, ceftizoxime, cefTRIAXone, cefuroxime, chloramphenicol, chlorproMAZINE, cimetidine, ciprofloxacin, cisatracurium, CISplatin, clindamycin, codeine, cyanocobalamin, cyclophosphamide, cycloSPORINE, cytarabine, DACTINomycin, DAPTOmycin, dexamethasone, dexmedetomidine, diltiazem, diphenhydrAMINE, DOBUTamine, DOCEtaxel, DOPamine, doripenem, doxacurium, doxycycline, enalaprilat, ePHEDrine, EPINEPHrine, epirubicin, epoetin alfa, eptifibatide, ertapenem, erythromycin, esmolol, etoposide, famotidine, fenoldopam, fentaNYL, fludarabine, fluorouracil, folic acid, furosemide, ganciclovir, gatifloxacin, gemcitabine, gentamicin, glycopyrrolate, granisetron, heparin, hydrocortisone, HYDROmorphone, hydrOXYzine, ifosfamide, imipenemcilastatin, indomethacin, irinotecan, isoproterenol, ketorolac, labetalol, levofloxacin, lidocaine, linezolid, LORazepam, LR, magnesium sulfate, mannitol, mechlorethamine, meperidine, meropenem, methicillin, methotrexate, methyldopate, methylPREDNISolone, metoclopramide, metoprolol, metroNIDAZOLE, mezlocillin, miconazole, midazolam, milrinone, morphine, multiple vitamins injection, mycophenolate mofetil, nafcillin, nalbuphine, naloxone, nesiritide, metilmicin, nitroglycerin, nitroprusside, norepinephrine, octreotide, ondansetron, oxacillin, oxaliplatin, oxytocin, palonosetron, pamidronate, pancuronium, pantoprazole, papaverine, PEMEtrexed, penicillin G potassium/sodium, pentazocine, PENTobarbital, PHENobarbital, phenylephrine, phytonadione, piperacillin, piperacillintazobactam, polymyxin B, potassium chloride, procainamide, prochlorperazine, promethazine, propofol, propranolol, protamine, pyridoxine, quiNIDine, ranitidine, remifentanil, Ringer's, ritodrine, riTUXimab, rocuronium, sodium acetate/ bicarbonate, succinylcholine, SUFentanil, tacrolimus, teniposide, theophylline, thiamine, thiotepa, ticarcillin, ticarcillin-clavulanate, tigecycline, tirofiban, TNA, tobramycin, tolazoline, TPN, trastuzumab, trimetaphan, urokinase, vancomycin, vasopressin, vecuronium, verapamil, vin-CRIStine, vinorelbine, vit B/C, vitamin B complex, voriconazole, zoledronic acid

Patient/family education

• Advise patient not to stop abruptly; teach all aspects of product
• Caution patient to avoid OTC medications including cough, cold, allergy preparations, antacids, since many adverse product interactions may occur; do not take antacid at same time or within 2 hr of this product
• Instruct patient to notify prescriber of any loss of appetite, lower stomach pain, diarrhea, weakness, drowsiness, headache, blurred or yellow-green vision, rash, depression; teach toxic symptoms of this product and when to notify prescriber
• Advise patient to maintain a sodium-restricted diet as ordered; to take potassium supplements as ordered to prevent toxicity
• Instruct patient to report shortness of breath, difficulty breathing, weight gain, edema, persistent cough
• Teach patient purpose of product is to regulate the heart's functioning
• Teach patient as outpatient to check and record pulse for 1 min before taking dose; if there is a change of >15 bpm from usual pulse, prescriber should be notified
• Teach patient to take medication at the same time each day, take missed doses within 12 hr; do not double doses; notify prescriber if doses are missed for 2 days or more; how to monitor heart rate
• Teach patient toxic symptoms and when to notify prescriber
• Advise patient to carry/wear emergency ID describing dosage and reason for digoxin
• Advise patient to use one brand consistently, to keep in original container
• Teach patient how to take pulse, when to notify prescriber
• Teach patient to carry ID stating condition treated, products taken
• Teach patient to notify prescriber if pregnancy is planned or suspected or if breastfeeding

Evaluation

Positive therapeutic outcome
• Decreased in heart failure, dysrhythmias
• Serum digoxin level 0.5-2 ng/ml

TREATMENT OF OVERDOSE:

Discontinue product, administer potassium, monitor ECG, administer an adrenergic blocking agent, digoxin immune FAB

⚠ HIGH ALERT

dilTIAZem (Rx)

(dil-tye'a-zem)
Cardizem, Cardizem CD, Cardizem LA, Cartia XT, Taztia XT, Tiazac, Tiazac XC ✤

Func. class.: Calcium channel blocker, antianginal, antiarrhythmic class IV, antihypertensive
Chem. class.: Benzothiazepine

Do not confuse: Cardizem/Cardene Tiazac/Ziac

ACTION: Inhibits calcium ion influx across cell membrane during cardiac depolarization, produces relaxation of coronary vascular smooth muscle, dilates coronary arteries, slows SA/AV node conduction times, dilates peripheral arteries

Therapeutic outcome: Decreased angina pectoris, dysrhythmias, B/P

USES

Oral: Angina pectoris due to hypertension, coronary artery spasm, improvement in exercise tolerance (chronic stable angina)

Parenteral: Atrial fibrillation, flutter; paroxysmal supraventricular tachycardia

Pharmacokinetics

Absorption	Well absorbed
Distribution	Not known
Metabolism	Liver, extensively
Excretion	Metabolites (96%)
Half-life	3½-9 hr

Pharmacodynamics

	PO	PO–sus rel	IV
Onset	½ hr	Unknown	Unknown
Peak	2-3 hr	Unknown	Unknown
Duration	6-8 hr	11-18 hr	Unknown

CONTRAINDICATIONS

Sick sinus syndrome, 2nd- or 3rd-degree heart block, hypotension less than 90 mm Hg systolic, acute MI, pulmonary congestion, cardiogenic shock

Precautions: Pregnancy, breastfeeding, children, HF, aortic stenosis, bradycardia, GERD, hepatic disease, hiatal hernia, ventricular dysfunction, elderly

---

DOSAGE AND ROUTES
Hypertension
Adult: PO 30 mg TID, increase to max 480 mg/day; EXT REL 120-240 mg qday, max 540 mg/day; SUS REL 60 mg bid, max 360 mg/day

Prinzmetal's or variant angina, chronic stable angina
Adult: PO 30 mg qid, increasing dose gradually to 180-360 mg/day in divided doses or EXT REL (LA, CD, XT, XR products) 180-360 mg, max 480-540 mg/day, depending on brand

Atrial fibrillation, flutter, paroxysmal supraventricular tachycardia
Adult: IV 0.25 mg/kg as BOL over 2 min initially, then 0.35 mg/kg may be given after 15 min; if no response, may give CONT INF 5-15 mg/hr for up to 24 hr

Available forms: Tabs 30, 60, 90, 120 mg; ext rel tab 120, 180, 240, 300, 360, 420 mg; ext rel caps 60, 90, 120, 180, 240, 300, 360, 420 mg; inj 5 mg/ml (5, 10 ml); powder for inj 100 mg

ADVERSE EFFECTS
CNS: Tremor, paresthesia
CV: Dysrhythmia, *edema*, HF, bradycardia, hypotension, palpitations, heart block
EENT: Blurred vision, epistaxis, tinnitus
ENDO: Hyperglycemia, gynecomastia,
HEMA: Anemia, leukopenia, thrombocytopenia
MS: Stiffness, muscle cramps
MISC: Gingival hyperplasia
GI: *Nausea*, vomiting, diarrhea, *constipation*
GU: Nocturia, polyuria, sexual dysfunction, dysuria
INTEG: *Rash*, pruritus, flushing, photosensitivity, burning, Stevens-Johnson syndrome, sweating
RESP: Dyspnea, cough

INTERACTIONS
Individual drugs
CarBAMazepine, lithium, methylPREDNISolone: increased effects of each specific product, monitor for increased action of each product
Cimetidine: increased AV node slowing
CycloSPORINE: increased cycloSPORINE effect
Digoxin: increased digoxin effect
Theophylline, lithium: increased effect, toxicity

Drug classifications
Anesthetics: increased effects of anesthetics
β-Adrenergic blockers: increased bradycardia, HF, increased β-blocker effect
NSAIDs, PHENobarbital, phenytoin: decrease: Antihypertensive effect
Benzodiazepines: increased effect of benzodiazepines
HMG-CoA reductase inhibitors: increased effects

Drug/food
Increase: dilTIAZem effect, grapefruit juice, avoid use

NURSING CONSIDERATIONS
Assessment
• **HF:** monitor for dyspnea, weight gain, edema, jugular vein distention, rales; monitor I&O ratios daily, weight
• **Angina:** location, duration, alleviating factors, activity when pain starts
• **Dysrhythmias:** monitor B/P and pulse, respiration, ECG and intervals (PR, QRS, QT); PCWP, CVP often during infusion; if B/P drops 30 mm Hg, stop infusion and call prescriber, monitor B/P, ECG continuously if using IV, report bradycardia, have emergency equipment nearby
• Monitor if refills are being purchased
• Monitor digoxin levels
• Monitor potassium baseline and periodically; LFTs and renal studies
• **Stevens-Johnson syndrome:** Assess for rash, fever, fatigue, mouth blistering, discontinue product, if severe
• **Beers:** Avoid extended-release capsule in older adults, promotes fluid retention, exacerbates heart failure
• **Pregnancy:** Identify if pregnancy is planned or suspected or if breastfeeding, use only if benefits outweigh fetal risk

Patient problem
Pain (uses)
Impaired cardiac output (adverse reactions)
Risk for injury (adverse reactions)

Implementation
PO route
• Not all products are interchangeable
• Store at room temperature
• **Cardizem LA ext rel tab 24 hr:** give daily, either AM or PM, without regard to meals
• **Dilacor XR/Diltia XT ext rel cap 24 hr** give daily, take on empty stomach, swallow whole, do not cut, crush, chew, open
• **Tiazac, Tiztia XT:** give daily without regard to meals
• **Conventional regular-rel tab:** give before meals and at bedtime
• **Cardizem CD or equivalent (Cartia XT) generic ext rel cap 24 hr:** give daily, without regard to meals
• Give with meals for GI symptoms; may crush and sprinkle (reg tab) on applesauce

Direct IV route
• Give direct **IV** undiluted over 2 min
Continuous IV infusion route
• **Dilute** 125 mg/100 ml (1.25 mg/ml) or 250 mg/250 ml (1 mg/ml) or 250 mg/500 ml (0.5 mg/ml) of D₅W, 0.9% NaCl, D₅/0.45% NaCl; give 10 mg/hr; may increase by 5 mg/hr to 15 mg/hr; may continue inf up to 24 hr max

Y-site compatibilities: Albumin, amikacin, amphotericin B, aztreonam, bretylium, bumetanide, ceFAZolin, cefotaxime, cefoTEtan, cefOXitin, cefTAZidime, cefTRIAXone, cefuroxime, cimetidine, ciprofloxacin, clindamycin, digoxin, DOBUTamine, DOPamine, doxycycline, EPINEPHrine, erythromycin, esmolol, fentaNYL, fluconazole, gentamicin, hetastarch, HYDROmorphone, imipenem-cilastatin, labetalol, lidocaine, LORazepam, meperidine, metoclopramide, metroNIDAZOLE, midazolam, milrinone, morphine, multivitamins, niCARdipine, nitroglycerin, norepinephrine, oxacillin, penicillin G potassium, pentamidine, piperacillin, potassium chloride, potassium phosphates, raNITIdine, sodium nitroprusside, theophylline, ticarcillin, ticarcillin/clavulanate, tobramycin, trimethoprim-sulfamethoxazole, vancomycin, vecuronium

Patient/family education
• Caution patient to avoid hazardous activities until stabilized on product and dizziness is no longer a problem
• Instruct patient to limit caffeine consumption; to avoid grapefruit juice; to avoid alcohol, to discuss OTC, Rx, herbals, supplements with provider
• Tell patient to comply in all areas of medical regimen; diet, exercise, stress reduction, product therapy; to notify prescriber of irregular heartbeat, shortness of breath, swelling of feet and hands, pronounced dizziness, constipation, nausea, hypotension
• Teach patient to use sunscreen, protective clothing to prevent photosensitivity
• Teach patient how to take pulse to report <50 bpm, how to take B/P
• Advise to rise or change positions slowly, orthostatic hypotension may occur
• **Angina:** To discuss other therapy including nitrates, beta blockers, and when to take
• Advise patient to use good oral hygiene and teeth cleanings, gingival hyperphagia occurs
• Teach patient to use as directed even if feeling better; may be taken with other cardiovascular products (nitrates, β-blockers); how to take pulse, B/P before taking product; to change position slowly

• Teach patient not to discontinue abruptly
• **Pregnancy:** Teach patient to report if pregnancy is planned or suspected or if breastfeeding

Evaluation
Positive therapeutic outcome
• Decreased anginal pain
• Decreased D/P
• Increased exercise tolerance
• Absence of dysrhythmias

TREATMENT OF OVERDOSE:
Atropine for AV block, vasopressor for hypotension

dimenhyDRINATE (OTC, Rx)
(dye-men-hye′dri-nate)
Dirate ✦, Dramamine, Driminate, TripTone, Wal-Dram
Func. class.: Antiemetic, antihistamine, anticholinergic
Chem. class.: H1-receptor antagonist, ethanolamine derivative

Do not confuse: dimenhyDRINATE/
diphenhydrAMINE

ACTION: Competes with histamine for H1 receptors in GI tract, blood vessels, respiratory tract; central anticholinergic activity, which results in decreased vestibular stimulation and blockade of chemoreceptor trigger zone

Therapeutic outcome: Absence of nausea, vomiting, or vertigo

USES: Motion sickness, nausea, vomiting, vertigo

Unlabeled uses: Hyperemesis gravidarum, Ménière's syndrome

Pharmacokinetics

Absorption	Unknown
Distribution	May cross placenta, enter breast milk
Metabolism	Liver
Excretion	Kidneys
Half-life	Unknown

Pharmacodynamics

Onset	PO 15-30 min
Peak	PO 2 hr
Duration	PO 4-6 hr

CONTRAINDICATIONS

Hypersensitivity, infants, neonates, tartrazine dye hypersensitivity

Precautions: Pregnancy, breastfeeding, children, geriatric patients, cardiac dysrhythmias, asthma, prostatic hypertrophy, bladder-neck obstruction, closed-angle glaucoma, stenosing peptic ulcer, pyloroduodenal obstruction

DOSAGE AND ROUTES

Adult: PO 50-100 mg q4hr; IM/IV 50 mg q4hr as needed (Canada only)
Child 6-12 yr: PO 25-50 mg q6-8hr prn, max 150 mg/day
Child 2-5 yr: PO 12.5-25 mg q6-8hr, max 75 mg/day

Available forms: Tabs 50 mg; inj 50 mg/ml; elixir 15 mg/5 ml; chew tabs 50 mg

ADVERSE EFFECTS

CNS: Drowsiness, restlessness, headache, dizziness, insomnia, confusion, nervousness, tingling, vertigo
CV: Hypertension, hypotension, palpitation
EENT: Dry mouth, blurred vision, diplopia, nasal congestion, photosensitivity, xerostomia
GI: Nausea, anorexia, vomiting, constipation
INTEG: Rash, urticaria, fever, chills, flushing
MISC: Anaphylaxis

INTERACTIONS

Individual drugs
Alcohol: increased effects

Drug classifications
Anticholinergics, tricyclics, MAOIs, opiates, sedative/hypnotics, other CNS depressants: increased effects

Drug/lab test
False negative: allergy skin testing

NURSING CONSIDERATIONS

Assessment
• Monitor VS, B/P; check patients with cardiac disease more often
• **Assess for signs of toxicity of other products or masking of symptoms of disease:** brain tumor, intestinal obstruction
• Observe for drowsiness, dizziness
• **Pregnancy/breastfeeding:** Use only if clearly needed, no well-controlled studies, do not breastfeed, excreted in breast milk

Patient problem
Nausea (uses)

Implementation
• Give IM inj in large muscle mass; aspirate to avoid IV administration (Canada only)
• Tablets may be swallowed whole, chewed, or allowed to dissolve

IV route (Canada only)
• After diluting 50 mg/10 ml of NaCl inj, give 50 mg over 2 min

Patient/family education
• Advise patient to avoid hazardous activities, activities requiring alertness because dizziness may occur; to request assistance with ambulation
• Advise to avoid alcohol, other CNS depressants
• **Beers:** Avoid use in older adults, highly anticholinergic

Evaluation

Positive therapeutic outcome
• Absence of nausea, vomiting, or vertigo

dimethyl fumarate (Rx)
(dahy-meth'ul fyoo'muh-reyt)
Tecfidera
Func. class.: Immunomodulator

ACTION: Has beneficial effects on inflammation and oxidative stress. Induces an antioxidant effect–related neuronal death, and damage to myelin in the CNS may also improve mitochondrial function

USES: Relapsing multiple sclerosis

Pharmacokinetics

Absorption	Rapidly
Distribution	Unknown
Metabolism	Converted to MMF, then TCA
Excretion	By lungs exhalation (60%), minimal feces, urine
Half-life	1 hr

Pharmacodynamics

Onset	Unknown
Peak	2½ hr
Duration	Unknown

CONTRAINDICATIONS
Hypersensitivity

Precautions: Pregnancy, breastfeeding, immunosuppression, infertility, male-mediated teratogenicity

DOSAGE AND ROUTES

Adult: PO 120 mg bid × 7 days, may increase to 240 mg bid for maintenance

Available forms: Caps, del rel 120, 240 mg

SIDE EFFECTS

CNS: *Flushing*, progressive multifocal leukoencephalopathy
GI: Nausea, dyspepsia, abdominal pain, diarrhea, vomiting
GU: Albuminuria
INTEG: Rash, pruritus
HEMA: Lymphopenia, leukopenia
SYST: Anaphylaxis, angioedema

INTERACTIONS

None known

NURSING CONSIDERATIONS

Assessment:

• **Multiple sclerosis:** Monitor for improved number and severity of spasms, chronic pain, fatigue and weakness, balance and dizziness
• Monitor CBC with differential baseline and every 6 months thereafter; leukopenia and lymphopenia may occur
• **Anaphylaxis:** Usually during first dose but may occur any time during treatment; monitor for difficulty breathing, urticaria, and swelling of the throat and tongue
• **Progressive multifocal leukoencephalopathy:** Assess for ataxia, vision changes, weakness, trouble using arms/legs, confusion; discontinue at first sign of PML
• **Pregnancy:** Identify if pregnancy is planned or suspected, or if breastfeeding; use only if benefit outweighs fetal risk; cautious use in breastfeeding, excretion is unknown; if pregnant, register by calling 866-810-1462 or by visiting www.tecfiderapregnancyregistry.com

Patient problems

Lack of knowledge of medication (teaching)

Implementation:

• Do not break, crush, or chew, do not open cap; give without regard to meals, use with food may decrease flushing

Teach patient/family:

• **Advise patient** to notify prescriber if pregnancy is planned or suspected; not to breastfeed
• Teach patient expected results, side effects
• **Anaphylaxis:** Teach patient to discontinue the drug and seek immediate medical treatment if patient experiences difficulty breathing, urticaria, or swelling of the throat/tongue
• Progressive multifocal leukoencephalopathy: Advise patient to notify prescriber

immediately of vision changes, confusion, ataxia, weakness, trouble using arms/legs

Evaluation: Positive therapeutic outcome: improved symptoms of multiple sclerosis

dinoprostone (Rx)

(dye-noe-prost′one)
Cervidil, Prepidil, Prostin E
Func. class.: Oxytocic, abortifacient
Chem. class.: Prostaglandin E$_2$

Do not confuse: Prepidil/bepridil

ACTION: Stimulates uterine contractions similar to labor by myometrium stimulation, causing abortion; acts within 30 hr for complete abortion

Therapeutic outcome: Beginning of labor, fetal expulsion

USES: Abortion during 2nd trimester, benign hydatidiform mole, expulsion of uterine contents in fetal deaths to 28 wk, missed abortion, cervical effacement and dilatation in term pregnancy when they have not occurred spontaneously

Pharmacokinetics

Absorption	Rapidly absorbed
Distribution	Unknown
Metabolism	Enzymes
Excretion	Kidneys
Half-life	Unknown

Pharmacodynamics

	Gel	Supp
Onset	Rapid	10 min
Peak	30-45 min	Unknown
Duration	Unknown	2-3 hr

CONTRAINDICATIONS

Hypersensitivity, C-section, surgery, fetal distress, multiparity, vaginal bleeding, cephalopelvic disproportion

Precautions: Pregnancy, renal/hepatic/cardiac disease, asthma, anemia, jaundice, diabetes mellitus, seizure disorders, hypertension, glaucoma, uterine fibrosis, cervical stenosis, pelvic surgery, PID, respiratory disease

> **BLACK BOX WARNING:** Requires a specialized setting and an experienced clinician

DOSAGE AND ROUTES

Abortifacient

Adult: VAG SUPP 20 mg; repeat q3-5hr until abortion occurs; max dose 240 mg

Cervical ripening
Adult: GEL 0.5 mg vag gel placed in cervical canal, may repeat after 6 hr, max 1.5 mg/24 hr; vag insert 10 mg high in vagina, remove at onset of active labor or within 12 hr

Available forms: Vag supp 20 mg; endocervical gel 0.5 mg/3 g (prefilled syringe); vag insert 10 mg

ADVERSE EFFECTS
CNS: *Headache,* drowsiness
CV: Hypotension, hypertension
EENT: Blurred vision
GI: *Nausea, vomiting, diarrhea*
GU: Vaginal pain, uterine rupture, UTI; warm-feeling vagina (Gel, insert)
INTEG: Rash, skin color changes
MS: *Leg cramps, back pain*
SYST: Anaphylactoid syndrome of pregnancy
Insert: Uterine hyperstimulation, fever, nausea, vomiting, diarrhea, abdominal pain
Gel: Uterine contractile abnormality, GI side effects, back pain, fever, amniotic fluid embolism
Fetal: Bradycardia (i.e., deceleration)
Suppository: Uterine rupture, anaphylaxis

INTERACTIONS
Individual drugs
Drug classifications
Other oxytocics: increased effect

NURSING CONSIDERATIONS
Assessment

> **BLACK BOX WARNING: Specialized setting, specialized clinician:** use only with emergency equipment nearby, by a clinician experienced with use in pregnancy termination; complete abortion should result within 17 hr (insert), use only in 12-20 wk or up to 28 wk for removal of remaining material after miscarriage

• **Abortifacient:** Monitor contractions for frequency, duration, force
• **Anaphylaxis: Monitor for rash, wheezing**
• **Cervical ripening:** assess dilation and effacement of the cervix, uterine contractions, fetal heart tones; watch for contractions lasting over 1 min, hypertonus, fetal distress; product should be slowed or discontinued
• Monitor B/P, during treatment
• Assess for fever that occurs approximately 30 min after supp insertion (abortion)
• Monitor for nausea, vomiting, diarrhea; these may require medication
• **Assess for hypersensitivity reaction:** dyspnea, rash, chest discomfort
• **Check amount of vaginal discharge;** itching, irritation indicates vaginal infection

Patient problem
Lack of Knowledge of medication (teaching)

Implementation
Suppository route
• Warm supp by running warm water over package; insert high in vagina, wear gloves to prevent absorption; have patient recumbent for at least 10 min
Gel route
• Do not allow to come in contact with skin; use soap and water to wash after use
• Gel should be at room temperature
• Place patient in dorsal or lithotomy position to insert gel into cervical canal; remove catheter; discard all items after use; keep supine 15-30 min
Vaginal insert (Cervidil)
• The vaginal insert is supplied in an individually wrapped aluminum/polyethylene package with a 'tear mark' on one side of the package; the package should only be opened by tearing the aluminum package along the tear mark. Do not use scissors or other sharp objects to open. This could result in cutting the knitted polyester pouch that serves as the retrieval system for the polymeric slab (contains active ingredient). An integral part of the knitted polyester retrieval system is a long tape designed to aid in retrieval of the insert at the end of the dosing interval or earlier if clinically indicated.
• The insertion of the vaginal insert does not require sterile conditions.
• Position vaginal insert securely between the index and middle fingers. Place insert transversely in the posterior fornix of the vagina immediately after removal from the package. Do not use vaginal insert without its retrieval system. A small amount of water-miscible lubricant may be used to assist in insertion; take care not to overcoat the insert with excess lubricant.
• The patient should remain recumbent for 2 hours following insertion; but thereafter may be ambulatory. However, ensure that the vaginal insert remains in place.
• Removal: To remove vaginal insert, pull tape slowly from vagina. It is essential to ensure that the slab has been removed. Visualization of the knitted polyester retrieval system as well as the slab is necessary to ensure proper removal. If the slab is not contained within the polyester retrieval system, a vaginal exam should be performed and the slab removed manually.
• Discard the vaginal insert once used.

Patient/family education
• Teach patient all aspects of treatment including purpose of medication and expected results
• **Cervical ripening:** Tell patient that gel may produce warmth in her vagina

---

- Caution patient that if contractions are longer than 1 min to notify nurse or prescriber
- Advise patient to notify prescriber of cramping, pain, increased bleeding, chills, increased temp, or foul-smelling discharge; these symptoms may indicate uterine infection
- Advise patient to remain supine 10-15 min after insertion of suppository, 2 hr after insert, 15-30 min after gel

Evaluation

Positive therapeutic outcome
- Progression of labor
- Abortion

RARELY USED

dinutuximab
(di-noo-tux'i-mab)
Unituxin
Func. class.: Antineoplastics

USES: High-risk neuroblastoma in patients who achieve at least a partial response to first-line multiagent, multimodality therapy in combination with isotretinoin, granulocyte-macrophage colony-stimulating factor (sargramostim), and interleukin-2 (aldesleukin)

CONTRAINDICATIONS:
Hypersensitivity, pregnancy, lactation

DOSAGE AND ROUTES
Children and Adolescents: IV Infusion 17.5 mg/m^2/dose over 10 to 20 hr on scheduled days for 5 cycles in combination with isotretinoin, sargramostim, and aldesleukin.

---

diphenhydrAMINE
(OTC, Rx)
(dye-fen-hye'dra-meen)
Allerdryl ♣, Allergy formula ♣, AllerMax ♣, Banophen, Benadryl, Benadryl Allergy, Benadryl Allergy Dye Free, Allergy, Benylin ♣, Buckley's Bedtime, Diphenhist, Calmex ♣, Dormex ♣, Silphen, Sominex, Unisom ♣
Func. class.: Antihistamine (1st generation, nonselective), antitussive
Chem. class.: Ethanolamine derivative, H$_1$-receptor antagonist

Do not confuse: diphenhydrAMINE/dicyclomine/dimenhyDRINATE

ACTION: Acts on blood vessels, GI, respiratory system by competing with histamine for H$_1$-receptor site; decreases allergic response by blocking histamine

Therapeutic outcome: Absence of allergy symptoms and rhinitis, decreased dystonic symptoms, absence of motion sickness, absence of cough, ability to sleep

USES: Allergy symptoms, rhinitis, motion sickness, antiparkinsonism, nighttime sedation, infant colic, nonproductive cough, insomnia in children, dystonic reactions

Pharmacokinetics

Absorption	Well absorbed (PO, IM); completely absorbed (**IV**)
Distribution	Widely distributed; crosses placenta
Metabolism	Liver (95%)
Excretion	Kidneys, breast milk
Half-life	2½-7 hr

Pharmacodynamics

	PO	IM	IV
Onset	15-60 min	30 min	Immediate
Peak	2-4 hr	2-4 hr	Unknown
Duration	4-8 hr	4-8 hr	4-8 hr

CONTRAINDICATIONS
Hypersensitivity to H$_1$-receptor antagonist, neonates

Precautions: Pregnancy, breastfeeding, children <6 yr, increased intraocular pressure, renal/cardiac disease, hypertension, bronchial asthma, seizure disorder, stenosed peptic ulcers, hyperthyroidism, prostatic hypertrophy, bladder neck obstruction

DOSAGE AND ROUTES
Antihistamine/antiemetic/antivertiginic
Adult and child >12 yr: PO 25-50 mg q4-6hr, max 300 mg/day; IM/**IV** 10-50 mg, max 300 mg/day
Child 6-12 yr: PO/IM/**IV** 5 mg/kg/day in 4 divided doses, max 300 mg/day

Nighttime sleep aid
Adult and child ≥12 yr: PO 25-50 mg at bedtime

Antitussive (syrup only)
Adult and child ≥12 yr: 25 mg q4hr, max 150 mg/24 hr
Child 6-12 yr: 12.5 mg q4hr, max 75 mg/24 hr

Available forms: Caps 25, 50 mg; tabs 25, 50 mg; chew tabs 12.5, 25 mg; elix 12.5 mg/5 ml; syr 12.5 mg/5 ml; inj 50 mg/ml; orally

---

disintegrating tabs 12.5 mg; orally disintegrating strips 12.5, 25 mg

ADVERSE EFFECTS
CNS: *Dizziness, drowsiness,* confusion, seizures, headache
CV: Hypotension, palpitations
EENT: Blurred vision, tinnitus, nasal stuffiness
GI: Nausea, anorexia, diarrhea
GU: *Retention,* dysuria, frequency
HEMA: Thrombocytopenia, agranulocytosis, hemolytic anemia
INTEG: Photosensitivity, rash
MISC: Anaphylaxis
RESP: Increased thick secretions, wheezing, chest tightness

INTERACTIONS
Individual drugs
Alcohol: increased CNS depression

Drug classifications
Antidepressants (tricyclic), barbiturates, CNS depressants, opiates, sedative/hypnotics: increased CNS depression
MAOIs: increased effect of diphenhydrAMINE

Drug/herb
Increase: CNS depression--chamomile, kava, valerian

Drug/lab test
False negative: skin allergy tests (discontinue antihistamines 3 days before testing)

NURSING CONSIDERATIONS
Assessment
• Assess respiratory status: rate, rhythm, increase in bronchial secretions, wheezing, chest tightness; provide fluids to 2 L/day to decrease secretion thickness
• Monitor I&O ratio: be alert for urinary retention, frequency, dysuria, especially geriatric; product should be discontinued if these occur
• Monitor CBC during long-term therapy; blood dyscrasias may occur but are rare
• **EPS:** If giving for dystonic reactions, assess type of involuntary movements and evaluate response to this medication
• **Cough:** Assess characteristics including type, frequency, thickness of secretions; evaluate response to this medication, increase fluids to 2 L/day unless contraindicated
• **Anaphylaxis:** Assess for rash, throat tightness, have emergency equipment nearby

Patient problem
Impaired sleep (uses)
Risk of injury (adverse reaction)

Implementation
• Avoid use in children <6 yr, death has occurred; overdose has occurred in topical gel taken orally (adult/child)
• Give 20 min before bedtime if using for sleep aid
PO route
• Give with meals if GI symptoms occur; absorption rate may be slightly decreased; cap may be opened and product mixed with food/fluids for patients with swallowing difficulties
IM route
• Give IM inj in large muscle mass; aspirate to avoid **IV** administration; rotate sites

Direct IV route
• Give **IV** undiluted ≤25 mg/min
Intermittent IV infusion route
May be diluted with 0.9% NaCl, D₅W, D₁₀W, 0.45% NaCl, D₅/0.9% NaCl, D₅/0.45% NaCl, D₅/0.25% NaCl, LR, Ringer's; give 25 mg/min or less

Y-site compatibilities: Acetaminophen, aldesleukin, alfentanil hydrochloride, amifostine, amikacin sulfate, aminocaproic acid, amphotericin B lipid complex (Abelcet), amphotericin B liposome (AmBisome), amsacrine, anidulafungin, argatroban, ascorbic acid injection, atenolol, atracurium besylate, atropine sulfate, azithromycin, benztropine mesylate, bivalirudin, bleomycin, bumetanide, buprenorphine, butorphanol, calcium chloride/gluconate, CARBOplatin, caspofungin, cefTAZidime, ceftizoxime, chlorproMAZINE, cimetidine, ciprofloxacin, cisatracurium, CISplatin, cladribine, clindamycin, codeine, cyanocobalamin, cyclophosphamide, cycloSPORINE, cytarabine, DACTINomycin, DAPTOmycin, digoxin, dilTIAZem, DOBUTamine, DOCEtaxel, DOPamine, doripenem, doxacurium, DOXOrubicin, DOXOrubicin liposomal, doxycycline, enalaprilat, ePHEDrine, EPINEPHrine, epiRUBicin, epoetin alfa, eptifibatide, ertapenem, erythromycin, esmolol, etoposide, famotidine, fenoldopam, fentaNYL, filgrastim, fluconazole, fludarabine, folic acid, gallium, gatifloxacin, gemcitabine, gemtuzumab, gentamicin, glycopyrrolate, granisetron, HYDROmorphone, hydrOXYzine, IDArubicin, ifosfamide, imipenem-cilastatin, irinotecan, isoproterenol, labetalol, levofloxacin, lidocaine, linezolid, LORazepam, LR, magnesium sulfate, mannitol, mechlorethamine, melphalan, meperidine, meropenem, metaraminol, methadone, methicillin, methotrexate, methoxamine, methyldopate, metoclopramide, metoprolol, metroNIDAZOLE, miconazole, midazolam, minocycline, mitoXANTRONE, morphine, multiple vitamins injection, mycophenolate, nalbuphine, naloxone, nesiritide, netilmicin, nitroglycerin, norepinephrine, octreotide, ondansetron, oxaliplatin, oxytocin, PACLitaxel, palonosetron, pamidronate, pancuronium, papaverine, PEMEtrexed, penicillin G potassium/sodium, pentamidine, pentazocine, phenylephrine, phytonadione, piperacillin, piperacillin-tazobactam, polymyxin B, potassium chloride, procainamide, prochlorperazine, promethazine, propofol, propranolol, protamine, pyridoxine, quiNIDine, quinupristin-dalfopristin, raNITIdine, remifentanil, Ringer's, ritodrine, riTUXimab, rocuronium, sargramostim, sodium acetate, succinylcholine, SUFentanil, tacrolimus, teniposide, theophylline, thiamine, thiotepa, ticarcillin, ticarcillin-clavulanate, tigecycline, tirofiban, TNA, tobramycin, tolazoline, TPN, trastuzumab, trimetaphan, urokinase, vancomycin, vasopressin, vecuronium, verapamil, vinCRIStine, vinorelbine, vitamin B complex/C, voriconazole, zoledronic acid

Patient/family education
• Teach patient product should be discontinued 4 days prior to skin allergy tests
• Tell patient that a false-negative result may occur with skin testing; these procedures should not be scheduled until 3 days after discontinuing use
• Inform patient to use sugarless gum, candy, frequent water for dry mouth
• Caution patient to avoid hazardous activities and activities requiring alertness, since dizziness may occur; instruct patient to request assistance with ambulation
• Teach patient to use sunscreen to prevent photosensitivity
• Teach all aspects of product uses; to notify prescriber if confusion, sedation, hypotension occur; to avoid driving and other hazardous activity if drowsiness occurs; to avoid alcohol or other CNS depressants that may potentiate effect
• **Pregnancy/breastfeeding:** Teach patient to report if pregnancy is planned or suspected or if breastfeeding, avoid breastfeeding
• Teach patient not to use in child <6 yr, deaths have occurred, do not use in any child for sleep

Evaluation

Positive therapeutic outcome
• Absence of motion sickness
• Absence of nausea, vomiting
• Ability to sleep
• Absence of cough
• Decrease in involuntary movements

TREATMENT OF OVERDOSE:
• Administer lavage, diazePAM, vasopressors, phenytoin **IV**

divalproex sodium
See valproate

⚠ HIGH ALERT
DOBUTamine (Rx)
(doe-byoo'ta-meen)
Func. class.: Adrenergic direct-acting β_1-agonist, inotropic agent, cardiac stimulant
Chem. class.: Catecholamine

Do not confuse: DOBUTamine/DOPamine

ACTION: Causes increased contractility, increased cardiac output without marked increase in heart rate by acting on β_1-receptors in heart; minor α/β_2 effects

Therapeutic outcome: Cardiac output increased with decreased fatigue and dyspnea

USES: Cardiac decompensation due to organic heart disease or cardiac surgery

Pharmacokinetics
Absorption	Complete
Distribution	Unknown
Metabolism	Liver
Excretion	Kidneys
Half-life	2 min

Pharmacodynamics
Onset	1-5 min
Peak	10 min
Duration	<10 min

CONTRAINDICATIONS
Hypersensitivity, idiopathic hypertrophic subaortic stenosis

Precautions: Pregnancy, breastfeeding, children, hypertension, CAD, MI, hypovolemia, dysrhythmias, sulfite hypersensitivity, renal failure, geriatrics

DOSAGE AND ROUTES
Adult and child: IV INF 0.5-1 mcg/kg/min; titrate to 2-20 mcg/kg/min; may increase to 40 mcg/kg/min if needed

Available forms: Inj 12.5 mg/ml, premixed infusion 250 mg/250 mL, 500 mg/500 mL, 500 mg/250 mL, 1000 mg/250 mL

ADVERSE EFFECTS
CNS: *Anxiety,* headache, dizziness, fatigue
CV: Palpitations, tachycardia, hypo/hypertension, PVCs, angina
ENDO: Hypokalemia
GI: Heartburn, nausea, vomiting
MS: Muscle cramps (leg)
RESP: Dyspnea

INTERACTIONS
Drug classifications
Anesthetics (general): increased dysrhythmias

Antidepressants (tricyclic), COMT inhibitors, MAOIs, oxytocics: increased pressor response, dysrhythmias

β-Blockers: decreased action of DOBUTamine

NURSING CONSIDERATIONS
Assessment
• **Assess for hypovolemia;** if present, correct before beginning treatment with DOBUTamine; avoid use in patients with atrial fibrillation before digitalization

• **Monitor ECG for dysrhythmias, ischemia** during treatment; some patients may not need continuous ECG monitoring; also monitor PCWP, CVP, CO_2, urinary output; notify prescriber if <30 ml/hr, may induce ectopic beats

• **Assess for heart failure:** bibasilar crackles, S_3 gallop, dyspnea, neck vein distention in patients with cardiomyopathy or HF

• **Assess for oxygenation or perfusion deficit:** decreased B/P, chest pain, dizziness, loss of consciousness

• Monitor serum electrolytes, urine output, correct electrolytes before use

• Monitor B/P and pulse q5min during infusion; if B/P drops 30 mm Hg, stop infusion and call prescriber

• Monitor for sulfite sensitivity, which may be life threatening

• **Pregnancy/breastfeeding:** No well-controlled studies, use only if benefits outweigh fetal risk, cautious use in breastfeeding, excretion unknown

Patient problem
Impaired cardiac output (uses)

Ineffective tissue perfusion (uses)

Risk of injury (adverse reaction)

Implementation
• Visually inspect parenteral products for particulate matter and discoloration prior to administration whenever solution and container permit

IV administration
NOTE: Infusions lasting up to 72 hr have been given without development of tolerance. However, β-receptor desensitization may occur with prolonged infusions of any β-adrenergic agonist, including DOBUTamine, or as a consequence of sympathetic compensatory mechanisms associated with advanced congestive heart failure, resulting in alterations in DOBUTamine pharmacodynamics. Experience with intravenous DOBUTamine in controlled trials does not extend beyond 48 hours of repeated boluses and/or continuous infusions

• Must be diluted before administration

• Infuse into a large vein

Dilution
• Concentrate for injection must be diluted with at least 50 ml of a compatible IV solution (strongly alkaline [i.e., sodium bicarbonate] solutions are incompatible). A common dilution is 500 mg (40 ml) in 210 ml D_5W or NS (withdraw 40 ml from a 250 ml bag) to produce a final concentration of 2000 mcg/ml; or 1000 mg (80 ml) in 170 ml D_5W or NS (withdraw 80 ml from a 250 ml bag) to produce a final concentration of 4000 mcg/ml. Max 5000 mcg/ml and should be adjusted according to the fluid requirements of the patient

Continuous Infusion
• Premixed bags of D_5W solutions may be a pink color that, if present, will increase with time; this color change is due to slight oxidation of the drug, but there is no significant loss of potency.

• Do not give DOBUTamine simultaneously with solutions containing sodium bicarbonate or strong alkaline solutions (incompatible)

• Infusion should be started at a low rate and titrated frequently to reach the optimal dosage; dosage titration is guided by the patient's response, including systemic blood pressure, urine flow, frequency of ectopic activity, heart rate, and measurements of cardiac output, central venous pressure, and/or pulmonary capillary wedge pressure

Y-site compatibilities: Alfentanil, alprostadil, amifostine, amikacin, aminocaproic acid, amiodarone, anidulafungin, argatroban, ascorbic acid injection, atenolol, atracurium, atropine, aztreonam, benztropine, bleomycin, bumetanide, buprenorphine, butorphanol, calcium chloride/gluconate, CARBOplatin, caspofungin, chlorproMAZINE, cimetidine, ciprofloxacin, cisatracurium, CISplatin, cladribine, clarithromycin, cloNIDine, codeine, cyanocobalamin, cyclophosphamide, cycloSPORINE, cytarabine, DACTINomycin, DAPTOmycin, dexmedetomidine, digoxin, dilTIAZem, diphenhydrAMINE, DOCEtaxel, DOPamine, doripenem, doxacurium, DOXOrubicin, DOXOrubicin liposomal, doxycycline, enalaprilat, ePHEDrine, EPINEPHrine, epiRUBicin, epoetin alfa, eptifibatide, erythromycin, esmolol, etoposide, famotidine, fenoldopam, fentaNYL, fluconazole, fludarabine, gatifloxacin, gemcitabine, gentamicin, glycopyrrolate, granisetron, HYDROmorphone, hydrOXYzine, IDArubicin, ifosfamide, irinotecan, isoproterenol, labetalol, levofloxacin, lidocaine, linezolid, LORazepam, LR, magnesium sulfate, mannitol, mechlorethamine, meperidine, meropenem, metaraminol,

methoxamine, methyldopa, methylPREDNISolone, metoclopramide, metoprolol, metroNIDA-
ZOLE, miconazole, milrinone, minocycline, mito-
XANtrone, morphine, multiple vitamins injection,
mycophenolate mofetil, nafcillin, nalbuphine,
naloxone, netilmicin, niCARdipine, nitroglycerin,
norepinephrine, octreotide, ondansetron, oxaliplatin, oxytocin, PACLitaxel, palonosetron, pami
dronate, pancuronium, papaverine, pentamidine,
pentazocine, phenylephrine, polymyxin B, potassium chloride, procainamide, prochlorperazine,
promethazine, propofol, propranolol, protamine,
pyridoxine, quiNIDine, raNITIdine, remifentanil,
Ringer's, ritodrine, riTUXimab, rocuronium, sodium acetate, succinylcholine, SUFentanil, tacrolimus, temocillin, teniposide, theophylline, thiamine, thiotepa, tigecycline, tirofiban, TNA,
tobramycin, tolazoline, TPN, trastuzumab,
trimetaphan, urokinase, vancomycin, vasopressin, vecuronium, verapamil, vinCRIStine, vinorelbine, voriconazole, zidovudine, zoledronic acid

Y-site incompatibilities: Acyclovir, alteplase, aminophylline, foscarnet, phytonadione

Patient/family education
• Teach patient reason for medication and
expected results, reason for all monitoring and
procedures
• Advise patient to report dyspnea, headache, **IV**
site discomfort, chest pain, numbness of extremities
• Advise patient, family, caregiver when to notify
health care professional, exercise intolerance,
shortness of breathe, inability to complete ADLs

Evaluation
Positive therapeutic outcome
• Increased cardiac output
• Decreased PCWP, adequate CVP
• Decreased dyspnea, fatigue, edema, ECG
• Increased urine output

TREATMENT OF OVERDOSE:
Discontinue product, support circulation

⚠ HIGH ALERT

DOCEtaxel (Rx)
(doe-se-tax'el)
Docefrez, Taxotere
Func. class.: Antineoplastic,
miscellaneous

Do not confuse: Taxotere/Taxol

ACTION: Inhibits the reorganization of the
microtubule network needed for interphase and
mitotic cellular functions; also causes abnormal
bundles of microtubules during cell cycle and
multiple esters of microtubules during mitosis

Therapeutic outcome: Prevention of
rapidly growing malignant cells

USES: Locally advanced or metastatic
breast cancer, non–small cell lung cancer,
androgen-independent metastatic prostate
cancer, postsurgery operable node-positive
breast cancer, induction treatment of locally
advanced squamous cell cancer of the head/
neck, adjuvant treatment of breast cancer with
CARBOplatin and trastuzumab, gastric adenocarcinoma

Pharmacokinetics

Absorption	Completely absorbed
Distribution	Unknown
Metabolism	Liver, extensively
Excretion	Fecal
Half-life	11.1 hr

Pharmacodynamics

Onset	Rapid
Peak	5-9 days
Duration	1 wk

CONTRAINDICATIONS
Pregnancy, breastfeeding, hypersensitivity to this
product, bilirubin exceeding upper normal limit

BLACK BOX WARNING: Hypersensitivity to
other products with polysorbate 80, neutropenia
(neutrophils <1500/mm³)

Precautions: Children, CV disease, pulmonary disorders, bone marrow depression, herpes
zoster, pleural effusion

BLACK BOX WARNING: Edema, hepatic
disease, lung cancer, taxane hypersensitivity

DOSAGE AND ROUTES
• Other regimens are used

Breast cancer
Adult: IV 60-100 mg/m² given over 1 hr q3wk;
if neutrophil count is <500/mm³ for >1 wk,
reduce dose by 25%

**Operable node-positive breast
cancer; adjuvant breast cancer**
Adult: IV (TAC regimen) 75 mg/m² 1 hr after
DOXOrubicin 50 mg/m² and cyclophosphamide
500 mg/m² q3wk for 6 cycles
Adult: IV (TAC) regimen DOCEtaxel 75 mg/m²
with cyclophosphamide 600 mg/m² q21day ×
4 cycles

Locally advanced or metastatic non–small cell lung cancer after failure of CISplatin chemotherapy
Adult: IV 75 mg/m^2 over 1 hr q3wk; if neutrophil count is <500/mm^3 for >1 wk, reduce dose to 55 mg/m^2; if patient develops grade 3 peripheral neuropathy, stop product
Adult: IV 75 mg/m^2 over 1 hr, then CISplatin 75 mg/m^2 **IV** given over 30-60 min q3wk; reduce dose to 65 mg/m^2 in those with hematologic or nonhematologic toxicities

Squamous cell cancer of head/neck
Adult: IV 75 mg/m^2 over 1 hr, then CISplatin 100 mg/m^2 over 1 hr on day 1, then 5-FU 1000 mg/m^2/day CONT INF × 5 days, repeat cycle q3wk

Available forms: Inj 10 mg/ml, 20 mg/ 0.5 ml, 20 mg/ml, 80 mg/2 ml, 80 mg/4 ml; 20, 80 mg powder for injection/vial

ADVERSE EFFECTS
CNS: Seizures
CV: *Hypotension, fluid retention, peripheral edema,* pericardial effusion, pulmonary edema
EENT: Altered hearing, cystoid macular edema
GI: *Nausea, vomiting, diarrhea,* hepatotoxicity, stomatitis, colitis
HEMA: Leukopenia, thrombocytopenia, anemia
INTEG: *Alopecia,* nail changes, rash, skin eruptions
MISC: Secondary malignancy, Stevens-Johnson syndrome
MS: *Arthralgia, myalgia,* back pain, weakness
NEURO: *Peripheral neuropathy*
RESP: Dyspnea, pulmonary edema, fibrosis, embolism, acute respiratory distress syndrome, interstitial lung disease
SYST: Hypersensitivity reactions, AML, death

INTERACTIONS
Drug classifications
Antineoplastics, radiation: increased myelosuppression
CYP3A4 inhibitors: anastrozole (high doses), aprepitant, clarithromycin, conivaptan, delavirdine, efavirenz, erythromycin, fluconazole, FLUoxetine, fluvoxaMINE, fosaprepitant, imatinib, itraconazole, ketoconazole, nefazodone, voriconazole

NURSING CONSIDERATIONS
Assessment
• **Assess CNS changes:** confusion, paresthesias, peripheral neuropathy, dysesthesia, pain, weakness: if severe, product should be discontinued or use pyridoxine

• Check buccal cavity for dryness, sores or ulceration, white patches, oral pain, bleeding, dysphagia; obtain prescription for viscous lidocaine (Xylocaine) to use in mouth

BLACK BOX WARNING: Assess symptoms indicating severe allergic reaction, anaphylaxis: rash, pruritus, urticaria, purpuric skin lesions, itching, flushing, monitor continuously when giving infusion, may occur during any infusion, but more common during first or second dose; if mild treat symptoms, if severe may require discontinuing, do not retreat those with severe reactions

BLACK BOX WARNING: Neutropenia: Monitor CBC, differential, platelet count weekly; withhold product if WBC is <1500/ mm^3 or platelet count is <100,000/mm^3, notify prescriber of results, nadir 8 days

BLACK BOX WARNING: Use of DOCEtaxel, polysorbate 80 are contraindicated, some products may contain polysorbate 80

BLACK BOX WARNING: Edema: oral corticosteroids should be given as premedication; assess for fluid retention, may be severe, is usually dose related

BLACK BOX WARNING: Lung cancer: increased mortality in those with increased LFTs and a history of platinum-based products

• **Monitor renal function tests:** BUN, creatinine, serum uric acid, urine CCr before, during therapy; check I&O ratio; report fall in urine output to <30 ml/hr

BLACK BOX WARNING: Hepatic disease: Monitor liver function tests before each cycle (bilirubin, AST, ALT, LDH) as needed or monthly; if LFTs are >5 × upper limit discontinue, check for jaundice of skin and sclera, dark urine, clay-colored stools, itchy skin, abdominal pain, fever, diarrhea

BLACK BOX WARNING: Assess for bone marrow depression/bleeding: hematuria, stool guaiac, bruising or petechiae, mucosa or orifices; check for inflammation of mucosa, breaks in skin, avoid IM injections, rectal temps if platelets are low

---

- Assess effects of alopecia on body image; discuss feelings about body changes

Patient problem

Risk for infection (adverse reaction)
Risk for injury (adverse reaction)

Implementation

- Top of systemic analgesics for pain to lessen effects of stomatitis
- Give liquid diet: carbonated beverages; gelatin may be added if patient is not nauseated or vomiting
- Confirm that dexamethasone was given 8 mg BID × 3 days starting 1 day before infusion; for prostate cancer give 8 mg 12 hr, 3 hr and 1 hr prior to infusion
- Store prepared sol up to 27 hr in refrigerator

Intermittent IV infusion route

- Use gloves and cytotoxic handling precautions
- Use non-PVC bag and use non-DEHP tubing
- Double-check all orders and products, errors can be fatal
- Solution is yellow to brown; do not use if particulate is present
- Allow vials to warm to room temperature, withdraw all diluent and inject in vial of DOCEtaxel, rotate gently to mix, allow to stand to decrease foaming, then withdraw the required amount (10 mg/ml) and inject in 250 ml of 0.9% NaCl or D5W, mix gently, give over 1 hr

Y-site compatibilities: Acyclovir, alfentanil, allopurinol, amifostine, amikacin, aminocaproic acid, aminophylline, amiodarone, amphotericin B lipid complex, ampicillin, ampicillin-sulbactam, anidulafungin, atenolol, atracurium, azithromycin, aztreonam, bivalirudin, bleomycin, bumetanide, buprenorphine, busulfan, butorphanol, calcium chloride/gluconate, CARBOplatin, carmustine, caspofungin, ceFAZolin, cefepime, cefonicid, cefotaxime, cefoTEtan, cefOXitin, cefTAZidime, ceftizoxime, cefTRIAXone, cefuroxime, chloramphenicol, chlorproMAZINE, cimetidine, ciprofloxacin, cisatracurium, CISplatin, clindamycin, codeine, cyclophosphamide, cycloSPORINE, cytarabine, dacarbazine, DACTINomycin, DAPTOmycin, dexamethasone, dexmedetomidine, dexrazoxane, diazePAM, digoxin, dilTIAZem, diphenhydrAMINE, DOBUTamine, DOPamine, doripenem, doxacurium, DOXOrubicin HCl, doxycycline, droperidol, enalaprilat, ePHEDrine, EPINEPHrine, epiRUBicin, ertapenem, erythromycin, esmolol, etoposide, famotidine, fenoldopam, fentaNYL, fluconazole, fludarabine, fluorouracil, foscarnet,

fosphenytoin, furosemide, ganciclovir, gatifloxacin, gemcitabine, gentamicin, glycopyrrolate, granisetron, haloperidol, heparin, hydrALAZINE, hydrocortisone, HYDROmorphone, hydrOXYzine, ifosfamide, imipenem-cilastatin, inamrinone, insulin (regular), irinotecan, isoproterenol, ketorolac, labetalol, leucovorin, levofloxacin, levorphanol, lidocaine, linezolid, LORazepam, LR, magnesium sulfate, mannitol, meperidine, meropenem, mesna, methotrexate, methyldopate, metoclopramide, metoprolol, metroNIDAZOLE, midazolam, milrinone, minocycline, mitoXANTRONE, mivacurium, morphine, nafcillin, naloxone, nesiritide, netilmicin, niCARdipine, nitroglycerin, nitroprusside, norepinephrine, octreotide, ofloxacin, ondansetron, oxaliplatin, palonosetron, pamidronate, pancuronium, pantoprazole, PEMEtrexed, pentamidine, pentazocine, PENTobarbital, PHENobarbital, phenylephrine, piperacillin, piperacillin-tazobactam, polymyxin B, potassium chloride/phosphates, procainamide, prochlorperazine, promethazine, propranolol, quiNIDine, quinupristin-dalfopristin, raNITIdine, remifentanil, riTUXimab, rocuronium, sodium acetate/bicarbonate/phosphates, succinylcholine, SUFentanil, sulfamethoxazole-trimethoprim, tacrolimus, teniposide, theophylline, thiopental, thiotepa, ticarcillin, ticarcillin-clavulanate, tigecycline, tirofiban, tobramycin, tolazoline, trastuzumab, trimethobenzamide, vancomycin, vasopressin, vecuronium, verapamil, vinCRIStine, vinorelbine, voriconazole, zidovudine, zoledronic acid

Patient/family education

- **Pregnancy/breastfeeding:** Inform patient that nonhormonal contraceptive measures are recommended during therapy and >4 mo after; teratogenic effects are possible
- Teach patient to avoid use of products containing aspirin or ibuprofen, razors, commercial mouthwash, since bleeding may occur; to report symptoms of bleeding (hematuria, tarry stools)
- Instruct patient to report signs of **anemia** (fatigue, headache, irritability, faintness, shortness of breath) and CNS reactions (confusion, psychosis, nightmares, seizures, severe headaches)
- Instruct patient to report signs of **infection:** fever, sore throat, flulike symptoms
- Inform patient that hair may be lost during treatment; a wig or hairpiece may make patient feel better; new hair may be different in color and texture
- Inform patient that receiving vaccinations during therapy may cause serious reactions

---

• Instruct patient to rinse mouth tid-qid with water, club soda; brush teeth bid-qid with soft brush or cotton-tipped applicators for stomatitis; use unwaxed dental floss
• Advise patient not to use alcohol
• Advise patient not to drive until effect is known

Evaluation
Positive therapeutic outcome
• Prevention of rapid division of malignant cells

---

docosanol topical
See Appendix B

docusate calcium (OTC)
(dok'yoo-sate cal'see-um)
Kao-Tin, Kaopectate Stool Softener
docusate sodium (OTC)
Colace, Correctol, Diocto, Docu DOK, Doculace, Dulcolax, Dulcolax Stool Softener, Enemeez, Fleet Pedialax, Fleet Sof-Lax, Phillips Liquid-Gels, Selex ✦, Silace, Soflax ✦
Func. class.: Laxative, emollient
Chem. class.: Anionic surfactant

Do not confuse: Colace/Cozaar, Dulcolax **(docusate)**/Dulcolax (biscodyl)

ACTION: Increases water, fat penetration in intestine; allows for easier passage of stool

Therapeutic outcome: Passage of softened stool, absence of constipation

USES: Prevent hard, dry stools, prevent constipation, soften fecal impaction (rectal route)

Pharmacokinetics

Absorption	Minimal (PO)
Distribution	Unknown
Metabolism	Not metabolized
Excretion	Bile
Half-life	Unknown

Pharmacodynamics

	PO	RECT
Onset	12-72 hr	2-15 min
Peak	Unknown	Unknown
Duration	Unknown	Unknown

CONTRAINDICATIONS
Hypersensitivity, obstruction, fecal impaction, nausea/vomiting

Precautions: Pregnancy, breastfeeding

DOSAGE AND ROUTES
Adult: PO 50-400 mg/day in divided doses (docusate sodium) or 240 mg q day (docusate calcium); Rectal: enema 4 ml (docusate sodium)
Child >12 yr: Enema 2 ml (docusate sodium)
Child 6-12 yr: PO 40-150 mg/day (docusate sodium) in divided doses
Child 3-6 yr: PO 20-60 mg/day (docusate sodium) in divided doses
Child <3 yr: PO 10-40 mg/day (docusate sodium) in divided doses
Infant: PO 5 mg/kg/day in divided doses

Available forms: Docusate calcium: caps 240 mg; **docusate sodium:** caps 50, 100, 250 mg; tabs 100 mg; syr 20 mg/5 ml, liquid 50 mg/5 ml, enema 283 mg/15 mL

ADVERSE EFFECTS
EENT: Bitter taste, throat irritation
GI: Nausea, anorexia, cramps, diarrhea
INTEG: Rash

INTERACTIONS
Individual drugs
Mineral oil: toxicity

Drug/herb
Flax, senna: increased laxative action

NURSING CONSIDERATIONS
Assessment
• Assess cramping, rectal bleeding, nausea, vomiting; if these symptoms occur, product should be discontinued; identify cause of constipation; identify fluids, bulk, or exercise is missing from lifestyle
• **Pregnancy/breastfeeding:** low risk of fetal harm in pregnancy, breastfeeding

Patient problem
Constipation (uses)

Implementation
PO route
• Dilute oral sol in juice or other fluid to disguise taste
• Give tabs or caps with 8 oz of liquid; give on empty stomach for increased absorption, results
• Store in cool environment; do not freeze

Patient/family education
• Discuss with patient that adequate fluid consumption is as necessary as bulk, exercise for adequate bowel function
• Teach patient that normal bowel movements do not always occur daily
• Advise patient not to use in presence of abdominal pain, nausea, vomiting; tell patient to notify prescriber if unrelieved constipation or if symptoms of electrolyte imbalance occur: muscle cramps, pain, weakness, dizziness, excessive thirst

---

- Advise patient that product may take up to 3 days to soften stools
- Instruct patient to take oral preparation with a full glass of water and increase fluid intake unless on fluid restrictions
- Caution patients with heart disease to avoid using the Valsalva maneuver to expedite evacuation

Evaluation
Positive therapeutic outcome
- Decreased constipation within 3 days

⚠ HIGH ALERT

dofetilide
(doff-ee-till'-lide)
Tikosyn
Func. class.: Antidysrhythmic (Class III)

ACTION: Blocks cardiac ion channel carrying the rapid component of delayed potassium current, no effect on sodium channels

Therapeutic outcome: Absence of atrial fibrillation

USES: Atrial fibrillation, flutter, maintenance of normal sinus rhythm

Pharmacokinetics

Absorption	>90%
Distribution	Steady state 2-3 days
Metabolism	Not metabolized
Excretion	Kidneys 80%
Half-life	10 hr

Pharmacodynamics

Onset	Unknown
Peak	3 hr
Duration	Up to 24 hr

CONTRAINDICATIONS
Hypersensitivity, digoxin toxicity, aortic stenosis, pulmonary hypertension, children, severe renal disease, QT prolongation, torsades de pointes, renal failure

Precautions: Pregnancy, breastfeeding, AV block, bradycardia, electrolyte imbalance, renal disease

> **BLACK BOX WARNING:** arrhythmias, ventricular **arrhythmias**/tachycardia, requires an experienced clinician, in a specialized care setting

DOSAGE AND ROUTES
Adult PO 500 mcg bid initially; maintenance 250 mcg bid, max 500 mcg bid; adjust doses based on QT and renal function

Renal dose
Adult: PO initial dose for CCr >60 mg/ml 500 mcg bid; CCr 40-60 mg/min 250 mcg bid; CCr 20-39 mg/min 125 mcg bid; CCr <20 mg/min do not use

Available forms: Caps 125, 250, 500 mcg

ADVERSE EFFECTS
CNS: *Dizziness,* headache
CV: QT prolongation, torsades de pointes, ventricular dysrhythmias, chest pain

INTERACTIONS
Individual drugs
AMILoride, entecavir, lamiVUDine, memantine, metFORMIN, procainamide, triamterene, trospium: increased toxicity

Arsenic trioxide, chloroquine, ciprofloxacin, clarithromycin, droperidol, erythromycin, halofantrine, haloperidol, levomethadyl, levofloxacin, methadone, pentamidine, ziprasidone: increased QT prolongation, torsades de pointes

Cimetidine, hydroCHLOROthiazide, ketoconazole, megestrol, metFORMIN, prochlorperazine, triamterene, trimethoprim/sulfamethoxazole, verapamil: do not use together

Drug classifications
Antiretroviral protease inhibitors: increased dofetilide levels

Class IA/III antidysrhythmics, some phenothiazines: increased QT prolongation, torsades de pointes

Diuretics, potassium depletion: increased hypokalemia

CYP3A4 inhibitors, SSRIs, macrolides, azoles, protease inhibitors, amiodarone, doltizem, quinine: Increase: dysrhythmias

Drug/food
- Do not use with grapefruit juice

NURSING CONSIDERATIONS
Assessment
- **Severe renal impairment:** CCr <20 ml/min: do not use for mild to moderate renal disease, monitor BUN/creatinine; adjust dose based on creatinine clearance
- AF patients should receive anticoagulation prior to cardioversion
- Nausea, vomiting, before and after use
- Assess all products taken by patient (OTC, Rx, herbals, supplements), many drug interactions
- **Pregnancy/breastfeeding:** No well-controlled studies, use only if benefits outweigh fetal risk, avoid breastfeeding, excretion unknown

Patient problem
Impaired cardiac output (uses)

Implementation
- Physician and pharmacy must be registered to use product
- With patient hospitalized for ≥ 3 days

BLACK BOX WARNING: Step 1: Assess cardiac conduction: Before first dose, the QTc interval must be determined using an average of 5-10 beats; if the QTc interval is >440 msec (or >500 msec in ventricular conduction abnormalities), do not use. If baseline heart rate is <60 bpm, then the QT interval should be used
Step 2: Assess renal function: Before first dose, determine renal function using the Cockroft-Gault equation, use actual body weight to calculate creatinine clearance
Step 3: Adjust starting dose according to renal function: Refer to the Renal dose section (above) to determine the appropriate initial dose
Step 4: ECG monitoring: Begin continuous ECG monitoring starting with the first dose
Step 5: Dose adjustments: Approximately 2-3 hr after the first dose, determine the QTc interval. If the QTc interval has increased by >15% (compared with baseline), or, if the QTc interval is >500 msec (>550 msec in patients with ventricular conduction abnormalities), the initial dosage should be reduced by half as follows:
- Decrease an initial dose of 500 mcg bid to 250 mcg bid
- Decrease an initial dose of 250 mcg bid to 125 mcg bid
- Decrease an initial dose of 125 mcg bid to 125 mcg daily
Step 6: Reassess QTc interval: Reassess the QTc interval 2-3 hr after each subsequent dose; if, the QTc interval lengthens to >500 msec (or >550 msec in patients with ventricular conduction abnormalities), **discontinue**
Step 7: ECG Monitoring: Monitor continuous ECG for a minimum of 3 days or for 12 hr after conversion to normal sinus rhythm, whichever is greater

Patient/family education
- Instruct patient to notify prescriber if fast heartbeats with fainting or dizziness occur
- Instruct patient to notify all prescribers of all medications and supplements taken
- Teach patient that if a dose is missed, do not double, take next dose at usual time, to take only as prescribed, not to use grapefruit juice
- Teach patient and provide "Medication Guide" prior to use; stress need for continued follow-up lab work
- Teach patient how to take pulse and when to report changes

Evaluation
Positive therapeutic outcome
- Increased control in atrial fibrillation

dolasetron (Rx)
(do-la′se-tron)
Anzemet
Func. class.: Antiemetic
Chem. class.: 5-HT receptor antagonist

ACTION: Prevents nausea, vomiting by blocking serotonin peripherally, centrally, and in the small intestine

Therapeutic outcome: Control of nausea, vomiting

USES: Prevention of postoperative nausea, vomiting

Pharmacokinetics
Absorption	Completely absorbed
Distribution	Unknown
Metabolism	Liver, extensively
Excretion	Kidneys
Half-life	Metabolite 8.1 hr

Pharmacodynamics
Onset	Unknown
Peak	1-2 hr
Duration	12-24 hr

CONTRAINDICATIONS
Hypersensitivity

Precautions: Pregnancy, breast-feeding, children, geriatric, hypokalemia, electrolyte imbalances, granisetron, ondansetron, palonosetron hypersensitivity, QT prolongation

DOSAGE AND ROUTES
Prevention of cancer chemotherapy nausea/vomiting
Adult: PO 100 mg 1 hr before chemotherapy
Child 2-16 yr: PO 1.8 mg/kg, 1 hr before chemotherapy, max 100 mg

Available forms: Tabs 50, 100 mg

ADVERSE EFFECTS
CNS: *Headache,* dizziness, fatigue, drowsiness, serotonin syndrome
CV: Dysrhythmias, ECG changes, hypo/hypertension, tachycardia, bradycardia, QT prolongation, torsades de pointes, ventricular tachycardia/fibrillation, cardiac arrest (IV)
GI: *Diarrhea,* constipation, increased AST, ALT, abdominal pain, anorexia

---

⚠ Nurse Alert   ✳ Key NCLEX® Drug   >> Drug Specifics

GU: Urinary retention, oliguria
MISC: Rash, bronchospasm

INTERACTIONS
Individual drugs
Arsenic trioxide, chloroquine, clarithromycin, droperidol, erythromycin, halofantrine, haloperidol, levomethadyl, methadone, pentamidine, ziprasidone: increased QT prolongation; occurs at higher dose of dolasetron
Cimetidine: increased dolasetron levels
RifAMPin: decreased dolasetron levels

Drug classifications
Antidysrhythmics: increased dysrhythmias
Class IA/III antidysrhythmics, some phenothiazines, loop diuretics, thiazide: increased QT prolongation

NURSING CONSIDERATIONS
Assessment
• **QT prolongation and QRS, PR prolongation:** do not use in those with congenital long QT syndrome, hypokalemia, hypomagnesemia, complete heart block (unless a pacemaker is in place); correct electrolytes before use; monitor ECG in the elderly, renal cardiac disease
• **Assess for hypersensitivity reaction:** rash, bronchospasm
• **Pregnancy/breastfeeding:** No well-controlled studies, use only if clearly needed, cautious use in breastfeeding, excretion unknown
• **Serotonin syndrome:** Usually when combined with SSRIs, SNRIs, MAOIs

Patient problem
Nausea (uses)

Implementation
PO route
• Do not mix product for oral administration in juice until immediately before administration; apple or apple-grape diluted can be kept for 2 hr at room temperature
• Store at room temp 48 hr after dilution

Patient/family education
• Instruct patient to report diarrhea, constipation, rash, nausea, vomiting, or changes in respirations; may cause headache; use analgesic
• Teach patient reason for medication and expected results

Evaluation
Positive therapeutic outcome
• Absence of nausea, vomiting during cancer chemotherapy

---

dolutegravir
(dole-oo-teg'ra-vir)
Tivicay
Func. class.: Antiretroviral
Chem. class.: HIV integrase strand transfer inhibitor (ISTIs)

D

ACTION: Inhibits catalytic activity of HIV integrase, which is an HIV-encoded enzyme needed for replication

Therapeutic outcome: Improvement in cell counts, T-cell counts

USES: HIV in combination with other antiretrovirals

Pharmacokinetics

Absorption	Unknown
Distribution	Steady state 5 days, 98% protein binding
Metabolism	Liver; ⚹⚕ some patients are poor metabolizers
Excretion	Feces 53%, urine 31%
Half-life	14 hr

Pharmacodynamics

Onset	Unknown
Peak	2-3 hr
Duration	Up to 24 hr

CONTRAINDICATIONS
Breastfeeding, hypersensitivity

Precautions: Pregnancy, children, geriatric patients, hepatic disease, immune reconstitution syndrome, hepatitis, antimicrobial resistance, lactase deficiency

DOSAGE AND ROUTES
Adult and child >12 yr and ≥40 kg (treatment-naïve or treatment-experienced but integrase strand transfer inhibitor–naïve): PO 50 mg/day; if given with efavirenz, fosamprenavir/ritonavir, tipranavir/ritonavir or RifAMPin give 50 mg bid
Child 30-39 kg: PO 35 mg/day; if using efavirenz, fosamprenavir/ritonavir, tipranavirl ritonavir or rifampin 35 mg bid

Available forms: Tabs 10, 25, 50 mg
ADVERSE EFFECTS
CNS: Fatigue, headache, insomnia
GI: Nausea, vomiting, diarrhea, *hepatotoxicity*
INTEG: Rash, pruritus
GU: Renal dysfunction
META: Hyperglycemia
SYST: Immune reconstitution syndrome

INTERACTIONS
Individual drugs
Efavirenz, RifAMPin tenofovir, tipranavir/ritonavir: decreased levels of each product

Drug classifications
Antacids, buffered products, laxatives/sucralfate, oral iron products, oral calcium products, buffered products: decreased effect of dolutegravir

Drug/herb
St. John's wort: avoid concurrent use

NURSING CONSIDERATIONS
Assessment
• **HIV infection:** monitor CD4, T-cell count, plasma HIV RNA, viral load; resistance testing before treatment, at treatment failure
• Perform drug resistance testing prior to use in treatment-naïve patients
• Immune reconstitution syndrome, usually during initial phase of treatment, may be antiinfective before starting
• Monitor total/HDL/LDL cholesterol baseline and periodically, all may be elected
• **Pregnancy/breastfeeding:** All HIV-positive women should receive antiretroviral therapy, report pregnancy to the Antiretroviral Pregnancy Registry (800-258-4263), glucose screening should be performed at 24-28 wk gestation, confirm gestation age in each trimester by ultrasound, avoid breastfeeding

Patient problem
Infection (uses)
Nonadherence (teaching)

Implementation
• May give without regard to meals, with 8 oz of water
• Store at room temperature
• Give 2 hr before or 6 hr after cation-containing antacids or laxatives, sucralfate, oral iron, oral calcium, or buffered products

Patient/family education
• Teach patient to take as prescribed; if dose missed to take as soon as remembered up to 1 hr before next dose; not to double dose; not to share with others
• Advise patient to discuss all OTC, herbals, supplements with health care professional
• Inform patient that continuing follow-up and lab work will be needed
• Teach patient that fat accumulation/redistribution may occur

• Teach patient that sexual partners need to be told that patient has HIV; that product does not cure infection, just controls symptoms, does not prevent infecting others
• Teach patient to report sore throat, fever, fatigue (may indicate superinfection)
• Teach patient to notify prescriber if pregnancy is planned or suspected; to avoid breastfeeding and to continue follow-up exams and work

Evaluation
Positive therapeutic outcome
• Improvement in cell counts, T-cell counts

RARELY USED
dolutegravir/rilpivirine
(doe-loo-teg'- ra- vir/ril-pi-vir'-een)
Juluca
Func. class.: Antiviral

USES: For the treatment of HIV-1 infection in adults

DOSAGES AND ROUTES
HIV infection
Adult: PO 1 tab (dolutegravir 50 mg; rilpivirine 25 mg) plus an additional 25 mg tablet of rilpivirine (total daily rilpivirine dose of 50 mg) qday with a meal. When rifabutin coadministration is stopped, reduce rilpivirine dose to 25 mg qday with a meal

Human immunodeficiency virus (HIV) infection without concurrent rifabutin
Adult: PO 1 tab (dolutegravir 50 mg; rilpivirine 25 mg) qday with a meal

---

donepezil (Rx)
(don-ep-ee'zill)
Aricept
Func. class.: Anti-Alzheimer's agent
Chem. class.: Reversible cholinesterase inhibitor

Do not confuse: Aricept/Aciphex/Azitect

ACTION: Elevates acetylcholine concentrations (cerebral cortex) by slowing degradation of acetylcholine released in cholinergic neurons; does not alter underlying dementia

---

Therapeutic outcome: Decreased symptoms of Alzheimer's disease

USES: Treatment of mild to severe dementia in Alzheimer's disease

Pharmacokinetics

Absorption	Well
Distribution	Protein binding 96%
Metabolism	Liver to metabolites by CYP2D6, CYP3A4
Excretion	Kidneys
Half-life	70 hr

Pharmacodynamics

Unknown

CONTRAINDICATIONS

Hypersensitivity to this product or piperidine derivatives

Precautions: Pregnancy, breastfeeding, children, sick sinus syndrome, history of ulcers, GI bleeding, hepatic disease, bladder obstruction, asthma, seizures, COPD, abrupt discontinuation, AV block, GI obstruction, Parkinson's disease, surgery

DOSAGE AND ROUTES

Adult: PO 5 mg/day at bedtime; may increase to 10 mg/day after 4-6 wk, may increase to 23 mg/day after 3 mo of 10 mg/day (moderate to severe); 5 mg q day, may be increased by 10 mg q d after 4-6 wk; after 3 mo may increase to 23 mg q day (severe)

Available forms: Tabs 5, 10, 23 mg

ADVERSE EFFECTS

CNS: Insomnia, headache, fatigue, abnormal dreams, syncope, seizures, drowsiness, depression, confusion, hallucinations
CV: Atrial fibrillation, hypo/hypertension
GI: *Nausea, vomiting,* anorexia, *diarrhea,* abdominal pain, weight gain, GI bleeding
GU: Frequency
INTEG: Rash, flushing, diaphoresis, bruising
MS: Cramps, arthritis, arthralgia, back pain

INTERACTIONS
Individual drugs

CarBAMazepine, dexamethasone, PHENobarbital, phenytoin, RifAMPin: decreased donepezil effect
Succinylcholine: synergistic effects

Drug classification

Anticholinergics: decreased activity
Cholinergic agonists, cholinesterase inhibitors: synergistic effects

Increase: QT prolongation: astemizole, cisapride, dofetilide, dronedarone, grepafloxacin, mesoridazine, pimozide, probucol, sparfloxacin, terfenadine, ziprasidone, do not use concurrently
NSAIDs: increased GI bleeding
CYP2D6, CYP3A4 inducers: decreased donepezil effects
CYP2D6, CYP3A4 inhibitors: increased donepezil effects

Drug/herb

St. John's wort: decreased donepezil effect

Drug/lab test

Increase: CK

NURSING CONSIDERATIONS
Assessment

• **Alzheimer's disease:** assess ability to perform some ADLs, memory, language, confusion baseline and during treatment
• Monitor B/P, heart rate: hypo/hypertension
• Assess mental status: affect, mood, behavioral changes, depression
• Assess GI status: nausea, vomiting, anorexia, diarrhea, active/occult GI bleeding
• Assess GU status: urinary frequency, incontinence
• **Beers:** Avoid use in older adults, increases risk of hyper/hypotension/bradycardia

Patient problem

Distorted thinking process (uses)
Risk for injury (uses)

Implementation
PO route

• Give between meals; may be given with meals for GI symptoms

Patient/family education

• Advise patient to report side effects: twitching, nausea, vomiting, sweating, dizziness; indicates overdose
• Advise patient to use product exactly as prescribed, not to use with other products, unless approved by prescriber
• Teach patient and family, caregiver dizziness may occur; be aware of possible falls
• Advise patient to notify prescriber of nausea, vomiting, diarrhea (dose increase or beginning treatment), or rash
• Advise patient not to increase or abruptly decrease dosage, serious consequences may result
• Instruct patient that product is not a cure but controls symptoms
• Teach patient to report if pregnancy is planned or suspected, avoid breastfeeding
• Advise patient and caregiver that continuing follow-ups will be needed

Evaluation
Positive therapeutic outcome
• Decrease in confusion; improved mood memory

> **⚠ HIGH ALERT**
>
> ## DOPamine (Rx)
> (dope′pa-meen)
> *Func. class.:* Agonist, vasopressor, inotropic agent
> *Chem. class.:* Catecholamine

Do not confuse: DOPamine/DOBUTamine

ACTION: Causes increased cardiac output; acts on β_1- and α-receptors, causing vasoconstriction in blood vessels; when low doses are administered, causes renal and mesenteric vasodilatation; β_1 stimulation produces inotropic effects with increased cardiac output

Therapeutic outcome: Increased B/P, cardiac output

USES: Shock; to increase perfusion; hypotension, cardiogenic/septic shock

Pharmacokinetics

Absorption	Complete
Distribution	Widely
Metabolism	Liver
Excretion	Kidney, plasma
Half-life	2 min

Pharmacodynamics

Onset	2-5 min
Peak	Unknown
Duration	<10 min

CONTRAINDICATIONS
Hypersensitivity, ventricular fibrillation, tachydysrhythmias, pheochromocytoma, hypovolemia

Precautions: Pregnancy, breastfeeding, geriatric, arterial embolism, peripheral vascular disease, sulfite hypersensitivity, acute MI

> **BLACK BOX WARNING:** Extravasation

DOSAGE AND ROUTES
Adult: **IV** INF 2-5 mcg/kg/min, titrate upward 5-10 mcg/kg/min, max 50 mcg/kg/min; titrate to patient's response
Child: **IV** 1-5 mcg/kg/min initially; usual dosage range 2-20 mcg/kg/min

HF
Adult: **IV** 3-10 mcg/kg/min

Available forms: Inj 40, 80, 160 mg/ml; conc for **IV** inf 0.8, 1.6, 3.2 mg/ml in 250, 500 ml D₅W

ADVERSE EFFECTS
CNS: *Headache,* anxiety
CV: *Palpitations,* ectopic beats, *angina,* wide QRS complex, peripheral vasoconstriction, hypotension
GI: *Nausea, vomiting, diarrhea*
INTEG: Necrosis, tissue sloughing with extravasation
RESP: Dyspnea

INTERACTIONS
Individual drugs
Phenytoin: bradycardia, hypotension

Drug classifications
α-Adrenergic blockers, β-adrenergic blockers: decreased action of DOPamine
Anesthetics (general): increased dysrhythmias
Antidepressants (tricyclic): increased pressor response
Ergots: severe hypertension
MAOIs: increased hypertension (severe), do not use within 2 wk; increased pressor effect; hypertensive crisis may result
Oxytocics: increased B/P

Drug/lab test
Increased: urinary catecholamine, serum glucose

NURSING CONSIDERATIONS
Assessment
• Monitor ECG for dysrhythmias, ischemia during treatment; some patients may not need continuous ECG monitoring; also monitor PCWP, CVP, CO₂, urinary output; notify prescriber if <30 ml/hr
• **Assess for heart failure:** crackles, dyspnea, neck vein distention in patients with cardiomyopathy or HF
• **Assess for oxygenation or perfusion deficit:** decreased B/P, chest pain, dizziness, loss of consciousness
• Monitor B/P and pulse during inf; if B/P drops 30 mm Hg, stop inf and call provider

Patient problem
Impaired cardiac output (uses)
Ineffective tissue perfusion (uses)

Implementation
• Correct volume depletion before use
• Store reconstituted sol for up to 24 hr if refrigerated
• Do not use discolored sol; protect from light

Continuous infusion route
• Dilute 200-400 mg/250-500 ml of D₅W, 0.9% NaCl, D₅/LR, D₅/0.45% NaCl, D₅/0.9% NaCl, LR; do not use discolored sol; sol is stable for 24 hr; give 0.5-5 mcg/kg/min; may increase by 1-4 mcg/kg/min q15-30min until desired patient response; use infusion pump, titrate as needed, decrease infusion gradually

BLACK BOX WARNING: Extravasation: if extravasation occurs, stop infusion, may inject area with phentolamine 10 mg/15 ml NS

Y-site compatibilities: Alfentanil, alprostadil, amifostine, amikacin, aminocaproic acid, aminophylline, amiodarone, anidulafungin, argatroban, ascorbic acid injection, atenolol, atracurium, atropine, aztreonam, benztropine, bivalirudin, bleomycin, bumetanide, buprenorphine, butorphanol, calcium chloride/gluconate, CARBOplatin, caspofungin, cefmetazole, cefonicid, cefotaxime, cefoTEtan, cefOXitin, cefTAZidime, ceftizoxime, cefTRIAXone, cefuroxime, chlorproMAZINE, cimetidine, ciprofloxacin, cisatracurium, CISplatin, cladribine, clarithromycin, clindamycin, cloNIDine, codeine, cyanocobalamin, cyclophosphamide, cycloSPORINE, cytarabine, DACTINomycin, DAPTOmycin, dexamethasone, dexmedetomidine, digoxin, dilTIAZem, diphenhydrAMINE, DOBUTamine, DOCEtaxel, doripenem, doxacurium, DOXOrubicin, DOXOrubicin liposomal, doxycycline, droperidol, enalaprilat, ePHEDrine, EPINEPHrine, epiRUBicin, epoetin alfa, eptifibatide, ertapenem, erythromycin, esmolol, etoposide, famotidine, fenoldopam, fentaNYL, fluconazole, fludarabine, fluorouracil, folic acid, foscarnet, gatifloxacin, gemcitabine, gemtuzumab, gentamicin, glycopyrrolate, granisetron, heparin, hydrocortisone, HYDROmorphone, hydrOXYzine, IDArubicin, ifosfamide, imipenem-cilastatin, irinotecan, isoproterenol, ketorolac, labetalol, levofloxacin, lidocaine, linezolid, LORazepam, LR, magnesium sulfate, mannitol, mechlorethamine, meperidine, methicillin, methyldopa, methylPREDNISolone, metoclopramide, metoprolol, metroNIDAZOLE, micafungin, miconazole, midazolam, milrinone, minocycline, mitoXANTRONE, morphine, multiple vitamins injection, mycophenolate, nafcillin, nalbuphine, naloxone, netilmicin, niCARdipine, nitroglycerin, nitroprusside, norepinephrine, octreotide, ondansetron, oxacillin, oxaliplatin, oxytocin, PACLitaxel, palonosetron, pamidronate, pancuronium, pantoprazole, papaverine, PEMEtrexed, penicillin G potassium/sodium, pentamidine, pentazocine, PENTobarbital, PHENobarbital, phenylephrine, phytonadione, piperacillin, piperacillin-tazobactam, polymyxin B, potassium chloride, procainamide, prochlorperazine, promethazine, propofol, propranolol, protamine, pyridoxine, quiNIDine, raNITIdine, remifentanil, Ringer's, ritodrine, riTUXimab, rocuronium, sargramostim, sodium acetate, succinylcholine, SUFentanil, tacrolimus, temocillin, teniposide, theophylline, thiamine, thiotepa, ticarcillin, ticarcillin-clavulanate, tigecycline, tirofiban, TPA, tobramycin, tolazoline, TPN, trastuzumab, trimetaphan, urokinase, vancomycin, vasopressin, vecuronium, verapamil, vinCRIStine, vinorelbine, vitamin B complex/C, voriconazole, warfarin, zidovudine, zoledronic acid

Patient/family education
• Teach patient reason for medication, expected results, reason for all monitoring and procedures
• Advise patient to report all side effects
• Teach patient to report immediately chest pain, SOB, numbness/tingling of extremities
• Teach patient to report immediately pain, burning, redness at IV site

Evaluation

Positive therapeutic outcome
• Increased cardiac output, increased B/P

TREATMENT OF OVERDOSE: Discontinue product, support circulation; give a short-acting α-blocker

---

dorzolamide ophthalmic
See Appendix B

doxazosin (Rx)
(dox-ay'zoe-sin)
Cardura, Cardura XL
Func. class.: Peripheral α-adrenergic blocker, antihypertensive
Chem. class.: Quinazoline

Do not confuse: Cardura/Coumadin/Cardene/Ridaura

ACTION: Peripheral blood vessels are dilated, peripheral resistance lowered; reduction in B/P results from peripheral α-adrenergic receptors being blocked

Therapeutic outcome: Decreased B/P, decreased symptoms of benign prostatic hypertrophy (BPH)

USES: Hypertension, urinary outflow obstruction, symptoms of benign prostatic hyperplasia

---

Pharmacokinetics

Absorption	Well absorbed
Distribution	Not known; 98% protein bound
Metabolism	Liver, extensively (<63%)
Excretion	Kidneys
Half-life	22 hr

Pharmacodynamics

	PO	PO XL
Onset	2 hr	5 wk
Peak	2-3 hr	Unknown
Duration	Up to 24 hr	Unknown

CONTRAINDICATIONS
Hypersensitivity to quinazolines

Precautions: Pregnancy, breastfeeding, children, hepatic disease, geriatrics

DOSAGE AND ROUTES
BPH
Adult: PO 1 mg/day at bedtime, may increase to 8 mg/day; XL 4 mg q day at breakfast, may increase q 3-4 wk to 8 mg/day

Hypertension
Adult: PO 1 mg/day at bedtime, increasing gradually q 2 wk up to 16 mg daily if required; usual range 4-16 mg/day
Geriatric: PO 0.5 mg nightly, gradually increase

Available forms: Tabs 1, 2, 4, 8 mg; ext rel tabs 4, 8 mg

ADVERSE EFFECTS
CNS: *Dizziness,* headache, drowsiness, anxiety, depression, vertigo, weakness, fatigue
CV: Palpitations, *orthostatic hypotension, edema,* dysrhythmias, chest pain
EENT: Epistaxis, tinnitus, dry mouth, pharyngitis, rhinitis, blurred vision
GI: *Nausea,* vomiting, diarrhea, constipation, abdominal pain
GU: Priapism, impotence, decreased libido
RESP: Dyspnea

INTERACTIONS
Individual drugs
Alcohol: increased hypotensive effects

Drug classifications
NSAIDs, estrogens, sympathomimetics: decrease: hypotensive effects
Other antihypertensives, nitrates, PDE-5 inhibitors, dose may need adjustment: increased hypotensive effects

NURSING CONSIDERATIONS
Assessment
• **Hypertension:** monitor B/P (lying, standing) and pulse, syncope; check for edema in feet, legs daily; I&O; monitor for weight daily; notify prescriber of changes
• **BPH:** urinary pattern changes (hesitancy, dribbling, incomplete bladder emptying, dysuria, urgency, nocturia, urgency incontinence, intermittency before and during treatment)
• Assess for orthostatic hypotension; tell patient to rise slowly from sitting or lying position; assess pulse, jugular venous distention q4hr, crackles, dyspnea, orthopnea with B/P

Patient problem
Impaired urination (uses)
Risk for injury (adverse reactions)

Implementation
PO route
• **Tabs** broken, crushed, or chewed; chewed tabs taste bitter; do not break, crush, chew **XL tabs**
• **Immediate release tab:** give without regard to meals; **EXT REL tabs:** give with breakfast; when switching from immediate release to EXT REL, the final evening dose of immediate release should be taken
• Store in tight container at room temperature (86° F [30° C] or less)
• May be used in combination with other antihypertensives
• May be given with food to prevent GI symptoms

Patient/family education
• Teach patient not to discontinue product abruptly; emphasize the importance of complying with dosage schedule, even if feeling better; if dose is missed take as soon as remembered; take at same time each day
• Teach patient not to use OTC products (cough, cold, allergy) unless directed by prescriber; also to avoid large amounts of caffeine
• Emphasize the need to rise slowly to sitting or standing position to minimize orthostatic hypotension
• Teach patient to notify prescriber of mouth sores, sore throat, fever, swelling of hands or feet, irregular heartbeat, chest pain
• Caution patient to report excessive perspiration, dehydration, vomiting, diarrhea; may lead to fall in B/P
• Caution patient that product may cause dizziness, fainting, light-headedness; may occur during 1st few days of therapy; to avoid hazardous activities
• Teach patient how to take B/P, and normal readings for age-group; to take B/P q7days
• Inform patient that fainting occasionally occurs after 1st dose; do not drive or operate

machinery for 4 hr after 1st dose or after dosage increase or take 1st dose at bedtime; may take 1-2 wk in BPH
• Teach patient to comply with hypertension regimen, low-sodium diet, exercise, weight reduction, stress management, not to smoke
• Teach patient how to take B/P to check at least once/wk
• Teach patient to notify all health care providers of all RX, OTC, and herbal supplements; not to add any products unless approved by prescriber
• Teach patient to avoid hazardous activities until response is known, dizziness or drowsiness may occur
• Teach patient to continue to take product even if feeling better, take at same time each day, do not take double doses

Evaluation
Positive therapeutic outcome
• Decreased B/P in hypertension
• Decreased symptoms of BPH

TREATMENT OF OVERDOSE:
Administer volume expanders or vasopressors; discontinue product; place in supine position

doxercalciferol
See Vitamin D

⚠ HIGH ALERT

DOXOrubicin
(dox-oh-roo'bi-sin)
Adriamycin, Caelyx ✦, Myocet ✦
Func. class.: Antineoplastic, antibiotic
Chem. class.: Anthracycline glycoside

Do not confuse: DOXOrubicin/DOXOrubicin liposomal/DAUNOrubicin

ACTION: Inhibits DNA synthesis primarily; replication is decreased by binding to DNA, which causes strand splitting; active throughout entire cell cycle; a vesicant

USES: Wilms' tumor; bladder, breast, lung, ovarian, stomach, thyroid cancer; Hodgkin's/non-Hodgkin's disease; acute lymphoblastic leukemia; myeloblastic leukemia; neuroblastomas; soft tissue/bone sarcomas

Pharmacokinetics

Absorption	Complete
Distribution	Crosses placenta
Metabolism	Liver by CYP2D6, CYP3A4
Excretion	Urine, bile, breast milk
Half-life	16.5 hr

Pharmacodynamics (blood counts)

Onset	10 days
Peak	14 days
Duration	Up to 21 days

CONTRAINDICATIONS: Pregnancy 1st trimester, breastfeeding, hypersensitivity, systemic infections, cardiac disorders, severe myelosuppression, lifetime dose of 550 mg/m^2

> **BLACK BOX WARNING:** Hepatic disease

Precautions: Accidental exposure, cardiac disease, dental work, electrolyte imbalance, infection, hyperuricemia

> **BLACK BOX WARNING:** Bone marrow suppression, extravasation, heart failure, secondary malignancy; requires an experienced clinician, IM/SUBCUT use

DOSAGE AND ROUTES
Adult: IV 60-75 mg/m^2 q3wk, or 25-30 mg/m^2 q day × 2-3 days, repeat q 3-4 wk or 20 mg/m2/wk; or may be used in combination with other antineoplastics with 40-75 mg/m^2 q21-28d, max cumulative dose 550 mg/m^2 or 450 mg/m^2 if prior DAUNOrubicin, cyclophosphamide, mediastinal radiation
Child: IV 30 mg/m2/day × 3 days q 4 wk

Hepatic dose
Adult: IV Bilirubin 1.2-3 mg/dl, give 50% of dose; bilirubin 3.1-5 mg/dl, give 25% of dose

Renal dose
Adult: IV CCr <10 ml/min give 75% of dose

Available forms: Powder for inj 10, 20, 50 mg/vial; solution for injection 2 mg/ml

ADVERSE EFFECTS
CV: Increased B/P, chest pain, ECG changes, cardiomyopathy
GI: *Nausea, vomiting,* anorexia, *mucositis,* hepatotoxicity
GU: Urine discoloration
HEMA: Thrombocytopenia, leukopenia, anemia
INTEG: *Rash,* necrosis at inj site, radiation recall, dermatitis, reversible *alopecia,* cellulitis, thrombophlebitis at inj site
RESP: Recall pnemonitis
SYST: Anaphylaxis, secondary malignancy

INTERACTIONS
Individual drugs
CycloSPORINE, mercaptopurine: increased toxicity

Fluconazole, posaconazole: increased life-threatening dysrhythmias: do not use together

Fosphenytoin, phenytoin: increased effect of these drugs

PACLitaxel: decreased clearance of DOXOrubicin

PHENobarbital: decreased DOXOrubicin effect

Progesterone: increased neutropenia, thrombocytopenia

Streptozocin: increased DOXOrubicin effect

Drug classifications

Antineoplastics, radiation: increased toxicity

Calcium channel blockers: increased cardiomyopathy

Drugs that increase QT prolongation: increased effect

Live virus vaccine: decreased antibody response

Drug/lab test

Increased: uric acid

NURSING CONSIDERATIONS
Assessment:

> **BLACK BOX WARNING: Bone marrow depression:** CBC, differential, platelet count weekly; withhold or reduce dose of product if WBC is <1500/mm^3 or platelet count is <50,000/mm^3; notify prescriber of these results

• Renal studies: BUN, serum uric acid, urine CCr, electrolytes before, during therapy
• I&O ratio: Report fall in urine output to <30 ml/hr
• **Hepatotoxicity:** hepatic studies before, during therapy: bilirubin, AST, ALT, alk phos as needed or monthly; check for jaundice of skin and sclera, dark urine, clay-colored stools, itchy skin, abdominal pain, fever, diarrhea

> **BLACK BOX WARNING: Dysrhythmias:** ECG; possible dysrhythmias (sinus tachycardia, heart block, PVCs), ejection fraction before treatment, signs of irreversible cardiomyopathy, can occur up to 6 mo after treatment begins

• **Bleeding:** hematuria, guaiac, bruising, petechiae of mucosa or orifices every 8 hr
• Effects of alopecia on body image; discuss feelings about body changes; almost total alopecia is expected

> **BLACK BOX WARNING: Secondary malignancy:** Assess for acute myelogenous leukemia (AML) and myelodysplastic syndrome (MDS)

• Buccal cavity every 8 hr for dryness, sores, ulceration, white patches, oral pain, bleeding, dysphagia

> **BLACK BOX WARNING: Extravasation:** local irritation, pain, burning at inj site; a vesicant; if extravasation occurs, stop drug, restart at another site, apply ice, elevate extremity to reduce swelling; if resolution does not occur, surgical debridement may be required

• GI symptoms: frequency of stools, cramping
• Rinsing of mouth tid-qid with water, club soda; brushing of teeth bid-tid with soft brush or cotton-tipped applicators for stomatitis; use unwaxed dental floss

Patient problem

Risk for infection (adverse reactions)
Impaired cardiac output (adverse reactions)
Risk for injury (adverse reactions)

Implementation
IV route

• Give antiemetic 30-60 min before product to prevent vomiting
• Give allopurinol or sodium bicarbonate to maintain uric acid levels, alkalization of urine
• **Use cytotoxic handling procedures:** inspect for particulate and discoloration before use

> **BLACK BOX WARNING:** Do not give IM, subcut

> **BLACK BOX WARNING:** If extravasation occurs, stop inf and complete via another vein, preferably in another limb, use dexrazoxane topically

• Aluminum needles may be used during administration; avoid aluminum during storage
• Rapid injection can cause facial flushing or erythema along the vein

Reconstitution:

• To avoid risks with reconstitution, the commercially available injection may be used; there are still risks involved in handling the injection
• Do not use diluents containing preservatives to reconstitute powder for injection
• Reconstitute 10, 20, 50, 100 mg of DOXOrubicin with 5, 10, 25, 50 ml, respectively, of nonbacteriostatic NS injection (2 mg/ml), shake until completely dissolved; use reconstituted solution within 24 hr; do not expose to sunlight
• **IV injection:** Inject reconstituted solution over 0.3-5 min via Y-site or 3-way stopcock into a free-flowing IV inf of NS or D$_5$W; a butterfly needle inserted into a large vein is preferred

---

• Increased fluid intake to 2-3 L/day to prevent urate, calculi formation
• Store at room temperature for 24 hr after reconstituting

Y-site compatibilities: Alemtuzumab, alfentanil, amifostine, amikacin, anidulafungin, argatroban, aztreonam, bivalirudin, bleomycin, bumetanide, buprenorphine, butorphanol, calcium chloride/gluconate, CARBOplatin, carmustine, caspofungin, ceftizoxime, chlorproMAZINE, cimetidine, ciprofloxacin, CISplatin, cladribine, clindamycin, cyclophosphamide, cycloSPORINE, cytarabine, DACTINomycin, DAPTOmycin, dexamethasone, dilTIAZem, diphenhydrAMINE, DOBUTamine, DOCEtaxel, dolasetron, DOPamine, doripenem, doxycycline, droperidol, enalaprilat, ePHEDrine, EPINEPHrine, erythromycin, esmolol, etoposide, etoposide phosphate, famotidine, fenoldopam, fentaNYL, filgrastim, fluconazole, fludarabine, gemcitabine, gentamicin, granisetron, haloperidol, hydrocortisone, HYDROmorphone, ifosfamide, imipenem cilastatin, inamrinone, isoproterenol, ketorolac, labetalol, leucovorin, levorphanol, lidocaine, linezolid, LORazepam, mannitol, mechlorethamine, melphalan, meperidine, mesna, methotrexate, metoclopramide, metoprolol, metroNIDAZOLE, midazolam, milrinone, mitoMYcin, morphine, nalbuphine, naloxone, nesiritide, niCARdipine, nitroglycerin, nitroprusside, octreotide, ofloxacin, ondansetron, oxaliplatin, PACLitaxel, palonosetron, pancuronium, phenylephrine, potassium chloride, procainamide, prochlorperazine, promethazine, propranolol, quinupristin-dalfopristin, raNITIdine, sargramostim, sodium acetate, tacrolimus, teniposide, theophylline, thiotepa, ticarcillin/clavulanate, tigecycline, tirofiban, tobramycin, topotecan, trastuzumab, trimethobenzamide, vancomycin, vasopressin, vecuronium, verapamil, vinBLAStine, vinCRIStine, vinorelbine, zidovudine, zoledronic acid

Patient/family education
• Instruct patient to add 2-3 L of fluids unless contraindicated before and for 24-48 hr after to decrease possible hemorrhagic cystitis
• Instruct patient to report any complaints, side effects to nurse or prescriber
• Advise patient that hair may be lost during treatment; that wig or hairpiece might make patient feel better; that new hair might be different in color, texture
• Instruct patient to avoid foods with citric acid, hot or rough texture
• Advise patient to discuss all OTC, Rx, herbals, supplements with health care professional

• Advise patient that body fluids should not be handled unless protective equipment is used
• Teach patient to notify health care professional of trouble breathing; swelling of hands, feet; increase in weight; change in heart rate
• Advise patient that continuing follow-ups and lab work will be needed
• Instruct patient to report any bleeding, white spots, ulcerations in mouth to prescriber; to examine mouth daily, not to use razors, be aware that bleeding can occur from any orifice
• Advise patient that urine, other body fluids may be red-orange for 48 hr
• Instruct patient to avoid crowds and persons with infections when granulocyte count is low
• Instruct patient to avoid live virus vaccinations
• **Pregnancy/breastfeeding:** Advise patient that barrier contraceptive measures are recommended during therapy and for 4 mo after to avoid breastfeeding

Evaluation
Positive therapeutic outcome
• Decreased tumor size, decreased spread of malignancy

⚠ HIGH ALERT

DOXOrubicin liposomal
(dox-oh-roo′bi-sin)
Doxil, Lipodox
Func. class.: Antineoplastic, antibiotic
Chem. class.: Anthracycline glycoside

Do not confuse: DOXOrubicin liposomal/
DOXOrubicin/DAUNOrubicin

ACTION: Inhibits DNA synthesis primarily; replication is decreased by binding to DNA, which causes strand splitting; active throughout entire cell cycle; a vesicant

USES: AIDS-related Kaposi's sarcoma, multiple myeloma, metastatic ovarian carcinoma

Pharmacokinetics

Absorption	Complete
Distribution	Crosses placenta
Metabolism	Liver
Excretion	Urine, bile, breast milk
Half-life	55 hr

Pharmacodynamics

Onset	Unknown
Peak	Unknown
Duration	Unknown

CONTRAINDICATIONS:
Pregnancy, breastfeeding, hypersensitivity

Precautions: Children, infection, leukopenia, stomatitis, thrombocytopenia, cardiotoxicity, inf reactions, myelosuppression, hepatic disease, systemic infections, cardiac disorders

DOSAGE AND ROUTES
Max lifetime cumulative dose 550 mg/m^2; 400 mg/m^2 for those who have received other cardiotoxics or mediastinal radiation

Kaposi's sarcoma
Adult: IV 20 mg/m^2 q3wk until disease progression or unacceptable toxicity

Multiple myeloma
Adult: IV 30 mg/m^2 IV inf on day 4 every 3 wk plus bortezomib 1.3 mg/m^2/dose IV bolus on days 1, 4, 8, 11 of each cycle; give DOXOrubicin liposomal after bortezomib receipt on day 4; administer up to 8 treatment cycles or until disease progression or unacceptable toxicity occurs

Ovarian cancer
Adult: IV 50 mg/m2 q 4 wk

Available forms: Liposomal dispersion for inj: 2 mg/ml

ADVERSE EFFECTS
CNS: Paresthesias, headache, depression, insomnia, fatigue, fever
CV: Chest pain, decreased B/P, cardiomyopathy, heart failure, dysrhythmias, tachycardia
EENT: Optic neuritis, rhinitis, pharyngitis, stomatitis
GI: *Nausea, vomiting,* anorexia, *mucositis,* hepatotoxicity, constipation, oral candidiasis, abdominal pain
HEMA: Thrombocytopenia, leukopenia, anemia, secondary malignancy
INTEG: *Rash,* necrosis at inj site, dermatitis, reversible *alopecia,* exfoliative dermatitis, palmar-plantar erythrodysesthesia, thrombophlebitis at inj site
RESP: Dyspnea, cough, respiratory infections

INTERACTIONS
Individual drugs
CycloSPORINE, mercaptopurine: increased toxicity
Fluconazole, posaconazole: increased life-threatening dysrhythmias: do not use together
Fosphenytoin, phenytoin: increased effect of these drugs
Hematopoietic progenitor cell: decreased antineoplastic effect; do not use 24 hr before or after treatment
PACLitaxel: decreased clearance of DOXOrubicin
PHENobarbital: decreased DOXOrubicin effect

Progesterone: increased neutropenia, thrombocytopenia
Streptozocin: increased DOXOrubicin effect

Drug classifications
Antineoplastics, radiation: increased toxicity
Calcium channel blockers: increased cardiomyopathy
Drugs that increase QT prolongation: increased effect
Live virus vaccine: decreased antibody response

Drug/lab test
Increased: uric acid

NURSING CONSIDERATIONS
Assessment

> **BLACK BOX WARNING: Bone marrow depression:** CBC, differential, platelet count weekly; withhold or reduce dose of product if WBC is <1500/mm^3 or platelet count is <50,000/mm^3; notify prescriber of these results

- Renal studies: BUN, serum uric acid, urine CCr, electrolytes before, during therapy
- I&O ratio: Report fall in urine output to <30 ml/hr
- **Hepatotoxicity:** hepatic studies before, during therapy: bilirubin, AST, ALT, alk phos as needed or monthly; check for jaundice of skin and sclera, dark urine, clay-colored stools, itchy skin, abdominal pain, fever, diarrhea

> **BLACK BOX WARNING: Dysrhythmias:** ECG; watch for ST-T wave changes, low QRS and T, possible dysrhythmias (sinus tachycardia, heart block, PVCs), ejection fraction before treatment, signs of irreversible cardiomyopathy, can occur up to 6 mo after treatment begins

- Bleeding: hematuria, guaiac, bruising, petechiae of mucosa or orifices every 8 hr
- Effects of alopecia on body image; discuss feelings about body changes; almost total alopecia is expected
- Buccal cavity for dryness, sores, ulceration, white patches, oral pain, bleeding, dysphagia

> **BLACK BOX WARNING: Extravasation:** local irritation, pain, burning at inj site; a vesicant; if extravasation occurs, stop drug, restart at another site, apply ice, elevate extremity to reduce swelling; if resolution does not occur, surgical debridement may be required

- **Secondary malignancy:** Assess for acute myelogenous leukemia and oral cancer
- GI symptoms: frequency of stools, cramping

- Rinsing of mouth tid-qid with water, club soda; brushing of teeth bid-tid with soft brush or cotton-tipped applicators for stomatitis; use unwaxed dental floss

Patient problem
Risk for infection (adverse reactions)
Impaired cardiac output (adverse reactions)
Risk for injury (adverse reactions)

Implementation
- Prepared liposomal DOXOrubicin is a translucent, red liposomal dispersion; visually inspect for particulate matter and discoloration before use
- Pegylated liposomal DOXOrubicin (Doxil) is for IV INF use only and should not be given IM/subcut, give under the supervision of a physician who is experienced in cancer chemotherapy

> **BLACK BOX WARNING:** Care should be taken to avoid extravasation because the drug is irritating to extravascular tissue

- Premedication with antiemetics is recommended

IV route
- **Reconstitution (Doxil):** dilute the appropriate dose, not to exceed 90 mg/250 ml D_5W; do not mix with any other diluent, drugs, or bacteriostatic agent, use aseptic technique; product contains no preservative or bacteriostatic agent; diluted solution must be refrigerated and used within 24 hr
- **IV INF (Doxil):** do not administer as a bolus injection or an undiluted solution; rapid injection can increase the risk of an inf-related reaction
- An acute inf reaction can occur during the first inf and is usually resolved by slowing the rate of inf; most patients can tolerate subsequent inf
- **Rate:** infuse at an initial rate of 1 mg/min; if no inf-related action, the rate can be increased to complete the inf over 1 hr; do not filter
- For hematologic toxicity in patients with ovarian cancer or HIV-related Kaposi's sarcoma: Grade 1 (ANC of 1500-1900/mm³, platelets ≥75,000/mm³): No dose reduction; Grade 2 (ANC of 1000-1499/mm³, platelets ≥50,000/mm³ and <75,000/mm³): Wait until ANC ≥1500 cells/mm³ and platelets ≥75,000 cells/mm³; redose with no dose reduction; Grade 3 (ANC of 500-999/mm³, platelets ≥25,000/ mm³ and <50,000/mm³): Wait until ANC ≥1500 cells/mm³ and platelets ≥75,000 cells/mm³; redose with no dose reduction; Grade 4 (ANC <500/mm³, platelets <25,000/mm³): Wait until ANC

≥1500 cells/mm³ and platelets ≥75,000 cells/mm³; reduce dose by 25% or continue with full dose with colony-stimulating factor
- Give antiemetic 30-60 min before product to prevent vomiting
- Use allopurinol or sodium bicarbonate to maintain uric acid levels, alkalinization of urine
- Avoid mixing with other products
- Increase fluid intake to 2-3 L/day to prevent urate, calculi formation
- Store refrigerated for 24 hr after reconstituting

Patient/family education
- Instruct patient to add 2-3 L of fluids unless contraindicated before and for 24-48 hr after to decrease possible hemorrhagic cystitis
- Instruct patient to report any complaints, side effects to nurse or prescriber
- Advise patient that hair may be lost during treatment; that wig or hairpiece might make patient feel better; that new hair might be different in color, texture
- Instruct patient to avoid foods with citric acid, hot or rough texture
- Instruct patient to report any bleeding, white spots, ulcerations in mouth to prescriber; to examine mouth daily
- Advise patient that urine, other body fluids may be red-orange for 48 hr
- Instruct patient to avoid crowds and persons with infections when granulocyte count is low
- Instruct patient to avoid vaccinations because reactions can occur; to avoid alcohol
- **Pregnancy/breastfeeding:** Advise patient that barrier contraceptive measures are recommended during therapy and for 4 mo after to avoid breastfeeding

Evaluation
Positive therapeutic outcome
- Decreased tumor size, decreased spread of malignancy

---

doxycycline (Rx)
(dox-i-sye'kleen)
Acticlate, Apprilon ✦, Atridox ✦ Doryx, Doxy, Doxycin ✦, Monodox, Oracea, Periostat, Vibramycin, Vibra-Tabs
Func. class.: Antiinfective
Chem. class.: Tetracycline

Do not confuse: doxycycline/doxepin/dicyclomine

ACTION: Inhibits protein synthesis, phosphorylation in microorganisms by binding to 30S ribosomal subunits, reversibly binding to 30S ribosomal subunits; bacteriostatic

---

Therapeutic outcome: Bactericidal action against the following: gram-positive pathogens: *Acinetobacter, Actinomyces israelii, Bacillus anthracis, Bacteroides, Balantidium coli, Bartonella bacilliformis, Borrelia recurrentis, Brucella, Campylobacter fetus, Chlamydia psittaci, Chlamydia trachomatis, Clostridium, Entamoeba histolytica, Enterobacter aerogenes, Enterococcus, Escherichia coli, Francisella tularensis, Fusobacterium fusiforme, Haemophilus ducreyi, Haemophilus influenzae* (beta-lactamase negative), *Haemophilus influenzae* (beta-lactamase positive), *Klebsiella granulomatis, Klebsiella, Leptospira, Listeria monocytogenes, Mycoplasma pneumoniae, Neisseria gonorrhoeae, Neisseria meningitidis, Orientia tsutsugamushi, Plasmodium falciparum, Propionibacterium acnes, Rickettsia akari, Rickettsia prowazekii, Rickettsia rickettsii, Shigella, Staphylococcus aureus* (MSSA), *Streptococcus pneumoniae, Streptococcus pyogenes* (group A beta-hemolytic streptococci), *Treponema pallidum, Treponema pertenue, Ureaplasma urealyticum, Vibrio cholerae,* viridans streptococci, *Yersinia pestis*

USES: Syphilis, gonorrhea, lymphogranuloma venereum, uncommon gram-negative or gram-positive organisms, malaria prophylaxis, many different interactions

Pharmacokinetics

Absorption	Well absorbed
Distribution	Widely distributed, crosses placenta
Metabolism	Some hepatic recycling, 90% protein binding
Excretion	Bile, feces; kidneys unchanged (20%-40%), enters breast milk
Half-life	1 day; increased in severe renal disease

Pharmacodynamics

	PO	IV
Onset	1½-4 hr	Immediate
Peak	1½-4 hr	Infusion's end
Duration	12 hr	12 hr

CONTRAINDICATIONS

Pregnancy, children <8 yr, esophageal ulceration, hypersensitivity to tetracyclines

Precautions: Hepatic disease, breastfeeding, pseudomembranous colitis, ulcerative colitis, sulfite hypersensitivity, excessive sunlight

DOSAGE AND ROUTES
Most infections

Adult: PO/IV 100 mg q12hr on day 1, then 100 mg/day; IV 200 mg in 1-2 INF on day 1, then 100-200 mg/day

Child >8 yr (≥45 kg): PO/IV 100 mg q12hr on day 1, then 100 mg/day; severe infections 100 mg q12hr; IV 200 mg on day 1, then 100-200 mg/day, give 200 mg dose as 1 or 2 infusions

Child >8 yr, <45 kg: PO 2.2 mg/kg q12hr on day 1, then 2.2 mg/kg/day, severe infections 2.2 mg/kg q12hr; IV 4.4 mg/kg divided on day 1, then 2.2-4.4 mg/kg/day in 1-2 divided doses

Gonorrhea (patients allergic to penicillin)

Adult: PO 100 mg q12hr × 7 days, or 300 mg followed 1 hr later by another 300 mg

Malaria prophylaxis

Adult: 100 mg/day 1-2 days before travel, daily during travel, and 4 wk after return

Adolescent/child ≥8 yr <45 kg: PO 2 mg/kg/day (up to 100 mg/day) begin 1-2 days before travel, continue for 4 wk after return

Chlamydia trachomatis

Adult: PO 100 mg bid × 7 days

Syphilis (early)

Adult: PO 100 mg bid × 14 days

Anthrax (postexposure)

Adult and child ≥45 kg: IV 100 mg q12hr, change to PO when able × 60 days

Adolescent/child ≥8 yr and <45 kg: PO 2.2 mg/kg q12hr × 60 days; IV 100 mg q12hr, change to PO when able × 60 days

Lyme disease

Adult: PO 100 mg bid × 14-21 days

Periodontitis

Adult: 20 mg bid after sealing and root planing for ≤9 mo; give close to meal AM or PM

Available forms: Cap 40 mg; susp 50 mg/5 ml; cap 20, 50, 100 mg; del rel tab 75, 100, 150 mg; del rel cap 75, 100 mg; inj 100 mg; tabs 20, 100, mg; caps 50, 100, 150 mg; tabs 50, 75, 100 mg; oral susp 25 mg/5 ml

ADVERSE EFFECTS
CNS: Fever, headache
CV: Pericarditis
EENT: Dysphagia, glossitis, decreased calcification of deciduous teeth, oral candidiasis, tooth discoloration
GI: *Nausea, abdominal pain, vomiting, diarrhea,* anorexia, enterocolitis, hepatotoxicity, flatulence, abdominal cramps, gastric burning, stomatitis

GU: *Increased BUN*
HEMA: Eosinophilia, neutropenia, thrombocytopenia, hemolytic anemia
INTEG: Rash, urticaria, photosensitivity, increased pigmentation, exfoliative dermatitis, pruritus, phlebitis, injection site reaction
MS: Bone growth retardation (child <8 yr), muscle, joint pain
RESP: Cough
SYST· *Stevens Johnson* syndrome, *angioedema, toxic epidermal necrolysis*

INTERACTIONS
Individual drugs
Bismuth, calcium, carBAMazepine, cimetidine, cholestyramine, colestipol, kaolin/pectin, magnesium, NaHCO₃, phenytoin, RifAMPin, sucralfate, zinc: decreased effect of doxycycline
Digoxin: increased or decreased effect of digoxin, sevelamer
Iron: forms chelates, decreased absorption
Penicillins: decreased effects of penicillins
Warfarin: increased effect of warfarin

Drug classifications
Alkali products, antacids, barbiturates: decreased effect of doxycycline
Anticoagulants (oral): increased effect of anticoagulants, methotrexate

Drug/food
Decreased: absorption with dairy products

Drug/lab test
Increased: BUN, alkaline phosphatase, bilirubin, amylase, ALT, AST, eosinophils, WBC
False increase: urinary catecholamines

NURSING CONSIDERATIONS
Assessment
• Assess patient for previous sensitivity reaction
• **Assess patient for signs and symptoms of infection** including characteristics of wounds, sputum, urine, stool, WBC >10,000/mm³, fever; obtain baseline information before, during treatment
• Obtain C&S before beginning product therapy to identify if correct treatment has been initiated
• **Assess for allergic reactions:** rash, urticaria, pruritus, chills, fever, joint pain; angioedema may occur a few days after therapy begins
• Assess bowel pattern daily; if severe diarrhea occurs, product should be discontinued
• Monitor for bleeding: ecchymosis, bleeding gums, hematuria, stool guaiac daily if on long-term therapy; blood dyscrasias may occur

• **Assess for overgrowth of infection:** perineal itching, fever, malaise, redness, pain, swelling, drainage, rash, diarrhea, change in cough, sputum

Patient problem
Infection (uses)
Risk for injury (adverse reactions)

Implementation
PO route
• Do not break, crush, or chew caps
• Give around the clock to maintain proper blood levels; give with food to increase absorption of product; do not give within 3 hr of other agents; product reactions may occur
• Give with 8 oz of water 1 hr before bedtime to prevent ulceration
• Shake liquid preparation well before giving; use calibrated device for proper dosing
• Do not give with iron, calcium, magnesium products or antacids, which decrease absorption and form insoluble chelate
• **Del rel cap:** swallow whole or open and sprinkle on applesauce
• **Susp:** shake well, use calibrated device, may give with food/milk for GI irritation, store at room temperature, discard after 14 days

Intermittent IV infusion route
• Check for irritation, extravasation, phlebitis daily
• Dilute each 100 mg/10 ml or 200 mg/20 ml of 0.9% NaCl, sterile water for inj; each 100 mg must be further dilute in at least 100 ml of 0.9% NaCl, D₅W, Ringer's, LR, D₅W/LR; give over 1-4 hr
• Avoid rapid use, extravasation
• Store in tight, light-resistant container at room temperature; **IV** sol stable for 12 hr at room temperature, 72 hr if refrigerated; discard if precipitate forms

Y-site compatibilities: Acyclovir, alemtuzumab, alfentanil, amifostine, amikacin, aminophylline, amiodarone, anidulafungin, ascorbic acid, atracurium, atropine, aztreonam, bivalirudin, bumetanide, buprenorphine, butorphanol, calcium chloride, calcium gluconate, CARBOplatin, caspofungin, cefonicid, cefotaxime, cefTRIAXone, chlorproMAZINE, cimetidine, cisatracurium, CISplatin, clindamycin, codeine, cyanocobalamin, cyclophosphamide, cycloSPORINE, cytarabine, DACTINomycin, DAPTOmycin, dexmedetomidine, digoxin, dilTIAZem, diphenhydrAMINE, DOBUTamine, DOCEtaxel, DOPamine, doxacurium, DOXOrubicin, enalapril, ePHEDrine, EPINEPHrine, epiRUBicin, epoetin alfa, eftifibitide, ertapenem, esmolol, etoposide, etoposide phosphate, famotidine, fenoldopam, fentaNYL, filgrastim, fluconazole, fludarabine, gemcitabine, gentamicin,

---

glycopyrrolate, granisetron, HYDROmorphone, IDArubicin, ifosfamide, imipenem/cilastatin, insulin, isoproterenol, labetalol, levofloxacin, lidocaine, linezolid, LORazepam, magnesium sulfate, mannitol, mechlorethamine, melphalan, meperidine, methyldopate, metoclopramide, metoprolol, metroNIDAZOLE, miconazole, midazolam, milrinone, mitoXANTRONE, morphine, multivitamins, nalbuphine, naloxone, nesiritide, netilmicin, nitroglycerin, nitroprusside, norepinephrine, octreotide, ondansetron, oxaliplatin, oxytocin, PACLitaxel, pancuronium, pantoprazole, papaverine, pentamidine, pentazocine, perphenazine, phentolamine, phenylephrine, phytonadione, potassium chloride, procainamide, prochlorperazine, promethazine, propofol, propranolol, protamine, pyridoxine, quinupristin/dalfopristin, raNITIdine, remifentanil, ritodrine, riTUXimab, rocuronium, sargramostim, sodium acetate, streptokinase, succinylcholine, SUFentanil, tacrolimus, telavancin, teniposide, theophylline, thiamine, thiotepa, tirofiban, tobramycin, tolazoline, TPN (2 in 1), trastuzumab, trimetaphan, urokinase, vancomycin, vasopressin, vecuronium, verapamil, vinCRIStine, vinorelbine, voriconazole, zoledronic acid

Patient/family education

• Teach patient to report sore throat, bruising, bleeding, joint pain; may indicate blood dyscrasias (rare)

• Advise patient to contact prescriber if vaginal itching, loose foul-smelling stools, furry tongue occur; may indicate superinfection; report itching, rash, pruritus, urticaria

• Instruct patient to take all medication prescribed for the length of time ordered; product must be taken around the clock to maintain blood levels; do not give medication to others

• Advise patient to notify prescriber of diarrhea with blood or pus

• Teach patient not to use with antacids, iron products, H_2 blockers, sevelamer, calcium (milk), magnesium, zinc

• Advise patient to take with full glass of water, if nausea occurs take with food

Evaluation
Positive therapeutic outcome

• Absence of signs/symptoms of infection (WBC $<10,000/mm^3$, temp WNL, absence of red draining wounds)

• Reported improvement in symptoms of infection

---

doxylamine/pyridoxine
(docks-ill'ah-meen/peer-rehdock'seen)
Diclegis
Func. class.: Antiemetic

ACTION
Doxylamine: Competes with free histamine for binding at the H_1-receptor sites; competitively antagonizes the effects of histamine on H_1-receptors in the GI tract, uterus, large blood vessels, and bronchial muscle

Pyridoxine: Needed for the metabolism of fat, protein, and carbohydrate; decarboxylation of amino acids, conversion of tryptophan to niacin or serotonin, deamination, and transamination of amino acids; conversion of glycogen to glucose-1-phosphate; essential for synthesis of gamma aminobutyric acid (GABA) in the CNS and synthesis of heme

USES:
Nausea and vomiting of pregnancy in women who do not respond to other treatment

Pharmacokinetics

Absorption	Well
Distribution	Unknown
Metabolism	Doxylamine: liver
Excretion	Urine inactive metabolites
Half-life	12.5 hr (doxylamine), 0.5 hr pyridoxine

Pharmacodynamics

Onset	Unknown
Peak	Unknown
Duration	Up to 24 hr

CONTRAINDICATIONS
Hypersensitivity

DOSAGE AND ROUTES
Adult pregnant females: PO 2 tabs (on an empty stomach) at bedtime, on day 1; if dose controls symptoms the next day, continue regimen. If symptoms persist on the afternoon of day 2, continue 2 tabs at bedtime, then take 3 tabs starting on day 3 (1 tab in AM and 2 tabs at bedtime); if symptoms are controlled, continue regimen. If symptoms persist, on day 4, take 4 tabs (1 tab in AM, 1 tab midafternoon, and 2 tabs at bedtime); max 4 tabs/day. Use only as needed

Available forms: Delayed release tabs doxylamine 10 mg/ pyridoxine 10 mg

ADVERSE EFFECTS
CNS
Drowsiness

INTERACTIONS
Drug classifications
CNS depressants: increased CNS effect

NURSING CONSIDERATIONS
Assessment
- **Nausea/vomiting:** Monitor times per day and amount, also baseline before dose and after

Patient Problems
- Nausea (uses)

Implementation
- Swallow whole, do not crush, break, chew, or split the tablets
- Give on an empty stomach with a glass of water

Patient/family education
- Teach patient not to drive or engage in other hazardous activities until response is known
- Advise patient to avoid alcohol and CNS depressants
- Advise patient not to breastfeed while taking this product

Evaluation
Positive therapeutic outcome
- Absence of nausea, vomiting in pregnancy

🛆 HIGH ALERT

dronedarone (Rx)
(drone-da-rone)
Multaq
Func. class.: Antidysrhythmic (Class III)
Chem. class.: Iodinated benzofuran derivative

ACTION: Prolongs action potential duration and effective refractory period, noncompetitive α- and β-adrenergic inhibition; increases PR and QT intervals, decreases sinus rate, decreases peripheral vascular resistance

Therapeutic outcome: Decreased amount and severity of ventricular dysrhythmias

USES: Atrial fibrillation, atrial flutter

Pharmacokinetics

Absorption	Slow, variable (PO) up to 65%
Distribution	Body tissues; crosses placenta (protein binding 98%)
Metabolism	Liver by CYP3A
Excretion	Bile, kidney (minimal)
Half-life	13-19 hr

Pharmacodynamics (antidysrhythmic action)

	PO
Onset	Unknown
Peak	Unknown
Duration	12 hr

CONTRAINDICATIONS:
Pregnancy, breastfeeding, severe sinus node dysfunction, 2nd- or 3rd-degree AV block; bradycardia, hypersensitivity, heart failure, hepatic disease, QT prolongation

> **BLACK BOX WARNING:** NYHA class IV heart failure or class II-III with recent decompensation requiring hospitalization, permanent atrial fibrillation (cannot restore sinus rhythm)

Precautions: Children, electrolyte imbalances, elderly, Asian patients, females, atrial fibrillation/flutter

DOSAGE AND ROUTES
Adult: PO 400 mg bid; max 800 mg/day
Available forms: Tabs 400 mg

ADVERSE EFFECTS
CNS: Weakness
CV: *Bradycardia,* heart failure, QT prolongation, torsades de pointes, atrial flutter
ENDO: Hypo/hyperthyroidism
GI: Nausea, vomiting, diarrhea, abdominal pain, severe hepatic injury, hepatic failure
INTEG: Rash, photosensitivity, angioedema
RESP: Interstitial pneumonitis, pulmonary fibrosis

INTERACTIONS
Individual drugs
CycloSPORINE, dextromethorphan, digoxin, disopyramide, flecainide, methotrexate, phenytoin, procainamide, quiNIDine, theophylline: increased blood levels, increased toxicity
Dabigatran, warfarin: increased anticoagulant effect

Drug classifications
β-Adrenergic blockers, calcium channel blockers: increased bradycardia
CYP3A4 inhibitors, CYP2D6 inhibitors: increased dronedarone levels
CYP3A, CYP2D6 inducers: decreased dronedarone levels

Drug/herb
St. John's wort: decreased effect
Yohimbine: increased anticoagulant effect

Drug/food
Grapefruit juice: increased dronedarone effect, avoid use

Drug/lab test
Increased: T4, LFTs, bilirubin, creatinine
Decreased: potassium, magnesium

NURSING CONSIDERATIONS
Assessment
- Monitor I&O ratio; monitor electrolytes: potassium, creatinine, magnesium

---

• Monitor liver function studies: AST, ALT, bilirubin, alkaline phosphatase

> **BLACK BOX WARNING:** NYHA Class IV heart failure or symptomatic heart failure with recent decomposition requiring hospitalization doubles risk of death

• Monitor **ECG** to determine product effectiveness; measure PR, QRS, QT intervals; check for PVCs, other dysrhythmias; monitor B/P continuously for hypo/hypertension; check for rebound hypertension after 1-2 hr
• Monitor serum creatine, potassium, magnesium
• Monitor for dehydration or hypovolemia
• **Assess for hypothyroidism:** lethargy, dizziness, constipation, enlarged thyroid gland, edema of extremities, cool, pale skin
• Monitor cardiac rate, respiration: rate, rhythm, character, chest pain, ventricular tachycardia, supraventricular tachycardia or fibrillation
• Assess sight and vision before treatment and throughout therapy; microdeposits on the cornea may cause blurred vision, halos, and photophobia

Patient problem
Impaired cardiac output (uses)

Implementation
• Start with patient hospitalized and monitored
PO route
• Give reduced dosage slowly with ECG monitoring only
• Give loading dose with food to decrease nausea

Patient/family education
• Instruct patient to report weight gain, edema, difficulty breathing, fatigue, peripheral edema immediately to prescriber
• Instruct patient to use sunscreen and protective clothing to prevent burning associated with photosensitivity
• Instruct patient to take medication as prescribed, in AM, PM with meals not to double doses, avoid use with all other products without approval of prescriber, do not use grapefruit juice
• Instruct patient to complete follow-up appointment with health care provider, including pulmonary function studies, chest x-ray
• Teach patient to take consistently with or without food
• Teach patient not to take double doses
• **Pregnancy/breastfeeding:** Teach patient to use effective contraception during treatment, do not breastfeed

Evaluation
Positive therapeutic outcome
• Decreased dysrhythmias

TREATMENT OF OVERDOSE:
Administer O_2, artificial ventilation, ECG, DOPamine for circulatory depression

> **⚠ HIGH ALERT**
> ## dulaglutide (Rx)
> (doo-la-gloo'-tide)
> **Trulicity**
> *Func. class.:* Antidiabetic
> *Chem. class.:* Incretin mimetic

ACTION: Binds and activates known human glucagon-like peptide-1 (GLP-1) receptor agonist, mimics natural physiology for self-regulating glycemic control

Therapeutic outcome: Decreased polyuria, polydipsia, polyphagia; improved Hgb A1C

USES: Type 2 diabetes mellitus, once-weekly dosing

Pharmacokinetics
Absorption	47%-65%
Distribution	Unknown
Metabolism	Protein catabolism
Excretion	Unknown
Half-life	5 days

Pharmacodynamics (Decrease in HbA1c)
Onset	Up to 4 wk
Peak	12-13 wk
Duration	Unknown

CONTRAINDICATIONS
Hypersensitivity

> **BLACK BOX WARNING:** Medullary thyroid carcinoma, multiple endocrine neoplasia syndrome type 2 (men-2), thyroid cancer

Precautions: Pregnancy, breastfeeding, children, geriatric patients, severe renal/hepatic/GI disease, pancreatitis, vit D deficiency, burns, colitis, diarrhea, fever, GI bleeding/perforation/obstruction, ileus, infection, pseudomembranous colitis, thyroid disease, trauma, surgery, type 1 diabetes mellitus, tobacco smoking, vomiting

DOSAGE AND ROUTES
Adult: SUBCUT 0.75 mg qwk, may increase to 1.5 mg qwk

Available forms: Solution for subcut Inj 0.75 mg/0.5 ml, 1.5 mg/0.5ml (single use pen); 1.5 mg/0.5 mL (single-dose prefilled syringe)

ADVERSE EFFECTS
CNS: Fatigue
ENDO: Hypoglycemia
GI: Nausea, vomiting, diarrhea, anorexia, gastroesophageal reflux, *pancreatitis*, flatulence, abdominal pain, constipation
SYST: Secondary malignancy
INTEG: Injection-site reactions, rash, urticaria

INTERACTIONS
Individual drugs
Alcohol, disopyramide: increased hypoglycemia
Dextrothyroxine, niacin, triamterene: decreased hypoglycemia efficacy

Drug classifications
ACE inhibitors, anabolic steroids, androgens, fibric acid derivatives, sulfonylureas: increased hypoglycemia
Corticosteroids, phenothiazines: increased hyperglycemia
Estrogens, MAOIs, oral contraceptives, progestins, thiazide diuretics: decreased hypoglycemia

NURSING CONSIDERATIONS
Assessment
• Monitor fasting blood glucose, A1C levels, postprandial glucose during treatment to determine diabetes control
• **Pancreatitis:** severe abdominal pain, with/without vomiting; product should be discontinued
• Assess for hypo/hyperglycemic reaction that can occur soon after meals; for severe hypoglycemia give **IV** D₅W, then **IV** dextrose solution
• Assess for nausea, diarrhea, vomiting, ability to tolerate product, may cause dehydration

Patient problem
Excess food intake (uses)
Nonadherence (teaching)

Implementation
SUBCUT route
• Do not use as first-line therapy for those who have inadequate glycemic control on diet and exercise
• Administer the dose at any time of day, with or without meals
• If a dose is missed, take as soon as remembered, as long as the next dose is due at least 3 days later. If it is more than 3 days after the missed dose, wait until the next regularly scheduled dose

• Give by **SUBCUT** only; do not give **IV** or **IM**; inject into the thigh, abdomen, or upper arm; rotate sites with each inj to prevent lipodystrophy
• Properly dispose of the pen or syringe
• Store in refrigerator for unopened pen; may store at room temperature after opening for up to 30 days, do not freeze
• When using concomitantly with insulin, give as separate injections. Never mix them together. The two injections may be injected in the same body region, but not adjacent to each other
• **Pre-filled pen administration:** Part of pen is glass; if dropped on a hard surface, do not use; uncap the pen after checking that it is locked; place base flat and firmly; unlock by turning the lock ring, press and hold green button, click will be heard; continue holding until another click is heard; inj is complete when the gray plunger is visible, remove the pen, dispose of used pen

Patient/family education
• Teach patient symptoms of hypo/hyperglycemia, what to do about each; to have glucagon emergency kit available; to carry a glucose source (candy, sugar cube) to treat hypoglycemia
• Advise patient that product must be continued on a weekly basis explain consequences of discontinuing product abruptly
• Teach patient that diabetes is a lifelong illness; product will not cure disease
• Advise patient to carry emergency ID
• Advise patient to continue weight control, dietary restrictions, exercise, hygiene
• Inform patient that regular blood glucose monitoring and A1C testing is needed
• Advise patient to notify prescriber if pregnant or intend to become pregnant
• **Pancreatitis:** if severe abdominal pain with or without vomiting occurs, seek medical attention immediately

Evaluation
Positive therapeutic outcome
• Decreased polyuria, polydipsia, polyphagia; improved Hgb A1C

DULoxetine (Rx)
(du-lox′uh-teen)
Cymbalta
Func. class.: Antidepressant, miscellaneous
Chem. class: Serotonin, norepinephrine reuptake inhibitor (SNRI)

Do not confuse: Cymbalta/Symbyax, DULoxetine/FLUoxetine

ACTION: Unknown, may potentiate serotoninergic, noradrenergic activity in the CNS. In studies DULoxetine is a potent inhibitor of neuronal serotonin and norepinephrine reuptake

Therapeutic outcome: Decreased depression, decreased neuropathic pain

USES: Major depressive disorder (MDD), neuropathic pain associated with diabetic neuropathy, generalized anxiety disorder, fibromyalgia, chronic low back pain, osteoarthritis pain

Pharmacokinetics

Absorption	Well absorbed
Distribution	90% protein binding
Metabolism	Extensively metabolized *Ῥₐ (CYP2D6, CYP1A2) in the liver to an active metabolite
Excretion	70% of product recovered in urine, 20% in feces
Half-life	12 hr

Pharmacodynamics

Onset	Unknown
Peak	6 hr
Duration	12 hr

CONTRAINDICATIONS:
Hypersensitivity, closed-angle glaucoma, alcohol intoxication, alcoholism, hepatic disease, hepatitis, jaundice

Precautions: Pregnancy, breastfeeding, geriatric, mania, hypertension, cardiac/renal/hepatic disease, seizures, increased intraocular pressure, anorexia nervosa, bleeding, dehydration, diabetes, hyponatremia, hypotension, hypovolemia, orthostatic hypotension, abrupt drug withdrawal

> **BLACK BOX WARNING:** Children, suicidal ideation

DOSAGE AND ROUTES NTI
Depression
Adult: PO 40-60 mg/day as a single dose or 2 divided doses

Diabetic neuropathy
Adult: PO 60 mg qday

Generalized anxiety disorder
Adult: PO 60 mg/day, may start with 30 mg/day × 1 wk, then increase to 60 mg/day, maintenance 60-120 mg/day

Fibromyalgia
Adult: PO 30 mg/day × 1 wk, then 60 mg/day

Chronic musculoskeletal pain
Adult: PO 60 mg/day or 30 mg/day × 1 wk, then 60 mg/day

Renal dose
Adult: PO Start with 20 mg, gradually increase; avoid use in severe renal disease

Available forms: Caps 20, 30, 60 mg

ADVERSE EFFECTS
CNS: Insomnia, anxiety, dizziness, tremor, somnolence, fatigue, decreased appetite, decreased weight, agitation, diaphoresis, hallucinations, neuroleptic malignant syndrome–like reaction, aggression, seizures, headache, abnormal dreams, flushing, hot flashes, chills
CV: Thrombophlebitis, peripheral edema, palpitations, hypertension, supraventricular dysrhythmia, orthostatic hypotension
EENT: *Abnormal vision*
ENDO: Hypoglycemia, SIADH
GI: Constipation, diarrhea, dysphagia, *nausea,* vomiting, anorexia, dry mouth, colitis, gastritis, abdominal pain, hepatic failure
GU: Abnormal ejaculation, urinary hesitation, ejaculation delayed, erectile dysfunction, urinary frequency/retention, gyn bleeding
INTEG: Photosensitivity, bruising, sweating, Stevens-Johnson syndrome
MS: Gait disturbances, muscle spasm, restless legs syndrome, myalgia
SYST: Anaphylaxis, angioedema, serotonin syndrome, Stevens-Johnson syndrome

INTERACTIONS
Individual drugs
Alcohol: increased ALT, bilirubin

Drug classifications
MAOIs: coadministration (or within 14 days of MAOIs use) is contraindicated: hyperthermia, rigidity, rapid fluctuations of VS, mental status changes, neuroleptic malignant syndrome
Anticoagulants, antiplatelets, salicylates, NSAIDs: increased bleeding risk
Opioids, antihistamines, sedative/hypnotics: increased CNS depression
CYP1A2 inhibitors (fluvoxaMINE, quinolone antiinfectives); CYP2D6 inhibitors (FLUoxetine, quiNIDine, PARoxetine): increased action of DULoxetine
CYP2D6 extensively metabolized products (flecainide, phenothiazines, propafenone, tricyclics, thioridazine): narrow therapeutic index
SSRIs serotonin receptor agonists: increased serotonin syndrome, neuroleptic malignant syndrome

Drug/herb
Kava: increased CNS depression
St. John's wort: Increase: serotonin syndrome

Drug/lab test
Increased: blood glucose

NURSING CONSIDERATIONS
Assessment

> **BLACK BOX WARNING: Depression:** Assess mental status: mood, sensorium, affect, **suicidal tendencies,** increase in psychiatric symptoms; depression, panic; monitor children weekly face to face during first 4 wk or dosage change, then every other wk for next 4 wk, then at 12 wk

- **Hypo/hyperglycemia:** Assess for each during treatment and before dosing
- Assess B/P lying, standing; pulse q4hr; if systolic B/P drops 20 mm Hg, hold product, notify prescriber; take VS q4hr in patients with CV disease
- Monitor hepatic studies: AST, ALT, bilirubin
- Monitor weight qwk; weight loss or gain; appetite may increase; peripheral edema may occur
- Offer sugarless gum, hard candy, frequent sips of water for dry mouth
- Assess for withdrawal symptoms: headache, nausea, vomiting, muscle pain, weakness; not usual unless product is discontinued abruptly
- Assess for neuroleptic malignant syndrome–like reaction
- **Serotonin syndrome:** assess for nausea, vomiting, dizziness, facial flushing, shivering, sweating
- **Sexual dysfunction:** ejaculation dysfunction, erectile dysfunction, decreased libido, orgasm dysfunction
- **Beers:** Use with caution in older adults, may exacerbate or cause SIADH
- **Pregnancy/breastfeeding:** No well-controlled studies, use only if benefits outweigh fetal risk, complications in late third trimester have occurred, pregnancy should be registered with the Cymbalta Pregnancy Registry 866-814-6975

Patient problem
Depression (uses)
Pain (uses)
Suicidal ideation (adverse reactions)

Implementation
- Swallow caps whole; do not break, crush, or chew; do not sprinkle on food or mix with liquid
- Give without regard to food
- Store in tight container at room temperature; do not freeze
- Provide assistance with ambulation during beginning therapy, since drowsiness, dizziness occur
- Check to see if PO medication was swallowed

Patient/family education
- Advise that product is dispensed in small amounts because of suicide potential, especially in the beginning of therapy
- Teach patient/family to use caution when driving or other activities requiring alertness because of drowsiness, dizziness, blurred vision
- Advise patient to avoid alcohol ingestion, other CNS depressants, MAOIs
- Teach patient to notify prescriber of nausea, vomiting, dizziness, facial flushing, shivering, sweating, confusion, hallucinations, incoordination; may indicate serotonin syndrome
- **Abrupt discontinuation:** Advise patient not to discontinue medication quickly after long-term use; may cause nausea, headache, malaise
- Advise patient to wear sunscreen or large hat, since photosensitivity may occur
- Advise patient to notify prescriber if pregnancy is planned or suspected or if breastfeeding
- Tell patient that improvement may occur in 4-8 wk; up to 12 wk (geriatric patients)

> **BLACK BOX WARNING:** Advise that clinical worsening and suicide risk may occur

Evaluation
Positive therapeutic outcome
- Decreased depression

RARELY USED

dupilumab
(doo-pil′-ue-mab)
Dupixent
Func. class.: Dermatologicals

USES: For the treatment of moderate-to-severe atopic dermatitis in patients whose disease is not adequately controlled with topical therapies or when those therapies are not advised

DOSAGE AND ROUTES
Adult: SUBCUT 600 mg initially (administered as two 300-mg injections), then 300 mg every other week

---

⚠ HIGH ALERT

durvalumab
(dur-val′-yoo-mab)
Imfinzi
Func. class.: Antineoplastic monoclonal antibodies

ACTION: A human IgG1 kappa (IgG1k) monoclonal antibody, produced in Chinese

---

hamster ovary, inhibits programmed death ligand interactions

USES: For the treatment of advanced or metastatic urothelial carcinoma

Pharmacokinetics

Absorption	Unknown
Distribution	Steady state 16 wk
Metabolism	Unknown
Excretion	Unknown
Half-life	17 days

CONTRAINDICATIONS

Pregnancy, hypersensitivity

Precautions: Adrenal insufficiency, aseptic meningitis, autoimmune disease, breastfeeding, colitis, contraception requirements, Crohn's disease, diabetes mellitus, diarrhea, hemolytic anemia, hepatic disease, hepatitis, hypophysitis, hypopituitarism, IBS, infusion-related reactions, keratitis, myocarditis, organ transplant, pneumonitis, pulmonary disease, reproductive risk, serious rash, SLE, thyroid disease, ulcerative colitis, uveitis

DOSAGE AND ROUTES
Urothelial carcinoma

Adult: **IV** 10 mg/kg over 60 min, q2wk until disease progression or unacceptable toxicity

Management of immune-mediated toxicities
Adrenal insufficiency:
Grade 2 to 4: Hold until patient is stable and start corticosteroids (1-2 mg/kg/day of predniSONE or equivalent). Begin hormone replacement therapy as needed. When adrenal insufficiency improves to grade 1 or less, begin a steroid taper over at least 1 mo

Colitis or diarrhea:
Grade 2: Hold and start corticosteroids (1-2 mg/kg/day of predniSONE or equivalent). If there is worsening or no improvement, increase corticosteroids and/or other systemic immunosuppressants. When colitis improves to grade 1 or less, begin a steroid taper over at least 1 mo. Treatment may be resumed without a dose reduction when colitis is less than or equal to grade 1 and the corticosteroid dose has been reduced to less than 10 mg of predniSONE or equivalent per day. *Grade 3 or 4:* Permanently discontinue and start corticosteroids (1-2 mg/kg/day of predniSONE or equivalent). If there is worsening or no improvement, consider increasing the dose of corticosteroids and/or other systemic immunosuppressants. When colitis improves to grade 1 or less, begin a steroid taper over at least 1 mo

Diabetes, Type 1:
Grade 2 to 4: Hold until patient is stable and start insulin as needed

Hypophysitis:
Grade 2 to 4: Hold until patient is stable and start corticosteroids (1-2 mg/kg/day of predniSONE or equivalent). Begin hormone replacement therapy as needed. When hypophysitis improves to grade 1 or less, begin a steroid taper over at least 1 mo

Infection:
Grade 3 or 4: Hold and initiate symptomatic management; treat with antiinfectives for suspected or confirmed infections

Infusion-related reactions:
Grade 1 or 2: Interrupt or slow the rate of the infusion. Consider premedications before subsequent dosing. *Grade 3 or 4:* Permanently discontinue

Pneumonitis/interstitial lung disease (ILD):
Grade 2: Hold and start corticosteroids (1-2 mg/kg/day of predniSONE or equivalent). If there is worsening or no improvement, increase the dose of corticosteroids, other systemic immunosuppressants. When pneumonitis improves to grade 1 or less, begin a steroid taper over at least 1 mo. Treatment may be resumed without a dose reduction when pneumonitis is less than or equal to grade 1 and the corticosteroid dose has been reduced to less than 10 mg of predniSONE or equivalent per day. *Grade 3 or 4:* Permanently discontinue and start corticosteroids (1 to 4 mg/kg/day of predniSONE or equivalent). If there is worsening or no improvement, consider increasing the dose of corticosteroids and/or other systemic immunosuppressants. When pneumonitis improves to grade 1 or less, begin a steroid taper over at least 1 mo

Rash:
Grade 2 for more than 1 week or grade 3: Hold and start corticosteroids (1-2 mg/kg/day of predniSONE or equivalent). If there is worsening or no improvement, consider increasing the dose of corticosteroids and/or other systemic immunosuppressants. When the rash improves to grade 1 or less, begin a steroid taper over at least 1 mo. Treatment may be resumed without a dose reduction when the rash is less than or equal to grade 1 and the corticosteroid dose has been reduced to less than 10 mg of predniSONE or equivalent per day. *Grade 4:* Permanently discontinue and start corticosteroids (1 to 2 mg/kg/day of predniSONE or equivalent). If there is worsening or no improvement, consider increasing the dose of corticosteroids and/or other systemic immunosuppressants. When the rash improves to grade 1 or less, begin a steroid taper over at least 1 mo

Thyroid disorders:

Hypothyroidism, grade 2 to 4: Initiate thyroid hormone replacement as needed. ***Hyperthyroidism, grade 2 to 4:*** Hold until patient is clinically stable. Manage patient symptomatically as clinically indicated

Other immune-mediated toxicities:

Grade 3: Hold and begin symptomatic management of the toxicity. Based on the severity of the reaction, may use of corticosteroids. If there is worsening or no improvement, consider increasing the dose of corticosteroids and/or other systemic immunosuppressants. When the toxicity improves to grade 1 or less, begin a steroid taper over at least 1 mo. Treatment may be resumed without a dose reduction when the toxicity is less than or equal to grade 1 and the corticosteroid dose has been reduced to less than 10 mg of predniSONE or equivalent per day. ***Grade 4:*** Permanently discontinue and start symptomatic treatment and corticosteroids (1 to 4 mg/kg/day of predniSONE or equivalent). If there is worsening or no improvement, consider increasing the dose of corticosteroids and/or other systemic immunosuppressants. When the toxicity improves to grade 1 or less, begin a steroid taper over at least 1 mo

Hepatic impairment dosing
Baseline hepatic impairment:

Mild hepatic impairment: No change. ***Moderate (bilirubin 1.5 to 3 times the upper limit of normal [ULN] and any AST) or severe (bilirubin greater than 3 times ULN and any AST):*** Specific guidelines unknown

Immune-mediated hepatitis:

ALT/AST 3.1 to 5 times the upper limit of normal (ULN) or total bilirubin 1.6 to 3 times ULN (grade 2): Hold and start treatment with corticosteroids (1 to 2 mg/kg/day of predniSONE or equivalent). If there is worsening or no improvement, consider increasing the dose of corticosteroids, other systemic immunosuppressants. When hepatitis improves to grade 1 or less, begin a steroid taper over at least 1 mo. ***ALT/AST less than or equal to 8 times ULN or total bilirubin less than or equal to 5 times ULN (grade 3a):*** Hold and start corticosteroids (1 to 2 mg/kg/day predniSONE or equivalent). If there is worsening or no improvement, increase corticosteroids, systemic immunosuppressants. When hepatitis improves to grade 1 or less, begin a steroid taper over at least 1 mo. ***ALT/AST greater than 8 times ULN or total bilirubin greater than***

5 times ULN (grade 3b): Permanently discontinue and start corticosteroids (1 to 2 mg/kg/day of predniSONE or equivalent). If there is worsening or no improvement, increase the dose of corticosteroids, systemic immunosuppressants. When hepatitis improves to grade 1 or less, begin a steroid taper over at least 1 mo. ***Concurrent ALT/AST greater than 3 times ULN and total bilirubin greater than 2 times ULN with no other cause:*** Permanently discontinue and start corticosteroids (1 to 2 mg/kg/day of predniSONE or equivalent). If there is worsening or no improvement, consider increase the dose of corticosteroids, systemic immunosuppressants. When hepatitis improves to grade 1 or less, begin a steroid taper over at least 1 mo

Renal dose
Mild to moderate renal impairment (Ccr greater than or equal to 30 ml/min): No change; severe renal impairment (Ccr 15 to 29 ml/min): Unknown

Available forms: Powder for injection 120 mg/2.4 ml, 500 mg/10 ml

ADVERSE EFFECTS
CNS: *Fatigue, fever*

GI: *Nausea, diarrhea, constipation, anorexia, abdominal pain,* colitis

HEMA: Anemia, hemolytic anemia, lymphopenia

RESP: Cough, dyspnea

META: Hyponatremia, hyperbilirubinemia, hypercalcemia, hypermagnesemia, hypoalbuminemia

ENDO: Hyperglycemia, hyper- or hypothyroidism

MISC: Infection, peripheral edema, infection, musculoskeletal pain, rash, antibody formation, aseptic meningitis, dehydration, infusion reactions, keratitis, myocarditis, uveitis

INTERACTIONS
None known

Drug/lab test
Increased: LFTs, blood glucose, serum creatinine/BUN, thyroid function tests
Decreased: Thyroid function tests

NURSING CONSIDERATIONS
Assessment
• Monitor baseline and periodically blood glucose, LFTs, serum creatinine/BUN

• **Serious infection**: Some may be fatal. Monitor patients for signs and symptoms of infection; use prophylactic anti-infectives as appropriate

• **Pregnancy/breastfeeding:** Product can cause fetal harm, females of reproductive potential should avoid becoming pregnant during and for 3 mo after final dose; obtain a pregnancy test before starting product, do not breastfeed during and for at least 3 mo after the last dose

• **Immune-mediated pneumonitis or interstitial lung disease (ILD):** May be fatal. Monitor for signs or symptoms (new or worsening chest pain or shortness of breath) of pneumonitis. If pneumonitis is suspected, obtain a chest x-ray; an interruption or discontinuation of therapy and treatment with high-dose corticosteroids (followed by a steroid taper) may be necessary. The median time to onset of immune-mediated pneumonitis was 55.5 days (range 24 to 423 days)

• **Immune-mediated hepatitis:** May be fatal. Monitor for abnormal liver tests before each cycle of treatment interruption or discontinuation of therapy may be needed with high-dose corticosteroids (followed by a steroid taper). The median time to onset of immune-mediated hepatitis was 51.5 days (range 15 to 312 days)

• **Diarrhea and immune-mediated colitis:** Monitor for signs and symptoms of colitis (diarrhea or severe abdominal pain). Treatment with antidiarrheal agents and high-dose corticosteroids (followed by a steroid taper), along with an interruption or discontinuation of therapy, may be necessary. The median time to onset of immune-mediated colitis was 73 days (range 13 to 345 days). Use with caution in those with inflammatory bowel disease such as ulcerative colitis or Crohn's disease

• **Thyroid disease/disorders (hypothyroidism/hyperthyroidism):** Monitor thyroid function tests (TFTs) at baseline and periodically during treatment. Asymptomatic patients with abnormal TFTs can receive treatment, manage these patients with hormone replacement and symptomatic management as needed. The median time to onset of hypothyroidism was 42 days (range 15 to 239 days), and the median time to first onset of hyperthyroidism was 43 days (range 14 to 71 days)

• **Immune-mediated adrenal insufficiency and hypophysitis/hypopituitarism:** Monitor for signs and symptoms of adrenal insufficiency (hypotension, decreased cortisol level, fatigue, weakness, and weight loss) and hypophysitis (decreased pituitary hormone levels, pituitary gland inflammation, severe intractable headache, and vision impairment) during and after treatment. An interruption of therapy, treatment with high-dose corticosteroids, and hormone replacement may be necessary

• **Immune-mediated nephritis:** Monitor renal function at baseline and before each cycle of treatment. No initial dose adjustment is recommended in patients with renal dysfunction; use with caution in patients with renal disease or renal impairment. If immune-mediated nephritis occurs, an interruption or discontinuation of therapy may be needed with treatment with high-dose corticosteroids

• **Immune-mediated reactions (aseptic meningitis, hemolytic anemia, immune thrombocytopenic purpura, myocarditis, myositis) and ocular inflammatory toxicity (uveitis and keratitis):** Monitor for signs and symptoms of immune-mediated reactions; confirm etiology or exclude other causes. Therapy may need to be temporarily withheld or permanently discontinued; administer corticosteroids as needed

• **Severe infusion-related reactions:** Monitor signs and symptoms of an infusion-related reaction. Interrupt or slow the rate of infusion in those with mild or moderate infusion reactions. Permanently discontinue in those with grade 3 or 4 infusion reactions

Patient problems
Risk for injury (adverse reactions)

Implementation
IV route
• Follow cytotoxic handling procedures
• Visually inspect for particulate matter and discoloration, product should be clear to opalescent, colorless to slightly yellow, free from particles. Discard if the solution is cloudy, discolored, or particles are observed
• Do not shake

Preparation
• **Withdraw** the required volume of drug and transfer into an intravenous container containing 0.9% sodium chloride injection or 5% dextrose injection, to prepare an infusion with a final concentration ranging from 1 mg/ml to 15 mg/ml
• **Mix** diluted solution by gentle inversion. Do not shake
• **Discard** partially used or empty vials of durvalumab

Storage of diluted solution
• Does not contain a preservative; give immediately after preparation
• If storage of the diluted solution is necessary, the total time from vial puncture to the start of administration should be less than 24 hr if refrigerated (2 to 8° C; 36 to 46° F), or less

than 4 hr at room temperature (up to 25° C; up to 77° F). Do not freeze

IV infusion
• **Give** diluted over 60 min through an IV line using a low-protein-binding 0.2 or 0.22 micron in-line filter
• Do not admix or give other products through the same line

Patient/family education
• Teach patient to report adverse reactions immediately, report diarrhea, hepatic, flulike symptoms, cough, trouble breathing
• Teach patient about reason for treatment, expected results
• **Pregnancy/breastfeeding:** Teach patient to notify provider if pregnancy is planned or suspected, to use effective contraception during treatment and for 3 mo after discontinuing treatment, breastfeeding or for 3 mo after final dose

Evaluation
Positive therapeutic outcome
• Lack of disease progression

dutasteride (Rx)
(doo-tass′ter-ide)
Avodart
Func. class.: Benign prostatic hyperplasia agent, androgen inhibitor
Chem. class.: Synthetic 4-azasteroid compound

ACTION: Inhibits both types 1 and 2 forms of a steroid enzyme that converts testosterone to 5 μ-dihydrotestosterone (DHT), which is responsible for the initial growth of prostatic tissue

Therapeutic outcome: Decreased symptoms of benign prostatic hyperplasia (BPH)

USES: Treatment of symptomatic BPH in men with an enlarged prostate gland, or may be used in combination with tamsulosis

Pharmacokinetics

Absorption	Absolute bioavailability ~60%
Distribution	Protein binding 99%
Metabolism	Liver (CYP3A4)
Excretion	Feces
Half-life	5 wk

Pharmacodynamics

Onset	Rapid
Peak	2-3 hr
Duration	Levels detectable 4-6 mo posttreatment

CONTRAINDICATIONS
Pregnancy, breastfeeding, children, women, hypersensitivity

Precautions: Hepatic disease

DOSAGE AND ROUTES
Benign prostatic hyperplasia (BPH)
Adult: PO 0.5 mg/day may use with tamsulosin

Available forms: Caps 0.5 mg

ADVERSE EFFECTS
GU: Decreased libido, impotence, gynecomastia, ejaculation disorders (rare), mastalgia, teratogenesis
INTEG: Serious skin infections

INTERACTIONS
Individual drugs
Cimetidine, ciprofloxacin, dilTIAZem, ketoconazole, ritonavir, verapamil: increased dutasteride concentrations

Drug classifications
Antiretroviral protease inhibitors or other CYP3A4-metabolized products: increased dutasteride concentrations

Drug/lab test
Decreased: PSA

NURSING CONSIDERATIONS
Assessment
• **Assess for decreasing symptoms in BPH:** decreasing urinary retention, frequency, urgency, nocturia, assess PSA levels, digital rectal exam, urinary obstruction; determine the absence of urinary cancer before starting treatment
• **Assess liver function tests:** ALT, AST, bilirubin; blood studies: CBC with differential, serum creatinine, serum electrolytes

Patient problem
Impaired urination (uses)

Implementation
• Swallow caps whole: do not break, crush, chew, or open
• May be given without regard to meals

Patient/family education
• Advise patient to notify prescriber if therapeutic response decreases, if edema occurs
• Caution patient not to discontinue product abruptly
• Inform patient about changes in sex characteristics, gynecomastia, breast tenderness, decreased libido after 6 mo
• Caution patient not to donate blood for at least 6 mo after last dose to prevent possible blood administration to pregnant woman

• Inform patient that ejaculate volume may decrease during treatment, that product rarely interferes with sexual function

• Advise patient to read patient information leaflet before starting therapy and reread it upon prescription renewal

• Teach patient product should not be used or handled by breastfeeding women

• Advise patient to swallow whole; do not crush, chew, or open caps

• Teach patient that drug may increase risk for developing high-grade prostate cancer

• **Pregnancy/breastfeeding:** Advise patient and family that caps should not be handled by pregnant women or those who may become pregnant since this product can be absorbed through the skin

Evaluation
Positive therapeutic outcome

• Decreased Urinary frequency, urinary retention, urinary urgency, nocturia

econazole topical
See Appendix B

RARELY USED

edaraone
(e-dar'-a-vone)
Radicava
Func. class.: CNS agents

USES: For the treatment of amyotrophic lateral sclerosis

Dosage and routes
Amyotrophic lateral sclerosis (ALS)
Adult: IV 60 mg qday × 14 days then a 14-day drug-free period for an initial treatment cycle. For subsequent cycles, give × 10 days out of 14-day periods followed by 14-day drug-free periods

edoxaban (Rx)
(e-dox'a-ban)
Lixiana ✦, Savaysa
Func. class.: Anticoagulant
Chem. class.: Selective factor
Xa inhibitor

ACTION: Inhibits factor Xa; interrupts blood coagulation and inhibits thrombin formation; does not inactivate thrombin (activated factor II) or affect platelets

Therapeutic outcome: Prevention of stroke

USES: Prevention of stroke in nonvalvular atrial fibrillation

Pharmacokinetics

Absorption	63%
Distribution	Unknown
Metabolism	Minimal
Excretion	Eliminated unchanged urine
Half-life	10-14 hr

Pharmacodynamics

Onset	Unknown
Peak	1-2 hr
Duration	Up to 24 hr

CONTRAINDICATIONS
Hypersensitivity to this product; bleeding

Precautions: Pregnancy, breastfeeding, children, geriatric, hepatic disease (severe), renal failure, surgery

BLACK BOX WARNING: Spinal/epidural anesthesia, lumbar puncture, abrupt discontinuation, nonvalvular atrial fibrillation with CCr >95mL/min

DOSAGE AND ROUTES
For reduction in risk of stroke and systemic embolism
Adults: PO 60 mg q day

Deep venous thrombosis (DVT) or pulmonary embolism
Adults >60 kg: PO 60 mg q day after 5 to 10 days of initial therapy with a parenteral anticoagulant
Adults ≤60 kg: PO 30 mg q day after 5 to 10 days of initial therapy with a parenteral anticoagulant

Available forms: Tablets 15, 30, 60 mg

ADVERSE EFFECTS
HEMA: Bleeding, anemia
GI: Increased LFTs

INTERACTIONS
Individual drugs: Abciximab, clopidogrel, dipyridamole, eptifibatide, quiNIDine, tirofiban, valproic acid, some cephalosporins: increased risk of bleeding

Drug classifications
NSAIDs, salicylates: increased risk of bleeding

Drug/herb
Feverfew, garlic, ginger, ginkgo, ginseng, green tea, horse chestnut, kava: increased risk of bleeding

NURSING CONSIDERATIONS
Assessment

BLACK BOX WARNING: Monitor patients who have received epidural/spinal anesthesia or lumbar puncture for neurological impairment, including spinal hematoma, may lead to permanent disability or paralysis

• **Hemorrhage:** Assess for hemorrhage if coadministered with other products that may cause bleeding
• Assess blood studies (Hct, CBC, coagulation studies, platelets, occult blood in stools), anti-Xa; if platelets <100,000/mm³, treatment should be discontinued; renal studies: BUN, creatinine
• **Beers:** Avoid in older adults, increased risk of bleeding, lower creatinine clearance

• Assess for bleeding: gums, petechiae, ecchymosis, black tarry stools, hematuria; notify prescriber
• **Pregnancy/breastfeeding:** Use in pregnancy only if benefits outweigh risks to the fetus; avoid use in breastfeeding, it is not known if product is excreted in breast milk

Implementation
• May be taken without regard to food
• May be crushed and mixed with 2 to 3 ounces of water and immediately given by mouth or gastric tube. Crushed tablets may also be mixed into applesauce for immediate use by mouth

Switching from another anticoagulant to edoxaban
• Converting from warfarin or other vitamin K antagonists to edoxaban: Discontinue warfarin and start edoxaban when the INR is 2.5 or less
• Converting from an oral anticoagulant other than warfarin or other vitamin K antagonists to edoxaban: Discontinue current oral anticoagulant and start edoxaban at the time of the next scheduled dose of the other oral anticoagulant
• Converting from a low molecular weight heparin (LMWH) to edoxaban: Discontinue LMWH and start edoxaban at the time of the next scheduled administration of LMWH
• Converting from unfractionated heparin to edoxaban: Discontinue the infusion and start edoxaban 4 hours later

Switching from edoxaban to another anticoagulant:
• Converting from edoxaban to warfarin:
  • Oral option: For patients taking edoxaban 60 mg, reduce the dose to 30 mg and begin warfarin concomitantly. For patients receiving edoxaban 30 mg, reduce the dose to 15 mg and begin warfarin concomitantly. Measure INR at least weekly and just prior to the daily dose of edoxaban to minimize the influence of edoxaban on INR measurements. Once a stable INR 2 or greater is achieved, discontinue edoxaban and continue warfarin
• Parenteral option: Discontinue edoxaban and administer a parenteral anticoagulant and warfarin at the time of the next scheduled edoxaban dose. Once a stable INR 2 or greater is achieved, discontinue the parenteral anticoagulant and continue warfarin

Patient/family education
• Advise patient to use soft-bristle toothbrush to avoid bleeding gums, to use electric razor

• Advise patient to report any signs of bleeding: gums, under skin, urine, stools
• Caution patient to avoid OTC products containing aspirin, NSAIDs

Evaluation
Positive therapeutic outcome
• Absence of deep vein thrombosis
• Absence of stroke

efavirenz (Rx)
(ef-ah-veer′enz)
Sustiva
Func. class.: Antiretroviral
Chem. class.: Nonnucleoside reverse transcriptase inhibitor (NNRTI)

ACTION: Binds directly to reverse transcriptase and blocks RNA polymerase and DNA polymerase, causing a disruption of the enzyme's site

Therapeutic outcome: Improvement of HIV-1 infection

USES: HIV-1 in combination with other antiretrovirals

Pharmacokinetics
Absorption	Well absorbed, ᴬᴰ꜀ concentrations higher in females, Africans, Asians, Hispanics
Distribution	Protein bound (99%)
Metabolism	Liver
Excretion	Kidneys, feces
Half-life	Terminal 40-76 hr

Pharmacodynamics
Onset	Rapid
Peak	3-5 hr
Duration	Up to 24 hr

CONTRAINDICATIONS
Pregnancy, hypersensitivity, moderate/severe hepatic disease

Precautions: Liver disease, breastfeeding, children <3 yr, renal disease, myelosuppression, depression, seizures

DOSAGE AND ROUTES
Adult and child >40 kg: PO 600 mg/day at bedtime
Child ≥3 mo, 5-<7.5 kg: PO 150 mg/day at bedtime;

3.5-5 kg: 100 mg/day at bedtime;
≤5 kg: PO 100 mg/day at bedtime;
7-14.9 kg: PO 200 mg/day at bedtime;
15-19.9 kg: PO 250 mg/day at bedtime;
20-24.9 kg: PO 300 mg/day at bedtime;
25-32.4 kg: PO 350 mg/day at bedtime;
32.5-39.9 kg: PO 400 mg/day at bedtime

Available forms: Caps 50, 100, 200 mg; tabs 600 mg

ADVERSE EFFECTS
CNS: Headache, dizziness, fatigue, impaired cognition, insomnia, abnormal dreams, depression, anxiety, drowsiness, odd feeling, suicidal thoughts/behaviors
GI: *Diarrhea*, abdominal pain, *nausea*, vomiting, hepatotoxicity, flatulence
GU: Hematuria, kidney stones
MISC: Fat accumulation/redistribution
ENDO: Hyperlipidemia
CV: QT prolongation
SYST: Immune reconstitution syndrome
INTEG: *Rash*, sweating, pruritus

INTERACTIONS
Individual drugs
Alcohol: increased CNS depression
Amprenavir, indinavir, itraconazole, ketoconazole, lopinavir, posaconazole, saquinavir, voriconazole, cycloSPORINE, tacrolimus, sirolimus, buPROPion, sertraline: decreased level of each specific product
CarBAMazepine: decreased efavirenz levels
Cisapride, midazolam, triazolam, pimozide: do not give together
Ritonavir: increased levels of both products

Drug classifications
Anticonvulsants, ergots, statins (except pravastatin, fluvastatin): increased levels of each specific product
Antidepressants, antihistamines, opioids: increased CNS depression
Benzodiazepines, ergots: do not give together
CYP3A4 inhibitors (conivaptan, ambrisentan, sorafenib): decreased efavirenz metabolism
CYP2B6 inhibitors, CYP2C19 substrates, CYP3A4 substrates: Decreased metabolism
CYP3A4 inducers (carBAMazepine, rifamycins): decreased efavirenz effect
Estrogens: increased level of both products
Oral contraceptives: decreased level of these products
Rifamycins: decreased efavirenz action

Drug/herb
St. John's wort: decreased efavirenz level; do not use together

Drug/food
Increased: absorption of high-fat foods

Drug/lab test
Increased: ALT
False positive: cannabinoids

NURSING CONSIDERATIONS
Assessment
• **HIV:** Assess CBC, with differential, plasma HIV RNA, absolute CD4$^+$/CD8$^+$/cell counts/%, serum β_2 microglobulin, serum ICD+24 antigen levels, cholesterol, hepatic enzymes, blood glucose, pregnancy test, bilirubin, urinalysis
• **Serious skin reactions:** Stevens-Johnson syndrome, toxic epidermal necrolysis, usually occurs during first 2 wk, mild rash may resolve within 30 days; severe skin reactions including blistering, fever, product should be discontinued immediately and corticosteroids started
• **CNS reactions:** assess for suicidal thoughts/behaviors, poor concentration, dizziness, inability to sleep, usually resolves after 4 wk; give at bedtime
• Assess bowel pattern before, during treatment; if severe abdominal pain with bleeding occurs, product should be discontinued; monitor hydration
• **Assess for signs of toxicity:** severe nausea/vomiting, maculopapular rash
• **Hepatotoxicity:** Monitor LFTs in those with liver disease, hold if LFTs are moderately elevated; if severe or if LFTs increase after product is restarted, discontinue permanently
• **Pregnancy:** Rule out pregnancy before starting treatment; oral/non-oral contraceptives are decreased, use barrier methods also; avoid use of this product during the first trimester (particular caution during first 8 weeks of pregnancy) and in females of child-bearing potential. Register pregnant women with the Antiretroviral Pregnancy Registry at 800-258-4263. To reduce the risk of postnatal transmission, HIV-infected mothers are advised to avoid breastfeeding.

Patient problems
Infection (uses)
Nonadherence (teaching)

Implementation
• Give at bedtime to decrease CNS side effects, give on empty stomach
• Cap may be opened and sprinkled on food, or if an infant, may be mixed in formula (2 tsp/10 mL); clear container used to mix with more formula or water so all contents are taken
• Do not cut/break caps

Patient/family education
• Advise patient to take as prescribed; if dose is missed, take as soon as remembered; do not double dose; take on empty stomach with water/juice, teach patient to take at same time of day, not to break tabs, to use with other antiretrovirals
• Instruct patient to make sure health care provider knows of all the medications being taken, supplements, herbs, OTC products
• Advise patient that if severe rash occurs, stop taking and notify health care provider
• Advise patient not to breastfeed or become pregnant if taking this product, use barrier method during and ≥ 3 months after last dose
• Advise patient that adverse reactions (rash, dizziness, abnormal dreams, insomnia) lessen after a month
• Teach patient to avoid hazardous activities if dizziness, drowsiness occurs
• Teach patient that product does not cure disease but controls symptoms; HIV can be transmitted to others even while taking this product
• Advise patient to continue safer-sex practices, that opportunistic infections can occur
• Teach patient to report all adverse reactions, insomnia, poor concentration, but usually are less in 2-4 wk
• Tell patient that CNS side effects of feeling "drunk" or "stoned" usually abate in several months

Evaluation
Positive therapeutic outcome
• Increased CD4, cell counts
• Decreased viral load
• Improvement in symptoms and progression of HIV-1 infection

efinaconazole topical
See Appendix B

elvitegravir/cobicistat/ emtricitabine/tenofovir alafenamide
(el-vi-teg′ra-vir/koe-bik′i-stat/em-trye-sye′ta-been/ten-oh-fohveer a-fen′a-mide)
Genvoya
Func. class.: Antiretroviral
Chem. class.: INSTI (integrase strand transfer inhibitors)

ACTION:
• **Elvitegravir:** Inhibits enzymes' need for HIV replication
• **Cobicistat:** Enhances elvitegravir
• **Emtricitabine:** Inhibits viral reverse transcriptase and acts as a DNA chain terminator

• **Tenofovir alafenamide:** Inhibits viral reverse transcriptase and acts as a DNA chain terminator

Therapeutic outcome: Improvement in CD4, HIV RNC counts, decreasing signs and symptoms of HIV

USES: HIV in treatment-naive patients and certain virologically stable (HIV RNA <50 copies/ml) treatment-experienced patients

Pharmacokinetics

Absorption	**Elvitegravir**: unknown; **cobicistat**: unknown; emtricitabine: rapid and extensively; **tenofovir alafenamide**: a prodrug bioavailability is increased with a high-fat meal
Distribution	**Elvitegravir**: protein binding 98%-99%, unknown; **cobicistat**: protein binding 97%-98%, unknown; **emvitegravir**: unknown; **tenofovir alafenamide**: unknown
Metabolism	**Elvitegravir**: by CYP3A4; **cobicistat**: by CYP3A4; **emtricitabine**: metabolized via oxidation to 3'-sulfoxide diastereomer (approximately 9% of dose) and via conjugation with glucuronic acid to 2'-O-glucuronide; **tenofovir**: undergoes phosphorylation to its active metabolite
Excretion	**Elvitegravir**: 95% (feces), 5% (urine); **cobicistat**: 86% (feces), 8% (urine); **emtricitabine**: excreted renally (86%) and via feces (14%); **tenofovir alafenamide**: eliminated by a combination of glomerular filtration and active renal tubular secretion, 70%-80% excreted unchanged in urine by 72 hr
Half-life	**Elvitegravir**: 13 hr; **cobicistat**: 3.5hr; **emtricitabine**: 10 hr: **tenofovir alafenamide**: 30 min

Pharmacodynamics

Onset	Unknown
Peak	**Elvitegravir**: 4 hr; **cobicistat**: 3 hr; **emtricitabine**: 1-2 hr; **tenofovir alafenamide**: 0.5 hr
Duration	Unknown

CONTRAINDICATIONS:
Hypersensitivity

Precautions: Alcoholism, autoimmune disease, bone fractures, breastfeeding, children, depression, females, Graves' disease, Guillain-Barré syndrome, hepatic disease, hepatitis, hepatitis B and HIV coinfection, hepatitis C and HIV coinfection, hepatomegaly, HIV resistance, hypercholesterolemia, hyperlipidemia, hypertriglyceridemia, hypophosphatemia, immune reconstitution syndrome, lactic acidosis, obesity, osteomalacia, osteoporosis, pregnancy, renal failure, renal impairment, serious rash, suicidal ideation, torsades de pointes

> **BLACK BOX WARNING:** Hepatitis B exacerbation, hepatotoxicity

DOSAGE AND ROUTES
HIV infection in antiretroviral treatment-naïve patients

Adults/children ≥25 kg: PO One tablet (elvitegravir 150 mg; cobicistat 150 mg; emtricitabine 200 mg; tenofovir AF 10 mg) q day with food

Available forms: Tablet 150-159-200-10 mg

ADVERSE EFFECTS
CNS: *Headache*, abnormal dreams, *depression*, dizziness, *insomnia*, neuropathy, paresthesia, asthenia, suicide, fatigue, drowsiness
GI: Nausea, vomiting, anorexia, diarrhea, abdominal pain, dyspepsia, hepatomegaly with stenosis (may be fatal), hyperbilirubinemia, hypercholesterolemia, pancreatitis
GU: Glomerulonephritis membranous/mesangial proliferative
INTEG: *Rash*, skin discoloration
MS: Arthralgia, myalgia, rhabdomyolysis
RESP: Cough
SYST: Change in body fat distribution, lactic acidosis

INTERACTIONS
Individual drugs
Efavirenz, lamivudine: Do not use with, treatment duplication will occur

Drug classifications
CYP3A4 inhibitors (aldesleukin IL-2, amiodarone, aprepitant, atazanavir, basiliximab, boceprevir, bromocriptine, chloramphenicol, clarithromycin, conivaptan, danazol, dalfopristin, darunavir, dasatinib, delavirdine, diltiazem, dronedarone, efavirenz, erythromycin, ethinyl estradiol, fluconazole, fluoxetine, fluvoxamine, fosamprenavir, fosaprepitant, imatinib, indinavir, isoniazid, itraconazole, ketoconazole, lanreotide, lapatinib, miconazole, nefazodone, nelfinavir, nicardipine, octreotide, posaconazole, quinine, ranolazine, rifaximin, tamoxifen, telaprevir, telithromycin, tipranavir, troleandomycin, verapamil, voriconazole, zafirlukast): increased level interferons: decreased emtricitabine level

Drug/food
Increased: Adverse reactions: grapefruit juice

Drug/lab test
Increased: AST/ALT, amylase, bilirubin, CK, glucose, lipase
Decreased: Neutrophils

NURSING CONSIDERATIONS
Assessment
• **HIV infection:** Assess symptoms of HIV, including opportunistic infections, before and during treatment, some may be life threatening; monitor plasma CD4+, CD8 cell counts, serum beta-2 microglobulin, serum ICD+24 antigen levels, treatment failures occur more often in those with baseline HIV-1 RNA concentrations >100,000 copies/ml than in those <100,000 copies/ml; monitor blood glucose, CBC with differential, serum cholesterol, lipid panel

> **BLACK BOX WARNING:** Hepatotoxicity/lactic acidosis: Monitor hepatitis B serology, LFTs, plasma hepatitis C RNA, lactic acidosis levels. If lab reports confirm these conditions, discontinue product. More common in females or those who are overweight. Avoid use in alcoholism

• Pregnancy: Obtain pregnancy testing before use, hepatitis B exacerbation; those with coexisting HBV and HIV infections who discontinue emtricitabine or tenofovir may experience severe acute hepatitis B exacerbation with some cases resulting in hepatic decompensation and hepatic failure
• Patients coinfected with HBV and HIV who discontinue this product should have transaminase concentrations monitored q6wk for the first 3 mo, and q3-6 mo thereafter
• Resumption of anti–hepatitis B treatment may be required. For patients who refuse a fully suppressive antiretroviral regimen but still require treatment for HBV, consider 48 wk of peginterferon alfa; do not administer HIV-active medications in the absence
• Periodically monitor serum bilirubin (total and direct), serum creatinine, urinalysis, LFTs, amylase, lipase

Patient problems:
Infection (uses)
Risk for injury (adverse reactions)
Nonadherence (teaching)

Implementation:
• Antiretroviral drug resistance testing (preferably genotypic testing) is recommended before use in treatment-naive patients and before changing therapy for treatment failure
• For pregnant women, therapy should begin immediately after HIV diagnosis, as early maternal viral suppression is associated with lower risk of perinatal infection
• Avoid use of tenofovir-containing regimens in those with renal disease and osteoporosis

Evaluate
Teach patient/family:
• That hepatitis and HIV coinfected patients should avoid consuming alcohol; offer vaccinations against hepatitis A/hepatitis B as appropriate
• That GI complaints resolve after 2-3 wk of treatment
• To report suspected or planned pregnancy; not to breastfeed
• To take at the same time of day to maintain blood level; not to crush, break, or chew
• That product controls the symptoms of HIV but does not cure; that patient is still able to infect others; that other products may be necessary to prevent other infections
    • **Lactic acidosis:** To notify prescriber of fatigue, muscle aches/pains, abdominal pain, difficulty breathing, nausea, vomiting, change in heart rhythm

> **BLACK BOX WARNING: Hepatotoxicity:** To notify prescriber of dark urine, yellowing skin or eyes, clay-colored stools, anorexia, nausea, vomiting

    • **Suicide:** To report severe depression, suicidal ideation to prescriber immediately

Evaluation
Improvement in CD4, HIV RNC counts; decreasing signs and symptoms of HIV

elvitegravir/cobicistat/emtricitabine/tenofovir
(el-vi-teg′ra-vir/koe-bik′i-stat/em-trye-sye′ta-been/ten-oh-fohveer)
Stribild
Func. class.: Antiretroviral
Chem. class.: INSTI (integrase strand transfer inhibitors)

ACTION:
• **Elvitegravir:** Inhibits enzymes' need for HIV replication
• **Cobicistat:** Enhances elvitegravir
• **Emtricitabine:** Inhibits viral reverse transcriptase and acts as a DNA chain terminator
• **Tenofovir:** Inhibits viral reverse transcriptase and acts as a DNA chain terminator

Therapeutic outcome: Improvement in CD4, HIV RNC counts; decreasing signs and symptoms of HIV

USES: HIV in treatment-naive patients and certain virologically stable (HIV RNA <50 copies/ml) treatment-experienced patients

Pharmacokinetics

Absorption	**Elvitegravir**: unknown; **cobicistat:** unknown; **emtricitabine:** rapid and extensively; **tenofovir:** a prodrug bioavailability is increased with a high-fat meal
Distribution	**Elvitegravir:** Protein binding 98%-99%, unknown; **cobicistat:** protein binding 97%-98%, unknown; **emtricitabine:** unknown; **tenofovir:** unknown
Metabolism	**Elvitegravir:** By CYP3A4; **cobicistat:** by CYP3A4; **emtricitabine:** metabolized via oxidation to 3'-sulfoxide diastereomer (approximately 9% of dose) and via conjugation with glucuronic acid to 2'-O-glucuronide; **tenofovir:** undergoes phosphorylation to its active metabolite

| Excretion | **Elvitegravir:** 95% (feces), 5% (urine); **cobicistat:** 86% (feces), 8% (urine); **emtricitabine:** excreted renally (86%) and via feces (14%); **tenofovir:** eliminated by a combination of glomerular filtration and active renal tubular secretion, 70%-80% excreted unchanged in urine by 72 hr |
| Half-life | **Elvitegravir:** 13 hr; **cobicistat:** 3.5hr; **emtricitabine:** 10 hr: **tenofovir:** 30 min |

Pharmacodynamics	
Onset	Unknown
Peak	Elvitegravir: 4 hr; cobicistat: 3 hr; emtricitabine: 1-2 hr; tenofovir: 2 hr
Duration	24 hr

CONTRAINDICATIONS
Hypersensitivity

Precautions: Alcoholism, autoimmune disease, bone fractures, breastfeeding, children, depression, females, Graves' disease, Guillain-Barré syndrome, hepatic disease, hepatitis, hepatitis B and HIV coinfection, hepatitis C and HIV coinfection, hepatomegaly, HIV resistance, hypercholesterolemia, hyperlipidemia, hypertriglyceridemia, hypophosphatemia, immune reconstitution syndrome, lactic acidosis, obesity, osteomalacia, osteoporosis, pregnancy, renal failure, renal impairment, serious rash, suicidal ideation, torsades de pointes

> **BLACK BOX WARNING:** Hepatitis B exacerbation, hepatotoxicity

DOSAGE AND ROUTES
HIV infection in antiretroviral treatment-naïve patients
Adults/child 12-17 yr and ≥35 kg: PO One tablet (elvitegravir 150 mg; cobicistat 150 mg; emtricitabine 200 mg; tenofovir disoproxil fumarate 300 mg) q day

Available forms: Tablet 150-150-200-300 mg

ADVERSE EFFECTS
CNS: *Headache*, abnormal dreams, *depression*, dizziness, *insomnia*, neuropathy, paresthesia, asthenia, suicide, fatigue, drowsiness
GI: Nausea, vomiting, anorexia, diarrhea, abdominal pain, dyspepsia, hepatomegaly with stenosis (may be fatal), hyperbilirubinemia, hypercholesterolemia, pancreatitis
GU: Glomerulonephritis membranous/mesangial proliferative
INTEG: *Rash*, skin discoloration
MS: Arthralgia, myalgia, rhabdomyolysis
RESP: Cough
SYST: Change in body fat distribution, lactic acidosis

INTERACTIONS
Individual drugs
Efavirenz, lamivudine: Do not use with, treatment duplication will occur

Drug classifications
CYP3A4 inhibitors (aldesleukin IL-2, amiodarone, aprepitant, atazanavir, basiliximab, boceprevir, bromocriptine, chloramphenicol, clarithromycin, conivaptan, danazol, dalfopristin, darunavir, dasatinib, delavirdine, diltiazem, dronedarone, efavirenz, erythromycin, ethinyl estradiol, fluconazole, fluoxetine, fluvoxamine, fosamprenavir, fosaprepitant, imatinib, indinavir, isoniazid, itraconazole, ketoconazole, lanreotide, lapatinib, miconazole, nefazodone, nelfinavir, nicardipine, octreotide, posaconazole, quinine, ranolazine, rifaximin, tamoxifen, telaprevir, telithromycin, tipranavir, troleandomycin, verapamil, voriconazole, zafirlukast): increased level interferons: decreased emtricitabine level

Drug/food
Increased: Adverse reactions: grapefruit juice

Drug/lab test
Increased: AST/ALT, amylase, bilirubin, CK, glucose, lipase
Decreased: Neutrophils

NURSING CONSIDERATIONS
Assessment
• **HIV infection:** Assess symptoms of HIV, including opportunistic infections, before and during treatment, some may be life threatening; monitor plasma CD4_, CD8 cell counts, serum beta-2 microglobulin, serum ICD _24 antigen levels, treatment failures occur more often in those with baseline HIV-1 RNA concentrations _100,000 copies/ml than in those _100,000 copies/ml; monitor blood glucose, CBC with differential, serum cholesterol, lipid panel

> **BLACK BOX WARNING:** Hepatotoxicity/lactic acidosis: Monitor hepatitis B serology, LFTs, plasma hepatitis C RNA, lactic acidosis levels. If lab reports confirm these conditions, discontinue product. More common in females or those who are overweight. Avoid use in alcoholism

• **Pregnancy:** Obtain pregnancy testing before use, hepatitis B exacerbation; those with coexisting HBV and HIV infections who discontinue emtricitabine or tenofovir may experience severe acute hepatitis B exacerbation with some cases resulting in hepatic decompensation and hepatic failure

• Patients coinfected with HBV and HIV who discontinue this product should have transaminase concentrations monitored q6wk for the first 3 mo, and q3-6 mo thereafter

• Resumption of anti–hepatitis B treatment may be required. For patients who refuse a fully suppressive antiretroviral regimen but still require treatment for HBV, consider 48 wk of peginterferon alfa; do not administer HIV-active medications in the absence

• Periodically monitor serum bilirubin (total and direct), serum creatinine, urinalysis, LFTs, amylase, lipase

Patient problems
Infection (uses)
Risk for injury (adverse reactions)
Nonadherence (teaching)

Implementation:
• Antiretroviral drug resistance testing (preferably genotypic testing) is recommended before use in treatment-naive patients and before changing therapy for treatment failure

• For adults, treatment is recommended in all patients to reduce the risk of disease progression and to prevent the transmission of HIV, including perinatal transmission and transmission to sexual partners. Conditions increasing the urgency for therapy include pregnancy, AIDS-defining conditions (including HIV-associated dementia), acute or early HIV infection, acute opportunistic infections, HIV-associated nephropathy, hepatitis B (HBV) or hepatitis C (HCV) coinfection, lower CD4 counts (_200 cells/mm^3), rapidly declining CD4 counts (_100 cells/mm^3 decrease per year), or higher viral loads (_100,000 copies/ml)

• For pregnant women, therapy should begin immediately after HIV diagnosis, as early maternal viral suppression is associated with lower risk of perinatal infection

• Virologic failures occurred more frequently in those with baseline HIV RNA concentrations _100,000 copies; CD4 counts _200 cells/mm^3

• Avoid use of tenofovir-containing regimens in those with renal disease and osteoporosis

Evaluate
Teach patient/family:
• That hepatitis and HIV coinfected patients should avoid consuming alcohol; offer

vaccinations against hepatitis A/hepatitis B as appropriate

• That GI complaints resolve after 2-3 wk of treatment

• To report suspected or planned pregnancy, not to breastfeed

• To take at the same time of day to maintain blood level; not to crush, break, or chew

• That product controls the symptoms of HIV but does not cure, that patient is still able to infect others, that other products may be necessary to prevent other infections

• **Lactic acidosis:** To notify prescriber of fatigue, muscle aches/pains, abdominal pain, difficulty breathing, nausea, vomiting, change in heart rhythm

> **BLACK BOX WARNING: Hepatotoxicity:** To notify prescriber of dark urine, yellowing skin or eyes, clay-colored stools, anorexia, nausea, vomiting

• **Suicide:** To report severe depression, suicidal ideation to prescriber immediately

Evaluation
Improvement in CD4, HIV RNC counts, decreasing signs and symptoms of HIV

emedastine ophthalmic
See Appendix B

empagliflozin
(em-pa-gli-floe′zin)
Jardiance
Func. class.: Antidiabetic
Chem. class.: Sodium-glucose cotransporter 2 (SGLT2) inhibitors

ACTION: An inhibitor of sodium-glucose cotransporter 2 (SGLT2), the transporter responsible for reabsorbing the majority of glucose filtered by the tubular lumen in the kidney

Therapeutic outcome: Decreased blood glucose, A1c′

USES: Type 2 diabetes mellitus with diet and exercise

Pharmacokinetics

Absorption	Well
Distribution	Protein binding 82.6%, RBCs
Metabolism	Minimal
Excretion	Feces (41.2%) unchanged; urine (54.4%) unchanged
Half-life	12.4 hr

Pharmacodynamics (decrease in A1C)	
Onset	Up to 6 wk
Peak	12 wk
Duration	Up to 24 hr

CONTRAINDICATIONS: Hypersensitivity, dialysis, renal failure

Precautions: Adrenal insufficiency, breastfeeding, children, dehydration, diabetic ketoacidosis, fever, geriatric patients, hypercholesterolemia, hypercortisolism, hyperglycemia, hyperthyroidism, hypoglycemia, hypotension, hypothyroidism, hypovolemia, malnutrition, pituitary insufficiency, pregnancy, renal impairment, type 1 diabetes mellitus, vaginitis

DOSAGE AND ROUTES
Adult: PO 10 mg daily, may increase to 25 mg daily

Available forms: Tabs 10, 25 mg

ADVERSE EFFECTS
CNS: Syncope
CV: *Hypotension, orthostatic hypotension*, volume depletion
ENDO: *Hypercholesterolemia, hyperlipidemia, hypoglycemia* (in combination)
GU: *Increased urinary frequency, nocturia, polyuria, cystitis, dehydration, diuresis*
GI: Nausea
MISC: Infection, ketoacidosis
MS: Arthralgia

INTERACTIONS
Drug classifications
Angiotensin II receptor antagonists, angiotensin-converting enzyme (ACE) inhibitors
NSAIDs: Increased renal dysfunction
Antihypertensives, diuretics: Increased hypotensive effect
Antidiabetics: Increased hypoglycemia

Drug/herb
Chromium, horse chestnut: increased hypoglycemia
Green tea: decreased hypoglycemia
Niacin: increased/decreased hypoglycemia

Drug/lab test
Hct, creatinine: Increase
GFR: Increase

NURSING CONSIDERATIONS
Assessment
• **Diabetes:** Monitor blood glucose, glycosylated hemoglobin A1c (HbA1c), serum cholesterol profile, serum creatinine/BUN, assess for polydipsia, other products taken by patient; assess for hypoglycemia, headache, drowsiness, hunger, weakness, sweating; have sugar source available

• **Renal studies:** Monitor serum creatinine, eGFR baseline and periodically, avoid in those with eGFR <45 mL/min/1.73 m^2
• **Ketoacidosis:** If patient presents with volume depletion, dehydration, discontinue and give insulin, glucose source
• **UTI:** Assess for and treat with antiinfectives

Patient problems
Excess food intake (uses)
Nonadherence (teaching)

Implementation
• Give every day without regard to food in the AM

Patient/family education
• Teach patient how to check blood glucose, to continue with diet and exercise changes, to avoid smoking, alcohol
• Instruct patient to avoid other products unless approved by prescriber
• Teach patient to take in the am, without regard to food; if dose is missed, take when remembered; do not take double dose, to read "medication guide" provided, that product controls symptoms but does not cure diabetes
• **Hypoglycemia:** Teach patient to report rapid heartbeat, dizziness, weakness, that lab testing will be needed including blood glucose monitoring, a dosage change may be needed, to carry a sugar source at all times, review signs and symptoms of hypoglycemia and hyperglycemia and what to do about each
• **Hypotension:** Teach patient to report vision changes, dizziness, fatigue, B/P should be checked regularly
• **Ketoacidosis:** Teach patient to report nausea, vomiting, abdominal pain, confusion, sleepiness
• **Infections:** Usually urinary tract infections, patient should report burning, cloudy, foul-smelling urine; fever; back pain, antibiotics will be needed, or mycotic infections including foul-smelling vaginal discharge or penis discharge and redness
• **Pregnancy/breastfeeding:** Teach patient to report if pregnancy is planned or suspected, to avoid breastfeeding

Evaluation
Positive therapeutic outcome
• Decreased blood glucose, A1c

---

emtricitabine (Rx)
(em-tri-sit′uh-bean)
Emtriva
Func. class.: Antiretroviral
Chem. class.: Nucleoside reverse transcriptase inhibitor (NRTI)

ACTION: Synthetic nucleoside analog of cytosine; inhibits replication of HIV virus by competing with the natural substrate and then becoming incorporated into cellular DNA by viral reverse transcriptase, thereby terminating cellular DNA chain

Therapeutic outcome: Decreasing symptoms of HIV

USES: HIV-1 infection with other antiretrovirals

Pharmacokinetics

Absorption	Rapidly, extensively absorbed
Distribution	Protein binding <4%
Metabolism	Unknown
Excretion	Excreted unchanged in urine (86%), feces (14%)
Half-life	10 hr

Pharmacodynamics

Onset	Unknown
Peak	1-2 hr
Duration	Up to 24 hr

CONTRAINDICATIONS
Hypersensitivity, lactic acidosis

Precautions: Pregnancy, breastfeeding, children, geriatric, renal disease

> **BLACK BOX WARNING:** Hepatic insufficiency, chronic hepatitis B virus (HBV) infection, more common in females or those that are overweight; monitor lactic acid levels, LFTs

DOSAGE AND ROUTES
Oral cap and sol are not interchangeable
Adult: PO (caps) 200 mg/day; oral SOL 240 mg (24 ml) daily
Adolescent/child >33 kg: PO (caps) 200 mg/day
Child 3 mo-17 yr: oral SOL 6 mg/kg/day, max 240 mg (24 ml)
Infant <3 mo: PO oral SOL 3 mg/kg daily, do not use caps

Renal dose
Adult: PO CCr 30-49 ml/min 200 mg q48hr, SOL 120 mg q24hr; caps CCr 15-29 ml/min 200 mg q72hr, SOL 80 mg q24hr; caps CCr ,15 ml/min 200 mg q96hr, SOL 60 mg q24hr

Available forms: Caps 200 mg; oral sol 10 mg/ml

ADVERSE EFFECTS
CNS: Headache, abnormal dreams, depression, dizziness, insomnia, neuropathy, paresthesia, *asthenia*, weakness

GI: *Nausea, vomiting, diarrhea, anorexia, abdominal pain, dyspepsia,* hepatomegaly with stenosis (may be fatal)
INTEG: Rash, skin discoloration
MS: Arthralgia, myalgia
RESP: Cough
SYST: Change in body fat distribution, lactic acidosis, immune reconstitution syndrome

INTERACTIONS
None known

Drug classifications
Interferons: Decreased emtricitabine level

Drug/Lab
Increase: AST/ALT, glucose, amylase, bilirubin, CK, lipase
Decrease: neutrophils

NURSING CONSIDERATIONS
Assessment
• **HIV:** Monitor for infections and improvement in symptoms of HIV
• Monitor liver, renal function tests: AST, ALT, bilirubin, amylase, lipase, triglycerides periodically during treatment
• **Pregnancy/breastfeeding:** Use if clearly needed, register pregnant woman at the Antiretroviral Pregnancy Registry at 800-258-4263. To reduce the risk of postnatal transmission, HIV-infected mothers are advised to avoid breastfeeding
• **Assess for lactic acidosis, severe hepatomegaly with steatosis;** if lab reports confirm these conditions, discontinue treatment; more common in females, obese; monitor serum lactate levels, liver function tests

> **BLACK BOX WARNING:** Confirm that patient is free of HBV (hepatitis B virus) before starting treatment

> **BLACK BOX WARNING: Hepatotoxicity:** Do not use in those with risk factors such as alcoholism; discontinue if hepatotoxicity occurs

Patient problems
Infection (uses)
Adherence (teaching)

Implementation
• Give without regard to meals
• Store at 25° C (77° F)
• Take at same time every day
• Oral cap and sol are not interchangeable

Patient/family education
• Teach that GI complaints resolve after 3-4 wk of treatment

• Instruct that product must be taken at same time of day to maintain blood level, solution and cap are not interchangeable

• Advise that product will control symptoms, but is not a cure for HIV; patient is still infectious, may pass HIV virus on to others

• Instruct that other products may be necessary to prevent other infections

• Advise that changes in body fat distribution may occur

• **Lactic acidosis:** Teach patient to notify prescriber immediately of fatigue, muscle aches/pains, abdominal pain, difficulty breathing, nausea, vomiting, change in heart rate

> **BLACK BOX WARNING:** Hepatotoxicity: Teach patient to notify prescriber of dark urine, yellowing of skin/eyes, clay-colored stools, anorexia, nausea, vomiting

• Instruct patient to avoid breastfeeeding to reduce postnatal HIV transmission

• Advise patient to report planned or suspected pregnancy, not to breastfeed while taking this product

Evaluation
Positive therapeutic outcome
• Decrease in signs/symptoms of HIV
• Decrease viral load, increase CD4 counts

emtricitabine/rilpivirine/tenofovir disoproxil fumarate
(em-tri-situh-bean/ril-pi-vireen/ten-oh-fohveer)
Complera
Func. class.: Antiretroviral
Chem. class.: Nucleoside reverse transcriptase inhibitor (NRTI)

ACTION:
• **Emtricitabine:** Inhibits viral reverse transcriptase and is active both on HIV-1 and HBV
• **Tenofovir:** Inhibits viral reverse transcriptase and acts as a DNA chain terminator
• **Rilpivirine:** Inhibits HIV-1 reverse transcriptase; it does not compete for binding, nor does it require phosphorylation to be active

Therapeutic outcome: Improvement in CD4, HIV RNC counts, decreasing signs and symptoms of HIV

USES: HIV in treatment-naive patients with HIV RNA ≤100,000 copies/ml at initiation and certain virologically stable (HIV RNA >50 copies/ml) treatment-experienced patients

Absorption	**Tenofovir:** bioavailability is increased with a high-fat meal
Distribution	**Rilpivirine:** Protein binding 99.7% to albumin; **tenofovir** <0.7%; emtricitabine <4%
Metabolism	**Emtricitabine:** metabolized via oxidation **Tenofovir:** undergoes phosphorylation to its active metabolite; **Rilpivirine:** Via oxidation by CYP3A system
Excretion	**Emtricitabine:** excreted renally (86%) and via feces (14%); **tenofovir:** eliminated by glomerular filtration and active renal tubular secretion, 70%-80% excreted unchanged in urine by 72 hr; **rilpivirine:** 85% feces, 6.1% urine
Half-life	**Emtricitabine:** 10 hr; **Tenofovir:** 17 hr; **Rilpivirine:** 50 hr

Onset	Unknown
Peak	**Emtricitabine:** Peak 1-2 hr postdose; **Rilpivirine:** Peak 4-5 hr
Duration	Up to 24 hr

CONTRAINDICATIONS
Hypersensitivity

PRECAUTIONS: Alcoholism, autoimmune disease, bone fractures, breastfeeding, children, depression, females, Graves' disease, Guillain-Barré syndrome, hepatic disease, hepatitis, hepatitis B and HIV coinfection, hepatitis C and HIV coinfection, hepatomegaly, HIV resistance, hypercholesterolemia, hyperlipidemia, hypertriglyceridemia, hypophosphatemia, immune reconstitution syndrome, obesity, osteomalacia, osteoporosis, pregnancy, QT prolongation, renal failure, renal impairment, serious rash, suicidal ideation, torsades de pointes

> **BLACK BOX WARNING:** Hepatitis B exacerbation, hepatotoxicity, lactic acidosis

DOSAGE AND ROUTES
Adult/adolescent/child 12 years and older weighing 35 kg or more: PO 1 tablet qday. Coadministration with rifabutin, the rilpivirine dose needs to be increased to 50 mg qday; give an additional 25 mg/day of rilpivirine with a meal

---

Renal dose
Adult: PO CCr <50 ml/min: Not recommended

Available forms: Tablet 200-25-300 mg

ADVERSE EFFECTS
CNS: *Headache,* abnormal dreams, *depression,* dizziness, *insomnia,* neuropathy, paresthesia, suicide, fatigue, drowsiness
GI: *Nausea, anorexia, diarrhea, abdominal pain, dyspepsia,* hepatomegaly with stenosis (may be fatal), pancreatitis
GU: Acute renal failure
Integ: *Rash,* skin discoloration
MS: Arthralgia, myalgia, rhabdomyolysis
Syst: Change in body fat distribution, lactic acidosis

INTERACTIONS
Individual drugs
Arsenic trioxide, chloroquine, droperidol, haloperidol, levomethadyl, pentamidine: increased QT prolongation
Efavirenz, lamivudine: Do not use with, treatment duplication will occur

DRUG CLASSIFICATIONS
Arsenic trioxide, beta agonists, class IA/III antidysrhythmics, CYP3A4 inhibitors (amiodarone, clarithromycin, erythromycin, levomethadyl, telithromycin, troleandomycin), CYP3A4 substrates (methadone, pimozide, quetiapine, quinidine, risperidone, ziprasidone), local anesthetics, some phenothiazines, tricyclics: increased QT prolongation
CYP3A4 inducers (barbiturates, bexarotene, bosentan, carbamazepine, dexamethasone, efavirenz, enzalutamide, etravirine, griseofulvin, modafinil, nafcillin, nevirapine, phenobarbital, phenytoin, primidone, rifabutin, rifampin, rifapentine), proton pump inhibitors: decreased rilpivirine effect, treatment failure
CYP3A4 inhibitors (aldesleukin IL-2, amiodarone, aprepitant, atazanavir, basiliximab, boceprevir, bromocriptine, chloramphenicol, clarithromycin, conivaptan, danazol, dalfopristin, darunavir, dasatinib, delavirdine, diltiazem, dronedarone, efavirenz, erythromycin, ethinyl estradiol, fluconazole, fluoxetine, fluvoxamine, fosamprenavir, fosaprepitant, imatinib, indinavir, isoniazid, itraconazole, ketoconazole, lanreotide, lapatinib, miconazole, nefazodone, nelfinavir, nicardipine, octreotide, posaconazole, quinine, ranolazine, rifaximin, tamoxifen, telaprevir, telithromycin, tipranavir, troleandomycin, verapamil, voriconazole, zafirlukast): increased rilpivirine level
Interferons: decreased emtricitabine level

Drug/food
Increased: Adverse reactions: grapefruit juice

Drug/lab test
Increased: AST/ALT, amylase, bilirubin, CK, glucose, lipase
Decreased: Neutrophils

NURSING CONSIDERATIONS
Assessment
• **HIV infection:** Assess symptoms of HIV, including opportunistic infections, before and during treatment, some may be life threatening; monitor plasma CD4+, CD8 cell counts, serum beta-2 microglobulin, serum ICD+24 antigen levels, treatment failures occur more often in those with baseline HIV-1 RNA concentrations >100,000 copies/ml than in those <100,000 copies/ml; monitor blood glucose, CBC with differential, serum cholesterol, lipid panel

BLACK BOX WARNING: Hepatotoxicity/lactic acidosis: Monitor hepatitis B serology, LFTs, plasma hepatitis C RNA, lactic acidosis levels. If lab reports confirm these conditions, discontinue product. More common in females or those who are overweight. Avoid use in alcoholism

• **Pregnancy:** Obtain pregnancy testing before use for Hepatitis B exacerbation: Those with coexisting HBV and HIV infections who discontinue emtricitabine or tenofovir may experience severe acute hepatitis B exacerbation. Patients coinfected with HBV and HIV who discontinue this product should have transaminase concentrations monitored q6wk for the first 3 mo, and q3-6 mo thereafter. Resumption of anti–hepatitis B treatment may be required. For patients who refuse a fully suppressive antiretroviral regimen but still require treatment for HBV, consider 48 wk of peginterferon alfa; do not administer HIV-active medications in the absence of a fully suppressive ARV regimen
• Periodically monitor serum bilirubin (total and direct), serum creatinine, urinalysis, LFTs, amylase, lipase

Patient problems
Infection (uses)
Nonadherence (teaching)

Implementation:
• Antiretroviral drug resistance testing is recommended
• For pregnant women, therapy should begin immediately after HIV diagnosis

---

• Before initiating therapy virologic failures occurred more frequently in those with baseline HIV RNA concentrations >100,000 copies; CD4 counts <200 cells/mm^3

Teach patient/family:
• Inform patient that hepatitis and HIV coinfected patients should avoid consuming alcohol; offer vaccinations against hepatitis A/hepatitis B as appropriate
• Inform patient that GI complaints resolve after 2-3 wk of treatment
• Inform patient to report suspected or planned pregnancy, not to breastfeed
• Advise patient to take at the same time of day to maintain blood level, not to crush, break, or chew
• Advise patient that product controls the symptoms of HIV but does not cure, that patient is still able to infect others, that other products may be necessary to prevent other infections

> **BLACK BOX WARNING: Lactic acidosis:**
> Teach patient to notify prescriber of fatigue, muscle aches/pains, abdominal pain, difficulty breathing, nausea, vomiting, change in heart rhythm

> **BLACK BOX WARNING: Hepatotoxicity:**
> Teach patient to notify prescriber of dark urine, yellowing skin or eyes, clay-colored stools, anorexia, nausea, vomiting

• **Suicide:** Teach patient to report severe depression, suicidal ideation to prescriber immediately

Evaluation: Positive therapeutic outcome; improvement in CD4, HIV RNC counts, decreasing signs and symptoms of HIV

enalapril/enalaprilat (Rx)
(e-nal′a-pril/e-nal′a-pril-at)
Epaned, Vasotec, Vasotec IV ✦
Func. class.: Antihypertensive
Chem. class.: Angiotensin-converting enzyme (ACE) inhibitor

Do not confuse: enalapril/Eldepryl/ramipril/Anafranil

ACTION: Selectively suppresses renin-angiotensin-aldosterone system; inhibits ACE; prevents conversion of angiotensin I to angiotensin II, resulting in dilatation of arterial and venous vessels

Therapeutic outcome: Decreased B/P in hypertension; decreased preload, afterload in HF

USES: Hypertension, HF, left ventricular dysfunction

Pharmacokinetics

Absorption	Well absorbed (PO), complete (**IV**)
Distribution	Crosses placenta
Metabolism	Liver (active metabolite—enalaprilat)
Excretion	Kidneys (60%—enalaprilat, 20%—enalapril)
Half-life	Enalaprilat 35 hr, increased in renal disease

Pharmacodynamics

	PO	IV
Onset	1 hr	5-15 min
Peak	4-6 hr	1-4 hr
Duration	24 hr	4-6 hr

CONTRAINDICATIONS
Hypersensitivity, history of angioedema

> **BLACK BOX WARNING:** Pregnancy

Precautions: Breastfeeding, renal disease, hyperkalemia, hepatic failure, dehydration, bilateral renal artery/aortic stenosis

DOSAGE AND ROUTES
Hypertension
Adult: PO 2.5-5 mg/day, may increase or decrease to desired response, range 10-40 mg/day; **IV** 0.625-1.25 mg q6hr over 5 min
Child: PO 0.08 mg/kg/day in 1-2 divided doses, max 0.58 mg/kg/day in 1-2 divided doses; **IV** 5-10 mcg/kg/dose q8-24hr

HF
Adult: PO 2.5-20 mg/day in 2 divided doses, max 40 mg/day in divided doses

Asymptomatic left ventricular dysfunction
Adult: PO 2.5 mg bid, titrate to 10 mg bid

Renal dose
Adult: PO/IV CCr <30 ml/min 2.5 mg/day, increase gradually; IV CCr >30 ml/min 1.25 mg q6hr; CCr <30 ml/min 0.625 mg as one-time dose, increase as per B/P
Child >1 mo: PO/IV CCr <30 mL/min concentrated

Available forms: Enalapril: tabs 2.5, 5, 10, 20 mg; oral solution 1 mg/mL; enalaprilat: inj 1.25 mg/ml

ADVERSE EFFECTS
CNS: *Insomnia, dizziness,* paresthesias, headache, fatigue, anxiety

CV: *Hypotension,* chest pain, tachycardia, dysrhythmias, syncope, angina, MI, orthostatic hypotension

EENT: *Tinnitus,* visual changes, sore throat, double vision, dry burning eyes

GI: Nausea, vomiting, colitis, cramps, diarrhea, constipation, flatulence, dry mouth, loss of taste, hepatotoxicity

GU: Proteinuria, renal failure, increased frequency of polyuria or oliguria

HEMA: Agranulocytosis, neutropenia

INTEG: Rash, purpura, alopecia, hyperhidrosis, photosensitivity

META: Hyperkalemia

RESP: Dyspnea, dry cough, crackles

SYST: Toxic epidermal necrolysis, Stevens-Johnson syndrome, angioedema

INTERACTIONS
Individual drugs
Alcohol: increased hypotension (large amounts)

Allopurinol: increased hypersensitivity

CycloSPORINE, NSAIDs: increased potassium levels

Digoxin, lithium: increased serum levels

Rifampin: decreased effects of enalapril

Drug classifications
Antacids: decreased effects of enalapril

Diuretics, general anesthesia, nitrates, other antihypertensives, phenothiazines: increased hypotension

Diuretics (potassium-sparing), potassium supplements, salt substitutes: increased potassium levels

Drug/lab test
Increased: ALT, AST, bilirubin, alkaline phosphatase, glucose, uric acid, BUN, creatinine

False positive: ANA titer

NURSING CONSIDERATIONS
Assessment
• **Bone marrow depression (rare):** monitor blood studies: neutrophils, decreased platelets with differential baseline and q3mo; if neutrophils <1000/mm³, discontinue treatment

• **Hypertension:** monitor B/P, orthostatic hypotension, syncope; if changes occur, dosage change may be required; maintain adequate hydration

• **HF:** monitor for increased weight, rales, jugular vein distention, edema, difficulty breathing

• Monitor electrolytes: K, Na, Cl during 1st 2 wk of therapy

• **Monitor renal studies:** urine baseline and periodically, protein, BUN, creatinine; in those with renal dysfunction monitor renal

symptoms: polyuria, oliguria, frequency, dysuria

• **Serious skin disorders, angioedema:** 🅰️🔍 Black patients are more likely to develop angioedema; also, product is less effective; if rash occurs, stop product and notify prescriber

Patient problems
Impaired cardiac output (uses)

Nonadherence (teaching)

Implementation
PO route
• Store in airtight container at 86° F (30° C) or less

• Severe hypotension may occur after 1st dose of this medication; hypotension may be prevented by reducing or discontinuing diuretic therapy 3 days before beginning benazepril therapy

• Give by IV inf of 0.9% NaCl (as ordered) to expand fluid volume if severe hypotension occurs

• Oral solution: may be used in those unable to swallow tabs

Direct IV route/ intermittent IV infusion
• Give undiluted over ≥5 min; use diluent provided or 50 ml D₅W, 0.9% NaCl, 0.9% NaCl in D₅W, or LR, give over ≥5 min, sol is stable for 24 hr

Y-site compatibilities: Acyclovir, alemtuzumab, alfentanil, allopurinol, amifostine, amikacin, aminophylline, amphotericin B liposome, anidulafungin, ascorbic acid, atracurium, atropine, azaTHIOprine, aztreonam, benztropine, bivalirudin, bretylium, bumetanide, buprenorphine, butorphanol, calcium chloride/gluconate, CARBOplatin, ceFAZolin, cefonicid, cefotaxime, cefoTEtan, cefOXitin, cefTAZidime, ceftizoxime, cefTRIAXone, cefuroxime, chloramphenicol, cimetidine, cisatracurium, cladribine, clindamycin, cyanocobalamin, cyclophosphamide, cycloSPORINE, cytarabine, DACTINomycin, DAPTOmycin, dexamethasone, dexmedetomidine, dextran 40, digoxin, diltiazem, diphenhydrAMINE, DOBUTamine, DOCEtaxel, DOPamine, doripenem, doxacurium, DOXOrubicin, DOXOrubicin liposome, doxycycline, ePHEDrine, EPINEPHrine, epirubicin, epoetin, ertapenem, erythromycin, esmolol, etoposide, etoposide phosphate, famotidine, fenoldopam, fentaNYL, filgrastim, fluconazole, fludarabine, fluorouracil, folic acid, furosemide, ganciclovir, gemcitabine, gentamicin, granisetron, heparin, hydrocortisone, HYDROmorphone, ifosfamide, imipenem/cilastatin, indomethacin, insulin, isoproterenol, ketorolac, labetalol, levofloxacin, lidocaine, linezolid, LORazepam, magnesium sulfate, mannitol, mechlorethamine, melphalan, meperidine, meropenem, metaraminol, methicillin, methotrexate, methoxamine, methyldopate, methylPREDNISolone, metoclopramide, metoprolol, metroNIDAZOLE, mezlocillin, miconazole, midazolam, milrinone, minocycline, mitoXANtrone, morphine, moxalactam, multiple vitamin infusion, nafcillin, nalbuphine, naloxone, netilmicin, niCARdipine, nitroglycerin, nitroprusside, norepinephrine, octreotide, ondansetron, oxacillin, oxaliplatin, oxytocin, PACLitaxel, palonosetron, papaverine, PEMEtrexed, penicillin G potassium, pentamidine, pentazocine, PENTobarbital, PHENobarbital, phentolamine, phenylephrine, phytonadione, piperacillin/tazobactam, potassium chloride/phosphate, procainamide, prochlorperazine, promethazine, propofol, propranolol, protamine, pyridoxine, quinupristin/dalfopristin, ranitidine, remifentanil, ritodrine, riTUXimab, rocuronium, sodium acetate, sodium bicarbonate, succinylcholine, SUFentanil, tacrolimus, teniposide, tetracycline, theophylline, thiamine, thiotepa, ticarcillin/clavulanate, tigecycline, tirofiban, tobramycin, tolazoline, trastuzumab, trimetaphan, urokinase, vancomycin, vasopressin, vecuronium, verapamil, vinCRIStine, vinorelbine, voriconazole

Patient/family education
• Advise patient not to discontinue product abruptly; advise patient to tell all persons associated with health care that product is being taken
• Teach patient not to use OTC products (cough, cold, allergy medications) unless directed by physician, to avoid potassium, salt substitutes; serious side effects can occur; xanthines, such as coffee, tea, chocolate, cola, can prevent action of product
• **Hypertension:** instruct patient on the importance of complying with dosage schedule, even if feeling better; to continue with medical regimen to decrease B/P: exercise, cessation of smoking, decreasing stress, diet modifications
• Emphasize the need to rise slowly to sitting or standing position to minimize orthostatic hypotension; not to exercise in hot weather, which can cause increased hypotension
• Advise patient to notify prescriber of mouth sores, sore throat, fever, swelling of hands or feet, irregular heartbeat, chest pain, coughing, shortness of breath, trouble breathing
• Caution patient to report excessive perspiration, dehydration, vomiting, diarrhea; may lead to fall in B/P
• Caution patient that product may cause skin rash or impaired perspiration; that angioedema may occur and to discontinue if it occurs

• Caution patient that product may cause dizziness, fainting, light-headedness; may occur during 1st few days of therapy; to avoid activities that may be hazardous
• Teach patient how to take B/P, normal readings for age-group

BLACK BOX WARNING: Teach patient to use contraception during treatment, pregnancy, to notify prescriber if pregnancy is planned or suspected, not to breastfeed

Evaluation
Positive therapeutic outcome
• Decreased B/P in hypertension

TREATMENT OF OVERDOSE:
Lavage, **IV** atropine for bradycardia; **IV** theophylline for bronchospasm, digoxin, O_2; diuretic for cardiac failure, hemodialysis

⚠ HIGH ALERT
RARELY USED

enasidenib
(en′-a-sid′-a-nib)
IDHIFA
Func. class.: Antineoplastic

USES: For the treatment of relapsed or refractory acute myeloid leukemia with IDH2 mutation

CONTRAINDICATIONS
Hypersensitivity, pregnancy

DOSAGE AND ROUTES
Relapsed or refractory AML with an isocitrate dehydrogenase-2 (IDH2) mutation
Adult: PO 100 mg qday until disease progression. Treat those without disease progression for a minimum of 6 mo to allow time for clinical response

enfuvirtide (Rx)
(en-fyoo′vir-tide)
Fuzeon
Func. class.: Antiretroviral
Chem. class.: Fusion inhibitor

ACTION: Inhibitor of the fusion of HIV-1 with CD4+ cells

Therapeutic outcome: Decreasing symptoms of HIV

USES: Treatment of HIV-1 infection in combination with other antiretrovirals in those who are treatment experienced only

Pharmacokinetics

Absorption	Well absorbed
Distribution	92% protein binding
Metabolism	Undergoes catabolism
Excretion	Unknown
Half-life	3.8 hr

Pharmacodynamics

Onset	Unknown
Peak	8 hrs
Duration	Unknown

CONTRAINDICATIONS
Breastfeeding, hypersensitivity

Precautions: Pregnancy, children <6 yr, liver disease, myelosuppression, infections

DOSAGE AND ROUTES
Adult: SUBCUT 90 mg (1 ml) bid
Child 6-16 yr and <42.6 kg: SUBCUT 2 mg/kg bid, max 90 mg bid; **11-15.5 kg** 27 mg/0.3 ml bid; **15.6-20 kg** 36 ml/0.4 ml bid; **20.1-24.5 kg** 45 mg/0.5 ml bid; **24.6-29 kg** 54 mg/0.6 ml bid; **29.1-33.5 kg** 63 mg/0.7 ml bid; **33.6-38 kg** 72 mg/0.8 ml bid; **38.1-42.5 kg** 81 mg/0.9 ml bid

Available forms: Powder for injection, lyophilized 108 mg (90 mg/ml when reconstituted)

ADVERSE EFFECTS
CNS: Anxiety, peripheral neuropathy, taste disturbance, insomnia, depression, fatigue, peripheral neuropathy
GI: Nausea, abdominal pain, anorexia, constipation, pancreatitis, dry mouth, weight loss
INTEG: *Inj site reactions, skin papilloma*
MISC: Influenza, cough, conjunctivitis, lymphadenopathy, myalgias, hyperglycemia, pneumonia, rhinitis, fatigue

INTERACTIONS
Drug/drug
Protease inhibitors: Increase effect of either product

Drug/lab
Increased: LFTs, lipase, CK triglycerides
Decreased: Hgb

NURSING CONSIDERATIONS
Assessment
HIV: CBC, blood chemistry, plasma HIV RNA, absolute CD4/CD8 cell counts/%, serum 12 microglobulin, serum ICD+24 antigen levels, cholesterol
• Assess for signs of infection, inj site reactions, use analgesics; bacterial pneumonia may occur if blood counts are low or viral load is high or low CD4 counts, IV drug user, lung disease

• **Monitor renal studies:** BUN, creatinine, renal failure may occur
• Monitor bowel pattern before, during treatment; if severe abdominal pain or constipation occurs, notify prescriber; monitor hydration
• **Hypersensitivity:** assess skin eruptions, rash, urticaria, itching
• **Peripheral neuropathy:** May occur and last for several months, administration sites where nerves are close to skin

Patient problems
Infection (uses)
Nonadherence (teaching)

Implementation
• Reconstitute vial/1 mL sterile water for injection, tap, then roll to prevent foam forming, let stand or roll vial to dissolve, inject after determining correct dose
• Give SUBCUT, bid; rotate sites; preferred sites are upper arm, anterior thigh, abdomen
• Storage: Use reconstituted product within 24 hr, refrigerated, let product come to room temperature before injecting

Patient/family education
• If pregnant register with the antiretroviral pregnancy registry 800-258-4263
• Advise that pneumonia may occur, to contact prescriber if cough, fever occur
• Teach that hypersensitive reactions may occur: rash, pruritus; stop product, contact health care professional
• Teach that this product is not a cure for HIV-1 infection but controls symptoms; HIV-1 can still be transmitted to others
• Teach that this product is to be used in combination only with other antiretrovirals
• Teach patient how to prepare and give using subcut injection, watch for site reactions, rotate sites, if more information is needed call 877-438-9366
• Teach patient that pneumonia may occur; to contact prescriber if cough, fever occur
• **Pregnancy:** Identify if pregnancy is planned or suspected, if breastfeeding; if pregnant register with the antiretroviral pregnancy registry 800-258-4263

Evaluation
Positive therapeutic outcome
• Increased CD4 cell counts; decreased viral load; slowing progression of HIV-1 infection

enoxaparin (Rx)

(ee-nox′a-par-in)

Lovenox

Func. class.: Anticoagulant
Chem. class.: low-molecular-weight heparin

Do not confuse: enoxaparin/enoxacin,
Lovenox/Totronex

ACTION: Binds to antithrombin III inactivating factors Xa/IIa resulting in higher ratio of anti-factor Xa to anti-factor IIa

Therapeutic outcome: Prevention of deep vein thrombosis

USES: Prevention of DVT (inpatient or outpatient), pulmonary emboli (inpatient) in hip and knee replacement, abdominal surgery at risk for thrombosis; unstable angina/non–Q-wave MI, acute MI, coronary artery thrombosis

Pharmacokinetics

Absorption	Well absorbed (90%)
Distribution	Unknown
Metabolism	Unknown
Excretion	Kidneys
Half-life	3-6 hr

Pharmacodynamics

Onset	Unknown
Peak	3-5 hr
Duration	12 hr

CONTRAINDICATIONS

Hypersensitivity to this product, heparin, or pork; hemophilia; leukemia with bleeding; thrombocytopenic purpura, heparin-induced thrombocytopenia, active major bleeding

Precautions: Pregnancy, breastfeeding, children, geriatric, severe renal/hepatic disease, blood dyscrasias, severe hypertension, subacute bacterial endocarditis, acute nephritis, recent burn, spinal surgery, indwelling catheters, low weight (men <57 kg, women <45 kg), hypersensitivity to benzyl alcohol

BLACK BOX WARNING: Lumbar puncture, epidural/spinal anesthesia, aneurysm, coagulopathy

DOSAGE AND ROUTES

DVT prevention before hip/knee surgery

Adult: SUBCUT 30 mg bid given 12-24 hr postoperatively for 7-10 days

DVT prevention before hip replacement

Adult: SUBCUT 40 mg/day started 12 hr preop or 30 mg q12hr started 12-24 hr postop, continued × 7-14 days, may continue up to 3 wk

DVT prophylaxis before abdominal surgery

Adult: SUBCUT 40 mg/day × 7-12 days to prevent thromboembolic complications, start 2 hr before surgery

Treatment of DVT/PE

Adult: SUBCUT (outpatient without PE) 1 mg/kg q12hr or 1.5 mg/kg/day (outpatient/inpatient); warfarin should be started within 72 hr and continued ≥5 days until INR is 2-3

Prevention of ischemic complications in unstable angina/non–Q-wave/non-ST MI with aspirin

Adult: SUBCUT/**IV** 1 mg/kg q12hr until stable with aspirin 100-325 mg/day × 2-8 days

Renal dose

Adult: SUBCUT CCr <30 ml/min: 30 mg q day (thrombosis prophylaxis in abdominal surgery, hip or knee replacement surgery, during acute illness); 1 mg/kg q day (concurrently with aspirin to treat unstable angina or non-Q-wave MI); 1 mg/kg q day (STEMI in those ≥75 yrs, 30 mg IV bolus plus 1 mg/kg SC then 1 mg/kg q day (STEMI in those <75 yrs, or 1 mg/kg q day (concurrently with warfarin for inpatient or outpatient treatment of acute deep vein thrombosis (with or without pulmonary embolism)

Available forms: Prefilled syringes 30 mg/0.3 ml, 40 mg/0.4 ml; graduated prefilled syringes 60 mg/0.6 ml, 80 mg/0.8 ml, 100 mg/1 ml, 120 mg/0.8 ml, 150 mg/ml; multidose vials 100 mg/ml (3 ml)

ADVERSE EFFECTS

CNS: Fever, confusion, dizziness, headache
GI: Nausea, vomiting, constipation
HEMA: Hemorrhage from any site, hypochromic anemia, thrombocytopenia, bleeding
INTEG: Ecchymosis, inj site hematoma, alopecia, pruritus, rash
META: Hyperkalemia in renal failure
MS: Osteoporosis
SYST: Edema, peripheral edema, angioedema, anaphylaxis

INTERACTIONS

Drug classifications

Anticoagulants, antiplatelets, NSAIDs, RU-486, SSRIs, monitor INR/PT salicylates, thrombolytics: increased bleeding

Drug/herb

Feverfew, garlic, ginger, ginkgo, horse chestnut: increased bleeding risk

Drug/lab test

Increased: AST/ALT
Decreased: platelets

NURSING CONSIDERATIONS
Assessment

• Monitor blood studies (Hct, CBC, coagulation studies, occult blood in stools), anti-Xa levels q3mo; platelet count q2-3day; thrombocytopenia may occur, PT, PTT, is not needed in those with adequate coagulation; discontinue and notify prescriber if platelets <100

• Assess patient for bleeding gums, petechiae, ecchymosis, black tarry stools, hematuria, epistaxis, decrease in B/P; indicate bleeding and possible hemorrhage; notify prescriber immediately

---

BLACK BOX WARNING: Assess for **neuro-symptoms** in patients who have received spinal anesthesia, may develop spinal hematoma, those who have had trauma, spinal surgery are at greater risk

---

• **Anaphylaxis, angioedema:** Assess for rash, fever, chills, swelling of face, lips, or tongue, dyspnea; stop product, initiate emergency procedures

• **Injection site reactions:** Assess for inflammation, redness, hematomas

• **Beers:** Reduce dose in older adults, increased bleeding risk, or if CCr ≤30 ml/min

Patient problem

Ineffective tissue perfusion (uses)
Risk for injury (adverse reactions)

Implementation

• Give at same time each day to maintain steady blood levels

SUBCUT route

• Administer SUBCUT deeply; do not give IM, begin 1 hr before surgery, do not aspirate, do not expel bubble from syringe before administration; sol is clear to yellow; do not use sol with precipitate; apply gentle pressure for 1 min, do not use products with benzyl alcohol in pregnant women

• Give to recumbent patient, rotate sites (left/right anterolateral, left/right posterolateral abdominal wall)

Direct IV route

• Use multidose vial for IV administration; use TB syringe or other graduated syringe to measure dose; give IV BOL through IV line; flush before and after

• If withdrawing from multidose vial, use TB syringe for proper measurement

• Prefilled syringes (30, 40 mg) are not graduated; do not use for partial doses

• Do not mix with other products or infusion fluids

• Give only this product when ordered; not interchangeable with heparin or other LMWHs

Patient/family education

• **Spinal anesthesia:** Teach patient to report numbness, weakness in lower extremities

• Warn patient to avoid OTC preparations unless directed by prescriber because they could cause serious product interactions, not to start any Rx, OTC, supplements, or herbal products unless approved by prescriber

• Instruct patient to use soft-bristled toothbrush to avoid bleeding gums; to avoid contact sports; to use electric razor; to avoid IM inj

• **Advise patient to report any signs of bleeding, bruising:** gums, under skin, urine, stools, dizziness, rash, breathing changes, do not rub injection site

Evaluation
Positive therapeutic outcome

• Absence or resolution of DVT/PE

---

entacapone (Rx)

(en-ta′ka-pone)
Comtan
Func. class.: Antiparkinsonian agent
Chem. class.: COMT (Catechol-O- methyltransferase inhibitor)

ACTION: Inhibits COMT (catechol *O*-methyltransferase) and alters the plasma pharmacokinetics of levodopa; given with levodopa/carbidopa

Therapeutic outcome: Decreased symptoms of Parkinson's disease (involuntary movements)

USES: Parkinsonism in those experiencing end of dose, decreased effect as an adjunct to levodopa/carbidopa

Pharmacokinetics

Absorption	35%
Distribution	Protein binding 98%
Metabolism	Liver extensively
Excretion	Kidneys, feces; breast milk
Half-life	0.5 hr initial, 2.5 hr second

Pharmacodynamics

Onset	Unknown
Peak	Unknown
Duration	≤8 hr

CONTRAINDICATIONS
Hypersensitivity

Precautions: Pregnancy, breastfeeding, children, renal/hepatic disease, affective disorders, psychosis

DOSAGE AND ROUTES
Adult: PO 200 mg given with carbidopa/levodopa, max 1600 mg/day; (8 times/day)

Available forms: Tabs 200 mg film coated

ADVERSE EFFECTS
CNS: *Confusion,* hallucinations, dizziness, neuroleptic malignant syndrome
CV: *Orthostatic hypotension*, pleural effusion
GI: *Nausea, vomiting, anorexia, abdominal distress, dry mouth, flatulence,* gastritis, GI disorder, *diarrhea, constipation,* bitter taste
INTEG: Rash, sweating, alopecia, melanoma
MISC: Rhabdomyolysis

INTERACTIONS
Individual drugs
Ampicillin, chloramphenicol, erythromycin, probenecid, rifampin: decreased excretion of entacapone
DOBUTamine, DOPamine, isoetharine, methyldopa, norepinephrine: increased CV reactions; avoid use

Drug classifications
MAOIs: prevent catecholamine metabolism; do not use together

Drug/herb
Kava: decreased effect
Ma huang: increased B/P

NURSING CONSIDERATIONS
Assessment
• **Assess for neuroleptic malignant syndrome:** high temp, increased CPK, rigidity, change in consciousness, usually during rapid withdrawal, do not combine with SSRIs or MAOIs
• **Diarrhea:** Occurs between 4 and 12 wk of treatment
• Monitor B/P, respiration during initial treatment; hypotension should be reported
• Monitor liver function enzymes: AST, ALT, alkaline phosphatase; also check LDH, bilirubin, CBC
• **Parkinsonism:** Assess for akinesia, tremors, staggering gait, muscle rigidity, drooling; these symptoms should improve with therapy when given with levodopa/carbidopa; assess affect, mood, behavioral changes, depression; complete suicide assessment
• **Rhabdomyolysis:** Assess for muscle pain, tenderness, weakness, swelling of affected muscles, may lead to decreased B/P, shock

Patient problem
Impaired mobility (uses)
Risk for injury (uses, adverse reactions)

Implementation
• Adjust dosage to patient response
• Give with meals to decrease GI upset; limit protein taken with product
• Give only after MAOIs have been discontinued for 2 wk
• Use with levodopa/carbidopa

Patient/family education
• Advise patient that hallucinations, mental changes, nausea, dyskinesia can occur
• Caution patient to change positions slowly to prevent orthostatic hypotension; not to drive or operate machinery until stabilized on medication and mental performance is not affected
• Instruct patient to use product exactly as prescribed; if dose is missed, take as soon as remembered, up to 2 hr before next dose, not to discontinue abruptly, withdraw gradually
• Inform patient that urine, sweat may darken
• **Pregnancy/breastfeeding:** Instruct patient to notify prescriber if pregnancy is suspected; if breastfeeding, product is excreted in breast milk

Evaluation
Positive therapeutic outcome
• Decreased akathisia, other involuntary movements when used with levodopa/carbidopa
• Increased mood when used with levodopa/carbidopa

entecavir (Rx)
(en-te′ka-veer)
Baraclude
Func. class.: Antiviral
Chem. class.: Nucleoside analog

ACTION: Inhibits hepatitis B virus DNA polymerase by competing with natural substrates and by causing DNA termination after its incorporation into viral DNA; causes viral DNA death

Therapeutic outcome: Improved liver function tests in chronic hepatitis B (HBV)

USES: Chronic hepatitis B (HBV)

Pharmacokinetics

Absorption	Well
Distribution	Extensively to tissues, protein binding 13%
Metabolism	Unknown
Excretion	Unchanged 62%-73% via kidneys
Half-life	Terminal 128-149 hr

Pharmacodynamics

Onset	Rapid
Peak	0.5-1.5 hr
Duration	Up to 24 hr

CONTRAINDICATIONS
Hypersensitivity

Precautions: Pregnancy, breastfeeding, child, geriatric, severe renal disease, liver transplant

> **BLACK BOX WARNING:** Hepatic disease, hepatitis, lactic acidosis, HIV

DOSAGE AND ROUTES
Chronic hepatitis B (nucleoside treatment–naive)
Adult and adolescent ≥16 yr: PO tab 0.5 mg/day
Adult: PO (solution) 0.5 mg qday
Child/adolescent ≥2 yr, >30 kg: 0.5 mg (10 mL) qday
Child ≥2 yr, 27 to 30 kg: 0.45 mg (9 mL) qday
Child ≥2 yr, 24 to 26 kg: 0.4 mg (8 mL) qday
Child ≥2 yr, 21 to 23 kg: 0.35 mg (7 mL) qday
Child ≥2 yr, 18 to 20 kg: 0.3 mg (6 mL) qday
Child ≥2 yr, 15 to 17 kg: 0.25 mg (5 mL) qday
Child ≥2 yr, 12 to 14 kg: 0.2 mg (4 mL) qday
Child ≥2 yr: 0.15 mg (3 mL) qday

Chronic hepatitis B with compensated liver disease
Adult and adolescent ≥16 yr: PO tab 1 mg/day
Adult: PO (solution) 1 mg qday
Child/adolescent ≥2 yr, >30 kg: 1 mg (20 mL) qday
Child ≥2 yr, 27 to 30 kg: 0.9 mg (18 mL) qday
Child ≥2 yr, 24 to 26 kg: 0.8 mg (16 mL) qday
Child ≥2 yr, 21 to 23 kg: 0.7 mg (14 mL)
Child ≥2 yr, 18 to 20 kg: 0.6 mg (12 mL) qday
Child ≥2 yr, 15 to 17 kg: 0.5 mg (10 mL) qday
Child ≥2 yr, 12 to 14 kg: 0.4 mg (8 mL) qday
Child ≥2 yr, 10 to 11 kg: 0.3 mg (6 mL) qday

Renal dose
Adult and child >16 yr: PO CCr ≥50 ml/min 0.5 mg/day; CCr 30-49 ml/min 0.25 mg daily, 0.5 mg/day or 1 mg q48hr for lamiVUDine refractory patient; CCr 10-29 ml/min 0.15/day, 0.3 for lamiVUDine refractory patient; CCr <10 ml/min 0.05 mg PO/day, 0.1 mg/day or 1 mg q7days for lamiVUDine refractory patient

Available forms: Tabs, film coated 0.5, 1 mg; oral sol 0.05 mg/ml

ADVERSE EFFECTS
CNS: *Headache*, fatigue, dizziness, insomnia
ENDO: Hyperglycemia
GI: *Dyspepsia*, nausea, vomiting, diarrhea, elevated liver function enzymes, hepatomegaly with steatosis
INTEG: Alopecia, rash
SYST: Lactic acidosis

INTERACTIONS
Drug/food
High-fat meal: decreased absorption

Drug/lab test
Increased: ALT, AST, total bilirubin, amylase, lipase, creatinine, blood glucose, urine glucose
Decreased: platelets, albumin

NURSING CONSIDERATIONS
Assessment

> **BLACK BOX WARNING:** Assess **for HIV** before beginning treatment because HIV resistance may occur in patients with chronic hepatitis B infection; monitor HIV RNA, do not use in those with HIV and HBV unless receiving antiretroviral treatment for both

> **BLACK BOX WARNING:** Assess for **lactic acidosis and severe hepatomegaly with stenosis:** increased serum lactate, increased hepatic enzymes, palpate liver; discontinue product if these occur, may be fatal

• Monitor geriatric patients more carefully; may develop renal, cardiac symptoms more rapidly

> **BLACK BOX WARNING:** Assess **for exacerbations of hepatitis** (jaundice, pruritus, fatigue, anorexia) after discontinuing treatment; and for several months monitor liver function tests

• Pregnancy/breastfeeding: Use if clearly needed, register pregnant woman at the Antiretroviral Pregnancy Registry at 800-258-4263. To reduce the risk of postnatal transmission, HIV-infected mothers are advised to avoid breastfeeding

Patient problem
Infection (uses)
Nonadherence (teaching)

Implementation
• After hemodialysis give by mouth on empty stomach 2 hr before or after food
• Tabs: Store at room temperature
• **Oral solution:** Use calibrated oral dosing spoon provided, may be used interchangeably with tabs, do not dilute
• Store in cool environment; protect from light

Patient/family education
• Teach patient not to take with food
• Teach patient to take exactly as prescribed, read the "Patient Information," take missed dose when remembered unless close to time of next dose, that compliance with dosage schedule is required, do not share product
• Advise patient not to stop medication without approval of prescriber
• Advise that optimal duration of treatment is unknown
• Teach patient to avoid use with other medications, supplements unless approved by prescriber
• Teach patient to notify prescriber of decreased urinary output, blood in urine

> **BLACK BOX WARNING: Teach patient symptoms of lactic acidosis:** muscle pain, severe tiredness, weakness, trouble breathing, stomach pain with nausea/vomiting, coldness in arms/legs, fast/irregular heartbeat, dizziness

> **BLACK BOX WARNING: Teach patient symptoms of hepatotoxicity:** eyes/skin turns yellow, dark urine, light bowel movements, no appetite for days, nausea, stomach pain, may be worsened after discontinuing treatment

• Advise patient that product does not cure, but lowers the amount of HBV in body
• Teach patient that product does not stop the spreading of HBV to others by sex, sharing needles, or being exposed to blood
• Teach patient not to operate machinery until effect is known, dizziness may occur
• Inform patient that regular follow-up and lab tests will be needed
• Teach patient to notify prescriber if pregnancy is planned or suspected, not to breastfeed

Evaluation
Positive therapeutic outcome
• Decreased symptoms of chronic hepatitis B, improving liver function tests

---

RARELY USED

enzalutamide
(en-zal-u′ta-mide)
Xtandi
Func. class.: Antineoplastic hormone
Chem. class.: Nonsteroidal antiandrogen

Therapeutic outcome: Decreased tumor size, decreased spread of malignancy in prostate cancer

USES: Metastatic castration-resistant prostate cancer in those who have received DOCEtaxel

CONTRAINDICATIONS
Pregnancy, women, hypersensitivity

DOSAGE AND ROUTES
Adult: PO 160 mg ($4 \times$ 40-mg caps) daily
A grade 3 or higher toxicity or an intolerable adverse effect, withhold dosing for 1 wk or until symptoms improve to grade 2 or less, then resume at the same or a reduced dosage (120 or 80 mg), if warranted
The concomitant use of strong CYP2C8 inhibitors 80 mg once daily; CYP3A4 inducers 240 mg once daily

Available forms: TABs 40 mg

epinastine ophthalmic
See Appendix B

A HIGH ALERT

EPINEPHrine (Rx, OTC)
(ep-i-nef′rin)
**Adrenaclick, Allerjet ✦, Anapen ✦,
Anapen Jr. ✦, Auvi-Q
Adrenalin, EpiPen, EpiPen Jr.**
Func. class.: Bronchodilator, nonselective adrenergic agonist, cardiac stimulant, vasopressor
Chem. class.: Catecholamine

Do not confuse: EPINEPHrine/ePHEDrine

ACTION: β_1- and β_2-agonist causing increased levels of cyclic AMP producing bronchodilatation, cardiac and CNS stimulation; large doses cause vasoconstriction via α-receptors; small doses can cause vasodilation via β_2-vascular receptors

Therapeutic outcome: Vasoconstrictor, cardiac stimulator, bronchodilator, decreased aqueous humor

---

USES: Acute asthmatic attacks, hemostasis, bronchospasm, anaphylaxis, allergic reactions, cardiac arrest, adjunct in anesthesia, shock

Pharmacokinetics

Absorption	Well absorbed (PO), complete (**IV**)
Distribution	Unknown, crosses placenta
Metabolism	Liver
Excretion	Breast milk
Half-life	Unknown

Pharmacodynamics

	SUB-CUT	IM	IV	INH
Onset	5-10 min	6-10 min	Immediate	1 min
Peak	20 min	Unknown	20 min	Unknown
Duration	1-4 hr	1-4 hr	1-4 hr	1-4 hr

CONTRAINDICATIONS

Hypersensitivity to sympathomimetics, sulfites, closed-angle glaucoma, nonanaphylactic shock during general anesthesia

Precautions: Pregnancy, breastfeeding, cardiac disorders, hyperthyroidism, diabetes mellitus, prostatic hypertrophy, hypertension, organic brain syndrome, local anesthesia of certain areas, labor, cardiac dilatation, coronary insufficiency, cerebral arteriosclerosis, organic heart disease

DOSAGE AND ROUTES
Anaphylaxis/severe asthma exacerbation
Adult: **IM/SUBCUT** 0.3-0.5 mg, may repeat q10-15 min (anaphylaxis) or q20min-4 hr (asthma)

Severe anaphylaxis
Adult: IV 0.1-0.25 mg q 5-15 min; then 1-4 mcg/min; continuous infusion if needed
Child: IV ≤0.1 mg, or less depending on age, then 0.1 mcg/kg/min continuous infusion if needed

Severe allergic reactions type 1
Adult/child ≥30 kg: IM 0.3 mg (EpiPen/EpiPen 2-Pak, 1:1000)
Child <30 kg: IM 0.15 mg (EpiPen Jr/EpiPen Jr 2-Pak 1:2000)

CPR (ACLS)
Adult: IV 1 mg q 3-5 min

Bradycardia (ACLS)
Adult: IV 2-10 mcg/min

Bradycardia/pulseless arrest (PALS)
Child: (IV) 0.01 mg/kg may repeat q 3-5 min, may increase to 0.1-0.2 mg/kg if needed

Available forms: Nasal spray (sol) 1 mg/ml; sol for inj 1 mg/ml (1:1000); 0.1 mg/mL (1:10,000); inh vapor (sol) 0.22 mg/actuation; pressurized inh (sol) 0.22 mg/actuation; sol for inj 0.15 mg/0.15 ml autoinjector, 0.3 mg/0.3 ml autoinjector, 0.15 mg/0.3 ml

ADVERSE EFFECTS
CNS: *Tremors, anxiety,* insomnia, headache, dizziness, weakness, drowsiness, confusion, hallucinations
CV: *Palpitations, tachycardia,* hypertension, *dysrhythmias*
GI: *Anorexia, nausea, vomiting*
MISC: Sweating, dry eyes
RESP: *Dyspnea,* paradoxical bronchospasm (inhalation)
META: Hypoglycemia

INTERACTIONS
Drug classifications
β-Adrenergic blockers: decreased hypertensive effects, stop β blocker 3 days before starting product
Antidepressants (tricyclics): increased chance of hypertensive crisis; do not use together
MAOIs: increased chance of hypertensive crisis, do not use together
Other sympathomimetics: toxicity
α blockers: Increase: hypotension-antihistamines, thyroid replacement hormones: Increased: cardiac effects
Cardiac glycosides: Increase: dysrhythmias

NURSING CONSIDERATIONS
Assessment
• **Asthma:** Monitor respiratory function: vital capacity, forced expiratory volume, ABGs, lung sounds, heart rate, rhythm (baseline); amount, color of sputum
• **Vasopressor:** Monitor during administration continuously; if B/P increases, product should be decreased; check B/P, pulse q5min after parenteral route; CVP, PCWP, SVR; inadvertent high arterial B/P can result in angina, aortic rupture, cerebral hemorrhage
• Check inj site for tissue sloughing; if this occurs, administer phentolamine mixed with 0.9% NaCl
• **Monitor for evidence of allergic reactions, paradoxical bronchospasm:** (swelling of face/lips/eyelids, rash, difficulty breathing) withhold dose, notify prescriber; sulfite sensitivity, which may be life threatening
• **Pregnancy/breastfeeding:** Identify if pregnancy is planned or suspected or if breastfeeding

Patient problem
Impaired airway clearance (uses)
Ineffective tissue perfusion (uses)
Risk for injury (adverse reactions)

Implementation

- Give subcut, IM, intraosseously, IV; suspensions are for subcut use only; do not give IV
- Visually inspect parenteral products for particulate matter and discoloration prior to use; do not use solutions that are pinkish to brownish in color or contain a precipitate
- Avoid extravasation during parenteral administration; if extravasation occurs, infiltrate the affected area with phentolamine diluted in NS
- Death has occurred from drug errors; make sure the right concentration is used
- Store reconstituted sol refrigerated 24 hr

Direct IV injection route
- 1:10,000 solution can be given directly without diluting; dilute 1:1000 1 mg/9 mL 0.9% NaCl (1:1000 solution)
- Inject EPINEPHrine directly into a vein over 5-10 min for adults or 1-3 min for children; may be given IV push in cardiac arrest
- In neonates, may administer via the umbilical vein
- During adult cardiopulmonary resuscitation (CPR): resuscitation drugs may be given IV by bolus injection into a peripheral vein, followed by an injection of 20 ml IV fluid; elevate the extremity for 10-20 sec to facilitate drug delivery to the central circulation

Continuous IV infusion route
- Dilute 1 mg EPINEPHrine in 250 or 500 ml of a compatible IV infusion solution to provide a concentration of 4 or 2 mcg/ml, respectively; give into a large vein, if possible
- More concentrated solutions (16-32 mcg/ml) may be used in fluid-restricted patients when administered through a central line

IM route
- Give in the deltoid or anterior thigh (vastus lateralis); do not administer into the gluteal muscle, may give through clothing in an emergency

Subcut route
- Do not inject intradermally
- Massage site well after use, can cause tissue irritation

Intraosseous infusion route (unlabeled)
- During CPR, the same EPINEPHrine dosage may be given via the intraosseous route when IV access is not available

Intracardiac route
- Should be reserved for extreme emergencies. Intracardiac injection should only be performed by properly trained medical personnel

Inhalation route
- Use 2.25% sol diluted in nebulizer/respirator
- Rinse mouth after inh
- 10 drops of a 1% sol should be placed in nebulizer
- Dilute racepinephrine 2.25% sol

Endotracheal route
- Per the ACLS or PALS guidelines, the EPINEPHrine parenteral product is administered via this route
- Endotracheal (ET) administration should only be used if access to IV or intraosseous routes is not possible
- **Adult:** Dilute dose in 5-10 ml NS or sterile distilled water; administer via ET tube; endotracheal absorption of EPINEPHrine may be improved by diluting with water instead of NS
- **Child:** After dose administration, flush the ET tube with a minimum of 5 ml NS

Y-site compatibilities: Alfentanil, amikacin, amiodarone, amphotericin B liposome, anidulafungin, ascorbic acid, atracurium, aztreonam, benztropine, bivalirudin, bleomycin, bumetanide, buprenorphine, butorphanol, calcium chloride/gluconate, CARBOplatin, caspofungin, ceFAZolin, cefotaxime, cefoTEtan, cefOXitin, cefTAZidime, ceftizoxime, cefTRIAXone, cefuroxime, chloramphenicol, chlorproMAZINE, cimetidine, cisatracurium, CISplatin, clindamycin, cyanocobalamin, cyclophosphamide, cycloSPORINE, cytarabine, DACTINomycin, DAPTOmycin, dexamethasone, dexmedetomidine, digoxin, diltiazem, diphenhydrAMINE, DOBUTamine, DOCEtaxel, DOPamine, DOXOrubicin, doxycycline, enalaprilat, epirubicin, epoetin, ertapenem, erythromycin, esmolol, etoposide, etoposide phosphate, famotidine, fenoldopam, fentaNYL, fluconazole, fludarabine, folic acid, furosemide, gemcitabine, gentamicin, glycopyrrolate, granisetron, heparin, hydrocortisone, HYDROmorphone, ifosfamide, imipenem/cilastatin, isoproterenol, ketorolac, labetalol, levofloxacin, lidocaine, linezolid, LORazepam, magnesium sulfate, mannitol, mechlorethamine, meperidine, metaraminol, methicillin, methotrexate, methoxamine, methyldopa, methylPREDNISolone, metoclopramide, metoprolol, metroNIDAZOLE, midazolam, milrinone, minocycline, mitoXANtrone, morphine, multiple vitamins, nafcillin, nalbuphine, naloxone, niCARdipine, nitroglycerin, nitroprusside, norepinephrine, octreotide, ondansetron, oxacillin, oxaliplatin, oxytocin, PACLitaxel, palonosetron, pancuronium, pantoprazole, PEMEtrexed, penicillin G potassium, pentamidine, pentazocine, phentolamine, phenylephrine, phytonadione, piperacillin-tazobactam, potassium chloride, procainamide, prochlorperazine, promethazine, propofol, propranolol, protamine, pyridoxine, quinupristin/dalfopristin, ranitidine, remifentanil, ritodrine, rocuronium, sodium acetate, streptomycin, succinylcholine, SUFentanil, tacrolimus, teniposide, theophylline, thiamine, thiotepa, ticarcillin/clavulanate, tigecycline, tirofiban, tobramycin, tolazoline, trimethaphan, urokinase, vancomycin, vasopressin, vecuronium, verapamil, vinCRIStine, vinorelbine, vitamin B complex with C, voriconazole, warfarin, zoledronic acid

Patient/family education

• Tell patient not to use OTC medications; extra stimulation may occur; to use this medication before other medications and allow at least 5 min between each, to prevent overstimulation

• Teach patient that paradoxical bronchospasm may occur and to stop product immediately and notify prescriber; to limit caffeine products such as chocolate, coffee, tea, and colas

• Teach patient to have adequate fluids

• Teach patient to use this product before other inhalation products, wait 5 min

• **Inhalation:** Patient should rinse mouth after inh, teach correct use

• Patient should report blurred vision, irritation with ophth preparations

• **Autoinjector:** Teach patient how to use for anaphylaxis, remove cap, place black tip on thigh at 45-degree angle, hold 10 sec, remove

Evaluation
Positive therapeutic outcome

• Absence of dyspnea, wheezing, relief of bronchospasm

• Improved airway exchange, improved ABGs

• Decreased aqueous humor (opthalmic)

• Stabilization of heart rate and cardiac output

TREATMENT OF OVERDOSE:
Administer a β_2-adrenergic blocker, vasodilators, α-blocker

EPINEPHrine nasal agent
See Appendix B

⚠ HIGH ALERT

epirubicin (Rx)
(ep-i-roo'bi-sin)
Ellence, Pharmorubicin PFS ❦
Func. class.: Antineoplastic, antibiotic
Chem. class.: Anthracycline

Do not confuse: epirubicin/DOXOrubicin/
DAUNOrubicin/eribulin/IDArubicin

ACTION: Inhibits DNA synthesis primarily; replication is decreased by binding to DNA, which causes strand splitting; maximum cytotoxic effects at S and G_2 phases; a vesicant

Therapeutic outcome: Prevention of rapidly growing malignant cells

USES: Breast cancer as an adjuvant therapy, with axillary node involvement, after resection

Absorption	Complete
Distribution	Widely distributed, RBCs cross placenta
Metabolism	Liver, extensively, tissues
Excretion	Bile (60%)
Half-life	30 hr

Pharmacodynamics
Unknown

CONTRAINDICATIONS
Pregnancy, breastfeeding, hypersensitivity to this product, anthracyclines, anthracenediones, baseline neutrophil count <1500 cell/mm³, severe myocardial insufficiency, recent MI, heart failure, cardiomyopathy

BLACK BOX WARNING: Severe hepatic disease, IM/subcut

Precautions: Children, geriatric, renal/hepatic/cardiac disease, previous anthracycline use, accidental exposure, angina, dental disease, herpes, hyperkalemia, hyperphosphatemia, hypertension, hyperuricemia, hypocalcemia, infection, infertility, tumor lysis syndrome, ventricular dysfunction

BLACK BOX WARNING: Bone marrow suppression (severe), heart failure, extravasation, secondary malignancy, requires an experienced clinician

DOSAGE AND ROUTES
Adult: IV 100 mg/m² on day 1 with fluorouracil and cyclophosphamide (FEC regimen) q21 days × 6 cycles or 60 mg/m² on days 1 and 8 with oral cyclophosphamide and fluorouracil q28 days × 6 cycles

Hepatic dose
Adult: IV Bilirubin 1.2-3 mg/dl or AST 2-4 × normal upper limit, 50% of starting dose; bilirubin >3 mg/dl or AST >4 × normal upper limit, 25% of starting dose

Available forms: Solution for Inj (2 mg/ml)

ADVERSE EFFECTS
CV: Increased B/P, sinus tachycardia, PVCs, chest pain, bradycardia, cardiomyopathy
GI: Nausea, vomiting, diarrhea, anorexia, mucositis
GU: *Hot flashes, amenorrhea, hyperuricemia,* red urine
HEMA: Thrombocytopenia, leukopenia, anemia, neutropenia, secondary AML

INTEG: *Rash, necrosis, pain at inj site, reversible alopecia*
MISC: Infection, febrile neutropenia, lethargy, fever, conjunctivitis, tumor lysis syndrome

INTERACTIONS
Individual drugs
Cimetidine, radiation: increased toxicity
PACLitaxel: give epirubicin before PACLitaxel if given concurrently
Trastuzumab: increased ventricular dysfunction, HF

Drug classifications
Antineoplastics: increased toxicity
Calcium channel blockers: increased heart failure
Live virus vaccines: decreased antibody response

NURSING CONSIDERATIONS
Assessment

BLACK BOX WARNING: Heart failure: monitor left ventricular ejection fraction, multigated acquisition scan (MUGA) or echocardiogram, watch for possible dysrhythmias may occur; assess tachypnea, ECG changes, dyspnea, edema, fatigue; cardiac status: B/P, pulse, character, rhythm, rate, ABGs; identify cumulative amount of anthracycline received (lifetime); reactions that follow may be delayed; assess for dyspnea, tachycardia, peripheral edema, rales/crackles, ascites

• **Assess symptoms indicating severe allergic reaction:** rash, pruritus, urticaria, purpuric skin lesions, itching, flushing; product should be discontinued

BLACK BOX WARNING: Bone marrow depression (severe): monitor CBC, differential, platelet count weekly; withhold product if baseline neutrophil count is <1500/mm³; notify prescriber of results if WBC <20,000/mm³, platelets <150,000/mm³; leukocyte nadir occurs 10-14 days after administration; recovery by 21st day; assess for bleeding: Hemanaturia, guaiac, bruising or petechiae in mucosa or orifices

• **Infection:** treat before receiving this product in regimens >120 mg/m²; prophylactic antibiotics should be given (trimethoprim-sulfamethoxazole or a quinolone)
• Assess for increased uric acid levels, swelling, joint pain, primarily extremities; patient should be well hydrated to prevent urate deposits
• Monitor renal function studies: BUN, creatinine, serum uric acid, urine CCr before, during

therapy; I&O ratio; report fall in urine output to <30 ml/hr; dosage adjustment is needed for serum creatinine >5 mg/dl

BLACK BOX WARNING: Severe hepatic disease: monitor liver function tests before, during therapy (bilirubin, AST, ALT, LDH) as needed or monthly; note jaundice of skin or sclera, dark urine, clay-colored stools, itchy skin, abdominal pain, fever, diarrhea

• Assess for bleeding: hematuria, stool guaiac, bruising or petechiae, mucosa or orifices q8hr; inflammation of mucosa, breaks in skin
• Identify effects of alopecia on body image; discuss feelings about body changes
• **Pregnancy/breastfeeding:** Women of reproductive potential should avoid becoming pregnant during therapy and should use effective contraceptive methods. If a woman becomes pregnant during therapy, she should be advised of the potential risks to the fetus, there is potential for male-mediated teratogenicity. Men with sexual partners of reproductive potential should use effective contraceptive methods during and after therapy. Men or women who receive this product may have a risk of infertility. Women treated may develop irreversible amenorrhea or premature menopause; discontinue breastfeeding or discontinue product

BLACK BOX WARNING: Extravasation (vesicant): Assess for local irritation, pain, burning, necrosis at injection site; discontinue and start at another site

• **Stomatitis:** Assess oral mucosa for ulceration, burning, bleeding, may lead to inability to eat and swallow

Patient problem
Risk of infection (adverse reactions)
Impaired cardiac output (adverse reactions)
Risk of injury (adverse reactions)

Implementation
• Avoid contact with skin; very irritating; wash completely to remove; give fluids **IV** or PO before chemotherapy to hydrate patient
• Give antiemetic 30-60 min before giving product to prevent vomiting and prn
• Administer prophylactic antibiotic with a fluoroquinolone or trimethoprim/sulfamethoxazole if dose of epirubicin is 120 mg/m²

BLACK BOX WARNING: To be used by a clinician experienced in giving cytotoxic products

> **BLACK BOX WARNING:** Do not use IM/subcut due to severe tissue necrosis

> **BLACK BOX WARNING:** Give IV, only, a vesicant: if extravasation occurs, stop and complete via another vein, preferably in another limb; avoid infusion into veins over joints or in extremities with compromised venous or lymphatic drainage

• Rapid injection may cause facial flushing or erythema along the vein; avoid administration time of less than 3 min
• Product should be given to those with neutrophils ≥1500/mm³, platelet count ≥100,000/mm³, and non-hematologic toxicities recovered to ≤Grade 1
• When refrigerated, the preservative-free, ready-to-use solution may form a gelled product; and will return to solution after 2-4 hr at room temperature
• Visually inspect for particulate matter and discoloration prior to use
• Double-check dose and product, fatalities have occurred with wrong dose or product
• Give antiinfectives before using this product

IV route
• Product should be prepared by experienced personnel using proper precautions; pregnant women must not handle product
• Reconstitute 50 mg and 200 mg powder for injection vials with 25 ml and 100 ml, respectively, of sterile water for injection (2 mg/ml), shake vigorously for up to 4 min; reconstituted solutions are stable for 24 hr when stored refrigerated and protected from light or at room temperature in normal light
• Solution can be further diluted with sterile water for injection

IV injection route
• Give doses of 100-120 mg/m² into tubing of a freely flowing 0.9% sodium chloride (NS) or D₅W IV infusion over 15-20 min; the infusion time may be decreased, proportionally, in those who require lower doses; infusion times <3 min are not recommended
• Direct injection into the vein is not recommended due to the risk of extravasation; avoid use with any solution of alkaline pH as hydrolysis will occur

IV infusion route
• Dilute dose in 0.9% sodium chloride (NS) or D₅W; infuse over 30-60 min
• Avoid use with any solution of alkaline pH as hydrolysis will occur

Y-site compatibilities: Alemtuzumab, alfentanil, amifostine, amikacin, aminocaproic acid, anidulafungin, argatroban, atracurium, aztreonam, bivalirudin, bleomycin, bumetanide, buprenorphine, butorphanol, calcium chloride/gluconate, CARBOplatin, caspofungin, ceFAZolin, cefotaxime, ceftizoxime, chlorproMAZINE, cimetidine, ciprofloxacin, cisatracurium, CISplatin, clindamycin, cyclophosphamide, cycloSPORINE, DAPTOmycin, dexrazoxane, digoxin, diltiazem, diphenhydrAMINE, DOBUTamine, DOCEtaxel, dolasetron, DOPamine, doxacurium, doxycycline, droperidol, enalaprilat, ePHEDrine, EPINEPHrine, ertapenem, erythromycin, etoposide, famotidine, fenoldopam, fentaNYL, fluconazole, gatifloxacin, gemcitabine, gentamicin, granisetron, haloperidol, hydrocortisone, HYDROmorphone, hydrOXYzine, ifosfamide, imipenemcilastatin, inamrinone, insulin (regular), isoproterenol, labetalol, levofloxacin, levorphanol, lidocaine, linezolid, LORazepam, mannitol, meperidine, mesna, methotrexate, metoclopramide, metoprolol, metroNIDAZOLE, midazolam, milrinone, minocycline, mitoMYcin, mivacurium, morphine, moxifloxacin, nalbuphine, naloxone, nesiritide, niCARdipine, nitroglycerin, nitroprusside, norepinephrine, octreotide, ofloxacin, ondansetron, oxaliplatin, PACLitaxel, palonosetron, pamidronate, pancuronium, pentamidine, pentazocine, phenylephrine, potassium chloride, procainamide, prochlorperazine, promethazine, propranolol, quinupristin-dalfopristin, ranitidine, remifentanil, rocuronium, sodium acetate, succinylcholine, SUFentanil, tacrolimus, teniposide, theophylline, thiotepa, tigecycline, tirofiban, tobramycin, trimethobenzamide, vancomycin, vasopressin, vecuronium, verapamil, vinBLAStine, vinCRIStine, vinorelbine, voriconazole, zidovudine, zoledronic acid

Patient/family education
• Advise patient to avoid use of products containing aspirin or NSAIDs, razors, commercial mouthwash, since bleeding may occur; to report symptoms of bleeding (hematuria, tarry stools)
• Instruct patient to report signs of anemia (fatigue, headache, irritability, faintness, shortness of breath)
• Inform patient that hair may be lost during treatment; a wig or hairpiece may make patient feel better; new hair may be different in color, texture, new hair growth occurs in ≤3 mo after treatment
• Caution patient not to have any vaccinations without the advice of the prescriber; serious reactions can occur

> **BLACK BOX WARNING:** Teach patient that irreversible myocardial damage, leukopenia, menopause may occur

- Advise patient that urine may appear red for 2 days
- Instruct patient to avoid crowds, persons with known infection
- Caution patient to avoid OTC medications, supplements unless approved by prescriber
- Teach patient to report rapid heartbeat, trouble breathing, fever, nausea, vomiting, oral sores
- To report pain at site immediately
- **Pregnancy/breastfeeding:** Advise patient to use contraception during treatment and 4 mo afterward; not to breastfeed

Evaluation
Positive therapeutic outcome
- Prevention of rapid division of malignant cells

eplerenone (Rx)
(ep-ler-ee′known)
Inspra
Func. class.: Antihypertensive
Chem. class.: Aldosterone antagonist

Do not confuse: Inspra/Spiriva

ACTION: Binds to mineralocorticoid receptor and blocks the binding of aldosterone, a component of the renin-angiotensin-aldosterone system (RAAS)

Therapeutic outcome: Absence of hypertension

USES: Hypertension, alone or in combination with thiazide diuretics, HF, post-MI

Pharmacokinetics

Absorption	Well
Distribution	Protein binding 50%
Metabolism	Liver (CYP3A4)
Excretion	Urine <5%, feces
Half-life	4-6 hr

Pharmacodynamics Antihypertension

Onset	Unknown
Peak	4 wk
Duration	Unknown

CONTRAINDICATIONS
Hypersensitivity, increased serum creatinine >2 mg/dl (male) or >1.8 mg/dl (female), potassium >5.5 mEq/L, type 2 diabetes with microalbuminuria, hepatic disease, CCr <30 ml/min, CCr <50 ml/min in hypertension

Precautions: Pregnancy, breastfeeding, children, geriatric, impaired renal/hepatic function, hyperkalemia

DOSAGE AND ROUTES
Hypertension
Adult: PO 50 mg/day initially, may increase to 50 mg bid after 4 wk, max 100 mg/day; start dose at 25 mg/day if patient is taking CYP3A4 inhibitors

HF/post-MI
Adult: PO 25 mg/day initially, may increase to 50 mg/day; with CYP3A4 inhibitors max 25 mg/day

Available forms: Tabs 25, 50 mg

ADVERSE EFFECTS
CNS: Headache, *dizziness, fatigue*
CV: Angina, MI
GI: Increased GGT *diarrhea*, abdominal pain, increased ALT
GU: Gynecomastia, mastodynia (males), abnormal vaginal bleeding
META: *Hyperkalemia,* hyponatremia, hypercholesteremia, hypertriglyceridemia, increased uric acid
RESP: *Cough*

INTERACTIONS
Individual drugs
Clarithromycin, imatinib, nelfinavir, nefazodone, ritonavir, troleandomycin: do not use concurrently
Erythromycin, fluconazole, verapamil: reduce dose of eplerenone; increased eplerenone levels
Itraconazole, ketoconazole, saquinavir, verapamil: increased levels of eplerenone; reduce dose of eplerenone
Lithium: increased serum lithium levels, monitor lithium level

Drug classifications
ACE inhibitors, angiotensin II antagonists, diuretics (potassium-sparing), do not use together, NSAIDs, potassium supplements: increased hyperkalemia
CYP3A4 inhibitors: increased levels of eplerenone; reduce dose of eplerenone
NSAIDs: decreased antihypertensive effect

Drug/herb
Decreased antihypertensive effect: ephedra, St. John's wort

Drug/food
Grapefruit, grapefruit juice: increased product level by 25%
- Do not use salt substitutes with potassium

Drug/lab test
Increased: BUN, creatinine, potassium, cholesterol, lipids, uric acid
Decreased: sodium

NURSING CONSIDERATIONS
Assessment
• **Hypertension:** monitor B/P at peak/trough level of product, orthostatic hypotension, syncope when used with diuretic; those on moderate CYP3A4 inhibitors should monitor potassium at baseline, within first wk, and at 1 month and more often in diabetes, renal disease
• Monitor renal studies: protein, BUN, creatinine; increased liver function tests; uric acid may be increased, contraindicated in CCr <30 ml/min
• Monitor potassium levels, hyperkalemia may occur
• **Pregnancy/breastfeeding:** Use in pregnancy only if clearly needed, may be excreted in breast milk, discontinue breastfeeding or discontinue product

Patient problem
Impaired cardiac output (uses)
Nonadherence (teaching)

Implementation
• Store in tight container at 86° F (30° C) or less
• **Dosage adjustments for those receiving moderate CYP3A4 inhibitors:** Potassium level 5 mEq/L, increase from 25 mg every other day to 25 mg/qday, or increase from 25 mg/qday to 50 mg qday.
• If potassium level is 5-5.4 mEq/L no adjustment; if potassium level is 5.5 to 5.9 mEq/L, decrease dose from 50 mg qday to 25 mg/qday to 25 mg every other day; withhold dose; If potassium level is >6 mEq/L withhold; may restart drug at 25 mg every other day when potassium level is <5.5 mEq/L

Patient/family education
• Advise patient not to discontinue product abruptly
• Advise patient not to use OTC products (cough, cold, allergy) unless directed by prescriber; do not use salt substitutes containing potassium without consulting prescriber
• Teach patient the importance of complying with dosage schedule, even if feeling better
• Teach patient that product may cause dizziness, fainting, light-headedness; may occur during first few days of therapy
• Teach patient how to take B/P, normal readings for age group

Evaluation
Positive therapeutic outcome
• Decrease in B/P

⚠ HIGH ALERT

epoetin (Rx)
(ee-poe′e-tin)
Epogen, Eprex ✦, Procrit
Func. class.: Antianemic, hormone
Chem. class.: Amino acid polypeptide

ACTION: Erythropoietin is a factor controlling rate of red cell production; product is developed by recombinant DNA technology

Therapeutic outcome: Decreased anemia with increased RBCs

USES: Anemia caused by reduced endogenous erythropoietin production, primarily end-stage renal disease; to correct hemostatic defect in uremia; anemia caused by AZT (zidovudine) treatment in HIV-positive patients; anemia caused by chemotherapy; reduction of allogeneic blood transfusion in surgery patients

Pharmacokinetics

Absorption	Well absorbed (SUBCUT), completely absorbed (**IV**)
Distribution	Increased RBC count 2-6 wk
Metabolism	Unknown
Excretion	Unknown
Half-life	5-14 hr

Pharmacodynamics

	SUBCUT/IV
Onset	Unknown
Peak	Immediate; SUBCUT: Peak 5-24 hr
Duration	Unknown

CONTRAINDICATIONS
Hypersensitivity to mammalian cell–derived products or human albumin; uncontrolled hypertension

Precautions: Pregnancy, breastfeeding, children <1 mo, seizure disorder, porphyria, CV disease, hemodialysis, latex allergy, hypertension, history of CABG; multidose preserved formulation contains benzyl alcohol and should not be used in premature infants

BLACK BOX WARNING: Hgb >11 g/dl, surgery, neoplastic disease

DOSAGE AND ROUTES
Anemia due to chronic kidney disease
Adult/adolescent ≥17 yr: SUBCUT/IV, initially, 50-100 units/kg 3×/wk. If Hgb ≥ 11 g/dl

(dialysis), reduce or interrupt the dose. Hgb is <10 g/dl (not on dialysis), if Hgb has not increased >1 g/dl after 4 wk of therapy, increase by 25%.

Adolescent ≤16 yr >1 mo /infant: SUBCUT/ IV 50 units/kg 3×/wk initially; for dosage adjustments, see adult dosage

Zidovudine-induced anemia

Adult: SUBCUT/IV initially, 100 units/kg 3×/ wk. If Hgb does not increase after 8 wk, increase by 50-100 units/kg at 4 to 8 wk intervals until Hgb is at a concentration to avoid RBC transfusions or a dose of 300 units/kg is reached. If the Hgb >12 g/dl, withhold, once Hgb <11 g/dl resume at a dose 25% below the previous dose

Anemia in chemotherapy

Adult: SUBCUT 150 units/kg 3×/wk or 40,000 units weekly only when the hemoglobin is <10 g/ dl and only until the chemotherapy course is completed.

Available forms: Inj 2000, 3000, 4000, 10,000, 20,000, 40,000 units/mL

ADVERSE EFFECTS

CNS: Seizures, coldness, sweating, headache, fatigue, dizziness
CV: *Hypertension*, hypertensive encephalopathy, HF, edema, DVT, MI, stroke
INTEG: Pruritus, rash, inj site reaction
MISC: Iron deficiency
MS: Bone pain, arthralgia, myalgia
RESP: Cough

INTERACTIONS
Drug classifications

Anticoagulants: need for increased heparin during hemodialysis

NURSING CONSIDERATIONS
Assessment

• Monitor renal studies: urinalysis, protein, blood, BUN, creatinine; I&O, electrolytes; report drop in output to <50 ml/hr

---

BLACK BOX WARNING: Blood studies:
Monitor blood studies: ferritin, transferrin monthly, transferrin sat ≥20%; ferritin ≥100 ng/ml; Hct 2 ×/wk until stabilized in target range (30%-36%), then at regular intervals; those with endogenous erythropoietin levels of <500 units/L respond to this agent; check for symptoms of anemia: fatigue, pallor, dyspnea; monitor Hct 2 ×/wk in chronic renal failure; cancer patients and those being treated with zidovudine should be monitored weekly, then periodically after stabilization; death may occur in Hgb >12 g/dl

---

• Assess for CNS symptoms: coldness, sweating, pain in long bones
• Assess CV status: B/P before, during treatment; hypertension may occur rapidly, leading to hypertension encephalopathy; antihypertensives may be needed
• Assess patient during hemodialysis for bruits, thrills, or shunts, product prevents severe anemia in chronic renal failure; clotting may need to be treated with increased anticoagulant
• **Seizures:** place on seizure precautions; assess for seizures if Hct is increased within 2 wk by 4 points, increased B/P, more common in chronic renal failure in the first 90 days of treatment
• **Anemia:** Monitor serum iron, ferritin, transferrin levels; iron therapy may be needed to prevent recurring anemia; assess for weakness, fatigue
• Monitor B/P, check for rising B/P as Hct rises, use of antihypertensive may be needed
• Monitor blood studies: uric acid, platelets, WBC, phosphorus, potassium, bleeding time; Hct, Hgb, RBCs, reticulocytes should be checked in chronic renal failure
• For hypersensitivity reactions: Skin rashes, urticaria (rare), antibody development does not occur
• For pure cell aplasia (PRCA) in absence of other causes, evaluate by testing serum for recombinant erythropoietin antibodies; any loss of response to epoetin should be evaluated

Patient problem

Fatigue (uses)
Nonadherence (teaching)

Implementation

• Do not use if discolored or particulates are present, should be clear
SUBCUT route
• Before injecting, preservative-free, single-dose formulation may be admixed by using 0.9% NaCl, USP, with benzyl alcohol 0.9% at a 1:1 ratio to reduce injection site discomfort, store solution in refrigerator, protect from light

Direct IV route
• Administer by direct route at end of dialysis by venous line, do not shake vial, can be undiluted or diluted in 0.9% NaCl (1000-40000 U/mL), give over ≥1 min
• If Hgb increases by 1 g/dl in 2 wk, decrease dose by 25%; increase dose if Hgb does not increase by 5-6 points after 8 wk of therapy; suggested target Hgb range 30%-36%
• Give additional heparin to lower chance of clots

Solution compatibilities: Do not dilute or administer with other solutions

---

Patient/family education
• Teach patient how to take B/P, have patient read the "Medication Guide"; a form must be signed before each cycle
• Teach patient to report immediately chest pain, pain in calves, confusion, inability to speak, numbness in face, arms, legs
• Advise patients to take iron supplements, vit B_{12}, folic acid as directed
• Teach patient to avoid driving or hazardous activity during treatment
• Teach patients with renal disease to include high-iron and low-potassium foods in their diets (meat, dark green leafy vegetables, eggs, enriched breads) to comply with treatment regimen
• Teach patient the reason for treatment, expected results, to notify health care professional of use
• Pregnancy/breastfeeding: Advise patient to use contraception, to report if pregnancy is planned or suspected or if breastfeeding
• Chronic renal failure (anemia): Teach patient that product does not cure condition, to maintain prescribed diet, medications, dialysis follow-up appointments

Evaluation
Positive therapeutic outcome
• Increased appetite
• Enhanced sense of well-being
• Increase in reticulocyte count in 2-6 wk, Hgb, Hct

eprosartan (Rx)
(ep-roe-sar′tan)
Teveten
Func. class.: Antihypertensive
Chem. class.: Angiotensin II receptor antagonist

ACTION: Blocks the vasoconstrictor and aldosterone-secreting effects of angiotensin II; selectively blocks the binding of angiotensin II to the AT_1 receptor found in tissues

Therapeutic outcome: Decreased B/P

USES: Hypertension, alone or in combination with other antihypertensives

Pharmacokinetics

Absorption	~13%; food delays absorption
Distribution	Protein binding 98%, crosses placenta
Metabolism	Moderate renal impairment increases levels by 30%, hepatic impairment increases levels by 40%
Excretion	Feces
Half-life	20 hr

Pharmacodynamics (antihypertensive effect)

Onset	1-2 hr
Peak	2-3 wk
Duration	Up to 24 hr

CONTRAINDICATIONS
Hypersensitivity

> **BLACK BOX WARNING:** Pregnancy

Precautions: Breastfeeding, children, geriatric, hypersensitivity to ACE inhibitors, renal/hepatic disease, angioedema, hyperkalemia

DOSAGE AND ROUTES
Adult: PO 600 mg/day; dose may be divided and given bid, with total daily doses ranging from 400-800 mg, max 800 mg/day

Renal dose
Adult: PO CCr ≤30 ml/min, max 600 mg/day

Available forms: Tabs 400, 600 mg

ADVERSE EFFECTS
CNS: *Dizziness*, depression, *fatigue,* headache
CV: Chest pain, palpitations
EENT: Sinusitis
GI: *Diarrhea, dyspepsia, abdominal pain*
GU: UTI
HEMA: Neutropenia
INTEG: Pruritus, angioedema
META: Hypertriglyceridemia
MS: *Myalgia*, arthralgia, rhabdomyolysis
RESP: *Cough, upper respiratory infection,* rhinitis, pharyngitis, viral infection
SYST: Anaphylaxis

INTERACTIONS
Drug classifications
Antidiabetics: Increase: hyperglycemia
ACE inhibitors, angiotensin II receptor antagonists, potassium sparing diuretics, potassium supplements: increased hyperkalemia
NSAIDs, salicylates: decreased antihypertensive effect
Other antihypertensives: increased antihypertensive effect

Drug/food
Salt substitutes: Increased potassium level

Drug/lab test
Increased: ALT, AST, alkaline phosphatase, potassium
Decreased: Hgb

NURSING CONSIDERATIONS
Assessment
• Assess B/P with position changes, pulse baseline, periodically; note rate, rhythm, quality

• Assess electrolytes: K, Na, Cl
• Assess baselines in renal, liver function tests before therapy begins
• **Heart failure:** Assess for edema, daily weight, rales/crackles, jugular vein distension, report significant findings
• **Hypersensitivity/anaphylaxis/angioedema:** Monitor for rash, dyspnea, throat tightness, if these occur, stop product, give antihistamine first, notify prescriber immediately
• **Pregnancy:** Identify if pregnancy is planned or suspected, if breastfeeding

Patient problem
Impaired cardiac output (uses)
Nonadherence (teaching)

Implementation
• May be given without regard to meals
• Correct volume depletion if needed before starting treatment

Patient/family education
• Advise patient to comply with dosage schedule, even if feeling better, take doses that were missed as soon as remembered, if within 1 hr of next dose, do not double, use at same time of day, not to discontinue without discussing with prescriber
• Advise patient to comply with treatment regimen, to avoid salt substitutes with potassium, other potassium products
• Advise patient to discuss all OTC, RX, herbals, supplements with health care professional
• **Angioedema/hypersensitivity:** Teach patient to notify health care professional immediately of swelling of face, throat, trouble breathing, itching rash
• Teach patient that follow-ups and lab work will be needed
• Advise patient to notify prescriber of fever, swelling of hands or feet, chest pain
• Inform patient that excessive perspiration, dehydration, diarrhea may lead to fall in blood pressure; consult prescriber if these occur, maintain adequate hydration
• Inform patient that product may cause dizziness; advise to avoid hazardous activities until effect is known, to rise slowly from sitting position
• Teach patient/family how to take B/P, report changes if significant

> **BLACK BOX WARNING:** Advise patient not to take this medication if pregnant or breastfeeding, or if allergic reaction to this product has occurred

Evaluation
Positive therapeutic outcome
• Decreased B/P

> **⚠ HIGH ALERT**

eptifibatide (Rx)
(ep-tih-fib′ah-tide)
Integrilin
Func. class.: Antiplatelet agent
Chem. class.: Glycoprotein IIb/IIIa inhibitor

ACTION: Platelet glycoprotein antagonist; reversibly prevents fibrinogen, von Willebrand factor from binding to the glycoprotein IIb/IIIa receptor, inhibiting platelet aggregation

Therapeutic outcome: Decreased platelets

USES: Acute coronary syndrome, including those undergoing percutaneous coronary intervention (PCI)

Pharmacokinetics

Absorption	Complete
Distribution	Protein binding 25%
Metabolism	Limited
Excretion	Kidneys 50%
Half-life	2.5 hr

Pharmacodynamics

Onset	Within 1 hr

CONTRAINDICATIONS
Hypersensitivity, active internal bleeding, recent history of bleeding, stroke within 30 days or any hemorrhagic stroke, major surgery with severe trauma, severe hypertension, history of intracranial bleeding, current or planned use of another parenteral GPIIb/IIIa inhibitor, dependence on renal dialysis, coagulopathy, AV malformation, aneurysm

Precautions: Pregnancy, breastfeeding, children, geriatric, bleeding, renal function impairment

DOSAGE AND ROUTES
Acute coronary syndrome
Adult: **IV BOL** 180 mcg/kg as soon as diagnosed, then **IV CONT INF** 2 mcg/kg/min × 72 hr or coronary artery bypass graft (CABG) discontinue ≥ 2-4 hr before procedure

PCI in patients without acute coronary syndrome
Adult: **IV BOL** 180 mcg/kg given immediately before PCI; then 2 mcg/kg/min × 18 hr by **CONT IV INF** and a 2nd 180 mcg/kg BOL, 10 min after 1st BOL; continue INF for up to 18-24 hr at a rate of 1 mcg/kg/min (minimum 12 hr)

Renal dose
Adult: IV BOL CCr <50 ml/min 2-4 mg/dl same loading dose, then ½ usual INF dose; CCr <10 ml/min contraindicated

---

Available forms: Sol for inj 2 mg/ml (10 ml), 0.75 mg/ml (100 ml)

ADVERSE EFFECTS
CV: Stroke, hypotension
GU: Hematuria
HEMA: Thrombocytopenia, platelet dysfunction
SYST: Major/minor bleeding from any site, anaphylaxis

INTERACTIONS
Individual drugs
Abciximab, aspirin, clopidogrel, dipyridamole, heparin, ticlopidine, valproate: increased bleeding

Drug classifications
Anticoagulants, NSAIDs, SSRIs, SNRIs, thrombolytics: increased bleeding
Platelet receptor inhibitors IIb, IIIa: do not give together

Drug/herb
Feverfew, garlic, ginger, ginkgo, ginseng

NURSING CONSIDERATIONS
Assessment
• **Thrombocytopenia:** Monitor platelets, Hgb, Hct, creatinine, APTT baseline, INR, within 6 hr of loading dose and daily thereafter; patients undergoing PCI should have ACT monitored; maintain APTT 50-70 sec unless PCI is to be performed; during PCI, ACT should be 200-300 sec; if platelets drop <100,000/mm³, obtain additional platelet counts; if thrombocytopenia is confirmed, discontinue product; also draw Hct, Hgb, serum creatinine
• **Assess for bleeding:** gums, bruising, ecchymosis, petechiae; from GI, GU tract, cardiac catheter sites, IM inj sites
• **Pregnancy/breastfeeding:** Use in pregnancy only if clearly needed, it is not known if product is excreted in breast milk, consider risks and benefits

Patient problem
Ineffective tissue perfusion (uses)
Risk for injury (adverse reactions)

Implementation
• Aspirin may be given with this product; check for bleeding
• Discontinue heparin before removing femoral artery sheath after PCI
• Do not give discolored solutions, those with particulates; discard unused amount, protect from light
• Discontinue product prior to CABG

Direct IV route
• After withdrawing the BOL dose from 20 mg/10mL (2 mg/mL) vial, give **IV** push over 1-2 min
• Do not use discolored sol or sol with particulate
Continuous IV infusion route
• Follow BOL dose with cont inf using infusion pump, give product undiluted directly from the 100-ml vial, spike the 100-ml vial with a vented infusion set; use caution when centering the spike on the circle of the stopper top, refrigerate vials, store vials ≤2 months at room temperature

Y-site compatibilities: Alfentanil, alteplase, amikacin, aminophylline, amphotericin B lipid complex, amphotericin B liposome, ampicillin, ampicillin-sulbactam, anidulafungin, argatroban, atenolol, atracurium, atropine, azithromycin, aztreonam, bivalirudin, bumetanide, buprenorphine, butorphanol, calcium chloride/gluconate, ceFAZolin, cefepime, cefotaxime, cefoTEtan, cefOXitin, cefTAZidime, ceftizoxime, cefTRIAXone, cefuroxime, cimetidine, ciprofloxacin, cisatracurium, clindamycin, cycloSPORINE, DAPTOmycin, dexamethasone, D₅/NaCl 0.9%, diazepam, diltiazem, diphenhydrAMINE, DOBUTamine, dolasetron, DOPamine, doxycycline, droperidol, enalaprilat, ePHEDrine, EPINEPHrine, ertapenem, erythromycin, esmolol, famotidine, fentaNYL, fluconazole, fosphenytoin, ganciclovir, gatifloxacin, gentamicin, granisetron, haloperidol, heparin, hydrocortisone, HYDROmorphone, hydrOXYzine, imipenem-cilastatin, inamrinone, isoproterenol, ketorolac, labetalol, leucovorin, levofloxacin, levorphanol, lidocaine, linezolid, LORazepam, magnesium sulfate, mannitol, meperidine, meropenem, methylPREDNISolone, metoclopramide, metoprolol, metroNIDAZOLE, micafungin, midazolam, milrinone, minocycline, mivacurium, morphine, nalbuphine, naloxone, niCARdipine, nitroglycerin, nitroprusside, NS, octreotide, ofloxacin, ondansetron, oxytocin, palonosetron, pancuronium, PEMEtrexed, PENTobarbital, PHENobarbital, phenylephrine, piperacillin, piperacillin-tazobactam, potassium chloride/phosphates, procainamide, prochlorperazine, promethazine, propranolol, ranitidine, remifentanil, rocuronium, sodium bicarbonate/phosphates, succinylcholine, SUFentanil, sulfamethoxazole-trimethoprim, teniposide, theophylline, ticarcillin, ticarcillin-clavulanate, tigecycline, tirofiban, tobramycin, trimethobenzamide, vancomycin, vecuronium, verapamil, zidovudine, zoledronic acid

Patient/family education
• Teach patient to report bruising, bleeding, chest pain immediately

- Teach patient not to use other Rx, OTC, supplements without prescriber approval
- Inform patient of reason for medication and expected results

Evaluation
Positive therapeutic outcome
- Decreased platelets

eravacycline
(er′a-va-sye′ kleen)
Xerava
Func. class.: Antiinfective-tetracycline
Chem. class.: Synthetic fluorocycline

ACTION: Disrupts bacterial protein synthesis by binding to the 30S ribosomal subunit and preventing the incorporation of amino acid residues into elongating peptide chains. Bacteriostatic against gram-positive bacteria and certain strains of *Escherichia coli* and *Klebsiella pneumoniae*

Therapeutic outcome: Resolution of the signs/symptoms of the infection

USES: Treatment of complicated intraabdominal infections caused by *Bacteroides caccae, Bacteroides fragilis, Bacteroides ovatus, Bacteroides thetaiotaomicron, Bacteroides uniformis, Bacteroides vulgatus, Citrobacter freundii, Citrobacter koseri, Clostridium perfringens, Enterobacter aerogenes, Enterobacter cloacae, Enterococcus faecalis, Enterococcus faecium, Escherichia coli, Klebsiella oxytoca, Klebsiella pneumoniae, Parabacteroides distasonis, Staphylococcus aureus (MRSA), Staphylococcus aureus (MSSA), Streptococcus anginosus, Streptococcus salivarius*

Pharmacokinetics

Absorption	Unknown
Distribution	Unknown
Metabolism	Primarily by CYP3A4- and FMO-mediated oxidation
Excretion	47% feces, 34% urine
Half-life	20 hr

Pharmacodynamics

Onset	Unknown
Peak	Unknown
Duration	Unknown

CONTRAINDICATIONS: Hypersensitivity to this product or tetracyclines

PRECAUTIONS: Breastfeeding, children, colitis, diarrhea, geriatric, GI/hepatic disease, increased intracranial pressure, inflammatory bowel disease/ulcerative colitis, papilledema, pregnancy, pseudomembranous colitis, UV exposure

DOSAGE AND ROUTES
Adult: **IV** 1 mg/kg q12 hr × 4 to 14 days

Available forms: Powder for injection 50 mg

ADVERSE EFFECTS
GI: Nausea, vomiting, diarrhea, pancreatitis, *Clostridium difficile*
SYST: Anaphylaxis, wound dehiscence
RESP: Pleural effusion
HEMA: Thrombosis
EENT: Tooth discoloration
INTEG: Rash
CV: Hypotension

INTERACTIONS
Drug classifications
Anticoagulants: Increased anticoagulation; anticoagulant may need dosage reduction
- Strong CYP3A inducers (clarithromycin, telithromycin, nefazodone, itraconazole, ketoconazole, atazanavir, darunavir, indinavir, lopinavir, nelfinavir, ritonavir, saquinavir, tipranavir); increased eravacycline effect
- Strong CYP3A inducers (carbamazepine, rifampin); decreased eravacycline effect

NURSING CONSIDERATIONS
Assessment
- **Infection:** Assess for fever, condition of wound, pain, vital signs, urine, stools; monitor WBC for increased levels indicating continued infection; obtain C&S before starting treatment, may start product before receiving results
- **Bowel function:** Assess for diarrhea with mucus, blood, which may indicate CDAD-*Clostridium difficile* diarrhea; report to healthcare professional immediately; may occur several weeks after last dose
- **Wound dehiscence:** Assess for fever, inflammation, bleeding, pain, wound opening; report any of these signs immediately
- **Anaphylaxis:** Assess for rash, dyspnea, swelling of lips/tongue; discontinue product; if severe, epinephrine is usually given; if allergic reaction is mild, discontinuing product and giving diphenhydramine may be sufficient
- **Tooth discoloration:** May occur if used in 2nd or 3rd trimester of pregnancy or in children <8 yr

Patient problems
Infection (uses)

Implementation
Intermittent IV infusion route
- Visually inspect for particulate matter and discoloration prior to use; reconstituted solution is clear, pale yellow to orange

Reconstitution
• Reconstitute each vial with 5 ml of sterile water for injection to a concentration of 10 mg/ml; swirl gently until powder has dissolved; avoid shaking or rapid movement
• **Do not give reconstituted solution by direct injection**
Dilution
• Withdraw the full or partial reconstituted content from each vial and add it into a 0.9% sodium chloride injection infusion bag to a concentration of 0.3 mg/ml (within a range of 0.2 to 0.6 mg/ml)
• Do not shake
• **Storage:** The diluted solution must be infused within 6 hr if stored at room temperature, max 25° C or 77° F) or within 24 hr if stored refrigerated at 2 to 8° C (36 to 46° F). Do not freeze.
Intermittent IV Infusion
• Infuse through a dedicated IV line or by Y-site. If the same IV line is used for sequential infusion of several drugs, flush the line before and after infusion with 0.9% sodium chloride injection
• Give over 60 min; assess IV site frequently

Patient/family education
• Advise patient to inform healthcare provider of all OTC, Rx, herbals, and supplements taken and not to change medications without prescriber's approval
• **Pregnancy/breastfeeding:** Teach patient to inform healthcare provider if pregnancy is planned or suspected or if breastfeeding; teach that this product may cause permanent tooth discoloration and reversible inhibition of bone growth when used in the 2nd and 3rd trimester of pregnancy; teach not to breastfeed during and for 4 days after last dose
• **Allergic reactions**: Teach patient to identify allergies; that allergic reactions, including serious ones, could occur; and that serious reactions require immediate treatment. Ask patient about any previous allergies
• **Diarrhea:** Inform patient that diarrhea is common and to report watery and bloody stools (with or without stomach cramps and fever), which may be a serious intestinal infection, even after 2 or more months after last dose
• Advise patient that this product is only used to treat bacterial infections, to take all of the medication even if feeling better, not to skip doses, and to complete the full course of therapy

Evaluation
Resolution of the signs/symptoms of the infection

erenumab
(e-ren' ue-mab)
Almovig
Func. class.: CNS analgesic; anti-migraine agent
Chem. class.: IgG2 monoclonal antibody

ACTION: A human immunoglobulin G2 (IgG2) monoclonal antibody that binds to the calcitonin gene-related peptide receptor (CGRP). CGRP is involved in migraine pathophysiology. CGRP modulates pain in the brainstem; CGRP concentrations are elevated during acute migraine attacks and may be chronically elevated in those with chronic migraines

Therapeutic outcome: Decreased in severity and amount of migraines

USES: For the preventive treatment of migraine in adults

Pharmacokinetics

Absorption	82%
Distribution	Unknown
Metabolism	Unknown
Excretion	Unknown
Half-life	28 days

Pharmacodynamics

Onset	Unknown
Peak	6 days
Duration	Unknown

CONTRAINDICATIONS: Hypersensitivity

PRECAUTIONS: Breastfeeding, latex hypersensitivity, pregnancy

DOSAGE AND ROUTES
Adults: SUBCUT 70 mg monthly; may use 140 mg monthly if needed

Available forms: SureClick 70mg/ml Autoinjector Solution for Injection; solution for injection single-use 70 mg/ml

ADVERSE EFFECTS
MISC: Antibody formation, injection site reaction, erythema

INTERACTIONS
None known

NURSING CONSIDERATIONS
Assessment
• Migraines: Assess time of day, aggravating and ameliorating effects, auras or halos, sensitivity to light, noise, diet

- Pregnancy/breastfeeding: Data is lacking. No adverse effects on offspring were observed when animals were given the product throughout pregnancy. Consider the developmental and health benefits of breastfeeding along with the mother's clinical need for the product and any potential adverse effects on the breastfed infant

Patient problem
Pain (uses)

Implementation
Subcut Route
- Visually inspect for particulate matter and discoloration prior to use; do not use if solution is cloudy or discolored or contains flakes or particles; product should be clear to opalescent, colorless to light-yellow solution
- Product is intended for patient self-administration. Provide proper training to patients and/ or caregivers on how to prepare and administer, including aseptic technique
- Prior to use allow to come to room temperature for at least 30 min, protected from direct sunlight. Do not warm using a heat source, such as hot water or microwave
- Do not shake.
- Clean injection site on the abdomen, thigh, or upper arm with an alcohol wipe, and allow skin to dry
- Do not leave cap off the autoinjector or prefilled syringe for more than 5 min; product will dry out
- Do not inject into skin that is tender, bruised, red, or hard. Avoid injecting directly into raised, thick, red, or scaly skin patch or lesion, or areas with scars or stretch marks
- If using the same body area for the two separate injections needed for the 140 mg dose, ensure the second injection is not at same location
- Discard the autoinjector or prefilled syringe in sharps disposal container. Do not discard in household trash
- *Storage:* After removing from the refrigerator, it can be stored at room temperature between 20 to 25° C (68 to 77° F) for up to 7 days. Do not return to the refrigerator after it has reached room temperature

Single-dose, Prefilled Sureclick Autoinjector
- Pull white cap straight off
- Stretch or pinch skin to create a firm injection site
- Firmly push the autoinjector down onto the skin
- When ready to inject, press the purple start button; a click will be heard. The injection could take about 15 seconds. When the injection is complete, a click may be heard or felt, and the window will turn yellow
- Remove the autoinjector

Single-dose, Prefilled Syringe
- Always hold syringe by the barrel
- Pull gray needle cap straight out
- Pinch injection site skin firmly between thumb and fingers
- Hold the pinch, and insert the syringe into skin at 45 to 90 degrees
- Push the plunger rod all the way down with thumb until the prefilled syringe stops moving
- When done, release thumb and gently lift syringe off the skin

Patient/family education
- Have the patient read the FDA-approved patient labeling (Patient Information and Instructions for Use)
- Advise patient on proper SUBCUT administration technique, including aseptic technique, and how to use the single-dose prefilled autoinjector or single-dose prefilled syringe
- Advise patient to read and follow the "Instructions for Use" each time of use
- Teach patient those prescribed 140 mg to administer the once monthly dosage as two separate SUBCUT injections of 70 mg each
- Teach latex-sensitive patients that the needle shield within the white cap of the autoinjector and gray needle cap of the prefilled syringe contain dry natural rubber (a derivative of latex) that may cause allergic reactions

Evaluation
- Decreased in severity and amount of migraines

ergocalciferol
See vitamin D

⚠ HIGH ALERT
erlotinib (Rx)
(er-loe'tye-nib)
Tarceva
Func. class.: Misc. antineoplastic
Chem. class.: Epidermal growth factor receptor inhibitor

ACTION: Not fully understood. Inhibits intracellular phosphorylation of cell surface receptors associated with epidermal growth factor receptors.

Therapeutic outcome: Decrease in tumor size

USES: Non–small cell lung cancer (NSCLC), maintenance, after failure of at least one chemotherapy regimen including EGFR exon 19 deletions or exon 21 substitution mutations, pancreatic cancer

Pharmacokinetics

Absorption	Slowly absorbed
Distribution	Unknown
Metabolism	Metabolized by CYP3A4 ↞⌀⌀, inhibits tyrosine kinase, which is a factor in epidermal growth factor receptor (EGFR)
Excretion	Feces (86%), urine (<4%)
Half-life	36 hr

Pharmacodynamics

Onset	Unknown
Peak	3-7 hr
Duration	Up to 24 hr

CONTRAINDICATIONS
Pregnancy, breastfeeding

Precautions: Renal, hepatic; ocular, pulmonary disorders; children; geriatric, diverticulitis

DOSAGE AND ROUTES
Non–small cell lung cancer (NSCLC)
Adult: PO 150 mg/day
Pancreatic cancer
Adult: PO 100 mg/day in combination with gemcitabine 1000 mg/m² cycle 1, days 1, 8, 15, 22, 29, 36, 43 of an 8-wk cycle; cycle 2 and subsequent cycles, days 1, 8, 15 of a 4-wk cycle, used with gemcitabine

CYP3A4 inducers concurrently (such as rifampin or phenytoin)
Increase dose by 50 mg q 2 wk (max 450 mg/day)

CYP3A4 inhibitors (atazanavir, clarithromycin, indinavir, itraconazole, ketoconazole, telithromycin, ritonavir, saquinavir, troleandomycin, nelfinavir) or CYP3A4 and CYP1A2 inhibitors concurrently (capofloxacin)
Decrease dose by 50 mg as needed

Available forms: Tabs 25, 100, 150 mg

ADVERSE EFFECTS
CNS: CVA, anxiety, depression, headache, rigors, insomnia
CV: MI/ischemia
EENT: Ocular changes, *conjunctivitis, eye pain,* hypertrichosis
GI: *Nausea, diarrhea, vomiting, anorexia, mouth ulceration,* hepatic failure, GI perforation
GU: Renal impairment/failure
HEMA: DVT, bleeding
INTEG: *Rash,* Stevens-Johnson–like skin reactions, toxic epidermal necrolysis
MISC: *Fatigue, infection*

RESP: Interstitial lung disease, *cough, dyspnea*
SYST: Hepatorenal syndrome

INTERACTIONS
Individual drugs
Metoprolol, warfarin: increased plasma concentrations
Smoking: decreased erlotinib level, dose may need to be increased

Drug classifications
CYP3A4 inducers (phenytoin, rifampin, carBAMazepine, phenobarbital), proton-pump inhibitors: decreased erlotinib levels
CYP3A4 inhibitors (clarithromycin, erythromycin, itraconazole, ketoconazole, telithromycin): increased erlotinib concentrations
HMG-CoA reductase inhibitors: increased myopathy
NSAIDs: GI bleeding may be fatal

Drug/herb
St. John's wort: decreased erlotinib levels

Drug/food
Grapefruit juice: increased effect of erlotinib

Drug/labs
Increase: INR, PT, AST, ALT, bilirubin

NURSING CONSIDERATIONS
Assessment
• **Serious skin toxicities:** toxic epidermal necrolysis, Stevens-Johnson syndrome, check for rash, blistering, discontinue treatment, may need corticosteroid, antiinfectives
• Assess for MI/ischemia, CVA in pancreatic cancer
• **Assess for pulmonary changes:** lung sounds, cough, dyspnea; interstitial lung disease may occur, may be fatal; discontinue therapy if confirmed
• **Assess for ocular changes:** eye irritation, corneal erosion/ulcer, aberrant eyelash growth discontinue if ulcers are present in the cornea, hold for keratitis grade 3 or 4
• Assess for GI symptoms: frequency of stools; if diarrhea is poorly tolerated, therapy may be discontinued for up to 14 days; monitor for dehydration, fluid status during period of vomiting and diarrhea, may use antidiarrheal
• Monitor blood studies: INR, LFTs, PT
• **Hepatic failure:** interrupt dosing if severe changes to liver function occur (total bilirubin >3× ULN and/or transaminases >5× ULN for normal pretreatment LFTs)
• **GI perforation/bleeding:** some cases have been fatal, usually occurs in those using NSAIDs, taxanes, or those with diverticulitis or peptic ulcer disease, discontinue if these occur

---

A Nurse Alert   ✳ Key NCLEX® Drug   >> Drug Specifics

- **Pregnancy/breastfeeding:** Patient should not become pregnant during treatment or for 1 mo after last dose, do not breastfeed during or for 2 wk after final dose

Patient problem
Impaired breathing (adverse reactions)
Risk for injury (adverse reactions)

Implementation
- Administer 1 hr before or 2 hr after food

Patient/family education
- **Teach patient to report adverse reactions immediately:** SOB, severe abdominal pain, persistent diarrhea or vomiting, ocular changes, skin eruptions (face, upper chest, back pain)
- Explain reason for treatment, expected results, to take on empty stomach 1 hr before or 2 hr after meals
- **Pregnancy/breastfeeding:** Advise patient to use contraception during treatment; pregnancy, avoid breastfeeding
- Advise patient to use sunscreen, protective clothing to prevent sunburn
- Instruct patient to avoid use with other products, herbs, or supplements unless approved by provider, not to use with grapefruit or grapefruit juice
- Instruct patient to avoid smoking; decreases effect of this product

Evaluation
Positive therapeutic outcome
- Decrease non–small cell lung or pancreatic cancer cells

ertapenem (Rx)
(er-tah-pen′em)
INVanz
Func. class.: Antiinfective, miscellaneous
Chem. class.: Carbapenem

Do not confuse: INVanz/Aninza

ACTION: Interferes with cell wall replication of susceptible organisms

Therapeutic outcome: Bactericidal action against susceptible bacteria

USES: Bacteremia, *Bacteroides distasonis, Bacteroides fragilis, Bacteroides ovatus, Bacteroides thetaiotaomicron, Bacteroides uniformis, Bacteroides vulgatus, Citrobacter freundii, Citrobacter koseri, Clostridium clostridioforme, Clostridium perfringens,* community-acquired pneumonia, diabetic foot ulcer, endomyometritis, *Enterobacter aerogenes, Enterobacter cloacae, Escherichia coli, Eubacterium lentum,* *Fusobacterium, Haemophilus influenzae* (beta-lactamase negative), *Haemophilus influenzae* (beta-lactamase positive), *Haemophilus parainfluenzae,* intraabdominal infections, *Klebsiella oxytoca, Klebsiella pneumoniae, Moraxella catarrhalis, Morganella morganii, Peptostreptococcus, Porphyromonas asaccharolytica, Prevotella bivia, Proteus mirabilis, Proteus vulgaris, Providencia rettgeri, Providencia stuartii, Serratia marcescens,* skin infections, *Staphylococcus aureus* (MSSA), *Staphylococcus epidermidis, Streptococcus agalactiae* (group B streptococci), *Streptococcus pneumoniae, Streptococcus pyogenes* (group A beta-hemolytic streptococci), surgical infection prophylaxis, urinary tract infections

Pharmacokinetics
Absorption	Almost completely absorbed (IM); completely absorbed (**IV**)
Distribution	85%-95% plasma protein bound
Metabolism	Liver (IM, **IV**)
Excretion	Urine (80%), feces (10%), breast milk (IM, **IV**)
Half-life	4 hr (**IV**)

Pharmacodynamics
	IM	IV
Onset	Rapid	Immediate
Peak	2.3 hr	Dose-dependent
Duration	Unknown	Up to 24 hr

CONTRAINDICATIONS
Hypersensitivity to this product or its components, to amide-type local anesthetics (IM only); anaphylactic reactions to β-lactams, other carbapenems

Precautions: Pregnancy, breastfeeding, children, geriatric, renal/hepatic/GI disease, seizures

DOSAGE AND ROUTES
Adult/child ≥13 yr: IM/IV 1 g q day × 14 days (IV), 7 days(IM)
Child 3 mo-12 yr: IM/IV 15 mg/kg q 12 h (max 1g/day) × up to 14 days (IV) or 7 days (IM)

Renal dose
Adult: IM/IV CCr ≤30 ml/min, 500 mg/day

Available forms: Powder, lyophilized, 1 g/vial

ADVERSE EFFECTS
CNS: Insomnia, seizures, dizziness, *headache,* confusion
CV: Tachycardia, seizures

GI: *Diarrhea, nausea, vomiting, Clostridium difficile*–associated diarrhea, abdominal pain
GU: *Vaginitis*
INTEG: *Rash,* pain at inj site, *phlebitis/ thrombophlebitis*, erythema at inj site
SYST: Anaphylaxis, angioedema

INTERACTIONS
Individual drugs
Probenecid: increased ertapenem plasma levels; do not coadminister
Valproic acid: decreased effect of valproic acid, monitor valproic levels, seizure control
Warfarin: Increase: INR

Drug/lab test
Increased: hepatic enzymes, albumin, alkaline phosphatase, bilirubin, creatinine, PT
Decrease: Hct, WBC

NURSING CONSIDERATIONS
Assessment
• Assess for renal disease: lower dose may be required
• **CDAD:** Assess bowel pattern daily: if severe diarrhea, abdominal pain, mucus or blood in stools occurs, product should be discontinued
• **Assess for infection:** temp, sputum, characteristics of wound, monitor WBC before, during, after treatment
• **Pregnancy/breastfeeding:** Use only when clearly needed, use caution in breastfeeding
• **Assess for allergic reactions, anaphylaxis:** rash, urticaria, pruritus may occur a few days after therapy begins; assess for sensitivity to carbapenem antibiotics, other β-lactam antibiotics, penicillins, have emergency equipment, epinephrine close by
• **Assess for overgrowth of infection:** perineal itching, fever, malaise, redness, pain, swelling, drainage, rash, diarrhea, change in cough or sputum

Patient problem
Infection (uses)

Implementation
IV route
• Visually inspect for particulate matter and discoloration before use: may be colorless to pale yellow; do not mix with other products; dextrose solutions are not compatible
• 1 g vial: For each gram reconstitute with 10 ml of either NS injection, sterile water for injection, or bacteriostatic water for injection to 100 mg/ml, shake

• 1 g dose: immediately transfer contents of the reconstituted vial to 50 ml of NS injection; for a dose <1 g (pediatric patients 3 mo to 12 yr): from the reconstituted vial, immediately withdraw a volume equal to 15 mg/kg of body weight (max 1 g/day) and dilute in NS injection to a concentration of 20 mg/ml or less
Intermittent IV infusion route
• Complete the infusion within 6 hr of reconstitution, infuse over 30 min; do not co-infuse with other medications
• The reconstituted IV solution may be stored at room temperature if used within 6 hr, or stored under refrigeration for 24 hr and used within 4 hr after removal from refrigeration; do not freeze

IM route
• Reconstitute 1 g vial of ertapenem with 3.2 ml of 1% lidocaine HCl injection (without EPINEPHrine) (280 mg/ml), agitate; the IM reconstituted formulation is not for IV use
• IM may be used as an alternative to IV administration in the treatment of infections where IM therapy is appropriate; only given via IM injection × 7 days
• For a 1 g dose: immediately withdraw the contents of the vial and inject deeply into a large muscle, aspirate prior to injection to avoid injection into a blood vessel
• For a dose <1 g for pediatric patients 3 mo to 12 yr): immediately withdraw a volume equal to 15 mg/kg (max 1 g/day) and inject deeply into a large muscle, aspirate prior to injection to avoid injection into a blood vessel; use the reconstituted IM solution within 1 hr after preparation

Y-site compatibilities: Acyclovir, alfentanil, amifostine, amikacin, aminocaproic acid, aminophylline, amphotericin B lipid complex, amphotericin B liposome, argatroban, arsenic trioxide, atenolol, atracurium, azithromycin, aztreonam, bivalirudin, bleomycin, bumetanide, buprenorphine, busulfan, butorphanol, calcium chloride/gluconate, CARBOplatin, carmustine, chloramphenicol, cimetidine, ciprofloxacin, cisatracurium, CISplatin, cyclophosphamide, cycloSPORINE, cytarabine, dacarbazine, DACTINomycin, DAPTOmycin, dexamethasone, dexmedetomidine, dexrazoxane, digoxin, diltiazem, diphenhydrAMINE, DOCEtaxel, dolasetron, DOPamine, doxacurium, doxycycline, enalaprilat, ePHEDrine, EPINEPHrine, eptifibatide, erythromycin, esmolol, etoposide, etoposide phosphate, famotidine, fenoldopam, fluconazole, fludarabine, fluorouracil, foscarnet, fosphenytoin, furosemide, ganciclovir, gatifloxacin, gemcitabine, gemtuzumab, gentamicin, glycopyrrolate, granisetron, haloperidol, heparin, hydrocortisone, HYDROmorphone, ifosfamide, inamrinone, insulin (regular), irinotecan, isoproterenol, ketorolac, labetalol, lepirudin, leucovorin, levofloxacin, lidocaine, linezolid, LORazepam, magnesium sulfate, mannitol, mechlorethamine, melphalan, meperidine, mesna, metaraminol, methotrexate, methyldopate, methylPREDNISolone, metoclopramide, metroNIDAZOLE, milrinone, mitoMYcin, mivacurium, morphine, moxifloxacin, nalbuphine, naloxone, nesiritide, nitroglycerin, nitroprusside, norepinephrine, octreotide, oxaliplatin, oxytocin, PAClitaxel, pamidronate, pancuronium, pantoprazole, PEMEtrexed, PENTobarbital, PHENobarbital, phentolamine, phenylephrine, polymixin B, potassium acetate/chloride/phosphates, procainamide, propranolol, ranitidine, remifentanil, rocuronium, sodium acetate/bicarbonate/phosphates, streptozocin, succinylcholine, SUFentanil, sulfamethoxazole-trimethoprim, tacrolimus, telavancin, teniposide, theophylline, thiotepa, tigecycline, tirofiban, tobramycin, trimethobenzamide, vancomycin, vasopressin, vecuronium, vinBLAStine, vinCRIStine, vinorelbine, voriconazole, zidovudine, zoledronic acid

Patient/family education

- Advise patient to report severe diarrhea; may indicate CDAD
- **Advise patient to report overgrowth of infection:** black, furry tongue, vaginal itching, foul-smelling stools
- Pregnancy/breastfeeding: Identify if pregnancy is planned or suspected or if breastfeeding

Evaluation

Positive therapeutic outcome

- Negative C&S, absence of signs and symptoms of infection

TREATMENT OF OVERDOSE:

Administer EPINEPHrine, antihistamines; resuscitate if needed (anaphylaxis)

RARELY USED

ertugliflozin

(er-too-gli-floe'-zin)

Steglatro

Func. class.: Antidiabetic

USES: For the treatment of type 2 diabetes mellitus

DOSAGE AND ROUTES

For the treatment of type 2 diabetes mellitus in combination with diet and exercise

Adult: PO 5 mg qday, in the morning, with or without food, max: 15 mg qday

---

ERYTHROMYCIN

erythromycin base (Rx)

(eh-rith-roh-my'sin)

Erybid ✦, Eryc, Ery-Tab, PCE

erythromycin ethylsuccinate (Rx)

EES, Ery Pod

erythromycin lactobionate (Rx)

Erythrocin

erythromycin stearate (Rx)

Erythrocin Stearate, Erythro-S ✦

erythromycin (topical)

Akne-Mycin, Erygel

Func. class.: Antiinfective

Chem. class.: Macrolide

Do not confuse: erythromycin/ azithromycin

ACTION: Binds to 50S ribosomal subunits of susceptible bacteria and suppresses protein synthesis

Therapeutic outcome: Bactericidal action against the following organisms: *Neisseria gonorrhoeae, Streptococcus pneumoniae, Mycoplasma pneumoniae, Corynebacterium diphtheriae, Bordetella pertussis, Borrelia burgdorferi, Listeria monocytogenes, Treponema pallidum;* streptococci, staphylococci; gram-negative pathogens: *Neisseria, Haemophilus influenzae* (when used with sulfonamides), *Legionella pneumophila, Chlamydia trachomatis*

USES: Mild to moderate respiratory tract, skin, soft tissue infections, Legionnaire's disease, syphilis

Pharmacokinetics

Absorption	Well absorbed (PO)
Distribution	Widely distributed; minimally distributed (CSF); crosses placenta
Metabolism	Liver, partially
Excretion	Bile, unchanged; kidneys (minimal), unchanged
Half-life	1-3 hr, neonates 2 hr

Pharmacodynamics

	PO	IV
Onset	1 hr	Rapid
Peak	1-4 hr	Infusion's end
Duration	6-12 hr	6-12 hr

CONTRAINDICATIONS
Hypersensitivity, preexisting liver disease (estolate)

Precautions: Pregnancy, breastfeeding, geriatric, hepatic/GI disease, QT prolongation, seizure disorder, myasthenia gravis

DOSAGE AND ROUTES
Acne
Adult/child >12 yr: Topical applied bid 2%

Most infections
Adults PO (base, stearate): 250 mg q 6 h or 333 mg q 8 h or 500 mg q 12 hr; (ethylsuccinate) 400 mg q 6 h or 800 mg q 12 h; IV 250-500 mg

Child >1mo PO (base, ethylsuccinate): 30-50 mg/kg/day divided q 6-8 hr, max 2 g/day (base), max 3.2 g/day (ethyl succinate); (stearate) 30-50 mg/kg/day divided q 6 h (max 2 g/day)

Neonates: PO (ethylsuccinate) 20-50 mg/kg/day divided q 6-8 hr

Available forms: Base: enteric-coated tab 250, 333, 500 mg; film-coated tab 250, 500 mg; enteric-coated caps, 250, 333 mg; stearate: film-coated tabs, 250 mg, granules for oral susp: 200, 400 mg/5 ml powder for inj 500 mg, 1 g (lactobionate); 1 g (as glucceptate)

ADVERSE EFFECTS
CNS: Seizures, rare
CV: Dysrhythmias, QT prolongation
GI: *Nausea, vomiting, diarrhea,* abdominal pain, stomatitis, heartburn, anorexia, pruritus ani, *Clostridium difficile*–associated diarrhea (CDAD), esophagitis, hepatotoxicity
GU: *Vaginitis, moniliasis*
INTEG: Rash, urticaria, pruritus, thrombophlebitis, injection-site reactions (**IV** site)
SYST: Anaphylaxis

INTERACTIONS
Individual drugs
Alfentanil, ALPRAZolam, bromocriptine, busPIRone, carBAMazepine, cilostazol, clindamycin, cloZAPine, cycloSPORINE, diazepam, digoxin, disopyramide, felodipine, ibrutinib, methylPREDNISolone, midazolam, quiNIDine, rifabutin, sildenafil, tacrolimus, tadalafil, theophylline, triazolam, vardenafil, vinBLAStine, warfarin: increased toxicity, increased action
Diltiazem, itraconazole, ketoconazole, nefazodone, pimozide, verapamil: increased serious dysrhythmias, do not use together

Drug classifications
Ergots: increased action, toxicity
HMG-CoA reductase inhibitors: increased action, toxicity

Products that increase QT prolongation: increased QT
Protease inhibitors: serious dysrhythmias
  rifamycins (rifabutin, rifAMPin, rifapentine)
  Decrease: erythromycin effect

Drug/food
Grapefruit juice, avoid using together
Decrease: Erythromycin metabolism

Drug/lab test
Increased: AST/ALT
Decreased: folate assay
False increase: 17-OHCS/17-KS

NURSING CONSIDERATIONS
Assessment
- Assess patient for previous sensitivity reaction
- **Assess patient for signs and symptoms of infection** including characteristics of wounds, sputum, urine, stool, WBC >10,000/mm^3, earache, fever; obtain baseline information before, during treatment
- Obtain C&S test results before beginning product therapy to identify if correct treatment has been initiated
- Assess for allergic reactions: rash, urticaria may occur a few days after therapy begins
- Monitor blood studies: AST, ALT, CBC, Hct, bilirubin, LDH, alkaline phosphatase, Coombs' test monthly if patient is on long-term therapy
- **Assess for overgrowth of infection:** perineal itching, fever, malaise, redness, pain, swelling, drainage, rash, diarrhea, change in cough, sputum
- **CDAD:** assess for diarrhea with blood, mucus, abdominal pain, fever, product should be discontinued immediately
- **Anaphylaxis:** assess for generalized hives, itching, flushing, swelling of lips/tongue/throat, wheezing; have emergency equipment nearby
- **QT prolongation:** may occur (IV >15 mg/min), those with electrolyte imbalances, congenital QT prolongation, and the elderly are at greater risk; correct electrolyte imbalances prior to treatment; monitor ECG

Patient problem
Infection (uses)

Implementation
- Store at room temp; store susp in refrigerator
- Adequate intake of fluids (2 L) during diarrhea episodes
PO route
- Give around the clock on an empty stomach, at least 1 hr before or 2 hr after meals; may be taken with food if GI upset occurs; do not take

---

with juices; take dose with a full glass of water: use calibrated measuring device for drops or susp; shake well
• Store susp in refrigerator
• Do not crush or chew enteric-coated tab

IV route
• Add 10 ml of sterile water for inj without preservatives to 250- or 500-mg vials and 20 ml to 1-g vial; sol is stable for 1 wk after reconstitution if refrigerated

Intermittent IV infusion route
• Dilute further in 100-250 ml of 0.9% NaCl or D₅W
• Give over 20-60 min to avoid phlebitis; assess for pain along vein; slow inf if pain occurs; apply ice to site and notify prescriber if unable to relieve pain

Continuous infusion route
• May also be administered as an inf in a dilution of 1 g/L of 0.9% NaCl, D₅W, over 4 hr

Erythromycin lactobionate

Y-site compatibilities: Acyclovir, alfentanil, amikacin, aminocaproic acid, aminophylline, amiodarone, anidulafungin, argatroban, atenolol, atosiban, atracurium, atropine, azaTHIOprine, benztropine, bivalirudin, bleomycin, bumetanide, buprenorphine, butorphanol, calcium chloride/gluconate, CARBOplatin, caspofungin, cefotaxime, cefTAZidime, cefTRIAXone, cefuroxime, chlorproMAZINE, cimetidine, CISplatin, cyanocobalamin, cyclophosphamide, cycloSPORINE, cytarabine, DACTINomycin, DAPTOmycin, dexmedetomidine, digoxin, diltiazem, diphenhydrAMINE, DOBUTamine, DOCEtaxel, DOPamine, doxacurium, doxapram, DOXOrubicin, enalaprilat, ePHEDrine, EPINEPHrine, epirubicin, epoetin, eptifibatide, ertapenem, esmolol, etoposide, famotidine, fenoldopam, fentaNYL, fluconazole, fludarabine, fluorouracil, folic acid, foscarnet, gatifloxacin, gemcitabine, gentamicin, glycopyrrolate, granisetron, hydrocortisone, HYDROMorphone, hydrOXYzine, IDArubicin, ifosfamide, imipenem-cilastatin, insulin (regular), irinotecan, isoproterenol, labetalol, levofloxacin, lidocaine, LORazepam, LR, mannitol, mechlorethamine, meperidine, methicillin, methotrexate, methoxamine, methyldopate, methylPREDNISolone, metoclopramide, metroNIDAZOLE, miconazole, midazolam, milrinone, mitoXANtrone, morphine, multiple vitamins injection, mycophenolate nafcillin, nalbuphine, naloxone, nesiritide, netilmicin, niCARdipine, nitroglycerin, norepinephrine, octreotide, ondansetron, oxacillin, oxaliplatin, oxytocin, PACLitaxel, palonosetron, pamidronate, pancuronium, papaverine, pentamidine, pentazocine, perphenazine, phenylephrine, phytonadione, piperacillin, piperacillin-tazobactam, polymyxin B, procainamide, prochlorperazine, promethazine, propranolol, protamine, pyridoxine, quiNIDine, ranitidine, Ringer's, ritodrine, sodium acetate/bicarbonate, succinylcholine, SUFentanil, tacrolimus, temocillin, teniposide, theophylline, thiamine, thiotepa, tigecycline, tirofiban, TNA, tobramycin, tolazoline, TPN, trimetaphan, urokinase, vancomycin, vasopressin, vecuronium, verapamil, vinCRIStine, vinorelbine, vitamin B complex/C, voriconazole, zidovudine, zoledronic acid

Patient/family education
• Advise patient to contact prescriber if vaginal itching, loose foul-smelling stools, furry tongue occur; may indicate superinfection
• Instruct patient to take all medication prescribed for the length of time ordered
• Teach patient to avoid use with other products unless approved by prescriber

Evaluation
Positive therapeutic outcome
• Absence of signs/symptoms of infection (WBC <10,000/mm³, temp WNL, absence of red, draining wounds, earache)
• Reported improvement in symptoms of infection

TREATMENT OF OVERDOSE: Withdraw product, maintain airway, administer EPINEPHrine, aminophylline, O₂, **IV** corticosteroids

erythromycin ophthalmic
See Appendix B

erythromycin topical
See Appendix B

escitalopram (Rx)
(es-sit-tal′oh-pram)
Cipralex ✦, **Cipralex Meltz** ✦, **Lexapro**
Func. class.: Antidepressant
Chem. class.: (SSRI) Selective serotonin reuptake inhibitor

Do not confuse Lexapro/Loxitane

ACTION: Inhibits CNS neuron uptake of serotonin but not of norepinephrine

Therapeutic outcome: Decreased symptoms of depression

USES: General anxiety disorder; major depressive disorder in adults/adolescents

Unlabeled uses: Panic disorder, social phobia, hot flashes related to menopause

Pharmacokinetics

Absorption	80%
Distribution	Unknown
Metabolism	Liver (CYP3A4, CYP2C19)
Excretion	Urine
Half-life	Unknown

Pharmacodynamics

Unknown

CONTRAINDICATIONS

Hypersensitivity to this product or citalopram, MAOIs

Precautions: Pregnancy, breastfeeding, geriatric, renal/hepatic disease, history of seizures, abrupt discontinuation, bleeding, anticoagulants

> **BLACK BOX WARNING:** Children ≤12 yr/ adolescents, suicidal ideation

DOSAGE AND ROUTES

Adult/adolescent: PO 10 mg/day may increase to 20 mg/day

Hepatic dose
Adult Child ≥12 yr: PO 10 mg q day

Available forms: Tabs 5, 10, 20 mg; oral sol 5 mg (as base)/5 ml (contains sorbitol)

ADVERSE EFFECTS

CNS: *Insomnia,* suicidal ideation, *drowsiness, anxiety, tremor, dizziness, fatigue, sedation, abnormal dreams,* neuroleptic malignant syndrome–like reactions
CV: Postural hypotension
GI: *Nausea, diarrhea, dry mouth, anorexia,* abdominal pain, *constipation, taste changes,* hepatitis
GU: *Decreased libido,* impotence, ejaculation disorder
INTEG: *Sweating, rash, pruritus*
SYST: Serotonin syndrome, Stevens-Johnson synrome

INTERACTIONS
Individual drugs

Alcohol: increased CNS depression
Amantadine, bromocriptine, busPIRone, cyclobenzaprine, lithium, linezolid, methylene blue, traMADol, tryptophan: increased serotonin syndrome
BusPIRone: increased symptoms of OCD
CarBAMazepine, lithium, phenytoin, warfarin: increased levels or toxicity of each specific product
Diazepam: increased half-life of diazepam
Haloperidol: increased effect of haloperidol

Drug classifications

Antidepressants, opioids, sedatives: increased CNS depression
Antidysrhythmics, antipsychotics: increased levels, toxicity
Highly protein-bound products: increased side effects of escitalopram
MAOIs: do not use with or 14 days before escitalopram
NSAIDs, salicylates, anticoagulants, SSRIs, platelet inhibitors: increased bleeding risk
Phenothiazines: increased levels of phenothiazines
SSRIs, SNRIs, serotonin-receptor agonists, amphetamines: increased serotonin syndrome
Tricyclics: increased levels of tricyclics

Drug/herb
Kava: increased CNS effect
SAMe, St. John's wort: do not use together, serotonin syndrome may occur

Drug/food
Grapefruit juice: increased escitalopram effect

Drug/lab test
Increased: serum bilirubin, blood glucose, alkaline phosphatase
Decreased: VMA, 5-HIAA
False increase: urinary catecholamines

NURSING CONSIDERATIONS
Assessment

> **BLACK BOX WARNING:** Assess mental status: mood, sensorium, affect, **suicidal tendencies,** increase in psychiatric symptoms, depression, panic, not approved for use in children <12 yr, provide a limited amount of product, continuing follow ups should be q wk × 4 wk, q 3 wk for next 4 wk

• Assess appetite in bulimia nervosa, weight daily, increase nutritious foods in diet, watch for bingeing and vomiting
• **Assess allergic reactions:** itching, rash, urticaria; product should be discontinued; may need to give antihistamine
• Monitor B/P (lying/standing), pulse; if systolic B/P drops 20 mm Hg, hold product, notify prescriber; take VS more often in patients with cardiovascular disease
• **Serotonin syndrome:** Assess for nausea, vomiting, sedation, dizziness, sweating, facial flushing, mental changes, shivering, increased B/P: discontinue, notify prescriber
• Monitor liver function tests: AST, ALT, bilirubin, creatinine; thyroid function studies

- Monitor weight qwk; appetite may decrease with product
- Monitor ECG for flattening of T wave, bundle branch, AV block, dysrhythmias in cardiac patients
- Monitor alcohol consumption; if alcohol is consumed, hold dose until AM

Patient problem

Depression (uses)
Impaired sexual functioning (adverse reactions)

Implementation
- Give with food or milk for GI symptoms; give with full glass of water, one a day in the AM
- Give crushed if patient is unable to swallow medication whole, scored tabs can be cut
- Give dose at bedtime if oversedation occurs during the day
- Give gum, hard candy, frequent sips of water for dry mouth
- **Oral sol:** measure with calibrated device
- Store at room temperature; do not freeze

Patient/family education
- Teach patient that therapeutic effect may take 1-4 wk, may have increased anxiety for first 5-7 days, do not abruptly discontinue
- **Serotonin syndrome:** To report immediately nausea, vomiting, sedation, dizziness, sweating, facial flushing, mental changes, shivering
- Advise patient to use caution in driving, other activities requiring alertness because of drowsiness, dizziness, blurred vision
- Advise patient to use sunscreen to prevent photosensitivity
- Advise patient to avoid alcohol ingestion, other CNS depressants
- Advise patient to change positions slowly; orthostatic hypotension may occur
- Teach patient to avoid all OTC, herbals, supplements products unless approved by prescriber, to take without regard to meals

BLACK BOX WARNING: Teach patient that clinical worsening and suicide risk may occur, especially in adolescents and young adults, worsening of depression, increased depression, thoughts of dying

- Teach patient using MedGuide provided
- Teach patient about drug interactions
- **Pregnancy/breastfeeding:** Identify if pregnancy is planned or suspected or if breastfeeding

Evaluation
Positive therapeutic outcome
- Decreased depression

△ HIGH ALERT

esmolol (Rx)
(ez'moe-lole)
Brevibloc
Func. class.: β-Adrenergic blocker
(antidysrhythmic II)

Do not confuse. Brevibloc/Brevital

ACTION: Competitively blocks stimulation of β_1-adrenergic receptors in the myocardium; produces negative chronotropic, inotropic activity (decreases rate of SA node discharge, increases recovery time), slows conduction of AV node, decreases heart rate, decreases O_2 consumption in myocardium; also decreases renin-aldosterone-angiotensin system at high doses; inhibits β_2-receptors in bronchial system at higher doses

Therapeutic outcome: Decreased supraventricular tachycardia

USES: Supraventricular tachycardias, noncompensatory sinus tachycardia, hypertensive crisis, intraoperative and postoperative tachycardia and hypertension, atrial fibrillation/flutter

Pharmacokinetics

Absorption	Complete
Distribution	Widely
Metabolism	Liver
Excretion	Kidneys
Half-life	9 min

Pharmacodynamics

Onset	Rapid
Peak	Unknown
Duration	1-15 min

CONTRAINDICATIONS
Heart block (2nd- or 3rd-degree), cardiogenic shock, HF, cardiac failure, hypersensitivity, severe bradycardia

Precautions: Pregnancy, breastfeeding, geriatric patients, hypotension, peripheral vascular disease, diabetes, hypoglycemia, thyrotoxicosis, renal disease, atrial fibrillation, bronchospasms, hyperthyroidism, myasthenia gravis, asthma, COPD, CV disease, pheochromocytoma, abrupt discontinuation

DOSAGE AND ROUTES
Atrial fibrillation/flutter
Adult: **IV** Loading dose 500 mcg/kg/min over 1 min; maintenance 50 mcg/kg/min for 4 min; if no response in 5 min, give 2nd loading dose; then increase INF to 100 mcg/kg/min for 4 min;

if no response, repeat loading dose, then increase maintenance INF by 50 mcg/kg/min (max of 200 mcg/kg/min); titrate to patient response
Child: IV A total loading dose of 600 mcg/kg over 2 min, maintenance **IV** INF 200 mcg/kg/min, titrate upward by 50-100 mcg/kg/min q5-10 min until B/P, heart rate reduced by >10%

Perioperative hypertension/tachycardia
Adult: IV immediate control 80 mg (bolus) over 30 seconds, then 150 mcg/kg/min, adjust to response, max 300 mcg/kg/min

Available forms: Inj 10 mg/mL vial; 10 mg/mL in 250 mL bag, 20 mg/mL in 100 mL bag

ADVERSE EFFECTS
CNS: Confusion, dizziness, fatigue, headache, drowsiness, weakness
CV: Hypotension, bradycardia, chest pain, peripheral ischemia
GI: *Nausea*, vomiting, anorexia
INTEG: Sweating, inflammation at injection site

INTERACTIONS
Individual drugs
Amphetamine, ePHEDrine, EPINEPHrine, norepinephrine, phenylephrine, pseudoephedrine: increased α-adrenergic stimulation
Clonidine: possibly fatal increased B/P
Digoxin: increased digoxin levels
DilTIAZem, verapamil:
Increase: potentiate suppressive effects of these products
Thyroid hormones: decreased action of thyroid hormone

Drug classifications
Antidiabetics: Increased: effect of antidiabetic
MAOIs, solatol: avoid use
General anesthetics: increased antihypertensive effect

Drug/herb
Ephedra, hawthorn: decreased antihypertensive effect

Drug/lab test
Interference: glucose/insulin tolerance test

NURSING CONSIDERATIONS
Assessment
• **Dysrhythmias:** Monitor B/P during beginning treatment, periodically thereafter; pulse; note rate, rhythm, quality; apical/radial pulse before administration; notify prescriber of any significant changes (pulse <50 bpm); if severe, slow or stop infusion, monitor ECG

• **HF:** Assess for edema in feet, legs daily; monitor I&O, daily weight; check for jugular vein distention, crackles bilaterally, dyspnea
• **Bronchospasm:** Assess breath sounds and respiratory patterns
• **Infusion site:** Monitor infusion site during infusion, do not use butterfly if irritation occurs, stop and start at another site

Patient problem
Impaired cardiac output (adverse reactions)

Implementation
IV route
• Check that correct concentration is being given
IV direct route
• The 10 mg/ml inj solution needs no dilution and may be used as an **IV** loading dose using handheld syringe
Continuous IV infusion route
• Ready-to-use bags premixed isotonic sol of 10 mg/ml and 20 mg/ml are available in 100, 250 ml bags; use controlled device, a central line is preferred, rate is based on patient's weight
• Store at room temperature for 24 hr; sol should be clear

Y-site compatibilities: Amikacin, aminophylline, ampicillin, amiodarone, atracurium, butorphanol, calcium chloride, ceFAZolin, cefmetazole, cefoperazone, cefTAZidime, ceftizoxime, chloramphenicol, cimetidine, cisatracurium, clindamycin, diltiazem, DOPamine, enalaprilat, erythromycin, famotidine, fentaNYL, gentamicin, heparin, hydrocortisone, regular insulin, labetalol, magnesium sulfate, methyldopate, metroNIDAZOLE, midazolam, morphine, nafcillin, nitroglycerin, norepinephrine, nitroprusside, pancuronium, penicillin G potassium, phenytoin, piperacillin, polymyxin B, potassium chloride, potassium phosphate, propofol, ranitidine, remifentanil, streptomycin, tacrolimus, tobramycin, trimethoprim/sulfamethoxazole, vancomycin, vecuronium, voriconazole, zoledronic acid

Patient/family education
• Teach patient not to drive or perform other hazardous activities if drowsiness occurs
• Teach patient to change positions slowly to prevent orthostatic hypotension
• Teach patient need for medication and expected results
• Caution patient to rise slowly to prevent orthostatic hypotension
• Advise patient to notify if pain, swelling occurs at **IV** site
• Teach patient to notify prescriber if chest pain, shortness of breath, wheezing, low B/P occur

• **Pregnancy/breastfeeding:** Identify if pregnancy is planned or suspected

Evaluation
Positive therapeutic outcome
• Absence of dysrhythmias

TREATMENT OF OVERDOSE:
Defibrillation, vasopressor for hypotension, IV glucagon if needed

esomeprazole (Rx)
(es′oh-mep′rah-zohl)
NexIUM, Nexium 24 hr
Func. class.: Antiulcer, proton pump inhibitor
Chem. class.: Benzimidazole

Do not confuse: NexIUM/NexAVAR

ACTION: Suppresses gastric secretion by inhibiting hydrogen/potassium ATPase enzyme system in the gastric parietal cell; characterized as gastric acid pump inhibitor, since it blocks final step of acid production

Therapeutic outcome: Absence of duodenal ulcers; decreased gastroesophageal reflux

USES: Gastroesophageal reflux disease (GERD), adult/child/infant; severe erosive esophagitis; treatment of active duodenal ulcers in combination with antiinfectives for *Helicobacter pylori* infection; long-term use in hypersecretory conditions

Pharmacokinetics

Absorption	Unknown
Distribution	97% plasma protein bound
Metabolism	Liver (metabolites), by CYP2C19, CYP3A4 ᴾᴰ Asian, Black and some Caucasians may be poor metabolizers
Excretion	Urine (metabolites), feces (metabolites); in geriatric, elimination rate decreased, bioavailability increased
Half-life	1-1½ hr

Pharmacodynamics

	PO	IV
Onset	Unknown	
Peak	1½ hr	Infusion's end
Duration	24 hr	24 hr

CONTRAINDICATIONS
Hypersensitivity to proton-pump inhibitors (PPIs)

Precautions: Pregnancy, breastfeeding, children, geriatric, hypomagnesemia, osteoporosis

DOSAGE AND ROUTES
Active duodenal ulcers associated with *H. pylori*
Adult: PO 40 mg/day × 10-14 days in combination with clarithromycin 500 mg bid × 10 days and amoxicillin 1000 mg bid × 10 days

GERD/erosive esophagitis
Adult: PO 20 or 40 mg/day × 4-8 wk; no adjustment needed in renal, liver failure, geriatric; IV 20 or 40 mg/day up to 10 days
Child and adolescent 12-17 yr: PO 20 or 40 mg/day 1 hr before meals up to 8 wk
Child 1-11 yr and ≥20 kg: PO 10 mg/day 1 hr before meals for up to 8 wk
Infant ≥1 mo: IV 0.5 mg/kg over 10-30 min
Infant 1-11 mo (>7.5-12 kg): PO 10 mg daily up to 6 wk
Infant 1-11 mo (5-7.5 kg): PO 5 mg daily up to 6 wk
Infant 1-11 mo (3-5 kg): PO 2.5 mg daily up to 6 wk

Hepatic dose
Adult: PO/IV max 20 mg/day (severe hepatic disease)

Available forms: Del rel caps 20, 40 mg; powder for **IV** inj 20, 40 mg/vial; del rel powder for oral susp 2.5, 5, 20, 40 mg

ADVERSE EFFECTS
CNS: *Headache, dizziness*
GI: *Diarrhea, flatulence,* abdominal pain, constipation, dry mouth, hepatic failure, hepatitis, microscopic colitis, *Clostridium difficile*–associated diarrhea (CDAD)
GU: Nephritis
MISC: Fractures, SLE, Vitamin B$_{12}$ deficiency
INTEG: *Rash,* dry skin
RESP: *Cough,* pneumonia
SYST: Stevens-Johnson syndrome, toxic epidermal necrolysis, exfoliative dermatitis

INTERACTIONS
Individual drugs
Atazanavir, Calcium carbonate, clopidogrel, dapsone, indinavir, iron, itraconazole, ketoconazole, mycophenolate, nelfinavir, vitamin B$_{12}$: decreased effect
Increase: effect of methotrexate, tacrolimus, warfarin
Cilostazol, clozapine, those drugs metabolized by CYP2C19, diazepam, digoxin, penicillins, saquinavir: increased effect, toxicity

Drug/lab test
Interference: sodium, Hgb, WBC, platelets, magnesium
False positive: CgA

NURSING CONSIDERATIONS
Assessment
• **Assess GI system:** bowel sounds, abdomen for pain, swelling, anorexia, bloody stools; CDAD may occur
• **Hepatic failure, hepatitis:** monitor AST, ALT, alkaline phosphatase during treatment
• **Serious skin disorders:** Stevens-Johnson syndrome, toxic epidermal necrolysis, exfoliative dermatitis

Patient problem
Pain (uses)

Implementation
PO route
• Swallow caps whole; do not crush or chew; cap may be opened and sprinkled over Tbsp of applesauce
• Same time daily, 1 hr before meal
• **Oral susp (del rel):** empty contents of packet into container with 1 Tbsp of water, let stand 2-3 min to thicken, restir, give within 30 min of mixing; any residual product should be flushed with more water, taken immediately
• **NG tube (del rel oral susp):** add ml water to contents of packet in syringe, shake, leave 2-3 min to thicken, shake, inject through NG tube within 30 min, make sure granules are dissolved

IV, direct route
• Reconstitute each vial with 5 ml 0.9% NaCl, D_5W, LR; give over 3 min
Intermittent IV INF route
• Dilute reconstituted sol to 50 ml, give over 30 min, do not admix, flush line with D_5W, 0.9% NaCl, LR after inf
Continuous IV route
Use 2 (40 mg vials/5 mL of 0.9% NaCl) for 80 mg/loading dose, further dilute in 100 mL 0.9% NaCl, give over 30 min, then infusion at 8 mg/hr × 71.5 hr

Y-site compatibility: ceftaroline, fentanyl, furosemide, regular insulin, nitroglycerin

Patient/family education
• Instruct patient to report severe diarrhea; product may have to be discontinued, rash
• Advise diabetic patients that hypoglycemia may occur
• Advise patient to avoid hazardous activities; dizziness may occur
• Teach patient to notify provider if pregnancy is planned or suspected, or if breastfeeding
• Advise patient to avoid alcohol, salicylates, ibuprofen; may cause GI irritation
• Teach patient to take ≥1 hr prior to meal; not to crush, chew delayed-release product, if missed, take as soon as remembered if not almost time for next dose, take full course prescribed "Patient Information"
• Teach patient if cap cannot be swallowed whole contents may be mixed with a tablespoon of applesauce
• Teach patient to notify all providers of all OTC/Rx or herbal products taken
• **Hypomagnesemia:** Teach patient if dizziness, fast heartbeat, tremors, weakness, spasm, cramps, notify health care professional
• **Pregnancy/breastfeeding:** Teach patient to notify provider if pregnancy is planned or suspected, or if breastfeeding

Evaluation
Positive therapeutic outcome
• Absence of epigastric pain, swelling, fullness, decreased GERD

---

estradiol (Rx)
(ess-tra-dye′ole)
Estrace
estradiol cypionate (Rx)
Depo-Estradiol
estradiol topical emulsion (Rx)
Estrasorb
estradiol valerate (Rx)
Delestrogen
estradiol transdermal system (Rx)
Alora, Climara, Estraderm, Estradot ✲, Minivelle, Menostar, Oesclim ✲, Vivelle
estradiol transdermal spray (Rx)
Evamist
estradiol vaginal tablet (Rx)
Vagifem
estradiol vaginal ring (Rx)
Estring, Femring
estradiol gel (Rx)
Divigel, Elestrin, Estrogel
Func. class.: Estrogen, progestin
Chem. class.: Nonsteroidal synthetic estrogen

ACTION: Needed for adequate functioning of female reproductive system; affects release of pituitary gonadotropins, inhibits ovulation, promotes adequate calcium use in bone structure

Therapeutic outcome: Decreased tumor size in prostatic cancer; increased estrogen levels in menopause, female hypogonadism

---

USES: Vasomotor symptoms associated with menopause, inoperable breast cancer (selected cases), prostatic cancer, atrophic vaginitis, kraurosis vulvae, hypogonadism, primary ovarian failure, prevention of osteoporosis, castration

Pharmacokinetics

Absorption	Well absorbed
Distribution	Widely distributed, crosses placenta
Metabolism	Liver, tissues, enterohepatic recirculation
Excretion	Breast milk
Half-life	Unknown

Pharmacodynamics

	PO	IM	IV
Onset	Rapid	Slow	Rapid
Peak	Unknown	Unknown	Unknown
Duration	Unknown	Unknown	Unknown

CONTRAINDICATIONS

Pregnancy, breastfeeding, reproductive cancer, genital bleeding (abnormal, undiagnosed), protein S or C deficiency, antithrombin deficiency, angioedema, MI, stroke

> **BLACK BOX WARNING:** Breast/endometrial cancer, thromboembolic disorders, MI, stroke

Precautions: Hypertension, asthma, blood dyscrasias, gallbladder disease, HF, diabetes mellitus, bone disease, depression, migraine headache, seizure disorders, renal/hepatic disease, family history of cancer of breast or reproductive tract, history of smoking, uterine fibroids, vaginal irritation/infection, history of angioedema, cardiac disease

> **BLACK BOX WARNING:** Dementia, accidental exposure pets/children (topical)

DOSAGE AND ROUTES
Hormone replacement/menopause symptoms
Adult: **TD** 1 patch delivering 0.025, 0.0375, 0.05, 0.075, or 0.1 mg/day 2×/wk (Alora, Estraderm, Vivelle-Dot); 1 patch delivering 0.025, 0.0375, 0.05, 0.06, 0.075, or 0.1 mg/day replace q7 days (Climara); **GEL** apply entire unit dose packet to 5- × 7-inch area of upper thigh/day, alternate thighs; **SPRAY** (Evamist) 1 spray to inner surface of forearm/day in AM

Menopause/hypogonadism/ castration/ovarian failure
Adult: PO 0.5-2 mg/day 3 wk on, 1 wk off or continuously; IM 1-5 mg q3-4wk (cypionate),

1-5 mg q3-4wk; 10-20 mg q4wk (valerate); TOP Estraderm 0.05 mg/24 hr applied 2 ×/wk, Climara 0.05 mg/hr applied 1 ×/wk in a cyclic regimen; women with hysterectomy may use continuously

Prostatic cancer
Adult: IM 30 mg q1-2wk **(valerate); PO** 1-2 mg tid (oral estradiol)

Breast cancer (palliative treatment)
Adult: PO 10 mg tid × 3 mo or longer

Atropic vaginitis/kraurosis vulvae
Adult: VAG cream 2-4 g/day × 1-2 wk, then 1 g 1-3 ×/wk cycled; VAG tab 1/day × 2 wk, maintenance 1 tab 2 ×/wk; VAG ring inserted and left in place continuously for 3 mo

Vasomotor symptoms
Adult: TOP after cleaning and drying skin on left thigh, calf, rub in contents of pouch using both hands until completely absorbed; wash hands

Available forms: Estradiol: tabs 0.5, 1, 2 mg; **valerate:** inj 10, 20, 40 mg/ml; **transdermal** 0.014, 0.025, 0.0375, 0.05, 0.075, 0.1 mg/24-hr release rate; **vag cream** 100 mcg/g; **vag ring** 2 mg/90 days; **vag tab** 10 mcg; **topical emulsion:** 2.5 mg; **gel** 0.1%, 0.06%, (Divigel); **spray** (Evamist) 1.53 mg/actuation

ADVERSE EFFECTS
CNS: Dizziness, headache
CV: Hypertension, edema, thromboembolism, MI
GI: *Nausea,* vomiting, diarrhea, anorexia, hepatic adenoma
GU: Amenorrhea, cervical erosion, breakthrough bleeding, dysmenorrhea, vaginal candidiasis, breast changes, *testicular atrophy, impotence;* changes in libido
INTEG: Rash, urticaria, acne, hirsutism, alopecia, oily skin, seborrhea, purpura, erythema, pruritus, melasma; site irritation (transdermal)
META: Hypercalcemia, hyperglycemia, sodium retention
MS: Leg cramps

INTERACTIONS
Drug classifications
Anticoagulants: decreased action of anticoagulants
Anticonvulsants, barbiturates: decreased estradiol action
Corticosteroids: increased action of corticosteroids, tricyclics
Hypoglycemics (oral): decreased action of hypoglycemics

Drug/herb
Black cohosh, DHEA: altered estrogen effect
Saw palmetto, St. John's wort: decreased estrogen effect
Smoking: Increased side effects

Drug/food
Grapefruit juice: increased estrogen level

Drug/lab test
Increased: HDL, lipids; T_4; serum sodium; platelet aggregation; thyroxine-binding globulin (TBS); prothrombin; factors VII, VIII, IX, X; triglycerides
Decreased: LDL, total cholesterol, serum folate, T_3, glucose tolerance test, antithrombin III, metyrapone test
False positive: LE prep, ANA titer

NURSING CONSIDERATIONS
Assessment

> **BLACK BOX WARNING:** Assess for previous breast/endometrial cancer, thromboembolic disorders, MI, stroke, dementia, use adequate screening for these conditions, estrogen increases the risk

• Monitor blood glucose in patient with diabetes; hyperglycemia may occur
• Monitor B/P baseline and periodically; watch for increase caused by water and sodium retention
• Monitor I&O ratio; be alert for decreasing urinary output and increasing edema; monitor weight daily; notify prescriber if weekly weight gain is >5 lb; if increased, diuretic may be ordered
• Assess edema, hypertension, cardiac symptoms, jaundice
• Assess female patient for intact uterus; if so, progesterone should be added to estrogen therapy to decrease risk of endometrial cancer
• **Beers:** Avoid oral and topical patch in older adults, evidence of carcinogenic potential (breast, endometrial)
• **Pregnancy/breastfeeding:** Do not use in pregnancy; estrogens decrease milk production, use only if clearly needed

Patient problem
Impaired sexual functioning (uses)

Implementation
PO route
• Give titrated dose, use lowest effective dose
• Give with food or milk to decrease GI symptoms
• Don't give with grapefruit juice
IM route
• Administer deeply in large muscle mass; product is painful
• Rotate syringe to mix oil and medication, never give IV

Transdermal route
• May contain aluminum or other metals in backing of patch, can overheat in MRI scan and burn patients
• Apply to area free of hair to ensure adhesion on trunk of body 2 ×/wk; press firmly and hold in place for 10 sec to ensure good contact; do not apply to breasts
• Start transdermal dose 7 days before last PO dose if routes are to be changed
Topical route spray (Evamist)
• Use daily in AM; spray to inner upper arm; may increase to 2-3 ×/day based on response; let dry for 2 min, do not wash site for 30 min, avoid secondary exposure to children, pets, caregivers
Vaginal route
• Place cream in applicator by attaching tube to applicator; squeeze cream into tube to mark; insert with patient reclining
• Use a new applicator daily

Patient/family education
• Tell patient to take exactly as prescribed; do not double doses, not to discontinue abruptly
• **Advise patient that increased weight gain and symptoms of fluid retention should be reported to prescriber:** edema of feet, ankles, sacral area; abnormal vaginal bleeding; breast lumps; hepatic disease (dark urine, clay-colored stools, jaundice of skin, sclera, pruritus); to report dermal rash with transdermal patch
• **Caution patient that thromboembolic symptoms should be reported:** tenderness in legs, chest pain, dyspnea, headaches, blurred vision
• Inform patient to use sunscreen and protective clothing because change in pigmentation may occur
• Advise patient to stop smoking; smokers have a greater chance of thromboembolic disorder
• Teach patient to avoid grapefruit or grapefruit juice (PO)
• Teach patient regular follow-up and lab work will be required
• **Osteoporosis:** Use of other recommendations should be used including exercise
• Advise patient to discuss all OTC, Rx, herbals, supplements with health care professional; to notify before surgery
• **Transdermal:** Teach patient to apply with clean, dry hands to abdomen, press to ensure sticking, change site with each dose
• **Vaginal ring:** Insert into upper portion of vagina, placement should not be uncomfortable, if MRI is needed notify before test, removal is needed
• Inform patient to report changes in blood glucose, if diabetic

• Advise patient to notify prescriber if pregnancy is planned or suspected, and not to become pregnant when using estrogen

Evaluation
Positive therapeutic outcome
• Reversal of menopausal symptoms
• Decrease in tumor size in prostatic or breast cancer
• Decrease in itching, inflammation of vagina
• Absence of symptoms of osteoporosis

⚠ HIGH ALERT

estrogens, conjugated, equine
C.E.S ✦, Congest ✦, Premarin
estrogens, conjugated (Rx) (synthetic A)
Cenestin
estrogens, conjugated (synthetic B) (Rx)
Enjuvia
Func. class.: Hormone—estrogen

Do not confuse: Premarin/Provera, Enjuvia/Januvia

ACTION: Needed for adequate functioning of female reproductive system; affects release of pituitary gonadotropins; inhibits ovulation; promotes adequate calcium use in bone structures

Therapeutic outcome: Decreased tumor size in prostatic cancer; increased estrogen levels in menopause, female hypogonadism

USES: Symptoms associated with menopause, inoperable breast cancer, prostatic cancer, abnormal uterine bleeding, hypogonadism, primary ovarian failure, prevention of osteoporosis, castration, atrophic vaginitis

Pharmacokinetics

Absorption	Well absorbed (PO), completely absorbed (**IV**)
Distribution	Widely distributed, crosses placenta
Metabolism	Liver, exclusively; hepatic recirculation
Excretion	Kidney
Half-life	Unknown

Pharmacodynamics

	PO	IM	IV
Onset	Rapid	Slow	Immediate
Peak	Unknown	Unknown	Unknown
Duration	Unknown	Unknown	Unknown

CONTRAINDICATIONS
Pregnancy, breastfeeding, thromboembolic disorders, reproductive cancer, genital bleeding (abnormal, undiagnosed), hypersensitivity, MI, stroke, phlebitis

BLACK BOX WARNING: Endometrial breast cancer, thromboembolic diseases

Precautions: Hypertension, asthma, blood dyscrasias, gallbladder disease, HF, diabetes mellitus, bone disease, depression, migraine headache, seizure disorders, renal/hepatic disease, family history of cancer of breast or reproductive tract, history of smoking, hypothyroidism, obesity, SLE

BLACK BOX WARNING: Dementia

DOSAGE AND ROUTES
≫ Estrogens, conjugated
Menopause
Adult: PO 0.3-1.25 mg/day 3 wk on, 1 wk off

Prevention of osteoporosis
Adult: PO 0.3 mg/day or in a cycle

Atrophic vaginitis
Adult: VAG cream 0.5 g/day × 21 days, off 7 days, repeat

Prostatic cancer
Adult: PO 1.25-2.5 mg tid

Advanced inoperable breast cancer
Adult: PO 10 mg tid × 3 mo or longer

Abnormal uterine bleeding
Adult: IV/IM 25 mg, repeat in 6-12 hr

Castration/primary ovarian failure
Adult: PO 1.25 mg/day 3 wk on, 1 wk off

Hypogonadism
Adult: PO 0.3 or 0.625 mg q day/3 wk on, 1 wk off; adjust to response

≫ Estrogens, conjugated synthetic B
Menopause
Adult: PO 0.625 mg/day initially, may increase based on response

Available forms: Tabs 0.3, 0.45, 0.625, 0.9, 1.25 mg; inj 25 mg/vial; vag cream 0.625 mg/g; **synthetic B:** tabs 0.625, 1.25 mg

ADVERSE EFFECTS
CNS: Dizziness, headache, depression
CV: Hypertension, edema, thromboembolism, MI
EENT: Contact lens intolerance, increased myopia, astigmatism
GI: *Nausea,* vomiting, anorexia, increased appetite, jaundice

---

GU: Amenorrhea, cervical erosion, breakthrough bleeding, dysmenorrhea, vaginal candidiasis, breast changes, *atrophy, impotence,* libido changes

INTEG: Rash, urticaria, acne, pigmentation, oily skin

META: Hypercalcemia, sodium retention

MS: Leg cramps

MISC: Anaphylaxis, angioedema

INTERACTIONS
Drug classifications
Anticoagulants: decreased action of anticoagulants

Anticonvulsants, barbiturates: decreased action of estrogens

Oral hypoglycemics: decreased action of hypoglycemics

Drug/food
Grapefruit juice: increased estrogen level

Drug/herb
Black cohosh, DHEA: altered estrogen effect

Saw palmetto, St. John's wort: decreased estrogen effect

Smoking: Increased side effects

Drug/lab test
Increased: HDL, lipids, T_4; serum sodium; platelet aggregation; thyroxine-binding globulin (TBG); prothrombin; factors VII, VIII, IX, X; triglycerides

Decreased: LDL, total cholesterol, T_3, glucose tolerance test, antithrombin III, metyrapone test

False positive: LE prep, ANA titer

NURSING CONSIDERATIONS
Assessment

> **BLACK BOX WARNING:** Breast, endometrial cancer: estrogens should not be used in known, suspected, or history of these disorders

> **BLACK BOX WARNING:** Stroke, thromboembolic disease of MI: should not be used in these conditions or known protein C deficiency, protein S deficiency or antithrombin in deficiency

• Monitor blood glucose in patient with diabetes; hyperglycemia may occur

• Monitor B/P; watch for increase caused by water and sodium retention

• Monitor I&O ratio; be alert for decreasing urinary output and increasing edema; monitor weight daily; notify prescriber if weekly weight gain is >5 lb; if increased, diuretic may be ordered

• Assess edema, hypertension, cardiac symptoms, jaundice

• Assess female patient for intact uterus; if so, progesterone should be added to estrogen therapy to decrease risk of endometrial cancer; abnormal uterine bleeding, breast exam

• **Beers:** Avoid oral and topical patch in older adults, evidence of carcinogenic potential (breast, endometrial)

• Pregnancy, estrogens decrease milk production, use only if clearly needed

Patient problem
Impaired sexual functioning (uses)

Implementation
PO route
• Give titrated dose, use lowest effective dose

• Give in 1 dose in AM for prostatic cancer, vaginitis, hypogonadism

• Give with food or milk to decrease GI symptoms

IM route
• Reconstitute after withdrawing at least 5 ml of air from container and inject sterile diluent on vial side, rotate to dissolve

• Give IM inj deeply in large muscle

Vaginal route
• Place cream in applicator by attaching tube to applicator, squeeze cream into tube to mark, insert with patient recumbent

• Applicator should be washed after each use

IV, direct route
• Reconstitute as for IM, inject into distal port of running **IV** line of D_5W, 0.9% NaCl, LR, at a rate of 5 mg/min or less

Y-site compatibilities: Heparin/hydrocortisone, potassium chloride, vit B/C

Patient/family education
• Caution patient to take exactly as prescribed and not to double doses, not to discontinue abruptly

> **BLACK BOX WARNING:** Advise patient that increased weight gain and symptoms of fluid retention should be reported to prescriber: edema of feet, ankles, sacral area; abnormal vaginal bleeding; breast lumps; hepatic disease (dark urine, clay-colored stools, jaundice of skin, sclera, pruritus)

• **Caution patient that thromboembolic symptoms should be reported:** pain, redness, tenderness in legs; chest pain, dyspnea, headaches, blurred vision

• Inform patient that change in pigmentation may occur and to use sunscreen and protective clothing

• Teach patient that regular follow-up and lab work will be required

---

Nurse Alert   Key NCLEX® Drug   >> Drug Specifics

- **Osteoporosis:** Use of other recommendations should be used including exercise
- Advise patient to discuss all OTC, Rx, herbals, supplements with health care professional; to notify before surgery
- Teach patient that premarin tablet may be visible in stools
- Vaginal: Teach patient how to insert, use of applicator, not to use tampon
- Advise patient to stop smoking; smokers have a greater chance of thromboembolic disorder
- Tell patient that vasomotor symptoms improve in 2 wk, max relief 8 wk
- Tell patient to use nonhormonal birth control and to notify prescriber if pregnancy is suspected

Evaluation
Positive therapeutic outcome
- Reversal of menopause symptoms
- Decrease in tumor size in prostatic, breast cancer
- Decrease in itching, inflammation of vagina
- Absence of symptoms of osteoporosis

⚠ HIGH ALERT

eszopiclone (Rx)
(es-zop′i-klone)
Lunesta
Func. class.: Sedative-hypnotic, non-benzodiazepine
Chem. class.: Cyclopyrrolone
Controlled substance schedule IV

Do not confuse: Lunesta/Neulasta

ACTION: Interacts with GABA receptors

Therapeutic outcome: Ability to sleep and stay asleep throughout the night

USES: Insomnia

Pharmacokinetics

Absorption	Unknown
Distribution	Unknown
Metabolism	Extensively in the liver by CYP3A4, CYP2E1; protein binding 52%-59%
Excretion	Via kidneys
Half-life	6 hr, geriatric 9 hr

Pharmacodynamics

Onset	Rapid
Peak	1 hr
Duration	6 hr

CONTRAINDICATIONS
Hypersensitivity

Precautions: Pregnancy, breastfeeding, children, geriatric, severe hepatic disease, abrupt discontinuation, COPD, depression, labor, sleep apnea, substance abuse, suicidal ideation, ethanol intoxication

DOSAGE AND ROUTES
Adult: PO 1 mg immediately before bed, may increase to 2-3 mg if needed, max 3 mg nightly

Hepatic dose/CYP3A4 inhibitors
Adult: PO 1 mg immediately before bed in severe hepatic disease, max 2 mg/day

Available forms: Tabs 1, 2, 3 mg

ADVERSE EFFECTS
CNS: Worsening depression, hallucinations, headache, *daytime drowsiness,* suicidal thoughts/actions, migraine, restlessness, anxiety, sleep driving, sleep walking
CV: Peripheral edema, chest pain
GI: *Dry mouth,* bitter taste (dysgeusia)
GU: Gynecomastia, dysmenorrhea
INTEG: Rash, angioedema

INTERACTIONS
Drug classifications
CNS depressants: increased CNS depression
CYP3A4 inducers (dexamethasone, barbiturates, carBAMazepine, OXcarbazepine, phenytoin, fosphenytoin, ethotoin): Decrease: eszopiclone effect
CYP3A4 inhibitors (clarithromycin, itraconazole, ketoconazole, nefazodone, nelfinavir, ritonavir, troleandomycin): increased toxicity due to decreased eszopiclone elimination

Drug/food
High-fat meal: decreased product action

Drug/herb
- St. John's wort: Decrease: eszopiclone effect

NURSING CONSIDERATIONS
Assessment
- **Assess sleep pattern:** ability to go to sleep, stay asleep; early morning awakenings; conservative methods used
- Mental status: Monitor for abuse of this or other products
- **Pregnancy/breastfeeding:** Use in pregnancy only if clearly needed, avoid breastfeeding
- **Beers:** Avoid in older adults with or at high risk for delirium

Patient problem
Impaired sleep (uses)

Implementation
- Do not break, crush, or chew tab
- For short-term use only
- Give immediately before bedtime
- Avoid use with a high-fat meal
- Check to see product is swallowed

Patient/family education
- Caution patient that daytime drowsiness may occur; not to engage in hazardous activities until effect is known, memory problems may occur
- Advise patient that all other medications and supplements should be avoided unless approved by prescriber
- Discuss alternative methods to improve sleep: reading, quiet environment, warm bath, milk
- Teach patient to avoid use after a high-fat meal
- Teach patient to swallow tab whole
- Teach patient to notify prescriber of facial swelling, rash, complex sleeping disorders (sleep driving, sleep eating) change in thinking or behavior
- Teach patient that tolerance and dependence may occur after extended use
- Teach patient to take immediately before going to bed
- Teach patient to be aware of CNS depression, sleep, driving, eating, walking, to avoid CNS depressants report at once
- **Pregnancy/breastfeeding:** Identify if pregnancy is planned or suspected, avoid breastfeeding

Evaluation
Positive therapeutic outcome
- Ability to sleep and stay asleep throughout the night

---

etanercept (Rx)
(eh-tan'er-sept)
Brenzys ✦, Enbrel, Ereizi
Func. class.: Antirheumatic agent (disease-modifying) (DMARDs)
Chem. class.: Anti-TNF agent

Do not confuse: Enbrel/Levbid

ACTION: Binds to tumor necrosis factor (TNF), which decreases inflammation and immune response

Therapeutic outcome: Decreased pain, inflammation

USES: Acute, chronic rheumatoid arthritis that has not responded to other disease-modifying agents; polyarticular course juvenile rheumatoid arthritis (JRA), ankylosing spondylitis, plaque psoriasis, psoriatic arthritis

Pharmacokinetics

Absorption	Rapidly absorbed (60%)
Distribution	Unknown
Metabolism	Unknown
Excretion	Unknown
Half-life	115 hr

Pharmacodynamics
Unknown

CONTRAINDICATIONS
Hypersensitivity

Precautions: Pregnancy, breastfeeding, children <4 yr, geriatric, malignancies, HF, seizures, multiple sclerosis, latex hypersensitivity

> **BLACK BOX WARNING:** Infection, lymphoma, neoplastic disease, TB

DOSAGE AND ROUTES
Rheumatoid/psoriatic arthritis, ankylosing spondylitis
Adult: SUBCUT 50 mg qwk or 25 mg 2×/wk, 3-4 days apart

Plaque psoriasis
Adult: SUBCUT 50 mg 2 ×/wk × 3 mo, then 50 mg q wk maintenance
Adolescent and child 4-17 yr (unlabeled): SUBCUT 0.8 mg/kg/wk, max 50 mg/wk

Juvenile rheumatoid arthritis (JRA)
Adolescent and child 2-17 yr: SUBCUT 0.8 mg/kg/wk, max 50 mg/wk

Available forms: Powder for subcut inj 25 mg/vial; inj 50 mg/ml; auto injector, single use; subcut solution for subcut injection 25 mg/0.5mL (prefilled syringe)

ADVERSE EFFECTS
CNS: Headache, dizziness, weakness
GI: Abdominal pain, dyspepsia
HEMA: Pancytopenia
INTEG: Rash, *inj site reaction*
SYST: Serious infections, malignancies, Stevens-Johnson syndrome, reactivation of hepatitis B virus, lupuslike syndrome

INTERACTIONS
Individual drugs
Anakinra, cyclophosphamide, rilonacept: avoid use, serious adverse reaction
Azathioprine, methotrexate: Increased HSTCL

Drug classifications
Immunizations: should be brought up to date before treatment

Drug/lab test
Increased: LFTs

NURSING CONSIDERATIONS
Assessment
- **Rheumatoid arthritis:** assess for pain; check ROM, inflammation of joints, characteristics of pain
- Assess inj site for pain, swelling; usually occurs after 2 inj (4-5 days)

> **BLACK BOX WARNING: Infection:** Monitor CBC with differential baseline and periodically; patients using immunosuppressives, corticosteroids, methotrexate are at greater risk, assess for fever, discontinue in those that develop a serious infection, do not use in active infection, obtain testing before use, TB must be treated before use

> **BLACK BOX WARNING:** Assess for hypersensitivity: to this product, latex needle cap, benzyl alcohol; usual reaction to this product lasts 3-5 days

> **BLACK BOX WARNING: Secondary malignancy:** Assess for lymphoma and other neoplastic diseases in children and adolescents, avoid in those with a history of malignancy

Patient problem
Impaired mobility (uses)
Pain (uses)

Implementation
Subcut route
- Administration of one 50 mg/ml prefilled syringe or autoinjector provides a dose equivalent to two, 25 mg prefilled syringes or two, 25 mg vials of lyophilized powder
- The needle cap on the prefilled syringe and on the SureClick autoinjector contain dry natural rubber (latex) and should not be handled by persons sensitive to this product
- Inspect for particulate matter and discoloration prior to use, solution should be clear and colorless, although small white particles may be in the autoinjector or prefilled syringe
- Injection sites front of the thigh; abdomen except the 2 inches around the navel; or outer area of the upper arm. Rotate injection sites. Do not use where skin is tender, bruised, red, or hard. Also, do not inject directly into any raised, thick, red, or scaly skin patches or lesions related to psoriasis
- A vial adaptor is supplied for use when reconstituting the powder. To reconstitute using the vial adaptor, slide the plunger into the flange

end of the syringe. Attach the plunger to the gray rubber stopper in the syringe by turning the plunger clockwise until a slight resistance is felt. Remove the twist-off cap from the prefilled diluent syringe by turning counterclockwise. Once the twist-off cap is removed, twist the vial adapter onto the syringe clockwise until a slight resistance is felt. Place the vial adaptor over the top of the vial; the plastic spike inside the vial adaptor should puncture the gray stopper. Push the plunger down gently swirl to dissolve the powder. Do not shake. Turn the vial upside down and slowly pull the plunger down to the unit markings on the side bubbles. Remove the syringe and attach the 27 gauge needle
- If the vial will be used for multiple doses, use a 25-gauge needle for reconstituting and withdrawing the solution. After the diluent is added, some foaming may occur. Do not shake. Remove the 25-gauge needle from the syringe. Attach a 27-gauge needle
- Use as soon as possible after reconstitution. Place reconstituted vials for multiple doses in the refrigerator at 2-8° C (36°-46° F) within 4 hr of reconstitution and may be stored up to 14 days. DO NOT FREEZE

Use of the SureClick autoinjector
- Allow to reach room temperature, do not shake. Immediately before use, remove the needle
- Stretch the skin under and around the prefilled autoinjector, place the open end against the injection site at a 90° angle. Without pushing the purple button on top, push the autoinjector firmly against the skin to unlock. Press the purple button on top once and release the button. Listen for the first click. Wait for the second click or wait 15 seconds, and remove the autoinjector from injection site. Do NOT rub the site

Use of the prefilled syringe
- **Single-use:** allow to come to room temperature, do not shake. If bubbles are seen, very gently tap the syringe. Turn the syringe so that the purple horizontal lines on the barrel are directly facing you.
- Insert the needle at a 45° angle to the pinched skin. Do NOT rub the site

Patient/family education
- Teach patient that product must be continued for prescribed time to be effective; to avoid aspirin, alcoholic beverages
- Instruct patient to use caution when driving; dizziness may occur
- Teach patient about self-administration, if appropriate: inj should be made in thigh,

abdomen, upper arm; rotate sites at least 1 in from old site, check for injection reactions, reactions usually last 3-5 days
• Teach patient to not have live virus vaccines during treatment, bring immunizations up-to-date before treatment
• **Pregnancy/breastfeeding:** Use only if clearly needed, use cautiously in breastfeeding, enroll in Amgen Pregnancy Surveillance Program 800-772-6436

Evaluation
Positive therapeutic outcome
• Decreased pain in arthritic conditions
• Decreased inflammation in arthritic conditions
• Reduced chronic plague psoriasis

RARELY USED

etelcalcetide
(e-tel-kal′-se-tide)
Parsabiv
Func. class.: Parathyroid analogs

USES: For the treatment of secondary hyperparathyroidism in adults with chronic kidney disease on hemodialysis

Dosage and routes
For the treatment of secondary hyperparathyroidism in patients with chronic kidney disease on hemodialysis
Adult: IV 5 mg 3 times/wk at the end of hemodialysis treatment

For patients switching from cinacalcet to etelcalcetide
Adult: IV 5 mg 3 times/wk at the end of hemodialysis treatment after discontinuing etelcacetide for at least 7 days

---

ethambutol (Rx)
(e-tham′byoo-tole)
Etibi ✦, **Myambutol**
Func. class.: Antitubercular
Chem. class.: Diisopropylethylene diamide derivative

Do not confuse: ethambutol/Ethmozine

ACTION: Inhibits RNA synthesis, decreases tubercle bacilli replication

Therapeutic outcome: Resolution of TB infection

USES: Pulmonary TB, as an adjunct, other mycobacterial infections

Absorption	Rapidly absorbed
Distribution	Widely distributed, crosses blood-brain barrier, placenta, protein binding 30%
Metabolism	Liver 50%
Excretion	Kidneys, unchanged
Half-life	3 hr, increased in liver, kidney disease

Pharmacodynamics

Onset	Rapid
Peak	2-4 hr
Duration	Up to 24 hr

CONTRAINDICATIONS
Hypersensitivity, optic neuritis, child <13 yr

Precautions: Pregnancy, breastfeeding, renal disease, diabetic retinopathy, cataracts, ocular defects, hepatic and hematopoietic disorders

DOSAGE AND ROUTES
Adult and child >13 yr: PO 15-25 mg/kg/day as a single dose or (treatment naive) or 25 mg/kg q day (treatment experienced)
Child 1 mo-13 yr: PO 15-20 mg/kg/day q day max 1 g/day or 50 mg/kg/dose 2x per wk, max 2.5 g/dose (HIV negative); 15-25 mg/kg/day max 2.5 g/day (HIV); 15-25 mg/kg/day max 2.5g/day in combination (MAC)

Renal dose
Adult: PO CCr 10-50 ml/min dose q24-36hr; CCr <10 ml/min dose q48hr

Retreatment
Adult: PO 25 mg/kg/day as single dose × 2 mo with at least 1 other product, then decrease to 15 mg/kg/day as single dose, max 2.5 g/day
Child: PO 15 mg/kg/day

Available forms: Tabs 100, 400 mg

ADVERSE EFFECTS
CNS: *Headache, confusion,* fever, malaise, dizziness, *disorientation,* hallucinations, peripheral neuropathy
EENT: Blurred vision, optic neuritis, photophobia
GI: *Abdominal distress, anorexia, nausea, vomiting,* hepatitis
INTEG: Dermatitis, pruritus
META: *Elevated uric acid*
MISC: Joint pain, anaphylaxis

INTERACTIONS
Drug classifications
Aluminum, antacids: decreased absorption, separate by 4 hr

Neurotoxic agents, other: increased neuro-toxicity

NURSING CONSIDERATIONS
Assessment
• **TB:** Obtain C&S tests including sputum tests before initiating treatment; monitor qmo to detect resistance; lung sounds, amount and characteristics of sputum baseline and periodically
• Monitor liver function tests baseline, periodically: ALT, AST, bilirubin; renal studies: before, BUN, creatinine output, specific gravity, urinalysis, uric acid; decreased appetite, jaundice, dark urine, fatigue
• Assess patient's mental status often: affect, mood, behavioral changes; psychosis may occur with hallucinations, confusion
• Assess patient for vision disturbance that may indicate optic neuritis: blurred vision, change in color perception; may lead to blindness
• **Serious skin reaction:** anaphylaxis

Patient problem
Infection (uses)

Implementation
• Give at same time of day as a daily dose, other regimens may be used, used in combination with other antituberculars
• Tablets may be crushed and mixed with food or juice, if patient is unable to swallow
• Give with meals to decrease GI symptoms, at same time each day to maintain blood level
• 4 hr between this product and antacids
• Give antiemetic if vomiting occurs

Patient/family education
• Advise patient that compliance with dosage schedule and duration is necessary to eradicate disease; to keep scheduled appointments, including ophthalmic appointments, or relapse may occur
• Caution patient to report weakness, fatigue, loss of appetite, nausea, vomiting, yellowing of skin or eyes, tingling/numbness of hands/feet, weight gain, or decreased urine output
• Instruct patient to report any vision changes; rash; hot, swollen, painful joints; numbness or tingling of extremities to physician
• Caution patient to inform prescriber if pregnancy is suspected
• Pregnancy/breastfeeding: notify prescriber if pregnancy is planned or suspected, or if breastfeeding

Evaluation
Positive therapeutic outcome
• Decreased symptoms of TB
• Decrease in acid-fast bacteria

---

etodolac (Rx)
(ee-toe-doe'lak)
Func. class.: Nonsteroidal antiinflammatory, nonopioid analgesic
Chem. class.: Pyranocarboxylic acid

ACTION: Unknown, analgesic, antiinflammatory properties

Therapeutic outcome: Decreased pain, inflammation

USES: Mild to moderate pain, osteoarthritis, rheumatoid arthritis, arthralgia, myalgia, juvenile rheumatoid arthritis

Pharmacokinetics
Absorption	Well absorbed
Distribution	99% protein binding
Metabolism	Liver
Excretion	Urine, unchanged
Half-life	7 hr

Pharmacodynamics
	PO	Ext Rel
Onset	½ hr	Unknown
Peak	1-2 hr	3-12 hr
Duration	4-12 hr	6-12 hr

CONTRAINDICATIONS
Hypersensitivity; patients in whom aspirin, iodides, or other NSAIDs have produced asthma, rhinitis, urticaria, nasal polyps, angioedema, bronchospasm; coronary artery bypass graft surgery (CABG)

Precautions: Pregnancy, breastfeeding, children, geriatric, bleeding, GI/cardiac/renal/hepatic disorders, bronchospasm, nasal polyps, alcoholism, bone marrow suppression, MI, hemophilia, neutropenia, ulcerative colitis

> **BLACK BOX WARNING:** GI bleeding, perforation, MI, stroke

DOSAGE AND ROUTES
Analgesia
Adult: PO 200-400 mg q6-8hr; max 1200 mg/day; patients <60 kg max 20 mg/kg

Osteoarthritis/RA
Adult: PO 300 mg bid-tid, or 400-500 mg bid initially, then adjust to 600-1200 mg/day in divided doses; max 1200 mg/day; ext rel 400-1000 mg/day

---

Juvenile RA
Child 6-16 yr and 20-30 kg: PO extended release 400 mg q day; 31-45 kg 600 mg q day; 46-60 kg 800 mg q day; >60 kg 1000 q day

Available forms: Caps 200, 300 mg; tabs 400, 500 mg; ext rel tabs 400, 500, 600 mg

ADVERSE EFFECTS
CNS: Dizziness, headache, drowsiness, insomnia, anxiety, malaise, syncope, weakness
CV: Tachycardia, peripheral edema, fluid retention, palpitations, dysrhythmias, HF, MI, stroke
EENT: Tinnitus, hearing loss, blurred vision, photophobia
GI: *Nausea, anorexia,* vomiting, diarrhea, constipation, flatulence, dry mouth, dyspepsia, GI bleeding, abdominal pain
GU: Nephrotoxicity, dysuria
HEMA: Anemia, thrombocytopenia, bleeding time
INTEG: Erythema, urticaria, purpura, rash, pruritus, sweating, Stevens-Johnson syndrome
SYST: Angioedema, anaphylaxis

INTERACTIONS
Individual drugs
Cidofovir, cycloSPORINE, digoxin, lithium, methotrexate, phenytoin: increased toxicity

Drug classifications
Aminoglycosides: Increased toxicity
Antacids: delayed etodolac effect
Anticoagulants, antiplatelets, salicylates, SSRIs: Increased bleeding risk
β-Adrenergic blockers: decreased effect
Diuretics: decreased effectiveness of diuretics

Drug/herb
Arnica, chamomile, chondrotin, clove, dong guai, feverfew, garlic, ginkgo, horse chestnut: bleeding risk
St. John's wort: severe photosensitivity

Drug/Lab
Increased: BUN, creatinine
Decreased: Hgb/Hct, WBC, uric acid

NURSING CONSIDERATIONS
Assessment
• Assess pain: location, frequency, characteristics; relief after medication

> **BLACK BOX WARNING:** Assess for GI bleeding: black stools, hematemesis

• Assess for asthma, aspirin hypersensitivity, nasal polyps that may be hypersensitive to etodolac
• **Stevens Johnson syndrome:** monitor for rash, fatigue, lesions on face, body, fever; product should be discontinued immediately

• Monitor blood counts during therapy; watch for decreasing platelets; if low, therapy may need to be discontinued, then restarted after hematologic recovery; watch for blood dyscrasia (thrombocytopenia): bruising, fatigue, bleeding, poor healing
• **Beers:** Avoid chronic use in older adults unless alternatives are not available, increased risk of GI bleeding/peptic ulcer disease

Patient problem
Pain (uses)

Implementation
• Do not break, crush, or chew ext rel tabs
• Administer with full glass of water to enhance absorption
• Administer with food or milk to decrease gastric symptoms; food will slow absorption slightly, will not decrease absorption

Patient/family education
• Inform patient that product must be continued for prescribed time to be effective

> **BLACK BOX WARNING:** avoid aspirin, alcoholic beverages, other NSAIDs

• Caution patient to report bleeding, bruising, fatigue, malaise because blood dyscrasias can occur
• Instruct patient to use caution when driving; drowsiness, dizziness may occur
• Teach patient to take with a full glass of water to enhance absorption
• Identify if pregnancy is planned or suspected

Evaluation
Positive therapeutic outcome
• Decreased pain
• Decreased inflammation
• Increased mobility

⚠ HIGH ALERT

everolimus (Rx)
(e-ve-ro′li-mus)
Afinitor, Afinitor Disperz, Certican ✤, Zortress
Func. class.: Antineoplastic (miscellaneous)
Chem. class.: Kinase inhibitor

Do not confuse: everolimus/sirolimus/tacrolimus

ACTION: Proliferation signal inhibitor that inhibits mammalian target of rapamycin (mTOR); this pathway is dysregulated in cancer

---

USES: Renal cell cancer in those with failed treatment with suritinib or sorafenib or SUNItinib, kidney transplant rejection prophylaxis with cycloSPORINE, subependymal giant cell astrocytoma, progressive pancreatic neuroendocrine tumor (PNET) with unresectable locally advanced metastatic disease, renal angiomyolipoma, tuberous sclerosis complex, breast cancer hormone receptor positive/HER-2 negative, liver transplant rejection prophylaxis

Therapeutic outcome: Decreasing tumor size, decreasing spread of malignancy

Pharmacokinetics

Absorption	Rapid, well
Distribution	Protein binding 74%
Metabolism	Extensively by CYP3A4, P-gp
Excretion	Feces 80%, urine 5%
Half-life	30 hr, reduced by high-fat meal

Pharmacodynamics

Onset	Unknown
Peak	1-2 hr
Duration	Up to 24 hr

CONTRAINDICATIONS
Breastfeeding; hypersensitivity to this product, Rapamune, and Torisel; pregnancy

Precautions: Children, renal/hepatic disease, diabetes mellitus, infection, hyperlipidemia, pleural effusion

BLACK BOX WARNING: Immunosuppression, infection, renal artery thrombosis, renal impairment, renal vein thrombosis, neoplastic disease, heart transplant

DOSAGE AND ROUTES
Advanced Renal Cell Carcinoma
Adult: PO 10 mg q day; **use of moderate CYP3A4, P-gp inhibitors** 2.5mg q day; **strong CYP3A4 inducers** increase to 20 mg q day in 5 mg increments

Hepatic Dose
Adult: PO Child-Pugh class A 7.5mg q day; **Child-Pugh class B** 5mg q day; **Child-Pugh class C** 2.5 mg q day

SEGA with TSC
Adult/Child ≥ 1 yr: PO 4.5 mg/m², titrate q 2 wk; **moderate CYP3A4, P-gp inhibitors 2.25 mg/m²; strong CYP3A4 inducers** 9 mg/m²

Hepatic Dose
Adult: PO Child-Pugh class C 2.5 mg q day

Liver Transplant
Adult: PO 1 mg bid with lower dose of tacrolimus, begin ≥ 30 days after transplant, titrate

Hepatic Dose
Adult: PO Child-Pugh class A decrease dose by 33%; **Child-Pugh class B or C** decrease dose by 50%

Kidney Transplant
Adult: PO 0.75 bid with lower dose cyclosporine, titrate

Hepatic Dose
Adult: PO Child-Pugh class A decrease dose by 33%; Child-Pugh class B or C decrease dose by 50%

Available forms: Tabs 0.25, 0.5, 0.75, 2.5 mg (Zortress); 2.5, 5, 7.5, 10 mg (Afinitor); tablets for oral suspension 2, 3, 5 mg (Afinitor Disperz)

ADVERSE EFFECTS
CNS: *Headache, insomnia, paresthesia, chills,* fever, seizure, personality changes, dizziness
CV: *Hypertension, peripheral edema,* weakness, fatigue
EENT: Blurred vision, photophobia, eyelid edema, epistaxis, sinusitis, cataracts, conjunctivitis
GI: Nausea, vomiting, diarrhea, constipation, stomatitis, anorexia, abdominal pain, dysgeusia, hepatic artery thrombosis
GU: Renal failure, infertility
HEMA: Anemia, leukopenia, thrombocytopenia, hemolytic uremic syndrome, thrombotic microangiopathy, thrombotic thrombocytopenic purpura
INTEG: *Rash,* vasculitis
META: Hyperglycemia, *hyperlipemia,* hypertriglyceridemia
RESP: Pleural effusion, PE, cough, dyspnea
SYST: Angioedema, anaphylaxis, lymphoma

INTERACTIONS
Individual drugs
Cimetidine, cycloSPORINE, danazol, erythromycin: increased everolimus effect
CarBAMazepine, PHENobarbital, phenytoin, rifamycin, rifapentine

Drug classifications

BLACK BOX WARNING: Immunosuppressants: increased nephrotoxicity

Antifungals, calcium channel blockers, CYP3A4 inhibitors (strong, moderate), HIV-protease inhibitors: increased everolimus effect

Vaccines: decreased effect of these products
Decrease: everolimus effect: CYP3A4 inducers

Drug/herb
St. John's wort: may decrease the effect of
everolimus

Drug/food
Alters bioavailability; use consistently with or
without food; do not use with grapefruit juice

Drug/lab test
Increased: bilirubin, calcium, cholesterol, glucose, potassium, lipids, phosphate, triglycerides, uric acid
Decreased: calcium, glucose, potassium, magnesium, phosphate

NURSING CONSIDERATIONS
Assessment
• Monitor lipid profile: cholesterol, triglycerides, a lipid-lowering agent may be needed;
blood glucose

> **BLACK BOX WARNING: Monitor immunosup-
> pression:** Hgb, WBC, platelets during treatment
> qmo; if leukocytes <3000/mm³ or platelets
> <100,000/mm³, product should be discontinued
> or reduced; decreased hemoglobulin level may
> indicate bone marrow suppression

• Monitor hepatic studies: alk phos, AST, ALT,
amylase, bilirubin, and for hepatotoxicity: dark
urine, jaundice, itching, light-colored stools;
product should be discontinued

> **BLACK BOX WARNING: Infection:** bacterial/
> fungal infections can occur and are more common
> with combination immunosuppression therapy;
> assess for fever, cough, dyspnea, fatigue

• **Pneumonitis:** Assess for continuing cough,
dyspnea, pleural effusion baseline and during
treatment, use corticosteroids if needed, if
severe reduce dose or discontinue
• **Renal studies:** Monitor BUN, creatinine,
protein in urine baseline and throughout therapy

> **BLACK BOX WARNING: Renal artery/vein
> thrombosis (Zortress):** may result in graft
> loss within 30 days after transplantation

Patient problem
Infection (adverse reactions)

Implementation
• Swallow tabs whole with a full glass of water;
do not chew, crush, or break
• **Afinitor:** take at same time of day, consistently with or without food; if unable to swallow,
disperse in 30 ml of water

• **Zortress:** must take consistently with or
without food, give at same time of day q12h with
cycloSPORINE
• **Oral suspension:** (Afinitor Disperz) wear
gloves when preparing use 10 mL syringe and
place dose in syringe; do not crush, chew,
break; using 5 mL water and 4 mL air draw into
syringe with dose, wait 3 min until in suspension
after use; use same amount of water and air,
swirl, give contents
• Follow procedure for proper handling of
antineoplastics
• Give all medications PO if possible, avoiding
IM inj; bleeding may occur
• Store protected from light, at room temperature
• **Trough (Zortress)** obtain routine trough
levels, therapeutic levels should be 3 to 8 ng/mL,
trough obtained 4 or 5 days after a previous
dosing change. If the trough concentration is
below 3 ng/mL, double the total daily dose using
the available tablet strengths; if the trough is
greater than 8 ng/mL on 2 consecutive
measures, decrease the dose by 0.25 mg bid.
For liver transplant patients, ensure that the
steady-state whole blood trough is at least 3 ng/
mL before reducing the tacrolimus dose. The
recommended tacrolimus whole blood trough
concentrations are 3 to 5 ng/mL by 3 weeks
after the first dose (approximately Month 2)
and through Month 12 after transplantation.
Ensure that the steady-state whole blood
trough concentration is at least 3 ng/mL
before reducing the cyclosporine dose. The
recommended cyclosporine therapeutic range
when administered with everolimus is 100 to
200 ng/mL through the first month after
transplantation, 75 to 150 ng/mL during months
2 and 3 after transplantation, 50 to 100 ng/mL
during month 4 after transplantation, and 25 to
50 ng/mL during months 6 through 12 after
transplantation.
• Trough **(Afinitor Disperz):** Determine
trough concentrations 1 to 2 wks after starting
treatment. Adjust dose using the equation: new
dose = current dose × (target concentration
divided by current concentration), max dose
increment at any titration must not exceed
5 mg; multiple dose titrations may be required.
Titrate the dose to obtain trough concentrations
of 5 to 15 ng/mL. If dose reduction is required
for patients receiving the lowest available
strength, use alternate day dosing. Assess trough
concentrations approximately 1 to 2 wks after
any change in dose or change in dosage form
(Afinitor tablets to Afinitor Disperz). Assess
trough concentrations approximately 2 weeks
after an initiation or change in coadministration
of CYP3A4 and/or P-gp inducers or inhibitors

or after any hepatic status change. After a stable dose is obtained, monitor trough concentrations every 6 to 12 mon in patients with stable body surface area (BSA) or every 3 to 6 mon in patients with changing BSA.

Patient/family education

BLACK BOX WARNING: Advise to report fever, rash, severe diarrhea, chills, sore throat, fatigue; serious infections may occur; clay-colored stools, cramping (hepatotoxicity)

• Advise to avoid crowds, persons with known infections to reduce risk of infection
• **Pregnancy/breastfeeding:** Use effective contraception, report exposure to the National Transplant Pregnancy Registry 877-955-6877, do not breastfeed
• Teach to use contraception before, during, and 12 wk after product has been discontinued, avoid breastfeeding
• Advise not to use with grapefruit juice
• Inform to avoid live virus vaccines, that frequent lab tests are required
• Advise to take up to 6 hr after normally scheduled time if dose is missed
• Advise that product may decrease male/female fertility
• Teach that drinking alcohol is not recommended
• Teach patient to take consistently with or without food
• Teach patient to report visual changes, weight gain, edema, shortness of breath, impaired wound healing

Evaluation
Positive therapeutic outcome

• Decreasing size of tumor, decreasing spread of malignancy

evolocumab (Rx)
(e'-voe-lok'-ue-mab)
Repatha
Func. class.: Antilipemic
Chem. class.: PCSK9 inhibitor

ACTION: Binds to low-density lipoproteins, a human monoclonal antibody (IgG1)

USES: Heterozygous, familial hypercholesterolemia, atherosclerotic disease

Pharmacokinetics

Absorption	40%
Distribution	Extensive
Metabolism	Liver, CYP3A4
Excretion	Urine, feces
Half-life	At steady state 17-20 days

Pharmacodynamics

Onset	Unknown
Peak	2-3 days
Duration	4-5 days

CONTRAINDICATIONS
Hypersensitivity

Precautions: Pregnancy, breastfeeding, latex sensitivity

DOSAGE AND ROUTES
Primary hyperlipidemia with established clinical atherosclerosis
Adults: SUBCUT 140 mg q2wk or 420 mg qmo.

Homozygous familial hypercholesterolemia in patients who require additional lowering of LDL-C:
Adults and adolescents: 420 mg qmo

Available forms: Auto injector 140 mg/ml, solutions for inj 140 mg/ml

ADVERSE EFFECTS
MS: *Myalgia*
INTEG: Pruritus, injection-site reaction, erythema

INTERACTIONS
Drug/lab test
Increased: LFTs

NURSING CONSIDERATIONS
Assessment
• **Hypercholesterolemia:** obtain diet history; monitor fat content, lipid levels (triglycerides, LDL, HDL, total cholesterol), LFTs baseline and periodically during treatment

Patient problem
Nonadherence (teaching)

Implementation
• Visually inspect for particulate matter and discoloration, solution is clear, colorless to pale yellow
SUBCUT route
• Prefilled syringe or SureClick autoinjector
• If stored in the refrigerator, warm to room temperature for ≥ 30 min before use. Do not shake
• Give into areas of the abdomen (except for a 2-in area around the umbilicus), thigh, or upper arm that are not tender, bruised, red, or indurated
• To use the 420-mg dose, give 3 injections consecutively within 30 min
• Rotate the site with each inj
• Do not administer with other injectable drugs at the same inj site
Prefilled syringe administration
• Do not pick up or pull the prefilled syringe by the plunger rod or gray needle cap. Hold the syringe by the barrel

• Pull the gray needle cap off. It is normal to see a drop of sol at the end of the needle. Do not remove any air bubbles in the syringe
• Pinch the skin inj site to create a firm surface approximately 2 in wide. Hold the pinch, and insert the needle into the skin using a 45- to 90-degree angle
• Push the plunger rod all the way down until the syringe is empty
• When done, release the plunger, and gently lift the syringe off skin

SureClick autoinjector administration
• Do not remove the orange cap until you are ready to inject
• Pull the orange cap off
• Stretch (thigh) or pinch (stomach or upper arm) the skin inj site to create a firm surface approximately 2 in wide. Hold the stretch or pinch, and place the autoinjector on the skin at 90 degrees
• Firmly push down onto the skin; when ready to inject, press the gray button. A click should be heard. Keep pushing on the skin and then lift the thumb. The inj could take about 15 sec. The window on the autoinjector will turn from clear to yellow when the inj is complete. A second click may be heard
• Remove the needle that will be automatically covered

Patient/family education
• Teach patient that compliance is needed
• Advise that risk factors should be decreased: high-fat diet, smoking, alcohol consumption, absence of exercise
• Advise patient to notify prescriber if pregnancy suspected, planned, or if breastfeeding
• Teach patient to report confusion, injection-site reactions

Evaluation
• Positive therapeutic response: Decreased cholesterol, LDL; increased HDL

RARELY USED

exemestane (Rx)
(x-ee-mes'tane)
Aromasin
Func. class.: Antineoplastic
Chem. class.: Aromatase inhibitor

Therapeutic outcome: Prevention of rapidly growing malignant cells

USES: Advanced breast carcinoma that has not responded to other therapy in estrogen receptor–positive patients (postmenopausal), estrogen receptor-positive early breast cancer that has received tamoxifen

CONTRAINDICATIONS
Pregnancy, breastfeeding, hypersensitivity, premenopausal women

DOSAGE AND ROUTES
Adult: PO 25 mg/day after meals; may need 50 mg/day if taken with a potent CYP3A4 inhibitor

---

⚠ HIGH ALERT

exenatide (Rx)
(ex-en'a-tide)
Bydureon, Byetta
Func. class.: Antidiabetic
Chem. class.: Incretin mimetic

ACTION: Binds and activates known human GLP-1 receptor, mimics natural physiology for self-regulating glycemic control

Therapeutic outcome: Decreased polyuria, polydipsia, polyphagia; improved Hgb A1c

USES: Type 2 diabetes mellitus given in combination with metformin, sulfonylurea, or a thiazolidinedione, insulin glargine

Pharmacokinetics	
Absorption	Well
Distribution	Unknown
Metabolism	Unknown
Excretion	Glomerular filtration
Half-life	

Pharmacodynamics 2.4 h	
Onset	Unknown
Peak	Immediate release: 2.1 hr; ext rel: 2 wk
Duration	Unknown

CONTRAINDICATIONS
Hypersensitivity

BLACK BOX WARNING: Medullary thyroid carcinoma, multiple endocrine neoplasia syndrome type 2 (MEN-2), thyroid cancer

Precautions: Pregnancy, geriatric, severe renal/hepatic/GI disease, vitamin D deficiency

DOSAGE AND ROUTES
Adult: SUBCUT 5 mcg bid 1 hr before morning and evening meal; may increase to 10 mcg bid after 1 mo; ext rel subcut (Bydureon) 2 mg q7 days; ext rel inj 2 mg q7 days

Renal dose
Adult: PO CCr 30-50 mL/min, use caution when increasing dose

Available forms: Inj 5, 10 mcg pen; ext rel powder for susp for inj 2 mg

ADVERSE EFFECTS

CNS: *Headache, dizziness,* jittery feeling, restlessness, weakness

ENDO: Hypoglycemia, thyroid hyperplasia

GI: Nausea, vomiting, diarrhea, dyspepsia, anorexia, gastroesophageal reflux, weight loss, pancreatitis

SYST: Angioedema, anaphylaxis

INTEG: Serious injection-site reactions (cellulitis, abscess, skin necrosis)

INTERACTIONS
Individual drugs

Acetaminophen: may decrease the effect of acetaminophen

Acetaminophen (elixir), digoxin, lovastatin: decreased action of these products

Alcohol, disopyramide: increased hypoglycemia

Dextrothyroxine, niacin, triamterene: decreased hypoglycemia efficacy

Erythromycin, metoclopramide: do not use with exenatide

Drug classifications

ACE inhibitors, anabolic steroids, androgens, fibric acid derivatives, sulfonylureas: increased hypoglycemia

Corticosteroids, phenothiazines: increased hyperglycemia

Estrogens, MAOIs, oral contraceptives, progestins, thiazide diuretics: decreased hypoglycemia

NURSING CONSIDERATIONS
Assessment

• Monitor fasting blood, glucose, A1c levels, postprandial glucose during treatment to determine diabetes control

• **Pancreatitis:** severe abdominal pain, with/without vomiting; product should be discontinued

• Assess for hypo/hyperglycemic reaction that can occur soon after meals; for severe hypoglycemia give **IV** D₅W, then **IV** dextrose solution

• **Anaphylaxis, angioedema:** product should be discontinued immediately

• Assess for nausea, diarrhea, vomiting, ability to tolerate product, may cause dehydration

• **Pregnancy/breastfeeding:** Use only if benefits clearly outweigh risks, if pregnant enroll in the Exenatide Pregnancy Registry 800-633-9081, do not breastfeed

Patient problem
Excess food intake (uses)

Implementation

• Store in refrigerator; unopened pen may be stored at room temperature after opening for up to 30 days

Subcut route (regular release—Byetta)

• Give SUBCUT only, do not give **IV/IM**

• Pen needles must be purchased separately and be compatible

• Prime prior to use

• Inject into thigh, abdomen, upper arm

Subcut route (extended release—Bydureon)

• Give 1× wk; the dose can be given at any time of day, without regard to meals

• Available as a single dose tray containing a vial of 2 mg, a prefilled syringe delivering 0.65 ml diluent, a vial connector, and two custom needles (23G, 5/16″) specific to this delivery system (one is a spare needle); do not substitute needles or any other components

• Inject immediately after the white/off-white powder is suspended in the diluent and transferred to the syringe

• Inject subcutaneously into the thigh, abdomen, or upper arm; rotate sites to prevent lipodystrophy

• Give 1 hr before meals, approximately 6 hr apart; if patient is NPO, may need to hold dose to prevent hypoglycemia

• Store in refrigerator; unopened pen may be stored at room temperature after opening for up to 30 days

• If added to insulin glargine, insulin detemir, a dosage reduction in these products may be required

Patient/family education

• Teach patient symptoms of hypo/hyperglycemia, what to do about each; to have glucagon emergency kit available; to carry a glucose source (candy, sugar cube) to treat hypoglycemia

• Advise patient that product must be continued on daily or weekly basis (ext rel); explain consequences of discontinuing product abruptly

• Teach patient that diabetes is a lifelong illness; product will not cure disease

• Advise patient to carry emergency ID with prescriber and medications

• Advise patient to continue weight control, dietary restrictions, exercise, hygiene

• Inform patient that regular blood glucose monitoring and A1c testing is needed

• Advise patient to notify prescriber if pregnant or intend to become pregnant

• Advise patient to read "Information for the Patient" and "Pen User Manual"; provide education on self-injection

• **Pancreatitis:** if severe abdominal pain with or without vomiting occurs, seek medical attention immediately

E

• Review injection procedure, to store product in refrigerator, room temperature after first use, discard 30 days after first use, do not freeze, protect from light (Byetta)

Evaluation
Positive therapeutic outcome
• Decrease in polyuria, polydipsia, polyphagia, clear sensorium; improved A1c, weight; absence of dizziness, stable gait

---

ezetimibe (Rx)
(ehz-eh-tim′bee)
Ezetrol ✦, Zetia
Func. class.: Antilipemic

ACTION: Inhibits absorption of cholesterol by the small intestine

Therapeutic outcome: Decreased cholesterol levels

USES: Hypercholesterolemia, homozygous familial hypercholesterolemia (HoFH), homozygous sitosterolemia

Pharmacokinetics

Absorption	Variable
Distribution	Unknown
Metabolism	Small intestine, liver
Excretion	Urine (11%), feces (78%)
Half-life	22 hr

Pharmacodynamics
Unknown

CONTRAINDICATIONS
Hypersensitivity, severe hepatic disease

Precautions: Pregnancy, breastfeeding, children, hepatic disease

DOSAGE AND ROUTES
Adult: PO 10 mg/day

Available forms: Tabs 10 mg

ADVERSE EFFECTS
CNS: Fatigue, dizziness, headache
GI: Diarrhea, abdominal pain
MISC: Chest pain
MS: *Myalgias, arthralgias,* back pain, myopathy, rhabdomyolysis

RESP: Pharyngitis, sinusitis, cough, URI
EENT: Sinusitis, nasopharyngitis

INTERACTIONS
Individual drugs
Cholestyramine: decreased ezetimibe action
CycloSPORINE: increased action of ezetimibe

Drug classifications
Antacids: decreased action of ezetimibe
Fibric acid derivatives, bile acid sequestrants: increased ezetimibe action

Drug/lab test
Increase: LFTs

NURSING CONSIDERATIONS
Assessment
• **Hypercholesterolemia:** obtain diet history; monitor fat content, lipid levels (triglycerides, LDL, HDL, total cholesterol), LFTs baseline and periodically during treatment
• **Myopathy/rhabdomyolysis:** monitor for increased CPK; myalgia, muscle cramps, musculoskeletal pain, lethargy, fatigue, fever; more common when combined with statins
• **Pregnancy/breastfeeding:** Do not use in pregnancy, breastfeeding

Patient problem
Nonadherence (teaching)

Implementation
• Give without regard to meals

Patient/family education
• Teach patient that compliance is needed
• Advise that risk factors should be decreased: high-fat diet, smoking, alcohol consumption, absence of exercise
• Advise patient to notify prescriber if pregnancy is suspected or planned or if breastfeeding
• Advise patient to notify prescriber if unexplained weakness, or muscle pain is present
• Teach patient to notify prescriber of dietary/herbal supplements

Evaluation
Positive therapeutic outcome
• Decreased cholesterol

---

famciclovir (Rx)

(fam-sye-klo'vir)

Famvir ✦

Func. class.: Antiviral
Chem. class.: Guanosine nucleoside

ACTION: Inhibits DNA polymerase and viral DNA synthesis by conversion of this guanosine nucleoside to penciclovir

Therapeutic outcome: Decreasing size and number of lesions

USES: Treatment of acute herpes zoster (shingles), genital herpes, recurrent mucocutaneous herpes simplex virus (HSV) in HIV patients, initial episodes of herpes genitalis, herpes labialis in the immunocompromised

Pharmacokinetics

Absorption	Well absorbed, 77%
Distribution	Protein binding 20%
Metabolism	Intestinal tissue, blood, liver
Excretion	Breast milk, kidney, bile
Half-life	2-3 hr

Pharmacodynamics

Onset	Rapid
Peak	1 hr
Duration	12 hrs

CONTRAINDICATIONS

Hypersensitivity to this product, penciclovir, acyclovir, ganciclovir, valacyclovir, or valganciclovir

Precautions: Pregnancy, breastfeeding, renal disease, lactose intolerance

DOSAGE AND ROUTES

Herpes zoster
Adult: PO 500 mg q8hr × 7 days

Renal dose
Adult: PO; CCr 40-59 ml/min 500 mg q12hr; 20-39 ml/min 500 mg q24hr; CCr <20 ml/min 250 mg q24hr

Suppression of recurrent herpes simplex
Adult: PO 250 mg q12hr up to 1 yr

Renal dose: CCr 60 ml/min or greater, usual dose; CCr 40 to 59 ml/min, 750 mg as a single dose; CCr 20 to 39 ml/min, 500 mg as a single dose; CCr less than 20 ml/min, 250 mg as a single dose; hemodialysis, 250 mg as a single dose after dialysis

Recurrent genital herpes simplex
Adult: PO 1000 mg bid in a single dose

Renal dose
Adult: PO CCr 40-59 ml/min 500 mg q12hr × 1 day; CCr 20-39 ml/min 500 mg as a single dose; CCr <20 ml/min 250 mg as a single dose

Available forms: Tabs 125, 250, 500 mg

ADVERSE EFFECTS

CNS: *Headache, fatigue, dizziness,* fever, seizures
GI: Nausea, vomiting, diarrhea, anorexia
GU: Decreased sperm count
INTEG: *Pruritus,* vasculitis
SYST: Anaphylaxis

INTERACTIONS

Individual drugs
Probenecid: increased effect of famciclovir
Zoster vaccine: decreased effect of vaccine, varicella virus

NURSING CONSIDERATIONS

Assessment
• **Herpes zoster:** assess number and severity of the breakout; also burning, itching, or pain (early symptoms of herpes infection); neuralgia during, after treatment; monitor for postherpetic neuralgia
• **Acute renal failure:** usually in high doses or in those >65 yr; monitor renal function tests: urine CCr, BUN before, during treatment if patient has decreased renal function; dosage may need to be lowered; hepatic studies: LFTs
• Monitor bowel pattern before, during treatment; diarrhea may occur
• Assess for posttherapeutic neuralgia during and after treatment
• **Pregnancy/breastfeeding:** Use only if benefits outweigh fetal risk, enroll pregnant patient in Fanvir Pregnancy Registry (888-689-6682), use if potential benefits to the mother outweigh risks to the infant

Patient problem
Infection (uses)

Implementation
• Give with or without meals; absorption does not appear to be lowered when taken with food
• Give within 72 hr of the appearance of rash in herpes zoster

Patient/family education
• Teach patient how to recognize signs of beginning of infection (pain, itching, tingling); use product within 48 hr of rash
• Teach patient how to prevent the spread of infection to others, that until crusting of lesions

---

has taken place, not to be around those who have not had the chicken pox vaccine or those who are immunocompromised, that product must be taken for whole course of treatment
• Teach patient reason for medication and expected results
• Teach patient to avoid driving or other hazardous activities until results are known, dizziness may occur
• Advise patient that this medication does not prevent spread of disease to others, that condoms should be used
• Advise women with genital herpes to have yearly Pap smears; cervical cancer is more likely

Evaluation
Positive therapeutic outcome
• Decreased size and spread of lesions
• Prevention of recurrence (genital herpes)
• Decreased time for healing

famotidine (Rx, OTC)
(fa-moe′ti-deen)
Acid Control ✤, Pepcid, Pepcid AC, Peptic Guard ✤, Ulcidine ✤
Func. class.: H$_2$-histamine receptor antagonist, antiulcer agent

ACTION: Inhibits histamine at H$_2$-receptor site in gastric parietal cells, which inhibits gastric acid secretion while pepsin remains at a stable level

Therapeutic outcome: Healing of duodenal ulcers or gastric ulcers; prevention of duodenal ulcers; decreases symptoms of gastroesophageal reflux disease or Zollinger-Ellison syndrome, heartburn

USES: Short-term treatment of duodenal ulcer, maintenance therapy for duodenal ulcer, Zollinger-Ellison syndrome, multiple endocrine adenomas, gastric ulcers, heartburn, gastroesophageal reflux disease

Unlabeled uses: GI disorders in those taking NSAIDs, urticaria, prevention of stress ulcers, aspiration pneumonitis, prevention of paclitaxel hypersensitivity reactions

Pharmacokinetics

Absorption	50% absorbed (PO)
Distribution	Plasma, protein binding (15%-20%), breast milk, CSF
Metabolism	Liver (30% active metabolizing)
Excretion	Kidneys (70%)
Half-life	2½-3½ hr

Pharmacodynamics

	PO	IV
Onset	60 min	Immediate
Peak	1-3 hr	1-4 hr
Duration	12 hr	8-12 hr

CONTRAINDICATIONS
Hypersensitivity

Precautions: Pregnancy, breastfeeding, children <12 yr, geriatric, severe renal/hepatic disease

DOSAGE AND ROUTES
Short-term treatment of gastric ulcer
Adult: PO 40 mg/day at bedtime × 4-8 wk, then 20 mg/day at bedtime if needed (maintenance); IV 20 mg q12hr if unable to take PO
Child 1-16 yr: PO/IV 0.25 mg/kg/dose q 12 hr, max 40 mg/day

Short-term treatment of duodenal ulcer
Adult: PO 40 mg at bedtime or 20 mg bid, maintenance 20 mg qday at bedtime

Pathologic hypersecretory conditions
Adult: PO 20 mg q6hr; up to 160 mg q6hr if needed; IV 20 mg q12hr if unable to take PO
Child 1-16 yr: PO 1 mg/kg/day in two divided doses, max 40 mg bid
Child 3 mo to <1 yr: PO 0.5 mg/kg/dose bid ≤ 8 wk; child <30 mo: PO 0.5 mg/kg/dose qday, ≤8 wk

GERD
Adult: PO 20 mg bid ≤ 6 wk; 40 mg bid ≤ 2 wk (ulcerative esophagitis)

Heartburn relief/prevention (OTC)
Adult: PO 10 mg with water, 15 min-1 hr before eating

Renal dose
Adult: PO CCr <50 ml/min; give 50% of dose or extend interval to q36-48hr

Available forms: Tabs 10, 20, 40 mg; powder for oral susp 40 mg/5 ml; inj 0.4 mg/ml premixed in normal saline, 10 mg/ml, 20 mg/ 50 ml 0.9% NaCl; orally disintegrating tabs (RPD) 20, 40 mg; chew tabs 10 mg

ADVERSE EFFECTS
CNS: *Headache, dizziness,* paresthesia, depression, anxiety, somnolence, insomnia, fever, seizures in renal disease
CV: Dysrhythmias, QT prolongation (impaired renal functioning)
EENT: Taste change, tinnitus, orbital edema

GI: *Constipation,* nausea, vomiting, anorexia, cramps, abnormal liver enzymes, diarrhea
HEMA: Thrombocytopenia, aplastic anemia
INTEG: Rash, toxic epidermal necrolysis, Stevens-Johnson syndrome
MS: Myalgia, arthralgia
RESP: Pneumonia

INTERACTIONS
Individual drugs
Cefditoren, cefpodoxime, itraconazole, ketoconazole: decreased absorption of each specific product
Atazanivir, delavirdine: decreased effects of each specific product

Drug classifications
Antacids: decreased absorption of famotidine

NURSING CONSIDERATIONS
Assessment
• **Assess patient with ulcers or suspected ulcers:** epigastric, abdominal pain, hematemesis, occult blood in stools, blood in gastric aspirate before treatment; throughout treatment, monitor gastric pH (maintain at pH 5)
• **Renal function:** Patients with decreased renal function are at risk for prolonged QT
• Monitor I&O ratio, BUN, creatinine, CBC with differential monthly
• **Beers:** Avoid in older adults with or at high risk of delirium, may induce or worsen delirium, assess for confusion, healing of duodenal ulcers, decreased gastroesophageal reflux

Patient problems
Pain (uses)

Implementation
PO route
• Administer oral susp after shaking well; discard unused sol after 1 mo
• Store in cool environment (oral)

Direct IV route
• Give **IV** direct after diluting 2 ml of product (10 mg/ml) in 0.9% NaCl to total volume of 5-10 ml; inject over 2 min to prevent hypotension
Intermittent IV infusion route
• Administer after diluting 20 mg of product in 100 ml of LR, 0.9% NaCl, D_5W, $D_{10}W$; run over 15-30 min
Continuous IV infusion route
• **Adults:** Dilute 40 mg/250 ml D_5W or NS, infuse over 24 hr, run at 11 ml/hr, use infusion device
• Store in cool environment (oral); **IV** sol is stable for 48 hr at room temperature; do not use discolored sol

Y-site compatibilities: Acyclovir, allopurinol, amifostine, aminophylline, amphotericin, ampicillin, ampicillin/sulbactam, inamrinone, amsacrine, atropine, aztreonam, bretylium, calcium gluconate, ceFAZolin, cefoperazone, cefotaxime, cefoTEtan, cefOXitin, cefTAZidime, ceftizoxime, cefTRIAXone, cefuroxime, cephalothin, cephapirin, chlorproMAZINE, CISplatin, cladribine, cyclophosphamide, cytarabine, dexamethasone, dextran 40, digoxin, diphenhydrAMINE, DOBUTamine, DOPamine, DOXOrubicin, droperidol, enalaprilat, EPINEPHrine, erythromycin lactobionate, esmolol, filgrastim, fluconazole, fludarabine, folic acid, gentamicin, granisetron, haloperidol, heparin, hydrocortisone, HYDROmorphone, hydrOXYzine, imipenem/cilastatin, regular insulin, isoproterenol, labetalol, lidocaine, LORazepam, magnesium sulfate, melphalan, meperidine, methotrexate, methylPREDNISolone, metoclopramide, mezlocillin, midazolam, morphine, nafcillin, nitroglycerin, nitroprusside, norepinephrine, ondansetron, oxacillin, PACLitaxel, perphenazine, phenylephrine, phenytoin, phytonadione, piperacillin, potassium chloride, potassium phosphate, procainamide, propofol, sargramostim, sodium bicarbonate, teniposide, theophylline, thiamine, thiotepa, ticarcillin, ticarcillin-clavulanate, verapamil, vinorelbine

Patient/family education
• Caution patient to avoid driving, other hazardous activities until stabilized on this medication; dizziness may occur
• Advise patient to avoid black pepper, caffeine, alcohol, harsh spices, NSAIDs, extremes in temperature of food; tell patient to avoid OTC preparations: aspirin, cough/cold preparations; condition may worsen
• Advise patient to avoid taking OTC and prescription preparations of this product concurrently, do not take for extended periods, risk of B_{12} malabsorption
• Tell patient that smoking decreases the effectiveness of the product; that smoking cessation should be considered
• Instruct patient that product must be continued for prescribed time to be effective and taken exactly as prescribed; doses are not to be doubled; take missed dose when remembered up to 1 hr before next dose
• Tell patient to report diarrhea, black tarry stools, sore throat, rash, dizziness, confusion, or delirium to prescriber immediately

Evaluation

Positive therapeutic outcome
• Decreased pain in abdomen
• Healing of ulcers, decreased gastroesophageal reflux

febuxostat (Rx)
(feb-ux'oh-stat)
Uloric
Func. class.: Antigout drug, antihyperuri-cemic
Chem. class.: Xanthine oxidase inhibitor

ACTION: Inhibits the enzyme xanthine oxidase, reducing uric acid synthesis; more selective for xanthine oxidase than allopurinol

Therapeutic outcome: Decreased signs/symptoms of gout, hyperuricemia

USES: Chronic gout, hyperuricemia

Pharmacokinetics

Absorption	50%
Distribution	Protein binding 99.2%, max lowering of uric acid 2 wk
Metabolism	Extensive liver
Excretion	Feces, urine
Half-life	5-8 hr

Pharmacodynamics (blood level)

Onset	Rapid
Peak	1-1.5 hr
Duration	Up to 24 hr

CONTRAINDICATIONS
Hypersensitivity

Precautions: Pregnancy, breastfeeding, children, renal/hepatic/cardiac/neoplastic disease, stroke, MI, organ transplant, Lesch-Nyhan syndrome

DOSAGE AND ROUTES
Adult: PO 40 mg daily, may increase to 80 mg daily if uric acid levels are >6 mg/dl after 2 wk of therapy

Available forms: Tabs 40, 80 mg

ADVERSE EFFECTS
CNS: Dizziness
CV: MI, atrial fibrillation, atrial flutter, AV block, bradycardia, hyper/hypotension, palpitations, sinus tachycardia, stroke, angina
GI: *Nausea*
GU: Renal failure, urinary urgency/frequency/incontinence, nephrolithiasis, hematuria
INTEG: Rash
MISC: Arthralgia, gout flare

INTERACTIONS
Individual drugs
AzaTHIOprine, didanosine, mercaptopurine: do not use together increased toxicity

Rasburicase: increased xanthine nephropathy, calculi

Drug classifications
Antineoplastics: increased xanthine nephropathy, calculi
Increase: Effect of theophylline

Drug/lab
Increase: LFTs, alkaline phosphatase, serum cholesterol, triglycerides, amylase, BUN, creatinine, aPTT, PT, CPK, creatine
Decrease: Hct/Hgb, RBC, platelets, lymphocytes, neutrophils, TSH, blood glucose

NURSING CONSIDERATIONS
Assessment
• **Hyperuricemia:** Monitor uric acid levels q2wk; uric acid levels should be 6 mg/dl or less
• Hepatic studies prior to use, then at 2, 4 mo, and then periodically; assess for fatigue, anorexia, right upper abdominal discomfort, dark urine, jaundice
• **Renal disease:** Monitor I&O ratio; increase fluids to 2 L/day to prevent stone formation and toxicity
• Assess for rash, hypersensitivity reactions; discontinue
• **Assess for gout:** joint pain, swelling; may use with NSAIDs for acute gouty attacks and gout flare (first 6 wk)

Patient problem
Pain (uses)

Implementation
PO route
• Give without regard to meals or antacid; may crush and add to foods or fluids

Patient/family education
• Inform patient that tabs may be crushed
• Teach patient to take as prescribed; if dose is missed, take as soon as remembered; do not double dose
• Teach patient to increase fluid intake to 2 L/day unless contraindicated
• Advise patient to avoid alcohol, caffeine; will increase uric acid levels
• Advise patient to report cardiovascular events to prescriber immediately (chest pain, dyspnea, slurred speech, weakness)
• **Gout:** teach patient that flares may occur during first 6 wk of treatment, continue and notify prescriber

Evaluation
Positive therapeutic outcome
• Decreased pain in joints, decreased stone formation in kidneys, decreased uric acid levels

felodipine (Rx)

(feh-loh'dih-peen)

Plenedil ✦

Func. class.: Calcium-channel blocker, antihypertensive, antianginal

Chem. class.: Dihydropyridine

ACTION: Inhibits calcium ion influx across cell membrane, resulting in inhibition of excitation/contraction of vascular smooth muscle

Therapeutic outcome: Decreased B/P in hypertension

USES: Essential hypertension, alone or with other antihypertensives

Pharmacokinetics

Absorption	Well absorbed
Distribution	Unknown; protein binding >99%
Metabolism	Liver, extensively
Excretion	Kidneys, unchanged, minimal
Half-life	11-16 hr

Pharmacodynamics

Onset	1 hr
Peak	2½-5 hr
Duration	<24 hr

CONTRAINDICATIONS

Hypersensitivity to this product or dihydropyridines, sick sinus syndrome, 2nd- or 3rd-degree heart block, hypotension <90 mm Hg systolic

Precautions: Pregnancy, breastfeeding, children, geriatric, HF, hepatic injury, renal disease, coronary artery disease

DOSAGE AND ROUTES

Adult: PO 5 mg/day initially, usual range 2.5-10 mg/day; max 10 mg/day; do not adjust dosage at intervals of <2 wk

Geriatric: PO 2.5 mg/day, max 10 mg/day

Hepatic dose

Adult: PO 2.5-5 mg/day, max 10 mg/day

Available forms: Ext rel tabs 2.5, 5, 10 mg

ADVERSE EFFECTS

CNS: *Headache*, fatigue, drowsiness, dizziness, anxiety, depression, nervousness, insomnia, light-headedness, paresthesia, tinnitus, psychosis, somnolence

CV: Dysrhythmias, *edema*, HF, hypotension, palpitations, MI, pulmonary edema, tachycardia, syncope, AV block, angina

GI: Nausea, vomiting, diarrhea, gastric upset, constipation, dry mouth

GU: Nocturia, polyuria, sexual dysfunction, decreased libido

HEMA: Anemia

INTEG: Rash, pruritus, peripheral edema

MISC: Flushing, sexual difficulties, cough, nasal congestion, shortness of breath, wheezing, epistaxis, respiratory infection, chest pain, angioedema, gingival hyperplasia, Stevens-Johnson syndrome

INTERACTIONS

Individual drugs

Alcohol, carBAMazepine, cimetidine, clarithromycin, conivaptan, cycloSPORINE, dalfopristin, delavirdine, dilTIAZem, erythromycin, itraconazole, ketoconazole, miconazole, phenytoin, propanolol, quiNIDine, quinupristin, zileuton: increased hypotension

Digoxin, disopyramide, phenytoin: increased bradycardia, increased HF

Drug classifications

β-Adrenergic blockers: increased bradycardia, HF

Nitrates: increased hypotension

NSAIDs: decreased antihypertensive effects

Drug/herb

Ginkgo, ginseng, hawthorn: increased antihypertensive effect

Ephedra, St. John's wort: decreased antihypertensive effect

Drug/food

Grapefruit juice: increased felodipine level

NURSING CONSIDERATIONS

Assessment

• **HF:** Assess fluid volume status: I&O ratio and record; weight; skin turgor; adequacy of pulses; moist mucous membranes; bilateral lung sounds; peripheral pitting edema; dehydration symptoms of decreasing output, thirst, hypotension, dry mouth, and mucous membranes should be reported; for HF: weight gain, crackles, dyspnea, edema, jugular venous distention

• Monitor ALT, AST, bilirubin often if these are elevated

• Monitor cardiac status: B/P, pulse, respiration, ECG periodically during prolonged treatment

• **Assess for anginal pain:** duration; intensity; ameliorating, aggravating factors; **Hypertension:** Check for compliance, number of refills

• **Pregnancy/breastfeeding:** Fetal anomalies have occurred, avoid use in pregnancy, do not breastfeed

Patient problem
Ineffective tissue perfusion (uses)
Pain (uses)

Implementation
PO route
• Do not break, crush, or chew ext rel tabs
• Give once a day with food for GI symptoms

Patient/family education
• Caution patient to avoid hazardous activities until stabilized on product and dizziness is no longer a problem
• Instruct patient to limit caffeine consumption; to avoid alcohol and OTC products unless directed by prescriber
• **Urge patient to comply in all areas of medical regimen:** diet, exercise, stress reduction, product therapy; to notify prescriber of irregular heartbeat, shortness of breath, swelling of feet and hands, pronounced dizziness, constipation, nausea, hypotension
• Advise patient to use protective clothing, sunscreen to prevent photosensitivity
• Teach patient to change positions slowly to prevent orthostatic hypotension
• Advise patient to obtain correct pulse; to contact prescriber if pulse is <50 bpm
• Teach patient to use as directed even if feeling better; may be taken with other CV products (nitrates, β-blockers); that capsules may appear in stools but are insignificant
• Teach patient to practice good oral hygiene to prevent gingival hyperplasia
• Advise patient not to stop medication abruptly
• Advise patient to avoid grapefruit juice

Evaluation

Positive therapeutic outcome
• B/P within normal limits
• Decreased anginal attacks
• Increase in activity tolerance

---

fenofibrate (Rx)
(fen-oh-fee′brate)
Antara, Lipidil EZ ✦, Lipidil ✦, Lipidil Supra ✦, Lipofem, Lipofen, Lofibra, Tricor, Triglide
Func. class.: Antilipemic
Chem. class.: Fibric acid derivative

Do not confuse: Tricor/Tracleer

ACTION: Increases lipolysis and elimination of triglyceride-rich particles from plasma by activating lipoprotein lipase, resulting in triglyceride change in size and composition of LDL, leading to rapid breakdown of LDL; mobilizes triglycerides from tissue; increases excretion of neutral sterols

Therapeutic outcome: Decreasing cholesterol levels and low-density lipoproteins, decreased pruritus

USES: Hypercholesterolemia, patients with types IV, V hyperlipidemia who do not respond to other treatment and who are at risk for pancreatitis; Fredrickson type IV, V hypertriglyceridemia

Pharmacokinetics

Absorption	60%
Distribution	Protein binding 99%
Metabolism	Liver to fenofibric acid
Excretion	Urine 60%, feces 25%
Half-life	20 hr

Pharmacodynamics (triglyceride lowered)

Onset	Unknown
Peak	2 wk
Duration	Unknown

CONTRAINDICATIONS
Hypersensitivity, severe renal/hepatic disease, primary biliary cirrhosis, preexisting gallbladder disease, breastfeeding

Precautions: Pregnancy, geriatric, peptic ulcer, pancreatitis, renal/hepatic disease, diabetes mellitus

DOSAGE AND ROUTES
Hypertriglyceridemia
Adult: PO (Antara) 30-90 mg/day; (Fenoglide) 40-120 mg/day; (Lofibra) 67-200 mg/day; (Tricor) 48-145 mg/day; (Triglide) 50-160 mg/day; Lipofen) 50 mg qday

Primary hypercholesterolemia/mixed hyperlipidemia
Adult: PO (Antara) 90 mg/day; (Lofibra) 200 mg/day; (Tricor) 145 mg/day; (Triglide) 160 mg/day; (Lipofen) 50 mg/day

Renal dose (geriatric)
Adult: PO (Tricor) CCr 30-80 ml/min 48 mg/day; CCr <30 ml/min contraindicated; (Triglide, Lipofem) CCr 11-49 ml/min 50 mg/day; (Antara) 30 mg/day; (Lofibra) 67 mg/day; (Antara, Lipofem, Lofibra, Triglide) CCr <30 ml/min, contraindicated

Available forms: Cap: **Antara** 30, 90 mg; **Lipofen** 50, 150 mg tab: **Triglide** 50, 160 mg; **Lofibra** 54, 160 mg; **Tricor** 48, 145 mg; **Fenoglide** 40, 120 mg

ADVERSE EFFECTS
CNS: Fatigue, headache, paresthesia, drowsiness, **dizziness**

CV: Angina, **hypertension**, hypotension
GI: Nausea, **vomiting**, **dyspepsia**, **flatulence**, **hepatomegaly**, **gastritis**, pancreatitis, cholelithiasis
GU: diarrhea, constipation
HEMA: Anemia, leukopenia, thrombosis, pulmonary embolism
INTEG: *Rash*, **pruritus**
MS: **Myalgias**, **arthralgias**, myopathy, rhabdomyolysis
RESP: Pharyngitis, bronchitis, cough

INTERACTIONS
Individual drugs
CycloSPORINE: increased nephrotoxicity

Drug classifications
Anticoagulants (oral): increased effect of anticoagulants
Bile acid sequestrants: decreased absorption
HMG-CoA reductase inhibitors: do not use together, rhabdomyolysis may occur

Drug/herb
Red yeast rice: increased effects

Drug/food
Increased absorption

Drug/lab test
Increase: ALT, AST, BUN, CK, creatinine
Decrease: WBC, uric acid, Hgb

NURSING CONSIDERATIONS
Assessment
• **Hypercholesterolemia:** Hyperlipidemia: Diet history, monitor lipid levels (triglycerides, LDL, HDL, total cholesterol), fat content
• Liver function tests, baseline and periodically during treatment; if >3 × ULN, discontinue CPK if muscle pain occurs, CBC, Hct, Hgh, protime with anticoagulant therapy, serum bilirubin (total and direct)
• Assess for pancreatitis, cholelithiasis, renal failure, rhabdomyolysis (when combined with HMG-CoA reductase inhibitors), myositis; product should be discontinued; assess often for muscle pain, weakness, fever
• Assess nutrition: Obtain fat, protein, carbohydrates, nutritional analysis should be completed by dietitian
• **Pregnancy/breastfeeding:** Avoid in pregnancy unless benefits outweigh risk to the fetus, do not breastfeed

Patient problem
Nonadherence (Teaching)

Implementation
• Do not break, crush, or chew tabs
• Give with evening meal; if dose is increased, give with breakfast and evening meal (Lipofen,

Lofibra); Triglide, Antara without regard to food; may increase q4-8wk
• Brands are not interchangeable; therapy should be discontinued if there is not adequate response after 2 mo
• Store in cool environment in tight, light-resistant container
• Caps must be swallowed whole
• Protect Lipofen, Triglide, from light, moisture

Patient/family education
• Inform patient that compliance is needed
• Instruct patient not to consume chipped or broken tabs (Triglide)
• Teach patient that risk factors—high-fat diet, smoking, alcohol consumption, absence of exercise—should be decreased
• Caution patient to notify prescriber if pregnancy is planned or suspected, not to breastfeed
• Teach patient to notify prescriber if the GI symptoms of diarrhea, abdominal or epigastric pain, nausea, or vomiting occur
• Advise patient to notify prescriber of muscle pain, weakness, fever, fatigue, epigastric pain

Evaluation
Positive therapeutic outcome
• Decrease in cholesterol to desired level after 8 wk

---

fenofibric acid (Rx)
(fen-oh-fye-brick)
TriLipix, Fibricor
Func. class.: Antilipemic
Chem. class.: Fibric acid derivative

ACTION: An active metabolite of fenofibrate; increases lipolysis and elimination of triglyceride-rich particles from plasma by activating lipoprotein lipase, resulting in triglyceride change in size and composition of LDL, leading to rapid breakdown of LDL; mobilizes triglycerides from tissue; increases excretion of neutral sterols

Therapeutic outcome: Triglyceride level returning to normal

USES: Hyperlipoproteinemia; hypertriglyceridemia

Pharmacokinetics

Absorption	Unknown
Distribution	Protein binding 99%
Metabolism	Liver, converted to fenofibric acid
Excretion	Urine 60%
Half-life	20 hr

Pharmacodynamics

Onset	Unknown
Peak	4-5 hr (del rel cap), 2.5 hr (tab)
Duration	Unknown

CONTRAINDICATIONS: Hypersensitivity, severe renal/hepatic disease, primary biliary cirrhosis, preexisting gallbladder disease, breastfeeding

Precautions: Pregnancy, geriatric, pancreatitis, thromboembolic disease

DOSAGE AND ROUTES
Combination with HMG-CoA reductase inhibitors to reduce triglycerides and increase HDL-C in those with mixed dyslipidemia or coronary heart disease
Adult: DEL REL cap PO 135 mg daily

Severe hypertriglyceridemia
Adult: DEL REL cap PO 45-135 daily; tabs 35-105 mg daily

Renal dose
Adult: PO CCr 30-80 ml/min 35 mg (Fibricor) or 45 mg (TriLipix) q day, initially; CCr <30 ml/min, do not use

Available forms: Tabs 35, 105 mg; cap (Fibricor), gastro-resistant pellet 45, 135 mg (TriLipix)

ADVERSE EFFECTS
CNS: Fatigue, weakness, drowsiness, dizziness, insomnia, depression, vertigo, asthenia, headache
CV: Hypertension
EENT: Blurred vision
GI: *Nausea*, vomiting, dyspepsia, increased liver enzymes, abdominal pain, cholecystitis, cholelithiasis, constipation, diarrhea, hepatitis, jaundice, pancreatitis
GU: Impotence, decreased libido
HEMA: Anemia, leukopenia, thrombosis/pulmonary embolism, agranulocytosis, eosinophilia
INTEG: *Rash*, urticaria, pruritus, Stevens-Johnson syndrome
MISC: Infection
MS: Myalgias, arthralgias, myopathy, back pain, MS pain, rhabdomyolysis
RESP: Pharyngitis, cough

INTERACTIONS
Individual drugs
CycloSPORINE: increased nephrotoxicity

Drug classifications
Monitor use with HMG-CoA reductase inhibitors; rhabdomyolysis may occur
Bile acid sequestrants: decreased absorption of fenofibrate
Oral anticoagulants: increased anticoagulant effect

Drug/herb
Glucomannan: increased effect
Gotu cola: decreased effect

Drug/food
Increase: absorption

NURSING CONSIDERATIONS
Assessment
• **Diet history:** monitor fat content, lipid levels (triglycerides, LDL, HDL, total cholesterol), LFTs baseline periodically during treatment, CBC with differential, CPK, serum bilirubin (direct/indirect)
• **Assess for pancreatitis, cholelithiasis, renal failure, rhabdomyolysis** (when combined with HMG CoA reductase inhibitors), myositis; product should be discontinued

Patient problems
Risk of injury (uses)
Nonadherence (teaching)
Lack of knowledge related to medication (teaching)

Implementation
• Give product with meals; may increase q4-8wk

Patient/family education
• Teach patient that compliance is needed
• Advise patient that risk factors should be decreased: high-fat diet, smoking, alcohol consumption, absence of exercise
• Advise patient to notify prescriber if pregnancy is suspected or planned
• Teach patient to report GU symptoms: decreased libido, impotence
• Advise patient to notify prescriber of muscle pain, weakness, fever, fatigue, epigastric pain

Evaluation:
Positive therapeutic outcome
• Decreased triglycerides

⚠ **HIGH ALERT**

fentaNYL (Rx) REMS
(fen′ta-nill)
RAN-Fentanyl ❋, **Sublimaze** ❋
fentaNYL transdermal (Rx)
Duragesic, Ionsys
Func. class.: Opioid analgesic
Chem. class.: Synthetic phenylpiperidine derivative

---

fentaNYL nasal spray (Rx)
Lazanda
fentaNYL SL spray (Rx)
Subsys
fentaNYL SL
Abstral
fentaNYL buccal
Fentora
fentaNYL lozenge
Actiq
Controlled substance schedule II

Do not confuse: fentaNYL/SUFentanil

ACTION: Inhibits ascending pain pathways in CNS, increases pain threshold, alters pain perception by binding to opiate receptors

Therapeutic outcome: Relief of pain, supplement to anesthesia

USES: Controls moderate to severe pain; preoperatively, postoperatively; adjunct to general anesthetic, adjunct to regional anesthesia; **FentaNYL:** for anesthesia as premedication, conscious sedation; **Actiq:** for breakthrough cancer pain

Pharmacokinetics

Absorption	Well absorbed (IM), completely absorbed (**IV**)
Distribution	Unknown, crosses placenta
Metabolism	Extensively, liver; 80% bound to plasma proteins
Excretion	Kidneys, up to 25% unchanged; breast milk
Half-life	IV 2-4 hr; transdermal 13-22 hr; transmucosal 7 hr; buccal 4-12 hr

Pharmacodynamics

	IM	IV	TD	TM
Onset	7-15 min	Rapid	6 hr	5-15 min
Peak	30 min	3-5 min	12-24 hr	30 min
Duration	1-2 hr	½-1 hr	72 hr	

	Intranasal	TD	Transmucosal
Onset	15-20 min	12-24 hr,	5-15 min
Peak	25-30 min	1-3 days,	30 min

CONTRAINDICATIONS
Hypersensitivity to opiates, myasthenia gravis

BLACK BOX WARNING: headache, migraine (Actiq), Astral, Fentora, Lazanda, Onsolis, emergency dept use (Abstral, Lazanda), outpatient surgeries (Duragesic TD), opioid-naïve patients, respiratory disorders, depression

Precautions: Pregnancy, breastfeeding, geriatric, increased ICP, seizure disorders, cardiac dysrhythmias, severe respiratory disorders

BLACK BOX WARNING: Children, accidental exposure, ambient temperature increase, fever, skin abrasion (TD patch), substance abuse, surgery, requires an experienced clinician

DOSAGE AND ROUTES
>> FentaNYL
Anesthetic (adjust to regional anesthesia)
Adult: IV 50-100 mcg/kg over 1-2 min, max 150 mcg/kg

Anesthesia supplement to general anesthesia
Adult and child >12 yr: Low dose 1-2 mcg/kg; (IV) **moderate dose** 2-20 mcg/kg; High dose 20-50 mcg/kg, then 25 mcg to half initial loading dose as needed

Induction and maintenance
Child 2-12 yr: IV 2-3 mcg/kg

Preoperatively
Adult and child >12 yr: IM/IV 50-100 mcg q30-60 min before surgery

Postoperatively
Adult and child >12 yr: IM/IV 50-100 mcg q1-2hr prn

Moderate/severe pain
Adult: IV/IM 50-100 mcg q1-2hr
Nasal: 100 mcg spray in one nostril, titrate stepwise

>> Actiq
Adult: Transmucosal 200 mcg, redose if needed 15 min after completion of 1st dose, max 2 doses during titration period, max 4 doses/day

>> Fentora
Adult: BUCCAL/SL 100 mcg placed above rear molar between upper cheek and gum, a second 100 mcg dose, if needed, may be started 30 min after first dose

>> ABSTRAL
Adult: SL 100 mcg, another dose may be taken 30 min after first, max 2 doses per episode of breakthrough pain, ≥2 hr must elapse before treating again, titrate stepwise over consecutive episodes

---

>> FentaNYL transdermal
Adult: Duragesic: 12.5-25 mcg/hr; may increase until pain relief occurs; apply patch to flat surface on upper torso and wear for 72 hr; apply new patch to different site for continued relief; **Ionsys:** Use only after patient has been titrated to acceptable level of analgesics, one dose activation = 40 mcg TD over 10 min, max 6 (40 mcg doses/hr)

>> FentaNYL nasal spray
Adult: 100 mcg (1 spray in 1 nostril), may re-treat after ≥2 hr, titrate upward to adequate analgesia, treat a max of 4 episodes q day

>> FentaNYL SL spray
Adult: SL 100 mcg sprayed under the tongue; titrate stepwise carefully

Available forms: Inj 0.05 mg/ml; lozenges 100, 200, 300, 400, 600, 800, 1200, 1600 mcg; lozenges on a stick 200, 400, 600, 800, 1200, 1600 mcg; buccal tab 100, 200, 400, 600, 800 mcg; transdermal patch 12, 25, 50, 75, 100 mcg/hr; SL tab (ABSTRAL) 100, 200, 300, 400, 600, 800 mcg; SL spray: 100, 200,400,600, 1200, 1600 mcg/spray; nasal spray 100, 400 mcg/actuation

ADVERSE EFFECTS
CNS: Dizziness, delirium, euphoria, sedation, confusion, weakness, dizziness, seizures
CV: Bradycardia, cardiac arrest, hypo/hypertension, DVT, PE
EENT: Blurred vision, miosis
GI: Nausea, vomiting, constipation
GU: Urinary retention
INTEG: Rash, diaphoresis
MS: Muscle rigidity
RESP: Respiratory depression, arrest, laryngospasm

INTERACTIONS
Individual drugs
Alcohol: increased respiratory depression, hypotension, increased sedation

> **BLACK BOX WARNING:** Cimetidine, conivaptan, cycloSPORINE, fluconazole, itraconazole, ketoconazole, nefazodone, ranolazine, zafirlukast, zileuton: increased fentaNYL effect, fatal respiratory depression, CYP3A4 inhibitors

diazePAM: increased CV depression
Droperidol: increased hypotension

Drug classifications
Antipsychotics, opioids, skeletal muscle relaxants: effects increased, protease inhibitors
CNS depressants, sedative/hypnotics: increased respiratory depression, hypotension

CYP3A4 inducers (carBAMazepine, PHENobarbital, phenytoin, rifampin): decreased fentaNYL effect
MAOIs: increased fatal reactions

Drug/herb
St. John's wort, valerian: increased fentaNYL action
Echinacea: decreased effect of fentaNYL

Drug/lab test
Increased: amylase, lipase

NURSING CONSIDERATIONS
Assessment
• Monitor VS after parenteral route (B/P, pulse, respiration); note muscle rigidity; take drug history before administering product; check renal/liver function tests

> **BLACK BOX WARNING:** Respiratory depression: Monitor character, rate, rhythm; notify prescriber if respirations <10/min

• Monitor CNS changes: dizziness, drowsiness, hallucinations, euphoria, LOC, pupil reaction
• Monitor allergic reactions: rash, urticaria; product should be discontinued
• **Assess for pain:** intensity, location, duration, type, before and 15 min after IM route or 3-5 min after **IV** route

> **BLACK BOX WARNING: Headache, migraine:** Abstral, Actiq, Fentora, Lazanda, Onsolis are not to be used for this condition; Abstral, Lazanda is not to be used in the ED; Duragesic TD is not to be used for outpatient surgery patients

> **BLACK BOX WARNING: Apnea, respiratory arrest in opioid-naïve patients:** Do not use Abstral, Actiq, Duragesic, Fentora, Lazanda, Onsolis, opioid tolerant are those using ≥60 ml/day oral morphine, ≥30 mg/day oxyCODONE PO, 8 mg/day HYDROmorphone, 25 mcg tid fentaNYL/hr

• **Pregnancy/breastfeeding:** Use in pregnancy only if potential benefit outweighs risks, not recommended in breastfeeding
• **Beers:** Avoid in older adults unless safer alternative is not available, may cause ataxia, impaired psychomotor function

Patient problem
Pain (uses)
Risk for injury (adverse reactions)

Implementation
• Store in light-resistant area at room temperature
• Overdose has been fatal when confusing products/dose; recheck both before using

---

Transmucosal route

• Remove foil just before administration; instruct patient to place between cheek and lower gum, moving it back and forth and sucking, not chewing (Actiq); place above rear molar (Fentora); place film on the inside of the cheek (Onsolis); all products not used or partially used should be flushed down the toilet; this product may be used SL

Transdermal route

Duragesic

• Apply patch to chest on a flat area with skin intact; for skin preparation, use clear water with no soap; clip hair, skin should be dry before applying patch; apply immediately after removing from package and press firmly in place with palm of hand; flush old patch down toilet immediately upon removal

Ionsys (iontophoretic transdermal system) route:

• Apply only one system at any given time. Always wear gloves when handling

• Remove the foil pouch and the controller from the tray. Remove the drug unit from the foil pouch and place on a hard, flat surface

• Assemble the system. Align the matching shapes of the controller and the unit. Press on both ends of the device to ensure that the snaps at both ends are fully engaged. One or two clicks will be heard when the snaps are engaged

• The digital display of the controller will complete a short self-test during which there is one audible beep, the red light will blink once, and the digital display will flash the number 88. Then the display will show 0 and a green light will blink

• Choose an application site of healthy, unbroken skin on the upper outer arm or chest only. Clip excessive hair. Do not shave, as this may irritate the skin

• Clean the site with alcohol and let dry. Do not use soaps, lotions, or other agents

• Peel off and discard the clear plastic liner covering the adhesive and hydrogels. Do not pull the red tab while preparing to apply the system; the red tab is only to be used during disposal

• Press and hold the system in place for ≥ 15 sec with sticky side facing the skin. Make sure the edges adhere to the skin

• If the system loosens from the skin, secure it by pressing the edges or use a nonallergenic tape to secure the edges. Do not apply tape if skin is blistered or broken. Apply tape along the long edges of the system. Do not tape over the button, light, or digital display. After taping if the system beeps again, remove it and apply a new system on a different skin site

• To initiate administration of a dose, the patient should press the recessed button on the top housing of the system twice within 3 sec. A single beep indicates the start of dose delivery that occurs over 10 min. During this time the system is locked out and another dose cannot be delivered. When dose delivery is complete, the display will show the number of doses delivered

• Each system will function for 24 hr or 80 doses, whichever comes first. At this time, the green light will turn off and the number of doses delivered will flash on and off. To turn off the digital display, press the dosing button for 6 sec

• Remove the system from the patient's skin. Ensure both hydrogels (one contains fentanyl) remain within the removed system. If a hydrogel becomes separated during removal, use gloves or tweezers to remove it from the skin and properly dispose of in accordance with state and federal regulations for controlled substances

• Do not touch exposed hydrogel compartments or adhesive. If a hydrogel is touched accidentally, rinse the area with water. Do not use soap

• If additional analgesia is needed, a new system must be applied to a different site on the upper outer arm or chest

• *Disposal:* With gloves on, pull the red tab to separate the red bottom housing containing fentanyl from the system. Fold the red housing in half with the sticky side facing in. Dispose of the red housing per policies for disposal of schedule II drugs or by flushing it down the toilet. Hold the dosing button down until the display goes blank, and then dispose of the remaining part of the system containing electronics in waste designated for batteries

Use pain dosing

• Dosage is titrated based on patient's report of pain; dosage is determined by calculating the previous 24-hr requirement and converting to equianalgesic morphine dose

• To convert to another opioid analgesic, remove transdermal patch and begin treatment with half the equal pain-controlling dose of the new analgesic in 12-18 hr

SL spray

• Open blister package with scissors immediately prior to use; spray contents under tongue; dispose of unit by placing it into disposable bags provided; seal bag, discard into trash container out of reach of children.

IV route

• Give by inj (IM, **IV**), only with resuscitative equipment available; give slowly to prevent rigidity

• Give **IV** undiluted by anesthesiologist or diluted with 5 ml or more sterile water or 0.9% NaCl given through Y-tube or 3-way stopcock given at 0.1 mg or less/1.2 min

• Muscular rigidity may occur with rapid IV administration

Y-site compatibilities: Abciximab, acyclovir, alemtuzumab, alfentanil, alprostadil, amikacin, aminocaproic acid, aminophylline, amiodarone, amphotericin B cholesteryl, amphotericin B lipid complex, amphotericin B liposome, anidulafungin, argatroban, ascorbic acid injection, atenolol, atracurium, atropine, azaTHIOprine, aztreonam, benztropine, bivalirudin, bleomycin, bumetanide, buprenorphine, butorphanol, calcium chloride/gluconate, CARBOplatin, caspofungin, ceFAZolin, cefmetazole, cefonicid, cefotaxime, cefoTEtan, cefOXitin, cefTAZidime, ceftizoxime, ceftobiprole, cefTRIAXone, cefuroxime, cephalothin, chloramphenicol, chlorproMAZINE, cimetidine, cisatracurium, CISplatin, clindamycin, cloNIDine, cyanocobalamin, cyclophosphamide, cycloSPORINE, cytarabine, DACTINomycin, DAPTOmycin, dexamethasone, dexmedetomidine, digoxin, dilTIAZem, diphenhydrAMINE, DOBUTamine, DOCEtaxel, DOPamine, doripenem, doxacurium, doxapram, DOXOrubicin, doxycycline, enalaprilat, ePHEDrine, EPINEPHrine, epirubicin, epoetin alfa, eptifibatide, erythromycin, esmolol, etomidate, etoposide, famotidine, fenoldopam, fluconazole, fludarabine, fluorouracil, folic acid, furosemide, ganciclovir, gatifloxacin, gemcitabine, gentamicin, glycopyrrolate, granisetron, heparin, hydrocortisone, HYDROmorphone, hydrOXYzine, IDArubicin, ifosfamide, imipenem-cilastatin, inamrinone, insulin (regular), irinotecan, isoproterenol, ketorolac, labetalol, lansoprazole, levofloxacin, lidocaine, linezolid, LORazepam, LR, magnesium sulfate, mannitol, mechlorethamine, meperidine, metaraminol, methicillin, methotrexate, methotrimeprazine, methoxamine, methyldopate, methylPREDNISolone, metoclopramide, metoprolol, metroNIDAZOLE, mezlocillin, miconazole, midazolam, milrinone, minocycline, mitoXANTRONE, mivacurium, morphine, moxalactam, multiple vitamins injection, mycophenolate, nafcillin, nalbuphine, naloxone, nesiritide, netilmicin, niCARdipine, nitroglycerin, nitroprusside, norepinephrine, octreotide, ondansetron, oxacillin, oxaliplatin, oxytocin, PAClitaxel, palonosetron, pamidronate, pancuronium, papaverine, PEMEtrexed, penicillin G potassium/sodium, pentamidine, pentazocine, PENTobarbital, PHENobarbital, phenylephrine, phytonadione, piperacillin, piperacillin-tazobactam, polymyxin B, potassium chloride, procainamide, prochlorperazine, promethazine, propofol, propranolol, protamine, pyridoxine, quiNIDine, quinupristin-dalfopristin, ranitidine, remifentanil, Ringer's, ritodrine, riTUXimab, rocuronium, sargramostim, scopolamine, sodium acetate/bicarbonate, succinylcholine, SUFentanil, tacrolimus, teniposide, theophylline, thiamine, thiopental, thiotepa, ticarcillin, ticarcillin-clavulanate, tigecycline, tirofiban, TNA, tobramycin, tolazoline, TPN, trastuzumab, trimetaphan, urokinase, vancomycin, vasopressin, vecuronium, verapamil, vinCRIStine, vinorelbine, vitamin B complex/C, voriconazole, zoledronic acid

Patient/family education

• Discuss the dangers of children or pets getting the product
• Advise patient to report any symptoms of CNS changes, allergic reactions
• Instruct patient to avoid CNS depressants: alcohol, sedative-hypnotics for at least 24 hr after taking this product
• Teach patient that dizziness, drowsiness, confusion are common, and to avoid getting up without assistance
• Discuss in detail with patient all aspects of the product
• Teach patient CNS changes: physical dependence; not to use with alcohol, other CNS depressants

Transdermal route

> **BLACK BOX WARNING: Ambient temperature increase:** Discuss with patient that excessive heat may increase absorption; excessive perspiration may alter adhesiveness; do not use with heating pads, electric blankets, heat/tanning lamps, saunas, hot tubs, heated waterbeds, sunbathing

• Discuss with patient that hair may need to be clipped before applying
• Teach patient how to dispose of patch: place sticky sides together and flush in toilet
• May add first aid tape around the edges if there is a problem with adhesion, always remove old patch before applying new patch, never cut patch in half

Evaluation
Positive therapeutic outcome
• Maintenance of anesthesia
• Decreased breakthrough cancer pain
• General pain relief

TREATMENT OF OVERDOSE:
Naloxone 0.2-0.8 **IV**, O_2, **IV** fluids, vasopressors

---

ferrous fumarate (Rx)
Femiron, Feostat, Ferrate, Ferretts, Ferrocite, Hemocyte, Palafer ✿
ferrous gluconate (Rx)
Fergon
ferrous sulfate (Rx) ▨
Feosol, Fer-Gen-Sol, Fer-In-Sol, FeroSul

---

carbonyl iron (OTC)
(kar'boh-nil)
ICAR Pediatric, Iron Chews
iron polysaccharide (OTC)
iFerex, Niferex, Nu-Iron
Func. class.: Hematinic
Chem. class.: Iron preparation

ACTION: Replaces iron stores needed for red blood cell development, energy and O_2 transport, utilization; fumarate contains 33% elemental iron; gluconate, 12%; sulfate, 20%; iron, 30%; ferrous sulfate exsiccated

Therapeutic outcome: Prevention and correction of iron deficiency

USES: Iron deficiency anemia, prophylaxis for iron deficiency in pregnancy, nutritional supplementation

Pharmacokinetics

Absorption	Up to 30%
Distribution	Bound to transferrin, crosses placenta
Metabolism	Recycled
Excretion	Feces, urine, skin, breast milk
Half-life	Unknown

Pharmacodynamics

Unknown

CONTRAINDICATIONS
Sideroblastic anemia, thalassemia, hemosiderosis/hemochromatosis

Precautions: Pregnancy; anemia (longterm), peptic ulcer disease, hemolytic anemia, cirrhosis, ulcerative colitis/regional enteritis, sulfite sensitivity

> **BLACK BOX WARNING:** Accidental exposure

DOSAGE AND ROUTES
Fumarate
Adult: PO 50-100 mg tid
Child: PO 3 mg/kg/day (elemental iron) tid-qid
Infant: PO 10-25 mg/day (elemental iron) in 3-4 divided doses, max 15 mg/day

Gluconate
Adult: PO 60 mg bid-qid
Child 6-12 yr: PO 3 mg/kg/day divided

Sulfate
Adult: PO 0.75-1.5 g/day in divided doses tid
Child 6-12 yr: 600 mg/day in divided doses

Pregnancy
Adult: PO 300-600 mg/day in divided doses

Iron polysaccharide
Adult: 100-200 mg tid
Child: PO 4-6 mg/kg/day in 3 divided doses (severe iron deficiency)

Available forms: Fumarate: tabs 90, 150, 200, 300, 324, 325 mg; chewable tabs 100 mg; extended release tabs 18 mg; **gluconate:** tabs 225, 240, 324, 325 mg; **sulfate:** tabs 195, 300, 325 mg; elixir 220 mg/5 ml; dried: tabs 200 mg; ext rel tabs 160 mg; ext rel caps 160 mg; **iron polysaccharide:** tabs 50 mg; caps 150 mg; sol 100 mg/5 ml

ADVERSE EFFECTS
GI: *Nausea, constipation, epigastric pain, black and red tarry stools,* vomiting, diarrhea
INTEG: Temporarily discolored tooth enamel and eyes
SYST: Hypersensitivity reactions (Ferrlecit)

INTERACTIONS
Individual drugs
Chloramphenicol, vit C: increased absorption of iron products
Cholestyramine, ʟ-thyroxine, levodopa, methyldopa, penicillamine, tetracycline, vitamin E: decreased absorption of each product

Drug classifications
Antacids, H_2 antagonists, proton pump inhibitors: decreased absorption of iron preparations
Fluoroquinolones: decreased absorption of fluoroquinolone

Drug/food
Caffeine, dairy products, eggs: decreased absorption

Drug/lab test
False positive: occult blood

NURSING CONSIDERATIONS
Assessment
• Monitor blood studies: Hct, Hgb, reticulocytes, bilirubin before treatment, at least monthly; iron studies (Fe, TIBC, ferritin), avoid use with blood transfusions, iron overload may occur
• **Assess for toxicity:** nausea, vomiting, diarrhea (green, then tarry stools) hematemesis, pallor, cyanosis, shock, coma
• Assess bowel elimination: if constipation occurs, increase water, bulk, activity before laxatives are required
• **Assess nutrition:** amount of iron in diet (meat, dark green leafy vegetables, dried beans, dried fruits, eggs); provide referral to dietitian if indicated

• **Pregnancy/breastfeeding:** Use in pregnancy only if benefit outweighs risks to fetus, excreted in breast milk, avoid use
• Identify cause of iron loss or anemia, including salicylates, sulfonamides, antimalarials, quiNIDine

Patient problem
Activity intolerance (uses)
Diarrhea (adverse reactions)

Implementation
PO route
• Swallow all tabs whole; do not break, crush, or chew
• Give between meals for best absorption; may give with juice; do not give with antacids or milk, delay at least 1 hr; if GI symptoms occur, give after meals even if absorption is decreased; eggs, milk products, chocolate, caffeine interfere with absorption; ferrous gluconate is less GI irritating than ferrous sulfate
• Give **liquid** preparations through plastic straw to avoid discoloration of tooth enamel; dilute thoroughly
• Store in tight, light-resistant container
• Give at least 1 hr before bedtime because corrosion may occur in stomach
• Give for <6 mo for anemia
• Store at room temperature; protect from moisture

Patient/family education
• Advise patient that iron will make stools black or dark green, stain teeth; that iron poisoning may occur if increased beyond recommended level
• **Accidental exposure:** advise patient to keep out of reach of children, pets
• Caution patient not to substitute one iron salt for another; elemental iron content differs (e.g., 300 mg ferrous fumarate contains about 100 mg elemental iron, whereas 300 mg ferrous gluconate contains only about 30 mg elemental iron)
• Caution patient to avoid reclining position for 15-30 min after taking product to avoid esophageal corrosion; to follow diet high in iron
• Caution patient to avoid taking iron, dairy products, calcium supplements, vit C together; they compete for absorption

Evaluation

Positive therapeutic outcome
• Decreased fatigue, weakness
• Improvement in Hct, Hgb, reticulocytes

TREATMENT OF OVERDOSE:
Induce vomiting; give eggs, milk until lavage can be done

fesoterodine (Rx)
(fess'oh-ter-oh-deen)
Toviaz
Func. class.: Overactive bladder product
Chem. class.: Muscarinic receptor antagonist

ACTION: Relaxes smooth muscles in urinary tract by inhibiting acetylcholine at postganglionic sites

Therapeutic outcome: Absence of urinary frequency, urgency, incontinence

USES: Overactive bladder (urinary frequency, urgency), urinary incontinence

Pharmacokinetics
Absorption	Rapid
Distribution	Protein binding 50%
Metabolism	⏳ Liver, CYP2D6, CYP3A4, converted to active metabolite
Excretion	Urine, feces
Half-life	7 hr

Pharmacodynamics (metabolite)
Onset	Rapid
Peak	5 hr
Duration	Up to 24 hr

CONTRAINDICATIONS
GI obstruction, ileus, pyloric stenosis, urinary retention, gastric retention, hypersensitivity, closed-angle glaucoma

Precautions: Pregnancy, breastfeeding, children, renal/hepatic disease, urinary tract obstruction, ambient temperature increase, autonomic neuropathy, constipation, contact lenses, hazardous activity, GERD, gastroparesis, myasthenia gravis, prostatic hypertrophy, toxic megacolon, ulcerative colitis, possible cross-sensitivity with tolterodine

DOSAGE AND ROUTES
Adult and geriatric: PO EXT REL 4 mg/day, may increase to 8 mg/day, max 4 mg/day in those taking potent CYP3A4 inhibitors

Renal dose
Adult: PO EXT REL CCr <30 ml/min max 4 mg

Available forms: Ext rel tabs 4, 8 mg

ADVERSE EFFECTS
CNS: Insomnia, headache, dizziness
CV: Chest pain, angina, QT prolongation, peripheral edema
EENT: Xerophthalmia

GI: *Nausea, vomiting,* abdominal pain, constipation, dry mouth
GU: Dysuria, urinary retention, urinary tract infection
INTEG: Rash, angioedema
MISC: Peripheral edema, insomnia
MS: Back pain
RESP: Cough, upper respiratory infection
SYST: Infection

INTERACTIONS
Drug classifications
Anticholinergics, antimuscarinics: increased anticholinergic effect
CYP3A4 inhibitors (antiretroviral protease inhibitors, azole antifungals), avoid use with doses >4 mg, not recommended, macrolide antiinfectives: increased action of fesoterodine

Drug/herb
Caffeine, green tea, guarana: decreased fesoterodine

Drug/lab test
Increase: ALT

NURSING CONSIDERATIONS
Assessment
• **Assess urinary patterns:** distention, nocturia, frequency, urgency, incontinence
• **Angioedema:** Assess for swelling of face, tongue, throat, may occur anytime during treatment, have emergency equipment nearby
• **Pregnancy/breastfeeding:** Avoid in pregnancy/breastfeeding unless benefits outweigh fetal risk, no controlled studies

Patient problem
Impaired urination (uses)

Implementation
• Do not break, crush, or chew ext rel product
• Give without regard to meals
• Store at room temperature; protect from moisture

Patient/family education
• Advise patient not to drink liquids before bedtime
• Instruct the patient on the importance of bladder maintenance
• Teach patient to avoid increased temperature
• Teach patient not to drive or operate machinery until response is known
• Teach patient to avoid alcohol; drowsiness may occur
• Teach patient to report immediately allergic reactions, including, rash, swelling of mouth, face, lips, trouble breathing
• Teach patient not to use new meds, herbs without prescriber approval

Evaluation
Positive therapeutic outcome
• Absence of urinary frequency, urgency, incontinence

fexofenadine (Rx, OTC)
(fex-oh-fin'a-deen)
Allegra, Children's Allegra Allergy, Children's Allegra Hives, Allegra ODT, Mucinex Allergy
Func. class.: Histamine antagonist, 2nd generation
Chem. class.: Piperidine, peripherally selective

Do not confuse: Allegra/Viagra

ACTION: Acts on blood vessels, GI, respiratory system by competing with histamine for H_1-receptor site

Therapeutic outcome: Absence of allergy symptoms and rhinitis

USES: Rhinitis, allergy symptoms, chronic idiopathic urticaria

Pharmacokinetics

Absorption	Well absorbed
Distribution	Unknown
Metabolism	Liver
Excretion	Kidneys (80%)
Half-life	14.4, increased renal disease

Pharmacodynamics (antihistamine action)

Onset	1 hr
Peak	2-3 hr
Duration	12-24 hr

CONTRAINDICATIONS
Breastfeeding, newborn or premature infants, hypersensitivity

Precautions: Pregnancy, children, geriatric, respiratory disease, closed-angle glaucoma, prostatic hypertrophy, bladder neck obstruction, asthma, renal failure

DOSAGE AND ROUTES
Adult and child >12 yr: PO ODT 60 mg bid or 180 mg/day
Children 6 to 11 years: ODT 30 mg BID; place on the tongue and allow to disintegrate
Child 2-11 yr: PO 30 mg bid
Child 6 mo-2 y: PO 15 mg bid

Renal dose
Adult and child ≥12 yr: PO CCr <80 ml/min 60 mg/day

Child 6-11 yr: PO CCr <80 ml/min 30 mg/day

Available forms: Caps 60 mg; tabs 30, 60, 180 mg; oral susp 6 mg/ml; orally disintegrating tab 30 mg

ADVERSE EFFECTS

CNS: Headache, stimulation, drowsiness, sedation, fatigue, confusion, blurred vision, tinnitus, restlessness, tremors, paradoxical excitation in children or geriatric

INTERACTIONS
Individual drugs
Erythromycin, ketoconazole: increased fexofenadine effect

Rifampin: decreased fexofenadine effect

Aluminum, antacids, magnesium: decreased fexofenadine effect

Drug/food
Apple, orange, grapefruit juice: decreased absorption

Drug/lab test
False negative: skin allergy tests (discontinue antihistamine 3 days before testing)

NURSING CONSIDERATIONS
Assessment
• **Allergy:** assess for itchy, runny, watery eyes; congested nose; before and during treatment

• Assess respiratory status: rate, rhythm, increase in bronchial secretions, wheezing, chest tightness; provide fluids to 2 L/day to decrease secretion thickness

• **Pregnancy/breastfeeding:** Avoid use in first trimester, no well-controlled studies, use only if benefits outweigh fetal risk, use cautiously in breastfeeding

Patient problem
Impaired airway clearance (uses)

Implementation
• Give without regard to meals; caps/tabs should not be given with or right before grapefruit, orange, or apple juice

• **Orally disintegrating tab:** allow to dissolve, swallow

• **Oral susp:** shake well, use calibrated measuring device

• Store in tight, light-resistant container

Patient/family education
• Teach all aspects of product uses; to notify prescriber if confusion, sedation, hypotension occur; to avoid driving or other hazardous activity if drowsiness occurs; to avoid alcohol or other CNS depressants that may potentiate effect

• Instruct patient to take 1 hr before or 2 hr after meals to facilitate absorption

• Teach patient that hard candy, gum, frequent rinsing of mouth may be used for dryness

• Teach patient to take with water, avoid fruit juices as they may decrease effectiveness

Evaluation
Positive therapeutic outcome
• Absence of running or congested nose, rashes

TREATMENT OF OVERDOSE:
Administer lavage, diazePAM, vasopressors, **IV** phenytoin

---

fidaxomicin (Rx)
(fye-dax-oh-mye′sin)
Dificid
Func. class.: Antiinfective-macrolide

ACTION: Bactericidal against *Clostridium difficile;* is a fermentation product obtained from *Dactylosporangium aurantiacum;* inhibits RNA synthesis by inhibiting transcription of bacterial RNA polymerases; may act at the early stages of transcription

Therapeutic outcome: Resolution of *C. difficile* based on stool culture

USES: Pseudomembranous colitis, *C. difficile*-associated diarrhea

Pharmacokinetics

Absorption	Minimal
Distribution	GI tract
Metabolism	P-glucoprotein
Excretion	Feces 92%; parent drug
Half-life	12 hr

Pharmacodynamics

Onset	<1 hr
Peak	1 hr
Duration	1-5 hr

CONTRAINDICATIONS
Hypersensitivity

Precautions: Pregnancy, breastfeeding, children

DOSAGE AND ROUTES
Adult: **PO** 200 mg bid × 10 days

Available forms: Tab 200 mg

ADVERSE EFFECTS
GI: Nausea, vomiting, abdominal pain, GI bleeding, intestinal obstruction
HEMA: Anemia, neutropenia
INTEG: Rash, pruritus
META: Metabolic acidosis, hyperglycemia

INTERACTIONS
Individual drugs
CycloSPORINE: Increased fidaxomicin action

Drug/lab test
Increased: glucose, LFTs, alk phos
Decreased: sodium bicarbonate, platelets

NURSING CONSIDERATIONS
Assessment
• **CDAD:** Assess for diarrhea, abdominal pain, fever, fatigue, anorexia, possible anemia, elevated WBC and low serum albumin; this product may be used in place of vancomycin (PO); monitor CBC with differential, and stool culture (*C. difficile*); not to be used for systemic infection; obtain C&S prior to use; monitor glucose (diabetic patients); monitor fluid, electrolyte depletion
• Pregnancy/breastfeeding: No harm to fetus in animal studies, no well-controlled studies in pregnant women, use only if clearly needed, use cautiously in breastfeeding

Patient problem
Infection (uses)
Diarrhea (adverse reactions)

Implementation:
• Give without regard to food
• Store at room temperature

Patient/family education
• Advise patient to report GI bleeding, severe abdominal pain, continuing diarrhea
• Teach patient to report if pregnancy is planned or suspected or if breastfeeding
• Teach patient to take without regard to food, to take as directed, must take all of the medication

Evaluation

Positive therapeutic outcome
• Resolution of *C. difficile*, decreased diarrhea

⚠ HIGH ALERT

filgrastim (Rx)
(fill-gras′stim)
Granix, Grastofil ✦, Neupogen, Zarxio
Func. class.: Biological modifier
Chem. class.: Granulocyte colony-stimulating factor

Do not confuse: Neupogen/Neumega

ACTION: Stimulates proliferation and differentiation of neutrophils; a glycoprotein

Therapeutic outcome: Absence of infection

USES: To decrease infection in patients receiving antineoplastics that are myelosuppressive; to increase WBC in patients with product-induced neutropenia; bone marrow depression, acute radiation exposure

Unlabeled uses: Neutropenia in HIV infection, aplastic anemia, ganciclovir-induced neutropenia, zidovudine-induced neutropenia

Pharmacokinetics

Absorption	Well absorbed (SUBCUT), completely absorbed (**IV**)
Distribution	Unknown
Metabolism	Unknown
Excretion	Unknown
Half-life	Unknown

Pharmacodynamics

	IV	SUBCUT
Onset	5-60 min	5-60 min
Peak	24 hr	2-8 hr
Duration	up to 1 wk	up to 1 wk

CONTRAINDICATIONS
Hypersensitivity to proteins of *Escherichia coli*

Precautions: Pregnancy, breastfeeding, children, myeloid malignancies, radiation therapy, sepsis, sickle cell disease, chemotherapy, respiratory disease

DOSAGE AND ROUTES
After myelosuppressive chemotherapy
Adult and child: IV/SUBCUT 5 mcg/kg/day in a single dose up to 14 days; may increase by 5 mcg/kg in each chemotherapy cycle

After myelosuppresive doses of radiation
Adult and child >7 mo: SUBCUT 10 mcg/kg/day, start as soon as possible after receiving ≥2 gray (Gy)

After bone marrow transplantation
Adult: IV/SUBCUT 10 mcg/kg as an INF (**IV**) over 4 or 24 hr, begin 24 hr after chemotherapy and 24 hr after bone marrow transplantation

Peripheral blood progenitor cell collection/therapy
Adult: 10 mcg/kg/day as a **BOL** or **CONT INF** × 4 days or more before leukapheresis, continue to last leukapheresis, may alter dose if WBC >100,000/mm³

Severe neutropenia (chronic), idiopathic/cyclical
Adult: SUBCUT 5 mcg/kg daily

Neutropenia in neonates
IV/SUBCUT: 5-10 mcg/kg/day × 3-5 days

Available forms: Inj 300 mcg/ml, 480 mcg/1.6 ml, 480 mcg/0.8 ml

ADVERSE EFFECTS
CNS: Fever, headache
GI: Nausea, vomiting, diarrhea, mucositis, anorexia, splenic rupture
HEMA: Thrombocytopenia, excessive leukocytosis
INTEG: Alopecia, exacerbation of skin conditions, urticaria, cutaneous vasculitis, allergic reactions
MS: Osteoporosis, skeletal pain
OTHER: Chest pain, hypotension
RESP: Acute respiratory distress syndrome, wheezing, alveolar hemorrhage

INTERACTIONS
Individual drugs
Lithium: do not use concurrently

Drug classifications
Antineoplastics: increased neutrophils, do not use together 24 hr before or after antineoplastics

Drug/lab test
Increase: uric acid, lactate dehydrogenase, alkaline phosphatase, WBC

NURSING CONSIDERATIONS
Assessment
• Monitor blood studies: CBC, platelet count before treatment and twice weekly; neutrophil counts (ANC) drop by 50% if filgrastim is discontinued the next day but treatment should continue until ANC >10,000/mm^3
• Assess for bone pain: frequency, intensity, duration; analgesics may be given; opiates should not be used
• Check B/P, heart rate, respiration; baseline, during treatment
• **Respiratory distress syndrome:** fever, dyspnea; withhold product if these occur
• **Allergic reactions:** rash, wheezing, facial edema, dyspnea may occur within 30 min of use; give antihistamines, bronchodilators and EPINEPHrine if needed
• **Splenic rupture:** severe left upper abdominal pain
• **Pregnancy/breastfeeding:** If used in pregnancy, enroll in the Amgen Surveillance Program (800-772-6436), use only if benefits outweigh risk to fetus, use caution in breastfeeding

Patient problem
Risk for Infection (uses)
Pain (adverse reactions)

Implementation
• Store in refrigerator; do not freeze; may store at room temp up to 24 hr
• Given by subcut injection, short IV infusion, continuous SC or IV infusion
• Avoid use within 24 hr before or after chemotherapy
• Do not shake commercial single-dose vials prior to withdrawing the dose. If the vial is shaken and froth or bubbles form, allow the vial to stand undisturbed for a few min until the froth or bubbles dissipate
• Prior to injection, filgrastim may be allowed to reach room temperature for a maximum of 24 hr. Any vial or syringe exposed to room temperature for more than 24 hr should be discarded
• Visually inspect for particulate matter and discoloration prior to use

IV route
• May be diluted with 5% dextrose. Do not dilute with NS; product may precipitate
• May be diluted to concentrations 5-15 mcg/ml; should be protected from absorption to plastic by the addition of albumin to a final albumin concentration of 2 mg/ml. Do not dilute filgrastim to a concentration <5 mcg/ml
IV infusion
• Infuse IV over 15-30 min or as a continuous infusion over 24 hr

SUBCUT route
• May divide into 2 injections if dose is >1 ml
• Subcut injection: no dilution is necessary; inject by rapid subcut injection taking care not to inject intradermally; inject into abdomen, upper outer buttock, upper outer arm, rotate sites
• Subcut continuous infusion: infuse subcut at a rate not to exceed 2 ml/hour

Y-site compatibilities: Acyclovir, allopurinol, amikacin, aminophylline, ampicillin, ampicillin/sulbactam, aztreonam, bleomycin, bumetanide, buprenorphine, butorphanol, calcium gluconate, CARBOplatin, carmustine, ceFAZolin, cefoTEtan, cefTAZidime, chlorproMAZINE, cimetidine, CISplatin, cyclophosphamide, cytarabine, dacarbazine, DAUNOrubicin, dexamethasone, diphenhydrAMINE, DOXOrubicin, doxycycline, droperidol, enalaprilat, famotidine, floxuridine, fluconazole, fludarabine, gallium, ganciclovir, granisetron, haloperidol, hydrocortisone, hydroMORPHONE, hydrOXYzine, IDArubicin, ifosfamide, leucovorin, LORazepam, mechlorethamine, melphalan, meperidine, mesna, methotrexate, metoclopramide, miconazole, minocycline, mitoXANTRONE, morphine, nalbuphine, netilmicin, ondansetron, plicamycin, potassium chloride, promethazine, ranitidine, sodium bicarbonate, streptozocin, ticarcillin, ticarcillin/clavulanate, tobramycin, trimethoprim-sulfamethoxazole, vancomycin, vinBLAStine, vinCRIStine, vinorelbine, zidovudine

Patient/family education
• Teach patient technique for self-administration: dose, side effects, disposal of containers and needles; provide instruction sheet
• Teach patient that bone pain is common

Evaluation
Positive therapeutic outcome
• Absence of infection

---

finasteride (Rx)
(fin-ass'te-ride)
Propecia, Proscar
Func. class.: Androgen hormone inhibitor, hair stimulant
Chem. class.: 5-α-Reductase inhibitor

Do not confuse: Proscar/ProSom/Prozac, **finasteride**/furosemide

ACTION: Inhibits 5-α-reductase and reduction in dihydrotestosterone (DHT); DHT induces androgenic effects by binding to androgen receptors in the cell nuclei of the prostate gland, liver, skin; prevents development of benign prostatic hypertrophy (BPH)

Therapeutic outcome: Reduced prostate size

USES: Symptomatic BPH; male-pattern baldness (Propecia)

Pharmacokinetics

Absorption	63%, readily
Distribution	Plasma protein binding 90%, crosses blood-brain barrier
Metabolism	Liver
Excretion	Kidneys, metabolites (39%); feces (57%)
Half-life	6-15 hr

Pharmacodynamics

Onset	Immediate
Peak	1-2 hr
Duration	14 days

CONTRAINDICATIONS
Pregnancy, breastfeeding, children, women who are pregnant or may become pregnant should not handle tabs, hypersensitivity

Precautions: Large residual urinary volume, severely diminished urinary flow, liver function abnormalities

DOSAGE AND ROUTES
BPH
Adult: PO 5 mg/day × 6-12 mo

Male-pattern baldness
Adult: PO 1 mg/day for 3 mo or more for results

Available forms: Tabs (Propecia) 1 mg, (Proscar) 5 mg

ADVERSE EFFECTS
GU: Impotence, decreased libido, decreased volume of ejaculate, sexual dysfunction, gynecomastia
INTEG: Rash
MISC: Breast tenderness, secondary malignancy

INTERACTIONS
Drug classifications
Anticholinergics, bronchodilators (adrenergic), theophylline: decreased effect of finasteride

Drug/lab test
Decreased: PSA levels (finasteride)

NURSING CONSIDERATIONS
Assessment
• **BPH:** Assess urinary patterns, residual urinary volume, severely diminished urinary flow; PSA levels and digital rectal exam results before initiating therapy and periodically thereafter
• Monitor liver function tests before initiating treatment; extensively metabolized in liver

Patient problem
Impaired urination (uses)

Implementation
• Administer without regard to meals; give for a minimum of 6 mo; not all patients will respond
• Store at temp <86° F (30° C); protect from light; keep container tightly closed

Patient/family education
• **Pregnancy/breastfeeding:** Contraindicated in pregnancy, breastfeeding, pregnant women or those trying to conceive should not handle crushed or broken tabs or come in contact with semen from male using product
• Inform patient that volume of ejaculate may be decreased during treatment; impotence and decreased libido may also occur and may continue after discontinuing treatment
• Inform patient that Propecia results may not occur for 3 mo

---

• Inform patient that Proscar results may not occur for 6-12 mo

Evaluation
Positive therapeutic outcome
• Decreased postvoiding dribbling, frequency, nocturia
• Increased urinary flow
• Regression of prostate size
• Hair growth within 3-6 mo

fingolimod (Rx)
(fin-go′li-mod)
Gilenya
Func. class.: Immunosuppressant
Chem. class.: Sphingosine 1-phosphate receptor modulator

ACTION: Binds with high affinity to sphingosine 1 phosphate receptors, blocks lymphocyte egress to lymph nodes, reducing the number of peripheral blood lymphocytes, may reduce lymphocyte migration into the CNS

Therapeutic outcome: Improved symptoms of multiple sclerosis and prevention of increasing disability

USES: To reduce frequency of exacerbation, to delay physical disability of relapsing forms of MS

Pharmacokinetics

Absorption	Protein binding (99.7%)
Distribution	Distributed to RBCs (86%)
Metabolism	Metabolized by CYP4F2 and CYP2D6 to a lesser extent
Excretion	Excreted in urine (81% inactive metabolites)
Half-life	Terminal half-life 6-9 days

Pharmacodynamics

Onset	Unknown
Peak	12-16 hr
Duration	Steady state 1-2 mo

CONTRAINDICATIONS
Hypersensitivity

Precautions: AIDS, asthma, AV block, bradycardia, breastfeeding, cardiac disease, children, COPD, diabetes mellitus, dysrhythmias, heart failure, hepatic disease, HIV, hypertension, immunosuppression, infants, leukemia, lymphoma, neonates, pregnancy, QT prolongation, respiratory insufficiency, sick sinus syndrome, syncope, uveitis

DOSAGE AND ROUTES
Adult: PO 0.5 mg/day

Hepatic dose
Adult: PO Child-Pugh C, total score >10: Closely monitor, fingolimod exposure is doubled

Available forms: Cap 0.5 mg

ADVERSE EFFECTS
CNS: Asthenia, depression, fatigue, headache, dizziness, progressive multifocal leukoencephalopathy, migraine, paresthesias, stroke
CV: AV block, bradycardia, chest pain, hypertension, palpitations, QT prolongation
EENT: Blurred vision, vision impairment, ocular pain, macular edema
GI: Abdominal pain, anorexia, diarrhea, jaundice, vomiting, weight loss, hepatotoxicity
HEMA: Leukopenia, lymphopenia, neutropenia
INTEG: Alopecia, pruritus
MS: Back pain
RESP: Dyspnea, cough
SYST: Infection, influenza, secondary malignancy

INTERACTIONS
Individual drugs
Digoxin: increased risk of heart block, serious bradycardia, avoid if possible
Ketoconazole: increased fingolimod effect

Drug classifications
Class Ia/III antidysrhythmics: increased risk of torsades de pointes
β-blockers, calcium channel blockers: increased risk of heart block, serious bradycardia
Antineoplastics, immunosuppressants, immune modulating therapies: increased immunosuppression
Inactive vaccines, toxoids: decreased effects
Live vaccines: increased infection risk

NURSING CONSIDERATIONS
Assessment
• **Multiple sclerosis:** Assess for improving paresthesia, muscle weakness, clonus, muscle spasms, difficulty in moving, difficulty in coordination in balance, speech, swallowing, vision problems, fatigue; prevention of increasing disability
• **Monitor laboratory values:** obtain before initial dose, CBC, LFTs, serum bilirubin, ophthalmologic exam, antibodies to VZV if there is not a history of chickenpox or without vaccination, may give VZV vaccination of antibody-negative patient before giving product, postpone for 1 month after vaccination; obtain ECG for evidence of bradycardia, or AV block

---

- **Progressive multifocal leukoencephalopathy (PML):** Assess for confusion, apathy, dizziness, unstable gait; may be fatal; discontinue product; contact prescriber
- **Bradycardia:** Monitor for ≥6 hr after beginning dose, ECG before and after 1st dose, if heart rate 45 bpm or new heart block (2nd degree) occurs, do not use until resolved
- Monitor for QT prolongation
- **Pregnancy/breastfeeding:** No well-controlled studies, may cause fetal harm, pregnant women should enroll in Gilenya Pregnancy Registry (877-598-7237), use contraception during and for 2 mo after final dose, do not breastfeed

Patient problem
Immunologic impairment (uses)
Fatigue (uses)
Lack of knowledge of medication (teaching)

Implementation
PO route
- Watch patient for 6 hr after initial dose or if product is not given for >2 wk for development of bradycardia. Give without regard to food
- Store at room temperature, protect from moisture

Patient/family education
- Provide med guide to patient and explain use of product and expected results
- Advise patient that continuing follow-up exams and laboratory tests will be required on a regular basis
- Advise patient to use contraception during and for 2 months after conclusion of treatment
- **Liver dysfunction:** Teach patient to report jaundice, nausea, vomiting, anorexia, abdominal pain, fatigue, dark urine
- **Cardiac changes:** Chest pain, palpitations

Evaluation
Positive therapeutic outcome
- Improved symptoms of multiple sclerosis and prevention of increasing disability

> ## fluconazole (Rx)
> (floo-kon′a-zole)
> **Diflucan Canesoral ✜, Diflucan One ✜, Monicure ✜**
> *Func. class.:* Antifungal, systemic
> *Chem. class.:* Triazole

Do not confuse: Diflucan/Diprivan

ACTION: Inhibits ergosterol biosynthesis, causes direct damage to membrane phospholipids in the cell wall of fungi

Therapeutic outcome: Fungistatic fungicidal against the following susceptible organisms: *Candida, Cryptococcus neoformans*

USES: Oropharyngeal candidiasis; chronic mucocutaneous candidiasis; systemic, vaginal, urinary candidiasis; cryptococcal meningitis; prevention of candidiasis in bone marrow transplant in those who receive chemotherapy and/or radiation therapy, cystitis, fungal prophylaxis, peritonitis, pneumonia, pyelonephritis

Pharmacokinetics

Absorption	Well absorbed (PO)
Distribution	Widely distributed (peritoneum, CSF), excreted in breast milk
Metabolism	<10%, liver
Excretion	80% kidneys (unchanged)
Half-life	30 hr (adult), increased in renal disease; child 19-25 hr (PO); premature neonates (46-74 hr)

Pharmacodynamics

	PO	IV
Onset	Unknown	Immediate
Peak	1-2 hr	Infusion's end
Duration	Unknown	Unknown

CONTRAINDICATIONS
Hypersensitivity to this product or azoles, pregnancy

Precautions: Breastfeeding, renal/hepatic disease, torsades de pointes

DOSAGE AND ROUTES
Vulvovaginal candidiasis
Adult: PO 150 mg as a single dose; prevention of recurrence (unlabeled) 150 mg/day × 3 days, then qwk × 6 mo

Serious fungal infections
Adult: PO/IV 400 mg initially, then 200-800 mg once daily for 4 wk
Child: PO/IV 6-12 mg/kg/day, ×28 days
Neonates <14 days, 30-36 wk gestation: PO/IV same as child except q 48 hr

Oropharyngeal candidiasis
Adult: PO/IV 200 mg initially, then 100 mg/day for at least 2 wk
Child >14 days: PO/IV 6 mg/kg initially, then 3 mg/kg/day for ≥2 wk
Neonates <14 days, 30-60 wk gestation: PO/IV 6 mg/kg/dose once then 3 mg/kg/dose once daily

Esophageal candidiasis

Adult: PO/IV 200 mg on 1st day, then 100 mg/day × ≥3 wk and for ≥2 wk after resolution of symptoms

Child: PO/IV 6 mg/kg on 1st day, then 3 mg/kg/day × ≥3 wk and for ≥2 wk after resolution of symptoms

Cryptococcal meningitis

Adult: PO/IV 400 mg on 1st day, then 200 mg/day × 10-12 wk after CSF culture negative, suppressive therapy 200 mg qday

Child/infant/neonate >14 days: PO/IV 12 mg/kg on 1st day, then 6-12 mg/kg/day × 10-12 wk after negative CSF culture, suppressive therapy 6 mg/kg/day

Neonate 0-14 days: PO/IV 12 mg/kg on 1st day, then 6-12 mg/kg q72hr × 10-12 wk after negative CSF culture

Prevention of candidiasis in bone marrow transplant

Adult: PO/IV 400 mg/day; those anticipated to have neutrophils <500/mm³, start several days prior to anticipated onset of neutropenia and continue for 7 days after rise of neutrophils >1000/mm³

Child >14 days: PO/IV 10-12 mg/kg/day, max 600 mg/day

Renal dose

Adult: PO CCr <50 ml/min after loading dose, give 50% of usual dose; hemodialysis give 100% of usual dose after dialysis treatment, give dose as per CCr on nondialyisis days

Available forms: Tabs 10, 40, 50, 100, 150, 200 mg; inj 2 mg/ml; powder for oral susp 50, 200 mg/ml

ADVERSE EFFECTS

CNS: *Headache,* seizures
CV: QT prolongation, torsades de pointes
GI: *Nausea, vomiting,* diarrhea, cramping, flatus, increased AST, ALT, hepatotoxicity, abdominal pain, cholestasis
HEMA: Agranulocytosis, eosinophilia, leukopenia, neutropenia, thrombocytopenia
INTEG: Stevens-Johnson syndrome, angioedema, anaphylaxis, exfoliative dermatitis, toxic epidermal necrolysis

INTERACTIONS
Individual drugs

Alfentanil, buprenorphine, ergot, fentaNYL, methadone, saquinavir, SUFentanil, zidovudine: increased effect of each specific drug
CycloSPORINE, phenytoin, rifabutin, sirolimus, tacrolimus, theophylline, zidovudine, zolpidem: increased plasma concentrations

Lovastatin, simvastatin: increased myopathy, rhabdomyolysis risk
Warfarin: increased anticoagulation

Drug classification

Calcium channel blockers: decreased effect
Oral sulfonylureas (glipiZIDE): hypoglycemia
Proton pump inhibitors: decreased fluconazole

Drug/herb

Gossypol: increased nephrotoxicity

Drug/lab test

Increased: alk phos, LFTs
Decreased: WBC, platelets

NURSING CONSIDERATIONS
Assessment

• **Assess for signs and symptoms of infection:** clearing of CSF culture during treatment, obtain C&S baseline and during treatment, product may be started as soon as culture is taken
• **QT prolongation:** Avoid with other products that cause QT prolongation
• **Monitor for hepatotoxicity:** increased AST, ALT, alkaline phosphatase, bilirubin; discontinue product if hepatotoxicity occurs
• **Pregnancy/breastfeeding:** Do not use in pregnancy for most indications, birth defects may occur, use cautiously in breastfeeding
• **Monitor for skin symptoms:** color, lesions, injection site reactions; if lesions progress, discontinue product; monitor rash, usually after second week of treatment and disappears in 2 wk if continuing product

Patient problem

Infection (uses)

Implementation

• Take with food to reduce GI effects

PO route
• Shake oral susp before each use; use within 2 wk

Intermittent IV infusion route
• Give after diluting according to package directions; run at 200 mg/hr or less; do not use plastic containers in connections
• Do not admix
• Administer **IV** using an in-line filter, using distal veins; check for extravasation and necrosis q2hr
• Give product only after C&S confirms organism, product needed to treat condition
• Store protected from moisture and light, diluted sol is stable for 24 hr

Y-site compatibilities: Acyclovir, aldesleukin, alfentanil, allopurinol, amifostine, amikacin, aminocaproic acid, aminophylline, amiodarone, anidulafungin, ascorbic acid injection, atenolol, atracurium, atropine, azaTHIOprine, aztreonam, benztropine, bivalirudin, bleomycin, bumetanide, buprenorphine, butorphanol, calcium chloride, CARBOplatin, caspofungin, ceFAZolin, cefepime, cefmetazole, cefonicid, cefoTEtan, cefOXitin, cefpirome, cefTAZidime, ceftizoxime, ceftobiprole, cephalothin, cephapirin, chlorproMAZINE, cimetidine, cisatracurium, CISplatin, codeine, cyanocobalamin, cyclophosphamide, cycloSPORINE, cytarabine, DACTINomycin, DAPTOmycin, dexamethasone, dilTIAZem, dimenhyDRINATE, diphenhydrAMINE, DOBUTamine, DOCEtaxel, DOPamine, doripenem, doxacurium, DOXOrubicin, DOXOrubicin liposomal, doxycycline, droperidol, drotrecogin alfa, enalaprilat, ePHEDrine, EPINEPHrine, epiRUBicin, epoetin alfa, eptifibatide, ertapenem, erythromycin, esmolol, etoposide, famotidine, fenoldopam, fentaNYL, filgrastim, fludarabine, fluorouracil, folic acid, foscarnet, gallium, ganciclovir, gatifloxacin, gemcitabine, gentamicin, glycopyrrolate, granisetron, heparin, hydrocortisone, HYDROmorphone, IDArubicin, ifosfamide, IV immune globulin, inamrinone, indomethacin, insulin (regular), irinotecan, isoproterenol, ketorolac, labetalol, lansoprazole, leucovorin, levofloxacin, lidocaine, linezolid, LORazepam, LR, magnesium sulfate, mannitol, mechlorethamine, melphalan, meperidine, meropenem, metaraminol, methicillin, methotrexate, methoxamine, methyldopate, methylPREDNISolone, metoclopramide, metoprolol, metroNIDAZOLE, mezlocillin, miconazole, midazolam, milrinone, minocycline, mitoXANTRONE, morphine, moxalactam, multiple vitamins injection, mycophenolate, nafcillin, nalbuphine, naloxone, nesiritide, nitroglycerin, nitroprusside, norepinephrine, octreotide, ondansetron, oxacillin, oxaliplatin, oxytocin, PACLitaxel, palonosetron, pamidronate, pancuronium, papaverine, PEMEtrexed, penicillin G potassium/sodium, pentazocine, PENTobarbital, PHENobarbital, phenylephrine, phenytoin, phytonadione, piperacillin-tazobactam, polymyxin B, potassium chloride, procainamide, prochlorperazine, promethazine, propofol, propranolol, protamine, pyridoxine, quiNIDine, quinupristin-dalfopristin, ranitidine, remifentanil, Ringer's, ritodrine, riTUXimab, rocuronium, sargramostim, sodium acetate/bicarbonate, succinylcholine, SUFentanil, tacrolimus, temocillin, teniposide, theophylline, thiotepa, ticarcillin-clavulanate, tigecycline, tirofiban, TNA, tobramycin, tolazoline, TPN, trastuzumab, trimetaphan, urokinase, vancomycin, vasopressin, vecuronium, verapamil, vinCRIStine, vinorelbine, voriconazole, zidovudine, zoledronic acid

Patient/family education

• Caution patient that long-term therapy may be needed to clear infection; to take entire course of medication; take in equal intervals (PO), not to add new meds, herbs without prescriber approval

• **Teach patient the signs and symptoms of hepatotoxicity:** nausea, vomiting, clay-colored stools, dark urine, anorexia, fatigue, jaundice, skin rash; prescriber should be notified immediately, abdominal pain, fever, bruising, bleeding

• Inform patient that medication may be taken with food to reduce GI effects

Evaluation
Positive therapeutic outcome

• Decreasing oral candidiasis, fever, malaise, rash

• Negative C&S for infecting organism

fludrocortisone (Rx)

(floo-droe-kor'ti-sone)

Florinef ✤

Func. class.: Synthetic corticosteroid

Do not confuse: Florinef/Floranex/Florastor

ACTION: Promotes increased reabsorption of sodium and loss of potassium, water, hydrogen from distal tubules

Therapeutic outcome: Correction of adrenal insufficiency

USES: Adrenal insufficiency, salt-losing adrenogenital syndrome, Addison's disease

Unlabeled uses: Idiopathic hypotension

Pharmacokinetics

Absorption	Well
Distribution	Widely, protein binding >80%
Metabolism	Liver
Excretion	Urine
Half-life	3.5 hr

Pharmacodynamics

Onset	Unknown
Peak	1.5 hr
Duration	Unknown

CONTRAINDICATIONS

Children <2 yr, hypersensitivity

Precautions: HF, hypertension, diabetes, acute glomerulonephritis, amebiasis, psychosis, Cushing's syndrome, fungal infections, pregnancy, breastfeeding, children >2 yrs, osteoporosis

DOSAGE AND ROUTES
Adrenocortical insufficiency
Adult: PO 100-200 mcg/day
Child: PO 50-100 mcg/day

Idiopathic hypotension (unlabeled)
Adult PO 50-200 mcg/day

Available forms: Tabs 100 mcg (0.1 mg)

ADVERSE EFFECTS
CV: Hypertension, circulatory collapse, thrombophlebitis, embolism, tachycardia, HF, edema
CNS: Flushing, sweating, headache, paralysis, dizziness, seizure
ENDO: Weight gain, adrenal suppression, hyperglycemia
META: Hypokalemia
MISC: Hypersensitivity, cataracts, GI ulcers, anaphylaxis, infection
MS: Fractures, osteoporosis, weakness

INTERACTIONS
Drug classifications
Barbiturates: decreased fludrocortisone action
Loop/thiazide diuretics, potassium-wasting products: increased potassium levels
Sodium-containing products: increased B/P

Drug/lab test
Increased: potassium, sodium
Decreased: HCT

NURSING CONSIDERATIONS
Assessment
• Assess weight daily, notify prescriber of weekly gain >5 lb
• Monitor I&O, be alert for decreasing output, increasing edema
• Monitor B/P, pulse, notify prescriber of chest pain
• Potassium depletion: assess for paresthesia, fatigue, nausea, vomiting, dysrhythmias, weakness, depression, polyuria
• Electrolytes: monitor sodium, potassium, chloride; hypokalemia is common
• **Beers:** Avoid in older adults with or at high risk of delirium

Patient problem
Fluid imbalance (uses)

Implementation
• Titrate to lowest dose
• Give with food or milk to decrease GI symptoms
• Tabs are scored and may be divided

Patient/family education
• Teach patient that emergency ID as corticosteroid user should be carried
• Teach patient not to discontinue abruptly
• Instruct patient to notify health care provider of muscle cramps, weight gain, edema, nausea, infection, trauma, stress
• Advise patient to avoid exposure to disease, trauma

Evaluation
Positive therapeutic outcome
• Correction of adrenal insufficiency

---

flumazenil (Rx)
(flu-maz′e-nil)
Anexate ✚, **Romazicon**
Func. class.: Antidote: benzodiazepine receptor antagonist
Chem. class.: Imidazobenzodiazepine derivative

Do not confuse: **flumazenil**/influenza virus vaccine

ACTION: Antagonizes the actions of benzodiazepines on the CNS, competitively inhibits the activity at the benzodiazepine receptor complex

Therapeutic outcome: Reversed benzodiazepine toxic effects

USES: Reversal of the sedative effects of benzodiazepines

Pharmacokinetics
Absorption	Complete
Distribution	Unknown, 50% protein binding (albumin)
Metabolism	Liver
Excretion	Unknown
Half-life	41-79 min (adult); 20-75 min (child)

Pharmacodynamics
Onset	1-2 min
Peak	10 min
Duration	1-2 hr

CONTRAINDICATIONS
Hypersensitivity to this product or benzodiazepines, serious tricyclic overdose, patients given benzodiazepine for control of life-threatening condition

Precautions: Pregnancy, breastfeeding, children, geriatric, ambulatory patients, renal/hepatic disease, status epilepticus, head injury,

---

labor and delivery, hypoventilation, panic disorder, drug/alcohol dependency, benzodiazepine dependence

> **BLACK BOX WARNING:** Benzodiazepine dependence, seizures

DOSAGE AND ROUTES
Reversal of conscious sedation or in general anesthesia
Adult: IV 0.2 mg (2 ml) given over 15 sec; wait 45 sec, then give 0.2 mg (2 ml) if consciousness does not occur; may be repeated at 60-sec intervals as needed (max 3 mg/hr) or 1 mg/5 min
Child: IV 10 mcg (0.01 mg)/kg; cumulative dose of 1 mg or less

Management of suspected benzodiazepine overdose
Adult: IV 0.2 mg (2 ml) given over 30 sec; wait 30 sec, then give 0.3 mg (3 ml) over 30 sec if consciousness does not occur; further doses of 0.5 mg (5 ml) can be given over 30 sec at intervals of 1 min up to cumulative dose of 3 mg
Child: IV 10 mcg (0.01 mg/kg); cumulative dose of less than 1 mg

Available forms: Inj 0.1 mg/ml

ADVERSE EFFECTS
CNS: Dizziness, agitation, emotional lability, confusion, *seizures*, somnolence, panic attacks
CV: Hypertension, palpitations, cutaneous vasodilatation, dysrhythmias, bradycardia, tachycardia, chest pain
EENT: Abnormal vision, blurred vision, tinnitus
GI: Nausea, vomiting, hiccups
SYST: Headache, inj site pain, increased sweating, fatigue, rigors

INTERACTIONS
Individual drugs
Zaleplon, zolpidem: antagonize action

Drug classifications
Benzodiazepines: antagonize action
Toxicity: mixed product overdosage

NURSING CONSIDERATIONS
Assessment
• Assess cardiac and respiratory status using continuous monitoring
• Assess for seizures, protect patient from injury; most likely in those who usually experience withdrawal from sedatives
• Assess for GI symptoms: nausea, vomiting; place in side-lying position to prevent aspiration
• **Assess for allergic reactions:** flushing, rash, urticaria, pruritus

• **Pregnancy/breastfeeding:** Use only if benefits outweigh risks to the fetus; use cautiously in breastfeeding, it is not known if product is excreted in breast milk

> **BLACK BOX WARNING: Seizures/benzodiazepine dependence:** Do not use in those who have used these products for interictal psychosis, status epilepticus, use in ICU cautiously where there may be unrecognized benzodiazepine dependence

• Teach patient not to use with alcohol or other medications for at least 24 hr
• Teach patient sedation may occur after treatment

Patient problem
Risk for injury (uses)

Implementation
Direct IV route
• Give directly undiluted or diluted in 0.9% NaCl, D5W, or LR; give over 15-30 sec into running IV, check for extravasation
• Use large vein
• Check airway and IV access before administration
• Stable for 24 hr if drawn into a syringe or mixed with other solutions

Teach patient/family
• Teach patient not to use alcohol or any products with alcohol for 18-24 hr
• Teach patient to avoid hazardous activities, such as driving until residual effects are gone
• Caution patient that amnesia may continue

Evaluation
Positive therapeutic outcome
• Decreased sedation, respiratory depression
• Absence of toxicity

flunisolide nasal agent
See Appendix B

fluocinolone topical
See Appendix B

fluorometholone ophthalmic
See Appendix B

A HIGH ALERT

fluorouracil (Rx)

(flure-oh-yoor′a-sil)
Adrucil, Carac, Efudex, Fluoroplex, Tolak
Func. class.: Antineoplastic, antimetabolite
Chem. class.: Pyrimidine antagonist

Do not confuse: Carac/Kuric

ACTION: Inhibits DNA, RNA synthesis; interferes with cell replication by competitively inhibiting thymidylate synthesis; cell cycle specific (S phase)

Therapeutic outcome: Prevention of rapidly growing malignant cells

USES: Systemic: cancer of breast, colon, rectum, stomach, pancreas; **Topical:** superficial basal cell carcinoma; multiple actinic keratoses

Pharmacokinetics

Absorption	Completely (**IV**), minimal (topical)
Distribution	Widely distributed, concentration in tumor
Metabolism	Liver, converted to active metabolite
Excretion	Lungs (60%-80%), kidneys (up to 15%)
Half-life	16 min (IV)

Pharmacodynamics

	IV	Top
Onset	1-9 days	2-3 days
Peak	9-21 days (nadir)	2-6 wk
Duration	30 days	1-2 month

CONTRAINDICATIONS

Pregnancy, breastfeeding, hypersensitivity, poor nutritional status, serious infections, dihydropyrimidine dehydrogenase deficiency (DPD), bone marrow suppression

Precautions: Children, renal/hepatic disease, angina, stomatitis, diarrhea, sunlight exposure, vaccination, occlusive dressing, GI bleeding

> **BLACK BOX WARNING:** Requires a specialized care setting and experienced clinician

DOSAGE AND ROUTES

Doses vary widely, doses are based on actual body weight, unless obese, then based on lean body weight

Colon, rectal, breast, stomach, pancreatic cancer

Adult: IV 12 mg/kg/day × 4 days (max 800 mg), then 6 mg/kg on days 6, 8, 10, 12 if no toxicity, then 10-15 mg/kg as a single dose weekly maintenance dose (max 1 g/wk); *poor-risk patients:* 6 mg/kg/day × 3 days, then 3 mg/kg on days 5, 7, 9 if no toxicity (max 400 mg/day)

Actinic/solar keratoses

Adult: TOP, (Carac) 1% cream/solution bid or 2%-5% SOL for hands

Superficial basal cell carcinoma

Adult: TOP, (Efudex) 5% cream/solution 2 ×/day × 3-12 wk

Available forms: Inj 50 mg/ml; cream 0.5%, 1%, 4%, 5%; topical solution, 2%, 5%

ADVERSE EFFECTS
SYSTEMIC USE

CNS: Lethargy, malaise, weakness, acute cerebellar dysfunction
EENT: Epistaxis, light intolerance, lacrimation
GI: *Anorexia, stomatitis,* diarrhea, nausea, vomiting, hemorrhage, enteritis, glossitis
HEMA: Thrombocytopenia, leukopenia, myelosuppression, anemia, agranulocytosis
INTEG: *Rash,* fever, photosensitivity, anaphylaxis, alopecia, hand-foot syndrome

INTERACTIONS
Individual drugs

Leucovorin: increased toxicity, bone marrow depression
MetroNIDAZOLE: increased toxicity, irinotecan
Phenytoin: decreased effect of phenytoin
Radiation: increased toxicity, bone marrow suppression

Drug classifications

Anticoagulants, NSAIDs, platelet inhibitors, thrombolytics: increased bleeding
Antineoplastics: increased toxicity, bone marrow depression
Live virus vaccines: decreased antibody response

Drug/lab test

Increased: AST, ALT, LDH, serum bilirubin, Hct, Hgb, WBC, platelets, 5-HIAA
Decreased: albumin

NURSING CONSIDERATIONS
Assessment

• Assess buccal cavity q8hr for dryness, sores or ulceration, white patches, oral pain, bleeding,

---

dysphagia; obtain prescription for viscous lidocaine (Xylocaine)

• **Bone marrow suppression:** Monitor daily during IV treatment: monitor CBC, differential, platelet count daily **(IV)**; withhold product if WBC is <4000/mm³ or platelet count is <100,000/mm³; notify prescriber of results if WBC <20,000/mm³, platelets <50,000/mm³; nadir of leukopenia within 2 wk, recovery 1 mo; if pretreatment of WBC <2000/mm³ or platelets <100,000/mm³, delay until recovery of counts above this level; nadir usually 9-14 days, recovery 30 days

BLACK BOX WARNING: Use only in a specialized care setting and with experienced clinician

• **Palmar-plantar erythrodysesthesia:** hand/foot tingling changing to pain, redness
• **Infiltration:** monitor frequently for pain, redness, inflammation at site; if present, stop infusion and start at new site; may use ice at site
• Monitor renal function studies: BUN, creatinine, serum uric acid, urine CCr before, during therapy; I&O ratio; report fall in urine output to <30 ml/hr
• Monitor liver function tests before, during therapy (bilirubin, AST, ALT, LDH) as needed or monthly; jaundice of skin, sclera, dark urine, clay-colored stools, itchy skin, abdominal pain, fever, diarrhea
• **Assess for bleeding:** hematuria, stool guaiac, bruising or petechiae, mucosa or orifices q8hr; avoid IM injections, rectal temperatures, inflammation of mucosa, breaks in skin
• **Pregnancy/breastfeeding:** Assess for pregnancy before starting therapy, do not use in pregnancy, breastfeeding
• **Assess for infection:** (fever, chills, cough, sore throat) those with current infections should be treated prior to receiving 5-FU, the dose reduced or discontinued if infection occurs
• **Toxicity:** Assess for hemorrhage, severe vomiting, severe diarrhea, stomatitis, WBC <3500/mm³, platelets <100,000 notify prescriber
• **Acute cerebellar dysfunction:** Monitor for dizziness, weakness

Patient problem

Infection (uses)
Risk for injury (adverse reactions)

Implementation

• Avoid contact with skin (very irritating); wash completely to remove
• Give fluids **IV** or PO before chemotherapy to hydrate patient
• Give antiemetic 30-60 min before giving product to prevent vomiting, and prn for several days thereafter; antibiotics for prophylaxis of infection
• Provide liquid diet: carbonated beverages; gelatin may be added if patient is not nauseated or vomiting
• Rinse mouth tid-qid with water, club soda; brush teeth bid-qid with soft brush or cotton-tipped applicators for stomatitis; use unwaxed dental floss

Topical route

• The 1% strength is used on face, other higher strengths are used on other parts of the body
• Wear gloves when applying; may use with a loose dressing; use a plastic or wooden applicator, do not use occlusive dressings; may use gauze dressing

IV route

• Prepare in biological cabinet using gloves, gown, mask
• Double-check all amounts and type of product to be used, fatalities have occurred
• **IV Direct:** undiluted; may inject through Y-tube or 3-way stopcock; give over 1-3 min
• May be diluted in 0.9% NaCl, D₅W; given as an **Intermittent infusion:** infusion in plastic containers over 2-8 hr; do not refrigerate/freeze; protect from light; discard unused portion, stable for 24 hr at room temperature; do not use discolored, cloudy solution; solution is pale yellow; for crystals, dissolve by warming slowly and shaking; cool to body temperature before use

Y-site compatibilities: Acyclovir, alatrofloxacin, alfentanil, allopurinol, amifostine, amikacin, amphotericin B lipid complex, amphotericin B liposome, ampicillin, ampicillin-sulbactam, anidulafungin, argatroban, atenolol, atracurium, azithromycin, aztreonam, bivalirudin, bleomycin, bumetanide, butorphanol, calcium gluconate, CARBOplatin, ceFAZolin, cefepime, cefotaxime, cefoTEtan, cefOXitin, cefTAZidime, ceftizoxime, cefTRIAXone, cefuroxime, cimetidine, cisatracurium, CISplatin, clindamycin, codeine, cyclophosphamide, cycloSPORINE, DAPTOmycin, dexamethasone, digoxin, DOCEtaxel, DOPamine, doripenem, DOXOrubicin liposomal, enalaprilat, ePHEDrine, ertapenem, erythromycin, esmolol, etoposide phosphate, famotidine, fenoldopam, fentaNYL, fluconazole, fludarabine, foscarnet, fosphenytoin, furosemide, ganciclovir, gatifloxacin, gemcitabine, gentamicin, granisetron, heparin, hydrocortisone, HYDROmorphone, ifosfamide, imipenem-cilastatin, inamrinone, isoproterenol, ketorolac, labetalol, leucovorin, levorphanol, lidocaine, linezolid, magnesium sulfate, mannitol, melphalan, meperidine, meropenem, mesna, methohexital, methotrexate, methylPREDNISolone, metoprolol, metroNIDAZOLE, milrinone, mitoMYcin, mitoXANTRONE, morphine sulfate, nalbuphine, naloxone, nesiritide, nitroglycerin, nitroprusside, octreotide, ofloxacin, PACLitaxel, palonosetron, pamidronate, pancuronium, pantoprazole, PEMEtrexed, PENTobarbital, PHENobarbital, phenylephrine, piperacillin, piperacillin-tazobactam, potassium chloride/phosphates, procainamide, propofol, propranolol, ranitidine, remifentanil, riTUXimab, sargramostim, sodium acetate/bicarbonate/phosphates, succinylcholine, SUFentanil, sulfamethoxazole-trimethoprim, teniposide, theophylline, thiopental, thiotepa, ticarcillin, ticarcillin-clavulanate, tigecycline, tirofiban, tobramycin, trastuzumab, vasopressin, vecuronium, vinBLAStine, vinCRIStine, vitamin B complex/C, voriconazole, zidovudine, zoledronic acid

Patient/family education

• Caution patient that contraceptive measures are recommended during therapy
• **Bleeding:** Teach patient to avoid using aspirin, NSAIDs, or ibuprofen-containing products, razors, commercial mouthwash because bleeding may occur; to report symptoms of bleeding (hematuria, tarry stools), IM injections if counts are low
• **Instruct patient to report signs of anemia** (fatigue, headache, irritability, faintness, SOB)
• **Instruct patient to report signs of stomatitis** (bleeding, white spots, ulcerations in the mouth); tell patient to examine mouth daily, to report symptoms; viscous lidocaine (Xylocaine) may be used
• Teach patient to avoid crowds, persons with known infections
• Advise patient to avoid vaccinations during therapy, to use sunscreen or stay out of the sun to prevent burns; about hair loss; explore use of wigs or other products until hair regrowth occurs

Evaluation
Positive therapeutic outcome
• Prevention of rapid division of malignant cells

FLUoxetine (Rx)
(floo-ox′uh-teen)
PROzac, PROzac Weekly, Sarafem, Selfemra
Func. class.: Antidepressant, selective serotonin reuptake inhibitor

Do not confuse: FLUoxetine/Loxitane, **PROzac**/Prograf/Provera/PriLOSEC, **Sarafem**/Serophene, **FLUoxetine**/DULoxetine/Loxitane, PARoxetine

ACTION: Inhibits CNS neuron uptake of serotonin but not of norepinephrine

Therapeutic outcome: Decreased symptoms of depression after 2-3 wk

USES: Major depressive disorder, obsessive-compulsive disorder (OCD), bulimia nervosa; *Sarafem:* premenstrual dysphoric disorder (PMDD), panic disorder

Unlabeled uses: Alcoholism, anorexia nervosa, ADHD, diabetic neuropathy, fibromyalgia, Raynaud's, obesity, posttraumatic stress disorder, social phobia

Pharmacokinetics

Absorption	Well absorbed
Distribution	Crosses blood-brain barrier, protein binding 95%
Metabolism	Liver, extensively to norfluoxetine ✏️ by CYP2D6 isoenzyme, some patients may be poor metabolizers
Excretion	Kidneys, unchanged (12%), metabolite (7%); steady state 28-35 days, protein binding 94%
Half-life	1-3 days metabolite up to 1 wk (antidepressant)

Pharmacodynamics

Onset	1-4 wk
Peak	Unknown
Duration	2 wk

CONTRAINDICATIONS
Hypersensitivity, MAOI therapy

Precautions: Pregnancy, breastfeeding, geriatric, diabetes mellitus, narrow-angle glaucoma, cardiac malformations in infants (exposed to FLUoxetine in utero), osteoporosis, QT prolongation

---

BLACK BOX WARNING: Children, suicidal ideation

DOSAGE AND ROUTES
Depression/OCD
Adult: PO 20 mg/day AM; after 4 wk if no clinical improvement is noted, dosage may be increased to 20 mg bid in AM, afternoon; max 80 mg/day; PO 90 mg weekly
Geriatric: PO 10 mg/day, increase as needed
Child 7-17 yr: PO 5-10 mg/day, max 20 mg/day

Alcoholism (unlabeled)
Adult: PO 20-80 mg/day

Anorexia nervosa (unlabeled)
Adult: PO 10 mg every other day-20 mg/day

Posttraumatic stress disorder (unlabeled)
Adult: PO 10-80 mg/day

Premenstrual dysphoric disorder (Sarafem)
Adult: PO 20 mg/day, may be taken daily 14 days before menses

Available forms: Caps 10, 20, 40 mg; tabs 10, 20, 60 mg; oral sol 20 mg/5 ml; del rel caps (PROzac Weekly) 90 mg

ADVERSE EFFECTS
CNS: *Headache, nervousness, insomnia, drowsiness, anxiety, tremor, dizziness, fatigue, sedation, poor concentration, abnormal dreams, agitation,* seizures, apathy, euphoria, hallucinations, delusions, psychosis, suicidal ideation, neuroleptic malignant syndrome–like reactions, serotonin syndrome
CV: *Hot flashes, palpitations,* angina pectoris, hemorrhage, hypertension, tachycardia, 1st-degree AV block, bradycardia, MI, thrombophlebitis, generalized edema, torsades de pointes
EENT: Visual changes, ear/eye pain, photophobia, tinnitus, increased intraocular pressure
GI: *Nausea, diarrhea, dry mouth, anorexia, dyspepsia, constipation,* taste changes, flatulence, decreased appetite
GU: *Dysmenorrhea, decreased libido, urinary frequency, urinary tract infection,* amenorrhea, cystitis, impotence, urine retention
INTEG: *Sweating, rash, pruritus,* acne, alopecia, urticaria; angioedema, exfoliative dermatitis, Stevens-Johnson syndrome, toxic epidermal necrolysis
MS: *Pain,* arthritis, twitching
RESP: *Pharyngitis, cough, dyspnea, bronchitis,* asthma, hyperventilation, pneumonia
SYST: *Asthenia,* serotonin syndrome, flulike symptoms, neonatal abstinence syndrome

INTERACTIONS
Individual drugs
Alcohol: increased CNS depression
Antidiabetics: increased levels or toxicity
Bosentan, budesonide, carBAMazepine, darifenacin, diazePAM, digoxin, donepezil, lithium, paricalcitol, phenytoin, thioridazine, vinBLAStine, warfarin: increased toxicity
Cyproheptadine: decreased FLUoxetine effect
BusPIRone, haloperidol, loxapine, selegiline, thiothixene, tryptophan: increased serotonin syndrome, do not use concurrently

Drug classifications
Increase: QT prolongation: pimozide, thioridazine, antidysrythmics class III
Anticoagulants, NSAIDs, platelet inhibitors, salicylates, thrombolytics: increased bleeding risk
Antidepressants, opioids, sedative/hypnotics: increased CNS depression
MAOIs, linezolid, methylene blue: hypertensive crisis, seizures; do not use with or 14 days prior to FLUoxetine
SSRIs, SNRIs, serotonin-receptor agonists, tricyclics: increased serotonin syndrome, do not use concurrently

Drug/herb
Hops, kava, lavender, valerian: increased CNS effect
St. John's wort, SAM-e: do not use together; increased risk of serotonin syndrome

NURSING CONSIDERATIONS
Assessment
• Monitor B/P (lying, standing), pulse; if systolic B/P drops 20 mm hg, hold product and notify prescriber; take VS q4hr in patients with CV disease
• Monitor **blood studies:** CBC, leukocytes, differential, cardiac enzymes if patient is receiving long-term therapy; check platelets, bleeding can occur; thyroid growth rate (children)
• Monitor **hepatic studies:** AST, ALT, bilirubin
• Check weight qwk; appetite may increase with product
• Assess ECG for flattening of T-wave, bundle branch block, AV block, dysrhythmias in cardiac patients
• **Pregnancy/breastfeeding:** Use in pregnancy only if benefits outweigh risks to the fetus, avoid use in breastfeeding, excreted in breast milk

BLACK BOX WARNING: Assess mental status: mood, sensorium, affect, suicidal tendencies; increase in psychiatric symptoms: depression, panic; monitor for seizures; seizure potential is increased; Sarafem is not approved for children

---

- **Beers:** Avoid use in older adults unless safer alternative is not available, may cause ataxia, impaired psychomotor function
- Monitor urinary retention, constipation; constipation is more likely to occur in children or geriatric
- Identify patient's alcohol consumption; if alcohol is consumed, hold dose until AM
- **QT prolongation:** May be more severe in those with history of QT prolongation, if thioridazine is being used discontinue for 5 wk before using this product
- **Neuroleptic malignant syndrome:** Fever, seizures, diaphoresis, dyspnea, hyper/hypotension, report immediately
- **Serotonin syndrome:** Symptoms can occur anytime after first dose, nausea/vomiting, sedation, dizziness, diaphoresis, mental changes, elevated B/P; if these occur product should be stopped, notify prescriber
- **Assess appetite in bulimia nervosa,** monitor weight daily, increase nutritious foods in diet, watch for bingeing and vomiting
- **Serious skin reactions:** angioedema, exfoliative dermatitis, Stevens-Johnson syndrome, toxic epidermal necrolysis
- **Assess allergic reactions:** itching, rash, urticaria, product should be discontinued; may need to give antihistamine

Patient problem
Risk for injury (adverse reactions)
Impaired sexual functioning (adverse reactions)
Nonadherence (teaching)

Implementation
- Give without regard to meals
- Give dose at bedtime if oversedation occurs during day; may take entire dose at bedtime; geriatric may not tolerate once/day dosing, crush if patient unable to swallow whole (tabs only), immediate-release product should be given in AM unless sedation occurs
- **PROzac Weekly:** Give on same day each week, swallow whole, do not crush, cut, chew
- Store at room temperature; do not freeze
- Sarafem is only used for premenstrual dysphoric disorder

Patient/family education
- Teach patient that therapeutic effects may take 1-4 wk, not to discontinue abruptly, that follow-up will be required
- Instruct patient to use caution in driving or other activities requiring alertness because of drowsiness, dizziness, blurred vision; to avoid rising quickly from sitting to standing, especially geriatric; to use sunscreen to prevent photosensitivity

- Caution patient to avoid alcohol ingestion, other CNS depressants
- Teach patient that decreased libido, erectile dysfunction may occur
- Advise patient not to discontinue medication quickly after long-term use: may cause nausea, headache, malaise
- Instruct patient to increase fluids, bulk in diet if constipation, urinary retention occur, especially geriatric
- Advise patient to take gum, hard sugarless candy, or frequent sips of water for dry mouth
- Teach patient to avoid all OTC products unless approved by prescriber
- Advise patient to notify prescriber if allergic reactions occur (rash, trouble breathing, itching)
- Advise patient to change positions slowly, orthostatic hypotension may occur
- Teach that suicidal thoughts, behavior may occur in young adults, children, usually during early treatment
- Inform patient to notify prescriber of worsening symptoms or if insomnia, anxiety, or depression continues
- **Serotonin syndrome:** Teach patient to report fever, sweating, diarrhea, poor coordination, nausea/vomiting, sedation, flushing, mental changes

Evaluation
Positive therapeutic outcome
- Decrease in depression
- Absence of suicidal thoughts
- Decreased symptoms of OCD
- Decreased symptoms of PMDD
- Decreased panic attacks

flurandrenolide topical
See Appendix B

flurbiprofen ophthalmic
See Appendix B

fluticasone (Rx)
(floo-tic'a-sone)
Arnuity Ellipta, Flonase, Flovent HFA, Flovent Diskus ✦, Veramyst (nasal spray)
Func. class.: Corticosteroids, inhalation; antiasthmatic

Do not confuse: Flonase/Flovent

ACTION: Decreases inflammation by inhibiting mast cells, macrophages, and leukotrienes; antiinflammatory and vasoconstrictor properties

Therapeutic outcome: Decreased severity of asthma

USES: Prevention of chronic asthma during maintenance treatment in those requiring oral corticosteroids; nasal symptoms of seasonal/perennial and allergic/nonallergic rhinitis

Pharmacokinetics

Absorption	30% aerosol, 13.5% powder
Distribution	Protein binding 91%
Metabolism	In liver after absorption in lung
Excretion	<5% in urine and feces
Half-life	7.8 hr

Pharmacodynamics

	Intranasal	INH
Onset	12 hr	24 hr
Peak	Several days	Several days
Duration	1-2 wk	1-2 wk

CONTRAINDICATIONS

Hypersensitivity to this product or milk protein, primary treatment in status asthmaticus, acute bronchospasm

Precautions: Pregnancy, breastfeeding, active infections, glaucoma, diabetes, immunocompromised patients, Cushing syndrome

DOSAGE AND ROUTES
Prevention of chronic asthma
>> Flovent HFA
Adult and child ≥12 yr: INH 88-440 mcg bid (in those previously taking bronchodilators alone); INH 88-220 mcg bid, max 440 mcg bid (in those previously taking inhaled corticosteroids); INH 440 mcg bid, max 880 mcg bid (in those previously taking oral corticosteroids)
Child 4-11 yr: INH 88 mg bid

>> Flovent Diskus ✦
Adult and child ≥12 yr: INH 100 mcg bid, max 500 mcg bid (in those previously taking bronchodilators alone); INH 100-250 mcg bid, max 500 mcg bid (in those previously taking inhaled corticosteroids); INH 500-1000 mcg bid, max 1000 mcg bid (in those previously taking oral corticosteroids)
Child 4-11 yr: INH initially 50 mcg bid, max 100 mcg bid (in those previously taking bronchodilators alone or inhaled corticosteroids)

>> Arnuity Ellipta
Adult, child ≥ 12 yr: INH 100 mcg via oral inhalation qday initially, may increase to 200 mcg qday after 2 wk, max 200 mcg/day

Seasonal, perennial allergic, nonallergic rhinitis
>> Flonase
Adult: Nasal 2 sprays initially, in each nostril per day or 1 spray bid, when controlled, lower to 1 spray in each nostril per day
Adolescent/child >4 yr: Nasal 1 spray in each nostril per day, may increase to 2 sprays in each nostril per day, when controlled, lower to 1 spray in each nostril per day

>> Veramyst (nasal spray)
Adult/child ≥12 yr: Nasal 2 sprays in each nostril per day
Child 2-11 yr: Nasal 1 spray in each nostril per day

Available forms: Oral inh aerosol 44, 110, 220 mcg; oral inh powder 50, 100, 250 mcg; nasal spray (Veramyst) 27.5 mcg/actuation, (propionate) 50 mcg/actuation, 27.5 mcg/spray (furoate); inhalation powder 100, 200 mcg/actuation (Arnuity Ellipta)

ADVERSE EFFECTS
CNS: Fever, headache, nervousness, dizziness, fatigue, migraines, numbness in fingers
EENT: *Pharyngitis,* sinusitis, rhinitis, laryngitis, hoarseness, dry eyes, cataracts, nasal discharge, epistaxis, blurred vision
GI: Diarrhea, abdominal pain, nausea, vomiting, *oral candidiasis,* gastroenteritis
GU: UTI
INTEG: Urticaria, dermatitis
META: Hyperglycemia, growth retardation in children, cushingoid features
MISC: Influenza, eosinophilic conditions, angioedema, Churg-Strauss syndrome, adrenal insufficiency (high doses), bone mineral density reduction
MS: Osteoporosis, muscle soreness, joint pain, arthralgia
RESP: *Upper respiratory infection,* dyspnea, cough, bronchitis, bronchospasm

INTERACTIONS
Individual drugs
Amprenavir, atazanavir, darunavir, delavirdine, fosamprenavir, nelfinavir, ritonavir, saquinavir: increased fluticasone levels
Isoproterenol (asthma patients): increased cardiac toxicity
Mecasermin: decreased effects of mecasermin

Drug classifications
CYP3A4 inhibitors (ketoconazole, itraconazole): increased fluticasone levels

NURSING CONSIDERATIONS
Assessment
• **Assess respiratory status:** lung sounds, pulmonary function tests during and several months after change from systemic to inhalation corticosteroids
• Assess for withdrawal symptoms from oral corticosteroids: depression, pain in joints, fatigue
• **Monitor adrenal insufficiency:** nausea, weakness, fatigue, hypotension, hypoglycemia, anorexia; may occur when changing from systemic to inhalation corticosteroids; may be life-threatening
• Monitor growth rate in children; blood glucose, serum potassium in all patients
• Monitor adrenal function tests periodically: hypothalamic-pituitary-adrenal axis suppression in long-term treatment
• **Pregnancy/breastfeeding:** Use in pregnancy only if benefits outweigh risks, avoid use in breastfeeding
• **Beers:** Avoid use in older adults with or at high risk of delirium; may worsen delirium

Patient problem
Impaired airway clearance (uses)
Risk for infection (adverse reactions)
Nonadherence (teaching)

Implementation
• Give at 1 min intervals
• Decrease dose to lowest effective dose after desired effect; decrease dose at 2- to 4-wk intervals
• Blow nose prior to use
Inhalation route: powder for oral inhalation (Flovent Diskus)
• Fill in the "Pouch opened" and "Use by" dates in the blank lines on the label. The "Use by" date for Flovent diskus 50 mcg is 6 wk from the date the pouch is opened. The "Use by" date for diskus 100 mcg and 250 mcg is 2 months from the date pouch is opened
• Open the diskus by holding in one hand and using the thumb of the other to push the thumbgrip away as far as it will go until the mouthpiece shows and snaps into place
• Hold and slide the lever away from the patient as far as it will go until it clicks. The number on the dose counter will count down by 1; the diskus is now ready to use
• Before inhaling the dose, have patient breathe out, hold the diskus level and away from the mouth. Breathe out into the mouthpiece
• Instruct the patient to put the mouthpiece to the lips and breathe in through the mouth quickly and deeply through the diskus. The patient should then remove the diskus from the mouth, hold breath for about 10 sec, and breathe out slowly
• After taking a dose, close the diskus by sliding the thumbgrip back as far as it will go. The diskus will click shut. The lever will automatically return to its original position
• The counter displays how many doses are left. The counter number will count down each time the patient uses the diskus. After 55 doses (23 doses from the sample pack), numbers 5 to 0 appear in red to warn that there are only a few doses left
• After use, instruct patient to rinse mouth with water and spit out the water; patient should not swallow it
• To avoid the spread of infection, do not use the inhaler for more than one person
Intranasal
• Prime before first use
• Shake well before each use
• Rinse tip after use, dry with tissue

Patient/family education
• **Teach patient to report immediately cushingoid symptoms:** no appetite, nausea, weakness, fatigue, decreased B/P
• Teach patient how to use and when it may be empty
• Advise patient to use bronchodilator first before using inhalation, if taking both
• Caution patient not to use for acute asthmatic attack; acute asthma may require oral corticosteroids
• Advise patient to avoid smoking, smoke-filled rooms, those with URIs, those not immunized against chickenpox or measles
• Advise patient to use medical ID identifying corticosteroid use

Evaluation
Positive therapeutic outcome
• Decreased severity of asthma, COPD, allergies

---

fluticasone topical
See Appendix B

fluvastatin (Rx)
(flu'vah-stay-tin)
Lescol, Lescol XL
Func. class.: Antilipidemic
Chem. class.: HMG-CoA reductase inhibitor

ACTION: Inhibits HMG-CoA reductase enzyme, which reduces cholesterol synthesis

Therapeutic outcome: Decreased cholesterol levels and LDLs, increased HDLs

---

USES: As an adjunct in primary hypercholesterolemia (types Ia, Ib), coronary atherosclerosis in CAD; secondary prevention of coronary events in patients with CAD; adjunct to diet to reduce LDL, total cholesterol, apo B levels in heterozygous familial hypercholesterolemia (LDL-C ≥190 mg/dl) or LDL-C >160 mg/dl with history of premature CV disease

Pharmacokinetics

Absorption	Unknown
Distribution	Steady state 4-5 wk
Metabolism	Liver
Excretion	Feces, kidneys
Half-life	9 hr

Pharmacodynamics

Unknown

CONTRAINDICATIONS

Pregnancy, breastfeeding, hypersensitivity, active liver disease

Precautions: Past liver disease, alcoholism, severe acute infections, trauma, hypotension, uncontrolled seizure disorders, severe metabolic disorders, electrolyte imbalance, myopathy, rhabdomyolysis

DOSAGE AND ROUTES

Adult: PO 20 mg/day in PM initially, max 80 mg/day; may increase q 4 wk, or 60 mg/day (extended release)

Renal dose
Adult: PO CCr <30 mL/min max 20 mg/day unless titrated
Child/adolescent 10-17: PO 10-40 mg/day (familial heterozygous hypercholesterolemia)

Available forms: Caps 20, 40 mg; ext rel tab 80 mg

ADVERSE EFFECTS

CNS: Headache, dizziness, insomnia, confusion
EENT: Lens opacities
GI: *Nausea, constipation, diarrhea, abdominal pain, cramps, dyspepsia, flatus,* liver dysfunction, pancreatitis
HEMA: Thrombocytopenia, hemolytic anemia, leukopenia
INTEG: Rash, pruritus
MISC: Fatigue, influenza, photosensitivity
MS: Myalgia, *arthritis, arthralgia,* myositis, rhabdomyolysis

INTERACTIONS
Individual drugs
Alcohol, cimetidine, ranitidine, omeprazole: increased fluvastatin effect, rifampin

Cholestyramine, colestipol: decreased fluvastatin effect; separate by ≥4 hr
Colchicine, cycloSPORINE, niacin: increased myopathy
Digoxin, phenytoin, warfarin: increased action, monitor closely
Fluconazole, itraconazole, ketoconazole: increased adverse reactions
TraMADol: increased serotonin syndrome

Drug classifications
Fibric acid derivatives, protease inhibitors: increased myopathy, erythromycin

Drug/herb
Red yeast rice: increased adverse reactions
Gotu kola, St. John's wort: decreased effect

Drug/lab test
Increased: LFTs, CK
Decreased: platelets, WBC

NURSING CONSIDERATIONS
Assessment
• **Hypercholesterolemia:** Assess nutrition: fat, protein, carbohydrates; nutritional analysis should be completed by dietitian before treatment
• Assess fasting lipid profile (cholesterol, LDL, HDL, triglycerides) q4-6wk, then q3-6mo when stable
• Monitor bowel pattern daily; diarrhea may occur
• **Hepatotoxicity/pancreatitis:** Monitor liver function studies q1-2mo during the first 1½ yr of treatment; AST, ALT, liver function test results may be increased
• Monitor renal studies in patients with compromised renal system: BUN, I&O ratio, creatinine
• Obtain ophth exam before, 1 mo after treatment begins, annually; lens opacities may occur
• **Myopathy, rhabdomyolysis:** Assess for muscle pain, tenderness; obtain baseline CPK, if elevated or if symptoms occur, product should be discontinued
• **Pregnancy/breastfeeding:** Do not use in pregnancy/breastfeeding

Patient problem
Diarrhea (adverse reactions)
Nonadherance (teaching)

Implementation
• Give without regard to food at any time of day (tab) or in the evening (cap)
• Do not break, cut, chew capsule
• Give at least 4 hr after bile acid sequestrant if used concurrently
• Store at room temperature, protected from light

Patient/family education
• Inform patient that compliance is needed for positive results to occur, not to double doses
• Advise patient to notify prescriber if GI symptoms of diarrhea, abdominal or epigastric pain, nausea, vomiting, or if chills, fever, sore throat occur; also muscle pain, weakness, tenderness
• Advise patient that blood studies and eye exam will be necessary during treatment, that effect may take ≥4 wk
• Instruct patient to report suspected pregnancy, not to use during pregnancy or breastfeeding
• Advise patient that previously prescribed regimen will continue, including diet, exercise, smoking cessation
• Instruct patient to notify all health care providers of products taken
• Teach patient to take without regard to meals, to take immediate release product in the evening, to separate by ≥4 hr with bile-acid product, not to cut, break, or chew capsule

Evaluation
Positive therapeutic outcome
• Decreased LDL, VLDL, total cholesterol levels
• Improved ratio of HDLs
• Prevention of CV disease

fluvoxamine (Rx)
(floo-voks′ a-meen)
Luvox
Func. class.: Antidepressant
Chem. class.: Selective serotonin reuptake inhibitor (SSRI)

ACTION: Inhibits CNS neuron uptake of serotonin but not of norepinephrine

Therapeutic outcome: Decreased symptoms of depression after 2-3 wk

USES: Obsessive-compulsive disorders Major depressive disorder

Unlabeled uses: Depression, panic disorder, social phobia, anxiety, PTSD

Pharmacokinetics

Absorption	Well absorbed
Distribution	Unknown
Metabolism	Liver, by CYP1A2, CYP2D6, several patients are poor metabolizers
Excretion	Kidneys, steady state 28-35 days
Half-life	Unknown

Pharmacodynamics
Unknown

CONTRAINDICATIONS
Hypersensitivity

Precautions: Pregnancy, breastfeeding, geriatric, renal/hepatic disease, seizure disorder, hypersensitivity to escitalopram, bradycardia, recent MI, abrupt discontinuation, QT prolongation

> **BLACK BOX WARNING:** Children, suicidal ideation

DOSAGE AND ROUTES
Adults: PO (**Immediate release**) Initially, 50 mg at bedtime, then adjust as needed; (**controlled release**) initially, 100 mg PO once daily at bedtime. Titrate as needed and tolerated in increments of 50 mg per week to a target range of 100 to 300 mg/day
Children and adolescents 6 years and older: PO (immediate release) Initiate at 25 mg/day at bedtime, may titrate by 25 mg increments every 4 to 7 days based on efficacy and tolerability. Max: 200 mg/day PO. Daily doses more than 50 mg should be divided

Available forms: Tabs 25, 50, 100 mg; controlled release capsules 100, 150 mg

ADVERSE EFFECTS
CNS: Headache, nervousness, insomnia, drowsiness, anxiety, tremor, dizziness, fatigue, sedation, poor concentration, abnormal dreams, agitation, seizures, apathy, euphoria, hallucinations, delusions, psychosis, suicidal attempts, malignant neuroleptic-like syndrome reactions
CV: *Palpitations*, hypertension, tachycardia, orthostatic hypotension
EENT: Sinusitis
GI: Nausea, diarrhea, dry mouth, anorexia, dyspepsia, constipation, cramps, vomiting, flatulence
GU: Decreased libido, impotence
INTEG: Sweating, rash,
MS: Twitching
RESP: Cough, dyspnea
SYST: Serotonin syndrome

INTERACTIONS
Individual drugs:
Alcohol: increased CNS depression
CarBAMazepine, cloNIDine: decreased citalopram levels
Lithium, linezolid, methylene blue, tricyclics, fentaNYL, busPIRone, triptans, traMADol, traZODone: increased serotonin syndrome

---

Pimoside, ziprasidone: increased QTc interval; do not use together

Drug classifications:

Anticoagulants, antiplatelets, NSAIDs, salicylates, thrombolytics: increased risk of bleeding

Antidepressants (tricyclics): increased effect, use cautiously

Antifungals (azole), macrolides: increased citalopram levels

Adrenergic blockers: increased plasma levels of adrenergic blockers

Barbiturates, benzodiazepines, CNS depressants, sedatives/hypnotics: increased CNS depression

MAOIs: hypertensive crisis, seizures, fatal reactions; do not use together within 14 days

Serotonin receptor agonists, SNRIs, SSRIs: increased serotonin syndrome

Drug/herb:

SAM-e, St. John's wort: serotonin syndrome; do not use with citalopram, fatal reaction may occur

Yohimbe: increased CNS stimulation

Drug/lab test:

Increased: serum bilirubin, blood glucose, alkaline phosphatase

Decreased: VMA, 5-HIAA

False increase: increased urinary catecholamines

NURSING CONSIDERATIONS
Assessment

• Monitor B/P (lying, standing), pulse q4hr; if systolic B/P drops 20 mm Hg, hold product and notify prescriber; take vital signs in patients with cardiovascular disease

• Monitor blood studies: CBC, leukocytes, differential, cardiac enzymes if patient is receiving long-term therapy; check platelets; bleeding can occur

• Monitor hepatic studies: AST, ALT, bilirubin

• Check weight qwk; appetite may increase with product

BLACK BOX WARNING: Assess mental status: mood, sensorium, affect, suicidal tendencies; increase in psychiatric symptoms: depression, panic, risk for suicide is greater in children and those < 24 yr, these patients should be evaluated q wk × 4 wks, and q3 wks × 4 wks

• Monitor constipation; constipation is more likely to occur in children or geriatric

• **Assess for serotonin syndrome:** increased heart rate, sweating, dilated pupils, tremors, twitching, hyperthermia, agitation, hyperreflexia,

nausea, vomiting, diarrhea, coma, hallucinations; may be worse in those taking SSRIs, SNRIs, triptans

• Identify patient's alcohol consumption; if alcohol is consumed, hold dose until am

• **Beers:** Avoid in older adults unless safer alternative is not available; may cause ataxia, impaired psychomotor function

• **Pregnancy/breastfeeding:** No well-controlled studies; use only if benefits outweigh fetal risk, excreted in breast milk, discontinue breastfeeding or product

Patient problems

Depression (uses)
Risk for injury (adverse reactions)
Nonadherence (teaching)

Implementation

• *Immediate-release tablets:* To minimize side effects, administer at bedtime. Administer doses >100 mg/day (or >50 mg/day in pediatric patients 8-17 years) in two divided doses; if doses are not equal, give the larger dose at bedtime.

• *Extended-release capsules:* Do not crush or chew. To minimize side effects, administer at bedtime. A combination of the 100 mg and 150 mg capsules may be required to attain the appropriate titration or maintenance dose. Once stabilized, prescribe the smallest combination of capsules needed to achieve the total daily dose.

Patient/family education

• Teach patient that therapeutic effects may take 4-6 wk, not to discontinue abruptly

• Instruct patient to use caution in driving or other activities requiring alertness because of drowsiness, dizziness, blurred vision; to avoid rising quickly from sitting to standing, especially geriatric patients

BLACK BOX WARNING: Advise that suicidal ideas, behavior may occur in children or young adults; to watch closely for suicidal thoughts, behaviors; notify prescriber immediately

• Caution patient to avoid alcohol ingestion, other CNS depressants

• Teach patient to notify prescriber if planned or suspected pregnancy and not to breastfeed

• Instruct patient to increase fluids, bulk in diet if constipation occurs, especially geriatric

• Advise patient to take gum, hard sugarless candy, or frequent sips of water for dry mouth

• **Teach patient to report serotonin syndrome:** sweating, dilated pupils, tremors, twitching, extreme heat, agitation

Evaluation
Positive therapeutic outcome
- Decrease in depression
- Absence of suicidal thoughts

folic acid (vitamin B₉) (PO, OTC; IM/IV, Ph)
(foe-lik a′sid)
Folvite
Func. class.: Vitamin B-complex group, water-soluble vitamin
Chem. class.: Supplement

ACTION: Needed for erythropoiesis; increases RBC, WBC, and platelet formation in megaloblastic anemias

Therapeutic outcome: Absence of macrocytic, megaloblastic anemias

USES: Megaloblastic or macrocytic anemia caused by folic acid deficiency; liver disease; alcoholism; hemolysis; intestinal obstruction; pregnancy; to reduce risk of neural tube defect

Unlabeled uses: Methotrexate toxicity prophylaxis in those receiving methotrexate for RA

Pharmacokinetics

Absorption	Well absorbed
Distribution	Liver, crosses placenta
Metabolism	Liver (converted to active metabolite)
Excretion	Kidneys (unchanged)
Half-life	Unknown

Pharmacodynamics

Onset	Unknown
Peak	½-1 hr
Duration	Unknown

CONTRAINDICATIONS
Hypersensitivity

Precautions: Pregnancy, anemias other than megaloblastic/macrocytic anemia, vit B₁₂ deficiency anemia, uncorrected pernicious anemia

DOSAGE AND ROUTES
RDA
Adult (pregnant/breastfeeding): PO 600 mcg/day
Adult and child ≥14 yr: PO 400 mcg
Child 9-13 yr: PO 300 mcg
Child 4-8 yr: PO 200 mcg
Child 1-3 yr: PO 150 mcg
Infant 6 mo-1 yr: PO 80 mcg
Neonate and infant <6 mo: PO 65 mcg

Megaloblastic/macrocytic anemia due to folic acid or nutritional deficiency
Pregnant/lactating: PO 800-1000 mcg

Therapeutic dose
Adult and child: PO/IM/SUBCUT/IV up to 1 mg/day

Maintenance dose
Adult and child >4 yr: PO/IM/IV/SUBCUT 0.4 mg/day
Child <4 yr: PO/IM/IV/SUBCUT up to 0.3 mg/day
Infant: PO/IM/IV/SUBCUT up to 0.1 mg/day
Pregnant/lactating: PO/IM/IV/SUBCUT 0.8-1 mg/day

Prevention of neural tube defects during pregnancy
Adult: PO 0.6 mg/day

Prevention of megaloblastic anemia during pregnancy
Adult: PO/IM/SUBCUT up to 1 mg/day during pregnancy

Tropical sprue
Adult: PO 3-15 mg/day

Methotrexate toxicity
Adult: PO/IM/Subcut 1 mg q day or 5 mg q wk

Available forms: Tabs 0.1, 0.4, 0.8, 1, 5 mg; inj 5, 10 mg/ml

ADVERSE EFFECTS
CNS: Confusion, depression, excitability, irritability
GI: Anorexia, nausea, bitter taste
INTEG: Flushing, pruritus, rash, erythema
RESP: Bronchospasm
SYST: Anaphylaxis (rare)

INTERACTIONS
Individual drugs
CarBAMazepine: increased need for folic acid
Fosphenytoin: decreased fosphenytoin levels, may increase seizures
Methotrexate, sulfaSALAzine, trimethoprim: decreased action of folic acid
Phenytoin: decreased phenytoin levels, may increase seizures

Drug classifications
Estrogens, glucocorticoids, hydantoins: increased need for folic acid
Sulfonamides: decreased action of folic acid

NURSING CONSIDERATIONS
Assessment
- **Megaloblastic anemia:** Assess patient for fatigue, dyspnea, weakness, activity intolerance (signs of megaloblastic anemia)

• Monitor Hgb, Hct, and reticulocyte count; folate levels: 6-15 mcg/ml baseline, throughout treatment
• Assess nutritional status: bran, yeast, dried beans, nuts, fruits, fresh vegetables, asparagus; if high folic acid foods are missing from the diet, a referral to a dietitian may be indicated
• Identify products currently taken: alcohol, oral contraceptives, estrogens, methotrexate, trimethoprim, carBAMazepine, hydantoins, trimethoprim; these products may cause increased folic acid use by the body and contribute to deficiency if taking other neurotoxic products
• **Pregnancy/breastfeeding:** May use in pregnancy, breastfeeding at recommended levels

Patient problem
Lack of knowledge of medication (teaching)

Implementation
SUBCUT route
• Do not inject intradermally
IM route
• Inject deeply in large muscle mass, aspirate

Direct IV route
• Give **IV** directly, undiluted 5 mg or less over 1 min or more
Continuous IV route
• May be added to most **IV** sol or TPN
• Store in light-resistant container

Patient/family education
• Advise patient to take product exactly as prescribed; not to double doses, toxicity may occur
• Instruct patient to notify prescriber of side effects; rash or fever may indicate hypersensitivity
• Advise patient that urine may become more yellow
• Instruct patient to increase intake of foods rich in folic acid in diet as recommended by dietitian or health care provider
• Advise patient to avoid breastfeeding

Evaluation
Positive therapeutic outcome
• Absence of fatigue, weakness, dyspnea
• Absence of symptoms of megaloblastic anemia
• Increase in reticulocyte count within 5 days
• Absence of fetal neural tube defect

⚠ HIGH ALERT

fondaparinux (Rx)
(fon-dah-pair'ih-nux)
Arixtra
Func. class.: Anticoagulant, antithrombotic
Chem. class.: Synthetic, selective factor Xa inhibitor

Do not confuse: Arixtra/Anti-Xa/Arista AH

ACTION: Inhibits factor Xa; interrupts blood coagulation and inhibits thrombin formation; does not inactivate thrombin (activated factor II) or affect platelets

Therapeutic outcome: Prevention of deep vein thrombosis

USES: Prevention/treatment of deep vein thrombosis, pulmonary emboli in hip and knee replacement, hip fracture or abdominal surgery, acute MI, unstable angina

Pharmacokinetics
Absorption	Rapidly, completely absorbed
Distribution	Blood; does not bind to plasma proteins except 94% to ATIII
Excretion	Eliminated unchanged in 72 hr in normal renal function
Half-life	17-21 hr

Pharmacodynamics
Onset	Rapid
Peak	3 hr
Duration	Up to 24 hr

CONTRAINDICATIONS
Hypersensitivity to this product; hemophilia, leukemia with bleeding, peptic ulcer disease, hemorrhagic stroke, surgery, thrombocytopenic purpura, weight <50 kg, severe renal disease (CCr <30 ml/min), active major bleeding, bacterial endocarditis

Precautions: Pregnancy, breastfeeding, children, geriatric, alcoholism, hepatic disease (severe), blood dyscrasias, heparin-induced thrombocytopenia, uncontrolled severe hypertension, acute nephritis, mild to moderate renal disease

BLACK BOX WARNING: Spinal/epidural anesthesia, lumbar puncture

---

DOSAGE AND ROUTES
Deep vein thrombosis/PE
Adult <50 kg: SUBCUT 5 mg/day × 5 days or more until INR is 2-3; give warfarin within 72 hr of fondaparinux
Adult 50-100 kg: SUBCUT 7.5 mg/day × 5 days or more until INR is 2-3; give warfarin within 72 hr of fondaparinux
Adult >100 kg: SUBCUT 10 mg/day × 5 days or more until INR is 2-3; give warfarin within 72 hr of fondaparinux

Prevention of deep vein thrombosis
Adult: SUBCUT 2.5 mg/day, given 6 hr after surgery (hemostasis established); continue for 5-9 days; hip surgery up to 32 days; abdominal surgery up to 24 days

Renal disease
Adult: Do not use if CCr <30 ml/min; CCr 30-50 ml/min, use cautiously

Available forms: Inj 2.5 mg/0.5 ml, 5 mg/0.4 ml, 7.5 mg/0.6 ml, 10 mg/0.8 ml prefilled syringes

ADVERSE EFFECTS
CNS: confusion, headache, dizziness, *insomnia*
HEMA: *Anemia,* purpura, hematoma, thrombocytopenia, postoperative hemorrhage, heparin-induced thrombocytopenia
INTEG: Local reaction—*rash,* pruritus, inj site bleeding, increased wound drainage, bullous eruption
META: Hypokalemia

INTERACTIONS
Do not mix with other products or inf fluids

Individual drugs
Abciximab, clopidogrel, dipyridamole, eptifibatide, quiNIDine, tirofiban, valproic acid, some cephalosporins: increased risk of bleeding

Drug classifications
NSAIDs, salicylates: increased risk of bleeding

Drug/herb
Feverfew, garlic, ginger, ginkgo, ginseng, green tea, horse chestnut, kava: increased risk of bleeding

NURSING CONSIDERATIONS
Assessment

> **BLACK BOX WARNING:** Monitor patients who have received epidural/spinal anesthesia or lumbar puncture for neurological impairment, including spinal hematoma, may lead to permanent disability or paralysis

• **Hemorrhage:** Assess for hemorrhage if coadministered with other products that may cause bleeding
• Assess blood studies (Hct, CBC, coagulation studies, platelets, occult blood in stools), anti-Xa; if platelets <100,000/mm³, treatment should be discontinued; renal studies: BUN, creatinine
• **Beers:** Avoid in older adults, increased risk of bleeding, lower creatinine clearance
• Assess for bleeding: gums, petechiae, ecchymosis, black tarry stools, hematuria; notify prescriber
• **Pregnancy/breastfeeding:** Use in pregnancy only if benefits outweigh risks to the fetus, avoid use in breastfeeding, it is not known if product is excreted in breast milk

Patient problem
Infective tissue perfusion (uses)
Risk for injury (adverse reactions)

Implementation
• Do not mix with other products or solutions; cannot be used interchangeably (unit to unit) with other anticoagulants
• Give only after screening patient for bleeding disorders
• Store at 77° F (25° C); do not freeze
SUBCUT route
• Administer SUBCUT only; do not give IM
• Check for discolored sol or sol with particulate; if present, do not give
• Administer to recumbent patient, rotate inj sites (left/right anterolateral, left/right posterolateral abdominal wall), administer 6-8 hr after surgery
• Wipe surface of inj site with alcohol swab, twist plunger cap and remove, remove rigid needle guard by pulling straight off needle, do not aspirate, do not expel air bubble from surface
• Insert whole length of needle into skin fold held with thumb and forefinger
• When product is injected, a soft click may be felt or heard
• Give at same time each day to maintain steady blood levels
• Avoid all IM inj that may cause bleeding
• Administer only this product when ordered; not interchangeable with heparin

---

Patient/family education
• Advise patient to use soft-bristle toothbrush to avoid bleeding gums, to use electric razor
• Advise patient to report any signs of bleeding: gums, under skin, urine, stools
• Caution patient to avoid OTC products containing aspirin, NSAIDs unless approved by health care professional

Evaluation

Positive therapeutic outcome
• Absence of deep vein thrombosis

formoterol (Rx)
(for-moh'ter-ahl)
Foradil Aerolizer ❦, Oxeze ❦,
Performist
Func. class.: Bronchodilator
Chem. class.: β-Adrenergic agonist

Do not confuse: Foradil/Toradol

ACTION: Has β_1 and β_2 action; relaxes bronchial smooth muscle and dilates the trachea and main bronchi by increasing levels of cyclic AMP, which relaxes smooth muscles; causes increased contractility and heart rate by acting on β-receptors in the heart

Therapeutic outcome: Bronchodilation, increased heart rate and cardiac output from action on β-receptors in heart

USES: Maintenance, treatment of asthma, COPD, prevention of exercise-induced bronchospasm

Pharmacokinetics

Absorption	Rapid (INH)
Distribution	Plasma protein binding 61%-64% at concentrations of 0.1-100 ng/mL; 31%-38% at concentrations of 5-500 ng/mL
Metabolism	Liver, lungs, GI tract
Excretion	Urine, feces
Half-life	10 hr

Pharmacodynamics bronchodilation

Onset	15 min
Peak	1-3 hr
Duration	12 hr

CONTRAINDICATIONS
Hypersensitivity to sympathomimetics, monotherapy for asthma, COPD, status asthmaticus

Precautions: Pregnancy, geriatric, cardiac disorders, hyperthyroidism, diabetes mellitus, prostatic hypertrophy, hypertension, ☛ African descendants

> **BLACK BOX WARNING:** Asthma-related death

DOSAGE AND ROUTES
Adult and child ≥ 5 yr: 20 mcg/2 mL bid by jet nebulizer

Available forms: INH powder in cap 12 mcg (Foradil Aerolizer); nebulizer sol for inhalation 20 mcg/2 ml (Performist); powder for oral inh (Oxeze Turbuhaler) 6 mcg/inh, 2 mcg/inh ❦

ADVERSE EFFECTS
CNS: Tremors, *anxiety*, insomnia, headache, dizziness, stimulation
CV: Palpitations, tachycardia, hypertension, chest pain
GI: Nausea, vomiting, xerostomia
RESP: Bronchial irritation, dryness of oropharynx, bronchospasms (overuse); infection, inflammatory reactions (child)

INTERACTIONS
Amoxapine, arsenic trioxide, chloroquine, clarithromycin, dasatinib, dolasetron, droperidol, erythromycin, halofantrine, levomethadyl, ondansetron, paliperidone, palonosetron, pentamidine, probucol, ranolazine, SUNItinib, vorinostat, pimozide, risperiDONE, ziprasidone: increased QT prolongation

Drug classifications
Class IA/III antidysrhythmics, phenothiazines, halogenated anesthetics, tricyclics, some quinolones: increase QT prolongation
β-blockers: decreased action of formoterol
MAOIs, antidepressants (tricyclics): serious dysrhythmias
Sympathomimetics, thyroid hormones, tricyclics, some quinolones: increased action of both products
Loop/thiazide diuretics: increased hypokalemia

NURSING CONSIDERATIONS
Assessment
• Assess respiratory function: B/P, pulse, lung sounds; be alert for bronchospasm, may occur with this patient
• Cardiac status: Assess for hypertension, palpitations, tachycardia; if CV reactions occur, product may need to be discontinued
• Assess I&O ratio; check for urinary retention, frequency, hesitancy

---

• Assess for paresthesias and coldness of extremities; peripheral blood flow may decrease
• **Pregnancy/breastfeeding:** Use in pregnancy only if benefits outweigh risk, use cautiously in breastfeeding

Patient problem
Impaired airway clearance (uses)
Impaired gas exchange (uses)

Implementation
• Store at room temperature; protect from heat, moisture
Inhalation route
• Place cap in aerolizer inhaler; the cap is punctured; do not wash aerolizer inhaler
• Pull off cover, twist mouthpiece to open, push buttons in; make sure the four pins are visible; remove cap from blister pack, place cap in chamber; twist to close, press (a click will be heard), release; patient should exhale, place inhaler in mouth, inhale rapidly

Patient/family education
• Review package insert with patient and inform about all aspects of product
• Teach correct use of inhaler; not to swallow caps
• Teach use of spacer device in children or geriatric
• Advise patient to avoid getting aerosol in eyes
• Advise patient to wash inhaler in warm water and dry daily
• Advise patient to avoid smoking, smoke-filled rooms, persons with respiratory infections

> **BLACK BOX WARNING:** Asthma-related death, severe asthma exacerbations: if wheezing worsens and cannot be relieved during an acute asthma attack, immediate medical attention should be sought

Evaluation
Positive therapeutic outcome
• Absence of dyspnea, wheezing
• Improved airway exchange
• Improved ABGs

TREATMENT OF OVERDOSE:
Administer β-blocker

---

foscarnet (Rx)
(foss-kar′net)
Foscavir
Func. class.: Antiviral
Chem. class.: Inorganic pyrophosphate organic analog

ACTION: Antiviral activity is produced by selective inhibition at the pyrophosphate binding site on virus-specific DNA polymerases and reverse transcriptases at concentrations that do not affect cellular DNA polymerases

Therapeutic outcome: Virostatic agents against CMV retinitis

USES: Treatment of CMV, retinitis in patients with AIDS acyclovir-resistant, herpes simplex virus (HSV) infections; used with ganciclovir for relapsing patients

Pharmacokinetics

Absorption	Complete (**IV**)
Distribution	14%-17% plasma protein binding, CSF
Metabolism	Not metabolized
Excretion	Kidneys (79%-92%) unchanged, breast milk
Half-life	3 hr; increased in renal disease

Pharmacodynamics

Onset	Rapid
Peak	Infusion end
Duration	Up to 24 hr

CONTRAINDICATIONS
Hypersensitivity, CCr <0.4 ml/min/kg

Precautions: Pregnancy, breastfeeding, children, geriatric, seizure disorders, severe anemia

> **BLACK BOX WARNING:** Nephrotoxicity electrolyte/mineral imbalances, seizures

DOSAGE AND ROUTES
CMV retinitis
Adult: IV 60 mg/kg q 8 hr or 90 mcg/kg q 12 hr × 2-3 wk, then 90-120 mg/kg/day as a single dose

HSV
Adult: IV 40 mg/kg q 8-12 hr × 2-3 wk or until resolution
Adult: IV CCr >1.4 ml/min/kg: no change; CCr >1-1.4 ml/min/kg: decrease to 30 mg/kg q12hr; CCr >0.8-1 ml/min/kg: decrease to 20 mg/kg q12hr; CCr >0.6-0.8 ml/min/kg: decrease to 35 mg/kg/day; CCr >0.5-0.6 ml/min/kg: decrease to 25 mg/kg/day; CCr ≥0.4-0.5 ml/min/kg: decrease to 20 mg/kg/day; CCr <0.4 ml/min/kg: not recommended

Available forms: Solution for injection 24 mg/mL

ADVERSE EFFECTS
CNS: *Fever,* dizziness, *headache,* seizures, *fatigue,* neuropathy, asthenia, encephalopathy,

malaise, meningitis, *paresthesia,* depression, *confusion, anxiety*
CV: ECG abnormalities, 1st-degree AV block, nonspecific ST-T segment changes, cerebrovascular disorder, cardiomyopathy, cardiac arrest, atrial fibrillation, HF, sinus tachycardia
GI: *Nausea, vomiting, diarrhea, anorexia,* abdominal pain, pancreatitis
GU: Acute renal failure, decreased CCr and increased serum creatinine, azotemia, diabetes mellitus
HEMA: Anemia, granulocytopenia, leukopenia, thrombocytopenia, thrombosis, lymphadenopathy, neutropenia
INTEG: *Rash,* sweating, pruritus, skin discoloration
RESP: *Coughing, dyspnea,* pneumonia, pulmonary infiltration, pneumothorax, hemoptysis
SYST: *Hypokalemia, hypocalcemia, hypomagnesemia,* hypophosphatemia

INTERACTIONS
Individual drugs
Acyclovir, cidofovir, CISplatin, tacrolimus, tenofovir, vancomycin, amphotericin B, cycloSPORINE, calcium products (decreases ionized calcium), lithium: increased nephrotoxicity
Pentamidine: increased hypocalcemia

Drug classifications

> **BLACK BOX WARNING:** Aminoglycosides, gold compounds, NSAIDs: increased nephrotoxicity

NURSING CONSIDERATIONS
Assessment
• **CMV retinitis:** Ophthalmic exam should confirm diagnosis, another exam at conclusion of induction and q 4 wk during treatment
• **General** culture should be done before treatment with foscarnet is begun; cultures of blood, urine, and throat may all be taken; CMV is not confirmed by this method
• **HSV:** Assess for characteristics of lesions baseline and daily during treatment

> **BLACK BOX WARNING: Renal tubular disorders:** Assess kidney: BUN, serum creatinine, creatinine clearance, if CCr <0.4 ml/min/kg, discontinue product, provide adequate hydration before and during infusion to prevent toxicity

• Blood counts should be done q2wk; watch for decreasing granulocytes, Hgb; if low, therapy may have to be discontinued and restarted after hematologic recovery; blood transfusions may be required

• Assess for GI symptoms: severe nausea, vomiting, diarrhea; severe symptoms may necessitate discontinuing product
• **Seizures:** May be caused by alterations in minerals and electrolytes, monitor electrolytes and minerals: calcium, phosphorous, magnesium, sodium, potassium; watch closely for tetany during first administration
• Assess for symptoms of blood dyscrasias (anemia, granulocytopenia); bruising, fatigue, bleeding, poor healing
• **Assess for symptoms of allergic reactions:** flushing, rash, urticaria, pruritus

Patient problem
Infection (uses)
Risk for injury (adverse reactions)

Implementation

Intermittent IV infusion route
• Administer increased fluids before, during product administration to induce diuresis and minimize renal toxicity
• Administer via inf pump, at no more than 1 mg/kg/min; do not give by rapid or bolus **IV;** give by central venous line or peripheral vein; standard 24 mg/ml sol may be used without dilution if using by central line; dilute the 24 mg/ml sol to 12 mg/ml with D_5W or 0.9% NaCl if using peripheral vein
• Monitor patient closely during therapy; if tingling, numbness, paresthesias occur, stop inf and obtain lab sample for electrolytes

Y-site incompatibilities: Manufacturer recommends that product not be given with other medications in syringe or admixed

Patient/family education
• Advise patient to notify prescriber if sore throat, swollen lymph nodes, malaise, fever occur; may indicate presence of other infections
• **Pregnancy/breastfeeding:** Use cautiously in pregnancy only if clearly needed, do not breastfeed
• Advise patient to report perioral tingling, numbness in extremities, and paresthesias; inf should be stopped and electrolytes should be requested
• Caution patient that serious product interactions may occur if OTC products are ingested; check first with prescriber
• Inform patient that product is not a cure but will control symptoms
• Advise patient that ophth exams must be continued

Evaluation
Positive therapeutic outcome
• Improvement in CMV retinitis
• Healing of HSV lesions

fosinopril (Rx)
(foss-in-o'pril)
Func. class.: Antihypertensive
Chem. class.: Angiotensin-converting
enzyme (ACE) inhibitor

ACTION: Selectively suppresses renin-angiotensin-aldosterone system; inhibits ACE; prevents conversion of angiotensin I to angiotensin II; results in dilatation of arterial, venous vessels

Therapeutic outcome: Decreased B/P in hypertension

USES: Hypertension, alone or in combination with thiazide diuretics, systolic HF

Pharmacokinetics

Absorption	30%
Distribution	Crosses placenta, protein binding 99%
Metabolism	Liver, converted to fosinoprilat
Excretion	50% kidneys (metabolites), 50% feces
Half-life	12 hr fosinoprilat

Pharmacodynamics

Onset	1 hr
Peak	2-6 hr
Duration	24 hr

CONTRAINDICATIONS
Breastfeeding, children, hypersensitivity to ACE inhibitors, history of ACE inhibitor–induced angioedema

> **BLACK BOX WARNING:** Pregnancy

Precautions: Geriatric, impaired liver function, hypovolemia, blood dyscrasias, HF, COPD, asthma, angioedema, hyperkalemia, renal artery stenosis, renal disease, aortic stenosis, autoimmune disorders, collagen vascular disease, febrile illness, Black patients ⚠🔑

DOSAGE AND ROUTES
Hypertension
Adult: PO 5-10 mg/day initially, then 20-40 mg/day divided bid or daily, max 80 mg/day

HF
Adult: PO 10 mg/day, then up to 40 mg/day, increased over several weeks; use lower dose in those undergoing diuresis before fosinopril
Child >50 kg: PO 5-10 mg q day initially, max 40 mg/day

Available forms: Tabs 10, 20, 40 mg

ADVERSE EFFECTS
CNS: *Headache, dizziness,* fatigue, syncope, stroke, drowsiness, insomnia, weakness
CV: *Hypotension,* orthostatic hypotension, tachycardia, chest pain, palpitations
GI: *Nausea,* constipation, *vomiting,* diarrhea, pancreatitis, hepatotoxicity
GU: Increased BUN, creatinine, azotemia, renal artery stenosis
HEMA: Decreased Hct, Hgb, eosinophilia, leukopenia, neutropenia, agranulocytosis
META: *Hyperkalemia*
RESP: *Cough,* bronchospasm
SYST: Anaphylaxis, angioedema
MS: Myalgia, arthralgia
INTEG: Rash, urticaria, photosensitivity, pruritus

INTERACTIONS
Individual drugs
Alcohol (acute ingestion): increased hypotension (large amounts)
Digoxin, hydrALAZINE, lithium, prazosin: increased toxicity

Drug classifications
Adrenergic blockers, antihypertensives, diuretics, ganglionic blockers, nitrates: increased hypotension
Antacids: decreased absorption
Diuretics (potassium-sparing), sympathomimetics, NSAIDs, vasodilators: increased toxicity
Salicylates: decreased antihypertensive effect

Drug/herb
Hawthorn: increased antihypertensive effect
Ephedra: decreased antihypertensive effect

Drug/lab test
Increased: AST, ALT, alkaline phosphatase, glucose, bilirubin, uric acid, BUN, potassium
Positive: ANA titer
False positive: urine acetone

NURSING CONSIDERATIONS
Assessment
• **Hypertension:** Monitor B/P, check for orthostatic hypotension, syncope; if changes occur, dosage change may be required
• **Collagen vascular disease:** Monitor blood studies: neutrophils, decreased platelets; obtain WBC with differential at baseline and qmo × 6 mo, then q2-3mo × 1 yr; if neutrophils <1000/mm³, discontinue
• Monitor renal studies: protein, BUN, creatinine; watch for increased levels that may indicate nephrotic syndrome and renal failure; monitor urine daily for protein; monitor renal symptoms: polyuria, oliguria, frequency, dysuria
• Establish baselines in renal, liver function tests before therapy begins

- Check potassium levels throughout treatment
- **HF:** Check for edema in feet, legs daily, monitor weight daily
- **Assess for allergic reactions:** rash, fever, pruritus, urticaria; product should be discontinued if antihistamines fail to help
- **Pregnancy/breastfeeding:** Do not use in pregnancy, breastfeeding

Patient problem
Impaired cardiac output (uses)
Nonadherence (teaching)

Implementation
- Store in tight container at 86° F (30° C)
- Severe hypotension may occur after 1st dose of this medication; hypotension may be prevented by reducing or discontinuing diuretic therapy 3 days before beginning benazepril therapy

Patient/family education
- Advise patient not to discontinue product abruptly; warn patient to tell all persons associated with his or her care
- Teach patient not to use OTC products (cough, cold, allergy) unless directed by prescriber because serious side effects can occur; xanthines such as coffee, tea, chocolate, cola can prevent action of product
- Teach patient the importance of complying with dosage schedule, even if feeling better; to continue with medical regimen to decrease B/P: exercise, smoking cessation, decreasing stress, diet modifications
- Emphasize the need to rise slowly to sitting or standing position to minimize orthostatic hypotension; not to exercise in hot weather or increased hypotension can occur
- Advise patient to notify prescriber of mouth sores, sore throat, fever, swelling of hands or feet, irregular heartbeat, chest pain, coughing, shortness of breath
- Instruct patient to report excessive perspiration, dehydration, vomiting, diarrhea; may lead to fall in B/P
- Caution patient that product may cause dizziness, fainting, light-headedness; may occur during 1st few days of therapy; to avoid activities that may be hazardous
- Teach patient how to take B/P, normal readings for age-group

> **BLACK BOX WARNING:** Advise patient to notify prescriber if pregnancy is planned or suspected, to use contraception during treatment

Evaluation
Positive therapeutic outcome
- Decreased B/P in hypertension
- Decreased signs in HF
- Prevention of early death due to MI, stroke

TREATMENT OF OVERDOSE:
0.9% NaCl IV inf, hemodialysis

fosphenytoin (Rx)
(foss-fen'i-toy-in)
Cerebyx
Func. class.: Anticonvulsant
Chem. class.: Hydantoin, phosphate phenytoin ester

ACTION: Inhibits spread of seizure activity in motor cortex by altering ion transport; increases AV conduction; prodrug of phenytoin

Therapeutic outcome: Decreased seizures, absence of dysrhythmias

USES: Generalized tonic-clonic seizures, status epilepticus, partial seizures

Pharmacokinetics

Absorption	Rapid, converted to phenytoin (IV)
Distribution	Protein binding 99%, CSF, tissues, crosses the placenta
Metabolism	Liver: converted to phenytoin
Excretion	Kidneys (minimal)
Half-life	15 min

Pharmacodynamics

	IM	IV
Onset	Unknown	15-45 min
Peak	30 min	15-60 min
Duration	24 hr	24 hr

CONTRAINDICATIONS
Pregnancy, hypersensitivity, bradycardia, SA and AV block, Stokes-Adams syndrome

Precautions: Breastfeeding, allergies, renal/hepatic disease, myocardial insufficiency, hypoalbuminemia, hypothyroidism, Asian patients positive for HLA-B 1502, abrupt discontinuation, agranulocytosis, alcoholism, carBAMazepine/barbiturate hypersensitivity, bone marrow suppression, CAD, geriatrics, hemolytic anemia, hyponatremia, methemoglobinemia, myasthenia gravis, psychosis, suicidal ideation

> **BLACK BOX WARNING:** Dysrhythmias, hypotension (rapid IV infusion)

DOSAGE AND ROUTES
All doses in PE (phenytoin sodium equivalent)

Status epilepticus
Adult and child: IV 15-20 mg PE/kg

Nonemergency/maintenance dosing

Adult and adolescent >16 yr: IM/IV 10-20 mg PE/kg 10 mg dose; 4-6 mg PE/kg/day (maintenance)

Available forms: Inj, 50 mg/ml vials

ADVERSE EFFECTS

CNS: *Drowsiness,* dizziness, insomnia, paresthesias, depression, suicidal tendencies, aggression, headache, confusion, paresthesia, emotional lability, syncope, cerebral edema

CV: Hypotension, hypertension, HF, shock, dysrhythmias

EENT: Nystagmus, diplopia, blurred vision

GI: Nausea, vomiting, diarrhea, constipation, anorexia, weight loss, hepatitis, jaundice, gingival hyperplasia

HEMA: Agranulocytosis, leukopenia, aplastic anemia, thrombocytopenia, megaloblastic anemia

INTEG: Rash, lupus erythematosus, Stevens-Johnson syndrome, hirsutism, hypersensitivity, pruritus

RESP: Bronchospasm, cough

SYST: Hyperglycemia, hypokalemia, toxic epidermal necrolysis ✖⊶ (Asian patients positive for HLA-B 1502), DRESS, purple glove syndrome, anaphylaxis

INTERACTIONS
Individual drugs

Alcohol: decreased effects of fosphenytoin (chronic use)

Amiodarone, chloramphenicol, cimetidine: increased fosphenytoin level

CarBAMazepine, folic acid, rifampin, theophylline, tramadol: decreased effects of fosphenytoin

Delavirdine: do not use concurrently; decreased virologic response, resistance

Drug classifications

Antacids, antihistamines, antineoplastics, CYP1A2 inducers: decreased effects of fosphenytoin

Antidepressants (tricyclics), CYP1A2 inhibitors, estrogens, H_2-receptor antagonists, phenothiazines, salicylates, sulfonamides: increased fosphenytoin level

Drug/herb

Ginseng, valerian: decreased anticonvulsant effect

Ginkgo: increased anticonvulsant effect

Drug/lab test

Increased: glucose, alkaline phosphatase

Decreased: dexamethasone, metyrapone test serum, PBI, urinary steroids, potassium

NURSING CONSIDERATIONS
Assessment

• Assess drug level: target level 10-20 mcg/ml; toxic level 30-50 mcg/ml, wait at least 2 hr after dose before testing, 4 hr after IM dose

• Assess seizure activity including type, location, duration, and character; provide seizure precaution

• Assess renal studies: urinalysis, BUN, urine creatinine

• Monitor hepatic studies: ALT, AST, bilirubin, creatinine

• Assess allergic reaction: red raised rash; if this occurs, product should be discontinued

• **Monitor for toxicity:** bone marrow depression, nausea, vomiting, ataxia, diplopia, cardiovascular collapse, slurred speech, confusion

• **Pregnancy/breastfeeding:** Do not use in pregnancy, birth defects have occurred, avoid breastfeeding

• Assess product level: toxic level 30-50 mcg/ml

• Assess for rash, discontinue as soon as rash develops, serious adverse reactions such as Stevens-Johnson syndrome can occur

• **Assess mental status:** mood, sensorium, affect, memory (long, short), especially geriatric; suicidal thoughts/behaviors

• **Serious skin reactions:** usually occurring within 28 days of treatment; if a rash develops, patient should be evaluated for DRESS

• **Assess for blood dyscrasias:** fever, sore throat, bruising, rash, jaundice, epistaxis (long-term treatment only)

• Monitor blood studies: RBC, Hct, Hgb, reticulocyte counts weekly for 4 wk, then monthly; also check thyroid function tests, serum calcium, albumin, phosphorus, potassium

Patient problem

Risk for injury (uses)

Lack of knowledge of medication (teaching)

Implementation
Injectable routes

• Give IM/IV; the dosage, concentration, and infusion rate of fosphenytoin should always be expressed, prescribed, and dispensed in phenytoin sodium equivalents (PE); exercise extreme caution when preparing and administering fosphenytoin; the concentration and dosage should be carefully confirmed; fatal overdoses have occurred in children when the per-ml concentration of the product (50 mg PE/mL) was misinterpreted as the total amount of drug in the vial

• Visually inspect for particulate matter and discoloration prior to use

IV infusion route

• Prior to infusion, dilute in 5% dextrose or 0.9% saline solution to a concentration ranging from 1.5-25 mg PE/ml

BLACK BOX WARNING: Because of the risk of hypotension, do not exceed recommended infusion rates. Continuous monitoring of ECG, B/P, and respiratory function is recommended, especially throughout the period when phenytoin concentrations peak (about 10-20 min after the end of the infusion)

• Loading doses should always be followed by maintenance doses of oral or parenteral phenytoin or parenteral fosphenytoin

BLACK BOX WARNING: Adult: Infuse IV at a rate max 150 mg PE/min

• Elderly or debilitated adult: infuse IV at a max 3 mg PE/kg/min or 150 mg PE/min, whichever is less

BLACK BOX WARNING: Child: Infuse IV at a rate of 0.5-3 mg PE/kg/min, max 150 mg PE/min, whichever is less

BLACK BOX WARNING: Infant, neonate: infuse IV at a rate max 0.5-3 mg PE/kg/min

Y-site compatibilities: Aminocaproic acid, amphotericin B lipid complex, amphotericin B liposome, anidulafungin, atenolol, bivalirudin, bleomycin, CARBOplatin, CISplatin, cyclophosphamide, cytarabine, DACTINomycin, DAPTOmycin, dexmedetomidine, dilTIAZem, DOCEtaxel, doxacurium, eptifibatide, ertapenem, etoposide, fludarabine, fluorouracil, gatifloxacin, gemcitabine, gemtuzumab, granisetron, ifosfamide, levofloxacin, linezolid, LORazepam, mechlorethamine, meperidine, methotrexate, metroNIDAZOLE, nesiritide, octreotide, oxaliplatin, oxytocin, PACLitaxel, palonosetron, pamidronate, pantoprazole, PEMEtrexed, PHENobarbital, piperacillin-tazobactam, rocuronium, sodium acetate, tacrolimus, teniposide, thiotepa, tigecycline, tirofiban, vinCRIStine, vinorelbine, voriconazole, zoledronic acid

Patient/family education

• Teach patient the reason for and expected outcome of treatment

• Instruct patient not to use machinery or engage in hazardous activity; drowsiness, dizziness may occur

• Advise patient to carry/wear emergency ID identifying product used, name of prescriber

• Advise patient to notify prescriber of rash, bleeding, bruising, slurred speech, jaundice of skin or eyes, joint pain, nausea, vomiting, severe headache, depression, suicidal ideation

• Advise patient to keep all medical appointments, including lab work, physical assessment

• Advise patient to notify prescriber if pregnancy is planned or suspected; to use contraception with this product; not to use in pregnancy, avoid breastfeeding

Evaluation

Positive therapeutic outcome

• Decreased seizure activity

frovatriptan (Rx)

(froh-vah-trip'tan)

Frova

Func. class.: Antimigraine agent
Chem. class.: 5-HT$_1$ receptor agonist

ACTION: Binds selectively to the vascular 5-HT$_{1B}$, 5-HT$_{1D}$ receptor subtypes, exerts antimigraine effect; binds to benzodiazepine receptor sites, causes vasoconstriction in cranium

Therapeutic outcome: Absence of migraines

USES: Acute treatment of migraine

Pharmacokinetics

Absorption	Absolute bioavailability of PO dose ~20% in males, 30% in females
Distribution	Protein binding 15%; reversibly bound to blood cells at equilibrium 60%
Metabolism	Liver, by CYP1A2
Excretion	Urine (32%), feces (62%)
Half-life	25-29 hr

Pharmacodynamics

Onset	10 min-2 hr
Peak	2-4 hr
Duration	Unknown

CONTRAINDICATIONS

Angina pectoris, history of MI, documented silent ischemia, Prinzmetal's angina, ischemic heart disease, concurrent ergotamine-containing preparations, uncontrolled hypertension, hypersensitivity, basilar or hemiplegic migraine; ischemic bowel disease; peripheral vascular disease, severe hepatic disease, prophylactic migraine treatment

Precautions: Pregnancy, breastfeeding, children, geriatric, postmenopausal women, men >40 yr, risk factors for CAD, hypercholesterolemia, obesity, diabetes, impaired hepatic function, seizure disorder

DOSAGE AND ROUTES
Adult: PO 2.5 mg; a 2nd dose may be taken after ≥2 hr; max 3 tabs/day (7.5 mg)

Available forms: Tabs 2.5 mg

ADVERSE EFFECTS
CNS: *Hot sensation,* paresthesia, *dizziness,* headache, fatigue, cold sensation, insomnia, anxiety, somnolence, seizures
CV: *Flushing,* chest pain, palpitation, coronary artery vasospasm, MI, myocardial ischemia, ventricular tachycardia, ventricular fibrillation
GI: Dry mouth, dyspepsia, abdominal pain, diarrhea, vomiting, nausea
MS: Skeletal pain

INTERACTIONS
Individual drugs
Estrogen, propranolol: increased effects of frovatriptan

Drug classifications
CYP1A2 inhibitors (cimetidine, ciprofloxacin, erythromycin), hormonal contraceptives: increased frovatriptan levels
Selective serotonin reuptake inhibitors, other serotonin agonists (dextromethorphan, antidepressants): increased toxicity, MAOIs

NURSING CONSIDERATIONS
Assessment
• **Migraine:** aura, alleviating/exacerbating factor, diet, character
• Assess for ingestion of tyramine-containing foods (pickled products, beer, wine, aged cheese), food additives, preservatives, colorings, artificial sweeteners, chocolate, caffeine, which may precipitate these types of headaches
• **Serious cardiac reactions:** May occur within a few hours of taking a 5-HT1 agonist, dysrhythmias, ventricular fibrillation leading to death
• **Serotonin syndrome:** Assess for agitation, confusion, diaphoresis, increased B/P, nausea, vomiting, diarrhea, product should be discontinued
• Assess B/P; signs/symptoms of coronary vasospasms
• Assess for stress level, activity, recreation, coping mechanisms
• Assess neurologic status: LOC, paresthesia, hot/cold sensations, dizziness, headache, fatigue

• **Pregnancy/breastfeeding:** Use only if benefits outweigh risk to the fetus, do not breastfeed

Patient problem
Pain (uses)

Implementation
• Ensure that tablets are swallowed whole
• Provide quiet, calm environment with decreased stimulation from noise, bright light, excessive talking

Patient/family education
• Instruct patient to report any side effects to prescriber
• Advise patient that photosensitivity may occur, to use sunscreen and wear protective clothing when outdoors
• Advise patient to have dark, quiet environment available
• **Serotonin syndrome:** Teach patient to report immediately agitation, confusion, sweating, nausea, vomiting, diarrhea
• **Serious cardiac reactions:** Advise patient to report immediately pain, chest tightness

Evaluation

Positive therapeutic outcome
• Decrease in frequency, severity of migraine

TREATMENT OF OVERDOSE:
No specific antidote; monitor patient closely for ≥48 hr, treat any symptoms as necessary

furosemide (Rx)
(fur-oh'se-mide)
Lasix
Func. class.: Loop diuretic
Chem. class.: Sulfonamide derivative

Do not confuse: furosemide/torsemide, **Lasix**/Lanoxin/Lomotil/Losec/Luvox

ACTION: Acts on the ascending loop of Henle in the kidney, inhibiting reabsorption of electrolytes sodium and chloride, causing excretion of sodium, calcium, magnesium, chloride, water, and some potassium; decreases reabsorption of sodium and chloride and increases excretion of potassium in the distal tubule of the kidney; responsible for slight antihypertensive effect and peripheral vasodilatation

Therapeutic outcome: Decreased edema in lung tissue, peripherally; decreased B/P

USES: Pulmonary edema, edema in HF, nephrotic syndrome, ascites, hepatic disease, hypertension

---

Pharmacokinetics

Absorption	GI tract (60%-70%)
Distribution	Crosses placenta, enters breast milk, protein binding 90%-99%
Metabolism	Liver (30%-40%)
Excretion	Breast milk, urine, feces
Half-life	½-1 hr

Pharmacodynamics

	PO	IM	IV
Onset	1 hr	½ hr	5 min
Peak	1-2 hr	Unknown	½ hr
Duration	6-8 hr	4-8 hr	2 hr

Unlabeled uses: Hypercalcemia in malignancy

CONTRAINDICATIONS

Anuria, hypovolemia

Precautions: Pregnancy, diabetes mellitus, dehydration, severe renal disease, cirrhosis, ascites, hypersensitivity to sulfonamides, breastfeeding, infants, electrolyte depletion

DOSAGE AND ROUTES
Edema
Adult: PO 20-80 mg/day in AM, may give another dose in 6 hr, up to 600 mg/day; IM/IV 20-40 mg, increased by 20 mg q2hr until desired response

Child: PO/IM/IV 1-2 mg/kg, may increase by 1-2 mg/kg/q6-8hr up to 6 mg/kg

Antihypercalcemia
Adult: IM/IV 80-100 mg q1-4hr or PO 120 mg/day or divided bid

Child: IM/IV 25-50 mg, repeat q4hr if needed

Acute/chronic renal failure
Adult: PO 80 mg/day, increase by 80-120 mg/day to desired response; IV 100-200 mg, max 600-800 mg

Available forms: Tabs 20, 40, 80 mg; oral sol 8 mg/ml, 10 mg/ml; inj IM, IV 10 mg/ml

ADVERSE EFFECTS

CNS: Headache, fatigue, weakness, vertigo, paresthesias

CV: Orthostatic hypotension, chest pain, ECG changes, circulatory collapse

EENT: *Loss of hearing*, ear pain, tinnitus, blurred vision

META: *Hypokalemia, hypochloremic alkalosis, hypomagnesemia, hyperuricemia, hypocalcemia, hyponatremia*, metabolic alkalosis

ENDO: *Hyperglycemia*

GI: *Nausea*, diarrhea, dry mouth, vomiting, anorexia, cramps, oral or gastric irritations, pancreatitis

GU: *Polyuria*, renal failure, *glycosuria*, bladder spasms

HEMA: Thrombocytopenia, agranulocytosis, leukopenia, neutropenia, anemia

INTEG: *Rash, pruritus, purpura*, sweating, photosensitivity, urticaria

MS: Cramps, stiffness

SYST: Toxic epidermal necrolysis, erythema muliforme, Stevens-Johnson syndrome

INTERACTIONS
Individual drugs
CISplatin, vancomycin: increased risk of ototoxicity

Digoxin: increased toxicity

Lithium: decreased renal clearance, causing increased toxicity

Probenecid: decreased furosemide effect

Drug classifications
Aminoglycosides: increased ototoxicity

Anticoagulants, salicylates: increased effects

Antihypertensives: increased antihypertensive effect

Nitrates: increased hypotensive action

Nondepolarizing skeletal muscle relaxants, salicylates, aminoglycosides, CISplatin: increased toxicity

Drug/lab test
Interference: GTT

Increase: LDL

NURSING CONSIDERATIONS
Assessment
• **HF:** Assess fluid volume status: I&O ratios and record, count or weigh diapers as appropriate, weight, distended red veins, crackles in lung, color, quality, and specific gravity of urine, skin turgor, adequacy of pulses, moist mucous membranes, bilateral lung sounds, peripheral pitting edema; dehydration symptoms of decreasing output, thirst, hypotension, dry mouth and mucous membranes should be reported

• Monitor electrolytes: potassium, sodium, chloride, magnesium; also include BUN, blood pH, ABGs, uric acid, CBC, blood glucose

• **Hypertension:** Assess B/P before and during therapy, lying, standing, and sitting as appropriate; orthostatic hypotension can occur rapidly

• **Ototoxicity:** Assess patient for tinnitus, hearing loss, ear pain; periodic testing of hearing is needed when high doses of this product are given by IV route

• **Hypokalemia:** acidic urine, reduced urine osmolality, nocturia, polyuria and polydipsia;

hypotension, broad T-wave, U-wave, ectopy, tachycardia, weak pulse; muscle weakness, altered LOC, drowsiness, apathy, lethargy, confusion, depression; anorexia, nausea, cramps, constipation, distention, paralytic ileus; hypoventilation, respiratory muscle weakness
• Monitor for CV, GI, neurologic manifestations of hyponatremia: increased B/P, cold, clammy skin, hypovolemia or hypervolemia; anorexia, nausea, vomiting, diarrhea, abdominal cramps; lethargy, increased ICP, confusion, headache, seizures, coma, fatigue, tremors, hyperreflexia
• Monitor for neurologic, respiratory manifestations of hyperchloremia: weakness, lethargy, coma; deep rapid breathing
• **Beers:** Use with caution in older adults, may exacerbate or cause syndrome of inappropriate antidiuretic hormone secretion or hyponatremia, monitor sodium level closely when changing dose
• **Serious rash:** Monitor for skin rash often, Stevens-Johnson syndrome, toxic epidermal necrolysis, erythema multiforme may occur and is life-threatening
• **Pregnancy/lactation:** Use only if benefits outweigh risks to the fetus, use cautiously in breastfeeding, excreted in breast milk

Patient problem
Fluid imbalance (uses, adverse reactions)

Implementation
• Give in AM to avoid interference with sleep
• Potassium replacement if potassium level is <3.0 mg/dl; product may be crushed if patient is unable to swallow
PO route
• With food or milk or use oral sol if nausea occurs; absorption may be reduced slightly

IV route
• Do not use sol that is yellow, has a precipitate or crystals
IV, direct route
• Give undiluted through Y-tube on 3-way stopcock; give 20 mg or less/min
Intermittent IV inf route
• May be added to 0.9% NaCl, D₅W, use within 24 hr to ensure compatibility; give through Y-tube or 3-way stopcock; give at 4 mg/min or less, use inf pump

Y-site compatibilities: Acyclovir, alfentanil, allopurinol, alprostadil, amifostine, amikacin, aminocaproic acid, aminophylline, amphotericin B cholesteryl/lipid complex/liposome, anidulafungin, argatroban, ascorbic acid, atenolol, atropine, azaTHIOprine, aztreonam, bivalirudin, bleomycin, bumetanide, calcium chloride/gluconate, CARBOplatin, cefamandole, ceFAZolin, cefepime, cefonicid, cefotaxime, cefoTEtan, cefOXitin, cefTAZidime, ceftizoxime, ceftobiprole, cefTRIAXone, cefuroxime, chloramphenicol, CISplatin, cladribine, clindamycin, cyanocobalamin, cyclophosphamide, cycloSPORINE, cytarabine, DACTINomycin, DAPTOmycin, dexamethasone, dexmedetomidine, digoxin, DOCEtaxel, doripenem, doxacurium, DOXOrubicin liposome, enalaprilat, ePHEDrine, EPINEPHrine, etoposide, fentaNYL, fludarabine, fluorouracil, folic acid, foscarnet, gallium nitrate, ganciclovir, granisetron, heparin, hydrocortisone, HYDROmorphone, ifosfamide, imipenemcilastatin, indomethacin, insulin (regular), isosorbide, kanamycin, leucovorin, lidocaine, linezolid, LORazepam, LR, mannitol, mechlorethamine, melphalan, meropenem, methicillin, methotrexate, methylPREDNISolone, metoprolol, metroNIDAZOLE, mezlocillin, micafungin, miconazole, mitoMYcin, moxalactam, multiple vitamins injection, nafcillin, naloxone, nitroprusside, octreotide, oxacillin, oxaliplatin, oxytocin, PACLitaxel, palonosetron, pamidronate, pantoprazole, PEMEtrexed, penicillin G, PENTObarbital, PHENobarbital, phytonadione, piperacillin, piperacillin-tazobactam, potassium chloride, procainamide, propofol, propranolol, ranitidine, remifentanil, Ringer's, ritodrine, sargramostim, sodium acetate/bicarbonate, succinylcholine, SUFentanil, temocillin, teniposide, theophylline, thiopental, thiotepa, ticarcillin, ticarcillin-clavulanate, tigecycline, tirofiban, TNA, tobramycin, urokinase, vit B/C, voriconazole, zoledronic acid

Patient/family education
• Teach patient to take the medication early in the day to prevent nocturia
• Instruct the patient to take with food or milk if GI symptoms of nausea and anorexia occur
• Teach patient to maintain a record of weight on a weekly basis and notify physician of weight loss of >5 lb
• Caution the patient that this product causes a loss of potassium, that food rich in potassium should be added to the diet; refer to a dietitian for assistance in planning
• Caution the patient to rise slowly from sitting or reclining positions, not to exercise in hot weather or stand for prolonged periods because orthostatic hypotension will be enhanced; lie down if dizziness occurs
• Advise patient to wear protective clothing and sunscreen to prevent photosensitivity
• Caution patient not to use alcohol or any OTC medications without physician's approval; serious product reactions may occur

• Emphasize the need to contact physician immediately if muscle cramps, weakness, nausea, dizziness, or numbness occurs
• Teach patient to take and record own B/P and pulse
• Advise patient to continue taking medication even if feeling better; this product controls symptoms but does not cure the condition
• Advise the patient with hypertension to continue other medical treatment (exercise, weight loss, relaxation techniques, cessation of smoking)

• Teach patient to contact prescriber if rash, cramps, nausea, dizziness, numbness, weakness occur

Evaluation
Positive therapeutic outcome
• Decreased edema
• Decreased B/P
• Lowered calcium level in malignancy
• Increased diuresis

F

gabapentin (Rx)
(gab´a-pen-tin)
Gralise, Horizant, Neurontin
Func. class.: Anticonvulsant
Chem. class.: GABA analogue

Do not confuse: Neurontin/Noroxin/
Neoral

ACTION: Mechanism unknown; may increase seizure threshold; structurally similar to GABA, but does not bind to GABAa or GABAb; gabapentin binding sites in neocortex, hippocampus

Therapeutic outcome: Decreased seizure activity

USES: Adjunct treatment of partial seizures, with or without generalization in patients >12 yr; adjunct in partial seizures in children 3-12 yr, postherpetic neuralgia, primary restless leg syndrome (RLS) in adults

Unlabeled uses: Neuropathic pain, bipolar disorder, migraine prophylaxis, fibromyalgia, anxiety

Pharmacokinetics

Absorption	Unknown
Distribution	Unknown
Metabolism	None
Excretion	Urine unchanged
Half-life	5-7 hr

Pharmacodynamics

	Immediate Release	Extended Release
Onset	Unknown	Unknown
Peak	2 hr	8 hr-Gralise, 5-7 hr-Horizant
Duration	Unknown	Unknown

CONTRAINDICATIONS
Hypersensitivity to this product

Precautions: Pregnancy, breastfeeding, children <3 yr, geriatric, renal disease, hemodialysis, suicidal thoughts, depression

DOSAGE AND ROUTES
Generalized tonic-clonic seizures (Neurontin only)
Adult and child >12 yr: PO 300 mg tid; may titrate to 1800 mg/day in 3 divided doses
Child 3-12 yr: PO 10-15 mg/kg/day in 3 divided doses, initially titrate dose upward over approximately 3 days; if >5 yr old, 40 mg/kg/day in 3 divided doses; all given in 3 divided doses

Postherpetic neuralgia
Adult: PO (Neurontin) 300 mg on day 1, 600 mg/day divided bid on day 2, 900 mg/day divided tid on day 3, may titrate to 1800-3600 mg divided tid if needed; **ext rel tab (Gralise only)** 300 mg on day 1, then 600 mg on day 2, 900 mg on days 3-6, 1200 mg on days 7-10, 1500 mg on days 11-14, 1800 mg on day 15 and thereafter; **Horizant only:** 600 mg in AM × 3 days, day 4 give 600 mg bid

Moderate to severe RLS (Horizant only)
Adult: PO ext rel tab 600 mg qd with food at about 5 PM; if dose is missed, take next day at 5 PM

Diabetic neuropathy pain (unlabeled)
Adult: PO 900 mg-3.6 g/day in divided doses tid

Fibromyalgia (unlabeled)
Adult: PO 300 mg at bedtime × 1 wk, then gradually increase (target dose 2400 mg), 300 mg bid × 1 wk, 300 mg bid and 600 mg at bedtime × 2 wk, then 600 mg tid × 2 wk with 1200 mg at bedtime; to discontinue, taper by 300 mg/day

Renal Dose
Adult and child >12 yr PO immediate release: CCr ≥ 60 ml/min: No change; **CCr >30-59 ml/min:** Total dose range 400-1400 mg/day given divided bid; **CCr >15-29 ml/min:** 200-700 mg/day PO given in a single daily dose; **CCr = 15 ml/min:** 100-300 mg/day given in one daily dose as 100, 125, 150, 200, or 300 mg; CCr <15 ml/min
Adult: PO ext rel tablets (Gralise tablets only): CCr ≥ 60 ml/min: No change; CCr 30-59 ml/min: 600-1800 mg/day as tolerated; CCr <30 ml/min: Do not use; **ext rel tablets (Horizant tablets only): CCr ≥ 60 ml/min:** No change; before discontinuing reduce the dose to 600 mg q daily × 1 wk before discontinuing; **CCr 30-59 ml/min:** for RLS, start at 300 mg/day, increase to 600 mg/day as needed; for PHN, start at 300 mg in the AM × 3 days, then increase to 300 mg bid, increase to 600 mg bid as needed; for dose tapering, reduce the maintenance dose to q daily in the AM × 1 wk before discontinuing; **CCr 15-29 ml/min:** for RLS, 300 mg/day; for PHN, 300 mg PO on day 1 and day 3, then 300 mg qday in the AM, increase dose to 300 mg bid as needed for dose tapering, if dose is 300 mg bid, reduce dose to 300 mg

qday in AM × 1 wk before discontinuation; if the dose is 300 qday, no taper is required; **CCr <15 ml/min:** for RLS and PHN, 300 mg every other day, for PHN, dose can be increased to 300 mg qday in AM, no dose taper is required before discontinuing

Available forms: Caps 100, 300, 400 mg; tabs 600, 800 mg; oral sol 250 mg/5 ml, Horizant: ext rel tab 300, 600 mg (Gralise)

ADVERSE EFFECTS

CNS: *Drowsiness, confusion,* dizziness, fatigue, anxiety, poor concentration, lability, hyperkinesia; emotional lability, aggression, hostility, seizures, suicidal ideation
CV: Vasodilatation, peripheral edema, hypotension, hypertension
EENT: Dry mouth, blurred vision, nystagmus, otitis media (child 3-12 yr)
GI: Constipation/diarrhea, weight gain, increased appetite, gingivitis; diarrhea (Gralise)
INTEG: Pruritus, abrasion, Stevens-Johnson syndrome, acne vulgaris
MS: Myalgia, back pain, gout, rhabdomyolysis
RESP: Rhinitis, pharyngitis, coughing; upper respiratory infection (child 3-12 yr)
SYST: Drug reaction with eosinophilia and systemic symptoms (DRESS); dehydration (child 3-12 yr)

INTERACTIONS
Individual drugs
Alcohol: increased CNS depression
Cimetidine, sevelamer, separate by 2 hr: decreased gabapentin levels
HYDROcodone, dosage reduction may be needed: increased effect of HYDROcodone

Drug classifications
Antacids: decreased gabapentin levels
Antihistamines, sedatives, all other CNS depressants: increased CNS depression

Drug/herb
Chamomile, kava, valerian: increased CNS depression

Drug/lab test
False positive: urinary protein using Ames N-multistix SG

NURSING CONSIDERATIONS
Assessment
• **Assess seizures:** aura, location, duration, frequency, activity at onset
• **Assess mental status:** mood, sensorium, affect, behavioral changes, suicidal thoughts/behaviors; if mental status changes, notify prescriber

• Monitor for drug reaction with eosinophilia and systemic symptoms
• Provide increased fluids, bulk in diet for constipation
• **Neuropathic pain:** Assess for type of pain, location, character baseline, and periodically
• **RLS:** Assess for restless leg syndrome characteristics baseline and periodically
• **Migraine:** Assess for characteristics baseline and periodically
• **Beers:** Avoid in older adults unless safer alternative is not available; ataxia, impaired psychomotor function may occur

Patient problem
Pain (uses)
Risk for injury (uses)
Suicidal ideation (adverse reactions)

Implementation
• Do not break, crush, or chew caps, ext rel tabs; cap may be opened and contents put in applesauce or dissolved in juice; scored tab may be cut in half
• Gradually withdraw over 7 days; abrupt withdrawal may precipitate seizures
• Give at least 2 hr apart when giving antacids; give without regard to meals (immediate release)
• Store at room temperature away from heat and light
• Provide assistance with ambulation during early part of treatment; dizziness occurs
• **Provide seizure precautions:** padded side rails, move objects that may harm patient
• **Oral sol:** measure with calibrated device, refrigerate
• **Ext release:** give with food at about 5 PM, bioavailability is increased with food; do not interchange Gralise with Horizant

Patient/family education
• Advise patient to carry/wear emergency ID stating patient's name, products taken, condition, prescriber's name and phone number
• Advise patient to avoid driving, other activities that require alertness, until response is known, dizziness, drowsiness are common, prescriber will approve or disapprove
• **Seizures:** Teach patient not to discontinue medication quickly after long-term use, withdrawal-precipitated seizures may occur, not to double dose; if dose is missed, take if 2 hr or more before next dose
• Teach patient to gradually withdraw over 7 days; abrupt withdrawal may precipitate seizures, those taking tid should not use >12 hr between dosing; take missed dose up to 2 hr prior to next dose
• Advise patient to notify caregivers of suicidal ideation, increasing depression, panic

attacks, hostility, confusion; that if these occur, to notify prescriber immediately
• Advise patient to notify health care professional before surgery
• Teach patient if tablet is to be broken in half, use half within 28 days or discard
• Teach patient to use hard candy, gum, and frequent rinsing of mouth for dry mouth
• Teach patient to increase fluids, bulk in diet for constipation
• Advise patient to notify prescriber if pregnancy is planned or suspected, avoid breastfeeding

Evaluation
Positive therapeutic outcome
• Decreased seizure activity; document on patient's chart

TREATMENT OF OVERDOSE:
Lavage, VS

---

galantamine (Rx)
(gah-lan'tah-meen)
Razadyne, Razadyne ER, Reminyl ✦
Func. class.: Anti-Alzheimer's agent
Chem. class.: Cholinesterase inhibitor

Do not confuse: Razadyne/Rozerem

ACTION: Enhances cholinergic functioning by increasing acetylcholine

Therapeutic outcome: Decreased signs and symptoms of Alzheimer's dementia

USES: Mild to moderate dementia of Alzheimer's disease, vascular dementia, dementia with Lewy bodies

Pharmacokinetics

Absorption	Rapidly and completely absorbed
Distribution	18% protein binding
Metabolism	Liver
Excretion	Kidneys; clearance decreased in geriatric, hepatic/renal disease, females (20% lower)
Half-life	7 hr

Pharmacodynamics

Onset	Unknown
Peak	1 hr (regular release), 4.5-5 hr (extended release)
Duration	12 hr

CONTRAINDICATIONS
Hypersensitivity to this product, children, GI bleeding, jaundice, renal failure

Precautions: Pregnancy, respiratory/renal/hepatic/cardiac disease, seizure disorder, peptic ulcer, asthma, bradycardia, heart block, geriatric patients, surgery, urinary tract obstruction, breastfeeding

DOSAGE AND ROUTES
Adult: PO 4 mg bid with morning and evening meals; after 4 wk or more may increase to 8 mg bid; after another 4 wk may increase to 12 mg bid; usual dose 16-24 mg/day in 2 divided doses; EXT REL 8 mg/day in AM; may increase to 16 mg/day after 4 wk, and 24 mg/day after another 4 wk

Hepatic dose
Adult: (Child-Pugh 7-9) PO max 16 mg/day
Adult: (Child-Pugh 10-15) avoid PO use

Renal dose
Adult: PO CCr 10-70 ml/min; max 16 mg/day; CCr <9 ml/min: PO avoid use

Available forms: Tabs 4, 8, 12 mg; ext rel caps 8, 16, 24 mg; oral sol 4 mg/ml

ADVERSE EFFECTS
CNS: *Tremors, insomnia,* dizziness, headache, fatigue
CV: Bradycardia, chest pain
GI: *Nausea, vomiting, anorexia, abdominal distress, flatulence,* diarrhea
GU: Urinary incontinence, bladder outflow obstruction
INTEG: Stevens-Johnson syndrome, acute generalized exanthematous pustulosis

INTERACTIONS
Drug classifications
Cholinesterase inhibitors, cholinomimetics: increased effect, avoid concurrent use before anesthesia
CYP3A4/CYP2D6 inducers (bosentan, carBAMazepine, fosphenytoin, nevirapine, OXcarbazepine, phenytoin, rifabutin, rifampin, rifapentine, troglitazone), anticholinergics: decreased galantamine effect, monitor for decreased effect
CYP3A4/CYP2D6 inhibitors (antiretroviral protease inhibitors, clarithromycin, conivaptan, delavirdine, diltiazem, efavirenz, fluconazole, fluvoxaMINE, imatinib, itraconazole, ketoconazole, nefazodone, niCARdipine, troleandomycin, verapamil, zafirlukast): increased galantamine effect, monitor for increased effect
Succinylcholine-like neuroblockers: increased neuromuscular blicking action

---

Drug/herb
St. John's wort: decreased galantamine effect, avoid concurrent use

NURSING CONSIDERATIONS
Assessment
• **Alzheimer's disease:** Assess mental status: affect, mood, behavioral changes, depression, memory, attention, confusion, cognitive func during baseline and periodically
• Assess B/P, heart rate, respiration during initial treatment, rash

Patient Problem
Distorted thinking process (uses)
Risk for injury (uses)

Implementation
• Give with meals, morning and evening, ext rel product can be opened and sprinkled on food; do not crush/chew
• Dose increase after minimum of 4 wk at prior dose; if dose is interrupted for several days, restart at lower dose, titrate to current dose
• Provide assistance with ambulation during beginning therapy
• Perform complete suicide assessment
• Oral solution: use pipette provided; put in liquid and have patient consume

Patient/family education
• Teach patient or caregiver correct procedure for giving oral sol, using instruction sheet provided
• Instruct patient or caregiver to notify prescriber of severe GI effects, nausea, vomiting
• Instruct patient or caregiver to report hypo/hypertension, slow heart rate
• Teach patient to take with food to minimize side effects
• Advise patient to notify health care professional of use before surgery
• Advise that follow-up exams will be needed
• Teach patient to notify prescriber immediately and stop taking product if rash occurs.

Evaluation

Positive therapeutic outcome
• Decreased symptoms of dementia
• Increased coherence, language, ability to perform ADLs
• Improved cognitive performance (memory, orientation, attention, reasoning, language)

TREATMENT OF OVERDOSE:
Administer **IV** atropine titrated to effect at an initial dose of 0.5-1 mg, with subsequent doses based on clinical response; provide general supportive measures

galcanezumab
(gal-kuh-nezz'-you-mab)
Emgality
Func. class.: Anti-migraine agent
Chem. class.: Calcitonin gene-related peptide (CGRP) antagonists

ACTION: Binds to the calcitonin gene-related peptide (CGRP) receptor and antagonizes CGRP receptor function

Therapeutic outcome: Prevention of migraine

USES: Migraine prophylaxis

Pharmacokinetics
Absorption	Unknown
Distribution	Unknown
Metabolism	Unknown
Excretion	Unknown
Half-life	27 days

Pharmacodynamics
Onset	Unknown
Peak	5 days
Duration	Unknown

CONTRAINDICATIONS:
Hypersensitivity

PRECAUTIONS: Breastfeeding, pregnancy

DOSAGE AND ROUTES
Adult: SUBCUT 240 mg once as a loading dose, then 120 mg monthly

Available forms: Prefilled pen 120 mg/ml solution for injection

ADVERSE EFFECTS
INTEG: Injection site reaction, rash, urticaria, pruritus, erythema
MISC: Antibody formation, dyspnea

INTERACTIONS
None known

NURSING CONSIDERATIONS
Assessment
• **Migraine:** Pain, location, intensity, duration, photophobia in the past; assess the response to preventing migraine after use of this product
• Injection site reaction, rash, urticaria, pruritus, erythema, may indicate allergic reactions
• **Pregnancy/breastfeeding:** Identify if pregnancy is planned or suspected or if breastfeeding; no adequate studies are available

Implementation
SUBCUT route
• Visually inspect for particulates, discoloration prior to use; do not use if the solution is cloudy, discolored, or contains particles; product is clear to opalescent, colorless to slightly yellow
• Allow to sit at room temperature ≥30 min; protect from direct sunlight; do not shake
• Clean injection site on the abdomen, thigh, or upper arm with an alcohol wipe, and allow skin to dry
• Do not inject into areas where the skin is tender, bruised, red, or hard. Avoid injecting directly into raised, thick, red, or scaly skin patch or lesion, or areas with scars or stretch marks
• If using the same body area for the two separate injections needed for the 240 mg dose, ensure the second injection is not at same location used for the first injection
• Do not coadminister with other injectable drugs at the same injection site
• If a dose is missed, give the next dose as soon as possible
• *Storage:* After removing from refrigerator, may be stored at room temperature up to 25° C (77° F) for ≤24 hr; discard if not used within 24 hr after removal from refrigerator

Single-dose, prefilled syringe
• Pinch injection site skin firmly between thumb and fingers
• Hold, insert the syringe at 45-90 degrees for administration

Patient/family education
• Teach patient how to self-administer product
• Advise patient not to double, skip doses; when switching between monthly and quarterly dosage options, give the first dose of the new regimen on the next scheduled date of administration
• Teach patient to report injection site reaction, rash, itching, which may indicate allergic reaction

Evaluation
• Prevention of migraine

ganciclovir (Rx)
(gan-sye′kloe-vir)
Cytovene, Zirgan
Func. class.: Antiviral
Chem. class.: Synthetic nucleoside analog

Do not confuse: Cytovene/Cytosar

ACTION: Inhibits replication of herpes viruses in vitro; competitively inhibits human cytomegalovirus (CMV) DNA polymerase and is incorporated, resulting in termination of DNA elongation

Therapeutic outcome: Decreased proliferation of virus responsible for CMV retinitis

USES: Cytomegalovirus (CMV) retinitis in immunocompromised persons, including those with AIDS, after indirect ophthalmoscopy confirms diagnosis; prophylaxis of CMV in transplantation

Pharmacokinetics
Absorption	Completely, increased bioavailability with fatty foods
Distribution	Crosses blood-brain barrier, CSF, minimal protein binding
Metabolism	Not metabolized
Excretion	Kidneys (90%) unchanged, breast milk
Half-life	3 hr

Pharmacodynamics
Onset	Rapid
Peak	Infusion end
Duration	Up to 24 hr

CONTRAINDICATIONS
Hypersensitivity to acyclovir, famciclovir, penciclovir, valacyclovir, valganciclovir, or ganciclovir

BLACK BOX WARNING: ANC <500/mm³, platelet count <25,000/mm³ (intravitreal)

Precautions: Pregnancy, breastfeeding, children <6 mo, geriatric, preexisting cytopenias, renal function impairment, radiation therapy

BLACK BOX WARNING: Secondary malignancy, bone marrow suppression, anemia, infertility, neutropenia, pregnancy, male-mediated teratogenicity

DOSAGE AND ROUTES
Induction treatment
Adult: **IV** 5 mg/kg/dose given over 1 hr q12hr × 2-3 wk

Maintenance treatment
Adult: **IV** INF 5 mg/kg/day given over 1 hr, daily × 7 days/wk; or 6 mg/kg/day × 5 days/wk; PO 1000 mg tid with food or 500 mg q3hr while awake; intravitreal 4.5-mg implant

Prevention of CMV infection
Adult: **IV** 5 mg/kg/dose over 1 hr q12hr × 1-2 wk, then 5 mg/kg/day × 7 days/wk, then 6 mg/kg/day × 5 days/wk; PO 1000 mg tid, starting 10 days posttransplant × 14 days

---

Renal dose

Adult: IV CCr 50-69 ml/min, reduce to 2.5 mg/kg q12hr (induction), 2.5 mg/kg q24hr (maintenance); PO 1500 mg/day or 500 mg tid; IV **CCr 25-49 ml/min** reduce to 2.5 mg q24hr (induction); 1.25 mg/kg q24hr (maintenance); PO 1000 mg/day or 500 mg bid; **IV CCr 10-24 ml/min** reduce to 1.25 mg/kg q24hr (induction); 0.625 mg/kg q24hr (maintenance), **PO** 500 mg/day; **IV CCr <10 ml/min** reduce to 1.25 mg/kg 3×/wk after hemodialysis (induction); 0.625 mg/kg 3×/wk after hemodialysis (maintenance); **PO** 500 mg 3×/wk after hemodialysis

Available forms: Powder for inj 500 mg/vial, caps 250, 500 mg

ADVERSE EFFECTS

CNS: *Fever,* coma, *confusion,* dizziness, bizarre dreams, *headache,* tremors, seizures, peripheral neuropathy, drowsiness
CV: Dysrhythmia, hypo/hypertension
EENT: Retinal detachment in CMV retinitis, cataracts, ocular hypertension, ocular pain, conjunctival scarring
GI: *Abnormal liver function tests, nausea, vomiting, anorexia, abdominal pain,* hemorrhage, perforation, pancreatitis
GU: Hematuria, *increased creatinine,* BUN
HEMA: Thrombocytopenia, irreversible neutropenia, anemia, eosinophilia
INTEG: *Rash,* alopecia, *pruritus,* pain at inj site, phlebitis
RESP: Dyspnea, pneumonia

INTERACTIONS
Individual drugs

Adriamycin, amphotericin B, cycloSPORINE, dapsone, DOXOrubicin, flucytosine, mycophenolate, pentamidine, probenecid, tacrolimus, trimethoprim/sulfa combinations, vinBLAStine, vinCRIStine: increased ganciclovir toxicity
Didanosine: increased didanosine effect
Imipenem with cilastatin: increased risk for seizures
Probenecid: decreased renal clearance of ganciclovir
Radiation, zidovudine: severe granulocytopenia; do not give together

Drug classifications

Antineoplastics: severe granulocytopenia; do not give together

NURSING CONSIDERATIONS
Assessment

• **CMV retinitis:** Cultures of blood, urine, and throat may all be taken; CMV is not confirmed

by this method; the diagnosis is made by an ophthalmic exam, these exams should be done baseline, q wk (induction), q 2 wk (maintenance)

• Assess kidney, liver function; increases in hemopoietic studies: BUN, serum creatinine, AST creatinine clearance, ALT, A:G ratio, baseline, and drip treatment; blood counts should be done q2wk; watch for decreasing granulocytes, Hgb; if low, therapy may have to be discontinued and restarted after hematologic recovery; blood transfusions may be required

• **Infection:** Assess for flu-like symptoms (fever, sore throat, cough)

• **Bleeding:** Assess for bleeding; thrombocytopenia may increase; gums; urine; emesis; avoid rectal temperature, vein punctures

• Assess for GI symptoms: severe nausea, vomiting, diarrhea; severe symptoms may necessitate discontinuing product

• Monitor electrolytes and minerals: calcium, phosphorus, magnesium, sodium, potassium; watch closely for tetany during 1st administration

• Assess for symptoms of allergic reactions: flushing, rash, urticaria, pruritus

> **BLACK BOX WARNING: Monitor for leukopenia/neutropenia/thrombocytopenia:** WBCs, platelets q2day during 2 ×/day dosing and qwk thereafter; check for leukopenia with daily WBC count in patients with prior leukopenia with other nucleoside analogs or for whom leukopenia counts are <1000 cells/mm³ at start of treatment; bruising, fatigue, bleeding, poor healing

• Assess for seizures, dysrhythmias

> **BLACK BOX WARNING:** Assess for secondary malignancy; avoid direct contact with powder in caps/solution; if skin contact occurs, wash thoroughly with soap and water; do not get in the eyes

• **Pregnancy/breastfeeding:** not to be used in pregnancy, confirm by pregnancy test

Patient problem
Infection (uses)

Implementation
PO route
• Give with food, do not open or crush caps

IV route
• Product should be mixed under strict aseptic conditions using gloves, gown, and mask and using precautions for antineoplastics, do not use if particulate matter is present

Intermittent IV inf route
• Administer **IV** after reconstituting 500 mg/10 ml of sterile water for inj (50 mg/ml); shake; further dilute in 100 ml of D$_5$W, 0.9% NaCl, LR, Ringer's and run over 1 hr; use inf pump, in-line filter, flush line well before and after product
• Check IV site frequently, rotate sites
• Provide adequate fluids during treatment
• Do not give by BOL **IV**, IM, SUBCUT inj
• Use reconstituted sol within 12 hr, do not refrigerate or freeze; do not use sol with particulate matter or discoloration, fludarabine, sargramostim

Y-site compatibilities: Allopurinol, CISplatin, cyclophosphamide, enalaprilat, etoposide, filgrastim, fluconazole, gatifloxacin, granisetron, linezolid, melphalan, methotrexate, PACLitaxel, propofol, tacrolimus, teniposide, thiotepa

Patient/family education
• **Infection:** Advise patient to notify prescriber if sore throat, swollen lymph nodes, malaise, fever occur; tell patient to avoid crowds, persons with respiratory infection
• Advise patient to report perioral tingling, numbness in extremities, and paresthesias
• Caution patient that serious product interactions may occur if OTC products are ingested; check first with prescriber
• Inform patient that product is not a cure, but will control symptoms
• Advise patient that regular blood tests, ophth exams must be continued
• Inform patient that major toxicities may necessitate discontinuing product
• Teach patient to take PO with food, do not open or crush caps
• Teach patient to report infection; blood dyscrasias; bruising, bleeding, petechiae
• Advise patient to use sunscreen to prevent burns
• Advise patient to report itching, redness, or eye pain (ophthalmic treatment)

> **BLACK BOX WARNING: Pregnancy:** Instruct patient to use contraception during treatment of males, females, and that infertility may occur and may be permanent; men should use barrier contraception for 90 days after treatment, women ≥30 days; not to breastfeed (IV)

Evaluation

Positive therapeutic outcome
• Decreased symptoms of CMV infection
• Prevention of CMV retinitis in transplant patients (if needed)

ganciclovir ophthalmic
See Appendix B

gatifloxacin ophthalmic
See Appendix B

gefitinib (Rx)
(ge-fi'tye-nib)
Iressa
Func. class.: Antineoplastic, miscellaneous
Chem. class.: Epidermal growth factor receptor inhibitor

ACTION: Not fully understood; inhibits intracellular phosphorylation of cell surface receptors associated with epidermal growth factor receptors

Therapeutic outcome: Decreased growth and spread of malignant cells

USES: Advanced/metastatic non–small cell lung cancer (NSCLC) in those who have not responded to platinum or docetaxel products

Pharmacokinetics	
Absorption	Slowly
Distribution	Unknown
Metabolism	Unknown
Excretion	In feces (86%), urine (<4%)
Half-life	Unknown

Pharmacodynamics	
Onset	Unknown
Peak	3-7 hr
Duration	Unknown

CONTRAINDICATIONS: Pregnancy, breastfeeding, children, hypersensitivity

Precautions: Renal/hepatic/ocular/pulmonary disorders, geriatric

DOSAGE AND ROUTES
Adult: PO 250 mg/day

CYP3A4 inducers concurrently (such as rifampin or phenytoin)
Adult: PO 500 mg/day

Available forms: Tabs 250 mg

ADVERSE EFFECTS
EENT: Amblyopia, conjunctivitis, eye pain, corneal erosion/ulcer
GI: Nausea, diarrhea, vomiting, anorexia, pancreatitis, mouth ulceration, hepatotoxicity
INTEG: Rash, pruritus, acne, dry skin, toxic epidermal neurolysis, angioedema

---

⚠ Nurse Alert   ✴ Key NCLEX® Drug   ≫ Drug Specifics

MISC: Peripheral edema, hemorrhage
RESP: Interstitial lung disease, cough, dyspnea, pneumonia

INTERACTIONS
Individual drugs
Cimetidine, phenytoin, ranitidine, rifampin, sodium bicarbonate: decreased levels
Clarithromycin, erythromycin, itraconazole, ketoconazole. Increased concentration
Clozapine: increased bone marrow suppression
Metoprolol, warfarin: increased plasma concentration

Drug/herb
St. John's wort: decreased gefitinib levels

NURSING CONSIDERATIONS
Assessment
• Assess pulmonary changes: lung sounds, cough, dyspnea; interstitial lung disease may occur, may be fatal; discontinue therapy if confirmed
• Assess ocular changes: eye irritation, corneal erosion/ulcer, aberrant eyelash growth
• Assess for pancreatitis: abdominal pain, levels of amylase, lipase
• Assess for toxic epidermal necrosis, angioedema
• Monitor GI symptoms: frequency of stools; if diarrhea is poorly tolerated, therapy may be discontinued for up to 14 days

Patient problems
• Risk for Infection (adverse reactions)
• Risk for Injury (adverse reactions)
• Lack of knowledge regarding medication (teaching)

Implementation
• Give without regard to food

Patient/family education
• Teach to report adverse reactions immediately: SOB, severe abdominal pain, ocular changes, skin eruptions
• Advise of reason for treatment, expected results
• Advise to use contraception during treatment

Evaluation
Positive therapeutic outcome
• Decreased non–small cell lung cancer cells

⚠ HIGH ALERT

gemcitabine (Rx)
(gem-sit'a-been)
Gemzar
Func. class.: Antineoplastic—miscellaneous
Chem. class.: Pyrimidine analog

Do not confuse: Gemzar/Zinecard

ACTION: Exhibits antitumor activity by killing cells undergoing DNA synthesis (S phase) and blocking G_1/S-phase boundary

Therapeutic outcome: Prevention of growth of tumor

USES: Adenocarcinoma of the pancreas (nonresectable stage II, III, or metastatic stage IV); in combination with CISplatin for inoperable, advanced, or metastatic non–small cell lung cancer; advanced breast cancer in combination with PACLitaxel; with CARBOplatin for ovarian cancer, biliary tract cancer

Pharmacokinetics

Absorption	Complete
Distribution	Crosses placenta
Metabolism	To active metabolites
Excretion	Kidney
Half-life	2.5-18 hr

Pharmacodynamics
Unknown

CONTRAINDICATIONS
Pregnancy, breastfeeding, hypersensitivity

Precautions: Children, geriatric, myelosuppression, radiation therapy, renal/hepatic disease

DOSAGE AND ROUTES
Pancreatic carcinoma
Adult: IV 1000 mg/m^2 given over ½ hr qwk × 7 wk, then 1 wk rest period; subsequent cycles should be infused once qwk × 3 wk out of every 4 wk depending on hematologic toxicity

Non–small cell lung cancer
4 wk schedule
Adult: IV 1000 mg/m^2 given over ½ hr on days 1, 8, 15 of each 28-day cycle; give CISplatin IV 100 mg/m^2 on day 1 after gemcitabine

---

3 wk schedule
Adult: IV 1250 mg/m² given over ½ hr on days 1, 8 of each 21-day cycle; give CISplatin 100 mg/m² after the INF of gemcitabine on day 1

Advanced breast cancer
Adult: IV 1250 mg/m² over ½ hr on days 1 and 8 of a 21-day cycle; give with PACLitaxel on day 1, 175 mg/m² over 3 hr prior to gemcitabine

Ovarian cancer
Adult: IV 1000 mg/m² on days 1 and 8 (21-day cycle)

Available forms: Lyophilized powder for inj 200 mg, 1 gm, 2 gm ❦; solution for inj 1 gm/26.3 ml, 200 mg/ 5.26 ml, 2 gm/52.6 ml

ADVERSE EFFECTS
CNS: Posterior reversible encephalopathy syndrome (PRES)
CV: Dysrhythmias, capillary leak syndrome, MI, hypertension
GI: Diarrhea, nausea, vomiting, anorexia, stomatitis, diarrhea, hepatotoxicity
GU: Proteinuria, hematuria, hemolytic uremic syndrome
HEMA: Leukopenia, anemia, neutropenia, thrombocytopenia
INTEG: Irritation at site, rash, alopecia
MISC: Fever, infection, flulike syndrome, paresthesia, peripheral edema, myalgia, dup
RESP: Dyspnea, bronchospasm, pneumonitis

INTERACTIONS
Individual drug
Alcohol: increased bleeding risk

Drug classifications
Anticoagulants, NSAIDs, salicylates: increased bleeding risk
Antineoplastics, radiation: increased myelosuppression, diarrhea
Live virus vaccines: decreased antibody response

Drug/lab test
Increased: BUN, AST, ALT, alkaline phosphatase, bilirubin, creatinine

NURSING CONSIDERATIONS
Assessment
• **Bone marrow depression:** monitor CBC, differential, platelet count before each dose; **single agent: absolute granulocyte count >1000, and platelets >100,000,** give complete dose; **absolute granulocyte count 500-999/mm³, platelets 50,000-99,999/mm³,** give 75%; **absolute granulocyte count <500 or platelets <50,000/mm³,** do not give; **combination with PACLitaxel in breast cancer: absolute granulocyte count >1200/mm³**

and platelets >75,000/mm³, give complete dose; **absolute granulocyte count 1000-1199/mm³ or platelets 50,000-75,000/mm³,** give 75%; **absolute granulocyte 700-999/mm³ or platelets ≥50,000/mm³,** give 50%; **granulocyte count <700/mm³ or platelets <50,000/mm³,** do not give; combination with CARBOplatin in ovarian cancer: **absolute granulocyte count >1500/mm³ and platelet count >100,000/mm³,** give complete dose; **absolute granulocyte count 1000-1499/mm3 or platelets 75,000-99,999/mm³,** give 75%; **absolute granulocyte count <1000/mm³ or platelets <75,000/mm³,** do not give
• **Assess for:** bruising, bleeding, petechiae
• Monitor renal/hepatic studies before, during treatment; may increase AST, ALT, alkaline phosphatase, bilirubin, BUN, creatinine; product may need to be discontinued for toxicity
• Assess food preferences: list likes, dislikes
• Assess buccal cavity for dryness, sores or ulceration, white patches, oral pain, bleeding, dysphagia
• Assess GI symptoms: frequency of stools; cramping
• **Capillary leak syndrome:** Monitor for hemoconcentration, decreased albumin, B/P; discontinue
• **Posterior reversible encephalopathy syndrome (PRES):** assess for hypertension, visual changes, headache, seizures discontinue if present, confirmed by MRI
• **Hemolytic uremic syndrome** (HUS) may occur more frequently when given with bleomycin, assess renal function before use and periodically, anemia with microangiopathic hemolysis, elevated bilirubin or LDH, reticulocytosis, severe thrombocytopenia, increased BUN/creatinine are indications of HUS; permanently discontinue this product; pneumonitis, pulmonary edema, acute respiratory distress syndrome (ARDs)
• **Pulmonary fibrosis or evidence of pulmonary toxicity,** may occur ≤ 2 wk after last dose

Patient problem
Risk for infection (uses)

Implementation
• Give increased fluid intake to 2-3 L/day to prevent dehydration, unless contraindicated
• Provide antiemetic agents before and after treatment

Intermittent IV route
• Prepare in biological cabinet using gown, mask, gloves; infusion-related reactions

including hypotension, severe flulike symptoms, myelosuppression, asthenia
• After reconstituting with 0.9% NaCl 5 ml/200 mg vial of product or 25 ml/1 g of product, shake (38 mg/ml); may be further diluted with 0.9% NaCl to concentrate as low as 0.1 mg/ml; discard unused portion, give over ½ hr, do not admix

Y-site compatibilities: Alemtuzumab, alfentanil, allopurinol, amifostine, amikacin, aminophylline, ampicillin, anidulafungin, argatroban, aztreonam, bivalirudin, bleomycin, bumetanide, butorphanol, calcium gluconate, caspofungin, cefOXitin, cefTAZidime, ceftizoxime, cefTRIAXone, chlorproMAZINE, cimetidine, ciprofloxacin, CISplatin, clindamycin, cyclophosphamide, cytarabine, DACTINomycin, DAUNOrubicin, diphenhydrAMINE, DOBUTamine, DOCEtaxel, DOPamine, DOXOrubicin, droperidol, enalaprilat, etoposide, famotidine, floxuridine, fluconazole, fludarabine, fluorouracil, gentamicin, granisetron, haloperidol, heparin, hydrocortisone, HYDROmorphone, IDArubicin, ifosfamide, leucovorin, linezolid, LORazepam, mannitol, meperidine, mesna, metoclopramide, metroNIDAZOLE, minocycline, mitoXANtrone, morphine, nalbuphine, ondansetron, PACLitaxel, promethazine, ranitidine, streptozocin, teniposide, thiotepa, ticarcillin, tigecycline, tobramycin, topotecan, trimethoprim/sulfamethoxazole, vancomycin, vinBLAStine, vinCRIStine, vinorelbine, voriconazole zidovudine, zoledronic acid

Patient/family education
• Teach patient to rinse mouth tid-qid with water, club soda; brush teeth bid-tid with soft brush or cotton-tipped applicator for stomatitis, use unwaxed dental floss
• Advise patient to report stomatitis; any bleeding, white spots, ulcerations in mouth; tell patient to examine mouth daily, report symptoms; advise patient to avoid foods with citric acid or hot or rough texture if stomatitis is present; to drink adequate fluids
• Advise patient to report signs of anemia: fatigue, headache, faintness, shortness of breath, irritability; hematuria, dysuria
• **Pregnancy/breastfeeding:** Advise patient to use contraception during therapy and for 4 mo after
• Bleeding: Instruct patient to avoid use with NSAIDs, salicylates, alcohol; not to receive vaccinations during treatment
• Teach about possible hair loss and what can be done
• Advise to report flulike symptoms, swelling of feet/legs, bruising; bleeding of gums, blood in urine, stools, emesis

• Teach to avoid crowds, persons with known upper respiratory infections
• Advise patient to use electric razor
• Teach patient that continuing exams and lab work will be needed

Evaluation

Positive therapeutic outcome
• Decrease in tumor size, decrease in spread of cancer, symptom relief

TREATMENT OF OVERDOSE:
Induce vomiting, provide supportive care

gemfibrozil (Rx)
(gem-fye′broe-zil)
Lopid
Func. class.: Antilipemic
Chem. class.: Fibric acid derivative

Do not confuse: Lopid/Levbid/Slo-bid

ACTION: Inhibits biosynthesis of VLDL, decreases triglyceride production in the liver, increases HDLs

Therapeutic outcome: Decreased hepatic triglyceride production, VLDL; accelerates removal of cholesterol from liver

USES: For use as an adjunct to diet for the treatment of hyperlipoproteinemia and for hypertriglyceridemia, including type IV (elevated triglycerides, VLDL) and type V (elevated triglycerides, chylomicrons, VLDL) in patients who have significant risk of coronary artery disease or pancreatitis and have not responded to diet

Pharmacokinetics
Absorption	Well absorbed
Distribution	Unknown, plasma protein binding >95%
Metabolism	Liver, minimal
Excretion	Kidney, unchanged (70%), feces (6%)
Half-life	1½ hr

Pharmacodynamics
Onset	1-2 hr
Peak	1-2 hr
Duration	2-4 months

CONTRAINDICATIONS
Severe renal/hepatic disease, preexisting gallbladder disease, primary biliary cirrhosis, hypersensitivity; use with dasabuvir, repaglinide, simvastatin

Precautions: Pregnancy, breastfeeding, renal disease, cholelithiasis, children

DOSAGE AND ROUTES
Adult: PO 600 mg bid 30 min before meals

Hepatic/renal dose
Avoid use

Available forms: Tabs 600 mg; caps 300 mg ✦

ADVERSE EFFECTS
CNS: Headache, paresthesia, dizziness
GI: Nausea, vomiting, *dyspepsia, diarrhea, abdominal pain*
HEMA: Leukopenia, anemia
INTEG: Rash, urticaria, pruritus, alopecia
MS: Myopathy, rhabdomyolysis

INTERACTIONS
Individual drugs
Do not use with repaglinide, simvastatin, dasabuvir cyclosporine: increase nephrotoxicity, monitor renal function

Repaglinide, metformin, glyburide, pioglitazone, other antidiabetic agents: increased hypoglycemic effect

Warfarin, avoid concurrent use: increased anticoagulant effect

Drug classifications
Bile acid sequestrants: decreased effect of gemfibrozil, separate by >2 hr

HMG-CoA reductase inhibitors: increased risk of myositis, myalgia, rhabdomyolysis

Sulfonylureas: increased hypoglycemic effect

CYP2C8, CYP2C9, CYP2C19: Increased levels, monitor for toxicities

Drug/lab test
Increased: liver function tests, CK, bilirubin, alkaline phosphatase
Decreased: Hgb, Hct, WBC, potassium

NURSING CONSIDERATIONS
Assessment
• **Hypercholesteremia:** Assess nutrition: fat, protein, carbohydrates; nutritional analysis should be performed by dietitian before treatment is initiated; monitor triglycerides, cholesterol, lipids baseline, during treatment; LDL and VLDL should be watched closely and if increased, product should be discontinued
• Assess renal, liver function tests, CBC, blood glucose if patient is on long-term therapy; if liver function test results increase, product should be discontinued; monitor hematologic and hepatic function
• Monitor bowel pattern daily; diarrhea may be a problem
• **Myopathy, rhabdomyolysis:** Assess for muscle pain, tenderness; obtain baseline CPK: if elevated or if these occur, product should be discontinued

Patient problem
Nonadherance (teaching)

Implementation
• Give 30 min before AM or PM meals

Patient/family education
• Inform patient that compliance is needed for positive results to occur; not to double doses, take missed dose as soon as remembered unless almost time for next dose; that product may be discontinued if no improvement in 3 mo
• Caution patient to decrease risk factors: high-fat diet, smoking, alcohol consumption, lack of exercise
• Advise patient to notify prescriber if GI symptoms of diarrhea, abdominal or epigastric pain, nausea, vomiting occur; or if chills, fever, sore throat occur; also occurrence of muscle cramps, abdominal cramps, severe flatulence
• Pregnancy/breastfeeding: identify if pregnancy is planned or suspected, or if breastfeeding

Evaluation
Positive therapeutic outcome
• Decreased cholesterol levels, serum triglyceride and improved ratio with HDLs

gemifloxacin (Rx)
(gem-ah-flox′a-sin)
Factive
Func. class.: Antiinfective
Chem. class.: Fluoroquinolone

ACTION: Inhibits DNA gyrase, which is an enzyme involved in replication, transcription, and repair of bacterial DNA

Therapeutic outcome: Negative C&S, decreasing symptoms of infection

USES: Acute bacterial exacerbation of chronic bronchitis caused by *Streptococcus pneumoniae, Haemophilus influenzae, Haemophilus parainfluenzae, Moraxella catarrhalis;* community-acquired pneumonia caused by *Streptococcus pneumoniae* including multi-product-resistant strains, *H. influenzae, M. catarrhalis, Mycoplasma pneumoniae, Chlamydia pneumoniae, Klebsiella pneumoniae*

Pharmacokinetics

Absorption	Rapidly, bioavailability 71%
Distribution	Widely
Metabolism	Minimal
Excretion	In urine as active product, metabolites
Half-life	4-12 hr

Pharmacodynamics

Onset	Unknown
Peak	$^1/_2$ hr
Duration	Up to 24 hr

CONTRAINDICATIONS
Hypersensitivity to quinolones

Precautions: Pregnancy, breastfeeding, children, geriatric, hypokalemia, hypomagnesemia, renal disease, seizure disorders, excessive exposure to sunlight, psychosis, increased intracranial pressure, history of QT interval prolongation, dysrhythmias, myasthenia gravis, torsades de pointes

> **BLACK BOX WARNING:** Tendon pain/rupture, tendinitis, neurotoxicity

DOSAGE AND ROUTES
Adult: PO 320 mg/day $\times$ 3-7 days depending on type of infection

Renal dose
Adult: PO CCr ≤40 ml/min 160 mg q24hr

Available forms: Tabs 320 mg

ADVERSE EFFECTS
CNS: *Dizziness, headache,* depression, insomnia, agitation, seizures, pseudotumor cerebri, suicidal ideation
CV: QT prolongation, vasodilatation, torsade de pointes
EENT: Visual disturbances, retinal detachment
GI: Diarrhea, *nausea,* vomiting, anorexia, flatulence, heartburn, dry mouth; increased AST, ALT; constipation, abdominal pain, *Clostridium difficile*–associated diarrhea
GU: Vaginitis
INTEG: Rash, pruritus, urticaria, *photosensitivity,* generalized exanthematous pustulosis
SYST: Anaphylaxis, Stevens-Johnson syndrome, toxic epidermal necrolysis, exfoliative dermatitis

INTERACTIONS
Individual drugs
Amiodarone, disopyramide, dofetilide, erythromycin, procainamide, sotolol: Increased torsade de pointes risk
Amoxapine, chloroquine, cloZAPine, dasatinib, dolasetron, dronedarone, droperidol, erythromycin, flecainide, haloperidol, lapatinib, maprotiline, methadone, octreotide, ondansetron, palonosetron, pentamidine, pimozide, propafenone, ranolazine, risperidone, sertindole, SUNItinib, tacrolimus, telithromycin, troleandomycin, vardenafil, vorinostat, ziprasidone: increased QT prolongation

Probenecid: may increase toxicity

> **BLACK BOX WARNING:** Corticosteroids: increase tendon rupture

Theophylline: toxicity; do not use concurrently

Drug classifications
Antacids containing aluminum, iron salts, magnesium, sucralfate, zinc salts: decreased absorption; give 2 hr before or 3 hr after meals
Antiarrhythmics (amiodarone, disopyramide, procainamide, quiNIDine, sotalol), antidepressants (tricyclics), b-blockers, halogenated/local anesthetics: may decrease effect, resulting in life-threatening dysrhythmias, QT prolongation
Antipsychotics, tricyclic antidepressants: increased torsade de pointes risk
NSAIDs: increased CNS stimulation

NURSING CONSIDERATIONS
Assessment
- **Infection:** Assess for flu-like symptoms (fever, chills, sore throat); characteristics of wounds, sputum, urine baseline and periodically
- Monitor renal, liver function tests: BUN, creatinine, AST, ALT, electrolytes
- Monitor I&O ratio; urine pH, <5.5 is ideal
- Assess CNS symptoms: insomnia, vertigo, headache, agitation, confusion

> **BLACK BOX WARNING: Tendon rupture**
> Assess for tendon pain, inflammation; if present discontinue use; more common with corticosteroids; discontinue immediately if tendon pain, inflammation occurs

- **Assess allergic reactions and anaphylaxis:** rash, flushing, urticaria, pruritus, chills, fever, joint pain; may occur a few days after therapy begins; EPINEPHrine and resuscitation equipment should be available for anaphylactic reaction
- **CDAD:** Monitor bowel pattern daily; if severe diarrhea, fever, abdominal pain occurs, product should be discontinued
- **Suicide:** Assess for suicidal ideation, increasing depression, agitation, panic attacks baseline and periodically
- **Assess for overgrowth of infection:** perineal itching, fever, malaise, redness, pain, swelling, drainage, rash, diarrhea, change in cough, sputum
- **QT prolongation:** Avoid use of quinolones in those with known QT prolongation; females and those with ongoing proarrhythmic conditions (TdP) are at greater risk; monitor ECG and/or Holter monitoring if product is used

G

• **Toxic psychosis/pseudotumor cerebri:**
Assess for headache, blurred vision, neck/
shoulder pain, nausea/vomiting, dizziness,
tinnitus; discontinue immediately, may occur
within hours to weeks after starting product
• **Pregnancy/breastfeeding:** Use only if
benefits outweigh fetal risk

Patient problem
Infection (uses)

Implementation
• Give with or without food
• Theophylline should not be used with this
product; toxicity may result
• Administer 2 hr before or 3 hr after antacids,
iron, zinc, or buffered products
• Provide adequate hydration

Patient/family education
• Advise patient that fluids must be increased to
2 L/day to avoid crystallization in kidneys
• Instruct patient that if dizziness or light-headedness occurs, to ambulate, perform activities
with assistance
• Instruct patient to complete full course of
product therapy
• Teach patient to contact prescriber if adverse
reactions occur
• Teach patient to avoid iron- or mineral-
containing supplements or aluminum/magnesium
antacids within 2 hr before or 3 hr after dosing
• Advise patient that photosensitivity may occur
and sunscreen should be used
• Advise patient to use frequent rinsing of
mouth, sugarless candy or gum for dry mouth
• **CDAD:** Teach patient to notify health care
professional immediately of diarrhea with
mucus, blood
• **Suicide:** Teach patient, caregivers to be
aware of signs of suicide, increased depression, to notify health care professional
immediately
• **Peripheral neuropathy:** Teach patient to
notify health care professional of tingling, pain
in extremities
• Teach patient to avoid other medication unless approved by prescriber
• **Tendon pain:** To immediately report pain,
inflammation in tendons, weakness, tingling
in extremities
• **Allergic reactions:** To report rash and stop
product if it occurs
• Identify if pregnancy is planned or suspected

Evaluation

Positive therapeutic outcome
• Negative C&S, absence of signs/symptoms of
infection

gentamicin (Rx)
(jen-ta-mye′sin)
Cidomycin ✦
Func. class.: Antiinfective
Chem. class.: Aminoglycoside

Do not confuse: gentamicin/kanamycin/
clindamycin/ tobramycin/erythromycin/
vancomycin

ACTION: Interferes with protein synthesis
in bacterial cell by binding to 30S ribosomal
subunit, causing misreading of genetic code; inaccurate peptide sequence forms in protein
chain, causing bacterial death

Therapeutic outcome: Bactericidal effects for the following organisms: *Pseudomonas
aeruginosa, Proteus, Klebsiella, Serratia, Escherichia coli, Enterobacter, Citrobacter, Staphylococcus, Shigella, Salmonella, Acinetobacter,
Bacillus anthracis*

USES: Severe systemic infections of CNS; respiratory, GI, and urinary tracts; bone; skin; soft
tissues; caused by susceptible strains

Pharmacokinetics

Absorption	Well absorbed (IM)
Distribution	Distributed in extracellular fluids, poorly distributed in CSF; crosses placenta
Metabolism	Liver, minimal
Excretion	Mostly unchanged (79%) kidneys
Half-life	2-3 hr; infants 6-7 hr; in-creased in renal disease

Pharmacodynamics

	IM	IV
Onset	Rapid	Immediate
Peak	30-90 min	Infusion end
Duration	Unknown	Unknown

CONTRAINDICATIONS
Hypersensitivity to this or other aminoglycosides

BLACK BOX WARNING: Pregnancy

Precautions: Breastfeeding, geriatric, neonates, pseudomembranous colitis

BLACK BOX WARNING: Myasthenia gravis,
Parkinson's disease, infant botulism, tinnitus,
nephrotoxicity, neurotoxicity, ototoxicity

DOSAGE AND ROUTES
Severe systemic infections
Adult: IV INF 3-6 mg/kg/day in 3 divided doses q8hr; IM 3-5 mg/kg/day in divided doses q8hr
Child: IV/IM 2-2.5 mg/kg q8hr

Neonate and infant: IV/IM 2.5 mg/kg q8-12hr

Neonate <1 wk: 2.5 mg/kg q12hr

Renal dose
Adult: IM/IV CCr 70-100 ml/min reduce dose by multiplying maintenance dose by 0.85, give q8-12hr; CCr 50-69 ml/min reduce dose as above, give q12hr; CCr 25-49 ml/min reduce as above, give q24hr; CCr <25 ml/min reduce as above, give based on serum concentrations

Renal dose: extend interval (unlabeled)
Adult: IV CCr 40-59 ml/min, 5-7 mg/kg q36hr; CCr 20-39 ml/min, 5-7 mg/kg q48hr; CCr <20 ml/min, 5-7 mg/kg once, then base on serial levels

Available forms: Inj 10, 40 mg/ml; premixed inj 40, 60, 70, 80, 90, 100, 120 mg/100 ml NS

ADVERSE EFFECTS
CNS: Dizziness, seizures, neurotoxicity, encephalopathy, headache
EENT: Ototoxicity, deafness, visual disturbances, tinnitus
GI: *Nausea, vomiting, anorexia,* increased ALT, AST, bilirubin, hepatomegaly, hepatic necrosis, splenomegaly
GU: Nephrotoxicity
INTEG: *Rash,* urticaria, photosensitivity, anaphylaxis
MS: Muscle paralysis (IV)
RESP: Apnea

INTERACTIONS
Individual drugs

> **BLACK BOX WARNING:** Acyclovir, amphotericin B, cidofovir, CISplatin, cycloSPORINE, ethacrynic acid, foscarnet, furosemide, ganciclovir, mannitol, methoxyflurane, pamidronate, polymyxin, tacrolimus, vancomycin, zoledronic acid: increased ototoxicity, neurotoxicity, nephrotoxicity

Drug classifications

> **BLACK BOX WARNING:** Aminoglycosides, cephalosporins, penicillins: increased ototoxicity, neurotoxicity, nephrotoxicity

Nondepolarizing neuromuscular blockers: increased neuromuscular blockade, respiratory depression
Penicillins: Do not use at the same time as or physically mix with penicillins

Drug/lab test
Increase: LDH, AST, ALT, bilirubin, BUN, creatinine, eosinophils
Decrease: Hgb, WBC, platelets, granulocytes

NURSING CONSIDERATIONS
Assessment
- Assess patient for previous sensitivity reaction
- **Assess patient for signs and symptoms of infection** including characteristics of wounds, sputum, urine, stool, WBC >10,000/mm³; obtain baseline, periodically during treatment

> **BLACK BOX WARNING: Neurotoxicity (myasthenia gravis, Parkinson's disease, infant botulism):** Assess for paresthesias, tetany, Chvostek's/Trousseau's signs, confusion (adults) tetany, muscle weakness (infants); correct electrolyte imbalance

- **Assess for allergic reactions:** rash, urticaria, pruritus, chills, fever, joint pain may occur a few days after therapy begins

> **BLACK BOX WARNING: Nephrotoxicity** Identify urine output; if decreasing, notify prescriber (may indicate nephrotoxicity); also, increased BUN, creatinine, urine CCr <80 ml/min; monitor I&O ratio; urinalysis daily for proteinuria, cells, casts; report sudden change in urine output; assess urine pH if product is used for UTI; urine should be kept alkaline

- Monitor blood studies: AST, ALT, CBC, Hct, bilirubin, LDH, alkaline phosphatase, Coombs' test monthly if patient is on long-term therapy
- Monitor electrolytes: potassium, sodium, chloride, magnesium if patient is on long-term therapy
- **Assess for overgrowth of infection:** perineal itching, fever, malaise, redness, pain, swelling, drainage, rash, diarrhea, change in cough, sputum
- Obtain weight before treatment; calculation of dosage is usually based on ideal body weight but may be calculated on actual body weight
- Monitor VS during inf, watch for hypotension, change in pulse
- Assess IV site for thrombophlebitis including pain, redness, swelling q30min, change site if needed; apply warm compresses to discontinued site

G

- Obtain serum peak, measured at 30-60 min after **IV** inf or 60 min after IM inj, trough level measured just before next dose; blood level should be 2-4 times bacteriostatic level (based on traditional dosing)

> **BLACK BOX WARNING: Ototoxicity: Assess for deafness** by audiometric testing, ringing, roaring in ears, vertigo; assess hearing before, during, after treatment

- Assess for dehydration: high specific gravity, decrease in skin turgor, dry mucous membranes, dark urine
- **Pregnancy/breastfeeding:** identify if pregnancy is planned or suspected, or if breastfeeding

Patient problem
Infection (uses)

Implementation
- Obtain C&S before starting treatment; treatment may be started before results are received

IM route
- Give inj deeply in large muscle mass; rotate sites

Intermittent IV route
- Give in even doses around the clock
- After diluting in 50-200 ml normal saline, D₅W, decrease volume of diluent in child; maintain 0.1% solution, run over ½-1 hr (adults), up to 2 hr (child). Give by intermittent inf, flush with 0.9% NaCl or D₅W after inf
- Separate aminoglycosides and penicillins by ≥1 hr
- Store in tight container

Y-site compatibilities: Alatrofloxacin, aldesleukin, alemtuzumab, alfentanil, alprostadil, amifostine, amikacin, aminocaproic acid, aminophylline, amiodarone, amsacrine, anidulafungin, argatroban, arsenic trioxide, ascorbic acid injection, asparaginase, atenolol, atracurium, atropine, aztreonam, benztropine, bivalirudin, bleomycin, bumetanide, buprenorphine, butorphanol, calcium chloride/gluconate, CARBOplatin, carmustine, caspofungin, cefamandole, ceFAZolin, cefepime, cefotaxime, cefOXitin, cefpirome, ceftaroline, cefTAZidime, ceftizoxime, cefTRIAXone, cefuroxime, chlorothiazide, chlorpheniramine, chlorproMAZINE, cimetidine, ciprofloxacin, cisatracurium, CISplatin, clarithromycin, clindamycin, cloxacillin, codeine, colistimethate, cyanocobalamin, cyclophosphamide, cycloSPORINE, cytarabine, DACTINomycin, DAPTOmycin, DAUNOrubicin citrate liposome, DAUNOrubicin hydrochloride, dexmedetomidine, dexrazoxane, digoxin, diltiazem, dimenhyDRINATE, diphenhydrAMINE, DOBUTamine, DOCEtaxel, dolasetron, DOPamine, doripenem, doxacurium, doxapram, DOXOrubicin hydrochloride, DOXOrubicin hydrochloride liposomal, doxycycline, edetate calcium disodium, edetate disodium, enalaprilat, EPHEDrine, EPINEPHrine, epirubicin, epoetin alfa, eptifibatide, ergonovine, ertapenem, erythromycin lactobionate, esmolol, etoposide, etoposide phosphate, famotidine, fenoldopam, fentaNYL, fluconazole, fludarabine, fluorouracil, foscarnet, gallamine, gallium, gatifloxacin, gemcitabine, glycopyrrolate, granisetron, HYDROmorphone, hydrOXYzine, ifosfamide, imipenemcilastatin, irinotecan, isoproterenol, ketamine, ketorolac, labetalol, lactated Ringer's injection, lansoprazole, lepirudin, leucovorin, levofloxacin, lidocaine, lincomycin, linezolid, LORazepam, magnesium sulfate, mannitol, mechlorethamine, melphalan, meperidine, mephentermine sulfate, meropenem, mesna, metaraminol, methyldopate, methylprednisolone sodium succinate, metoclopramide, metoprolol, metroNIDAZOLE, midazolam, milrinone, minocycline, mitoXANtrone, mivacurium, morphine, multiple vitamins injection, mycophenolate mofetil, nafcillin, nalbuphine, nalorphine, naloxone, netilmicin, niCARdipine, nitroglycerin, nitroprusside, norepinephrine, octreotide, ondansetron, oritavancin, oxacillin, oxaliplatin, oxytocin, PACLitaxel (solvent/surfactant), palonosetron, pamidronate, pancuronium, papaverine, penicillin G potassium/sodium, pentazocine, perphenazine, PHENobarbital, phentolamine, phenylephrine, phytonadione, piperacillin, polymyxin B, posaconazole, potassium acetate/chloride, procainamide, prochlorperazine, promazine, promethazine, propranolol, protamine, pyridoxine, quiNIDine gluconate, ranitidine, remifentanil, Ringer's injection, riTUXimab, rocuronium, sargramostim, sodium acetate/bicarbonate/citrate, streptomycin, succinylcholine, SUFentanil, tacrolimus, telavancin, temocillin, teniposide, theophylline, thiamine, thiotepa, ticarcillin, ticarcillin-clavulanate, tigecycline, tirofiban, TNA (3-in-1), tobramycin, tolazoline, topotecan, TPN (2-in-1), trastuzumab, trimetaphan, tubocurarine, urokinase, vancomycin, vasopressin, vecuronium, verapamil, vinBLAStine, vinCRIStine, vinorelbine, vitamin B complex with C, voriconazole, zidovudine, zoledronic acid

Patient/family education
- Teach patient to report sore throat, bruising, bleeding, joint pain; may indicate blood dyscrasias (rare)
- Advise patient to contact prescriber if vaginal itching, loose foul-smelling stools, furry tongue occur; may indicate superimposed infection
- Teach patient to drink adequate fluids

• Teach patient to avoid hazardous activities until reaction is known

BLACK BOX WARNING: Advise patient to report loss of hearing, ringing, roaring in ears; feeling of fullness in the head

Evaluation
Positive therapeutic outcome
• Absence of signs/symptoms of infection (WBC <10,000/mm³, temp WNL, absence of red, draining wounds)
• Reported improvement in symptoms of infection

TREATMENT OF OVERDOSE:
Withdraw product, hemodialysis

gentamicin ophthalmic
See Appendix B

gentamicin topical
See Appendix B

glecaprevir/pibrentasvir
(glek-a′ pre-vir brent′ as-vir)
Mavyret
Func. class.: antivirals, anti-hepatitis
Chem. class.: HCV NS3/4A protease inhibitor-HCV NS5A inhibitor

ACTION: Glecaprevir: is an inhibitor of the HCV NS3/4A protease, which is necessary for viral replication
Pibrentasvir: prevents hepatitis C viral replication by inhibiting the HCV NS5A protein

Therapeutic outcome: Decreased levels of HCV and lessened chronic HCV infection

USES: Treatment of most strains of hepatitis C

Pharmacokinetics

Absorption	Unknown
Distribution	>98% protein binding
Metabolism	Affected cytochrome P450 isoenzymes and drug transporters: CYP3A4, P-glycoprotein (P-gp), breast cancer resistance protein (BCRP), organic anion transporting polypeptide (OATP) 1B1/3
Excretion	Unknown
Half-life	Glecaprevir 6 hr, pibrentasvir 13 hr

Pharmacodynamics

Onset	Unknown
Peak	5 h
Duration	Unknown

CONTRAINDICATIONS: Hypersensitivity, severe hepatic disease (Child-Pugh C)

PRECAUTIONS: Anticoagulant therapy, breastfeeding, hepatitis C and HIV coinfection, pregnancy

BLACK BOX WARNING: Hepatitis B exacerbation

DOSAGE AND ROUTES
Treatment-naïve (chronic HCV genotype 1, 2, 3, 4, 5, 6, without cirrhosis)
Adult: PO 3 tablets q day × 8 wks Treatment-naïve (chronic HCV genotype 1, 2, 3, 4, 5, 6, with compensated cirrhosis) (Child-Pugh A)
Adult: PO 3 tablets q day × 12 wks HCV genotype 1 with or without compensated cirrhosis (Child-Pugh A); previously treated with HCV NS5A inhibitor but lacking a NS3/4A protease inhibitor
Adult: PO 3 tablets q day × 16 wks HCV genotype 1 with or without compensated cirrhosis (Child-Pugh A), previously treated with HCV NS3/4A inhibitor but lacking a NS5A protease inhibitor
Adult: PO 3 tablets q day X 12 wks HCV genotypes 1, 2, 4, 5, 6 without cirrhosis that have received interferon, pegylated interferon, ribavirin, or sofosuvir, but treatment-naïve with HCV NS3/4A protease inhibitor or NS5A inhibitor
Adult: PO 3 tablets q day × 8 wks HCV genotypes 1, 2, 4, 5, 6 with compensated cirrhosis (Child-Pugh A), which have previously received interferon, pegylated interferon, ribavirin, or sofosuvir, but treatment-naïve with HCV NS3/4A protease inhibitor or NS5A inhibitor
Adult: PO 3 tablets q day × 12 wks HCV genotype 3 with or without cirrhosis (Child-Pugh A) that has previously received interferon, pegylated interferon, ribavirin, or sofosuvir, but treatment-naïve with HCV NS3/4A protease inhibitor or NS5A inhibitor

Available forms: Tablets 100 mg glecaprevir/40 mg pibrentasvir

ADVERSE EFFECTS

CNS: Headache, fatigue, asthenia

GI: *Nausea,* diarrhea, hyperbilirubinemia

INTEG: *Pruritus*

INTERACTIONS
Drug classifications
Decreased glecaprevir effect: CYP3A4 inducers
Increased pibrentasvir effect: P-gp

Drug/lab test
Increase: Bilirubin

Drug/herb
Decreased medication effect: St. John's wort, avoid using together

NURSING CONSIDERATIONS
Assessment

> **BLACK BOX WARNING: HBV infection:**
> Obtain hepatitis B surface antigen (HBsAg), hepatitis B core antibody (anti-HBc); for those with HBV infection, a baseline HBV DNA concentration should be obtained prior to treatment. Continue to monitor coinfected patients during and after treatment for clinical and laboratory signs of hepatitis B exacerbation (HBsAg, HBV DNA, hepatic enzymes, bilirubin); may cause hepatic failure and death

• **Concurrent anticoagulant therapy (warfarin):** Closely monitor for changes in INR both during and after discontinuation of the HCV treatment regimen.
• **HIV/hepatitis C coinfection:** All should be tested for hepatitis C, with annual screening advised for those at high risk for acquiring hepatitis C. If hepatitis C and HIV coinfection is present, both viral infections should be treated concurrently

Implementation
• Give with food
• Do not split
• *Storage:* At or below 30° C (86° F)

Patient problem
Infection (uses)

Patient/family education
• **Pregnancy/breastfeeding:** Identify if pregnancy is planned or suspected; pregnancy should be avoided during treatment, or if breastfeeding, consider risk to infant
• Teach patient to report all OTC, Rx, herbal, and supplements currently taken and not to start new products without prescriber approval; serious drug interactions may occur
• Advise patient to take as prescribed, not to skip or double doses, not to split tablet
• Teach patient to immediately report any signs of liver toxicity (yellow eyes or skin, fatigue, weakness, loss of appetite, nausea, vomiting, or light-colored stools) to their healthcare provider

Evaluation
• Decreased levels of HCV and lessened chronic HCV infection

> **⚠ HIGH ALERT**
> ## glimepiride (Rx)
> (gly-meh′pih-ride)
> **Amaryl**
> ## glipiZIDE (Rx)
> (glip-i′zide)
> **Glucotrol, Glucotrol XL**
> *Func. class.:* Antidiabetic
> *Chem. class.:* Sulfonylurea (2nd generation)

Do not confuse: glipiZIDE/glucotrol/glyBURIDE

ACTION: Causes functioning β cells in pancreas to release insulin, leading to drop in blood glucose levels; may improve insulin binding to insulin receptors or increase the number of insulin receptors with prolonged administration; may also reduce basal hepatic glucose secretion; not effective if patient lacks functioning β cells

Therapeutic outcome: Decrease in polyuria, polydipsia, polyphagia, clear sensorium, absence of dizziness, stable gait

USES: Type 2 diabetes mellitus

Pharmacokinetics
Absorption	Well absorbed, GI tract
Distribution	Bile, protein binding 99%
Metabolism	Liver
Excretion	Via kidneys
Half-life	2-4 hr glipizide; 5 hr glimepiride

Pharmacodynamics
	glipiZIDE	glimepiride
Onset	1-1.5 hr	unknown
Peak	1-2 hr	2-3 hr
Duration	10-12 hr	24 hr

CONTRAINDICATIONS
Hypersensitivity to sulfonylureas/sulfonamides, type 1 diabetes, diabetic ketoacidosis

Precautions: Pregnancy, geriatric, cardiac disease, severe renal/hepatic disease, G6PD deficiency

DOSAGE AND ROUTES
Glimepiride
Adult: PO 1-2 mg/day with breakfast, then increase by ≤2 mg/day at q1-2wk, max 8 mg/day
Geriatric: PO 1 mg/day, may increase if needed

Renal/Hepatic dose
Adult: PO 1 mg/day with breakfast, may titrate upward as needed

GlipiZIDE
Adult: PO 5 mg initially before breakfast, then increase by 2.5-5 mg after several days, to desired response; max 40 mg/day in divided doses or 15 mg/dose; (XL) PO 5 mg/day with breakfast, may increase to 10 mg/day; max 20 mg/day
Geriatric: PO 2.5 mg/day, may increase if needed

Hepatic dose
Adult: PO 2.5 mg initially, then increase to desired response; max 40 mg/day in divided doses or 15 mg/dose

Available forms: Glimepiride: tabs 1, 2, 4 mg; **glipiZIDE:** tabs 5, 10 mg scored; EXT REL tabs 2.5, 5, 10 mg

ADVERSE EFFECTS
CNS: *Headache, weakness, dizziness, drowsiness*
ENDO: Hypoglycemia
GI: Hepatotoxicity, cholestatic jaundice, nausea, vomiting, diarrhea, weight gain
HEMA: Leukopenia, thrombocytopenia, agranulocytosis, aplastic anemia, pancytopenia, hemolytic anemia
INTEG: Rash, pruritus, photosensitivity, erythema
SYST: Serious hypersensitivity

INTERACTIONS
Individual drugs
Cholestyramine, diazoxide, isoniazid, rifampin: possible decreased action of glipiZIDE
Chloramphenicol, cimetidine, clarithromycin, clofibrate, fenfluramine, fluconazole, gemfibrozil, guanethidine, insulin, methyldopa, phenylbutazone, probenecid, sulfinpyrazone, voriconazole: increased hypoglycemia, monitor blood glucose
Digoxin: increased action of digoxin, cycloSPORINE

Drug classifications
Androgens, anticoagulants, fibric acid derivatives, H$_2$-antagonists, magnesium salts, MAOIs, NSAIDs, salicylates, sulfonamides, tricyclics, urinary acidifiers: increased hypoglycemia
β-Blockers: may mask symptoms of hypoglycemia
Diuretics (thiazide), corticosteroids, hydantoins, colesevelam, urinary alkalinizers: possible decreased action of glipiZIDE
Glycosides: increased action of glycosides

Drug/herb
Garlic, horse chestnut: increased antidiabetic effect
Chromium: decreased antidiabetic effect
Chromium, coenzyme Q10, fenugreek, ginseng: increased or decreased hypoglycemic effect
Green tea: decreased hypoglycemic effect

Drug/lab test
Increase: AST, ALT, LDH, BUN, creatinine
Decrease: Platelets, WBC, sodium

NURSING CONSIDERATIONS
Assessment
• **Assess for hypoglycemic/hyperglycemic reactions** that can occur soon after meals; hypoglycemic reactions (sweating, weakness, dizziness, anxiety, tremors, hunger); hyperglycemic reactions; A1c (baseline, q3mo) during treatment
• **Blood dyscrasias:** Monitor CBC baseline and periodically

Patient Problems
Excess food intake (uses)
Nonadherence (teaching)

Implementation
• Do not break, crush, or chew ext rel tabs
• Convert from other oral hypoglycemic agents or insulin dosage of <40 units/day; change may be made without gradual dosage change
• Patients taking >40 units/day of insulin convert gradually by receiving oral hypoglycemic agents and 50% of previous insulin dosage for 3-5 days
• Monitor serum or urine glucose and ketones 3 ×/day during conversion
• **GlipiZIDE:** Give 30 min before meals (regular release); with breakfast (ext rel)
• **Glimepiride:** with breakfast; if patient is NPO, may need to hold dose to prevent hypoglycemia
• Give tab crushed and mixed with meal or fluids for patients with difficulty swallowing
• For severe hypoglycemia give **IV** D$_{50}$W, then **IV** dextrose solution
• Store in tight container in cool environment

Patient/family education
• **Teach patient to check for symptoms of cholestatic jaundice:** dark urine, pruritus, yellow sclera; if these occur, prescriber should be notified
• Teach patient to use capillary blood glucose test
• Teach patient to report bleeding, bruising, weight gain, edema, SOB, weakness, sore throat, swelling in ankles, rash
• Teach patient symptoms of hypo/hyperglycemia, what to do about each
• Instruct patient that product must be continued on daily basis; explain consequence of discontinuing product abruptly
• Advise patient to notify health care professional of use prior to surgery

• Teach patient not to operate machinery or drive until response is known; dizziness may occur
• Advise patient that continuing follow-up exams and lab work will be needed
• Caution patient to avoid OTC medications unless approved by a prescriber
• Teach patient that diabetes is a lifelong illness; that this product is not a cure
• Teach patient to avoid alcohol; inform about disulfiram reaction (nausea, headache, cramps, flushing, hypoglycemia)
• Instruct patient that all food included in diet plan must be eaten to prevent hypoglycemia
• Advise patient to use sunscreen or stay out of the sun to prevent burns
• Advise patient to carry/wear emergency ID and carry a glucagon emergency kit for emergency purposes; also prescriber name, phone number, and medications taken
• Teach patient ext rel tab may appear in stool
• **Pregnancy/breastfeeding:** Identify if pregnancy is planned or suspected; breastfed infant may be hypoglycemic

Evaluation
Positive therapeutic outcome
• Decrease in polyuria, polydipsia, polyphagia; clear sensorium; absence of dizziness; stable gait
• Improved serum glucose, A1c

glucagon
(gloo′ka-gon)
GlucaGen
Func. class.: Antihypoglycemic

ACTION: Increases in blood glucose, relaxation of smooth muscle of the GI tract, and a positive inotropic and chronotropic effect on the heart; increases in blood glucose are secondary to stimulation of glycogenolysis

USES: Hypoglycemia, used to temporarily inhibit movement of GI tract

Unlabeled uses: Beta blocker, calcium channel toxicity

Pharmacokinetics

Absorption	Complete (IV), well (IM/SUBCUT)
Distribution	Unknown, protein binding >99%
Metabolism	Not metabolized
Excretion	97% feces
Half-life	8-18 min

Pharmacodynamics

	IV	IM/SUBCUT
Onset	Immediate	5-10 min
Peak	30 min	13-20 min
Duration	1 hr	Up to 90 min

CONTRAINDICATIONS
Hypersensitivity, pheochromocytoma, insulinoma

Precautions: Pregnancy, breastfeeding, cardiac disease, adrenal insufficiency

DOSAGE AND ROUTES
Hypoglycemia in those with diabetes mellitus
Adult/adolescent/child 55 lb (25 kg): IM/IV/SUBCUT (GlucaGen) 1 mg (1 IU)
Child <55 lb (25 kg) or <6-8 yr: IM/IV/**SUBCUT** (Glucagon) 0.5 mg (0.5 IU)
Adult/adolescent/child ≥44 lb (20 kg): IM/IV/SUBCUT (Glucagon) 1 mg (1 IU)
Child <44 lb (20 kg): IM/IV/SUBCUT (Glucagon) 0.5 mg (0.5 IU) or 0.02-0.03 mg/kg (IU/kg)

Severe hypoglycemia
Neonate: IM/IV/SUBCUT 0.2 mg/kg/dose, max 1 mg/dose; **CONT INFUSION** (unlabeled): 0.5-1 mg/day

Available forms: Powder for injection 1 mg vial

SIDE EFFECTS
CNS: Dizziness, headache
CV: Hypotension
GI: Nausea, vomiting
SYST: Hypersensitivity

INTERACTIONS
Anticoagulants: Increase: bleeding risk
Antidiabetics: Decrease: effect of antidiabetics
Beta blockers: Increase: B/P and heart rate

NURSING CONSIDERATIONS
Assessment:
• **Hypoglycemia:** monitor glucose levels before and after product use; use other products to control hypoglycemia if patient is conscious

Patient problem
Risk for injury (uses)
Nonadherence (teaching)

Implementation:
• Visually inspect for particulate matter and discoloration before use

Reconstitution: Reconstitute with 1 mL of sterile water for injection or with diluent supplied by the manufacturer; the reconstituted

---

injection should be clear and of waterlike consistency (1 mg/mL); discard any unused portion

IM route
• Inject into a large muscle mass; aspirate before injection to avoid injection into a blood vessel

SUBCUT route
• Inject, taking care not to inject intradermally

IV route
• Inject directly into a vein at a rate ≤1 mg/ min; may be given through line running D5W or given at the same time as a bolus of dextrose

Patient/family education
• Teach patient how to use this product, symptoms of hypoglycemia; instruct patient in use of oral glucose when hypoglycemia occurs; use this product only when patient is unable to swallow
• Advise patient not to use outdated product
• Teach patient to carry a sugar source at all times

Evaluation
Positive therapeutic outcome
• Decreased hypoglycemia

▲ HIGH ALERT

glyBURIDE (Rx)
(glye′byoor-ide)
DiaBeta ✦, **Euglucon** ✦, **Glynase PresTab**
Func. class.: Antidiabetic
Chem. class.: Sulfonylurea
(2nd generation)

Do not confuse: glyBURIDE/Glucotrol/ glipiZIDE, **DiaBeta**/Zebeta

ACTION: Causes functioning β cells in pancreas to release insulin, leading to drop in blood glucose levels; may improve insulin binding to insulin receptors and increase number of insulin receptors with prolonged administration; may also reduce basal hepatic glucose secretion; not effective if patient lacks functioning β cells

Therapeutic outcome: Decrease in polyuria, polydipsia, polyphagia, clear sensorium, absence of dizziness, stable gait

USES: Type 2 diabetes mellitus

Pharmacokinetics
Absorption	Well-absorbed GI tract
Distribution	99% plasma protein binding, crosses placenta
Metabolism	Liver
Excretion	Urine, feces (metabolites)
Half-life	10 hr

Pharmacodynamics
Onset	45-60 min
Peak	2-4 hr
Duration	24 hr

CONTRAINDICATIONS
Hypersensitivity to sulfonylureas, type 1 diabetes, diabetic ketoacidosis, renal failure

Precautions: Pregnancy, geriatric, cardiac/ thyroid disease, severe renal/hepatic disease, severe hypoglycemic reactions, sulfonamide/ sulfonylurea hypersensitivity, G6PD deficiency

DOSAGE AND ROUTES
To replace insulin
Adults: PO if insulin was <40 U/day, switch directly when glyBURIDE is stopped; if insulin <20 U/day give 2.5-5 mg or (1.5-3 mg micronized); if insulin was 20-40 U/day give 5 mg or (3 mg micronized); if insulin >40 U/day, give 5 mg (3 mg micronized) initially with 50% insulin dose, gradually taper insulin and increase glyBURIDE

DiaBeta
Adult: PO 1.25-5 mg initially, then increased to desired response at weekly intervals up to 20 mg/day; may be given as a single or divided dose
Geriatric: PO 1.25 mg initially, then increased to desired response; max 20 mg/day, maintenance 1.25-20 mg/day

Renal dose
Adult: PO CCr 50 ml/min, use conservative dose
Geriatric: PO 0.75-3 mg/day, may increase by 1.5 mg/wk

Glynase PresTab (micronized)
Adult: PO 1.5-3 mg/day initially, may increase by 1.5 mg/wk, max 12 mg/day
Geriatric: PO 0.75-3 mg/day, may increase by 1.5 mg/wk

Available forms: Tabs (DiaBeta) 1.25, 2.5, 5 mg; tabs micronized (Glynase PresTab) 1.5, 3, 6 mg

ADVERSE EFFECTS
CNS: *Headache, weakness,* paresthesia, tinnitus, fatigue, vertigo
EENT: Blurred vision
ENDO: Hypoglycemia
GI: Nausea, hepatoxicity, cholestatic jaundice, vomiting, diarrhea
HEMA: Leukopenia, thrombocytopenia, agranulocytosis, aplastic anemia
INTEG: Rash, allergic reactions, pruritus, photosensitivity, erythema
SYST: Serious hypersensitivity

INTERACTIONS
Individual drugs
Bosentan: increased LFTs, avoid concurrent use

Charcoal, cholestyramine, isoniazid, rifampin thyroid: decreased action of glyBURIDE

Clarithromycin, chloramphenicol, fenfluramine, fluconazole, gemfibrozil, guanethidine, insulin, methyldopa, phenylbutazone, probenecid, sulfinpyrazone: increased hypoglycemia

Colesevelam: increased triglyceride levels

CycloSPORINE: increased action of cycloSPORINE

Diazoxide: both products may have action decreased

Digoxin: increased level

Drug classifications
Androgens, anticoagulants, antidepressants (tricyclics), β-blockers, H_2-antagonists, magnesium salts, MAOIs, NSAIDs, salicylates, sulfonamides, urinary acidifiers: increased hypoglycemia; voriconazole, monitor blood glucose

β-Adrenergic blockers: increased masking of symptoms of hypoglycemia

Diuretics (thiazide), hydantoins, urinary alkalinizers, corticosteroids, phenothiazines, oral contraceptives, estrogens: decreased action of glyBURIDE; monitor blood glucose

Drug/herb
Garlic, horse chestnut: increased antidiabetic effect

Green tea: decreased hypoglycemic effect

Drug/lab test
Increased: AST, ALT, LDH, BUN, creatinine, alkaline phosphatase

Decrease: Hgb, sodium, glucose, platelets, WBC

NURSING CONSIDERATIONS
Assessment
• Assess for hypo/hyperglycemic reactions that can occur soon after meals; hypoglycemic reactions (sweating, weakness, dizziness, anxiety, tremors, hunger); hyperglycemic reactions; A1c (baseline, q3mo) during treatment

• **Blood dyscrasias:** Monitor CBC, check liver function tests periodically, AST, LDH, and renal studies: BUN, creatinine during treatment

• **Beers:** Avoid in older adults, severe prolonged hypoglycemia

Patient problem
Excess food intake (uses)

Nonadherence (teaching)

Implementation
• Conversion from other oral hypoglycemic agents or insulin dosage of <40 units/day; change may be made without gradual dosage change

• Patients taking >40 units/day of insulin convert gradually by receiving oral hypoglycemic agents and 50% of previous insulin dosage for 3-5 days

• Monitor serum or urine glucose and ketones 3 ×/day during conversion

• Give product 30 min before breakfast; if large dose is required, may be divided into two; give with meals to decrease GI upset and provide best absorption; if patient is NPO, may need to hold dose to avoid hypoglycemia, take at same time each day

• Give tab crushed and mixed with meal or fluids for patients with difficulty swallowing

• For severe hypoglycemia, give **IV** $D_{50}W$, then **IV** dextrose sol

• Store in tight container in cool environment

Patient/family education
• **Teach patient to check for symptoms of cholestatic jaundice:** dark urine, pruritus, yellow sclera; if these occur, prescriber should be notified

• Teach patient to use capillary blood glucose test

• **Teach patient symptoms of hypo/hyperglycemia,** what to do about each

• Instruct patient that product must be continued on daily basis; explain consequence of discontinuing product abruptly

• Teach patient to report bleeding, bruising, weight gain, edema, shortness of breath, weakness, sore throat

• Teach patient to take product in AM to prevent hypoglycemic reactions at night

• Caution patient to avoid OTC medications unless approved by a prescriber

• Teach patient that diabetes is a lifelong illness; that this product is not a cure

• Instruct patient that all food included in diet plan must be eaten to prevent hypoglycemia

• Advise patient to carry/wear emergency ID and carry a glucagon emergency kit for emergency purposes: have sugar packets available; also prescriber name, phone number, and medications

• Advise patient to notify health care professional of use prior to surgery

• Teach patient not to operate machinery or drive until response is known; dizziness may occur

• Advise patient that continuing follow-up exams and lab work will be needed

• Advise patient to use sunscreen or stay out of the sun to prevent burns

• **Pregnancy/breastfeeding:** Identify if pregnancy is planned or suspected; insulin is usually used in pregnancy; breastfed infant may be hypoglycemic

Evaluation
Positive therapeutic outcome
• Decrease in polyuria, polydipsia, polyphagia; clear sensorium; absence of dizziness; stable gait
• Improved serum glucose, A1c

golimumab (Rx)

(goal-lim′yu-mab)

Simponi, Simponi Aria

Func. class.: Antirheumatic agent (disease modifying), immunomodulator

Chem. class.: Monoclonal antibody, DMARDS, tumor necrosis factor (TNF) modifier

ACTION: Monoclonal antibody specific for human tumor necrosis factor (TNF); elevated levels of TNF are found in patients with rheumatoid arthritis

Therapeutic outcome: Decreased pain, decreased inflammation in joints, better ROM

USES: Rheumatoid arthritis, ankylosing spondylitis, psoriatic arthritis, ulcerative colitis

Pharmacokinetics

Absorption	Well
Distribution	Circulation
Metabolism	Unknown
Excretion	Unknown
Half-life	2 wk

Pharmacodynamics

	IV	Subcut
Onset	Unknown	Unknown
Peak	2-7 days	Unknown
Duration	Unknown	Unknown

CONTRAINDICATIONS

Hypersensitivity active infections

Precautions: Pregnancy, breastfeeding, children, geriatric patients, CNS demyelinating disease, Guillain-Barré syndrome, HF, hepatitis B carriers, blood dyscrasias, surgery, MS, neurological disease, diabetes, immunosuppression

BLACK BOX WARNING: Infection

DOSAGE AND ROUTES
Rheumatoid arthritis
Adult: SUBCUT 50 mg qmo; for RA give with methotrexate; IV (Simponi Aria only) 2 mg/kg over 30 min, repeat in 4 wk, then q8wk; give with methotrexate

Ankylosing spondylitis/psoriatic arthritis
Adult: SUBCUT 50 mg monthly

Ulcerative colitis
Adult: SUBCUT 200 mg for 1 dose, then 100 mg in 2 wk; maintenance 100 mg q4wk starting at wk 6

Available forms: Inj 50 mg/0.5 ml, 100 mg/ml prefilled syringe, SmartJect Auto Injector; inj 50 mg/4 ml single-use vial

ADVERSE EFFECTS

CNS: Dizziness, paresthesia, CNS demyelinating disorder, weakness, Guillain-Barré syndrome, MS

CV: Hypertension, HF

GI: Hepatitis

HEMA: Agranulocytosis, aplastic anemia, leukopenia, polycythemia, thrombocytopenia, pancytopenia

INTEG: Psoriasis

MISC: Increased risk of cancer, antibody development to this drug, risk of infection (TB, invasive fungal infections, other opportunistic infections); may be fatal, inj site reactions, anaphylaxis

INTERACTIONS
Individual drugs
Abatacept, adalimumab, anakinra, etanercept, immunosuppressants, inFLIXimab, rilonacept, riTUXimab: increased infection, avoid concurrent use

Warfarin, cycloSPORINE, theophylline: dosage change may be needed

Drug classifications
Live vaccines: do not give concurrently or within 3 mo; immunization should be brought up to date before treatment

Drug/lab tests
Increase: LFTs
Decrease: platelets, WBC

NURSING CONSIDERATIONS
Assessment
• **Assess for pain,** stiffness, ROM, swelling of joints during treatment
• Check for inj site pain, swelling; usually occur after 2 inj (4-5 days)

BLACK BOX WARNING: Infections Assess for fever, flulike symptoms, dyspnea, change in urination, redness/swelling around any wounds, stop treatment if present; some serious infections including sepsis may occur, may be fatal; patients with active infections should not be started on this product

• **HBV:** Test before use; reactivation of HBV may also occur; discontinue if reactivation occurs
• **Blood dyscrasias:** CBC, differential before and periodically during treatment; discontinue if present

> **BLACK BOX WARNING: TB:** Obtain TB skin test before starting treatment; treat latent TB before starting therapy, continue to monitor for TB, even if TB test is negative

> **BLACK BOX WARNING: Neoplastic disease:** May occur in those <18 yr; avoid use in those with known malignancies, monitor for secondary malignancies during treatment

• **Pregnancy/breastfeeding:** Use only if benefits outweigh fetal risk; do not breastfeed, excretion unknown
• **Anaphylaxis:** assess for rash, dyspnea, wheezing; emergency equipment should be nearby; if present discontinue product immediately, notify health care professional
• **HF:** Monitor B/P, pulse, edema, shortness of breath, may occur or worsen with treatment
• **Psoriasis:** May occur or worsen; monitor LFTs, hepatitis B serology, may reactivate HBV

Patient problem
Pain (uses)
Risk for infection (adverse reactions)
Risk for injury (adverse reactions)

Implementation
SUBCUT route
• Refrigerate; do not freeze; allow to warm to room temp before using
• Visually inspect solution for particulate or discoloration, solution should be clear to slightly opalescent and colorless to slightly yellow; there may be tiny white particles; do not shake
• *SmartJect autoinjector:* Allow to reach room temperature for 30 min prior to use, remove cap, inject within 5 min of removing cap, do not put cap back on, place the open end against the inj site at a 90-degree angle, without pushing button, push the injector firmly against the skin, press the button once and release, listen for the first click, wait for the second click or 15 sec, and remove the injector; do not rub site
• *Prefilled syringe:* Allow to warm to room temperature for 30 min, remove needle cover by pulling straight off, do not twist or recap, inject within 5 min of needle cover removal, hold the syringe in one hand like a pencil and use the other to pinch the skin, inject needle at a 45-degree angle, push plunger down as far as it will go, keep pressure on the plunger head and remove needle from skin, remove pressure from

the plunger head, the needle guard will cover the needle, do not rub site

IV route (Simponi Aria)
• Calculate number of vials needed; do not shake; dilute total volume of product in NS to yield 100 ml for infusion, slowly add product, mix gently
• Infuse over 30 min; use infusion set with in-line, sterile, non-pyrogenic, low-protein binding filter (≤0.22 mm pore size)

Patient/family education
• Teach patient about self-administration if appropriate: inj should be made in thigh, abdomen, upper arm; rotate sites at least 1 inch from old site; do not inject in areas that are bruised, red, hard
• Advise patient to discuss all Rx, OTC, herbals, supplements with health care professional
• Teach patient to report infection, flu-like symptoms, dyspnea
• Advise patient that if medication is not taken when due, inject next dose as soon as remembered and inject next dose as scheduled

> **BLACK BOX WARNING:** Teach patient to report signs, symptoms of infection, allergic reaction, or lupuslike syndrome

• **HBV infection:** Test for HBV before starting treatment, HBV can be fatal in HBV carriers; monitor to report clay-colored stools, fatigue, yellow skin or eyes
• Identify if pregnancy is planned or suspected, or if breastfeeding

Evaluation
Positive therapeutic outcome
• Decreased inflammation, pain in joints

goserelin (Rx)
(goe'se-rel-lin)
Zoladex
Func. class.: Gonadotropin-releasing hormone, antineoplastic
Chem. class.: Synthetic decapeptide analog of LHRH

ACTION: Inhibitor of pituitary gonadotropin secretion; initially increases LH and FSH, with increases in testosterone, reduction in sex steroid levels (substitute serum testosterone levels)

Therapeutic outcome: Decrease in tumor size and spread of malignant cells

USES: Advanced prostate cancer Stage B2-C (10.8 mg); endometriosis, advanced breast cancer, endometrial thinning (3.6 mg)

Pharmacokinetics

Absorption	Well absorbed
Distribution	Unknown
Metabolism	Liver
Excretion	Kidneys
Half-life	4½ hr

Pharmacodynamics

Onset	Unknown
Peak	14-28 days
Duration	Treatment length

CONTRAINDICATIONS

Pregnancy, breastfeeding, nondiagnosed vaginal bleeding, children, 10.8 mg dose in women, hypersensitivity to LHRH, LHRH-agonist analogs

Precautions: Spinal cord decompression, renal disease, bone mineral density loss

DOSAGE AND ROUTES

Adult: SUBCUT 3.6 mg q4wk (implant) or 10.8 mg q12wk

Endometrial thinning

Adult: SUBCUT 1-2 depot inj (usually 1 depot, surgery performed at 4 wk); (if 2 depots, surgery performed 2-4 wk after 2nd depot)

Available forms: Depot inj 3.6, 10.8 mg

ADVERSE EFFECTS

CNS: Headaches, fatigue, weakness, anxiety, depression, dizziness, insomnia, lethargy, stroke, seizures

CV: Dysrhythmia, prolonged QT, hypertension, MI, chest pain, HF

ENDO: Gynecomastia, breast tenderness, hot flashes; hyperglycemia, diabetes

GI: Nausea, vomiting, constipation, diarrhea, ulcer

GU: *Spotting, breakthrough bleeding, decreased libido,* renal insufficiency, urinary obstruction, impotence

INTEG: Rash, pain at injection site, diaphoresis

MS: Bone pain, arthralgia, decreased bone density

INTERACTIONS

Drug/lab test

Increased: alkaline phosphatase, estradiol, FSH, LH
Decreased: progesterone

NURSING CONSIDERATIONS

Assessment

• **Reproductive studies:** monitor pelvic ultrasound, pelvic exam, PSA, serum estradiol/testosterone, pregnancy test prior to therapy

• Monitor I&O ratios; palpate bladder for distention in urinary obstruction

• **Cancer metastases:** monitor for relief of bone pain (back pain), change in motor function

• Blood studies: monitor acid phosphatase; calcium in breast/prostate cancer, hypercalcemia may occur

• **Endometriosis:** Assess for pain, excessive menstrual period, bleeding between periods baseline and periodically

• **Pregnancy/breastfeeding:** Do not use in pregnancy, breastfeeding

Patient problem

Impaired sexual functioning (adverse reactions)

Implementation

Depot

• Give SUBCUT using implant, inserted by qualified person into upper subcutaneous tissue in abdominal wall q28days or q12wk (10.8 mg), do not attempt to remove air bubbles from syringe, assess for injection site reaction

Patient/family education

• Caution patient that gynecomastia and postmenopausal symptoms may occur but will decrease after treatment is discontinued; that bone pain may increase, then decrease, may use analgesics

• Explain reason for product, expected results; to use q3mo, to notify health care professional characteristics of periods (endometriosis)

• Teach patient to contact prescriber for difficulty urinating, hot flashes occur during treatment

• **Pregnancy/breastfeeding:** Advise patient not to breastfeed while taking product; use effective nonhormonal contraception

• Advise patient to notify prescriber if chest pain, weakness, difficulty breathing occur; may indicate MI or stroke

Evaluation

Positive therapeutic outcome

• Decreased endometriosis symptoms

• Decreased symptoms in breast cancer

• More normal levels of PSA, acid phosphatase, alkaline phosphatase; testosterone level of <25 mg/dl

---

granisetron (Rx)

(grane-iss'e-tron)
Granisol, Kytril ✚, Sancuso, Sustol
Func. class.: Antiemetic
Chem. class.: 5-HT₃ receptor antagonist

ACTION: Prevents nausea, vomiting by blocking serotonin peripherally, centrally, and in the small intestine

Therapeutic outcome: Absence of nausea and vomiting

USES: Prevention of nausea, vomiting associated with cancer chemotherapy including high-dose CISplatin, radiation

Unlabeled uses: Acute nausea, vomiting after surgery

Pharmacokinetics

Absorption	PO 50%
Distribution	Erythrocytes, protein binding 65%
Metabolism	Liver
Excretion	Kidney
Half-life	10-12 hr

Pharmacodynamics

	PO	IV	TD
Onset	Rapid	Immediate	Unknown
Peak	60 min	30 min	48 hr
Duration	24 hr	24 hr	Unknown

CONTRAINDICATIONS
Hypersensitivity to this product or benzyl alcohol

Precautions: Pregnancy, breastfeeding, children, geriatric, ondansetron/palonosetron/dolasetron hypersensitivity, cardiac dysrhythmias, cardiac/hepatic disease/GI, electrolyte imbalances

DOSAGE AND ROUTES
Nausea, vomiting in chemotherapy
Adult and child ≥2 yr: IV 10 mcg/kg over 5 min, 30 min before the start of cancer chemotherapy, **TD** apply 1 patch (3.1 mg/24 hr) to upper arm 24-48 hr before chemotherapy; patch may be worn up to 7 days
Adult: PO 1 mg bid, give 1st dose 1 hr before chemotherapy and next dose 12 hr after 1st or 2 mg as a single dose anytime within 1 hr prior to chemotherapy or radiation

Nausea, vomiting in radiation therapy
Adult: PO 2 mg/day 1 hr prior to radiation

Available forms: Inj 0.1 mg/ml, 1 mg/ml; tabs 1 mg, oral sol 2 mg/10 ml; patch TD 3.1 mg/24 hr

ADVERSE EFFECTS
CNS: *Headache, asthenia,* anxiety, dizziness, stimulation, insomnia, drowsiness
CV: Hypertension, QT prolongation
GI: Diarrhea, *constipation, nausea*
MISC: Rash, serotonin, serotonin syndrome

INTERACTIONS
Individual drugs
Amoxapine, arsenic, chloroquine, cloZAPine, dasatinib, dolasetron, dronedarone, droperidol, erythromycin, flecainide, fluconazole, haloperidol, lapatinib, maprotiline, methadone, octreotide, ondansetron, palonosetron, pentamidine, pimozide, posaconazole, propafenone, ranolazine, risperiDONE, sertindole, SUNItinib, tacrolimus, telithromycin, troleandomycin, vardenafil, voriconazole, vorinostat, ziprasidone: increased QT prolongation

Drug classifications
β-blockers, class I, III antidysrhythmics, halogenated/local anesthetics, phenothiazines, tricyclics: increased QT prolongation

NURSING CONSIDERATIONS
Assessment
• Assess patient for absence of nausea, vomiting during chemotherapy
• **Assess patient for hypersensitive reaction:** rash, bronchospasm
• **Extrapyramidal symptoms:** Assess for grimacing, shuffling gait, tremors, involuntary movements, rare
• **QT prolongation:** Monitor ECG in those with heart disease, renal disease, or the elderly
• **Serotonin syndrome:** Assess for hallucinations, seizures, diaphoresis, dizziness, flushing, hyperthermia, nausea, vomiting, diarrhea

Patient problem
Nausea (uses)

Implementation
PO route
• Give dose 1 hr prior to chemotherapy/radiation and another dose 12 hr after the first
• **Transdermal:** Apply to clean, dry skin on upper arm q24-48hr prior to chemotherapy
• Do not cut in pieces
• Apply immediately after opening pouch

IV route
• May give undiluted over 30 sec via Y-site
IV intermittent infusion route
• Dilute in 0.9% NaCl for inj or D₅W (20-50 ml), give over 5-15 min, ½ hr prior to chemotherapy
• Store at room temp for 24-hr dilution, do not freeze vials
• Do not admix

Y-site compatibilities: Acetaminophen, alemtuzumab, alfentanil, allopurinol, amifostine, amikacin, aminophylline, amphotericin B cholesteryl, ampicillin, ampicillin/sulbactam, amsacrine, aztreonam, bleomycin, bumetanide, buprenorphine, butorphanol, calcium gluconate, CARBOplatin, carmustine, ceFAZolin, cefepime, cefonicid, cefotaxime, cefoTEtan, cefOXitin, cefTAZidime, ceftizoxime, cefTRIAXone, cefuroxime, chlorproMAZINE, cimetidine, ciprofloxacin, CISplatin, cladribine, clindamycin, cyclophosphamide, cytarabine, dacarbazine, DACTINomycin, DAUNOrubicin, dexamethasone, diphenhydrAMINE, DOBUTamine, DOPamine, DOXOrubicin, DOXOrubicin liposome, doxycycline, droperidol, enalaprilat, etoposide, famotidine, filgrastim, floxuridine, fluconazole, fluorouracil, fludarabine, furosemide, gallium, ganciclovir, gentamicin, haloperidol, heparin, hydrocortisone, HYDROmorphone, hydrOXYzine, IDArubicin, ifosfamide, imipenemcilastatin, leucovorin, LORazepam, magnesium sulfate, melphalan, meperidine, mesna, methotrexate, methylPREDNISolone, metoclopramide, metroNIDAZOLE, mezlocillin, miconazole, minocycline, mitoMYcin, mitoXANtrone, morphine, nalbuphine, netilmicin, ofloxacin, PACLitaxel, piperacillin, piperacillin/tazobactam, plicamycin, potassium chloride, prochlorperazine, promethazine, propofol, ranitidine, sargramostim, sodium bicarbonate, streptozocin, teniposide, thiotepa, ticarcillin, ticarcillin/clavulanate, tobramycin, trimethoprim/sulfamethoxazole, vancomycin, vinBLAStine, vinCRIStine, vinorelbine, voriconazole, zidovudine, zoledronic acid

Solution compatibilities: D_5W, 0.9% NaCl

Transdermal route

• Apply to dry, clean, intact skin of upper, outer arm 24 hr prior to chemotherapy; firmly press on skin; keep on during chemotherapy; can bathe; avoid swimming, whirlpool; remove ≥24 hr after chemotherapy

Patient/family education

• Advise patient to report diarrhea, constipation, rash, or changes in respirations
• Teach patient to take second dose of PO 12 hr after first dose
• Teach patient that allergic reactions can occur up to 7 days after use (ext rel) or later (SUBCUT)
• **Serotonin syndrome:** Teach patient to report mental changes, including, agitation, hallucinations, dizziness, sweating, flushing, tremors, seizures, discontinue immediately and notify prescriber
• Teach patient to use as prescribed, not to double or skip doses
• Advise patient not to drive, operate machinery until response is known; drowsiness, dizziness may occur

• Advise patient to notify health care professional of change in heartbeat or if feeling faint
• **TD:** Not to use near heat such as heating pad or expose to sunlight, tanning; not to cut patch or use in MRI
• **Pregnancy/breastfeeding:** Identify if pregnancy is planned or suspected or if breastfeeding

Evaluation

Positive therapeutic outcome

• Absence of nausea, vomiting during cancer chemotherapy

---

guaiFENesin (Rx, OTC)

(gwye-fen'e-sin)

Alfen, Altarussin, Balminil ✦, Benylin Chest Congestion Extra Strength ✦, Benylin E ✦, Bidex, Bismutal ✦, Bronchophan, Expectorant ✦, Calmylin Expectorant ✦, Cough Syrup Expectorant ✦, Diabetic Tussin, Expectorant Syrup ✦, Guiatuss, Jack & Jill ✦, Miltuss EX, Mucinex, Naldecon Senior EX, Organidin NR, Robitussin GuaiFENesin ✦, Scot-Tussin Expectorant, Siltussin DAS, Siltussin SA, Vicks Chest Congestion Relief ✦, Vicks DayQuil Mucus Control ✦

Func. class.: Expectorant

Do not confuse: guaiFENesin/guanFACINE Mucinex/Mucomyst

ACTION: Increases the volume and reduces the viscosity of secretions in the trachea and bronchi to facilitate secretion removal

Therapeutic outcome: Decreased cough

USES: Productive and nonproductive cough

Pharmacokinetics

Absorption	Well absorbed
Distribution	Unknown
Metabolism	Unknown
Excretion	Unknown
Half-life	Unknown

Pharmacodynamics

	PO	PO–EXT REL
Onset	½ hr	Unknown
Peak	Unknown	Unknown
Duration	4-6 hr	12 hr

CONTRAINDICATIONS
Hypersensitivity, chronic persistent cough

Precautions: Pregnancy, breastfeeding, HF, asthma, emphysema, fever

DOSAGE AND ROUTES
Adult and child ≥12 yr: PO 200-400 mg q4hr, or EXT REL 600-1200 mg q12hr; max 2.4 g/day
Child 6-11 yr: PO 100-200 mg q4hr or EXT REL 600 mg q12hr; max 1.2 g/day
Child 2-5 yr: PO: 50-100 mg q4hr; max 600 mg/day, EXT REL 300 mg q12hr, max 600 mg/day

Available forms: Tabs 100, 200, 400 mg; ext rel tabs 600, 1200 mg; syr 100 mg/5 ml; oral sol 100 mg/5 ml; oral granules 50, 100 mg/packet; caps 200 mg; liquid 100, 200 mg/5 ml

ADVERSE EFFECTS
CNS: Drowsiness, headache, dizziness
GI: Nausea, anorexia, vomiting, diarrhea

NURSING CONSIDERATIONS
Assessment
• **Assess cough:** type, frequency, character, including characteristics of sputum; lung sounds bilaterally; fluids should be increased to 2 L/day to decrease secretion viscosity (thickness)

Patient problem
Impaired airway clearance (uses)

Implementation
• Store at room temperature; provide room humidification to assist with liquefying secretions
• Avoid fluids for ½ hr after administration

Patient/family education
• Caution patient to avoid driving, other hazardous activities if drowsiness occurs (rare)
• Advise patient to avoid smoking, smoke-filled rooms, perfumes, dust, environmental pollutants, cleansers
• Instruct patient to notify prescriber if dry, nonproductive cough lasts over 7 days
• Pregnancy/breastfeeding: Identify if pregnancy is planned or suspected, or if breastfeeding
• Advise patient to avoid in child <2 yr

Evaluation

Positive therapeutic outcome
• Absence of dry cough
• Thinner, more productive cough that raises secretions

---

guanfacine
(gwahn-fa-seen)
Intuniv, Intuniv ❖, Tenex
Func. class.: Antihypertensive, centrally acting antiadrenergics

USES: Hypertension in combination with a thiazide diuretic, ADHD

CONTRAINDICATIONS
Hypersensitivity

DOSAGE AND ROUTES
Hypertension
Adult: PO 1 mg q day at bedtime, may increase after 3-4 wk

ADHD
Adult/child ≥6 yr: PO 1 mg in AM and PM, may increase by 1 mg/day weekly

guselkumab (Rx)
(gus-elk'-ue-mab)
Tremfya
Func. class.: Antirheumatic agent (disease modifying), immunomodulator, anti-TNF
Chem. class.: Recombinant human IgG1 monoclonal antibody, DMARD

ACTION: A form of human IgG1 monoclonal antibody selectively binds to the p19 subunit of interleukin 23 (IL-23) cytokine, inhibiting its interaction with the IL-23 receptor. A naturally occurring cytokine, IL-23 is involved in normal inflammatory and immune responses. By inhibiting the interaction of IL-23 with its receptor, blocks the release of proinflammatory cytokines and chemokines

USES: For the treatment of moderate to severe plaque psoriasis in those who are candidates for phototherapy or systemic therapy

Pharmacokinetics
Absorption	49%
Distribution	Unknown
Metabolism	Unknown
Excretion	Unknown
Half-life	15-18 days

Pharmacodynamics
Onset, peak duration	Unknown

CONTRAINDICATIONS
Hypersensitivity

Precautions: Pregnancy, breastfeeding, children, geriatric patients, infection, vaccination

DOSAGE AND ROUTES
Adult: SUBCUT 100 mg at week 0, week 4, and every 8 wk thereafter

Available forms: Prefilled syringe 100 mg/ml

ADVERSE EFFECTS
CNS: Headache
EENT: Sinusitis
GI: Diarrhea
MS: Arthralgia
INTEG: Erythema, pruritus, skin discoloration
HEMA: Bleeding
MISC: Infection, injection site reactions, antibody formation, pharyngitis, edema, TB

INTERACTIONS
Avoid use with CYP2D6 substrates
Do not give concurrently with live virus vaccines; immunizations should be brought up to date before treatment

Drug/lab test
Increased: ALT, AST

NURSING CONSIDERATIONS
Assessment
• Assess for injection site pain, swelling, redness—use cold compress to relieve pain/swelling, give at 45-degree angle using abdomen, thighs; rotate injection sites; discard unused portions
• **Infection**: Assess for infections (fever, flu-like symptoms, dyspnea, change in urination, redness/swelling around any wounds), stop treatment if present; some serious infections, including sepsis, may occur, may be fatal; patients with active infections should not be started on this product
• **TB:** Obtain a TB test before starting this product, do not use in active TB; for latent TB, give antituberculosis therapy before use of this product, monitor closely for signs and symptoms of active tuberculosis infection during and after treatment
• **Pregnancy/breastfeeding**: Use only if benefits outweigh fetal risk; cautious use in breastfeeding, excretion unknown

Patient problem
Impaired skin integrity (uses)

Implementation
SUBCUT route
• Remove prefilled syringe from refrigerator and allow to reach room temperature (about 30 min) without removing the needle cap
• Do not shake the prefilled syringe

• Visually inspect for particulate matter and discoloration, the solution should be colorless to slightly yellow and may contain a few small translucent particles. Do not use if discolored, cloudy, or if foreign particulate matter is present
• Only an individual trained in subcutaneous drug delivery should administer the injection. A patient who is properly trained in injection technique may self-inject using the prefilled syringe or vial, if his or her prescriber deems the action appropriate. However, the first injection needs to be under the supervision of a qualified health care professional
• Use front part of the middle thigh, the gluteal or abdominal region, and the outer area of the upper arm. For injection sites, rotate injection sites. Do not use where skin is tender, bruised, red, hard, thick, scaly, or affected by psoriasis
• Gently pinch the cleaned area of skin and insert the needle at about a 45-degree angle subcutaneously using a quick, dartlike motion. Push the plunger slowly and evenly to deliver the dose, remove the needle, and release the pinched skin. Do not rub the injection site; slight bleeding may occur
• Each single-use prefilled syringe contains 100 mg/ml of product. Inject the entire 1 ml contents of the syringe. No preservatives are present; discard any unused portion
• Protect from light, do not freeze

Patient/family education
• Teach patient about self-administration if appropriate: injection should be made in thigh, abdomen, upper arm; rotate sites at least 1 inch from old site; do not inject in areas that are bruised, red, hard
• Teach patient that if medication is not taken when due, inject dose as soon as remembered and inject next dose as scheduled
• Teach patient not to take any live virus vaccines during treatment
• Teach patient to report signs of infection (fever, sweats, or chills; muscle aches; weight loss; cough; warm, red, or painful skin or sores on body different from psoriasis; diarrhea or stomach pain; shortness of breath; blood in phlegm (mucus); burning when urinate or urinating more often than normal); allergic reactions (itching, rash)
• Advise patient to tell provider of all prescription, OTC, herbals, and supplements currently taken

Evaluation
Positive therapeutic outcome
• Decrease in lesions

halcinonide topical
See Appendix B

haloperidol (Rx)
(hal-oh-pehr'ih-dol)
Haldol, Haldol Decanoate
Func. class.: Antipsychotic/neuroleptic
Chem. class.: Butyrophenone

Do not confuse: haloperidol/Halotestin

ACTION: Depresses cerebral cortex, hypothalamus, limbic system, which control activity and aggression; blocks neurotransmission produced by dopamine at synapse; exhibits strong α-adrenergic, anticholinergic blocking action; mechanism for antipsychotic effects unclear

Therapeutic outcome: Decreased signs and symptoms of psychosis; decreased effects of Tourette's syndrome (child)

USES: Psychotic disorders, control of tics, vocal utterances in Tourette's syndrome, short-term treatment of hyperactive children showing excessive motor activity, prolonged parenteral therapy in chronic schizophrenia, organic mental syndrome with psychotic features, emergency sedation of severely agitated or delirious patients, ADHD

Unlabeled uses: Nausea, vomiting in chemotherapy

Pharmacokinetics

Absorption	Well absorbed (PO, IM); decanoate (IM) absorbed slowly
Distribution	High concentrations in liver, crosses placenta, protein binding 92%
Metabolism	Liver, extensively
Excretion	Kidneys, breast milk
Half-life	12-36 hr metabolites

Pharmacodynamics

	PO	IM	IM (decanoate)
Onset	Erratic	½ hr	3-9 days
Peak	2-6 hr	30-45 min	4-11 days
Duration	8-12 hr	4-8 hr	3 wk

CONTRAINDICATIONS
Children <3 yr, hypersensitivity, coma, Parkinson's disease, CNS depression

Precautions: Pregnancy, breastfeeding, geriatric, seizure disorders, hypertension, hepatic/cardiac/pulmonary disease, prostatic hypertrophy, hyperthyroidism, thyrotoxicosis, blood dyscrasias, brain damage, bone marrow depression, alcohol and barbiturate withdrawal states, angina, epilepsy, urinary retention, closed-angle glaucoma

> **BLACK BOX WARNING:** Dementia; increased mortality in elderly patients with dementia-related psychosis

DOSAGE AND ROUTES
Acute psychosis
Adult and child >12 yr: IM/IV 2-10 mg, may repeat q1hr, convert to **PO** as soon as possible, **PO** should be 150% of total parenteral dose required
Child 6-12 yr: IM/IV (unlabeled) 1-3 mg q4-8hr, max 0.15 mg/kg/day, switch to **PO** as soon as possible

Chronic psychosis
Adult: IM (decanoate) 50-200 mg

Tourette's syndrome
Adult and adolescent: PO 0.5-2 mg bid-tid, increased until desired response occurs
Elderly: PO 0.5-2 mg bid-tid; may increase gradually
Child 3-12 yr or weighing 15-40 kg: PO 0.25-0.5 mg/day in 2-3 divided doses, increase by 0.05-0.075 mg q5-7days, max 0.15 mg/kg/day

Nonpsychotic behavior disorders
Child: 3-12 yr PO 0.05-0.075 mg/kg in 2-3 divided doses, max 6 mg/day

Available forms: Tabs 0.5, 1, 2, 5, 10, 20 mg; **lactate:** oral sol 2 mg/ml; inj 5 mg/ml; **decanoate:** 50 mg/ml, 100 mg/ml

ADVERSE EFFECTS
CNS: *EPS, pseudoparkinsonism, akathisia, dystonia, tardive dyskinesia, drowsiness, headache,* seizures, neuroleptic malignant syndrome, confusion
CV: *Orthostatic hypotension,* ECG changes, tachycardia, QT prolongation, dysrhythmias,
EENT: Blurred vision, glaucoma, dry eyes
GI: *Dry mouth, anorexia, constipation,* weight gain, ileus, hepatitis
GU: Urinary retention, urinary frequency, impotence
INTEG: *Rash,* photosensitivity, dermatitis
HEMA: Agranulocytosis, anemia, neutropenia, leukopenia
RESP: Laryngospasm, dyspnea, respiratory depression
SYST: Risk of death (dementia), hypersensitivity, hyperpyrexia

INTERACTIONS
Individual drugs
Alcohol: increased effects of both products, oversedation

Amoxapine, chloroquine, cloZAPine, dasatinib, dolasetron, dronedarone, droperidol, erythromycin, flecainide, lapatinib, maprotiline, methadone, octreotide, ondansetron, palonosetron, pentamidine, pimozide, propafenone, ranolazine, risperiDONE, sertindole, SUNItinib, tacrolimus, telithromycin, troleandomycin, vardenafil, vorinostat, ziprasidone: increased QT prolongation, usually with IV use

CarBAMazepine: decreased effects of haloperidol

EPINEPHrine: increased toxicity

Levodopa: decreased effects of levodopa

Lithium: increased toxicity; decreased effects of lithium

PHENobarbital: decreased effects of haloperidol

Drug classifications
Anticholinergics: increased anticholinergic effects

Barbiturate anesthetics, CNS depressants: oversedation

β-Adrenergic blockers: increased effects of both products

Class IA, III antidysrhythmics, halogenated/local anesthetics, phenothiazines, tricyclics, β-blockers: increased QT prolongation

SSRIs, SNRIs: increased serotonin syndrome, increased neuroleptic malignant syndrome

Drug/herb
Chamomile, kava: increased CNS depression

Drug/lab test
Increased: liver function tests

NURSING CONSIDERATIONS
Assessment

> **BLACK BOX WARNING:** Assess for dementia, affect, orientation, LOC, reflexes, gait, coordination, sleep pattern disturbances; risk for death in dementia-related psychosis

• Assess mental status: orientation, mood, behavior, presence and type of hallucinations before initial administration and monthly; this product should significantly reduce psychotic behavior

• Monitor I&O ratio; palpate bladder if low urinary output occurs, especially in geriatric; urinalysis is recommended before, during prolonged therapy

• Monitor bilirubin, CBC, liver function tests monthly

• Assess affect, orientation, LOC, reflexes, gait, coordination, sleep pattern disturbances

• Monitor B/P with patient sitting, standing, and lying; take pulse and respirations q4hr during initial treatment; establish baseline before starting treatment; report drops of ≥30 mm Hg; QT prolongation may occur

• Check for dizziness, faintness, palpitations, tachycardia on rising; severe orthostatic hypotension is common

• **Assess for neuroleptic malignant syndrome:** hyperpyrexia, muscle rigidity, increased CPK, altered mental status; product should be discontinued immediately; if seizures, hypo/hypertension, tachycardia occur, notify prescriber immediately

• **Dehydration:** I&O, daily weight, lethargy, decreased thirst, low intake

• **Assess for EPS** including akathisia (inability to sit still, no pattern to movements), tardive dyskinesia (bizarre movements of the jaw, mouth, tongue, extremities), pseudoparkinsonism (ragged tremors, pill rolling, shuffling gait); an antiparkinsonian product should be prescribed

• Assess for constipation and urinary retention daily; if these occur, increase bulk, water in diet

• **Abrupt discontinuation:** Do not withdraw abruptly, taper

• **QT prolongation:** More common with IV use at high doses; monitor ECG in those with CV disease

• **Beers:** Avoid use in older adults except for schizophrenia, bipolar disorder, increased risk of stroke and cognitive decline, mortality

• **Pregnancy/breastfeeding:** No well-controlled studies, use in third trimester results in infant extrapyramidal symptoms, avoid breastfeeding

Patient problem
Distorted thinking process (uses)
Risk of injury (adverse reactions)

Implementation
PO route—oral liquid
• Give product in liquid form mixed in glass of juice or caffeine-free cola if hoarding is suspected; do not mix in caffeine drinks, tannics, pectins

• Give decreased dosage in geriatric because of slower metabolism

• Give PO with full glass of water, milk; or give with food to decrease GI upset

• Give antacids 2 hr before or after this product

• Store in tight, light-resistant container; oral sol in amber bottle

• Avoid skin contact with oral susp or sol: may cause contact dermatitis

IM route

• Inject in deep muscle mass, do not give SUBCUT; use 21-gauge 2-in needle; do not administer sol with a precipitate; give <3 ml per inj site; give slowly, may be painful

• Patient should remain lying down after IM inj for at least 30 min

IV route (lactate) (unlabeled)

• Give undiluted for psychotic episode at 5 mg/min

• Only use lactate for IV

• Closely monitor ECG for QT prolongation

• Switch to oral as soon as possible if needed; give first PO dose within 12-24 hr of last parenteral dose

Y-site compatibilities: alcohol 10%, dextrose 5%, alemtuzumab, amifostine, aminocaproic acid, amiodarone, amphotericin B liposome (AmBisome), amsacrine, anidulafungin, argatroban, Arsenic trioxide, asparaginase, atenolol, azithromycin, bleomycin, Cangrelor, CARBOplatin, carmustine, Caspofungin, ceftaroline, cisatracurium, CISplatin, Cladribine, cloNIDine, codeine phosphate, cyclophosphamide, cytarabine, DACTINomycin, DAPTOmycin, DAUNOrubicin liposome, DAUNOrubicin, Dexmedetomidine, Dexrazoxane, diltiazem, DOCEtaxel, dolasetron, Doxacurium, DOXOrubicin, DOXOrubicin liposomal, epirubicin, eptifibatide, ertapenem, etoposide, etoposide phosphate, fenoldopam, filgrastim, Fludarabine, gatifloxacin, gemcitabine, granisetron, HYDROmorphone, IDArubicin, ifosfamide, irinotecan, Ketamine, lepirudin, leucovorin, levofloxacin, linezolid, LORazepam, mechlorethamine, melphalan, Mesna, methadone, metroNIDAZOLE, milrinone, MitoXANtrone, Mivacurium, morphine, moxifloxacin, mycophenolate mofetil, nesiritide, niCARdipine, octreotide, oritavancin, oxaliplatin, PACLitaxel (solvent/surfactant), palonosetron, pamidronate, pancuronium, PEMEtrexed, potassium acetate, propofol, Quinupristin-Dalfopristin, remifentanil, riTUXimab, rocuronium, Sodium acetate, tacrolimus, Teniposide, Thiotepa, tigecycline, tirofiban, topotecan, TPN (2-in-1), vecuronium, vinBLAStine, vinCRIStine, vinorelbine, voriconazole, zoledronic acid

Patient/family education

• Teach patient to use good oral hygiene; use frequent rinsing of mouth, sugarless gum for dry mouth; oral candidiasis may occur

• Advise patient to avoid hazardous activities until product response is determined and effects are known; dizziness, blurred vision are common

• Inform patient that orthostatic hypotension occurs often and to rise from sitting or lying position gradually; tell patient that in hot weather

heat stroke may occur; take extra precautions to stay cool

• Instruct patient to avoid abrupt withdrawal of this product, or EPS may result; product should be withdrawn slowly

• Caution patient to avoid OTC preparations (cough, hay fever, cold) unless approved by prescriber, since serious product interactions may occur; avoid use with alcohol, CNS depressants since increased drowsiness may occur

• Teach patient to use sunscreen, protective clothing, to minimize photosensitivity, avoid being overheated

• Teach patient to take as prescribed, not to use OTC, herbal products unless directed by prescriber

• Teach patient to use good oral hygiene, frequent sips of water, sugarless gum, candy for dry mouth

Evaluation

Positive therapeutic outcome

• Decrease in emotional excitement, hallucinations, delusions, paranoia, reorganization of patterns of thought, speech; improvement in specific behaviors

TREATMENT OF OVERDOSE: Lavage if orally ingested; provide airway; *do not induce vomiting*

⚠ HIGH ALERT

heparin (Rx)

(hep'a-rin)

Hepalean ✦, Hep-Lock, Hep-Lock U/P

Func. class.: Anticoagulant, antithrombotic

Do not confuse: heparin/Hespan

ACTION: Prevents conversion of fibrinogen to fibrin and prothrombin to thrombin by enhancing inhibitory effects of antithrombin III

Therapeutic outcome: Prevention of new thrombi formation, prevention growth of current thrombi

USES: Prevention and treatment in MI, open heart surgery, disseminated intravascular clotting syndrome, atrial fibrillation with embolization; as an anticoagulant in transfusion and dialysis procedures; to maintain patency of indwelling venipuncture devices; diagnosis, treatment of disseminated intravascular coagulation (DIC)

Pharmacokinetics

Absorption	Well absorbed (SUBCUT)
Distribution	Protein binding high
Metabolism	Partially in kidney, liver
Excretion	Lymph, spleen, in urine (<50% unchanged)
Half-life	1-2 hr (dose dependent)

Pharmacodynamics

	SUBCUT	IV
Onset	½-1 hr	5 min
Peak	2 hr	10 min
Duration	8-12 hr	2-6 hr

CONTRAINDICATIONS

Bleeding, hypersensitivity to this product, corn, porcine protein (pork product)

Precautions: Pregnancy C, children, geriatric, alcoholism, hyperlipidemia, diabetes, renal disease, heparin-induced thrombocytopenia (HIT), hemophilia, leukemia with bleeding, peptic ulcer disease, severe thrombocytopenic purpura, renal/hepatic disease (severe), blood dyscrasias, severe hypertension, subacute bacterial endocarditis, acute nephritis; benzyl alcohol products in neonates, infants, pregnancy, lactation

DOSAGE AND ROUTES
Anticoagulation

Adult IV bolus (Intermittent) 10,000 units, then 5000-10,000 q 4-6 hr; **continuous IV infusion**: 5000 units, then 20,000-40,000 units given over 24 hr; **subcut** 5000 units, then 10,000-20,000 units; then 8000-10,000 units q8hr

Child >1 yr IV bolus (intermittent) 50-100 units/kg q 4 hr; **continuous IV infusion** 75 units/kg, then 20 units/kg/hr, adjusted to aPTT of 65-85 sec

Neonates, infants <1 yr Continuous IV infusion 75 units/kg, then 28 units/kg/hr, adjusted to a PTT of 65-85 sec

Thromboembolism prevention
Adult Subcut 5000 units q 8-12 hr

CV surgery
Adult IV ≥150 units/kg, 300 units/kg <60 min, 400 units/kg for procedure ≥60 min

Line flush
Adult/child IV 10-100 units/mL (10 units-infants) to fill heparin lock

TPN
Adult/Child IV 0.5-1 unit/mL

Available forms: Sol for inj 10, 100, 1000, 2000, 5000, 7500, 10,000, 20,000, 40,000 units/ml; premixed 1000 units/500 ml, 2000 units/1000 ml, 12,500 units/250 ml, 25,000 units/250 ml, 25,000 units/500 ml; lock flush preparations 10 units/ml

ADVERSE EFFECTS
CNS: *Fever,* chills, headache
GI: Elevated hepatic studies
MS: Osteoporosis (pediatrics)
GU: Hematuria
HEMA: Hemorrhage, thrombocytopenia, anemia, heparin-induced thrombocytopenia (HIT)
INTEG: *Rash,* dermatitis, urticaria, pruritus, delayed transient alopecia, hematoma, cutaneous necrosis (SUBCUT), injection site reactions
META: Rebound hyperlipidemia, vitamin D deficiency
SYST: Hypersensitivity

INTERACTIONS
Individual drugs
Dextran, dipyridamole, ticlopidine, clopidogrel, presgrel: increased action of heparin
Digoxin: decreased action of heparin
Nicotine: decreased action of heparin

Drug classifications
Anticoagulants (oral), cephalosporins, NSAIDs, penicillins, platelet inhibitors, salicylates, antineoplastics, SSRIs, SNRIs: increased action of heparin, quinidine, valproic acid
Antihistamines, tetracyclines, cardiac glycosides: decreased action of heparin, nitroglycerin
Corticosteroids: decreased action of corticosteroids

Drug/herb
Anise, arnica, chamomile, clove, dong quai, feverfew, garlic, ginger, ginkgo, green tea, horse chestnut: increased bleeding risk

Drug/lab test
Increased: ALT, AST, INR, pro-time, PTT, potassium
Decreased: platelets

NURSING CONSIDERATIONS
Assessment
• **Thrombosis:** Monitor for increased thrombosis daily in affected areas
• Monitor blood studies assess for (Hct, occult blood in stools) q3mo if patient is on long-term therapy; monitor PPT, which should be 1½-2 × control, PTT; often done daily, APTT, ACT, PTT 1.5-2.5 × control; monitor platelet count q2-3day; thrombocytopenia may occur on fourth day of treatment and resolve, or continue to fifth to tenth day of treatment
• **Bleeding, hemorrhage:** Assess for bleeding gums, petechiae, ecchymosis, black

tarry stools, hematuria, epistaxis, decrease in Hct, B/P; notify prescriber immediately
• **HIT (heparin-induced thrombocytopenia):** may occur after product is discontinued; check periodically for signs of decreasing thrombi
• **Monitor for hypersensitivity:** fever, skin rash, urticaria; notify prescriber immediately
• **Pregnancy/breastfeeding:** Use only if benefits outweigh fetal risk, cautious use in breastfeeding, do not use products with benzyl alcohol in pregnancy, breastfeeding

Patient problem
Ineffective tissue perfusion (uses)
Risk of injury (adverse reactions)

Implementation
• Heparin and low-molecular-weight heparins are not interchangeable
• Give at same time each day to maintain steady blood levels
• Store at room temperature
SUBCUT route
• Give SUBCUT with at least 25-G ³/₈-in needle; do not massage area or aspirate fluid when giving SUBCUT inj; give in abdomen between pelvic bones, inject at 45- or 90-degree angle, rotate sites; apply gentle pressure for 1 min
• Do not give IM
Heparin lock route
• Do not mistake heparin sodium injection 10,000 units/ml and Hep-Lock U/P 10 units/ml; they have similar blue labeling; deaths in pediatric patients have occurred when heparin sodium injection vials were confused with heparin flush vials
• Inject 10-100 units/0.5-1 ml after each inf or q8-12hr
• Inject to prevent clots in heparin lock, inject dilute heparin solution (10-100 units) 0.5-1 ml after each injection of q8hr, flush lock before and after each use with sterile water or 0.9% NaCl, to prevent drug interactions

Direct IV route
• Give loading dose undiluted over ≥1 min; use before continuous infusion
IV route
• Obtain baseline coagulation tests before use
• Use infusion pump, make sure pressure dressings are used after drawing blood
• Draw coagulation studies 30 min before next dose, never draw from tubing or from infused vein, use other
Continuous IV infusion route
• Dilute 25,000 units/250-500 ml 0.9% NaCl or D₅W (50-100 units/ml); some solutions are premixed and ready for use

• When product is added to inf sol for cont **IV**, invert container at least 6 × to ensure adequate mixing

Y-site compatibilities: acetaminophen, acetylcysteine, acyclovir, Alcohol 10%, dextrose 5%, alemtuzumab, alfentanil, allopurinol, Amifostine, Aminocaproic acid, aminophylline, amphotericin B lipid complex, Amphotericin B liposome, anidulafungin, argatroban, Arsenic trioxide, ascorbic acid injection, asparaginase, atenolol, atropine, azaTHIOprine, azithromycin, Aztreonam, Benztropine, Betamethasone, Bivalirudin, bleomycin, Bretylium, bumetanide, buprenorphine, butorphanol, Caffeine, calcium chloride/gluconate, Cangrelor, CARBOplatin, carmustine, Cefamandole, ceFAZolin, Cefoperazone, cefotaxime, cefoTEtan, Cefotiam, cefOXitin, ceftaroline, cefTAZidime, ceftizoxime, Ceftobiprole, cefTRIAXone, cefuroxime, Cephapirin, chloramphenicol succinate, chlordiazePOXIDE, chlorothiazide, chlorpheniramine, cimetidine, CISplatin, Cladribine, clindamycin, Cloxacillin, codeine, Colistimethate, Cyanocobalamin, cyclophosphamide, cycloSPORINE, cytarabine, DACTINomycin, DAPTOmycin, DAUNOrubicin citrate liposome, dexamethasone, Dexmedetomidine, Dexrazoxane, digoxin, DOCEtaxel, DOPamine, doripenem, Doxacurium, Doxapram, DOXOrubicin liposomal, Edetate calcium disodium, Edrophonium, enalaprilat, Ephedrine sulfate, EPINEPHrine, epoetin alfa, eptifibatide, Ergonovine, ertapenem, esmolol, estrogens conjugated, Ethacrynate, etoposide, etoposide phosphate, famotidine, fenoldopam, fentaNYL, flecainide, fluconazole, Fludarabine, fluorouracil, folic acid (as sodium salt), foscarnet, Gallamine, Gallium, ganciclovir, gemcitabine, Gemtuzumab, Glycopyrrolate, granisetron, hydrocortisone, HYDROmorphone, ibuprofen lysine, ifosfamide, imipenem-cilastatin, indomethacin, irinotecan, Isoproterenol, ketorolac, Lactated Ringer's Injection, lansoprazole, leucovorin, lidocaine, Lincomycin, linezolid, LORazepam, magnesium sulfate, mannitol, mechlorethamine, melphalan, Mephentermine, meropenem, Mesna, Metaraminol, methadone, Methohexital, methotrexate, Methoxamine, Methyldopa, methylergonovine, metoclopramide, metoprolol, metroNIDAZOLE, micafungin, midazolam, milrinone, minocycline, mitoMYcin, Mivacurium, morphine, moxifloxacin, Multiple vitamins injection, nafcillin, Nalbuphine, Nalorphine, naloxone, neostigmine, nitroglycerin, nitroprusside, norepinephrine, octreotide, ondansetron, oxacillin, oxaliplatin, oxytocin, PACLitaxel (solvent/surfactant), palonosetron, pamidronate, pancuronium, PEMEtrexed, penicillin G potassium/sodium,

PENTobarbital, Phenobarbital, phentolamine, phenylephrine, phytonadione, piperacillin sodium, piperacillin-tazobactam, potassium acetate/chloride, procainamide, prochlorperazine, Promazine, propofol, propranolol, pyridostigmine, pyridoxine, ranitidine, remifentanil, Ringer's injection, riTUXimab, rocuronium, sargramostim, scopolamine, Sodium acetate/Bicarbonate/fusidate, succinylcholine, Sufentanil, tacrolimus, theophylline, thiamine, Thiopental, Thiotepa, Ticarcillin, ticarcillin-clavulanate, tigecycline, tirofiban, Tolazoline, topotecan, TPN (2-in-1), Tranexamic acid, trastuzumab, Trimetaphan, trimethobenzamide, Tubocurarine, urokinase, vasopressin, vecuronium, verapamil, vinBLAstine, vinCRIStine, voriconazole, warfarin, zidovudine, zoledronic acid.

Patient/family education
• Advise patient to avoid OTC preparations that may cause serious product interactions unless directed by prescriber; may contain aspirin or other anticoagulants, notify all health care persons of heparin use
• Tell patient that product may be withheld during active bleeding (menstruation), depending on condition
• Caution patient to use soft-bristle toothbrush to avoid bleeding gums; avoid contact sports; use electric razor; avoid IM inj
• Instruct patient to carry/wear emergency ID or other identification identifying product taken and condition treated
• **Advise patient to report any signs of bleeding:** gums, under skin, urine, stools; or unusual bruising even after discontinuing product
• Teach patient how to prepare and give this medication if receiving at home; use exactly as directed; do not stop using unless directed by health care professional

Evaluation
Positive therapeutic outcome
• Prevention of new clots
• PTT of 1.5-2.5 × control
• Free-flowing **IV**, prevention of DVT and pulmonary emboli

TREATMENT OF OVERDOSE:
Withdraw product, give protamine sulfate 1 mg protamine/100 units heparin

homatropine ophthalmic
See Appendix B

hydrALAZINE (Rx)
(hye-dral′a-zeen)
Apresoline ✦
Func. class.: Antihypertensive, direct-acting peripheral vasodilator
Chem. class.: Phthalazine

Do not confuse: hydrALAZINE/hydrOXYzine

ACTION: Vasodilates arterioles in smooth muscle by direct relaxation; reduces B/P with reflex increases in heart rate, stroke volume, cardiac output

Therapeutic outcome: Decreased B/P in hypertension, decreased afterload in HF

USES: Essential hypertension, hypertensive emergency/urgency, eclampsia

Unlabeled uses: Heart failure not responsive to cardiac glycosides and diuretics

Pharmacokinetics
Absorption	Rapidly absorbed (PO); well absorbed (IM); completely absorbed (**IV**)
Distribution	Widely distributed; crosses placenta, protein binding 89%
Metabolism	GI mucosa, liver extensively ⚘ ; half of Mexicans, Blacks, South Indians, and Caucasians are at risk for toxicity
Excretion	Kidneys, urine (12%-14%)
Half-life	3-7 hr

Pharmacodynamics
	PO	IM	IV
Onset	½ hr	10-30 min	5-20 min
Peak	1-2 hr	1 hr	10-80 min
Duration	6-12 hr	2-6 hr	Up to 12 hr

CONTRAINDICATIONS
Hypersensitivity to hydrALAZINEs, mitral valvular rheumatic heart disease, CAD

Precautions: Pregnancy, breastfeeding, geriatric, CVA, advanced renal disease, liver disease, SLE, dissecting aortic aneurysm

DOSAGE AND ROUTES
Hypertension
Adult: PO 10 mg qid 2-4 days, then 25 mg qid for rest of 1st wk, then 50 mg qid individualized to desired response; max 300 mg/day
Child: PO 0.75-1 mg/kg/day in 2-4 divided doses; max 25 mg/dose, increase over 3-4 wk to max 7.5 mg/kg/day or 200 mg, whichever is less

Hypertensive crisis
Adult: IV BOL 10-20 mg q4-6hr; administer PO as soon as possible; IM 10-50 mg q4-6hr
Child: IV BOL 0.1-0.6 mg/kg q4hr; IM 0.1-0.6 mg/kg q4-6hr, max 1.7-3.5 mg/kg/day

HF
Adult: PO 10-25 mg bid, max 75 mg tid

Eclampsia
Adult IM/IV 5 mg q 15-20 min

Available forms: Inj 20 mg/ml; tabs 10, 25, 50, 100 mg

ADVERSE EFFECTS
CNS: *Headache, dizziness,* drowsiness
CV: *Palpitations, tachycardia, angina,* orthostatic hypotension, edema
GI: *Nausea, vomiting, anorexia, diarrhea*
INTEG: Rash, pruritus
MISC: Lupuslike symptoms

INTERACTIONS
Individual drugs
Alcohol: increased hypotension
Indomethacin: decreased effects of hydrALAZINE

Drug classifications
β-Adrenergic blockers: metoprolol, propranolol; increased effects
MAOIs: severe hypotension
Other antihypertensives, thiazide diuretics: increased hypotension
Sympathomimetics (EPINEPHrine, norepinephrine): increased tachycardia, angina
NSAIDs, estrogens: decreased hydrALAZINE effects

Drug/Food
Increase: drug absorption; have patient take with food

NURSING CONSIDERATIONS
Assessment
• **Assess cardiac status:** B/P q15min for 2 hr, then qhr for 2 hr, then q4hr after IV dose, pulse, jugular venous distention q4hr decreased after level
• Monitor electrolytes, blood studies: potassium, sodium, chloride, carbon dioxide, CBC, serum glucose; LE prep, ANA titer before starting treatment
• Monitor weight daily, I&O; check for edema in feet, legs daily; for hydration status

• Assess for crackles, dyspnea, orthopnea; peripheral edema, fatigue, weight gain, jugular vein distention (HF)
• For fever, joint pain, rash, sore throat (lupuslike symptoms), notify prescriber, number of refills to determine compliance
• **Beers:** Use with caution in older adults, may exacerbate syncope in those with a history of syncope
• **Pregnancy/breastfeeding:** Use only if benefits outweigh fetal risk, third-trimester toxicity has occurred; cautious use in breastfeeding

Patient problems
Ineffective tissue perfusion (uses)
Nonadherence (teaching)

Implementation
PO route
• Give with meals to enhance absorption
• Store protected from light and heat
IM route
• Do not admix; switch to PO as soon as possible; use only in those that cannot use PO

Direct IV route
• Give by **IV** undiluted through Y-tube or 3-way stopcock, give each 10 mg over 1 min or more
• Administer with patient in recumbent position; keep in that position for 1 hr after administration

Y-site compatibilities: Heparin, hydrocortisone, potassium chloride, verapamil, vit B/C

Patient/family education
• Teach patient to take with food to increase bioavailability (PO)
• Teach patient to avoid OTC herbals, supplements, preparations unless directed by prescriber
• Advise patient to notify prescriber if chest pain, severe fatigue, fever, muscle or joint pain, rash, sore throat occur; tingling, pain in hands and feet, pyridoxine can be used
• Advise patient to rise slowly to prevent orthostatic hypertension
• Advise patient to notify prescriber if pregnancy is suspected, or planned, or if breastfeeding
• Teach patient to notify health care professional of product use prior to surgery
• Advise patient to avoid driving or other hazardous activities until response is known; drowsiness, dizziness may occur
• Inform patient to weigh 2x per wk and check lower extremities for swelling
• Teach patient to take as prescribed, not to skip or double doses, to take at same time of day; if dose is missed, take when remembered, do not abruptly discontinue

---

• Advise patient that follow up will be needed, to comply with other requirements such as exercise, weight loss, avoiding smoking

Evaluation
Positive therapeutic outcome
• Decreased B/P, decreased afterload in hypertension

TREATMENT OF OVERDOSE:
Administer vasopressors, volume expanders for shock; if PO, lavage

---

hydrochlorothiazide (Rx)
(hye-droe-klor-oh-thye′a-zide)
Apo-Hydro ✤**, Microzide, Neo-Codema** ✤**, Oretic, Urozide** ✤
Func. class.: Diuretic, antihypertensive
Chem. class.: Thiazide, sulfonamide derivative

ACTION: Acts on the distal tubule in the kidney, increasing excretion of sodium, water, chloride, and potassium

Therapeutic outcome: Decreased B/P, decreased edema in lung tissues peripherally

USES: Edema, hypertension, diuresis, HF; idiopathic lower extremity edema therapy

Pharmacokinetics

Absorption	Variable
Distribution	Extracellular spaces; crosses placenta
Metabolism	Excreted unchanged in urine
Excretion	Breast milk
Half-life	6-15 hr

Pharmacodynamics

Onset	2 hr
Peak	4 hr
Duration	6-12 hr

CONTRAINDICATIONS
Hypersensitivity to thiazides or sulfonamides, anuria, renal decompensation, pregnancy (D) preeclampsia

Precautions: Pregnancy, breastfeeding, hypokalemia, renal/hepatic disease, gout, COPD, lupus erythematosus, diabetes mellitus, hyperlipidemia, CCr <30 ml/min, hypomagnesemia

DOSAGE AND ROUTES
Hypertension
Adult/adolescent: PO 12.5-25 mg/day, may increase to 50 mg/day in 1-2 divided doses, max 100 mg/day

Child >6 mo: PO 1-2 mg/kg/day in divided doses; max 37.5 mg/day for 6 mo-2 yr; max 37.5 mg/day
Child <6 mo: PO up to 2-3.3 mg/kg/day in divided doses
Geriatric: PO 12.5 mg qday

Renal dose
Adult: PO CCr <30 ml/min, do not use, not effective

Available forms: Tabs 12.5, 25, 50, 100 ✤ mg; caps 12.5 mg

ADVERSE EFFECTS
CNS: Drowsiness, paresthesia, depression, headache, *dizziness, fatigue, weakness,* fever
CV: Irregular pulse, *orthostatic hypotension,* palpitations, volume depletion, allergic myocarditis
EENT: Blurred vision
ELECT: *Hypokalemia,* hypercalcemia, hyponatremia, hypochloremia, hypomagnesemia
GI: *Nausea, vomiting, anorexia,* constipation, diarrhea, cramps, pancreatitis, GI irritation, hepatitis
GU: *Frequency,* polyuria, uremia, glucosuria, hyperuricemia, jaundice, erectile dysfunction
HEMA: Aplastic anemia, hemolytic anemia, leukopenia, agranulocytosis, thrombocytopenia, neutropenia
INTEG: *Rash,* urticaria, purpura, photosensitivity, alopecia, erythema multiforme
META: *Hyperglycemia, hyperuricemia,* renal failure, increased creatinine, BUN
SYST: Stevens-Johnson syndrome

INTERACTIONS
Individual drugs
Amphotericin B, piperacillin, ticarcillin: increased hypokalemia
Cholestyramine, colestipol: decreased absorption of hydrochlorothiazide
Diazoxide: increased hyperglycemia, hyperuricemia, hypotension
Lithium: increased toxicity

Drug classifications
Antidiabetics: decreased effect of antidiabetic agent
Cardiac glycosides, nondepolarizing skeletal muscle relaxants: increased toxicity
Diuretics (loop): increased effects of diuretic
Corticosteroids: increased hypokalemia
NSAIDs: decreased thiazide effect

Drug/food
Licorice: increased severe hypokalemia

H

Drug/lab test

Increased: parathyroid test, uric acid, calcium, glucose, cholesterol, triglycerides

Decreased: potassium, sodium, Hgb, WBC, platelets

NURSING CONSIDERATIONS

Assessment

• Check for rashes, temp elevation daily

• Assess for confusion, especially in geriatric patients; take safety precautions if needed

• Monitor for acidic urine, reduced urine, osmolality, nocturia; hypotension, broad T-wave, U-wave, ectopy, tachycardia, weak pulse; muscle weakness, altered LOC, drowsiness, apathy, lethargy, confusion, depression; anorexia, nausea, cramps, constipation, distention, paralytic ileus; hypoventilation, respiratory muscle weakness

• **Beers:** Use with caution in older adults, may exacerbate or cause syndrome of inappropriate antidiuretic hormone secretion or hyponatremia

• Assess fluid volume status: I&O ratios, electrolytes baseline and periodically record, count, or weigh diapers as appropriate; weight; distended red veins; crackles in lungs; color, quality, and specific gravity of urine; skin turgor; adequacy of pulses; moist mucous membranes; bilateral lung sounds; peripheral pitting edema; assess for dehydration: symptoms of decreasing output, thirst, hypotension; dry mouth and mucous membranes should be reported

• Monitor electrolytes: potassium, sodium, calcium, magnesium; also include BUN, blood pH, ABGs, uric acid, CBC, blood glucose, renal function

• Assess **hypertension** B/P before, during therapy with patient lying, standing, and sitting as appropriate; orthostatic hypotension can occur rapidly

• **Hypersensitivity to sulfonamides:** rash, discontinue; fatal Stevens-Johnson syndrome may occur, if skin rash occurs discontinue product

• Pregnancy, breastfeeding: May affect fetus, crosses placenta barrier, do not breastfeed

Patient Problems
Implementation
PO route

• Give in AM to avoid interference with sleep

• Provide potassium replacement if potassium level is ≤3.0 mg/dl; give whole tab or use oral sol lightly; product may be crushed if patient is unable to swallow, replace magnesium if needed

• Administer with food; if nausea occurs, absorption may be increased

Patient/family education

• Teach patient to take the medication early in the day at same time of day to prevent nocturia

• Instruct patient to take with food or milk if GI symptoms of nausea and anorexia occur

• Teach patient to maintain a weekly record of weight and notify prescriber of weight loss >5 lb

• Caution patient that this product causes a loss of potassium and that food rich in potassium should be added to the diet; refer to a dietitian for assistance in planning

• Caution patient to rise slowly from sitting or reclining positions, not to exercise in hot weather or stand for prolonged periods since orthostatic hypotension will be enhanced; lie down if dizziness occurs to prevent postural hypotension

• Teach patient not to use alcohol or any OTC medications without prescriber's approval; serious product reactions may occur

• Emphasize the need to contact prescriber immediately if muscle cramps, weakness, nausea, dizziness, or numbness occurs; rash

• Teach patient to take own B/P and pulse and record findings

• Teach patient to continue taking medication even if feeling better; this product controls symptoms but does not cure the condition

• Advise patient with hypertension to continue other medical treatment (exercise, weight loss, relaxation techniques, cessation of smoking)

• Discuss dietary potassium requirements

• Advise patient that follow-ups and routine lab tests will be required

• Teach patient how to take B/P, to continue with other medical regimens (weight loss, exercise)

Evaluation
Positive therapeutic outcome

• Decreased edema

• Decreased B/P if patient is hypertensive

• Increased diuresis

TREATMENT OF OVERDOSE:

Lavage if taken orally, monitor electrolytes, administer dextrose in saline, monitor hydration, CV, renal status

⚠ HIGH ALERT

HYDROcodone (Rx) REMS
(hye-droe-koe′done)
Hysingla ER, Zohydro ER ✦
HYDROcodone/
acetaminophen (Rx)
Anexsia, NorCo
HYDROcodone/ibuprofen
(Rx)
Reprexain, Vicoprofen
Func. class.: Antitussive opioid analgesic/
nonopioid analgesic
Controlled substance schedule II

Do not confuse: HYDROcodone/
hydrocortisone, oxyCODONE, Reprexain/ZyPREXA

ACTION: Acts directly on cough center in
medulla to suppress cough; binds to opiate receptors in the CNS to reduce pain

Therapeutic outcome: Pain relief, decreased cough, decreased diarrhea

USES: Moderate/severe pain

Pharmacokinetics

Absorption	Well absorbed
Distribution	Unknown; crosses placenta
Metabolism	Liver, extensively
Excretion	Kidneys
Half-life	3½-4½ hr

Pharmacodynamics

	PO (analgesic)	PO (antitussive)
Onset	10-20 min	Unknown
Peak	30-60 min	Unknown
Duration	4-6 hr	4-6 hr

CONTRAINDICATIONS
Abrupt discontinuation, hypersensitivity to this
product or benzyl, GI obstruction, status asthmaticus

BLACK BOX WARNING: Respiratory depression

Precautions: Pregnancy, breastfeeding, neonates, addictive personality, increased ICP, MI
(acute), severe heart disease, respiratory, renal/
hepatic disease, bowel impaction, urinary retention, viral infection, ulcerative colitis, seizures,
sulfite hypersensitivity, psychosis, hypertension,
hyperthyroidism

**BLACK BOX WARNING: Accidental expo-
sure:** Neonatal opioid withdrawal syndrome,
potential for overdose or poisoning, substance
abuse, ethanol ingestion

DOSAGES AND ROUTES
Analgesic
Adults PO 2.5-10 mg q 5-6 hr as needed; if
using with acetaminophen, max acetaminophen
4 g/day, total of 5 tablets with ibuprofen combination tablets; ext rel (zohydro ER) 10 mg q 12 hr,
may increase by 10 mg q 12 hr q 3-7 days as
needed; ext rel (Hysingla) 20 mg q day, may increase by 10-20 mg q 3-5 days
Child 1-13 yr PO 0.1-0.2 mg/kg q 3-4 hr

Antitussive
Adult PO 5 mg q 4-6 hr as needed
Child PO 0.6 mg/kg/day divided q 6-8 hr, max
<2 yr 1.25 mg/dose, 2-12 yr 5 mg/dose, >12 yr
10 mg/dose

Renal dose
Adult PO CCr <45 mL/min–Hysingla decrease dose by 50% initially

Hepatic dose
Adult PO Hysingla decrease dose by 50%
initially

**Available forms: HYDROcodone/acet-
aminophen:** tablet 15 mg HYDROcodone/325
acetaminophen, 10 mg HYDROcodone/325 acetaminophen (Norco); elixir/oral solution 7.5 mg
hydrocodone/325 acetaminophen/15 mL, 10 mg
hydrocodone/325 acetaminophen/15 mL;
HYDROcodone/ibuprofen: tabs 7.5 mg
HYDROcodone/200 mg ibuprofen (Vicoprofen), 2.5 mg HYDROcodone/200 mg ibuprofen, 5 mg HYDROcodone/200 mg ibuprofen,
10 mg HYDROcodone/200 mg ibuprofen

ADVERSE EFFECTS
CNS: *Drowsiness,* dizziness, confusion, head-
ache, sedation, euphoria, dysphoria, disorienta-
tion, mood changes, dependence
CV: Tachycardia, bradycardia; QT prolongation
(Hysingla)
EENT: Blurred vision, miosis, diplopia
GI: *Nausea, vomiting, anorexia, constipation,*
esophageal obstruction, choking
GU: Dysuria, urinary retention
INTEG: Rash, sweating
RESP: Respiratory depression

INTERACTIONS
Individual drugs
Alcohol: increased CNS depression

Drug classifications

Antidepressants (tricyclics), CNS depressants, general anesthetics, opioids, phenothiazines, sedative/hypnotics, skeletal muscle relaxants: increased CNS depression

MAOIs: increased severe reactions, separate by ≥14 days

CYP3A4 inducers (barbituates cabamazepine, corticosteroids, phenytoin, rifbutins): decreased hydrocodone effect

> **BLACK BOX WARNING:** CYP3A4 inhibitors (erythromycin, ketoconazole, nefazodone, protease inhibitors): Increase HYDROcodone effect

Drug/herb

Chamomile, kava, Lavender, valerian: increased CNS depression

Drug/lab test

Increase: amylase, lipase

NURSING CONSIDERATIONS
Assessment

• **Assess pain:** intensity, type, location, duration, precipitating factor before and 1 hr after giving product, titrate upward by 25%; assess need for pain medication, physical dependency

• Monitor VS after parenteral route; note muscle rigidity; product history; liver; renal function tests; cough; and respiratory dysfunction: respiratory depression, character, rate, rhythm; notify prescriber if respirations are <10/min

• **Opioid addiction:** Identify opioid addiction or use before starting product, if product has been used by snorting, fatal reactions have occurred

• **Monitor CNS changes:** dizziness, drowsiness, hallucinations, euphoria, LOC, pupil reaction

• Monitor allergic reactions: rash, urticaria

> **BLACK BOX WARNING: Neonatal opioid withdrawal syndrome:** Monitor neonate for withdrawal (irritability, hyperactivity, abnormal sleep patterns, high-pitched crying, tremor, vomiting, diarrhea)

• **Bowel status:** constipation; provide fluids, fiber in diet, may need stimulant laxative if opioid use exceeds 3 days

> **BLACK BOX WARNING: Respiratory depression:** Do not use in those with respiratory depression; monitor for decreased respiratory rate, urge to breathe, sighing breathing pattern; carbon dioxide retention from respiratory depression may worsen sedation; an opioid antagonist may be needed

> **BLACK BOX WARNING: Ethanol ingestion:** Warn patients use with ethanol can lead to serious overdose and death, do not use with other medications containing ethanol, unless directed by prescriber

• **Beers:** Avoid use in older adults, unless safer alternative is not available, may cause ataxia, impaired psychomotor function

• **Pregnancy/breastfeeding:** May affect fetus, crosses placental barrier; do not breastfeed

Patient problems

Pain (uses)
Risk for injury (adverse reactions)

Implementation
PO route

Check product carefully before using; fatalities have occurred by using wrong dose, wrong product

• Give with antiemetic if nausea, vomiting occur

• Give when pain is beginning to return; determine dosage interval by patient response; continuous dosing of medication is more effective than given prn

• Medication should be slowly withdrawn after long-term use to prevent withdrawal symptoms

> **BLACK BOX WARNING:** Max 4 g acetaminophen with combination product

• Store in light-resistant container at room temperature

• May be given with food or milk to lessen GI upset

• Do not break, crush, or chew tabs; only scored tabs may be broken

Extended release route

• May need short- or rapid-acting opioid for breakthrough pain

• Swallow caps whole; do not crush/chew

Patient/family education

• Instruct patient to report any symptoms of CNS changes, allergic reactions; to avoid CNS depressants: alcohol, sedative/hypnotics for at least 24 hr after taking this product

• Teach patient that dizziness, drowsiness, and confusion are common and to avoid getting up without assistance, driving, or other hazardous activities

• Discuss in detail all aspects of the product; to take as directed; not to double doses, exceed recommended doses; not to discontinue abruptly, taper; that there is a high abuse potential

• Advise patient for dry mouth, use sugarless gum, frequent sips of water; to use good oral hygiene

---

BLACK BOX WARNING: Advise patient not to exceed 4000 mg in combination product with acetaminophen, check all other products that may contain acetaminophen

- Teach patient to notify health care professional if pain is not controlled adequately

Evaluation
Positive therapeutic outcome
- Decreased pain
- Decreased cough
- Teach patient to notify prescriber if pregnancy is planned or suspected or if breastfeeding

TREATMENT OF OVERDOSE:
Naloxone HCl (Narcan) 0.2-0.8 **IV**, O₂, **IV** fluids, vasopressors

---

hydrocortisone (Rx)
(hy-droh-kor'tih-sone)
Cortef, Cortenema
hydrocortisone cypionate
Cortef
hydrocortisone sodium succinate (Rx)
A-Hydrocort, Solu-Cortef
Func. class.: Short-acting glucocorticoid
Chem. class.: Natural nonfluorinated, group IV potency (valerate), group VI potency (acetate and plain)

Do not confuse: hydrocortisone/ HYDROcodone

ACTION: Decreases inflammation by suppressing migration of polymorphonuclear leukocytes and fibroblasts and reversing increased capillary permeability and lysosomal stabilization (systemic); antipruritic, antiinflammatory (topical)

Therapeutic outcome: Decreased inflammation

USES: Severe inflammation, septic shock, adrenal insufficiency, ulcerative colitis, collagen disorders, asthma, COPD, SLE, Stevens-Johnson syndrome, ulcerative colitis, TB

Pharmacokinetics

Absorption	Well absorbed (PO); systemic (topical)
Distribution	Crosses placenta
Metabolism	Liver, extensively
Excretion	Kidney
Half-life	3-5 hr, adrenal suppression 3-4 days

Pharmacodynamics

	PO	IM	IV	TOPICAL
Onset	1-2 hr	20 min	Rapid	Min to hr
Peak	1 hr	4-8 hr	1-2 hr	Hr to days
Duration	1½ days	1½ days	1½ days	Hr to days

CONTRAINDICATIONS
Hypersensitivity, fungal infections

Precautions: Pregnancy, breastfeeding, diabetes mellitus, glaucoma, osteoporosis, seizure disorders, ulcerative colitis, HF, myasthenia gravis, renal disease, esophagitis, peptic ulcer, metastatic carcinoma, septic shock, Cushing syndrome, hepatic disease, hypothyroidism, coagulopathy, thromboembolism, children <2 yr, psychosis, idiopathic thrombocytopenia (IM), acute glomerulonephritis, amebiasis, nonasthmatic bronchial disease, AIDS, TB, recent MI (associated with left-ventricular rupture)

DOSAGE AND ROUTES
Most disorders
Adult: PO 20-240 mg daily in divided doses; IM/**IV** 100-500 mg (succinate), may repeat q2-6hr, then 50-100 mg IM as needed

Septic shock treatment
Adult: Cont IV 200 mg/day, taper when vasopressors are discontinued

Adrenocortical insufficiency:
Child: PO 0.56 mg/kg/day (15-20 mg/m²/day) as a single or divided dose; IM/IV 0.186-0.28 mg/kg/day (10-12 mg/m²/day) in three divided doses
Child: PO 2-8 mg/kg/day (60-240 mg/m²/day) as a single or divided dose; IM/IV 0.666-4 mg/kg (20-120 mg/m²) q12-24hr

Available forms: Hydrocortisone: enema 100 mg/60 ml; tabs 5, 10, 20 mg; **acetate:** rectal suppository: 25, 30 mg: 10%; **cypionate:** tabs 5, 10, 20 mg; **succinate:** inj 100, 250, 500, 1000 mg vial

ADVERSE EFFECTS
CNS: Depression, flushing, sweating, headache, mood changes, *pseudotumor cerebri*, euphoria, insomnia, *seizures*, psychosis
CV: Hypertension, edema
EENT: Increased intraocular pressure, blurred vision, cataracts
GI: Diarrhea, nausea, abdominal distention, GI hemorrhage, *pancreatitis*, vomiting, anorexia
HEMA: *Thrombophlebitis, thromboembolism*
INTEG: Acne, poor wound healing, ecchymosis, petechiae

MISC: Adrenal insufficiency (after stress/withdrawal), pheochromocytoma
MS: Fractures, osteoporosis, weakness

INTERACTIONS
Individual drugs
Alcohol, amphotericin B, cycloSPORINE, digoxin: increased side effects

Bosentan, carBAMazepine, cholestyramine, colestipol, ePHEDrine, phenytoin, rifampin, theophylline: decreased action of hydrocortisone

Drug classifications
Acetaminophen, NSAIDs, salicylates: increased risk of GI bleeding

Anticoagulants, calcium supplements, toxoids, vaccines: decreased action of each specific drug

Anticonvulsants: decreased effects of anticonvulsant
Antidiabetics: decreased effects of antidiabetics
Barbiturates: decreased action of hydrocortisone
Diuretics: increased side effects
Live virus vaccines/toxoids: increased neurologic reactions

Drug/herb
Ephedra: decreased hydrocortisone levels

Drug/lab test
Increase: cholesterol, sodium, blood glucose, uric acid, calcium, urine glucose
Decrease: calcium, potassium, T_4, T_3, thyroid ^{131}I uptake test, urine 17-OHCS, 17-KS
False negative: skin allergy tests

NURSING CONSIDERATIONS
Assessment
• **Adrenal insufficiency (cushingoid symptoms):** nausea, anorexia, shortness of breath, moon face, fatigue, dizziness, weakness, joint pain before and during treatment; monitor plasma cortisol levels during long-term therapy (normal level is 138-635 nmol/L when obtained at 8 AM); check adrenal function periodically for hypothalamic-pituitary-adrenal axis suppression
• Monitor potassium, blood glucose, urine glucose while patient is on long-term therapy; hypokalemia and hyperglycemia may occur
• Monitor I&O ratio; be alert for decreasing urinary output and increasing edema; weigh daily; notify prescriber of weekly gain >5 lb or edema, hypertension, cardiac symptoms
• **Assess for infection:** increased temp, WBC even after withdrawal of medication; product masks infection symptoms; if fever develops, product should be discontinued
• Check for potassium depletion: paresthesias, fatigue, nausea, vomiting, depression, polyuria, dysrhythmias, weakness

• Assess mental status: affect, mood, behavioral changes, aggression
• Check nasal passages during long-term treatment for changes in mucus (nasal)
• Assess for systemic absorption: increased temp, inflammation, irritation (topical)
• GI effects: nausea, vomiting, anorexia or appetite stimulation, diarrhea, constipation, abdominal pain, hiccups, gastritis, pancreatitis, GI bleeding/perforation with long-term treatment
• **Beers:** Avoid in older adults with or at high risk for delirium

Patient problems
Risk for infection (adverse reactions)
Risk for injury (adverse reactions)

Implementation
PO route
• Give with food or milk to decrease GI symptoms
• Do not use acetate or susp for IV, salts are not interchangeable

Topical route
• Apply only to affected areas; do not get in eyes
• Cleanse and dry area before applying medication, then cover with occlusive dressing (only if prescribed); seal to normal skin; change q12hr; systemic absorption may occur; use only on dermatoses; do not use on weeping, denuded, or infected area
• Use for a few days after area has cleared
• Store at room temperature

IM route
• Give deeply in large muscle mass; rotate sites; avoid deltoid; use 21-gauge needle

IV route
• **Succinate:** IV in mix-o-vial or reconstitute 250 mg or less/2 ml bacteriostatic water for injection, mix gently; give direct IV over 1 min or more; may be further diluted in 100, 250, 500, or 1000 ml of D_5W, D_5/0.9% NaCl, 0.9% NaCl given over ordered rate

Sodium succinate

Y-site compatibilities: Acetaminophen, acyclovir, alemtuzumab, alfentanil, allopurinol, amifostine, ampicillin, amphotericin B cholesteryl, amsacrine, atracurium, atropine, aztreonam, betamethasone, calcium gluconate, cefepime, cefmetazole, cephalothin, chlordiazePOXIDE, chlorproMAZINE, cisatracurium, cladribine, cyanocobalamin, cytarabine, dexamethasone, digoxin, diphenhydrAMINE, DOPamine, DOXOrubicin liposome, droperidol, edrophonium, enalaprilat, EPINEPHrine, esmolol, conjugated estrogens, ethacrynate, famotidine, fentaNYL, fentaNYL/droperidol, filgrastim, fludarabine, fluorouracil, foscarnet, furosemide, gallium, granisetron, heparin, hydrALAZINE, inamrinone, regular insulin, isoproterenol, kanamycin, lidocaine, LORazepam, magnesium sulfate, melphalan, menadiol, meperidine, methicillin, methoxamine, methylergonovine, minocycline, morphine, neostigmine, norepinephrine, ondansetron, oxacillin, oxytocin, PACLitaxel, pancuronium, penicillin G potassium, pentazocine, phytonadione, piperacillin/tazobactam, prednisoLONE, procainamide, prochlorperazine, propofol, propranolol, pyridostigmine, remifentanil, scopolamine, sodium bicarbonate, succinylcholine, tacrolimus, teniposide, theophylline, thiotepa, trimethaphan, trimethobenzamide, vecuronium, vinorelbine, zoledronic acid

Patient/family education

• Teach patient all aspects of product use, including cushingoid symptoms
• Advise patient to carry/wear emergency ID as corticosteroid user; not to discontinue abruptly; adrenal crisis can result
• Instruct patient to notify prescriber if therapeutic response decreases; dosage adjustment may be needed
• Instruct patient to notify prescriber of signs of infection
• Teach patient that product can mask infections and cause hyperglycemia (diabetic)
• Teach patient to avoid live-virus vaccines if using steroids long term
• Teach patient not to discontinue abruptly, adrenal crisis can result; product should be tapered
• Caution patient to avoid OTC, herbals, supplements products unless directed by prescriber: salicylates, alcohol in cough products, cold preparations
• **Teach patient symptoms of adrenal insufficiency:** nausea, anorexia, fatigue, dizziness, dyspnea, weakness, joint pain; and when to notify prescriber
• Advise patient that long-term therapy may be needed to resolve infection (1-2 mo depending on type of infection)
• Teach patient to report immediately abdominal pain, black tarry stools, as GI bleeding/perforation can occur; if received by epidural route, report immediately change in vision, severe headache, seizures, weakness (emergency response needed)
• Advise patient not to discontinue abruptly or adrenal crisis can result; product should be tapered

• **Epidural use:** Assess for vision changes, seizures, stroke, paralysis, brain edema and death may occur (rare)

Evaluation
Positive therapeutic outcome
• Decreased inflammation
• Absence of severe itching, patches on skin, flaking (top)
• Decreased GI symptoms

hydrocortisone topical
See Appendix B

> **⚠ HIGH ALERT**

HYDROmorphone (Rx) REMS
(hye-droe-mor'fone)
Dilaudid, Dilaudid-HP, Exalgo, Hydromorph Contin, Jurnista ✦
Func. class.: Antitussive, opioid analgesic agonist
Chem. class.: Phenanthrene derivative, guaifenesin
Controlled substance schedule II

Do not confuse: HYDROmorphone/meperidine/morphine, **Dilaudid**/Demerol

ACTION: Inhibits ascending pain pathways in CNS, increases pain threshold, alters pain perception

Therapeutic outcome: Decreased cough, decreased pain

USES: As an antitussive to suppress cough; moderate to severe pain

Pharmacokinetics

Absorption	Well absorbed (PO), complete (**IV**)
Distribution	Unknown; crosses placenta
Metabolism	Liver, extensively
Excretion	Kidneys
Half-life	Varied

Pharmacodynamics

	PO/IM/SUBCUT	IV	RECT
Onset	15-30 min	10-15 min	15-30 min
Peak	30-60 min	15-30 min	30-90 min
Duration	4-5 hr	2-3 hr	4-5 hr

CONTRAINDICATIONS
Hypersensitivity to this product, sulfite, COPD, cor pulmonale, emphysema, GI obstruction, ileus, increased intracranial pressure, obstetric delivery, status asthmaticus

> **BLACK BOX WARNING:** Respiratory depression, opioid-naïve patients

Precautions: Pregnancy, breastfeeding, children <18 yr, increased ICP, addictive personality, renal/hepatic disease, MI (acute), abrupt discontinuation, adrenal insufficiency, angina, asthma, biliary tract disease, bladder obstruction, hypothyroidism, hypovolemia, hypoxemia, IBD, IV use, labor, latex hypersensitivity, myxedema, seizure disorders, sleep apnea

> **BLACK BOX WARNING:** Substance abuse, accidental exposure, potential for overdose/poisoning, neonatal opioid withdrawal syndrome

DOSAGE AND ROUTES
Analgesic
Adult ≥50 kg PO Immediate release 4-8 mg q 3-4 hr initially or IM/IV/subcut 1.5 mg q 3-4 hr as needed
Renal dose
Adult PO moderate impairment (ext rel) decrease dose by 50%; severe impairment (ext rel) decrease dose by 75%
Hepatic dose
Adult **PO** moderate impairment (ext rel) decrease dose by 75%
Antitussive
Adult/child >12 yr PO 1 mg q 3-4 hr
Child 6-12 yr PO 0.5mg q 3-4 hr
Adult/Child <50 kg PO 0.06 mg/kg q 3-4 hr initially IM/IV/subcut 0.015 mg/kg q 3-4 hr initially

Available forms: Powder of injection 250 mg; inj 1, 2, 4, 10 mg/ml; tabs 2, 4, 8 mg; oral sol 5 mg/5 ml; supp 3 mg, ext rel tab 8, 12, 16, 32 mg

ADVERSE EFFECTS
CNS: Dizziness, drowsiness, *sedation, confusion,* headache, euphoria, mood changes, seizures
CV: *Hypotension, bradycardia*
EENT: Miosis, diplopia, blurred vision, tinnitus
GI: *Nausea, constipation, vomiting, anorexia,* dry mouth, cramps, paralytic ileus
GU: Urinary retention
INTEG: Rash, flushing, diaphoresis
RESP: Respiratory depression
MISC: Physical/psychological dependence

INTERACTIONS
Individual drugs
Alcohol: increased respiratory depression, hypotension, sedation

Drug classifications
Antipsychotics, opiates, sedative/hypnotics, skeletal muscle relaxants: increased effects
MAOIs: increased severe reactions, separate by ≥14 days
Opiate antagonists: decreased HYDROmorphone effects

Drug/herb
Chamomile, hops, kava, lavender, St. John's wort, valerian: increased action

Drug/lab test
Increased: amylase

NURSING CONSIDERATIONS
Assessment
• **Assess pain control,** sedation by scoring on 0-10 scale or developmentally appropriate pain scale for children; around-the-clock dosing is best for pain control
• Monitor VS after parenteral route; note muscle rigidity

> **BLACK BOX WARNING: Respiratory dysfunction;** respiratory depression; monitor character, rate, rhythm; notify prescriber if respirations are <10/min

> **BLACK BOX WARNING: Substance abuse; Opioid addiction;** assess for previous or current substance abuse, risk of abuse will be increased in these patients, assess for misuse of medication

• Monitor CNS changes: dizziness, drowsiness, hallucinations, euphoria, LOC, pupil reaction
• Monitor allergic reactions: rash, urticaria; bowel function, constipation
• **Pregnancy/breastfeeding:** Use only if benefits outweigh fetal risk, neonatal opioid withdrawal syndrome can occur if used for prolonged periods in pregnancy, do not use in breastfeeding, excretion unknown
• **Beers:** Avoid in older adults unless safer alternative is unavailable, may cause ataxia, impaired psychomotor function

Patient problems
Pain (uses)
Risk for injury (adverse reactions)

Implementation
- Give with antiemetic if nausea, vomiting occur
- Give when pain is beginning to return; determine dosage interval by patient response; continuous dosing of medication is more effective given prn; explain analgesic effect
- Withdraw medication slowly after long-term use to prevent withdrawal symptoms
- Store in light-resistant container at room temperature

PO route
- May be given with food or milk to lessen GI upset

Extended release

BLACK BOX WARNING: Do not use extended-release products in opioid-naïve patients or with other extended-release opioids; do not use with other extended-release HYDROmorphone products, may be fatal

- **Converting from oral opioids;** conversion ratios are approximate; initiate ext rel tabs at 50% of calculated total daily equivalent dose of ext rel, give q24hr; max increase q2-3days, consider titration increases of 25%-50% in each step
- **Converting from transdermal patch (fentaNYL)** initiate ext rel tabs 18 hr after removal of patch; for each 25 mcg/hr dose of transdermal fentaNYL the dose is 12 mg q24hr, start dose at 50% of calculated HYDROmorphone ext rel dose q24hr; titrate no more often than q3-4days, consider dose increases of 25%-50% with each step; if more than 2 rescue doses are required in 24 hr, consider titration

SUBCUT route
- Do not give if sol is cloudy or a precipitate has formed; rotate inj sites
- Use short 30-G needle, make sure not to inject intradermally

Direct IV route
- Give after diluting with 5 ml or more of sterile water or 0.9% NaCl for inj
- Give slowly at 2 mg over 3-5 min or less through Y-connector or 3-way stopcock

IV infusion route
- Dilute each 0.1-1 mg/ml in 0.9% NaCl, deliver by opioid syringe infusion; may be diluted in D₅W, D₅/NaCl, 0.45% NaCl or 0.9% NaCl for larger amounts and through an infusion pump

Y-site compatibilities: Acyclovir, allopurinol, amifostine, amikacin, amsacrine, aztreonam, cefamandole, cefepime, cefoperazone, cefotaxime, cefOXitin, cefTAZidime, ceftizoxime, cefuroxime, chloramphenicol, CISplatin, cladribine, clindamycin, cyclophosphamide, cytarabine, diltiazem, DOBUTamine, DOPamine, DOXOrubicin, doxycycline, EPINEPHrine, erythromycin lactobionate, famotidine, fentaNYL, filgrastim, fludarabine, foscarnet, furosemide, gentamicin, granisetron, heparin, kanamycin, labetalol, LORazepam, magnesium sulfate, melphalan, methotrexate, metroNIDAZOLE, midazolam, milrinone, morphine, nafcillin, niCARdipine, nitroglycerin, norepinephrine, ondansetron, oxacillin, PACLitaxel, penicillin G potassium, piperacillin, piperacillin/tazobactam, propofol, ranitidine, teniposide, thiotepa, ticarcillin, tobramycin, trimethoprim/sulfamethoxazole, vancomycin, vecuronium, vinorelbine

Patient/family education

BLACK BOX WARNING: Substance abuse: Instruct patient to report any symptoms of CNS changes, allergic reactions; to avoid CNS depressants: alcohol, sedative-hypnotics for at least 24 hr after taking this product

- Advise patient that dizziness, drowsiness, and confusion are common and to avoid getting up without assistance, driving, or other hazardous activities
- Teach patient to notify health care professional if pain is not controlled adequately
- Discuss in detail all aspects of the product, to take with food if nausea occurs
- Advise patient for dry mouth, use sugarless gum, frequent sips of water; to use good oral hygiene

BLACK BOX WARNING: Teach patient that extended-release products must be taken whole, not to use with alcohol, medications with alcohol content

Evaluation
Positive therapeutic outcome
- Decreased pain
- Decreased cough

TREATMENT OF OVERDOSE:
Naloxone HCl (Narcan) 0.2-0.8 **IV**, O₂, **IV** fluids, vasopressors

RARELY USED

hydroxyprogesterone caproate
(hye-drox-ee-pro-jess'-te-rone kap'-roe-ate)
Func. class: Hormone, progestin

USES: To decrease preterm birth risk in history of singleton preterm birth

CONTRAINDICATIONS: Hypersensitivity to this product or castor oil, thrombosis, hormone-sensitive cancers, liver disease, unexplained vaginal bleeding

DOSAGE AND ROUTES
Adult: IV 250 mg q wk, used between 16 wk and 20 wk 6 day, continue to wk 37 gestation or delivery

hydroxocobalmin
See vitamin B-12 products

hydroxychloroquine (Rx)
(hye-drox-ee-klor'oh-kwin)
Plaquenil
Func. class.: Antimalarial, antirheumatic (DMARDs)
Chem. class.: 4-Aminoquinoline derivative

ACTION: Impairs complement-dependent antigen-antibody reactions

Therapeutic outcome: Resolution of infection

USES: Malaria caused by *Plasmodium vivax, P. malariae, P. ovale, P. falciparum* (some strains); LE, rheumatoid arthritis

Pharmacokinetics
Absorption	Well absorbed
Distribution	Widely distributed, crosses placenta
Metabolism	Liver
Excretion	Urine/feces
Half-life	40 days

Pharmacodynamics
Onset	Rapid
Peak	1-2 hr
Duration	Days-weeks

CONTRAINDICATIONS
Hypersensitivity to this product or chloroquine, retinal field changes

Precautions: Pregnancy, breastfeeding, blood dyscrasias, severe GI disease, neurologic disease, alcoholism, hepatic disease, G6PD deficiency, psoriasis, eczema, children, ocular disease

BLACK BOX WARNING: Requires an experienced clinician

DOSAGE AND ROUTES
Malaria
Adult: PO **suppression or prevention** 400 mg qwk, begin 2 wk before travel to endemic area, continue 4 wk after returning; **treatment** 800 mg, then 400 mg after 6-8 hr, then 400 mg/day on 2nd and 3rd day, total dose 2 g
Child: PO **suppression or prevention** 6.4 mg/kg (5 mg/kg base) qwk, begin 2 wk before travel to endemic area, continue 4 wk after returning; **treatment** 10 mg/kg, 6.4 mg/kg (5 mg/kg base), at 6, 24, 48 hr after 1st dose

Lupus erythematosus
Adult: PO 400 mg (310 mg base) daily-bid; length depends on patient response; **maintenance** 200-400 mg/day

Rheumatoid arthritis
Adult: PO 400 mg/day for 4-12 wk; then 200-400 mg/day after good response

Available forms: Tabs 200 mg

ADVERSE EFFECTS
CNS: Headache, fatigue, irritability, seizures, bad dreams, dizziness, confusion, psychosis, anxiety, suicidal ideation
CV: HF, torsade de pointes, QT prolongation
EENT: *Blurred vision, corneal changes, retinal changes, difficulty focusing,* tinnitus, vertigo, nystagmus, corneal deposits
GI: *Nausea, vomiting, anorexia,* diarrhea, cramps
HEMA: Thrombocytopenia, agranulocytosis, leukopenia, aplastic anemia
INTEG: Pruritus, exfoliative dermatitis, alopecia, Stevens-Johnson syndrome, photosensitivity, DRESS, rash, pruritus

INTERACTIONS
Individual products
Magnesium, aluminum products: decreased malarial action
Digoxin: increased levels
Methotrexate: decreased levels
Rabies vaccine: increased antibody titer

Drug classifications
Live-virus vaccines, botulinum toxoids: decreased effects

NURSING CONSIDERATIONS
Assessment
• **Assess for lupus erythematosus, malaria symptoms** before treatment and daily
• **Assess for rheumatoid arthritis:** pain, swelling, ROM, temp of joints, for decreased reflexes: knee, ankle

• Assess ophthalmic exam baseline, q6mo if long-term treatment or product dosage >150 mg/day

• Assess hepatic studies qwk: AST, ALT, bilirubin

• **Bone marrow suppression:** Assess blood studies: CBC, platelets; WBC, RBC, platelets may be decreased; if severe, product should be discontinued, malaise, fever, bruising, bleeding (rare)

• Assess for decreased reflexes: knee, ankle

• Assess ECG during therapy

• Assess for depression of T waves, widening of QRS complex

• **Assess allergic reactions:** pruritus, rash, urticaria

• **Assess for ototoxicity** (tinnitus, vertigo, change in hearing); audiometric testing should be done before, after treatment

• **Assess for toxicity:** blurring vision, difficulty focusing, headache, dizziness, knee, ankle reflexes; product should be discontinued immediately

Patient problems
Infections (uses)

Implementation
PO route

> **BLACK BOX WARNING:** Only to be prescribed by experienced clinician

• Give before or after meals with milk, at same time each day to maintain product level

• Tabs may be crushed and mixed with food, fluids

• Malaria prophylaxis should be started 2 wk prior to exposure and 4-6 wk after leaving exposure area

• Store in tight, light-resistant container at room temperature; keep inj in cool environment

Patient/family education
• Teach patient to use sunglasses in bright sunlight to decrease effects of photophobia

• Teach patient that urine may turn rust or brown

• Teach patient to report hearing, vision problems; fever, fatigue, bruising, bleeding, which may indicate blood dyscrasias

• **Pregnancy/breastfeeding:** Identify if pregnancy is planned or suspected or if breastfeeding

• **RA:** Advise patient to report to health care professional if there is no change in condition; may need several months for results

• **Malaria prevention:** Discuss how to prevent mosquitoes in the environment

• Teach patient not to use with alcohol

Evaluation
Positive therapeutic outcome
• Decreased symptoms of malaria, LE, rheumatoid arthritis

TREATMENT OF OVERDOSE:
Induce vomiting; gastric lavage; administer barbiturate (ultra–short-acting), vasopressor, ammonium chloride; tracheostomy may be necessary

ibandronate (Rx)
(eye-ban'dro-nate)
Boniva
Func. class.: Bone-resorption inhibitor, electrolyte modifier
Chem. class.: Bisphosphonate

ACTION: Inhibits bone resorption, apparently without inhibiting bone formation and mineralization; absorbs calcium phosphate crystals in bone and may directly block dissolution of hydroxyapatite crystals of bone; more potent than other products

Therapeutic outcome: Increased bone mineral density

USES: Postmenopausal Osteoporosis and prophylaxis

Pharmacokinetics

Absorption	Poor
Distribution	Taken up primarily by bones, 91%-99% protein binding
Metabolism	Unknown
Excretion	Primarily by kidneys (60%)
Half-life	IV (4.5-25.5 hr), PO 1.5-6.5 days

Pharmacodynamics

	PO	IV
Onset	Unknown	Unknown
Peak	0.5-2 hr	3 hr
Duration	Up to 1 mo	Up to 3 mo

CONTRAINDICATIONS
Achalasia, esophageal stricture, hypocalcemia, intraarterial administration, renal failure, hypersensitivity to bisphosphonates, inability to stand or sit upright

Precautions: Pregnancy, breastfeeding, children, geriatric, anemia, chemotherapy, coagulopathy, dental disease, diabetes mellitus, dysphagia, GI/renal disease, GERD, hypertension, infection, multiple myeloma, phosphate hypersensitivity, vitamin D deficiency

DOSAGE AND ROUTES
Postmenopausal osteoporosis/ prophylaxis
Adult: PO 150 mg qmo; **IV** BOL 3 mg q3mo

Renal dose
Adult: PO CCr <30 ml/min, avoid use

Available forms: Tabs 150 mg; sol for inj 3 mg/ml

ADVERSE EFFECTS
CNS: Fever, insomnia, dizziness, headache
CV: Hypertension, atrial fibrillation
EENT: Ocular pain/inflammation, uveitis, esophageal ulceration
GI: Constipation, nausea, vomiting, diarrhea, dyspepsia, esophageal/GI ulcer
INTEG: Rash, inj site reaction
META: *Hypomagnesemia, hypophosphatemia, hypocalcemia,* hypercholesterolemia
MS: Bone pain, myalgia, osteonecrosis of the jaw
SYST: Stevens-Johnson syndrome, erythema multiforme, dermatitis bullous, anaphylaxis

INTERACTIONS
Individual drugs
Calcium, vitamin D, iron, aluminum, magnesium salts: decreased ibandronate effect, separate by 1 hr
Increased: GI irritation: NSAIDs, salicylates

Drug/food
• Do not take with food, calcium; give product on empty stomach

Drug/lab test
Decreased: alk phos, magnesium, calcium, phosphate
Increased: cholesterol

NURSING CONSIDERATIONS
Assessment
• **Osteoporosis:** before and during treatment; monitor DEXA scan for bone mineral density, correct electrolyte imbalances (calcium, magnesium, phosphate) before starting therapy
• **Anaphylaxis:** swelling of face, lips, mouth, rash, sweating, wheezing, trouble breathing, discontinue immediately, provide supportive treatment (IV)
• Assess dental health; before dental extraction, may require drug holiday for up to 2 mo; osteonecrosis of the jaw may occur
• **Assess for bone pain;** use analgesics; may begin within 24 hr, or even years after treatment, pain usually subsides after treatment is discontinued
• **Esophageal irritation/ulceration:** Assess for heart burn, painful swallowing, avoid use in those with swallowing difficulties

Patient problems
Risk for injury (adverse reactions)

Implementation
PO route
• Give early AM with a glass of water; if qmo, give on same day of each month

- Patient to remain upright for ≥ 1 hr after taking
- Not to suck/chew, throat ulcers may occur
- Store at room temperature

Direct IV route
- Use single-dose prefilled syringe; discard unused portion; give over 15-30 sec
- Store at room temperature
- Do not use if discolored or if sol contains particulates
- Do not admix

Patient/family education
- Teach patient to report hypercalcemic relapse: nausea, vomiting, bone pain, thirst; unusual muscle twitching, muscle spasms, severe diarrhea, constipation, chest pain, pain while chewing/swallowing
- Advise patient to continue with dietary recommendations, including calcium and vit D, calcium, alk phosphatase
- Instruct patient to obtain an analgesic from provider for bone pain that may occur rapidly or within months
- Advise patient that if nausea/vomiting occur, small, frequent meals may help
- Teach patient to report vision symptoms: blurred vision, edema, inflammation; report to prescriber
- Encourage to exercise regularly, to stop smoking, and decrease alcohol
- Teach patient to notify health care professional of osteonecrosis of the jaw after dental procedures pain, drainage, swelling, to notify dentist before dental procedures
- Advise to take in AM at least 60 min before other meds, food, beverages, to take monthly dose on same day; do not double or skip doses; if dose is missed take next regularly scheduled time; do not discontinue without discussing with health care professional; if IV dose is missed reschedule as soon as able, reschedule subsequent doses on new time schedule, not to receive IV dose more than once in 3 mo
- Teach to sit upright ≥60 min after PO dose, to swallow tab whole, not to chew or suck, to prevent irritation; contact provider of irritation, painful swallowing
- Teach to report if pregnancy is planned or suspected or if planning to breastfeed; pregnancy

Evaluation
Positive therapeutic outcome
- Increased bone mineral density
- Decrease symptoms of osteoporosis

ibuprofen (OTC, Rx)
(eye-byoo-proe'fen)
Advil, Advil Infants, Advil Junior, Advil Migraine, Children's Advil, Children's Europrofen ✦, Children's Motrin, Ibuprohm, Ibutab, Midol, Motrin ✦, Motrin IB (injection), Motrin Infant, Motrin Junior, Pamprin IB ✦, Profen, Tab-Profen
ibuprofen lysine (injection) (Rx)
Caldolor NeoProfen
Func. class.: NSAID

Do not confuse: Motrin/neurontin

ACTION: Inhibits COX-1, COX-2 by blocking arachidonate; analgesic, antiinflammatory, antipyretic

Therapeutic outcome: Decreased pain, inflammation, fever

USES: Rheumatoid arthritis, osteoarthritis, primary dysmenorrhea, dental pain, musculoskeletal disorders, fever, migraine, patent ductus arteriosus

Unlabeled uses: Cystic fibrosis

Pharmacokinetics
Absorption	Well absorbed
Distribution	Not known; crosses placenta, protein binding 99%
Metabolism	Liver, extensively
Excretion	Kidneys, unchanged (10%)
Half-life	1.8-2 hr (adult), 1-2 hr (child)

Pharmacodynamics
	PO	IV
Onset	½ hr	Unknown
Peak	1-2 hr	Unknown
Duration	4-6 hr	4-6 hr

CONTRAINDICATIONS
Avoid pregnancy 3rd trimester, hypersensitivity to this product, NSAIDs, salicylates, asthma, severe renal/hepatic disease, perioperative pain in CABG

Precautions: Pregnancy (1st and 2nd trimester), breastfeeding, children, geriatric, bleeding disorders, GI disorders, cardiac disorders, hypersensitivity to other antiinflammatory agents, HF, CCr <25 ml/min

BLACK BOX WARNING: GI bleeding, MI, stroke

DOSAGE AND ROUTES
Self-treatment of minor aches/pain
Adult/adolescent: PO (OTC product) 200 mg q4-6hr, may increase to 400 mg q4-6hr; max 1200 mg/day
Child 11 yr (72-95 lb): PO 300 mg q 6-8 hr
Child 9-10 yr (60-71 lb): PO 250 mg q 6-8 hr
Child 6-8 yr (48-59 lb): PO 200 mg q 6-8 hr
Child 4-5 yr (36-47 lb): PO 150 mg q 6-8 hr
Child 2-3 yr (24-35 lb): PO 100 mg q 6-8 hr
Child 12-23 mo (18-23 lb): PO 75 mg q 6-8 hr
Child 6-11 mo (12-17 lb): PO 50 mg q 6-8 hr

Analgesia
Adult: PO 200-400 mg q4-6hr; max 3.2 g/day; OTC use max 1200 mg/day
Child: PO 4-10 mg/kg/dose q6-8hr

Moderate to severe pain (hospitalized patients) (Caldolor)
Adult: IV 400-800 mg q6hr as an adjunct to opiate agonist therapy

Dysmenorrhea
Adult: PO 400 mg q4-6hr; max 1200 mg/day

Antipyretic
Child 6 mo-12 yr: PO 5 mg/kg (temp <102.5° F or 39.2° C), 10 mg/kg (temp >102.5° F), may repeat q6-8hr; max 40 mg/kg/day

Antiinflammatory
Adult: PO 400-800 mg tid-qid; max 3.2 g/day
Child: PO 30-40 mg/kg/day in 3-4 divided doses; max 50 mg/kg/day

Juvenile arthritis
Child: PO 30-40 mg/kg/day (oral suspension) in 3-4 divided doses

Cystic fibrosis (unlabeled)
Child 6 mo-12 yr: 20-30 mg/kg/day divided bid

Patent ductus arteriosus (PDA) (Neoprofen)
Premature neonate ≤32 wk gestation who weighs 500-1500 g: IV 10 mg/kg initially, then if needed, 2 doses 5 mg/kg at 24 hr intervals; if oliguria occurs, hold dose

Available forms: caps 200 mg, tabs 100, 200, 300, 400, 600, 800 mg; liqui-gel caps 200 mg; oral susp 40 mg/ml, 100 mg/5 ml; liquid 100 mg/5 ml; chew tabs 50, 100 mg; oral drops 50 mg/1.25 ml; inj 10 mg/ml (NeoProfen)

ADVERSE EFFECTS
CNS: *Headache,* dizziness, drowsiness, fatigue, tremors, confusion, insomnia, anxiety, depression
CV: Tachycardia, peripheral edema, palpitations, dysrhythmias, CV thrombotic events, MI, stroke
EENT: Tinnitus, hearing loss, blurred vision

GI: *Nausea, anorexia,* vomiting, diarrhea, jaundice, hepatitis, constipation, flatulence, cramps, dry mouth, peptic ulcer, GI bleeding, ulceration, necrotizing enterocolitis, GI perforation
GU: Nephrotoxicity, dysuria, hematuria, oliguria, azotemia
HEMA: Blood dyscrasias, increased bleeding time
INTEG: Purpura, rash, pruritus, sweating, urticaria, necrotizing fasciitis, photosensitivity, photophobia, toxic epidermal necrolysis, exfoliative dermatitis
META: Hyperkalemia, hyperuricemia, hypoglycemia, hyponatremia
SYST: Anaphylaxis, Stevens-Johnson syndrome

INTERACTIONS
Individual drugs
Alcohol, aspirin: increased GI reactions
Aspirin: decreased ibuprofen action
CycloSPORINE, lithium, methotrexate: increased toxicity
Furosemide: decreased effect of furosemide
Radiation: increased risk of blood dyscrasias
Valproic acid, warfarin: increased risk of bleeding

Drug classifications
Anticoagulants, antiplatelet agents, salicylates, SSRIs, thrombolytics: increased risk of bleeding
Anticoagulants (oral): increased toxicity
Antidiabetics (oral): increased hypoglycemia
Antihypertensives: decreased effect of antihypertensives
Antineoplastics: increased risk of blood dyscrasias
Corticosteroids, NSAIDs: increased GI reactions
Diuretics: decreased effectiveness of diuretics (thiazides)

Drug/herb
Feverfew, garlic, ginger, ginkgo, ginseng *(Panax),* horse chestnut, red clover: increased risk of bleeding

Drug/lab test
Increased: BUN, creatinine, LFTs, potassium
Decreased: Hgb/Hct, blood glucose, WBC, platelets

NURSING CONSIDERATIONS
Assessment

> **BLACK BOX WARNING: GI bleeding/perforation:** chronic use can cause gastritis with or without bleeding; in those with a prior history of peptic ulcer disease or GI bleeding, initiate treatment at lower dose; geriatrics are at greater risk, as are those who consume >3 alcohol drinks/day

---

⚠ Nurse Alert   ✷ Key NCLEX® Drug   >> Drug Specifics

• **Assess for infection;** may mask symptoms
• **Assess pain:** location, duration, type, intensity before dose, 1 hr after
• Assess musculoskeletal status: ROM before dose, 1 hr after
• Monitor liver function tests: AST, ALT, bilirubin, creatinine if patient is on long-term therapy, monitor electrolytes as needed, make sure patient is well hydrated
• **Perioperative pain in CABG:** MI and stroke can result for 10-14 days, can be fatal, those taking NSAIDs are at greater risk of MI and stroke, even in first few weeks of therapy
• **Serious skin disorders:** For skin rash, swelling of lips, face, tongue, discontinue immediately, provide supportive care
• **Nephrotoxicity:** Monitor renal function tests: BUN, urine creatinine if patient is on long-term therapy
• Assess cardiac status: edema (peripheral), tachycardia, palpitations; monitor B/P, pulse for character, quality, rhythm
• Monitor blood studies: CBC, Hct, Hgb, pro-time if patient is on long-term therapy
• Check I&O ratio; decreasing output may indicate renal failure if patient is on long-term therapy
• Assess for history of peptic ulcer disorder; asthma, aspirin, hypersensitivity, check closely for hypersensitivity reactions
• **PDA closure:** Monitor for bleeding, oliguria, infection in preterm neonates, use only doses needed for ductus arteriosus closure; hold dose if renal output <0.6 mL/kg/hr on second/third dose
• **Dysmenorrhea:** Give at onset of menses
• **Assess for allergic reactions:** rash, urticaria; if these occur, product may have to be discontinued
• Assess for vision changes: blurring, halos; may indicate corneal, retinal damage
• Identify prior product history; there are many product interactions
• **Identify fever:** length of time in evidence and related symptoms
• **Beers:** Avoid chronic use in older adults unless other alternatives are not effective, increased risk of GI bleeding
• **Pregnancy:** Identify if pregnancy is planned or suspected, if breastfeeding

Patient problem
Pain (uses)
Impaired motility (uses)

Implementation
PO route
• Administer to patient crushed or whole; 800-mg tab may be dissolved in water

• Give with food or milk to decrease gastric symptoms; give 2 hr before or 30 min after meals; absorption may be slowed
• Shake susp well before use
• Store at room temperature
• Do not use in pregnancy after 30 wk gestation

IV route
• Must be well hydrated prior to administration
• Dilute to ≤4 mg/ml (0.9% NaCl, LR, D$_5$W); infuse over ≥30 min
• Discard unused portion
Intermittent IV infusion route
• Visually inspect for particulate
• Ibuprofen lysine: dilute with dextrose or saline to appropriate volume (10 mg/ml of ibuprofen is recommended) given within 30 min of preparation: give via port that is nearest insertion site; give over 15 min
• Check for extravasation; do not give in same line with TPN, interrupt TPN for 15 min before and after product administration

Patient/family education
• Teach patient to use sunscreen, sunglasses, and protective clothing to prevent photosensitivity, photophobia
• Advise patient to read label on other OTC products
• Inform patient that the therapeutic response takes 1 mo (arthritis)
• Teach patient to take with a full glass of water, sit upright for 30 min after use
• Caution patient to avoid alcohol ingestion, salicylates, NSAIDs; GI bleeding may occur
• Advise patient with allergies that allergic reactions may develop
• Advise patient to report use of this product to all health care providers
• **Nephrotoxicity:** advise to report change in urinary pattern, weight increase, edema, increased pain in joints, fever, blood in urine; monitor fluid status, BUN, creatinine
• Teach patient to avoid driving or other hazardous activities until effect is known

> **BLACK BOX WARNING:** MI/stroke: Teach patient to report signs/symptoms of MI/stroke immediately and discontinue product, seek emergency medical treatment

• **Pregnancy:** notify prescriber if pregnancy is planned or suspected; avoid during third trimester

Evaluation
Positive therapeutic outcome
• Decreased pain

- Decreased inflammation
- Decreased fever
- Increased mobility

TREATMENT OF OVERDOSE:
Lavage, induce diuresis

RARELY USED

idarucizumab
(eye-da-roo-siz'ue-mab)
Praxbind
Func. class.: Antidote

USES: For dabigatran reversal during emergency surgery, urgent procedures, or for life-threatening or uncontrolled bleeding

CONTRAINDICATIONS: Hypersensitivity

DOSAGE AND ROUTES
Adults IV 5 g once

⚠ HIGH ALERT

ifosfamide (Rx)
(i-foss'fa-mide)
Ifex
Func. class.: Antineoplastic alkylating agent
Chem. class.: Nitrogen mustard

Do not confuse: ifosfamide/cyclophosphamide

ACTION: Alkylates DNA, RNA; inhibits enzymes that allow synthesis of amino acids in proteins; also responsible for cross-linking DNA strands; activity is not cell cycle stage-specific

Therapeutic outcome: Prevention of rapidly growing malignant cells

USES: Germ cell testicular cancer in combination

Pharmacokinetics

Absorption	Complete
Distribution	Saturation at high dosages
Metabolism	Liver
Excretion	Breast milk
Half-life	15 hr, depends on dose

Pharmacodynamics

Onset	Unknown
Peak	1-2 wk
Duration	3 wk

CONTRAINDICATIONS
Pregnancy, hypersensitivity

BLACK BOX WARNING: Bone marrow suppression

Precautions: Renal/hepatic disease, breastfeeding, children, accidental exposure, dehydration, dental disease, infection, IM injection, ocular exposure, varicella

---

BLACK BOX WARNING: Coma, hemorrhagic cystitis

DOSAGE AND ROUTES
Germ Cell Testicular Cancer
Adult: IV 1.2-2 g/m^2/day × 5 days; repeat course q3wk; give with mesna, in combination with 1-2 other antineoplastic agents

Renal dose
Adult: IV CCr 31-60 ml/min give 75% of dose; CCr 10-30 ml/min give 50% of dose; CCr <10 ml/min, do not give

Available forms: Inj 1, 3 g vials

ADVERSE EFFECTS
CNS: Facial paresthesia, fever, malaise, somnolence, confusion, depression, hallucinations, dizziness, disorientation, seizures, coma, cranial nerve dysfunction, encephalopathy
GI: Nausea, vomiting, anorexia, hepatotoxicity, stomatitis, constipation, diarrhea, dyslipidemia, hyperglycemia
GU: Hematuria, nephrotoxicity, hemorrhagic cystitis, dysuria, urinary frequency, retrograde ejaculation
HEMA: Thrombocytopenia, leukopenia, anemia
INTEG: Dermatitis, alopecia, pain at inj site, hyperpigmentation
META: Metabolic acidosis

INTERACTIONS
Individual drugs
Allopurinol, phenobarbitol: increased toxicity
Radiation: increased bone marrow suppression

Drug classifications
Anticoagulants, NSAIDs, salicylates, thrombolytics: increased bleeding risk
Antineoplastics: increased bone marrow suppression
CYP3A4 inducers (barbiturates, carbamazepine, phenytoin, rifampin): increased toxicity
CYP3A4 inhibitors (fluconazole, ketoconazole, itraconazole): decreased ifosfamide effect
Live virus vaccines: decreased antibody response

Drug/food
Increased: levels of product, avoid with grapefruit juice

NURSING CONSIDERATIONS
Assessment

> **BLACK BOX WARNING: Bone Marrow Suppression:** Monitor CBC, differential, platelet count weekly; withhold product if WBC is <2000 mm^3 or platelet count is <50,000; notify prescriber of results if WBC <10,000/mm^3, platelets <100,000/mm^3, severe myelosuppression; nadir of leukopenia/thrombocytopenia 7-14 days, recovery 21 days; assess for bleeding: hematuria, guaiac, bruising or petechiae, mucosa or orifices; no rect temp, avoid IM injections

• Monitor renal function studies: BUN, serum uric acid, urine CCr before, during therapy; I&O ratio; report fall in urine output of 30 ml/hr
• Monitor for cold, fever, sore throat (may indicate beginning of infection); identify edema in feet and joints, stomach pain, shaking; prescriber should be notified
• Monitor B/P, pulse respirations baseline and periodically during treatment

> **BLACK BOX WARNING: Hemorrhagic cystitis:** I&O ratio; monitor for hematuria; hemorrhagic cystitis can occur; increase fluids to 3 L/day; urinalysis prior to each dose; do not give at night, given with mesna to prevent this condition

• Monitor liver function tests before, during therapy (ALT, AST, LDH); jaundice of skin, sclera, dark urine, clay-colored stools, itching, abdominal pain, fever, diarrhea that may indicate liver involvement

> **BLACK BOX WARNING: Neurotoxicity:** Assess for neurologic symptoms: Hallucinations, confusion, disorientation, coma; product should be discontinued; usually resolves within 3-4 days

• **Pregnancy/breastfeeding:** Do not use in pregnancy, breastfeeding

Patient problem
Risk for injury (adverse reactions)

Implementation
• Administer antiemetic 30-60 min before product to prevent vomiting
• Visually inspect parenteral products for particulate matter and discoloration prior to use
• Store powder at room temperature

Intermittent/continuous IV infusion route
• Give as an intermittent infusion or continuous infusion
• Well hydrate with at least 2 L/day of oral or IV fluids; should be given to prevent bladder toxicity
• Must be given in combination with mesna to prevent hemorrhagic cystitis
• Close hematologic monitoring is recommended. WBC count, platelet count, and hemoglobin should be obtained prior to each use and periodically thereafter
• A urinalysis should be performed prior to each dose to monitor for hematuria

Reconstitution and further dilution
• Reconstitute 1 or 3 g with 20 or 60 ml, respectively, of sterile water for injection or bacteriostatic water for injection containing parabens or benzyl alcohol to give IV solutions containing 50 mg/ml
• Solutions may be diluted further to achieve concentrations of 0.6-20 mg/ml in the following solutions: D$_5$W, NS, LR
• Infuse slowly over at least 30 min
• Diluted and reconstituted solutions refrigerated and used within 24 hours

Y-site compatibilities: Acyclovir, Alatrofloxacin, alemtuzumab, alfentanil, allopurinol, Amifostine, amikacin, Aminocaproic acid, aminophylline, amiodarone, amphotericin B cholesteryl (Amphotec), amphotericin B conventional colloidal, amphotericin B lipid complex (Abelcet), amphotericin B liposome (AmBisome), ampicillin, ampicillin-sulbactam, anidulafungin, argatroban, Arsenic trioxide, atenolol, Atracurium, azithromycin, Aztreonam, bivalirudin, bleomycin, bumetanide, buprenorphine, Butorphanol, Calcium chloride/gluconate, CARBOplatin, Caspofungin, ceFAZolin, Cefoperazone, cefotaxime, cefoTEtan, cefOXitin, cefTAZidime, cefTAZidime (L-arginine), ceftizoxime, cefTRIAXone, cefuroxime, chlorproMAZINE, cimetidine, ciprofloxacin, cisatracurium, CISplatin, clindamycin, codeine, cycloSPORINE, cytarabine, DACTINomycin, DAPTOmycin, DAUNOrubicin liposome, dexamethasone phosphate, dexmedetomidine, Dexrazoxane, digoxin, diltiazem, diphenhydrAMINE, DOBUTamine, DOCEtaxel, dolasetron, DOPamine, doripenem, Doxacurium, DOXOrubicin, DOXOrubicin liposomal, doxycycline, droperidol, enalaprilat, Ephedrine, EPINEPHrine, epirubicin, ertapenem, erythromycin, esmolol, etoposide, etoposide phosphate, famotidine, fenoldopam, fentaNYL, filgrastim, fluconazole, Fludarabine, fluorouracil, foscarnet, fosphenytoin, furosemide, Gallium nitrate, ganciclovir, gatifloxacin, gemcitabine, Gemtuzumab, gentamicin, granisetron, haloperidol, heparin, hydrocortisone phosphate/succinate,

HYDROmorphone, hydrOXYzine, IDArubicin, imipenem-cilastatin, inamrinone, insulin, regular, Isoproterenol, ketorolac, labetalol, lansoprazole, lepirudin, leucovorin, levofloxacin, Levorphanol, lidocaine, linezolid, LORazepam, magnesium sulfate, mannitol, melphalan, meperidine, meropenem, Mesna, Methohexital, methylPREDNISolone, metoclopramide, metoprolol, metroNIDAZOLE, midazolam, milrinone, minocycline, mitoMYcin, mitoXANtrone, Mivacurium, morphine, moxifloxacin, Nalbuphine, naloxone, nesiritide, niCARdipine, nitroglycerin, nitroprusside, norepinephrine, octreotide, ofloxacin, ondansetron, oxaliplatin, PAClitaxel (solvent/surfactant), palonosetron, pamidronate, pancuronium, PEMEtrexed, pentamidine, PENTobarbital, Phenobarbital, phenylephrine, piperacillin, piperacillin-tazobactam, potassium acetate/chloride, procainamide, prochlorperazine, promethazine, propofol, propranolol, Quinupristin-Dalfopristin, ranitidine, Rapacuronium, remifentanil, riTUXimab, rocuronium, sargramostim, sodium acetate/bicarbonate/phosphates, succinylcholine, Sufentanil, sulfamethoxazole-trimethoprim, tacrolimus, Teniposide, theophylline, Thiopental, Thiotepa, ticarcillin, ticarcillin-clavulanate, tigecycline, tirofiban, TNA (3-in-1), tobramycin, topotecan, TPN (2-in-1), trastuzumab, vancomycin, vasopressin, vecuronium, verapamil, vinBLAStine, vinCRIStine, vinorelbine, voriconazole, zidovudine, zoledronic acid

Additive compatibilities: CARBOplatin, CISplatin, epirubicin, etoposide, fluorouracil, mesna

Patient/family education
• Bleeding: teach patient to avoid use of products containing aspirin or NSAIDs, razors, commercial mouthwash, since bleeding may occur; to report symptoms of bleeding (hematuria, tarry stools)
• Instruct patient to report signs of anemia (fatigue, headache, irritability, faintness, shortness of breath)
• Advise patient to report any changes in breathing or coughing even several mo after treatment; to avoid crowds and persons with respiratory tract or other infections
• Teach patient that hair loss is common; discuss the use of wigs or hairpieces; that hair may be a different texture when regrowth occurs
• Caution patient not to have any live virus vaccinations without the advice of the prescriber; serious reactions can occur for 3 months–1 yr, to discuss encephalopathy, neurotoxicity

• Advise patient to report confusion, hallucinations, extreme drowsiness, numbness, tingling; avoid use of alcohol for ≥4 months after treatment
• Teach patient to avoid driving, hazardous activities until reaction is known

> **BLACK BOX WARNING:** Instruct patient to drink extra fluids in order to urinate often to prevent hemorrhagic cystitis, to report pink or red urine

• Teach patient to notify prescriber if pregnancy is planned or suspected; advise patient that contraception is needed during treatment and for several mo after completion of therapy

Evaluation
Positive therapeutic outcome
• Prevention of rapid division of malignant cells

iloperidone (Rx)
(ill-o-pehr′ih-dohn)
Fanapt
Func. class.: Antipsychotic; second-generation atypical: benzisoxazole derivative

Do not confuse: Fanapt/Xanax

ACTION: Unknown; may be mediated through both dopamine type 2 (D_2) and serotonin type 2 (5-HT_2) antagonism; high receptor binding affinity for norepinephrine (alpha 1)

Therapeutic outcome: Decreased signs/symptoms of schizophrenia

USES: Schizophrenia ⚕⚕

Pharmacokinetics
Absorption	Well
Distribution	Unknown, protein binding 95%
Metabolism	Extensively, liver (major metabolite) ⚕⚕ CYP2D6, CYP3A4
Excretion	Urine, feces
Half-life	18 hr extensive, feces metabolizers; 33 hr poor metabolizers

Pharmacodynamics
Onset	Unknown
Peak	2-4 hr
Duration	Unknown

CONTRAINDICATIONS
Breastfeeding, hypersensitivity

Precautions: Pregnancy, children, geriatric patients, renal/hepatic disease, breast cancer, Parkinson's disease, dementia with Lewy bodies, seizure disorder, QT prolongation, bundle branch block, acute MI, ambient temperature increase, AV block, stroke, substance abuse, suicidal ideation, tardive dyskinesia, torsades de pointes, blood dyscrasias, dysphagia

> **BLACK BOX WARNING:** Increased mortality in elderly patients with dementia-related psychosis

DOSAGE AND ROUTES
Adult: PO 1 mg bid, may increase to target dose of 6-12 mg bid with daily dose adjustment of max 2 mg bid; titrate slowly; max 24 mg/day in two divided doses; reduce dose by 50% in poor metabolizer of CYP2D6 or when used with strong CYP2D6/CYP3A4 inhibitors

Available forms: Tabs 1, 2, 4, 6, 8, 10, 12 mg; titration pack

ADVERSE EFFECTS
CNS: *EPS, pseudoparkinsonism, akathisia, dystonia, tardive dyskinesia; drowsiness,* seizures, neuroleptic malignant syndrome, dizziness, delirium, depression, paranoia, tremor, drowsiness
CV: Orthostatic hypotension, QT prolongation, tachycardia
EENT: Blurred vision, nasal congestion
GI: *Nausea,* vomiting, *anorexia, constipation,* jaundice, weight gain/loss, abdominal pain, stomatitis, xerostomia, dry mouth
GU: Urinary retention/incontinence, priapism
HEMA: Agranulocytosis, leukopenia, neutropenia
ENDO: Hyperglycemia
MS: Decreased bone density
SYST: Anaphylaxis, angioedema

INTERACTIONS
Individual drugs
Alcohol: increased sedation
Chloroquine, clarithromycin, droperidol, erythromycin, haloperidol, methadone, pentamidine: increased QT prolongation

Drug classifications
CYP2D6, CYP3A4 inducers (carBAMazepine, barbiturates, phenytoins, rifampin): iloperidone action
CYP2D6 (fluoxetine, paroxetine), CYP3A4 inhibitors (delavirdine, indinavir, itraconazole, dalfopristin, ritonavir, tipranavir): increased iloperidone effect, decreased clearance, reduce dose

Class IA/ III antidysrhythmics, some phenothiazines, β-agonists, local anesthetics, tricyclics: increased QT prolongation
Other CNS depressants: increased sedation

Drug/lab test
Increased: prolactin levels, cholesterol, glucose, lipids, triglycerides
Decreased: potassium

NURSING CONSIDERATIONS
Assessment
• Assess AIMS assessment, lipid panel, blood glucose, CBC, glycosylated hemoglobin A1C, LFTs, neurologic function, pregnancy test, serum creatinine, electrolytes, prolactin, thyroid function studies, weight; fasting blood sugar baseline, periodically in diabetic patients
• Assess affect, orientation, LOC, reflexes, gait, coordination, sleep pattern disturbances
• Monitor B/P standing and lying; also pulse, respirations; take these often during initial treatment; establish baseline before starting treatment; report drops of 30 mm Hg; watch for ECG changes; QT prolongation may occur
• Monitor that patient swallows the medication
• Assess for dizziness, faintness, palpitations, tachycardia on rising
• **Assess for EPS,** including akathisia, tardive dyskinesia (bizarre movements of the jaw, mouth, tongue, extremities), pseudoparkinsonism (rigidity, tremors, pill rolling, shuffling gait)

> **BLACK BOX WARNING:** Assess for serious reactions in the geriatric patient: fatal pneumonia, heart failure, sudden death, not to be used in the elderly with dementia

• **Assess for neuroleptic malignant syndrome:** hyperthermia, increased CPK, altered mental status, muscle rigidity, seizures, diaphoresis, discontinue immediately, notify prescriber
• Assess for constipation, urinary retention daily; if these occur, increase bulk and water in diet
• Monitor weight gain, BMI, waist circumference, hyperglycemia, metabolic changes in diabetes
• **Beers:** Avoid in older adults except for schizophrenia, bipolar disorder, or short-term use as an antiemetic during chemotherapy; increased risk of stroke
• **Pregnancy/breastfeeding:** Use only if benefits outweigh fetal risk, infant exposed to product during third trimester may exhibit extrapyramidal symptoms; do not breastfeed, excretion unknown
• Advise patient to take as prescribed, not to sip or double doses; if medication is missed >3 days, start as initial dose

Patient problem
Distorted thinking process (uses)
Risk for injury (adverse reactions)

Implementation
• Give reduced dose in geriatric patients
• Give anticholinergic agent on order from prescriber, to be used for EPS
• Avoid use with CNS depressants
• Provide decreased stimulus by dimming lights, avoiding loud noises
• Provide supervised ambulation until patient is stabilized on medication; do not involve in strenuous exercise program because fainting is possible; patient should not stand still for a long time
• Give increased fluids to prevent constipation
• Provide sips of water, candy, gum for dry mouth
• Store in tight, light-resistant container (PO); store unopened vials in refrigerator; protect from light; do not freeze

Patient/family education
• Teach that orthostatic hypotension may occur and to rise from sitting or lying position gradually
• Advise to avoid hot tubs, hot showers, tub baths; hypotension may occur
• Teach to avoid abrupt withdrawal of this product; EPS may result; product should be withdrawn slowly; to review symptoms of neuroleptic malignant syndrome
• Teach to avoid OTC preparations (cough, hay fever, cold, herbals, supplements) unless approved by prescriber; serious product interactions may occur; avoid use of alcohol; increased drowsiness may occur
• Advise to avoid hazardous activities if drowsiness or dizziness occurs
• Teach to report impaired vision, tremors, muscle twitching
• Advise patient that continuing follow-up exams will be needed
• Advise to use contraception; inform prescriber if pregnancy is planned or suspected, if pregnant should enroll in the Atypical Antipsychotic National Pregnancy Registry (1-866-961-2388)
• Advise patient to use gum, lozenges for dry mouth

Evaluation

Positive therapeutic outcome
• Decrease in emotional excitement, hallucinations, delusions, paranoia; reorganization of patterns of thought, speech

TREATMENT OF OVERDOSE:
Lavage if orally ingested; provide airway; *do not induce vomiting*

⚠ HIGH ALERT

imatinib (Rx)
(im-ah-tin′ib)
Gleevec
Func. class.: Antineoplastic—miscellaneous
Chem. class.: Protein-tyrosine kinase inhibitor

ACTION: Inhibits Bcr-Abl tyrosine kinase created in chronic myeloid leukemia (CML), also inhibits tyrosine kinases including EGF, FGF, PDGF, SCF, VEGF, NGF

Therapeutic outcome: Decreased tumor size, prevention of spread of cancer

USES: Treatment of chronic myeloid leukemia (CML), Philadelphia chromosome positive in blast cell crisis or chronic failure; gastrointestinal stromal tumors (GIST), positive for C-KIT; chronic eosinophilic leukemia, Philadelphia chromosome positive (PH+), acute lymphocytic leukemia, dermatofibrosarcoma protuberans, myelodysplastic syndrome, systemic mastocytosis

Pharmacokinetics

Absorption	Well absorbed; bound to plasma protein (98%)
Distribution	Unknown
Metabolism	Liver (metabolites) by CYP3A4
Excretion	Feces, primarily (metabolites)
Half-life	18-40 hr

Pharmacodynamics

Onset	Unknown
Peak	2-4 hr
Duration	24 hr (imatinib), 40 hr (metabolite)

CONTRAINDICATIONS
Pregnancy, hypersensitivity

Precautions: Breastfeeding, children, geriatric, cardiac/renal/hepatic/dental disease, GI bleeding, bone marrow suppression, infection, thrombocytopenia, neutropenia, immunosuppression

DOSAGE AND ROUTES
Chronic myelogenous leukemia (CML)
Adult: PO (chronic phase) 400 mg/day; may increase to 600 mg/day; accelerated phase/blast crisis 600 mg q day, may increase to 800 mg q day divided bid

---

Adolescent/child >2 yr: PO 340 mg/m²/day, max 600 mg/day

Ph+ acute lymphocytic leukemia (ALL)
Adult: PO 600 mg/day, continue as long as is beneficial

Child: PO 340 mg/m² q day, max 600 mg

GIST
Adult: PO 400-600 mg/day, may increase to 400 mg bid

Adjuvant treatment GIST after complete gross resection
Adult: PO 400 mg/day

Hypereosinophilic syndrome (HES) and/or chronic eosinophilic leukemia (CEL)
Adult: PO 400 mg/day in those who are FIPL1L-PDGFR alpha fusion kinase negative or unknown; for HES/CEL patients with demonstrated FIP1L1-PDGFR alpha fusion kinase, 100 mg/day, may increase to 400 mg

Myelodysplastic syndrome (MDS)/myeloproliferative disease (MPD)
Adult: PO 400 mg/day

Aggressive systemic mastocytosis (ASM)
Adult: PO 400 mg/day

Dermatofibrosarcoma protuberans (DFSP)
Adult: PO 400 mg bid (800 mg/day)

Hepatic dose
Adult: PO total bilirubin 1.5-3 × ULN and any AST, decrease initial dose to 400 mg/day; total bilirubin >3 × ULN and any AST, decrease initial dose to 300 mg/day

Renal dose
Adult: PO CCr 40-59 ml/min, max 600 mg/day; CCr 20-39 ml/min decrease initial dose by 50%, max 400 mg/day; CCr <20 ml/min use with caution 100 mg/day

Available forms: Tabs 100, 400 mg

ADVERSE EFFECTS
CNS: Headache, dizziness, insomnia, subdural hematoma
CV: Heart failure, cardiac toxicity
EENT: Blurred vision
GI: *Nausea*, hepatotoxicity, *vomiting, dyspepsia, anorexia*, abdominal pain, GI perforation, diarrhea
HEMA: Neutropenia, thrombocytopenia, bleeding

INTEG: *Rash, pruritus,* alopecia, photosensitivity, drug rash with eosinophilia and systemic symptoms (DRESS)
META: Edema, fluid retention, hypokalemia
MISC: Fatigue, epistaxis, pyrexia, night sweats, increased weight, flulike symptoms, hypothyroidism, tumor lysis syndrome
MS: Cramps, pain, arthralgia, myalgia
RESP: Cough, dyspnea, nasopharyngitis, pneumonia

INTERACTIONS
Individual drugs
Simvastatin: increased plasma concentrations of simvastatin
Warfarin: increased plasma concentration of warfarin; avoid coadministration; use low-molecular-weight anticoagulants instead

Drug classifications
Calcium channel blockers, ergots: increased plasma concentrations
CYP3A4 inducers (carBAMazepine, dexamethasone, PHENobarbital, phenytoin, rifampin): decreased imatinib concentrations
CYP3A4 inhibitors (clarithromycin, erythromycin, ketoconazole, itraconazole): increased imatinib concentrations

Drug/herb
St. John's wort: decreased imatinib concentration

Drug/food
Increased effect: grapefruit juice, avoid use

Drug/lab test
Increased: bilirubin, amylase, LFTs
Decreased: albumin, calcium, potassium, sodium, phosphate, platelets, neutrophils, leukocytes, lymphocytes

NURSING CONSIDERATIONS
Assessment
• **Bone marrow suppression:** Assess ANC and platelets; in chronic phase if ANC <1 × 10⁹/L and/or platelets <50 × 10⁹/L, stop until ANC >1.5 × 10⁹/L and platelets >75 × 10⁹/L; in accelerated phase/blast crisis if ANC <0.5 × 10⁹/L and/or platelets <10 × 10⁹/L, determine whether cytopenia is related to biopsy/aspirate; if not, reduce dose by 200 mg; if cytopenia continues, reduce dose by another 100 mg; if cytopenia continues for 4 wk, stop product until ANC ≥1 × 10⁹/L
DRESS: Assess for rash, swelling of face, fever; later hepatitis, myocarditis may occur; discontinue if present
• **Assess for hepatotoxicity:** monitor liver function tests before treatment, and qmo, if

liver transaminases are >5 × IULN, with-hold imatinib until transaminase levels return to <2.5 × IULN
- **Renal toxicity:** monitor bilirubin, if >3 × IULN, withhold imatinib until bilirubin levels return to <1.5 × IULN
- Assess GI symptoms: frequency of stools
- Assess signs of fluid retention, edema: weigh, monitor lung sounds, 50-ml fluid retention is dose dependent
- Monitor CBC for first month, biweekly next month, and periodically thereafter; neutropenia (2-3 wk), thrombocytopenia (3-4 wk) and anemia may occur, may need dosage decrease or discontinuation

Patient problem
Risk for infection (adverse reactions)
Risk for injury (adverse reactions)

Implementation
PO route
- Give with meal and large glass of water to decrease GI symptoms, doses of 800 mg should be given 400 mg bid
- Tab may be dispersed in a glass of water or apple juice, use 50 ml of liquid for 100 mg tab, 200 ml/400 mg
- Store at 25° C (77° F)
- Continue as long as is beneficial
- Use low-molecular weight or heparin for anticoagulant if needed

Patient/family education
- **Instruct patient to report adverse reactions immediately:** shortness of breath, swelling of extremities, bleeding
- Teach patient reason for treatment, expected result
- Instruct patient to eat a nutritious diet with iron, vit supplement, low fiber, few dairy products
- Teach patient not to stop or change dose; to avoid hazardous activities until response is known, dizziness may occur
- **Pregnancy/breastfeeding:** Do not use in pregnancy, breastfeeding; teach patient to notify prescriber if pregnancy is planned or suspected; use effective contraception; do not breastfeed
- Teach patient to take with food and water; for those unable to swallow tabs, to mix in liquid (30 ml for 100 mg or 200 ml for 400 mg); after dissolved, stir and consume, avoid grapefruit juice
- Advise patient to avoid OTC products unless approved by prescriber

Evaluation
Positive therapeutic outcome
- Decrease in leukemic cells, size of tumors

imipenem/cilastatin (Rx)
(i-me-pen'em sye-la-stat'in)
Primaxin IM, Primaxin IV
Func. class.: Antiinfective, miscellaneous penicillin
Chem. class.: Carbapenem

ACTION: Interferes with cell wall replication of susceptible organisms; osmotically unstable cell wall swells and bursts from osmotic pressure; addition of cilastatin prevents renal inactivation that occurs with high urinary concentrations of imipenem

Therapeutic outcome: Bactericidal action against the following: *Streptococcus pneumoniae*, group A β-hemolytic streptococci, *Staphylococcus aureus*, enterococcus; gram-negative organisms: *Klebsiella, Proteus, Escherichia coli, Acinetobacter, Serratia, Pseudomonas aeruginosa; Salmonella, Shigella, Haemophilus influenzae, Listeria* spp.

USES: Serious infections caused by gram-positive or gram-negative organisms

Pharmacokinetics
Absorption	Complete (**IV**)
Distribution	Widely distributed; crosses placenta
Metabolism	Liver
Excretion	Kidneys, unchanged (70%-80%); breast milk
Half-life	1 hr; increased in renal disease

Pharmacodynamics
	IM	IV
Onset	Unknown	Rapid
Peak	1-2 hr	20 min-1 hr
Duration	12 hr	6-8 hr

CONTRAINDICATIONS
Hypersensitivity, IM hypersensitivity to local anesthetics of the amide type, or carbapenems, AV block, shock (IM)

Precautions: Pregnancy, breastfeeding, children, geriatric, hypersensitivity to cephalosporins, penicillins, seizure disorders, renal disease, head trauma, pseudomembranous colitis, ulcerative colitis, diabetes mellitus

DOSAGE AND ROUTES
Doses based on imipenem content
Most infections
Adult ≥70 kg: IV 250 mg q6hr (mild infections); 500 mg q6-8hr (moderate infections); 500 mg q6hr (severe life-threatening infections)

Adult 60-<70 kg: IV 250 mg q8hr (mild infections); 250 mg q6hr (moderate or severe life-threatening infections)

Adult 50-<60 kg: IV 125 mg q6hr (mild infections) 250 mg q6hr (moderate or severe life-threatening infections)

Adult 40-<50 kg: IV 125 mg q6hr (mild infections); 250 mg q6-8hr (moderate infections); 250 mg q6hr (severe life-threatening infections)

Adult 30-<40 kg: IV 125 mg q8hr (mild infections); 125 mg q6hr or 250 mg q8hr (moderate infections); 250 mg q8hr (severe life-threatening infections)

Adolescent/child/infant ≥3 mo: IV 15-25 mg/kg q6hr

Infant 1-3 mo weighing ≥1500 g: IV 25 mg/kg q6hr

Neonate 1-4 wk weighing ≥1500 g: IV 25 mg/kg q8hr

Neonate <7 days weighing ≥1500 g: IV 25 mg/kg q12hr

Imipenem renal dose
Adults 70 kg or more: IV If 70-kg dose is 1 g/day, reduce dose to: CCr 41 to 70 ml/min/1.73 m^2: 250 mg q 8 hr; CCr 6 to 40 ml/min/1.73 m^2: 250 mg q 12 hr; CCr 5 ml/min/1.73 m^2 or less: do not use unless hemodialysis is instituted within 48 hr; If 70-kg dose is 1.5 g/day reduce dose to: CCr 41 to 70 m/min/1.73 m^2: 250 mg q 6 hr; CCr 21 to 40 ml/min/1.73 m^2: 250 mg q 8 hr; CCr 6 to 20 ml/min/1.73 m^2: 250 mg q 12 hr; CCr 5 ml/min/1.73 m^2 or less: do not use unless hemodialysis is instituted within 48 hr; If 70-kg dose is 2 g/day, reduce dose to: CCr 41 to 70 ml/min/1.73 m^2: 500 mg q 8 hr; CCr 21 to 40 ml/min/1.73 m^2: 250 mg q 6 hr; CCr 6 to 20 ml/min/1.73 m^2: 250 mg q 12 hr; CCr 5 ml/min/1.73 m^2 or less: do not use unless hemodialysis is instituted within 48 hr; If 70-kg dose is 3 g/day, reduce dose to: CCr 41 to 70 ml/min/1.73 m^2: 500 mg q 6 hr; CCr 21 to 40 ml/min/1.73 m^2: 500 mg q 8 hr; CCr 6 to 20 ml/min/1.73 m^2: 500 mg q 12 hr; CCr 5 ml/min/1.73 m^2 or less: do not use unless hemodialysis is instituted within 48 hr; If 70-kg dose is 4 g/day, reduce dose to: CCr 41 to 70 ml/min/1.73 m^2: 750 mg q 8 hr; CCr 21 to 40 ml/min/1.73 m^2: 500 mg q 6 hr; CCr 6 to 20 ml/min/1.73 m^2: 500 mg q 12 hr;

CCr 5 ml/min/1.73 m^2 or less: do not use unless hemodialysis is instituted within 48 hr

Available forms: Powder for inj sol 250, 500; powder for inj susp 500, 750 mg

ADVERSE EFFECTS
CNS: Fever, somnolence, seizures, confusion, dizziness, weakness, myoclonus, drowsiness
CV: Hypotension, palpitations, tachycardia
GI: *Diarrhea, nausea, vomiting, Clostridium difficile*–associated diarrhea (CDAD), hepatitis, glossitis, gastroenteritis, abdominal pain, jaundice
HEMA: Eosinophilia
INTEG: Rash, urticaria, pruritus, pain at inj site, phlebitis, erythema at inj site, erythema multiforme
MISC: Hearing loss, tinnitus
SYST: Anaphylaxis, Stevens-Johnson syndrome, toxic epidermal necrolysis, angioedema

INTERACTIONS
Individual drugs
Aminophylline, cycloSPORINE, ganciclovir, theophylline: increased risk of seizures
Probenecid: increased imipenem plasma levels
Valproic acid: decreased effect of valproic acid

Drug classifications
Aminoglycosides: inactivation if admixed

Drug/lab test
Increased: AST, ALT, LDH, BUN, alkaline phosphatase, bilirubin, creatinine, potassium, chloride
Decreased: sodium
False positive: direct Coombs' test

NURSING CONSIDERATIONS
Assessment
• Assess patient for previous penicillin sensitivity reaction or sensitivity to other β-lactams, may have sensitivity to this product
• **Assess patient for signs and symptoms of infection,** including characteristics of wounds, sputum, urine, stool, WBC $>10,000/$ mm^3, fever; obtain baseline information before, during treatment
• Complete C&S tests before beginning product therapy to identify if correct treatment has been initiated, may start before results are recieved
• **Seizures:** Product decreases seizure threshold and may decrease effectiveness of seizure medications, monitor closely
• **Assess for allergic reactions, anaphylaxis:** rash, urticaria, pruritus, chills, wheezing, laryngeal edema, fever, joint pain; angioedema

---

may occur a few days after therapy begins; epiNEPHrine, resuscitation equipment should be available for anaphylactic reaction
• Monitor blood studies: AST, ALT, CBC, Hct, bilirubin, LDH, alkaline phosphatase, Coombs' test monthly if patient is on long-term therapy
• Monitor electrolytes: potassium, sodium, chloride monthly if patient is on long-term therapy
• CDAD: Assess bowel pattern daily; if severe diarrhea occurs, product should be discontinued
• **Monitor for bleeding:** ecchymosis, bleeding gums, hematuria, stool guaiac daily if patient is on long-term therapy
• Assess for overgrowth of infection: perineal itching, fever, malaise, redness, pain, swelling, drainage, rash, diarrhea, change in cough, sputum
• **Pregnancy/breastfeeding:** Use only if benefits outweigh fetal risk, cautious use in breastfeeding, excretion unknown

Patient problem
Infection (uses)

Implementation
IM route
• Reconstitute 500 mg/2 ml lidocaine without epiNEPHrine; shake well, withdraw and administer entire vial; give inj deep in large muscle mass, aspirate, product for IM is not for IV use

Intermittent IV infusion route
• Only IV form is for IV use
• Reconstitute each 250 or 500 mg/10 ml of compatible diluent; shake well; transfer the resulting susp to ≥100 ml of compatible diluent; add 10 ml to each previously reconstituted vial and shake to ensure all medication is used; transfer the remaining contents of the vial to the inf container; do not administer susp by direct inj
• Give each 250- or 500-mg dose over 20-30 min, and each 1-g dose over 40-60 min; administer over 15-20 min for pediatric patients; do not administer direct **IV**; do not admix with other antibiotics, separate ≥1 hr (aminoglycosides)

Y-site compatibilities: Acyclovir, alfentanil, amifostine, amikacin, aminocaproic acid, anidulafungin, argatroban, ascorbic acid, atenolol, atracurium, atropine, benztropine, bivalirudin, bleomycin, bumetanide, buprenorphine, butorphanol, CARBOplatin, caspofungin, ceFAZolin, cefotaxime, cefoTEtan, cefOXitin, cefTAZidime, ceftizone, cefuroxime, chloramphenicol, cimetidine, CISplatin, clindamycin, codeine, cyanocobalamin, cyclophosphamide, cycloSPORINE, cytarabine, DACTINomycin, dexamethasone, dexrazoxane, digoxin, diltiazem,

diphenhydrAMINE, DOCEtaxel, dolasetron, DOPamine, doxacurium, DOXOrubicin, DOXOrubicin liposomal, doxycycline, enalaprilat, famotidine, fludarabine, foscarnet, granisetron, IDArubicin, regular insulin, melphalan, methotrexate, ondansetron, propofol, tacrolimus, teniposide, thiotepa, vinorelbine, zidovudine

Patient/family education
• Advise patient to contact prescriber if vaginal itching, loose foul-smelling stools, furry tongue occur; may indicate superinfection
• CDAD: advise patient to notify prescriber of diarrhea with blood or pus
• Instruct patient to report seizures immediately

Evaluation
Positive therapeutic outcome
• Absence of signs/symptoms of infection (WBC <10,000/mm^3, temp WNL, absence of red, draining wounds)
• Reported improvement in symptoms of infection

Treatment of anaphylaxis: EPINEPHrine, antihistamines, resuscitate if needed

imipramine (Rx)
(im-ip'ra-meen)
Impril ✦, Tofranil, Tofranil PM
Func. class.: Antidepressant, tricyclic
Chem. class.: Dibenzazepine, tertiary amine

Do not confuse: imipramine/desipramine

ACTION: ✎ Blocks reuptake of norepinephrine and serotonin into nerve endings, increasing action of norepinephrine and serotonin in nerve cells; has anticholinergic effects

Therapeutic outcome: Decreased symptoms of depression after 2-3 wk; decreased bedwetting in children

USES: Depression, enuresis in children

Unlabeled uses: Chronic pain, migraine headaches, cluster headaches as adjunct, incontinence

Pharmacokinetics	
Absorption	Well absorbed
Distribution	Widely distributed; crosses placenta, protein binding 90%-95%
Metabolism	Liver by ✎ CYP2D6, extensively
Excretion	Kidneys, breast milk
Half-life	8-16 hr

Pharmacodynamics

	PO
Onset	1 hr
Peak	Unknown
Duration	Unknown

CONTRAINDICATIONS

Pregnancy, hypersensitivity to this product or carBAMazepine; acute MI

Precautions: Suicidal patients, severe depression, increased intraocular pressure, closed-angle glaucoma, urinary retention, cardiac/hepatic disease, hyperthyroidism, electroshock therapy, elective surgery, breastfeeding, geriatric, seizure disorders, prostatic hypertrophy, MI, hypersensitivity to tricyclics, AV block, bundle-branch block, ileus, QT prolongation

> **BLACK BOX WARNING:** Children other than for enuresis; suicidal ideation

DOSAGE AND ROUTES
Depression
Adult: PO 75-100 mg/day in divided doses; may increase by 25-50 mg up to 200 mg, 200 mg/day (outpatients), 300 mg/day (inpatients); may give daily dose at bedtime

Geriatric: PO 25 mg at bedtime, may increase to 100 mg/day in divided doses

Child ≥6 yr (unlabeled): PO 1.5 mg/kg/day in divided doses; max 2.5 mg/kg/day

Enuresis
Child 6-12 yr: PO 25 mg at bedtime, max 50 mg

Available forms: Tabs 10, 25, 50, 75 ✦ mg; caps 75, 100, 125, 150 mg

ADVERSE EFFECTS

CNS: *Dizziness, drowsiness,* confusion, headache, anxiety, paresthesia, seizures, suicidal ideation

CV: *Orthostatic hypotension, ECG changes,* dysrhythmias

EENT: Blurred vision, tinnitus, mydriasis

ENDO: Hyperglycemia, hypothyroidism/hyperthyroidism

GI: *Diarrhea, dry mouth,* nausea, vomiting, paralytic ileus, increased appetite

GU: *Retention,* decreased libido

HEMA: Agranulocytosis, thrombocytopenia, eosinophilia, leukopenia

INTEG: Rash, urticaria, pruritus, photosensitivity

INTERACTIONS
Individual drugs
Alcohol: increased effects

Bupropion, cyclobenzaprine, trazadone, tramodil: Increased serotonin syndrome

CloNIDine: hyperpyretic crisis, seizures, hypertensive episode

CloNIDine, guanethidine: decreased effects

Gatifloxacin, levofloxacin, moxifloxacin, ziprasidone: increased QT interval

Drug classifications
MAOIs: hyperpyretic crisis, hypertensive episode, seizures

SSRIs, SNRIs, serotonin-receptor agonists, tricyclic antidepressants: increased serotonin syndrome, increased neuroleptic malignant syndrome; avoid concurrent use

Sympathomimetics (direct acting [EPINEPHrine]), barbiturates, benzodiazepines, CNS depressants: increased effects

Sympathomimetics (indirect acting [ePHEDrine]): decreased effects

Tricyclic antidepressants, class IA/III antidysrhythmics: increased QT interval

Drug/herb
Chamomile, kava, valerian: Increased sedation
St. John's wort: serotonin syndrome

Drug/lab test
Increased: serum bilirubin, blood glucose, alkaline phosphatase, LFTs

NURSING CONSIDERATIONS
Assessment
• **Depression:** Assess mood, behavior, sleep, meta status, lability, suicidal ideation; report changes

• **Enuresis:** Assess bedwetting frequency, stressors

• Monitor B/P (with patient lying, standing), pulse q4hr; if systolic B/P drops 20 mm Hg, hold product, notify prescriber; take vital signs q4hr in patients with CV disease

• Monitor blood studies: CBC, leukocytes, differential, cardiac enzymes if patient is receiving long-term therapy

• Monitor hepatic studies: AST, ALT, bilirubin

• Check weight weekly; appetite may increase with product

• **QT prolongation:** Assess ECG for flattening of T wave, bundle branch block, AV block, dysrhythmias in cardiac patients

• Assess for EPS primarily in geriatric: rigidity, dystonia, akathisia

> **BLACK BOX WARNING: Suicidal Ideation;** assess mental status: mood, sensorium, affect, suicidal tendencies especially in children, young adults; increase in psychiatric symptoms: depression, panic; monitoring should occur q wk for 1 mo, then q 3 wk; give in limited amounts

• Monitor urinary retention, constipation; constipation is more likely to occur in children or geriatric
• **Assess for withdrawal symptoms:** headache, nausea, vomiting, muscle pain, weakness, diarrhea, insomnia, restlessness; do not usually occur unless product was discontinued abruptly
• Identify alcohol consumption; if alcohol is consumed, hold dose until AM
• **Beers:** Avoid in older adults, highly anticholinergic, high risk of delirium

Patient problem
Depression (uses)
Impaired sexual functioning (adverse reaction)

Implementation
PO route
• Do not break, crush, or chew caps
• Give with food or milk to prevent GI upset
• Do not discontinue abruptly; taper 50% ×3 days, another 50% x3 days, then stop
• Give increased doses at bedtime to prevent sleepiness
• Store in tight container at room temp; do not freeze

Patient/family education

> **BLACK BOX WARNING:** Teach patient to report suicidal thoughts, behaviors immediately; more common in children, young adults

• Teach patient that therapeutic effects may take 2-3 wk
• Teach patient to use caution in driving and other activities requiring alertness because of drowsiness, dizziness, blurred vision; to avoid rising quickly from sitting position, especially geriatric; orthostatic hypotension may occur
• Teach patient to avoid alcohol ingestion, other CNS depressants during treatment, sedation may occur
• Teach patient not to discontinue medication quickly after long-term use: may cause nausea, headache, malaise
• Teach patient to wear sunscreen or large hat, since photosensitivity occurs
• Teach patient to increase fluids, bulk in diet if constipation, urinary retention occur, especially geriatric
• Teach patient to take gum, hard sugarless candy, frequent sips of water for dry mouth
• **Pregnancy/breastfeeding:** Identify if pregnancy is planned or suspected or if breastfeeding

Evaluation
Positive therapeutic outcome
• Decreased depression
• Absence of suicidal thoughts
• Decreased enuresis in children
• Decreased neurogenic pain

TREATMENT OF OVERDOSE:
ECG monitoring, lavage, administer anticonvulsant; sodium bicarbonate (cardiac effects), antidysrhythmias

---

indacaterol
(in-da-kat′er-ol)
Arcapta Neohaler, Onbrez Breezhal ER ✹
Func. class.: β₂-agonist, long-acting

ACTION: An agonist at β₂-receptors. Stimulation of β₂-receptors in the lung causes relaxation of bronchial smooth muscle, which produces bronchodilation and an increase in bronchial airflow. These effects may be mediated, in part, by increased activity of adenyl cyclase, an intracellular enzyme responsible for the formation of cyclic-3′,5′-adenosine monophosphate (cAMP); has >24 times greater agonist activity at β₂-receptors (primarily in the lung) than at β₁-receptors (primarily in the heart)

USES: Bronchitis, chronic obstructive pulmonary disease (COPD), emphysema

Pharmacokinetics

Absorption	Poor
Distribution	Widely, protein binding 94%-96%
Metabolism	By CYP3A4, CYP1A1, CYP2D6, UTG1A1
Excretion	54% (urine), 23% (feces)
Half-life	45.5-126 hrs

Pharmacodynamics

Onset	5 min
Peak	15 min
Duration	24 hr

CONTRAINDICATIONS
Acute bronchospasm, acute asthma attack, status asthmaticus, acute respiratory insufficiency, monotherapy of asthma

Precautions: Cardiac arrhythmias, congenital long QT syndrome, diabetes mellitus, hypertension, hyperthyroidism (thyrotoxicosis, thyroid disease), hypokalemia, ischemic cardiac disease (coronary artery disease), milk protein hypersensitivity, pheochromocytoma, QT prolongation, seizure disorder, severe hepatic disease, tachycardia, torsades de pointes history, unusual

---

responsiveness to other sympathomimetic amines; not indicated for neonates, infants, children, or adolescents under the age of 18 years, pregnancy, breastfeeding

> **BLACK BOX WARNING:** Asthma-related deaths

DOSAGE AND ROUTES
Adult: INH 75 mcg (contents of 1 capsule) inhaled once daily; max 1 dose in 24 hours

Available forms:
Powder in capsules for inhalation: 75 mcg

ADVERSE EFFECTS
CNS: Headache, dizziness
CV: Tachycardia, palpitations, peripheral edema
ENDO: Hyperglycemia
GI: Nausea, dry mouth
MS: Muscle cramps/spasm, musculoskeletal pain
INTEG: Rash, pruritus
RESP: Cough, dyspnea, upper respiratory tract infection

INTERACTIONS
Individual drugs
Amoxapine, some antipsychotics (phenothiazines, pimozide, haloperidol, risperiDONE, sertindole, ziprasidone), arsenic trioxide, astemizole, bepridil, cisapride, citalopram, chloroquine, clarithromycin, dasatinib, dolasetron, dronedarone, droperidol, erythromycin, flecainide, halofantrine, levomethadyl, maprotiline, methadone, ondansetron, paliperidone, palonosetron, pentamidine, probucol, propafenone, some quinolones (ofloxacin, gatifloxacin, gemifloxacin, grepafloxacin, levofloxacin, moxifloxacin, sparfloxacin), ranolazine, sunitinib, terfenadine, thioridazine, troleandomycin, vorinostat, tetrabenazine: increased QT prolongation

Drug classifications
B2 agonists: increase effect, overdose
Beta blockers: decrease effect
Class IA/III antiarrhythmics, halogenated anesthetics, tricyclic antidepressants: increased QT prolongation
Corticosteroids: increased hypokalemia
MAOIs: increased cardiovascular reactions

NURSING CONSIDERATIONS
Assessment

> **BLACK BOX WARNING:** Asthma-related death; not to be used in asthma

• **COPD, emphysema, bronchospasm:** Monitor pulmonary function tests; respiratory status

(dyspnea, rate, breath sounds) before and during treatment; if paradoxical bronchospasm occurs, discontinue this medication immediately; use a short-acting beta-agonist for rescue therapy, as appropriate
• **QT prolongation:** Monitor ECG for QT prolongation

Patient problem
Impaired air clearance (uses)
Activity intolerance (uses)

Implementation
Inhalation route
• For oral inhalation use only; *not* to swallow the capsules; always use the Neohaler inhaler; do *not* use with a spacer
• To administer, use dry hands to remove a capsule from the blister pack immediately before use and place into the capsule chamber of the Neohaler inhaler; click the inhaler closed; then, holding upright, depress buttons fully one time to pierce capsule; a click will be heard; have patient breathe out fully away from inhaler; place inhaler in the mouth with lips closed around the mouthpiece and buttons positioned to the left and right, then breathe deeply, in through the inhaler. A whirring sound should be heard; if no sound repeat inhalation steps until no powder remains. Most patients can empty the capsule in one or two inhalations. After administration, discard capsule

Patient/family education
• Teach patient/family to report dyspnea, wheezing, bronchospasm
• Teach patient/family not to use with other products unless approved by prescriber; there are many interactions, it is always prescribed with a short-acting beta 2 or steroidal inhaler
• Teach patient how to use neoinhaler, not to stop treatment unless approved by prescriber
• Teach patient to discuss with health care professional if Rx, OTC, herbals, supplements taken
• Teach patient about allergic reactions and not to be used for severe breathing problems
• Advise patient to inform other providers of use

> **BLACK BOX WARNING:** Not to use for asthma

• **Pregnancy/breastfeeding:** Use only if benefits outweigh fetal risk, cautious use in breastfeeding

---

indomethacin (Rx)

(in-doe-meth′a-sin)

Indocin, Tivorbex ✤

Func. class.: NSAID (nonsteroidal antiinflammatory), antirheumatic

Chem. class.: Acetic acid derivative

Do not confuse: Indocin/Endocet, minocin/Vicodin

ACTION: Inhibits prostaglandin synthesis by decreasing enzyme needed for biosynthesis; analgesic, antiinflammatory, antipyretic

Therapeutic outcome: Decreased pain, inflammation; closure of patent ductus arteriosus (premature infants)

USES: Rheumatoid arthritis, ankylosing spondylitis, osteoarthritis, bursitis, tendinitis, acute gouty arthritis; closure of patent ductus arteriosus in premature infants (**IV**)

Pharmacokinetics

Absorption	Well absorbed (PO); erratic (RECT); complete (**IV**)
Distribution	Crosses blood-brain barrier; placenta, 99% protein binding
Metabolism	Liver, extensively
Excretion	Breast milk; urine 60%, feces 33%
Half-life	2.6-11.2 hr

Pharmacodynamics

	PO	PO–ext rel	IV
Onset	30 min	½ hr	2 day
Peak	2 hr	Unknown	Unknown
Duration	4-6 hr	4-6 hr	Unknown

CONTRAINDICATIONS

Pregnancy (3rd trimester) hypersensitivity, asthma, aortic coarctation, bleeding, salicylate/NSAID hypersensitivity, GI bleeding

> **BLACK BOX WARNING:** Perioperative pain in CABG

Precautions: Pregnancy (1st trimester), breastfeeding, children, bleeding disorders, GI disorders, cardiac disorders, asthma, diabetes, acute bronchospasm, ulcerative colitis, seizures, Parkinson's disease, renal/hepatic disease, depression, neonates

> **BLACK BOX WARNING:** Stroke, GI bleeding, MI, those taking NSAIDs are at greater risk of MI and stroke, even in first few weeks of therapy

DOSAGE AND ROUTES

Arthritis/antiinflammatory

Adult: PO 25-50 mg bid-tid, max 200 mg/day; SUS REL 75 mg daily; may increase to 75 mg bid

Acute gouty arthritis

Adult: PO 50 mg tid; use only for acute attack, then reduce dosage

Mild-moderate pain (Tivorbex)

Adult: PO 20 mg tid or 40 mg bid-tid

Child >2 yr: PO 1-2 mg/kg/day in 2-4 divided doses, max 4 mg/kg/day or 150-200 mg/day

Patent ductus arteriosus

Longer or repeated treatment courses may be necessary for very premature infants

Infant <2 days: IV 0.2 mg/kg, then 0.1 mg/kg × 2 doses at 12, 24 hr

Infant 2-7 days: IV 0.2 mg/kg, then 0.2 mg/kg × 2 doses at 12, 24 hr

Infant >7 days: IV 0.2 mg/kg, then 0.25 mg/kg × 2 doses at 12, 24 hr

Available forms: Caps 25, 50 mg; cap (Tivorbex) 20, 40 mg; sus rel caps 75 mg; oral susp 5 mg/ ml; powder for inj 1-mg vials; supp 50 mg

ADVERSE EFFECTS

CNS: Dizziness, drowsiness, fatigue, confusion, insomnia, anxiety, depression, *headache*

CV: Peripheral edema, hypertension, CV thrombotic events, MI, stroke

EENT: Tinnitus, hearing loss, blurred vision

GI: *Nausea,* anorexia, *vomiting,* diarrhea, jaundice, cholestatic hepatitis, *constipation,* flatulence, cramps, dry mouth, peptic ulcer, ulceration, perforation, GI bleeding

GU: Nephrotoxicity (dysuria, hematuria, oliguria, azotemia) (IV)

HEMA: Blood dyscrasias, prolonged bleeding

INTEG: Purpura, rash, pruritus, sweating, phlebitis at IV site

INTERACTIONS

Individual drugs

Abciximab, aspirin, clopidogrel, eptifibatide, plicamycin, ticlopidine, tirofiban: increased bleeding risk

Cidofovir, cycloSPORINE, lithium, methotrexate, probenecid: increased toxicity

Digoxin, penicillamine, phentoin: increased effect of each specific product

---

⚠ Nurse Alert   ✸ Key NCLEX® Drug   ≫ Drug Specifics

Drug classifications

Aminoglycosides: increased effects of aminoglycosides

Anticoagulants, SNRIs, SSRIs, thrombolytics:
increased risk of bleeding

Antihypertensives diuretics: decreased effect of
antihypertensives diuretics

Diuretics (potassium sparing): increased hyperkalemia

Drug/herb

Chamomile, clove, dong quai, garlic, ginger,
ginko: Increased bleeding risk

NURSING CONSIDERATIONS
Assessment

• **Assess for patent ductus arteriosus:**
respiratory rate, character, heart sounds

• **Assess for joint pain** (duration, intensity,
ROM), baseline and during treatment

• Assess for confusion, mood changes, hallucinations, especially in geriatric

• Assess renal, liver, blood studies: BUN, creatinine, AST, ALT, Hgb before treatment, periodically
thereafter; if renal function decreases, do not
give subsequent doses

> **BLACK BOX WARNING:** Assess for cardiac
> disease, CV, thrombotic events (MI, stroke)
> prior to administration, not to be used for
> perioperative pain in CABG surgery

> **BLACK BOX WARNING:** GI bleeding/perforation:
> chronic use can lead to GI bleeding: use cau-
> tiously in those with a history of active GI disease

> **BLACK BOX WARNING:** MI, stroke: risk may
> be greater with longer-term use and in those
> with CV risk factors

• **Beers:** Avoid use in older adults; more likely
to cause CNS effects

• **Pregnancy/breastfeeding:** Do not use
after 30 wk gestation, use only if benefits
outweigh fetal risk, <30 wk gestation, do
not breastfeed, excreted in breast milk

Patient problem

Pain (uses)
Impaired mobility (uses)

Implementation
PO route

• Swallow sus rel cap whole; do not break,
crush, or chew sus rel cap

• Give with food or milk to decrease gastric
symptoms and prevent ulceration

• Shake susp; do not mix with other liquids

Rectal route

• Have patient retain rect supp for 1 hr after
insertion

• Store at room temperature

IV route

• Give after diluting 1 mg with 1 or 2 ml saline
or sterile water for inj without preservative;
give 1 or 0.5 mg/ml, respectively, do not
dilute further; give over 20-30 min; avoid
extravasation

• Do not give by umbilical catheter into vessels
near superior mesenteric artery, do not give
intra-arterially

• Hold dose in patent ductus arterious in
oliguria <0.6 ml/kg/hr

Patient/family education

• Advise patient to report change in vision, blurring, rash, tinnitus, black stools

• Tell patient not to use for any other condition
than prescribed

• Advise patient to avoid use with OTC, herbals, supplements, medications for pain unless
approved by prescriber, to report use to all
providers

• Advise patient to avoid hazardous activities,
since dizziness or drowsiness can occur

• Instruct patient to use sunscreen, protective
clothing, and a hat to prevent photosensitivity

• Advise to take with food for GI upset; to use as
prescribed; not to skip or double doses; to take
with 8 oz of water

• Teach patient to report signs of GI bleeding:
dark stools, hematemesis

• Teach patient to report hepatotoxicity (diarrhea, dark stools, yellowing of eyes, skin, nausea
occur)

• Teach patient to notify providers of product
use before surgery

> **BLACK BOX WARNING:** MI/stroke: Teach
> patient to immediately report and seek medical
> attention for signs/symptoms of MI/stroke,
> discontinue product

Evaluation
Positive therapeutic outcome

• Decreased stiffness
• Increased joint mobility
• Decreased pain
• PDA closure

inFLIXimab (Rx)

(in-fliks'ih-mab)

Inflectra ✦, **Remicade, Remsima** ✦, **Renflexis**

Func. class.: Antirheumatic (DMRDs), GI antiinflammatory, immunoglobulin

Chem. class.: Tumor necrosis factor modifiers

Do not confuse: inFLIXimab/riTUXimab, **Remicade**/Renacidin

ACTION: Monoclonal antibody that neutralizes the activity of tumor necrosis factor α (TNFα) that has been found in Crohn's disease; decreased infiltration of inflammatory cells

Therapeutic outcome: Decreased cramping and blood in stools

USES: Crohn's disease, fistulizing, moderate to severe; rheumatoid arthritis given with methotrexate, plaque psoriasis, ankylosing spondylitis, ulcerative colitis, psoriatic arthritis, psoriasis

Pharmacokinetics

Absorption	Complete
Distribution	Vascular compartment
Metabolism	Unknown
Excretion	Unknown
Half-life	9½ days

Pharmacodynamics

Unknown

CONTRAINDICATIONS

Hypersensitivity to murines, moderate to severe HF (NYHA class III/IV)

Precautions: Pregnancy, breastfeeding, children, geriatric, COPD, hepatotoxicity, hematologic abnormalities, hepatitis B, Guillain-Barré syndrome, seizures, multiple sclerosis

> **BLACK BOX WARNING:** Infection, neoplastic disease, TB

DOSAGE AND ROUTES
Rheumatoid arthritis

Adult: IV 3 mg/kg initially, and 2, 6 wk and q8wk thereafter, max 10 mg/kg/dose

Crohn's disease/ankylosing spondylitis

Adult/adolescent/child ≥6 yr: IV INF 5 mg/kg initially, then repeat dose 2, 6 wk, then q8wk; q6wk (ankylosing spondylitis); may increase to 10 mg/kg if needed (adults)

Ulcerative colitis/plaque psoriasis

Adult/adolescent/child ≥ 6 yr: IV infusion 5 mg/kg initially and at 2, 4 wk, then 5 mg/kg q8wk

Available forms: Powder for inj 100 mg

ADVERSE EFFECTS

CNS: *Headache, dizziness, depression, vertigo, fatigue, anxiety, fever,* seizures, chills, *flulike symptoms,* demyelinating disease

CV: Chest pain, hypo/hypertension, tachycardia, HF, acute coronary syndrome

GI: *Nausea, vomiting, abdominal pain, stomatitis, constipation, dyspepsia, flatulence*

GU: Dysuria, frequency

HEMA: Anemia, leukopenia, thrombocytopenia, pancytopenia

INTEG: *Rash, dermatitis, urticaria,* dry skin, sweating, flushing, hematoma, pruritus, keratoderma blennorrhagicum

MS: Myalgia, back pain, arthralgia

RESP: URI, pharyngitis, bronchitis, cough, dyspnea, sinusitis

SYST: Anaphylaxis, fatal infections, sepsis, malignancies, immunogenicity, Stevens-Johnson syndrome, toxic epidermal necrolysis, sarcoidosis

INTERACTIONS
Drug classifications

Live virus vaccines: do not administer live vaccines concurrently

TNF blockers (abatacept, anakinra, golimumab, rilonacept): increased infections, neutropenia; avoid concurrent use

NURSING CONSIDERATIONS
Assessment

• **RA:** Assess for characteristics of pain, joints involved, aggravating/ameliorating actions, ROM, baseline and periodically

• **Ulcerative colitis/Crohn's disease:** Assess for characteristics of pain; symptoms including abdominal pain, diarrhea; inability to participate in activities, baseline and periodically

• **Plaque psoriasis:** Assess characteristics of lesions, body area affected baseline and periodically

• Assess GI symptoms: nausea, vomiting, abdominal pain

• **Blood dyscrasias:** Take periodic blood counts: CBC with differential baseline and periodically, may cause blood dycriasis, discontinue if present

• Assess CV status: B/P, pulse, chest pain

• **Assess for allergic reaction, anaphylaxis:** rash, dermatitis, urticaria, fever, chills, dyspnea, hypotension; discontinue if severe; administer epinephrine, corticosteroids, antihistamines; assess for allergy to murine proteins before starting therapy

---

BLACK BOX WARNING: Fatal infections: discontinue if infection occurs, do not administer to patients with active infections; identify TB before beginning treatment, a TD test should be obtained; if present, TB should be treated before giving inFLIXimab; exercise caution when switching one DMARD to another

---

BLACK BOX WARNING: Assess for neoplastic disease in those <18 yr, including hepatosplenic T-cell lymphoma, usually occurs in those with inflammatory bowel disease

---

• **Pregnancy/breastfeeding:** Does not cross the placenta during first trimester, but does second and third trimester, discontinue 8-10 wk before birth, do not breastfeed

Patient problem
Pain (uses)
Diarrhea (uses)

Implementation
Intermittent IV infusion route
• Administer immediately after reconstitution; reconstitute each vial with 10 ml of sterile water for inj, further dilute total dose/250 ml of 0.9% NaCl inj to a total conc of between 0.4 and 4 mg/ml; use 21-G or smaller needle for reconstitution, direct sterile water at glass wall of vial, gently swirl, do not shake, may foam; allow to stand for 5 min, give within 3 hr
• Give over ≥2 hr, use polyethylene-lined inf with in-line, sterile, low-protein-bind filter
• Do not admix
• Provide refrigerated storage, do not freeze

Patient/family education
• Instruct patient to report infusion reaction immediately
• Instruct patient to notify prescriber immediately if infection occurs
• Advise patient to notify prescriber of GI symptoms, hypersensitivity reactions
• Advise patient not to operate machinery or drive if dizziness, vertigo occurs
• Teach patient to avoid live virus vaccinations, bring up to date prior to use
• **Malignancy:** Teach patient to check for changes in skin, growths or color changes
• **Pregnancy/breastfeeding:** Identify if pregnancy is planned or suspected or if breastfeeding

Evaluation
Positive therapeutic outcome
• Absence of blood in stool
• Reported improvement in comfort
• Weight gain

inotuzumab ozogamicin
(ih noh too' zoo mab oh'-zoh-ga-MIH-sin)
Besponsa
Func. class.: Antineoplastic monoclonal antibodies

ACTION: A CD22-directed antibody-drug conjugate, CD22 is expressed on pre-B-cells and mature B-cells. Consists of a cytotoxic agent; it induces double-strand DNA breaks, resulting in cell cycle arrest and apoptotic cell death

USES: For the treatment of adults with relapsed or refractory B-cell precursor acute lymphoblastic leukemia

Pharmacokinetics

Absorption, metabolism, excretion, half-life	Unknown
Distribution	Protein binding 97%

Pharmacodynamics

Onset, peak, duration	Unknown

CONTRAINDICATIONS
Pregnancy, hypersensitivity

Precautions: Alcoholism, bleeding, breastfeeding, contraception requirements, diabetes mellitus, electrolyte imbalances, females, geriatric patients, infertility, male-mediated teratogenicity, neutropenia, bone marrow suppression, infection, reproductive risk, thrombocytopenia, thyroid disease, QT prolongation

---

BLACK BOX WARNING: Hepatic disease, hepatotoxicity, mortality, sinusoidal obstructive disease, venoocclusive disease

---

DOSAGE AND ROUTES
B-cell precursor ALL
Adult: IV 0.8 mg/m² day 1 and 0.5 mg/m² days 8 and 15 (cycle 1). Length of cycle 1 is 21 days, may extend to 28 days in those who achieve a complete remission (CR) or a complete remission with incomplete hematologic recovery (CRi) or to allow for recovery from toxicity. In patients who do not achieve a CR or CRi, give product at the same dosage (0.8 mg/m² on day 1 and 0.5 mg/m² on days 8 and 15) repeated

q8days; discontinue if a CR or CRi is not achieved after 3 cycles. In patients who achieve a CR or CRi, give product 0.5 mg/m² on days 1, 8, and 15 repeated q28days. In patients who proceed to hematopoietic stem cell transplant (HSCT), administer 2 cycles of therapy; consider a third cycle in patients who do not achieve CR or CRi and minimal residual disease (MRD) negativity after 2 cycles. Patients not proceeding to HSCT should receive a maximum of 6 cycles of therapy.

Management of treatment-related toxicity

Do not interrupt doses within a treatment cycle (day 8 or day 15 dose) for neutropenia or thrombocytopenia. Dosing interruptions within a cycle are recommended for nonhematologic toxicity. If a dose reduction is necessary, do not re-escalate the dose

Hematologic toxicity:

Absolute neutrophil count (ANC) of 1 × 10⁹ cells/L or greater before starting therapy: If the ANC decreases, hold the next cycle of therapy until recovery of the ANC to 1 × 10⁹ cells/L or greater. Discontinue therapy if low ANC lasts longer than 28 days and is suspected to be due to inotuzumab ozogamicin. *Platelet count of 50 × 10⁹ cells/L or greater before starting therapy:* If platelet count decreases, hold the next cycle of therapy until the platelet count recovers to 50 × 10⁹ cells/L or greater. Discontinue therapy if low platelet count lasts longer than 28 days and is suspected to be due to inotuzumab ozogamicin. *ANC was less than 1 × 109 cells/L and/or platelet count was less than 50 X 10⁹ cells/L before starting therapy:* If the ANC or platelet count decreases, hold the next cycle until at least 1 of the following occurs: the ANC and platelet counts recover to baseline or better for the prior cycle; the ANC recovers to 1 × 10⁹ cells/L or greater and the platelet count recovers to 50 × 10⁹ cells/L or greater; the patient has stable or improved disease (based on most recent bone marrow assessment) and the ANC and platelet count decrease is considered to be due to the underlying disease and not product-related toxicity

Infusion-related reactions:

Mild to moderate reactions: Hold infusion and start medical management. Consider discontinuing or give steroids and antihistamines depending on the severity; *severe or life-threatening reactions:* Stop infusion, permanently discontinue

Nonhematologic toxicity:

Evaluate for toxicity before each dose. For grade 2 or higher toxicity, hold until toxicity recovers to grade 1 or less (or pretreatment grade level).

Dose modifications depend on duration of dosing interruption as follows: *Less than 7 days (within a cycle):* Hold the next dose; maintain a minimum of 6 days between doses; *7 days or greater:* omit the next dose within the cycle; *14 days or greater:* After recovery, decrease the total dose by 25% for the subsequent cycle. If further dose modification is required, reduce the number of doses to 2 per cycle for subsequent cycles. If a 25% decrease in the total dose followed by a decrease to 2 doses per cycle is not tolerated, permanently discontinue therapy; *greater than 28 days:* consider permanent discontinuation

Hepatic dose

Baseline hepatic impairment: No change

Treatment-related hepatotoxicity:

Evaluate for toxicity before each dose. Dosing interruptions within a cycle are recommended for hepatic impairment. If a dose reduction is necessary, do not re-escalate the dose. *Total bilirubin level of 1.5 times the upper limit of normal (ULN) or less and AST/ALT level of 2.5 times the ULN or less:* No dose adjustment is necessary. *Total bilirubin level greater than 1.5 times the ULN and AST/ALT level greater than 2.5 times the ULN:* Hold therapy until the total bilirubin level is 1.5 times the ULN or less and the AST/ALT level is 2.5 times the ULN or less unless hyperbilirubinemia is due to Gilbert's syndrome or hemolysis. Dose modifications depend on duration of dosing interruption as follows: *Less than 7 days (within a cycle):* Hold the next dose; maintain a minimum of 6 days between doses. *7 days or greater:* Omit the next dose within the cycle; *14 days or greater:* After recovery, decrease the total dose by 25% for the subsequent cycle. If further dose modification is required, reduce the number of doses to 2 per cycle for subsequent cycles. If a 25% decrease in the total dose followed by a decrease to 2 doses per cycle is not tolerated, permanently discontinue; *greater than 28 days:* Permanently discontinue

Hepatic venoocclusive disease (VOD)/ sinusoidal obstruction syndrome (SOS) or other severe liver toxicity: Permanently discontinue

Available forms: Powder for injection 0.9 mg

ADVERSE EFFECTS

CNS: *Fatigue, fever, headache, migraine, chills*
GI: *Nausea, vomiting, diarrhea, stomatitis, constipation, anorexia, abdominal pain,* hepatotoxicity

HEMA: Anemia, thrombocytopenia, *bleeding, hematoma, hematuria, ecchymosis, venoocculsive disease*

MISC: Infection, asthenia, QT prolongation, tumor lysis syndrome, sinusoidal obstruction syndrome

INTERACTIONS
Other products that increase QT prolongation: Increased QT prolongation

Drug/lab test
Increased: LFTs

NURSING CONSIDERATIONS
Assessment
• **Serious infection**: Some may be fatal. Monitor patients for signs and symptoms of infection; use prophylactic antiinfectives as appropriate

• **Severe myelosuppression/bone marrow suppression:** Assess for thrombocytopenia, neutropenia; obtain a CBC before each dose, therapy interruption or permanent discontinuation may be necessary in patients who develop severe myelosuppression

• **Pregnancy/breastfeeding:** Product can cause fetal harm, females of reproductive potential should avoid becoming pregnant during and for 8 mo after final dose; obtain a pregnancy test before starting product, do not breastfeed during and for at least 2 mo after the last dose; men with female partners of reproductive potential should avoid fathering a child and use effective contraception during and for at least 5 mo after therapy

• **QT prolongation**: Obtain an electrocardiogram (ECG) and monitor serum electrolytes before the start of treatment and periodically during therapy as needed. Use with caution in patients with a history of QT prolongation or who have an electrolyte imbalance. Avoid concomitant use with other drugs known to prolong the QT interval; if coadministration is unavoidable, monitor ECGs and serum electrolytes after starting the other QT-prolonging drug. Females, geriatric patients, patients with diabetes mellitus, thyroid disease, malnutrition, alcoholism, hepatic dysfunction, or patients who have received high-cumulative-dose anthracycline therapy may also be at increased risk for QT prolongation

---

BLACK BOX WARNING: Severe or life-threatening hepatotoxicity, including venoocclusive disease (VOD)/sinusoidal obstruction syndrome (SOS): Monitor liver function tests (LFTs), total bilirubin, alkaline phosphatase levels before and after each dosage change; therapy interruption, dose reduction, or permanent discontinuation may be necessary in those who develop liver function test abnormalities. Closely monitor for VOD/SOS (hepatomegaly, rapid weight gain, and ascites). Permanently discontinue in those who develop VOD/SOS; in those who undergo a hematopoietic stem cell transplant (HSCT), monitor LFTs frequently during the first month post-HSCT; then continue to monitor LFTs but less often. Time from HSCT to onset of VOD/SOS was 15 days (range 3 to 57 days). The risk of VOD/SOS may be greater in patients who receive an HSCT or a conditioning regimen that contains 2 alkylating agents before HSCT and in patients who have an increased total bilirubin level before a HSCT; other risk factors include hepatic disease (e.g., cirrhosis, nodular regenerative hyperplasia, active hepatitis), a prior HSCT, increased age, later salvage lines, and a larger number of treatment cycles

BLACK BOX WARNING: Mortality: Those who underwent a hematopoietic stem cell transplant (HSCT) may have a higher 100-day post-HSCT nonrelapse mortality; monitor closely for post-HSCT toxicity. The most common causes of post-HSCT death were venoocclusive disease/sinusoidal obstruction syndrome and infectious complications

Patient problem
Risk for injury (adverse reactions)

Implementation
IV route
• Visually inspect for particulate matter and discoloration before use
• Follow cytotoxic handling procedures
• Available as a single-dose, preservative-free, 0.9-mg lyophilized powder vial
• Premedication with a corticosteroid, an antipyretic agent (acetaminophen), and an antihistamine before each dose is recommended; observe patients during and for at least 1 hr after the end of the infusion for symptoms of infusion-related reactions

Reconstitution
• After calculating the number of vials needed, add 4 ml of sterile water for injection to each vial for a final vial concentration of 0.25 mg/ml (0.9 mg/3.6 ml); gently swirl the vial to dissolve powder, do not shake

---

• The reconstitution solution should be clear to opalescent, colorless to slightly yellow, and free of visible foreign matter
• **Storage of reconstituted vials:** If not further diluted immediately, vials may be stored in the refrigerator (at 2 to 8° C or 36 to 46° F) for up to 4 hr after reconstitution; protect from light, do not freeze

Dilution
• Add the required dose/volume from the reconstituted vials to an infusion container made of polyvinyl chloride (PVC) or non-DEHP-containing polyolefin (polypropylene and/or polyethylene), or ethylene vinyl acetate (EVA); discard any unused portion
• Add 0.9% sodium chloride injection to the infusion container for a final total volume of 50 ml; gently invert to mix, do not shake
• **Storage of admixture:** If not infused immediately, the diluted solution may be stored at room temperature (20 to 25° C or 68 to 77° F) for up to 4 hr or refrigerated (2 to 8° C or 36 to 46° F) for up to 3 hr; protect from light and do not freeze

IV infusion
• Allow refrigerated admixtures to warm to room temperature for 1 hr before use
• Give admixture (protected from light) as an IV infusion over 1 hr through an infusion line made of PVC, polyolefin (polypropylene and/or polyethylene), or polybutadiene
• Complete infusion within 8 hr of reconstitution
• The diluted solution does not need to be filtered; if it is filtered, use polyethersulfone (PES)-, polyvinylidene fluoride (PVDF)-, or hydrophilic polysulfone (HPS)-based filters
• Do not use filters made of nylon or mixed cellulose ester (MCE)
• Do not mix with or administer as an infusion with other drugs

Patient/family education
• Teach patient to report adverse reactions immediately, bleeding; report diarrhea, hepatic, hematologic symptoms/toxicity, flulike symptoms
• Teach patient about reason for treatment, expected results
• **Pregnancy/breastfeeding:** Teach patient to notify provider if pregnancy is planned or suspected, to use effective contraception during treatment and for 8 mo after discontinuing treatment, breastfeeding or for 2 mo after final dose; men with female partners of reproductive potential should be cautioned to avoid fathering a child and use effective contraception during and for at least 5 mo after therapy

Evaluation
Positive therapeutic outcome
• Improving blood counts

⚠ HIGH ALERT

INSULINS

RAPID ACTING

insulin aspart (Rx)
Fiasp, NovoLOG, NovoRapid ✢
insulin glulisine (Rx)
Apidra, Apidra SoloStar
insulin (Human)
Afreeza
insulin lispro (Rx)
HumaLOG

SHORT ACTING

insulin, regular (OTC)
Humulin R ✢, NovoLIN R, ReliOn R
insulin, regular concentrated (Rx)
Humulin R, Novolin ge Toronto ✢, Novolin R, Humulin RU-500

INTERMEDIATE ACTING

insulin, isophane suspension (NPH) (OTC)
Humulin N, NovoLIN N

LONG ACTING

insulin degludec
Tresiba
insulin detemir (Rx)
Levemir
insulin glargine (Rx)
Basaglar, Lantus, Toujeo Solostar

MIXTURES

insulin degludec, insulin aspart
Ryzodez 70/30
insulin, isophane suspension and regular insulin (Rx)
HumaLIN 70/30, NovoLIN 70/30
isophane insulin suspension (NPH) and insulin mixtures (Rx)
Humulin 50/50
NPH/regular insulin mixture
Aumatin 70/30, Novolin 70/30
insulin lispro mixture (Rx)
HumaLOG Mix 75/25, HumaLOG Mix 50/50

---

insulin aspart mixture (Rx)
NovoLOG 70/30, Novolog Mix Flexpen Prefilled Syringe 70/30
insulin, inhaled
(in'soo-lin)
Afrezza
Func. class.: Antidiabetic, pancreatic hormone
Chem. class.: Modified structures of endogenous human insulin

Do not confuse: Novolog Flexipen/ Novolog/Humalog

ACTION: Decreases blood glucose; by transport of glucose into cells and the conversion of glucose to glycogen, indirectly increases blood pyruvate and lactate, decreases phosphate and potassium; insulin may be human (processed by recombinant DNA technologies)

Therapeutic outcome: Decreased blood glucose levels in diabetes mellitus

USES: Type 1 diabetes mellitus, type 2 diabetes mellitus, gestational diabetes, insulin lispro may be used in combination with sulfonylureas in children >3 yr

Pharmacokinetics

Absorption	Rapidly absorbed (SUBCUT)
Distribution	Widely distributed
Metabolism	Liver, muscle, kidney
Excretion	Kidneys
Half-life	Regular 3-5 min; NPH 10 min

Pharmacodynamics

Rapid acting	
Insulin glulisine	Onset 15-30 min, peak ½-1½ hr, duration 3-4 hr
Insulin aspart	Onset 10-20 min, peak 1-3 hr, duration 3-5 hr
Insulin lispro	Onset 15-30 min, peak ½-1½ hr, duration 3-4 hr
Short acting	
Insulin regular	Onset 30 min, peak 2.5-5 hr, duration up to 6 hr
Intermediate acting	
Insulin, isophane suspension (NPH)	Onset 1.5-4 hr, peak 4-12 hr, duration up to 24 hr
Long acting	
Insulin detemir	Onset 0.8-2 hr, peak unknown, duration up to 24 hr (concentration dependent)
Insulin glargine	Onset 1.5 hr, no peak identified, duration ≥ 24 hr
Insulin degludec	Peak 12 hr, duration 42 hr after 8 doses
Mixtures	
Insulin, isophane suspension and regular insulin (70/30)	Onset 10-20 hr, peak 2.4 hr, duration up to 24 hr
Isophane insulin suspension (NPH) and insulin mixtures (50/50)	Onset ½-1 hr, peak dual, duration 10-16 hr

CONTRAINDICATIONS
Hypersensitivity to protamine; creosol (aspart)

Precautions: Pregnancy

DOSAGE AND ROUTES
>> Insulin glulisine
Adult/adolescent/child ≥4 yr: SUBCUT dosage individualized, give within 15 min before or 20 min after starting a meal
Adult: IV dilute to 1 unit/ml in INF systems with 0.9% NaCl, using PVC Viaflex INF bags and PVC tubing, use dedicated line

>> Insulin aspart
Adult/adolescent/child ≥6 yr: Intermittent SUBCUT total daily dose is given as 2-4 inj/day just prior to beginning of a meal; in general, 50%-70% of total daily insulin may be given as insulin aspart, the remainder should be intermediate or long-acting insulin; CONTINUOUS SUBCUT used with external insulin pump via cont SUBCUT insulin INF (CSII), the insulin dose should be based on the insulin dose from the previous regimen

>> Insulin lispro
Adult/adolescent/child ≥3 yr: SUBCUT 15 min before meals; **continuous subcut infusion (external insulin pump)** the total daily dose should be based on the insulin dose in previous regimen, 50% of total dose can be given as meal-related boluses and the remainder as basal infusion

>> Human regular
Adult: SUBCUT ½-1 hr before meals

Insulin, isophane suspension
Adult: SUBCUT dosage individualized by blood, urine glucose; usual dose 7-26 units; may increase by 2-10 units/day if needed

>> insulin degludec
Adult: SUBCUT dose individualized

>> Insulin detemir
Adult/adolescent/child ≥2 yr: SUBCUT 1 or 2 times/day; if 1 time, give with evening meal

>> Insulin glargine
Adult and child ≥6 yr: SUBCUT 10 international units/day, range 2-100 international units/day, but may go much higher

>> Insulin, inhaled
Adult: INH: (type 1) the average initial dose is 0.5-0.6 unit/kg/day, usually ≥ 3 administrations/day; (type 2) the average initial dose is 0.2-0.6 unit/kg/day. When used in combination with oral hypoglycemic agents, may only need a single dose of a longer acting insulin at a dosage of 10 units or 0.2 units/kg/day.

>> Regular insulin (ketoacidosis)
Adult: IV 5-10 units, then 5-10 units/hr until desired response, then switch to SUBCUT dose; **IV/INF** 2-12 units (50 units/500 ml of normal saline)
Child: IV 0.1 units/kg

>> Replacement
Adult and child: SUBCUT 0.5-1 units/kg/day qid given 30 min before meals
Adolescent: SUBCUT 0.8-1.2 mg/kg/day; this dosage is used during rapid growth

Available forms: NPH inj 100 units/ml; **regular** inj 100 units/ml, cartridges 100 units/ml; **insulin analog** inj 100 units/ml; **isophane insulin** inj 100 units/ml, cartridges 100 units/ml; **insulin lispro** 100 units/ml, 1.5-ml cartridges; Humalog KwikPen sol for inj 100 units/ml, Humalog KwikPen 200 units/ml prefilled pen solution for injection; **insulin glulisine** inj 100 units/ml; **insulin glargine** inj 100, 300 units/ml; **insulin degludec** Solution for INJ 100 units/ml (u-100), 200 units/ml (u-200); **insulin detemir** inj 100 units/ml in 10 vials, 3-ml cartridges; **insulin aspart** inj 100 mg/ml (Flexpen, PenFill); **insulin inhaled** 4 units powder for inh

ADVERSE EFFECTS
EENT: Blurred vision, dry mouth
INTEG: Flushing, rash, urticaria, warmth, *lipodystrophy,* lipohypertrophy, swelling, redness
META: *Hypoglycemia,* rebound hyperglycemia (Somogyi effect 12-72 hr or longer)
MISC: Peripheral edema
SYST: Anaphylaxis

INTERACTIONS
Individual drugs
Alcohol: increased hypoglycemia
DOBUTamine: increased insulin need
EPINEPHrine: decreased hypoglycemia
Sulfinpyrazone, tetracycline: decreased insulin need

Drug classifications
Anabolic steroids, β-adrenergic blockers, hypoglycemics (oral), salicylates: increased hypoglycemia
Contraceptives (oral), corticosteroids, diuretics (thiazide), thyroid hormones: decreased hypoglycemia
Estrogens: increased insulin need
MAOIs: decreased insulin need

Drug/lab test
Increased: VMA
Decreased: potassium, calcium
Interference: liver, thyroid function tests

NURSING CONSIDERATIONS
Assessment
• Fasting blood glucose, also Hgb A1c may be tested to identify treatment effectiveness q3mo
• Urine ketones during illness; insulin requirements may increase during stress, illness, surgery
• For hypoglycemic reaction that can occur during peak time (sweating, weakness, dizziness, chills, confusion, headache, nausea, rapid weak pulse, fatigue, tachycardia, memory lapses, slurred speech, staggering gait, anxiety, tremors, hunger)
• For hyperglycemia: acetone breath, polyuria, fatigue, polydipsia, flushed, dry skin, lethargy
• **Pregnancy/breastfeeding:** Use if clearly needed, product of choice for pregnancy, monitor blood glucose levels, cautious use in breastfeeding
• **Beers:** Avoid use of short- or rapid-acting insulin in older adults, sliding-scale insulin poses a higher risk of hypoglycemia without improvement in hyperglycemia management

---

A Nurse Alert   ✳ Key NCLEX® Drug   >> Drug Specifics

Patient problem
Nonadherence (teaching)
Lack of knowledge of medication (teaching)

Implementation
• Store at room temperature for <1 mo (some insulins); keep away from heat and sunlight; refrigerate all other supply; NPH, premixed insulins are cloudy; regular, rapid-acting analogs, long-acting analogs are clear; do not freeze—**IV** route, regular only

INHALED route
• Give by inhalation only; use at beginning of a meal (blue cartridge = 4 units of regular insulin, green cartridge = 8 units of regular insulin); multiple cartridges may be needed; for single-use only; inhaler should be discarded after 15 days; store unopened cartridge packages in refrigerator, if not refrigerated, use within 10 days
• Sealed (unopened) blister cards and strips must be used within 10 days. Cartridges left over in an opened strip must be used within 3 days. Remove a blister card from the foil package. Tear along a perforation to remove one strip. Press the clear side of the strip to push the cartridge out. To load the cartridge, hold the inhaler level in one hand with the white mouthpiece on the top and purple base on the bottom; open the inhaler by lifting the white mouthpiece to a vertical position. Before placing the cartridge in the inhaler, both the cartridge and the inhaler should be at room temperature for 10 minutes. Hold the cartridge with the cup facing down, and line up the cartridge with the opening in the inhaler. The pointed end of the cartridge should line up with the pointed end in the inhaler. The cartridge can be placed into the inhaler; ensure that the cartridge lies flat in the inhaler. Once the cartridge is loaded, keep level.
• Remove the purple mouthpiece cover. Hold the inhaler away from the mouth and fully exhale. While keeping the head level, place the mouthpiece in the mouth and tilt the inhaler down toward the chin. Close lips around the mouthpiece to form a seal. Inhale deeply through the inhaler. Hold breath for as long as is comfortable, and at the same time remove the inhaler from the mouth. Exhale and continue to breathe normally.

SUBCUT route
• Give after warming to room temperature by rotating in palms to prevent injecting cold insulin; use only insulin syringes with markings or syringe matching units/ml; rotate inj sites within one area: abdomen, upper back, thighs, upper arm, buttocks; keep record of sites
• Give increased dosages if tolerance occurs
• Premixed insulins and NPH are cloudy suspensions
• Regular human insulin, rapid-acting analogs, and long-acting analogs are clear; do not use if cloudy, thick, or discolored

CONT SUBCUT route (insulin infusion CSII)
• Do not mix with other insulins when using a pump
• Insulin lispro 3 ml cartridges are to be used in Disetronic H-TRON plus V100 pump using Disetronic rapid inf sets; the inf set and the cartridge adapter should be changed q3day; replace 3 ml cartridge q6days

IV route (insulin glulisine only)
• Dilute to 1 international unit/ml in infusion systems with 0.9% NaCl using PVC viaflex inf bags and PVC tubing; use dedicated line; do not admix

IV route (regular only)
• When regular insulin is administered IV, monitor glucose, potassium often to prevent fatal hypoglycemia, hypokalemia
• **IV** direct, undiluted via vein, **Y**-site, 3-way stopcock; give at 50 units/min or less
• Give by cont inf after diluting with **IV** sol and run at prescribed rate; use **IV** inf pump for correct dosing; give reduced dose at serum glucose level of 250 mg/100 ml

Y-site compatibilities: Amiodarone, ampicillin, ampicillin/sulbactam, aztreonam, ceFAZolin, cefoTEtan, DOBUTamine, esmolol, famotidine, gentamicin, heparin, heparin/hydrocortisone, imipenem/cilastatin, indomethacin, magnesium sulfate, meperidine, meropenem, midazolam, morphine, nitroglycerin, oxytocin, PENTobarbital, potassium chloride, propofol, ritodrine, sodium bicarbonate, sodium nitroprusside, tacrolimus, terbutaline, ticarcillin, ticarcillin/clavulanate, tobramycin, vancomycin, vit B/C

Patient/family education
• Advise patient that blurred vision occurs; not to change corrective lens until vision is stabilized 1-2 mo
• Advise patient to keep insulin, equipment available at all times; carry a glucagon kit, candy, or lump sugar to treat hypoglycemia
• Inform patient that product does not cure diabetes but controls symptoms

• Advise patient to carry emergency ID as diabetic
• Instruct patient to recognize hypoglycemia reaction: headache, tremors, fatigue, weakness
• Instruct patient to recognize hyperglycemia reaction: frequent urination, thirst, fatigue, hunger
• Teach patient the dosage, route, mixing instructions, any diet restrictions, disease process
• **Teach patient the symptoms of ketoacidosis:** nausea, thirst, polyuria, dry mouth, decreased B/P, dry, flushed skin, acetone breath, drowsiness, Kussmaul respirations
• Advise patient that a plan is necessary for diet, exercise; all food on diet should be eaten; exercise routine should not vary
• Teach patient about blood glucose testing; make sure patient is able to determine glucose level
• Advise patient to avoid OTC products unless directed by prescriber

Evaluation

Positive therapeutic outcome
• Decrease in polyuria, polydipsia, polyphagia; clear sensorium; absence of dizziness; stable gait
• Blood glucose HBA1c within normal limits

TREATMENT OF OVERDOSE:
Glucose 25 g **IV,** via dextrose 50% sol, 50 ml, or glucagon 1 mg

---

⚠ HIGH ALERT
RARELY USED

insulin degludec/liraglutide
(in'su-lin de-gloo'dek/lir'a-gloo'tide)
Xultophy
Func. class.: Antidiabetic combination

USES: Type 2 diabetes mellitus, in combination with diet and exercise, for adults who are inadequately controlled on basal insulin (less than 50 units daily) or liraglutide (less than or equal to 1.8 mg daily)

CONTRAINDICATIONS
Angioedema, hypoglycemia, medullary thyroid carcinoma (MTC), multiple endocrine neoplasia syndrome type 2 (MEN 2)

DOSAGE AND ROUTES
Adult: SUBCUT: 16 dose units (16 units of insulin degludec and 0.58 mg of liraglutide) subcut qday at the same time each day, with or without food. DOSE TITRATION: Titrate the dosage upward or downward by 2 dose units (2 units of insulin degludec and 0.072 mg of liraglutide) q3-4 days

based on the metabolic needs, blood glucose monitoring results, and glycemic control goal until the desired fasting plasma glucose is achieved.

⚠ HIGH ALERT
RARELY USED

insulin glargine/ lixisenatide
(in'su-lin glar'gine/lix'i-sen'a-tide)
Soliqua
Func. class.: Antidiabetic

USES: Type 2 diabetes mellitus in combination with diet and exercise in adults inadequately controlled on basal insulin or lixisenatide

CONTRAINDICATIONS
Angioedema, hypoglycemia

DOSAGE AND ROUTES
Adult: SUBCUT: In those inadequately controlled on less than 30 units of basal insulin or on lixisenatide, initiate with 15 units (15 units insulin glargine and 5 mcg lixisenatide) subcut qday within the hour before the first meal of the day. In those inadequately controlled on 30-60 units of basal insulin or on lixisenatide, initiate with 30 units (30 units insulin glargine and 10 mcg lixisenatide) subcut qday within the hour before the first meal of the day. TITRATION: Titrate the dosage upward or downward by 2-4 units qwk based on response

---

Interferons beta
interferon beta-1a (Rx)
(in-ter-feer'on)
Avonex, Rebif
interferon beta-1b (Rx)
Betaseron, Extavia
Func. class.: Multiple sclerosis agent, immune modifier
Chem. class.: Interferon, *Escherichia coli* derivative

ACTION: Antiviral, immunoregulatory; action not clearly understood; biologic response-modifying properties mediated through specific receptors on cells, inducing expression of interferon-induced gene products

Therapeutic outcome: Decreased symptoms of multiple sclerosis

USES: Ambulatory patients with relapsing or remitting multiple sclerosis

---

Pharmacokinetics

Absorption	50% is absorbed
Distribution	Unknown
Metabolism	Unknown
Excretion	Unknown
Half-life	8 min-4½ hr (beta-1b), 8.6 hr (beta-1a)

Pharmacodynamics

	Beta-1a	Beta-1b
Onset	Up to 12 hr	Rapid
Peak	16 hr	2-8 hr
Duration	4 days	Unknown

CONTRAINDICATIONS

Hypersensitivity to natural or recombinant interferon-beta or human albumin, hamster protein, rotavirus vaccine

Precautions: Pregnancy, breastfeeding, children <18 yr, chronic progressive multiple sclerosis, depression, mental disorders, seizure disorders, latex allergy, autoimmune disorders, bone marrow suppression, hepatotoxicity, cardiac disease, alcoholism, chickenpox, herpes zoster

DOSAGE AND ROUTES

>> Interferon beta-1a
Multiple sclerosis
Adult: IM (Avonex) 30 mcg qwk; SUBCUT (Rebif) 22 or 44 mcg 3 ×/wk with each dose 48 hr apart, titrate to full dose over 4-wk period

>> Interferon beta-1b
Multiple sclerosis
Adult: SUBCUT 0.0625 mg every other day for wk 1 and 2; then 0.125 mg every other day for wk 3 and 4; then 0.1875 mg every other day for wk 5 and 6; then 0.25 mg every other day thereafter; higher doses should not be used

Available forms: Beta-1a (Avonex): 33 mcg (6.6 million international units/vial) (auto-injector pen); (Rebif) 22 mcg, 44 mcg/0.5 ml; beta-1b: powder for inj 0.3 mg (9.6 m international units)

ADVERSE EFFECTS

CNS: *Headache, fever, pain, chills, mental changes,* depression, hypertonia, suicide attempts, seizures
CV: *Migraine, palpitations, hypertension,* tachycardia, peripheral vascular disorders
EENT: Conjunctivitis, blurred vision
GI: *Diarrhea, constipation, vomiting, abdominal pain*
GU: *Dysmenorrhea, irregular menses, metrorrhagia,* cystitis, breast pain
HEMA: Decreased lymphocytes, ANC, WBC, *lymphadenopathy,* anemia
INTEG: *Sweating, inj site reaction*
MS: *Myalgia,* myasthenia
RESP: *Sinusitis,* dyspnea

INTERACTIONS
Individual drugs
Zidovudine: decreased clearance

Drug classifications
Antiretrovirals (NNRTIs, NRTIs, protease inhibitors): increased hepatic damage
Antineoplastics: increased myelosuppression

Drug/herb
Astragalus, echinacea, melatonin: change in immunomodulation

Drug/lab test
Increased: liver function tests
Interference: vaccines, toxoids; avoid concurrent use

NURSING CONSIDERATIONS
Assessment
• Monitor blood, renal, liver function tests: CBC, differential, platelet counts, BUN, creatinine, ALT, urinalysis; if neutrophil count is <750/mm³, or if AST, ALT is 10 × greater than ULN, or if bilirubin is 5 × greater than ULN, discontinue product; when neutrophil count exceeds 750/mm³ and liver function or renal studies return to normal, treatment may resume at 50% original dosage
• Assess for CNS symptoms: headache, fatigue, depression; if depression occurs and is severe, product should be discontinued
• Assess for multiple sclerosis symptoms
• Assess mental status: depression, depersonalization, suicidal thoughts, insomnia
• Monitor GI status: diarrhea or constipation, vomiting, abdominal pain
• Monitor cardiac status: increased B/P, tachycardia
• Assess for lupuslike symptoms

Patient problem
Lack of knowledge of medication (teaching)

Implementation
• Reconstitute 0.3 mg (9.6 million international units)/1.2 ml of supplied diluent (0.2 mg or 8 million international units concentration); rotate vial gently, do not shake; withdraw 1 ml using a syringe with 27-G needle; administer SUBCUT only into hip, thigh, arm; discard unused portion

>> Interferon beta-1a

- Reconstitute with 1.1 ml of diluent, swirl, give within 6 hr
- Store in refrigerator; do not freeze
- Visually inspect parenteral products for particulate matter and discoloration prior to use

IM route

- Premedication with acetaminophen or ibuprofen and give at bedtime to lessen flulike symptoms
- Interferon beta-1a (Avonex) 30 mcg is equivalent to 6 million IU
- If a dose is missed, give it as soon as possible; continue the regular schedule but do not give 2 injections within 2 days of each other; all products are for single-use only. Do not re-use needles, syringes, prefilled syringes, or autoinjectors; rotate injection sites
- Check site to minimize injection site reactions
- Do not inject into an area of the body where skin is irritated, reddened, bruised, infected, or scarred
- The injection site should be checked after 2 hours for redness, edema, or tenderness
- The manufacturer of Avonex offers free training on IM use for patients and health care partners. Contact MS ActiveSource for more information (800-456-2255)

Reconstitution and administration of Avonex lyophilized powder for IM route

- Use aseptic technique for preparation of solution
- Sites for injection include the thigh or upper arm
- Slowly add 1.1 ml sterile water for injection, preservative-free (supplied by manufacturer) to the vial. Rapid addition of the diluent may cause foaming
- Gently swirl; do not shake. Final concentration should be 30 mcg/ml (6 million IU/ml)
- The solution should be clear to slightly yellow without particles. Discard if the reconstituted product contains particulate matter or is discolored
- Withdraw 1 ml of reconstituted solution into a syringe. Attach the sterile needle and inject IM
- A 25-gauge, 1″ needle for IM may be substituted for the 23-gauge, 1¼″ needle provided
- *Storage:* Use within 6 hours of reconstitution; store reconstituted solution refrigerated; do NOT freeze. Discard any unused solution; both drug and diluent vials are single-use only

Administration of Avonex prefilled syringe

- The first injection should be performed under the supervision of an appropriately qualified person
- If self-injecting, rotate between thighs.

- Wash hands prior to handling the Dose Pack
- Remove prefilled syringe from the refrigerator to warm to room temperature (usually 30 min before use)
- Attach the needle by pressing it onto the syringe and turning it clockwise until it locks in place
- Inject IM at a 90-degree angle into the thigh or upper arm as directed by the provider
- Dispose of used needles and syringes
- *Storage:* Store refrigerated; if refrigeration is unavailable, may store at 77° F or less for up to 7 days; after removal from refrigerator, do not store product above 25° C. Do not freeze. Protect from light

Administration of Avonex prefilled autoinjector

- The first injection should be performed under the supervision of provider
- Remove one Administration Dose Pack from the refrigerator to warm to room temperature (about 30 min before use). Do not use external heat sources such as hot water to warm the syringe Dose Pack
- Wash hands prior to handling Dose Pack contents
- Grasp the cap and bend it at a 90-degree angle until it snaps off. Pull off the sterile foil from the needle cover
- Hold the Avonex pen with the glass syringe tip pointing up. Press the needle onto the glass syringe tip. Gently turn the needle clockwise until firmly attached. Do not remove plastic cover from the needle
- Hold pen with one hand and using other hand, hold onto the injector shield (grooved area) tightly and quickly pull up on the injector shield until the injector shield covers the needle all the way. The plastic needle cover will pop off after the injector shield has been fully extended
- When the injector shield is extended the right way, there will be a small blue rectangular area next to the oval medication display window. Check the display window and make sure the Avonex is clear and colorless
- Do not use the injection if the liquid is colored, cloudy, or has lumps or particles. Air bubbles will not affect your dose
- Avonex pen should be injected into the upper, outer thigh
- Hold pen at 90-degree angle to the injection site. Firmly push the body of the pen down against the thigh to release the safety lock. Push down on blue activation button with thumb and count to 10. You will hear a click if the injection is given the right way

- The circular display window on the pen will be yellow if you have received the full dose
- Dispose of used needles and syringes
- Refer to the Patient Medication Guide for detailed instructions for preparing and giving a dose
- *Storage:* Store at 36°-46° F (2°-8° C). If refrigeration is unavailable, may store at 77° F (25° C) or less for up to 7 days. After removal from refrigerator, do not store product above 77° F (25° C). Do not freeze. Protect from light

Subcutaneous administration

- Give at the same time (preferably late in the afternoon or evening) on the same days of the week at least 48 hr apart
- Do not give on two consecutive days. If a dose is missed, administer the dose as soon as possible then skip the following day. Return to the regular schedule the following week
- Premedication with acetaminophen or ibuprofen may lessen the severity of flulike symptoms
- Interferon beta-1a (Rebif) 44 mcg is equivalent to 12 million IU
- Rotate injection sites.
- A "Starter Pack" containing a lower dose of Rebif syringes is available for the initial titration period
- The manufacturer offers complimentary services including injection training and reimbursement support. Contact MS LifeLines at 877-44-REBIF

Injection (Rebif)

- Interferon beta-1a (Rebif) is available in a prefilled syringe with a 29-gauge needle
- Subcut into the outer surface of the upper arm, abdomen, thigh, or buttock. Do not inject the area near the navel or waistline. Take care not to inject intradermally
- Discard any unused solution. Prefilled syringes do not contain preservatives and are single-use only

>> Interferon beta-1b

- Reconstitute by injecting diluent provided (1.2 ml) into vial, swirl (8 million international units/ml), use 27-G needle for inj
- Give acetaminophen for fever, headache; use SUBCUT route only; do not give IM or **IV**
- Store reconstituted sol in refrigerator; do not freeze; do not use sol that contains precipitate or is discolored

Subcut route

- The manufacturers of Betaseron and of Extavia offer materials to assist with training on subcut use: call 1-800-788-1467 (Betaseron), 1-888-669-6682 (Extavia)

- Premedication with acetaminophen or ibuprofen and use of product at bedtime may lessen the severity of flulike symptoms
- Visually inspect parenteral products for particulate matter and discoloration prior to use. Do not use if particulate matter is present

Reconstitution

- Add 1.2 ml of 0.54% sodium chloride injection (supplied by the manufacturer) to the vial by using the vial adapter to attach the prefilled syringe that contains the diluent.
- If not used immediately, store in the refrigerator for up to 3 hr; do not freeze; discard any unused portion after 3 hr

Injection

- Withdraw the desired amount of the reconstituted solution into the syringe. Twist the vial adapter to remove it and the vial
- Choose an injection site on the upper, back arms; abdomen; buttocks; or front thighs. Do not inject within 2 in of the navel or in a site where the skin is red, bruised, infected, broken, painful, uneven, or scabbed; rotate injection sites
- Inject subcut. Take care not to inject intradermally

Patient/family education

- Provide patient or family member with written, detailed instructions about the product; provide initial and return demonstrations on inj procedure; give information on use and disposal of product
- Inform patient that blurred vision, hearing loss, sweating may occur
- Teach patient to use sunscreen as drug causes photosensitivity
- Teach patient inj technique and care of equipment
- Instruct patient to notify prescriber of increased temp, chills, muscle soreness, fatigue
- Advise female patients that irregular menses, dysmenorrhea, or metrorrhagia, as well as breast pain, may occur; use contraception during treatment; product may cause spontaneous abortion; instruct patient to notify prescriber if pregnancy is suspected

Evaluation

Positive therapeutic outcome

- Decreased symptoms of multiple sclerosis

⚠ HIGH ALERT

ipilimumab
(ip-i-lim'ue-mab)
Yervoy
Func. class.: Antineoplastic; biologic response modifier

ACTION: A recombinant, human monoclonal antibody that binds to the cytotoxic T-lymphocyte–associated antigen 4 (CTLA-4); action is indirect, possibly through T-cell–mediated antitumor immune responses

Therapeutic outcome: Decreased spread of malignant cells

USES: Treatment of unresectable or metastatic malignant melanoma

Pharmacokinetics

Absorption	Unknown
Distribution	Steady state (end of 3rd dose)
Metabolism	Unknown
Excretion	Unknown
Half-life	Terminal 15.4 days

Pharmacodynamics

Onset	Unknown
Peak	Unknown
Duration	Unknown

CONTRAINDICATIONS
Hypersensitivity

Precautions: Pregnancy, breastfeeding, Crohn's disease, hepatitis, immunosuppression, inflammatory bowel disease, iritis, ocular disease, organ transplant, pancreatitis, renal disease, rheumatoid arthritis, sarcoidosis, systemic lupus erythematosus, thyroid disease, ulcerative colitis, uveitis

> **BLACK BOX WARNING:** Adrenal insufficiency, diarrhea, Guillain-Barre syndrome, hepatic disease, myasthenia gravis, hypo/hyperthyroidism, hypopituitarism, peripheral neuropathy, serious rash, hypophysitis

DOSAGE AND ROUTES
Unresectable, metastatic melanoma
Adult: IV 3 mg/kg over 90 min q3wk × 4 doses.

Melanoma adjuvant treatment
Adult/Child ≥12 yr 10 mg/kg q 3 wk x 4 doses, then 10 mg/kg q 12 wk for up to 3 yr

Available forms: Solution for inj 50 mg/10 ml, 200 mg/40 ml

ADVERSE EFFECTS
CNS: Severe and fatal immune-mediated neuropathies, fatigue, fever, headache
EENT: Episcleritis, iritis, uveitis
ENDO: Severe and fatal immune-mediated endocrinopathies
GI: Severe and fatal immune-mediated enterocolitis, hepatitis; pancreatitis, abdominal pain, colitis, constipation, decreased appetite, diarrhea, nausea, vomiting
INTEG: Severe and fatal immune-mediated dermatitis, pruritus, rash, urticaria
MISC: Anemia, cough, dyspnea, eosinophilia, nephritis
SYST: Antibody formation, Stevens-Johnson syndrome, toxic epidermal necrolysis

> **BLACK BOX WARNING:** Adrenal insufficiency, diarrhea, Guillain-Barré syndrome, hepatic disease, myasthenia gravis, hyper/hypothyroidism, hypopituitarism, peripheral neuropathy, serious rash

NURSING CONSIDERATIONS
Assessment
• **Serious skin disorders:** Stevens-Johnson syndrome, toxic epidermal necrolysis: permanently discontinue in these or rash complicated by full thickness dermal ulceration or necrotic, bullous, or hemorrhagic manifestations like bullous rash; give systemic corticosteroids at a dose of 1-2 mg/kg/day of predniSONE or equivalent; when dermatitis is controlled, taper corticosteroids over a period of at least 1 month. Withhold in those with moderate to severe reactions; for mild to moderate dermatitis (localized rash and pruritus), give topical or systemic corticosteroids

> **BLACK BOX WARNING: Immune-mediated reactions:** Assess for enterocolitis, hepatitis, dermatitis, neuropathy, endocrinopathy, before starting treatment, take LFTs, ACTH, and thyroid function tests, permanently discontinue if these occur

• **Hepatotoxicity:** Monitor baseline and before each dose; rule out infectious or malignant causes and increase the frequency of liver function test monitoring until resolution; permanently discontinue in those with Grade 3-5, give systemic corticosteroids at a dose of 1-2 mg/kg/day of prednisone or equivalent

---

⚠ Nurse Alert　　　✺ Key NCLEX® Drug　　　≫ Drug Specifics

• **Neuropathy:** Monitor for motor or sensory neuropathy (unilateral or bilateral weakness, sensory alterations, or paresthesias) before each dose; permanently discontinue if severe neuropathy (interfering with daily activities) such as Guillain-Barré-like syndromes occur

• **Endocrinopathy:** Monitor thyroid function tests at baseline and before each dose; monitor hypophysitis, adrenal insufficiency, adrenal crisis, hyperthyroidism, hypothyroidism (fatigue, headache, mental status changes, abdominal pain, unusual bowel habits, hypotension, or nonspecific symptoms that may resemble other causes)

Patient problem
Impaired skin integrity (uses)
Risk for injury (adverse reactions)

Implementation

Intermittent IV infusion route
• Visually inspect parenteral products for particulate matter and discoloration before using whenever solution and container permit; solution may have a pale yellow color and have translucent-to-white, amorphous particles; discard the vial if the solution is cloudy, if there is pronounced discoloration, or if particulate matter is present

• Allow vials to stand at room temperature for 5 min before infusion preparation; withdraw the required volume and transfer into an IV bag. Discard partially used vials or empty vials; dilute with 0.9% sodium chloride injection, or 5% dextrose injection, to a final concentration (1-2 mg/ml); mix diluted solution by gentle inversion; do not admix

• Give infusion over 90 min through an IV line with a low-protein binding in-line filter, do not give with other products; after each infusion, flush the line with 0.9% sodium chloride injection, or 0.5% dextrose injection

• Store once diluted; store for no more than 24 hr refrigerated or at room temperature

Patient/family education
• Instruct patient/family to report immediately allergic reaction, skin rash, severe abdominal pain, yellowing of skin, eyes; tingling of extremities, change in bowel habits
• Discuss reason for treatment and expected results, to read medication guide
• **Vision changes:** Assess eyes for uveitis, iritis, episcleritis, corticosteroids may be used
• **Pregnancy:** Notify prescriber if pregnancy is planned or suspected, if breastfeeding to use contraception during and for 3 mo after final dose

Evaluation

Positive therapeutic outcome
• Decreasing spread of malignant melanoma

ipratropium (Rx)
(i-pra-troe′pee-um)
Atrovent ✦, Atrovent HFA
Func. class.: Anticholinergic, bronchodilator
Chem. class.: Synthetic quaternary ammonium compound

ACTION: Inhibits interaction of acetylcholine at receptor sites on the bronchial smooth muscle, resulting in decreased cyclic guanosine monophosphate (cyclic GMP) and bronchodilatation

Therapeutic outcome: Bronchodilatation

USES: Bronchospasm, COPD; rhinorrhea (nasal spray)

Pharmacokinetics
Absorption	Minimal
Distribution	Does not cross blood-brain barrier
Metabolism	Liver, minimal
Excretion	Unknown
Half-life	2 hr

Pharmacodynamics
Onset	5-15 min
Peak	1-1½ hr
Duration	3-6 hr

CONTRAINDICATIONS
Hypersensitivity to this product, atropine, bromide, soybean, or peanut products

Precautions: Pregnancy, breastfeeding, children <12 yr, angioedema, heart failure, surgery, acute bronchospasm, closed-angle glaucoma, prostatic hypertrophy, bladder neck obstruction, urinary retention

DOSAGE AND ROUTES
Bronchospasm in chronic bronchitis/emphysema
Adult: INH 2 sprays (17 mcg/spray) 3-4×/day, max 12 INH/24 hr, SOL 500 mcg (1 unit dose) given 3-4×/day by nebulizer; nasal spray: 2 sprays (42 mcg/spray) 3-4×/day
Child 5-12 yr: NASAL 2 sprays in each nostril 3×/day

Rhinorrhea perennial rhinitis
Adult/child ≥6 yr: INTRANASAL 2 sprays (43 mcg)/nostril bid or tid

Child 5-12 yr: INTRANASAL 2 sprays (0.03%) in each nostril 3×/day

Available forms: Aerosol 17 mcg/actuation; nasal spray 0.03%, 0.06%; sol for inh 0.0125% 🍁, 0.02%

ADVERSE EFFECTS

CNS: *Anxiety, dizziness, headache,* nervousness
CV: Palpitations
EENT: Dry mouth, blurred vision, nasal congestion
GI: *Nausea, vomiting, cramps*
INTEG: Rash
RESP: *Cough, worsening of symptoms,* bronchospasm

INTERACTIONS
Individual drugs
Disopyramide: increased anticholinergic action

Drug classifications
Antihistamines, phenothiazines: increased anticholinergic action
Bronchodilators (other): increased toxicity

Drug/herb
Belladonna: increased anticholinergic effect
Green tea (large amounts), guarana: increased bronchodilator effect

NURSING CONSIDERATIONS
Assessment
• Monitor respiratory function: vital capacity, FEV, ABGs/VBGs, lung sounds, heart rate, rhythm (baseline, during treatment); if severe bronchospasm is present, a more rapid medication is required
• Monitor for evidence of allergic reactions, paradoxical bronchospasm; withhold dose and notify prescriber; identify if patient is allergic to belladonna products or atropine; allergy to this product may occur
• **Pregnancy/breastfeeding:** Use only if benefits outweigh fetal risk, cautious use in breastfeeding, excretion unknown

Patient problem
Impaired airway clearance (uses)
Activity intolerance (uses)

Implementation
• Give after shaking container; have patient exhale, place mouthpiece in mouth, inhale slowly, hold breath, remove, exhale slowly; allow at least 1 min between inhalations
• Give this medication before other medications and allow at least 5 min between each

Nebulizer route
• Use solution in nebulizer with a mouthpiece rather than a face mask
Intranasal route
• Prime pump, initially requires 7 actuations of the pump, priming again is not necessary if used regularly; tilt head backward after dose
• Store in light-resistant container; do not expose to temperature over 86° F (30° C)

Patient/family education
• Advise patient not to use OTC medications unless approved by prescriber; extra stimulation may occur; to use this medication before other medications and allow at least 5 min between each to prevent overstimulation
• Teach patient that compliance is necessary with number of inhalations/24 hr, or overdose may occur
• Instruct geriatric patients to use spacer device
• Teach patient the proper use of the inhaler; review package insert with patient; to avoid getting aerosol in eyes, blurring may result; to wash inhaler in warm water daily and dry; to avoid smoking, smoke-filled rooms, persons with respiratory tract infections
• Teach patient if paradoxical bronchospasm occurs to stop product immediately and notify prescriber; to limit caffeine products such as chocolate, coffee, tea, and colas
• Instruct patient on administration of dose, not to use more than prescribed; serious side effects may occur; if dose is missed, take when remembered; space other doses on new time schedule; do not double doses
• Use spacer to improve drug delivery if required

Evaluation

Positive therapeutic outcome
• Absence of dyspnea, wheezing after 1 hr
• Improved airway exchange
• Improved ABGs/VBGs

irbesartan (Rx)
(er-be-sar′tan)
Avapro
Func. class.: Antihypertensive
Chem. class.: Angiotensin II receptor (type AT_1)

Do not confuse: Avapro/Anaprox

ACTION: Blocks the vasoconstrictor and aldosterone-secreting effects of angiotensin II;

⚠ Nurse Alert   ✼ Key NCLEX® Drug   ≫ Drug Specifics

selectively blocks the binding of angiotensin II to the AT_1 receptor found in tissues

Therapeutic outcome: Decreased B/P

USES: Hypertension, alone or in combination, nephropathy in patients with type 2 diabetes mellitus; proteinuria

Unlabeled uses: Heart failure

Pharmacokinetics

Absorption	Well absorbed
Distribution	Bound to plasma proteins (90%)
Metabolism	Liver (minimal) by CYP2C9
Excretion	Feces, urine
Half-life	11-15 hr

Pharmacodynamics

Unknown

CONTRAINDICATIONS
Hypersensitivity

BLACK BOX WARNING: Pregnancy (2nd/3rd trimesters)

Precautions: Pregnancy (1st trimester), breastfeeding, children <6 yr, geriatric, renal/hepatic disease, renal artery stenosis, hypersensitivity to ACE inhibitors, African descent, angioedema

DOSAGE AND ROUTES
Hypertension
Adult: PO 150 mg/day; may be increased to 300 mg/day; volume-depleted patients: start with 75 mg/day

Nephropathy in patients with type 2 diabetes mellitus
Adult: PO maintenance dose 300 mg/day, start 75 mg/day

Available forms: Tabs 75, 150, 300 mg

ADVERSE EFFECTS
CNS: Dizziness, anxiety, *headache, fatigue,* syncope
CV: Hypotension
GI: *Diarrhea, dyspepsia,* hepatitis, cholestasis
HEMA: Thrombocytopenia
MISC: Edema, chest pain, rash, tachycardia, UTI, angioedema, hyperkalemia
RESP: *Cough, upper respiratory infection,* rhinitis, pharyngitis, sinus disorder

INTERACTIONS
Drug classifications
CYP2C9 inhibitors (amiodarone, delavirdine, fluconazole, FLUoxetine, fluvastatin, fluvoxaMINE, imatinib, sulfonamides, sulfinpyrazone, voriconazole, zafirlukast): increased irbesartan level
Diuretics (potassium sparing), ACE inhibitors, potassium salt substitutes: increased hyperkalemia
NSAIDs: decreased antihypertensive effect

Drug/herb
Astragalus, cola tree: increased or decreased antihypertensive effect
Black cohosh, garlic, goldenseal, hawthorn, kelp: increased antihypertensive effect
Guarana, khat, licorice, yohimbe: decreased antihypertensive effect

NURSING CONSIDERATIONS
Assessment
• **Hypotension:** For severe hypotension, place in supine position and give IV infusion of NS; drug may be continued after B/P is restored
• Assess B/P, pulse q4hr; note rate, rhythm, quality
• Monitor electrolytes: potassium, sodium, chloride
• Obtain baselines for renal, liver function tests before therapy begins
• Monitor for edema in feet, legs daily
• Assess for skin turgor, dryness of mucous membranes for hydration status

Patient problem
Risk for injury (adverse reactions)
Nonadherence (teaching)

Implementation
• Administer without regard to meals
• May be used with other antihypertensives, diuretic
• Volume depletion should be done before use

Patient/family education
• Advise patient to comply with dosage schedule, even if feeling better
• Inform patient that product may cause dizziness, fainting, light-headedness
• Caution patient to rise slowly to sitting or standing position to minimize orthostatic hypotension
• Teach patient not to stop product abruptly
• Teach patient to take without regard to food

BLACK BOX WARNING: Advise patient to notify prescriber if pregnancy is suspected; pregnancy (D) 2nd/3rd trimester, (C) 1st trimester

Evaluation
Positive therapeutic outcome
• Decreased B/P

> **⚠ HIGH ALERT**
>
> # irinotecan (Rx)
> (ear-een-oh-tee'kan)
> **Camptosar**
> *Func. class.:* Antineoplastic hormone
> *Chem. class.:* Topoisomerase inhibitor

ACTION: Cytotoxic by producing damage to single-strand DNA during DNA synthesis, binds to topoisomerase I

Therapeutic outcome: Prevention in growth of tumor

USES: Metastatic carcinoma of colon or rectum, or 1st-line treatment in combination with fluorouracil (5-FU) and leucovorin for metastatic carcinoma of colon or rectum

Pharmacokinetics

Absorption	Complete
Distribution	Widely, 30%-68% bound to plasma proteins, increased risk of toxicity in those homozygous for UGT1A128
Metabolism	Unknown
Excretion	Urine/bile
Half-life	6-12 hr

Pharmacodynamics

Unknown

CONTRAINDICATIONS
Pregnancy, hypersensitivity

Precautions: Breastfeeding, children, geriatric, irradiation, hepatic disease

> **BLACK BOX WARNING:** Myelosuppression, diarrhea

DOSAGE AND ROUTES
Colorectal cancer in combination with 5-fluorouracil: IV dosage (with bolus 5-FU/leucovorin)
Adult: IV 125 mg/m² over 90 min followed by leucovorin (20 mg/m² IV bolus) and then 5-FU (500 mg/m² IV bolus) on days 1, 8, 15, and 22; the next course begins on day 43 or when toxicity has recovered to NCI grade 1 or less

IV dosage (with infusional 5-FU/ leucovorin)
Adult: IV 180 mg/m² over 90 min followed by leucovorin (200 mg/m² IV over 2 hr) then 5-FU bolus and continuous infusion (400 mg/m² IV bolus, then 600 mg/m² IV infusion over 22 hr); give days 1, 15, and 29, while leucovorin and

5-FU are given on days 1, 2, 15, 16, 29, and 30; the next course begins on day 43 or when toxicity has recovered to NCI grade 1 or less

Available forms: Inj 20 mg/ml

ADVERSE EFFECTS
CNS: Fever, headache, chills, dizziness
CV: Vasodilatation, edema, thromboembolism
GI: Severe diarrhea, *nausea, vomiting,* anorexia, constipation, cramps, flatus, stomatitis, dyspepsia, hepatotoxicity
HEMA: Leukopenia, anemia, neutropenia
INTEG: Irritation at site, rash, sweating, alopecia
MISC: Asthenia, weight loss, back pain
RESP: Dyspnea, increased cough, rhinitis

INTERACTIONS
Individual products
CarBAMazepine, PHENobarbital, phenytoin: decreased irinotecan levels
Dexamethasone: increased lymphocytopenia, hyperglycemia
Fluorouracil: increased toxicity
Prochlorperazine: increased akathisia
Radiation: increased myelosuppression, diarrhea

Drug classifications
Anticoagulants, NSAIDs: increased bleeding risk
Antineoplastics: increased myelosuppression, diarrhea
CYP3A4 inhibitors (ketoconazole): increased irinotecan levels
CYP3A4 inducers (phenytoin, carBAMazepine, PENTobarbital): decreased irinotecan levels
Diuretics: increased dehydration

Drug/herb
St. John's wort: decreased product level; avoid concurrent use

Drug/lab test
Increased: ALK phos, AST, LFTs, bilirubin
Decreased: platelets, WBC, neutrophils, Hgb/Hct

NURSING CONSIDERATIONS
Assessment
• Assess for CNS symptoms: fever, headache, chills, dizziness

> **BLACK BOX WARNING: Myelosuppression:**
> Assess CBC, differential, platelet count weekly; use colony-stimulating factor if WBC is <2000/mm³, platelet count is <100,000/mm³, Hgb ≤9 g/dl, neutrophils ≤1000/mm³; notify prescriber of these results, product should be discontinued

---

• Assess buccal cavity for dryness, sores or ulceration, white patches, oral pain, bleeding, dysphagia

> **BLACK BOX WARNING:** Assess GI symptoms: frequency of stools; cramping; severe life-threatening diarrhea may occur with fluid and electrolyte imbalances; treat diarrhea within 24 hr of use with 0.25-1 mg atropine IV; treat diarrhea >24 hr of use with loperamide; diarrhea >24 hr (late diarrhea) can be fatal

• Assess early diarrhea and other cholinergic symptoms, treat with atropine; late diarrhea can be life-threatening, must be treated promptly with loperamide
• **Assess signs of dehydration:** rapid respirations, poor skin turgor, decreased urine output; dry skin, restlessness, weakness
• **Assess for bone marrow depression:** bruising, bleeding, blood in stools, urine, sputum, emesis

Patient problem
Risk for infection (adverse reactions)
Risk for injury (adverse reactions)

Implementation
• Use cytotoxic handling precautions

IV route
• Premedicate with antiemetic, dexamethasone plus another antiemetic agent, such as a 5-HT$_3$ blocker, given at least 30 min before use
• Prior to beginning a course of therapy, the granulocyte count should be ≥1500, the platelet count ≥100,000 and treatment-related diarrhea should be fully resolved
Dilution
• Dilute appropriate dose in D$_5$W (preferred) or NS injection to a final concentration of 0.12-2.8 mg/ml
• Store up to 24 hr at room temperature and room lighting; because of possible microbial contamination during preparation, an admixture prepared with D$_5$W or NS should be used within 6 hr; solutions prepared with D$_5$W, refrigerated and protected from light, can be stored for up to 48 hr; avoid refrigeration if prepared with NS
Intravenous infusion
• Infuse over 90 min

Y-site compatibilities: alemtuzumab, alfentanil, amifostine, amikacin, aminocaproic acid, aminophylline, amiodarone, ampicillin, ampicillin-sulbactam, anidulafungin, argatroban, atenolol, atracurium, azithromycin, aztreonam, bivalirudin, bleomycin, bretylium, bumetanide, buprenorphine, butorphanol, calcium chloride/gluconate, capreomycin, CARBOplatin, caspofungin, cefazolin, cefoTEtan, cefOXitin, cefTAZidime, ceftazidime (L-arginine), ceftizoxime, cefuroxime, cimetidine, ciprofloxacin, cisatracurium, CISplatin, clindamycin, cyclophosphamide, cyclosporine, cytarabine, dacarbazine, daptomycin, daunorubicin, daunorubicin liposome, dexamethasone, dexrazoxane, digoxin, diltiazem, diphenhydramine, dobutamine, DOCEtaxel, dolasetron, dopamine, doxacurium, doxorubicin, doxorubicin liposomal, doxycycline, enalaprilat, ePHEDrine, EPINEPHrine, ertapenem, erythromycin, esmolol, etoposide, etoposide phosphate, famotidine, fenoldopam, fentaNYL, fluconazole, foscarnet, gallium, garenoxacin, gatifloxacin, gemtuzumab, gentamicin, granisetron, haloperidol, heparin, hydrALAZINE, hydrocortisone, HYDROmorphone, hydrOXYzine, IDArubicin, imipenem-cilastatin, inamrinone, insulin regular, isoproterenol, ketorolac, labetalol, lepirudin, leucovorin, levofloxacin, levoleucovorin, levorphanol, lidocaine, linezolid, lorazepam, magnesium sulfate, mannitol, meperidine, meropenem, mesna, metaraminol, methadone, methyldopa, metoclopramide, metoprolol, metroNIDAZOLE, midazolam, milrinone, minocycline, mitoxantrone, mivacurium, morphine, moxifloxacin, nalbuphine, naloxone, nesiritide, niCARdipine, nitroglycerin, norepinephrine, octreotide, ondansetron, oxaliplatin, PACLitaxel (solvent/surfactant), palonosetron, pancuronium, pantoprazole, pentamidine, pentazocine, PENTobarbital, PHENobarbital, phentolamine, phenylephrine, polymyxin b, potassium acetate/chloride/phosphates, procainamide, prochlorperazine, promethazine, propranolol, quiNIDine, quinupristin-dalfopristin, raNITIdine, remifentanil, riTUXimab, rocuronium, sodium acetate/bicarbonate/phosphates, succinylcholine, SUFentanil, sulfamethoxazole-trimethoprim, tacrolimus, teniposide, theophylline, thiotepa, ticlidine, ticarcillin-clavulanate, tigecycline, tirofiban, tobramycin, tolazoline, trimethobenzamide, vancomycin, vasopressin, vecuronium, verapamil, vinblastine, vinorelbine, voriconazole, zidovudine, zoledronic acid

Patient/family education
• Advise patient to avoid foods with citric acid or hot or rough texture if stomatitis is present; to drink adequate fluids
• Advise patient to report stomatitis; any bleeding, white spots, ulcerations in mouth; tell patient to examine mouth daily, report symptoms
• Advise patient to report signs of anemia: fatigue, headache, faintness, shortness of breath, irritability, infection, rash
• Advise patient to avoid vaccinations while taking this product

---

> **BLACK BOX WARNING:** Instruct patient to report diarrhea that occurs 24 hr after administration; severe dehydration can occur rapidly

- Teach patient to avoid salicylates, NSAIDs, alcohol; bleeding may occur; to avoid all of these products unless approved by prescriber
- Teach patient to report immediately injection site pain, irritation
- Teach patient to report vomiting, dizziness
- Teach patient that regular lab exams will be needed
- Advise patient to use contraception during therapy; to report if pregnancy is planned or suspected

Evaluation

Positive therapeutic outcome
- Decrease in tumor size, decrease in spread of cancer

iron, carbonyl
See ferrous fumarate

iron dextran (Rx)
DexFerrum, Dexiren ✤, InFed, Infufer ✤
Func. class.: Hematinic
Chem. class.: Ferric hydroxide complex with dextran

Do not confuse: Imferon/Imuran/Roferon-A/Interferon

ACTION: Iron is carried by transferrin to the bone marrow, where it is incorporated into hemoglobin

Therapeutic outcome: Prevention and resolution of iron-deficiency anemia

USES: Iron-deficiency anemia

Pharmacokinetics

Absorption	Well absorbed; lymphatics over wk or mo
Distribution	Crosses placenta
Metabolism	Slow; blood loss, desquamation
Excretion	Breast milk, feces, urine, bile
Half-life	6 hr

Pharmacodynamics

Unknown

CONTRAINDICATIONS

> **BLACK BOX WARNING:** Hypersensitivity

Precautions: Pregnancy, breastfeeding, infants <4 mo, children, acute renal disease, asthma, rheumatoid arthritis (**IV**), all anemias excluding iron-deficiency anemia, hepatic/cardiac/renal disease, neonates, ankylosing spondylitis, lupus, hypotension

DOSAGE AND ROUTES
Adult and child: IM 0.5 ml as a test dose by Z-track, then no more than the following total dose including test dose per day:
Adult/adolescent/child (>15 kg):
Total iron dextran dose in ml =
$[0.0442 \times (\text{Desired Hb} - \text{observed Hb}) \times \text{LBW}]$
$+ (0.26 \times \text{LBW})$,
max of undiluted is 100 mg (2 ml)/day

Child (10-15 kg):
Total iron dextran dose in ml =
$[0.0442 \times (\text{Desired Hb} - \text{observed Hb}) \times \text{LBW}]$
$+ (0.26 \times \text{ABW})$,
max of undiluted iron dextran is 100 mg (2 ml)/day

Child/Infant >4 mo (5-9.9 kg):
Total iron dextran dose in ml =
$[0.0442 \times (\text{Desired Hb} - \text{observed Hb}) \times \text{LBW}]$
$+ (0.26 \times \text{ABW})$

Infants >4 mo (<5 kg):
Total iron dextran dose in ml =
$[0.0442 \times (\text{Desired Hb} - \text{observed Hb}) \times \text{LBW}]$
$+ (0.26 \times \text{ABW})$

Available forms: Inj **IM/IV** 50 mg/ml (2 ml, 10 ml vials)

ADVERSE EFFECTS
CNS: Headache, paresthesia, dizziness, shivering, weakness, seizures
CV: Chest pain, shock, hypotension, tachycardia
GI: *Nausea*, vomiting, metallic taste, abdominal pain
HEMA: Leukocytosis
INTEG: Rash, pruritus, urticaria, fever, sweating, chills, brown skin discoloration, pain at inj site, necrosis, sterile abscesses, phlebitis
MISC: Anaphylaxis
RESP: Dyspnea

INTERACTIONS
Individual drugs
Chloramphenicol: decreased reticulocyte response
Oral iron: do not use together, increased toxicity

Drug/lab test
False increase: serum bilirubin
False decrease: serum calcium
False positive: ^{99m}Tc diphosphate bone scan, iron test (large doses >2 ml)

NURSING CONSIDERATIONS
Assessment
• Observe for 1 hr after test dose
• Monitor blood studies: Hct, Hgb, reticulocytes, transferrin, plasma iron concentrations, ferritin, total iron-binding bilirubin before treatment, at least monthly

> **BLACK BOX WARNING:** Assess for allergic reaction and anaphylaxis; rash, pruritus, fever, chills, wheezing; notify prescriber immediately, keep emergency equipment available

• Assess cardiac status: anginal pain, hypotension, tachycardia
• Assess for nutrition: amount of iron in diet (meat, dark green leafy vegetables, dried fruits, eggs); cause of iron loss or anemia, including salicylates, sulfonamides
• Monitor pulse, B/P during **IV** administration
• Assess for toxicity: nausea, vomiting, diarrhea, fever, abdominal pain (early symptoms); cyanotic lips, nailbeds, seizures, CV collapse (late symptoms)
• **Pregnancy/breastfeeding:** Use only if benefits outweigh fetal risk, cautious use in breastfeeding, trace amounts appear in breast milk

Patient problem
Fatigue (uses)
Activity intolerance (uses)

Implementation
IM route
• Discontinue oral iron before parenteral; give only after test dose of 25 mg by preferred route; wait at least 1 hr before giving remaining portion
• Give IM inj deep in large muscle mass; use Z-track method and 19-G, 20-G 2-, 3-inch needle; ensure needle is long enough to place product deep in muscle; change needles after withdrawing medication and injecting to prevent skin and tissue staining

IV route
• Give **IV** after flushing tubing with 10 ml of 0.9% NaCl; give undiluted; give 1 ml (50 mg) or less over 1 min or more; flush line after use with 10 ml of 0.9% NaCl; patient should remain recumbent for 30-60 min to prevent orthostatic hypotension
• **IV** inj requires single-dose vial without preservative; verify on label **IV** use is approved
• Give by cont inf after diluting in 50-250 ml of 0.9% NaCl for inf; administer over 4-5 hr

• Give only with epinephrine available in case of anaphylactic reaction during dose
• Store at room temperature in cool environment

Patient/family education
• Caution patient that iron poisoning may occur if increased beyond recommended level; to not take oral iron preparation or vitamins containing iron unless approved by prescriber
• Advise patient that delayed reaction may occur 1-2 days after administration and last 3-4 days (IV) or 3-7 days (IM); report fever, chills, malaise, muscle/joint aches, nausea, vomiting, backache
• Advise patient to avoid breastfeeding
• Advise patient that stools may become dark

Evaluation
Positive therapeutic outcome
• Increased serum iron levels, Hct, Hgb

TREATMENT OF OVERDOSE:
Discontinue product, treat allergic reaction, give diphenhydrAMINE or EPINEPHrine as needed for anaphylaxis; give iron-chelating product in acute poisoning

iron polysaccharide
See ferrous fumarate

iron sucrose (Rx)
Venofer
Func. class.: Hematinic
Chem. class.: Ferric hydroxide complex with dextran

ACTION: Iron is carried by transferrin to the bone marrow, where it is incorporated into hemoglobin

Therapeutic outcome: Improved signs/symptoms of iron deficiency anemia; iron levels improved

USES: Iron deficiency anemia, hyperphosphatemia in chronic kidney disease on dialysis

Pharmacokinetics	
Absorption	Unknown
Distribution	Unknown
Metabolism	Unknown
Excretion	Urine
Half-life	6 hr

Pharmacodynamics
Unknown

CONTRAINDICATIONS
Hypersensitivity, all anemias excluding iron deficiency anemia, iron overload

Precautions: Pregnancy, breastfeeding (**IV**), children, geriatric, abdominal pain, anaphylactic shock, arthralgia, chest pain, cough, diarrhea, dizziness, dyspnea, edema, increased LFTs, fever, headache, heart failure, hyper/hypotension, infection, MS pain, nausea/vomiting, seizures, weakness

DOSAGE AND ROUTES
Adult: IV 5 ml (100 mg of elemental iron) given during dialysis, most will need 1000 mg of elemental iron over 10 sequential dialysis sessions

Hyperphosphatemia in chronic kidney disease
Adult: PO 500 mg tid

Available forms: Inj 20 mg/ml; chew tab 500 mg

ADVERSE EFFECTS
CNS: Headache, dizziness
CV: Chest pain, hypo/hypertension, hypervolemia, heart failure
GI: *Nausea, vomiting, abdominal pain*
INTEG: Rash, pruritus, urticaria, fever, sweating, chills
MISC: Anaphylaxis, hyperglycemia
RESP: Dyspnea, pneumonia, cough

INTERACTIONS
Individual drugs
Chloramphenicol: decreased iron sucrose
Dimercaprol, iron (oral): increased toxicity; do not use together

Drug/lab test
Increased: glucose

NURSING CONSIDERATIONS
Assessment
• Monitor blood studies: Hct, Hgb, reticulocytes, transferrin, plasma iron concentrations, ferritin, total iron binding, bilirubin before treatment, at least monthly
• **Assess for allergy:** anaphylaxis, rash, pruritus, fever, chills, wheezing; notify prescriber immediately, keep emergency equipment available
• Assess cardiac status: hypotension, hypertension, hypervolemia
• **Assess for toxicity:** nausea, vomiting, diarrhea, fever, abdominal pain (early symptoms), cyanotic-looking lips and nailbeds, seizures, CV collapse (late symptoms)

• **Pregnancy/breastfeeding:** Use only if clearly needed, cautious use in breastfeeding

Patient problem
Fatigue (uses)
Activity intolerance (uses)

Implementation
• Give only with epinephrine, Solu-MEDROL in case of anaphylactic reaction during dose
• Do not use if particulate is present, or if sol is discolored

IV route
• Give directly in dialysis line by slow inj or inf; give by slow inj at 1 ml/min (5 min/vial); inf dilute each vial exclusively in a maximum of 100 ml of 0.9% NaCl, give at rate of 100 mg of iron/15 min, discard unused portions
• Store at room temperature in cool environment, do not freeze
• Do not use with other IV products

Patient/family education
• Teach patient that iron poisoning may occur if increased beyond recommended level; not to take oral iron preparations
• Teach patient to report itching, rash, chest pain, headache, vertigo, nausea, vomiting, abdominal pain, joint/muscle pain, numbness, tingling

Evaluation
Positive therapeutic outcome
• Increased serum iron levels, Hct, Hgb

TREATMENT OF OVERDOSE:
Discontinue product, treat allergic reaction, give diphenhydrAMINE or epinephrine as needed, give iron-chelating product in acute poisoning

isavuconazonium (Rx)
(eye′ sa-vue-koe′ na-zoe′ nee-um)
Cresemba
Func. class.: Antifungal, systemic
Chem. class.: Azole

ACTION: Exerts antifungal activity by inhibiting the synthesis of ergosterol, an essential component of the fungal cell membrane. The depletion of ergosterol within the fungal cell membrane results in increased cellular permeability causing leakage of cellular content

Therapeutic outcome: Decreasing signs, symptoms of infection

USES: *Aspergillus flavus, Aspergillus fumigatus, Aspergillus niger, Rhizopus oryzae,* Rucormycetes species; do NOT use for infections of *Candida, Blastomyces, Histoplasma* V

Pharmacokinetics

Absorption	Unknown
Distribution	Chinese patients (levels 40% lower), protein binding >99%
Metabolism	By CYP3A4, CYP3A5, UGT, P-gp, OCT2 enzymes
Excretion	Eliminated in urine/feces
Half-life	Unknown

Pharmacodynamics

Onset	Unknown
Peak	2 hrs (**PO**)
Duration	Unknown

CONTRAINDICATIONS

Hypersensitivity, short QT syndrome

Precautions: Azole hypersensitivity, pregnancy, breastfeeding, infusion-related reactions, hepatic disease

DOSAGE AND ROUTES

Adults: PO loading dose of 2 caps (372 mg) q8hr X 6 doses. Then, 2 caps (372 mg) qday. Start maintenance dosing 12-24 hr after the last loading dose; **IV** loading dose of 372 mg q8hr X 6 doses, then 372 mg day; then 12-24 hr after the last loading dose give over 1 hr, use a 0.2- to 1.2-micron in-line filter and be administered over a minimum of 1 hr, an additional loading dose is not needed when switching to PO

Available forms: Caps 186 mg; powder for inj 382 mg

ADVERSE EFFECTS

CNS: *Headache,* paresthesias, peripheral neuropathy, *hallucinations,* depression, insomnia, dizziness, fever, vertigo, tremor, confusion
CV: tachypnea, supraventricular tachycardia, atrial fibrillation/flutter
EENT: Tinnitus
GI: *Nausea, vomiting, anorexia, diarrhea,* cramps, hepatitis, stomatitis
GU: *Hypokalemia,* renal failure
HEMA: Anemia, eosinophilia, hypomagnesemia, thrombocytopenia, leukopenia
INTEG: *Burning, irritation,* pain, necrosis at injection site with extravasation, rash
MISC: Cough

INTERACTIONS
Individual drugs

CycloSPORINE, pimozide, quiNIDine, predniso-LONE, sirolimus, tacrolimus, warfarin, rifabutin, phenytoin: increased effects of each

Drug classifications

Benzodiazepines, calcium channel blockers, ergots, HMG-CoA reductase inhibitors, sulfonylureas, vinca alkaloids, proton pump inhibitors, NNRTIs, protease inhibitors: increased effects of each
CYP3A4 substrates: increased effect of these
CYP3A4 inhibitors: decreased effect of these

Drug/herb

• Do not use with St. John's wort

Drug/lab test

Increased: AST/ALT, alk phos, creatinine, bilirubin
Decreased: Hgb/Hct, platelets, WBC

NURSING CONSIDERATIONS
Assessment

• **Short QT syndrome:** Do not use in this condition
• Monitor VS q15-30min during first infusion; note changes in pulse, B/P
• Blood studies: Obtain CBC, potassium, sodium, calcium, magnesium, q2wk
• **Hepatotoxicity:** Identify increasing AST, ALT, alk phos, bilirubin, baseline and periodically
• **Allergic reaction:** Assess for dermatitis, rash; product should be discontinued, antihistamines (mild reaction) or epinephrine (severe reaction) administered
• **Hypokalemia:** Assess for anorexia, drowsiness, weakness, decreased reflexes, dizziness, increased urinary output, increased thirst, paresthesias
• **Ototoxicity:** Assess for tinnitus (ringing, roaring in ears), vertigo
• **Pregnancy:** Test for pregnancy before starting treatment, do not breastfeed

Patient problem

Infection (uses)

Implementation
PO route

• Swallow whole, do not chew, crush, dissolve, open the capsules; may be used without regard to food

IV route

• Visually inspect for particulate matter and discoloration. The diluted solution may contain translucent to white particulates which will be removed by the in-line filter

Reconstitution

• Reconstitute the dry powder with 5 mL sterile water for inj, gently shake until dissolved
• Storage: The reconstituted solution may be stored below 25° C (77° F) for a maximum of 1 hr before further dilution

Dilution

• Remove 5 mL of the reconstituted solution and add it to 250 mL of either 0.9% NaCI or D₅W (1.5 mg /mL)

- Gently mix the solution or roll the bag. DO NOT shake. Do not place in a pneumatic transport system
- Apply an in-line filter (0.2-1.2 micron), adhere an in-line filter reminder sticker to the infusion bag
- Give over ≤ 6 hr of dilution
- Storage: May be stored immediately after dilution at 2 to 8 degrees C (36 to 46 degrees F); administration MUST be completed within 24 hr of the time of dilution. Do NOT freeze
- Use product only after C&S confirms organism, product needed to treat condition; make sure product used in life-threatening infections
- Flush IV lines with 0.9% sodium chloride or 5% dextrose in water before and after administration of the infusion
- Must be administered through a 0.2-1.2 micron filter; give over ≥ 1 hr. Do not give by bolus. *Do not admix*

Patient/family education
- Teach patient that long-term therapy may be needed to clear infection (2 wk-3 mo, depending on type of infection)
- Advise patient to notify prescriber of bleeding, bruising, soft-tissue swelling, dark urine, persistent nausea or diarrhea, headache, rash, yellow skin/eyes
- Women of childbearing age should use effective contraceptive

Evaluation
- Therapeutic response: Resolution of fungal infection, negative C&S

isoniazid (Rx)
(eye-soe-nye′a-zid)
Isotamine ✤
Func. class.: Antitubercular
Chem. class.: Isonicotinic acid hydrazide

ACTION: Bactericidal interference with lipid, nucleic acid biosynthesis

Therapeutic outcome: Resolution of TB infection

USES: Treatment, prevention of TB

Pharmacokinetics

Absorption	Well absorbed
Distribution	Widely, protein binding 15%
Metabolism	Liver ⬥ 50% of patients may metabolize slowly, increasing toxicity;
Excretion	Kidneys
Half-life	1-4 hr (slow acetylators); 0.5-1.5 hr (fast acetylators)

Pharmacodynamics

	PO	IM
Onset	Rapid	Rapid
Peak	1-2 hr	45-60 min
Duration	6-8 hr	6-8 hr

CONTRAINDICATIONS
Hypersensitivity

BLACK BOX WARNING: Acute liver disease

Precautions: Pregnancy, diabetic retinopathy, cataracts, ocular defects, renal disease, **IV** drug users, people >35 yr, postpartum period, HIV, neuropathy

BLACK BOX WARNING: ⬥ Female (African descent, Hispanic), alcoholism

DOSAGE AND ROUTES
Adult/adolescent: PO/IM 5 mg/kg/day up to 300 mg/day or 15 mg/kg 2-3 times per week, max 900 mg 2-3 times per week
Child and infant HIV positive: PO/IM 10-15 mg/kg/day; max 300 mg/day

Available forms: Tabs 100, 300 mg; inj 100 mg/ml; oral sol 10 mg/ml

ADVERSE EFFECTS

CNS: *Peripheral neuropathy, dizziness,* seizures, psychosis
EENT: Blurred vision, optic neuritis
GI: *Nausea, vomiting,* fatal hepatitis
HEMA: Agranulocytosis, hemolytic anemia, aplastic anemia, thrombocytopenia, eosinophilia, methemoglobinemia
MISC: Stevens-Johnson syndrome, DRESS, toxic epidermal necrolysis, rash, fever

INTERACTIONS
Individual drugs
Alcohol, carBAMazepine, cycloSERINE, ethionamide, meperidine, phenytoin, rifampin, warfarin: increased toxicity
BCG vaccine, ketoconazole: decreased effectiveness

Drug classifications
Antacids, aluminum: decreased absorption
Benzodiazepines: increased toxicity
SSRIs, SNRIs: increased serotonin syndrome

Drug/food
Tyramine foods: increased toxicity

Drug/lab test
Increased: LFTs, bilirubin, glucose
Decreased: platelets, granulocytes

NURSING CONSIDERATIONS
Assessment
• Obtain C&S tests, including sputum tests, before treatment; monitor every mo to detect resistance, may start treatment before results are received

> **BLACK BOX WARNING:** Monitor liver function tests weekly; obtain baseline in all patients, those >35 yr and all women should be monitored periodically; monitor ALT, AST, bilirubin; increased results may indicate hepatitis; renal studies during treatment, monthly: BUN, creatinine, output, specific gravity, urinalysis, uric acid; those with fast acetylation (genetic) may metabolize product more than 5 times faster (Black, Asian, and some Caucasians are at greater risk); fatal hepatitis is a greater risk in Blacks/Hispanics after birth

• **DRESS:** Assess for fever, flu-like symptoms, rash, lymphadenopathy, facial swelling; may involve other organ systems
• **Stevens-Johnson syndrome, toxic epidermal necrolysis:** Assess for rash, fever, fatigue, blistering; discontinue immediately if these occur
• 🐾 Susceptibility tests before and periodically, half of Mexicans, Blacks, Caucasians, and Indians may be slow acetylators, fast acetylators may be Asians, Eskimos
• Assess mental status often: affect, mood, behavioral changes; psychosis may occur with hallucinations, confusion
• Assess hepatic status: decreased appetite, jaundice, dark urine, fatigue
• Assess for visual disturbance that may indicate optic neuritis: blurred vision, change in color perception; may lead to blindness
• **Pregnancy/breastfeeding:** Use during pregnancy even in first trimester for active TB, use only if benefits outweigh fetal risk for other indications, compatible with breastfeeding

Patient problem
Infection (uses)
Nonadherence (teaching)

Implementation
• Give antiemetic for vomiting
• Provide a list of foods to avoid while taking this product
PO route
• Give with meals to decrease GI symptoms; absorption is better when taken on empty stomach, 1 hr before or 2 hr after meals
IM route
• Give inj deep in large muscle mass, massage; rotate inj sites, warm inj to room temperature to dissolve crystals

Patient/family education
• Instruct patient that compliance with dosage schedule for duration is necessary; not to skip or double doses; that scheduled appointments must be kept or relapse may occur
• Caution patient to avoid alcohol while taking product or hepatotoxicity may result; to avoid ingestion of aged cheeses, fish or hypertensive crisis may result; give patient written directions on which foods to avoid while taking this medication
• **Tell patient to report peripheral neuritis:** weakness, tingling/numbness of hands/feet, fatigue; hepatotoxicity: loss of appetite, nausea, vomiting, jaundice of skin or eyes

> **BLACK BOX WARNING: Fatal hepatitis:** teach patient to notify prescriber immediately of yellow skin/eyes, dark urine, loss of appetite

Evaluation
Positive therapeutic outcome
• Decreased symptoms of TB
• Culture negative for TB

TREATMENT OF OVERDOSE:
Pyridoxine

> ### isosorbide dinitrate (Rx)
> (eye-soe-sor′bide)
> **Dilatrate-SR, Isordil**
> ### isosorbide mononitrate (Rx)
> **Imbur ✦, Monoket**
> *Func. class.:* Antianginal
> *Chem. class.:* Nitrate

Do not confuse: Imdur/Imuran/Inderal/K-Dur

ACTION: Relaxation of vascular smooth muscle, which leads to decreased preload, afterload, thus decreasing left ventricular end-diastolic pressure, and systemic vascular resistance and reducing cardiac O_2 demand

Therapeutic outcome: Relief and prevention of angina pectoris

USES: Treatment, prevention of chronic stable angina pectoris

Unlabeled
Chronic HF

Pharmacokinetics

Absorption	Well absorbed
Distribution	Unknown
Metabolism	Liver
Excretion	Urine, metabolites
Half-life	Dinitrate 1 hr, mononitrate 5 hr

Pharmacodynamics

	Sus rel	PO
Onset	Up to 4 hr	15-30 min
Peak	Unknown	Unknown
Duration	5 hr	5-6 hr

CONTRAINDICATIONS

Hypersensitivity to this product or nitrates, severe anemia, closed-angle glaucoma

Precautions: Pregnancy, breastfeeding, children, orthostatic hypotension, MI, HF, severe renal/hepatic disease, increased ICP, cerebral hemorrhage, acute MI, geriatrics, GI disease, syncope

DOSAGE AND ROUTES
Dinitrate
Adult: PO 5-20 mg bid-tid, initially, maintenance 10-40 mg bid-tid; SL buccal tab 2.5-5 mg; may repeat q5-10min × 3 doses; ext rel 40-80 mg q8-12hr, max 160 mg/day

Mononitrate
Adult: PO (Monoket) 10-20 mg bid, 7 hr apart; (Imdur) initiate at 30-60 mg/day as a single dose, increase q3day as needed; may increase to 120 mg/day; max 240 mg/day

Available forms: Dinitrate: sus rel caps 40 mg; ext rel tabs 40 mg; tabs 5, 10, 20, 30, 40 mg; mononitrate: tabs (Monoket) 10, 20 mg; ext rel tabs (Imdur) 30, 60, 120 mg

ADVERSE EFFECTS

CNS: *Vascular headache, flushing, dizziness,* weakness
CV: *Orthostatic hypotension,* tachycardia, collapse, syncope
GI: Nausea, vomiting
INTEG: Pallor, sweating, rash
MISC: Twitching, hemolytic anemia, methemoglobinemia, tolerance, xerostomia

INTERACTIONS
Individual drugs
Alcohol: increased hypotension
Rosiglitazone: increased myocardial ischemia; avoid concurrent use
• **Avanafil, Sildenafil, tadalafil, vardenafil:** fatal hypotension, do not use together

Drug classifications
Antihypertensives, β-adrenergic blockers, calcium channel blockers, diuretics, phenothiazines: increased hypotension
Sympathomimetics: increased heart rate, B/P

NURSING CONSIDERATIONS
Assessment
• **Assess for angina pain:** duration, time started, activity being performed, character, intensity
• Monitor for orthostatic B/P, pulse at baseline, during treatment and periodically thereafter
• **Beers:** Use with caution in older adults, may exacerbate episodes of syncope

Patient problem
Ineffective tissue perfusion (uses)
Activity intolerance (uses)

Implementation
PO route
• Swallow sus rel cap and ext rel tab whole; do not break, crush, or chew
• Do not swallow SL tab; tab should be dissolved under tongue
• Give 1 hr before or 2 hr after meals with 8 oz of water

Patient/family education
• Teach patient that tolerance may occur if taken over long periods; to prevent, allow intervals of 12-14 hr/day without product
• Advise patient to treat headache with OTC analgesics
• Instruct patient to not skip or double doses; if dose is missed take when remembered if 2 hr before next dose (dinitrate), 6 hr before next dose (sus rel), or 8 hr before next dose (mononitrate)
• Caution patient to avoid alcohol and OTC medications unless approved by prescriber
• Inform patient that product may be taken before stressful activity: exercise, sexual activity
• Advise patient that SL tab may sting mucous membranes
• Caution patient to avoid driving and hazardous activities if dizziness occurs
• Advise patient to comply with complete medical regimen
• Caution patient to make position changes slowly to prevent orthostatic hypotension
• Teach patient not to use with avanafil, sildenafil, tadalafil, vardenafil with nitrates; may cause serious drop in B/P
• Teach patient not to discontinue abruptly; may cause heart attack
• Teach patient to use at beginning of angina symptoms, may repeat every 15 min;

if no relief seek medical attention immediately

Evaluation
Positive therapeutic outcome
• Decrease in, prevention of anginal pain

RARELY USED

isotretinoin
(eye-soe-tret'i-noyn)
Absorica, Accutane ✦, Amnesteem, Claravis, Clarus ✦, Epuris ✦, Myorisan, Sotret, Zenatane
Func. class.: Antiacne agent

USES: For the treatment of severe recalcitrant cystic acne vulgaris (nodular acne)

CONTRAINIDCATIONS: Hypersensitivity to this product or glycerin, parabens, retinoids, soybean oil, breastfeeding, blood donation

BLACK BOX WARNING: Pregnancy

DOSAGE AND ROUTES
Adults/child ≥12 yr: PO 0.5 to 1 mg/kg/day PO, given in two divided doses with food, for 15 to 20 wk or until the total cyst count decreases by 70%

ivabradine (Rx)
(eye-vab'ra-deen)
Corlanor, Lancora ✦
Func. class.: Cardiovascular agent
Chem. class.: Hyperpolarization-activated cyclic nucleotide-gated channel blocker

ACTION: Selectively and specifically inhibits the cardiac pacemaker I_f current in the sinoatrial node, resulting in a dose-dependent reduction in heart rate

Therapeutic outcome: Lowered heart rate in heart failure

USES: Stable symptomatic heart failure

Pharmacokinetics

Absorption	40%, food decreases absorption
Distribution	Unknown
Metabolism	Liver, extensively by CYP3A4 to active metabolite
Excretion	Urine 4% unchanged
Half-life	6 hr

Pharmacodynamics

Onset	Unknown
Peak	1 hr
Duration	12 hr

CONTRAINDICATIONS
Hypersensitivity, sick sinus syndrome, second/third degree heart block, pregnancy, breastfeeding, acute heart block, pacemaker dependence, bradycardia, hypotension

Precautions: Contraception requirements, bundle branch block, hepatic disease

DOSAGE AND ROUTES
Adults: PO 5 mg bid initially. Initiate at 2.5 mg bid in patients with a history of conduction defects or in those whom bradycardia could lead to hemodynamic compromise. After 2 wk, adjust the dose to achieve a resting heart rate between 50 and 60 bpm, max: 7.5 mg bid
Children and Adolescents <40 kg: PO 0.05 mg/kg/dose bid. Adjust the dose by 0.05 mg/kg at 2 wk intervals to a target heart rate reduction of at least 20% based on tolerability. Max: 0.3 mg/kg/dose bid or 7.5 mg bid, whichever is less
Infants 6 to 11 mo: PO 0.05 mg/kg/dose bid. Adjust the dose by 0.05 mg/kg at 2 wk intervals to a target heart rate reduction of at least 20% based on tolerability

Available forms: Tablets 5, 7.5 mg; oral solution 5 mg/5mL

ADVERSE EFFECTS
CNS: *Headache*, drowsiness, apathy, confusion, disorientation, fatigue, depression, hallucinations
CV: Dysrhythmias, hypotension, bradycardia, AV block, torsade de pointes
EENT: Blurred vision, yellow-green halos, photophobia, diplopia
GI: Nausea, vomiting, anorexia, abdominal pain, diarrhea

INTERACTIONS
Individual drugs
Drug classifications
CYP3A4 inhibitors—strong (azoles, macrolides, protease inhibitors); increase effects, do not use together
CYP3A4 inhibitors—moderate (aprepitant, calcium channel blockers, verapamil, diltiazem, fluconazole, cimetidine, ciprofloxacin, cyclosporine): increased effects, avoid using together
CYP3A4 inducers (antiandrogens, phenytoin, carbamazepine, phenytoin, barbiturates, rifampicin): decrease effects, avoid using together

---

Drug/herb
St. John's wort: Decreased product effect, avoid concurrent use

Drug/food
Grapefruit juice: Increased effect, avoid concurrent use

NURSING CONSIDERATIONS
Assessment
• Assess and document heart rate baseline, after 2 wk and periodically thereafter, if pulse >60 bpm, dose should be increased by 2.5 mg bid, max 7.5 mg bid; if pulse is 50-60 bpm keep dose at same level; if pulse <50 bpm, decrease dose by 2.5 mg bid
• Monitor ECG baseline and periodically during treatment, discontinue if significant changes occur or atrial fibrillation

Patient problems
Impaired cardiac output (uses)
Risk for injury (adverse reactions)

Implementation
PO route
• Give with food; avoid ingestion of grapefruit juice
• If a dose is missed or spit out, do not give another dose, give the next dose at the usual time
• *Oral solution:* Empty contents of the ampule(s) into a medication cup, measure with a calibrated oral syringe
• *Storage:* Discard unused oral solution; do not store or reuse any solution left in the medication cup or ampule

Patient/family education
• Caution patient to discuss all OTC, Rx, herbals, supplements with provider; avoid use of grapefruit juice
• Teach patient purpose of product, expected results, how to use tablet or oral solution
• **Pregnancy/breastfeeding:** Identify if pregnancy is planned or suspected or if breastfeeding; use adequate contraception if pregnant, as fetal harm may occur

Evaluation
Positive therapeutic outcome
• Decrease in heart rate in heart failure

---

ivacaftor/lumacaftor (Rx)
(eye-va-kaf′tor/loo-ma-kaf′tor)
Orkambi
Func. class.: Respiratory agent, cystic fibrosis agent

ACTION: A modulator of the cystic fibrosis protein; a chloride channel present at the surface of epithelial cells in multiple organs with the F508del mutation in the CFTR gene

Therapeutic outcome: Improved respiratory function, including breathing and decreased cystic fibrosis symptoms

USES: Cystic fibrosis with the F508del mutation in the CFTR gene

Pharmacokinetics

Absorption	Fatty food increases absorption
Distribution	Unknown, protein binding 99%
Metabolism	Liver, extensively by CYP3A4 to active metabolite
Excretion	Urine 4% unchanged
Half-life	9 hr (ivacaftor), 26 hr (lumacaftor)

Pharmacodynamics

Onset	Unknown
Peak	4 hr
Duration	12 hr

CONTRAINDICATIONS
Hypersensitivity, use of CYP3A4 inducers

Precautions: CYP3A4 inhibitors, pregnancy, breastfeeding, children, severe renal disease/hepatic disease, cataracts, severe lung dysfunction

DOSAGE AND ROUTES
Adults: PO tablet 2 tablets (lumacaftor 200 mg and ivacaftor 125 mg) q12hr with fatty food
Children and adolescents ≥12 yr: PO tablet 2 tablets (lumacaftor 200 mg and ivacaftor 125 mg) q12hr with fatty food
Children 6 to 11 years: PO tablet 2 tablets (lumacaftor 100 mg and ivacaftor 125 mg) q12hr with fatty food
Children 2 to 5 years, ≥ 14 kg: PO granules One packet of oral granules (lumacaftor 150 mg and ivacaftor 188 mg) q12hr with fatty
Children 2 to 5 years, <14 kg: PO granules One packet of oral granules (lumacaftor 100 mg and ivacaftor 125 mg) q12hr with fatty food

Hepatic dose
Moderate impairment (Child-Pugh Class B):
Child 2 to 5 yr, reduce to 1 packet of oral granules in AM and 1 packet every other day in the PM; **child** >6 yr, reduce the dosage to 2 tablets in AM, 1 tablet in PM
Severe impairment (Child-Pugh Class C):
Child 2 to 5 yr, reduce to 1 packet of oral granules q day in the AM or less frequently;

child ≥6 yr, reduce to 1 tablet q12hr or less frequently

Available forms: Tablets 100-200, 125-200 mg, **granules** 100-125 mg

ADVERSE EFFECTS
CNS: Fatigue, headache
CV: Hypertension
EENT: Cataracts, rhinorrhea
GU: Amenorrhea
GI: Nausea, flatulence, vomiting, abdominal pain, diarrhea, *hepatic encephalopathy*, increased LFTs, hyperbilirubin
RESP: Dyspnea, chest pain

INTERACTIONS
Drug classifications
CYP3A4 inhibitors—strong (azoles, macrolides, protease inhibitors); increase effects, do not use together

CYP3A4 inhibitors—moderate (aprepitant, calcium channel blockers, verapamil, diltiazem, fluconazole, cimetidine, ciprofloxacin cyclosporine): increase effects, avoid using together

CYP3A4 inducers (antiandrogens, barbiturates, phenytoin, carbamazepine, phenytoin, rifampicin): decrease effects, avoid using together

Drug/herb
St. John's wort: decreased product effect, avoid concurrent use

NURSING CONSIDERATIONS
Assessment
• **Cystic fibrosis:** Assess respiratory status, including dyspnea, chest tightness, cough, wheezing, bronchitis baseline and periodically
• **Hypertension:** Monitor B/P baseline and periodically; report significant changes to provider
• **Cataracts:** Obtain baseline and follow-up ophthalmological examinations in pediatric patients

Patient Problems
Ineffective airway clearance (uses)

Implementation
PO route
• Give with food (eggs, avocados, nuts, butter, peanut butter, cheese pizza, whole-milk dairy products)
• If a dose is missed within 6 hr of the time it is usually taken, the dose should be taken with fat-containing food as soon as possible. If more than 6 hr have passed since the dose is usually taken, skip that dose and resume with the usual dosing schedule

• **Oral granules:** Mix granules with 5 mL of soft food (pureed fruits, flavored yogurt, pudding) or liquid (milk or juice); the mixture should be completely consumed. Food should be at room temperature or below. Each packet is for single use only. Once mixed, the product is stable for 1 hr and should be consumed during that time

Patient/family education
• Caution patient/family to discuss all OTC, Rx, herbals, supplements with provider
• Teach patient purpose of product, expected results, how to use tablet or oral solution

Evaluation
Positive therapeutic outcome
• Decreased symptoms of cystic fibrosis, ease of breathing

⚠ HIGH ALERT

ixabepilone (Rx)
(ix-ab-ep'i-lone)
Ixempra
Func. class.: Antineoplastic—miscellaneous
Chem. class.: Epothilone B analogue

ACTION: Microtubule stabilizing agent; microtubules are needed for cell division

Therapeutic outcome: Decreased tumor size, decreased spread of malignancy

USES: Breast cancer

Pharmacokinetics

Absorption	Unknown
Distribution	Unknown
Metabolism	Liver by CYP3A4
Excretion	Feces 65%, urine 21%
Half-life	Terminal 52 hr

Pharmacodynamics
Unknown

CONTRAINDICATIONS
Pregnancy, hypersensitivity to products with polyoxyethylated castor oil, breastfeeding, neutropenia <1500/mm³, thrombocytopenia <100,000/mm³

BLACK BOX WARNING: Hepatic disease

Precautions: Children, geriatric, alcoholism, bone marrow suppression, cardiac dysrhythmias, cardiac/renal disease, diabetes mellitus, peripheral neuropathy, ventricular dysfunction

---

DOSAGE AND ROUTES
Adult: IV INF 40 mg/m^2 over 3 hr q3wk

Hepatic dose
Adult: IV moderate 20 mg/m^2 q 3 wk, max 30 mg/m^2

Dosage reduction in those taking a strong CYP3A4 inhibitor
Adult: IV INF 20 mg/m^2 over 3 hr q3wk

Available forms: Powder for inj 15, 45 mg, vial

ADVERSE EFFECTS
CNS: *Peripheral neuropathy,* chills, fatigue, fever, flushing, headache, insomnia, impaired cognition, asthenia
CV: Bradycardia, *hypotension,* abnormal ECG, angina, atrial flutter, cardiomyopathy, chest pain, edema, MI, vasculitis
GI: *Nausea, vomiting, diarrhea,* abdominal pain, anorexia, colitis, constipation, gastritis, jaundice, GERD, hepatic failure, trismus
GU: Renal failure
HEMA: Neutropenia, thrombocytopenia, anemia, infections, coagulopathy
INTEG: *Alopecia,* rash, hot flashes
META: Hypokalemia, metabolic acidosis
MS: *Arthralgia, myalgia*
RESP: Bronchospasm, cough, dyspnea
SYST: *Hypersensitivity reactions,* anaphylaxis, dehydration, radiation recall reaction

INTERACTIONS
Drug classifications
CYP3A4 inducers (aminoglutethimide, barbiturates, bexarotene, bosentan, carBAMazepine, dexamethasone, efavirenz, griseofulvin, modafinil, nafcillin, nevirapine, OXcarbazepine, phenytoin, rifamycin, topiramate): decreased ixabepilone levels

CYP3A4 inhibitors (amiodarone, amprenavir, aprepitant, atazanavir, chloramphenicol, clarithromycin, conivaptan, cycloSPORINE, danazol, darunavir, dalforpristan, delavirdine, diltiazem, erythromycin, estradiol, fluconazole, fluvoxaMINE, fosamprenavir, imatinib, indinavir, isoniazid, itraconazole, ketoconazole, lopinavir, miconazole, nefazodone, nelfinavir, propoxyphene, ritonavir, RU-486, saquinavir, tamoxifen, telithromycin, troleandomycin, verapamil, voriconazole, zafirlukast): increased ixabepilone level

Drug/herb
St. John's wort: avoid use

Drug/food
Grapefruit products: avoid use

Drug/lab test
Increased: LFTs, bilirubin
Decreased: platelets, neutrophils, RBC, potassium

NURSING CONSIDERATIONS
Assessment
• Monitor CBC, differential, platelet count prior to therapy, qwk; withhold product if WBC is <1500/mm^3 or platelet count is <100,000/mm^3, notify prescriber
• Monitor temp (may indicate beginning infection)

> **BLACK BOX WARNING:** Monitor liver function tests before, during therapy (bilirubin, AST, ALT, LDH) prn or qmo; check for jaundiced skin and sclera, dark urine, clay-colored stools, itchy skin, abdominal pain, fever, diarrhea

• Monitor VS during 1st hr of inf; check IV site for signs of infiltration
• **Cardiac ischemia:** Monitor cardiac function in those with cardiac function that is impaired; chest pain, ECG changes may occur
• Assess for hypersensitive reactions, anaphylaxis including hypotension, dyspnea, angioedema, generalized urticaria; discontinue inf immediately; keep emergency equipment available
• Assess effects of alopecia on body image; discuss feelings about body changes
• **Pregnancy/breastfeeding:** Do not use in pregnancy, breastfeeding

Patient problem
Risk of infection (adverse reactions)
Risk of injury (adverse reactions)

Implementation
• Premedicate with histamine antagonists 1 hr prior to use, prevents hypersensitivity
• Give antiemetic 30-60 min before giving product and prn

IV route
• Let kit stand at room temperature for 30 min; to reconstitute, withdraw supplied diluent (8 ml for 15 mg vials, 23.5 ml for 45 mg vials); slowly inject solution into vial; gently swirl and invert to mix, final conc 2 mg/ml; further dilute in LR in DEHP-free bags; final conc should be 0.2-0.6 mg/ml; after added, mix by manual rotation
• Diluted sol is stable for 6 hr at room temperature; inf must be completed within 6 hr
• Use in-line filter 0.2-1.2 mcm
• Give over 3 hr

Patient/family education
• Teach patient to report signs of infection: fever, sore throat, flulike symptoms

---

- Teach patient to report signs of anemia: fatigue, headache, faintness, shortness of breath
- Teach patient to report any complaints or side effects to nurse or prescriber
- Caution patient that hair may be lost during treatment; a wig or hairpiece may make patient feel better; new hair may be different in color, texture
- Advise patient that pain in muscles and joints 2-5 days after inf is common
- Advise patient to use nonhormonal type of contraception
- Instruct patient to avoid receiving vaccinations while on this product

Evaluation
Positive therapeutic outcome
- Decreased tumor size, decreased spread of malignancy

RARELY USED

ixazomib
(ix-az-oh-mib)
Ninlaro
Func. class.: Antineoplastic, proteasome inhibitor

USES: Multiple myeloma in patients who have received at least one prior therapy, in combination with lenalidomide and dexamethasone

CONTRAINDICATIONS: Hypersensitivity, pregnancy, lactation, with strong CYP3A4 inducers

DOSAGE AND ROUTES
Adults: PO 4 mg orally on days 1, 8, and 15 in combination with lenalidomide 25 mg orally daily on days 1 through 21 and dexamethasone 40 mg orally on days 1, 8, 15, and 22. Repeat treatment cycles every 28 days until disease progression

Renal dose
Adult: PO Baseline mild or moderate renal impairment (creatinine clearance [CrCl] of 30 mL/min or greater): *no change;* baseline severe renal impairment (CrCl less than 30 mL/min): *reduce starting dosage to 3 mg on days 1, 8, and 15 repeated q 28 days*

Hepatic dose
Adult: PO mild hepatic impairment (AST level greater than the upper limit of normal [ULN] or a total bilirubin level of 1 to 1.5 times the ULN and any AST level): no change; baseline moderate (total bilirubin level greater than 1.5 to 3 times the ULN) or severe (total bilirubin level greater than 3 times the ULN)

hepatic impairment: reduce starting dosage to 3 mg PO on days 1, 8, and 15 repeated every 28 days; treatment-related grade 3 and 4 hepatotoxicity: hold until the toxicity recovers to baseline or grade 1 or less; resume at a reduced dose (from 4 mg to 3 mg or from 3 mg to 2.3 mg)

ixekizumab
(ix'e-kiz'ue-mab)
Taltz
Func. class.: Immunosuppressive

ACTION: A human IgG4 monoclonal antibody that selectively binds to the interleukin 17A (IL-17A) cytokine, inhibiting its interaction with the IL-17 receptor
  Treatment inhibits the release of proinflammatory cytokines and chemokines

USES: The treatment of moderate to severe plaque psoriasis in adults who are candidates for systemic therapy or phototherapy

Pharmacokinetics
Absorption	60% to 81%, injection in the thigh achieved higher bioavailability
Distribution	Minimal
Metabolism	Catabolism
Excretion	Unknown
Half-life	13 days

Pharmacodynamics
Onset	Unknown
Peak	4 days
Duration	Unknown

CONTRAINDICATIONS: Risk of serious hypersensitivity reactions or anaphylaxis

Precautions: Breastfeeding, children, Crohn's disease, immunosuppression, infection, inflammatory bowel disease, pregnancy, tuberculosis, ulcerative colitis, vaccination

DOSAGE AND ROUTES
Adult: SUBCUT 160 mg at week 0 (administered as two 80 mg injections) followed by 80 mg at weeks 2, 4, 6, 8, 10, and 12, then 80 mg q4wk

Available forms: Solution for injection 80 mg/mL, autoinjector 80 mg/mL

SIDE EFFECTS
SYST: antibody formation, infection, angioedema
INTEG: injection site reaction, urticaria
HEMA: neutropenia

INTERACTIONS
• Do not use concurrently with vaccines; immunizations should be brought up-to-date before treatment
• Avoid use with immunosuppressives

NURSING CONSIDERATIONS
Assessment:
• **TB:** TB testing should be done before use
• Assess for injection-site reactions, redness, swelling, pain
• Bring immunizations up-to-date before use
• **Infection:** monitor for fever, sore throat, cough; do not use in active infections

Patient problems
Risk for infection (uses)
Risk for injury (adverse reactions)

Implementation:
Subcut route
• Administer by subcutaneous injection only
• Visually inspect for particulate matter and discoloration before administration whenever solution and container permit. The solution should be free of visible particles, clear, and colorless to slightly yellow
• Available as a prefilled syringe and as an autoinjector; each device contains 80 mg
• Patients may use the prefilled syringe or autoinjector after proper training
• Use upper arms, thighs, and any quadrant of the abdomen for injection sites
• Do not use where skin is tender, bruised, erythematous, indurated, or affected by psoriasis; rotate sites with each dose

• Does not contain preservatives; discard any unused product remaining in the prefilled syringe or autoinjector. Discard the single-dose autoinjector or syringe after use in a proper puncture-resistant container
• **Missed doses:** If a dose is missed, give as soon as possible, then resume dosing at the regular scheduled time
• **Preparation for use of the prefilled syringe or autoinjector:** Remove prefilled syringe or autoinjector from refrigerator and allow to warm 30 minutes at room temperature; inspect syringe or autoinjector for particulate matter and discoloration before administration
• **Storage of unopened prefilled syringes and autoinjectors:** Protect from light; store refrigerated at 2°-8° C (36°-46° F) until time of use. Do not freeze and do not use the injection if it has been frozen. Do not shake

Teach Patient/Family:
• Teach patient that product must be continued for prescribed time to be effective and to use as prescribed
• Advise patient not to receive live virus vaccinations during treatment
• **Infection:** Advise patient to notify prescriber of possible infections, respiratory or other, or of allergic reactions
• Teach patient injection techniques and disposal of equipment and not to reuse needles, syringes

Evaluation
Positive therapeutic outcome: decreased psoriasis

ketoconazole topical
See Appendix B

ketoprofen (OTC, Rx)
(ke-to-proe′fen)
Func. class.: NSAID; nonopioid analgesic, antirheumatic
Chem. class.: Propionic acid derivative

ACTION: May inhibit prostaglandin synthesis; analgesic, antiinflammatory, antipyretic

Therapeutic outcome: Decreased pain, inflammation

USES: Mild to moderate pain; osteoarthritis; rheumatoid arthritis; dysmenorrhea; OTC relief of minor aches, pains

Pharmacokinetics

Absorption	Well absorbed
Distribution	Not known, protein binding 99%
Metabolism	Liver 60%
Excretion	Kidneys
Half-life	2-4 hr; 5.4 hr (ext rel)

Pharmacodynamics

Onset	Onset 2-3 hr
	Peak 7 hr
Peak	1-2 hr; 1-2 hr (ext rel)
Duration	Unknown

CONTRAINDICATIONS
Pregnancy, 2nd/3rd trimesters; hypersensitivity to this product, NSAIDs, salicylates

BLACK BOX WARNING: Perioperative pain in CABG

Precautions: Pregnancy (1st trimester), breastfeeding, children, geriatric, bleeding/GI/cardiac disorders, hypersensitivity to other antiinflammatory agents, asthma, severe renal/hepatic disease, ulcer disease

BLACK BOX WARNING: GI bleeding, MI, stroke

DOSAGE AND ROUTES
Analgesic
Adult: PO 25-50 mg q6-8hr, max 300 mg/day

Rheumatoid arthritis, osteoarthritis
Adult: PO 50 mg qid or 75 mg tid, max 300 mg/day or ext rel 100, 150, 200 mg/day

Renal dose/hepatic dose
Adult: PO GFR <25 ml/min/1.73 m², albumin <3.5 g/dl, decreased hepatic function, or ESRD, max 100 mg qday

Available forms: Caps 25, 50, 75 mg; ext rel caps 100, 150, 200 mg

ADVERSE EFFECTS
CNS: Dizziness, drowsiness, insomnia, depression, headache
CV: Tachycardia, peripheral edema, palpitations, dysrhythmias, hypertension, CV thrombotic events, MI, stroke
GI: *Nausea, anorexia, vomiting, diarrhea,* jaundice, hepatitis, constipation, flatulence, cramps, dry mouth, peptic ulcer, GI bleeding, *dyspepsia*
GU: Nephrotoxicity: cystitis
HEMA: Blood dyscrasias
INTEG: Purpura, rash, pruritus, sweating, photosensitivity
SYST: Anaphylaxis, exfoliative dermatitis, Stevens-Johnson syndrome, toxic epidermal necrosis

INTERACTIONS
Individual drugs
Alcohol, cidofovir: increased adverse GI reactions, toxicity
Aspirin: increased ketoprofen levels, increased adverse GI reactions
Clopidogrel, eptifibatide, ticlopidine, tirofiban: increased risk of bleeding
CycloSPORINE, lithium, methotrexate, phenytoin: increased ketoprofen levels, increased toxicity
Insulin: increased hypoglycemia
Probenecid: increased ketoconazole levels

Drug classifications
Anticoagulants, thrombolytics: increased risk of bleeding
Antihypertensives: decreased effect of antihypertensives
Antineoplastics: increased hematologic toxicity
Corticosteroids: increased adverse GI reactions
Diuretics: decreased effectiveness of diuretics
NSAIDs: increased adverse GI reactions
Sulfonylureas: increased hypoglycemia

Drug/herb
Feverfew, Dong quai, garlic, ginger, ginkgo, horse chestnut, ginseng *(Panax):* increased risk of bleeding

Drug/lab test
Increased: bleeding time, BUN, alkaline phosphatase, AST, ALT, creatinine, LDH

K

NURSING CONSIDERATIONS
Assessment
- **Assess for pain:** type, location, intensity; ROM before and 1-2 hr after treatment
- **Fever:** Monitor temperature baseline and periodically
- **Aspirin sensitivity asthma:** These patients may be more likely to develop hypersensitivity to NSAIDs
- Monitor renal, liver function tests: AST, ALT, bilirubin, creatinine, BUN, urine creatinine, CBC Hct, Hgb, pro-time if patient is on long-term therapy and q6mo
- **Assess hepatotoxicity:** dark urine, clay-colored stools, jaundice of skin and sclera, itching, abdominal pain, fever, diarrhea if patient is on long-term therapy
- **Assess for allergic reactions:** rash, urticaria; if these occur, product may have to be discontinued
- Check edema in feet, ankles, legs
- Identify prior product history; there are many product interactions

> **BLACK BOX WARNING: Assess for CV thrombotic events:** MI, stroke, this product or other NSAIDs may increase the risk

> **BLACK BOX WARNING: For GI bleeding:** blood in sputum, emesis, stools

- **Beers:** Avoid chronic use in older adults unless other alternatives are not available, increased risk of GI bleeding, peptic ulcer disease

Patient problems
Pain (uses)
Impaired mobility (uses)

Implementation
- Store at room temperature
- Swallow whole; do not break, crush, chew, or open ext rel cap
- Give with 8 oz of water and sit upright for 30 min after dose to prevent ulceration
- Give with a full glass of water 2 hr after meals
- Give with food or milk, antacids to decrease gastric symptoms; give 30 min before or 2 hr after meals; absorption may be slowed

Patient/family education
- Teach patient to report any symptoms of hepatotoxicity, allergic reactions, bleeding (long-term therapy)
- Advise patient to take with 8 oz of water and sit upright for 30 min after dose to prevent ulceration, not to crush or chew ext rel products
- Caution patient not to exceed recommended dosage, acute poisoning may result; to take as prescribed; do not double dose
- Advise patient to read label on other OTC products; many contain other antiinflammatories
- Advise patient to use sunscreen, protective clothing to prevent photosensitivity
- Inform patient that the therapeutic response takes 2 wk (arthritis)
- Teach patient to report diarrhea, sweating, fever, joint aches
- Caution patient to avoid alcohol ingestion; GI bleeding may occur
- Teach patient to report use to all providers
- Teach patient to report immediately rash, itching
- **Pregnancy, breastfeeding:** Teach patient to report planned or suspected; avoid breastfeeding

Evaluation
Positive therapeutic outcome
- Decreased pain
- Decreased inflammation
- Increased mobility
- Decreased fever

ketorolac (systemic, nasal) (Rx)
(kee′toe-role-ak)
Acular, Sprix, Toradol ✤
Func. class.: Nonsteroidal antiinflammatory (NSAID), nonopioid analgesic
Chem. class.: Acetic acid

Do not confuse: Toradol/tramadol

ACTION: Inhibits prostaglandin synthesis by decreasing an enzyme needed for biosynthesis; analgesic, antiinflammatory, antipyretic effects

Therapeutic outcome: Decreased pain, inflammation, ocular itching

USES: Mild to moderate pain (short term); decreased ocular itching in seasonal allergic conjunctivitis (ophthalmic)

Pharmacokinetics

Absorption	Rapidly, completely absorbed
Distribution	Bound to plasma proteins (99%)
Metabolism	Liver (<50%)
Excretion	Kidney, metabolites (92%); breast milk (6%); feces
Half-life	6 hr (IM); increased in renal disease

K

Pharmacodynamics

	IM	Ophth/PO
Onset	Up to 10 min	Unknown
Peak	50 min IM; 2-3 hr PO; 0.5-2 hr nasal	Unknown; 6-8 hr nasal
Duration	4-6 hr PO	Unknown

CONTRAINDICATIONS

Pregnancy (3rd trimester), hypersensitivity, asthma, hepatic disease, peptic ulcer disease, CV bleeding

> **BLACK BOX WARNING:** Breastfeeding, severe renal disease, labor and delivery, perioperative pain in CABG, prior to major surgery, epidural/intrathecal administration, GI bleeding, hypovolemia

Precautions: Pregnancy, GI/cardiac disorders, hypersensitivity to other antiinflammatory agents, CCr <25 ml/min

> **BLACK BOX WARNING:** Children, geriatric, bleeding, MI, stroke

DOSAGE AND ROUTES

Adult/adolescent >17 yr and ≥50 kg: PO continuation from **IM/IV** only 20 mg, then 10 mg q4-6hr prn, max 40 mg/day; nasal 1 spray (15.75 mg/spray) in each nostril (31.5 mg/spray) q6-8hr, max 4 doses/day × 5 days

Adult/adolescent >17 yr and <50 kg: IM (single dose) 30-60 mg, **IV** 15-30 mg; **IM/IV** (multiple dosing) 15-30 mg q6hr, max 60 mg/day × 5 day combined either **PO/IM/IV;** nasal 1 spray (15.75 mg/spray) in one nostril q6-8hr, max 4 doses/day × 5 days

Child 2-16 yr, <50 kg PO 1 mg/kg as a single dose; IM 0.4-1 mg/kg max 30 mg/dose (single dose), 0.5 mg/kg q 6 hr (multiple doses); IV 0.4 mg-1 mg/kg max 15 mg/dose (single dose), 0.5 mg/kg q 6 hr (multiple doses)

Renal dose
Do not use in advanced renal disease

Ophthalmic route
Adult: 1 gtt (0.25 mg) qid × 7 days

Available forms: Inj 15, 30 mg/ml (prefilled syringes); ophth 0.5% sol; tabs 10 mg; nasal spray 15.75 mg/spray

ADVERSE EFFECTS

CNS: Dizziness, *drowsiness,* tremors, seizures
CV: Hypertension, flushing, syncope, pallor, edema, vasodilatation, CV thrombotic events, MI, stroke
EENT: Tinnitus, hearing loss, blurred vision, transient burning/stinging
GI: Nausea, anorexia, vomiting, diarrhea, constipation, flatulence, cramps, dry mouth, peptic ulcer, GI bleeding, perforation, taste change, hepatitis, hepatic failure
GU: Nephrotoxicity: dysuria, hematuria, oliguria, azotemia
HEMA: Blood dyscrasias, prolonged bleeding
INTEG: Purpura, rash, pruritus, sweating, angioedema, Stevens-Johnson syndrome, toxic epidermal necrolysis

INTERACTIONS
Individual drugs
Alcohol, aspirin: increased GI effects
Aspirin: increased ketorolac levels, contraindicated
Cefamandole, cefoperazone, cefoTEtan, clopidogrel, eptifibatide, plicamycin, ticlopidine, tirofiban, valproic acid: increased risk of bleeding
CycloSPORINE, lithium, methotrexate, pentoxifylline, probenecid: increased toxicity

Drug classifications
ACE inhibitors: increased renal impairment
Anticoagulants: increased effects
Antihypertensives: decreased antihypertensive effect
Salicylates, SNRIs, SSRIs, thrombolytics: increased risk of bleeding
Corticosteroids, NSAIDs, potassium products, steroids: increased GI effects
Diuretics: decreased diuretic effect
NSAIDs (other): increased ketorolac levels; contraindicated

Drug/lab test
Increased: AST, ALT, LDH, bleeding time

NURSING CONSIDERATIONS
Assessment

> **BLACK BOX WARNING:** Monitor renal, hepatic, blood studies: BUN, creatinine, AST, ALT, Hgb before treatment, periodically thereafter, check for dehydration

• **Monitor for aspirin sensitivity, asthma;** these patients may be more likely to develop hypersensitivity to NSAIDs
• **Monitor for pain:** type, location, intensity, ROM before and 1 hr after treatment
• **Assess for CV thrombotic events:** MI, stroke; do not use for perioperative pain in CABG

> **BLACK BOX WARNING: Assess for GI bleeding:** blood in sputum, emesis, stools

> **BLACK BOX WARNING:** Do not use epidurally, intrathecally; alcohol is present in the solution

• **Beers:** Avoid in older adults, increased risk of GI bleeding/peptic ulcer disease

Patient problem
Pain (uses)

Implementation
PO route
• Administer to patient crushed or whole
• Max 5 days
• Give with full glass of water; give with food or milk to decrease gastric symptoms; give 30 min before or 2 hr after meals; absorption may be slowed

Nasal route
• Prime pump before using for the first time, point away from person/pets, pump activator 5 times, no need to re-prime
• For single use only, discard 24 hr after opening if not used
• Do not share with others
• Have patient blow nose, sit upright to spray

IM/IV route
• **IV** give undiluted ≥15 sec
• Give IM inj deeply into large muscle mass
• Store at room temperature, protect from light

Y-site compatibilities: Cisatracurium, remifentanil, SUFentanil

Solution compatibilities: D₅W, 0.9% NaCl, LR, D₅, plasmalyte

Patient/family education
• Teach patient that product must be continued for prescribed time to be effective; to avoid aspirin, alcoholic beverages, other NSAIDs, acetaminophen
• Caution patient to report bleeding, bruising, fatigue, malaise, since blood dyscrasias do occur
• Instruct patient to use caution when driving; drowsiness, dizziness may occur
• Instruct patient to take with a full glass of water to enhance absorption
• Caution patient that this product may cause eye redness, burning if soft contact lenses are worn
• Advise to report use to all health care providers, not to use with other products unless approved by prescriber; use for ≤5 days
• Instruct patient to report change in urine pattern, weight increase, edema; pain in joints, fever, blood in urine (indicates nephrotoxicity); bruising, black tarry stools (indicates bleeding)
• Caution patient not to breastfeed
• **Pregnancy/breastfeeding:** Teach patient to report if pregnancy is planned or suspected, not to breastfeed
• **Nasal:** Instruct patient to discard within 24 hr of opening; may cause irritation; may drink water after dose

> **BLACK BOX WARNING:** Instruct patient to report change in urine pattern, weight increase, edema, increased joint pain, fever, blood in urine (indicates nephrotoxicity); bruising, black tarry stools (indicates bleeding); pruritus, jaundice, nausea, right upper quadrant pain, abdominal pain (hepatotoxicity); to notify prescriber immediately

Evaluation
Positive therapeutic outcome
• Decreased pain
• Decreased inflammatory response
• Increased mobility
• Decreased ocular itching

ketorolac ophthalmic
See Appendix B

ketotifen ophthalmic
See Appendix B

⚠ Nurse Alert   ✴ Key NCLEX® Drug   ≫ Drug Specifics

RARELY USED

L-glutamine
Endari
Func. class.: Functional bowel agents, hematological agents

USES: For the treatment of short bowel syndrome in patients receiving specialized nutritional support in conjunction with recombinant human growth hormone; for the treatment of sickle cell disease

DOSAGE AND ROUTES
Short bowel syndrome
Adult: PO 5 g (1 packet) 6 times/day for up to 16 wk given in conjunction with a specialized diet adjusted for individual patient requirements and preferences. Recombinant human growth hormone (rh-GH) should be given during the first 4 wk of therapy

To reduce the acute complications of sickle cell disease
Adult: >65 kg PO 15 g (3 packets) bid; 30 to 65 kg 10 g (2 packets) bid
Child and Adolescent: 5 to 17 yr and >65 kg 15 g (3 packets) **bid**; 30 to 65 kg 10 g (2 packets) **bid**; <30 kg 5 g (1 packet) **bid**

⚠ HIGH ALERT

labetalol (Rx)
(la-bet'a-lole)
Trandate ✦
Func. class.: Antihypertensive, antianginal
Chem. class.: α- and β-blocker

Do not confuse: Labetalol/Lamictal

ACTION: Produces decreases in B/P without reflex tachycardia or significant reduction in heart rate through mixture of α-blocking, β-blocking effects; elevated plasma resins are reduced

Therapeutic outcome: Decreased B/P

USES: Mild to moderate hypertension; treatment of severe hypertension (**IV**), hypertensive emergency in pregnancy, subarachnoid hemorrage

Pharmacokinetics
Absorption	Bioavailability 25% (PO); complete (**IV**)
Distribution	Crosses placenta, CNS, protein binding 50%
Metabolism	Liver, extensively
Excretion	Breast milk, kidneys, bile
Half-life	3-8 hr

Pharmacodynamics
	PO	IV
Onset	30 min	2-5 min
Peak	1 hr	5-15 min
Duration	24 hr	2-4 hr

CONTRAINDICATIONS
Hypersensitivity to β-blockers, cardiogenic shock, heart block (2nd or 3rd degree), sinus bradycardia, HF, bronchial asthma

Precautions: Pregnancy breastfeeding, geriatric, major surgery, diabetes mellitus, thyroid/renal/hepatic disease, COPD, well-compensated heart failure, CAD, nonallergic bronchospasm, peripheral vascular disease

BLACK BOX WARNING: Abrupt discontinuation

DOSAGE AND ROUTES
Hypertension
Adult: PO outpatient 100 mg bid; may be given with diuretic; may increase to 200 mg bid after 2 days; may continue to increase q1-3 days; max 2400 mg/day in divided doses; **inpatient** 200 mg then 200-400 mg in 6-12 hr, depends on response; may increase by 200 mg bid at 1-day intervals
Child/adolescent (unlabeled): PO 1-3 mg/kg/day, titrate to max 10-12 mg/kg/day based on B/P; IV 0.2-1 mg/kg over 2 min, max 40 mg/dose; IV INF 0.25-3 mg/kg/hr

Hypertensive crisis
Adult: IV direct 20 mg over 2 min; may repeat 20-80 mg over 2 min q10min, max 300 mg; IV **Cont INF** after loading dose give 1-2 mg/min until desired response or max 300 mg

Available forms: Tabs 100, 200, 300 mg; INJ 5 mg/ml, 20-, 40-ml vials

ADVERSE EFFECTS
CNS: *Dizziness,* mental changes, drowsiness, *fatigue,* headache, depression, anxiety, nightmares, paresthesias, lethargy
CV: *Orthostatic hypotension,* bradycardia, HF, chest pain, dysrhythmias, pulmonary edema

EENT: *Tinnitus,* vision changes, sore throat, double vision, dry burning eyes, floppy iris syndrome, nasal congestion
ENDO: Hyperkalemia
GI: *Nausea, vomiting, diarrhea,* dyspepsia, taste distortion, hepatotoxicity, constipation
GU: Impotence, dysuria, ejaculatory failure
INTEG: Rash, pruritus, fever
RESP: Bronchospasm, dyspnea, wheezing

INTERACTIONS
Individual drugs
Alcohol (large amounts), cimetidine, nitroglycerin: increased hypotension
Lidocaine: decreased effect
Verapamil: increased myocardial depression

Drug classifications
Antidepressants, tricyclics: increased tremor
Antidiabetics: increased or decreased effect, monitor blood glucose
Antihypertensives: increased hypotension
β-Blockers, bronchodilators, sympathomimetics, xanthines: decreased effects
Diuretics: increased hypotension
General anesthetics, hydantoins, class IC antidysrhythmics: increased myocardial depression
MAOIs: do not use within 2 wk
NSAIDs, salicylates: decreased antihypertensive effect
Theophyllines: decreased bronchodilatation

Drug/herb
Hawthorn: increased antihypertensive effect
Ephedra: decreased antihypertensive effect

Drug/lab test
Increased: ANA titer, blood glucose, alkaline phosphatase, LDH, AST, ALT, uric acid
False increase: urinary catecholamines

NURSING CONSIDERATIONS
Assessment
• **Hypertension:** monitor B/P at beginning of treatment, periodically thereafter; pulse; note rate, rhythm, quality: apical/radial pulse before administration; notify prescriber of any significant changes (pulse <50 bpm)
• Check for baselines in renal, liver function tests before therapy begins
• **HF:** assess for edema in feet, legs daily; monitor I&O, daily weight; check for jugular vein distention, crackles bilaterally, dyspnea; report weight gain >5 lb

> **BLACK BOX WARNING: Abrupt discontinuation:** Product should be tapered to prevent adverse reactions

Patient problem
Impaired cardiac functioning (uses)
Nonadherence

Implementation
• Store in dry area at room temp; do not freeze
PO route
• Give before meals, or with meals; tab may be crushed or swallowed whole; give with food to prevent GI upset, increase absorption
• Do not discontinue prior to surgery
• When discontinuing IV and starting PO when B/P rises start at 200 mg, then 200-400 mg in 6-12 hr, adjust as needed
• Take apical pulse before use; if <50 bpm, withhold; notify prescriber
• Store protected from light, moisture; place in cool environment

> **Direct IV route**
> • Give undiluted (5 mg/ml) over 2 min
> **Continuous IV infusion route**
> • Give at a rate of 2 mg/min after diluting in LR, D_5W, D_5 in 0.2%, 0.9%, 0.33% NaCl or Ringer's; infusion is titrated to patient's response; 200 mg of product/160 ml sol (1 mg/ml); 300 mg of product/240 ml sol (1 mg/ml); 200 mg of product/250 ml sol (2 mg/3 ml); use inf pump
> • Keep patient recumbent during and for 3 hr after inf, monitor VS q5-15min q10min as needed

Y-site compatibilities: Alemtuzumab, alfentanil, amikacin, aminocaproic acid, aminophylline, amiodarone, anidulafungin, argatroban, arsenic trioxide, ascorbic acid injection, atracurium, atropine, azithromycin, aztreonam, benztropine, bivalirudin, bleomycin, bretylium, bumetanide, buprenorphine, butorphanol, calcium chloride/gluconate, CARBOplatin, carmustine, caspofungin, ceFAZolin, cefotaxime, cefoTEtan, cefOXitin, ceftaroline, cefTAZidime, ceftizoxime, chlorproMAZINE, cimetidine, CISplatin, cloNIDine, cyanocobalamin, cyclophosphamide, cycloSPORINE, cytarabine, DACTINomycin, DAPTOmycin, DAUNOrubicin liposome, dexmedetomidine, dexrazoxane, digoxin, diltiazem, diphenhydrAMINE, DOBUTamine, DOCEtaxel, dolasetron, DOPamine, doripenem, doxacurium, DOXOrubicin, DOXOrubicin liposomal, doxycycline, enalaprilat, ePHEDrine, EPINEPHrine, epirubicin, epoetin alfa, eptifibatide, ertapenem, erythromycin lactobionate, esmolol, etoposide, etoposide phosphate, famotidine, fenoldopam, fentaNYL, fluconazole, fludarabine, fluorouracil, folic acid, gallium, ganciclovir, gatifloxacin, gemcitabine, gentamicin, glycopyrrolate, granisetron, HYDROmorphone, hydroxyzine, IDArubicin, ifosfamide, imipenem-cilastatin, inamrinone, irinotecan, iso-proterenol, lactated Ringer's injection, lepirudin, leucovorin, levofloxacin, lidocaine, linezolid injection, LORazepam, magnesium sulfate, mannitol, mechlorethamine, meperidine, meta-raminol, methyldopa, methyl-PREDNISolone, metoclopramide, metoprolol, metroNIDAZOLE, midazolam, milrinone, minocycline, mitoXAN-trone, morphine, moxifloxacin, multiple vitamins injection, mycophenolate, nalbuphine, naloxone, netilmicin, niCARdipine, nitroglycerin, nitroprus-side, norepinephrine, octreotide, ondansetron, oxacillin, oxaliplatin, oxytocin, palonosetron, pamidronate, pancuronium, papaverine, PEMEtrexed, pentamidine, pentazocine, PENTobarbital, PHENobarbital, phentolamine, phenylephrine, phytonadione, polymyxin B, potassium acetate/chloride/phosphates, procainamide, prochlor-perazine, promethazine, propofol, propranolol, protamine, pyridoxine, quiNIDine, quinupristin-dalfopristin, ranitidine, Ringer's injection, ro-curonium, sodium acetate/bicarbonate, succinyl-choline, SUFentanil, tacrolimus, telavancin, teniposide, theophylline, thiamine, thiotepa, ticarcillin-clavulanate, tigecycline, tirofiban, to-bramycin, tolazoline, urokinase, vancomycin, va-sopressin, vecuronium, verapamil, vinBLAStine, vinCRIStine, vinorelbine, voriconazole, zole-dronic acid

Patient/family education

BLACK BOX WARNING: Teach patient not to discontinue product abruptly, precipitate angina might occur; taper over 2 wk

• Teach patient not to use OTC products containing α-adrenergic stimulants (such as nasal decongestants, cold preparations); to avoid alcohol, smoking; to limit sodium intake as prescribed
• Teach patient that product may mask symptoms of hypoglycemia; monitor blood glucose closely in diabetes
• Teach patient how to take pulse and B/P at home; advise when to notify prescriber
• **Hypertension:** Instruct patient to comply with weight control, dietary adjustments, modi-fied exercise program
• Advise patient to carry/wear emergency ID to identify products being taken, allergies; that product controls symptoms but does not cure the condition
• **Teach patient to report symptoms of HF:** difficulty breathing, especially on exertion or when lying down, night cough, swelling of extremities, bradycardia, dizziness, confu-sion, depression, fever, difficulty breathing, cold extremities, confusion, rash, sore throat

• Teach patient to take product as prescribed, not to double or skip doses; take any missed doses as soon as remembered if at least 4 hr until next dose
• Advise patient to avoid driving or other hazardous activities until response is known; dizziness, drowsiness occurs
• Teach patient to advise providers of product use before surgery
• Teach patient to avoid hot baths, showers

Evaluation

Positive therapeutic outcome
• Decreased B/P in hypertension (after 1-2 wk)
• Absence of dysrhythmias

TREATMENT OF OVERDOSE:
Lavage, **IV** glucagon or atropine for bradycardia, **IV** theophylline for bronchospasm, digoxin, O₂, diuretic for cardiac failure, hemodialysis, **IV** glucose for hyperglycemia, **IV** diazepam (or phenytoin) for seizures

lacosamide (Rx)
(la-koe′sa-mide)
Vimpat
Func. class.: Anticonvulsant
Chem. class.: Functionalized amino acid
Schedule V

ACTION: May act through action at sodium channels; exact action is unknown

Therapeutic outcome: Decrease in se-verity of seizures

USES: Partial-onset seizures

Pharmacokinetics

Absorption	100%
Distribution	Protein binding <15%
Metabolism	Liver
Excretion	Kidneys (40%)
Half-life	13 hr (PO)

Pharmacodynamics

	PO	IV
Onset	Unknown	Unknown
Peak	1-4 hr (PO)	30-60 min
Duration	Unknown	Unknown

CONTRAINDICATIONS
Hypersensitivity

Precautions: Pregnancy, breastfeeding, al-lergies, renal/hepatic disease, geriatric patients, child <17 yr, acute MI, atrial fibrillation/flutter,

AV block, bradycardia, cardiac disease, congenital heart disease, dehydration, depression, dialysis, hazardous activity, electrolyte imbalance, heart failure, labor, PR prolongation, sick sinus syndrome, substance abuse, suicidal ideation, syncope, torsades de pointes

DOSAGE AND ROUTES
Adjunctive therapy
Adult and child ≥17 yr: PO 50 mg bid, may increase qwk by 100 mg bid to 200-400 mg/day; **IV** 50 mg 2×/day, infuse over 30-60 min, may be increased 100 mg/day weekly, up to 200-400 mg/day maintenance

Monotherapy
Adult: PO 100 mg bid, may increase qwk by 100 mg/day in two divided doses, increase 300-400 mg/day in two divided doses

Renal/hepatic dose
Adult: PO/IV max 300 mg/day in mild to moderate hepatic disease or CCr ≤30 ml/min; do not use in severe hepatic disease; reduce dose in renal/hepatic disease in those taking strong CYP3A4, CYP2C9 inhibitors

Available forms: Film-coated tabs 50, 100, 150, 200 mg; solution for injection **IV** 20 ml single-use vials (200 mg/20 ml), oral sol 10 mg/ml

ADVERSE EFFECTS
CNS: Dizziness, syncope, tremor, drowsiness, fever, paresthesias, depression, fatigue, headache, confusion, suicidal ideation
CV: Atrial fibrillation/flutter, bradycardia, orthostatic hypotension, palpitations
EENT: Diplopia, blurred vision
GI: Nausea, constipation, vomiting, hepatitis, diarrhea, dyspepsia
HEMA: Anemia, neutropenia, agranulocytosis
INTEG: Rash, erythema, inj site reaction, pruritus
SYST: Drug reaction with eosinophilia and systemic symptoms (DRESS), Stevens-Johnson syndrome, toxic epidermal necrolysis

INTERACTIONS
Individual drugs
Atazanavir, dronedarone, digoxin, lopinavir, ritonavir: increase PR prolongation

Drug classifications
β-blockers, calcium-channel blockers: increase PR prolongation
CYP2C19 inhibitors (fluconazole, isoniazid, miconazole): increase lacosamide effect

Drug/lab test
Increased: LFTs

NURSING CONSIDERATIONS
Assessment
• **Assess for seizures:** duration, type, intensity, precipitating factors
• Monitor for renal function: albumin concentration
• **Assess CV status:** orthostatic hypotension, PR prolongation; monitor cardiac status throughout treatment; ECG before therapy (IV), AV block may occur
• **Assess mental status:** mood, sensorium, affect, memory (long, short), depression, suicidal ideation, psychological dependence
• **Pregnancy:** Pregnant patient should enroll in UCB Antiepileptic Drugs Registry 888-233-2334, use only if benefits outweigh fetal risk, do not breastfeed, excretion unknown
• **Serious skin reactions:** Assess for rash, discontinue product at first sign of rash, DRESS, Stevens-Johnson syndrome, toxic epidermal necrolysis may occur
• **Beers:** Avoid in older adults unless safer alternatives are not available, may cause ataxia, impaired psychomotor function

Patient problem
Risk for injury (uses, adverse reactions)

Implementation
• Store PO products/IV vials at room temp; sol is stable for 24 hr when mixed with compatible diluents in glass or PVC bags at room temp
PO route
• **Tablet:** give without regard to meals
• **Oral sol:** measure with calibrated measuring device

IV route
• May give undiluted or mixed in 0.9% NaCl, D_5W, or LR
• Infuse over 30-60 min
• Do not use if discolored or particulates are present; discard unused portions, stable at room temperature, discard unused portion

Patient/family education
• Caution patient not to discontinue product abruptly, taper over 1 wk; seizures may occur
• Teach patient to report blurred vision, nausea, dizziness, syncope; Advise patient to avoid hazardous activities until stabilized on product
• Teach patient to report rash, fever, fatigue, yellowing of skin, eyes, dark urine, may be hypersensitivity
• Instruct patient to carry emergency ID stating product use

- Advise patient to notify prescriber immediately of suicidal thoughts or actions, syncope, cardiac changes
- Teach patient that interactions with other medications may occur, to report all OTC, Rx, herbals, supplements taken, not to use alcohol
- Give patient MediGuide for proper use and risks and review with patient
- **Pregnancy/breastfeeding:** Identify if pregnancy is planned or suspected or if breastfeeding; if so, enroll in pregnancy registry at 888-233-2334, www.aedpregnancyregistry.com

Evaluation
Positive therapeutic outcome
- Increased seizure control

lactulose (Rx)
(lak′tyoo-lose)
Cholac, Constilac, Constulose, Enulose, Generlac, Kristalose
Func. class.: Laxative (hyperosmotic/ammonia detoxicant)
Chem. class.: Lactose synthetic derivative

Do not confuse: lactulose/lactose

ACTION: Prevents absorption of ammonia in colon by acidifying stool; increases water, softens stool

Therapeutic outcome: Decreased constipation, decreased blood ammonia level (PSE)

USES: Chronic constipation, portal-systemic encephalopathy (PSE) in patients with hepatic disease

Pharmacokinetics

Absorption	Poorly absorbed
Distribution	Not known
Metabolism	Colonic bacteria to acids
Half-life	Unknown
Excretion	Urine unchanged

Pharmacodynamics constipation resolution

Onset	24-28 hr
Peak	Unknown
Duration	Unknown

CONTRAINDICATIONS
Hypersensitivity, low-galactose diet

Precautions: Pregnancy, breastfeeding, geriatric and debilitated patient, diabetes mellitus

DOSAGE AND ROUTES
Constipation
Adult: PO 15-30 ml/day (10-20 g), may increase to 60 ml/day prn
Child: PO 7.5 ml/day after breakfast

Hepatic encephalopathy
Adult: PO 30-45 ml (20-30 g) tid or qid until stools are soft, retention enema 300 ml diluted
Child: PO (unlabeled) 40-90 ml/day in divided doses given 3-4 ×/day
Infant: PO (unlabeled) 2.5-10 ml/day in divided doses

Available forms: Oral sol 10 g/15 ml; packets: 10, 20 g; rectal sol: 10 g/15 ml

ADVERSE EFFECTS
GI: *Nausea, vomiting, anorexia, abdominal cramps, diarrhea,* flatulence, *distention, belching*
META: Hypernatremia, hypokalemia; hyperglycemia (diabetes)

INTERACTIONS
Drug classifications
Antiinfectives (oral), antacids: decreased lactulose effect
Laxatives: do not use together (hepatic encephalopathy)

Drug/herb
Flax, senna: increased laxative effect

Drug/lab test
Blood glucose (diabetic patients): increase
Blood ammonia: decrease

NURSING CONSIDERATIONS
Assessment
- **Stool:** Assess for amount, color, consistency, abdominal pain/distention bowel sound prior to use and after use
- Monitor glucose levels in diabetic patients (increases)
- **Cause of constipation:** Determine whether fluids, bulk, or exercise is missing from lifestyle
- Monitor blood, urine, electrolytes if used often by patient; may cause diarrhea, hypokalemia, hypernatremia; check I&O ratio to identify fluid loss
- Assess cramping, rectal bleeding, nausea, vomiting; if these symptoms occur, product should be discontinued; identify cause of constipation
- **Hepatic encephalopathy:** Monitor blood ammonia level 15-45 mcg/dl or 35-65 umol/L is normal range; monitor for clearing of confusion, lethargy, restlessness, irritability (hepatic encephalopathy); may decrease ammonia level by 50%, monitor sodium in higher doses

Patient problem
Constipation (uses)
Diarrhea (adverse reactions)

Implementation
PO route
• Give with full glass of fruit juice, water, milk to increase palatability of oral form; for rapid effect, give on empty stomach; increase fluids by 2 L/day; do not give with other laxatives; if diarrhea occurs, reduce dosage
• **Kristalose:** dissolve contents of packet in 4 oz of water
Rectal route
• Administer retention enema (no commercial product) by diluting 300 ml of lactulose/700 ml of water or of 0.9% NaCl; administer by rect balloon catheter; retain for 30-60 min; repeat if evacuated too quickly

Patient/family education
• Discuss with patient that adequate fluid consumption is necessary
• Teach patient that normal bowel movements do not always occur daily
• Teach patient not to use in presence of abdominal pain, nausea, vomiting; tell patient to notify prescriber of unrelieved constipation or if symptoms of electrolyte imbalance occur: muscle cramps, pain, weakness, dizziness, excessive thirst
• Teach patient not to use laxatives for long-term therapy; bowel tone will be lost
• Do not give at bedtime as a laxative; may interfere with sleep
• Notify prescriber if diarrhea occurs; may indicate overdosage

Evaluation
Positive therapeutic outcome
• Decreased constipation
• Decreased blood ammonia level
• Clearing of mental state

lamiVUDine (3TC) (Rx)
(lam-i′vue-dine)
Epivir, Epivir-HBV, Heptovir ✦
Func. class.: Antiretroviral
Chem. class.: Nucleoside reverse transcriptase inhibitor (NRTI)

Do not confuse: lamiVUDine/ LamoTRIgine

ACTION: Inhibits replication of HIV virus by incorporating into cellular DNA by viral reverse transcriptase, thereby terminating the cellular DNA chain

Therapeutic outcome: Improved symptoms of HIV infection

USES: HIV-1–related infection in combination with at least 2 other antiretrovirals; chronic hepatitis B (Epivir-HBV)

Unlabeled uses: Prophylaxis of HIV postexposure with indinavir and zidovudine

Pharmacokinetics

Absorption	Rapidly absorbed
Distribution	Extravascular space
Metabolism	Protein binding <36%
Excretion	Unchanged in urine
Half-life	Half-life 4 hr; child 2 hr

Pharmacodynamics

Peak	3.2 hr

CONTRAINDICATIONS
Hypersensitivity

Precautions: Pregnancy, breastfeeding, children, geriatric, granulocyte count <1000/mm^3 or Hgb <9.5 g/dl, renal disease, pancreatitis, peripheral neuropathy

> **BLACK BOX WARNING:** Severe hepatic dysfunction, lactic acidosis

DOSAGE AND ROUTES
HIV
Adult and adolescent >16 yr and ≥ 50 kg: PO 150 mg bid or 300 mg/day; <50 kg 2 mg/kg bid
Child 3 mo-16 yr: PO 4 mg/kg bid; max 150 mg bid

Renal dose
Adult: PO CCr 30-49 ml/min: Epivir 150 mg/day; **Epivir HBV** 100 mg 1st dose, then 50 mg/day; **CCr 15-29 ml/min: Epivir** 150 mg 1st dose, then 100 mg/day; **Epivir HBV** 100 mg 1st dose, then 25 mg/day; **CCr 5-14 ml/min: Epivir** 150 mg 1st dose, then 50 mg/day; **Epivir HBV** 35 mg 1st dose, then 15 mg/day; **CCr <5 ml/min: Epivir** 50 mg 1st dose, then 25 mg/day; **Epivir HBV** 35 mg 1st dose, then 10 mg/day

Chronic hepatitis B
Adult: PO 100 mg/day
Child/adolescent 2-17 yr: PO 3 mg/kg/day, max 100 mg

Available forms: Oral sol **(Epivir)** 10 mg/ml, tabs 150, 300/mg; oral sol **(Epivir-HBV)** 5 mg/ml, tabs 100 mg

ADVERSE EFFECTS

CNS: *Fever, headache, malaise, dizziness, insomnia, depression, fatigue, chills,* seizures, peripheral neuropathy, paresthesia

EENT: Taste change, hearing loss, photophobia

GI: *Nausea, vomiting, diarrhea,* anorexia, cramps, dyspepsia, hepatomegaly with steatosis, pancreatitis (more common in children)

HEMA. Neutropenia, anemia, thrombocytopenia

INTEG: *Rash*

MS: *Myalgia, arthralgia, pain*

RESP: *Cough*

SYST: Lactic acidosis, anaphylaxis, Stevens-Johnson syndrome, immune reconstitution syndrome

INTERACTIONS

Individual drugs

AMILoride, dofetilide, entecavir, metFORMIN, memantine, procainamide, trospium, trimethoprim/sulfamethoxazole: increased level of lamiVUDine

Emtricitabine: do not combine, duplication

Other products that cause pancreatitis: increase: pancreatitis

Sulfamethoxazole/trimethoprim: increase: lamotrigine level

Zalcitabine: decreased both products, avoid concurrent use

Drug/lab test

Increased: ALT, bilirubin, lipase, CK

Decreased: Hgb, neutrophil, platelet count

NURSING CONSIDERATIONS

Assessment

• **HIV:** Test for HIV before starting treatment; monitor blood counts q2wk; watch for neutropenia, thrombocytopenia, Hgb, CD4, viral load, lipase, triglycerides periodically during treatment; if low, therapy may have to be discontinued and restarted after hematologic recovery; blood transfusions may be required; assess for lessening of symptoms; if HBV is present, a higher dose of Epivir-HBV is needed

• Hepatitis B: Assess for fatigue, anorexia, pruritus, jaundice during and for several months after discontinuation; monitor liver function tests: AST, ALT, bilirubin; amylase; bilirubin; triglycerides, lipase

• **Monitor children for pancreatitis:** abdominal pain, nausea, vomiting, neuropathy, discontinuing may be required; monitor amylase, lipase; use cautiously in children

> **BLACK BOX WARNING: Assess for lactic acidosis, severe hepatomegaly with steatosis:** obtain baseline liver function tests; if elevated, discontinue treatment; discontinue even if liver function tests are normal and symptoms of lactic acidosis, severe hepatomegaly develops; may be fatal, especially in women

• **Pregnancy/breastfeeding:** Epivir is a drug that is used in pregnancy to treat HIV, enroll in the Antiretroviral Pregnancy Registry at 800-258-4263, do not breastfeed

Patient problems

Infection (uses)

Risk for injury (adverse reactions)

Implementation

• Epivir and Epivir-HBV are not interchangeable

• Administer PO daily, bid without regard to meals

• Give with other antiretrovirals only, do not triple antiretrovirals with abacavir or didanosine, resistance may occur

• Store in cool environment; protect from light

Patient/family education

• Teach patient that GI complaints and insomnia resolve after 3-4 wk of treatment

• Tell patient that product is not a cure for AIDS but will control symptoms; compliance is needed, take as directed, to complete full course of treatment even if feeling better

• Teach patient to notify prescriber of sore throat, swollen lymph nodes, malaise, fever, peripheral neuropathy; other infections may occur

• Teach patient to report pancreatitis, immune reconstitution syndrome immediately

• Teach patient that virus is still infective, may pass AIDS virus to others

• Encourage patient to continue follow-up visits since serious toxicity may occur; blood counts must be done q2wk

• Tell patient that other products may be necessary to prevent other infections

• Teach patient that product may cause fainting or dizziness

• **Pregnancy/breastfeeding:** To enroll in the Antiretroviral Pregnancy Registry at 800-258-4263, not to breastfeed

Evaluation

Positive therapeutic outcome

• Absence of infection, symptoms of HIV infection

---

lamoTRIgine (Rx)

(lam-o-trye'geen)

LaMICtal, Lamictal CD, Lamictal ODT, Lamictal XR

Func. class.: Anticonvulsant—miscellaneous

Chem. class.: Phenyltriazine

Do not confuse: lamoTRIgine/lamiVUDine, **LaMICtal**/LamISIL/Lomotil

ACTION: May inhibit voltage-sensitive sodium channels, decreasing seizures

Therapeutic outcome: Decrease in intensity and number of seizures

USES: Adjunct in the treatment of partial, tonic-clonic seizures, children with Lennox-Gastaut syndrome, bipolar disorder

Pharmacokinetics

Absorption	Well absorbed, rapid
Distribution	Protein binding 55%, crosses placenta
Metabolism	Glucuronic acid conjunction
Excretion	Excreted in breast milk
Half-life	15-27 hr with enzyme inducers

Pharmacodynamics

Onset	Unknown
Peak	1.4-2.3 hr, XR 4-10 hr
Duration	Unknown

CONTRAINDICATIONS

Hypersensitivity, mania

Precautions: Pregnancy (cleft lip/palate in 1st trimester), breastfeeding, geriatric, renal/hepatic/cardiac disease, severe depression, suicidal ideation, blood dyscrasias, children <16 yr, serious rash

DOSAGE AND ROUTES

Seizures: monotherapy

Adult and adolescent ≥16 yr: PO 50 mg/day for wk 1 and 2, then increase to 100 mg divided bid for wk 3 and 4; **maintenance** 300-500 mg/day; **receiving enzyme inducing AEDs (carBAMazepine, PHENobarbital, phenytoin, primidone but not valproic acid);** ext rel 50 mg/day × 1-2 wks, then 100 mg/day during wk 3-4, then 200 mg/day during wk 5, then 300 mg/day during wk 6, then 400 mg/day during wk 7; after wk 7 range is 400-600 mg/day

Adolescent <16 yr and child: PO 0.3 mg/kg/day wk 1 and 2, then 0.6 mg/kg/day wk 3 and 4;

depends on use of AED; usual dosage 4.5-7.5 mg/kg/day, max 300 mg/day

Monotherapy for patients taking valproate

Adult/adolescent ≥16 yr: receiving lamoTRIgine and valproate, without enzyme-inducing drug PO (immediate-release) stabilize on valproate and target dose of 200 mg/day lamoTRIgine; if patient is not taking lamoTRIgine 200 mg/day, increase dose by 25-50 mg/day q1-2wk to reach 200 mg/day; while maintaining lamoTRIgine 200 mg/day, decrease valproate to 500 mg/day by ≤500 mg/day/wk, maintain valproate at 500 mg/day × 1 wk, then increase lamoTRIgine to 300 mg/day, while decreasing valproate 250 mg/day × 1 wk, then discontinue valproate and increase lamoTRIgine by 100 mg/day qwk to maintenance dosage of 500 mg/day

Seizures: multiple therapy with valproate

Adult and adolescent ≥16 yr: PO 25 mg every other day, then 25 mg/day wk 3-4, increase by 25-50 mg q1-2wk; maintenance 100-500 mg/day

Adolescent <16 yr and child: PO 0.1-0.2 mg/kg/day initially, then increase q2wk as needed to 1.5 mg/kg/day or 200 mg/day

Hepatic dose

Adult (moderate hepatic impairment or severe without ascites): PO reduce by 25%

Adult (severe hepatic impairment with ascites): PO reduce by 50%

Available forms: Tabs 25, 100, 150, 200 mg; chew tabs 5, 25 mg; oral disintegrating tab 25, 50, 100, 200 mg; oral disintegrating 25-50, 50-100, 25-50-100 mg titration kit; PO ext rel 25-50-100, 50-100-200 mg titration kit; PO 25-100 mg starter kit, ext rel 25, 50, 100, 250, 300 mg

ADVERSE EFFECTS

CNS: Fever, insomnia, tremor, depression, anxiety, *dizziness*, ataxia, *headache*, suicidal ideation, seizures, poor concentration

EENT: Nystagmus, *diplopia*, *blurred vision*

GI: *Nausea, vomiting, anorexia*, abdominal pain, hepatotoxicity

GU: *Dysmenorrhea*

HEMA: Anemia, DIC, leukopenia, thrombocytopenia

INTEG: Rash (potentially life-threatening), alopecia, photosensitivity

CV: chest pain, palpitations

MS: neck pain, myalgias

SYST: Stevens-Johnson syndrome, angioedema, toxic epidermal necrolysis, DRESS

INTERACTIONS
Individual drugs
Acetaminophen, carBAMazepine, OXcarbazepine, PHENobarbital, phenytoin, primidone: decreased lamoTRIgine serum concentration
Valproic acid: decreased metabolic clearance of lamoTRIgine

Drug classifications
CYP3A4 inhibitors: decreased metabolic clearance of lamoTRIgine

Drug/herb
Ginkgo: increased anticonvulsant effect
Ginseng, santonica: decreased anticonvulsant effect

Drug/lab
False positive: PCP (rapid drug screen)

NURSING CONSIDERATIONS
Assessment
• Assess for rash (Stevens-Johnson syndrome or toxic epidermal necrolysis) in pediatric patients; product should be discontinued at first sign of rash, more common in those taking multiple products for seizures, rash usually occurs during 2-8 wk of therapy
• **Assess for seizure activity: Assess for** duration, type, intensity, halo before seizure, baseline and periodically
• Assess for hypersensitive reactions
• **Bipolar disorder:** assess for suicidal thoughts/behaviors
• **DRESS:** Monitor for fever, rash, lymphadenopathy, may be with hepatitis, nephritis, myocarditis, discontinue immediately, may involve multiple organ systems

Patient problem
Risk for injury (uses, adverse reactions)
Impaired skin integrity (adverse reactions)

Implementation
PO route
• Extended-release product is not to be used for conversion to monotherapy from ≥ 2 antiepileptic products
• **Orange Starter Kit:** for those **NOT** taking carBAMazepine, phenytoin, PHENobarbital, primidone, rifampin, or valproate
• **Green Starter Kit:** for those taking carBAMazepine, phenytoin, PHENobarbital, primidone, rifampin but **NOT** valproate
• **Blue Starter Kit:** for those taking valproate
• Discontinue all products gradually ≥2 wk, abrupt discontinuation can increase seizures
• All forms may be given without regard to meals
• **Chewable dispersible tab:** may be swallowed whole, chewed, mixed in water or fruit juice; to mix, add to small amount of liquid in a glass or spoon, tabs will dissolve in 1 min, then mix in more liquid and swirl and swallow immediately
• **Orally disintegrating tabs:** place on tongue, move around in mouth, when disintegrated, swallow; examine blister pack before use, do not use if blisters are torn or missing; do not cut tabs in half
• **Extended-release tabs:** swallow whole; do not cut, break, chew
• Give correct starter kit: severe side effects have occurred from incorrect starter kit
• Give in divided doses with or after meals to decrease adverse effects

Patient/family education
• Caution patient not to discontinue product abruptly; seizures may occur
• Caution patient to avoid hazardous activities until stabilized on product
• Advise patient to notify prescriber of skin rash or increased seizure activity
• Teach patient to use sunscreen and protective clothing; photosensitivity occurs
• Advise patient to carry/wear emergency ID stating product use
• Advise patient, caregiver to notify prescriber immediately of suicidal thoughts, behaviors
• **Rash:** Teach patient to notify prescriber immediately if rash, fever, or swollen lymph nodes occur
• Teach patient to notify prescriber if pregnancy is planned or suspected, use a nonhormonal contraceptive; enroll with the North American Antiepileptic Drug Pregnancy Registry at 888-233-2334 (www.aedpregnancyregistry.org), product decreases folate; avoid breastfeeding

Evaluation
Positive therapeutic outcome
• Decrease in severity of seizures or severity of bipolar symptoms

lansoprazole (Rx, OTC)
(lan-soe′prah-zole)
Prevacid, Prevacid 24 hr, Prevacid SoluTab
Func. class.: Proton-pump inhibitor
Chem. class.: Benzimidazole

Do not confuse: Prevacid/Pravachol/Prinivil

ACTION: Suppresses gastric secretion by inhibiting hydrogen/potassium ATPase enzyme system in gastric parietal cell; characterized as gastric acid pump inhibitor since it blocks final step of acid production

Therapeutic outcome: Reduction in gastric pain, swelling, fullness

USES: Gastroesophageal reflux disease (GERD), severe erosive esophagitis, poorly responsive systemic GERD, pathologic hypersecretory conditions (Zollinger-Ellison syndrome, systemic mastocytosis, multiple endocrine adenomas); possibly effective for treatment of duodenal, gastric ulcers, maintenance of healed duodenal ulcers

Pharmacokinetics

Absorption	Rapid after granules leave stomach
Distribution	Protein binding 97%
Metabolism	Liver extensively
Excretion	Urine, feces; clearance decreased in geriatric, renal/hepatic disease
Half-life	1.5 hr

Pharmacodynamics

Onset	1-3 hr
Peak	1.7 hr
Duration	24 hr

CONTRAINDICATIONS
Hypersensitivity

Precautions: Pregnancy, breastfeeding, children, hypomagnesemia, osteoporosis

DOSAGE AND ROUTES
Frequent heartburn
Adult: PO 15 mg qd up to 14 days

Duodenal ulcer
Adult: PO 15 mg/day before meals for 4 wk, then 15 mg/day to maintain healing of ulcers; ulcers associated with **Helicobacter pylori:** 30 mg lansoprazole bid, 1 g amoxicillin bid, clarithromycin 500 mg bid, × 10-14 days or 30 mg lansoprazole tid with 1 g amoxicillin tid × 14 day

Pathologic hypersecretory conditions
Adult: PO 60 mg/day, may give up to 90 mg bid, administer >120 mg/day in divided doses

NSAID-related ulcer (continuing use)
Adult PO 30 mg q d × 8 wk

GERD/esophagitis
Adult/adolescent: PO 15-30 mg/day × 8 wk
Child 1-11 yr (>30 kg): PO 30 mg/day ≤12 wk
Child 1-11 yr (≤30 kg): 15 mg/day ≤12 wk

Stress gastric prophylaxis
Adult: NG use 30 mg oral cap or 300 mg disintegrating tab

Available forms: del rel caps 15, 30 mg; orally disintegrating tabs 15, 30 mg

ADVERSE EFFECTS
CNS: *Headache,* dizziness
GI: Diarrhea, abdominal pain, vomiting, nausea, *constipation,* flatulence, acid regurgitation, anorexia, *Clostridium difficile*–associated diarrhea

INTERACTIONS
Individual products
Calcium carbonate, iron salts, itraconazole, ketoconazole, atazanavir, ampicillin: decreased absorption of each specific product
Warfarin: increased bleeding risk
Sucralfate: delayed absorption of lansoprazole

Drug/herb
• Avoid use with red yeast rice, St. John's wort

Drug/food
• Food decreases rate of absorption; use before food

Drug classifications
Loop/thiazide diuretics: increased hypomagnesemia
Antimuscarinics, H_2 blockers: decreased lansoprazole effect

NURSING CONSIDERATIONS
Assessment
• **CDAD:** monitor bowel sounds q8hr, abdomen for pain, swelling, anorexia, blood in stool, may occur even after completion of therapy
• Monitor liver enzymes (AST, ALT, alkaline phosphatase) during treatment
• Monitor INR and pro-time when taking warfarin
• Monitor for low magnesium levels, including palpitations, muscle spasm, tremor
• **Beers:** Avoid scheduling use for >8 wk unless for high-risk patients (oral corticosteroids/chronic NSAIDs use)
• Teach patient the route used and how to take; take 30-60 min prior to eating
• Teach symptoms of low magnesium levels

Patient problem
Pain (uses)
Diarrhea (adverse reactions)

Implementation
PO route
• Swallow del rel cap whole; do not break, crush, chew, or open
• Administer before eating
• **Delayed Release Capsules:** Swallow intact, do not chew or crush; may be opened and

contents sprinkled on 1 tbs applesauce or other soft food, swallow immediately, or contents may be put into a small volume of juice, mixed, and swallowed; rinse with 2 or more volumes of liquid and have patient take

• **Oral cap:** Open cap and pour ¼ of granules into NG feeding syringe with plunger removed, slowly add water and depress plunger, repeat until all granules are used, flush tube with 15 ml water

• Place on tongue, allow to dissolve, use without regard to water

• **Oral syringe:** Dissolve 15 mg/4 ml or 30 mg/10 ml water; use extra water in syringe to remove all of the product

NG tube

• **Oral disintegrating tab:** Mix 30 mg tab in 10 ml water, give via NG tube, flush tube with 10 ml sterile water, clamp for 60 min

Patient/family education

• Instruct patient to report severe diarrhea, cramping, blood in stools, fever product may have to be discontinued

• Inform diabetic patient that hypoglycemia may occur, to monitor blood glucose

• Encourage patient to avoid hazardous activities; dizziness may occur

• Tell patient to avoid alcohol, salicylates, ibuprofen; may cause GI irritation

• Teach patient that if using OTC for heartburn, it may take 1-4 days to see full benefit

• **Pregnancy:** Teach patient to notify provider if pregnancy is planned or suspected; if breastfeeding, do not breastfeed

Evaluation

Positive therapeutic outcome

• Absence of gastric pain, swelling, fullness

RARELY USED

lanthanum (Rx)
(lan'-tha-num)
Fosrenol
Func. class.: Phosphate binder

USES: End-stage renal disease

CONTRAINDICATIONS: Hypophosphatemia, hypersensitivity

DOSAGE AND ROUTES
Adult: **PO** 750-1500 mg/day in divided doses with meals; titrate dose q2-3wk until an acceptable phosphate level is reached; tabs should be chewed completely before swallowing; intact tabs should not be swallowed; maintenance dose 1500-3000 mg/day divided with meals; max 3750 mg/day

---

RARELY USED

lapatinib (Rx)
(la-pa'tin-ib)
Tykerb
Func. class.: Antineoplastic—miscellaneous
Chem. class.: Biologic response modifier, signal transduction inhibitor (STIs)

Therapeutic outcome: Decrease in breast cancer progression

USES: Advanced/metastatic breast cancer patients with tumor that overexpresses HER2 protein and who have received previous chemotherapy

CONTRAINDICATIONS
Pregnancy, hypersensitivity, breastfeeding

DOSAGE AND ROUTES
Advanced/metastatic breast cancer with HER2
Adult: **PO** 1250 mg (5 tabs)/day 1 hr before or after food on days 1-21 plus capecitabine 2000 mg/m²/day in 2 divided doses on days 1-14 in a repeating 21-day cycle; continue until therapeutic response or toxicity occurs

Metastatic breast cancer with HER2 overexpression for whom hormonal therapy is indicated
Adult: **PO** 1500 mg (6 tabs) 1 hr before food with letrozole 2.5/day

Hepatic dose
Adult (Child-Pugh C): **PO** 750 mg/day (with capecitabine); 1000 mg/day (with letrozole)

---

latanoprost ophthalmic
See Appendix B

⚠ HIGH ALERT

ledipasvir/sofosbuvir
(le-dip'as-vir/soe-fos'bue-veer)
Harvoni
Func. class.: Antiviral antihepatitis agent
Chem. class.: N55A inhibitor

ACTION: A combination product with a HCV NS5A inhibitor (ledipasvir) and a nucleotide analog HCV NS5B polymerase inhibitor (sofosbuvir)

Therapeutic outcome: Hepatitis C RNA reduction

USES: Chronic hepatitis C virus (HCV) genotype 1 infection in patients with compensated liver disease

---

Absorption	Rapid
Distribution	Ledipasvir: >99.8% protein binding, Sofosbuvir: 61%-65% protein binding
Metabolism	Extensively
Excretion	Ledipasvir: biliary; Sofosbuvir: kidneys 80% recovered in the urine
Half-life	Half-life sofosbuvir 0.4 hr, metabolite 27 hr

Onset	Unknown
Peak	Ledipasvir peak 4-5 hr, Sofosbuvir peak 0.8-1 hr
Duration	24 hr

CONTRAINDICATIONS: Hypersensitivity

Precautions: Decompensated hepatic disease, decompensated cirrhosis, severe renal impairment (eGFR <30 ml/min/1.73 m²), endstage renal failure requiring dialysis, pregnancy, breastfeeding

DOSAGE AND ROUTES

Adults genotype 1 (treatment-naive) with compensated (Child-Pugh A) cirrhosis: 1 tablet (90 mg ledipasvir; 400 mg sofosbuvir) PO once daily with or without food × 12 wk

Adults genotype 1 (treatment-experienced) without cirrhosis: 1 tablet (90 mg ledipasvir; 400 mg sofosbuvir) PO once daily with or without food × 12 wk

Adults genotype 1 (treatment-experienced) with compensated (Child-Pugh A) cirrhosis: 1 tablet (90 mg ledipasvir; 400 mg sofosbuvir) PO once daily with or without food × 24 wk. Alternatively, treatment duration may be reduced to 12 wk if ledipasvir; sofosbuvir is administered in combination with ribavirin. Ribavirin must be administered with food in two divided doses, and the dose is based on weight as follows: less than 75 kg give 500 mg PO twice daily; 75 kg or more give 600 mg PO twice daily. Recommendation includes patients coinfected with HIV

Adults genotype 1 (treatment-naive and experienced) with decompensated (Child-Pugh B or C) cirrhosis: 1 tablet (90 mg ledipasvir; 400 mg sofosbuvir) PO once daily with ribavirin (600 mg PO once daily) × 12 wk. Ribavirin must be administered with food

Adults genotype 1 (treatment-naive and experienced) liver transplantation and are without cirrhosis or have compensated (Child-Pugh A) cirrhosis: 1 tablet (90 mg ledipasvir; 400 mg sofosbuvir) PO once daily with ribavirin for 12 wk. Ribavirin must be administered with food

Children and adolescent 12 to 17 yr genotype 1 (treatment-naive) without cirrhosis or with compensated (Child-Pugh A) cirrhosis: 1 tablet (90 mg ledipasvir; 400 mg sofosbuvir) PO once daily with or without food × 12 wk

Children and adolescent 12 to 17 yr (treatment-experienced) without cirrhosis: 1 tablet (90 mg ledipasvir; 400 mg sofosbuvir) PO once daily with or without food × 12 wk

Children and adolescent 12 to 17 yr genotype 1 (treatment-experienced) with compensated (Child-Pugh A) cirrhosis: 1 tablet (90 mg ledipasvir; 400 mg sofosbuvir) PO once daily with or without food × 24 wk

For the treatment of chronic hepatitis C virus (HCV) genotype 4, 5, 6 infection
Oral dosage

Adult (treatment-naive and experienced) without cirrhosis or who have compensated (Child-Pugh A) cirrhosis: 1 tablet (90 mg ledipasvir; 400 mg sofosbuvir) PO once daily with or without food × 12 wk

Adult (treatment-naive and experienced) who have undergone liver transplantation and are without cirrhosis or have compensated (Child-Pugh A) cirrhosis: 1 tablet (90 mg ledipasvir; 400 mg sofosbuvir) PO once daily with ribavirin for 12 wk. Ribavirin must be administered with food in two divided doses

Children and adolescent 12 to 17 yr (treatment-naive and experienced) without cirrhosis or who have compensated (Child-Pugh A) cirrhosis: 1 tablet (90 mg ledipasvir; 400 mg sofosbuvir) PO once daily with or without food. The recommended duration of treatment is 12 wk

Available forms: Tab 90 mg ledipasvir/400 mg sofosbuvir

ADVERSE EFFECTS
CNS: *Fatigue, headache,* insomnia
GI: Nausea, vomiting, diarrhea

INTERACTIONS
Drug classifications

Digoxin: Increased digoxin level: Anticonvulsants, antimycobacterials (rifabutin, rifAMPin, rifapentine), p-glycoprotein inducers, avoid using together

Decrease: ledipasvir/sofosbuvir level

H2 receptor antagonists (famotidine): Decrease: Ledipasvir level, separate by ≤12 hr, max dose of H2 receptor antagonist should not exceed famotidine 40 mg bid equivalent

Avoid use with products that increase P-glycoprotein

Drug/lab test
Increased: bilirubin, lipase, CK

NURSING CONSIDERATIONS
Assessment
• **Hepatitis C:** monitor hepatitis C RNA, serum bilirubin, creatinine
• **Pregnancy/breastfeeding:** Use only if benefits outweigh fetal risk, cautious use in breastfeeding, excretion unknown

Patient problem
Infection (uses)

Implementation
• Use without regard to food

Patient/family education
• Instruct patient to report effects to the prescriber
• Teach patient to take at the same time each day and use for full course even if feeling better, to take missed doses when remembered on the same day, do not take double doses
• Identify if pregnancy is planned or suspected or if breastfeeding
• Teach patient if antacids (magnesium, aluminum) are needed, take 4 hr before or after this product
• Teach patient will not decrease transmission of infection of others
• Teach patient to notify all providers of product
• CHC decreased

Evaluation
Positive therapeutic outcome
• Hepatitis C RNA reduction

leflunomide (Rx)
(leh-floo'noh-mide)
Arava
Func. class.: Antirheumatic (DMARDs)
Chem. class.: Immune modulator, pyrimidine synthesis inhibitor

ACTION: Inhibits an enzyme involved in pyrimidine synthesis and has antiproliferative, antiinflammatory effect

Therapeutic outcome: Decreased pain, joint swelling, increased mobility

USES: Rheumatoid arthritis, to reduce disease process as well as symptoms

Unlabeled uses: Juvenile rheumatoid arthritis

Pharmacokinetics
Absorption	Well
Distribution	Protein binding 99%, crosses placenta
Metabolism	Liver
Excretion	Kidneys
Half-life	14-18 days

Pharmacodynamics RA effect
Onset	Up to 1 mo
Peak	Up to 6 mo
Duration	Unknown

CONTRAINDICATIONS
Breastfeeding, hypersensitivity

> **BLACK BOX WARNING:** Pregnancy

Precautions: Children, renal disorders, vaccinations, infection, alcoholism, immunosuppression, jaundice, lactase deficiency, hepatic disease

DOSAGE AND ROUTES
Adult: **PO loading dose** 100 mg/day × 3 days, **maintenance** 20 mg/day; may be decreased to 10 mg/day if not well tolerated

Juvenile rheumatoid arthritis (unlabeled)
Adolescent and child >40 kg: PO 20 mg/day
Adolescent and child 20-40 kg: PO 15 mg/day
Adolescent and child 10-19.9 kg: PO 10 mg/day

Available forms: Tabs 10, 20, 100 mg

ADVERSE EFFECTS
CNS: Dizziness, insomnia, depression, paresthesia, anxiety, migraine, neuralgia, headache
CV: Palpitations, hypertension, chest pain, angina pectoris, peripheral edema
EENT: Pharyngitis, oral candidiasis, stomatitis, dry mouth, blurred vision
GI: *Nausea, anorexia, vomiting, constipation, flatulence, diarrhea, increased liver function tests,* hepatotoxicity, weight loss
HEMA: Anemia, ecchymosis, hyperlipidemia
INTEG: Rash, pruritus, alopecia, acne, hematoma, herpes infections
RESP: Pharyngitis, rhinitis, bronchitis, cough, respiratory infection, pneumonia, sinusitis, interstitial lung disease
SYST: Opportunistic/fatal infections, Stevens-Johnson syndrome, toxic epidermal necrolysis, DRESS

INTERACTIONS
Individual drugs
Cholestyramine: decreased effect of leflunomide, use for overdose

Methotrexate: increased hepatotoxicity
Rifampin: increased leflunomide levels
Warfarin: increased bleeding risk

Drug classifications
Hepatotoxic agents: increased side effects of
leflunomide
Live virus vaccines: decreased antibody reaction
NSAIDs: increased NSAID effect

NURSING CONSIDERATIONS
Assessment
• **Assess arthritic symptoms:** ROM, mobility,
swelling of joints, baseline, during treatment
• **Assess for infection:** fatal opportunistic
infections can occur

> **BLACK BOX WARNING: Hepatic necrosis/
> failure: Hepatic studies:** Monitor liver
> function studies, if ALT elevations are >2×
> baseline, reduce dose to 10 mg/day, monitor
> monthly or more frequently

• Screen for latent TB before starting treatment;
if TB is present, treat before using this product
• **Interstitial lung disease:** assess for
worsening cough, dyspnea, fever; may need
to be discontinued, and drug elimination
procedure initiated (rare)
• Obtain CBC with differential qmo × 6 mo,
then q6-8wk thereafter, pregnancy test,
electrolytes

> **BLACK BOX WARNING: Pregnancy:** Determine
> that patient is not pregnant before treatment;
> not to be given to women of childbearing
> potential who are not using reliable contra-
> ception

• **Stevens-Johnson syndrome, toxic epidermal necrolysis:** Monitor for rash during treatment, if rash with fever, fatigue, joint aches,
blisters are present discontinue immediately,
initiate drug elimination procedure

Patient problem
Impaired mobility (uses)
Pain (uses)

Implementation
• Give with full glass of water to enhance
absorption
• Give PO with food, milk, or antacids for GI
upset, give same time each day; loading dose is
recommended
• **Drug elimination:** to eliminate product
give cholestyramine 8 g tid × 11 days, check
levels <0.02 mg/L × 2, 2 wk apart, may still be
elevated, retreatment may be needed

Patient/family education
• Teach patient that product must be continued
for prescribed time to be effective, that up to a
month may be required for improvement, that
continuing monitoring will be needed
• Instruct patient to take with food, milk, or
antacids to avoid GI upset, take at same time
of day
• Advise patient to use caution when driving;
drowsiness, dizziness may occur
• Teach patient effect may take up to 1 mo, that
other treatment may continue, corticosteroids,
NSAIDs
• Advise patient to discuss with health care
professional all Rx, OTC, herbals, supplements
used
• Advise patient to take with a full glass of
water to enhance absorption, may continue
with correct prescribed treatment with other
antiinflammatories
• Inform patient that hair loss may occur,
review alternatives
• Advise patient to avoid live virus vaccinations
during treatment

> **BLACK BOX WARNING: Pregnancy:** Advise
> patient not to become pregnant while taking
> this product

Evaluation
Positive therapeutic outcome
• Increased joint mobility without pain
• Decreased joint swelling

TREATMENT OF OVERDOSE:
Give cholestyramine 8 g tid × 11 days

---

lenalidomide (Rx)
(len-a-lid-o-mide)
Revlimid
Func. class.: Antianemic, biologic
response modifier, hormone
Chem. class.: Thalidomide derivative/TNF
modifier

ACTION: Decreases secretion of inflammatory cytokines and increases secretion of antiinflammatory cytokines, also inhibits COX-2

Therapeutic outcome: Increase in
reticulocyte count

USES: Transfusion-dependent anemia due
to low- or intermediate-1-risk myelodysplastic
syndrome (MDS); multiple myeloma in combination with dexamethasone

---

Pharmacokinetics	
Absorption	Rapid
Distribution	Unknown
Metabolism	Unknown
Excretion	Unknown
Half-life	Elimination 3 hr

Pharmacodynamics	
Onset	Unknown
Peak	Unknown
Duration	Unknown

CONTRAINDICATIONS: Breast-
feeding, hypersensitivity

> **BLACK BOX WARNING:** Pregnancy, females

Precautions: Accidental exposure, bone marrow suppression, children, dental disease, uterine bleeding, geriatric, fungal/viral infections, smoking

> **BLACK BOX WARNING:** Neutropenia/thrombocytopenia, thromboembolic disease

DOSAGE AND ROUTES
Transfusion-dependent anemia due to low- or intermediate-1-risk MDS associated with a deletion 5q cytogenetic abnormality with or without additional cytogenetic abnormalities

Adult: PO 10 mg/day; continue/adjust based on clinical toxicity/lab findings

Multiple myeloma
Adult: PO 25 mg/day on days 1-21 with dexamethasone 40 mg/day PO on days 1-4, 9-12, 17-20 of each 28-day cycle for the first 4 therapy cycles; starting with cycle 5, the lenalidomide dose stays the same, but only give dexamethasone 40 mg/day PO on days 1-4 q28day; continue/adjust dosing based on clinical and laboratory findings

Dosage adjustments for hematologic toxicities associated with MDS
Thrombocytopenia or neutropenia within 4 wk of starting at 10 mg/day
PO: Reduce dose from 10 mg/day PO to 5 mg/day PO; withhold lenalidomide if platelet count <50,000/mm³ from a baseline of at least 100,000/mm³, if platelet count falls to 50% of the baseline value, if the baseline is <100,000/mm³, if absolute neutrophil count (ANC) <750/mm³ from a baseline of at least 1000/mm³, or if <500/mm³ from a baseline of <1000/mm³; the

new dose of 5 mg/day PO may begin once the platelet count is at least 50,000/mm³ (30,000/mm³ if the baseline <60,000/mm³), and the ANC returns to at least 1000/mm³ or 500/mm³ for patients with a baseline <1000/mm³

Thrombocytopenia or neutropenia after 4 wk of starting at 10 mg/day
PO: Reduce dose from 10 mg/day PO to 5 mg/day PO; withhold lenalidomide if platelet count <30,000/mm³, if platelet count <50,000/mm³ and a platelet transfusion, if neutrophils <500/mm³ for at least 7 days, or if <500/mm³ and a temp of at least 38.5° C are present; the new dose of 5 mg/day PO may begin once the platelet count is at least 30,000/mm³ without hemostatic failure and the ANC is at least 500/mm³

Thrombocytopenia or neutropenia that develops while taking 5 mg/day
PO: Reduce dose from 5 mg/day PO to 5 mg PO every other day; withhold lenalidomide if platelet count <30,000/mm³, platelet count <50,000/mm³ and a platelet transfusion, neutrophils <500/mm³ for at least 7 days, or if <500/mm³ and a temp of at least 38.5° C are present; the new dose of 5 mg PO every other day may begin once the platelet count is at least 500/mm³

Dosage adjustments for toxicities (multiple myeloma)
Thrombocytopenia: Reduce dose from 25 mg/day PO to 15 mg/day PO; withhold lenalidomide if platelet count <30,000/mm³; check CBC qwk; the new dose of 15 mg/day PO may begin once the platelet count is at least 30,000/mm³; withhold lenalidomide each time the platelet count is <30,000/mm³; a new dose of 5 mg less than the previous dose should be started once the platelet count is at least 30,000/mm³; do not dose below 5 mg/day PO

Neutropenia without other toxicity: Hold dose; withhold lenalidomide and add G-CSF if neutrophils <1000/mm³; check CBC weekly; resume lenalidomide at 25 mg/day PO once neutrophils are at least 1000/mm³, and neutropenia is the only toxicity

Neutropenia with other toxicity: Reduce dose from 25 mg/day PO to 15 mg/day PO; withhold lenalidomide and add G-CSF if neutrophils <1000/mm³; check CBC qwk; resume lenalidomide at 15 mg/day PO once neutrophils are at least 1000/mm³; withhold lenalidomide and add G-CSF each time the neutrophils are <1000/mm³; if other toxicity is present, a new dose of 5 mg less than the previous dose should be started

L

once the neutrophils are at least 1000/mm³; do not dose below 5 mg/day PO

Other grade 3 or 4 toxicity related to lenalidomide: Reduce dosage from 25 mg/day PO to 15 mg/day PO; withhold lenalidomide and resume lenalidomide at 15 mg/day PO once the toxicity has resolved to grade 2 or less; withhold lenalidomide each time a grade 3 or 4 toxicity occurs; a new dose of 5 mg less than the previous dose should be started once the toxicity has resolved to grade 2 or less; do not dose below 5 mg/day

NURSE ALERT
Renal dose
Adult: PO CCr 30-59 ml/min, 5 mg q24hr (MDS), 10 mg q24hr (multiple myeloma); CCr <30 ml/min (not requiring dialysis), 5 mg q48hr (MDS), 15 mg q48hr (multiple myeloma)

Available forms: Caps 5, 10, 15, 25 mg

ADVERSE EFFECTS
CNS: Depression, dizziness, fatigue, fever, headache, sweating, peripheral neuropathy
CV: Chest pain, hypotension, palpitations
GI: Abdominal pain, anorexia, constipation, diarrhea, nausea/vomiting, dysgeusia, xerosis
HEMA: Anemia, leukopenia, pancytopenia, thrombocytopenia, neutropenia
META: Hypokalemia, hypomagnesemia
MS: Arthralgia, back pain, myalgia
RESP: Cough, dyspnea, pulmonary embolism, epistaxis, rhinitis
SYST: Angioedema, secondary malignancy

INTERACTIONS
Drug classifications
Anticoagulants, NSAIDs, platelet inhibitors, salicylates, thrombolytics: increased bleeding risk
Toxoids, vaccines: decreased immune response

NURSING CONSIDERATIONS
Assessment

> **BLACK BOX WARNING:**

- Monitor blood tests: HCT, Hgb, electrolytes
- Monitor B/P for hypotension
- Assess blood dyscrasias

> **BLACK BOX WARNING:** Assess for hypersensitivity reactions: skin rashes, urticaria (rare)

> **BLACK BOX WARNING:** Assess for pregnancy before use

Patient problems
- Lack of knowledge of medication (teaching)

Implementation
- Give PO, with dexamethasone for multiple myeloma
- Do not crush or open caps
- All persons involved must comply with the condition of rev assist program

Patient/family education
- Advise patient to avoid driving or hazardous activity during beginning of treatment

Evaluation
Positive therapeutic outcome
- Increase in reticulocyte count

> **⚠ HIGH ALERT**
> **RARELY USED**
> ## lenvatinib
> (len-va'-ti-nib)
> **Lenvima**
> *Func. class.:* Antineoplastic

USES: Locally recurrent or metastatic, progressive, radioactive iodine refractory differentiated thyroid cancer (DTC)

CONTRAINDICATIONS: Hypersensitivity

DOSAGE AND ROUTES
Thyroid cancer
Adult: PO 24 mg (two 10-mg capsules and one 4-mg capsule) daily. Advanced renal cell carcinoma after one prior treatment, used with everolimus
Adult: PO 18 mg/day with everolimus 5 mg/day

> ## lesinurad/allopurinol (Rx)
> (le-sin'-ure-ad/al-oh-pure'i-nole)
> **Duzallo**
> *Func. class.:* Antigout agent, antihyperuricemic
> *Chem. class.:* Xanthine oxidase inhibitor

ACTION: Inhibits the enzyme xanthine oxidase, reducing uric acid synthesis

USES: For the treatment of hyperuricemia associated with gout

Absorption	Unknown
Distribution	Allopurinol: Protein binding <1 %; lesinurad: highly bound to plasma proteins

Metabolism: **Lesinurad:** Metabolized via oxidation CYP2C9

Excretion	Allopurinol: Excreted in feces, urine
Half-life	Allopurinol: 1-2 hr; lesinurad: 5 hr

Pharmacodynamic

Onset, duration	Unknown
Peak	Allopurinol: 1.5 hr

CONTRAINDICATIONS
Hypersensitivity

Precautions: Pregnancy, breastfeeding, children, renal/hepatic disease

DOSAGE AND ROUTES
Hyperuricemia associated with gout
Adult: PO 1 tablet (lesinurad 200 mg; allopurinol 300 mg) qday in those who have not achieved target serum uric acid on allopurinol 300 mg/day or more

Renal dose
Adult: CCr less than 45 ml/min: Use not recommended

Available forms: Tabs 200 mg-200 mg, 200 mg-300 mg

INTERACTIONS
Individual drugs
Ammonium chloride, vit C, potassium/sodium phosphate: Increase: kidney stone formation—
Ampicillin, amoxicillin: Increase: rash, avoid concurrent use
Rasburicase: Increase xanthine nephropathy, calculi

Drug categories
Oral anticoagulants, oral antidiabetics, theophylline: Increased action of each product
ACE inhibitors, thiazides: Increased hypersensitivity, toxicity
Antineoplastics (mercaptopurine, azaTHIOprine): Increased bone marrow depression

SIDE EFFECTS
CNS: Headache
GI: Nausea, vomiting, malaise, cramps, diarrhea
INTEG: Rash
MS: Acute gouty attack

NURSING CONSIDERATIONS
Assessment
• **Gout: Assess** for joint pain, swelling; may use with NSAIDs for acute gouty attacks; uric acid levels q2wk; uric acid levels should be ≤6 mg/dl, effect may take several weeks
• Monitor CBC, AST, BUN, creatinine, prothrombin time/INR, before starting treatment, periodically; prothrombin time/INR should be reassessed periodically in patients receiving coumarin anticoagulant therapy
• Monitor I&O ratio; increase fluids to 2 L/day prevent stone formation and toxicity
• Assess for rash, hypersensitivity reactions, discontinue product
• **Hepatic disorder:** Monitor LFTs baseline and periodically; assess for abdominal pain, jaundice of skin, eyes
• **Bone marrow suppression:** Usually in those who have received concomitant drugs that may cause this reaction, may occur 6 wk to 6 yr after starting allopurinol
• **Pregnancy/breastfeeding:** Use only if needed, no well-controlled studies, use cautiously in breastfeeding

Patient problem
Pain (uses)

Implementation
PO route
• Give in the a.m. with food and water
• To provide adequate hydration (drink 2 liters [68 ounces] of fluid daily)
• Do not discontinue if a gout flare occurs during treatment; the flare can be managed concurrently as appropriate for the individual patient
• Missed dose: Do not take a missed dose later in the day. Wait to take on the next day; do not double the dose

Patient/family education
• Teach patient to avoid hazardous activities if drowsiness or dizziness occurs
• Teach patient to avoid alcohol, caffeine; will increase uric acid levels
• Teach patient to avoid large doses of vit C; kidney stone formation may occur
• Teach patient to reduce dairy products, refined sugars, sodium, meat if taking for calcium oxalate stones
• Advise patient to take as prescribed; if dose is missed, take as soon as remembered; do not double dose; tabs may be crushed
• Advise patient to increase fluid intake to 2 L/day
• Teach patient to report skin rash, stomatitis, malaise, fever, aching; product should be discontinued

L

Evaluation
Positive therapeutic outcome
• Decreased pain in joints, decreased stone formation in kidneys, decreased uric acid levels

---

RARELY USED

letermovir
(le- term- oh- vir)
Prevymis
Func. class.: Antiviral

USES: For the prevention of cytomegalovirus after allogenic hematopoietic stem cell transplant

Dosage and routes
For cytomegalovirus (CMV) disease prophylaxis without concurrent cyclosporine
Adult: PO/IV 480 mg qday started between day 0 and day 28 posttransplantation (before or after engraftment) and continued through day 100 posttransplantation

For cytomegalovirus (CMV) disease prophylaxis with concurrent cyclosporine
Adult: PO/IV 240 mg qday started between day 0 and day 28 posttransplantation (before or after engraftment) and continued through day 100 posttransplantation.

⚠ HIGH ALERT

letrozole (Rx)
(let'tro-zohl)
Femara
Func. class.: Antineoplastic, nonsteroidal aromatase inhibitor

---

Do not confuse: Femoral/Femhrt

ACTION: Binds to the heme group of aromatase; inhibits conversion of androgens to estrogens to reduce plasma estrogen levels

Therapeutic outcome: Decreased spread of malignancy

USES: Early, advanced, or metastatic breast cancer in postmenopausal women who are hormone receptor positive

---

Pharmacokinetics

Absorption	Well absorbed
Distribution	Widely distributed, steady state 2-6 wk
Metabolism	Liver
Excretion	Kidneys
Half-life	Terminal 48 hr

Pharmacodynamics

Onset	Unknown
Peak	2 days
Duration	Unknown

CONTRAINDICATIONS
Pregnancy, hypersensitivity, premenopausal females

Precautions: Hepatic disease, respiratory disease, osteoporosis

DOSAGE AND ROUTES
Adult: PO 2.5 mg/day

Available forms: Tabs 2.5 mg

ADVERSE EFFECTS
CNS: Somnolence, dizziness, depression, anxiety, *headache, lethargy*
CV: Angina, MI, CVA, thromboembolic events, peripheral edema, hypertension
GI: *Nausea, vomiting, anorexia,* constipation, heartburn, diarrhea
GU: Endometrial cancer, vaginal bleeding, endometrial proliferation disorder
INTEG: *Rash, pruritus,* alopecia, sweating
MISC: Hot flashes, night sweats, second malignancies, anaphylaxis, angioedema, infections
MS: Arthralgia, arthritis, bone fracture, myalgia, osteoporosis
RESP: Dyspnea, cough

INTERACTIONS
Drug classifications
Estrogens, oral contraceptives: decreased letrozole effect

NURSING CONSIDERATIONS
Assessment
• **Pain:** Assess for pain baseline and periodically
• Monitor temperature; may indicate beginning of infection
• Monitor LFTs before, during therapy (bilirubin, AST, ALT, LDH) as needed or monthly

Patient problem
Pain (uses)

Implementation
- May administer bisphosphonates to increase bone density
- Give with food or fluids for GI upset
- Give in equal intervals q6hr

Patient/family education
- Tell patient that product may be taken without regard to meals
- Teach patient to report vaginal bleeding, diarrhea, chest/bone pain
- Advise patient to use adequate contraception in perimenopausal, recently menopausal women
- Advise patient to avoid driving or other hazardous activities until response is known, as dizziness may occur

Evaluation

Positive therapeutic outcome
- Prevention of rapid division of malignant cells, postmenopausal cancer

RARELY USED

leucovorin (Rx)
(loo-koe-vor′in)
Func. class.: Vitamin/folic acid antagonist antidote
Chem. class.: Tetrahydrofolic acid derivative

USES: Megaloblastic or macrocytic anemia caused by folic acid deficiency, overdose of folic acid antagonist, methotrexate toxicity, toxicity caused by pyrimethamine/trimethoprim/trimetrexate, pneumocystosis, toxoplasmosis

CONTRAINDICATIONS
Hypersensitivity to this product or folic acid, benzyl alcohol, anemias other than megaloblastic not associated with vit B_{12} deficiency

DOSAGE AND ROUTES
Methotrexate toxicity—leucovorin rescue
Adult and child: PO/IM/**IV (normal elimination)** given 6 hr after dose of methotrexate 10 mg/m^2 until methotrexate is $<5 \times 10^{-8}$ m, CCr has increased 50% above prior level, or methotrexate level is 5×10^{-8} m at 24 hr or at 48 hr level is $>9 \times 10^{-8}$ m; give leucovorin 100 mg/m^2 q3hr until level drops to $<10^{-8}$ m

Megaloblastic anemia caused by enzyme deficiency
Adult and child: PO/IM/**IV** up to 6 mg/day

Advanced colorectal cancer
Adult: IV 200 mg/m^2, then 5-fluorouracil 370 mg/m^2; or leucovorin 20 mg/m^2, then 5-fluorouracil 425 mg/m^2; give daily $\times$ 5 days q4-5wk

Pyrimethamine/trimethoprim toxicity prevention
Adult and child: PO/IV 5-15 mg/day

⚠ HIGH ALERT

leuprolide (Rx)
(loo-proe′lide)
Eligard, Lupron ✦, Lupron Depo, Lupron Depot-Ped
Func. class.: Antineoplastic hormone
Chem. class.: Gonadotropin-releasing hormone

Do not confuse: Lupron/Lopurin/Nuprin

ACTION: Causes initial increase in circulating levels of LH, FSH; continuous administration results in decreased LH, FSH; in men testosterone is reduced to castration levels; in premenopausal women estrogen is reduced to menopausal levels

Therapeutic outcome: Prevention of rapidly growing malignant cells in prostate cancer, decreased pain in endometriosis, resolution of central precocious puberty (CPP)

USES: Metastatic prostate cancer (inj implant), management of endometriosis (depot), CPP, uterine leiomyomata (fibroids)

Pharmacokinetics
Absorption	Rapidly absorbed (SUBCUT)
Distribution	Unknown
Metabolism	Unknown
Excretion	Unknown
Half-life	3-4 hr

Pharmacodynamics
Onset	Unknown
Peak	4 hr
Duration	Up to 12 wk

CONTRAINDICATIONS
Pregnancy, breastfeeding, hypersensitivity to GnRH or analogs, thromboembolic disorders, undiagnosed vaginal bleeding; Viadur implant or Eligard should not be used in women or children

Precautions: Edema, hepatic disease, CVA, MI, seizures, hypertension, diabetes mellitus, HF, depression, osteoporosis, spinal cord compression, urinary tract obstruction

DOSAGE AND ROUTES
Advanced prostate cancer
Adult: SUBCUT 1 mg/day; IM depot 7.5 mg/dose qmo; or IM depot 22.5 mg q3mo; or IM depot 30 mg q4mo; or IM depot 45 mg q6mo

Endometriosis/fibroids
Adult: IM 3.75 mg qmo for 6 mo, 11.25 mg q3mo for 6 mo, or IM 30 mg q4mo

Anemia related to uterine fibroids
Adult: IM 3.75 mg depot qmo × 3 mo or 11.25 mg depot as a single dose

Central precocious puberty
Child: SUBCUT 50 mcg/kg/day; increase as needed by 10 mcg/kg/day
Child >37.5 kg: IM Lupron Depot-Pcd 15 mg q4wk
Child 25-37.5 kg: IM Lupron Depot-Pcd 11.25 mg q4wk
Child ≤25 kg: Lupron Depot-Pcd 7.5 mg q4wk

Available forms: Lupron Depot inj: 3.75, 7.5, 11.25, 15, 22.5, 30, 45 mg; Solution for subcut Inj: 5 mg/ml (2.8-ml multidose vials)

ADVERSE EFFECTS
CNS: Memory impairment, depression, seizures
CV: MI, pulmonary emboli, dysrhythmias, peripheral edema
GI: Anorexia, diarrhea, GI bleeding, nausea, vomiting
GU: Edema, hot flashes, impotence, decreased libido, amenorrhea, vaginal dryness, gynecomastia, profuse vaginal bleeding
INTEG: Alopecia
MS: Bone pain
RESP: Dyspnea, pulmonary fibrosis, interstitial lung disease

INTERACTIONS
Individual drugs
Flutamide, megestrol: increased antineoplastic action

Drug classifications
SSRIs: Increased seizure risk

NURSING CONSIDERATIONS
Assessment
• **Prostate cancer:** Assess for increased bone pain during first 4 wk of treatment, those with metastasis in the spinal column may exhibit severe back pain
• **Assess for symptoms of endometriosis/fibroids** including lower abdominal pain, excessive vaginal bleeding, bloating if product is given for the diagnosis of endometriosis
• **For central precocious puberty (CPP):** the diagnosis should have been confirmed by development of secondary sex characteristics in children <9 yr; also included to confirm the diagnosis of CPP is estradiol/testosterone, GnRH test, tomography of head, adrenal steroid, chorionic gonadotropin, wrist x-ray, height, weight; patients with CPP display the signs of testicular growth, facial, body hair (boys), breast development, menses (girls)
• Monitor liver function tests before, during therapy (bilirubin, AST, ALT, LDH) as needed or monthly; prostate-specific antigen in prostate cancer; calcium, testosterone, bone mineral density, blood glucose, HbA1c
• Monitor pituitary gonadotropic and gonadal function during therapy and 4-8 wk after therapy is decreased; check LH, FSH, acid phosphate at beginning of treatment
• **QT prolongation:** Depot: monitor ECG in those CV patients using the depot route
• **Tumor flare:** monitor worsening of signs and symptoms (normal during beginning therapy): fatigue, increased pulse, pallor, lethargy, edema in feet, joints, stomach pain, shaking
• Monitor renal status: I&O ratio, check for bladder distention daily during beginning therapy (renal obstruction)
• **Severe allergic reaction:** rash, pruritus, urticaria, purpuric skin lesions, itching, flushing

Patient problems
Impaired sexual functioning (adverse reactions)
Risk of injury (adverse reactions)

Implementation
• Never give IV
• Store in tight container at room temp
• Use depot only IM; never give SUBCUT
• Unused vials may be stored at room temperature
Subcut route
• No dilution needed; if patient is self-administering make sure patient uses syringes provided by manufacturer
• **Eligard subcut:** Bring to room temp, once mixed give within 30 min; prepare the 2 syringes for mixing, join the 2 syringes by pushing in and twisting until secure; mix the product by pushing the contents of both syringes back and forth between syringes until uniform, should be light tan to tan; hold syringes vertically with syringe B on the bottom, draw entire mixed product into syringe B (short, wide syringe) by depressing the syringe A plunger and slightly withdrawing syringe B plunger, uncouple syringe A while pushing down on syringe A plunger, small air bubbles will remain; hold syringe B upright, remove pink cap, attach needle cartridge to the end of syringe B, remove needle cover, give by subcut route

---

⚠ Nurse Alert　　　✖ Key NCLEX® Drug　　　>> Drug Specifics

IM route
- Never give IV
- **Give monthly:** reconstitute single-use vial with 1 ml of diluent; if multiple vials are used, withdraw 0.5 ml and inject into each vial (1 ml), withdraw all and inject at 90-degree angle (3.75 mg)
- **Give 3 month:** reconstitute microspheres using 1.5 ml of diluent and inject in vial, shake, withdraw, and inject
- **12-month:** inserted into upper arm; at the end of 12 months, implant must be removed
- Use syringe and product packaged together; give deep in large muscle mass; rotate sites

Patient/family education
- Advise patient to notify prescriber if menstruation continues (menstruation should stop); to use a nonhormonal method of contraception during therapy
- Instruct patient to report any complaints, side effects to nurse or prescriber; hot flashes may occur; record weight, report gain of 2 lb/day
- Teach patient how to prepare, administer; to rotate sites for SUBCUT/IM inj; use only syringe provided by manufacturer; to store depot at room temperature, refrigerate unopened vials, to protect all from heat; to keep accurate records of dosing (prostate cancer)
- Instruct patient that tumor flare may occur: increase in size of tumor, increased bone pain; tell patient that bone pain disappears after 1 wk; may take analgesics for pain, usually in prostate cancer
- Advise the patient not to breastfeed while taking this product
- Inform patient that voiding problems may increase in beginning of therapy, but will decrease in several weeks
- Teach patient that ongoing treatment is needed to control precocious puberty
- **Pregnancy/breastfeeding:** Teach patient to notify prescriber if pregnancy is planned or suspected, avoid breastfeeding, to use a nonhormonal form of contraception (women of childbearing potential)

Evaluation
Positive therapeutic outcome
- Decreased size, spread of malignancy
- Decreased pain in endometriosis, fibroids
- Decreased signs of CPP
- Increased follicle maturation

levalbuterol (Rx)
(lev-al-bute'er-ole)
Xopenex, Xopenex HFA
Func. class.: Bronchodilator
Chem. class.: Adrenergic β₂-agonist

ACTION: Causes bronchodilatation by action on β_2 (pulmonary) receptors by increasing levels of cyclic adenosine monophosphate (AMP), which relaxes smooth muscle; produces bronchodilatation; CNS, cardiac stimulation, increased diuresis, and increased gastric acid secretion

Therapeutic outcome: Increased ability to breathe because of bronchodilatation

USES: Treatment or prevention of bronchospasm (reversible obstructive airway disease), asthma

Pharmacokinetics
Absorption	Unknown
Distribution	Unknown
Metabolism	Liver extensively, tissues
Excretion	Unknown, breast milk
Half-life	3¼-4 hr

Pharmacodynamics
	INH SOL	INH AEROSOL
Onset	5-15 min	4.5-10.2 min
Peak	1½ hr	76-78 min
Duration	5-6 hr	6 hr

CONTRAINDICATIONS
Hypersensitivity to sympathomimetics, this product, or albuterol

Precautions: Pregnancy, breastfeeding, hyperthyroidism, diabetes mellitus, hypertension, prostatic hypertrophy, closed-angle glaucoma, seizures, renal disease, QT prolongation, tachydysrhythmias, severe cardiac disease, hypokalemia, children

DOSAGE AND ROUTES
Bronchospasm in reversible obstructive airway disease
Adult and child ≥12 yr: INH 0.63 mg tid, q6-8hr by nebulization; may increase to 1.25 mg q8hr
Adult/adolescent/child >4 yr: (HFA, metered dose) 90 mcg (2 INH) q4-6hr
Child 6-11 yr: INH 0.31 mg tid via nebulization, max 0.63 mg tid

Available forms: Inh pediatric 0.31 mg/3 ml; sol 0.63/3 ml, 1.25 mg/3 ml, 125 mg/0.5 ml, 45 mcg per actuation (HFA)

ADVERSE EFFECTS

CNS: *Tremors, anxiety,* headache, nervousness, dizziness
CV: Tachycardia
EENT: Dry nose, irritation of nose and throat
GI: Diarrhea, dyspepsia
INTEG: Rash
META: Hypokalemia, hyperglycemia
MS: Muscle cramps
RESP: Cough, dyspnea, asthma, bronchospasm
SYST: Anaphylaxis, angioedema
MISC: Flu-like syndrome, lymphadenopathy, infections

INTERACTIONS
Individual drugs
Digoxin: Decreased digoxin effect

Drug classifications
β-Adrenergic blockers: decreased levalbuterol action, severe bronchospasm may occur
Bronchodilators (aerosol): increased action of bronchodilator
Loop/thiazide diuretics: increased hypokalemia
MAOIs: tricyclics, other adrenergics, increased levalbuterol action

Drug/herb
Cola nut, guarana, tea (black/green), coffee, yerba maté: increased stimulation

NURSING CONSIDERATIONS
Assessment
• Assess cardiac status: palpitations, increased or decreased B/P, dysrhythmias
• **Assess respiratory function:** vital capacity, pulse oximetry, forced expiratory volume, ABGs, lung sounds, heart rate, rhythm (baseline, during therapy); character of sputum: color, consistency, amount
• Monitor for evidence of allergic reactions; paradoxic bronchospasm, withhold dose; notify prescriber, if these occur hold dose, notify prescriber at once, bronchospasm may occur with new canister or vial
• **Pregnancy/breastfeeding:** Avoid use in pregnancy, do not breastfeed, unknown reaction

Patient problems
Ineffective airway clearance (uses)

Implementation
• Give by nebulization q6-8hr; wait at least 1 min between inhalation of aerosols
• Use this medication before other medications and allow 5 min between each to prevent overstimulation

• Keep unopened until ready for use, after opening, use within 2 wk, protect from light, heat
Inhalation route
• Shake well before use, use a spacer device, prime with 4 test sprays in new canister or when not used for >3 days
Nebulizer route
• Dilute conc sol with normal sterile saline (1.25 mg/0.5ml) before use

Patient/family education
• Tell patient not to use OTC medications before consulting prescriber; extra stimulation may occur; instruct patient to use this medication before other medications and allow at least 5 min between each to prevent overstimulation; to limit caffeine products such as chocolate, coffee, tea, and cola or herbs such as cola nut, guarana, yerba maté
• Teach patient that if paradoxical bronchospasm occurs to stop product immediately and notify prescriber
• Teach patient to use this product first, if using other inhalers, wait 5 min or more between products; rinse mouth with water after each dose to prevent dry mouth
• **Inhaler:** Teach patient to shake well before using and to breathe normally while using and mist goes into the reservoir, to spray × 4 before first use or if not used for 3 days, wash at least weekly
• **Diabetes:** Teach patient that diabetes may be exacerbated, use other products for diabetes in addition if needed

Evaluation
Positive therapeutic outcome
• Absence of dyspnea and wheezing after 1 hr
• Improved airway exchange
• Improved ABGs/VBGs

TREATMENT OF OVERDOSE:
Administer a β_1-adrenergic blocker

---

levETIRAcetam (Rx)
(lev-ee-tye′ra-see-tam)
Keppra, Keppra XR, Spirtam
Func. class.: Anticonvulsant
Chem. class.: Pyrrolidine derivative

Do not confuse: levETIRAcetam/
lamoTRIgine/levOCARNitine/levoFLOXacin
Keppra/Kareltra

ACTION: Unknown; may inhibit nerve impulses by limiting influx of sodium ions across cell membrane in motor cortex

---

Therapeutic outcome: Absence of seizures

USES: Adjunctive therapy in partial-onset seizures, primary generalized tonic-clonic seizures, myoclonic seizures in juvenile patients

Pharmacokinetics

Absorption	Rapidly absorbed
Distribution	Widely distributed, not protein bound
Metabolism	Liver, small amount
Excretion	Kidneys, 66% unchanged
Half-life	6-8 hr, longer in renal disease/geriatric

Pharmacodynamics

	Immediate release	Ext rel
Onset	1 hr	Unknown
Peak	1 hr	4 hr
Duration	12 hr	Unknown

CONTRAINDICATIONS

Hypersensitivity, breastfeeding

Precautions: Pregnancy, children, geriatric, cardiac/renal disease, psychosis

DOSAGE AND ROUTES
Adjunctive treatment of partial onset seizures

Adult and adolescent ≥16 yr: IV 500 mg bid, may titrate by 1000 mg/day q2wk; max 3000 mg/day in divided doses; ext rel 1000 mg/day, may increase q2wk, max 3000 mg/day

Adolescent <16 yr/child/infant: PO 10 mg/kg bid, increase the daily dose q2wk, by 20 mg/kg to 30 mg/kg bid; if unable to tolerate, may reduce dose

Myoclonic seizures/tonic-clonic seizures/partial seizures

Adult and adolescent >16 yr: PO/IV 500 mg bid, may increase by 1000 mg/day q2wk; max 3000 mg/day, in 2 divided doses

Adjunctive treatment of partial-onset seizure in those with epilepsy (Spirtam)

Adult/child ≥4 yr and >40 kg: PO 500 mg bid, may increase q2wk by 500 mg bid, max 1500 mg bid

Renal dose

Adult: PO CCr 50-80 ml/min, 500-1000 mg q12hr, ext rel 1000-2000 q24hr, max 2000 mg/day; CCr 30-49 ml/min, 250-750 mg q12hr, ext rel 500-1500 mg q24hr, max 1500 mg/day; CCr <30 ml/min 250-500 mg q12hr, ext rel 500-1000 mg q24hr, max 1000 mg/day

Available forms: Tabs 250, 500, 750, 1000; oral sol 100 mg/ml; SOL for inj 100 mg, 5 ml, ext rel tab 500, 750 mg; premixed solutions 1000 mg/100 ml 0.75% NaCl, 1500 mg/100 ml 0.54% NaCl, 500 mg/100 ml 0.82% NaCl tabs for oral suspension (Spirtam) 250, 500, 750, 1000 mg

ADVERSE EFFECTS

CNS: Dizziness, somnolence, asthenia, psychosis, suicidal ideation, non-psychotic behavioral symptoms, headache, ataxia
EENT: Diplopia, conjunctivitis
GI: Nausea, vomiting, anorexia, diarrhea, constipation, hepatitis
HEMA: Infection, leukopenia
INTEG: Pruritus, rash
MISC: Abdominal pain, pharyngitis, infection
SYST: Stevens-Johnson syndrome, toxic epidermal necrolysis; dehydration (child <4 yr)

INTERACTIONS
Drug classifications

Antihistamines, benzodiazepines, other CNS depressants, tricyclic antidepressants: increased sedation

Drug/lab test

Decreased: Hct/Hgb, WBC, RBC

NURSING CONSIDERATIONS
Assessment

• Assess seizure activity including type, location, duration, and character, intensity, precipitating factors; provide seizure precautions
• Monitor urine function tests (BUN, urine protein) periodically during treatments
• Assess blood studies: CBC, LFTs
• **Assess mental status:** mood, sensorium, affect, behavioral changes, suicidal thoughts/behaviors
• **Beers:** Avoid in older adults unless safer alternatives are not available, may cause ataxia, impaired psychomotor function
• **Pregnancy/breastfeeding:** Use only if benefits outweigh fetal risk, if used in pregnancy patient should enroll in the Antiepileptic Drug Pregnancy Registry 888-233-2334, do not breastfeed

Patient problems

Risk for injury (uses, adverse reactions)

Implementation
PO route
- Ext rel product should not be used in dialysis patients
- Give with food, milk to decrease GI symptoms (rare)
- **Child <20 kg:** give oral sol, use calibrated device
- Store at room temperature (PO); diluted preparation stable for 24 hr at room temperature in polyvinyl bags

Tablets for oral suspension (Spirtam)
- Give only whole tabs
- Peel foil from blister, do not push through foil
- Place on tongue and follow with a sip of liquid, do not swallow
- Tab can be added to a tablespoon of liquid, swirl gently, consume

Intermittent IV route
- Single-use vials: dilute in 100 mg of 0.9% NaCl, D_5W, LR; give over 15 min, discard unused vial contents, do not use product with particulates or discoloration
Child: Max concentration of product to be used 15 mg/ml (diluted solution) infuse over 15 min
- Store vials at room temperature

Patient/family education
- Teach patient to carry/wear emergency ID stating patient's name, products taken, condition, prescriber's name, phone number
- Caution patient to avoid driving, other activities that require alertness until stabilized on medication, until response is known, drowsiness occurs during first month
- Teach patient not to discontinue medication quickly after long-term use
- Instruct patient to report suicidal thoughts, behaviors immediately, mood changes, hostility, thoughts of death/dying
- Teach patient to take exactly as prescribed, do not double or omit doses
- **Pregnancy/breastfeeding:** Identify if pregnancy is planned or suspected or if breastfeeding

Evaluation
Positive therapeutic outcome
- Decreased seizure activity

levobetaxolol ophthalmic
See Appendix B

levobunolol ophthalmic
See Appendix B

levocabastine ophthalmic
See Appendix B

levodopa-carbidopa (Rx)
(lee-voe-doe′pa kar-bi-doe′pa)
Duopa, Duodopa ✦, Rytary, Sinemet, Sinemet CR
Func. class.: Antiparkinsonism agent
Chem. class.: Catecholamine

ACTION: Decarboxylation of levodopa in periphery is inhibited by carbidopa; more levodopa is made available for transport to brain and conversion to dopamine in the brain

Therapeutic outcome: Absence of involuntary movements

USES: Parkinson's disease, parkinsonism resulting from carbon monoxide, chronic manganese intoxication, cerebral arteriosclerosis, motor fluctuations in those with advanced Parkinson's disease

Pharmacokinetics

Absorption	Well absorbed (PO); ER dose slowly absorbed
Distribution	Widely distributed
Metabolism	Liver, extensively
Excretion	Kidneys, metabolites
Half-life	Levodopa (1 hr); carbidopa (1-2 hr)

Pharmacodynamics

	PO	PO-ER	Enteral
Onset	Unknown	Unknown	
Peak	1 hr	2½ hr	2.5 hr
Duration	6-24 hr	Unknown	

CONTRAINDICATIONS
Hypersensitivity, malignant melanoma, history of malignant melanoma, or undiagnosed skin lesions resembling melanoma

Precautions: Pregnancy, breastfeeding, diabetes, renal/cardiac/hepatic/respiratory disease, MI with dysrhythmias, open-angle glaucoma, seizures, peptic ulcer, depression

DOSAGE AND ROUTES
Idiopathic Parkinson's disease, postencephalitic parkinsonism, and symptomatic parkinsonism
Adult: PO (immediate-release tablets): Initial treatment: 1 carbidopa 25 mg/levodopa 100 mg tablet tid, may increase by 1 tablet qday or every other day max of 8 tablets/day. If carbidopa 10 mg/levodopa 100 mg is used, may start with 1 tablet three or four times a day. **MAINTENANCE**

TREATMENT: Individualize and adjust according to response and tolerability. At least 70 mg to 100 mg of carbidopa per day should be used. When a greater proportion of carbidopa is required, 1 tablet of carbidopa 25 mg/levodopa 100 mg may be substituted for each carbidopa 10 mg/levodopa 100 mg tablet. **PO (extended-release tablets – Sinemet CR): Initial Treatment:** carbidopa 50 mg/levodopa 200 mg tablet bid, most have been use extended-release tablets 400 mg to 1600 mg of levodopa/ day. The dosing intervals should be 4 to 8 hr apart during the waking day, adjust dose at 3-day intervals. **Patients From Levodopa To Carbidopa-Levodopa:** Initiate at 25% of the previous dose of levodopa alone; in those with mild to moderate disease, the usual initial dosage is carbidopa 50 mg/levodopa 200 mg extended-release tablet twice daily.

For the treatment of motor fluctuations in patients with advanced Parkinson's disease

Adults: Enteral suspension dosage (nasojejunal tube for short-term administration or PEG-J for long-term administration) Before initiating the enteral suspension on day 1, convert patients from all other forms of levodopa to oral immediate-release carbidopa/levodopa tablets (1:4 ratio). DAY 1 CONTINUOUS DOSING: Determine the amount of oral immediate-release levodopa that the patient received from oral immediate-release carbidopa-levodopa doses throughout the previous day (16 waking hr), in milligrams (mg). Do not include the doses of oral immediate-release carbidopa-levodopa taken at night when calculating the levodopa amount. Subtract the first oral levodopa dose in milligrams (mg) taken by the patient on the previous day from the total oral levodopa dose in milligrams (mg) taken over 16 waking hr. Divide the result by 20 mg/ml. This is the dose of carbidopa/levodopa suspension administered as a continuous dose (in ml) over 16 hr. The hourly infusion rate (ml per hour) is obtained by dividing the continuous dose by 16 hr. The hourly infusion rate will be programmed into the pump as the continuous rate. If persistent or numerous "off" periods occur during the 16-hr infusion, consider increasing the continuous dose or using the extra dose function.

Available forms: Tabs 10 mg carbidopa/100 mg levodopa, 25 mg carbidopa/100 mg levodopa, 25 mg carbidopa/250 mg levodopa; ext rel tab 25 mg/100 mg, 50 mg/200 mg carbidopa/levodopa (Sinemet CR); oral disintegrating tab (Parcopa) 10 mg carbidopa/100 mg levodopa, 25 mg carbidopa/100 mg levodopa, 25 mg carbidopa/250 mg levodopa; ext rel caps (Rytary) 23.75 mg/95 mg, 36.25 mg/145 mg, 48.75/195 mg, 61.25/245 mg; enteral suspension (Duopa) levodopa 20 mg/ml/4.63 mg/ml carbidopa

ADVERSE EFFECTS
CNS: *Involuntary choreiform movements, hand tremors, fatigue, headache, anxiety, twitching, numbness, weakness, confusion, agitation, insomnia, nightmares,* psychosis, hallucination, hypomania, severe depression, dizziness, impulsive behaviors, neuroleptic malignant syndrome, suicidal ideation
CV: *Orthostatic hypotension,* tachycardia, hypertension, palpitation, MI
EENT: Blurred vision, diplopia, dilated pupils
GI: *Nausea, vomiting, anorexia, abdominal distress, dry mouth, flatulence, dysphagia, bitter taste, diarrhea, constipation,* GI bleeding
HEMA: Hemolytic anemia, leukopenia, agranulocytosis, thrombocytopenia
INTEG: Rash, sweating, alopecia
MISC: Urinary retention, incontinence, weight change, dark urine, increased libido, hypersensitivity, dark sweat

INTERACTIONS
Individual drugs
Metoclopramide: increased effects of levodopa
Papaverine, pyridoxine: decreased effects of levodopa

Drug classifications
Antacids: increased effects of levodopa
Anticholinergics, antipsychotics, benzodiazepines, hydantoins: decreased effects of levodopa
Antihypertensives: Increased: Hypotension
MAOIs: hypertensive crisis

Drug/food
Protein: decreased absorption of levodopa

Drug/lab test
Increased: AST, ALT, bilirubin, LDH, alkaline phosphatase, BUN, serum glucose
Decreased: BUN, creatinine, uric acid
False increase: urine protein
False positive: urine ketones (dipstick), Coombs' test
False negative: urine glucose

NURSING CONSIDERATIONS
Assessment
• **Parkinsonism:** Assess for shuffling gait, muscle rigidity, involuntary movements, pill rolling, muscle spasms, drooling before and during treatment
• Assess B/P, respiration, orthostatic B/P

• Monitor I&O ratio; retention commonly causes decreased urinary output, distention, frequency, incontinence; palpate bladder if retention occurs
• Assess for muscle twitching, blepharospasm that may indicate toxicity
• Monitor renal, liver, hematopoietic studies; also for diabetes, acromegaly during long-term therapy
• Monitor for constipation, cramping, pain in abdomen, abdominal distention; increase fluids, bulk, exercise if this occurs
• Assess for tolerance over long-term therapy; dose may have to be increased or changed
• Assess for mental status: affect, mood, CNS depression, worsening of mental symptoms during early therapy

Patient problems
Impaired mobility (uses)
Risk for injury (uses)

Implementation
PO route
• Swallow **ext rel tabs** whole; do not break, crush, or chew
• **Oral disintegrating tab:** gently remove from bottle, place on tongue, swallow with saliva; after it dissolves, liquid is not necessary
• Give product until NPO before surgery; check with prescriber for continuing product
• Adjust dosage depending on patient response
• Give with meals or after meals to prevent GI symptoms; limit protein taken with product
• Give only after MAOIs have been discontinued for 2 wk; if previously on levodopa, discontinue for at least 8 hr before change to levodopa-carbidopa

Enteral route
• Fully thaw in refrigerator, remove one cassette from refrigerator, 20 min before to use, give through NG tube or a percutaneous endoscopic gastronomy tube connected to the CADD - Legacy 1400 pump, disconnect after use and flush with water, cassettes are single use only, label in order to be used based on date

Patient/family education
• Teach patient to change positions slowly to prevent orthostatic hypotension, especially during beginning of treatment
• Teach patient to report side effects: twitching, eye spasms, grimacing, protrusion of tongue, personality changes that indicate overdose
• Instruct patient to use product exactly as prescribed; if product is discontinued abruptly, parkinsonian crisis may occur; do not double doses; take missed dose as soon as remembered up to 2 hr before next dose
• Teach patient that urine, sweat may darken and is harmless
• Advise patient to use physical activities to maintain mobility and lessen spasms
• Instruct patient that OTC medications should not be used unless approved by prescriber
• Advise patient that drowsiness, dizziness are common; to avoid hazardous activities until response is known
• Explain that sips of water, hard candy, or gum may lessen dry mouth
• Teach patient to take with meals to prevent GI symptoms; to limit protein intake, which impairs product's absorption
• Teach patient not to chew, crush extended-release product
• Teach patient to immediately report nausea, vomiting, abdominal pain, ongoing constipation if using enteral product
• Teach patient to use ODT immediately after removing from container, to dissolve on tongue, swallow with saliva
• Teach patient to take as prescribed, not to take double doses

Evaluation
Positive therapeutic outcome
• Decrease in akathisia
• Improved mood
• Decreased involuntary movements

levofloxacin (Rx)
(lev-o-floks′a-sin)
Levaquin
Func. class.: Antiinfective
Chem. class.: Fluoroquinolone antibacterial

Do not confuse: Levaquin/Larium, levoFLOXacin/levetiracetam

ACTION: Interferes with conversion of intermediate DNA fragments into high molecular weight DNA in bacteria; DNA gyrase inhibitor; inhibits topoisomerase IV

Therapeutic outcome: Bacteriocidal action against the following: *Streptococcus pneumoniae, Streptococcus pyogenes, Haemophilus influenzae, Haemophilus parainfluenzae, Moraxella catarrhalis, Klebsiella pneumoniae, Mycoplasma pneumoniae, Escherichia coli, Serratia marcescens, Chlamydia pneumoniae, Legionella pneumophila, Enterococcus faecalis, Staphylococcus* epidermidis, Staphylococcus pyogenes, Staphylococcus aureus, Bacillus anthracis

USES: Acute sinusitis, acute chronic bronchitis, community-acquired pneumonia, uncomplicated skin infections, UTI, cellulitis, prostatitis, inhalational anthrax (postexposure), acute pyelonephritis, inhalation anthrax in children

Pharmacokinetics

Absorption	Unknown
Distribution	Unknown
Excretion	Kidneys unchanged
Half-life	6-8 hr

Pharmacodynamics

Onset	Immediate
Peak	Infusion's end
Duration	Unknown

CONTRAINDICATIONS
Hypersensitivity to quinolones

Precautions: Pregnancy, breastfeeding, children; photosensitivity, acute MI, atrial fibrillation, colitis, dehydration, diabetes, QT prolongation, myasthenia gravis, renal disease, seizure disorder, syphilis

> **BLACK BOX WARNING:** Tendon pain/rupture, tendinitis, myasthenia gravis, neurotoxicity

DOSAGE AND ROUTES
Most infections
Adult PO/IV 250-750 mg q 24 hr

Inhaled anthrax-postexposure
Adult PO/IV 500 mg q day × 60 days
Child >50 kg PO/IV 500 mg q day × 60 days
Child <50 kg, ≥6 mo PO/IV 8 mg/kg q 12 hr × 60 days, max 250 mg/dose

Plague
Adult PO/IV 500 mg q 24 hr × 10-14 days
Child >50 kg PO/IV 500 mg qday × 10-14 days
Child <50 kg, ≥6 mo PO/IV 8 mg/kg q 12 hr × 10-14 days, max 250 mg/dose

Renal disease
Adult: PO/IV CCr 20-49 ml/min: for 750-mg dose, give 750 mg q48hr; for 500-mg dose, give 500 mg once, then 250 mg q24hr; for 250-mg dose, no adjustment; CCr 10-19 ml/min: for 750-mg dose, give 750 mg once, then 500 mg q48hr; for 500-mg dose, give 500 mg once, then 250 mg q48hr; for 250-mg dose, give 250 mg q48hr, except when treating complicated UTI, then no dose adjustment

Available forms: Single-use vials (500, 750 mg), premixed flexible container; 250 mg/50 ml D$_5$W, 500 mg/100 ml D$_5$W, 750 mg/150 ml D$_5$W; tabs 250, 500, 750 mg; oral sol 25 mg/ml

ADVERSE EFFECTS
CNS: *Headache*, dizziness, *insomnia*, anxiety, seizures, *encephalopathy*, paresthesia, pseudotumor cerebri
CV: Chest pain, palpitations, vasodilatation, QT prolongation, hypotension (rapid infusion)
EENT: Dry mouth, visual impairment, tinnitus
GI: *Nausea*, flatulence, *vomiting*, diarrhea, abdominal pain, *Clostridium difficile*–associated diarrhea (CDAD), hepatotoxicity, esophagitis, pancreatitis
GU: Vaginitis, crystalluria
HEMA: Eosinophilia, hemolytic anemia, lymphopenia
INTEG: Rash, pruritus, photosensitivity, epidermal necrolysis, injection site reaction, edema
MISC: Hypoglycemia, hypersensitivity, tendon rupture, rhabdomyolysis
RESP: Pneumonitis
SYST: Anaphylaxis, multisystem organ failure, Stevens-Johnson syndrome, angioedema, toxic epidermal necrolysis

INTERACTIONS
Individual drugs
Calcium, iron, sucralfate, zinc: decreased absorption of levofloxacin, give 2 hr before or after products
Foscarnet: increased CNS stimulation, seizures
Haloperidol, chloroquine, droperidol, pentamidine, arsenic trioxide, levomethadyl: increased QT prolongation
Magnesium: decreased levofloxacin absorption; do not use in same **IV** line
Probenecid: increased levofloxacin levels
Theophylline: decreased theophylline clearance; toxicity may result
Warfarin: increased bleeding, monitor coagulation studies (INR/PT)

Drug classifications
Antacids (magnesium, aluminum): decreased absorption of levofloxacin

> **BLACK BOX WARNING:** Corticosteroids: increased tendon rupture, assess for tendon pain

Class IA/III antidysrhythmics, some phenothiazines, beta agonists, local anesthetics, tricyclics, CYP3A4 inhibitors (amiodarone, clarithromycin, erythromycin, telithromycin, troleandomycin), CYP3A4 substrates (methadone, pimozide, QUEtiapine, quiNIDine, risperiDONE, ziprasidone): increased QT prolongation, avoid using together

NSAIDs, cycloSPORINE: increased CNS stimulation, seizures

Drug/lab test
Increased: PT, INR
Decreased: glucose, lymphocytes

Drug/herb
Increase: Photosensitivity: St. John's wort

NURSING CONSIDERATIONS
Assessment
• Assess patient for previous sensitivity reaction to quinolones
• **Infection:** Assess patient for signs and symptoms of infection, including characteristics of wounds, sputum, urine, stool, WBC >10,000/mm³, fever; baseline, during treatment
• Obtain C&S before beginning product therapy to identify if correct treatment has been initiated
• **QT prolongation:** Monitor for QT prolongation, ejection fraction; assess for chest pain, palpitations, dyspnea
• **CDAD:** Assess for diarrhea, abdominal pain, fever, fatigue, anorexia; possible anemia, elevated WBC and low serum albumin; stop product and give usually either vancomycin or IV metroNIDAZOLE
• **Assess for allergic reactions and anaphylaxis:** rash, urticaria, pruritus, chills, fever, joint pain; may occur a few days after therapy begins; EPINEPHrine and resuscitation equipment should be available for anaphylactic reaction
• Determine urine output; if decreasing, notify prescriber (may indicate nephrotoxicity); also check for increased BUN, creatinine
• **Peripheral neuropathy:** tingling, pain, burning in extremities, can be permanent

> **BLACK BOX WARNING: Myasthenia gravis:** Do not use this product, may lead to life-threatening weakness of the respiratory muscles

> **BLACK BOX WARNING: Neurotoxicity:** May occur within hours to weeks after starting use, may be irreversible, avoid use in those who have experienced peripheral neuropathy, numbness, tingling, burning in extremities report immediately to prescriber

• Monitor blood tests: AST, ALT, CBC, Hct, bilirubin, LDH, alkaline phosphatase, Coombs' test monthly if patient is on long-term therapy
• Monitor electrolytes: potassium, sodium, chloride monthly if patient is on long-term therapy
• Monitor for bleeding: ecchymosis, bleeding gums, hematuria, stool guaiac daily if on long-term therapy
• **Assess for overgrowth of infection:** perineal itching, fever, malaise, redness, pain, swelling, drainage, rash, diarrhea, change in cough, sputum

> **BLACK BOX WARNING: Tendon rupture:** Discontinue product at first sign of tendon pain or inflammation; usually the Achilles tendon is affected, can occur up to a few months after treatment and may require surgical repair; steroids may increase risk, elderly transplant patients

Patient problem
Infection (uses)
Risk for infection (uses)

Implementation
• Obtain C&S before treatment and periodically to determine resistance to this product, treatment can start before results are obtained
• Give PO 2 hr before or 2 hr after antacids, iron, calcium, zinc, sucralfate; give fluids
• Check for irritation, extravasation, phlebitis daily

Oral solution
• Give 1 hr prior to or 2 hr after food

Intermittent IV infusion route
• Discard any unused sol in the single-dose vial
• Visually inspect for particulate matter/discoloration prior to use

IV (single use vial)
• **500 mg/20 ml vials:** To prepare a dose of 500 mg, withdraw 20 ml from a 20-ml vial and dilute with a compatible IV solution (D₅W, NS) to a total volume of 50 ml. To prepare a 500-mg dosage, withdraw all 20 ml from the vial and dilute with a compatible IV solution to a total volume of 100 ml
• **750 mg/30 ml vials:** To prepare a dose of 750 mg, withdraw 30 ml from a 30-ml vial and dilute with a compatible intravenous solution (D₅W, NS) to a total volume of 150 ml
• The concentration of the diluted solution should be 5 mg/ml prior to administration. Solutions contain no preservatives; any unused portions must be discarded

---

- **Storage:** The diluted solution may be stored for up to 72 hours when stored at or below 25° C (77° F) or for 14 days when stored under refrigeration at 5° C (41° F) in plastic containers. Solutions may be frozen for up to 6 months (−20° C or −4° F) in glass bottles or plastic containers. Thaw frozen solutions at room temperature (25° C or 77° F) or in a refrigerator (8° C or 46° F). Do not force thaw by microwave or water bath immersion. Do not refreeze after initial thawing
- Reconstituted product is stable for 72 hr at room temperature, 14 days refrigerated, 6 mo frozen
- Do not admix

Premixed IV solution
- No dilution is necessary

Intermittent IV injection
- Infuse doses of ≤500 mg IV over 60 minutes and doses of 750 mg IV over 90 minutes. Shorter infusions or bolus injections should be avoided because of the risk of hypotension

Y-site compatibilities: Alemtuzumab, alfentanil, amifostine, amikacin, aminocaproic acid, aminophylline, ampicillin, ampicillin-sulbactam, anidulafungin, argatroban, atenolol, atracurium, aztreonam, bivalirudin, bleomycin, bumetanide, buprenorphine, busulfan, butorphanol, caffeine citrate, calcium gluconate, CARBOplatin, carmustine, caspofungin, cefepime, cefoTEtan, ceftaroline, cefTAZidime, ceftizoxime, cefTRIAXone, cefuroxime, chlorproMAZINE, cimetidine, cisatracurium, CISplatin, clindamycin, codeine, cyclophosphamide, cycloSPORINE, cytarabine, dacarbazine, DACTINomycin, DAPTOmycin, DAUNOrubicin liposomal, dexamethasone, dexrazoxane, digoxin, diltiazem, diphenhydrAMINE, DOBUTamine, DOCEtaxel, dolasetron, DOPamine, doripenem, doxacurium, doxycycline, droperidol, enalaprilat, ePHEDrine, EPINEPHrine, epirubicin, ertapenem, erythromycin, esmolol, etoposide, etoposide phosphate, famotidine, fenoldopam, fentaNYL, filgrastim, floxuridine, fluconazole, fludarabine, foscarnet, fosphenytoin, gallium, gemcitabine, gemtuzumab, gentamicin, granisetron, haloperidol, hydrocortisone, HYDROmorphone, IDArubicin, ifosfamide, imipenem-cilastatin, irinotecan, isoproterenol, labetalol, lepirudin, leucovorin, levorphanol, lidocaine, linezolid, mannitol, mechlorethamine, meperidine, mesna, methylPREDNISolone, metoclopramide, metroNIDAZOLE, midazolam, milrinone, minocycline, mitoMYcin, mitoXANtrone, mivacurium, morphine, mycophenolate mofetil, nalbuphine, naloxone, nesiritide, netilmicin, niCARdipine, octreotide, ondansetron, oxacillin, oxaliplatin, oxytocin, PACLitaxel, palonosetron, pamidronate, pancuronium, PEMEtrexed, penicillin G sodium, pentamidine, phenylephrine, plicamycin, potassium acetate/chloride, promethazine, propranolol, quinupristin-dalfopristin, ranitidine, romiFentanil, rOcuronium, sargramostim, sodium bicarbonate, succinylcholine, SUFentanil, sulfamethoxazole-trimethoprim, tacrolimus, teniposide, theophylline, thiotepa, ticarcillin, ticarcillin-clavulanate, tigecycline, tirofiban, tobramycin, topotecan, trimethobenzamide, vancomycin, vasopressin, vecuronium, verapamil, vinBLAStine, vinCRIStine, vinorelbine, voriconazole, zidovudine, zoledronic acid

Solution compatibilities: 0.9% NaCl, D₅W, D₅/0.9% NaCl, D₅LR, D₅/0.45% NaCl, sodium lactate, plasma-lyte 56/D₅W

Patient/family education
- Teach patient to report sore throat, bruising, bleeding, joint pain; may indicate **blood dyscrasias (rare)**
- **Superinfection:** Advise patient to contact prescriber if vaginal itching, loose foul-smelling stools, furry tongue occur, purulent discharge in stool
- Instruct patient to take all medication prescribed for the length of time ordered; product must be taken around the clock to maintain blood levels; do not give medication to others
- **CDAD:** Advise patient to notify prescriber of diarrhea with blood or purulent discharge in stool
- Instruct patient to take 2 hr before antacids, iron, calcium, zinc products
- Tell patient to complete full course of therapy; to increase fluid intake to 2 L/day to prevent crystalluria
- Advise patient to avoid hazardous activities, driving until response to product is known, as dizziness may occur
- Instruct patient to rinse mouth frequently and use sugarless candy or gum for dry mouth
- Instruct patient to avoid taking other medications unless approved by prescriber
- Teach patient to monitor glucose (diabetes), notify provider of changes
- Advise patient to avoid sun exposure or use sunscreen to prevent phototoxicity

BLACK BOX WARNING: Teach patient to notify prescriber of tendon pain, inflammation, avoid corticosteroids with this product

• **Pregnancy/breastfeeding:** Identify if pregnancy is planned or suspected or if breastfeeding

Evaluation
Positive therapeutic outcome
• Absence of signs/symptoms of infection (WBC <10,000/mm³, temp WNL)
• Reported improvement in symptoms of infection

levofloxacin ophthalmic
See Appendix B

levomilnacipran
(lee'voe-mil-na'si-pran)
Fetzima
milnacipan
Savella
Chem. class.: Antidepressant
Func. class.: Serotonin norepinephrine reuptake inhibitor (SNRI)

Do not confuse Fetzima/Farxiga

ACTION: May potentiate serotonergic, andrenergic activity in the CNS; is a potent inhibitor of adrenal serotonin and norepinephrine reuptake

Therapeutic outcome: Decreased depression

USES: Major depressive disorder in adults

Pharmacokinetics

Absorption	Well
Distribution	22% protein binding, widely
Metabolism	By CYP2D6 in the liver
Excretion	58% (urine)
Half-life	12 hr (levomilnapran), 6-10 (milnacipran)

Pharmacodynamics

	Levomilnacipran	Milacipran
Onset	Unknown	Unknown
Peak	6-8 hr	2-4 hr
Duration	Unknown	36-48 hr

CONTRAINDICATIONS
Alcohol intoxication, alcoholism, closed angle glaucoma, hepatic disease, hepatitis, jaundice, hypersensitivity

Precautions: Pregnancy, breastfeeding, geriatric patients, mania, hypertension, renal/cardiac disease, seizures, increased intraocular pressure, anorexia, bleeding, dehydration, diabetes, hypotension, hypovolemia, orthostatic hypotension, abrupt product withdrawal

> **BLACK BOX WARNING:** Children, suicidal ideation

DOSAGE AND ROUTES
Major depressive disorder (levomilnacipran)
Adult: PO 20 mg/day × 2 days, then 40 mg/day, may increase in increments of 40 mg at intervals of at least 2 days, max 120 mg/day; max 80 mg/day (strong CYP3A4 inhibitors therapy)

Major depressive disorder (milnacipran)
Adult: PO 12.5-25 mg bid, may titrate up to 100 mg bid, max 200 mg/day

Renal dose
Adult: PO CCr 30-59 ml/min, max 80 mg/day; 15-29 ml/min, max 40 mg/day; <15 ml/min, avoid use

Fibromyalgia (levomilnacipran)
Adult/adolescent ≥17 yr: PO 12.5 mg once on day 1, then 12.5 mg bid on days 2-3, then 25 mg bid on days 4-7 and 50 mg bid thereafter

Fibromyalgia (Sarella) (milnacipran)
Adult: PO 12.5 mg qday, increase by 12.5 mg bid on days 4 to 7, increase to 50 mg bid after day 7, may increase to 100 mg bid as needed

Available forms: Ext rel caps 20, 40, 80, 120 mg; tabs 12.5, 25, 50, 100 mg

ADVERSE EFFECTS
CNS: Dizziness, agitation, hallucinations, seizures, drowsiness, mania, migraine, paresthesias, suicidal ideation, syncope
CV: Hypertension, palpitations, dysrhythmia, sinus tachycardia
EENT: Teeth grinding, blurred vision
GI: Constipation, diarrhea, nausea, vomiting, anorexia, dry mouth, abdominal pain
GU: Urinary retention
SYST: Serotonin syndrome, Stevens-Johnson syndrome

INTERACTIONS
Individual drugs
Linezolid, methylene blue IV: do not use concurrently

Drug classifications
Anticoagulants, antiplatelets, NSAIDs, salicylates: increased bleeding risk

---

Antipsychotics, dopamine antagonists: Increased neuroleptic malignant syndrome, avoid using together

CYP34A inhibitors: increased levomilnacipran effect

MAOIs: Coadministration contraindicated within 14 days of MAOI

SSRIs, serotonin receptor agonists, SNRIs: increased serotonin syndrome

Drug/herb
Alfalfa, feverfew, dong quai, fish oil: Increased bleeding risk

NURSING CONSIDERATIONS
Assessment
• **Serotonin syndrome:** assess for nausea/vomiting, dizziness, facial flush, shivering, sweating

> **BLACK BOX WARNING: Depression:** assess mood, sensorium, affect, suicidal tendencies, increase in psychiatric symptoms, depression, panic; monitor children qwk face to face during first 4 wk or dosage change, then every other week for the next 4 wk, then at 12 wk

• Monitor B/P lying, standing; pulse more often; if systolic B/P drops 20 mm Hg, hold product, notify prescriber; take VS more often in patients with CV disease
• Hepatic studies: monitor AST ALT, bilirubin baseline and periodically
• Withdrawal symptoms: assess for headache, nausea, vomiting, muscle pain, weakness; not common unless product is discontinued abruptly
• **Beers:** Use with caution in older adults, may exacerbate or cause SIADs, monitor for hyponatremia
• **Pregnancy/breastfeeding:** Use only if benefits outweigh fetal risk, SSRIs should not be used in the third trimester, do not breastfeed

Patient problem
Depression (uses)
Suicidal ideation (adverse reactions)

Implementation
• Swallow cap whole; do not break, crush, or chew; do not sprinkle on food or mix with liquid
• Give without regard to food
• Give at the same time of day

Patient/family education
• Teach patient signs and symptoms of bleeding (GI bleeding, nosebleed, ecchymoses, bruising)
• Instruct patient to use caution when driving and in other activities requiring alertness because of drowsiness and blurred vision
• Instruct patient to avoid alcohol ingestion, MAOIs, other CNS depressants, to notify all providers of use of this product; advise not to use within 14 days of MAOIs
• Instruct patient not to discontinue medication quickly after long-term use; may cause headache, malaise; taper

> **BLACK BOX WARNING:** Teach patient that clinical worsening and suicidal risk may occur, to notify prescriber immediately if suicidal thoughts/behaviors, aggression, panic attacks occur

• **Serotonin syndrome:** Teach patient to report immediately nausea, vomiting, dizziness, facial flush, shivering, sweating
• Teach patient improvement may occur in 4-8 wk or up to 12 wk (geriatric patients)
• Teach patient to swallow caps whole; do not break, crush, chew
• Advise patient that product may be used without food
• Teach patient to notify prescriber if pregnancy is planned or suspected, or if breastfeeding

Evaluation
Positive therapeutic outcome
• Decreased depression

levothyroxine (Rx)
(lee-voe-thye-rox'een)
Eltroxin ✦, Euthyrox ✦, Levo-T, Levo-TB, Levoxyl, Synthroid, Tirosint, Unithroid
Func. class.: Thyroid hormone
Chem. class.: Levoisomer of thyroxine

Do not confuse: Synthroid/Symmetrel, **levothyroxine**/lamatrigine/Lanoxin/liothyronine

ACTION: Controls protein synthesis; increases metabolic rate, cardiac output, renal blood flow, O_2 consumption, body temp, blood volume, growth, development at cellular level via action on thyroid hormone receptors

Therapeutic outcome: Correction of lack of thyroid hormone

USES: Hypothyroidism, myxedema coma, thyroid hormone replacement, thyrotoxicosis, congenital hypothyroidism, some types of thyroid cancer, pituitary TSH suppression

Pharmacokinetics

Absorption	Erratic (PO); complete (**IV**)
Distribution	Widely distributed, protein binding 99%
Metabolism	Liver; enterohepatic recirculation
Excretion	Feces via bile; breast milk (small amounts)
Half-life	6-7 days

Pharmacodynamics

	PO	IV
Onset	24 hr	6-8 hr
Peak	12-48 hr	12-48 hr
Duration	Unknown	Unknown

CONTRAINDICATIONS

Adrenal insufficiency, recent MI, thyrotoxicosis, hypersensitivity to beef, alcohol intolerance (inj only)

> **BLACK BOX WARNING:** Obesity treatment

Precautions: Pregnancy, breastfeeding, geriatric, angina pectoris, hypertension, ischemia, cardiac disease, diabetes

DOSAGE AND ROUTES NTI
Severe hypothyroidism
Adult ≤50 yr: PO 1.6 mcg/kg/day, 6-8 wk, average dose 100-200 mcg/day; IM/**IV** 50-100 mcg/day as a single dose or 50% of usual oral dosage
Adult >50 yr without heart disease or <50 yr with heart disease: PO 25-50 mcg/day, titrate q6-8wk
Adult >50 yr with heart disease: PO 12.5-25 mcg/day, titrate by 12.5-25 mcg q6-8wk
Child: PO (puberty complete) 1.7 mcg/kg/day
Child >12 yr: PO (incomplete puberty) 2-3 mcg/kg/day given as a single dose AM
Child 6-12 yr: PO 4-5 mcg/kg/day given as a single dose AM
Child 1-5 yr: PO 5-6 mcg/kg/day given as a single dose AM
Child 6-12 mo: PO 6-8 mcg/kg/day given as a single dose AM
Child 3-6 mo: PO 8-10 mcg/kg/day given as a single dose AM

Myxedema coma
Adult: IV 300-500 mcg; may increase by 100-300 mcg after 24 hr; give oral medication as soon as possible

Subclinical hypothyroidism
Adult: PO 1 mcg/kg/day may be sufficient

Available forms: Powder for inj 100, 200, 500 mcg/vial; tabs 25, 50, 88, 100, 112, 125, 137, 150, 175, 200, 300; cap (Tirosint) (liquid filled) 13, 25, 50, 75, 88, 100, 112, 125, 137, 150 mcg

ADVERSE EFFECTS
CNS: *Anxiety, insomnia, tremors,* headache, thyroid storm, excitability
CV: *Tachycardia, palpitations, angina, dysrhythmias,* hypertension, cardiac arrest
GI: Nausea, diarrhea, increased or decreased appetite, cramps
MISC: Menstrual irregularities, weight loss, sweating, heat intolerance, fever, alopecia, decreased bone mineral density

INTERACTIONS
Individual drugs
Aluminum, calcium, iron, magnesium, sucralfate, rifampin, rifabutin: decreased levothyroxine effects
Orlistat, ferrous sulfate: decreased absorption of levothyroxine

Drug classifications
Antacids: decreased levothyroxine effects
Anticoagulants (oral): increased anticoagulant effect, monitor coagulation studies (INR, PT)
Antidiabetics, insulin: Increased or decreased glucose levels, adjust levels
Bile acid sequestrants: decreased levothyroxine absorption
EPINEPHrine products: increased cardiac insufficiency risk
Estrogens: decreased thyroid hormone effects
Selective serotonin reuptake inhibitors, antileptics (carBAMazepine, OXcarbazepine, PHENobarbital, primidone, phenytoin); antimicrobials (rifAMPin, efavirenz, nevirapine, rifabutin, rifapentine): decreased levothyroxine effects
Sympathomimetics: increased sympathomimetic effect
Tricyclic/tetracyclic antidepressants: Increased effects of both products

Drug/food
Fiber, walnuts: decreased product absorption, avoid concurrent use or adjust dose

Drug/herb
Horseradish, Soy: decreased thyroid hormone effect

Drug/lab test
Increased: CPK, LDH, AST, blood glucose
Decreased: thyroid function tests

NURSING CONSIDERATIONS
Assessment

• **Hypothyroidism:** Determine if the patient is taking anticoagulants, antidiabetic agents; document on chart

• Take B/P, pulse before each dose; monitor I&O ratio and weight every day in same clothing, using same scale, at same time of day

• Monitor height, weight, psychomotor development, and growth rate if given to a child

• **Hypothyroidism:** Monitor T_3, T_4, which are decreased; radioimmunoassay of TSH, which is increased; radioactive iodine uptake (RAIU), which is increased if patient's dosage of medication is too low; assess for increased nervousness, excitability, irritability, which may indicate a too-high dosage of medication, usually after 1-3 wk of treatment

• Monitor pro-time (may require decreased anticoagulant); check for bleeding, bruising

• Assess cardiac status: angina, palpitations, chest pain, change in VS; the geriatric patient may have undetected cardiac problems and baseline ECG should be completed before treatment

• **Anticoagulants:** Should be tested and dose adjusted as needed

• **CAD:** Monitor for coronary insufficiency, also watch for cardiac changes in those receiving high, rapid doses

• **Bone density:** Patient bone density testing baseline and periodically, bone loss may occur with long-term therapy

• **Pregnancy/breastfeeding:** May be used in pregnancy, breastfeeding

Patient problems
Lack of knowledge of medication (teaching)
Nonadherence (teaching)

Implementation
• Store in tight, light-resistant container; sol should be discarded if not used immediately

• Withdraw medication 4 wk before RAIU test

PO route
• Give in AM if possible as a single dose to decrease sleeplessness; give at same time each day to maintain product level

• Give crushed and mixed with water, nonsoy formula (decreased absorption), or breast milk for infants/children, give by spoon or dropper, may crush and sprinkle over food

• Give only for hormone imbalances; not to be used for obesity, male infertility, menstrual conditions, lethargy; give lowest dosage that relieves symptoms; lower dosage for geriatric and in cardiac disease

• Use 8 oz of water on empty stomach

• Separate antacids, iron, calcium products by 4 hr

Direct IV route
• Give IV after reconstituting with 5 ml normal saline injection (0.9% NaCl), 500 mcg/5 ml, 200 mcg/2 ml; shake well; give through Y-tube or 3-way stopcock; give 100 mcg or less over 1 min, do not add to IV infusion; considered incompatible in syringe with all other products

Patient/family education
• Teach patient that product is not a cure but controls symptoms and that treatment is long term

• Instruct patient to report excitability, irritability, anxiety, sweating, heat intolerance, chest pain, palpitations, which indicate overdose

• Advise patient not to switch brands unless approved by prescriber; bioavailability may differ; do not take with food; absorption will be decreased

• Teach patient that product may be discontinued after giving birth; thyroid panel will be evaluated after 1-2 mo

• Teach patient or parent that hyperthyroid child will show almost immediate behavior/personality change; that hair loss will occur in child but is temporary

• Caution patient that product is not to be taken to reduce weight

• Caution patient to avoid OTC preparations with iodine; read labels; other medications should not be used unless approved by prescriber, not to switch brands, protect from light, moisture

• Teach patient to avoid iodine-rich food: iodized salt, soybeans, tofu, turnips, high-iodine seafood, some bread, products

• **Pregnancy/breastfeeding**: Teach patient to continue using in pregnancy, breastfeeding

Evaluation
Positive therapeutic outcome
• Absence of depression

• Weight loss, increased diuresis, pulse, appetite

• Absence of constipation, peripheral edema, cold intolerance, pale, cool dry skin, brittle nails, alopecia, coarse hair, menorrhagia, night blindness, paresthesias, syncope, stupor, coma, rosy cheeks

• Improved levels of T_3, T_4 by laboratory tests

• Child: age-appropriate weight, height, and psychomotor development

TREATMENT OF OVERDOSE:
Withhold dose for up to 1 wk; acute overdose: gastric lavage or induced emesis, provide supportive treatment to control symptoms

> **⚠ HIGH ALERT**

lidocaine, parenteral (Rx)
(lye'doe-kane)
LidoPen Auto-Injector, Xylocaine, Xylocard ✦
Func. class.: Antidysrhythmic (class IB)
Chem. class.: Aminoacyl amide

ACTION: Increases electrical stimulation threshold of ventricle and His-Purkinje system, which stabilizes cardiac membrane and decreases automaticity

Therapeutic outcome: Decreased ventricular dysrhythmia

USES: Ventricular tachycardia, ventricular dysrhythmias during cardiac surgery, MI, digoxin toxicity, cardiac catheterization

Pharmacokinetics

Absorption	Complete bioavailability (**IV**)
Distribution	Erythrocytes, cardiovascular endothelium
Metabolism	Liver
Excretion	Kidneys
Half-life	Biphasic 8 min, 1-2 hr

Pharmacodynamics

	IV	IM
Onset	2 min	5-15 min
Peak	Unknown	½ hr
Duration	20 min	1½ hr

CONTRAINDICATIONS
Hypersensitivity to amides, severe heart block, supraventricular dysrhythmias, Adams-Stokes syndrome, Wolff-Parkinson-White syndrome

Precautions: Pregnancy, breastfeeding, children, geriatric, renal/hepatic disease, HF, respiratory depression, malignant hyperthermia, myasthenia gravis, weight <50 kg

DOSAGE AND ROUTES
Ventricular arrythmias caused by MI, cardiac manipulation, glycosides
Adult: IV BOL 50-100 mg (1-1.5 mg/kg) 25-50 mg/min, repeat 5min, until arrythmias are controlled, max 300 mg in 1 hr; begin **IV** INF 1-4 mg/min (20-50 mcg/kg/min)
Child: IV/intraosseous bolus: 1 mg/kg, start infusion at 30 mcg/kg/min

Available forms: **IV** inf 0.2% (2 mg/ml), 0.4% (4 mg/ml), 0.8% (8 mg/ml); **IV** admixture 4% (40 mg/ml), 10% (100 mg/ml), 20% (200 mg/ml); **IV direct** 1% (10 mg/ml), 2% (20 mg/ml); inj (to IV admixture) 20% (200 mg/ml)

ADVERSE EFFECTS
CNS: *Headache, dizziness,* involuntary movement, confusion, tremor, *drowsiness,* euphoria, seizures, shivering
CV: *Hypotension, bradycardia,* heart block, cardiovascular collapse, arrest
EENT: Tinnitus, blurred vision
GI: Nausea, vomiting, anorexia
HEMA: Methemoglobinemia
INTEG: Rash, urticaria, edema, swelling, petechiae, pruritus
MISC: Febrile response, phlebitis at inj site
RESP: Dyspnea, respiratory depression

INTERACTIONS
Individual drugs
Amiodarone, phenytoin, procainamide, propranolol, quiNIDine: increase cardiac depression, toxicity
Cimetidine, metoprolol, phenytoin: increased lidocaine effects
CycloSPORINE: decreased effect of cycloSPORINE

Drug classifications
Antihypertensives, MAOIs: increased hypotensive effects
β-blockers, protease inhibitors: increased lidocaine effects, toxicity
Barbiturates: decreased lidocaine effects
Ergots: Increased hypotension, avoid concurrent use
Neuromuscular blockers: increased neuromuscular blockade, monitor for effects

NURSING CONSIDERATIONS
Assessment
• Assess for oxygenation or perfusion deficit: decreased B/P, chest pain, dizziness, loss of consciousness
• Assess respiratory status: auscultate lung fields for bibasilar crackles in patients with advanced HF
• Assess for urinary retention: check for pain, abdominal absorption, palpate bladder; check males with benign prostatic hypertrophy; anticholinergic reaction may cause retention
• Monitor I&O ratio, electrolytes (potassium, sodium, chloride); watch for decreasing urinary output, possible retention
• Monitor liver function tests: AST, ALT, bilirubin, alk phos
• Monitor ECG continuously to determine product effectiveness, measure PR, QRS, QT intervals, check for PVCs, other dysrhythmias; monitor B/P continuously

for hypo/hypertension; check for rebound hypertension after 1-2 hr, prolonged PR/QT intervals, QRS complex; if QT or QRS increases by 50% or more, withhold next dose, notify prescriber

• Monitor for CNS symptoms: confusion, numbness, depression, involuntary movements; if these occur, product should be discontinued

• Monitor drug levels (therapeutic level 1.5-5 mcg/ml), notify prescriber of abnormal results

• **Malignant hyperthermia:** Monitor for tachypnea, tachycardia, changes in B/P, increased temperature

• **Toxicity:** Monitor for seizures, confusion, tremors, if these occur discontinue immediately, notify prescriber, keep emergency equipment nearby

• **Pregnancy/breastfeeding:** Use only if clearly needed, cautious use in breastfeeding, excreted in breast milk

Patient problem
Impaired cardiac output (uses)
Pain (uses)
Risk for injury (uses, adverse reactions)

Implementation
IM route
• Administer in deltoid, aspirate to prevent **IV** administration, usually used if ECG monitoring cannot be done

• Check site daily for extravasation, do not use in shock

Direct IV route
• Give undiluted (1%, 2% only); give 6 mg or less over 1 min; if using an **IV** line, use port near insertion site, flush with 0.9% NaCl (50 ml)

• Store at room temperature; sol should be clear

Continuous IV infusion route
• Give after adding 1 g/250-1000 ml of D_5W; give 1-4 mg/min; use infusion pump for correct dosage; pediatric inf is 120 mg of lidocaine/100 ml of D_5W; 1-2.5 ml/kg/hr = 20-50 mcg/kg/min

• Use cardiac monitor

• Additive syringes/single-use vials are for infusing and must be diluted

Solution compatibilities: D_5W, D_5/0.9% NaCl, D_5/0.45% NaCl, D_5/LR, LR, 0.9% NaCl, 0.45% NaCl

Y-site compatibilities: Acetaminophen, alemtuzumab, alfentanil, alteplase, amikacin, aminocaproic acid, aminophylline, amiodarone, amphotericin B lipid/liposome, anidulafungin, argatroban, ascorbic acid injection, atenolol, atracurium, atropine, azithromycin, aztreonam, benztropine, bivalirudin, bleomycin, bumetanide, buprenorphine, butorphanol, calcium chloride/gluconate, CARBOplatin, carmustine, ceFAZolin, cefotaxime, cefoTEtan, cefOXitin, ceftaroline, cefTAZidime, ceftizoxime, cefTRIAXone, cefuroxime, chloramphenicol, chlorproMAZINE, cimetidine, ciprofloxacin, cisatracurium, CISplatin, clarithromycin, clindamycin, cyanocobalamin, cyclophosphamide, cycloSPORINE, cytarabine, DACTINomycin, DAPTOmycin, DAUNOrubicin, dexamethasone, dexmedetomidine, dexrazoxane, digoxin, diltiazem, diphenhydrAMINE, DOBUTamine, DOCEtaxel, dolasetron, DOPamine, doxacurium, DOXOrubicin, DOXOrubicin liposomal, doxycycline, enalaprilat, EPINEPHrine, epirubicin, epoetin alfa, eptifibatide, ertapenem, erythromycin, esmolol, etomidate, etoposide, etoposide phosphate, famotidine, fenoldopam, fentaNYL, fluconazole, fludarabine, fluorouracil, folic acid, furosemide, gentamicin, granisetron, haloperidol, heparin, hydrocortisone, imipenem/cilastatin, inamrinone, insulin, isoproterenol, ketorolac, labetalol, levofloxacin, linezolid, LORazepam, magnesium sulfate, meperidine, methylPREDNISolone, metoclopramide, metoprolol, metroNIDAZOLE, micafungin, midazolam, morphine, nafcillin, niCARdipine, nitroglycerin, nitroprusside, norepinephrine, ondansetron, palonosetron, penicillin G potassium, phenylephrine, phytonadione, piperacillin/tazobactam, potassium chloride, procainamide, prochlorperazine, promethazine, propofol, propranolol, protamine, quinupristin/dalfopristin, ranitidine, remifentanil, sodium bicarbonate, tacrolimus, theophylline, ticarcillin/clavulanate, tigecycline, tirofiban, tobramycin, vancomycin, vasopressin, verapamil, vitamin B complex with C, voriconazole, warfarin

Patient/family education
• Teach patient or family reason for use of medication and expected results

• Instruct patient in at-home use of Lidopen Auto-Injector; patient should call prescriber before use if heart attack is imminent

Evaluation
Positive therapeutic outcome
• Decreased B/P, dysrhythmias
• Decreased heart rate
• Normal sinus rhythm

TREATMENT OF OVERDOSE:
Oxygen, artificial ventilation, ECG, administer DOPamine for circulatory depression, diazepam or thiopental for seizures; decreased product or discontinuation may be required

lidocaine/prilocaine
(lye'doe-kane pri'loe-kane)
EMLA, Oraqix
Func. class.: Topical anesthetic

ACTION: Produces the analgesic effects by diminishing nerve membrane permeability to sodium, which decreases the rate of membrane depolarization. The threshold for electrical excitability is increased. The resulting reversible nerve conduction blockade affects all nerve fibers in the following sequence: autonomic, sensory, and motor, with effects diminishing in reverse order

USES: Use as local anesthesia to provide topical anesthesia

Pharmacokinetics

Absorption	Minimal
Distribution	Minimal, cross placenta, blood-brain barrier
Metabolism	Liver and kidneys
Excretion	Unknown
Half-life	Unknown

Pharmacodynamics

Onset	1 hr (EMLA)
Peak	3 hr (EMLA)
Duration	Unknown

CONTRAINDICATIONS: Hypersensitivity to this product, local anesthetics, broken skin, methoglobulemia

Precautions: Breastfeeding, pregnancy, use on large areas

DOSAGE AND ROUTES
Application to intact skin prior to minor dermal procedures (IV cannulation and venipuncture)
Adults, adolescents, and children: Topical cream/disc (EMLA): Apply 2.5 g cream over area for at least 1 hr. Cover cream with an occlusive dressing. Dermal analgesia can be expected to increase for up to 3 hr under occlusive dressing and persist for 1-2 hr after removal of the cream, max duration 4 hr
Infants 4-12 months weighing 5-10 kg: Apply no more than 2 g EMLA cream over a max 20 cm² surface area at least 1 hr before the procedure. Cover cream with an occlusive dressing
Neonates ≥37 weeks gestation and infants 1-3 mo or weighing <5 kg: Apply no more than 1 g of cream ≥1 hr before the procedure. Cover cream with an occlusive dressing

Application to intact skin for major dermal procedures (split thickness skin graft harvesting)
Adults, adolescents, and children >10 kg: Topical cream (EMLA) apply 2 g cream, cover with an occlusive dressing, and remain in contact with the skin for at ≥2 hr
Children and infants 4-12 mo, 5-10 kg: Topical cream (EMLA) apply no more than 2 g EMLA cream over a max 20 cm² surface area at least 2 hr before the procedure. Cover cream with an occlusive dressing
Neonates ≥37 weeks gestation and infants 1-3 months or weighing <5 kg: Topical cream (EMLA) apply no more than 1 g of EMLA cream to a max 10 cm² surface area at least 2 hr before the procedure. Cover cream with an occlusive dressing

Application to male genital mucous membranes as a pretreatment to local anesthetic infiltration
Male adults, adolescents, children, infants, and neonates ≥37 weeks gestation: Topical cream (EMLA) apply a thick layer of EMLA cream to skin surface for 15 min

Application to adult female external genitalia prior to minor procedures (removal of condylomata acuminata) or prior to infiltration anesthesia
Adult and adolescent (unlabeled) females: Topical cream (EMLA) apply a thick layer (5-10 g) of EMLA cream for 5-10 min

Application to periodontal pockets during scaling and/or root planing
Adults: Topical GEL (Oraqix) apply the liquid to the gingival margin; after 30 sec, fill the periodontal pockets until the gel is visible at the gingival margin. Max anesthetic effect is obtained 30 sec after application; reapply

Available forms: Topical cream 2.5%; **periodontal gel** 2.5% in a dental cartridge

SIDE EFFECTS
INTEG: Rash, itching, hypersensitivity reactions

INTERACTIONS
None significant

NURSING CONSIDERATIONS
Assessment:
• **Pain:** Assess for level of pain after application and before procedure; assess for numbness after procedure

Patient problems
Pain (uses)

⚠ Nurse Alert ✴ Key NCLEX® Drug ≫ Drug Specifics

Implementation
• Cover cream with an occlusive dressing. Local anesthetic infiltration should begin immediately after removal of EMLA cream.
• Occlusion is not necessary for absorption but may be helpful to keep the cream in place. Patients should be lying down during application of the cream, especially if no occlusion is used. The procedure or local anesthetic infiltration should begin immediately after removal of the cream.

Patient/family education
• Explain reason for product and expected result
• Explain to caregiver how to apply cream and how long to leave on the area

lidocaine topical
See Appendix B

⚠ HIGH ALERT

linagliptin
(lin-a-glip'tin)
Tradjenta, Trajenta ✦
Func. class.: Antidiabetic
Chem. class.: Dipeptidyl peptidase-4 inhibitor

ACTION: Slows the inactivation of incretin hormones. Concentrations of the active, intact hormones are increased by linagliptin, thereby increasing and prolonging the action of these hormones. Incretin hormones are released by the intestine throughout the day, and levels are increased in response to a meal.

Therapeutic outcome: Decreasing blood glucose level, A1C; decreasing polydipsia, polyphagia

USES: Type 2 diabetes mellitus with diet and exercise

Pharmacokinetics
Absorption	Rapidly, bioavailability 30%
Distribution	Extensive, tissues; protein binding concentration dependent
Metabolism	Weak CYP3A4 inhibitor
Excretion	90% unchanged, 80% enterohepatic, urine 5%
Half-life	>100 hr

Pharmacodynamics
Onset	Rapid
Peak	1.5 hr
Duration	Unknown

CONTRAINDICATIONS
Hypersensitivity to linagliptin, type 1 diabetes mellitus, diabetic ketoacidosis (DKA)

Precautions: Pregnancy, breast-feeding, adolescents or children <18 years old, debilitated physical condition, malnutrition, uncontrolled adrenal insufficiency, pituitary insufficiency, hypothyroidism, diarrhea, gastroparesis, GI obstruction, ileus, female hormonal changes, high fever, severe psychological stress, uncontrolled hypercortisolism, hyperthyroidism

DOSAGE AND ROUTES
Adult: PO 5 mg/day; when used with a sulfonylurea, a lower dose of the sulfonylurea or insulin may be necessary to minimize the risk of hypoglycemia

Available forms: Tab 5 mg

ADVERSE EFFECTS
CNS: Headache
EENT: Nasopharyngitis
ENDO: Hyperuricemia, hypoglycemia, hypertriglyceridemia
GI: Body weight loss, pancreatitis
INTEG: Serious angioedema, exfoliative dermatitis, hypersensitivity reactions, urticaria
MISC: Arthralgia, back pain
RESP: Bronchial hyperreactivity (with bronchospasm), cough, nasopharyngitis

INTERACTIONS
Individual drugs
Alcohol, cisapride, lithium, metoclopramide, tegaserod: increased need for dosing change
Bumetanide, dextrothyroxine, ethacrynic acid, ethotoin, fosphenytoin, furosemide, glucagon, niacin (nicotinic acid), phenothiazine, phenytoin, torsemide, triamterene: decreased hypoglycemic effect
CloNIDine, dexfenfluramine, disopyramide, fenfluramine, FLUoxetine, guanethidine, octreotide: increased hypoglycemia
Reserpine, β-blockers: increased masking the signs and symptoms of hypoglycemia

Drug classifications
Beta blockers, ACE inhibitors, angiotensin II receptor antagonists, fibric acid derivatives, monoamine oxidase inhibitors (MAOIs), salicylates, sulfonylureas: increased or prolonged hypoglycemia
Atypical antipsychotics (ARIPiprazole, cloZAPine, OLANZapine, QUEtiapine, risperiDONE, and ziprasidone), carbonic anhydrase inhibitors, estrogens, glucocorticoids, oral contraceptives, progestins, thiazide diuretics, thyroid hormones: decreased hypoglycemic effect

Androgens, quinolones: increased need for dosing change

CYP3A4 inducers (topiramate, rifabutin, pioglitazone, OXcarbazepine, carBAMazepine, nevirapine, modafinil, metyrapone, etravirine, efavirenz, bosentan, barbiturates, aprepitant, fosaprepitant): decreased effect of linagliptin

Drug/lab test
Increased: uric acid
Decrease: HbA1C level, fasting blood glucose

NURSING CONSIDERATIONS
Assessment
• **Diabetes:** Monitor blood glucose, A1C, during treatment to determine diabetes control; monitor for hypoglycemia: confusion, sweating, tachycardia, anxiety; hyperglycemia, polydipsia, polyuria, polyphagia
• Monitor CBC baseline and periodically during treatment, report decreased blood counts

Patient problems
Excess food intake (uses)
Nonadherence (teaching)

Implementation
• Given once daily; may give without regard to food
• May require an increased dose in stress, fever, surgery, trauma
• Store at room temperature

Patient/family education
• Teach patient the symptoms of hypo/hyperglycemia and what to do about each; to have glucagon emergency kit available, carry sugar packets
• Advise patient that product must be continued on a daily basis, explain consequences of discontinuing product abruptly; to take only as directed
• Direct patient to avoid OTC products unless approved by prescriber
• Teach patient that diabetes is a life-long illness, product will not cure diabetes
• Advise patient to carry emergency ID with prescriber, condition and medications taken
• Report immediately, skin disorders, swelling, difficulty breathing, or severe abdominal pain
• **Pancreatitis (rare):** Teach patient to report immediately severe abdominal pain, vomiting may be fatal, discontinue product immediately, use supportive therapy, monitor amylase, lipase electrolytes
• **Arthralgia:** May be severe, but temporary
• **Pregnancy:** Teach patient to notify provider if pregnancy is planned or suspected, or if breastfeeding

Evaluation
Positive therapeutic outcome
• Improving blood glucose level, A1C; decreasing polydipsia, polyphagia, polyuria, clear sensorium, absence of dizziness

lindane (OTC)
(lin-dane)
Hexit ✽
Func. class.: Scabicide/pediculicide
Chem. class.: Chlorinated hydrocarbon (synthetic)

ACTION: Stimulates nervous system of arthropods, resulting in seizures, death of organism

Therapeutic outcome: Resolution of infestation

USES: Scabies, lice (head/pubic/body), nits in those intolerant to or who do not respond to other agents

Pharmacokinetics
Absorption	20%
Distribution	Fat
Metabolism	Liver
Excretion	Kidneys
Half-life	18 hr

Pharmacodynamics
Onset	3 hr
Peak	Rapid
Duration	3 hr

CONTRAINDICATIONS
Hypersensitivity; patients with known seizure disorders; Norwegian (crusted) scabies

> **BLACK BOX WARNING:** Premature neonate; inflammation of skin, abrasions, or breaks in skin; seizure disorder

Precautions: Pregnancy, breastfeeding, infants, children <10 yr; avoid contact with eyes

DOSAGE AND ROUTES
Lice
Adult and child: Shampoo using 30 ml, work into lather, rub for 5 min, rinse, dry with towel; use fine-toothed comb to remove nits; most require 1 oz, max 2 oz

Scabies
Adult and child: TOP cream/lotion wash area with soap and water, remove visible crusts; apply to skin surfaces; remove with soap, water 8-12 hr

---

after application; may reapply in 1 wk if needed; TOP apply 1% cream/lotion to skin from neck to bottom of feet, toes; repeat in 1 wk if necessary; most require 1 oz, max 2 oz

Available forms: Lotion, shampoo, cream (1%)

ADVERSE EFFECTS
CNS: Seizures, stimulation, dizziness
INTEG: *Pruritus, rash, irritation, contact dermatitis*

INTERACTIONS
Oil-based hair dressing: increased absorption; wash, rinse, and dry hair before using lindane

NURSING CONSIDERATIONS
Assessment

> **BLACK BOX WARNING:** Skin with abrasions, breaks, inflammation; do not use on these areas

• **Infestation:** Assess head, hair for lice and nits before, after treatment; if scabies are present, check all skin surfaces
• Identify source of infection: school, family members, sexual contacts
• **Pregnancy/breastfeeding:** Avoid in pregnancy, breastfeeding

Patient problems
Impaired skin integrity (uses)

Implementation
• Apply to body areas, scalp only; do not apply to face, lips, mouth, eyes, any mucous membrane, anus, or meatus
• Give topical corticosteroids as ordered to decrease contact dermatitis; provide antihistamines
• Apply menthol or phenol lotions to control itching
• Give topical antibiotics for infection
• Provide isolation until areas on skin, scalp have cleared and treatment is completed
• Remove nits by using a fine-toothed comb rinsed in vinegar after treatment; use gloves
• Caregivers applying these products to another person should wear gloves less permeable to lindane, thoroughly clean hands after application, avoid natural latex gloves
Cream/ointment/lotion
• Use for scabies only; skin should be clean without other products on it, wait 1 hr after bathing or showering before application, shake well, apply under fingernails after trimming, a toothbrush can be used to apply; after application wrap toothbrush in paper and discard, use only a single application, apply as a thin layer over all

skin from neck down, close bottle with leftover and discard
• Do not cover, wash off after 8-12 hr using warm (not hot) water, do not leave on >12 hr
Shampoo
• For lice only, do not use other hair products before use, shake well, hair should be completely dry, use only enough shampoo to lightly wet the hair and scalp, work into hair, do not use water, allow to remain only 4 min, rinse and lather away, towel briskly

Patient/family education
• Advise patient to wash all inhabitants' clothing, using insecticide; preventive treatment may be required for all persons living in same house, using lotion or shampoo to decrease spread of infection; use rubber gloves when applying product
• Instruct patient that itching may continue for 4-6 wk; that product must be reapplied if accidentally washed off, or treatment will be ineffective; remove after specified time to prevent toxicity
• Advise patient not to apply to face; if contact with eyes occurs, flush with water
• Advise patient that sexual contacts should be treated simultaneously
• **Inform the patient of CNS toxicity:** dizziness, cramps, anxiety, nausea, vomiting, seizures

Evaluation
Positive therapeutic outcome
• Decreased crusts, nits, brownish trails on skin, itching papules in skinfolds
• Decreased itching after several wk

TREATMENT OF INGESTION:
Gastric lavage, saline laxatives, **IV** diazepam (Valium) for seizures (if taken orally)

---

linezolid (Rx)
(lih-nee'zoh-lid)
Zyvox, Zyvoxom ✦
Func. class.: Broad-spectrum antiinfective
Chem. class.: Oxazolidinone

Do not confuse: Zyvox/Vioxx/Zovirax

ACTION: Inhibits protein synthesis by interfering with translation; binds to bacterial 23S ribosomal RNA of the 50S subunit, preventing formation of the bacterial translation process in primarily gram-positive organisms

Therapeutic outcome: Negative blood cultures, absence of signs/symptoms of infection

USES: Vancomycin-resistant *Enterococcus faecium* infections, nosocomial pneumonia

---

caused by *Staphylococcus aureus* or *Streptococcus pneumoniae*, uncomplicated or complicated skin and skin structure infections, community-acquired pneumonia, *Pasteurella multocida*, viridans Streptococcus, *E. faecium* infections *S. aureus, S. pyogenes;* can be used for MSSA/MSRA/MDRSP/ strains

Pharmacokinetics

Absorption	Rapid, excessive
Distribution	Protein binding 31%
Metabolism	Oxidation of the morpholine ring
Excretion	Unknown
Half-life	Unknown

Pharmacodynamics

Unknown

CONTRAINDICATIONS
Hypersensitivity

Precautions: Pregnancy, breastfeeding, children, thrombocytopenia, bone marrow suppression, hypertension, hyperthyroidism, pheochromocytoma, seizure disorder, ulcerative colitis, MI, PKU, renal/GI disease

DOSAGE AND ROUTES
Vancomycin-resistant *E. faecium* infections
Adult/adolescent/child ≥12 yr: IV/PO 600 mg q12hr × 14-28 days; max 1200 mg/day
Child <12 yr/infant/term neonate: IV/PO 10 mg/kg q8hr × 14-28 days

Pneumonia/complicated skin infections
Adult/child ≥12 yr: IV/PO 600 mg q12hr × 10-14 days; max 1200 mg/day
Child birth-11 yr: PO 10 mg/kg q8hr × 10-14 days

Uncomplicated skin infections caused by *S. aureus* (MSSA only) or *S. pyogenes*
Adult: IV/PO 400 mg q12hr × 10-14 days; max 1200 mg/day
Adolescent: PO 600 mg q12hr × 10-14 days, max 1200 mg/day
Child 5-11 yr: PO 10 mg/kg q12hr × 10-14 days
Neonate ≥7 days old/infant/child <5 yr old: PO 10 mg/kg q8hr × 10-14 days
Infant, preterm <7 days old: PO 10 mg/kg q12hr × 10-14 days

Available forms: Tabs 600 mg; oral susp 100 mg/5 ml; premixed infusion 200 mg/100 mg, 400 mg/200 ml, 600 mg/300 ml, (2 mg/ml)

ADVERSE EFFECTS
CNS: *Headache,* dizziness, insomnia
GI: *Nausea, diarrhea,* increased ALT, AST, *vomiting,* taste change, tongue color change, *Clostridium difficile*–associated diarrhea (CDAD)
EENT: Optic neuropathy
HEMA: Myelosuppression
MISC: Vaginal moniliasis, fungal infection, oral moniliasis, lactic acidosis, anaphylaxis, angioedema, Stevens-Johnson syndrome, serotonin syndrome

INTERACTIONS
Individual drugs
Amoxapine, cyclobenzaprine, maprotiline, methyldopa, mirtazapine, traZODone: increased hypertensive crisis, seizures, coma
Bupropion, cyclobenzeprine, tramadol, trazadone: increased serotonin syndrome

Drug classifications
Adrenergic blockers (dopamine, EPINEPHrine, pseudoePHEDrine): increased effects of adrenergics, monitor B/P
Antidepressants (tricyclics): increased hypertensive crisis, seizures, coma
MAOIs or those that possess MAOI-like action (furazolidone, isoniazid, procarbazine): do not use together; hypertensive crisis may occur
SSRIs, SNRIs: increased serotonin syndrome, notify prescriber immediately
Serotoninergic agents: increased effect

Drug/herb
Green tea, valerian, ginseng, yohimbe, kava: avoid use

Drug/lab test
Increase: LFTs, alkaline phosphatase, amylase, lipase, BUN
Decrease: WBC, platelets, blood glucose

Drug/food
Tyramine foods: avoid; increased pressor response

NURSING CONSIDERATIONS
Assessment
• **Infection:** Assess vital signs, wounds, sputum, stool, urine emesis, WBC baseline and periodically
• Assess for change in vision; optic neuropathy may occur
• Assess CNS symptoms: headache, dizziness
• Monitor liver function tests: AST, ALT
• Monitor CBC weekly, assess for myelosuppression (anemia, leukopenia, pancytopenia, thrombocytopenia)
• **CDAD:** Assess for diarrhea, abdominal pain, fever, fatigue, anorexia; possible

anemia, elevated WBC, and low serum albumin; stop product and usually give either vancomycin or IV metroNIDAZOLE
• **Serotonin syndrome:** at least 2 wk should elapse between continuing linezolid and start of serotonergic agents; assess for increased heart rate, shivering, sweating, dilated pupils, tremor, high B/P, hyperthermia, headache, confusion; if these occur stop linezolid; administer a serotonin antagonist if needed
• **Lactic acidosis:** Assess for repeated nausea/vomiting, unexplained acidosis, low bicarbonate level: notify prescriber immediately
• **Anaphylaxis/angioedema/Stevens-Johnson syndrome:** rash, pruritus, difficulty breathing, fever: have emergency equipment nearby
• **Diabetes mellitus:** Monitor those receiving insulin or oral antidiabetics for increased hypoglycemia
• **Pregnancy/breastfeeding:** Avoid in pregnancy, breastfeeding

Patient problem
Infection (uses)
Diarrhea (adverse reactions)

Implementation
• Obtain culture and sensitivity before starting treatment; may give before results are received
PO route
• Store reconstituted oral susp at room temperature, use within 3 wk
• Give over 30-120 min; do not use **IV** inf bag in series connections, do not use with additives in sol, do not use with another product, administer separately, flush line before and after use

Intermittent IV infusion route
• Do not use if particulate is present; yellow color is normal
• Premixed solutions are ready to use (2 mg/ml)
• Store at room temperature in original packaging

Y-site compatibilities: Acyclovir, alfentanil, amikacin, aminophylline, ampicillin, aztreonam, bretylium, buprenorphine, butorphanol, calcium gluconate, CARBOplatin, ceFAZolin, cefoperazone, cefoTEtan, cefOXitin, cefTAZidime, ceftizoxime, cefTRIAXone, cefuroxime, cimetidine, ciprofloxacin, cisatracurium, CISplatin, clindamycin, cyclophosphamide, cycloSPORINE, cytarabine, HYDROmorphone, ifosfamide, labetalol, leucovorin, levofloxacin, lidocaine, LORazepam, magnesium sulfate, mannitol, meperidine, meropenem, mesna, methotrexate, methylPREDNISolone, metoclopramide, metroNIDAZOLE, midazolam, minocycline, mitoXANtrone, morphine, nalbuphine, naloxone, nitroglycerin,

ofloxacin, ondansetron, PACLitaxel, PENTobarbital, piperacillin, potassium chloride, prochlorperazine, promethazine, propranolol, ranitidine, remifentanil, theophylline, ticarcillin, tobramycin, vancomycin, vecuronium, verapamil, vinCRIStine, zidovudine

Solution compatibilities: D$_5$W, 0.9% NaCl, LR

Patient/family education
• Advise patient if dizziness occurs, to ambulate and perform activities with assistance
• Advise patient to complete full course of product therapy, to use as directed, not to skip or double doses, take missed dose when remembered unless close to next dose
• Advise patient to contact prescriber if adverse reaction occurs
• Advise patient to avoid large amounts of tyramine-containing foods (give list)
• **Serotonin syndrome:** Notify provider immediately of fever, sweating, diarrhea, confusion
• Teach patient that tab and suspension may be taken with or without food
• Advise patient to notify health care professional of change in vision
• Advise patient to avoid foods with large amounts of tyramine (cured meats, pickled products, beer, wine, chocolate)
• Advise patient to discuss with health care professional all Rx, OTC, herbals, supplements used
• **Pregnancy/breastfeeding:** Identify if pregnancy is planned or suspected or if breastfeeding

Evaluation
Positive therapeutic outcome
• Decreased symptoms of infection, blood cultures negative

⚠ HIGH ALERT
liraglutide (Rx)
(lir'a-gloo'tide)
Saxenda, Victoza
Func. class.: Antidiabetic agent
Chem. class.: Incretin mimetics

ACTION: Improved glycemic control and potential weight loss via activation of the glucagon-like peptide-1 (GLP-1) receptor

Therapeutic outcome: Stable and improved serum glucose, HbA1C, weight loss

USES: Type 2 diabetes mellitus in combination with diet and exercise, obesity

Pharmacokinetics

Absorption	Protein binding (98%)
Distribution	Binds to albumin, then released into circulation
Metabolism	Unknown
Excretion	Unknown
Half-life	12-13 hr

Pharmacodynamics

Onset	Unknown
Peak	Peak 8-12 hr
Duration	Unknown

CONTRAINDICATIONS

Hypersensitivity, pancreatitis, pregnancy

Precautions: Alcoholism, breastfeeding, children, cholelithiasis, ketoacidosis, diarrhea, elderly, fever, gastroparesis, hepatic disease, hypoglycemia, infection, renal disease, surgery, thyroid disease, trauma, vomiting, medullary thyroid carcinoma (MTC), multiple endocrine neoplasia syndrome type 2 (MEN 2), thyroid cancer

> **BLACK BOX WARNING:** Thyroid C-cell tumors

DOSAGE AND ROUTES

Adult: SUBCUT (Victoza) 0.6 mg/day × 1 wk, then increase to 1.2 mg/day, max 1.8 mg/day; (Saxenda) 0.6 mg/day × 1 wk, then 1.2 mg/day × 1 wk, then 1.8 mg/day × 1 wk, then 2.4 mg/day × 1 wk, then 3 mg/day

Available forms: Solution for injection 0.6, 1.2, 1.8 mg prefilled pen; solution for injection (Saxenda) 0.6, 1.2, 1.8, 2.4, 3 mg prefilled pen

ADVERSE EFFECTS

CNS: Dizziness, headache
CV: Hypertension
ENDO: Hypoglycemia
EENT: Sinusitis
GI: Abdominal pain, anorexia, constipation, diarrhea, dyspepsia, nausea, vomiting, pancreatitis
INTEG: Angioedema, erythema, injection site reaction, urticaria
MS: Back pain
SYST: Antibody formation, infection, influenza, secondary thyroid malignancy, anaphylaxis, angioedema

INTERACTIONS
Individual drugs

Atorvastatin, acetaminophen, griseofulvin: increased or decreased effects of each specific drug

Baclofen, cycloSPORINE, tacrolimus, dextrothyroxine, diazoxide, phenytoin, fosphenytoin, ethotoin, isoniazid, niacin, nicotine: increased hyperglycemic reactions

Bortezomib, cloNIDine, alcohol, lithium, pentamidine: increased or decreased hypoglycemic reactions

Dexfenfluramine, fenfluramine, disopyramide, FLUoxetine, mecasermin, octreotide, pegvisomant, salicylates: increased hypoglycemic reactions

Digoxin: decreased digoxin levels

Drug classifications

Angiotensin II receptor antagonists, ACE inhibitors, other antidiabetics, β-blockers, fibric acid derivatives, MAOIs, salicylates: increased hypoglycemic reactions

Protease inhibitors, phenothiazines, atypical antipsychotics, corticosteroids, carbonic anhydrase inhibitors, estrogens, progestins, oral contraceptives, growth hormones, sympathomimetics: increased hyperglycemic reactions

Androgens, quinolones: decreased liraglutide effect

Drug/lab test

Increase: Calcitonin, lipase
Decrease: Glucose

NURSING CONSIDERATIONS
Assessment

• **Diabetes:** hypoglycemic reactions that can occur soon after meals: hunger, sweating, weakness, dizziness, tremors, restlessness, tachycardia; monitor serum glucose, A1C, CBC during treatment

• Assess for hypersensitivity to this product

• **Assess for stress:** diabetic patients exposed to stress, surgery, fever, infections may require insulin administration temporarily

• **Assess for serious skin reactions:** angioedema; also pancreatitis, secondary thyroid malignancy

• **Insulin use with Victoza:** monitor for hypoglycemic reactions

• **Pancreatitis:** Monitor for nausea, vomiting, severe abdominal pain, product should be discontinued, give supportive care, monitor amylase, lipase, electrolytes

> **BLACK BOX WARNING: Thyroid C-cell tumors:** monitor during treatment; if calcitonin is elevated or if nodules can be felt, a referral is needed, do not use in those with a family history of MTC and those with multiple endocrine neoplasia syndrome type 2

Patient problem

Excess food intake (uses)
Nonadherence (teaching)

⚠ Nurse Alert   ✴ Key NCLEX® Drug   ≫ Drug Specifics

Implementation
SUBCUT route

- Use safe handling procedures
- Give by SUBCUT only, inspect for particulate matter or discoloration, do not use if unusually viscous, cloudy, discolored, or if particles are present; give daily at any time without regard to meals; pen needles must be purchased separately, use Novo Nordisk needles, prime before first use, see manual for directions; give in thigh, abdomen, or upper arm; lightly pinch fold of skin, insert needle at 90-degree angle or 45-degree angle if thin, release skin, aspiration is not needed, give over 6 seconds, rotate injection sites
- Storage: do not store pen with needle attached; avoid direct heat and sunlight, discard 30 days after first use, after first use may be stored at room temperature or refrigerated, do not freeze; if >3 days have elapsed since last dose, reinitiate at 0.6 mg, titrate
- If dose is missed, resume once daily dosing at next scheduled dose

Patient/family education

- Teach patient the symptoms of hypo/hyperglycemia and what to do about each, to have glucagon emergency kit available, carry a carbohydrate source at all times
- Teach patient about side effects associated with therapy such as nausea and vomiting; upward dose titration can be delayed or ignored depending on tolerance
- Teach patient that diabetes is a lifelong illness, product does not cure disease and must be continued on a daily basis
- Instruct patient to carry emergency ID with prescriber's phone number and medications taken
- Advise patient to continue with other recommendations: diet, exercise, hygiene
- Advise continuing follow-up exams will be needed
- Teach patient to test blood glucose using a blood glucose meter
- Advise patient to avoid other medications, herbs, supplements unless approved by prescriber
- Advise patient to report serious skin effects, abdominal pain with nausea/vomiting
- Provide patient with written instructions if self-administration is ordered, to discard pen after 30 days, teach patient how to use pen
- **Hypersensitivity:** Teach patient to report any allergic symptoms
- Teach patient not to share product with other, infections may occur
- Teach patient that secondary malignancy is possible, that routing monitoring may be needed, to report trouble breathing, continuous hoarseness, lump in neck to report immediately

- **Pregnancy/breastfeeding:** Teach patient that product is not to be used in pregnancy or breastfeeding, that insulin is usually used in pregnancy, to notify health care professional if pregnancy is planned or suspected or if breastfeeding

Evaluation
Positive therapeutic outcome

- Stable and improved serum glucose, A1C, weight loss

lisinopril (Rx)

(lyse-in′oh-pril)

Zestril

Func. class.: Antihypertensive, angiotensin converting enzyme (ACE) I inhibitor

Chem. class.: Enalaprilat lysine analog

Do not confuse: lisinopril/Risperdal/Lipitor, **Zestril**/Zetia/Zipexa

ACTION: Selectively suppresses renin-angiotensin-aldosterone system; inhibits ACE; prevents conversion of angiotensin I to angiotensin II

Therapeutic outcome: Decreased B/P in hypertension, decreased preload, afterload in HF

USES: Mild to moderate hypertension, adjunctive therapy of systolic HF, acute MI

Unlabeled uses: Diabetic nephropathy/retinopathy, proteinuria, post MI

Pharmacokinetics

Absorption	Variable
Distribution	Unknown
Metabolism	Not metabolized
Excretion	Kidneys, unchanged
Half-life	12 hr

Pharmacodynamics

Onset	1 hr
Peak	6-8 hr
Duration	24 hr

CONTRAINDICATIONS

Hypersensitivity, angioedema

BLACK BOX WARNING: Pregnancy

Precautions: Pregnancy (1st trimester), breastfeeding, renal disease, hyperkalemia, renal artery stenosis, HF, aortic stenosis

DOSAGE AND ROUTES
Hypertension

Adult: PO initially 10 mg, 10-40 mg/day; may increase to 80 mg/day if required

Child ≥6 yr: PO 0.7 mg/kg/day, up to 5 mg/day; titrate q1-2wk up to 0.6 mg/kg/day or 40 mg/day
Geriatric: PO 2.5-5 mg/day, increase q7day

Renal dose
Adult: PO CCr <30 ml/min reduce dose by 50%, initially 5 mg/day, max 40 mg/day; CCr <10 ml/min 2.5 mg/day, max 40 mg/day

Heart failure
Adult: PO 5 mg/day, increase if needed to max 20 mg/day or 40 mg/day (Zestril): in hyponatremia <130 mEq/L or creatinine >3 mg/dl or CCr <30 ml/min use 2.5 mg/day initially

Myocardial infarction
Adults: PO give 5 mg within 24 hr of onset of symptoms, then 5 mg after 24 hr, 10 mg after 48 hr, then 10 mg/day

Available forms: Tabs 2.5, 5, 10, 20, 30 40 mg

ADVERSE EFFECTS
CNS: *Vertigo,* depression, stroke, insomnia, paresthesias, *headache,* fatigue, asthenia, *dizziness*
CV: Chest pain, *hypotension,* sinus tachycardia
EENT: Blurred vision, nasal congestion
GI: Nausea, vomiting, anorexia, constipation, flatulence, GI irritation, diarrhea, hepatic failure, hepatic necrosis, pancreatitis
GU: Proteinuria, renal insufficiency, sexual dysfunction, impotence
HEMA: Neutropenia, agranulocytosis
INTEG: Rash, pruritus
MISC: Muscle cramps, *hyperkalemia*
RESP: Dry cough, dyspnea
SYST: Angioedema, anaphylaxis, toxic epidermal necrolysis

INTERACTIONS
Individual drugs
Alcohol (large amounts), probenecid: increased hypotension
Allopurinol: increased hypersensitivity
Aspirin: decreased lisinopril effect
CycloSPORINE: increased hyperkalemia
Indomethacin: decreased antihypertensive effect
Lithium: increased levels of lithium, toxicity

Drug classifications
Antihypertensives, diuretics, nitrates, phenothiazines: increased hypotension
Diuretics, potassium-sparing, potassium salt substitutes, potassium supplements: increased hyperkalemia
NSAIDs: decreased lisinopril effect, adjust dose as needed

Drug/food
High-potassium diet (bananas, orange juice, avocados, broccoli, nuts, spinach), salt substitutes should be avoided; hyperkalemia may occur, monitor potassium

Drug/lab test
Interference: glucose/insulin tolerance tests, LFTs, BUN, creatinine

NURSING CONSIDERATIONS
Assessment
• **Hypertension:** monitor B/P, check for orthostatic hypotension, syncope; if changes occur, dosage change may be required
• **Acute MI:** can be used in combination with salicylates, beta blockers, thrombolytics
• **HF:** check for edema in feet, legs daily, weight daily, dyspnea, wet crackles
• **Assess blood studies:** platelets, WBC with differential: baseline, q3mo; if neutrophils are <1000/mm³, discontinue treatment

> **BLACK BOX WARNING:** Determine pregnancy before starting, if breastfeeding

• Monitor renal/liver function tests baseline and periodically: protein, BUN, creatinine; watch for increased levels that may indicate nephrotic syndrome and renal failure; monitor renal symptoms: polyuria, oliguria, frequency, dysuria
• Check potassium levels throughout treatment, although hyperkalemia rarely occurs
• Assess for anaphylaxis, toxic epidermal necrolysis, angioedema, allergic reactions: rash, fever, pruritus, urticaria; facial swelling, dyspnea, tongue swelling (rare), have emergency equipment nearby, may be more common in Black patients; product should be discontinued if antihistamines fail to help

> **BLACK BOX WARNING:** Pregnancy/breastfeeding: Do not use in pregnancy, breastfeeding

Patient problem
Impaired cardiac output (uses, adverse reactions)
Nonadherence (teaching)

Implementation
• Store in airtight container at 86° F (30° C) or less
• Severe hypotension may occur after 1st dose of this medication; may be prevented by reducing or discontinuing diuretic therapy 3 days before beginning lisinopril therapy
• Without regard to food

Patient/family education
• Caution patient not to discontinue product abruptly; advise patient to inform all health care providers about taking this product

---

- Teach patient not to use OTC products (cough, cold, allergy) unless directed by prescriber; serious side effects can occur
- Teach patient the importance of complying with dosage schedule, even if feeling better; to continue with medical regimen to decrease B/P: exercise, cessation of smoking, decreasing stress, diet modifications
- Teach patient to notify prescriber of mouth sores, sore throat, fever, swelling of hands or feet, irregular heartbeat, chest pain, coughing, shortness of breath
- Caution patient to report excessive perspiration, dehydration, vomiting, diarrhea; may lead to fall in B/P
- Emphasize the need to rise slowly to sitting or standing position to minimize orthostatic hypotension; not to exercise in hot weather or increased hypotension can occur
- Caution patient that product may cause dizziness, fainting, light-headedness; may occur during 1st few days of therapy; to avoid activities that may be hazardous
- Teach patient how to take B/P, and normal readings for age-group; advise patient to take B/P regularly
- Instruct patient to avoid increasing potassium in the diet

BLACK BOX WARNING: Advise patient to report if pregnancy is planned or suspected, do not breastfeed, not to use in pregnancy

Evaluation
Positive therapeutic outcome
- Decreased B/P in hypertension
- Decreased HF symptoms

TREATMENT OF OVERDOSE:
0.9% NaCl **IV** inf, hemodialysis

lithium (Rx)
(li'thee-um)
Carbolith ✦, Lithane ✦, Lithmax ✦, Lithobid
Func. class.: Antimanic, antipsychotic
Chem. class.: Alkali metal ion salt

Do not confuse: lithium/lanthanum

ACTION: May alter sodium, potassium ion transport across cell membrane in nerve, muscle cells; may balance biogenic amines of norepinephrine, serotonin in CNS areas involved in emotional responses

Therapeutic outcome: Stable mood

USES: Bipolar disorder (manic phase), prevention of bipolar manic-depressive psychosis

Pharmacokinetics
Absorption	Completely absorbed
Distribution	Reabsorbed by renal tubules (80%); crosses blood-brain barrier; crosses placenta
Metabolism	Unknown
Excretion	Urine, unchanged
Half-life	18-36 hr depending on age

Pharmacodynamics
Onset	Rapid
Peak	½-3 hr
Duration	Unknown

CONTRAINDICATIONS
Pregnancy, breastfeeding, children <12 yr, hepatic disease, brain trauma, organic brain syndrome, schizophrenia, severe cardiac/renal disease, severe dehydration

Precautions: Geriatric, thyroid disease, seizure disorders, diabetes mellitus, systemic infection, urinary retention, QT prolongation

BLACK BOX WARNING: Lithium level >1.5 mmol/L is toxic

DOSAGE AND ROUTES NTI
Bipolar disorder (mania)
Adult: PO 600 mg tid; maintenance 300 mg tid or qid; EXT REL 900 mg q12hr; dosage should be individualized to maintain blood levels at 0.5-1.5 mEq/L or 0.6-1.2 mEq/L (maintenance)
Geriatric: PO 300 mg bid, increase q7day by 300 mg to desired dose
Child: PO 15-20 mg/kg/day in 3-4 divided doses; increase as needed; do not exceed adult doses; maintain blood levels at 0.4-0.5 mEq/L

Renal dose
Adult: PO CCr 10-50 ml/min 50%-75% of dose; CCr <10 ml/min 25%-50% of dose

Available forms: Caps 150, 300, 600 mg; tabs 300 mg; ext rel tabs 300, 450 mg; syr 300 mg/5 ml (8 mEq/5 ml)

ADVERSE EFFECTS
CNS: *Headache, drowsiness, dizziness, tremors,* twitching, ataxia, seizures, slurred speech, restlessness, *confusion,* stupor, memory loss, clonic movements, *fatigue*
CV: *Hypotension,* ECG changes, dysrhythmias, circulatory collapse, edema, Brudaga syndrome, QT prolongation
EENT: Tinnitus, blurred vision
ENDO: Hypothyroidism, goiter, hyperglycemia, hyperthyroidism, hyponatremia
GI: *Dry mouth, anorexia, nausea, vomiting, diarrhea,* incontinence, abdominal pain, metallic taste

GU: Polyuria, glycosuria, proteinuria, albuminuria, urinary incontinence, polydipsia
HEMA: Leukocytosis
INTEG: Drying of hair, alopecia, rash, pruritus, hyperkeratosis, *acneiform rash, folliculitis*
MS: *Muscle weakness*

INTERACTIONS
Individual drugs
AcetaZOLAMIDE, aminophylline, mannitol, sodium bicarbonate: increased renal clearance
Calcium iodide, iodinated glycerol, potassium iodide: increased hypothyroid effect
CarBAMazepine, FLUoxetine, methyldopa, probenecid: increased lithium effect/toxicity

Drug classifications
ACE inhibitors: Increase: Lithium level
Antiarrhythmics, other products that prolong the QT interval: Increase GT interval
Antithyroid agents: increased hypothyroid effects
β-Blockers used for lithium tremor: increase masking of lithium toxicity
Calcium channel blockers: decreased effect of lithium
Neuromuscular blocking agents: increased effect of neuromuscular blocking effects
NSAIDs, thiazides: increased lithium toxicity

Drug/herb
Guarana, tea (black/green): decreased lithium effect
• Avoid use with kava, St. John's wort, valerian

Drug/food
Caffeine: Decrease lithium level, adjust dose
Sodium: Significant changes in sodium intake will alter lithium excretion

Drug/lab test
Increased: potassium excretion, urine glucose, blood glucose, protein, BUN
Decreased: VMA, T_3, T_4, PBI, ^{131}I

NURSING CONSIDERATIONS
Assessment
• **Bipolar disorder:** manic symptoms, mood, behavior before and during treatment

> **BLACK BOX WARNING: Assess for lithium toxicity:** Vomiting, diarrhea, poor coordination, fine motor tremors, weakness, lassitude; major toxicity: coarse tremors, severe thirst, tinnitus, dilute urine. Monitor serum lithium levels weekly initially, then q2mo (therapeutic level: 0.5-1.5 mEq/L; toxic level >1.5 mcg/L; twitching; toxicity and therapeutic levels are very close; toxicity may occur rapidly; blood levels are measured before the AM dose, there is a narrow therapeutic index (NTI)

• Assess weight daily; check for edema in legs, ankles, wrists; report if present; check skin turgor at least daily
• Monitor sodium intake; decreased sodium intake with decreased fluid intake may lead to lithium retention; increased sodium and fluids may decrease lithium retention
• Monitor urine for albuminuria, glycosuria, uric acid during beginning treatment, q2mo thereafter, specific gravity any level <1.005 may indicate diabetes insipidus and should be reported to the provider
• Assess neurologic status: LOC, gait, motor reflexes, hand tremors
• ECG in those >50 yr with CV disease; cardiology consult is recommended in those with risk factors, QT prolongation may occur

Patient problems
Disturbed thinking process (uses)
Excess food intake (adverse reactions)

Implementation
• Do not break, crush, or chew caps
• Administer reduced dosage to geriatric; give with meals to avoid GI upset
• Provide adequate fluids (2-3 L/day) to prevent dehydration during initial treatment, 1-2 L/day during maintenance
• Give list of products that interact with lithium

Patient/family education
• **Provide patient with written information on symptoms of minor toxicity:** vomiting, diarrhea, poor coordination, fine motor tremors, weakness, lassitude; major toxicity: coarse tremors, severe thirst, tinnitus, dilute urine, seek medical care immediately
• Advise patient to monitor urine specific gravity; emphasize need for follow-up care to determine lithium effects
• Caution patient not to operate machinery until lithium levels are stable and response determined; that beneficial effects may take 1-3 wk
• Provide to the patient a list of products that interact with lithium and discuss need for adequate, stable intake of salt and fluid
• Advise patient to have lithium levels monitored to ensure effectiveness
• Teach patient to use an emergency ID with diagnosis, product used
• Advise patient that contraception is necessary, since lithium may harm fetus

Evaluation
Positive therapeutic outcome
• Decrease in excitement, poor judgment, insomnia (manic phase)
• Decreased mood swings and lability

TREATMENT OF OVERDOSE:

Induce emesis or lavage, maintain airway, respiratory function; dialysis for severe intoxication

---

⚠ HIGH ALERT

lixisenatide

(lixi cona tide)
Adlyxin
Func. class.: Antidiabetic
Chem. class.: Incretin mimetic

ACTION: An incretin mimetic; a glucagon-like peptide-1 (GLP-1) receptor agonist; binds and activates the GLP-1 receptor. GLP-1 is an important, gut-derived, glucose homeostasis regulator that is released after the oral ingestion of carbohydrates or fats.

Therapeutic outcome: Decreasing polydipsia, polyuria, polyphagia, clear sensorium, improving A1c, weight

USES: Treatment of type 2 diabetes mellitus in combination with diet and exercise

Pharmacokinetics

Absorption	Unknown
Distribution	Unknown
Metabolism	Unknown
Excretion	Eliminated through glomerular filtration and proteolytic degradation; elimination prolonged in renal disease with mild (CCr 60-89 ml/min), moderate (CCr 30-59 ml/min), and severe renal impairment (CCr 15-29 ml/min) was increased by approximately 34%, 69%, and 124%, respectively; use with caution in renal disease
Half-life	1-3 hr

Pharmacodynamics

Onset	Unknown
Peak	1-3½ hr
Duration	Unknown

CONTRAINDICATIONS

Angioedema

Precautions: Alcoholism, breastfeeding, children, cholelithiasis, diabetic ketoacidosis, gastroparesis, hypoglycemia, pancreatitis, pregnancy, renal failure, renal impairment, risk of serious hypersensitivity reactions or anaphylaxis, type 1 diabetes mellitus

DOSAGE AND ROUTES

Adult: SUBCUT Initially, 10 mcg qday within 1 hr before the morning meal. If a dose is missed, give within 1 hr before the next meal. Continue 10 mcg qday × 14 days; on day 15, increase the dose to the maintenance dose of 20 mcg qday, max 20 mcg/day

Renal dose

Adult: eGFR 30-89 ml/min/1.73 m² : No dosage adjustment needed; eGFR 15-29 ml/min/1.73 m² : Monitor closely for adverse reactions, especially hypoglycemia, nausea, and vomiting, and for changes in renal function. Dehydration and acute renal failure and worsening of chronic renal failure may occur in these patients; eGFR less than 15 ml/min/1.73 m² : Do not use

Available forms: Solution for injection 10 mcg, 20 mcg prefilled pen starter pack, maintenance pack

ADVERSE EFFECTS

CNS: Dizziness, headache
GI: Nausea, vomiting, diarrhea, constipation, abdominal pain, dyspepsia, pancreatitis (rare)
MISC: Antibody formation, hypoglycemia, injection-site reactions, hypotension, anaphylactoid reaction, bronchospasm, renal failure, laryngeal edema

INTERACTIONS

Drug classifications

Antidiabetics: hypoglycemic risk
Sulfonylureas: increased hypoglycemia risk
Hormonal contraceptives: may alter effect, take at least 1 hr before

NURSING CONSIDERATIONS

Assessment

• **Diabetes:** monitor fasting blood glucose, A1c level during treatment to determine diabetic control; check for reaction, which can occur soon after meals; for severe hypoglycemia give IV D50W, IV dextrose solution
• **Pancreatitis:** Severe abdominal pain with or without nausea and vomiting, product should be discontinued immediately

---

- **Renal disease:** Monitor BUN, creatinine in mild renal disease, do not use in severe renal disease
- **Pregnancy:** If pregnant or planning to become pregnant, take oral contraceptive 1 hr before this product

Patient problem
Excess food intake (uses)
Nonadherence (teaching)

Implementation
- May be used as monotherapy or with other antidiabetic medications. Dose adjustment of metformin or a thiazolidinedione is not usually required. A reduction in the dose of a sulfonylurea may be needed to reduce the risk of hypoglycemia
- Give subcut injection only. Do not give IV/IM
- Visually inspect for particulate matter and discoloration before use; do not use if unusually viscous, cloudy, discolored, or if particles are present
- Available as a prefilled pen. Each pen must be activated before the first use
- Administer qday within 1 hr before the first meal of the day, preferably the same meal each day. If a dose is missed, give within 1 hr before the next meal
- Inject subcut into the thigh, abdomen, or upper arm
- Double-check dosage before use
- Rotate sites with each injection to prevent lipodystrophy
- Storage: The pen should be protected from light and kept in its original packaging, discard pen 14 days after its first use

Patient/family education
- Not to share among patients. Even if the disposable needle is changed, sharing may result in transmission of hepatitis viruses, HIV, or other bloodborne pathogens. Do not share pens among multiple patients in an inpatient setting; use multidose vials, if available, or reserve the use of any pen to 1 patient only
- For patients and caregivers, give instruction on the preparation and use of the pen, include a practice injection
- About the signs and symptoms of hypo/hyperglycemia and what to do about each; to have emergency glucagon kit available at all times, to carry glucose source (sugar, candy)
- That product must be taken on a continuing basis, not to discontinue without prescriber's approval
- That diabetes is a lifelong condition, product will not cure condition, to carry emergency ID with condition, products taken, prescriber's phone number and name

- To continue weight control, dietary restrictions, exercise, hygiene
- That regular lab testing and A1c will be necessary
- **Pancreatitis:** If severe abdominal pain occurs with or without nausea, vomiting, seek medical care immediately
- **Pregnancy:** To notify prescriber if pregnant or planning to become pregnant, if taking oral contraceptives, take at least 1 hr before this product

Evaluation
Therapeutic response: Decreasing polydipsia, polyuria, polyphagia, clear sensorium, improving A1c, weight

Iodoxamide ophthalmic
See Appendix B

Iofexidine
(loe FEX i deen)
Lucemyra
Func. class.: Opioid withdrawal agent
Chem. class.: Central alpha-2 agonist

ACTION: A central alpha-2 agonist that binds to adrenergic receptors, resulting in a reduction in the release of norepinephrine and a decrease in sympathetic tone

Therapeutic outcome: Opioid discontinuation with minimal withdrawal symptoms

USES: For the mitigation of opioid withdrawal symptoms to facilitate abrupt opioid discontinuation in adults

Pharmacokinetics

Absorption	Unknown
Distribution	Protein binding 55%
Metabolism	30% of a dose is converted to inactive metabolites during first pass metabolism by CYP2D6, CYP1A2, and CYP2C19
Excretion	Kidney 15%-20%
Half-life	17-22 hr after repeated dosing

Pharmacodynamics

Onset	Unknown
Peak	3-5 hr
Duration	Unknown

CONTRAINDICATIONS: Hypersensitivity

PRECAUTIONS: Abrupt discontinuation, acute MI, alcoholism, bradycardia, breastfeeding, cardiac dysrhythmias, CV disease, children, coadministration with other CNS depressants, coronary artery disease, dehydration, diabetes mellitus, dialysis, driving or operating machinery, electrolyte imbalance, ethanol ingestion, females, geriatrics, heart failure, hepatic disease, hypertension, hypocalcemia, hypomagnesaemia, hypotension, infertility, long QT syndrome, malnutrition, poor metabolizers, pregnancy, renal disease, syncope, thyroid disease

DOSAGE AND ROUTES

Adult: PO Usual initial dose is 0.54 mg (3 × 0.18 mg tablets) 4 × daily during peak withdrawal symptoms (the first 5 to 7 days following the last use of an opioid) up to14 days. There should be 5 to 6 hr between each dose, max 2.88 mg/day (16 tablets/day) max 0.72 mg/dose (4 tablets/dose) as a single dose; DISCONTINUATION: gradually taper over 2 to 4 days (reduce by 1 tablet per dose q1 to 2 days)

Available forms: Tablet 0.18 mg

ADVERSE EFFECTS

CV: Bradycardia, hypotension, orthostatic hypotension

CNS: Dizziness, drowsiness, insomnia

MISC: Withdrawal, xerostomia

INTERACTIONS
Drug classifications

Type IA, IC, III antidysrhythmics, antihistamines, antidepressants: Increased QT prolongation, monitor ECG if used concurrently

Other CNS depressants, if used concurrently: Increased CNS effects and sedation; monitor for increased sedation

Antihypertensives: Increased hypotension; avoid concurrent use if possible

CYP2D6 inhibitors: Increased hypotension, bradycardia

NURSING CONSIDERATIONS
Assessment

• **QT prolongation:** This product can cause QT prolongation and should be avoided in those with congenital long QT syndrome. Use with caution in those with cardiac disease, cardiac dysrhythmias, heart failure, bradycardia, MI, hypertension, coronary artery disease, hypomagnesemia, hypokalemia, hypocalcemia, or in patients receiving medications known to prolong the QT interval or cause an electrolyte imbalance. Monitor ECG in heart failure, bradyarrhythmias, liver or kidney impairment, or during concurrent use of other medications that lead to QT prolongation

• **Electrolyte imbalances:** (hypokalemia, hypomagnesemia) should be corrected prior to use, monitor electrolytes for changes

• **Somnolence and sedation** are common and may cause impairment of cognitive and motor skills; may be increased when coadministered with other CNS depressants (benzodiazepines, ethanol, and barbiturates)

• **Abrupt discontinuation**: Monitor B/P during tapering, a significant increase in B/P may occur with abrupt discontinuation. May also cause diarrhea, insomnia, anxiety, chills, hyperhidrosis, and extremity pain

• **Hepatic disease:** May reduce the clearance of the drug; reduce dose in hepatic impairment

• **Renal impairment:** product may reduce the clearance of the drug; reduce dose in renal disease

• **Geriatric patients:** Caution is recommended when administering to geriatric patients over 65 years of age. Dose adjustments may be needed

• **Fertility:** Infertility has been noted in some animal studies

• **Pregnancy/breastfeeding:** Safety not established. In animal studies, use resulted in a reduction in fetal weights, increases in fetal resorptions, and litter loss at exposures below human exposure. Consider the benefits of breastfeeding, the risk of potential infant drug exposure, and the risk of an untreated or inadequately treated condition

Patient problem
Excess food intake (uses)

Implementation
• May administer orally without regard to meals

Patient/family education
• Teach patient self-monitoring for hypotension, bradycardia, and related symptoms. Instruct that moving from a supine to upright position may increase the risk for hypotension or orthostatic effects

• Teach patient to stay hydrated, be able to recognize symptoms of hypotension, and know how to minimize the risk of serious consequences if hypotension occurs (sit or lie down, carefully rise from a sitting or lying position)

• Advise patient to withhold doses when experiencing hypotension or bradycardia and to contact their health care provider for guidance on dose adjustments

• Inform patient to use caution or avoid performing activities that require mental alertness, such as driving or operating machinery, until they know effect of product

• Teach patient not to discontinue without consulting their health care provider. When discontinuing the drug, a gradual reduction in dose is recommended

• Teach patient to inform their health care provider of other medications they are taking, including ethanol ingestion; those who complete opioid discontinuation are at an increased risk of fatal overdose should they resume opioid use; and inform patients and caregivers of increased risk of overdose

Evaluation
• Opioid discontinuation with minimal withdrawal symptoms

---

loperamide (OTC, Rx)
(loe-per'a-mide)
Imodium, Imodium A-D
Func. class.: Antidiarrheal
Chem. class.: Piperidine derivative

Do not confuse: Imodium/Indocin, **Loperamide**/furosemide

ACTION: Direct action on intestinal muscles to decrease GI peristalsis; reduces volume, increases bulk; electrolytes are not lost

Therapeutic outcome: Absence of diarrhea

USES: Diarrhea (cause undetermined), chronic diarrhea, to decrease amount of ileostomy discharge, traveler's diarrhea

Pharmacokinetics

Absorption	Poor
Distribution	Protein binding 97%
Metabolism	Liver
Excretion	Feces, unchanged; small amount in urine
Half-life	9-14 hr

Pharmacodynamics

Onset	½-1 hr
Peak	Unknown
Duration	24 hr

CONTRAINDICATIONS
Hypersensitivity, pseudomembranous colitis, constipation, dysentery, GI bleeding/obstruction/perforation, ileus, vomiting

Precautions: Pregnancy, breastfeeding, children <2 yr, hepatic disease, gastroenteritis, toxic megacolon, geriatric patients, dehydration, bacterial disease, AIDS, severe ulcerative colitis

DOSAGE AND ROUTES
Adult: PO 4 mg, then 2 mg after each loose stool, max 16 mg/24 hr
Child 9-11 yr: PO 2 mg, then 1 mg after each loose stool, max 6 mg/24 hr
Child 6-8 yr: PO 2 mg, then 0.1 mg/kg after each loose stool, max 4 mg/day
Child 2-5 yr: PO 1 mg, then 0.1 mg/kg after each loose stool, max 4 mg/24 hr

Traveler's diarrhea (unlabeled)
Adult: PO 4 mg, then 2 mg after each diarrhea stool, max 16 mg/day

Available forms: Caps 2 mg; liquid 1 mg/5 ml; tabs 2 mg; chew tabs 2 mg

ADVERSE EFFECTS
CNS: Dizziness, drowsiness, fatigue
GI: *Nausea, dry mouth, vomiting, constipation,* abdominal pain, anorexia, toxic megacolon, bacterial enterocolitis, flatulence
INTEG: Rash
MISC: Hyperglycemia
SYST: Anaphylaxis, angioedema, toxic epidermal necrolysis

INTERACTIONS
Individual drugs
Alcohol: increased CNS depression

Drug classifications
Antihistamines, analgesics (opioids), sedative/hypnotics: increased CNS depression

Drug/herb
Chamomile, hops, kava, skullcap, valerian: increased CNS depression
Nutmeg: increased antidiarrheal effect

NURSING CONSIDERATIONS
Assessment
• Monitor electrolytes (potassium, sodium, chloride) if patient is on long-term therapy; check fluid status, skin turgor
• **Stools:** Assess bowel pattern before, during treatment; check for rebound constipation after termination of medication; check bowel sounds
• Check response after 48 hr; if no response, product should be discontinued and other treatment initiated
• Assess for abdominal distention, toxic megacolon, which may occur in ulcerative colitis
• Assess for dehydration, CNS symptoms in children or those with hepatic disease

Patient problem
Diarrhea (uses)
Risk for injury (adverse reactions)

Implementation
- Do not break, crush, or chew caps
- Store in airtight containers
- Do not mix oral sol with other sol

Patient/family education
- Caution patient to avoid alcohol and OTC products unless directed by prescriber; may cause increased CNS depression
- Advise patient not to exceed recommended dosage; product may be habit forming; ileostomy patient may take this product for extended time
- Advise patient that product may cause drowsiness and to avoid hazardous activities until response to product is determined
- Teach patient that dry mouth can be decreased by frequent sips of water, hard candy, sugarless gum

Evaluation

Positive therapeutic outcome
- Decreased diarrhea

lopinavir/ritonavir
(low-pin'ah-ver/ri-toe'na-veer)
Kaletra
Func. class.: Antiretroviral
Chem. class.: Protease inhibitor

ACTION: Inhibits human immunodeficiency virus (HIV-1) protease and prevents maturation of the infectious virus

USES: HIV-1 in combination with or without other antiretrovirals

Pharmacokinetics

Absorption	Well
Distribution	98% protein binding
Metabolism	Liver by CYP3A4 and CYP2D6
Excretion	3.5% unchanged in urine
Half-life	3-6 hr

Pharmacodynamics

Onset	Unknown
Peak	4 hr
Duration	Up to 12 hr

CONTRAINDICATIONS: Hypersensitivity to this product or polyoxyethylated castor oil (oral solution), CYP3A4 metabolized products

Precautions: Pregnancy, breastfeeding, hepatic disease, pancreatitis, diabetes, hemophilia, AV block, hypercholesterolemia, immune reconstitution syndrome, neonates, cardiomyopathy, congenital long-QT prolongation, hypokalemia, elderly patients, Graves' disease, polymyositis, Guillain-Barré syndrome, children, HBV/HCV coinfection

DOSAGE AND ROUTES
HIV infection
Adult: PO 400 mg lopinavir/100 mg ritonavir bid or 800 mg lopinavir/200 mg ritonavir per day

Pregnant adult: PO 400 mg lopinavir/100 mg ritonavir bid, may need 600 mg lopinavir/150 mg ritonavir bid in the second/third trimesters; once-daily dosing is not recommended

Adult receiving concomitant efavirenz, nelfinavir, or nevirapine: PO TABS, 500 mg lopinavir/125 mg ritonavir bid; CAPS/SOL, 533 mg lopinavir/133 mg ritonavir bid

Adolescent/child/infant >6 mo: 300 mg lopinavir/75 mg ritonavir/m²/dose bid. The once-daily regimen is not recommended in pediatric patients; capsules are not recommended for use in patients ≤40 kg

Available forms: Oral solution 400 mg lopinavir/100 mg ritonavir/5 mL; tablets 100 mg lopinavir/25 mg ritonavir, 200 mg lopinavir/50 mg ritonavir

SIDE EFFECTS
CNS: Paresthesia, *headache, seizures,* fever, *dizziness, insomnia,* asthenia, intracranial bleeding, encephalopathy
CV: QT, PR interval prolongation, deep vein thrombosis
EENT: Blurred vision, otitis media, tinnitus
GI: *Diarrhea,* buccal mucosa ulceration, abdominal pain, *nausea,* taste perversion, dry mouth, vomiting, anorexia
MISC.: Asthenia, angioedema, anaphylaxis, Stevens-Johnson syndrome, increased lipids, lipodystrophy
MS: Pain, rhabdomyolysis, myalgias

INTERACTIONS
Individual Drugs
Atovaquone, divalproex, ethinyl estradiol, lamoTRIgine, phenytoin, sulfamethoxazole, theophylline, voriconazole, zidovudine: **decrease:** levels

Amiodarone, avanafil, buPROPion, cloZAPine, desipramine, dihydroergotamine, encainide, ergotamine, flecainide, interleukins, meperidine, midazolam, pimozide, piroxicam, propafenone, quiNIDine, ranolazine, rivaroxaban, saquinavir, triazolam, zolpidem: increase: toxicity

Haloperidol, chloroquine, droperidol, pentamidine: increase: QT prolongation

Fluconazole: increase: ritonavir levels

Clarithromycin, ddI: increase: level of both products

Bosentan: increase: levels of bosentan

Rifamin, nevirapine, barbiturates, phenytoin, budesonide, prednisone: decrease: ritonavir levels

Drug classifications

Azole antifungals, benzodiazepines, HMG-CoA reductase inhibitors: increase-toxicity

Class IA/III Antidysrhythmics, some phenothiazines, β-agonists, local anesthetics, tricyclics, CYP3A4 inhibitors (amiodarone, clarithromycin, erythromycin, telithromycin, troleandomycin), arsenic trioxide, levomethadyl, CYP3A4 substrates (methadone, pimozide, QUEtiapine, quiNIDine, risperiDONE, ziprasidone): increase: QT prolongation

Drug/lab test

Increase: AST, ALT, CPK, cholesterol, GGT, triglycerides, uric acid, glucose

Decrease: Hct, Hgb, RBC, neutrophils, WBC

Drug/herb

Decrease: ritonavir levels—St. John's wort; avoid concurrent use

• Avoid use with red yeast rice, evening primrose oil

NURSING CONSIDERATIONS
Assess:

• **HIV:** Monitor viral load, CD4 at baseline, throughout therapy; blood glucose, plasma HIV RNA, serum cholesterol/lipid profile; resistance testing before starting therapy and after treatment failure

• Assess for signs of infection, anemia

• Monitor hepatic studies: ALT, AST

• Monitor bowel pattern before, during treatment; if severe abdominal pain with bleeding occurs, discontinue product; monitor hydration

• Assess for skin eruptions, rash

• Rhabdomyolysis: Assess for muscle pain, increased CPK, weakness, swelling of affected muscles, tea-colored dark urine; if these occur and if confirmed by CPK, product should be discontinued

• QT prolongation: Monitor ECG for QT prolongation, ejection fraction; assess for chest pain, palpitations, dyspnea

• Serious skin disorders: Assess for Stevens-Johnson syndrome, angioedema, anaphylaxis

• **Pregnancy/breastfeeding:** all pregnant women who experience adverse reactions should have provider report the reactions to Antiretroviral Pregnancy Registry, 800-258-4263; avoid breastfeeding

Patient Problems

Infection (uses)

Nonadherence (teaching)

Implementation:
PO route

• **TAB:** take without regard to food; swallow whole; do not crush, break, chew

• **ORAL SOL:** shake well, use calibrated measuring device

• Drug resistance testing should be done before beginning therapy in antiretroviral-naive patients and before changing therapy for treatment failure

Teach patient/family:

• Advise patient to take as prescribed; if dose is missed, to take as soon as remembered up to 1 hr before next dose; not to double dose

• Tell patient that product is not a cure for HIV; that opportunistic infections can continue to be acquired

• Advise patient that redistribution of body fat or accumulation of body fat may occur

• Teach patient that others can continue to contract HIV from patient

• Inform patient to avoid OTC, prescription medications, herbs, supplements unless approved by prescriber; not to use St. John's wort because it decreases product's effect; that taking this product with ED drugs may increase adverse reactions

• Advise patient that regular follow-up exams and blood work will be required

• Advise patient to report a change in heart rhythm or abnormal heartbeats

Evaluation:
Positive therapeutic outcome

• Improvement in HIV symptoms

• Improving viral load, CD4+ T cells

loratadine (Rx, OTC)
(lor-a'ti-deen)
Alavert, Claritin, Children's Claritin RediTabs, Dimetapp, Triaminic Allerchews
Func. class.: Antihistamine (2nd generation)
Chem. class.: Selective histamine (H_1) receptor antagonist

Do not confuse: loratadine/lovastatin/LORazepam/losartan

ACTION: Binds to peripheral histamine receptors, which provides antihistamine action without sedation

Therapeutic outcome: Decreased nasal stuffiness, itching, swollen eyes

USES: Seasonal rhinitis, chronic idiopathic urticaria for those ≥2 yr

Pharmacokinetics

Absorption	Well absorbed
Distribution	Unknown
Metabolism	Liver, extensively, to active metabolite desloratadine
Excretion	Kidneys
Half-life	17-28 hr

Pharmacodynamics

Onset	1-3 hr
Duration	>24 hr

CONTRAINDICATIONS

Hypersensitivity, acute asthma attacks, lower respiratory tract disease

Precautions: Pregnancy, increased intraocular pressure, bronchial asthma, breastfeeding, hepatic/renal disease

DOSAGE AND ROUTES

Adult and child ≥6 yr: PO 10 mg/day
Child 2-5 yr: PO 5 mg/day

Renal dose
Adult: PO CCr <30 ml/min 10 mg every other day
Child 2-5 yr: PO GFR <50 ml/min 5 mg every other day

Hepatic dose
Adult: PO 10 mg every other day

Available forms: Tabs 10 mg; rapid-disintegrating tabs 10 mg; orally disintegrating tabs 10 mg; syr 1 mg/ml; susp 5 mg/ml; ext rel tabs 10 mg

ADVERSE EFFECTS

CNS: Sedation (more common with increased dosages), headache, fatigue, restlessness
EENT: Dry mouth

INTERACTIONS

Individual drugs
Alcohol: increased CNS depression

Drug classifications
Antidepressants, antihistamines (other), MAOIs, sedative-hypnotics: increased CNS depression

Drug/herb
Chamomile, kava, valerian: Increased CNS depression

Drug/lab test
False negative: skin allergy tests (discontinue antihistamine 3 days before testing)

NURSING CONSIDERATIONS
Assessment
• **Assess allergy:** hives, rash, rhinitis
• Assess respiratory status: rate, rhythm, increase in bronchial secretions, wheezing, chest tightness
• **Beers:** avoid in older men, may decrease urinary flow and cause urinary retention

Patient problem
Impaired skin integrity (uses)
Impaired airway clearance (uses)
Risk for injury (adverse reactions)

Implementation
• Give on an empty stomach, 1 hr before or 2 hr after meals to facilitate absorption
• **Rapid-disintegrating tabs:** Place rapidly disintegrating tabs on tongue, then swallow after disintegrated with or without water
• Use within 6 mo of opening pouch; immediately after opening blister pack
• Store in airtight, light-resistant container
• **Ext rel tab:** Do not break, crush, or chew

Patient/family education
• Teach all aspects of product uses; to notify prescriber if confusion, sedation, hypotension occur; to avoid driving and other hazardous activity if drowsiness occurs; to avoid alcohol and other CNS depressants that may potentiate effect
• Teach patient to take 1 hr before or 2 hr after meals to facilitate absorption
• Advise patient to use sunscreen or stay out of the sun to prevent burns
• Caution patient not to exceed recommended dosage; dysrhythmias may occur
• Teach patient that hard candy, gum, frequent rinsing of mouth may be used for dryness

Evaluation
Positive therapeutic outcome
• Absence of runny or congested nose, other allergy symptoms

⚠ HIGH ALERT

LORazepam (Rx)
(lor-az′e-pam)
Ativan
Func. class.: Sedative-hypnotic, antianxiety agent
Chem. class.: Benzodiazepine, short acting
Controlled substance schedule IV

Do not confuse: LORazepam/ALPRAZolam/clonazePAM

ACTION: Potentiates the actions of GABA, an inhibitory neurotransmitter, especially in the

---

limbic system and reticular formation, which depresses the CNS

Therapeutic outcome: Decreased anxiety, relaxation

USES: Anxiety, irritability in psychiatric or organic disorders, preoperatively; adjunct in endoscopic procedures, status epilepticus, insomnia

Pharmacokinetics

Absorption	Well absorbed (PO); completely absorbed (IM)
Distribution	Widely distributed; crosses placenta, blood-brain barrier; 91% protein bound
Metabolism	Liver, extensively
Excretion	Kidneys, breast milk
Half-life	12 hr, 91% protein bound

Pharmacodynamics

	PO	IM	IV
Onset	1 hr	15-30 min	5 min
Peak	1-2 hr	1-1½ hr	1-1.5 hr
Duration	12-24 hr	6-8 hr	6-8 hr

CONTRAINDICATIONS
Pregnancy, breastfeeding, hypersensitivity to benzodiazepines/benzyl alcohol, closed-angle glaucoma, psychosis, history of drug abuse, COPD, sleep apnea

Precautions: Geriatric, debilitated patients, children <12 yr, renal/hepatic disease, addiction, suicidal ideation, abrupt discontinuation

> **BLACK BOX WARNING:** Coadministration with other CNS depressants

DOSAGE AND ROUTES
Anxiety
Adult/adolescent ≥12 yr: PO 2-3 mg/day in divided doses, max 10 mg/day
Child <11 yr (unlabeled): PO 0.025-0.05 mg/kg/dose (max q4hr)
Geriatric: PO 1-2 mg/day in divided doses, or 0.5-1 mg at bedtime

Insomnia
Adult: PO 2-4 mg at bedtime; only minimally effective after 2 wk continuous therapy
Geriatric: PO 0.5-1 mg initially

Preoperatively for sedation
Adult: IM 50 mcg/kg 2 hr before surgery; **IV** 44 mcg/kg 15-20 min before surgery, max 2 mg 15-20 min before surgery

Status epilepticus
Adult IM/IV: 4 mg, may repeat after 10-15 min

Available forms: Tabs 0.5, 1, 2 mg; inj 2, 4 mg/ml; oral sol 2 mg/ml

ADVERSE EFFECTS
CNS: *Dizziness, drowsiness,* confusion, headache, anxiety, tremors, stimulation, fatigue, depression, insomnia, hallucinations, weakness, unsteadiness
CV: *Orthostatic hypotension,* ECG changes, tachycardia, hypotension, apnea, cardiac arrest (IV, rapid)
EENT: *Blurred vision,* tinnitus, mydriasis
GI: Constipation, dry mouth, nausea, vomiting, anorexia, diarrhea
INTEG: Rash, dermatitis, itching
MISC: Acidosis

INTERACTIONS
Individual drugs

> **BLACK BOX WARNING:** Alcohol: increased CNS depression

Clozapine: increased delirium, sedation
Hormonal contraceptives, valproic acid: decreased LORazepam effects
Probenecid, Valproate: increased lorazepam effect, reduce dose by 50%

Drug classifications

> **BLACK BOX WARNING:** CNS depressants, opioids: increased LORazepam effects

Drug/herb
Chamomile, hops, kava, lavender, valerian: increased CNS depression

Drug/lab test
Increased: AST, ALT

NURSING CONSIDERATIONS
Assessment
• Assess degree of anxiety; what precipitates anxiety and whether product controls symptoms; other signs of anxiety: dilated pupils, inability to sleep, restlessness, inability to focus
• Assess for alcohol withdrawal symptoms, including hallucinations (visual, auditory), delirium, irritability, agitation, fine to coarse tremors

> **BLACK BOX WARNING:** Coadministration with other CNS depressants (especially opioids) should be avoided, if used together, use lower dose

---

- Monitor B/P (with patient lying/standing), pulse; check respiratory rate; if systolic B/P drops 20 mm Hg, hold product, notify prescriber; respirations q5-15min if given **IV**
- Monitor for seizure control; type, duration, and intensity of seizures; what precipitates seizures
- Monitor hepatic studies: AST, ALT, bilirubin, creatinine, LDH, alkaline phosphatase
- Assess mental status: mood, sensorium, affect, sleeping pattern, drowsiness, dizziness, suicidal tendencies, and ability of product to control these symptoms; check for tolerance, withdrawal symptoms: headache, nausea, vomiting, muscle pain, weakness after long-term use
- **Beers:** Avoid in older adults; may increase cognitive impairment, delirium

Patient problem
Anxiety (uses)
Risk for injury (uses, adverse reactions)

Implementation
PO route
- Give largest dose before bedtime if giving in divided dose
- **Oral solution:** use calibrated dropper; add to food/drink, consume immediately
- Give with food or milk for GI symptoms; crush tab if patient is unable to swallow medication whole; provide sugarless gum, hard candy, frequent sips of water for dry mouth

SUBCUT route
- Use by SUBCUT route for rapid response (investigational use)

IM route
- Give deep in muscle mass; if using for preoperative sedation, give 2 hr or more before surgical procedure
- Use this route when IV route is not feasible

Direct IV route
- Prepare immediately before use; short stability time
- Dilute with sterile water for inj, 0.9% NaCl, or D5W just before using; give by Y-site or 3-way stopcock at 2 mg/min
- Do not use sol that is discolored or contains a precipitate

Y-site compatibilities: Acetaminophen, acyclovir, albumin, allopurinol, amifostine, amikacin, amoxicillin, amoxicillin/clavulanate, amphotericin B cholesteryl, amsacrine, atenolol, atracurium, bivalirudin, bleomycin, bumetanide, butorphanol, calcium chloride/gluconate, CARBOplatin, ceFAZolin, cefepime, cefotaxime, cefoTEtan, cefOXitin, cefTAZidime, ceftizoxime, ceftobiprole, cefTRIAXone, cefuroxime, chloramphenicol, chlorproMAZINE, cimetidine, ciprofloxacin, cisatracurium, CISplatin, cladribine,

clindamycin, cloNIDine, cyclophosphamide, cycloSPORINE, cytarabine, DACTINomycin, DAPTOmycin, dexamethasone, dexmedetomidine, diltiazem, DOBUTamine, DOCEtaxel, DOPamine, doripenem, DOXOrubicin, DOXOrubicin liposomal, droperidol, enalaprilat, ePHEDrine, EPINEPHrine, epirubicin, eptifibatide, erythromycin, *esmolol*, etomidate, *famotidine*, fenoldopam, fentaNYL, filgrastim, fluconazole, fludarabine, fosphenytoin, furosemide, ganciclovir, gatifloxacin, gemcitabine, gentamicin, glycopyrrolate, granisetron, haloperidol, heparin, hydrocortisone, HYDROmorphone, hydrOXYzine, ifosfamide, inamrinone, insulin (regular), irinotecan, isoproterenol, ketorolac, labetalol, lidocaine, linezolid, magnesium sulfate, mannitol, mechlorethamine, melphalan, meropenem, metaraminol, methadone, methotrexate, methyldopate, methylPREDNISolone, metoclopramide, metoprolol, metroNIDAZOLE, micafungin, midazolam, milrinone, minocycline, mitoXANtrone, morphine, mycophenolate, nafcillin, nalbuphine, naloxone, nesiritide, niCARDipine, nitroglycerin, nitroprusside, norepinephrine, octreotide, oxaliplatin, oxytocin, PACLitaxel, palonosetron, pamidronate, pancuronium, PEMEtrexed, pentamidine, PENTobarbital, PHENobarbital, piperacillin, piperacillin-tazobactam, polymyxin B, potassium chloride, propofol, ranitidine, remifentanil, tacrolimus, teniposide, theophylline, thiotepa, ticarcillin, ticarcillin-clavulanate, tigecycline, tirofiban, tobramycin, TPN, trastuzumab, trimethobenzamide, trimethoprim-sulfamethoxazole, vancomycin, vasopressin, vecuronium, verapamil, vinCRIStine, vinorelbine, voriconazole, zidovudine

Patient/family education
- Teach patient to notify prescriber if pregnancy is planned or suspected; do not breastfeed, use contraception
- Advise patient that product may be taken with food; to take no more than prescribed amount; may be habit forming, not to discontinue abruptly, taper, withdrawl may occur

> **BLACK BOX WARNING:** Caution patient to avoid OTC preparations unless approved by prescriber; to avoid alcohol, other psychotropic medications unless prescribed by physician, notify prescriber immediately if trouble breathing, dizziness, coma, no response; not to discontinue medication abruptly after long-term use

- Inform patient to avoid driving and activities that require alertness; drowsiness may occur; to rise slowly or fainting may occur, especially in geriatric

- Inform patient that drowsiness may worsen at beginning of treatment
- Teach patient/family to report suicidal ideation

Evaluation

Positive therapeutic outcome
- Decreased anxiety, restlessness, insomnia

TREATMENT OF OVERDOSE:
Lavage, VS, supportive care

lorcaserin
(lor-ca-ser'in)
Belviq, Belviq XR
Func. class.: Appetite suppressant
Chem. class.: Serotonin 2C (5-HT$_{2C}$) receptor agonist
Controlled substance IV

ACTION: Decreases food consumption and decreases hunger by selectively activating 5-HT$_{2C}$ receptors

Therapeutic outcome: Decrease in weight

USES: Obesity management

Pharmacokinetics

Absorption	Unknown
Distribution	70% protein binding
Metabolism	Unknown
Excretion	Unknown
Half-life	11 hr

Pharmacodynamics

Onset	Unknown
Peak	Unknown
Duration	Unknown

CONTRAINDICATIONS
Pregnancy, breastfeeding, hypersensitivity, severe renal impairment

Precautions: Children, other organic causes of obesity, anemia, AV block, bradycardia, bundle branch block, depression, dialysis, liver/kidney disease, multiple myeloma, neutropenia, suicidal ideation, Peyronie's disease, pulmonary hypertension, sick sinus syndrome

DOSAGE AND ROUTES
Adult: PO 10 mg bid, discontinue if at 12 wk <5% of weight loss has occurred; extended release 20 mg qday

Renal dose
Adult: PO 10 mg bid; do not exceed recommended dosage; discontinue after 12 wk if weight loss has not been achieved

Available forms: Tabs, film-coated 10 mg; extended release tablets 20 mg

ADVERSE EFFECTS
CNS: Insomnia, depression, serotonin syndrome, anxiety, suicidal ideation, dizziness, headache, fatigue
CV: Bradycardia, hypertension
GI: Diarrhea, constipation, nausea
HEMA: Neutropenia, leukopenia, lymphopenia
INTEG: Rash
MS: Back pain

INTERACTIONS
Individual drugs
Linezolid, buPROPion, lithium, sibutramine, traMADol: increased life-threatening serotonin syndrome
Insulin: increased risk of hypoglycemia with this product

Drug classifications
SSRIs, SNRIs, serotonin receptor agonists, MAOIs, tricyclic antidepressants: increased life-threatening serotonin syndrome
Sulfonylureas: increased risk of hypoglycemia with this product

Drug/lab test
Increase: Prolactin
Decrease: Glucose, Hct, WBC, RBC

Drug/herb
St. John's wort: increased serotonin syndrome

NURSING CONSIDERATIONS
Assessment
- Monitor weight weekly; oral hypoglycemic dosage might need to be reduced in diabetic patients
- Monitor blood glucose, CBC with differential, Hct/Hgb, serum prolactin
- **Suicidal ideation:** use caution in psychiatric disorders with emotional lability; assess for depression, suicidal thoughts/behaviors, hostility, irritability
- **Serotonin syndrome:** Assess for nausea, vomiting, diarrhea, confusion, tachycardia, hyperthermia, if these occur stop product, notify prescriber

Patient problem
Excess food intake (uses)
Lack of knowledge of medication (teaching)

Implementation
• Identify obesity if patient is on weight reduction program that includes dietary changes, exercise
• May give without regard to food

Patient/family education
• Advise patient to avoid hazardous activities until stabilized on medication
• Inform patient to discuss unpleasant side effects
• Teach patient to notify prescriber if pregnancy is planned or suspected, do not use in pregnancy, breastfeeding
• Teach patient to use in conjunction with diet, exercise

Evaluation
Positive therapeutic outcome
• Decrease in weight

losartan (Rx)
(low-sar'tan)
Cozaar
Func. class.: Antihypertensive
Chem. class.: Angiotensin II receptor (type AT_1)

Do not confuse: losartan/valsartan, Cozaar/Zocor

ACTION: Blocks the vasoconstrictor and aldosterone-secreting effects of angiotensin II; selectively blocks the binding of angiotensin II to the AT_1 receptor found in tissues

Therapeutic outcome: Decreased B/P

USES: Hypertension, alone or in combination; nephropathy in type 2 diabetes, proteinuria, stroke prophylaxis in hypertensive patients with left ventricular hypertrophy

Pharmacokinetics

Absorption	Well absorbed
Distribution	Bound to plasma proteins
Metabolism	Extensive
Excretion	Feces, urine
Half-life	Biphasic, 2 hr, 6-9 hr

Pharmacodynamics

Unknown

CONTRAINDICATIONS
Hypersensitivity

BLACK BOX WARNING: Pregnancy (2nd/3rd trimesters), pregnancy (1st trimester), breast-feeding, children, geriatric, hypersensitivity to ACE inhibitors, hepatic disease, angioedema, renal artery stenosis, ✱⊕✱ African descent, hyperkalemia, hypotension

DOSAGE AND ROUTES
Hypertension
Adult: PO 50 mg/day alone or 25 mg/day when used in combination with diuretic; maintenance 25-100 mg/day
Child ≥6 yr: PO 0.7 mg/kg/day, max 50 mg/day

Hepatic dose
Adult: PO 25 mg/day as starting dose/volume depletion

Hypertension with left ventricular hypertrophy (benefit does not apply to those of African descent)
Adult: PO 50 mg/day, add hydrochlorothiazide 12.5 mg/day and/or increase losartan to 100 mg/day, then increase hydrochlorothiazide to 25 mg/day

Nephropathy in type 2 diabetes patients
Adult: PO 50 mg/day, may increase to 100 mg/day

Available forms: Tabs 25, 50, 100 mg

ADVERSE EFFECTS
CNS: *Dizziness, insomnia,* anxiety, confusion, abnormal dreams, migraine, tremor, vertigo, headache, malaise, depression, fatigue
CV: Angina pectoris, 2nd-degree AV block, CVA, *hypotension,* MI, dysrhythmias
EENT: Blurred vision, burning eyes, conjunctivitis
GI: *Diarrhea, dyspepsia,* anorexia, constipation, dry mouth, flatulence, gastritis, vomiting
GU: Impotence, nocturia, urinary frequency, urinary tract infection, renal failure
HEMA: Anemia, thrombocytopenia
INTEG: Alopecia, dermatitis, dry skin, flushing, photosensitivity, rash, pruritus, sweating, angioedema
META: Gout, hyperkalemia, hypoglycemia
MS: Cramps, myalgia, pain, stiffness
RESP: *Cough, upper respiratory infection,* congestion, dyspnea, bronchitis
MISC: Diabetic vascular disease

INTERACTIONS
Individual drugs
Lithium: increased toxicity

Drug classifications
ACE inhibitors, diuretics (potassium-sparing), potassium supplements: increased hyperkalemia
NSAIDs: decreased antihypertensive effect

Drug/lab test
Increase: AST/ALT, bilirubin

Drug/herb
Garlic: Increased antihypertensive effect
Black licorice, Ma huang: Decrease antihypertensive effects

NURSING CONSIDERATIONS
Assessment
• Assess B/P with position changes, pulse q4hr; note rate, rhythm, quality ✖⊛, Black patients should use combination therapy for better control of B/P
• Monitor electrolytes: potassium, sodium, chloride
• Obtain baselines for renal, electrolyte, liver function tests before therapy begins
• **HF:** assess for jugular vein distention, weight daily, edema in feet, legs daily
• **Angioedema:** facial swelling, dyspnea, wheezing, may occur rapidly, tongue swelling (rare)
• **Blood dyscrasias:** thrombocytopenia, anemia (rare)

> **BLACK BOX WARNING:** Pregnancy before starting treatment; not to use in pregnancy, breastfeeding

Patient problem
Risk for injury (adverse reactions)
Nonadherence (teaching)

Implementation
• Administer without regard to meals
• If product is compounded into a suspension, store in refrigerator and shake well before use
• May use alone or in combination

Patient/family education
• Teach patient to avoid sunlight or wear sunscreen if in sunlight; photosensitivity may occur
• Advise patient to comply with dosage schedule, even if feeling better
• Teach patient to notify prescriber of mouth sores, fever, swelling of hands or feet, irregular heartbeat, chest pain
• Advise patient that excessive perspiration, dehydration, vomiting, diarrhea may lead to fall in blood pressure, consult prescriber if these occur
• Inform patient that product may cause dizziness, fainting; light-headedness may occur, to avoid hazardous activities until reaction is known

• Caution patient to rise slowly to sitting or standing position to minimize orthostatic hypotension

> **BLACK BOX WARNING:** Advise patient to use contraception while taking this product, pregnancy not to breastfeed

Evaluation
Positive therapeutic outcome
• Decreased B/P

loteprednol ophthalmic
See Appendix B

lovastatin (Rx)
(loe´va-sta-tin)
Altoprev
Func. class.: Antilipemic
Chem. class.: HMG-CoA reductase inhibitor

Do not confuse: lovastatin/Lotensin

ACTION: By inhibiting HMG-CoA reductase, which reduces cholesterol synthesis

Therapeutic outcome: Decreased cholesterol levels and LDL, increased HDL

USES: As an adjunct in primary hypercholesterolemia (types IIa, IIb), atherosclerosis, heterozygous familial hypercholesterolemia (adolescents)

Pharmacokinetics

Absorption	Poorly absorbed, erratic
Distribution	Crosses placenta, blood-brain barrier
Metabolism	Liver, extensively
Excretion	Feces (83%); kidneys, urine (10%)
Half-life	3-4 hr

Pharmacodynamics

Onset	Unknown
Peak	2-4 hr
Duration	Unknown

CONTRAINDICATIONS
Pregnancy, breastfeeding, hypersensitivity, active liver disease

Precautions: Past liver disease, alcoholism, severe acute infections, trauma, hypotension, uncontrolled seizure disorders, severe metabolic disorders, electrolyte imbalances, visual condition, children

---

⚠ Nurse Alert   ✴ Key NCLEX® Drug   ≫ Drug Specifics

DOSAGE AND ROUTES
To prevent/treat CAD, hyperlipidemia
Adult: PO 20 mg/day with evening meal; may increase to 20-40 mg/day in single or divided doses at 4-wk intervals; max 40 mg/day; ext rel 20-60 mg/day at bedtime; max 40 mg/day

Heterozygous familial hypercholesterolemia 🐭⚠
Adolescent 10-17 yr: PO 10-40 mg with evening meal

Primary prevention of CV disease
Adult 45-75 yr with type 1 or 2 diabetes: PO 40 mg immediate-release

Secondary prevention of CV disease
Adult >75 yr (not a candidate for high-intensity use): 40 mg immediate-release qday

Renal dose
Adult: PO CCr <30 mg/min max 20 mg/day unless titrated

Available forms: Tabs 10, 20, 40 mg; ext rel tab 10, 20, 40, 60 mg

ADVERSE EFFECTS
CNS: Dizziness, headache, tremor, insomnia, paresthesia
EENT: Blurred vision, lens opacities
GI: Nausea, constipation, diarrhea, dyspepsia, *flatus,* abdominal pain, heartburn, liver dysfunction, vomiting, acid regurgitation, dry mouth, dysgeusia
HEMA: Thrombocytopenia, hemolytic anemia, leukopenia
INTEG: Rash, pruritus, photosensitivity
MS: Muscle cramps, myalgia, myositis, rhabdomyolysis; leg, shoulder, or localized pain

INTERACTIONS
Individual drugs
Amiodarone: Decreased lovastatin metabolism, avoid combining with >40 mg/day amiodarone
Clarithromycin, clofibrate, cycloSPORINE, danazol, diltiazem, erythromycin, gemfibrozil, niacin, quinupristin-dalfopristin, telithromycin, verapamil: increased myalgia, myositis, rhabdomyolysis; avoid concurrent use
Warfarin: increased bleeding

Drug classifications
Azole antifungals, protease inhibitors: increased myositis, myalgia, rhabdomyolysis
Bile acid sequestrants: decreased lovastatin effects

Drug/herb
Pectin, St. John's wort: decreased effect
Red yeast rice: increased adverse reactions

Drug/food
Increased levels of lovastatin with food, must be taken with food
Grapefruit juice: increased toxicity
Oat bran: decreased absorption

Drug/lab test
Increased: CPK, liver function tests
Interference: T3, T4, T7, TSH

NURSING CONSIDERATIONS
Assessment
• Assess nutrition: fat, protein, carbohydrates; nutritional analysis should be completed by dietitian before treatment
• Monitor bowel pattern daily; diarrhea may be a problem
• Monitor triglycerides, fasting cholesterol LDL, HDL at baseline, throughout treatment; watch LDL and VLDL closely; if increased, product should be discontinued
• Assess for muscle pain, tenderness, obtain CPK; if these occur, product may need to be discontinued
• **Rhabdomyolysis:** muscle pain, increased CPK, weakness, swelling of affected muscles; if these occur and if confirmed by CPK, product should be discontinued

Patient problem
Nonadherence (teaching)

Implementation
• Give with evening meal; if dosage is increased, take with breakfast and evening meal (immediate release); use at bedtime
• Altroprev is not equivalent to Mevacor
• Store in cool environment in airtight, light-resistant container
• Do not crush or chew ext rel tab

Patient/family education
• Inform patient that compliance is needed for positive results to occur; not to double doses
• Inform patient that blood work and ophthalmic exam will be necessary during treatment
• Teach patient that risk factors should be decreased: high-fat diet, smoking, alcohol consumption, absence of exercise
• Advise patient to notify prescriber if the GI symptoms of diarrhea, abdominal or epigastric pain, nausea, vomiting occur; or if chills, fever, sore throat, blurred vision, dizziness, headache, muscle pain, weakness occur
• Advise patient to stay out of the sun or use sunscreen to prevent burns
• Instruct patient that product should be taken with food; not to crush, chew ext rel product; to take immediate-release product in the AM and extended-release product at bedtime

- Teach patient not to use with grapefruit juice, large amounts of alcohol
- Teach patient to protect from light, moisture
- Advise patient to report if pregnancy is suspected, do not breastfeed, do not use in pregnancy

Evaluation
Positive therapeutic outcome
- Decreased cholesterol, serum triglyceride levels
- Improved level of HDL

lurasidone (Rx)
(loo-ras'i-done)
Latuda
Func. class.: Atypical antipsychotic
Chem. class.: Dopamine-serotonin receptor antagonist

Do not confuse: Latuda/Lantus

ACTION: May modulate central dopaminergic and serotoninergic activity, high affinity for dopamine-D_2 receptors, serotonin 5-HT_{2A} receptors, and partial agonist at serotonin 5-HT_{1A} receptor

Therapeutic outcome: Decreasing hallucinations, delusions, agitation, social withdrawal

USES: Schizophrenia, depression associated with bipolar disorder I

Pharmacokinetics

Absorption	9%-19%
Distribution	99% protein binding
Metabolism	Unknown
Excretion	80% feces, 9% urine
Half-life	18 hr

Pharmacodynamics

Onset	Unknown
Peak	1-3 hr
Duration	Steady state 7 days

CONTRAINDICATIONS
Hypersensitivity

Precautions: Abrupt discontinuation, ambient temperature increase, breast cancer, breastfeeding, cardiac disease, children, dehydration, diabetes, ketoacidosis, driving/operating machinery, dysphagia, geriatrics, heart failure, hematological/hepatic/renal disease, hypotension, hypovolemia, MI, infertility, obesity, Parkinson's disease, pregnancy, seizures, strenuous exercise, stroke, substance abuse, suicidal ideation, syncope, tardive dyskinesia

BLACK BOX WARNING: Dementia: antipsychotics, such as lurasidone, are not approved for the treatment of dementia-related psychosis in geriatric patients and may increase the risk of death in this population, children, suicidal ideation

DOSAGE AND ROUTES
Schizophrenia
Adult: PO 40 mg/day, range 40-160 mg/day, those receiving CYP3A4 inhibitors max 80 mg/day, do not use with strong CYP3A4 inducers/inhibitors
Child: 13-17 yr: PO 40 mg qday, may increase to max 80 mg qday

Bipolar disorder I
Adult: PO 20 mg qday, max 120 mg/day

Hepatic/renal dose
Adult: PO CCr <50 ml/min, hepatic disease CTPA start dose 20 mg/day, max 80 mg/day; hepatic disease CTP B start dose 20 mg/day, max 40 mg/day

Available forms: 20, 40, 80, 120 mg tabs

ADVERSE EFFECTS
CNS: Agitation, akathisia, anxiety, dizziness, drowsiness, fatigue, hyperthermia, insomnia, dystonic reactions; pseudoparkinsonism, restlessness, seizures, suicidal ideation, syncope, tardive dyskinesia, vertigo
CV: Angina, bradycardia, hypertension, orthostatic hypotension, tachycardia, stroke
EENT: Blurred vision
ENDO: Diabetes mellitus, ketoacidosis, hyperglycemia, hyperprolactinemia
GI: Abdominal pain, diarrhea, dyspepsia, nausea, vomiting, gastritis, weight gain/loss
GU: Amenorrhea, breast enlargement, dysmenorrhea, impotence, dysuria, renal failure
HEMA: Agranulocytosis, anemia, leucopenia, neutropenia
INTEG: Pruritus, rash
MS: Back pain, dysarthria; rhabdomyolysis (rare)
SYST: Angioedema

INTERACTIONS
Individual drugs
Metoclopramide: do not use concurrently

Drug classifications
Antihypertensives: increased hypotensive risk
Other CNS depressants, alcohol: increased sedation
Opioids: increased respiratory depression, sedation, death; avoid using together

Strong CYP3A4 inducers: (carbamazepine, rifampin): decreased lurasidone effect, do not use together

Drug/herb
St. John's wort: decrease: product effect, do not use together

Drug/food
Not to use with grapefruit/grapefruit juice

NURSING CONSIDERATIONS
Assessment
• **Assess for schizophrenia:** hallucinations, delusions, agitation, social withdrawal; monitor orientation, behavior, mood prior to and periodically during therapy
• Assess AIMS assessment, thyroid function tests, LFTs, lipid panel, electrolytes
• **Assess for EPS:** restlessness, difficulty speaking, loss of balance, pill rolling, masklike face, shuffling gait, rigidity, tremors, muscle spasms; monitor prior to and periodically during therapy; report tardive dyskinesia immediately

> **BLACK BOX WARNING: Dementia:** This product is not approved for the elderly with dementia-related psychosis

• Monitor for weight gain, hyperglycemia, metabolic changes in diabetes
• Coadministration with other CNS depressants (opioids). If given together, assess for excessive sedation, slow breathing, avoid concurrent use

> **BLACK BOX WARNING: Suicidal ideation/children:** Avoid use in children, may be risk of suicide in young adults (<24 yr) and children; assess for worsening depression, suicidal thoughts/behaviors, product should be dispensed in small quantities

• **Beers:** Avoid in older adults except for schizophrenia, bipolar disorder, short-term use as an antiemetic for chemotherapy, increased risk of stroke, cognitive decline

Patient problem
Distorted thinking process (uses)
Risk for injury (adverse reactions)

Implementation
• Give with a meal of at least 350 calories
• Store at room temperature, protect from moisture

Patient/family education
• Explain reason for treatment and expected results
• **Teach patient to report EPS, blood dyscrasias:** sore throat, fever, unusual bleeding/bruising
• Teach patient that lab work will be needed regularly
• Advise patient to avoid hazardous activities until response is known
• Teach patient to avoid OTC products unless approved by prescriber, serious reaction may occur, not to use grapefruit juice, alcohol
• Teach patient to report fast heartbeat, extra beats, trouble breathing, sweating, stiffness

> **BLACK BOX WARNING: Suicidal ideation/children:** Teach patient/family to be aware and report immediately worsening depression, suicidal thoughts/behaviors, hostility, irritability

Evaluation
Positive therapeutic outcome
• Decreasing hallucinations, delusions, agitation, social withdrawal

luliconazole topical
See Appendix B

---

mafenide topical
See Appendix B

magaldrate (OTC)
(mag′al-drate)
Riopan Plus
Func. class.: Antacid
Chem. class.: Aluminum/magnesium
hydroxide

magnesium hydroxide/ aluminum hydroxide
**Alamag, Dioval Plus ✦, Maalox,
Rulox**

ACTION: Neutralizes gastric acidity; product is dissolved in gastric contents; this product is a combination of aluminum and magnesium

Therapeutic outcome: Decreased pain of ulcers

USES: Antacid, hiatal hernia, indigestion/ heartburn, hyperacidity

Unlabeled uses: Duodenal and gastric ulcers, peptic ulcer disease (adjunct), reflex esophagitis

Pharmacokinetics

Absorption	Not absorbed
Distribution	Not distributed, crosses placenta
Metabolism	Not metabolized
Excretion	Kidneys
Half-life	Unknown

Pharmacodynamics

Onset	Unknown
Peak	½ hr
Duration	1 hr

CONTRAINDICATIONS
Hypersensitivity to this product or benzyl alcohol

Precautions: Pregnancy, geriatric, fluid restriction, decreased GI motility, GI obstruction, dehydration, renal disease, sodium-restricted diets, bone disease, hypertension, appendicitis, diverticulitis, ulcerative colitis, neonates/infants, hypermagnesemia, hypophosphatemia

DOSAGE AND ROUTES
Magaldrate
Adult/child/geriatric: Magnesium hydroxide/ aluminum hydroxide SUSP 5-10 ml (480-1080 mg) with water between meals, at bedtime

Magnesium hydroxide/aluminum hydroxide
Adult/child ≥12 yr: PO 5-30 mL or 1-2 tablets 1-3 hr after meals, bedtime

Available forms: Magaldrate: SUSP 540 mg/ 5 ml, 1080 mg/5 ml; **magnesium hydroxide/ aluminum hydroxide chew tabs** 300 mg/ 150 mg, suspension 225 mg/200 mg/5 ml

ADVERSE EFFECTS
GI: Constipation, diarrhea, anorexia
META: Hypermagnesemia, hypophosphatemia

INTERACTIONS
Individual drugs
ChlordiazePOXIDE, cimetidine, isoniazid, ketoconazole, phenytoin, tetracycline: decreased absorption of each specific product
Flecainide, quiNIDine: increased action when taken in large amounts

Drug classifications
Amphetamines: increased action when taken in large amounts
Anticholinergics, corticosteroids, fluoroquinolones, iron salts, phenothiazines, salicylates: decreased absorption of each specific product
Salicylates: decreased action when taken in large amounts

NURSING CONSIDERATIONS
Assessment
• **Antacid:** Assess for location of pain, intensity, characteristics, what aggravates, ameliorates pain; heartburn/indigestion; hematemesis
• Monitor serum magnesium, calcium, phosphate, potassium if using long term or with impaired renal function
• Assess for constipation: increase bulk in diet if needed or obtain order for stool softener

Patient problem
Pain (uses)

Implementation
• Take antacids 2 hr before or 2 hr after taking enteric-coated products
• Give laxatives or stool softeners if constipation occurs
• Give SUSP after shaking; give between meals and at bedtime
• Give when stomach is empty after meals and at bedtime

Patient/family education
• Advise patient to separate ingestion of enteric-coated products and antacid by 2 hr

---

• Advise patient to use product 2 wk or less; product should not be used for long periods
• Teach patient to notify prescriber immediately if coffee-ground emesis, emesis with frank blood, or black tarry stools occur

Evaluation

Positive therapeutic outcome
• Absence of abdominal pain
• Decreased acidity

magnesium salts
(mag-neez′ee-um)
magnesium chloride (Rx)
(12% Mg, 9.8 mEq Mg/g) Chloromag, Slo-mag
magnesium citrate (OTC)
(16.2% Mg, 4.4 mEq Mg/g) Citrate of magnesia, Citroma, Citromag ✦
magnesium gluconate (OTC)
(5.4% Mg, 4.4 mEq Mg/g) Magtrate, Magonate
magnesium hydroxide (OTC)
(41.7% Mg; 34.3 mEq Mg/g) Dulcolax, Magnesia Tablets, Phillips Milk of Magnesia, MOM
magnesium oxide (OTC)
(60.3% Mg; 49.6 mEq Mg/s) Mag-Ox 400, Uro-Mag

⚠ HIGH ALERT

magnesium sulfate (OTC, Rx)
(9.9% Mg; 8.1 mEq Mg/g) (IV)
Func. class.: Electrolyte; anticonvulsant, laxative, saline; antacid

ACTION: Increases osmotic pressure, draws fluid into colon, neutralizes HCl

Therapeutic outcome: Magnesium levels WNL, absence of constipation

USES: Constipation, dyspepsia, bowel preparation before surgery or exam, electrolyte, anticonvulsant, in preeclampsia, eclampsia (magnesium sulfate); cardiac glycoside-induced arrhythmias, nutritional supplement

Pharmacokinetics

Absorption	Unknown
Distribution	Unknown
Metabolism	Unknown
Excretion	Kidneys

Half-life	Unknown
	effective anticonvulsant levels 2.5-7.5 mEq/L

Pharmacodynamics

	PO	IM	IV
Onset	3-6 hr	1 hr	Unknown
Peak	Unknown	Unknown	Unknown
Duration	Unknown	4 hr	½ hr

CONTRAINDICATIONS
Hypersensitivity, abdominal pain, nausea/vomiting, obstruction, acute surgical abdomen, rectal bleeding, heart block, myocardial damage

Precautions: Pregnancy (magnesium sulfate), renal disease/cardiac disease

DOSAGE AND ROUTES
Laxative
Adult: PO 15-60 ml at bedtime (Milk of Magnesia)
Adult and child >12 yr: PO 15 g in 8 oz of H_2O (magnesium sulfate); PO 5-30 ml (Concentrated Milk of Magnesia); PO 5-10 oz at bedtime (magnesium citrate)
Child 2-6 yr: 5-15 ml/day (Milk of Magnesia)

Prevention of magnesium deficiency (Mg of magnesium)
Adult and child ≥10 yr: PO (male): 350-400 mg/day; (female): 280-300 mg/day; (breastfeeding): 335-350 mg/day; (pregnancy): 320 mg/day
Child 8-10 yr: PO 170 mg/day
Child 4-7 yr: PO 120 mg/day

Magnesium sulfate deficiency (Mg of magnesium)
Adult: PO 200-400 mg in divided doses tid-qid; IM 1 g q6hr × 4 doses; **IV** 5 g (severe)
Child 6-12 yr: 3-6 mg/kg/day in divided doses tid-qid

Preeclampsia/eclampsia magnesium sulfate
Adult: IM/IV INF 4-5 g; with 5 g IM in each gluteus, then 5 g q4hr or 4 g **IV** INF, then 1-3 g/hr cont INF, max 40 g/24 hr or 20 g/48 hr in severe renal disease

Available forms: Chloride: sus rel tabs 535 mg (64 mg Mg); enteric tabs 833 mg (100 mg Mg); **hydroxide:** liquid 400 mg/5 ml (164 mg Mg/5 ml); conc liquid 800 mg/5 ml (328 mg Mg/5 ml); chew tabs 300, 600 mg; **Gluconate:** tabs 500 mg; liquid 54 mg/5 ml; **oxide:** tabs 400 mg (241.3 mg Mg); caps 140 mg (84.5 mg Mg); **sulfate:** 500 mg/ml; premixed infusion 1g/100 ml, 2 g/100 ml, 4 g/50 ml, 4 g/100 ml, 20 g/500 ml, 40 g/1000 ml; **citrate:** oral sol 240, 296, 300 ml bottles (77 mEq/100 ml)

M

ADVERSE EFFECTS

CNS: Muscle weakness, flushing, sweating, confusion, sedation, depressed reflexes, flaccid paralysis, hypothermia

CV: Hypotension, heart block, circulatory collapse, vasodilatation

GI: *Nausea, vomiting, anorexia, cramps,* diarrhea

HEMA: Prolonged bleeding time

META: Electrolyte, fluid imbalances

RESP: Respiratory depression/paralysis

INTERACTIONS
Individual products
Digoxin: decreased effect of digoxin
Nitrofurantoin: decreased absorption

Drug classifications
Antihypertensives: increased hypotension, calcium channel blockers

Antiinfectives (fluoroquinolones), tetracyclines: decreased absorption

Neuromuscular blockers: increased effect

NURSING CONSIDERATIONS
Assessment
• Assess I&O ratio; check for decrease in urinary output
• **Laxative:** assess cause of constipation; lack of fluids, bulk, exercise
• Assess cramping, rectal bleeding, nausea, vomiting; product should be discontinued
• **Assess magnesium toxicity:** thirst, confusion, decrease in reflexes
• Assess visual changes: blurring, halos, corneal and retinal damage
• Assess edema in feet, ankles, legs
• Assess prior product history; there are many product interactions
• **Eclampsia:** seizure precautions, BP, ECG (magnesium sulfate)

Patient problem
Constipation (uses)
Risk for injury (IV) (uses, adverse reactions)

Implementation
PO route
• Administer with 8 oz of water
• Refrigerate magnesium citrate before administration
• Shake susp before using
• Administer to patient crushed or whole; chewable tablets may be chewed
• Administer with food or milk to decrease gastric symptoms; give 30 min before or 2 hr after antacids
• Tablets should be chewed thoroughly before swallowing, give 4 oz of water afterward

• **Laxative:** give on empty stomach, give full glass of liquid, do not give at bedtime

IM route (magnesium sulfate)
• Give deeply in gluteal site

IV route (magnesium sulfate)
• Only when calcium gluconate available for magnesium toxicity

Direct IV route
• Dilute 50% solution to 20% or less give at ≤150 mg/min

Continuous IV INF route
• May dilute to 20% sol, infuse over 3 hr
• IV at less than 125 mg/kg/hr; circulatory collapse may occur; use inf pump

Y-site compatibilities: Acyclovir, aldesleukin, alemtuzumab, alfentanil, amifostine, amikacin, aminocaproic acid, argatroban, arsenic trioxide, ascorbic acid injection, asparaginase, atenolol, atosiban, atracurium, atropine, azithromycin, aztreonam, benztropine, bivalirudin, bleomycin, bumetanide, buprenorphine, butorphanol, calcium gluconate, cangrelor, CARBOplatin, carmustine, caspofungin, cefotaxime, cefoTEtan, cefOXitin, cefTAZidime, ceftizoxime, cephapirin, chloramphenicol, chlorproMAZINE, cimetidine, cisatracurium, CISplatin, clindamycin, cloNIDine, codeine, cyanocobalamin, cyclophosphamide, cytarabine, DACTINomycin, DAPTOmycin, DAUNOrubicin liposome, DAUNOrubicin, dexmedetomidine, dexrazoxane, digoxin, diltiazem, dimenhyDRINATE, diphenhydrAMINE, DOBUTamine, DOCEtaxel, dolasetron, DOPamine, doripenem, doxacurium chloride, DOXOrubicin liposomal, doxycycline, enalaprilat, EPHEDrine, EPINEPHrine, epoetin alfa, eptifibatide, ertapenem, esmolol, etoposide, etoposide phosphate, famotidine, fenoldopam, fentaNYL, fluconazole, fludarabine, fluorouracil, folic acid (as sodium salt), foscarnet, gallium, gatifloxacin, gemcitabine, gemtuzumab, gentamicin, glycopyrrolate, granisetron, heparin, HYDROmorphone, hydrOXYzine, IDArubicin, ifosfamide, imipenemcilastatin, insulin, regular, irinotecan, isoproterenol, kanamycin, ketamine, ketorolac, labetalol, lactated ringer's injection, lepirudin, leucovorin, lidocaine, linezolid, LORazepam, mannitol, mechlorethamine, mesna, metaraminol, methotrexate, methyldopate, metoclopramide, metoprolol, metroNIDAZOLE, micafungin, midazolam, milrinone, minocycline, mitoMYcin, mitoXANtrone, mivacurium, morphine, moxifloxacin, multiple vitamins injection, mycophenolate mofetil, nafcillin, nalbuphine, nesiritide, netilmicin, niCARdipine, nitroglycerin, nitroprusside, norepinephrine, octreotide, ondansetron, oxaliplatin, oxytocin, PACLitaxel, palonosetron, pamidronate, pancuronium, papaverine, PEMEtrexed, penicillin G potassium/sodium, pentazocine, PENTobarbital, PHENobarbital, phentolamine, phenylephrine, piperacillin, piperacillin tazobactam, polymyxin B, potassium acetate/chloride, procainamide, prochlorperazine, promethazine, propranolol, protamine, pyridoxine, quiNIDine, quinupristin-dalfopristin, ranitidine, remifentanil, ringer's injection, riTUXimab, rocuronium, sargramostim, sodium acetate/bicarbonate, succinylcholine, SUFentanil, tacrolimus, telavancin, teniposide, theophylline, thiamine, thiotepa, ticarcillin, ticarcillin-clavulanate, tigecycline, tirofiban, TNA (3-in-1), tobramycin, tolazoline, topotecan, TPN (2-in-1), trastuzumab, urokinase, vancomycin, vasopressin, vecuronium, verapamil, vinBLAStine, vinCRIStine, vinorelbine, vitamin B complex with C, voriconazole, zoledronic acid

Patient/family education
PO route

• Teach not to use laxatives for long-term therapy; bowel tone will be lost
• Teach that chilling helps the taste of magnesium citrate
• Teach to shake suspension well
• Teach to not use at bedtime as a laxative; may interfere with sleep; MOM is usually given at bedtime
• Teach to give citrus fruit after administering to counteract unpleasant taste
• Teach reason for product, expected result
• **Pregnancy/breastfeeding:** Identify if pregnancy is planned or suspected or breastfeeding

Evaluation

Positive therapeutic outcome
• Decreased constipation; absence of seizures (eclampsia), normal serum calcium levels

---

mannitol (Rx)
(man′i-tole)
Osmitrol, Resectisol
Func. class.: Diuretic-osmotic
Chem. class.: Hexahydric alcohol

ACTION: Increases osmolarity of glomerular filtrate, which raises osmotic pressure of fluid in renal tubules; there is a decrease in reabsorption of water, electrolytes; increases in urinary output, sodium, chloride, potassium, calcium, phosphorus, uric acid, urea, magnesium

USES: Edema; promote systemic diuresis in cerebral edema, decrease intraocular pressure,

improve renal function in acute renal failure, chemical poisoning, urinary bladder irrigation, kidney transplant

Pharmacokinetics

Absorption	Complete
Distribution	Extracellular spaces
Metabolism	Minimal
Excretion	Renal
Half-life	100 min

Pharmacodynamics

Onset	½-1 hr
Peak	1 hr
Duration	6-8 hr

CONTRAINDICATIONS
Active intracranial bleeding, hypersensitivity, anuria, severe pulmonary congestion, edema, severe dehydration, progressive heart disease, renal failure, acute MI, aneurysm, stroke

Precautions: Pregnancy, breastfeeding, geriatric, dehydration, severe renal disease, HF, electrolyte imbalances

> **BLACK BOX WARNING:** Acute bronchospasm, asthma

DOSAGE AND ROUTES
Oliguria, prevention in acute renal failure
Adult: **IV** after initial test dose and if urine output is 30-50 mg/hr × 2 hr, give 20-100 g of a 15% or 20% SOL in a 24-hr period

Oliguria, treatment
Adult: **IV** after initial test dose, give balance of 50 g of a 20% SOL over 1 hr, then 5% via CONT IV INF to maintain output at 50 ml/hr
Child (unlabeled): **IV** 0.5-2 g/kg as a 15%-20% SOL, run over 30-60 min; maintenance 0.25-0.5 g/kg q4-6hr

Edema
Adult: **IV** after dose, use product 10%-20% at a rate of 25-75 ml/hr, give loop diuretics prior to mannitol
Child: **IV** (unlabeled) 0.5-2 g/kg of 15%-20% mannitol over 2-6 hr

Intraocular pressure
Adult: **IV** 1.5-2 g/kg of a 15%-20% SOL over 30-60 min

ICP
Adult: **IV** 1-2 g/kg, then 0.25-1 g/kg q4hr

M

Diuresis in product intoxication
Adult and child >12 yr: 5%-25% SOL continuously up to 200 g **IV**, while maintaining 100-500 ml urine output/hr

Available forms: Inj 5%, 10%, 15%, 20%, 25%; GU irrigation 5%; Inhalation cap challenge kit

ADVERSE EFFECTS
CNS: *Dizziness, headache,* confusion
CV: Edema, hypotension, hypertension, tachycardia, HF, thrombophlebitis, angina-like chest pains, fever, chills, circulatory overload
ELECT: Fluid, electrolyte imbalances, electrolyte loss, dehydration, hyper/hypokalemia
GI: *Nausea, vomiting,* dry mouth
GU: Marked diuresis, urinary retention, thirst
INTEG: Injection site reaction

INTERACTIONS
Individual drugs
Digoxin: increased hypokalemia
Lithium: increased elimination of mannitol, monitor lithium level
Imipramine: increased excretion of imipramine

Drug/food
Potassium foods: increased hyperkalemia

Drug/lab test
Interference: inorganic phosphorus, ethylene glycol
Decrease: ANC
Increase or decrease: sodium, potassium, magnesium

NURSING CONSIDERATIONS
Assessment
• Assess neurologic status: LOC, ICP reading, pupil size and reaction when product is given for increased ICP
• Assess for vision changes or eye discomfort or pain before, during treatment (increases intraocular pressure); neurologic checks, ICP during treatment (increased ICP)

> **BLACK BOX WARNING: Bronchospasm/asthma:** Test for bronchial hyperresponsiveness should not be performed in any person with asthma or baseline pulmonary function test FEV1<1-1.5L or <70% of predicted values

• Assess patient for tinnitus, hearing loss, ear pain; periodic testing of hearing is needed when high doses of this product are given by **IV** route
• Assess fluid volume status: check I&O ratios and record hourly urine values, breath sounds, weight, distended red veins, crackles in lungs; color, quality, and specific gravity of urine, skin turgor, adequacy of pulses, moist mucous membranes (provide adequate fluids), bilateral lung sounds, peripheral pitting edema
• Assess for dehydration; symptoms of decreasing output, thirst, hypotension, dry mouth and mucous membranes should be reported, provide frequent mouth care
• Monitor electrolytes: potassium, sodium, calcium, magnesium; also include BUN, PAP, qday; regularly monitor serum and urine levels of sodium and potassium
• Assess B/P before, during therapy with patient lying, standing, and sitting as appropriate; orthostatic hypotension can occur rapidly
• Monitor for rebound ICP: headache, confusion
• **Beers:** Use with caution in older adults, may cause or exacerbate SIADH

Patient problem
Fluid imbalance (uses, adverse reactions)

Implementation
Irrigation
• Use 100 ml of 25%/900 ml of sterile water for inj (2.5% sol)
• Administer potassium replacement if potassium level is <3 mg/ml

Intermittent/continuous IV route
• Change IV set q24hr
• May warm solution to dissolve crystals
• Precipitate may occur with PVC
• Use an in-line filter for 15%, 20%, 25%; give with inf pump; check **IV** patency at inf site before, during administration; do not use sol that is yellow or has a precipitate or crystals, use in-line filter, do not give as direct injection; to redissolve, run bottle under hot water and shake vigorously; cool to body temp before giving
• Run at 30-50 ml/hr in **oliguria**; run over 30-60 min in increased **ICP**; run over 30 min for **intraocular pressure**; 60-90 min after **surgery**
• Monitor for infiltration, potency during use
• Give 20 mEq NaCl/L of product solution if blood is given concurrently
• **Test dose** with severe oliguria, 0.2 g/kg over 3-5 mins; if continued oliguria, give 2nd test dose; if no response, reassess patient

Y-site compatibilities: Acetaminophen, acyclovir, alemtuzumab, amifostine, amikacin, ampicillin, atropine, asparaginase, aztreonam, bivalirudin, bumetanide, calcium gluconate, caspofungin, ceFAZolin, cefotaxime, cefOXitin, cefTAZidime, ceftizoxime, chloramphenicol, cimetidine, cisatracurium, clindamycin, DAPTOmycin, dexmedetomidine, digoxin, diltiazem, diphenhydrAMINE, DOBUTamine, DOPamine,

DOXOrubicin liposome, doxycycline, enalaprilat, EPINEPHrine, ertapenem, esmolol, famotidine, fenoldopam, fentaNYL, fluconazole, fludarabine, gentamicin, granisetron, heparin, HYDROmorphone, hydrOXYzine, IDArubicin, imipenem/cilastatin, insulin, isoproterenol, ketorolac, labetalol, levofloxacin, lidocaine, linezolid, LORazepam, meperidine, metoclopramide, metoprolol, metroNIDAZOLE, micafungin, midazolam, milrinone, morphine, nafcillin, niCARdipine, nitroglycerin, nitroprusside, norepinephrine, ondansetron, oxaliplatin, PACLitaxel, palonosetron, pantoprazole, penicillin G potassium, phenylephrine, piperacillin/tazobactam, potassium chloride, procainamide, prochlorperazine, promethazine, propofol, propranolol, protamine, quinupristin/dalfopristin, ranitidine, remifentanil, sargramostim, sodium bicarbonate, tacrolimus, thiotepa, ticarcillin/clavulanate, tirofiban, tobramycin, trimethoprim/sulfamethoxazole, vancomycin, vasopressin, verapamil, vinCRIStine, vitamin B complex with C, voriconazole, zoledronic acid

Patient/family education
• Teach patient reason for and method of treatment, pain at injection site, hearing loss, blurred vision

Evaluation
Positive therapeutic outcome
• Decreased intraocular pressure
• Prevention of hypokalemia (diuretic use)
• Decreased edema
• Decreased ICP
• Increased diuresis of >30 ml/hr
• Increased excretion of toxic substances

TREATMENT OF OVERDOSE:
Discontinue infusion; correct fluid, electrolyte imbalances; hemodialysis; monitor hydration, CV, renal function

---

meclizine (OTC, Rx)
(mek′li-zeen)
Bonine, Dramamine Less Drowsy Formula
Func. class.: Antiemetic, antihistamine, anticholinergic
Chem. class.: H₁-receptor antagonist, piperazine derivative

ACTION: Suppresses vestibular end-organ receptors and inhibits activation of cholinergic pathways

Therapeutic outcome: Decreased nausea in motion sickness; decreased vertigo

---

USES: Vertigo, motion sickness

Pharmacokinetics
Absorption	Well absorbed
Distribution	Unknown
Metabolism	Unknown
Excretion	Unknown
Half-life	6 hr

Pharmacodynamics
Onset	1 hr
Peak	Unknown
Duration	8-24 hr

CONTRAINDICATIONS
Hypersensitivity to cyclizines, shock

Precautions: Pregnancy, breastfeeding, children, geriatric, closed-angle glaucoma, glaucoma, prostatic hypertrophy, hypertension, urinary retention, GI obstruction, contact lenses

DOSAGE AND ROUTES
Vertigo
Adult/adolescent: PO 25-100 mg/day in divided doses

Motion sickness
Adult/adolescent: PO 25-50 mg 1 hr before traveling; repeat dose q24hr prn

Available forms: Tabs 12.5, 25, 50 mg

ADVERSE EFFECTS
CNS: *Drowsiness,* fatigue
CV: Hypotension
EENT: blurred vision
GI: Dry mouth

INTERACTIONS
Individual drugs
Alcohol: increased effects
Atropine: increased anticholinergic effects

Drug classifications
Antihistamines, antidepressants, phenothiazines: increased anticholinergic effect
CNS depressants, opioids: increased CNS depression

Drug/herb
Hops, valerian, kava: increased sedative effect

Drug/lab test
False negative: allergy skin testing (allergen extracts)

NURSING CONSIDERATIONS
Assessment
• **Vertigo/motion sickness:** nausea, vomiting after 1 hr, assess vertigo periodically
• Monitor VS, B/P

M

• **Assess for signs of toxicity of other products or masking of symptoms of disease:** brain tumor, intestinal obstruction
• Observe for drowsiness, dizziness, LOC

Patient problem
Nausea (uses)
Risk for injury (adverse reactions)

Implementation
• May give without regard to food
• **Chew tab:** Give without regard to water or may be swallowed whole with water
• Give lowest possible dose in geriatric, anticholinergic effects

Patient/family education
• Teach patient that a false-negative result may occur with skin testing for allergies; these procedures should not be scheduled for 4 days after discontinuing use
• Advise patient to use sugarless gum, frequent sips of water for dry mouth
• Teach patient to avoid hazardous activities, activities requiring alertness; dizziness may occur; instruct patient to request assistance with ambulation
• Teach patient to avoid alcohol, other depressants, breastfeeding, report severe side effects
• **Motion sickness prophylaxis:** Teach patient to take ≥ 1 hr before event that may cause motion sickness

Evaluation

Positive therapeutic outcome
• Absence of dizziness, vomiting

⚠ HIGH ALERT

medroxyPROGESTERone (Rx)
(me-drox-ee-proe-jess′te-rone)
Depo-Provera, Depo-subQ Provera 104, Medroxy ❋, Provera
Func. class.: Hormone: progestogen, contraceptive, antineoplastic
Chem. class.: Progesterone derivative

Do not confuse: medroxyPROGESTERone/ methylPREDNISolone, **Provera**/Premarin/Covera

ACTION: Inhibits secretion of pituitary gonadotropins, which prevents follicular maturation and ovulation; antineoplastic action against endometrial cancer

Therapeutic outcome: Decreased abnormal uterine bleeding, absence of amenorrhea

USES: Uterine bleeding (abnormal), secondary amenorrhea, contraceptive, prevention of endometrial changes associated with estrogen replacement therapy (ERT), inoperable, recurrent, metastatic endometrial/renal cancer

Pharmacokinetics
Absorption	10% (PO)
Distribution	Breast milk
Metabolism	Liver
Excretion	Unknown
Half-life	14.5 hr

Pharmacodynamics
	PO	SC	IM
Onset	Unknown	Unknown	Unknown
Peak	Unknown	1 wk	Unknown
Duration	2-4 hr	3 mo	Unknown

CONTRAINDICATIONS
Pregnancy, hypersensitivity, reproductive cancer, genital bleeding (abnormal, undiagnosed), missed abortion, stroke, cerebrovascular disease, cervical cancer, hepatic disease, uterine/vaginal cancer

> **BLACK BOX WARNING:** Breast cancer, MI, stroke, thromboembolic disease, thrombophlebitis

Precautions: Breastfeeding, hypertension, asthma, blood dyscrasias, gallbladder disease, HF, diabetes mellitus, bone disease, depression, migraine headache, seizure disorders, renal/hepatic disease, family history of cancer of breast or reproductive tract, bone mineral density loss, ocular disorders, AIDS/HIV, alcoholism, children, hyperlipidemia, cardiac disease

> **BLACK BOX WARNING:** Use of this product has been shown to increase dementia in women ≥65 yr old; use may increase osteoporosis in long-term treatment, those at greater risk also smoke, adequate calcium and vitamin D should be taken

DOSAGE AND ROUTES
Secondary amenorrhea
Adult: PO 5-10 mg/day × 5-10 days, start during any time of the menstrual cycle

Uterine bleeding
Adult: PO 5-10 mg/day × 5-10 days starting on 16th or 21st day of menstrual cycle

---

With ERT
Adult: PO 5-10 mg qd × 10-14 or more days/mo (sequential estrogen); 2.5-5 mg qd (continuous estrogen)

Contraceptive
Adult (women): IM 150 mg q12wk (Depo-Provera); SUBCUT (depot SUBCUT 104 inj) 104 mg q3mo, give first dose during first 5 days of the menstrual period, only within the first 5 days postpartum (no breastfeeding), only sixth postpartum week (breastfeeding)

Endometrial/renal cancer inoperable recurrent metastatic
Adult: IM 400 mg-1 g (using 400 mg/ml depot inj susp) qwk

Endometriosis pain
Adult: SUBCUT 104 mg q12-14 wk, begin on day 5 of normal menses, avoid use >2 yr

Available forms: Tabs 2.5, 5, 10 mg; inj susp 50, 150, 400 mg/ml; 104 mg/0.65 ml

ADVERSE EFFECTS
CNS: Dizziness, *headache*, migraine, depression, fatigue, nervousness
CV: Thrombophlebitis, edema, thromboembolism, stroke, pulmonary embolism, MI
EENT: Diplopia
GI: *Nausea, increased weight*, cholestatic jaundice, *abdominal pain*
GU: *Amenorrhea*, cervical erosion, breakthrough bleeding, dysmenorrhea, vaginal candidiasis, breast changes, vaginitis, increased/decreased libido
INTEG: Acne, injection site reaction
META: Hyperglycemia
MS: Decreased bone density
SYST: Angioedema, anaphylaxis, breast cancer

INTERACTIONS
Individual drugs
Aminoglutethimide, carBAMazepine, phenytoin, PHENobarbital, rifampin: decreased contraceptive effect

Drug categories
Anticoagulants, corticosteroids: decreased bone mineral density
Strong CYP3A4 inhibitors (clarithromycin, ketoconazole, itraconazole, ritonavir, indinavir, voriconazole: Increased: medroxyprogesterone, avoid using together

Drug/herb
St. John's wort: Decreased levels, avoid using together

Drug/lab test
Increased: LFTs, HDL, triglycerides, coagulation tests, alkaline phosphatase, LDL
Decreased: GTT, pregnanediol, HDL

NURSING CONSIDERATIONS
Assessment
• **Menstrual history:** assess for duration of menses, bleeding, spotting, age of menstruation, regularity; start on any day in those with amenorrhea, or day 16 or 21 in dysfunctional bleeding
• Assess for symptoms indicating severe allergic reaction, angioedema; have EPINEPHrine and resuscitative equipment available
• Monitor B/P at beginning of treatment and periodically; check weight daily; notify prescriber of weekly weight gain >5 lb; bone mineral density
• Assess liver function tests: ALT, AST, bilirubin, baseline and periodically during long-term therapy

> **BLACK BOX WARNING:** Use of product shown to increase dementia in women ≥65 yr old; use may increase osteoporosis in long-term treatment; those who smoke also at greater risk; adequate calcium and vitamin D should be taken

> **BLACK BOX WARNING:** This product should not be given to those with breast cancer, MI, stroke, thromboembolic disorders

• **Bone mineral density loss:** Assess in those taking anticoagulants, corticosteroids with Depo-Provera or Depo-subQ Provera
• Assess mental status: affect, mood, behavioral changes, depression
• **Ectopic pregnancy:** Assess for severe abdominal pain, if patient becomes pregnant, may indicate ectopic pregnancy, which is a medical emergency

Patient problem
Impaired sexual functioning (uses)
Risk for injury (adverse reactions)

Implementation
PO route
• Give without regard to food
IM route
• Visually inspect particulate matter and discoloration prior to use
• Give titrated dose; use lowest effective dose; give oil sol deep in large muscle mass (IM); rotate sites; use after warming to dissolve crystals
Depo-Provera Contraceptive injection suspension:
• IM only, NEVER IV, use only 150 mg/ml vial

- Instruct patient on risks and warnings associated with hormonal contraceptives (see Patient Information)
- The possibility of pregnancy should be excluded prior to giving the first dose of medroxyprogesterone or whenever more than 14 weeks have passed since the last dose
- Do not dilute
- Shake vigorously immediately before administration
- Inject deeply into the gluteal or deltoid muscle. Aspirate prior to injection to avoid injection into a blood vessel

Depo-Provera Sterile Aqueous Suspension, preserved:
- IM only, NEVER IV
- Instruct patient on risks and warnings associated with progestin use (see Patient Information)
- Shake vigorously immediately before use
- When multidose vials are used, take special care to prevent contamination
- Inject deeply into the gluteal or deltoid muscle. Aspirate prior to injection

SUBCUT route
Depo-subQ Provera 104 Contraceptive Injection Suspension ONLY:
- For SUBCUT use only; NEVER give IM or IV
- Instruct patient on risks and warnings associated with hormonal contraceptives (see Patient Information)
- Shake vigorously for at least 1 min before use
- Inject the entire contents of the prefilled syringe subcut into the anterior thigh or abdomen, avoiding bony areas and the umbilicus. Gently grasp and squeeze a large area of skin in the chosen injection area, ensuring that the skin is pulled away from the body. Insert the needle at a 45-degree angle. Inject until the syringe is empty; this usually requires 5-7 seconds. Following use, press lightly on the injection site with a clean cotton pad for a few seconds; do not rub the area

Patient/family education
- Advise patients to avoid sunlight or use sunscreen; photosensitivity and melasma (brown patches on the face) can occur
- Teach patient about cushingoid symptoms: weight gain, moon face, buffalo hump, acne
- Teach women patients to report breast lumps, vaginal bleeding, edema, jaundice, dark urine, clay-colored stools, dyspnea, headache, blurred vision, abdominal pain, sudden changes in speech/coordination, numbness or stiffness in legs, chest pain; teach men to report impotence or gynecomastia

> **BLACK BOX WARNING:** Long-term use decreases bone density; exercise, calcium, vitamin D supplements can help lessen osteoporosis

- Advise patient that product doesn't protect against sexually transmitted disease, including HIV
- Advise patient that injection (SUBCUT) must be given every 3 mo for contraception, if dose is missed, pregnancy can occur
- Teach patient how to perform a breast self-exam, that if lumps are detected notify provider immediately
- Teach patient to take with food if nausea occurs
- Teach patient to have complete physical exam with reproductive exam, including mammogram, yearly
- Review package insert with patient, patient must understand all possible reactions
- Teach patient to report suspected pregnancy immediately; fertility returns in 6-12 mo after discontinuing; do not use in pregnancy, breastfeeding

Evaluation
Positive therapeutic outcome
- Decreased abnormal uterine bleeding
- Absence of amenorrhea
- Prevention of pregnancy
- Arrested spread of malignant cells

⚠ HIGH ALERT

megestrol (Rx)
(me-jess′trole)
Megace, Megace ES, Megase OS ✦
Func. class.: Antineoplastic hormone
Chem. class.: Progestin

ACTION: Affects endometrium by antiluteinizing effect; this is thought to bring about cell death, stimulates appetite by unknown action

Therapeutic outcome: Prevention of rapidly growing malignant cells; weight gain, increased appetite in AIDS

USES: Breast, endometrial cancer; increased weight, decreased cachexia and anorexia associated with AIDS

Pharmacokinetics

Absorption	Well absorbed; food increases oral sol
Distribution	Unknown
Metabolism	Liver, completely
Excretion	Feces, urine
Half-life	13-105 hr

Pharmacodynamics

Onset	Several wk to mo
Peak	Unknown

CONTRAINDICATIONS
Pregnancy, hypersensitivity

Precautions: Diabetes, thrombosis, adrenal insufficiency

DOSAGE AND ROUTES
Endometrial/ovarian carcinoma (palliative)
Adult: PO 40-320 mg/day in divided doses

Breast carcinoma
Adult: PO 40 mg qid or 160 mg/day

Available forms: Tabs 20, 40, 160 ✦ mg; oral susp 40, 125 mg/ml

ADVERSE EFFECTS
CNS: Mood swings, insomnia, fever, lethargy, depression
CV: Thrombophlebitis, thromboembolism, hypertension
ENDO: Adrenal insufficiency
GI: Nausea, vomiting, *diarrhea*, abdominal cramps, *weight gain*, flatus, indigestion
GU: Gynecomastia, fluid retention, vaginal bleeding, discharge, *impotence*, decreased libido, menstruation disorders
INTEG: Alopecia, *rash*, pruritus
MISC: Tumor flare, leukopenia

INTERACTIONS
Individual drugs
Dofetilide: Serious arrhythmias, avoid using concurrently
Indinavir: Decrease effect of indinavir, may need to increase dose

Drug/lab test
Increased: glucose

NURSING CONSIDERATIONS
Assessment
• PSA levels in men (prostate cancer); blood glucose, liver function studies, serum calcium, weight
• Monitor effects of alopecia on body image; discuss feelings about body changes
• Monitor for frequency of stools, characteristics, cramping, acidosis, signs of dehydration (poor skin turgor, decreased urine output, dry skin, restlessness, weakness, rapid respirations)
• In AIDS patients monitor calorie counts, weight, appetite
• **Assess for thrombophlebitis:** Pain, redness, swelling in calf, thigh; notify prescriber immediately if these occur
• **Pregnancy/breastfeeding:** Do not use in pregnancy, breastfeeding
• Beers: Avoid in older adults for an appetite stimulant, minimal effect on weight, increased risk of thrombotic events

Patient problem
Excess food intake (uses)

Implementation
• Administer with meals for GI symptoms
• Oral susp is usually used for AIDS patients; shake well
• Give tablets for carcinoma
• Give without regard to food

Patient/family education
• Teach patient to report any complaints or side effects to prescriber
• Explore with patient the need for wig or a hairpiece for hair loss
• Caution patient to report vaginal bleeding to prescriber
• Review with patient the need to comply with dosage schedule, not to miss or double doses; missed doses may be taken up to 1 hr before next dose
• Teach patient how to recognize signs of fluid retention, thromboembolism and report immediately
• Teach that gynecomastia and alopecia can occur; reversible after discontinuing treatment
• Advise to monitor blood glucose if diabetic
• Advise patient that contraceptive measures must be used during and 4 mo after treatment; product is teratogenic

Evaluation
Positive therapeutic outcome
• Decreased spread of malignant cells
• Weight gain, increased appetite in AIDS patients
• Resolved dysfunctional uterine bleeding

meloxicam (Rx)

(mel-ox′ i-kam)
Mobic, Mobicox
Func. class.: Nonsteroidal antiinflammatory/nonopioid analgesic (NSAIDs)
Chem. class.: Oxicam

ACTION: Inhibits COX-1, COX-2 by blocking arachidonate; analgesic, antiinflammatory, antipyretic effects

Therapeutic outcome: Decreased pain, swelling of joints, improved mobility

USES: Osteoarthritis, rheumatoid arthritis, juvenile arthritis

Pharmacokinetics

Absorption	Unknown
Distribution	Protein binding 99.4%
Metabolism	Liver 50%
Excretion	Breast milk, kidneys, feces
Half-life	15-20 hr

Pharmacodynamics

	PO	IM
Onset	Unknown	Unknown
Peak	4-5 hr	50 min
Duration	Unknown	Unknown

CONTRAINDICATIONS

Labor and delivery, breastfeeding, hypersensitivity, asthma, severe renal/hepatic disease, peptic ulcer disease, CV bleeding

> **BLACK BOX WARNING:** Perioperative pain in CABG surgery

PRECAUTIONS: Pregnancy, children, geriatric, bleeding/GI/cardiac disorders, hypersensitivity to other antiinflammatory agents, CCr <25 ml/min

> **BLACK BOX WARNING:** GI bleeding, MI, stroke

DOSAGE AND ROUTES

Adult: PO 7.5 mg/day, may increase to 15 mg/day; max 15 mg/day

Juvenile rheumatoid arthritis
Child >2 yr: PO 0.125 mg/kg, max 7.5 mg q Day

Available forms: Tabs 7.5, 15 mg; susp 7.5 mg/5 ml

ADVERSE EFFECTS

CNS: Dizziness, drowsiness, tremors, headache, nervousness, malaise, fatigue, insomnia, depression, seizures
CV: Hypertension, angina, cardiac failure, MI, hypotension, palpitations, dysrhythmias, tachycardia, stroke
EENT: Tinnitus, hearing loss, blurred vision
GI: Pancreatitis, nausea, colitis, GERD, vomiting, diarrhea, constipation, flatulence, cramps, dry mouth, peptic ulcer, GI bleeding, perforation, jaundice
GU: Nephrotoxicity: dysuria, hematuria, oliguria, azotemia
HEMA: Blood dyscrasias, anemia, prolonged bleeding
INTEG: Rash, urticaria, photosensitivity
SYST: Angioedema, anaphylaxis, Stevens-Johnson syndrome, toxic epidermal necrolysis

INTERACTIONS

Individual drugs
Cholestyramine: decreased action of meloxicam
CycloSPORINE, tacrolimus: increased nephrotoxicity
Lithium, methotrexate: increased action of each of these

Drug classifications
Aminoglycosides, anticoagulants, diuretics: increased action of each specific product
Adrenergic blockers, ACE inhibitors, thiazides, other antihypertensives: decreased action of β-blockers
Salicylates, sulfonamides: increased action of meloxicam

Drug/herb
Feverfew, ginko: decreased meloxicam effect
Garlic: increased bleeding risk

NURSING CONSIDERATIONS

Assessment
• Monitor renal, liver, blood tests: BUN, creatinine, AST, ALT, Hgb before treatment, periodically thereafter

> **BLACK BOX WARNING:** Check for GI bleeding, perforation, stool guaiac

Assess for anaphylaxis and angioedema; emergency equipment should be nearby
Fatal fulminant hepatitis, hepatic necrosis, hepatic failure: Assess for jaundice, yellow sclera and skin, clay-colored stools; monitor for liver function studies; hepatic reactions are more common in those with liver disease

---

- Assess for audiometric, ophth exam before, during, after treatment

> **BLACK BOX WARNING:** Assess for hypertension, MI, stroke, cardiac conditions

Patient problems
- Lack of knowledge of medication (teaching)
- Impaired mobility (uses)
- Pain (uses)

Implementation
- May take without regard to meals; take with food for GI upset
- Take with full glass of water and sit upright for 1/2 hr
- Store at room temperature

Patient/family education
- Advise patient to report blurred vision or ringing, roaring in ears (may indicate toxicity)
- Advise patient to avoid driving, other hazardous activities if dizziness or drowsiness occurs
- Teach patient to report change in urine pattern, weight increase, edema, pain increase in joints, fever, blood in urine (indicates nephrotoxicity); to report rash, black stools, or continuing headache
- Teach patient to not use alcohol, aspirin, acetaminophen without consulting prescriber
- Advise to report use to all health care providers

Evaluation
Positive therapeutic outcome
- Decreased pain, stiffness, swelling in joints; able to move more easily

> ### ⚠ HIGH ALERT
>
> # melphalan (Rx)
> (mel′fa-lan)
> **Alkeran, Evomela**
> *Func. class.:* Antineoplastic, alkylating agent
> *Chem. class.:* Nitrogen mustard

Do not confuse: melphalan/myleran, **Alkeran**/LeuKeran

ACTION: Responsible for cross-linking DNA strands leading to cell death; activity is not cell cycle phase specific

Therapeutic outcome: Prevention of rapidly growing malignant cells

USES: Multiple myeloma, advanced ovarian cancer

Absorption	Variable; incompletely absorbed
Distribution	Rapidly distributed, protein binding ≤ 30%
Metabolism	Bloodstream
Excretion	Kidneys, unchanged (10%)
Half-life	2 hr

	PO	IV
Onset	5 days	Unknown
Peak	2-3 wk	2-3 wk
Duration	Up to 6 wk	Up to 6 wk

CONTRAINDICATIONS
Pregnancy, breastfeeding, hypersensitivity to this product

Precautions: Children, radiation therapy, infection, renal disease

> **BLACK BOX WARNING:** Bone marrow depression, secondary malignancy, radiation therapy: requires an experienced clinician, bleeding, infection, risk of serious hypersensitivity reactions

DOSAGE AND ROUTES
Multiple myeloma (palliative)
Adult: PO 6 mg qday × 2-3 wk, or 10 mg qday × 7-10 days, stop for ≤ 4 wk or until WBC/platelets begin to rise, maintenance 2 mg qday then 2 mg/day when WBC >4000 cells/mm³ and platelets >100,000 cells/mm³, adjust daily between 1 and 3 mg/day based on response or 0.15 mg/kg/day × 7 days, then a rest period of ≥ 14 days, maintenance ≤ 0.05 mg/kg/day or 0.25 mg/kg/day × 4 days repeat q4-6 wk
Adult: IV INF 16 mg/m²; give over 15-20 min; give at 2-wk intervals × 4 doses, then at 4-wk intervals

Ovarian carcinoma (palliative)
Adult: PO 0.2 mg/kg/day × 5 days repeat q4-5wk depending on blood counts

Available forms: Tabs 2 mg; powder for inj 50 mg

Multiple myeloma conditioning treatment before stem cell transplantation (Evomela only)
Adult: IV infusion 100 mg/m²/day over 30 min for 2 days before stem cell transplantation (day 3, day 2; day 0 (transplant); >130% of ideal body weight or renal disease BUN >30 mg/day, reduce dose by 50%

ADVERSE EFFECTS

GI: *Nausea, vomiting, stomatitis, diarrhea,* hepatotoxicity, abdominal pain, anorexia, *constipation*

GU: *Amenorrhea,* hyperuricemia, gonadal suppression, infertility

HEMA: Thrombocytopenia, neutropenia, leukopenia, anemia

INTEG: Pruritus, necrosis, extravasation, alopecia, rash

RESP: Dyspnea, *pneumonitis,* bronchospasm

SYST: Anaphylaxis, allergic reaction, secondary malignancies, edema

CNS: Fatigue, fever, dizziness

META: *Hypokalemia, hypophosphatemia*

ENDO: Menstrual irregularities

INTERACTIONS
Individual drugs
CycloSPORINE: increased renal failure risk, monitor renal studies

Radiation: increased toxicity

Drug classifications
Anticoagulants, NSAIDs, salicylates, thrombolytics, platelet inhibitors: increased bleeding risk, avoid concurrent use

Antineoplastics: increased toxicity

Live virus vaccines: increased adverse reactions; decreased antibody reaction, bring up to date before use

Drug/lab test
Increase: uric acid 5-HIAA

Decrease: Hgb, RBC, WBC, platelets

False-positive: direct Coombs test

NURSING CONSIDERATIONS
Assessment

> **BLACK BOX WARNING: Bone marrow suppression:** Monitor full nadir 2-3 wk; CBC, differential, platelet count weekly; notify prescriber; withhold product if WBC is <3000/mm^3 or platelet count is <100,000/mm^3; notify prescriber; recovery usually occurs in 6 wk, IV product causes more myelosuppression

> **BLACK BOX WARNING:** Requires an experienced clinician; product should be used only by clinician knowledgeable in use of chemotherapy

> **BLACK BOX WARNING: Infection:** monitor for cold, fever, chills, sore throat, notify health care professional if these occur

• **Assess for bleeding:** hematuria, guaiac, bruising or petechiae, from mucosa or orifices; no rectal temp or IM injections if possible

> **BLACK BOX WARNING:** Assess for symptoms indicating severe allergic reaction: rash, pruritus, urticaria, purpuric skin lesions, itching, flushing; assess allergy to chlorambucil; cross-sensitivity may occur

• **Gout:** Assess for increased uric acid, joint pain especially in extremities; provide fluids to 2 L/day; may use anti-gout medications such as allopurinol

• **Secondary malignancy:** May cause acute leukemia, myeloproliferative syndrome, may occur due to chromosomal change, risk in long-term use

• **Pregnancy/breastfeeding:** Do not use in pregnancy/breastfeeding

Patient problems
Risk of infection (adverse reactions)

Risk for injury (adverse reactions)

Implementation
• Give fluids **IV** or PO before chemotherapy to hydrate patient

• Give antacid before oral agent; give product after evening meal, before bedtime; provide antiemetic 30-60 min before giving product and prn to prevent vomiting; give antibiotics for prophylaxis of infection

• Give in AM so product can be eliminated before bedtime

PO route
• Give 1 hr before or 2 hr after meals to prevent nausea/vomiting

• Protect from light, store refrigerated

Intermittent IV INF route
• Use gloves during administration; if skin exposure occurs, wash immediately with soap and water, use cytotoxic handling procedures

Evomela
Reconstitution:
• Add 8.6 ml of 0.9% sodium chloride injection to the vial for a final vial concentration of 5 mg/ml

• Negative pressure should be present in the vial; discard any vial that does not have a vacuum present during reconstitution

• **Storage after reconstitution:** Store at room temperature for up to 1 hr or refrigerated up to 24 hr

IV infusion:
• Dilute the appropriate dose with 0.9% sodium chloride to a final concentration not to exceed 0.45 mg/ml

• The diluted solution may be stored at room temperature for up to 4 hr (in addition to 1 hr after reconstitution)

• Administer IV over 30 min when used as conditioning treatment before an autologous stem

cell transplant or IV over 15 to 20 min when used as palliative treatment in multiple myeloma patients
• Infuse into an injection port or by injecting slowly into a fast-running IV infusion via a central venous line to avoid extravasation

Alkeran and generic melphalan
Reconstitution:
• Using a 20-gauge or larger needle, rapidly inject 10 ml of the supplied diluent into a 50-mg vial for a final vial concentration of 5 mg/ml
• Immediately shake the vial well until the solution becomes clear and all material is dissolved
• Dilute the reconstituted vial immediately; the solution is unstable
• Do NOT refrigerate the reconstituted vial; a precipitate forms if the solution is stored at 5° C
IV infusion:
• Dilute the appropriate dose in 0.9% sodium chloride to a final concentration not to exceed 0.45 mg/ml
• Administer IV over 15 to 20 min; do NOT give over less than 15 min, and complete the infusion within 60 min from vial reconstitution
• The diluted solution is unstable; about 1% of the labeled dose hydrolyzes every 10 min after dilution with sodium chloride
• Infuse through a central line to avoid extravasation

Y-site compatibilities: Acyclovir, amikacin, aminophylline, ampicillin, aztreonam, bleomycin, bumetanide, buprenorphine, butorphanol, calcium gluconate, CARBOplatin, carmustine, ceFAZolin, cefepime, cefoperazone, cefotaxime, cefoTEtan, cefTAZidime, ceftizoxime, cefTRIAXone, cefuroxime, cimetidine, CISplatin, clindamycin, cyclophosphamide, cytarabine, dacarbazine, DACTINomycin, DAUNOrubicin, dexamethasone, diphenhydrAMINE, DOXOrubicin, doxycycline, droperidol, enalaprilat, etoposide, famotidine, floxuridine, fluconazole, fludarabine, fluorouracil, furosemide, gallium, ganciclovir, gentamicin, granisetron, haloperidol, heparin, hydrocortisone sodium phosphate, hydromorphone, hydrOXYzine, IDArubicin, ifosfamide, imipenem-cilastatin, LORazepam, mannitol, mechlorethamine, meperidine, mesna, methylPREDNISolone, metoclopramide, methotrexate, metroNIDAZOLE, miconazole, minocycline, mitoMYcin, mitoXANtrone, morphine, nalbuphine, netilmicin, ondansetron, pentostatin, piperacillin, plicamycin, potassium chloride, prochlorperazine, promethazine, ranitidine, sodium bicarbonate, streptozocin, teniposide, thiotepa, ticarcillin, ticarcillin/clavulanate, tobramycin, trimethoprim/sulfamethoxazole, vancomycin, vinBLAStine, vinCRIStine, vinorelbine, zidovudine

Patient/family education
• Teach patient to avoid use of products containing aspirin or ibuprofen; nausea/vomiting, dehydration, decreased urine output; to report symptoms of bleeding (hematuria, tarry stools)
• Instruct patient to report signs of anemia (fatigue, headache, irritability, faintness, shortness of breath)
• **Hepatotoxicity:** Teach patient to report immediately yellowing of skin, eyes; dark urine; clay-colored stools; itchy skin; abdominal pain; fever; diarrhea
• Instruct patient to report any changes in breathing or coughing even several mo after treatment; to avoid crowds and persons with respiratory tract or other infections
• Tell patient hair loss is common; discuss the use of wigs or hairpieces
• Caution patient not to have any vaccinations without the advice of the prescriber, serious reactions can occur
• Advise patient to report suspected pregnancy, that contraception is needed during treatment and for several mo after the completion of therapy

Evaluation
Positive therapeutic outcome
• Decreased size of tumor
• Decreased spread of malignancy

M

memantine (Rx)
(me-man′teen)
Ebixa ✦, **Namenda, Namenda XR**
Func. class.: Anti–Alzheimer's disease agent
Chem. class.: N-methyl-D-aspartate receptor antagonist

ACTION: Antagonist action of CNS NMDA receptors that may contribute to the symptoms of Alzheimer's disease

Therapeutic outcome: Improved mood, orientation, decreasing confusion

USES: Moderate to severe dementia in Alzheimer's disease

Pharmacokinetics

Absorption	Rapidly absorbed PO
Distribution	44% protein binding
Metabolism	Very little
Excretion	57%-82% excreted unchanged in urine
Half-life	60-80 hr

Pharmacodynamics

| Peak | 3-7 hr (tab) |
| | 9-12 hr (caps) |

CONTRAINDICATIONS
Hypersensitivity, children

Precautions: Pregnancy, breastfeeding, renal disease, seizures, severe hepatic disease, GU conditions that raise urine pH, renal failure

DOSAGE AND ROUTES
Adult: PO 5 mg/day, may increase dose in 5-mg increments ≥1-wk intervals over a 3-wk period; recommended target dose as 10 mg bid at week 4; **ext rel** 7 mg/day, increased by 7 mg ≥1 wk up to target dose of 28 mg/day

Renal dose
Adult: PO CC 5-29 ml/min, a target of 5 mg bid immediate release or 14 mg/day extended release

Available forms: Tabs 5, 10 mg; tab titration pak 5, 10 mg; oral sol 2 mg/ml, 10 mg/5 ml; cap ext rel 7, 14, 21, 28 mg

ADVERSE EFFECTS
CNS: *Dizziness, confusion,* headache
CV: Hypertension
GI: Vomiting, constipation, diarrhea
HEMA: Anemia
INTEG: Rash
MISC: Back pain, fatigue

INTERACTIONS
Individual drugs
Cimetidine, hydrochlorothiazide, nicotine, quiNIDine, ranitidine, triamterene: increased/decreased levels of both products, monitor for adverse reactions
Ergot, levodopa: increased effect of each, monitor for adverse reactions

Drug classifications
Drugs that make the urine alkaline (sodium bicarbonate, carbonic anhydrase inhibitors): decreased clearance
Use cautiously with amantadine, dextromethorphan, ketamine: reaction unknown

Drug/lab test
Increase: alkaline phosphatase
Decrease: HCT

NURSING CONSIDERATIONS
Assessment
• **Alzheimer's dementia:** Assess affect, mood, behavioral changes; hallucinations, confusion, attention, orientation, memory; monitor serum creatinine

Patient problems
Distorted thinking process (uses)
Risk for injury (adverse reactions)

Implementation
• Can be taken without regard to meals
• Give twice a day if dose >5 mg
• Dosage is adjusted to response no more than q1wk
• Provide assistance with ambulation during beginning therapy; dizziness may occur
• **Extended Release Caps:** Do not crush, chew, divide; swallow whole or open and sprinkle on applesauce
• When switching from immediate release product begin the ext rel the day after the last dose of immediate release product. Those on 10 mg bid should be switched to ext rel 28 mg q day

Patient/family education
• Advise to report side effects: restlessness, psychosis, visual hallucinations, stupor, loss of consciousness; indicate overdose
• Advise patient to avoid alcohol, nicotine
• Advise to use product exactly as prescribed; product is not a cure
• Teach patient to avoid OTC, herbal products unless approved by prescriber
• Teach patient that product doesn't cure Alzheimer's disease, but controls symptoms
• **Adverse reactions:** Patient may not be able to verbalize reactions

Evaluation

Positive therapeutic outcome
• Decrease in confusion, improved mood or ability to maintain function, even with no improvement in symptoms

---

⚠ HIGH ALERT

meperidine (Rx)
(me-per′i-deen)
Demerol
Func. class.: Opioid analgesic
Chem. class.: Phenylpiperidine derivative
Controlled substance schedule II

Do not confuse: meperidine/
HYDROmorphone/meprobamate/morphine,
Demerol/Dilaudid

ACTION: Depresses pain impulse transmission at the spinal cord level by interacting with opioid receptors

Therapeutic outcome: Relief of pain

USES: Moderate to severe pain, preoperatively, postoperatively, general anesthesia maintenance, sedation induction

Pharmacokinetics

Absorption	Well absorbed (IM, SUBCUT); 50% (PO), complete IV
Distribution	Widely distributed; crosses placenta; protein binding 65%-75%; toxic by-product accumulation can result from regular use or in renal disease
Metabolism	Liver, extensively to active/inactive metabolites
Excretion	Kidneys; breast milk
Half-life	3-4 hr

Pharmacodynamics

	PO	IM/SUBCUT	IV
Onset	15 min	10 min	immediate
Peak	1 hr	½-1 hr	5-7 min
Duration	2-4 hr	2-4 hr	2 hr

CONTRAINDICATIONS

Hypersensitivity, severe respiratory insufficiency, GI obstruction, ileus

Precautions: Pregnancy, breastfeeding, children, geriatric, addictive personality, increased ICP, respiratory depression, renal/hepatic disease, seizure disorder, abrupt discontinuation, chronic pain, cardiac disease, adrenal insufficiency, alcoholism, angina, anticoagulant therapy, asthma, atrial flutter, biliary tract disease, bladder obstruction, cardiac dysrhythmias, COPD, CNS depression, coagulopathy, constipation, cor pulmonale, dehydration, diarrhea, driving epidural use, geriatrics, GI obstruction, head trauma, heart failure, hypotension, hypothyroidism, ileus, IBS, IM/intrathecal/IV use, labor, myxedema/thrombocytopenia, MAOI therapy

> **BLACK BOX WARNING:** Coadministration with other CNS depressants, respiratory depression

DOSAGE AND ROUTES
Moderate to severe pain
Adult: PO/SUBCUT/IM 50-150 mg q3-4hr prn; IV cont. inf 15-35 mg/hr
Child: PO/SUBCUT/IM 1-1.8 mg/kg q3-4hr prn, max single dose 150 mg; IV cont. inf 0.5-1 mg/kg loading dose then 0.3 mg/kg/hr

Preoperative analgesia
Adult: IM/SUBCUT 50-100 mg 30-90 min before surgery

Child: IM/SUBCUT 1-2 mg/kg 30-90 min before surgery, max 100 mg

PCA
Adult: **IV** 10 mg, range 1-5 mg increments, lockout interval 6-10 min

Coadministration with other CNS depressants
Adult: PO/IM/SUBCUT/IV Reduce dose by 25%-50%

Renal dose
Adult: PO/SUBCUT/IM/IV, CCr 10-50 ml/min give 75% of dose; CCr <10 ml/min give 25%-50% of dose

Labor analgesia
Adult: SUBCUT/IM 50-100 mg given when contractions are regularly spaced, repeat q1-3hr prn

Available forms: Inj 10, 25, 50, 75, 100 mg/ml; tabs 50, 100 mg; oral solution 50 mg/5 ml

ADVERSE EFFECTS
CNS: Drowsiness, dizziness, confusion, headache, sedation, euphoria, increased ICP, seizures, serotonin syndrome
CV: Palpitations, bradycardia, hypotension, change in B/P, tachycardia (IV)
EENT: Tinnitus, blurred vision, miosis, diplopia, depressed corneal reflex
GI: Nausea, vomiting, anorexia, constipation, cramps, biliary spasm, paralytic ileus
GU: Urinary retention, dysuria
INTEG: Rash, urticaria, bruising, flushing, diaphoresis, pruritus
RESP: Respiratory depression
SYST: Anaphylaxis

INTERACTIONS
Individual drugs
Alcohol: increased respiratory depression, hypotension, sedation
Phenytoin: decreased meperidine effect
Procarbazine: fatal reaction, do not use together within 14 days

Drug classifications
CNS depressants, opioids, sedative/hypnotics, antipsychotics, skeletal muscle relaxants: increased effects, severe respiratory depression
CYP3A4 inhibitors (fluconazole, ketoconazole, itraconazole, clarithromycin, erythromycin, nefazodone, verapamil): Increased opioid toxicity, avoid using together
SSRIs, SNRIs, serotonin-receptor agonists, tricyclics, 5HT3 receptor antagonists: increased serotonin syndrome, increased neuroleptic malignant syndrome

> **BLACK BOX WARNING:** MAOIs: do not use for 2 wk before taking meperidine; may cause fatal reaction

Protease inhibitor antiretrovirals: increased adverse reactions

Drug/herb
Kava, hawthorn, lavender, valerian: Increased sedation

St. John's wort: increased CNS depression, avoid using together

Drug/lab test
Increased: amylase, lipase

NURSING CONSIDERATIONS
Assessment
• **Assess pain:** location, duration, intensity before and 1 hr (IM, SUBCUT, PO), 5-10 min **(IV)** after administration
• Assess that patient has not taken an MAOI within 14 days
• **Sex hormone change:** Assess for libido, changes in menstrual cycle, erectile dysfunction, infertility, if suspected, obtain androgen levels
• **Adrenal insufficiency:** Assess for anorexia, nausea, vomiting, decreased B/P, weakness; if suspected, obtain cortisol, sodium, potassium levels; if present do not abruptly withdraw, taper
• **Abrupt discontinuation:** Withdraw slowly, if stopped abruptly, assess for withdrawal
• Monitor BUN, serum creatinine
• **Opioids/benzodiazepine:** Use only if alternative products cannot be used, excessive sedation and death may occur
• Monitor B/P, pulse, respirations baseline and during use
• Assess renal function before initiating therapy; poor renal function can lead to accumulation of toxic metabolite and seizures
• **Serotonin syndrome:** When given with SSRI, SNRIs, and serotonin receptor agonists; monitor for hyperthermia, hypertension, rigidity, delirium, coma, symptoms may occur rapidly after a long period
• **Monitor VS after parenteral route; note muscle rigidity, product history, liver, kidney function tests, respiratory dysfunction:** respiratory depression, character, rate, rhythm; notify prescriber if respirations are <12/min, dose may need to be reduced by 25% or more
• Monitor CNS changes: dizziness, drowsiness, hallucinations, euphoria, LOC, pupil reaction; these are due to metabolite produced; CNS stimulation occurs with chronic or high doses
• Monitor allergic reactions: rash, urticaria

• **Bowel function:** Assess for constipation; increase fluids, bulk in diet; give stimulant laxatives if needed
• **Children:** Monitor for restlessness, changes in respirations may occur more frequently than in adult
• **Serotonin syndrome:** Report symptoms immediately
• Teach patient not to be used long term
• Pregnancy: Do not use in pregnancy until use in labor; do not breastfeed
• **Beers:** Avoid in older adults, especially in those with chronic disease; may cause neurotoxicity; monitor for delirium frequently

Patient problem
Pain (uses)
Risk for injury (adverse reactions)

Implementation
• Doses that are given regularly before pain returns are more effective
• Give with antiemetic if nausea, vomiting occur
• Administer when pain is beginning to return; determine dosage interval by patient response; continuous dosing of medication is more effective given prn
• Medication should be slowly withdrawn after long-term use to prevent withdrawal symptoms
• Store in light-resistant container at room temperature
PO route
• May be given with food or milk to lessen GI upset
• Syr should be mixed with 4 oz of water
• Do not use in severe respiratory insufficiency (PO)
• **Oral solution:** dilute in 4 oz water
IM/SUBCUT route
• Do not give if cloudy or a precipitate has formed
• Patient should remain recumbent for 1 hr after administration
• Inject IM into a large muscle mass; IM is preferred route for multiple injections

Direct IV route
• Give after diluting to 10 mg/ml or less with sterile water, 0.9% NaCl for inj; give slowly at ≤25 mg/min, over at least 5 min; rapid administration may cause respiratory depression, hypotension, circulatory collapse
• Have emergency equipment and opiate antagonist on hand
Intermittent IV infusion route
• Give after diluting to 1 mg/ml with D_5W, $D_{10}W$, dextrose/saline combinations, dextrose/Ringer's, inj combinations, 0.45% NaCl, 0.9% NaCl, Ringer's, LR; give by inf pump over 10-15 min; titrate according to response

Y-site compatibilities: Abelcet, acetaminophen, amifostine, amikacin, anidulafungin, atenolol, aztreonam, bumetanide, cefamandole, ceFAZolin, cefmetazole, cefotaxime, cefOXitin, cefoperazone, cefTAZidime, ceftizoxime, cefTRIAXone, cefuroxime, cladribine, clindamycin, diltiazem, diphenhydrAMINE, DOBUTamine, DOPamine, doxycycline, droperidol, erythromycin lactobionate, famotidine, filgrastim, fluconazole, fludarabine, gallium, gentamicin, granisetron, hydrocortisone, IDArubicin, regular insulin, imipenem/cilastatin, kanamycin, labetalol, lidocaine, melphalan, methyldopa, metoclopramide, metoprolol, metroNIDAZOLE, mezlocillin, minocycline ondansetron, oxytocin, PACLitaxel, penicillin G potassium, piperacillin, potassium chloride, propofol, propranolol, ranitidine, sargramostim, teniposide, thiotepa, ticarcillin, ticarcillin/clavulanate, tobramycin, vancomycin, verapamil, vinorelbine

Continuous intrathecal infusion route
• Use controlled-infusion device, an implantable controlled-microinfusion device is used for highly concentrated infusion, monitor for several days after implantation
• Infusion reservoir should only be filled by those fully qualified
• To prevent pain, depletion of reservoir should be avoided

Patient/family education
• Advise patients to avoid CNS depressants (alcohol, sedative/hypnotics) for at least 24 hr after taking this product
• Discuss with patient that dizziness, drowsiness, and confusion are common; to avoid getting up without assistance
• Discuss in detail with patient all aspects of the product, including its purpose and what to expect
• Caution patient to make position changes carefully to lessen orthostatic hypotension

Evaluation

Positive therapeutic outcome
• Decreased pain

TREATMENT OF OVERDOSE:
Naloxone 0.2-0.8 mg **IV** (caution in physically dependent patients), O_2, **IV** fluids, vasopressors

---

meropenem (Rx)
(mer-oh-pen′em)
Merrem IV
Func. class.: Antiinfective—miscellaneous
Chem. class.: Carbapenems

ACTION: Interferes with cell wall replication of susceptible organisms

Therapeutic outcome: Bactericidal action against the following: *Streptococcus pneumoniae,* group A β-hemolytic streptococci, *viridans* group streptococci, enterococcus; gram-negative organisms *Klebsiella, Proteus, Escherichia coli, Pseudomonas aeruginosa, Bacteroides fragilis, Bacteroides thetaiotaomicron,* bacterial meningitis (>3 mo old)

USES: *Acinetobacter, Aeromonas hydrophila, Bacteroides distasonis, Bacteroides fragilis, Bacteroides ovatus, Bacteroides thetaiotaomicron, Bacteroides uniformis, Bacteroides ureolyticus, Bacteroides vulgatus, Campylobacter jejuni, Citrobacter diversus, Citrobacter freundii, Clostridium difficile, Clostridium perfringens, Enterobacter cloacae, Enterococcus faecalis, Escherichia coli, Eubacterium lentum, Fusobacterium, Haemophilus influenzae* (beta-lactamase negative), *Haemophilus influenzae* (beta-lactamase positive), *Hafnia alvei, Klebsiella oxytoca, Klebsiella pneumoniae, Moraxella catarrhalis, Morganella morganii, Neisseria meningitidis, Pasteurella multocida, Peptostreptococcus, Porphyromonas asaccharolytica, Prevotella bivia, Prevotella intermedia, Prevotella melaninogenica, Propionibacterium acnes, Proteus mirabilis, Proteus vulgaris, Pseudomonas aeruginosa, Salmonella, Serratia marcescens, Shigella, Staphylococcus aureus* (MSSA), *Staphylococcus epidermidis, Streptococcus agalactiae* (group B streptococci), *Streptococcus pneumoniae, Streptococcus pyogenes* (group A beta-hemolytic streptococci), *Viridans streptococci, Yersinia enterocolitica;* appendicitis, bacteremia, intraabdominal infections, meningitis, peritonitis, skin/skin structure infections

Pharmacokinetics

Absorption	Complete
Distribution	Widely distributed to tissue, CSF
Metabolism	Liver
Excretion	Kidneys, unchanged 75%
Half-life	1 hr adult, child >2 yr; increased in renal disease

M

Pharmacodynamics

Onset	Rapid
Peak	Dose dependent
Duration	8 hr

CONTRAINDICATIONS

Hypersensitivity to meropenem, carbapenems: hypersensitivity to cephalosporins, penicillins

Precautions: Pregnancy, breastfeeding, geriatric, renal disease, seizure disorder, gram-negative infection, pneumonia, hypersensitivity to pneumonia

DOSAGE AND ROUTES

Intraabdominal infections (complicated appendicitis, peritonitis)
Adult/adolescent/child >50 kg: IV 1 g q8hr or 500 mg q6hr
Adolescent/child ≤50 kg/infant ≥3 mo: IV 20 mg/kg q8hr

Complicated skin and skin structure infections
Adult/adolescent/child >50 kg: IV 500 mg q8hr, 1 g q8hr for *Pseudomonas aeruginosa*, max 500 mg
Adolescent/child ≤50 kg/infant ≥3 mo: IV 10 mg/kg q8hr or 20 mg/kg q8hr for *Pseudomonas aeruginosa*, max 1 g

Bacterial meningitis
Adult: IV 2 g q8hr
Adolescent/child ≤50 kg/infant: IV 40 mg/kg q8hr, max 2 g

Renal dose
Adult: IV CCr 26-50 ml/min give dose q12hr; CCr 10-25 ml/min give ½ dose q12hr; CCr <10 ml/min give ½ dose q24hr

Available forms: Powder for inj 500 mg, 1 g

ADVERSE EFFECTS

CNS: Fever, somnolence, *seizures,* dizziness, *headache,* myoclonia, confusion
CV: Hypotension, tachycardia
ENDO: Hypoglycemia
GI: *Diarrhea, nausea, vomiting,* CDAD, hepatitis; thrush (pediatrics)
HEMA: Thrombocytopenia (renal disease)
INTEG: *Rash,* urticaria, *pruritus,* pain at inj site, phlebitis, erythema at inj site, DRESS
RESP: Apnea
SYST: Anaphylaxis, Stevens-Johnson syndrome, angioedema

INTERACTIONS
Individual drugs
Probenecid: increased meropenem levels, avoid concurrent use

Valproic acid: decreased effect of valproic acid, monitor for seizures

Drug/herb
Do not use acidophilus with antiinfectives; separate by several hours

Drug/lab test
Increased: AST, ALT, LDH, BUN, alkaline phosphatase, bilirubin, creatinine
Increase or decrease: INR, platelets, PT, PTT
False positive: direct Coombs' test, urine glucose

NURSING CONSIDERATIONS
Assessment
• **Infection:** Appearance of wound, urine, sputum, temperature, WBC, vital signs, stool baseline and periodically
• Complete C&S tests before beginning product therapy to identify if correct treatment has been initiated, may start treatment before results are received
• **Seizures:** may occur in those with brain lesions, seizure disorder, bacterial meningitis, or renal disease; stop product, notify prescriber if seizures occur, seizure threshold is lowered
• **Assess for allergic reactions, anaphylaxis:** rash, urticaria, pruritus, chills, fever, joint pain; angioedema may occur a few days after therapy begins; EPINEPHrine and resuscitation equipment should be available for anaphylactic reaction; identify if there has been hypersensitivity to penicillins, cephalosporins, beta-lactams: cross-sensitivity may occur, have emergency equipment nearby
• **DRESS:** Assess for rash, fever, swelling of face, lymphadenopathy; may lead to another organ system
• Monitor blood studies: AST, ALT, CBC, Hct, BUN, bilirubin, LDH, alkaline phosphatase, Coombs' test baseline and periodically if patient is on long-term therapy
• Assess bowel pattern daily; if severe diarrhea occurs, product should be discontinued; may indicate CDAD
• Monitor for bleeding: ecchymosis, bleeding gums, hematuria, stool guaiac daily if on long-term therapy
• **Assess for overgrowth of infection:** perineal itching, fever, malaise, redness, pain, swelling, drainage, rash, diarrhea, change in cough, sputum

Patient problem
Infection (uses)

Implementation

Direct IV route

• Monitor injection site for redness, inflammation, phlebitis periodically

• Reconstitute 500 mg or 1 g vials with 10, 20 ml of sterile water for inj respectively, shake to dissolve and let stand until clear (average conc 50 mg/ml) reconstituted sol may be stored for 3 hr at room temperature or 13 hr refrigerated, inject up to 1 g in 5-20 ml over 3-5 min

Intermittent IV infusion route

• Vials may be directly constituted with compatible inf fluid (NS, D_5W) to 2.5-50 mg/ml vials; vials with 0.9% NaCl can be stored up to 2 hr at room temperature, or 18 hr refrigerated, D_5W may be stored up to 1 hr at room temperature or up to 15 hr refrigerated, infuse over 15-30 min

Continuous IV infusion route (unlabeled)

• **3 g/day continuous IV infusion:** Constitute a 1 g vial according to manufacturer's recommendations; further dilute in 50 ml or 250 ml of NS and run over 8 hr for cont inf, administer a new infusion bag q8hr

• **4 g/day continuous IV infusion:** Constitute a 1 g vial according to manufacturer recommendations. Further dilute in 100 ml of NS and administer over 6 hr. For cont inf, administer a new infusion bag q6hr

• **3 g/day IV continuous infusion in ambulatory infusion pump with freezer packs:** Reconstitute 1 g vial according to manufacturer recommendations by adding 20 ml of NS into each vial. Add 3 g (60 ml) to a 100-ml medication cassette reservoir and bring the final volume to 100 ml (final concentration, 30 mg/ml) run over 24 hr

Y-site compatibilities: Alemtuzumab, aminocaproic acid, aminophylline, anidulafungin, argatroban, atenolol, atropine, azithromycin, bivalirudin, bleomycin, CARBOplatin, carmustine, caspofungin, cimetidine, CISplatin, cyclophosphamide, cycloSPORINE, cytarabine, DACTINomycin, DAPTOmycin, dexamethasone, dexmedetomidine, dexrazoxane, digoxin, diltiazem, diphenhydrAMINE, DOCEtaxel, doxacurium, DOXOrubicin liposomal, enalaprilat, eptifibatide, etoposide, etoposide phosphate, fluconazole, fludarabine, fluorouracil, foscarnet, furosemide, gallium, gatifloxacin, gemcitabine, gemtuzumab, gentamicin, granisetron, heparin sodium, HYDROmorphone, ifosfamide, insulin (regular), irinotecan, lepirudin, leucovorin, linezolid injection, LORazepam, mechlorethamine, methotrexate, metoclopramide, metroNIDAZOLE, milrinone, mitoXANtrone, morphine, nesiritide, norepinephrine, octreotide, oxaliplatin, oxytocin, PACLitaxel, palonosetron, pamidronate, pancuronium, PEMEtrexed, PHENobarbital, potassium acetate/chloride, rocuronium, teniposide, thiotepa, tigecycline, tirofiban, TNA (3-in-1) Total Nutrient Admixture, vancomycin, vasopressin, vecuronium, vinBLAStine, vinCRIStine, vinorelbine, voriconazole, zoledronic acid

Patient/family education

• Teach patient to report sore throat, bruising, bleeding, joint pain; may indicate blood dyscrasias (rare)

• Advise patient to contact prescriber if vaginal itching, loose foul-smelling stools, furry tongue occur; may indicate superinfection

• Advise patient to notify prescriber of diarrhea with blood or pus; may indicate CDAD

• Advise patient to avoid driving or other hazardous activities until response is known; dizziness may occur

• Teach patient to discuss with health care professional all OTC, Rx, herbals, supplements taken

• Pregnancy/breastfeeding: Identify if pregnancy is planned or suspected or if breastfeeding

Evaluation

Positive therapeutic outcome

• Absence of signs/symptoms of infection (WBC $<10,000/mm^3$, temp WNL, absence of red draining wounds)

• Reported improvement in symptoms of infection

• Negative C and S

TREATMENT OF ANAPHYLAXIS: EPINEPHrine, antihistamines, resuscitate if needed

---

mesalamine (Rx)

(me-sal'a-meen)
Apriso, Asacol ✦, Ascol 800 ✦, Asacol HD, Canasa, Delzicol, Lialda, Mesasal ✦, Mezavant ✦, Pentasa, Rowasa, Salofalk ✦, sfRowasa, Teva 5-ASA ✦

Func class.: GI antiinflammatory
Chem. class.: 5-Aminosalicylic acid

Do not confuse: Asacol/Os-Cal

ACTION: May diminish inflammation by blocking cyclooxygenase, inhibiting prostaglandin production in colon, local action only

Therapeutic outcome: Decreased cramping, pain in GI conditions

USES: Mild to moderate active distal ulcerative colitis, proctitis

Pharmacokinetics

Absorption	20%-30% (PO), 10%-25% (RECT)
Distribution	Unknown
Metabolism	Unknown
Excretion	Feces, unchanged
Half-life	PO 12 hr, rectal 1/2-1 1/2 hr

Pharmacodynamics

	PO	ER	Rectal
Onset	Unknown	2 hr	Up to 21 days
Peak	Unknown	8-12 hr	Unknown
Duration	Up to 8 hr	24 hr	24 hr

CONTRAINDICATIONS
Hypersensitivity to this product or salicylates, 5-aminosalicylates

Precautions: Pregnancy, breastfeeding, children, geriatric, renal disease, sulfite sensitivity, pyloric stenosis, GI obstruction

DOSAGE AND ROUTES
Treatment of ulcerative colitis
Adult: RECT 60 ml (4 g) at bedtime, retained for 8 hr × 3-6 wk; **del rel tab (Lialda)** 2.4-4.8 g/day × 8 wk; **del rel tab (Asacol)** 1.6 g × 6 wk; **cont rel cap (Pentasa)** 1 g qid up to 8 wk; **RECT SUPP** 500 mg bid retained for 1-3 hr × 3-6 wk until remission, may increase to tid if needed; **del rel cap (Delzicol)** 800 mg tid ×6 wk
Child ≥5 yr and 54-90 kg: PO Delzicol 27-44 mg/kg/day in divided doses × 6 wk, max 2.4 g/day
Child ≥5 yr and 33-53 kg: PO Delizocol 37-61 mg/kg/day in 2 divided doses × 6 wk, max 2 g/day
Child ≥5 yr and 17-32 kg: PO Delzicol 36-71 mg/kg/day in 2 divided doses × 6 wk, max 1.2 g/day

Maintenance of remission
Adult: PO (delayed release tabs: Asacol) 800 mg bid or 400 mg qid; **(delayed release caps: Apriso)** 1500 mg (4 caps) each AM; **(delayed release tabs: Lialda)** 2.4 g (2 tabs)/day with a meal; del rel cap **(Delzicol)** 800 mg bid

Treatment of ulcerative proctosig-moiditis
Adult: Rect Rowsa 4 g enema (60 ml) at bedtime retained for 8 hr × 3-6 wk

Treatment of Ulcerative Proctitis
Adult: Rect Rowsa 4 g enema (60 ml) at bedtime retained for 8 hr × 3-6 wk; **canasa insert** 1 suppository at bedtime, retain for 1-3 hr × 3-6 wk

Available forms: Rectal Susp 4 g/60 ml (Rowasa, ss Rowasa); del rel tabs 400 mg (Asacol); 800 mg (Asacol HD); ext rel tab 500 mg; ext rel cap 250 mg, 500 mg (Pentasa); del rel tab (Lialda) 1.2 g; 0.375 g (Apriso); rect supp 1000 mg; del rel cap (Delzicol) 400 mg; enema suspension 4 g/60 ml (sfRowasa)

ADVERSE EFFECTS
CNS: *Headache, fever, dizziness,* insomnia, asthenia, weakness, fatigue
CV: Chest pain, palpitations, pericarditis
GI: *Cramps, gas, nausea, diarrhea,* rectal pain, constipation, vomiting, pancreatitis
GU: Nephrotoxicity, interstitial nephritis
INTEG: *Rash, itching,* acne, Stevens-Johnson syndrome, hair loss
SYST: Anaphylaxis, acute intolerance syndrome, angioedema, DRESS

INTERACTIONS
Individual drugs
Azathioprine, mercaptopurine, thioguanine: increased action of each product
Lactulose: decreased mesalamine absorption

Drug/lab test
Increased: AST, ALT, alkaline phosphatase, LDH, GGTP, amylase, lipase, BUN, serum creatinine

NURSING CONSIDERATIONS
Assessment
• **Assess for GI symptoms:** cramping, gas, nausea, diarrhea, rectal pain, abdominal pain baseline and periodically; if severe, the product should be discontinued
• Assess for allergy to salicylates, sulfonamides, sulfites; if allergic reactions occur, discontinue product
• Assess renal function before, during treatment: BUN, creatinine periodically; increase fluids to maintain urine at ≥1200 ml/day to prevent crystalluria

Patient problems
Pain (uses)
Diarrhea (adverse reactions)

Implementation
PO route
• Give with full glass of water
• Do not break, crush, or chew del rel tabs
• **Lialda:** take with a meal
• **Apriso caps:** without regard to meals in AM
• **Delzicol caps:** give ≥1 hr before a meal or 2 hr after a meal
Rectal route (susp)
• Give at bedtime, retained until AM; empty bowel before insertion
• Store at room temperature

- Usual course of therapy is 3-6 wk
- Give after shaking bottle well

Patient/family education
- Teach patient that usual, initial course of therapy is 3-6 wk; to notify provider if symptoms do not improve after 2 mo of treatment, to continue to take even if feeling better, do not miss or take double doses, if a dose is missed take when remembered, if almost time for next dose skip it
- Advise patient to notify prescriber if abdominal pain, cramping, diarrhea with blood, headache, fever, rash, chest pain occur; product should be discontinued, rash, bruising, bleeding, fever, mouth sores
- Teach patient to notify health care professional of trouble breathing, rash, hives
- Advise patient to use rectal dose at bedtime, teach how to use
- Teach patient that follow-up exams and blood work will be needed, including possible proctoscopy or sigmoidoscopy
- Advise patient not to drive or engage in hazardous activities until response is known, dizziness may occur
- **Pregnancy/breastfeeding:** Identify if pregnancy is planned or suspected or if breastfeeding

Evaluation

Positive therapeutic outcome
- Absence of pain, bleeding from GI tract

mesna (Rx)
(mes' na)
Mesnex, Uromitexan ✤
Func. class.: Antidote
Chem class: Ifosfamide antidote

ACTION: Mesna forms bonds with urotoxic metabolites ifosfamide.

USES: For prophylaxis of ifosfamide-induced or cyclophosphamide-induced (unlabeled) hemorrhagic cystitis

Therapeutic response: Prevention of hemorrhagic cystitis

Pharmacokinetics

Absorption	Complete
Distribution	Unknown
Metabolism	Converted to mesna metabolite, binds to toxic metabolities
Excretion	Kidney (90%)
Half-life	0.36 hr (IV)

Pharmacodynamics

Onset	Rapid
Peak	Unknown
Duration	4 hr

CONTRAINDICATIONS
Hypersensitivity to this product of thiols

Precautions: Pregnancy, breastfeeding, children

DOSAGE AND ROUTES
Adults, adolescents, and children (unlabeled): IV Give mesna at a dosage of at least 20% of the ifosfamide dosage 15 minutes before ifosfamide use, then give the same dose 4 and 8 hr after ifosfamide use. Total daily mesna dosage is at least 60% of the ifosfamide dosage
Adults, adolescents, and children (unlabeled): IV, PO At the time of ifosfamide use, give a single dose of mesna IV at a dose of 20% of the ifosfamide dose, then mesna tablets equal to 40% of the ifosfamide dose 2 and 6 hr after each dose of ifosfamide. The total daily dose of mesna is 100% of the ifosfamide dose

Available forms: Tablets 400 mg, injection 100 mg/ml

SIDE EFFECTS
CNS: Drowsiness, dizziness, vertigo, headache
GI: Nausea, vomiting, anorexia, diarrhea
INTEG: Flushing, injection site reactions, flu-like symptoms
Interactions None known

Drug/lab test
False-positive: Urine ketones

NURSING CONSIDERATIONS
Assessment:
- **Hemorrhagic cystitis:** Assess for dysuria, hematuria, hemorrhage

Patient problems
Lack of knowledge of medication (uses)

Implementation
PO route
- Use at 2 and 6 hr after IV if used PO
- Patients who vomit within 2 hr of oral mesna should repeat the oral dose or receive an IV dose
- Give without regard to meals or food
- Mesna injection may be diluted 1:1 to 1:10 in carbonated cola drinks or chilled fruit juice, such as apple, grape, tomato, or orange juice for oral administration. Plain or chocolate milk has also been used. Because of the sulfur odor (rotten eggs) of the mesna injection, more dilute solutions may be better tolerated

IV route
- Visually inspect for particulate matter and discoloration prior to use
- Dilute to obtain a final concentration of 20 mg/ml
- May be given as a rapid IV infusion/bolus or as a continuous infusion
- Compatible with cyclophosphamide and ifosfamide in the same infusion fluid and may be admixed for continuous infusion
- Diluted solutions are stable for 24 hr at room temperature, 77° F (25° C). Multidose vials may be stored and used for up to 8 days

Patient/family education
- Discuss reason for product and expected results
- Each patient to report nausea, vomiting, diarrhea, painful urination, or blood in the urine
- Inform patient to be well-hydrated to clear product
- **Pregnancy/breastfeeding:** Identify if pregnancy is planned or suspected, or if breastfeeding

Evaluation
Positive therapeutic outcome
- Prevention of dysuria, hematuria, or hemorrhage

---

metaxalone (Rx)
(me-tax′ a-lone)
Skelaxin
Func. class.: Skeletal muscle relaxant, central acting

ACTION: May be related to sedative properties

Therapeutic outcome: Decreased spasticity of muscles

USES: Relaxation of skeletal muscles in musculoskeletal conditions

Pharmacokinetics

Absorption	Good (PO)
Distribution	Unknown
Metabolism	Liver, to metabolites
Excretion	Kidney
Half-life	2-3 hr

Pharmacodynamics

Onset	1 hr
Peak	2-3 hr
Duration	4-6 hr

CONTRAINDICATIONS
Hypersensitivity, severe hepatic/renal disease, drug-induced hemolytic anemia or other anemias

Precautions: Pregnancy, breastfeeding, renal/hepatic disease, children <12 yr, seizure disorder, geriatrics

DOSAGE AND ROUTES
Adult: PO 800 mg tid-qid

Available forms: Tabs 800 mg

ADVERSE EFFECTS
CNS: *Dizziness, weakness, fatigue, drowsiness,* headache, disorientation, insomnia, paresthesias, tremors, CNS depression, impaired cognition, memory loss, insomnia, somnolence
CV: Hypotension, bradycardia, flushing, orthostatic edema, mydriasis, tinnitus
GI: *Nausea,* constipation, vomiting, abdominal pain, dry mouth, anorexia, weight gain
GU: Urinary frequency, hematuria
INTEG: Rash, pruritus
RESP: Dyspnea

INTERACTIONS

Individual drugs
Alcohol: CNS depression

Drug classifications
Antidepressants (tricyclics), antihistamines, barbiturates, MAOIs, opioids, sedative/hypnotics: increased CNS depression, avoid concurrent use
Antihypertensives: increased hypotension

Drug/herb
Kava, valerian, chamomile: increased CNS depression

Drug/lab test
Increased: AST, ALT, alkaline phosphatase, blood glucose, CK

NURSING CONSIDERATIONS
- **Multiple sclerosis:** spasms, spasticity, ataxia, mobility, improvement should occur
- Monitor B/P, weight, blood glucose, and hepatic function periodically
- **Withdrawal symptoms:** Agitation, tachycardia, insomnia, hyperpyrexia
- Check for increased seizure activity in patients with epilepsy; this product decreases seizure threshold; monitor ECG

• Check I&O ratio; check for urinary retention, frequency, hesitancy
• Allergic reactions: rash, fever, respiratory distress; severe weakness, numbness in extremities
• Assess CNS depression: dizziness, drowsiness, psychiatric symptoms
• Check dosage, as individual titration is required
• Assess for CNS depression, dizziness, drowsiness, psychiatric symptoms
• **Pregnancy/breastfeeding:** Use in pregnancy only if benefits outweigh fetal risk, avoid breastfeeding, excretion unknown

Patient problems
Pain (uses)
Impaired mobility (uses)

Implementation
PO route
• Give without regard to meals. Use with food may enhance CNS depression

Patient/family education
• Advise patient not to discontinue medication quickly; hallucinations, spasticity, tachycardia will occur; product should be tapered off over 1-2 wk, especially intrathecal form
• Advise patient not to take with alcohol, other CNS depressants
• Teach patient to avoid hazardous activities if drowsiness, dizziness occurs; to rise slowly to prevent orthostatic hypotension
• Teach patient to avoid using OTC medications: cough preparations, antihistamines, unless directed by prescriber; to take with food or milk
• Teach patient to notify prescriber if nausea; headache; tinnitus; insomnia; confusion; constipation; or inadequate, painful urination continues
• **Pregnancy/breastfeeding:** To notify if pregnancy is planned or suspected, avoid breastfeeding
• May require 1-2 mo for full response

Evaluation
Positive therapeutic outcome
• Decreased pain, spasticity, ability to perform ADLs

TREATMENT OF OVERDOSE:
Induce emesis of conscious patient, dialysis, physostigmine to reduce life-threatening CNS side effects

▲ HIGH ALERT

metFORMIN (Rx)
(met-for'min)
Fortamet, Glucophage, Glucophage XR, Glumetza, Glycon ✤, Riomet
Func. class.: Antidiabetic, oral
Chem. class.: Biguanide

Do not confuse: metFORMIN/metroNI-DAZOLE

ACTION: Inhibits hepatic glucose production and increases sensitivity of peripheral tissue to insulin

Therapeutic outcome: Blood glucose at normal levels

USES: Type 2 diabetes mellitus

Pharmacokinetics

Absorption	Unknown
Distribution	Unknown
Metabolism	Unknown
Excretion	Kidneys, unchanged (35%-50%)
Half-life	1½-6 hr

Pharmacodynamics

Onset	Unknown
Peak	1-2 hr (immediate rel); 7 hr (ext rel); 2.5 hr (sol)
Duration	Unknown

CONTRAINDICATIONS
Creatinine ≥1.5 mg/ml (males); diabetic ketoacidosis, metabolic acidosis, renal failure, radiographic contrast use

Precautions: Pregnancy, breastfeeding, geriatric, thyroid disease, previous HF, hypersensitivity; hepatic disease; alcoholism; cardiopulmonary disease; acidemia; acute MI; cardiogenic shock; renal disease, heart failure

BLACK BOX WARNING: Lactic acidosis

DOSAGE AND ROUTES
Type 2 diabetes mellitus
Adult: PO 500 mg bid or 850 mg/day initially, then 500 mg weekly or 850 mg q2wk up to 2000 mg/day in divided doses; dosage adjustment q2-3wk or 850 mg/day with morning meal with dosage increased every other week, max 2550 mg/day; ext rel (Glucophage XR) 500 mg qd with evening meal; may increase by 500 mg qwk, max

2000 mg/day; (Glumetza) 1000 mg qd with food, preferably with the PM meal, may increase by 500 mg qwk, max 2000 mg/day; (Fortamet) 500-1000 mg qd with PM meal, may increase by 500 mg qwk, max 2550 mg/day

Renal dose
Adult: PO eGFR 30-45 ml/min/1.73 m^2 avoid use, if >45 ml/min/1.73 m^2 then falls <45 ml/min/1.73 m^2 assess benefits/risks of treatment; discontinue if falls <30 ml/min/1.73m^2

Available forms: Tabs 500, 850, 1000 mg; ext rel tabs 500, 750, 850, 1000 mg; oral sol (Riomet) 500 mg/5 ml

ADVERSE EFFECTS
ENDO: Lactic acidosis
GI: Nausea, vomiting, diarrhea, heartburn, anorexia, metallic taste
MISC: Decreased vitamin B12

INTERACTIONS
Individual drugs
Cimetidine, digoxin, morphine, procainamide, quiNIDine, ranitidine, triamterene, vancomycin: increased metFORMIN level, monitor blood glucose
β-blockers, phenytoin: increased hyperglycemia
Digoxin: increased digoxin levels, monitor digoxin levels
Dofetilide: increased lactic acidosis, do not use together

Drug classifications
Calcium channel blockers, contraceptives (oral), corticosteroids, diuretics, estrogens, phenothiazines, sympathomimetics: increased hypoglycemia, monitor blood glucose

Drug/herb
Chromium, coenzyme Q-10 Garlic, green tea: increased hypoglycemia
Glucosamine: increased hyperglycemia

Drug/lab test
Decreased: Vitamin B$_{12}$

NURSING CONSIDERATIONS
Assessment
• Assess for hypoglycemic reactions (sweating, weakness, dizziness, anxiety, tremors, hunger), hyperglycemic reactions soon after meals; these occur rarely with this product, may occur when combined with other antidiabetics
• Monitor CBC (baseline, q3mo) during treatment; check liver function tests (AST, LDH) and renal tests (BUN, creatinine) periodically during treatment; glucose, A1c; folic acid, vitamin B$_{12}$ q1-2yr

• **Surgery:** product should be discontinued temporarily for surgical procedures when patient is NPO, or if contrast media is used; resume when patient is eating

> **BLACK BOX WARNING:** Monitor for **lactic acidosis:** malaise, myalgia, abdominal distress; risk increases with age, poor renal function; monitor electrolytes, lactate, pyruvate, blood pH, ketones, glucose; suspect in any diabetic patient with metabolic acidosis, with ketoacidosis; immediately stop product if hypoxemia, or significant renal dysfunction occurs; do not use in those >80 yr unless CCr is normal, alcohol use may increase lactic acidosis risk

Patient problem
Excess food intake (uses)
Nonadherence (teaching)

Implementation
• Monitor eGFR at least annually
• Do not use in dialysis
• Conversion from other oral hypoglycemic agents; change may be made without gradual dosage change; monitor serum or urine glucose and ketones tid during conversion
• **Immediate rel:** give twice a day with meals to decrease GI upset and provide best absorption
• Give immediate rel tabs crushed and mixed with meal or fluids for patients with difficulty swallowing
• **Extended release product:** may also be taken as a single dose; titrate slowly to therapeutic response, side-effect tolerance
• Do not break, crush, or chew ext rel tabs
• May be given with evening meal
• Store in tight container in cool environment
• **Oral solution:** Use calibrated spoon, oral syringe, or container to measure, give with meals

Patient/family education
• Teach patient to regularly self-monitor blood glucose using blood glucose meter
• Teach patient symptoms of hypo/hyperglycemia, what to do about each (rare)
• Advise patient that product must be continued on daily basis; explain consequence of discontinuing product abruptly
• Advise patient to take product in morning to prevent hypoglycemic reactions at night
• Advise patient to avoid OTC medications, alcohol unless approved by the prescriber
• Teach patient that diabetes is a lifelong illness; that this product controls symptoms, but does not cure the condition

---

- Teach patient to report adverse reactions if GI upset occurs, it decreases over time

> **BLACK BOX WARNING: Teach patient symptoms of lactic acidosis**—hyperventilation, fatigue, malaise, myalgia, chills, somnolence—and to stop product/notify prescriber immediately, not to use in excess with chronic alcohol intake

- Teach patient to carry/wear emergency ID and glucagon emergency kit for emergencies
- Advise patient that glucophage XR tab may appear in stool
- Advise patient to take with meals; not to break, crush, chew ext rel product
- **Pregnancy:** Teach patient that PCOS patients with insulin resistance may be at risk of pregnancy; to use adequate contraception if pregnancy is not desired, avoid using in pregnancy, do not breastfeed

Evaluation

Positive therapeutic outcome
- Decrease in polyuria, polydipsia, polyphagia; clear sensorium; absence of dizziness; stable gait; blood glucose, A1C at normal level

---

⚠ HIGH ALERT

methadone REMS (Rx)
(meth'a-done)
Dolophine, Metadol ✿, Metadol-D ✿, Methadose
Func. class.: Opioid analgesic
Chem. class.: Synthetic diphenylheptane derivative
Controlled substance schedule II

Do not confuse: methadone/methylphenidate

ACTION: Depresses pain impulse transmission at the spinal cord level by interacting with opioid receptors; produces CNS depression

Therapeutic outcome: Relief of pain; successful opioid withdrawal

USES: Severe pain, opiate withdrawal

Pharmacokinetics

Absorption	Well absorbed (PO, SUBCUT, IM)
Distribution	Widely distributed; crosses placenta, half as active PO, as inj, protein binding 90%
Metabolism	Liver, extensively
Excretion	Kidneys, breast milk
Half-life	15-25 hr; extended interval with continued dosing

Pharmacodynamics

	PO	IM/SUBCUT
Onset	½-1 hr	20 min
Peak	1-1.5 hr	1½-2 hr
Duration	4-12 hr	4-6 hr

CONTRAINDICATIONS
Hypersensitivity to this product, or hypersensitivity to chlorobutanol (inj route), asthma, ileus

> **BLACK BOX WARNING:** Respiratory depression

Precautions: Pregnancy, breastfeeding, children <18 yr, geriatric, addictive personality, increased ICP, MI (acute), severe heart disease, respiratory depression, renal/hepatic disease, respiratory insufficiency, torsades de pointes, pulmonary disease, COPD, seizures

> **BLACK BOX WARNING:** QT prolongation, pain, coadministration with other CNS depressants, IV use, pregnancy, requires an experienced clinician

DOSAGE AND ROUTES
Severe pain
Adult: PO 2.5 mg q8-12hr in opioid-naive, titrate; IV/IM/SUBCUT 2.5-10 mg q8-12hr in opioid-naive

Opiate withdrawal
Adult including pregnant women: PO 20-30 mg initially, unless low opioid tolerance is expected, additional 5-10 mg q2-4hr as needed after initial dose, if symptoms continue may give for up to 5 days

Opiate dependency
Adult, child <50 kg: PO 0.05-0.1 mg/kg/dose until withdrawal controlled, after 1-2 days lengthen dosing interval to q 12-24 hr, taper by 0.05 mg/kg/day; ≥50 kg IM/IV/subcut 15-40 mg q day, decreased dose q 1-2 days

Available forms: Inj 10 mg/ml; tabs 5, 10 mg; oral sol 5, 10 mg/5 ml/(concentrate); 10 mg/ml/(concentrate); dispersible tabs 40 mg

M

ADVERSE EFFECTS

CNS: *Drowsiness, dizziness, confusion, headache, sedation,* euphoria, seizures

CV: Change in B/P, hypotension, torsades de pointes, QT prolongation

EENT: Blurred vision, miosis, diplopia

GI: *Nausea, vomiting, anorexia, constipation*

GU: Urinary retention

ENDO: Adrenal insufficiency

INTEG: *Rash,* flushing, diaphoresis

RESP: Respiratory depression

MISC: Dependence, tolerance

INTERACTIONS
Individual drugs

Alcohol: increased respiratory depression, hypotension, sedation

Linezolid, methylene blue, mirtazapine, tramadol, trazodone: Increased serotonin syndrome

Nalbuphine, pentazocine, phenytoin, rifampin: decreased analgesia

Selegiline: do not use within 2 wk of methadone

Drug classifications

Antipsychotics, opiates, sedative/hypnotics, skeletal muscle relaxants: increased respiratory depression, hypotension

Benzodiazepines: Increased fatal reactions

Class IA antiarrhythmics (disopyramide, procainamide, quiNIDine), class III antiarrhythmics (amiodarone, bretylium, dofetilide, ibutilide, sotalol), astemizole, arsenic trioxide, bepridil, cisapride, chloroquine, clarithromycin, levomethadyl, pentamidine, some phenothiazines, pimozide, probucol, sparfloxacin, terfenadine: increased QT prolongation

CYP2C9 inducers, CYP2C19 inducers, CYP3A4 inducers (barbiturates, bosentan, carBAMazepine, efavirenz, phenytoins, nevirapine, rifabutin, rifampin): decreased methadone effect, withdrawal symptoms may occur

CYP2C9 inhibitors, CYP2C19 inhibitors, CYP2D6 inhibitors, CYP3A4 inhibitors (aprepitant, antiretroviral protease inhibitors, clarithromycin, danazol, delavirdine, diltiazem, erythromycin, fluconazole, FLUoxetine, fluvoxaMINE, imatinib, ketoconazole, mibefradil, nefazodone, telithromycin, voriconazole): increased toxicity

MAOIs: do not use for 2 wk before taking methadone: unpredictable reactions

SSRIs, SNRIs, MAOIs, tricyclics, 5-HT3 receptor antagonists: Increased serotonin syndrome

Drug/food

Avoid use with grapefruit juice

Drug/herb

Chamomile, hops, kava, valerian: increased CNS depression

St. John's wort: avoid use, withdrawal may result

Drug/lab test

Increased: amylase, lipase

NURSING CONSIDERATIONS
Assessment

• **Assess for pain:** type, location, intensity, grimacing before and 1½-2 hr after administration; use pain scoring

• Monitor VS after parenteral route; note muscle rigidity, product history, liver, kidney function tests

• Monitor CNS changes: dizziness, drowsiness, hallucinations, euphoria, LOC, pupil reaction

• Monitor allergic reactions: rash, urticaria

• Monitor opioid detoxification: no analgesia occurs, only prevention of withdrawal symptoms

> **BLACK BOX WARNING:** Monitor B/P, pulse, ECG: hypotension, palpitations may occur

• Monitor bowel changes; bulk, fluids, laxatives should be used for constipation

> **BLACK BOX WARNING: Respiratory dysfunction:** respiratory depression, character, rate, rhythm; notify prescriber if respirations <10/min, avoid use with other CNS depressants (benzodiazepines)

> **BLACK BOX WARNING: QT prolongation:** may be dose related or use with other products that increase QT, titrate dose carefully

> **BLACK BOX WARNING: Accidental exposure:** make sure product is not accessible to children, pets, may be fatal

> **BLACK BOX WARNING: Overdose, poisoning:** advise persons involved in correct use

> **BLACK BOX WARNING: Substance abuse:** may occur but has less psychological dependence than other opiate agonists

• **Beers:** Avoid in older adults unless safer alternatives are not available; may cause ataxia, impaired psychomotor function

Patient problem

Pain (uses)

Risk for injury (adverse reactions)

Implementation
• Medication should be slowly withdrawn after long-term use to prevent withdrawal symptoms
PO route
• When using during a methadone maintenance program, use only PO according to NATA guidelines
• May be given with food or milk to lessen GI upset
• Store in light-resistant container at room temperature
• PO is half as potent as parenteral
IM/SUBCUT route
• Do not give if cloudy or a precipitate has formed
• Give deeply in large muscle mass (IM); rotate inj sites
• Pain and induration may occur at site
• Protect from light
IV route
• Used as PCA
• Protect from light

Patient/family education
• Instruct patient to report any symptoms of CNS changes, allergic reactions, extreme sedation, trouble breathing; to avoid CNS depressants (alcohol, sedative-hypnotics) for at least 24 hr after taking this product
• Discuss with patient that dizziness, drowsiness, and confusion are common; to avoid getting up without assistance
• Discuss in detail with patient all aspects of the product
• Caution patient to make position changes slowly to prevent orthostatic hypotension
• Teach patient withdrawal symptoms may occur: nausea, vomiting, cramps, fever, faintness, anorexia
• Advise patient to maintain proper hydration, avoid alcohol use
• Teach patient to avoid use with other products without approval of prescriber; many drug interactions
• Teach patient to use exactly as directed, do not increase unless directed by prescriber
• Teach patient that drowsiness, dizziness may occur, not to perform hazardous tasks until effect is known, to ask for assistance when getting out of bed
• Teach patient that regular ECGs will be needed
• Teach patient to advise all providers of product taken
• **Pregnancy/breastfeeding:** Caution the patient not to use in pregnancy, breastfeeding

Evaluation
Positive therapeutic outcome
• Decreased pain
• Successful opioid withdrawal

TREATMENT OF OVERDOSE:
Naloxone (Narcan) 0.2-0.8 mg **IV**, O_2, **IV** fluids, vasopressors

mothimazole (℞)
(meth-im′a-zole)
Tapazole
Func. class.: Thyroid hormone antagonist
Chem. class.: Thioamide

Do not confuse: methimazole/metoprolol/minoxidil

ACTION: Inhibits synthesis of thyroid hormones by decreasing iodine use in the manufacture of thyroglobin and iodothyronine; does not affect already formed hormones, does not affect circulatory T_4, T_3

Therapeutic outcome: Decreased T_4 levels, hyperthyroid symptoms

USES: Hyperthyroidism, preparation for thyroidectomy

Pharmacokinetics

Absorption	Rapidly absorbed
Distribution	Crosses placenta
Metabolism	Liver, extensively
Excretion	Kidneys, unchanged; breast milk
Half-life	5-13 hr

Pharmacodynamics

Onset	Rapid
Peak	Peak 1-2 hr
Duration	4-6 hr

CONTRAINDICATIONS
Pregnancy, breastfeeding, hypersensitivity

Precautions: Infection, bone marrow depression, hepatic disease, bleeding disorders

DOSAGE AND ROUTES
Hyperthyroidism
Adult: PO 15 mg/day (mild hyperthyroidism); 30-40 mg/day (moderate-severe); 60 mg/day (severe); maintenance dosage 5-15 mg/day, may be divided
Child: PO 0.4 mg/kg/day in divided doses q8hr; continue until euthyroid; maintenance dosage 0.2 mg/kg/day in divided doses q8hr, max 30 mg/24 hr, may be divided

M

Preparation for thyroidectomy
Adult and child: PO same as above; iodine may be added for 10 days before surgery

Thyrotoxic crisis
Adult and child: 15-20 mg q 4 hr $\times$ 24 hr with other products

Available forms: Tabs 5, 10 mg

ADVERSE EFFECTS
CNS: *Drowsiness, headache, vertigo, fever,* paresthesias, neuritis
ENDO: *Enlarged thyroid*
GI: *Nausea, diarrhea, vomiting, jaundice,* hepatitis, loss of taste
GU: Nephritis
HEMA: Agranulocytosis, leukopenia, thrombocytopenia, hypothrombinemia, lymphadenopathy, bleeding, vasculitis
INTEG: *Rash, urticaria, pruritus, alopecia, hyperpigmentation,* lupuslike syndrome
MS: Myalgia, arthralgia, nocturnal muscle cramps

INTERACTIONS
Individual drugs
Amiodarone, potassium iodide: decreased effectiveness, methimazole dose may need to be increased
Digoxin: increased response, monitor digoxin level
Radiation: increased bone marrow depression
Warfarin: decreased anticoagulant effect, monitor coagulation studies

Drug classifications
Antineoplastics: increased bone marrow depression

Drug/lab test
Increased: pro-time, AST, ALT, alkaline phosphatase

NURSING CONSIDERATIONS
Assessment
• **Hyperthyroidism:** Assess for palpitations, nervousness/loss of hair, insomnia, heat intolerance, weight loss, diarrhea
• **Hypothyroidism:** Assess for constipation, dry skin, weakness, fatigue, headache, intolerance to cold, weight gain; adjustment may be needed
• Monitor pulse, B/P, temp; check I&O ratio; check for edema (puffy hands, feet, periorbititis); indicates hypothyroidism
• Check weight daily; same clothing, scale, time of day
• Monitor T_3, T_4, which are increased; serum TSH, which is decreased; free thyroxine index, which is increased if dosage is too low; discontinue product 3-4 wk before radioactive iodine uptake

• **Monitor blood studies:** CBC for blood dyscrasias (leukopenia, thrombocytopenia, agranulocytosis); if these occur, product should be discontinued and other treatment initiated; LFTs, may occur at higher doses >40 mg/day
• **Assess for hypersensitivity** (rash, enlarged cervical lymph nodes); product may have to be discontinued
• **Assess for hypoprothrombinemia** (bleeding, petechiae, ecchymosis)
• Monitor clinical response: after 3 wk should include increased weight, pulse, decreased T_4
• **Assess for bone marrow depression:** sore throat, fever, fatigue
• Check weight daily, same clothing, time of day, scale; weight increase or decrease is a sign of product need for adjustment
• **Pregnancy/breastfeeding:** May cause fetal harm, do not use in pregnancy, avoid use in breastfeeding

Patient problems
Risk for Injury
Nonadherence (teaching)

Implementation
• Give with meals to decrease GI upset; give at same time each day to maintain product level
• Give lowest dosage that relieves symptoms
• Store in light-resistant container
• Increase fluids to 3-4 L/day, unless contraindicated

Patient/family education
• Advise patient to abstain from breastfeeding after delivery; product appears in breast milk
• Instruct patient to take pulse daily; to keep graph of weight, pulse, mood
• Advise patient to report redness, swelling, sore throat, mouth lesions, which indicate blood dyscrasias
• Caution patient to avoid OTC products that contain iodine; that seafood and other iodine-containing products may be restricted by prescriber
• Caution patient not to discontinue this medication abruptly; thyroid crisis may occur; stress patient compliance
• Advise patient that response may take several mo if thyroid is large
• **Teach patient symptoms/signs of overdose:** periorbital edema, cold intolerance, mental depression; notify prescriber at once
• **Teach patient symptoms of inadequate dosage:** tachycardia, diarrhea, fever, irritability; prescriber should be notified to adjust

---

⚠ Nurse Alert   ✴ Key NCLEX® Drug   ≫ Drug Specifics

• Teach patient to take medication exactly as prescribed, not to skip or double doses; missed doses should be taken when remembered up to 1 hr before next dose
• Instruct patient to carry ID describing medication taken and condition being treated
• Teach patient to report yellowing of skin/legs, dark urine, anorexia, right upper abdominal pain, may indicate hepatic dysfunction

Evaluation

Positive therapeutic outcome
• Decreased weight gain
• Decreased pulse
• Decreased T_4
• Decreased B/P

methocarbamol (Rx)

(meth-oh-kar' ba-mole)
Robaxin, Robaximol ✚
Func. class.: Skeletal muscle relaxant, central acting
Chem. class.: Carbamate derivative

ACTION: Depresses multisynaptic pathways in the spinal cord, causing skeletal muscle relaxation

Therapeutic outcome: Decreased pain, spasm, resolution of tetanic spasms

USES: Adjunct for relief of spasm and pain in musculoskeletal conditions, tetanus

Pharmacokinetics

Absorption	Rapidly absorbed (PO)
Distribution	Widely distributed; crosses placenta
Metabolism	Liver, partially
Excretion	Kidney, unchanged
Half-life	1-2 hr

Pharmacodynamics

	PO	IM	IV
Onset	1/2 hr	Rapid	Rapid
Peak	1-2 hr	Unknown	Inf end
Duration	<8 hr	Unknown	Unknown

CONTRAINDICATIONS: Hypersensitivity to this product or PEG300 (inj), children <12 yr, intermittent porphyria, renal disease (IM/IV)

Precautions: Pregnancy, renal/hepatic disease, addictive personalities, myasthenia gravis, epilepsy

DOSAGE AND ROUTES

Muscle spasm
Adult: PO 1.5 g qid × 2-3 days, then 1 g qid; IM 500 mg in each gluteal region; may repeat q8hr; **IV** BOL 1-3 g/day max at 3 ml/min; **IV** INF 1 g/250 ml D5W or 0.9% NaCl, max 3 g/day
Geriatric: PO 500 mg qid, titrate to needed dose

Tetanus management
Adult: IV DIRECT 1-2 g or **IV** INF 1-3 g q6hr, max 3 g
Child: IV 15 mg/kg q6hr prn, max 1-8 g/m^2/day for 3 consecutive days, max 3 ml/min **IV**

Available forms: Tabs 500, 750 mg; inj 100 mg/ml

ADVERSE EFFECTS

CNS: *Dizziness*, *weakness*, *drowsiness*, syncope, flushing, headache, tremor, depression, insomnia, seizures (IV, IM only)
CV: Postural hypotension, *bradycardia*
EENT: Diplopia, temporary loss of vision, conjunctivitis, nasal congestion, blurred vision, nystagmus
GI: *Nausea*, vomiting, hiccups, anorexia, metallic taste, dyspepsia, jaundice
GU: Brown, black, green urine
HEMA: Hemolysis, increased hemoglobin, leukopenia (IV only)
INTEG: Rash, pruritus, fever, facial flushing, urticaria, phlebitis, extravasation
MISC: Anaphylaxis, angioneurotic edema (IM, IV)

INTERACTIONS

Individual drugs
Alcohol: increased CNS depression

Drug classifications
Antidepressants (tricyclic), barbiturates, opioids, sedative-hypnotics: increased CNS depression

Drug/herb
Chamomile, hops, kava, skullcap, St. John's wort, valerian: increased CNS depression

Drug/lab test
False increase: VMA, urinary 5-HIAA

NURSING CONSIDERATIONS

Assessment
• Assess for pain and spasm: location, duration, intensity, range of motion
• Assess blood studies: CBC, WBC differential, blood dyscrasias may occur

M

• Assess hepatic studies: AST, ALT, alk phos; hepatitis may occur; renal studies: BUN, creatinine with **IV** use

• Monitor during and after inj: CNS effects, rash, conjunctivitis, and nasal congestion may occur

• Monitor EEG in epileptic patients; poor seizure control has occurred in patients taking this product

• Assess allergic reactions: rash, fever, respiratory distress; check for severe weakness, numbness in extremities

• Assess for tolerance: increased need for medication, more frequent requests for medication, increased pain

• Assess for CNS depression: dizziness, drowsiness, psychiatric symptoms

Patient problems

• Risk for injury (adverse reactions)
• Lack of knowledge of medication (teaching)
• Impaired mobility(uses)

Implementation

• Methocarbamol incompatible with any product in sol or syringe

PO route

• Give with meals if GI symptoms occur
• Store in airtight container at room temperature

IM route

• Give inj deep in large muscle mass; rotate sites
• Do not give SUBCUT

Direct IV route

• Give undiluted over 1 min or more; give 300 mg or less 1 min or longer

Intermittent IV infusion route

• May be diluted in 250 ml or less D5 or isotonic NaCl sol for slow **IV** inf
• Give by slow **IV** to prevent phlebitis; keep recumbent during and for 15 min after to prevent orthostatic hypotension; check for extravasation

Patient/family education

• Advise patient not to discontinue medication quickly; insomnia, nausea, headache, spasticity, tachycardia will occur; product should be tapered off over 1-2 wk

• Inform patient that urine may turn green, black, or brown

• Caution patient not to take with alcohol, other CNS depressants; increased CNS depression can occur

• Advise patient to avoid altering activities while taking this product

• Caution patient to avoid hazardous activities if drowsiness, dizziness occur; driving should be avoided until product response is known

• Advise patient to avoid using OTC medications that are CNS depressants (cough preparations, antihistamines) unless directed by prescriber; CNS depression can occur

Evaluation

Positive therapeutic outcome

• Decreased pain, spasticity

TREATMENT OF OVERDOSE:
Dialysis; have EPINEPHrine, antihistamines, and corticosteroids available; enhance elimination with osmotic diuresis; **IV** fluids for hypotension

---

⚠ HIGH ALERT

methotrexate (Rx)

(meth-oh-trex′ate)
Metoject ✤, Rheumatrex, Trexall, Otrexup, Xatmep, Rasuvo
Func. class.: Antineoplastic, antimetabolite
Chem. class.: Folic acid antagonist

Do not confuse: methotrexate/ metolazone/MTX patch

ACTION: Inhibits an enzyme that reduces folic acid, which is needed for nucleic acid synthesis in all cells; cell cycle specific (S phase); immunosuppressive

Therapeutic outcome: Prevention of rapidly growing malignant cells; immunosuppression

USES: Acute lymphocytic leukemia, in combination for breast, lung, head, neck carcinoma, lymphoma, sarcoma, gestational choriocarcinoma, hydatidiform mole, psoriasis, rheumatoid arthritis, mycosis fungoides, osteosarcoma

Pharmacokinetics

Absorption	Well absorbed (GI)
Distribution	Widely distributed; crosses placenta
Metabolism	Not metabolized
Excretion	Kidneys, unchanged; breast milk (minimal)
Half-life	Terminal 10-12 hr; increased in renal disease

Pharmacodynamics

	PO	IM/IV	IT
Onset	Unknown	Unknown	Unknown
Peak	1-4 hr	½-2 hr	Unknown
Duration	Unknown	Unknown	Unknown

CONTRAINDICATIONS

Hypersensitivity, leukopenia ($<3500/mm^3$), thrombocytopenia ($<100,000/mm^3$), anemia, psoriatic patients with severe renal disease, alcoholism, HIV infection, AIDS

> **BLACK BOX WARNING:** Pregnancy, exfoliative dermatitis, bone marrow suppression

Precautions: Breastfeeding, children

> **BLACK BOX WARNING:** Renal disease, ascites, diarrhea, infection, intrathecal administration, lymphoma, pleural effusion, pulmonary toxicity, radiation therapy, stomatitis, tumor lysis syndrome, ascites, stomatitis, gastroenteritis, GI bleeding, perforation, hepatotoxicity, intrauterine fetal death, neurotoxicity, requires experienced clinician

DOSAGE AND ROUTES

Acute lymphocytic leukemia

Adult and child: PO/IM/IV 3.3 mg/m^2/day × 4-6 wk until remission with prednisone 60 mg/m^2/day, then 20-30 mg/m^2 PO/IM qwk in 2 divided doses or 2.5 mg/kg IV q2wk; **IT adult** 12 mg/m^2; **child ≥3 yr** 12 mg; **2 yr** 10 mg; **1 yr** 8 mg; **<1 yr** 6 mg

Burkitt's lymphoma (stages I, II, III) (unlabeled)

Adult: PO 10-25 mg/day × 4-8 days with 7-day rest period

Child ≥3 yr: intrathecally 12 mg q2-5days; **child 2-3 yr** 10 mg q2-5days; **child 1-2 yr:** 8 mg q2-5days

Meningeal leukemia

Adult: 12 mg/m^2 IT q2-5days until CSF is normal, then one additional dose, max 15 mg

Choriocarcinoma, hydatidiform mole

Adult and child: PO/IM 15-30 mg/kg/day × 5 days, then off 1 wk; may repeat 1 wk × 5 courses

Breast cancer

Adult: IV 40-60 mg/m^2 on day 1 of every 21-28 days with other antineoplastics

Epidermal head/neck cancer

Adult/child: IV 40 mg/m^2 on days 1 and 15, q21 days alone or in combination with bleomycin, CISplatin

Adult: PO 25-50 mg/m^2 q7 days

Child: PO 7.5-30 mg/m^2 q7-14 days

Rheumatoid arthritis

Adult: PO 7.5 mg/wk or divided doses of 2.5 mg q12hr × 3 dose qwk, max 20 mg/wk

Polyarticular-course juvenile RA

Child: PO/IM 10 mg/m^2 qwk

Osteosarcoma

Adult and child: IV 12 g/m^2 given over 4 hr, then leucovorin rescue is given

Mycosis fungoides

Adult: PO 2.5-10 mg/day until cleared (may be many mo); IM 50 mg qwk or 15-37.5 mg 2 ×/wk

Psoriasis

Adult: PO/IM/IV 10-25 mg qwk or 2.5 mg PO q12hr × 3 doses qwk; may increase to 25 mg qwk, max 30 mg/wk

Renal/hepatic dose

Adult: PO/IM/IV

CCr 46-60 ml/min give 65% of standard dose; CCr 31-45 ml/min give 50% of standard dose; CCr ≤30 ml/min not recommended

Available forms: Tabs 2.5, 5, 7.5, 10, 15 mg; inj 25 mg/ml (2, 4, 8, 10, 20, 40 vials); 25 mg/ml (2,10 ml vials with benzyl alcohol); lyophilized powder: 2.5 mg/ml, 2.5 mg/ml in 1000 mg preservative-free vials; oral solution 2.5 mg/ml; autoinjector: 7.5/0.15 ml, 7.5/0.4 ml, 10 mg/0.2 ml, 10 mg/0.4 ml, 12.5 mg/0.25 ml, 15 mg/0.3 ml, 15 mg/0.4 ml, 17.5 mg/0.35 ml, 20 mg/0.4 ml, 22.5 mg/0.45 ml, 25 mg/0.4 ml, 25 mg/0.5 ml, 27.5 mg/0.55 ml, 30 mg/0.6 ml

ADVERSE EFFECTS

CNS: Dizziness, seizures, headache, confusion, encephalopathy, hemiparesis, malaise, fatigue, chills, fever, leukoencephalopathy; arachnoiditis (intrathecal)

EENT: Blurred vision, optic neuropathy

GI: *Nausea, vomiting, anorexia, diarrhea, ulcerative stomatitis,* hepatotoxicity, cramps, ulcer, gastritis, GI hemorrhage, abdominal pain, hematemesis, hepatic fibrosis, acute toxicity

GU: Urinary retention, renal failure, menstrual irregularities, defective spermatogenesis, hematuria, azotemia, uric acid nephropathy

HEMA: Leukopenia, thrombocytopenia, myelosuppression, anemia

INTEG: *Rash, alopecia,* dry skin, urticaria, photosensitivity, folliculitis, vasculitis, petechiae, ecchymosis, acne, alopecia, severe fatal skin reactions

RESP: Methotrexate-induced lung disease

SYST: Sudden death, *Pneumocystis jiroveci* pneumonia, tumor lysis syndrome, secondary malignancy

INTERACTIONS

Individual drugs

Alcohol, phenylbutazone, probenecid, radiation, theophylline: increased toxicity

Digoxin (PO), fosphenytoin, phenytoin: decreased effect of each specific product

---

Folic acid: decreased effect of methotrexate, asparaginase

Radiation: increased bone marrow suppression

Drug classifications

Anticoagulants (oral): increased hypoprothrombinemia

Antineoplastics, NSAIDs, penicillins, salicylates, sulfa products: increased toxicity

Live virus vaccines: decreased antibodies

Proton pump inhibitors: do not use concurrently

NURSING CONSIDERATIONS
Assessment

• Assess buccal cavity q8hr for dryness, sores or ulceration, white patches, oral pain, bleeding, dysphagia; obtain prescription for viscous lidocaine (Xylocaine)

• **Assess symptoms indicating severe allergic reaction:** rash, pruritus, urticaria, purpuric skin lesions, itching, flushing

• Assess tachypnea, ECG changes, dyspnea, edema, fatigue; identify dyspnea, crackles, unproductive cough, chest pain, tachypnea

> **BLACK BOX WARNING: Infection:** those with active infections should be treated for infection prior to product use; monitor temperature, fever may indicate beginning of infection, more common during neutropenia

• **Bone marrow suppression:** Monitor CBC, differential, platelet count weekly; avoid use until WBC is >1500/mm³ or platelet count is >75,000/mm³, neutrophils >200/mm³, notify prescriber of results if WBC <20,000/mm³, platelets <150,000/mm³; WBC, platelet nadirs occur on day 7; monitor

• Assess for increased uric acid levels, swelling, joint pain primarily in extremities; patient should be well hydrated to prevent urate deposits

• Make sure drug-drug interacting products are discontinued prior to therapy, and do not resume until methotrexate level is safe

> **BLACK BOX WARNING: Nephrotoxicity:** avoid use in renal failure; monitor renal function studies: BUN, creatinine, serum uric acid, urine CCr before, during therapy; check I&O ratio; report fall in urine output to <30 ml/hr

> **BLACK BOX WARNING: Hepatotoxicity:** monitor liver function tests before, during therapy (bilirubin, AST, ALT, LDH) as needed or monthly; check for jaundice of skin and sclera, dark urine, clay-colored stools, itchy skin, abdominal pain, fever, diarrhea (hepatotoxicity)

• **Bleeding:** Assess for bleeding: blood in emesis hematuria, stool guaiac, bruising or petechiae, mucosa or orifices; check for inflammation of mucosa, breaks in skin, avoid IM injections, rectal temperature when platelets are low

• Identify effects of alopecia on body image; discuss feelings about body changes

• Identify edema in feet, joint and stomach pain, shaking; prescriber should be notified

• Monitor methotrexate levels, adjust leucovorin dose based on the level

• Monitor vital signs during use, report changes if significant

• Monitor for stomatitis, diarrhea, abdominal cramping or pain, if severe discontinue product

• **Anemia:** Assess for extreme fatigue, increased heartbeat, dyspnea, headache, dizziness, pale skin

• Gout: Assess for joint warmth, pain, edema, increased uric acid level, use allopurinol and alkalinization of urine will decrease uric acid

> **BLACK BOX WARNING: Pulmonary toxicity:** those with ascites or pleural effusions are at greater risk for toxicity, fluid should be removed before treatment, monitor plasma methotrexate level, may start with dry, nonproductive cough

> **BLACK BOX WARNING: Tumor lysis syndrome:** hyperkalemia, hyperphosphatemia, hyperuricemia, hypocalcemia, decreased urine output; use aggressive hydration and allopurinol to correct severe electrolyte imbalances, renal toxicity

> **BLACK BOX WARNING: Serious skin reaction:** Stevens-Johnson syndrome, exfoliative dermatitis, skin necrosis, erythema multiforme may occur within days of receiving product by any route; product should be discontinued

• **Strokelike encephalopathy:** common in high-dose therapy; assess for confusion, hemiparesis, seizures, coma; usually transient

• **Rheumatoid arthritis:** ROM, pain, joint swelling, prior to and during treatment

• **Psoriasis:** assess skin lesions prior to and during treatment

Patient problem

Risk for infection (adverse reactions)

Risk for injury (adverse reactions)

Implementation

• Avoid contact with skin, since product is very irritating; wash completely to remove

---

- **Leucovorin rescue:** Administer leucovorin calcium within 24 hr of giving this product to prevent tissue damage; check agency policy; continue until methotrexate level $<10^{-8}$ m
- Give antiemetic 30-60 min before giving product and prn to prevent vomiting; administer antibiotics for infection prophylaxis
- Give in AM so product can be eliminated before bedtime
- Provide liquid diet: carbonated beverages; gelatin may be added if patient is not nauseated or vomiting

PO route
- Give 1 hr before or 2 hr after meals to prevent vomiting
- Make sure product is taken weekly in RA, JRA

IM route
- Give deeply in large muscle mass
- Store in tightly closed container in cool environment; store inj, powder for inj in dark, dry area
- Use safe handling procedures for chemo-therapeutic agents

PO route
- This route is preferred for low-dose therapy
- Methotrexate absorption is dose dependent; absorption of single doses more than 40 mg/m^2 is significantly less than that of lower doses
- Weekly therapy with Rheumatrex Dose Packs is not intended for doses more than 15 mg PO/wk

Oral liquid formulations
- Instruct patients and caregivers that the recommended dose should be taken weekly as directed. Mistaken daily use of the recommended dose has led to fatal toxicity
- Measure using a calibrated oral measuring device for accurate dosage administration
- **Storage:** Store at room temperature (68 to 77° F) for up to 60 days

Injectable routes
- Visually inspect parenteral products for particulate matter and discoloration before use
- The preserved solutions contain benzyl alcohol and should not be used for intrathecal, intermediate-, or high-dose therapy
- **Reconstitution of lyophilized powders:** Reconstitute each vial with an appropriate sterile, preservative-free solution such as 5% dextrose injection or 0.9% sodium chloride injection. Reconstitute the 25-mg vial to a concentration no greater than 25 mg/ml. The 1-g vial should be reconstituted with 19.4 ml to a concentration of 50 mg/ml; prepare immediately before use. Discard any unused portions

IV route
Direct IV injection: Inject as a slow push via Y-site or three-way stopcock into a free-flowing IV infusion

Intermittent/continuous IV infusion: Further dilute solution in 5% dextrose injection, 5% dextrose, and 0.9% sodium chloride injection, or 0.9% sodium chloride injection; before infusion, check vein patency by flushing with 5 to 10 ml of 5% dextrose injection or 0.9% sodium chloride injection; infuse at a rate recommended by the prescriber. After infusion, flush the IV tubing.

IV infusion of intermediate- or high-dose methotrexate (500 mg/m^2 over less than 4 hr or more than 1 g/m^2 over more than 4 hr):
- Before use, the following laboratory parameters should be confirmed: WBC >1,500/mm^3, neutrophil count >200/mm^3, platelet count >75,000/mm^3, serum bilirubin <1.2 mg/dl, normal serum creatinine, and SGPT <450 U. Creatinine clearance should be >60 ml/min. If serum creatinine has increased by 50% or more compared with a prior value, creatinine clearance should be measured and documented as more than 60 ml/min even if the serum creatinine is still within normal limits
- Previous mucositis should be healed and persistent effusions should be drained before use
- Give 1 L/m^2 of IV over 6 hr before initiation of the methotrexate infusion; continue hydration at 125 ml/m^2/hr during the methotrexate infusion and for 2 days after the infusion has been completed
- Alkalinize the urine using sodium bicarbonate to maintain the urine pH more than 7 during the methotrexate infusion and leucovorin therapy. This can be done orally or by incorporating the sodium bicarbonate in the intravenous fluids.
- Repeat serum creatinine and methotrexate serum level determinations 24 hr after starting methotrexate and at least daily until the methotrexate level is below 5×10^{-8} mol/L (0.05 micro-M)

IM route
- Inject deeply into a large muscle
- Aspirate before injection to avoid injection into a blood vessel

SUBCUT route
- Otrexup and Rasuvo are methotrexate formulations for SUBCUT use only
- Both Otrexup and Rasuvo are single-use autoinjectors. Otrexup is available in 5-mg increments for doses between 10 and 25 mg; Rasuvo is available in 2.5-mg increments for doses between 7.5 and 30 mg. Otrexup is yellow in color, and Rasuvo is yellow to brown in color. Neither formulation should have lumps or particles floating in it

---

• Administer Otrexup and Rasuvo in the abdomen or thigh; do NOT administer within 2 inches of the navel; on the arms; on any other areas of the body; or on skin that is tender, bruised, red, scaly, hard, or has scars or stretch marks

• If self-injection is deemed appropriate, patients or caregivers should practice injections using a training device with guidance from a health care professional.

Use of the Otrexup autoinjector

• Immediately before use, twist cap to remove; flip the safety clip

• Place the needle end of Otrexup against the thigh or stomach (abdomen) at a 90-degree angle and firmly push until you hear a click; hold for 3 sec before removing

• Press a cotton ball or gauze on the area for 10 sec; do not rub

• After use, the viewing window will be blocked to show that the medicine was given.

Use of the Rasuvo autoinjector

• Pull the yellow cap straight off. Do not twist

• Pinch a pad of skin surrounding a cleaned injection site (thigh or abdomen) with the thumb and forefinger. Position the uncapped end of the autoinjector at a 90-degree angle to the skin. Without pressing the button, push firmly onto the skin until the stop point is felt, which will unlock the yellow injection button

• Press the yellow injection button until a click is heard. Hold Rasuvo against the skin until all medication is injected. This can take up to 5 sec.

• To avoid incomplete injection, do not remove Rasuvo from the skin before the end of the injection. Look at the transparent control zone while injecting to make sure the entire dose is injected.

• Pull straight up to remove Rasuvo from the injection site.

• Visually inspect the transparent control zone to ensure no liquid is left in the syringe.

Intrathecal administration

• Use preservative-free solutions. The preserved solutions contain benzyl alcohol and should NOT be used for intrathecal therapy

• Reconstitute the preservative-free powder for injection with preservative-free 0.9% sodium chloride injection. The desired dose should be drawn into a 5- to 10-ml syringe

• After lumbar puncture is complete, withdraw an amount of CSF equivalent to the volume of methotrexate injection to be administered. If the puncture was traumatic, wait 2 days before attempting to administer methotrexate intrathecally

• Allow CSF (approximately 10% of estimated CSF total volume) to flow into the syringe and mix with the product

• Inject intrathecally over 15 to 30 sec with the bevel of the needle directed upward

Y-site compatibilities: Acyclovir, alemtuzumab, alfentanye, allopurinol, amifostine, aminophylline, asparaginase, aztreonam, bleomycin, cefepime, cefTRIAXone, cimetidine, CISplatin, cyclophosphamide, cytarabine, DAUNOrubicin, dexchlorpheniramine, diphenhydrAMINE, doripenem, DOXOrubicin, etoposide, famotidine, filgrastim, fludarabine, fluorouracil, furosemide, gallium, ganciclovir, granisetron, heparin, HYDROmorphone, imipenem-cilastatin, leucovorin, LORazepam, melphalan, mesna, methylPREDNISolone, metoclopramide, mitoMYcin, morphine, ondansetron, oxacillin, PACLitaxel, piperacillin/tazobactam, prochlorperazine, ranitidine, sargramostim, teniposide, thiotepa, vinBLAStine, vinCRIStine, vinorelbine, zoledronic acid

Solution compatibilities: Amino acids, 4.25%/D$_{25}$, D$_5$W, sodium bicarbonate 0.05 mol/L, 0.9% NaCl

---

BLACK BOX WARNING: Intrathecal route:
use preservative-free solutions, reconstitute with normal saline, the dose should be drawn into a 5 to 10-ml syringe after lumbar puncture, the volume of CSF should be withdrawn equal to volume of methotrexate, allow CSF to flow into syringe and mix, inject over 15-30 sec with bevel of needle upward

---

Patient/family education

• Encourage patient to rinse mouth tid-qid with water, club soda; brush teeth bid-qid with soft brush or cotton-tipped applicators for stomatitis; use unwaxed dental floss

---

BLACK BOX WARNING: Teach patient to avoid use of products containing aspirin or NSAIDs, razors, commercial mouthwash, since bleeding may occur; to report symptoms of bleeding (hematuria, tarry stools)

• Caution patient to report signs of anemia (fatigue, headache, irritability, faintness, shortness of breath); seizures

• **Pulmonary toxicity:** Advise patient to report any changes in breathing or coughing even several mo after treatment; to avoid crowds and persons with respiratory tract or other infections

• Advise patient to report stomatitis: any bleeding, white spots, ulcerations in mouth to prescriber; tell patient to examine mouth daily, report symptoms, use good oral hygiene

- Teach patient that hair may be lost during treatment; a wig or hairpiece may make patient feel better; new hair may be different in color, texture
- Caution patient not to have any vaccinations without the advice of the prescriber; serious reactions can occur
- Advise patient to use sunblock or protective clothing to prevent burns
- Teach patient to use good dental care, to prevent overgrowth of infection in the mouth, to use soft bristle toothbrush
- Teach patient how to use this product with leucovorin rescue
- Teach patient to continue leucovorin until told it is safe to stop
- Teach patient to report CNS symptoms, vision changes
- Teach patient to report fever, other symptoms of infection
- Teach patient to report decreased urine output
- Teach patient to advise all providers that methotrexate is being used, not to take Rx, OTC, herbs, supplements unless approved by prescriber
- **SUBCUT route:** Teach patient self-injection technique and use, disposal of equipment

> **BLACK BOX WARNING: Pregnancy, breastfeeding:** Advise patient that contraceptive measures for women and men are recommended during therapy; product is teratogenic; contraception should be used for 3 mo (male) and 4-6 wk (female); to discontinue breastfeeding, as toxicity to infant may occur

Evaluation
Positive therapeutic outcome
- Prevention of rapid division of malignant cells
- Decreased joint inflammation in RA

⚠ HIGH ALERT

methyldopa/methyldopate (Rx)
(meth-ill-doe′pa)
Func. class.: Antihypertensive
Chem. class.: Centrally acting α-adrenergic inhibitor

Do not confuse: methyldopa/L-dopa (levodopa)

ACTION: Stimulates central inhibitory α₂-adrenergic receptors or acts as false transmitter, resulting in reduction of arterial pressure

Therapeutic outcome: Decreased B/P in hypertension

USES: Hypertension, hypertensive crisis

Pharmacokinetics
Absorption	50% (PO)
Distribution	Crosses placenta, blood-brain barrier
Metabolism	Liver, moderately
Excretion	Kidneys, unchanged (partially)
Half-life	1½ hr

Pharmacodynamics
	PO	IV
Onset	Onset 4-6 hr	Unknown
Peak	4-6 hr	Onset 4-6 hr
Duration	24-48 hr	10-16 hr

CONTRAINDICATIONS
Active hepatic disease, hypersensitivity, MAOI therapy

Precautions: Pregnancy, geriatric patients, cardiac disease, autoimmune disease, depression, dialysis, hemolytic anemia, Parkinson's disease, pheochromocytoma, sulfite hypersensitivity

DOSAGE AND ROUTES
Hypertension/hypertensive crisis
Adult: PO 250-500 mg bid or tid, then adjusted q2day prn, 0.5-2 g/day in 2-4 divided doses (maintenance), max 3 g/day; IV 250-500 mg in 100 ml D₅W q6hr, run over 30-60 min, max 1 g q6hr, switch to PO as soon as possible
Child: PO 10 mg/kg/day in 2-4 divided doses, max 65 mg/kg or 3 g/day, whichever is less; IV 20-40 mg/kg/day in 4 divided doses, max 65 mg/kg or 3 g, whichever is less

Renal dose
Adult: PO CCr 10-50 ml/min dose q8-12hr; CCr <10 ml/min dose q12-24hr

Available forms: Methyldopa: tabs 125, ✚ 250, 500 mg; methyldopate: inj 50 mg/ml (250 mg/5 ml)

ADVERSE EFFECTS
CNS: *Drowsiness, weakness, dizziness, sedation, headache*, depression, psychosis, paresthesias, parkinsonism, Bell's palsy, nightmares, drug fever
CV: Bradycardia, myocarditis, orthostatic hypotension, angina, edema, weight gain, HF, paradoxical pressor response (**IV** use)
EENT: Nasal congestion
ENDO: Breast enlargement, gynecomastia, amenorrhea

M

GI: Nausea, vomiting, diarrhea, constipation, hepatic dysfunction, sore or "black" tongue, pancreatitis, colitis, flatulence
GU: Impotence, failure to ejaculate
HEMA: Leukopenia, thrombocytopenia, hemolytic anemia, granulocytopenia, positive Coombs' test
INTEG: Lupuslike syndrome, rash, toxic epidural necrolysis

INTERACTIONS
Individual drugs
Alcohol: CNS depression
Haloperidol: increased psychosis
Iron: decreased methyldopa absorption
Levodopa: increased CNS toxicity, hypotension
Lithium: increased lithium toxicity
TOLBUTamide: increased hypoglycemia

Drug classifications
Amphetamines, antidepressants (tricyclics), barbiturates, NSAIDs, phenothiazines: decreased antihypertensive effect
Analgesics, antidepressants, antihistamines, sedative/hypnotics: increased CNS depression
Antihypertensives, diuretics: increased hypotension
β-Adrenergic blockers: increased B/P
MAOIs: increased pressor effect, do not use concurrently
Sympathomimetic amines: increased pressor effect

Drug/lab test
Increased: creatinine, LFTs
Decreased: platelets, WBC, Hgb/Hct
Interference: urinary uric acid, serum creatinine, AST
False increase: urinary catecholamines

NURSING CONSIDERATIONS
Assessment
• **Hemolytic anemia:** monitor blood tests: CBC, neutrophils, decreased platelets; direct Coombs' test before, after 6, 12 mo of therapy; a positive test may indicate hemolytic anemia; usually reverses within weeks to months after discontinuing treatment, monitor Hgb/Hct and RBC, do not start therapy in those with hemolytic anemia
• Monitor renal studies: protein, BUN, creatinine; watch for increased levels that may indicate nephrotic syndrome: polyuria, oliguria, frequency; report weight gain >5 lb
• **Drug-induced hepatitis/drug fever:** usually subsides within 3 months of discontinuing therapy
• **Product tolerance:** may occur within 3 mo of starting treatment; dosage change and other products may be needed

• Obtain baselines in renal, liver function tests before therapy begins; check potassium levels, although hyperkalemia rarely occurs
• Monitor B/P, pulse if the product is being used for hypertension; notify prescriber of changes
• Monitor edema in feet, legs daily; monitor I&O; check weight for decreasing output
• Assess for allergic reaction: rash, fever, pruritus, urticaria; product should be discontinued if antihistamines fail to help
• Monitor CNS symptoms, especially in the geriatric; depression; change in mental status
• **Beers:** Avoid in older adults, high risk of CNS effects; may cause bradycardia and orthostatic hypotension
• **Pregnancy/breastfeeding:** Use cautiously in pregnancy, breastfeeding; has been used for pregnancy-induced hypertension

Patient problem
Risk for injury (uses, adverse reactions)
Nonadherence (teaching)

Implementation
PO route
• Give before meals
• Shake susp before using
• Store in airtight container at room temperature
• Product should not be withdrawn abruptly
• Increase in dose should be done in the evening to minimize drowsiness

Intermittent IV infusion route
• Give after diluting in 100 ml of 0.9% NaCl, D_5W, D_5/0.9% NaCl, 5% sodium bicarbonate, Ringer's; administer over 30-60 min

Y-site compatibilities: Alemtuzumab, alfentanil, amikacin, aminophylline, anidulafungin, ascorbic acid, atenolol, atracurium, atropine, aztreonam, benztropine, bivalirudin, bleomycin, bumetanide, buprenorphine, butorphanol, calcium chloride/gluconate, caspofungin, cefamandole, ceFAZolin, cefmetazole, cefonicid, cefotaxime, cefoTEtan, cefOXitin, cefTAZidime, ceftizoxime, cefTRIAXone, cefuroxime, cephalothin, chlorproMAZINE, cimetidine, clindamycin, cyanocobalamin, cycloSPORINE, DACTINomycin, DAPTOmycin, dexamethasone, digoxin, diltiazem, diphenhydrAMINE, DOCEtaxel, DOPamine, doxycycline, enalaprilat, ePHEDrine, EPINEPHrine, epoetin alfa, ertapenem, erythromycin, esmolol, etoposide, etoposide phosphate, famotidine, fenoldopam, fentaNYL, fluconazole, fludarabine, gatifloxacin, gemcitabine, gentamicin, glycopyrrolate, granisetron, heparin, hydrocortisone, HYDROmorphone, hydrOXYzine, IDArubicin, insulin(regular), irinotecan, isoproterenol, labetalol, lidocaine, linezolid, LORazepam, magnesium sulfate, mannitol, mechlorethamine, meperidine, metaraminol, methicillin, methoxamine, methylPREDNISolone, metoclopramide, metoprolol, metroNIDAZOLE, mezlocillin, miconazole, midazolam, milrinone, minocycline, mitoXANtrone, morphine, moxalactam, multiple vitamins, mycophenolate mofetil, nafcillin, nalbuphine, naloxone, netilmicin, nitroglycerin, nitroprusside, norepinephrine, octreotide, ondansetron, oxacillin, oxaliplatin, oxytocin, PACLitaxel, palonosetron, pamidronate, pancuronium, pantoprazole, papaverine, PEMEtrexed, penicillin G potassium/sodium, pentazocine, phentolamine, phenylephrine, phytonadione, piperacillin, polymyxin B, potassium chloride, procainamide, prochlorperazine, promethazine, propranolol, protamine, pyridoxine, quiNIDine, ranitidine, ritodrine, sodium bicarbonate, succinylcholine, SUFentanil, tacrolimus, teniposide, theophylline, thiamine, thiotepa, ticarcillin, ticarcillin-clavulanate, tigecycline, tirofiban, tobramycin, tolazoline, trimetaphan, urokinase, vancomycin, vasopressin, vecuronium, verapamil, vinorelbine, voriconazole, zoledronic acid

Solution compatibilities: D₅W, D₅/0.9% NaCl, Ringer's, sodium bicarbonate 5%, 0.9% NaCl, amino acids 4.25%/D₂₅, Dextran₆/0.9% NaCl, Normosol R, Normosol M/D₅W

Patient/family education
• Instruct patient not to discontinue product abruptly, or withdrawal symptoms may occur: anxiety, increased B/P, headache, insomnia, increased pulse, tremors, nausea, sweating
• Caution patient not to use OTC (cough, cold, or allergy) products unless directed by prescriber
• Teach patient about excessive perspiration, dehydration, vomiting, diarrhea; may lead to fall in B/P; consult prescriber if these occur
• Advise patient that product may cause dizziness, fainting; light-headedness may occur during 1st few days of therapy; that product may cause dry mouth, use hard candy, saliva product, or frequent rinsing of mouth; caution patient to change position slowly, to rise slowly to sitting or standing position to minimize orthostatic hypotension, especially geriatric
• Caution patient that compliance is necessary; not to skip or stop product unless directed by prescriber
• Teach patient that product may cause skin rash
• Teach patient to avoid hazardous activities, since product may cause drowsiness, dizziness

Evaluation

Positive therapeutic outcome
• Decreased B/P

TREATMENT OF OVERDOSE: Gastric evacuation, sympathomimetics may be indicated if severe; hemodialysis

methylergonovine (Rx)
(meth-ill-er-goe-noe'veen)
Methergine
Func. class.: Oxytocic
Chem. class.: Ergot alkaloid

ACTION: Stimulates uterine and vascular smooth muscle, causing contractions, decreased bleeding, arterial vasoconstriction

Therapeutic outcome: Absence of hemorrhage

USES: Prevention, treatment of hemorrhage postpartum or after abortion, uterine contractions

Pharmacokinetics

Absorption	Well absorbed (PO, IM)
Distribution	Unknown
Metabolism	Liver, possibly
Excretion	Unknown
Half-life	½-2 hr

Pharmacodynamics

	PO	IM	IV
Onset	5-15 min	5 min	Immediate
Peak	Unknown	Unknown	Unknown
Duration	3 hr	3 hr	Unknown

CONTRAINDICATIONS
Pregnancy (4th stage of labor [other than obstetric delivery/abortion]), hypersensitivity to ergot preparations, preeclampsia, eclampsia, elective induction of labor

Precautions: Severe renal/hepatic disease, jaundice, diabetes mellitus, seizure disorders, sepsis, CAD, last stage of labor

DOSAGE AND ROUTES
Adult: PO 200 mcg tid-qid up to 7 days; IM/IV 200 mcg q2-4hr for 1-5 doses

Available forms: Inj 200 mcg/ml; tabs 200 mcg

ADVERSE EFFECTS
CNS: *Headache, dizziness,* seizures, hallucinations, stroke (IV)
CV: Hypotension, chest pain, palpitations, *hypertension,* dysrhythmias; CVA **(IV)**
EENT: Tinnitus
GI: *Nausea, vomiting*

GU: Cramping
INTEG: Sweating, rash, allergic reactions
MS: Leg cramps
RESP: *Dyspnea*

INTERACTIONS
Individual drugs
Smoking: increased vasoconstriction

Drug classifications
CYP3A4 inhibitors: increased ergot toxicity, do not use together
Vasopressors, ergots, anesthetics (regional): increased vasoconstriction

NURSING CONSIDERATIONS
Assessment
• Monitor B/P, pulse; watch for change that may indicate hemorrhage
• Assess fundal tone, nonphasic contractions; check for relaxation or severe cramping
• **Assess for ergotism or overdose:** nausea, vomiting, weakness, muscular pain, insensitivity to cold, paresthesia of extremities; product should be decreased or infusion discontinued
• Before administering ergonovine, check calcium levels; if hypocalcemia is present, correction should be made to increase effectiveness of this product
• Monitor prolactin levels and for decreased breast milk production
• **Pregnancy/breastfeeding:** Do not use in pregnancy except after obstetric delivery or abortion to reduce hemorrhage risk, may breastfeed 1 wk postpartum to control uterine bleeding

Patient problem
Risk for injury (uses)

Implementation
PO route
• PO is the preferred route
• Do not exceed dosage limits
• Store tabs at room temperature
• Give with water
IM route
• Give inj deeply in large muscle mass, aspirate
• Protect from light

Direct IV route
• Give by this route for severe, life-threatening hemorrhage
• Give directly undiluted or diluted with 5 ml of 0.9% NaCl given through Y-site or 3-way stopcock; give 0.2 mg/min; use clear, colorless sol
• Store up to 2 mo if unused

Y-site compatibilities: Heparin, hydrocortisone sodium succinate, potassium chloride, vit B/C

Patient/family education
• Inform patient that abdominal cramps are a side effect of this medication
• Instruct patient to notify prescriber if chest pain, nausea, vomiting, headache, muscle pain, weakness, or cold, numb extremities occur

Evaluation
Positive therapeutic outcome
• Prevention of postpartum hemorrhage

methylnaltrexone (Rx)
(meth-il-nal-trex′one)
Relistor
Chem. class.: Opioid antagonist
Func. class.: GI agent

ACTION: Peripheral mu-opioid receptor antagonist that reduces constipation associated with opiate agonists

Therapeutic outcome: Decreased constipation

USES: Treatment of opioid-induced constipation in patients with advanced illness who are receiving palliative care when response to laxative therapy has been insufficient, opioid-induced constipation in chronic noncancer pain

Pharmacokinetics

Absorption	Unknown
Distribution	Protein binding 11%-15.3%
Metabolism	Unknown
Excretion	Unknown
Half-life	Terminal 8 hr

Pharmacodynamics

Onset	Unknown
Peak	30 min (SUBCUT)
Duration	Unknown

CONTRAINDICATIONS
Hypersensitivity, GI obstruction, **IV** route, eclampsia, elective induction of labor, hypertension, preeclampsia, pregnancy

Precautions: Pregnancy, breastfeeding, renal disease, children, diarrhea, driving, operating machinery, geriatric patients, neoplastic disease, Crohn's disease, peptic ulcer, ulcerative colitis

DOSAGE AND ROUTES
Opiate-agonist induced constipation
Adult >114 kg: SUBCUT 0.15 mg/kg every other day prn

Adult 62-114 kg: SUBCUT 12 mg every other day prn, max 12 mg/24 hr
Adult 38-62 kg: SUBCUT 8 mg every other day prn, max 8 mg/24 hr
Adult <38 kg: SUBCUT 0.15 mg/kg every other day prn, max 0.15 mg/kg/24 hr

Opioid-induced constipation with noncancer pain
Adult: PO 450 mg q day in the AM; SUBCUT 12 mg qday, discontinue laxative before starting this product

Renal dose
Adult: SUBCUT CCr <60 ml/min, reduce normal adult dose by 50%

Available forms: Solution for inj 12 mg/0.6 ml, (single-use vials) 8 mg/0.4 ml (prefilled syringes); tab 150 mg

ADVERSE EFFECTS
CNS: Dizziness
GI: Nausea, vomiting, diarrhea, flatulence, abdominal pain, GI perforation
INTEG: Hyperhidrosis

NURSING CONSIDERATIONS
Assessment
• Monitor serum creatinine
• **Opioid-induced constipation:** assess for stool characteristics: amount, consistency; bowel sounds during treatment
• Teach patient to notify prescriber before taking all other OTC, Rx, or herbal products
• Teach patient not to drive or perform other hazardous activities until response is known, dizziness may occur
• Teach patient to continue other products for constipation unless directed by prescriber not to
• **Pain:** Monitor characteristics of pain, this product does not effect analgesics
• **Beers:** Avoid in older adults unless safer alternatives are not available, may cause ataxia, impaired psychomotor function
• **Opioid withdrawal:** Teach patient to report severe diarrhea, abdominal pain, chills
• **Beers:** Avoid in older adults unless safer alternatives are not available; may cause ataxia, impaired psychomotor function

Patient problem
Constipation (uses)
Diarrhea (adverse reactions)

Implementation
PO route
• Take on empty stomach, at least 30 min before first meal of the day

Subcut route
• Do not give **IV**; IV dosing for urinary retention is investigational
• Store at 15°-30° C (59°-86° F); do not freeze
• Store away from light
• Inspect the solution before use; it should be a clear, colorless to pale yellow aqueous solution; do not use if particulate matter or discoloration are present
• Withdraw the needed amount of solution into a sterile syringe; if immediate administration is impossible, the syringe may be kept at room temperature for up to 24 hr; the syringe does not need to be kept away from light during the 24-hr period; immediately discard any unused portion in the vial; no preservatives are present
• Administer into the upper arm, abdomen, or thigh no more than 1 ×/24 hr; rotate inj sites; do not inject the same spot each time; do not inject into areas where skin is tender, bruised, red, or hard; avoid areas with scars or stretch marks
• If using with retractable needle, slowly push down on the plunger past the resistance point until the syringe is empty and a click is heard

Patient/family education
• Teach patient that after 30 min, toilet facilities should be nearby, bowel relaxation occurs, not to use more than one dose in 24 hr
• Advise patient to notify prescriber of abdominal pain, continuous or severe diarrhea, nausea or vomiting
• Teach patient to avoid use in pregnancy unless absolutely necessary; avoid in breastfeeding

Evaluation
Positive therapeutic outcome
• Decreased constipation

---

methylphenidate (Rx)
(meth-ill-fen'i-date)
Aptensio XR, Biphentin ✦, Concerta, Daytrana, Metadate CD, Metadate ER, Methylin, Methylin ER, QuillChew ER, Quillivant XR, Ritalin, Ritalin LA, Ritalin SR
Func. class.: Cerebral stimulant
Chem. class.: Piperidine derivative
Controlled substance schedule II

Do not confuse: methylphenidate/methadone, Metadate ER/methadone, Ritalin/Ritalin LA/ritodrine

ACTION: Increases release of norepinephrine and dopamine in cerebral cortex to reticular activating system; exact action not known

Therapeutic outcome: Increased alertness, decreased fatigue, ability to stay awake (narcolepsy), increased attention span, decreased hyperactivity (ADHD)

USES: Attention deficit disorder with hyperactivity (ADHD), narcolepsy (except Concerta, Metadate CD, Ritalin LA), attention deficit disorder (ADD)

Unabeled uses: Management of depression

Pharmacokinetics

Absorption	Well absorbed (PO); delayed (ext rel)
Distribution	Widely distributed; crosses placenta
Metabolism	Liver
Excretion	Kidneys
Half-life	1-3 hr

Pharmacodynamics

	PO	PO–ext rel
Onset	Varies with formulation	2 hr
Peak	1-3 hr	4 hr
Duration		6-8 hr

CONTRAINDICATIONS

Hypersensitivity, anxiety, history of Tourette's syndrome, glaucoma, hereditary fructose intolerance, glaucoma

Precautions: Pregnancy, breastfeeding, hypertension, depression, seizures, abrupt discontinuation, acute MI, aortic stenosis, arteriosclerosis, bipolar disorder, cardiac dysrhythmias, cardiomyopathy, chemical leukoderma, child depression, dysphagia, esophageal stricture, growth inhibition, heart failure, hepatic disease, hypertension, hyperthyroidism, ileus, mania, peripheral vascular disease, PKU, psychosis, Raynaud's, schizophrenia, stroke, suicidal ideation, visual disturbances

> **BLACK BOX WARNING:** Substance abuse, alcoholism

DOSAGE AND ROUTES
Attention-deficit/hyperactivity disorder (ADHD) initial treatment (not currently on methylphenidate)
>> Regular release: Ritalin, Methylin, Methylin oral sol, Methylin chew tabs
Adult: PO 20-30 mg/day, range 10-60 mg/day in 2-3 divided doses, 30-45 min before meals

Child ≥6 yr: PO 5 mg bid initially, increase 5-10 mg/day qwk, usual dose 0.3-2 mg/kg/day, max 60 mg/day

>> Extended release: Ritalin SR, Metadate ER, Methylin ER
Adult/adolescent/child ≥6 yr: PO max 20-30 mg tid

>> Extended-release once-daily tabs: Concerta
Adult: PO 18-36 mg/day initially, then adjust by 18 mg q wk, max 72 mg/day
Adolescent: PO 18 mg/day initially, then adjust by 18 mg q wk, max 72 mg/day
Child ≥6 yr: PO 18 mg/day initially, then adjust by 18 mg q wk, max 54 mg/day

>> Extended-release once-daily capsules: Ritalin LA
Adult/adolescent/child ≥6 yr: PO 10-20 mg/day in AM initially, adjust by 10 mg qwk, max 60 mg/day

>> Transdermal: Daytrana
Adolescent/child ≥6 yr: TD wk 1: 10 mg/day (9-hr patch); wk 2: 15 mg/day (9-hr patch); wk 3: 20 mg/day (9-hr patch); wk 4: 30 mg/day (9-hr patch)

Conversion to once-daily from other forms for ADHD
>> Extended-release once-daily capsules: Ritalin LA
Adult/adolescent/child ≥6 yr: PO give no more than total daily dose of other forms, may adjust by 10 mg qwk, max 60 mg/day

>> Extended-release once-daily tablets: Concerta
Adult/adolescent/child ≥6 yr (currently receiving 10-15 mg/day): PO 18 mg q AM initially, adjust by 18 mg qwk, max 72 mg/day (adult); max 72 mg/day, 2 mg/kg/day (adolescent); 54 mg/day (child)
Adult/adolescent/child ≥6 yr (currently receiving 20-30 mg/day): PO 36 mg q AM, adjust by 18 mg qwk, max 72 mg/day (adult); 72 mg/day, 2 mg/kg/day (adolescent); 54 mg/day (child)
Adult/adolescent/child ≥6 yr (currently receiving 30-45 mg/day): PO 54 mg q AM, adjust by 18 mg qwk, max 72 mg/day (adult); 72 mg/day, 2 mg/kg/day (adolescent); 54 mg/day (child)
Adult/adolescent/child ≥6 yr (currently receiving 40-60 mg/day): PO 72 mg q AM, 72 mg/day

>> **Extended-release once daily tabs: Quillivant XR**

Child > 6 yr/adolescent: PO 20 mg/day in AM, may increase by 10-20 mg qwk

>> **Transdermal: Daytrana**

Adolescent and child ≥6 yr: TD wk 1: 10 mg/day (9-hr patch); wk 2: 15 mg/day (9-hr patch); wk 3: 20 mg/day (9-hr patch); wk 4: 30 mg/day (9-hr patch)

Narcolepsy

>> **Immediate release: Ritalin, Methylin oral sol, Methylin chew tabs**

Adult: PO 20-30 mg/day, range 10-60 mg/day in 2-3 divided doses

Child ≥6 yr: PO 5 mg bid, may increase by 5-10 mg qwk, max 60 mg/day

>> **Extended-release tabs: Ritalin SR, Metadate ER**

Adult/adolescent/child ≥6 yr: PO max 20 mg tid

Poststroke depression; major depression (unlabeled)

Adult and geriatric: PO (immediate rel tabs) 2.5 mg bid morning/noon, may increase by 2.5-5 mg q2-3days

Available forms: Tabs 5, 10, 20 mg; ext rel tabs 10, 20, mg; ext rel tabs (Concerta) 18, 27, 36, 54 mg; ext rel caps 10, 20, 30, 40 mg; oral sol 5 mg, 10 mg/ml; chew tabs (Methylin) 2.5, 5, 10 mg; transdermal patch 12.5 cm² (10 mg), 18.75 cm² (15 mg), 25 cm² (20 mg), 37.5 cm² (30 mg)

ADVERSE EFFECTS

CNS: *Hyperactivity, insomnia, restlessness, talkativeness,* dizziness, headache, akathisia, dyskinesia, masking or worsening of Tourette's syndrome, seizures, drowsiness, toxic psychosis, hallucinations, neuroleptic malignant syndrome, aggression, cerebral vasculitis, hemorrhage, stroke (rare)
CV: *Palpitations, tachycardia,* B/P changes, angina, dysrhythmias, sudden death
ENDO: Growth retardation
GI: Nausea, anorexia, dry mouth, weight loss, abdominal pain
HEMA: Leukopenia, anemia, thrombocytopenic purpura
INTEG: Exfoliative dermatitis, urticaria, rash, erythema multiforme, hypersensitivity reactions; patch: permanent loss of skin color, anaphylaxis, angioedema
MISC: Fever, arthralgia, scalp hair loss, rhabdomyolysis

INTERACTIONS
Individual drugs
Guanethidine: decreased effect of guanethidine

Drug classifications
Anticonvulsants, antidepressants (tricyclics), SNRIs, CNS stimulants, selective serotonin reuptake inhibitors (SSRIs): increased effects, monitor for adverse effects
MAOIs (or within 14 days of MAOIs), vasopressors: increased hypertensive crisis
Antihypertensives: decreased effects of antihypertensives

Drug/herb
Cola nut, guarana, horsetail, yerba maté, yohimbe: increased CNS stimulation
Melatonin: synergistic effect

Drug/food
Caffeine: increased stimulation

NURSING CONSIDERATIONS
Assessment
• **ADHD:** In children or adults with ADHD, monitor for improved organizational skills, attention span, attending to tasks, impulse control, socialization, and ability to get along better with others

> **BLACK BOX WARNING: Substance abuse:** there is a high potential for abuse, use caution in those with history of substance abuse

• Monitor VS, B/P, since this product may reverse antihypertensives; check patients with cardiac disease more often for increased B/P
• Perform CBC, urinalysis; for diabetic patients monitor blood glucose, urine glucose; insulin changes may be required, since eating will decrease, but decreased growth will resume when product is discontinued
• Monitor height and weight q3mo since growth rate in children may be decreased; appetite is suppressed, weight loss is common during the first mo of treatment
• Monitor mental status: mood, sensorium, affect, stimulation, insomnia; aggressiveness may occur; depression with crying spells may occur after product has worn off, may produce euphoria, rebound depression after product wears off
• Assess for tolerance; should not be used for extended time except in ADHD; dosage should be discontinued gradually to prevent withdrawal symptoms
• Assess for narcoleptic symptoms before medication and after; ability to stay awake should increase significantly

M

• **Assess for withdrawal symptoms:** headache, nausea, vomiting, muscle pain, weakness; product tolerance will develop after long-term use; dosage should not be increased if tolerance develops, usually not associated with drug holidays
• Assess appetite, sleep, speech patterns
• Skin pigmentation when using TD product, may cause loss of pigmentation around site
• **Pregnancy/breastfeeding:** Use only if benefits outweigh fetal risk, no well-controlled studies, cautious use in breastfeeding
• Beers: Avoid use in older adults, CNS stimulant effects

Patient problem

Distorted thinking process (uses)
Risk for injury (adverse reactions)

Implementation
PO route

• **Methylin chewable tablets:** Give with at least 8 oz of fluid to avoid choking
• **Immediate-release dosage forms (Ritalin, Methylin, Metadate):** Give 30 to 45 min before meal; depending on the patient's needs, twice-daily dosages may be used in the morning and around noon. Individualized timing of the midday dose is usually necessary, as determined by the loss of positive drug effect, which occurs in a range of 2 to 6 hr after the AM dose
• **Extended-release tablets (Ritalin SR, Metadate ER):** May be given without regard to meals. Give whole; do not cut, crush, or chew. Give the last dose of the day several hours before bedtime. Extended-release tablets may be used when the determined 8-hr dose of immediate-release methylphenidate tablets equals the 8-hr dosage of the extended-release tablets
• **Once-daily extended-release tablets (Concerta):** May be given without regard to meals. Give whole; do not cut, crush, or chew; a portion of this tablet may appear intact in the stool; this is normal
• **Once-daily extended-release capsules (Ritalin LA, Aptensio XR):** May be given without regard to meals; however, patients should establish a routine pattern with regard to meals. Give with an adequate amount of fluid. Do not cut, crush, or chew. If swallowing is difficult, capsule may be opened and the contents sprinkled on one Tbsp of applesauce and swallowed immediately. The capsule contents (beads) should not be crushed or chewed. Instruct the patient to drink fluids (water, milk, or juice) after taking sprinkles with applesauce
• **Once-daily extended-release chewable tablets (QuilliChew ER):** Give qday in the morning with or without food. The tablet may be broken in half for 10-mg and 15-mg doses

Immediate-release oral solution (Methylin)
• Measure dose with an oral syringe or calibrated measuring device
• Give 30 to 45 min before meals in divided doses two to three times/day. Twice-daily dosages may be administered in the morning and around noon. Individualized timing of the midday dose is usually necessary, as determined by the loss of positive drug effect, which occurs 2 to 6 hr after the morning dose. Give the last dose of the day before 6 PM

Once-daily extended-release oral suspension (Quillivant XR)
• Vigorously shake before use, measure dose with the calibrated oral dosing dispenser provided
• Give in the morning without regard to meals

Reconstitution of once-daily extended-release oral suspension (Quillivant XR)
• Review the manufacturer's reconstitution instructions for the particular product and package size
• Before reconstitution, tap the bottle several times to loosen the powder
• To prepare the suspension, add the specified amount of water to the bottle, fully insert the bottle adapter into the bottle neck, replace the cap, and vigorously shake the bottle for at least 10 sec
• **Storage:** Store reconstituted suspension at 77° F; dispense in original packaging (bottle in container). The reconstituted suspension is stable for 4 mo from date of reconstitution

Topical route
Daytrana transdermal system:
• Patch should be applied 2 hr before the effect is needed
• Do not cut or trim patch
• Apply patch immediately after opening. Do not use if pouch seal is broken. Do not touch the adhesive side of the patch during application to avoid absorption. Wash hands immediately if adhesive side of the patch is touched. Discard the patch if difficulty is encountered in separating the patch from the release liner or if tearing or other damage occurs. Discard patch if adhesive containing medication has transferred to the liner during removal of the patch from the liner
• Place on a dry, clean area of the hip and hold in place for 30 sec with the palm of the hand. Do not apply to oily, damaged, or irritated skin. Do not apply topical preparations to the application site immediately before patch application. Avoid the waistline area where the patch could be rubbed by clothing

• Applications sites should be alternated from one hip to the next each day, avoiding sites where a patch was recently placed, when possible

• Avoid exposing the application site to hair dryers, heating pads, electric blankets, heated water beds, or other direct external heat sources. The rate and extent of absorption of methylphenidate are significantly increased during application of heat to the patch during use. Temperature-dependent increases in absorption may be greater than twofold, potentially resulting in overdose

• Do not apply or reapply the patch with dressings, tape, or adhesives. If the patch is not fully adhered to the skin during application or wear time, discard the patch according to disposal instructions and apply a new patch

• The total daily wear time should not exceed 9 hr, regardless of patch replacement

• Patches should be peeled off slowly. Patch removal may be aided by applying an oil-based product (petroleum jelly, mineral oil, olive oil) to the patch edges and gently working the oil underneath the edges of the patch

• **Disposal:** Instruct patient and/or caregiver to fold used patches so that the adhesive side of the patch adheres to itself, and then flush it down the toilet or dispose of in an appropriate lidded container. If the patient stops using the prescription, each unused patch should be removed from its pouch, separated from the protective liner, folded onto itself, and flushed down the toilet or disposed of in an appropriate lidded container. Do not flush pouch and protective liner down the toilet. Instead, dispose of them in an appropriate container with a lid

Patient/family education

• Teach patient to decrease caffeine consumption (coffee, tea, cola, chocolate); not to use guarana, cola nut, yerba maté, which may increase irritability and stimulation; to avoid OTC preparations unless approved by prescriber; to avoid alcohol ingestion; these may cause serious product interactions, to always use dosing dispenser provided for oral suspension dose

• Advise patient to taper off product over several wk, or depression, increased sleeping, lethargy may occur

• Notify prescriber if skin irritation or rash occurs if patch comes off, use a new one on a different skin site, tell child not to remove or share with others

• Instruct patient not to double doses if medication is missed; prescriber may suggest product holidays (ADHD) during the school year to assess progress and determine continued product necessity

• Instruct patient/family to notify prescriber if significant side effects occur: tremors, insomnia, palpitations, restlessness; product changes may be needed

• Inform patient that if dry mouth occurs to use frequent sips of water, sugarless gum, hard candy during beginning therapy; dry mouth lessens with continued treatment

• Encourage patient to get needed rest, patient will feel more tired at end of day; to take last dose at least 6 hr before bedtime to avoid insomnia

• Advise patient that shell of Concerta tab may appear in stools

Evaluation

Positive therapeutic outcome

• Decreased hyperactivity in ADHD
• Improved attention span in ADHD
• Absence of sleeping during day in narcolepsy

TREATMENT OF OVERDOSE:
Administer fluids, hemodialysis, peritoneal dialysis, antihypertensives for increased B/P; administer short-acting barbiturate before lavage

M

methylPREDNISolone (Rx)
(meth-ill-pred-niss′oh-lone)
A-Methapred, Depo-Medrol, Medrol, Solu-MEDROL
Func. class.: Corticosteroid, synthetic
Chem. class.: Glucocorticoid, intermediate acting

Do not confuse: methylPREDNISolone/ medroxyPROGESTERone/predniSONE/ methylTESTOSTERone/predniSONE/Methylprednisone

ACTION: Decreases inflammation by suppression of migration of polymorphonuclear leukocytes, fibroblasts; reverses increased capillary permeability and lysosomal stabilization

Therapeutic outcome: Decreased inflammation

USES: Severe inflammation, shock, adrenal insufficiency, collagen disorders, management of acute spinal cord injury, multiple sclerosis

Pharmacokinetics

Absorption	Well absorbed (PO); systemic (topical)
Distribution	Crosses placenta
Metabolism	Liver, extensively
Excretion	Kidney
Half-life	3-5 hr (plasma) 18-36 hr (tissue); adrenal suppression 3-4 days

Pharmacodynamics

	PO	IM	IV	Topical
Onset	Un-known	Un-known	Rapid	Min to hr
Peak	2 hr	4-8 days	Un-known	Hr to days
Duration	1½ days	1-4 wk	Un-known	Hr to days

CONTRAINDICATIONS
Hypersensitivity, intrathecal use, neonates

Precautions: Pregnancy, breastfeeding, diabetes mellitus, glaucoma, osteoporosis, seizure disorders, ulcerative colitis, HF, myasthenia gravis, renal disease, esophagitis, peptic ulcer; tartrazine, benzyl alcohol, corticosteroid hypersensitivity; viral infection, TB, traumatic brain injury, Cushing's syndrome, measles, varicella, fungal infections

DOSAGE AND ROUTES
Adrenal insufficiency/inflammation
Adult: PO 4-48 mg in 4 divided doses; IM 10-120 mg (acetate); IM/IV 10-40 mg (succinate); intraarticular 4-80 mg (acetate)
Child: IV 0.5-1.7 mg/kg in 3-4 divided doses (succinate)

Multiple sclerosis
Adult: PO/IM/IV 160 mg/day × 1 wk, then 64 mg every other day × 30 days

Most uses (succinate)
Adult: IM/IV 40-250 mg q 4-6 hr; pulse therapy IV 2 mg/kg, then 0.5-1 mg/kg q6hr for up to 5 days

Acute spinal cord injury (succinate)
Adult/child: IV 30 mg/kg over 15 min, then continuous infusion after 45 min, 5.4 mg/kg/hr × 23 hr

Pneumocystis jirovecii (succinate) (AIDS)
Adult: IV 30 mg bid × 5 days, then 30 mg q day × 5 days, then 15 mg q day × 10 days

Available forms: Tabs 2, 4, 6, 8, 16, 32 mg; inj 20, 40, 80 mg/ml acetate; inj 40, 125, 500, 1000, 2000 mg/vial succinate

ADVERSE EFFECTS
CNS: Depression, flushing, sweating, headache, mood changes
CV: Hypertension, circulatory collapse, thrombophlebitis, embolism, tachycardia
EENT: Fungal infections, increased intraocular pressure, blurred vision, cataracts
GI: Diarrhea, nausea, abdominal distention, GI hemorrhage, increased appetite, pancreatitis
HEMA: Thrombocytopenia
INTEG: Acne, poor wound healing, ecchymosis, petechiae
MS: Fractures, osteoporosis, weakness
MISC: Hyponatremia

INTERACTIONS
Individual drugs
Amphotericin B: increased side effects
Insulin: increased need for insulin
Phenytoin, rifampin: decreased action; increased metabolism
Somatrem: decreased effect

Drug classifications
Contraceptives, oral: increased methylPREDNISolone action
CYP3A4 inducers (barbiturates, bosentan, carBAMazepine, efavirenz, phenytoins, nevirapine, rifabutin, rifampin): decreased methylPREDNISolone effect
CYP3A4 inhibitors (aprepitant, antiretroviral protease inhibitors, clarithromycin, danazol, delavirdine, diltiazem, erythromycin, fluconazole, FLUoxetine, fluvoxaMINE, imatinib, ketoconazole, mibefradil, nefazodone, telithromycin, voriconazole): increased adrenal suppression
Diuretics: increased side effects
Hypoglycemic agents: increased need for hypoglycemic agents
Vaccines: decreased effects of vaccines

Drug/herb
St. John's wort: avoid use

Drug/food
Grapefruit juice: increased methylPREDNISolone level; do not use concurrently

Drug/lab test
Increased: cholesterol, blood glucose
Decreased: calcium, potassium, T_4, T_3, thyroid radioactive iodine uptake test, urine 17-OHCS, 17-KS
False negative: skin allergy tests

NURSING CONSIDERATIONS
Assessment
• **Adrenal insufficiency:** assess for weight loss, nausea, vomiting, confusion, anxiety, hypotension, weakness
• Monitor plasma cortisol levels during long-term therapy (normal level 138-635 nmol/L when drawn at 8 AM)
• Monitor potassium, blood glucose, urine glucose while patient is on long-term therapy; hypokalemia and hyperglycemia
• Monitor weight daily; notify prescriber of weekly gain >5 lb

---

- Monitor B/P q4hr, pulse; notify prescriber if chest pain occurs
- Monitor I&O ratio; be alert for decreasing urinary output and increasing edema
- Monitor adrenal function periodically for hypothalamic-pituitary-adrenal axis suppression
- **Assess for infection:** increased temp, WBC even after withdrawal of medication; product masks infection symptoms
- **Assess for potassium depletion:** paresthesias, fatigue, nausea, vomiting, depression, polyuria, dysrhythmias, weakness
- Assess for edema, hypertension, cardiac symptoms
- Assess mental status: affect, mood, behavioral changes, aggression
- Check temp; if fever develops, product should be discontinued
- Assess for systemic absorption: increased temp, inflammation, irritation (topical)
- Beers: Avoid in older adults with or at high risk for delirium; assess for confusion, delirium frequently

Patient problem
Risk for infection (adverse reactions)
Risk for injury (adverse reactions)

Implementation
PO route
- Give with food or milk to decrease GI symptoms
- Single daily dose should be given in AM to coincide with body's normal cortisol secretion
IM route
- Give IM inj deep in large muscle mass; rotate sites; avoid deltoid; use 21-G needle; injection site reaction may occur (induration, pain at site, atrophy)
- Give in one dose in AM to prevent adrenal suppression; avoid SUBCUT administration; may damage tissue

IV route
- Use only methylPREDNISolone sodium succinate (Solu-MEDROL) IV, never use methylPREDNISolone acetate suspension IV
- Give after diluting with provided diluent, agitate slowly; give directly over 3-15 min; doses ≥2 mg/kg or 250 mg should be given by intermittent IV infusion unless potential benefits outweigh potential risks
Intermittent/continuous IV infusion route
- Dilute further in D5W, 0.9% NaCl, D5NS, haze may form, give over 15-60 min, large doses (≥500 mg) give over 30-60 min

- Give after shaking susp (parenteral)
- Give titrated dosage; use lowest effective dosage

Y-site compatibilities: Acetaminophen, acyclovir, amifostine, aztreonam, cefepime, CISplatin, cladribine, cyclophosphamide, cytarabine, DOPamine, DOXOrubicin, enalaprilat, famotidine, fludarabine, granisetron, heparin, inamrinone, melphalan, meperidine, methotrexate, metroNIDAZOLE, midazolam, morphine, piperacillin/tazobactam, sodium bicarbonate, tacrolimus, teniposide, theophylline, thiotepa, vit B with C

Patient/family education
- Teach patient that emergency ID as corticosteroid user should be carried/worn
- Advise patient to notify prescriber if therapeutic response decreases; dosage adjustment may be needed
- Caution patient not to discontinue abruptly; adrenal crisis can result
- Teach patient to take PO with food, milk, to decrease GI symptoms
- Caution patient to avoid OTC products: salicylates, alcohol in cough products, cold preparations unless directed by prescriber
- Teach patient all aspects of product use including cushingoid symptoms
- Teach patient symptoms of **adrenal insufficiency:** nausea, anorexia, fatigue, dizziness, dyspnea, weakness, joint pain
- Inform patient that long-term therapy may be needed to clear infection (1-2 mo depending on type of infection)
- Teach patient to recognize **cushingoid symptoms:** buffalo hump, moon face, rapid weight gain, excess sweating
- **Infection:** Teach patient to avoid persons with known infections; corticosteroids can mask symptoms of infection
- **Pregnancy/breastfeeding:** Use only if benefits outweigh fetal risk; do not breastfeed, excreted in breast milk

Evaluation
Positive therapeutic outcome
- Ease of respirations, decreased inflammation
- Absence of severe itching, patches on skin, flaking (top)

metipranolol ophthalmic
See Appendix B

metoclopramide (Rx)
(met-oh-kloe-pra′mide)
Metonia ❋, Metozolv ODT, Reglan
Func. class.: Cholinergic, antiemetic
Chem. class.: Central dopamine receptor antagonist

Do not confuse: metoclopramide/metolazone, **Reglan**/Megace/Renagel

ACTION: Enhances response to acetylcholine of tissue in upper GI tract, which causes contraction of gastric muscle, relaxes pyloric, duodenal segments, increases peristalsis without stimulating secretions, blocks dopamine in chemoreceptor trigger zone of CNS

Therapeutic outcome: Decreased symptoms of delayed gastric emptying, decreased nausea, vomiting

USES: Prevention of nausea, vomiting induced by chemotherapy, radiation; delayed gastric emptying, gastroesophageal reflux

Pharmacokinetics

Absorption	Well absorbed (PO)
Distribution	Widely distributed; crosses blood-brain barrier, placenta
Metabolism	Liver, minimally
Excretion	Kidneys, breast milk
Half-life	2.5-6 hr

Pharmacodynamics

	PO	IM	IV
Onset	½-1 hr	10-15 min	1-3 min
Peak	Unknown	Unknown	Unknown
Duration	1-2 hr	1-2 hr	1-2 hr

CONTRAINDICATIONS
Hypersensitivity to this product or procaine or procainamide, seizure disorder, pheochromocytoma, GI obstruction

Precautions: Pregnancy, breastfeeding, GI hemorrhage, Parkinson's disease, abrupt discontinuation, cardiac disease, children, depression, diabetes mellitus, G6PD deficiency, geriatrics, heart failure, hypertension, infertility, malignant hyperthermia, methemoglobinemia, procainamide/paraben hypersensitivity, renal impairment, breast cancer (prolactin dependent)

BLACK BOX WARNING: Tardive dyskinesia

DOSAGE AND ROUTES
Nausea/vomiting (chemotherapy)
Adult: IV 1-2 mg/kg 30 min before administration of chemotherapy, then q2hr × 2 doses, then q3hr × 3 doses
Child (unlabeled): IV 1-2 mg/kg/dose

Facilitation of small bowel intubation in radiologic exams
Adult and child >14 yr: IV 10 mg over 1-2 min
Child 6-14 yr: IV 2.5-5 mg
Child <6 yr: IV 0.1 mg/kg

Diabetic gastroparesis
Adult: PO 10 mg 30 min before meals, at bedtime × 2-8 wk
Geriatric: PO 5 mg ½ hr before meals, at bedtime, increase to 10 mg if needed

Gastroesophageal reflux
Adult: PO 10-15 mg qid 30 min before meals and at bedtime
Child: PO 0.4-0.8 mg/kg/day divided in 4 doses

Renal dose
Adult: PO/IV CCr ≥40 ml/min, no change; CCr <40 ml/min: Reduce initial recommended dose by 50%. Thereafter dose may be increased or decreased as needed or CCr >50 ml/min: Give 100% of the normal dose; CCr 10 to 50 ml/min: Give 75% of the normal dose; CCr <10 ml/min: Give 50% of the normal dose
Child: PO/IV CCr 30 to 50 ml/min: Give 75% of the normal dose; CCr 10 to 29 ml/min: Give 50% of the normal dose; CCr <10 ml/min: Give 25% of the normal dose

Available forms: Tabs 5, 10 mg; syr 5 mg/5 ml; solution for inj 5 mg/ml; orally disintegrating tab 5, 10 mg; oral sol 5 mg/5 ml

ADVERSE EFFECTS
CNS: *Sedation, fatigue, restlessness, headache, sleeplessness, dystonia,* dizziness, drowsiness, suicidal ideation, seizures, EPS, neuroleptic malignant syndrome; tardive dyskinesia (>3 mo, high doses)
CV: Hypotension, supraventricular tachycardia
GI: Dry mouth, constipation, nausea, anorexia, vomiting, diarrhea
GU: Decreased libido, prolactin secretion, amenorrhea, galactorrhea
HEMA: Neutropenia, leukopenia, agranulocytosis
INTEG: Urticaria, rash

INTERACTIONS
Individual drugs
Alcohol: increased sedation
Haloperidol: increased extrapyramidal reaction

Drug classifications
Anticholinergics, opiates: decreased action of metoclopramide
CNS depressants: increased sedation
MAOIs: avoid use
Phenothiazines: increased extrapyramidal reaction

Drug/lab test
Increased: prolactin, aldosterone, thyrotropin

NURSING CONSIDERATIONS
Assessment
• Assess GI complaints: nausea, vomiting, anorexia, constipation, abdominal distention before, after administration

> **BLACK BOX WARNING: Assess for EPS and tardive dyskinesia** (more likely to occur in treatment >3 mo, geriatric): rigidity, grimacing, shuffling gait, tremors, rhythmic involuntary movements of tongue, mouth, jaw, feet, hands; these side effects should be reported to prescriber immediately; some effects may be irreversible; assess for involuntary movements frequently

• Assess mental status: depression, anxiety, irritability during treatment
• **Neuroleptic malignant syndrome:** assess for hyperthermia, change in B/P, pulse, tachycardia, sweating, rigidity, altered consciousness
• **Pregnancy/breastfeeding:** Use only if clearly needed, do not breastfeed, excreted in breast milk
• **Beers:** Avoid in older adults unless for gastroparesis, can cause extrapyramidal effects, monitor for EPS frequently

Patient problem
Nausea (uses)
Risk for injury (adverse reactions)

Implementation
PO route
• Use gum, hard candy, frequent rinsing of mouth for dryness of oral cavity
• Give ½-1 hr before meals for better absorption
• **Oral disintegrating:** place on tongue, allow to dissolve, swallow, remove from bottle immediately before use
IM route
• Give for postop nausea and vomiting before end of surgery

Direct IV route
• Give **IV** undiluted if dose is ≤10 mg; give over 2 min
• Give diphenhydrAMINE **IV** or benztropine IM for EPS
• Discard open ampules
Intermittent IV infusion route
• Dilute more than 10 mg in 50 ml or more D₅W, NaCl, Ringer's, LR and give over 15 min or more

Y-site compatibilities: Acetaminophen, acyclovir, aldesleukin, alfentanil, amifostine, amikacin, aminophylline, ascorbic acid, atracurium, atropine, azaTHIOprine, aztreonam, bivalirudin, bleomycin, bumetanide, buprenorphine, butorphanol, calcium chloride/gluconate, CARBOplatin, caspofungin, ceFAZolin, cefonicid, cefoperazone, cefotaxime, cefoTEtan, cefOXitin, cefTAZidime, ceftizoxime, cefTRIAXone, cefuroxime, chloramphenicol, chlorproMAZINE, cimetidine, ciprofloxacin, cisatracurium, CISplatin, cladribine, clindamycin, cyanocobalamin, cyclophosphamide, cycloSPORINE, cytarabine, DACTINomycin, DAPTOmycin, dexamethasone, dexmedetomidine, digoxin, diltiazem, diphenhydrAMINE, DOBUTamine, DOCEtaxel, DOPamine, doripenem, doxapram, DOXOrubicin hydrochloride, doxycycline, droperidol, enalaprilat, ePHEDrine, EPINEPHrine, epirubicin, epoetin alfa, ertapenem, erythromycin, esmolol, etoposide, etoposide phosphate, famotidine, fenoldopam, fentaNYL, filgrastim, fluconazole, fludarabine, folic acid, foscarnet, gallium nitrate, gemcitabine, gentamicin, glycopyrrolate, granisetron, heparin, hydrocortisone, HYDROmorphone, IDArubicin, ifosfamide, imipenem/cilastatin, indomethacin, insulin, isoproterenol, ketorolac, labetalol, leucovorin, levofloxacin, lidocaine, linezolid, LORazepam, magnesium sulfate, mannitol, mechlorethamine, melphalan, meperidine, meropenem, metaraminol, methadone, methotrexate, methoxamine, methyldopate, methylPREDNISolone, metoprolol, metroNIDAZOLE, miconazole, midazolam, milrinone, minocycline, mitoMYcin, morphine, moxalactam, multiple vitamins, nafcillin, nalbuphine, naloxone, nesiritide, nitroglycerin, nitroprusside, norepinephrine, octreotide, ondansetron, oxaliplatin, oxytocin, PACLitaxel, palonosetron, pantoprazole, papaverine, PEMEtrexed, penicillin G, pentamidine, pentazocine, PENTobarbital, PHENobarbital, phentolamine, phenylephrine, phytonadione, piperacillin/tazobactam, potassium chloride, procainamide, prochlorperazine, promethazine, propranolol, protamine, pyridoxine, quinupristin/dalfopristin, ranitidine, remifentanil, riTUXimab, rocuronium,

M

sargramostim, sodium acetate/bicarbonate, suc-cinylcholine, SUFentanil, tacrolimus, teniposide, theophylline, thiamine, thiotepa, ticarcillin/cla-vulanate, tigecycline, tirofiban, tobramycin, to-lazoline, topotecan, trastuzumab, trimethaphan, urokinase, vancomycin, vasopressin, ve-curonium, verapamil, vinBLAStine, vinCRIStine, vinorelbine, voriconazole, zidovudine

Patient/family education
• Instruct patient to avoid driving, other hazard-ous activities until stabilized on this medication
• Advise patient to avoid alcohol and other CNS depressants that enhance sedating properties of this product
• Advise patient to notify prescriber if involun-tary movements occur

Evaluation

Positive therapeutic outcome
• Absence of nausea, vomiting, anorexia, fullness, decreased GERD

---

metolazone (Rx)
(me-tole′a-zone)
Func. class.: Diuretic, antihypertensive
Chem. class.: Thiazide-like quinazoline derivative

Do not confuse: metolazone/methotrexate/metoclopramide

ACTION: Acts on the distal tubule and corti-cal thick ascending limb of the loop of Henle in the kidney, increasing excretion of sodium, wa-ter, chloride, magnesium, potassium, and bicar-bonate, decreases GFR

Therapeutic outcome: Decreased B/P, decreased edema in lung tissue and peripherally

USES: Edema, hypertension

Pharmacokinetics
Absorption	GI tract (10%-20%)
Distribution	Crosses placenta; protein binding 33%
Metabolism	Urine, unchanged
Excretion	Breast milk
Half-life	8 hr (extended); 14 hr (prompt)

Pharmacodynamics
Onset	Unknown
Peak	8 hr
Duration	12-24 hr

CONTRAINDICATIONS
Pregnancy (preeclampsia, intrauterine growth retardation), hypersensitivity to thiazides or sulfonamides, anuria, coma, hepatic encepha-lopathy

Precautions: Pregnancy, breastfeeding, geri-atric, hypokalemia, renal/hepatic disease, gout, COPD, lupus erythematosus, diabetes mellitus, hypotension, history of pancreatitis, hypersensi-tivity to sulfonamides, thiazides, electrolyte imbalance

DOSAGE AND ROUTES
Edema
Adult: PO 5-10 mg/day; max 20 mg/day

Hypertension
Adult: PO 2.5-5 mg/day
Child: PO 0.2-0.4 mg/kg/day in divided doses q12-24hr

Available forms: Tabs 2.5, 5, 10 mg

ADVERSE EFFECTS
CNS: Drowsiness, lethargy
CV: *Orthostatic hypotension,* palpitations, chest pain, hypotension
ELECT: *Hypokalemia,* hypercalcemia, hypo-natremia *hyperuricemia, hypomagnesemia, hypophosphatemia, hypovolemia*
GI: *Nausea, vomiting, anorexia,* constipation, diarrhea, cramps, pancreatitis, GI irritation, dry mouth, jaundice, hepatitis
GU: *Frequency,* polyuria, uremia, glucosuria, nocturia, impotence, *hyperuricemia*
HEMA: Aplastic anemia, hemolytic ane-mia, leukopenia, agranulocytosis, neutro-penia
INTEG: *Rash,* urticaria, purpura, photosensi-tivity, fever, dry skin, toxic epidermal necroly-sis, Stevens-Johnson syndrome
META: *Hyperglycemia,* increased creatinine, BUN
MS: Muscle cramps

INTERACTIONS
Individual drugs
Alcohol: increased hypotension (large amounts)
Amphotericin B, digoxin, mezlocillin, piperacil-lin: increased hypokalemia
Lithium: increased toxicity

Drug classifications
Antidiabetics: increased hyperglycemia
Antihypertensives: increased antihypertensive effect
Barbiturates, nitrates, opioids: increased hypo-tension
Diuretics (loop): increased metolazone effect

Glucocorticoids, laxatives (stimulant): increased hypokalemia

NSAIDs, salicylates: decreased action of metolazone

Drug/food
Licorice: increased severe hypokalemia

Drug/herb
Ephedra (ma huang): decreased antihypertensive effect

Hawthorn: increased antihypertensive effect

Drug/lab test
Increased: calcium, cholesterol, glucose, triglycerides

Decreased: potassium, sodium, chloride, magnesium

NURSING CONSIDERATIONS
Assessment
• **Hypertension:** assess B/P before, during therapy with patient lying, standing, and sitting as appropriate; orthostatic hypotension can occur rapidly

• **HF:** assess for improvement in feet, legs, sacral area daily if medication is being used

• Monitor blood glucose if patient is diabetic

• Check for rashes, temp elevation daily

• Monitor patients receiving cardiac glycosides for increased hypokalemia

• **Hypokalemia:** assess for postural hypotension, malaise, fatigue, tachycardia, leg cramps, weakness

• **Hepatic encephalopathy:** do not use in hepatic coma or precoma, fluctuations in electrolytes can occur rapidly and precipitate hepatic coma, use caution in those with impaired hepatic function

• Assess and record fluid volume status: I&O ratios; monitor weight, distended red veins, crackles in lung, color, quality, and specific gravity of urine; skin turgor, adequacy of pulses, moist mucous membranes, bilateral lung sounds, peripheral pitting edema; dehydration symptoms of decreasing output, thirst, hypotension, dry mouth and mucous membranes should be reported

• Monitor electrolytes: potassium, sodium, calcium, magnesium; also include BUN, blood pH, ABGs, uric acid, CBC, blood glucose

• **Beers:** Use with caution in older adults, may exacerbate or cause SIADH, monitor sodium level frequently

• **Pregnancy/breastfeeding:** Use in pregnancy only if needed; do not breastfeed, excreted in breast milk

Patient problem
Fluid imbalance (uses, adverse reactions)

Risk for injury (uses, adverse reactions)

Implementation
• Give in AM to avoid interference with sleep

• Provide potassium replacement if potassium level is 3.0; product may be crushed if patient is unable to swallow

• Give with food; if nausea occurs, absorption may be increased

Patient/family education
• Teach patient to take the medication early in the day at same time of day to prevent nocturia, not to double or skip doses, to take when remembered if not close to next dose

• Instruct patient to take with food or milk if GI symptoms of nausea and anorexia occur

• Teach patient to maintain a weekly record of weight and notify prescriber of weight loss >5 lb

• Caution patient that this product causes a loss of potassium, so foods rich in potassium should be added to the diet; refer to a dietitian for assistance in planning

• Caution the patient to rise slowly from sitting or reclining positions, not to exercise in hot weather or stand for prolonged periods, since orthostatic hypotension will be enhanced; lie down if dizziness occurs

• Teach patient not to use alcohol or any OTC medications without prescriber's approval; serious product reactions may occur

• Emphasize the need to contact prescriber immediately if muscle cramps, weakness, nausea, dizziness, or numbness occur

• Teach patient to take own B/P and pulse and record

• Advise patient to use sunscreen, protective clothing to prevent burns

• Teach patient to continue taking medication even if feeling better; this product controls symptoms but does not cure the condition

• Advise patient with hypertension to continue other medical regimen (exercise, weight loss, relaxation techniques, smoking cessation)

• Do not stop product abruptly

Evaluation
Positive therapeutic outcome
• Decreased edema

• Decreased B/P

TREATMENT OF OVERDOSE:
Lavage if taken orally, monitor electrolytes; administer dextrose in saline; monitor hydration, CV, renal status

M

⚠ HIGH ALERT

metoprolol (Rx)

(met-oh-proe′lole)

BEtaloc ✦, Lopressor ✦, Lopressor SR ✦, Nu-Metop ✦, Toprol-XL

Func. class.: Antihypertensive, antianginal
Chem. class.: β₁-Adrenergic blocker

Do not confuse: Lopressor/Lyrica
Toprol-XL/Topamax

ACTION: Lowers B/P by β-blocking effects; reduces elevated renin plasma levels; blocks β₂-adrenergic receptors in bronchial, vascular smooth muscle only at high doses, negative chronotropic effect

Therapeutic outcome: Decreased B/P, heart rate, AV conduction

USES: Mild to moderate hypertension, acute MI to reduce cardiovascular mortality, angina pectoris, New York Heart Association class II, III heart failure, cardiomyopathy

Pharmacokinetics

Absorption	Well absorbed (PO); completely absorbed (**IV**)
Distribution	Crosses blood-brain barrier, placenta
Metabolism	Liver, extensively ⅋ℚ⍺ by CYP2D6, some may be poor metabolizers
Excretion	Kidneys, breast milk
Half-life	3-7 hr

Pharmacodynamics

	PO	IV
Onset	15 min	Immediate
Peak	2-4 hr	20 min
Duration	6-19 hr	5-8 hr

CONTRAINDICATIONS

Hypersensitivity to β-blockers, cardiogenic shock, heart block (2nd and 3rd degree), sinus bradycardia, pheochromocytoma, sick sinus syndrome

Precautions: Pregnancy, breastfeeding, geriatric, major surgery, diabetes mellitus, thyroid/renal/hepatic disease, COPD, CAD, nonallergic bronchospasm, HF, bronchial asthma, CVA, children, depression, vasospastic angina

BLACK BOX WARNING: Abrupt discontinuation

DOSAGE AND ROUTES
Hypertension

Adult: PO 50 mg bid, or 100 mg/day; may give 100-450 mg in divided doses; ext rel 25-100 mg qday, titrate at weekly intervals, max 400 mg/day

Child/adolescent 6-16 yr: PO ext rel 1 mg/kg up to 50 mg qday

Geriatric: PO 25 mg/day initially, increase weekly as needed

Myocardial infarction

Adult: IV BOL (early treatment) 5 mg q2min × 3 doses, then 50 mg PO 15 min after last dose and q6hr × 48 hr (late treatment); PO maintenance 50-100 mg bid for 1-3 yr

Heart failure (NYHA class II/III)

Adult: PO ext rel 25 mg qd × 2 wk (class II); 12.5 mg qd (class III)

Angina

Adult: PO 100 mg/day as a single dose or in 2 divided doses, increase qwk as needed, or 100 mg ext rel tab daily, max 400 mg/day ext rel

Migraine prevention (unlabeled)

Adult: PO 25-100 mg bid-qid; 50-200 mg daily (XL)

Available forms: Tabs 25, 50, 100 mg; inj 1 mg/ml; ext rel tabs (tartrate) 100 mg; ext rel tabs (succinate) (XL) 25, 50, 100, 200 mg

ADVERSE EFFECTS

CNS: *Insomnia, dizziness,* mental changes, hallucinations, depression, anxiety, headaches, nightmares, confusion, fatigue, weakness
CV: HF, *palpitations,* dysrhythmias, cardiac arrest, *hypotension,* bradycardia, pulmonary/peripheral edema, chest pain
EENT: Blurred vision
GI: *Nausea, vomiting,* colitis, cramps, *diarrhea,* constipation, flatulence, dry mouth, *hiccups*
GU: Impotence, urinary frequency
HEMA: Agranulocytosis, eosinophilia, thrombocytopenic purpura
INTEG: Rash, purpura, alopecia, dry skin, urticaria, pruritus
RESP: Bronchospasm, dyspnea, wheezing
ENDO: Hyper/hypoglycemia

INTERACTIONS
Individual drugs

Cimetidine: increased metoprolol level
Digoxin, diltiazem, EPINEPHrine, hydrALAZINE, methyldopa prazosin, verapamil: increased hypotension, bradycardia
Insulin: increased hypoglycemia
Dopamine, theophylline: Decreased effect of each

Drug classifications

Antidiabetics (oral): increased hypoglycemia

Amphetamines, calcium channel blockers, histamine H_2 antagonists: increased hypotension, bradycardia

Barbiturates: decreased metoprolol level

MAOIs: do not use together

NSAIDs, salicylates: decreased antihypertensive effect

Xanthines: decreased effects of xanthines

Drug/food

Increased: absorption with food

Drug/lab test

Increased: BUN, potassium, ANA titer, serum lipoprotein, triglycerides, uric acid, alkaline phosphatase, LDH, AST, ALT, blood glucose

NURSING CONSIDERATIONS
Assessment

> **BLACK BOX WARNING: Abrupt withdrawal:** may cause MI, ventricular dysrhythmias, myocardial ischemia; taper dose over 7-14 days

• **Hypertension/angina:** monitor ECG directly when giving IV during initial treatment

• Monitor B/P during beginning treatment, periodically thereafter; pulse; note rate, rhythm, quality; check apical/radial pulse before administration; notify prescriber of any significant changes (pulse <40 bpm), if cardiac output is decreased, atropine may be needed; ECG q 5-15 min during and after use

• Check for baselines in renal, liver function tests before therapy begins and periodically thereafter

• Assess for edema in feet, legs daily; monitor I&O, daily weight; check for jugular vein distention, crackles bilaterally, dyspnea (HF)

• **Pregnancy/breastfeeding:** Use only if clearly needed, excreted in breast milk in small quantities, the American Academy of Pediatrics considers this product to be compatible with breastfeeding

Patient problems
Impaired cardiac output (uses)
Nonadherence (teaching)

Implementation
PO route

• Take apical pulse before giving, if <50 bpm hold and notify prescriber

• Do not break, crush, or chew ext rel tabs

• Give regular release tab before meals, at bedtime; tab may be crushed or swallowed whole; give with food to prevent GI upset; reduced

dosage in renal dysfunction; give at same time each day

• Store in dry area at room temp; do not freeze

Direct IV route

• Check dose with another person to prevent errors that could be fatal

• Give 1 mg/ml over 1 min

Y-site compatibilities: Abciximab, acyclovir, alemtuzumab, alfentanil, alteplase, amikacin, aminophylline, amiodarone, amphotericin B liposome, anidulafungin, argatroban, ascorbic acid, atracurium, atropine, azaTHIOprine, aztreonam, benztropine, bivalirudin, bleomycin, bumetanide, buprenorphine, butorphanol, calcium chloride/gluconate, CARBOplatin, caspofungin, ceFAZolin, cefonicid, cefoperazone, cefotaxime, cefoTEtan, cefOXitin, cefTAZidime, ceftizoxime, cefTRIAXone, cefuroxime, chloramphenicol, chlorproMAZINE, cimetidine, CISplatin, clindamycin, cyanocobalamin, cyclophosphamide, cycloSPORINE, cytarabine, DACTINomycin, DAPTOmycin, dexamethasone, dexmedetomidine, digoxin, diltiazem, diphenhydrAMINE, DOBUTamine, DOCEtaxel, DOPamine, doxacurium, DOXOrubicin, doxycycline, enalaprilat, ePHEDrine, EPINEPHrine, epirubicin, epoetin alfa, eptifibatide, esmolol, etoposide, etoposide phosphate, famotidine, fenoldopam, fentaNYL, fluconazole, fludarabine, fluorouracil, folic acid, furosemide, ganciclovir, gemcitabine, gentamicin, glycopyrrolate, granisetron, heparin, hydrocortisone, HYDROmorphone, IDArubicin, ifosfamide, imipenem/cilastatin, indomethacin, insulin, isoproterenol, ketorolac, labetalol, linezolid, LORazepam, magnesium sulfate, mannitol, mechlorethamine, meperidine, metaraminol, methotrexate, methoxamine, methyldopa, methylPREDNISolone, metoclopramide, metroNIDAZOLE, midazolam, milrinone, mitoXANtrone, morphine, multivitamins, nafcillin, nalbuphine, naloxone, nitroprusside, norepinephrine, octreotide, ondansetron, oxacillin, oxaliplatin, oxytocin, PACLitaxel, palonosetron, pancuronium, papaverine, PEMEtrexed, penicillin G, pentamidine, pentazocine, PENTobarbital, PHENobarbital, phentolamine, phenylephrine, phytonadione, piperacillin/tazobactam, potassium chloride, procainamide, prochlorperazine, promethazine, propranolol, protamine, pyridoxine, quinupristin/dalfopristin, ranitidine, rocuronium, sodium bicarbonate, succinylcholine, SUFentanil, tacrolimus, teniposide, theophylline, thiamine, thiotepa, ticarcillin/clavulanate, tigecycline, tirofiban, tobramycin, tolazoline, trimetaphan, urokinase, vancomycin, vasopressin, vecuronium, verapamil, vinCRIStine, vinorelbine, voriconazole

M

Patient/family education

> **BLACK BOX WARNING:** Teach patient not to discontinue product abruptly; taper over 2 wk; may cause precipitate angina if stopped abruptly

• Teach patient not to use OTC products containing α-adrenergic stimulants (such as nasal decongestants, cold preparations); to avoid alcohol, smoking and to limit sodium intake as prescribed
• Teach patient how to take pulse and B/P at home; advise when to notify prescriber
• Teach patient to rise from sitting slowly to decreased orthostatic hypotension
• Instruct patient to comply with weight control, dietary adjustments, modified exercise program
• Tell patient to carry/wear emergency ID to identify product being taken, allergies; tell patient product controls symptoms but does not cure
• Caution patient to avoid hazardous activities if dizziness, drowsiness is present, to avoid driving until product response is known
• Teach patient to report symptoms of HF; difficult breathing, especially with exertion or when lying down, night cough, swelling of extremities or bradycardia, dizziness, confusion, depression, fever, decreased vision
• Teach patient to take product as prescribed, not to double doses or skip doses; take any missed doses as soon as remembered if at least 4 hr until next dose
• Advise patient to monitor blood glucose closely if diabetic, monitor for hypo/hyperglycemia
• Advise patient to report Raynaud's symptoms

Evaluation

Positive therapeutic outcome
• Decreased B/P in hypertension (after 1-2 wk)
• Absence of dysrhythmias
• Decreased anginal pain

TREATMENT OF OVERDOSE:

Lavage, **IV** atropine for bradycardia, digoxin, O₂, diuretic for cardiac failure, hemodialysis, **IV** glucose for hyperglycemia, **IV** diazepam (or phenytoin) for seizures

---

metroNIDAZOLE (Rx)

(me-troe-ni′da-zole)
Flagyl, Flagyl ER, MetroCream, MetroGel, MetroGel Vaginal, Metro Lotion, Metro IV, Nidagel ✹, Noritate, Nuvessa, Vandazole
Func. class.: Antiinfective, miscellaneous
Chem. class.: Nitroimidazole derivative

Do not confuse: Metronidazole/Metformin

ACTION: Direct-acting amebicide/trichomonacide; binds, degrades DNA structure, inhibiting bacterial nucleic acid synthesis

Therapeutic outcome: Trichomonacidal, amebicidal, bactericidal for the following susceptible organisms: *Bacteroides, Clostridium, Trichomonas vaginalis, Giardia lamblia, Entamoeba histolytica*

USES: Intestinal amebiasis, amebic abscess, trichomoniasis, refractory trichomoniasis, bacterial anaerobic infections, giardiasis; septicemia, endocarditis, bone, joint, and lower respiratory tract infections, rosacea

Unlabeled uses: Crohn's disease

Pharmacokinetics

Absorption	80% (PO)
Distribution	Widely distributed, crosses placenta
Metabolism	Liver
Excretion	Urine, unchanged; feces
Half-life	6-11 hr

Pharmacodynamics

	PO	IV
Onset	Rapid	Immediate
Peak	1-2 hr	Infusion's end
Duration	Unknown	Unknown

CONTRAINDICATIONS

Pregnancy (1st trimester), breastfeeding, hypersensitivity to this product

Precautions: Pregnancy (2nd/3rd trimesters), candidal infections, heart failure, fungal infection, geriatric, dental disease, bone marrow suppression, hematologic disease, renal/hepatic/GI disease, contracted visual or color fields, blood dyscrasias, CNS disorders

> **BLACK BOX WARNING:** Secondary malignancy

DOSAGE AND ROUTES
Trichomoniasis
Adult: PO 500 mg bid × 7 days or 2 g in single dose; do not repeat treatment for 4-6 wk
Child ≥45 kg (unlabeled): PO 2 g once
Child <45 kg (unlabeled): PO 15 mg/kg/day divided in 3 doses × 7-10 days

Amebic hepatic abscess
Adult: PO 750 mg tid × 7-10 days
Child: PO 35-50 mg/kg/day in 3 divided doses × 7-10 days

Intestinal amebiasis
Adult: PO 750 mg tid × 7-10 days
Child: PO 35-50 mg/kg/day in 3 divided doses × 7-10 days; then oral iodoquinol

Anaerobic bacterial infections
Adult: **IV** INF 15 mg/kg/over 1 hr, then 7.5 mg/kg **IV** or PO q6hr, max 4 g/day; first maintenance dose should be administered 6 hr after loading dose

Bacterial vaginosis
Adult: PO reg rel 500 mg bid or 250 mg tid × 7 days; ext rel 750 mg/day × 7 days; Vaginal MetroGel Vaginal, apply 1 applicatorful of 0.75% gel 1-2 times per day × 5 days; Nuvessa: 1 applicatorful of 1.3% gel dose at bedtime; Vandazole: 1 applicatorful of 0.75% gel q day × 5 day

Acne rosacea
Adult: Top apply a small, thin layer bid

Giardiasis (unlabeled)
Adult: PO 250 mg tid × 5-7 days
Child: PO 5 mg/kg divided tid × 5 days

Antibiotic-associated CDAD
Adult (unlabeled): PO 250-500 mg 3 times per day × 10-14 days
Child: PO 20 mg/kg/day (max 2 g) divided q6hr

Available forms: Tabs 250, 500 mg; ext rel tabs 750 mg; caps 375 mg; inj sol 5 mg/ml

ADVERSE EFFECTS
CNS: *Headache, dizziness,* confusion, irritability, restlessness, ataxia, depression, fatigue, drowsiness, insomnia, paresthesia, peripheral neuropathy, seizures, incoordination, depression, encephalopathy, aseptic meningitis (IV)
CV: Flat T-waves
EENT: Blurred vision, sore throat, retinal edema, dry mouth, metallic taste, furry tongue, glossitis, stomatitis, photophobia, optic neuritis
GI: *Nausea, vomiting, diarrhea,* epigastric distress, *anorexia,* constipation, *abdominal cramps, Clostridium difficile* (CDAD), xerostomia, metallic taste, abdominal pain, pancreatitis
GU: Genital Candida infection
HEMA: Leukopenia, bone marrow depression, aplasia, thrombocytopenia
INTEG: Rash, pruritus, urticaria, flushing, phlebitis at injection site, toxic epidermal necrolysis

INTERACTIONS
Individual drugs
Alcohol, oral ritonavir, any product with alcohol: increased disulfiram-like reaction
AzaTHIOprine, fluorouracil: increased leukopenia
Amprenavir, disulfiram: do not use bortezomib; norfloxacin, zalcitabine: avoid use

Busulfan: increased busulfan toxicity, avoid concurrent use
Cholestyramine: decreased metroNIDAZOLE, toxicity
Fosphenytoin, lithium, phenytoin, warfarin: increased action of these drugs

Drug classifications
Barbiturates: decreased metroNIDAZOLE half life
CYP3A4 substrates: increased levels

Drug/lab test
Altered: AST, ALT, LDH
Decrease: WBC, neutrophils
False decrease: triglycerides

NURSING CONSIDERATIONS
Assessment
• **Assess patient for signs and symptoms of infection** including characteristics of wounds, WBC $>10,000/mm^3$, vaginal secretions, fever; obtain baseline information and during treatment
• Obtain C&S before beginning product therapy to identify if correct treatment has been initiated, product can be started before results are received
• **Assess for allergic reactions:** rash, urticaria, pruritus; if fever, facial swelling, blisters, discontinue immediately
• Identify urine output; if decreasing, notify prescriber **(may indicate nephrotoxicity)**; also check for increased BUN, creatinine
• Assess bowel pattern daily; if severe diarrhea occurs, product should be discontinued
• Assess for overgrowth of infection: perineal itching, fever, malaise, redness, pain, swelling, drainage, rash, diarrhea, change in cough, sputum

> **BLACK BOX WARNING: Secondary malignancy:** use only when indicated, avoid unnecessary use

• **Giardiasis:** Obtain stools before starting treatment to confirm diagnosis, then 3-4 wk after treatment
• Monitor I&O, weight, sodium, and other electrolytes; product contains sodium

Patient problem
Infection (uses)
Diarrhea (uses)
Risk for injury (adverse reactions)

Implementation
Acne rosacea
• Adult top: apply thin film to area bid
• Store in light-resistant container; do not refrigerate

M

PO route

• Give with or after a meal to avoid GI symptoms, metallic taste; crush tab if needed, give on empty stomach

Topical route

• A thin coating should be applied to affected area after cleaning with soap and water and patting dry

Intermittent IV infusion route

• Give intermittent **IV** prediluted; 500 mg/100 ml (5 mg/ml) give over 30-60 min

Y-site compatibilities: Acyclovir, alemtuzumab, alfentanil, allopurinol, amifostine, amikacin, aminophylline, amiodarone, ampicillin, ampicillin/sulbactam, anidulafungin, atracurium, bivalirudin, bumetanide, buprenorphine, busulfan, butorphanol, calcium acetate/chloride/gluconate, CARBOplatin, ceFAZolin, cefepime, cefoperazone, cefoTEtan, cefotaxime, cefTRIAXone, cefuroxime, chloramphenicol, chlorproMAZINE, cimetidine, ciprofloxacin, cisatracurium, CISplatin, clindamycin, codeine, cyclophosphamide, cycloSPORINE, cytarabine, DACTINomycin, dexamethasone, dexmedetomidine, dexrazoxane, digoxin, diltiazem, dimenhyDRINATE, diphenhydrAMINE, DOBUTamine, DOCEtaxel, DOPamine, doripenem, doxacurium, doxapram, DOXOrubicin, DOXOrubicin liposome, doxycycline, droperidol, enalaprilat, ePHEDrine, EPINEPHrine, epirubicin, eptifibatide, ertapenem, erythromycin, esmolol, etoposide, etoposide phosphate, famotidine, fenoldopam, fentaNYL, fluconazole, fludarabine, fluorouracil, foscarnet, fosphenytoin, furosemide, gemcitabine, gentamicin, glycopyrrolate, granisetron, haloperidol, heparin, hydrALAZINE, hydrocortisone, HYDROmorphone, IDArubicin, ifosfamide, imipenem/cilastatin, inamrinone, insulin, isoproterenol, ketorolac, labetalol, leucovorin, levofloxacin, lidocaine, linezolid, LORazepam, magnesium sulfate, mannitol, mechlorethamine, melphalan, meperidine, meropenem, mesna, metaraminol, methotrexate, methyldopate, methylPREDNISolone, metoclopramide, metoprolol, midazolam, milrinone, mitoXANtrone, morphine, nafcillin, nalbuphine, naloxone, nesiritide, niCARdipine, nitroglycerin, nitroprusside, norepinephrine, octreotide, ondansetron, oxaliplatin, oxytocin, PACLitaxel, palonosetron, pancuronium, pentamidine, pentazocine, PENTobarbital, perphenazine, PHENobarbital, phentolamine, phenylephrine, piperacillin/tazobactam, potassium chloride/phosphates, prochlorperazine, promethazine, propranolol, ranitidine, remifentanil, riTUXimab, rocuronium, sargramostim, sodium acetate/bicarbonate/phosphates, streptozocin, succinylcholine, SUFentanil, tacrolimus, teniposide, theophylline, thiopental, thiotepa, ticarcillin/clavulanate, tigecycline, tirofiban, tobramycin, trastuzumab, trimethobenzamide, trimethoprim/sulfamethoxazole, vancomycin, vasopressin, vecuronium, verapamil, vinCRIStine, vinorelbine, voriconazole, zidovudine, zoledronic acid

Patient/family education

• Teach patient to report sore throat, bruising, bleeding, joint pain; may indicate blood dyscrasias (rare)

• Advise patient to contact prescriber if vaginal itching, loose foul-smelling stools, furry tongue occur; may indicate superinfection

• Advise patient to avoid driving or other hazardous activities until response is known; dizziness may occur

• Teach patient to notify health care professional of rash, fever, facial swelling, blisters

• Advise patient to discuss with professional all OTC, Rx, herbals, supplements taken

• Instruct patient incorrect use of vaginal or topical products

• Advise patient to notify physician of numbness or tingling of extremities

• Teach trichomoniasis patient that both partners need to be treated; condoms should be used during intercourse to prevent reinfection

• **Pregnancy/breastfeeding:** Not to be used in breastfeeding or first trimester of pregnancy

• Advise patient of disulfiram-like reaction to alcohol ingestion; alcohol should not be used within 48 hr of this product

• Inform patient product has a metallic taste and urine may turn dark

• Advise patient to contact prescriber if pregnancy is suspected

• Advise patient to use sips of water, sugarless gum, candy for dry mouth

Evaluation

Positive therapeutic outcome

• Decreased symptoms of infection

metroNIDAZOLE topical
See Appendix B

micafungin (Rx)
(my-ca-fun'gin)
Mycamine
Func. class.: Antifungal, systemic
Chem. class.: Echinocandin

ACTION: Inhibits an essential component in fungal cell walls; causes direct damage to fungal cell wall

Therapeutic outcome: Prevention of *Candida* infection in hematopoietic stem cell transplantation (HSCT); or decreased symptoms of *Candida* infection, negative culture

USES: Treatment of esophageal candidiasis; prophylaxis of *Candida* infections in patients undergoing HSCT; susceptible *Candida* species: *C. albicans, C. glabrata, C. krusei, C. parapsilosis, C. tropicalis,* prophylaxis of HIV-related esophageal candidiasis

Pharmacokinetics

Absorption	Unknown
Distribution	Protein binding 99%
Metabolism	Liver
Excretion	Feces (70%), urine
Half-life	14-17.2 hr

Pharmacodynamics

Onset	Rapid
Peak	Infusion's End
Duration	up to 24 hr

CONTRAINDICATIONS
Hypersensitivity to this product or other echinocandins

Precautions: Pregnancy, breastfeeding, children, geriatric, severe hepatic disease, renal impairment, hemolytic anemia

DOSAGE AND ROUTES
Candidemia/acute disseminated candidiasis, abscess, peritonitis
Adult: IV 100 mg/day over 1 hr × 15 days
Child ≥4 mo and >30 kg: IV 2 mg/kg/day, max 100 mg/day; **≥4 mo and <30 kg** 2 mg/kg/day

Esophageal candidiasis
Adult: IV 150 mg/day, given over 1 hr × 15 days
Child ≥4 mo and >30 kg: IV 2.5 mg/kg/day, max 150 mg/day; **≥4 mo and ≤30 kg** 3 mg/kg/day

Prophylaxis of *Candida* infections
Adult: IV 50 mg/day, given over 1 hr × 6-50 days
Child ≥4 mo and >30 kg: IV 1 mg/kg/day, max 50 mg/day; **≥4 mo and ≤30 kg** 1 mg/kg/day

Available forms: Powder for injection 50 mg, in single-dose vials; 50, 100 mg vial

ADVERSE EFFECTS
GI: Abdominal pain, *nausea, anorexia, vomiting, diarrhea,* hepatitis
GU: Renal failure
HEMA: Hemolytic anemia
INTEG: *Rash, pruritus, inj site pain*
MISC: Allergic reactions

INTERACTIONS
Individual drugs
Itraconazole, sirolimus, NIFEdipine: increased plasma concentrations; may need dosage reduction

Drug/lab test
Increased: ALT/AST, alk phos, bilirubin, LDH, BUN, creatinine
Decreased: blood glucose, potassium sodium, platelets, Hgb, WBCs

NURSING CONSIDERATIONS
Assessment
• Assess for signs and symptoms of infection, clearing of cultures during treatment; obtain culture baseline, throughout; product may be started as soon as culture is taken (esophageal candidiasis); monitor cultures during HSCT, for prevention of *Candida* infections
• Monitor CBC (RBC, Hct, Hgb), differential, platelet count baseline, periodically; notify prescriber of results
• Monitor renal studies: BUN, urine CCr, electrolytes before, during therapy
• Monitor hepatic studies before, during treatment: bilirubin, AST, ALT, alkaline phosphatase, as needed
• Assess for hypersensitivity: rash, pruritus, facial swelling; also for phlebitis
• Assess for hemolytic anemia
• **Pregnancy/breastfeeding:** Use cautiously in breastfeeding, in pregnancy use only if benefits outweigh fetal risk

Patient problem
Infection (uses)

Implementation
• Protect diluted sol from light
• Do not use if cloudy or precipitated; do not admix product
• Flush line before, after administration with 0.9% NaCl

Intermittent IV infusion route

• Visually inspect parenteral products for particulate matter and discoloration prior to use
• Reconstitute each 50 mg vial or 100 mg vial with 5 ml of either 0.9% Sodium Chloride Injection, USP, or 5% Dextrose Injection, USP. Neither the NS nor the D5W should have a bacteriostatic agent. Each reconstituted 50 mg micafungin vial will yield a solution containing 10 mg/ml, and each 100 mg micafungin vial will yield a solution containing 20 mg/ml.
Gently dissolve the powder by swirling the vial. In order to minimize excessive foaming, do not vigorously shake the vial.
• Reconstituted micafungin may be stored in the original vial for up to 24 hr at room temperature (25° C or 77° F). Do not mix or co-infuse micafungin with other medications.
• Adults: Transfer the needed amount of reconstituted micafungin to an IV bag containing 100 ml of 0.9% sodium chloride or 5% Dextrose Injection.
• Pediatric patients: Calculate the total dose needed by multiplying recommended dose (mg/kg) by the patient's weight (kg). Calculate the volume of reconstituted micafungin needed by dividing the calculated dose (mg) from step one by the final concentration of the reconstituted vial (either 10 mg/ml for the 50 mg vial or 20 mg/ml for the 100 mg vial). Withdraw the calculated volume of reconstituted micafungin and add to an IV bag or syringe containing 0.9% sodium chloride or 5% Dextrose Injection. Ensure the final concentration of the diluted solution is between 0.5-4 mg/ml. Infusion bags/syringes containing micafungin concentrations >1.5 mg/ml should be labeled for administration through a central catheter only.
• Discard partially used vials; micafungin is preservative-free. The final diluted solution should be protected from light and may be stored for up to 24 hr at room temperature (25° C or 77° F). Coverage of the infusion drip chamber or the tubing to protect them from light is not necessary. If an existing IV line will be used, flush the line with 0.9% sodium chloride before infusing micafungin.
• Infusion: Give over 1 hr. If administered more rapidly, more frequent histamine-mediated reactions may occur. Do not administer as an IV bolus injection. To minimize the risk of infusion reactions, solutions with micafungin concentrations >1.5 mg/ml should be administered via a central catheter

Y-site compatibilities: Aminophylline, bumetanide, calcium chloride/gluconate, cyclo-SPORINE, DOPamine, eptifibatide, esmolol, fenoldopam, furosemide, heparin, HYDROmorphone, lidocaine, LORazepam, magnesium sulfate, milrinone, nitroglycerin, nitroprusside, norepinephrine, phenylephrine, potassium chloride, potassium phosphate, tacrolimus, vasopressin

Patient/family education

• Teach patient to report bleeding, facial swelling, wheezing, difficulty breathing, itching, rash, hives, increasing warmth, flushing
• Instruct patient to report signs of infection: increased temp, sore throat, flulike symptoms
• Advise patient to notify prescriber if pregnancy is suspected or planned or if breastfeeding

Evaluation
Positive therapeutic outcome

• Prevention of *Candida* infection in HSCT; decreased symptoms of *Candida* infection, negative culture

---

miconazole (Rx, OTC)

(mi-kon′a-zole)
Oravig
miconazole nitrate
Baza, Desenex, Micaderm, Fungold, Lotrimin AF, Micozole ✹, Monistat 1, Monistat 3, Monistat 7: Micatin, Micatin, Vagistat 3, Zeasorb-AF, M-zole 3, Tetterine
Func. class.: Antifungal
Chem. class.: Imidazole

ACTION: Alters cell membranes, inhibits fungal enzymes, inhibits sterols so intracellular contents are lost, prevents biosynthesis of phospholipids/triglycerides

Therapeutic outcome: Fungistatic/fungicidal against *Aspergillus, Coccidioides, Cryptococcus, Candida, Dermatophytes, Histoplasma*

USES: Coccidioidomycosis, candidiasis, cryptococcosis, paracoccidioidomycosis, chronic mucocutaneous candidiasis, fungal meningitis; **IV** used for severe infections only; topical for tinea pedis, tinea cruris, tinea corporis, tinea versicolor, vaginal or vulva candidal infections

Pharmacokinetics

Absorption	Poorly absorbed (PO)
Distribution	Bound to serum proteins (90%)
Metabolism	Liver, extensively
Excretion	Unknown
Half-life	Triphasic: 0.4, 2.1, 24 hr

Pharmacodynamics

	Topical	Vag
Onset	Unknown	Unknown
Peak	Unknown	Unknown
Duration	Unknown	Unknown

CONTRAINDICATIONS
Hypersensitivity

Precautions: Pregnancy, renal/hepatic disease

DOSAGE AND ROUTES
Oropharyngeal candidiasis (thrush)
Adult/adolescent ≥16 yr: Buccal apply 1 tab (50 mg) to upper gum region just above incisor tooth q day × 14 days
Adult and child: TOP apply to affected area bid × 2-4 wk
Adult: Intravaginal 200 mg SUPP at bedtime × 3 days or 100 mg SUPP × 1 wk

Available forms: Inj 10 mg/ml; aerosol 2%; cream 2%; lotion 2%; powder 2%; spray 2%; vag cream 2%; vag supp 100, 200 mg; buccal tab 50 mg

ADVERSE EFFECTS
CNS: Drowsiness, headache, fatigue, pain
CV: Tachycardia
GI: Nausea, vomiting (buccal), anorexia, diarrhea, cramps, dry mouth
GU: Vulvovaginal burning, itching, hyponatremia, pelvic cramps (topical forms)
HEMA: Anemia, lymphopenia, neutropenia
INTEG: Pruritus, rash, fever, flushing, hives

INTERACTIONS
Individual drugs
Progesterone: Decreased progesterone effect (vaginal)
Warfarin: increased anticoagulant effect (buccal), monitor PT, INR

Drug/lab test
Decrease: WBC, RBC (buccal)

NURSING CONSIDERATIONS
Assessment
• Assess for signs and symptoms of **infection**: drainage, sore throat, urinary pain, hematuria, fever
• Monitor bowel pattern before, during treatment; diarrhea may occur
• Monitor blood studies: WBC, RBC, Hgb, Hct, bleeding time; patients taking anticoagulants may need a decreased dosage; monitor liver and renal studies periodically for patients on long-term therapy
• Monitor for allergies before initiation of treatment and reaction to each medication; highlight allergies on chart; check for allergic reaction: burning, stinging, swelling, redness (topical); observe for skin eruptions after administration of product to 1 wk after discontinuing product

Patient problem
Infection (uses)

Implementation
Transmucosal use (adhesive buccal tablet)
• Apply tab in the morning after brushing the teeth; use dry hands
• Place the rounded surface of the tab against the upper gum just above the incisor tooth; hold in place with a slight pressure over the upper lip for 30 seconds to ensure adhesion
• Although the tab is rounded on one side for comfort, the flat side may also be applied to the gum
• The tab will gradually dissolve
• Administration of subsequent tabs should be made to alternating sides of the mouth
• Before applying the next tab, clear away any remaining tab material
• Do not crush, chew or swallow; food and drink can be taken normally; avoid chewing gum
• If tab does not adhere or falls off within the first 6 hr, the same tab should be repositioned immediately. If the tab still does not adhere, a new tab should be used
• If the tab falls off or is swallowed after it was in place for 6 hr or more, a new tab should not be applied until the next regularly scheduled dose
Topical route
• Apply after cleansing area with soap and water before each application; use enough medication to cover lesions completely; dry well
• Store at room temperature in dry place
Vaginal route
• Administer 1 applicator full every night high into the vagina
• Store at room temperature in dry place

Patient/family education
• Advise patient to notify nurse of diarrhea, symptoms of candidal vaginitis
Topical route
• Teach patient to use medical asepsis (hand washing) before, after each application; to apply with glove to prevent further infection; to avoid contact with eyes; not to use occlusive dressings
• Caution patient to avoid use of OTC creams, ointments, lotions unless directed by prescriber
• Instruct patient to notify prescriber if condition does not improve in 4 wk or if symptoms return in 2 mo; pregnancy or a serious medical condition may be the cause
• Teach patient to use for full prescribed treatment time, or reinfection may occur

M

Vaginal route
- Instruct patient in asepsis (hand washing) before, after each application
- Teach patient to apply with applicator only; to avoid use of any other vaginal product unless directed by prescriber; sanitary napkin may prevent soiling of undergarments; to abstain from sexual intercourse until treatment is completed or reinfection and irritation may occur; not to use tampons, douches, spermicides; not to engage in sexual activity; product may damage condoms, diaphragms, cervical caps
- Instruct patient to notify prescriber if symptoms persist

Evaluation

Positive therapeutic outcome
- Decreasing oral candidiasis, fever, malaise, rash
- Negative C&S for infectious organism
- Decrease in size, number of lesions
- Decrease in itching or white discharge (vaginal)

TREATMENT OF OVERDOSE:
Withdraw product; maintain airway; administer EPINEPHrine, aminophylline, O₂, **IV** corticosteroids for anaphylaxis

---

⚠ HIGH ALERT

midazolam (Rx)
(mid′ay-zoe-lam)
Func. class.: Sedative/hypnotic, Anxiolytic
Chem. class.: Benzodiazepine, short-acting
Controlled substance schedule IV

ACTION: Depresses subcortical levels in CNS; may act on limbic system, reticular formation; may potentiate GABA by binding to specific benzodiazepine receptors

Therapeutic outcome: Sedation for anesthesia induction and procedures

USES: Preoperative sedation, general anesthesia induction, sedation for diagnostic endoscopic procedures, intubation, anxiety

Unlabeled uses: Refractory status epilepticus

Pharmacokinetics

Absorption	Well absorbed
Distribution	Crosses placenta, blood-brain barrier; protein binding 97%
Metabolism	Liver; by CYP3A4 to metabolites excreted in urine
Excretion	Kidneys, breast milk
Half-life	1-5 hr

Pharmacodynamics

	PO	IM	IV
Onset	10-30 min	15 min	1.5-5 min
Peak	Unknown	½-1 hr	Unknown
Duration	Unknown	2-3 hr	<2 hr

CONTRAINDICATIONS
Pregnancy, hypersensitivity to benzodiazepines, acute closed-angle glaucoma, epidural/intrathecal use

Precautions: Breastfeeding, children, geriatric, COPD, HF, chronic renal failure, chills, debilitated, hepatic disease, shock, coma, alcohol intoxication, status asthmaticus

> **BLACK BOX WARNING:** Neonates (contains benzyl alcohol), **IV** administration, respiratory depression/insufficiency, specialized care setting, experienced clinician, coadministration with other CNS depressants

DOSAGE AND ROUTES
Preoperative sedation/amnesia induction
Adult and child ≥12 yr: IM 0.07-0.08 mg/kg 30-60 min before general anesthesia
Child 6 mo-5 yr: IV 0.05-0.1 mg/kg, a total dose of 0.6 mg/kg may be needed
Child 6-12 yr: IV 0.025-0.05 mg/kg, a total dose of 0.4 mg/kg may be needed

Induction of general anesthesia
Adult >55 yr: (ASA I/II) IV 150-300 mcg/kg over 30 sec; (ASA III/IV) limit dose to 250 mcg/kg (nonpremedicated) or 150 mcg/kg (premedicated)
Adult <55 yr: IV 200-350 mcg/kg over 20-30 sec; if patient has not received premedication, may repeat by giving 20% of original dose; if patient has received premedication reduce dosage by 50 mcg/kg
Child: No safe and effective dosage is established; however, doses of 50-200 mcg/kg **IV** have been used

Continuous infusion for mechanical ventilation (critical care)
Adult: IV 0.01-0.05 mg/kg over several min; repeat at 10-15 min intervals until adequate sedation, then 0.02-0.10 mg/kg/hr maintenance; adjust as needed

---

Child: IV 0.05-0.2 mg/kg over 2-3 min, then 0.06-0.12 mg/kg/hr by CONT INF; adjust as needed

Neonate: IV 0.03 mg/kg/hr titrate using lowest dose

Status epilepticus (unlabeled) (seizures >5 min)

Adult: IM 10 mg or 0.2 mg/kg once, max 10 mg

Child ≥1 yr >40 kg: IM 10 mg once; **13-40 kg** 5 mg once

Available forms: Inj 1, 5 mg/ml, (preservative free); injection 1 mg/ml, 5 mg/ml; syr 2 mg/ml

ADVERSE EFFECTS

CNS: Retrograde amnesia, headache, slurred speech, paresthesia, tremors, weakness, chills, agitation, paradoxical reactions

CV: Hypotension, PVCs

EENT: Nystagmus

GI: *Nausea, vomiting*

INTEG: Urticaria, pain/swelling at injection site

RESP: Coughing, apnea, respiratory depression

INTERACTIONS
Individual drugs

Alcohol: increased respiratory depression

Cimetidine, erythromycin, ranitidine, theophylline: decreased midazolam metabolism

FluvoxaMINE, indinavir, ritonavir, verapamil, protease inhibitors: increased respiratory depression, use caution

Drug classifications

Antihypertensives, nitrates, opiates: increase in hypotension

> **BLACK BOX WARNING:** Barbiturates, opiate analgesics, other CNS depressants: increased respiratory depression, dosage adjust may be needed

CYP3A4 inducers (azole antifungals, theophylline): increased half-life of midazolam, adjust dose if needed

CYP3A4 inhibitors (fluconazole, itraconazole, ketoconazole, macrolide antiinfectives, calcium channel blockers): increased levels of midazolam, avoid using together

Drug/herb

Kava, valerian: increased sedation

St. John's wort: decreased midazolam, don't use together

Drug/food

Grapefruit juice: increased midazolam effect (PO); don't use together

NURSING CONSIDERATIONS
Assessment

• **Respiratory depression/insufficiency:** assess for apnea, respiratory depression, which may be increased in the geriatric population

• Monitor B/P, pulse, respiration during **IV**; O_2 and emergency equipment should be nearby

• Monitor inj site for redness, pain, swelling

• Assess degree of amnesia in geriatric; may be increased

• **Beers:** Avoid in older adults with or at high risk for delirium, assess frequently for confusion, delirium

Patient problem

Impaired breathing (adverse reactions)

Risk for injury (adverse reactions)

Implementation

• Store at room temperature; protect from light

PO route (syrup)

• **Press-in bottle adaptor (PIBA):** Remove cap of press-in bottle adaptor and push adaptor into neck of bottle; close with cap, remove cap, and insert tip of dispenser and insert into adaptor; turn upside-down and withdraw correct dose; place in mouth

IM route

• Give inj deep into large muscle mass

IV route

• Give **IV** undiluted or after diluting with D_5W or 0.9% NaCl (1 mg/ml or 5 mg/ml undiluted or 0.03-3 ml diluted); give over 2-5 min

• Ensure immediate availability of resuscitation equipment, O_2 to support airway; do not give by rapid bol

Continuous IV infusion route

• Dilute in 0.9% NaCL or D5W, to 0.5-1 mg/ml, dose is calculated on patient's weight and use

Y-site compatibilities: Abciximab, acetaminophen, alemtuzumab, alfentanil, amikacin, amiodarone, anidulafungin, argatroban, atracurium, atropine, aztreonam, benztropine, calcium gluconate, ceFAZolin, cefotaxime, cefOXitine, cefTRIAXone, cimetidine, ciprofloxacin, CISplatin, clindamycin, cloNIDine, cyanocobalamin, cycloSPORINE, DACTINomycin, digoxin, diltiazem, diphenhydrAMINE, DOCEtaxal, DOPamine, doxycycline, enalaprilat, EPINEPHrine, erythromycin, esmolol, etomidate, etoposide, famotidine, fentaNYL, fluconazole, folic acid, gatifloxacin, gemcitabine, gentamicin, glycopyrrolate, granisetron, heparin, hetastarch, HYDROmorphone, hydrOXYzine, inamrinone, isoproterenol, labetalol, lactated Ringer's, levofloxacin, lidocaine, linezolid, LORazepam, magnesium, mannitol, meperidine, methadone, methyldopa, methylPREDNISolone, metoclopramide, metoprolol, metroNIDAZOLE, milrinone, morphine, nalbuphine, naloxone, niCARdipine, nitroglycerin, nitroprusside, norepinephrine, ondansetron, oxacillin, oxytocin, PACLitaxel, palonosetron, pancuronium, papaverine, phentolamine, phytonadione, piperacillin, potassium chloride, propanolol, protamine, pyridoxine, ranitidine, remifentanil, sodium nitroprusside, streptokinase, succinylcholine, SUFentanil, teniposide, theophylline, thiotepa, ticarcillin, tobramycin, vancomycin, vasopressin, vecuronium, verapamil, voriconazole, zoledronic acid

Patient/family education
- Inform patient that amnesia occurs; events might not be remembered
- Caution patient to avoid CNS depressants including alcohol for 24 hr after taking this product
- Pregnancy/breastfeeding: Identify if pregnancy is planned or suspected or if breastfeeding
- Advise patient to ask for assistance in getting up as dizziness, drowsiness occurs

Evaluation

Positive therapeutic outcome
- Induction of sedation, amnesia

TREATMENT OF OVERDOSE:
O_2, flumazenil

⚠ HIGH ALERT
RARELY USED

midostaurin
(mye-doe-staw'-rin)
Rydapt
Func. class.: Antineoplastic

USES: For the treatment of newly diagnosed, FLT3 mutation-positive AML in combination with standard cytarabine and daunorubicin induction and consolidation therapy and for the treatment of aggressive systemic mastocytosis, systemic mastocytosis with associated hematological neoplasm, or mast cell leukemia

DOSAGE AND ROUTES
Newly diagnosed, FLT3 mutation-positive AML
Adult: **PO** 50 mg bid on days 8 to 21 of each cycle of induction therapy with cytarabine and daunorubicin; additionally, give midostaurin 50 mg bid on days 8 to 21 of each cycle of consolidation with high-dose cytarabine therapy

Aggressive systemic mastocytosis, systemic mastocytosis with associated hematological neoplasm, or mast cell leukemia
Adult: **PO** 100 mg bid until disease progression

mifepristone (Rx)
(mif-ee-press' tone)
Mifeprex
Func. class.: Abortifacient
Chem. class.: Antiprogestational

ACTION: Stimulates uterine contractions, causing complete abortion

Therapeutic outcome: Termination of pregnancy

USES: Abortion through 49 days of gestation

Pharmacokinetics

Absorption	Rapidly
Distribution	98% protein binding, albumin, glycoprotein
Metabolism	Unknown
Excretion	Feces, urine
Half-life	Unknown

Pharmacodynamics

Onset	Unknown
Peak	90 min
Duration	Unknown

CONTRAINDICATIONS: Hypersensitivity to this product, misoprostol, or prostaglandins; severe renal/hepatic disease, PID, respiratory/cardiac disease, IUD, ectopic pregnancy, chronic adrenal failure, bleeding disorder, inherited porphyrias

Precautions: Pregnancy, women >35 yr smoking 10 cigarettes/day, asthma, anemia, jaundice, diabetes mellitus, seizure disorders, past uterine surgery

> **BLACK BOX WARNING:** Infection, sepsis, vaginal bleeding

DOSAGE AND ROUTES
Coadministration of mifepristone/misoprostol
Adult: Day 1: PO single dose 600 mg mifepristone, 400 mcg misoprostol day 3 if needed (unless complete termination is confirmed)

Available forms: Tabs 200 mg

ADVERSE EFFECTS
CNS: Dizziness, insomnia, anxiety, syncope, fainting, headache
GI: Nausea, vomiting, diarrhea, dyspepsia
GU: Uterine cramping, uterine hemorrhage, vaginitis, pelvic pain
MISC: Fatigue, back pain, fever, viral infections, chills, sinusitis

INTERACTIONS
Individual drugs
Erythromycin, itraconazole, ketoconazole: decreased metabolism of each specific product

Drug classifications
Anticoagulants, long-term corticosteroids: do not use together

Drug/herb
St. John's wort: decreased mifepristone action

Drug/food
Grapefruit juice: decreased metabolism of mifepristone

NURSING CONSIDERATIONS
Assessment
• Monitor B/P, pulse; watch for change that may indicate hemorrhage
• Monitor respiratory rate, rhythm, depth; notify prescriber of abnormalities
• Assess for length, duration of contraction; notify prescriber of contractions lasting >1 min or absence of contractions
• **Assess for incomplete abortion;** pregnancy must be terminated by another method; product is teratogenic

Patient problems
• Lack of knowledge of medication (teaching)
• Pain (adverse reactions)

Implementation
• Provide emotional support before and after abortion

Patient/family education
• **Sepsis:** advise patient to report increased blood loss, abdominal cramps, increased temp, foul-smelling lochia
• Teach patient some methods of comfort control and pain control
• Advise patient to continue with follow-up
• Advise patient that cramping and vaginal bleeding will occur

Evaluation
Positive therapeutic outcome
• Expulsion of fetus

⚠ HIGH ALERT
milrinone (Rx)
(mill-re′none)
Func. class.: Inotropic/vasodilator agent with phosphodiesterase activity
Chem. class.: Bipyridine derivative

ACTION: Positive inotropic agent with vasodilator properties; increases contractility of cardiac muscle; reduces preload and afterload by direct relaxation of vascular smooth muscle; increases myocardial contractility

Therapeutic outcome: Increased inotropic effect resulting in increased cardiac output

USES: Short-term management of advanced HF that has not responded to other medication

Pharmacokinetics
Absorption	Completely absorbed
Distribution	Unknown
Metabolism	Liver (50%)
Excretion	Kidney, unchanged (83%), metabolites (12%)
Half-life	2.4 hr; increased in HF

Pharmacodynamics
Onset	2-5 min
Peak	10 min
Duration	Variable

CONTRAINDICATIONS
Hypersensitivity to this product, severe aortic disease, severe pulmonic valvular disease, acute MI

Precautions: Pregnancy, breastfeeding, children, geriatric, renal/hepatic disease, atrial flutter/fibrillation

DOSAGE AND ROUTES
Adult: IV BOL 50 mcg/kg given over 10 min; start INF of 0.375-0.75 mcg/kg/min; reduce dosage in renal impairment

Renal dose
Adult: IV CCr 41-50 ml/min 0.43 mcg/kg/min, titrate up; CCr 31-40 ml/min 0.38 mcg/kg/min, titrate up; CCr 21-30 ml/min 0.33 mcg/kg/min, titrate up; CCr 11-20 ml/min 0.28 mcg/kg/min; CCr 6-10 ml/min 0.23 mcg/kg/min; CCr <6 ml/min 0.20 mcg/kg/min; max all dosages 0.75 mcg/kg/min

Available forms: Inj 1 mg/ml; premixed inj 200 mcg/ml in D_5W

M

ADVERSE EFFECTS
CNS: Headache
CV: Dysrhythmias, hypotension, chest pain, PVCs
HEMA: Thrombocytopenia
MISC: Hypokalemia, injection site reactions

INTERACTIONS

NURSING CONSIDERATIONS
Assessment
• Monitor B/P and pulse, ECG continuously during IV; ventricular dysrhythmia can occur; PCWP, CVP, index often during inf; if B/P drops 30 mm Hg, stop inf and call prescriber
• Monitor for hypokalemia: acidic urine, reduced urine, osmolality, nocturia; hypotension, broad T-wave, U-wave, ectopy, tachycardia, weak pulse; muscle weakness, altered LOC, drowsiness, apathy, lethargy, confusion, depression; anorexia, nausea, cramps, constipation, distention, paralytic ileus; hypoventilation, respiratory muscle weakness
• Assess fluid volume status: complete I&O ratio and record; note weight, distended red veins, crackles in lung; color, quality, and specific gravity of urine; skin turgor, adequacy of pulses, moist mucous membranes, bilateral lung sounds, peripheral pitting edema; dehydration symptoms of decreasing output, thirst, hypotension, dry mouth and mucous membranes should be reported
• Monitor electrolytes: potassium, sodium, calcium, magnesium; also include BUN, blood pH, ABGs
• Monitor ALT, AST, bilirubin daily; if these are elevated, hepatotoxicity is suspected
• Monitor platelets; if <150,000/mm³, product is usually discontinued and another product started
• Assess for extravasation: change site q48hr

Patient problem
Impaired cardiac output (uses)
Risk for injury (adverse reactions)

Implementation
Direct IV route
• Give **IV** loading dose undiluted over 10 min; use controlled-rate device
• Administer by direct **IV** into inf through Y-connector or directly into tubing
Continuous IV infusion route
• Dilute 20 mg vial with 80, 112, 180 ml of 0.45% NaCl, 0.9% NaCl, or D₅W to a concentration of 200, 150, 100 mcg/ml respectively
• Do not mix directly with glucose sol (chemical reaction occurs over 24 hr) precipitate forms if milrinone and furosemide come into contact

• Titrate rate based on hemodynamic and clinical response, use controlled device
• Administer potassium supplements if ordered for potassium levels <3.0 mg/dl

Y-site compatibilities: Acyclovir, alfentanil, allopurinol, amifostine, amikacin, aminocaproic acid, aminophylline, amiodarone, amphotericin B liposome, ampicillin, ampicillin-sulbactam, anidulafungin, argatroban, atenolol, atracurium, aztreonam, bivalirudin, bleomycin, bumetanide, buprenorphine, busulfan, butorphanol, calcium chloride/gluconate, CARBOplatin, caspofungin, ceFAZolin, cefepime, cefotaxime, cefoTEtan, cefOXitin, cefTAZidime, ceftizoxime, cefTRIAXone, cefuroxime, chloramphenicol, chlorproMAZINE, cimetidine, ciprofloxacin, cisatracurium, CISplatin, clindamycin, cyclophosphamide, cycloSPORINE, cytarabine, DACTINomycin, DAPTOmycin, dexamethasone, digoxin, diltiazem, DOBUTamine, DOCEtaxel, DOPamine, doripenem, doxacurium, DOXOrubicin, doxycycline, droperidol, enalaprilat, ePHEDrine, EPINEPHrine, epirubicin, eptifibatide, ertapenem, erythromycin, etoposide, famotidine, fenoldopam, fentaNYL, fluconazole, fludarabine, fluorouracil, gallium, ganciclovir, gatifloxacin, gemcitabine, gentamicin, glycopyrrolate, granisetron, haloperidol, heparin, hydrALAZINE, hydrocortisone, HYDROmorphone, IDArubicin, ifosfamide, insulin (regular), irinotecan, isoproterenol, ketorolac, labetalol, levofloxacin, linezolid, LORazepam, magnesium sulfate, mannitol, mechlorethamine, melphalan, meperidine, meropenem, methohexital, methotrexate, methyldopa, methylPREDNISolone, metoclopramide, metoprolol, metroNIDAZOLE, micafungin, midazolam, mitoXANtrone, morphine, mycophenolate, nafcillin, nalbuphine, naloxone, nesiritide, norepinephrine, octreotide, oxacillin, oxaliplatin, oxytocin, PACLitaxel, palonosetron, pamidronate, pancuronium, PEMEtrexed, pentamidine, pentazocine, PENTobarbital, PHENobarbital, phenylephrine, piperacillin, piperacillin-tazobactam, polymyxin B, potassium chloride/phosphates, prochlorperazine, promethazine, propofol, propranolol, quiNIDine, quinupristin-dalfopristin, ranitidine, remifentanil, rocuronium, sodium acetate/bicarbonate/phosphates, streptozocin, succinylcholine, SUFentanil, sulfamethoxazole-trimethoprim, tacrolimus, teniposide, theophylline, thiopental, thiotepa, ticarcillin, ticarcillin-clavulanate, tigecycline, tirofiban, tobramycin, torsemide, vancomycin, vasopressin, vecuronium, verapamil, vinCRIStine, vinorelbine, voriconazole, zidovudine, zoledronic acid

Patient/family education
• Teach patient reason for medication and expected results

- Instruct patient to make position changes slowly; orthostatic hypotension may occur
- Teach patient signs and symptoms of hypersensitivity reactions and hypokalemia

Evaluation

Positive therapeutic outcome
- Increased cardiac output
- Decreased PCWT, adequate CVP
- Decreased dyspnea, fatigue, edema

TREATMENT OF OVERDOSE:
Discontinue product, support circulation

RARELY USED

milnacipran
(mil-na-sip′ ran)
Savella
Func. class.: Antifibromyalgia agent

USES: Fibromyalgia

CONTRAINDICATIONS: Hypersensitivity, MAOIs

BLACK BOX WARNING: Children, suicidal ideation

DOSAGE AND ROUTES
Adult: PO 50 mg bid after titration; titrate using this schedule: 12.5 mg on day 1, then 12.5 mg bid on days 2 and 3, then 25 mg bid (days 4 to 7). Give 50 mg bid

Renal Dose
Adult PO CCr 5 to 29 mL/min: Reduce maintenance dose by 50%; **CCr <5 mL/min and those with end-stage renal disease:** Do not use

---

minocycline (Rx)
(min-oh-sye′kleen)
Dynacin, Minolira, Minocin, Solodyn
Func. class.: Broad-spectrum antiinfective
Chem. class.: Tetracycline

ACTION: Inhibits protein synthesis and phosphorylation in microorganisms by binding to 30S ribosomal subunits and reversibly binding to 50S ribosomal subunits; bacteriostatic

Therapeutic outcome: Bactericidal action against susceptible organisms, including *Neisseria meningitidis, Neisseria gonorrhoeae, Treponema pallidum, Chlamydia trachomatis, Ureaplasma urealyticum, Mycoplasma pneumoniae, Nocardia, Rickettsia*

USES: Syphilis, chlamydial infection, gonorrhea, lymphogranuloma venereum, rickettsial infections, inflammatory acne, meningitis carriers, periodontitis, methicillin-resistant *Staphylococcus aureus* (MRSA) infections, nonnodular moderate to severe acne vulgaris, *Rickettsia* sp.

Pharmacokinetics

Absorption	Well absorbed (PO)
Distribution	Widely distributed; some distribution in CSF, crosses placenta
Metabolism	Liver, some
Excretion	Kidneys, unchanged (20%), bile, feces
Half-life	11-17 hr

Pharmacodynamics

	PO	IV
Onset	Rapid	Rapid
Peak	2-3 hr	Infusion's end
Duration	Unknown	Unknown

CONTRAINDICATIONS
Pregnancy, hypersensitivity to tetracyclines, children <8 yr

Precautions: Breastfeeding, hepatic disease

DOSAGE AND ROUTES
Most infections
Adult: PO/IV 200 mg, then 100 mg q12hr, max 400 mg/24 hr **IV**
Child >8 yr: PO/IV 4 mg/kg then 4 mg/kg/day PO in divided doses q12hr

Rickettsial infections
Adult: PO/IV 200 mg, then 100 mg q12hr
Adolescent/child ≥8 yr: PO/IV 4 mg/kg, then 2 mg kg q12hr, max adult dose

Gonorrhea
Adult: PO 200 mg, then 100 mg q12hr × 4 days or more

Syphilis
Adult: PO 200 mg, then 100 mg q12hr × 10-15 days

Uncomplicated gonococcal urethritis in men
Adult: PO 100 mg q12hr × 5 days

Acne vulgaris (solodyn only)
Adult/adolescent/child ≥12 yr: ext rel 1 mg/kg/day × 12 wk or those weighing 126-136 kg: 135 mg/day; 111-125 kg: 115 mg/day; 97-110 kg: 105 mg/day; 85-96 kg: 90 mg/day; 72-84 kg: 80 mg/day; 60-71 kg: 65 mg/day; 50-59 kg: 55 mg/day; 45-49 kg: 45 mg/day

Acne vulgaris (all except solodyn)
Adult/adolescent/child ≥12 yr: ext rel 1 mg/kg × 12 wk or 91-136 kg/135 mg/day; 60-90 kg 90 mg/day; 45-59 kg 45 mg/day

Available forms: Caps 50, 75, 100 mg; powder for inj 100 mg; tabs 50, 75, 100 mg; ext rel tabs 45, 55, 65, 80, 90, 105, 115, 135 mg

ADVERSE EFFECTS
CNS: *Dizziness,* fever, light-headedness, vertigo, seizures, increased intracranial pressure, headache
CV: Pericarditis, thrombophlebitis
EENT: Dysphagia, glossitis, decreased calcification, permanent discoloration of teeth, tinnitus
GI: *Nausea, vomiting, diarrhea,* anorexia, hepatotoxicity
GU: Renal failure
HEMA: Eosinophilia, neutropenia, thrombocytopenia, hemolytic anemia, pancytopenia
INTEG: *Rash, urticaria, photosensitivity, increased pigmentation,* exfoliative dermatitis, pruritus, blue-gray color of skin and mucous membranes
MS: Myalgia, arthritis, bone growth retardation (<8 yr)
SYST: Angioedema, Stevens-Johnson syndrome
RESP: Bronchospasm, cough, dyspnea

INTERACTIONS
Drug classifications
Alkali products, antacids, laxatives (calcium, aluminum, magnesium), antidiarrheals: decreased minocycline effect
Anticoagulants increased effect, monitor INR, PT
Barbiturates, penicillins: decreased effect
Contraceptives hormonal: Decreased effect, use another form of contraception
Iron products: Decreased minocycline absorption, give 2 hr prior to or 3 hr after iron
Live virus vaccines: Decreased effect of vaccine, bring up-to-date before use
Retinoids: increased chance of pseudomotor cerebri, do not use concurrently

Drug/lab test
False negative: urine glucose with Clinistix, Tes-Tape
Increase: BUN, LFTs, eosinophils
Decrease: Hb, platelets, neutrophils

NURSING CONSIDERATIONS
Assessment
• Assess patient for previous sensitivity reaction
• **Assess patient for signs and symptoms of infection** including characteristics of wounds, sputum, urine, stool, WBC >10,000/mm³, fever; obtain baseline information before, during treatment

• Obtain C&S before beginning product therapy to identify if correct treatment has been initiated, may start before results are received
• **Assess for allergic reactions:** rash, urticaria, pruritus, angioedema
• Monitor blood studies: AST, ALT, CBC, Hct, bilirubin, alkaline phosphatase, amylase monthly if patient is on long-term therapy
• **Pseudomembranous colitis:** assess bowel pattern daily; if severe diarrhea occurs, product should be discontinued
• Monitor for bleeding: ecchymosis, bleeding gums, hematuria, stool guaiac daily if on long-term therapy; blood dyscrasias may occur
• **Assess for overgrowth of infection:** perineal itching, fever, malaise, redness, pain, swelling, drainage, rash, diarrhea, change in cough, sputum; black, furry tongue

> **BLACK BOX WARNING: Cardiac disease:** May cause reflex increase in heart rate and decrease B/P

• **Beers:** Avoid use in older adults, may exacerbate syncope, monitor frequently for syncope
• **Pregnancy/breastfeeding:** Do not use in pregnancy, can cause fetal harm, if pregnancy occurs, stop immediately, do not breastfeed, excreted in breast milk

Patient problem
Infection (uses)

Implementation
• Store in airtight, light-resistant container at room temp
PO route
• Give around the clock to maintain proper blood levels; give with food to increase absorption of product; do not give within 3 hr of other agents; product interactions may occur
• Give with 8 oz of water 1 hr before bedtime to prevent ulceration
• Do not give with iron, calcium, magnesium products, or antacids, which decrease absorption and form insoluble chelate

IV route
• Check for irritation, extravasation, phlebitis daily; change site q72hr
• For intermittent inf, dilute each 100 mg/10 ml of 0.9% NaCl, sterile water for inj; further dilute in 100-1000 ml of 0.9% NaCl, D₅W, or 250-1000 ml with Ringer's or lactated Ringer's; give over 1-6 hr, do not give rapidly
• Do not admix

Patient/family education
- Teach patient to use sunscreen when outdoors to decrease photosensitivity reaction
- Teach patient to report sore throat, bruising, bleeding, joint pain; may indicate blood dyscrasias (rare)
- Teach patient to avoid driving or other hazardous activities until response is known, dizziness may occur
- Advise patient to take ext rel product at same time of day without regard to food; not to crush, chew, split ext rel tab
- Advise patient to report diarrhea, which can occur several months after discontinuing product
- Advise patient to contact prescriber if vaginal itching, loose foul-smelling stools, furry tongue occur; may indicate superinfection; report itching, rash, pruritus, urticaria
- Instruct patient to take all medication prescribed for the length of time ordered; product must be taken around the clock to maintain blood levels; do not give medication to others; take with a full glass of water; may take with food; not to use outdated product, Fanconi's syndrome may occur
- **Pregnancy/breastfeeding:** Identify if pregnancy is planned or suspected, to use as a nonhormonal type of contraception

Evaluation

Positive therapeutic outcome
- Absence of signs/symptoms of infection (WBC <10,000/mm^3, temp WNL, absence of red, draining wounds)
- Reported improvement in symptoms of infection

mirabegron
(mir′a-beg′ron)
Myrbetriq
Func. class.: Bladder antispasmodic
Chem. class.: β$_3$-Adrenergic receptor agonist

ACTION: Relaxes smooth muscles in urinary tract, increases bladder capacity

Therapeutic outcome: Decreasing dysuria, frequency, nocturia, incontinence

USES: Overactive bladder (urinary frequency, urgency), urinary incontinence

Pharmacokinetics

Absorption	Unknown
Distribution	71% protein binding
Metabolism	Unknown
Excretion	25% unchanged in urine
Half-life	50 hr

Pharmacodynamics

Onset	Unknown
Peak	3.5 hr
Duration	Unknown

CONTRAINDICATIONS
Hypersensitivity

Precautions: Pregnancy, breastfeeding, children, kidney/liver disease, bladder obstruction, dialysis, hypertension

DOSAGE AND ROUTES
Adult: PO 25 mg/day, may increase to 50 mg/day if needed

Hepatic/renal dose
Adult: PO Child–Pugh B or (CCr 15-29 ml/min, max 25 mg/day; Child–Pugh C or CCr 15 ml/min, not recommended

Available forms: Tabs ext rel 25, 50 mg

ADVERSE EFFECTS
CNS: Fatigue, dizziness, headache
CV: *Hypertension*
EENT: Xerophthalmia, blurred vision, dry mouth
GI: Anorexia, abdominal pain, constipation, diarrhea
GU: Urinary retention, frequency, UTI, bladder discomfort
SYST: Stevens–Johnson syndrome, angioedema

INTERACTIONS
Individual drugs
Digoxin, warfarin, desipramine: increased effect of these agents

Drug classifications
CYP2D6 substrates (desipramine, felcainide, metoprolol, thioridazine): increased effect of these substrates

Drug/lab
Increase: LFTs, INR, LDH, digoxin levels

NURSING CONSIDERATIONS
Assessment
- **Urinary patterns:** Assess for distention, nocturia, frequency, urgency, incontinence
- Monitor LFTs at baseline, periodically
- Monitor B/P baseline and periodically, B/P may increase

• Angioedema, Stevens-Johnson syndrome: Assess for facial swelling, dyspnea, discontinue immediately, provide airways

Patient problem
Impaired urination (uses)

Implementation
• Give whole; take with liquids; do not crush, chew, or break ext rel product; use without regard to meals

Patient/family education
• Teach patient to avoid hazardous activities; dizziness can occur, may take up to 8 wk for full effect
• Advise patient not to drink liquids before bedtime
• Advise patient to take as prescribed, not to skip or double doses; if dose is missed, give regularly scheduled next day; provide "Patient Information" materials
• Teach patient to check B/P as B/P may increase
• Teach patient to discuss all OTC, Rx, herbals, supplements taken with health care professional
• Advise patient not to drive or engage in other hazardous activities until response is known
• Inform patient about the importance of bladder maintenance
• **Pregnancy/breastfeeding:** Use only if benefits outweigh fetal risk, discontinue breastfeeding or product, excretion unknown

Evaluation

Positive therapeutic outcome
• Decreasing dysuria, frequency, nocturia, incontinence

---

mirtazapine (Rx)
(mer-ta′za-peen)
Remeron, Remeron RD ✽, Remeron Soltab
Func. class.: Antidepressant
Chem. class.: Tetracyclic

ACTION: Blocks reuptake of norepinephrine, serotonin into nerve endings, increasing action of norepinephrine, serotonin in nerve cells; antagonist of central α_2-receptors, blocks histamine receptors; has anticholinergic action

Therapeutic outcome: Decreased symptoms of depression after 2-3 wk

USES: Depression, dysthymic disorder, bipolar disorder: depression, agitated depression

Unlabeled uses: Panic disorder, PTSD, generalized anxiety disorder (GAD)

Absorption	Slow, complete
Distribution	Widely distributed; crosses placenta
Metabolism	Liver, extensively
Excretion	Feces; breast milk
Half-life	20-40 hr

Onset	Unknown
Peak	2 hr
Duration	Unknown

CONTRAINDICATIONS
Hypersensitivity to tricyclics, recovery phase of MI, agranulocytosis, jaundice, MAOIs

Precautions: Pregnancy, geriatric, suicidal patients, severe depression, increased intraocular pressure, closed-angle glaucoma, urinary retention, cardiac/renal/hepatic disease, hypo/hyperthyroidism, electroshock therapy, elective surgery, seizure disorder, bone marrow suppression, thrombocytopenia

> **BLACK BOX WARNING:** Suicidal ideation, children

DOSAGE AND ROUTES
Adult: PO 15 mg/day at bedtime, maintenance to continue for 6 mo, titrate up to 45 mg/day; orally disintegrating tabs open blister pack, place tab on tongue, allow to disintegrate, swallow
Geriatric: PO 7.5 mg nightly, increase by 7.5 mg q1-2wk to desired dose, max 45 mg/day

Available forms: Tabs 15, 30, 45 mg; orally disintegrating tabs (Soltab) 15, 30, 45 mg

ADVERSE EFFECTS
CNS: *Dizziness, drowsiness,* confusion, anxiety, weakness, nightmares, abnormal dreams, neuroleptic malignant syndrome, suicidal ideation, twitching
CV: *Orthostatic hypotension, ECG changes, tachycardia, hypertension,* palpitations
EENT: Sinusitis
GI: *Dry mouth,* nausea, vomiting, paralytic ileus, increased appetite, cramps, epigastric distress, jaundice, hepatitis, stomatitis, constipation, weight gain
GU: Urinary frequency
HEMA: Agranulocytosis
INTEG: Rash, urticaria, sweating, pruritus, photosensitivity

META: Hyponatremia, hypercholesterolemia
MS: Back pain, myalgia
RESP: Cough, dyspnea
SYST: Flulike symptoms, serotonin syndrome

INTERACTIONS
Individual drugs
Alcohol: increased CNS depression
CloNIDine: decreased effects
Buspiron, fentanyl, kinezolid, methylene blue, nefazodone: increased serotonin syndrome

Drug classifications
Barbiturates, benzodiazepines, CNS depressants (other): increased effects
MAOIs: Increased hypertensive episode, seizures, hyperpyretic crisis, do not use within 14 days
SSRIs, SNRIs, serotonin-receptor agonists: increased serotonin syndrome

Drug/herb
St. John's wort, SAM-e: serotonin syndrome

Drug/lab test
Increased: Cholesterol, LFTs

NURSING CONSIDERATIONS
Assessment
• Assess mental status: mood, sensorium, affect, suicidal tendencies; assess increase in psychiatric symptoms: depression, panic
• Monitor B/P (with patient lying, standing), pulse during beginning treatment; if systolic B/P drops 20 mm Hg, hold product, notify prescriber; take VS more often in patients with CV disease
• **Serotonin syndrome, neuroleptic malignant syndrome:** assess for increased heart rate, shivering, sweating, dilated pupils, tremors, high B/P, hyperthermia, headache, confusion; if these occur, stop product, administer a serotonin antagonist if needed; at least 2 wk should elapse between discontinuation of serotoninergic agents and start of this product
• Monitor blood studies: CBC, LFTs if patient is receiving long-term therapy
• Suicidal ideation: Assess for suicidal thoughts, behaviors
• Seizures: Assess for seizures in those with seizures, may be increased, provide seizure precautions

• Check weight weekly; product may increase appetite
• Identify alcohol consumption; if alcohol is consumed, hold dose until AM
• **Pregnancy/breastfeeding:** Use only if clearly needed, excreted in breast milk, discontinue product or breastfeeding

Patient problem
Depression (uses)
Anxiety (uses)

Implementation
• Administer without regard to meals; crush if patient is unable to swallow medication whole
• Give dose at bedtime if oversedation occurs during day; may take entire dose at bedtime; geriatric may not tolerate once/day dosing
• Store in tight container at room temperature; do not freeze
• Allow **orally disintegrating tablets** to dissolve on tongue; no water needed; do not split; contain phenylalanine

Patient/family education
• Inform patient that therapeutic effects may take 2-3 wk; take at bedtime, do not discontinue abruptly
• Advise patient to use caution in driving and other activities requiring alertness because of drowsiness, dizziness, blurred vision; to avoid rising quickly from sitting to standing, especially geriatric
• Advise patient that follow-up will be needed
• Inform patient to discuss all OTC, RX, herbals, supplements taken with health care professional
• **Serotonin syndrome:** Teach patient to notify health care professional immediately of fever, nausea, vomiting, diarrhea, mental changes
• Caution patient to avoid alcohol ingestion, other CNS depressants
• Teach patient to increase fluids, bulk in diet if constipation, urinary retention occur, especially geriatric
• Teach patient to use gum, hard sugarless candy, or frequent sips of water for dry mouth
• Advise not to use within 14 days of MAOIs

BLACK BOX WARNING: Notify prescriber of suicidal thoughts, behavior immediately

Evaluation
Positive therapeutic outcome
- Decrease in depression
- Absence of suicidal thoughts, behaviors
- Increased interest in activities

TREATMENT OF OVERDOSE:
ECG monitoring, lavage, administer anticonvulsant

misoprostol (Rx)
(mye-soe-prost'ole)
Cytotec
Func. class.: Gastric mucosa protectant; antiulcer
Chem. class.: Prostaglandin E$_1$ analog

Do not confuse: misoprostol/metoprolol

ACTION: Inhibits gastric acid secretion; may protect gastric mucosa; can increase bicarbonate, mucus production

Therapeutic outcome: Prevention of gastric ulcers

USES: Prevention of NSAID-induced gastric ulcers

Unlabeled uses: Duodenal ulcers, labor induction, cervical ripening

Pharmacokinetics
Absorption	Well absorbed
Distribution	Unknown
Metabolism	Liver
Excretion	Kidneys
Half-life	½-1 hr

Pharmacodynamics
Onset	½ hr
Peak	Unknown
Duration	3 hr

CONTRAINDICATIONS
Hypersensitivity to this product or prostaglandins

BLACK BOX WARNING: Pregnancy, females

Precautions: Breastfeeding, children, geriatric, renal disease, CV disease, abnormal fetal position, cardiac/renal/inflammatory bowel disease, C-section, dehydration, diarrhea, fever, ectopic pregnancy, fetal distress, sepsis, vaginal bleeding

DOSAGE AND ROUTES
Adult: PO 200 mcg qid with food for duration of NSAID therapy with last dose at bedtime; if 200 mcg is not tolerated, 100 mcg may be given

Termination of pregnancy
Adults: PO 400 mg q dx2 days after mifepistone if abortion did not occur; vaginal 25 mcg, may repeat q 3-6 hr

Available forms: Tabs 100, 200 mcg

ADVERSE EFFECTS
GI: *Diarrhea,* nausea, vomiting, flatulence, constipation, dyspepsia, abdominal pain
GU: Spotting, cramps, hypermenorrhea, menstrual disorders

INTERACTIONS
Drug/drum
Antacids, magnesium: Increased diarrhea
Drug/food
Maximum concentrations when taken with food

NURSING CONSIDERATIONS
Assessment
- **NSAID-induced ulcer prophylaxis:** monitor patient for GI symptoms: hematemesis, occult or frank blood in stools, also severe abdominal pain, cramping, severe diarrhea
- **Abortion:** Assess for uterine pain, cramping, and bleeding periodically
- **Cervical ripening:** measure dilation periodically

BLACK BOX WARNING: Pregnancy: obtain a negative pregnancy test in women of childbearing age before starting medication; miscarriages are common, start 3rd day after mentrual period after confirmation that patient is not pregnant

Patient problem
Pain (uses) (ulcers)

Implementation
- Give with meals for prolonged product effect; avoid use of magnesium antacids
- Store at room temp

Patient/family education
- Advise patient to avoid black pepper, caffeine, alcohol, harsh spices, extremes in temperature of food, which may aggravate condition
- Caution patient to avoid OTC preparations: aspirin, cough, cold preparations; condition may worsen
- Teach patient that product must be continued for prescribed time to be effective and taken exactly as prescribed; doses are not to be doubled
- Instruct patient to report to prescriber diarrhea, black tarry stools, abdominal pain, cramping, menstrual disorders

---

BLACK BOX WARNING: Caution patient to prevent pregnancy while taking this product; spontaneous abortion may occur

Evaluation
Positive therapeutic outcome
- Prevention of ulcers

⚠ HIGH ALERT

mitoMYcin (Rx)
(mye-toe-mye′sin)
Func. class.: Antineoplastic, antibiotic

Do not confuse: mitoMYcin/mitoXANtrone

ACTION: Inhibits DNA synthesis, primarily; derived from *Streptomyces caespitosus;* appears to cause cross-linking of DNA; a vesicant

Therapeutic outcome: Prevention of rapidly growing malignant cells

USES: Pancreas, stomach, colorectal, bladder cancer

Unlabeled uses: Carcinoma--colon, breast, head and neck, biliary, lung, cervical squamous cell (advanced)

Pharmacokinetics

Absorption	Complete bioavailability
Distribution	Widely distributed; concentrates in tumor
Metabolism	Liver, extensively
Excretion	Kidneys, unchanged
Half-life	1 hr

Pharmacodynamics

Unknown

CONTRAINDICATIONS
Pregnancy, breastfeeding, hypersensitivity, as a single agent, coagulation disorders

BLACK BOX WARNING: Thrombocytopenia

Precautions: Accidental exposure, acute bronchospasm, anemia, children, dental disease/work, extravasation, females, hemolytic-uremic syndrome, infection, radiation therapy, surgery, vaccines, renal/respiratory disease

BLACK BOX WARNING: Bone marrow suppression, hemolytic uremic syndrome, leukopenia, requires a specialized care setting/experienced clinician

DOSAGE AND ROUTES
Adult: IV 20 mg/m^2 q6-8wk

Available forms: Inj 5, 20, 40 mg/vial

ADVERSE EFFECTS
CNS: Fever, headache, confusion, drowsiness, syncope, fatigue
CV: Edema
EENT: Blurred vision
GI: *Nausea, vomiting, anorexia, stomatitis,* hepatotoxicity, diarrhea
GU: Urinary retention, renal failure, infertility
HEMA: Thrombocytopenia, leukopenia, anemia
INTEG: *Rash,* alopecia, extravasation, nail discoloration
MISC: Hemolytic uremic syndrome
RESP: Fibrosis, pulmonary infiltrate

INTERACTIONS
Individual drugs
Radiation: increased toxicity

Drug classifications
Antineoplastics: increased toxicity
Vaccines: avoid concurrent use

Drug/herb
Black cohosh: avoid use

NURSING CONSIDERATIONS
Assessment

BLACK BOX WARNING: Assess for **fatal hemolytic uremic syndrome**: hypertension, thrombocytopenia, microangiopathic hemolytic anemia; occurs during long-term therapy

- Assess buccal cavity q8hr for dryness, sores or ulceration, white patches, oral pain, bleeding, dysphagia; obtain prescription for viscous lidocaine (Xylocaine)
- **Assess symptoms indicating severe allergic reaction:** rash, pruritus, urticaria, purpuric skin lesions, itching, flushing

BLACK BOX WARNING: Bone marrow suppression: Monitor CBC, differential, platelet count weekly; withhold product if WBC is <4000/mm^3 or platelet count is <100,000/mm^3, nadir of leukopenia, thrombocytopenia is 4-8 wk; recovery within 10 wk; serum creatinine >1.7 mg/dl; notify prescriber; bleeding: hematuria, guaiac, bruising, petechiae, mucosa, or orifices; avoid IM injections when platelets are low

M

• **Nepharotoxicity:** Monitor renal function tests: BUN, creatinine, serum uric acid, urine CCr before, during therapy; check I&O ratio; report fall in urine output to <30 ml/hr; adjust dose based on renal function

• **Assess for pulmonary fibrosis, bronchospasm,** dyspnea, crackles, unproductive cough, chest pain, tachypnea, fatigue, increased pulse, pallor, lethargy

• **Hepatotoxicity:** Monitor liver function tests before, during therapy (bilirubin, AST, ALT, LDH) as needed or monthly; check for jaundiced skin and sclera, dark urine, clay-colored stools, itchy skin, abdominal pain, fever, diarrhea

• Assess for bleeding: hematuria, stool guaiac, bruising or petechiae, mucosa or orifices q8hr

• Identify effects of alopecia on body image; discuss feelings about body changes

• Identify edema in feet, joint pain, stomach pain, shaking; check for inflammation of mucosa, breaks in skin

• **Pregnancy/breastfeeding:** Do not use in pregnancy or breastfeeding

Patient problem
Risk for infection (adverse reactions)
Risk for injury (adverse reactions)

Implementation
Direct IV route
• Use cytotoxic handling procedures
• Give antiemetic 30-60 min before product to prevent vomiting
• Use port or central line if possible, product is very irritating to tissues
• Reconstitute 5 mg/10 ml; 20 mg/40 ml; 40 mg/80 ml of sterile water for injection (0.5 mg/ml); shake to dissolve, let stand until completely dissolved; stable for 1 wk at room temperature, 2 wk refrigerated, can be further diluted to 20-40 mcg/ml
• Inject reconstituted injection slowly over 5-10 min **IV** push into free-flowing **IV** infusion of 0.9% NaCl or D₅W
• Avoid excessive heat, store unreconstituted product at room temp

Y-site compatibilities: Allopurinol, amifostine, amphotericin B lipid complex, amphotericin B liposome, anidulafungin, argatroban, atenolol, bivalirudin, bleomycin, caspofungin, CISplatin, cyclophosphamide, DACTINomycin, dolasetron, DOXOrubicin, droperidol, epirubicin, ertapenem, fluorouracil, furosemide, granisetron, heparin, leucovorin, melphalan, methotrexate, metoclopramide, nesiritide, octreotide, ondansetron, oxaliplatin, PACLitaxel, palonosetron, PEMEtrexed, riTUXimab, teniposide, thiotepa, tigecycline, tirofiban, trastuzumab, vinBLAStine, vinCRIStine, voriconazole, zoledronic acid

Patient/family education
• Advise patient to get adequate fluids 2-3 L/day unless contraindicated
• Encourage patient to rinse mouth tid-qid with water, club soda, brush teeth bid-qid with soft brush or cotton-tipped applicators for stomatitis, use unwaxed dental floss
• Teach patient to avoid use of products containing aspirin or ibuprofen, razors, commercial mouthwash, since bleeding may occur; to report symptoms of bleeding (hematuria, tarry stools)
• Caution patient to report signs of anemia (fatigue, headache, irritability, faintness, shortness of breath)
• Advise patient to report any changes in breathing or coughing even several mo after treatment; to avoid crowds and persons with respiratory tract or other infections
• Teach patient to report signs of IV site reaction, redness, inflammation, burning, pain
• Inform patient that hair may be lost during treatment; a wig or hairpiece may make patient feel better; new hair may be different in color, texture
• **Infection:** teach patient to report fever, flulike symptoms, sore throat
• Advise patient not to have any vaccinations without the advice of the prescriber; serious reactions can occur
• Teach patient to report immediately urine retention, absence of urine, dyspnea, bleeding, jaundice, signs of pulmonary toxicity
• **Pregnancy/breastfeeding:** Teach patient that contraception is needed during treatment and for several months after completion of therapy

Evaluation
Positive therapeutic outcome
• Prevention of rapid division of malignant cells

> **⚠ HIGH ALERT**

mitoXANtrone (Rx)

(mye-toe-zan'trone)
Func. class.: Antineoplastic-antibiotic, immunomodulator
Chem. class.: Synthetic anthraquinone

Do not confuse: mitoXANtrone/mitoMYcin/mithramycin/mitotane

ACTION: DNA reactive agent; cytocidal effect on both proliferating and nonproliferating cells; topoisomerase II inhibitor; a vesicant

Therapeutic outcome: Prevention of rapidly growing malignant cells

USES: Acute myelogenous leukemia (adult), relapsed leukemia, breast cancer, multiple sclerosis; used with steroids to treat bone pain (advanced prostate cancer); multiple sclerosis

Unlabeled uses: Liver malignancies, non-Hodgkin's lymphoma, breast cancer

Pharmacokinetics

Absorption	Completely absorbed
Distribution	Widely distributed, protein binding 78%
Excretion	Bile; kidneys, unchanged ($<$10%)
Half-life	23-215 hr

Pharmacodynamics

Unknown

CONTRAINDICATIONS

Pregnancy, hypersensitivity

Precautions: Breastfeeding, children, myelosuppression, cardiac/renal/hepatic disease, gout

> **BLACK BOX WARNING:** Secondary malignancy, neutropenia, intrathecal administration, extravasation, heart failure

DOSAGE AND ROUTES
Acute nonlymphatic leukemia/induction

Adult: IV INF 12 mg/m^2/day on days 1-3, and 100 mg/m^2 cytosine arabinoside $\times$ 7 days as a CONT 24-hr INF, may use 2nd induction

Consolidation

Adult: IV INF 12 mg/m^2 given as a short 5-15 min INF for 2 days with cytarabine $\times$ 5 days, use 6 wk after induction, and another course after 4 wk

Advanced prostate cancer

Adult: IV 12-14 mg/m^2 as a single dose or short INF q21day

Multiple sclerosis, relapsing

Adult: IV INF 12 mg/m^2 as a 5-15 min INF q3mo, cumulative lifetime dose 140 mg/m^2

Available forms: Solution for Inj 2 mg/ml

ADVERSE EFFECTS

CNS: Headache, seizures, fatigue
CV: Cardiotoxicity, dysrhythmias
EENT: Conjunctivitis, blue-green sclera, blurred vision
GI: *Nausea, vomiting, diarrhea, anorexia, stomatitis*, hepatotoxicity, abdominal pain, constipation
GU: Amenorrhea, menstrual disorders, blue-green urine, renal failure
HEMA: Thrombocytopenia, leukopenia, myelosuppression, anemia, secondary leukemia
INTEG: *Rash*, necrosis at inj site, alopecia, dermatitis, thrombophlebitis at inj site
MISC: Fever, hyperuricemia, infections
RESP: Cough, dyspnea
SYST: Tumor lysis syndrome, sepsis

INTERACTIONS
Individual drugs

Cyclosporine: increased effect
Natalizumab: increased infection, avoid using together
Palifermin: increased oral mucositis; do not use within 24 hr of mitoxantrone
Tofacitinib: increased immunosuppression, avoid using together
Radiation: increased toxicity, bone marrow suppression
Trastuzumab: increased cardiac adverse reactions, monitor CV status

Drug classifications

Antineoplastics: increased toxicity, bone marrow suppression
Live virus vaccines: increased adverse reactions

Drug/lab test

Increased: LFTs, uric acid
Decreased: Hct/Hgb, platelets, WBC, calcium, sodium, granulocytes

NURSING CONSIDERATIONS
Assessment

• **Multiple sclerosis:** obtain baseline multigated angiogram, left ventricular ejection fraction (LVEF) if symptoms of HF occur, repeat LVEF or if cumulative dose is $>$100 mg/m^2; do not administer to patients who have received

M

a lifetime dose of ≥140 mg/m² or if LVEF is <50% or significant decrease in LVEF; do not administer in multiple sclerosis if neutrophils <1500/mm³
• Obtain pregnancy test in all women of child-bearing age

> **BLACK BOX WARNING: Cardiotoxicity**
> Monitor ECG; watch for ST-T wave changes, low QRS and T, possible dysrhythmias (sinus tachycardia, heart block, PVCs); also monitor ECHO, MUGA, chest x-ray, RAI angiography to assess ejection fraction before, during treatment; product is cardiotoxic: may develop during treatment or months to years after treatment; risk is greater in cumulative dose >140 mg/m²

• Assess buccal cavity q8hr for dryness, sores or ulceration, white patches, oral pain, bleeding, dysphagia; obtain prescription for viscous lidocaine (Xylocaine)
• **Assess symptoms indicating severe allergic reaction:** rash, pruritus, urticaria, purpuric skin lesions, itching, flushing
• Assess tachypnea, ECG changes, dyspnea, edema, fatigue
• **Bone marrow depression:** Monitor CBC, differential, platelet count weekly; withhold product if WBC is <1500/mm³; leukopenia, neutropenia, thrombocytopenia are expected—leukocyte nadir 10-14 days, recovery in 2-3 wk
• Assess for increased uric acid levels, swelling, joint pain primarily in extremities; patient should be well hydrated to prevent urate deposits
• Monitor renal function tests: BUN, creatinine, urine CCr before, during therapy; determine I&O ratio
• **Hepatotoxicity:** monitor liver function tests before, during therapy (bilirubin, AST, ALT, LDH) as needed or monthly; dose reduction needed in hepatic disease; check for jaundiced skin and sclera, dark urine, clay-colored stools, itchy skin, abdominal pain, fever, diarrhea
• **Assess for bleeding:** hematuria, stool guaiac, bruising or petechiae, mucosa or orifices q8hr; check for inflammation of mucosa, breaks in skin
• Identify effects of alopecia on body image; discuss feelings about body changes

> **BLACK BOX WARNING:** Assess for secondary acute myelogenous leukemia (AML), which can develop after taking this product

• **Pregnancy/breastfeeding:** Do not use in pregnancy or breastfeeding

Patient problem
Risk for infection (adverse reactions)
Risk for injury (adverse reactions)

Implementation
• Do not mix with any other product
• Give fluids **IV** or PO before chemotherapy to hydrate patient
• Provide antiemetic 30-60 min before giving product and prn to prevent vomiting
• Give topical or systemic analgesics for pain
• Sol should be prepared by qualified personnel only under controlled conditions in a biological cabinet using mask, gloves, gown
• Use Luer-Lok tubing to prevent leakage; do not let sol come in contact with skin; if contact occurs, wash well with soap and water

Direct IV route
• Give after diluting with 50 ml or more of 0.9% NaCl or D₅W; give over 3-5 min into running **IV** of D₅W or 0.9% NaCl
Intermittent IV infusion route
• May be diluted further in D₅W, 0.9% NaCl (0.02-0.5 mg/ml) and run over 15-30 min; check for extravasation
Continuous IV infusion route
• Give over 24 hr

Y-site compatibilities: Acyclovir, alemtuzumab, alfentanil, allopurinol, amikacin, aminocaproic acid, aminophylline, amiodarone, anidulafungin, argatroban, arsenic trioxide, atracurium, bivalirudin, bleomycin, bretylium, bumetanide, buprenorphine, butorphanol, calcium chloride, calcium gluconate, CARBOplatin, carmustine, caspofungin, cefoTEtan, ceftizoxime, chloramphenicol, chlorproMAZINE, cimetidine, ciprofloxacin, cisatracurium, CISplatin, cladribine, codeine, cyclophosphamide, cycloSPORINE, cytarabine, DACTINomycin, DAPTOmycin, DAUNOrubicin citrate liposome, dexmedetomidine, dexrazoxane, diltiazem, diphenhydrAMINE, DOBUTamine, DOCEtaxel, dolasetron, DOPamine, doxacurium, doxycycline, droperidol, enalaprilat, ePHEDrine, EPINEPHrine, erythromycin l, esmolol, etoposide, etoposide phosphate, famotidine, fenoldopam, fentaNYL, filgrastim, fluconazole, fludarabine, fluorouracil, ganciclovir, gatifloxacin, gemcitabine, gentamicin, glycopyrrolate, granisetron, haloperidol, hydrALAZINE, hydrocortisone sodium succinate, HYDROmorphone, hydrOXYzine, ifosfamide, imipenemcilastatin, inamrinone, insulin, regular, irinotecan, isoproterenol, ketorolac, labetalol, leucovorin, levofloxacin, levorphanol, lidocaine, linezolid, LORazepam, magnesium sulfate, mannitol, melphalan, meperidine, meropenem, mesna, metaraminol, methohexital, methotrexate, methyldopate, metoclopramide, metoprolol, metroNIDAZOLE, midazolam, milrinone, minocycline, mivacurium, morphine sulfate, nalbuphine, naloxone, nesiritide, niCARdipine, nitroglycerin, norepinephrine, octreotide, ondansetron, oxaliplatin, palonosetron, pamidronate, pancuronium, pentamidine, pentazocine, PENTobarbital, PHENobarbital, phentolamine, phenylephrine, polymyxin B, potassium acetate, potassium chloride, procainamide, prochlorperazine, promethazine hydrochloride, propranolol, quiNIDine gluconate, quinupristin-dalfopristin, ranitidine, remifentanil, riTUXimab, rocuronium, sargramostim, sodium acetate, sodium bicarbonate, succinylcholine, SUFentanil, sulfamethoxazole-trimethoprim, tacrolimus, teniposide, theophylline, thiopental, thiotepa, tigecycline, tirofiban, tobramycin, tolazoline, trastuzumab, trimethobenzamide, vancomycin, vasopressin, vecuronium, verapamil, vinCRIStine, vinorelbine, zidovudine, zoledronic acid

Solution compatibilities: D₅/0.9 NaCl, D₅W, 0.9% NaCl

Patient/family education

• Provide the patient package insert, review with patient
• Teach patient to report to health care professional immediately yellow eyes, skin, clay-colored stools, dark urine, diarrhea
• Inform patient that follow-up exams and blood work will be needed
• Encourage patient to rinse mouth tid-qid with water, club soda; brush teeth bid-qid with soft brush or cotton-tipped applicators for stomatitis; use unwaxed dental floss
• Teach patient to avoid use of products containing aspirin or NSAIDs, razors, commercial mouthwash, since bleeding may occur; to report symptoms of bleeding (hematuria, tarry stools)
• Caution patient to report signs of anemia (fatigue, headache, irritability, faintness, shortness of breath)
• Inform patient that hair may be lost during treatment; a wig or hairpiece may make patient feel better; new hair may be different in color, texture
• Caution patient not to have any vaccinations without the advice of the prescriber; serious reactions can occur
• Advise patient that sclera, urine may turn blue or green
• Advise patient to increase fluids to 2-3 L/day unless contraindicated
• Teach patient to avoid crowds, persons with infections

• Teach patient to report immediately bleeding, dyspnea, possible infections, seizure, jaundice, fever, cough or dyspnea
• **Pregnancy/breastfeeding:** Advise patient that contraception is needed during treatment and for several months after completion of therapy; teach patient to notify prescriber if pregnancy is planned or suspected

Evaluation

Positive therapeutic outcome
• Prevention of relapse in multiple sclerosis
• Prevention of rapid division of malignant cells

modafinil (Rx)
(mo-daf′i-nil)
Alertec ✦, Provigil
Func. class.: CNS stimulant
Chem. class.: Racemic compound
Controlled substance IV

ACTION: Similar action as sympathomimetics; does not alter release of dopamine, norepinephrine

Therapeutic outcome: Ability to stay awake

USES: Narcolepsy, shift work sleep disturbance, obstructive sleep apnea

Pharmacokinetics

Absorption	Rapid
Distribution	60% protein binding
Metabolism	Liver (90%)
Excretion	Unknown
Half-life	15 hr

Pharmacodynamics

Onset	Unknown
Peak	2-4 hr
Duration	Unknown

CONTRAINDICATIONS
Hypersensitivity, ischemic heart disease, left ventricular hypertrophy, chest pain, dysrhythmias

Precautions: Pregnancy, breastfeeding, child <16 yr, geriatric, unstable angina, history of MI, severe hepatic disease

DOSAGE AND ROUTES
Adult/adolescent ≥16 yr: PO 200 mg qd

Hepatic dose (severe hepatic disease)
Adult: PO 100 mg qd

Available forms: Tabs 100, 200 mg

ADVERSE EFFECTS
CNS: *Headache,* anxiety, cataplexy, depression, dizziness, insomnia, amnesia, confusion, ataxia, tremors, paresthesia, dyskinesia, suicidal ideation
CV: Dysrhythmias, hyper/hypotension, chest pain, vasodilation
EENT: Change in vision, *rhinitis,* pharyngitis, epistaxis
GI: Nausea, vomiting, changes in LFTs, anorexia, diarrhea, thirst, mouth ulcers
GU: Ejaculation disorder, urinary retention, albuminuria
HEMA: Eosinophilia
INTEG: Rash, dry skin, herpes simplex, Stevens-Johnson syndrome
MISC: Infection, hyperglycemia, neck pain
RESP: *Dyspnea,* lung changes

INTERACTIONS
Individual drugs
CycloSPORINE, theophylline: decreased effects of these drugs
Dextroamphetamine, methylphenidate: delayed effect of modafinil by 1 hr, dose should be separated

Drug classifications
Antidepressants (tricyclics): increased effects, reduce dose if needed
CYP3A4 inhibitors (azole antibiotics): altered levels of these agents, reaction difficult to predict
CYP2C19 substrates (diazepam, phenytoin, some tricyclics): increased levels of these agents, adjust dose if required
CYP3A4 inducers (carBAMazepine, phenytoin, rifampin; cycloSPORINE, theophylline): altered levels of these agents
Hormonal contraceptives: decreased effects, use alternative contraception

Drug/herb
Coffee, cola nut, guarana, mate, tea: increased stimulation

Drug/lab test
Increased: eosinophils, glucose, LFTs

NURSING CONSIDERATIONS
Assessment
• For narcolepsy, shift work, history of sleep apnea
• For depression, suicidal ideation
• Monitor B/P in those with hypertension
• **Stevens-Johnson syndrome:** Assess for rash, fever, fatigue, blisters; discontinue immediately if these occur, provide supportive therapy
• **Beers:** Avoid in older adults, CNS stimulant effects

Patient problem
Impaired sleep (uses)
Lack of knowledge of medication (teaching)

Implementation
• Give 1 hr before start of shift work, or in the AM for those with narcolepsy or sleep apnea
• Store at room temperature
• Give without regard to food

Patient/family education
• Advise patient to take only as directed; may be taken with or without food
• Advise patient to notify prescriber of allergic reaction, tremors, confusion
• Teach patient to avoid all OTC medications unless approved by prescriber
• Teach patient to avoid hazardous activities until drug effect is known
• Pregnancy/breastfeeding: Advise patient to use other form of contraception during and at least 30 days after discontinuing medication, if using hormonal birth control; advise patient to notify prescriber if pregnancy is planned or suspected or if breastfeeding

Evaluation
Positive therapeutic outcome
• Ability to stay awake

montelukast (Rx)
(mon-teh-loo′kast)
Singulair
Func. class.: Bronchodilator
Chem. class.: Leukotriene antagonist

Do not confuse: Singulair/SINEquan

ACTION: Inhibits leukotriene (LTD$_4$) formation; leukotrienes exert their effects by increasing neutrophil, eosinophil migration; aggregation of neutrophils, monocytes; smooth muscle contraction, capillary permeability; these actions further lead to bronchoconstriction, inflammation, edema

Therapeutic outcome: Ability to breathe with ease

USES: Chronic asthma in adults and children, seasonal allergic rhinitis, bronchospasm prophylaxis

Pharmacokinetics
Absorption	Rapidly absorbed
Distribution	Protein binding 99%
Metabolism	Liver
Excretion	Bile
Half-life	2.7-5.5 hr

Pharmacodynamics

Onset	Unknown
Peak	3-4 hr
Duration	Unknown

CONTRAINDICATIONS
Hypersensitivity

Precautions: Pregnancy, breastfeeding, children <6 yr, acute attacks of asthma, alcohol consumption, severe hepatic disease, corticosteroid withdrawal, phenylketonuria, suicidal ideation, depression

DOSAGE AND ROUTES
Asthma allergic rhinitis
Adult and child ≥15 yr: PO 10 mg/day PM
Child 6-14 yr: PO 5 mg chew tabs/day PM
Child 2-5 yr: PO (chew tabs, granules) 4 mg/day
Child 6-23 months (alergic rhinitis only): PO one packet of 4 mg oral granules PM

Exercise-induced bronchoconstriction prevention
Adult/child ≥6 yr: PO 10 mg 2 hr prior to exercise; do not take another dose within 24 hr

Available forms: Tabs 10 mg; chewable tabs 4, 5 mg; oral granules 4 mg/packet

ADVERSE EFFECTS
CNS: Dizziness, fatigue, headache, behavior changes, seizures, agitation, anxiety, depression, fever, hallucinations, drowsiness, suicidal ideation, memory impairment, hostility, somnambulism
GI: Abdominal pain, dyspepsia, nausea, vomiting, diarrhea, pancreatitis
HEMA: Thrombocytopenia
INTEG: Rash, pruritus, erythema
MS: Asthenia, myalgia, muscle cramps
RESP: Influenza, cough, nasal congestion
SYST: Churg-Strauss syndrome, Stevens-Johnson syndrome, toxic epidermal necrolysis

INTERACTIONS
Individual drugs
Rifabutin, rifapentine, rifampin: decreased montelukast levels

Drug classifications
Barbiturates: decreased montelukast levels

Drug/herb
Tea (green, black), guarana: increased stimulation

Drug/lab test
Increased: ALT, AST

NURSING CONSIDERATIONS
Assessment
• Assess adult patients carefully for symptoms of Churg-Strauss syndrome (rare), including eosinophilia, vasculitic rash, worsening pulmonary symptoms, cardiac complications and/or neuropathy
• Assess for behavior changes and suicidal ideation, other neuropsychiatric reactions
• **Severe hepatic disease:** use cautiously
• **Stevens-Johnson syndrome:** Assess for rash, fever, blisters, fatigue, muscle/joint aches, if these occur discontinue, provide supportive therapy

Patient problem
Impaired airway clearance (uses)

Implementation
PO route
• Give PO in PM daily for all uses except exercise-induced bronchoconstriction; then take 2 hr prior to exercise
• Granules may be given directly in mouth or mixed with a spoonful of soft food (carrots, applesauce, ice cream, rice); do not open packet until ready to use; mix whole dose, give within 15 min

Patient/family education
• Advise patient to avoid hazardous activities; dizziness may occur
• Teach patient that product is not to be used for acute asthma attacks
• Advise patient to continue to use inhaled β-agonists if exercise-induced asthma occurs
• **Granules:** instruct patient to take directly by mouth or mixed in a spoonful of room temperature soft food (use only applesauce, carrots, rice, or ice cream); use within 15 min of opening packet, discard used portions

Evaluation
Positive therapeutic outcome
• Increased ease of breathing
• Decreased bronchospasm

M

⚠ HIGH ALERT

morphine (Rx)

(mor'feen)

Arymo ER, Doloral ✦, Duramorph PF, Infumorph PF, Kadian, M-Eslon ✦, M Eslon IR ✦, MorphaBond, Morphine LP Epidural ✦, MS Contin, MS IR ✦, Ratio-morphine ✦, Statex ✦

Func. class.: Opioid analgesic

Chem. class.: Alkaloid

Controlled substance schedule II   ✴

Do not confuse: morphine/
HYDROmorphone, **MS Contin**/oxyCONTIN

ACTION: Depresses pain impulse transmission at the spinal cord level by interacting with opioid receptors

Therapeutic outcome: Decreased pain

USES: Moderate to severe pain

Pharmacokinetics

Absorption	Variably absorbed (PO); well absorbed (IM, SUBCUT, RECT); completely absorbed (IV)
Distribution	Widely distributed; crosses placenta
Metabolism	Liver, extensively
Excretion	Kidneys
Half-life	1½-2 hr; IM 3-4 hr; AVINza 24 hr; Kadian 11-13 hr

Pharmacodynamics

	PO	PO EXT REL
Onset	Variable	Unknown
Peak	1 hr	Unknown
Duration	4-5 hr	8-12 hr
	IM	**SUBCUT**
Onset	10-30 min	20 min
Peak	30-60 min	1-1½ hr
Duration	4-5 hr	4-5 hr
	RECT	**IV**	**IT**
Onset	Unknown	Rapid	Rapid
Peak	½-1 hr	20 min	Unknown
Duration	3-7 hr	4-5 hr	Ext

CONTRAINDICATIONS

Hypersensitivity, addiction (opioid/alcohol), hemorrhage, bronchial asthma, increased ICP, paralytic ileus, hypovolemic shock, MAOI therapy

BLACK BOX WARNING: Respiratory depression

Precautions: Pregnancy, breastfeeding, children <18 yr, geriatric, addictive personality, acute MI, severe heart disease, renal/hepatic disease, bowel impaction, abrupt discontinuation, seizures

BLACK BOX WARNING: Accidental exposure, epidural/intrathecal/IM/subcut administration, opioid-naive patients, substance abuse

DOSAGE AND ROUTES

Acute and chronic moderate pain or severe pain

>> PO Route (regular-release)

Adults: Initially, 10 to 30 mg q 4 hrs as needed in opioid-naive patients. Titrate to pain relief, only use the concentrated oral morphine solution (20 mg/mL) in opioid-tolerant patients. When converting parenteral to oral morphine, an oral dose that is 3 times the parenteral dose is generally sufficient. When converting from extended-release morphine, give the same 24-hour total as a divided regimen given at appropriate intervals. When converting from other oral or parenteral opioids, calculate the 24-hour total dose of the current opioid and consult published relative potency information for conversion.

Infants, Children, and Adolescents ages 6 months to 17 yrs (unlabeled) Initially, 0.2 to 0.3 mg/kg/dose q 3 to 6 hrs as needed; max initial dose of 5 mg/dose for children or the adult initial dose of 10 mg/dose for larger adolescents. Titrate to pain relief.

>> Intermittent IV, IM, or SUBCUT

Adults: Initially, 2 to 10 mg/70 kg q 3 to 4 hrs as needed, titrated to pain relief. Higher doses (10 mg) are recommended for IM or subcut; dosage may range from 5 to 20 mg IM or subcutaneously every 4 hours depending on patient requirements and response

Infants 6 months and older, Children, and Adolescents 0.05 to 0.2 mg/kg/dose q 2 to 4 hrs as needed; begin at the lower end of dosage range and titrate to effect (usual Max dose: 4 mg for children or 8 mg for adolescents)

Neonates (unlabeled) and Infants<6 months Initially, 0.03 to 0.1 mg/kg/dose q 3 to 4 hrs as needed. Titrate upward as needed for adequate pain relief

>> Continuous IV Infusion dosage (unlabeled)

Continuous infusions should only be used in acute care settings (ICU) where trained personnel are continuously monitoring the patient and emergency medications and equipment are readily available

Adults: Loading dose by slow IV infusion at a rate of 2 mg/minute. Loading doses of 15 to 20 mg may be required; higher doses may be needed in opioid-tolerant patients. Initial infusion rates of 2 to 5 mg/hour have been used, with usual rates of 2 to 30 mg/hour used in critically ill patients. Higher infusion rates may be required in opioid-tolerant patients. Titrate dose to pain relief

• **Infants, Children, and Adolescents:** A bolus of 0.05 to 0.2 mg/kg IV (or 5 to 10 mg for patients weighing more than 60 kg) followed by a continuous infusion. Initial infusion rates of 0.01 to 0.03 mg/kg/hour, but initial doses up to 0.06 mg/kg/hour may be appropriate for some patients. Alternatively, rates of 0.8 to 3 mg/hour IV may be used for patients over 60 kg. Titrate to pain relief

Neonates: 0.01 to 0.02 mg/kg/hour and titrate to effect. May increase up to 0.03 mg/kg/hour if needed

›› Continuous subcut infusion dosage (unlabeled)

Adults: Initial infusion rates of 2 to 5 mg/hr may be used, with usual rates of 2 to 30 mg/hr used in critically ill patients

Infants, Children, and Adolescents: Initial rate of 0.03 mg/kg/hr. The mean infusion rate was 0.0175 mg/kg/hour over the first 24 hours after surgery in 60 patients (aged 7 months to 20 years) and decreased to 0.011 to 0.0133 mg/kg/hour over the next 48 hoursTitrate dose to pain relief.

›› IV dosage (Patient Controlled Analgesia (PCA))

• **Adults:** Starting dose should be based on the patient's recent exposure to opioids. Titrate the regimen to patient response. Larger doses may be needed in opioid-tolerant patients. For OPIOID NAIVE patients, start with a demand dose of 1 mg (range: 0.5 to 2.5 mg) and lockout interval of 6 minutes (range: 5 to 10 minutes), with a maximal dosing rate of 10 mg/hour. For OPIOID TOLERANT patients, start with a demand dose of 2 to 5 mg IV and lockout interval of 6 minutes (range: 5 to 10 minutes), with a maximal dosing rate of 30 mg/hr

• **Children 7 years and older and Adolescents**

Demand dose: 0.01 to 0.025 mg/kg IV (max: 1 mg/dose)

Lockout interval: 5 to 10 minutes

Doses per hour: 5

›› Epidural dosage (morphine sulfate injection, but NOT DepoDur)

• **Adults:** Initially, inject 5 mg epidurally in the lumbar region and assess the patient in

1 hour; if pain relief is not adequate at that time, administer incremental doses of 1 to 2 mg, with sufficient time between injections to appropriately assess for efficacy. Max 10 mg per 24 hrs. For continuous epidural infusion, initiate at 2 to 4 mg per 24 hrs, with additional doses of 1 to 2 mg given if pain relief is not initially achieved

›› Intrathecal dosage (morphine sulfate injection, but NOT DepoDur)

Adults: 0.2 to 1 mg in the lumbar area as a single dose or to establish dosage for continuous intrathecal infusion

›› Rectal dosage

Adults

10 to 20 mg q 4 hrs, as needed

›› PO [extended-release tablets (Arymo ER, Morphabond, MS Contin) or capsules (Kadian, Avinza)] in opioid non-tolerant adult patients

• **Adults:** 15 mg q 8 or 12 hrs (Arymo ER, Morphabond, or MS Contin) or 30 mg q 24 hours (Avinza) for use as the first opioid analgesic. Do not use Kadian capsules as a first opioid analgesic; initiate with an immediate-release formulation and then convert patients to Kadian. For opioid non-tolerant patients, initiate with 15 mg q 12 hrs (MS Contin), 15 mg q 8 or 12 hrs (Arymo ER or Morphabond), or 30 mg q 24 hrs (Avinza or Kadian). With the exception of Avinza, adjust the dose every 1 to 2 days based upon the total daily morphine requirements (extended-release dose plus breakthrough doses). Adjust the dose of Avinza q 3 to 4 days in increments of 30 mg or less.

›› PO dosage [extended-release tablets (Arymo ER, Morphabond, MS Contin) or capsules (Kadian, Avinza)] in adult patients receiving other opioid agonist therapy

Adults: Discontinue all other around-the-clock opioids. To convert from other morphine formulations, calculate the morphine 24-hour oral requirement; in general, the 24-hour oral requirement is 3 times the 24-hour parenteral requirement. Initiate dosing, using the 24-hour oral requirement (round down to the closest available tablet/capsule strength), for: Arymo ER, Morphabond, or MS Contin at one-half of the requirement every 12 hours or one-third every 8 hours; Avinza at the total requirement once every 24 hours; and Kadian at one-half every 12 hours or the total once every 24 hours. When initiating

M

extended-release morphine, anticipate and treat breakthrough pain with adequate doses of immediate-release morphine as needed. When converting from other opioids, established conversion ratios to extended-release formulations have not been defined by clinical trials. Initiate dosing for: Arymo ER, Morphabond, or MS Contin at 15 mg q 8 or 12 hrs; and Avinza or Kadian at 30 mg q 24 hrs. Alternatively, initiate with one-half of the calculated morphine 24-hour oral requirement estimate, anticipating breakthrough pain and providing adequate doses of immediate-release morphine as needed.

Available forms: Immediate release tablets 15, 30 mg; extended release tablets (Arymo ER) 15, 30, 60 mg; extended release tablets (MS Contin) 15, 30, 60, 100, 200 mg; extended release tablets (Morphabond ER) 15, 30, 60, 100 mg; extended release capsules (Kadian) 10, 20, 30, 40, 50, 60, 70, 80, 100, 130, 150, 200 mg; extended release capsules 30, 45, 60, 75, 90, 120 mg; oral solution 1 mg/ml ❦, 2 mg/ml, 4 mg/ml, 5 mg/ml ❦, 20 mg/ml; rectal suppositories 5, 10, 20, 30 mg; solution for injection (IM, IV, subcut) 1 mg/ml, 2 mg/ml, 4 mg/ml, 5 mg/ml, 8 mg/ml, 10 mg/ml, 15 mg/ml, 25 mg/ml, 50 mg/ml; solution for epidural, IV (no preservative) 0.5 mg/ml, 1 mg/ml; solution for IT or epidural, continuous microinfusion device no preservative 10 mg/ml, 25 mg/ml; solution for IV (PCA device) 1 mg/ml, 2 mg/ml, 3 mg/ml, 5 mg/ml

ADVERSE EFFECTS

CNS: Drowsiness, dizziness, *confusion*, headache, *sedation*, euphoria, insomnia, seizures
CV: Palpitations, bradycardia, change in B/P, shock, cardiac arrest, chest pain, hyper/hypotension, edema, tachycardia
EENT: Blurred vision, miosis, diplopia
ENDO: Gynecomastia
GI: Nausea, vomiting, anorexia, *constipation*, cramps, biliary tract pressure
GU: Urinary retention, impotence, gonadal suppression
HEMA: Thrombocytopenia
INTEG: Rash, urticaria, bruising, flushing, diaphoresis, pruritus
RESP: Respiratory depression, respiratory arrest, apnea

INTERACTIONS
Individual drugs
Alcohol: increased effects with other CNS depressants
Rifampin: decreased analgesic action

Drug classifications
Antipsychotics, opiates, sedative-hypnotics, skeletal muscle relaxants: increased effects with other CNS depressants
MAOIs: unpredictable reaction may occur; avoid use

Drug/herb
Chamomile, hops, kava, St. John's wort, valerian: increased CNS depression

Drug/lab test
Increased: amylase

NURSING CONSIDERATIONS
Assessment
• Assess pain: location, type, character, intensity; give dose before pain becomes extreme
• Monitor I&O ratio; check for decreasing output; may indicate urinary retention; check for constipation; increase fluids, bulk in diet if needed, or stimulant laxatives may be prescribed; monitor serum sodium

> **BLACK BOX WARNING:** Abrupt discontinuation: gradually taper to prevent withdrawal symptoms; decrease by 50% q1-2 days, avoid use of narcotic antagonist

• Monitor CNS changes: dizziness, drowsiness, hallucinations, euphoria, LOC, pupil reactions
• Monitor allergic reactions: rash, urticaria

> **BLACK BOX WARNING:** Accidental exposure: if Duramorph or Infamorph gets on skin, remove contaminated clothing and rinse affected area with water

> **BLACK BOX WARNING:** Assess respiratory dysfunction: depression, character, rate, rhythm; notify prescriber if respirations are <12/min; accidental overdose has occurred with high-potency oral sol

• **Pregnancy/breastfeeding:** Only use if benefits outweigh fetal risk, use can result in opioid withdrawal syndrome, do not use in breastfeeding

Patient problem
Pain (uses)
Risk for injury (adverse reactions)

Implementation
>> **PO route**
• Give with food or milk to minimize GI effects
Immediate-release cap
• May swallow whole, or opened and contents sprinkled on cool food (pudding or applesauce), or added to juice (given immediately)

or delivered via gastric or NG tube by either adding to or following with liquid

Extended-release and controlled-release tabs
• Swallow whole; do not crush, break, dissolve, or chew.
• The use of MS Contin 100 mg or 200 mg tabs should be limited to opioid-tolerant patients requiring oral doses equivalent to ≥200 mg/day. Use of the 100 mg or 200 mg tablet is only recommended for patients who have already been titrated to a stable analgesic regimen using lower strengths of MS Contin or other opioids

Sustained-release caps
• Swallow; do not chew, crush, or dissolve
• Caps may be opened and contents sprinkled on applesauce (at room temperature or cooler) immediately prior to ingestion. Do not chew, crush, or dissolve the pellets/beads inside the cap. The applesauce should be swallowed without chewing. If the pellets/beads are chewed, an immediate release of a potentially fatal morphine dose may be delivered. Rinse mouth to ensure all the pellets/beads have been swallowed. Do not separate applesauce into separate doses; the entire portion should be taken. Discard unused portion
• Kadian caps may be given through a 16 French gastrostomy tube; flush with water, and sprinkle the cap contents into 10 ml of water. Using a funnel and a swirling motion, pour the pellets and water into the tube. Rinse the beaker with 10 ml of water, and pour the water into the funnel. Repeat until no pellets remain in the beaker
• Do NOT administer Kadian through a nasogastric tube
• Consumption of alcohol while taking the ext rel capsules may result in the rapid release and absorption of a potentially fatal dose of morphine
• Kadian 100 mg, 130 mg, 150 mg or 200 mg caps should be given only to opioid tolerant patients
• Begin with immediate release products and titrate to correct dose and convert to a sustained release product

Oral liquid
• Check dose prior to use; many concentrations of oral sol are available; may be diluted in fruit juice; protect from light

>> Injectable administration
• Visually inspect for particulate matter and discoloration before use; do not use if a precipitate is present after shaking; do not use the Duramorph solution if a precipitate is present or if the color is darker than pale yellow

IV route
• Prior to use, an opiate antagonist and emergency facilities should be available
• Do not use the highly concentrated morphine injections (i.e., 10-25 mg/ml) for IV, IM, or SC administration of single doses. These injection solutions are intended for use via continuous, controlled-microinfusion devices

Direct IV route
• Dilute dose with ≥5 ml of sterile water for injection or NS injection
• Inject 2.5-15 mg directly into a vein or into the tubing of a freely flowing IV solution over 4-5 min; do not give rapidly

Continuous IV infusion
• Dilute in 5% dextrose; use a controlled-infusion device
• Adjust dose and rate based on patient response

Patient-controlled analgesia (PCA)
• A compatible patient-controlled infusion device must be used
• Dilute solutions to obtain a concentration of 1 or 10 mg/ml for ease in calculations and programming of PCA pumps
• Adjust dose and rate based on patient response. Consult the patient-controlled infusion device manual for directions on rate of infusion

Subcut route
• Inject taking care not to inject intradermally

Continuous SC infusion
• Morphine is not approved by the FDA for subcut use
• Dilute to an appropriate concentration in D_5W; administer using a portable, controlled, subcut device; adjust rate based on patient response and tolerance
• Max subcut rate 2 ml/hr/site

Intrathecal/epidural route
• Morphine sulfate injection is not interchangeable with morphine sulfate extended-release liposome injection (DepoDur), DepoDur is only for epidural administration
• Do not use Infumorph (10 mg/ml or 25 mg/ml) for single-dose neuraxial injection because lower doses can be more reliably administered with Duramorph (0.5 mg/ml or 1 mg/ml)

>> Rectal route
• Moisten the suppository with water prior to insertion. If suppository is too soft, chill in the refrigerator for 30 min or run cold water over it before removing the wrapper

>> Oral solid formulations
Immediate-release capsules administration
• May be swallowed whole or opened and the contents sprinkled on cool food such as pudding or applesauce

M

• Capsule contents may be added to juice and administered immediately or delivered via gastric or NG tube by either adding to or following with liquid

>> Extended-release and controlled-release tablets administration

• Swallow whole; do not crush, break, dissolve, or chew
• The use of MS Contin 100 mg or 200 mg tablets should be limited to opioid-tolerant patients requiring oral doses equivalent to ≥200 mg/day. Use of the 100 mg or 200 mg tablet is only recommended for patients who have already been titrated to a stable analgesic regimen using lower strengths of MS Contin or other opioids

Sustained-release capsule administration

• Capsules should be swallowed; do not chew, crush, or dissolve
• Capsules may be opened and the contents sprinkled on applesauce (at room temperature or cooler) immediately prior to ingestion; no other food has been tested. Do not chew, crush, or dissolve the pellets/beads inside the capsule. The applesauce needs to be swallowed without chewing. If the pellets/beads are chewed, an immediate release of a potentially fatal morphine dose may be delivered. Rinse mouth to ensure all the pellets/beads have been swallowed. Do not separate applesauce into separate doses; the entire portion should be taken. Discard any unused portion of the capsules after the contents have been sprinkled on the applesauce
• Kadian capsules may be administered through a 16 French gastrostomy tube. Flush the tube with water, and sprinkle the capsule contents into 10 ml of water. Using a funnel and a swirling motion, pour the pellets and water into the tube. Rinse the beaker with 10 ml of water, and pour the water into the funnel. Repeat until no pellets remain in the beaker
• Do NOT administer Kadian through a nasogastric tube
• Consumption of alcohol while taking the extended-release capsules may result in the rapid release and absorption of a potentially fatal dose of morphine
• Kadian 100 mg, 130 mg, 150 mg or 200 mg capsules should be limited to opioid tolerant patients

>> Oral liquid formulations

Oral solution administration

• Carefully check dose prior to dispensing medication as many concentrations of morphine oral solution are available

• May be diluted in fruit juice prior to administration
• Protect from light

Injectable administration

• Visually inspect parenteral products for particulate matter and discoloration prior to administration whenever solution and container permit. Unopened solutions should be discarded if a precipitate is present that does not disappear with shaking. Do not use the Duramorph solution if a precipitate is present or if the color is darker than pale yellow

>> Intravenous administration

• Prior to administration, an opiate antagonist and facilities for administration of oxygen and control of respiration should be available
• Do not use the highly concentrated morphine injections (i.e., 10-25 mg/ml) for IV, IM, or SC administration of single doses. These injection solutions are intended for use via continuous, controlled-microinfusion devices

Direct IV injection

• Dilute appropriate dose with at least 5 ml of sterile water for injection or NS injection
• Inject 2.5-15 mg directly into a vein or into the tubing of a freely flowing IV solution over 4-5 minutes. Rapid IV injection of morphine may result in an increased frequency of adverse effects. For example, the maximum CNS effects occur 30 minutes after administration. Rapid intravenous administration could result in an overdose

Continuous IV infusion

• Dilute in 5% dextrose
• Administer using a controlled-infusion device
• Adjust dose and rate based on patient response

Patient-controlled analgesia (PCA)

• A compatible patient-controlled infusion device must be used
• Dilute solutions to obtain morphine concentration of 1 or 10 mg/ml for ease in calculations and programming of PCA pumps
• Adjust dose and rate based on patient response. Consult the patient-controlled infusion device operator's manual for directions on administering the drug at the desired rate of infusion

>> Subcutaneous administration

• Inject subcutaneously taking care not to inject intradermally

Continuous SC infusion

• Morphine is not approved by the FDA for subcutaneous administration
• Dilute to an appropriate concentration in D_5W and administer using a portable, controlled, subcutaneous infusion device. Adjust rate based on patient response and tolerance
• Maximum SC rate of infusion is 2 ml/hour/site

>> Intrathecal administration

• Intrathecal dose is approximately one-tenth (1/10) the epidural dose

• Morphine sulfate injection is not interchangeable with morphine sulfate extended-release liposome injection (DepoDur). DepoDur is only for epidural administration (see below)

• Do not use Infumorph (10 mg/ml or 25 mg/ml) for single-dose neuraxial injection because lower doses can be more reliably administered with Duramorph (0.5 mg/ml or 1 mg/ml)

• Epidural or intrathecal administration should only be used by specially trained healthcare professionals

• May be given as intermittent bolus, continuous infusion, or as patient-controlled epidural analgesia. Infumorph is only indicated for intrathecal or epidural infusion; Infumorph is not recommended for single-dose intravenous, intramuscular, or subcutaneous administration because of the very large amount of morphine in the ampul and the associated overdosage risk

• Prior to administration, an opiate antagonist and facilities for administration of oxygen and control of respiration should be available. The patient should be in a setting where adequate monitoring is possible. Immediate availability of naloxone injection and resuscitative equipment is also needed during Infumorph reservoir refilling or reservoir manipulation

• Placement of epidural catheter and administration should be at a site near the dermatomes covering the field of pain to decrease dose requirements and increase specificity. For example, for thoracic surgery placement at T2-T8, upper abdominal surgery, T4-L1, lower abdominal surgery, T10-L3, upper extremity surgery, C2-C8 and lower extremity surgery, T12-L3

• Visually inspect parenteral products for particulate matter and discoloration prior to administration whenever solution and container permit. Unopened Infumorph solution should be discarded if a precipitate is present that does not disappear with shaking or if it is not colorless or pale yellow. Do not use the Duramorph solution if a precipitate is present or if the color is darker than pale yellow

Intrathecal injection (morphine sulfate injection)

• No more than 2 or 1 ml of the injection containing 0.5 or 1 mg/ml, respectively, should be injected intrathecally

• After ensuring proper placement of the needle or catheter, inject appropriate dose intrathecally. Monitor patient in a fully equipped and staffed environment for at least 24 hr after each dose,

as severe respiratory depression may occur up to 24 hr after drug administration. Repeated intrathecal injections are not recommended other than for establishing initial intrathecal dosage for continuous intrathecal infusion

Continuous intrathecal infusion (morphine sulfate injection)

• Intrathecal dose is approximately one-tenth (1/10) the epidural dose. Epidural dose is usually considered to be one-tenth (1/10) the IV dose

• A controlled-infusion device must be used. For highly concentrated injections, an implantable controlled-microinfusion device is used. Patients should be monitored in a fully equipped and staffed environment for several days following implantation of the device

• If dilution of the injection is necessary, NS injection is recommended

• The infusion device reservoir should only be filled by fully trained and qualified healthcare professionals. Strict aseptic technique must be used. Withdraw dose from the ampul through a 5-μm (or smaller pore diameter) microfilter to avoid contamination with glass or other particles. Ensure proper placement of the needle when filling the reservoir to avoid accidental overdosage

• To avoid exacerbation of severe pain and/or reflux of CSF into the reservoir, depletion of the reservoir should be avoided

>> Other injectable administration

Epidural administration

• Intrathecal dose is approximately one-tenth (1/10) the epidural dose. Epidural dose is usually considered to be one-tenth (1/10) the IV dose

• Morphine sulfate injection is not interchangeable with morphine sulfate extended-release liposome injection (DepoDur). DepoDur is only for epidural administration (see below)

• Do not use Infumorph (10 mg/ml or 25 mg/ml) for single-dose neuraxial injection because lower doses can be more reliably administered with Duramorph (0.5 mg/ml or 1 mg/ml)

• Epidural administration should only be used by specially trained healthcare professionals

• May be given as intermittent bolus, cont inf, or as patient-controlled epidural analgesia. Infumorph is only indicated for intrathecal or epidural infusion; Infumorph is not recommended for single-dose intravenous, intramuscular, or subcutaneous administration because of the very large amount of morphine in the ampul and the associated overdosage risk

• Prior to administration, an opiate antagonist and facilities for administration of oxygen and control of respiration should be available. The patient should be in a setting where adequate monitoring is possible. Immediate availability of naloxone injection and resuscitative equipment is also needed during Infumorph reservoir refilling or reservoir manipulation

• Placement of epidural catheter and administration should be at a site near the dermatomes covering the field of pain to decrease dose requirements and increase specificity. For example, for thoracic surgery placement at T2-T8, upper abdominal surgery, T4-L1, lower abdominal surgery, T10-L3, upper extremity surgery, C2-C8 and lower extremity surgery, T12-L3

Epidural injection (morphine sulfate injection)

• After ensuring proper placement of the needle or catheter, inject appropriate dose into the epidural space. Monitor patient in a fully equipped and staffed environment for at least 24 hr after each dose, as severe respiratory depression may occur up to 24 hr after drug administration

Continuous epidural infusion (morphine sulfate injection)

• Intrathecal dose is approximately one-tenth (1/10) the epidural dose. Epidural dose is usually considered to be one-tenth (1/10) the IV dose

• A controlled-infusion device must be used. For highly concentrated injections, an implantable controlled-microinfusion device is used. Patients should be monitored in a fully equipped and staffed environment for several days following implantation of the device

• If dilution of the injection is necessary, NS injection is recommended

• The infusion device reservoir should only be filled by fully trained and qualified healthcare professionals. Strict aseptic technique must be used. Withdraw dose from the ampul through a 5-µm (or smaller pore diameter) microfilter to avoid contamination with glass or other particles. Ensure proper placement of the needle when filling the reservoir to avoid accidental overdosage

• To avoid exacerbation of severe pain and/or reflux of CSF into the reservoir, depletion of the reservoir should be avoided

>> Epidural administration (morphine sulfate extended-release liposome injection [DepoDur] ONLY)

• Morphine sulfate ext rel liposome injection (DepoDur) is not interchangeable with other morphine sulfate injections

• DepoDur is only for epidural administration. Do not administer by any other parenteral route

• Epidural administration should only be used by specially trained healthcare professionals

• Prior to administration, an opiate antagonist and facilities for administration of oxygen and

control of respiration should be available. The patient should be in a setting where adequate monitoring is possible. Monitor patient in a fully equipped and staffed environment for at least 48 hr after each dose, as severe respiratory depression may occur

• Invert the vial to resuspend particles immediately before withdrawal. Administer DepoDur within 4 hr after withdrawal from the vial when kept at controlled room temperature 59-86° F (15-30° C). The product does not contain any bacteriostatic agents or preservatives. Do not heat- or gas-sterilize

Epidural injection [morphine sulfate extended-release liposome injection (DepoDur)]

• Placement of epidural needle or catheter and administration should be at the lumbar level. Due to lack of study data, administration of DepoDur at the thoracic level or higher is not recommended

• Determine proper needle or catheter placement by aspiration to check for blood or cerebrospinal fluid and/or by administration of a test dose of 3 ml of 1.5% preservative-free lidocaine and EPINEPHrine (1:200,000). If tachycardia or sudden onset of segmental anesthesia occurs, the needle or catheter is in the intrathecal space and thus, needs to be repositioned. If a test dose is given, flush the catheter with 1 ml of preservative-free normal saline injection and wait at least 15 minutes after test dose administration before administration of DepoDur

• Inject DepoDur at the lumbar level undiluted or diluted up to 5 ml total volume with preservative-free normal saline. During administration, do not use an inline filter or mix DepoDur with any medication. Additionally, do not administer any medication into the epidural space within 48 hr of DepoDur receipt

>> Rectal administration

• Instruct patient on proper use of suppository (see Patient Information)

• Moisten the suppository with water prior to insertion. If suppository is too soft because of storage in a warm place, chill in the refrigerator for 30 minutes or run cold water over it before removing the wrapper

Y-site compatibilities: Acetaminophen, aldesleukin, allopurinol, amifostine, amikacin, aminophylline, amiodarone, atenolol, atracurium, aztreonam, bumetanide, calcium chloride, cefamandole, ceFAZolin, cefotaxime, cefoTEtan, cefOXitin, cefTAZidime, ceftizoxime, cefTRIAXone, cefuroxime, cephalothin, chloramphenicol, cladribine, clindamycin, cyclophosphamide, cytarabine, dexamethasone, digoxin, diltiazem, DOBUTamine, DOPamine, doxycycline, enalaprilat, EPINEPHrine, erythromycin, esmolol, etomidate, famotidine, fentaNYL, filgrastim, fluconazole, fludarabine, foscarnet, genta-micin, granisetron, heparin, hydrocortisone, HYDROmorphone, kanamycin, labetalol, lidocaine, LORazepam, magnesium sulfate, melphalan, me-ropenem, methotrexate, methyldopate, methyl-PREDNISolone, metoclopramide, metoprolol, met-roNIDAZOLE, midazolam, milrinone, nafcillin, niCARdipine, nitroglycerin, norepinephrine, ondan-setron, oxacillin, oxytocin, PACLitaxel, pancuronium, penicillin G potassium, piperacillin, piperacillin/tazobactam, potassium chloride, propranolol, raniti-dine, sodium bicarbonate, teniposide, thiotepa, ti-carcillin, ticarcillin/clavulanate, tigecycline, tobra-mycin, vancomycin, vecuronium, vinorelbine, vit B/C, warfarin, zidovudine, zoledronic acid

Patient/family education
• Advise patient to report any symptoms of CNS changes, allergic reactions
• Caution patients to avoid CNS depressants (alcohol, sedative/hypnotics) for at least 24 hr after taking this product
• Discuss with patient that dizziness, drowsi-ness, and confusion are common; to avoid getting up without assistance
• Discuss in detail all aspects of the product and expected response

Evaluation

Positive therapeutic outcome
• Decreased pain

TREATMENT OF OVERDOSE:
Naloxone (Narcan) 0.2-0.8 **IV** (caution with opioid-tolerant individuals), O_2, **IV** fluids, vaso-pressors

moxifloxacin (Rx)
(mocks-ah-flox′a-sin)
Avelox, Avelox IV, Moxeza, Vigamox
Func. class.: Antiinfective
Chem. class.: Fluoroquinolone

Do not confuse: moxifloxacin/gatifloxacin/ciprofloxacin/levoFLOXacin

ACTION: Interferes with conversion of in-termediate DNA fragments into high molecular weight DNA in bacteria; DNA gyrase inhibitor

Therapeutic outcome: Bactericidal action against the following: *Staphylococcus aureus, Streptococcus pneumoniae, Haemophilus in-fluenzae, Haemophilus parainfluenzae, Morax-ella catarrhalis, Klebsiella pneumoniae, Myco-plasma pneumoniae, Chlamydia pneumoniae; Streptococcus pyogenes, Escherichia coli, Bacteroides fragilis, Streptococcus anginosus, Streptococcus constellatus, Enterococcus*

faecalis, Proteus mirabilis, Clostridium per-fringens, Bacteroides thetalomicron, Pepto-streptococcus, Enterobacter cloacae

USES: Acute bacterial sinusitis, acute bacterial exacerbation of chronic bronchitis, community-acquired pneumonia (mild to moderate), un-complicated skin/skin structure infections, com-plicated intraabdominal infections including polymicrobial infections, complicated skin/skin structure infections

Unlabeled uses: Anthrax treatment/prophy-laxis, gastroenteritis, MAC, nongonococcal urethri-tis, shigellosis, surgical infection prophylaxis, TB

Pharmacokinetics

Absorption	Well absorbed (75%) (PO)
Distribution	Widely distributed
Metabolism	Liver
Excretion	Kidneys
Half-life	Increased in renal disease

Pharmacodynamics

	PO	IV
Onset	Rapid	Unknown
Peak	1 hr	1-3 hr
Duration	Unknown	Unknown

CONTRAINDICATIONS
Hypersensitivity to quinolones

Precautions: Pregnancy, breastfeeding, chil-dren, renal/hepatic/cardiac disease, epilepsy, uncorrected hypokalemia, prolonged QT inter-val, patients receiving class IA, III antidysrhyth-mics, GI disease, seizure disorder, pseudomem-branous colitis, diabetes mellitus

> **BLACK BOX WARNING:** Tendon pain/rupture, tendinitis, myasthenia gravis

DOSAGE AND ROUTES
Acute bacterial sinusitis
Adult: PO/**IV** 400 mg q24hr × 10 days

Acute bacterial exacerbation of chronic bronchitis
Adult: PO/**IV** 400 mg q24hr × 5 days

Community-acquired pneumonia
Adult: PO/**IV** 400 mg q24hr × 7-14 days

Uncomplicated skin/skin structure infections
Adult: PO/**IV** 400 mg q24hr × 7 days

Complicated intraabdominal infections
Adult: **IV** 400 mg/day × 7-21 days

M

Complicated skin/skin structure infections
Adult: PO/IV 400 mg/day × 7-21 days

Plague
Adult: PO/IV 400 mg q 24 hr × 10-14 day

Bacterial conjunctivitis
Adult/child ≥1 yr: (Vigamox) 1 drop into affected eye tid x 7 days
Adult/child ≥4 months: (Moxeza) 1 drop in affected eye bid 7 days

Available forms: Tabs 400 mg; inj premix 400 mg/250 ml; ophthalmic solution 0.5%

ADVERSE EFFECTS
CNS: Headache, dizziness, fatigue, insomnia, depression, restlessness, seizures, confusion, increased intracranial pressure, peripheral neuropathy, pseudotumor cerebri, fever
CV: Prolonged QT interval, dysrhythmias, torsades de pointes, tachycardia
EENT: Blurred vision, tinnitus, taste changes
GI: Nausea, increased ALT, AST, flatulence, heartburn, vomiting, diarrhea, oral candidiasis, dysphagia, pseudomembranous colitis, abdominal pain, dyspepsia, constipation, gastroenteritis, xerostomia
GU: Renal failure
INTEG: Rash, pruritus, urticaria, photosensitivity, flushing, fever, chills, injection site reactions
MISC: Candidiasis vaginitis
MS: Tremor, arthralgia, tendon rupture, myalgia
SYST: Anaphylaxis, Stevens-Johnson syndrome, angioedema, toxic epidermal necrolysis

INTERACTIONS
Individual drugs
Aluminum hydroxide, calcium, didanosine, iron, sucralfate, zinc sulfate: decreased absorption of moxifloxacin
CycloSPORINE: increased cycloSPORINE effect
Haloperidol, chloroquine, droperidol, pentamidine; arsenic trioxide, levomethadyl: increased QT prolongation
Probenecid: increased blood levels
Warfarin: increased warfarin effect

Drug classifications
Antacids (magnesium), iron salts: decreased absorption of moxifloxacin
Class IA/III antidysrhythmics, some phenothiazines, β-agonists, local anesthetics, tricyclics, CYP3A4 inhibitors (amiodarone, clarithromycin, erythromycin, telithromycin, troleandomycin), CYP3A4 substrates (methadone, pimozide, QUEtiapine, quiNIDine, risperiDONE, ziprasidone): increased QT prolongation
NSAIDs: increased seizure risk, monitor

> **BLACK BOX WARNING:** Corticosteroids: increased tendon rupture

Drug/food
Enteral feeding: decreased absorption of moxifloxacin

Drug/lab test
Increased: glucose, lipids, triglycerides, uric acid, LDH, ALT, ionized calcium, chloride, globulin, albumin PT, INR, WBC
Decreased: potassium glucose, amylase, RBC, eosinophils, Hb, HCT

NURSING CONSIDERATIONS
Assessment
• Assess patient for previous sensitivity reaction
• Assess patient for signs and symptoms of infection including characteristics of wounds, sputum, urine, stool, WBC >10,000/mm³, fever baseline, during treatment
• Obtain C&S before beginning product therapy to identify if correct treatment has been initiated
• **Assess for allergic reactions, Stevens-Johnson syndrome, toxic epidermal necrolysis, and anaphylaxis:** rash, urticaria, pruritus, chills, fever, joint pain; may occur a few days after therapy begins; EPINEPHrine and resuscitation equipment should be available for anaphylactic reaction
• Assess for CNS symptoms: headache, dizziness, fatigue, insomnia, depression, **seizures**
• Identify urine output; if decreasing, notify prescriber (may indicate nephrotoxicity); also check for increased BUN, creatinine, electrolytes
• Monitor blood tests: AST, ALT, CBC, Hct, bilirubin, LDH, alkaline phosphatase, Coombs' test monthly if patient is on long-term therapy
• Monitor electrolytes: potassium, sodium chloride monthly if patient is on long-term therapy
• **CDAD:** assess for diarrhea, abdominal pain, fever, fatigue, anorexia; possible anemia, elevated WBC and low serum albumin; stop product and usually give either vancomycin or IV metroNIDAZOLE
• Monitor for bleeding: ecchymosis, bleeding gums, hematuria, stool guaiac daily if on long-term therapy
• Assess for overgrowth of infection: perineal itching, fever, malaise, redness, pain, swelling, drainage, rash, diarrhea, change in cough, sputum

---

BLACK BOX WARNING: Assess for tendon pain, rupture, tendinitis; if tendon becomes inflamed, drug should be discontinued, more common in achilles tendon

• **QT prolongation:** Monitor ECG for QT prolongation, ejection fraction; assess for chest pain, palpitations, dyspnea

Patient problem
Infection (uses)

Implementation
• Do not use theophylline with this product; may cause toxicity
PO route
• Give once a day for 5-10 days depending on condition
• Give without regard to food
• Store at room temperature

IV route
• Do not use if particulate matter is present
• Flush line with D5W, 0.9% NaCl, lactated Ringer's before and after use; give PO 4 hr before or 8 hr after antacids, sucralfate, multivitamins
• Discontinue primary **IV** while administering moxifloxacin, give over 60 min
• Do not give SUBCUT, IM
• Available as premixed sol, may be diluted at ratios from 1:10 to 10:1, do not refrigerate, give by direct infusion or through Y-type infusion set, do not add other medications to sol or infuse through same IV line at same time
• Do not refrigerate
• Do not admix

Opthalmic route: after instilling, use gentle pressure on lacrinal duct for 2 min

Solution compatibilities: 0.9% NaCl, D₅, D₁₀, LR, sterile water for inj

Patient/family education

BLACK BOX WARNING: Notify prescriber of tendon pain, inflammation, stop drug

• Teach patient to report sore throat, bruising, bleeding, joint pain; may indicate blood dyscrasias (rare)
• Advise patient to contact prescriber if vaginal itching, loose foul-smelling stools, furry tongue occur; may indicate superinfection; report itching, rash, pruritus, urticaria
• Instruct patient to take all medication prescribed for the length of time ordered; not to give medication to others
• Advise patient to notify prescriber of diarrhea with blood or pus
• Advise patient to rinse mouth frequently, use sugarless candy or gum for dry mouth

• Advise patient to take as prescribed, not to double or miss doses
• Pregnancy/breastfeeding: Identify if pregnancy is planned or suspected or if breastfeeding

Evaluation
Positive therapeutic outcome
• Absence of signs/symptoms of infection (WBC <10,000/mm³, temp WNL)
• Reported improvement in symptoms of infection

moxifloxacin ophthalmic
See Appendix B

mupirocin topical
See Appendix B

mycophenolate (Rx)
(mie-koe-feen'oh-late)
CellCept

mycophenolate acid
Myfortic (Rx)
Func. class.: Immunosuppressant

ACTION: Inhibits inflammatory responses that are mediated by the immune system; prolongs survival of allogenic transplants

Therapeutic outcome: Absence of graft rejection

USES: Organ transplants to prevent rejection (renal); prophylaxis of rejection in allogenic cardiac, hepatic, renal transplants

Unlabeled uses: Nephrotic syndrome

Pharmacokinetics

Absorption	Rapid and complete
Distribution	Crosses placenta, enters breast milk
Metabolism	To active metabolite (MPA)
Excretion	Urine, feces
Half-life	8-18 hr (MPA)

Pharmacodynamics
Unknown

CONTRAINDICATIONS
Hypersensitivity to this product or mycophenolic acid

BLACK BOX WARNING: Pregnancy

Precautions: Breastfeeding, lymphomas, neutropenia, renal disease, accidental exposure, anemia

BLACK BOX WARNING: Infection, neoplastic disease, requires a specialized care setting, requires an experienced clinician

DOSAGE AND ROUTES
Renal transplant (to prevent organ rejection)
Adult: PO mycophenolate mofetil 1 g or 720 mg mycophenolate sodium mg bid given to renal transplant patients in combination with corticosteroids and cycloSPORINE
Child: SUSP 600 mg bid or PO cap 750 mg bid body surface area (BSA) of 1.25 to 1.5 m² or 1 g bid BSA >1.5 m²

Renal dose
Adult: PO/IV GFR <25 ml/min, max 2 g/day

Cardiac transplant (to prevent organ rejection)
Adult: PO/**IV** 1.5 g bid, **IV** can be started ≤24 hr after transplant, switch to PO when able

Hepatic transplant (to prevent organ rejection)
Adult: PO 1.5 g bid, **IV** 1 g over ≥2 hr

Available forms: Caps 250 mg; tabs 500 mg; inj (powder) 500 mg/20 ml vial; powder for oral susp 200 mg/ml; delayed rel tab (Myfortic) 180, 360 mg

ADVERSE EFFECTS
CNS: *Tremor, dizziness, insomnia, headache, fever,* progressive multifocal leukoencephalopathy, asthenia, paresthesia, anxiety, pain
CV: *Hypertension, chest pain,* hypotension, edema
GI: *Nausea, vomiting,* stomatitis, *diarrhea, constipation,* GI bleeding, abdominal pain, anorexia, dyspepsia
GU: *UTI, hematuria,* renal tubular necrosis, polyomavirus-associated nephropathy
HEMA: Leukopenia, thrombocytopenia, anemia, pancytopenia, pure red cell aplasia, neutropenia
INTEG: *Rash*
META: *Peripheral edema, hypercholesterolemia, hypophosphatemia, edema, hypo/hyperkalemia, hyperglycemia,* hypocalcemia, hypomagnesemia
MS: Arthralgia, muscle wasting, back pain, weakness
RESP: *Dyspnea, respiratory infection, increased cough, pharyngitis, bronchitis, pneumonia,* pleural effusion, pulmonary fibrosis
SYST: Lymphoma, nonmelanoma skin carcinoma, sepsis

INTERACTIONS
Individual drugs
Acyclovir, ganciclovir, valacyclovir: increased toxicity
AzaTHIOprine: increased bone marrow suppression
Cholestyramine, cycloSPORINE, rifamycin: decreased levels of mycophenolate
Phenytoin: increased effects; decreased protein binding of phenytoin
Probenecid: increased levels of mycophenolate
Theophylline: increased effects; decreased protein binding of theophylline

Drug classifications
Antacids (magnesium, aluminum): decreased levels of mycophenolate
Anticoagulants, NSAIDs, thrombolytics, salicylates: increased risk of bleeding
Contraceptives (oral), live attenuated vaccines: decreased effects
Immunosuppressives, salicylates: increased levels of mycophenolate

Drug/herb
Astragalus, echinacea, melatonin: interferes with immunosuppression

Drug/food
Decreased absorption if taken with food

Drug/lab test
Increased: serum creatinine, BUN, potassium, cholesterol, glucose, abnormal LFTs
Decreased: WBC, platelets, neutrophils

NURSING CONSIDERATIONS
Assessment
• **Progressive multifocal leukoencephalopathy; may be fatal:** ataxia, confusion, apathy, hemiparesis, visual problems, weakness; side effects should be reported to the FDA

BLACK BOX WARNING: Infection/lymphoma: may occur from immunosuppressives, increased infections including BK virus, and may cause kidney graft loss

• Monitor blood tests: CBC monthly during treatment
• Monitor liver function tests: alkaline phosphatase, AST, ALT, bilirubin
• Monitor renal studies: BUN, CCr, electrolytes
• **Pregnancy:** obtain pregnancy test within 1 wk prior to initiation of treatment; confirm negative pregnancy test, do not use in pregnancy

Patient problem
Immunologic impairment (uses)
Risk for infection (adverse reactions)

Implementation
- May be given in combination with corticosteroids and cycloSPORINE

PO route
- Do not crush, chew tabs; do not open caps; avoid inhalation or direct contact with skin, mucous membranes; teratogenic in animals
- Give alone for better absorption
- Delayed rel tabs and caps; oral **susp** and tab are not interchangeable

Intermittent IV infusion route
- Reconstitute each vial with 14 ml D$_5$W, shake gently, further dilute to 6 mg/ml, dilute 1-g doses in 140 ml D$_5$W, and 1.5-g doses in 210 ml D$_5$W, give by slow **IV** infusion $\geq$2 hr, never give by bolus or rapid **IV** injection
- Do not give with other medications or solutions, do not use if particulates are present

Y-site compatibilities: Alemtuzumab, alfentanil, amikacin, anidulafungin, argatroban, bivalirudin, caspofungin, cefepime, DAPTOmycin, DOPamine, norepinephrine, octreotide, oxytocin, tacrolimus, tigecycline, tirofiban, vancomycin, zoledronic acid

Patient/family education
- Advise patient that repeated lab tests are necessary

BLACK BOX WARNING: Advise patient that infection and lymphomas may occur

- Teach patient to take on empty stomach, not to crush, chew, break ext rel caps

BLACK BOX WARNING: Infection: Teach patient to report fever, chills, sore throat, fatigue, serious infection may occur, avoid crowds, persons with known infections

BLACK BOX WARNING: Neoplastic disease: Teach patient lymphoma and other neoplastic diseases may occur, particularly skin cancer, limit UV exposure by wearing protective clothing, sunscreen

- Pregnancy/breastfeeding: Instruct patient to notify prescriber if pregnancy is planned or suspected (D); to use two forms of contraception before, during, and 6 wk after therapy

Evaluation

Positive therapeutic outcome
- Absence of graft rejection

M

nadolol (Rx)

(nay-doe'lole)

Corgard, Syn-Nadol ✚

Func. class.: Antihypertensive, antianginal

Chem. class.: β-Adrenergic receptor blocker

Do not confuse: Corgard/Cognex/Coreg

ACTION: Long-acting, nonselective β-adrenergic receptor blocking agent, blocks β_1 in the heart and β_2 in the lungs, uterus, and circulatory system; mechanism is similar to that of propranolol

Therapeutic outcome: Decreased B/P, heart rate

USES: Chronic stable angina pectoris, mild to moderate hypertension, atrial fibrillation

Unlabeled uses: Tachydysrhythmias, anxiety, tremors, esophageal varices (rebleeding only), migraines, reduction of intraocular pressure

Pharmacokinetics

Absorption	Variably absorbed
Distribution	Crosses placenta; minimal concentration in CNS, protein binding 30%
Metabolism	Unknown
Excretion	Kidneys, unchanged 70%
Half-life	10-24 hr; increased in renal disease

Pharmacodynamics

Onset	Variable
Peak	3-4 hr
Duration	10-24 hr

CONTRAINDICATIONS

Hypersensitivity to this product, cardiac failure, cardiogenic shock, 2nd- or 3rd-degree heart block, bronchospastic disease, sinus bradycardia, HF, COPD, asthma

Precautions: Pregnancy, breastfeeding, diabetes mellitus, renal disease, hyperthyroidism, peripheral vascular disease, myasthenia gravis, major surgery, nonallergic bronchospasm

> **BLACK BOX WARNING:** Abrupt discontinuation

DOSAGE AND ROUTES

Angina pectoris/hypertension

Adult: PO 40 mg/day; increase by 40-80 mg 7 days; maintenance 40-240 mg/day for angina, 40-320 mg/day for hypertension

Geriatric: PO 20 mg/day, may increase by 20 mg until desired dose

Renal dose

Adult: PO CCr 31-50 ml/min give q24-36hr; CCr 10-30 ml/min give q24-48hr; CCr <10 ml/min give q40-60hr

Esophageal varices (unlabeled)

Adult: PO 40 mg qday

Available forms: Tabs 20, 40, 80, 160 ✚ mg

ADVERSE EFFECTS

CNS: Anxiety, drowsiness, depression, *dizziness,* fatigue, lethargy, paresthesia, headache, *weakness,* insomnia, memory loss, nightmares

CV: *Bradycardia, hypotension,* HF, palpitations, chest pain, peripheral ischemia, flushing, edema, vasodilatation

EENT: Blurred vision, dry eyes, nasal congestion

ENDO: Hyperglycemia, hypoglycemia

GI: Nausea, vomiting, diarrhea, constipation, cramps, dry mouth, flatulence, taste distortion

GU: *Impotence,* decreased libido

INTEG: Rash, pruritus, fever, alopecia

RESP: Bronchospasm, cough, wheezing

INTERACTIONS

Individual drugs

CloNIDine, EPINEPHrine: increased hypotension, bradycardia, monitor for bradycardia

Digoxin: increased bradycardia

Thyroid: decreased β-blocking effect

Drug classifications

Antidiabetics, insulins: Increase: lack of dose stability

Antihypertensives: increased hypotension

Ergots: peripheral ischemia

MAOIs: increased orthostatic hypotension, monitor B/P

NSAIDs: decreased antihypertensive effect

Phenothiazines, general anesthetics: increased hypotensive effects

Drug/herb

Dong quai, garlic, ginseng, yohimbe: increased hypertension, avoid concurrent use

Drug/lab test

Increased: serum potassium, serum uric acid, ALT, AST, alkaline phosphatase, LDH, blood glucose, cholesterol, ANA, triglycerides

NURSING CONSIDERATIONS

Assessment

• **Hypertension:** check that prescriptions have been filled; monitor B/P at beginning of treatment, periodically thereafter; note rate, rhythm, quality of apical/radial pulse before administration; notify prescriber of any significant changes (pulse 60 bpm), orthostatic hypotension; if severe hypotension occurs, may use vasopressors to raise B/P

• **Pregnancy/breastfeeding:** Use only if benefits outweigh fetal risk, discontinue product or breastfeeding, excreted in breast milk

• **Angina:** monitor frequency of angina, alleviating factors

• Assess for edema in feet, legs daily; monitor I&O, daily weight; check for jugular vein distention and crackles bilaterally, dyspnea (HF)

• Assess for headache, light-headedness, decreased B/P; may indicate a need for decreased dosage

> **BLACK BOX WARNING. Abrupt discontinuation:** can result in MI, myocardial ischemia, ventricular dysrhythmias, severe hypertension; withdraw slowly by tapering over 1-2 wk; if symptoms return, restart

Patient problem
Impaired cardiac output (uses)
Nonadherence (teaching)

Implementation
• Give at bedtime; tab may be crushed or swallowed whole; give with food to prevent GI upset; give reduced dosage in renal dysfunction; check apical pulse prior to use, if <50 bpm, withhold dose and notify prescriber

• Store protected from light, moisture; place in cool environment

> **BLACK BOX WARNING:** Taper over 1-2 wk to discontinue, do not stop abruptly

Patient/family education

> **BLACK BOX WARNING:** Teach patient not to discontinue product abruptly; taper over 1-2 wk; may cause precipitate angina, serious dysrhythmias if stopped abruptly

• Teach patient not to use OTC products containing α-adrenergic stimulants (such as nasal decongestants, cold preparations); to avoid alcohol and smoking and to limit sodium intake as prescribed, to take as prescribed at same time each day; do not double; take missed dose as soon as remembered if before 8 hr prior to next dose

• Teach patient how to take pulse and B/P at home; to hold dose if pulse is ≤50 bpm, systolic B/P <90 mm Hg; advise when to notify

• **Hypertension:** instruct patient to comply with weight control, dietary adjustments,

modified exercise program; to report weight gain >5 lb, swelling, unusual bruising, bleeding

• Advise patient to carry/wear emergency ID to identify product being taken, allergies; teach patient product controls symptoms but does not cure condition

• Caution patient to avoid hazardous activities if dizziness, drowsiness are present, to rise slowly to prevent orthostatic hypotension

• **Teach patient to report symptoms of HF:** difficult breathing, especially on exertion or when lying down, night cough, swelling of extremities or bradycardia, dizziness, confusion, depression, fever

Evaluation

Positive therapeutic outcome
• Decreased B/P in hypertension
• Decreased angina episodes

> **RARELY USED**
>
> ## nafarelin
> (na-fare' e-lin)
> **Synarel**
> *Func. class:* Hormone, gonadotropin-releasing

USES: Central precocious puberty, endometriosis

CONTRAINDICATIONS: Hypersensitivity, this product, GnRH analogues, abnormal vaginal bleeding

DOSAGE AND ROUTES

Endometriosis
Adult females Nasal 400 mcg/day, one spray (note 1 spray = 200 mcg) into one nostril in the morning and one spray (200 mcg) into the other nostril in the evening. Treatment should be started between days 2 and 4 of the menstrual cycle. For those patients that do not achieve amenorrhea after 2 months of 400 mcg/day, the dose may be increased to 800 mcg/day, as one spray (200 mcg) in both nostrils every morning and every evening

Precocious puberty
Children Nasal 1600 mcg/ day, two sprays (total of 400 mcg) into each nostril every morning and every evening. If adequate suppression cannot be achieved, the dosage may be increased to 1800 mcg/day as three sprays (total of 600 mcg) into alternating nostrils tid

N

nafcillin (Rx)
(naf-sill'in)
Func. class.: Antiinfective, broad-spectrum
Chem. class.: Penicillinase-resistant penicillin

ACTION: Interferes with cell wall replication of susceptible organisms; osmotically unstable cell wall swells, bursts from osmotic pressure

Therapeutic outcome: Bactericidal effects for gram-positive cocci *Staphylococcus aureus, Streptococcus viridans, Streptococcus pneumoniae* and infections caused by penicillinase-producing *Staphylococcus*

USES: Infections caused by penicillinase-producing staphylococci, streptococci; respiratory tract, skin, skin structure, urinary tract, bone, joint infections; sinusitis; endocarditis; septicemia; meningitis

Pharmacokinetics

Absorption	Well absorbed (IM);
Distribution	Widely distributed; crosses placenta, 90% protein bound
Metabolism	Liver; 70%
Excretion	Kidneys, unchanged; breast milk
Half-life	30-90 min; increased in renal disease

Pharmacodynamics

	IM	IV
Onset	½ hr	Immediate
Peak	1-2 hr	Infusion end
Duration	Unknown	Unknown

CONTRAINDICATIONS
Hypersensitivity to penicillins

Precautions: Pregnancy, breastfeeding, neonates, GI disease, asthma, hypersensitivity to cephalosporins or carbapenems, electrolyte imbalances, hepatic/renal disease, pseudomembranous colitis

DOSAGE AND ROUTES
Adult: IV 500-1000 mg q4hr; IM 500-1000 mg q6-8hr, max 12 g/day
Infant and child >1 mo: IV/IM 150-200 mg/kg/day in divided doses q4-6hr
Neonate >7 days (weight >2 kg): IV 25 mg/kg q6hr
Neonate ≤7 days (weight ≤2 kg): IV 25 mg/kg q8hr

Available forms: Powder for inj 1 g/vial, 2 g/vial, 10 g/vial

ADVERSE EFFECTS
CNS: Lethargy, hallucinations, anxiety, depression, muscle twitching, seizures
GI: *Nausea, vomiting, diarrhea, clostridium difficile*–associated diarrhea (CDAD), hepatitis
GU: Interstitial nephritis
HEMA: Neutropenia
INTEG: Tissue necrosis, extravasation at injection site
SYST: Anaphylaxis, serum sickness, Stevens-Johnson syndrome

INTERACTIONS
Individual drugs
CycloSPORINE: decreased effect of cycloSPORINE
Probenecid: increased nafcillin levels

Drug classifications
Live virus vaccines: Decreased effect, do not use together
Hormonal contraceptives: decreased effect, use additional contraception
Tetracyclines, aminoglycosides: avoid use

Drug/food
Food, carbonated drinks, citrus fruit juices: decreased absorption

Drug/lab test
False positive: urine glucose, urine protein
Decreased: potassium, Hgb/Hct, neutrophils

NURSING CONSIDERATIONS
Assessment
• Assess patient for previous sensitivity reaction to penicillins or other cephalosporins; cross-sensitivity between penicillins and cephalosporins may occur
• **Infection:** Assess patient for signs and symptoms of infection including characteristics of wounds, sputum, urine, stool, WBC >10,000/mm³, earache, fever; obtain information baseline, during treatment
• Obtain C&S before beginning product therapy to identify if correct treatment has been initiated, may start treatment before receiving results
• **Assess for allergic reactions, anaphylaxis:** rash, urticaria, pruritus, chills, fever, dyspnea, laryngeal edema, joint pain; angioedema may occur a few days after therapy begins; cross-sensitivity with cephalosporins may occur; EPINEPHrine, resuscitation equipment should be available for anaphylactic reaction
• **CDAD:** assess for diarrhea, abdominal pain, fever, fatigue, anorexia; possible anemia, elevated WBC and low serum albumin; stop

product and usually give either vancomycin or IV metroNIDAZOLE

• Assess for overgrowth of infection: perineal itching, fever, malaise, redness, pain, swelling, drainage, rash, diarrhea, change in cough, sputum

• **IV site:** assess for redness, swelling, pain at site

• **Pregnancy/breastfeeding:** Use only if clearly needed, cautious use in breastfeeding

Patient problem
Infection (uses)

Implementation
IM route

• Reconstitute vials: Add 1.7 (1.8 Nafcil), 3, 4, or 6.4 ml (6.6 ml NaCl) (sterile water for INJ, 0.9% NaCl, bacteriostatic water for INJ with benzyl alcohol or parabens) to vials with 1 g, 2g of nafcillin, respectively (250 mg/ml)

• No further dilution needed; after reconstitution, inject in deep muscle mass

IV route

• Reconstitute vials: add 3.4 mL/1 g vial or 6.8 mL/2g vial (250 mg/ml)

Direct IV INJ route

• Further dilute the reconstituted sol with 15-30 ml of sterile water for inj, 0.45% NaCl, 0.9% NaCl (100 mg/mL); inj slowly over 5-10 min into the tubing of a free-flowing compatible IV solution

Intermittent IV route

• Vials, further dilute reconstituted solution to 2-40 mg/ml, for peripheral vein inf ≤20 mg/ml (preferred); piggyback unit no further dilution needed; infuse ≥30-60 min, make sure entire dose is given before 10% or more of solution is inactivated

• **Extravasation management:** stop infusion and disconnect; gently aspirate extravasated solution; do not flush line; use hyaluronidase; remove cannula/needle; apply dry cold compresses; elevate extremity

Y-site compatibilities: Acyclovir, alfentanil, amikacin, aminophylline, amphotericin B lipid complex (Abelcet), anidulafungin, argatroban, ascorbic acid injection, atenolol, atracurium, atropine, aztreonam, benztropine, bivalirudin, bleomycin, bretylium, bumetanide, buprenorphine, butorphanol, calcium chloride/gluconate, CARBOplatin, carmustine, cefamandole, ceFAZolin, cefoperazone, cefotaxime, cefoTEtan, cefOXitin, cefTAZidime, ceftizoxime, cefTRIAXone, cefuroxime, chlorproMAZINE, cimetidine, CISplatin, clindamycin, cyanocobalamin, cyclophosphamide, cycloSPORINE, DACTINomycin, DAPTOmycin, DAUNOrubicin

liposome, dexamethasone, digoxin, DOBUTamine, DOCEtaxel, DOPamine, DOXOrubicin liposomal, enalaprilat, ePHEDrine, EPINEPHrine, epoetin alfa, erythromycin, etoposide, etoposide phosphate, famotidine, fenoldopam, fentaNYL, fluconazole, fludarabine, foscarnet, furosemide, gallium, ganciclovir, gatifloxacin, gemtuzumab, gentamicin, glycopyrrolate, granisetron, heparin, hydrocortisone, HYDROmorphone, Imipenem cilastatin, indomethacin, isoproterenol, ketorolac, lactated Ringer's, lepirudin, leucovorin, lidocaine, linezolid injection, LORazepam, magnesium sulfate, mannitol, methyldopate, methylPREDNISolone, metoclopramide, metoprolol, metroNIDAZOLE, milrinone, morphine, multiple vitamins injection, naloxone, niCARdipine, nitroglycerin, nitroprusside, norepinephrine, octreotide, ondansetron, oxacillin, oxaliplatin, oxytocin, PACLitaxel (solvent/surfactant), pamidronate, pancuronium, pantoprazole, PEMEtrexed, penicillin G potassium/sodium, PENTobarbital, perphenazine, PHENobarbital, phentolamine, phenylephrine, phytonadione, piperacillin, polymyxin B, potassium acetate/chloride, procainamide, prochlorperazine, propofol, propranolol, ranitidine, Ringer's injection, sodium bicarbonate, SUFentanil, tacrolimus, teniposide, theophylline, thiamine, thiotepa, ticarcillin, ticarcillin-clavulanate, tigecycline, tirofiban, TNA (3-in-1), tobramycin, tolazoline, TPN (2-in-1), urokinase, vasopressin, vinBLAStine, voriconazole, zidovudine, zoledronic acid

Patient/family education

• Advise patient to contact prescriber if vaginal itching, loose foul-smelling stools, furry tongue occur; may indicate superinfection

• Instruct patient to take all medication prescribed for the length of time ordered

• Advise patient to notify prescriber of diarrhea with blood or pus, which may indicate CDAD

• Advise patient to carry/wear emergency ID if allergic to penicillins

• Teach patient to avoid use with other products unless approved by prescriber

Evaluation

Positive therapeutic outcome

• Absence of signs/symptoms of infection (WBC <10,000/mm^3, temp WNL, absence of red, draining wounds, earache)

• Reported improvement in symptoms of infection

TREATMENT OF ANAPHYLAXIS: Withdraw product, maintain airway, administer EPINEPHrine, aminophylline, O$_2$, IV corticosteroids

naftifine
(naff′ ti-feen)
Naftin
Func. class.: Topical antifungal

USES: Active against: *Candida albicans, Candida sp., Epidermophyton floccosum, Microsporum audouinii, Microsporum canis, Microsporum gypseum, Trichophyton mentagrophytes, Trichophyton rubrum, Trichophyton tonsurans;* may also have activity against the following: *Aspergillus flavus, Aspergillus fumigatus, Sporothrix schenckii, Trichophyton verrucosum*

For the treatment of *tinea cruri*
Adults Topical gel 1% Gently massage into the affected area and surrounding skin bid (morning and evening); topical dosage (1% cream); gently massage into the affected area and surrounding skin q day; topical dosage (2% cream): gently massage into the affected area and approximately 0.5 inches of surrounding skin q day × 2 wk.

nalbuphine (Rx)
(nal′byoo-feen)
Nubain ✦
Func. class.: Opioid analgesic
Chem. class.: Synthetic opioid agonist/ antagonist

Do not confuse: **nalbuphine**/naloxone

ACTION: Depresses pain impulse transmission at the spinal cord level by interacting with opioid receptors

Therapeutic outcome: Relief of pain

USES: Moderate to severe pain, supplement to anesthesia, sedation prior to surgery

Pharmacokinetics

Absorption	Well absorbed (SUBCUT, IM); completely absorbed (**IV**)
Distribution	Crosses placenta
Metabolism	Liver, extensively
Excretion	Feces, kidneys, unchanged (small amounts); breast milk
Half-life	3-6 hr

Pharmacodynamics

	IM	SUBCUT	IV
Onset	Up to 15 min	Up to 15 min	2-3 min
Peak	1 hr	Unknown	½ hr
Duration	3-6 hr	3-6 hr	3-6 hr

CONTRAINDICATIONS
Hypersensitivity to this product or parabens, addiction (opioid)

Precautions: Pregnancy, breastfeeding, addictive personality, increased ICP, MI (acute), severe heart disease, respiratory depression, renal/ hepatic disease, bowel impaction, abrupt discontinuation

DOSAGE AND ROUTES
Analgesic
Adult: SUBCUT/IM/**IV** 10 mg q3-6hr prn, max 160 mg/day, 20 mg/dose

Balanced anesthesia adjunct
Adult: **IV** 0.3-3 mg/kg given over 10-15 min; may give 0.25-0.5 mg/kg as needed (maintenance)

Available forms: Solution for inj 10, 20 mg/ml

ADVERSE EFFECTS
CNS: *Drowsiness, dizziness, confusion, headache, sedation, euphoria,* dysphoria (high doses), hallucinations, increased dreaming, tolerance, physical and psychological dependency
CV: Bradycardia, change in B/P
EENT: Blurred vision, miosis, diplopia
GI: *Nausea, vomiting, anorexia, constipation, cramps,* abdominal pain, dyspepsia, xerostomia, bitter taste
GU: Urinary urgency
INTEG: *Rash,* urticaria, flushing, *diaphoresis,* pruritus
RESP: Respiratory depression, pulmonary edema

INTERACTIONS
Individual drugs
Alcohol: increased respiratory depression, hypotension, sedation

Drug classifications
Antipsychotics, CNS depressants, sedative/hypnotics, skeletal muscle relaxants: increased respiratory depression, hypotension
Opiates: increased effects with other CNS depressants
MAOIs: increase: severe reactions, decrease dose to 25%

Drug/herb
Increase: CNS depression, kava, valerian, hops, chamomile

NURSING CONSIDERATIONS
Assessment
• **Assess pain characteristics** (location, intensity, type) before medication administration, 30 60 min after treatment, titrate upward by 25%-50% until pain is reduced by 50%, can repeat if initial dose is not adequately effective; not for long-term use

• Assess bowel status; constipation is common, may need laxative or stool softener

• Monitor VS, B/P, pulse baseline and periodically after parenteral route; note muscle rigidity, product history, liver, kidney function tests

• **Monitor CNS changes:** dizziness, drowsiness, hallucinations, euphoria, LOC, pupil reaction

• Monitor allergic reactions: rash, urticaria

• Monitor withdrawal reactions in opiate-dependent individuals: PE, vascular occlusion, abscesses, ulcerations, nausea, vomiting, seizures; low potential for dependence may lead to physical/physiological dependencies if used for extended time

• **Opioid addition:** Assess for abuse or addition of opioids or other substances before use, may lead to dependence if used long term

• **Respiratory dysfunction:** Monitor respiratory depression, character; rate, rhythm; notify prescriber if respirations <10/min

Patient problem
Pain (uses)
Risk for injury (adverse reactions)

Implementation
• Give by inj (IM, **IV**), only with resuscitative equipment available; give slowly to prevent rigidity

• Store in light-resistant area at room temperature
IM route
• Give inj deeply in large muscle mass; rotate inj sites; protect vial from light

Direct IV route
• Give direct **IV** undiluted 10 mg or less over 3-5 min or more into free-flowing IV line of D$_5$W, NS, LR

Patient/family education
• Instruct patient to report any symptoms of CNS changes, allergic reactions

• Teach patient that physical dependency can result from long-term use, although there is a low potential for dependency, profuse sweating, twitching, nausea, vomiting, cramps, fever, faintness, anorexia; without treatment, symptoms

resolve in 5-14 days; chronic abstinence syndrome may last 2-6 mo

• Caution patients to avoid CNS depressants: alcohol, sedative/hypnotics for at least 24 hr after taking this product

• Discuss with patient that dizziness, drowsiness, confusion are common; to avoid getting up without assistance

• Discuss in detail all aspects of the product; reason for taking product and expected results

• Instruct patient to change position slowly to prevent orthostatic hypotension

• **Pregnancy/breastfeeding:** Identify if pregnancy is planned or suspected or if breastfeeding

Evaluation

Positive therapeutic outcome
• Relief of pain without respiratory depression

TREATMENT OF OVERDOSE:
Naloxone (Narcan) 0.2-0.8 **IV**, O$_2$, **IV** fluids, vasopressors

---

RARELY USED

naldemedine
(nal-dem′ e-deen)
Symproic
Func. class.: Laxative, opioid antagonist

USES: Opioid-induced constipation

CONTRAINDICATION
Hypersensitivity, GI obstruction, severe hepatic disease, breastfeeding

DOSAGE AND ROUTES
Adult PO 0.2 mg q day

RARELY USED

naloxegel
(nal-ox′ ee-gol)
Movantik
Func. class.: laxative, opioid antagonist

USES: Opioid-induced constipation

CONTRAINDICATIONS
Hypersensitivity, GI obstruction, severe hepatic disease, strong CYP3A4 inducers, breastfeeding

DOSAGE AND ROUTES
Adult PO 25 mg q day, may reduce to 12.5 mg q day if needed; strong CYP3A4 inducers use 12.5 mg q day

naloxone (Rx)
(nal-oks'one)
Evzio, Narcan
Func. class.: Opioid antagonist, antidote
Chem. class.: Thebaine derivative

Do not confuse: naloxone/naltrexone, nalbuphine, Narcan/Norcuron

ACTION: Competes with opioids at opioid-receptor sites

Therapeutic outcome: Absence of opioid overdose

USES: Respiratory depression induced by opioids; refractory circulatory shock, asphyxia neonatorum, coma, hypotension, opiate agonist overdose

Unlabeled uses: IBS, opiate agonist dependence, opiate agonist-induced constipation, pruritus

Pharmacokinetics

Absorption	Well absorbed (SUBCUT, IM); completely absorbed (**IV**)
Distribution	Rapidly distributed; crosses placenta
Metabolism	Liver
Excretion	Kidneys
Half-life	1 hr; up to 3 hr (neonates)

Pharmacodynamics

	IV	IM/SUBCUT
Onset	1 min	2-5 min
Peak	Unknown	Unknown
Duration	45 min	30-81 min

CONTRAINDICATIONS
Hypersensitivity

Precautions: Pregnancy, breastfeeding, neonates, children, CV disease, opioid dependency, seizure disorder, drug dependency, hepatic disease

DOSAGE AND ROUTES
Opioid-induced respiratory depression (known or suspected opiate agonist overdose)
Adult: **IV**/SUBCUT/IM 0.4-2 mg; repeat q2-3min if needed, max 10 mg; **IV** infusion loading dose 0.005 mg/kg, then 0.0025 mg/kg/hr; nasal spray 1 spray, may repeat q2-3min in alternate nostril if needed
Child <5 yr or ≤20 kg: **IV**/intraosseous 0.01 mg/kg slowly followed by 0.1 mg/kg if needed;

IV infusion (PALS) 0.04-0.16 mg/kg/hr, titrate; nasal spray 1 spray, may repeat q2-3min in alternate nostril if needed

Postoperative opioid-induced respiratory depression
Adult: **IV** 0.1-0.2 mg q2-3min prn
Child: **IV** 0.005-0.01 mg/kg q2-3min prn
Neonates: **IM/IV** subcut 0.01 mg/kg, repeat q 2-3 min until adequate response

Nausea/vomiting from continuous morphine infusion/urinary retention (unlabeled)
Adult: **IV** 0.2 mg

Opioid-induced pruritus (unlabeled)
Child: Cont IV inf 2 mcg/kg/hr q4hr may increase by 0.5 mcg/kg/hr q4h

Available forms: Inj 0.4 mg/0.4 mL; auto injector; 1 mg/ml; nasal spray 4 mg/0.1 ml

ADVERSE EFFECTS
CV: Rapid pulse, ventricular tachycardia, fibrillation, hypo/hypertension
GI: Nausea, vomiting

INTERACTIONS
Drug classifications
Analgesics (opioids): decreased effects of opioid analgesics

Drug/lab test
Interference: urine VMA, 5-HIAA, urine glucose

NURSING CONSIDERATIONS
Assessment
• **Assess for signs of opioid withdrawal** in drug-dependent individuals: cramping, hypertension, anxiety, vomiting; may occur up to 2 hr after administration, severity depends on length of time opioids were taken, naloxone dose
• **Assess for pain:** duration, intensity, location before, after administration; may be used for respiratory depression, analgesia will be decreased
• **Assess for respiratory dysfunction:** respiratory depression, character, rate, rhythm; if respirations are <10/min, probably due to opioid overdose, administer naloxone; monitor LOC, ECG, B/P
• **Acute opioid reversal:** Patients may become very agitated and violent after use

Patient problem
Impaired breathing (uses)
Risk for injury (adverse reactions)

Implementation
• Store at room temperature and protect from light
• Double-check dose; those taking opioids (>1 wk) are sensitive to this product

Direct IV route
• Give undiluted (suspected opioid overdose); give 0.4 mg or less over 15 sec or titrate inf to response; (respiratory depression) dilute with sterile water for injection (0.1/mg/mL) <40 kg body weight

Continuous IV infusion route
• Dilute 2 mg/500 ml 0.9% NaCl or D_5W (4 mcg/ml), titrate to response
• Give only with resuscitative equipment, O_2 nearby
• Use only sol prepared within 24 hr
• Do not admix with bisulfite, sulfite

Y-site compatibilities: Acyclovir, alfentanil, amikacin, aminocaproic acid, aminophylline, anidulafungin, ascorbic acid, atenolol, atracurium, atropine, azaTHIOprine, aztreonam, benztropine, bivalirudin, bleomycin, bumetanide, buprenorphine, butorphanol, calcium chloride/gluconate, CARBOplatin, caspofungin, cefamandole, ceFAZolin, cefmetazole, cefonicid, cefoperazone, cefotaxime, cefoTEtan, cefOXitin, cefTAZidime, ceftizoxime, cefTRIAXone, cefuroxime, cephalothin, cephapirin, chloramphenicol, chlorproMAZINE, cimetidine, CISplatin, clindamycin, cyanocobalamin, cyclophosphamide, cycloSPORINE, cytarabine, DACTINomycin, DAPTOmycin, dexamethasone, digoxin, diltiazem, diphenhydrAMINE, DOBUTamine, DOCEtaxel, DOPamine, doxacurium, DOXOrubicin, doxycycline, enalaprilat, ePHEDrine, EPINEPHrine, epirubicin, epoetin alfa, eptifibatide, ertapenem, erythromycin, esmolol, etoposide, etoposide phosphate, famotidine, fenoldopam, fentaNYL, fluconazole, fludarabine, fluorouracil, folic acid, furosemide, ganciclovir, gatifloxacin, gemcitabine, gentamicin, glycopyrrolate, granisetron, heparin, hydrocortisone, hydrOXYzine, IDArubicin, ifosfamide, imipenem-cilastatin, inamrinone, indomethacin, insulin (regular), irinotecan, isoproterenol, ketorolac, labetalol, levofloxacin, lidocaine, linezolid, LORazepam, mannitol, mechlorethamine, meperidine, metaraminol, methicillin, methotrexate, methyldopate, methylPREDNISolone, metoclopramide, metoprolol, metroNIDAZOLE, mezlocillin, miconazole, midazolam, milrinone, minocycline, mitoXANtrone, morphine, multiple vitamins, mycophenolate, nafcillin, nalbuphine, nesiritide, netilmicin, nitroglycerin, nitroprusside, norepinephrine, octreotide, ondansetron, oxacillin, oxaliplatin, oxytocin, PACLitaxel, palonosetron, pamidronate, pancuronium, papaverine, PEMEtrexed, penicillin G potassium/sodium, pentamidine, pentazocine, PENTobarbital, PHENobarbital, phentolamine, phenylephrine, phytonadione, piperacillin, piperacillin-tazobactam, polymyxin B, potassium chloride, procainamide, prochlorperazine, promethazine, propofol, propranolol, protamine, pyridoxine, quiNIDine, quinupristin-dalfopristin, ranitidine, rocuronium, sodium acetate/bicarbonate, succinylcholine, SUFentanil, tacrolimus, teniposide, theophylline, thiamine, ticarcillin, ticarcillin-clavulanate, tigecycline, tirofiban, tobramycin, tolazoline, urokinase, vancomycin, vasopressin, vecuronium, verapamil, vinCRIStine, vinorelbine, voriconazole, zoledronic acid

Patient/family education
• Explain reason for and expected results of medication when patient is alert

Evaluation

Positive therapeutic outcome
• Reversal of respiratory depression
• LOC: alert

naphazoline ophthalmic
See Appendix B

naproxen
(na-prox'en)
Aleve, Anaprox, Anaprox DS, EC-Naprosyn, Naprelan, Naprosyn, Maxidol ✦
Func. class.: Nonsteroidal antiinflammatory, nonopioid analgesic
Chem. class.: Propionic acid derivative

ACTION: Completely inhibits COX-1, COX-2 by blocking arachidonate; analgesic, antiinflammatory, antipyretic

Therapeutic outcome: Decreased pain, inflammation

USES: Mild to moderate pain, osteoarthritis, rheumatoid arthritis, gouty arthritis, primary dysmenorrhea, tendinitis, ankylosing spondylitis, bursitis, myalgia, dental pain, juvenile rheumatoid arthritis

Pharmacokinetics

Absorption	Completely absorbed
Distribution	Crosses placenta, 99% protein binding
Metabolism	Liver, extensively
Excretion	Breast milk
Half-life	10-20 hr

Pharmacodynamics

Onset	1 hr
Peak	2-4 hr
Duration	<7 hr

CONTRAINDICATIONS

Pregnancy, hypersensitivity to NSAIDs, salicylates, perioperative pain in CABG surgery/MI/stroke

Precautions: Pregnancy (1st trimester), breastfeeding, children <2 yr, geriatric, bleeding disorders, GI/cardiac disorders, hypersensitivity to other antiinflammatory agents, CCr <30 ml/min, asthma, renal failure, hepatic disease

> **BLACK BOX WARNING:** GI bleeding, stroke

DOSAGE AND ROUTES

200 mg base = 220 mg naproxen sodium

Antiinflammatory/analgesic/antidysmenorrheal

Adult: PO 250-500 mg bid, max 1250 mg/day; DEL REL TAB 375-500 mg bid
Child ≥2 yr: PO 7 mg/kg/12 hr

Antigout

Adult: PO 750 mg, then 250 mg q8hr

OTC use

Adult: PO 220 mg q8-12hr or 440 mg, then 220 mg q12hr, max 660 mg/24 hr, taken no longer than 10 days
Geriatric >65 yr: PO max 220 mg q12hr

Available forms: Naproxen: tabs: 250, 375, 500 mg; del rel tabs (EC-Naprosyn, Naprosyn-E) 250 ✱, 375, 500 mg; oral susp 125 mg/5 ml; ext rel tabs (CR) 375, 500, 750 mg ✱; **naproxen sodium;** tabs 220, 275, 550 mg

ADVERSE EFFECTS

CNS: Dizziness, drowsiness, fatigue, tremors, confusion, insomnia, anxiety, depression
CV: Tachycardia, peripheral edema, palpitations, dysrhythmias, MI, stroke
EENT: Blurred vision, tinnitus
GI: Nausea, anorexia, vomiting, diarrhea, jaundice, hepatitis, constipation, flatulence, cramps, peptic ulcer, GI bleeding
GU: Nephrotoxicity: dysuria, hematuria, oliguria, azotemia
HEMA: Blood dyscrasias
INTEG: Purpura, rash, pruritus, sweating, photosensitivity
SYST: Anaphylaxis, Stevens-Johnson syndrome

INTERACTIONS

Individual drugs

Alcohol, aspirin: increased risk of GI side effects
Clopidogrel, eptifibatide, plicamycin, ticlopidine, tirofiban: increased bleeding risk
Lithium, methotrexate, probenecid, radiation: increased toxicity
Cholestyramine, sucralfate: decreased/delayed absorption of naproxen

Drug classifications

ACE inhibitors, angiotensin II antagonists: possible renal impairment
Antacids: decreased/delayed absorption of naproxen
Anticoagulants, SSRIs, SNRIs, thrombolytics, tricyclics: increased risk of bleeding
Antihypertensives: decreased effect of antihypertensives
Antineoplastics: increased risk of hematologic toxicity
Corticosteroids, NSAIDs: increased risk of GI adverse reactions
Loop/thiazide diuretics: decreased effectiveness of diuretics

Drug/herb

Alfalfa, anise, bilberry, fenugreek, feverfew, garlic, ginger, ginkgo, ginseng *(Panax),* licorice: increased bleeding risk

Drug/lab test

Increased: BUN, alkaline phosphatase, LFTs, potassium, glucose, cholesterol
Decreased: potassium, sodium
False: increased 5-HIAA, 17KS

NURSING CONSIDERATIONS

Assessment

• **Monitor pain:** location, frequency, duration, characteristics, type, intensity before dose and 1 hour after
• **Arthritis:** Assess ROM, pain, swelling before and 1-2 hr after use
• **Fever:** Assess before use and 1 hr after use
• **Cardiac status:** CV thrombotic events, MI, stroke; may be fatal; not to be used in CABG

> **BLACK BOX WARNING: GI status:** ulceration, bleeding, perforation; may be fatal

• Monitor liver function, renal function, other blood tests: AST, ALT, bilirubin, creatinine, BUN, CBC, Hct, Hgb, pro-time, LDH, blood glucose, WBC, platelets; if patient is on long-term therapy
• Check I&O ratio; decreasing output may indicate renal failure (long-term therapy)

- **Assess hepatotoxicity:** dark urine, clay-colored stools, yellowing of the skin and sclera, itching, abdominal pain, fever, diarrhea if patient is on long-term therapy
- Assess for allergic reactions: rash, urticaria; if these occur, product may have to be discontinued
- Monitor B/P baseline and periodically; Check for edema in feet, ankles, legs
- Identify prior product history; there are many product interactions
- Assess for asthma, aspirin hypersensitivity, or nasal polyps, increased risk of hypersensitivity
- **Beers:** Avoid chronic use in older adults unless other alternatives are not available, increased GI, bleeding risk, peptic ulcer disease

Patient problem
Pain (uses)
Impaired mobility (uses)
Risk for injury (adverse reactions)

Implementation
- Administer to patient crushed or whole (**regular release**); do not crush, break, or chew **extended rel tab**
- Give OTC for 10 days or less unless approved by prescriber
- Adequately hydrate those taking angiotensin receptor blockers/angiotensin-converting enzyme inhibitors
- Give with food or milk to decrease gastric symptoms; give ½ hr before or 2 hr after meals for better absorption
- Patient should take with 8 oz of water and sit upright for 30 min after dose to prevent ulceration
- Store at room temperature

Patient/family education
- Teach patient to report any symptoms of renal/hepatic toxicity, allergic reactions, bleeding (long-term therapy); to report use to all health care providers, **signs of MI, stroke**
- Caution patient not to exceed recommended dosage; acute poisoning may result; to take as prescribed, do not double dose

> **BLACK BOX WARNING:** Teach patient to read label on other OTC products; many contain other antiinflammatories; caution patient to avoid alcohol ingestion; GI bleeding may occur

- Inform patient that the therapeutic response takes 2 wk (arthritis)
- Teach patient to report tinnitus confusion, diarrhea, sweating, hyperventilation, fever, joint aches, black stools, flulike symptoms

- Advise patient to use sunscreen, protective clothing to prevent photosensitivity
- Teach patient to notify prescriber if pregnancy is planned or suspected, or if breastfeeding

Evaluation
Positive therapeutic outcome
- Decreased pain
- Decreased inflammation
- Increased mobility

naratriptan (Rx)
(nair′ah-trip-tan)
Amerge
Func. class.: Antimigraine agent
Chem. class.: 5-HT₁-like receptor agonist

ACTION: Binds selectively to the vascular 5-HT₁ receptor subtype, exerts antimigraine effect; causes vasoconstriction in cranial arteries

Therapeutic outcome: Decreased intensity and incidence of migraines

USES: Acute treatment of migraine with or without aura

Pharmacokinetics
Absorption	Unknown
Distribution	28%-31% protein binding
Metabolism	Liver (metabolite)
Excretion	Urine/feces
Half-life	6 hr

Pharmacodynamics
Onset	Unknown
Peak	2-3 hr
Duration	Unknown

CONTRAINDICATIONS
Angina pectoris, history of MI, documented silent ischemia, ischemic heart disease, concurrent ergotamine-containing preparations, uncontrolled hypertension, hypersensitivity, severe renal disease (CCr <15 ml/min), severe hepatic disease (Child-Pugh grade C), CV syndromes, hemiplegic or basilar migraines

Precautions: Pregnancy, breastfeeding, children, geriatric, postmenopausal women, men >40 yr, risk factors for CAD, hypercholesterolemia, obesity, diabetes, impaired renal/hepatic function, peripheral vascular disease

DOSAGE AND ROUTES
Adult: PO 1 or 2.5 mg with fluids; if headache returns, repeat once after 4 hr, max 5 mg/24 hr

Renal/hepatic dose
Adult: PO CCr 15-39 ml/min Max 2.5 mg/24 hr

Available forms: Tabs 1, 2.5 mg

ADVERSE EFFECTS
CNS: Dizziness, sedation, fatigue
CV: Increased B/P, palpitations, tachydys-rhythmias, PR and QT_C prolongation, ST/T wave changes, PVCs, atrial flutter, fibrillation, coronary vasospasm
EENT: EENT infections, photophobia
GI: *Nausea, vomiting*
MISC: Temp change sensations, tightness, pressure sensations
MS: *Weakness, neck stiffness,* myalgia

INTERACTIONS
Individual drugs
Sibutramine: increased serotonin syndrome risk

Drug classifications
$5\text{-}HT_1$ agonists, ergot derivatives: increased vasospastic effect
MAOIs: increased risk of adverse reactions, do not use together
SSRIs (FLUoxetine, fluvoxaMINE, PARoxetine, sertraline), SNRIs, serotonin receptor agonists, sibutramine: increased serotonin syndrome, neuroleptic malignant syndrome

Drug/herb
SAMe, St. John's wort: increased serotonin syndrome

NURSING CONSIDERATIONS
Assessment
• **Migraines:** assess for aura, duration, effect of lifestyle, aggravating/alleviating factors
• **Serotonin syndrome, neuroleptic malignant syndrome:** assess for increased heart rate, shivering, sweating, dilated pupils, tremors, high B/P, hyperthermia, headache, confusion; if these occur, stop product, administer a serotonin antagonist if needed; at least 2 wk should elapse between discontinuing serotoninergic agents and starting this product
• Cardiac status: ECG, increased B/P, dysrhythmias in those with cardiac disease
• Assess for stress level, activity, recreation, coping mechanisms
• Assess neurologic status: LOC, blurred vision, nausea, tics preceding headache

Patient problem
Pain (uses)

Implementation
• Do not use product if another $5\text{-}HT_1$ agonist or an ergot preparation has been used in past 24 hr

• Give with fluids as soon as symptoms appear; may take another dose after 4 hr; max 5 mg in any 24-hr period
• Provide a quiet, calm environment with decreased stimulation, including noise, bright light, excessive talking

Patient/family education
• Teach patient to report pain, tightness in chest, neck, throat, or jaw; notify prescriber immediately if sudden, severe abdominal pain occurs
• Teach patient to use contraception while taking product, to notify prescriber not to use if pregnancy is planned or suspected or if breastfeeding
• Teach patient not to use if another $5\text{-}HT_1$ agonist or an ergot preparation has been used in the past 24 hr; avoid using >2 days/wk, rebound headache may occur
• Advise patient to discuss all OTC, Rx, herbals, supplements with health care professional; to avoid alcohol
• Teach patient to use as soon as headache is starting, to only use to treat, not prevent a migraine
• Advise patient that dizziness, drowsiness may occur, not to drive or perform other hazardous activities until response is known

Evaluation

Positive therapeutic outcome
• Absence of migraine headaches

natamycin ophthalmic
See Appendix B

⚠ HIGH ALERT
nebivolol (Rx)
(ne-biv'oh-lol)
Bystolic
Func. class.: Antihypertensive
Chem. class.: β_1-Blocker, selective

ACTION: Competitively blocks stimulation of β-adrenergic receptors within vascular smooth muscle; decreases rate of SA node discharge, increases recovery time, slows conduction of AV node resulting in decreased heart rate (negative chronotropic effect), which decreases O_2 consumption in myocardium due to β_1-receptor antagonism

Therapeutic outcome: Decreased B/P after 1-2 wk

USES: Hypertension alone or in combination

Pharmacokinetics

Absorption	Unknown
Distribution	Protein binding 98%
Metabolism	In liver by CYP2D6
Excretion	38% excreted in urine, 44% in feces
Half-life	12 hr

Pharmacodynamics

Onset	Unknown
Peak	1.5-4 hr
Duration	Unknown

CONTRAINDICATIONS

Cardiogenic shock, acute sick sinus syndrome, AV heart block, hypersensitivity to this agent or β-blockers, heart failure, severe hepatic disease, severe bradycardia

Precautions: Pregnancy, breastfeeding, children, major surgery, peripheral vascular disease, diabetes mellitus, thyrotoxicosis, COPD, asthma, well-compensated heart failure, renal/hepatic disease, abrupt discontinuation, acute bronchospasm

DOSAGE AND ROUTES
Hypertension
Adult: PO 5 mg/day, may be increased to desired response q2wk; max 40 mg/day
Geriatric: PO max 40 mg/day

Renal dose
Adult: PO CCr <30 ml/min, 2.5 mg/day; may increase cautiously

Hepatic dose
Adult: PO (Child-Pugh class B) 2.5 mg qd; use dose escalation cautiously

Available forms: Tabs 2.5, 5, 10, 20 mg

ADVERSE EFFECTS
CNS: *Insomnia, fatigue, dizziness, headache*
CV: Bradycardia, edema, chest pain
GI: *Nausea, diarrhea,* abdominal pain
MISC: Hyperuricemia, hypercholesterolemia, withdrawal symptoms

INTERACTIONS
Individual drugs
Cimetidine: increased nebivolol action
Mefloquine: do not give
Sildenafil: decreased nebivolol action

Drug classifications
β-blockers, others: do not use concurrently
Calcium channel blockers (nondihydropyridine), CYP2D6 inhibitors (amiodarone, buPROPion, chloroquine, chlorpheniramine, chlorproMAZINE, cinacalcet, diphenhydrAMINE, DULoxetine, FLUoxetine, haloperidol, imatinib, PARoxetine, promethazine, propoxyphene, quiNIDine, quiNINE, ritonavir, terbinafine, thioridazine), SSRIs: increased nebivolol action
CYP2D6 inducers (rifampin): decreased nebivolol action

Drug/herb
Hawthorn: may increase nebivolol effect
Ephedra: decreased nebivolol effect

Drug/lab test
Increased: serum lipoprotein levels, BUN, potassium, triglyceride, uric acid, LDH, AST, ALT, alkaline phosphatase
Decreased: platelets

NURSING CONSIDERATIONS
Assessment
• **Hypertension:** monitor B/P pulse, ECG during beginning treatment, periodically thereafter; assess apical/radial pulse before administration; notify prescriber of any significant changes (pulse <50 bpm); **signs of HF** (dyspnea, crackles, weight gain, jugular vein distention)
• Assess baselines in renal/hepatic studies before therapy begins and periodically, do not use in Child-Pugh class C
• Monitor I&O, edema in feet, legs, weight daily
• Assess blood glucose in diabetics

Patient problem
Impaired cardiac output (adverse reactions)

Implementation
PO route
• Give without regard for meals; tab may be crushed or swallowed whole; give with food to prevent GI upset
• Taper over 1-2 wk when discontinuing; minimize physical exertion; if angina recurs give nebivolol
• Store protected from light, moisture; place in cool environment

Patient/family education
• Caution patient not to discontinue product abruptly; severe cardiac reactions may occur; taper over 2 wk; do not double dose; if a dose is missed, take as soon as remembered up to 4 hr before next dose
• Inform patient product may mask signs of hypoglycemia or alter blood glucose levels
• Advise patient not to use OTC products containing α-adrenergic stimulants (such as nasal decongestants, OTC cold preparations) unless directed by prescriber

N

• Instruct patient to report low pulse, dizziness, confusion, depression, fever
• Teach patient to take pulse, B/P at home; advise when to notify prescriber
• Advise patient to comply with weight control, dietary adjustments, modified exercise program
• Instruct patient to carry emergency ID to identify product, allergies
• Caution patient to avoid hazardous activities if dizziness, drowsiness are present
• **Instruct patient to report symptoms of HF:** difficulty breathing, especially on exertion or when lying down, night cough, swelling of extremities
• Teach patient to continue with required lifestyle changes (exercise, diet, weight loss, stress reduction)

Evaluation

Positive therapeutic outcome
• Decreased B/P after 1-2 wk
• Decreased dysrhythmias

TREATMENT OF OVERDOSE:
Lavage, **IV** atropine for bradycardia, **IV** theophylline for bronchospasm, digoxin, O₂, diuretic for cardiac failure, **IV** glucose for hypoglycemia, **IV** diazepam (or phenytoin) for seizures, **IV** fluids, **IV** pressors

---

neomycin (Rx)
(nee-oh-mye´sin)
Neo-Fradin
Func. class.: Antiinfective—aminoglycoside

ACTION: Inhibits bacterial protein synthesis through irreversible binding to the 30 S ribosomal subunit of susceptible bacteria, actively transported into the bacterial cell where it binds to receptors present on the 30 S ribosomal subunit. This binding interferes with the initiation complex between the messenger RNA (mRNA) and the subunit. As a result, abnormal, nonfunctional proteins are formed due to misreading of the bacterial DNA

USES: Severe systemic infections of CNS, respiratory, GI, urinary tract, eye, bone, skin, soft tissues; hepatic coma, preoperatively to sterilize bowel, infectious diarrhea

Therapeutic response: Bacterial action against *Enterobacter sp.*, *Escherichia coli*, *Klebsiella sp.*; may be active against *Acinetobacter sp.*, *Bacillus anthracis*, *Citrobacter sp.*, *Haemophilus influenzae* (beta-lactamase negative), *Haemophilus influenzae* (beta-lactamase positive), *Neisseria sp.*, *Proteus mirabilis*, *Proteus vulgaris*, *Providencia sp.*, *Salmonella sp.*, *Serratia sp.*, *Shigella sp.*, *Staphylococcus aureus* (MSSA), *Staphylococcus epidermidis*

Pharmacokinetics

Absorption	Minimal
Distribution	Widely, crosses placenta
Metabolism	Unknown
Excretion	Kidney (90%)
Half-life	2-4 hr

Pharmacodynamics

Onset	Unknown
Peak	1-4 hr
Duration	Unknown

CONTRAINDICATIONS: Hypersensitivity to aminoglycosides, bisulfites, neonates, GI obstruction, IBS, colitis

Precautions: CDAD, respiratory depression, myasthenia gravis, GI disease

> **BLACK BOX WARNING:** Nephrotoxicity, neurotoxicity, neuromuscular blockade, ototoxicity, renal impairment

DOSAGE AND ROUTES

Hepatic encephalopathy
Adult: PO 4-12 g/day in divided doses q6hr × 5-6 days
Child: PO 50-100 mg/kg/day in divided doses q6hr × 5-6 days

Preoperative intestinal antisepsis
Adult: PO 1 g/hr × 4 hr, then 1 g q4hr for remaining 24 hr

Available forms: Tablets 500 mg

SIDE EFFECTS

CNS: Confusion, depression, numbness, tremors, seizures, muscle twitching, neurotoxicity, dizziness, vertigo, tinnitus, neuromuscular blockade with respiratory paralysis
EENT: Ototoxicity, deafness
GI: Nausea, vomiting, anorexia, bilirubin
GU: Oliguria, hematuria, renal damage, azotemia, renal failure, nephrotoxicity
HEMA: Eosinophilia, anemia
INTEG: *Rash*, burning, urticaria, dermatitis, alopecia

Individual drugs

> **BLACK BOX WARNING:** Acyclovir, amphotericin B, cidofovir, cycloSPORINE, vancomycin: nephrotoxicity

---

BLACK BOX WARNING: DimenhyDRINATE, ethacrynic acid: increased masking of ototoxicity

Drug classifications

BLACK BOX WARNING: Anesthetics, nondepolarizing neuromuscular blockers: increased neuromuscular blockade, respiratory depression

BLACK BOX WARNING: Increased: Ototoxicity-IV loop diuretics

Drug/lab test
Increased: BUN, creatinine

NURSING CONSIDERATIONS
Assessment:
• Assess patient for previous sensitivity reaction
• **Infection:** Assess patient for signs and symptoms of infection, including characteristics of wounds, sputum, urine, stool, WBC >10,000/mm³, earache, temp; obtain baseline information before and during treatment
• Assess for allergic reactions: rash, urticaria, pruritus

BLACK BOX WARNING: Nephrotoxicity: Assess renal impairment; obtain urine for CCr, BUN, serum creatinine; lower dosage should be given in renal impairment; nephrotoxicity may be reversible if product is stopped at first sign

• Notify prescriber of increased BUN and creatinine, urinalysis daily for protein, cells, casts
• Monitor blood studies: AST, ALT, CBC, Hct, bilirubin, LDH, alkaline phosphatase
• Assess for **overgrowth of infection:** perineal itching, fever, malaise, redness, pain, swelling, drainage, rash, diarrhea, change in cough, sputum

BLACK BOX WARNING: Ototoxicity: Assess for deafness by audiometric testing, ringing, roaring in ears, vertigo; assess hearing before, during, after treatment

BLACK BOX WARNING: Neuromuscular blockade; respiratory paralysis may occur, more common in those receiving anesthetics, neuromuscular blockers, use of calcium salts may reverse effect

• **Dehydration:** Monitor for high specific gravity, decrease in skin turgor, dry mucous membranes, dark urine

• **Vestibular dysfunction:** Assess for nausea, vomiting, dizziness, headache; product should be discontinued if severe
• **Pregnancy/breastfeeding:** Identify if pregnancy is planned or suspected or if breastfeeding; do not use in pregnancy or breastfeeding

Patient Problems
Infection (uses)
Impaired hearing (adverse reactions)

Implementation
• Give without regard to meals

Patient/family education
• Advise patient to contact prescriber if vaginal itching, loose foul-smelling stools, furry tongue occur; may indicate superinfection
• Advise patient to report hypersensitivity: rash, itching, trouble breathing, facial edema, notify prescriber

BLACK BOX WARNING: Neuromuscular blockade: respiratory paralysis may occur; more common in those receiving anesthetics, neuromuscular blockers; use of calcium salts may reverse effect

Evaluation
Positive therapeutic outcome
• Absence of signs/symptoms of infection: WBC <10,000/mm³, temp WNL; absence of red draining wounds; absence of earache
• Reported improvement in symptoms of infection

TREATMENT OF OVERDOSE:
Withdraw product; administer EPINEPHrine, O², hemodialysis

nepafenac ophthalmic
See Appendix B

neratinib
(ne-ra′-ti-nib)
Nerlynx
Func. class.: Antineoplastic
Chem. class.: Protein kinase inhibitors

ACTION: It is an irreversible inhibitor of the epidermal growth factor receptor (EGFR) and the human epidermal receptor type 2 (HER2) and HER4. It is a protein kinase inhibitor

USES: For the extended adjuvant treatment of early-stage HER2-positive breast cancer after completion of adjuvant trastuzumab

Pharmacokinetics

Absorption	Well, increased by fatty foods
Distribution	Protein binding >99%
Metabolism	Liver by CYP3A4
Excretion	Feces (97.1%)
Half-life	7-17 days

Pharmacodynamics

Onset	Unknown
Peak	2-4 hr
Duration	Up to 24 hr

CONTRAINDICATIONS: Hypersensitivity

Precautions: Breastfeeding, contraception requirements, geriatric patients, hepatic disease, hepatotoxicity, infertility, pregnancy, pregnancy testing, reproductive risk

DOSAGE AND ROUTES
For the extended adjuvant treatment of early-stage HER2-positive breast cancer after completion of adjuvant trastuzumab-based therapy
Adult: PO 240 mg/day with food × 1 yr

Hepatic dose
• **Adult:** PO Child-Pugh A or B: no change; Child-Pugh C: reduce starting dose to 80 mg/day; grade 3 elevations in ALT (5-20× UNL) or bilirubin (3-10× UNL): hold and evaluate causes; first occurrence, if LFTs resolve to grade ≤1 (ALT ≤3× UNL or bilirubin ≤1 to 1.5× UNL) in ≤3 wk, resume at the next lower dose; discontinue if hepatotoxicity does not recover to ≤1, if hepatotoxicity results in a treatment delay of >3 wk, or if grade 3 ALT or bilirubin occurs again despite one dose reduction

Available forms: Tabs 40 mg

SIDE EFFECTS
GI: Diarrhea, abdominal pain, anorexia, nausea, vomiting
MS: Muscle cramps
INTEG: Rash
GU: Renal failure (rare)
MISC: Infection

INTERACTIONS
Drug classifications
Gastric acid–reducing agents: **Decrease:** neratinib effect
Proton pump inhibitors (PPI), H2-receptor antagonists; avoid concomitant use: separate by 3 hr after antacid dosing strong or moderate CYP3A4 inhibitors; avoid concomitant use: **Increase:** neratinib effect

Strong or moderate CYP3A4 inducers; avoid concomitant use: **Decrease:** neratinib effect
P-glycoprotein (P-gp) substrates; monitor for adverse reactions of narrow therapeutic agents that are P-gp substrates: **Increase:** CNS and CV adverse reactions

NURSING CONSIDERATIONS
Assess
• Hepatotoxicity: use with caution in those with preexisting hepatic disease; a dose reduction is required for patients with severe (Child-Pugh C) hepatic disease at baseline. Monitor LFTs (total bilirubin, AST, ALT, alkaline phosphatase) baseline, q month ×3 mo and then q3mo thereafter and as needed. Monitor LFTs (including fractionated bilirubin and prothrombin time) in those experiencing grade 3 diarrhea or any signs of hepatotoxicity (fatigue, nausea, vomiting, right upper quadrant tenderness, fever, rash, eosinophilia)
• **Geriatric patients** >65 yr: monitor geriatric patients more closely for toxicities (vomiting, diarrhea, renal failure, dehydration) during treatment
• **Infection:** may occur after completion of adjuvant trastuzumab-based therapy; assess for urinary tract infection, cellulitis, and erysipelas
• Pregnancy/breastfeeding: avoid drug in females of reproductive potential; use contraception during treatment and for at least 1 mo after the last dose; can cause fetal harm or death; discontinue breastfeeding during treatment and for 1 mo after the final dose. Presence in breast milk unknown. Obtain a pregnancy test before starting treatment. Males with female partners of reproductive potential should avoid pregnancy, use effective contraception during treatment and ≥3 mo after last dose
• Risk for injury (adverse reactions)

Implementation:
• Use with food at the same time every day
• Swallow tablets whole; do not chew, crush, or split
• If a dose is missed, do not replace the missed dose. Resume with the next scheduled daily dose
• Antidiarrheal prophylaxis is recommended during the first two cycles (56 days) of treatment and should be initiated with the first dose of neratinib; loperamide should be taken as directed below, titrating to one to two bowel movements/day; additional antidiarrheal agents may be required to manage patients with loperamide-refractory diarrhea
• Weeks 1 to 2 (days 1 to 14): take loperamide 4 mg tid

⚠ Nurse Alert   ✴ Key NCLEX® Drug   >> Drug Specifics

• Weeks 3 to 8 (days 15 to 56): take loper-amide 4 mg bid
• Weeks 9 to 52 (days 57 to 365): take loper-amide 4 mg as needed (max 16 mg/day)

Patient /family education
• Teach patient that infection may occur; to report urinary pain, hesitancy; skin redness, pain, heat; fever, shaking, chills
• **Diarrhea:** Advise patient to report number of loose stools per day or change in stools to provider
• **Pregnancy/breastfeeding:** Teach patient not to use in pregnancy, breastfeeding; to use contraception during treatment and for at least 1 mo after last dose; men with a partner who may become pregnant should use contraception during treatment and for at least 3 mo after last dose

Evaluation:
• Positive therapeutic outcome: decrease in size of cancerous tumor

---

RARELY USED

netupitant/palonosetron
(ne-too′pi-tant pa-lone- o′se-tron)
Akynzeo
Func. class.: Antiemetic, neurokinin antagonist

USES: Nausea/vomiting associated with chemotherapy

CONTRAINDICATIONS: Hypersensitivity, severe hepatic/renal disease, breastfeeding, 5HT3 antagonists (cross-sensitivity)

DOSAGE AND ROUTES
Adult: PO 1 capsule, 1 hr prior to chemotherapy

RARELY USED

niacin (Rx, OTC)
(nye′a-sin)
Equaline Niacin, Niaspan, Ni-Odan ✦, Slo-Niacin
niacinamide (Rx, OTC)
(nye-a-sin′a-mide)
Func. class.: Vitamin B$_3$ lipid-lowering product
Chem. class.: Water-soluble vitamin

Therapeutic outcome: Decreasing cholesterol and LDL levels, B$_3$ supplementation

USES: Pellagra, hyperlipidemias (types IV, V), peripheral vascular disease that presents a risk for pancreatitis

CONTRAINDICATIONS
Breastfeeding, hypersensitivity, peptic ulcer, hepatic disease, hemorrhage, severe hypotension

DOSAGE AND ROUTES
Niacin deficiency
Adult: PO 100-500 mg/day in divided doses; IM/SUBCUT 50-100 mg 5 or more times a day; **IV** 25 100 mg bid or tid
Child: PO up to 300 mg/day in divided doses

Adjunct in hyperlipidemia
Adult: 250 mg after evening meal, may increase dosage at 1-4 wk intervals to 1-2 g tid, max 6 g/day; ext rel 500 mg at bedtime, ×4 wk, then 1000 mg at bedtime for wk 5-8, do not increase by more than 500 mg q4wk, max 2000 mg/day

Pellagra
Adult: PO 300-500 mg/day in divided doses, IM 50-100 mg 5 ×/day or IV 25-100 mg bid by slow IV INF
Child: PO 100-300 mg/day in divided doses; IV up to 300 mg/day by slow IV/INF

---

niCARdipine (Rx)
(nye-card′i-peen)
Cardene IV
Func. class.: Calcium channel blocker, antianginal, antihypertensive
Chem. class.: Dihydropyridine

Do not confuse: niCARdipine/NIFEdipine, **Cardene/**Cardizem

ACTION: Inhibits calcium ion influx across cell membrane during cardiac depolarization, produces relaxation of coronary vascular smooth muscle and peripheral vascular smooth muscle, dilates coronary arteries, increases myocardial oxygen delivery in patients with vasospastic angina

Therapeutic outcome: Decreased angina pectoris, decreased B/P in hypertension

USES: Chronic stable angina pectoris, hypertension

Pharmacokinetics

Absorption	Well absorbed (PO); bioavailability poor
Distribution	Unknown
Metabolism	Liver, extensively
Excretion	Kidneys 60%, feces 35%
Half-life	2-5 hr

N

Pharmacodynamics

	PO	PO SUS REL	IV
Onset	20 min	Unknown	1 min
Peak	1-2 hr		45 min
Duration	8 hr	10-12 hr	

CONTRAINDICATIONS

Sick sinus syndrome, 2nd- or 3rd-degree heart block, hypersensitivity to this product or dihydropyridine, advanced aortic stenosis

Precautions: Pregnancy, breastfeeding, children, geriatric, HF, hypotension, hepatic injury, renal disease

DOSAGE AND ROUTES
Hypertension
Adult: PO 20 mg tid initially; may increase after 3 days (range 20-40 mg tid) may increase to 60 mg bid **IV** 5 mg/hr; may increase by 2.5 mg/hr q15min; max 15 mg/hr

Angina
Adult: PO 20 mg tid, may be adjusted q3day, may use 20-40 mg tid

Renal dose
Adult: PO 20 mg tid or SUS REL 30 mg bid

Hepatic dose
Adult: PO 20 mg bid

Available forms: Caps 20, 30 mg; inj 2.5 mg/ml, premixed 20 mg/200 ml, 40 mg/200 ml

ADVERSE EFFECTS
CNS: *Headache, dizziness,* paresthesia
CV: Edema, hypotension, palpitations, chest pain, tachycardia, angina
GI: Nausea, vomiting, abdominal cramps, dry mouth
INTEG: Rash, infusion site discomfort, Stevens-Johnson syndrome
MISC: Myalgia (IV)

INTERACTIONS
Individual drugs
Alcohol: increased hypotension
CarBAMazepine, cycloSPORINE, prazosin, propranolol, quiNIDine: increased risk of toxicity
Cimetidine: increased niCARdipine effects
Digoxin, quiNIDine, theophylline: increased effects
Rifampin: decreased antihypertensive effect

Drug classifications
Antihypertensives, neuromuscular blocking agents, nitrates, protease inhibitors: increased hypotension
NSAIDs: decreased antihypertensive effect

Drug/herb
Ginkgo, ginseng, hawthorn: increased effect
Ephedra, melatonin, St. John's wort, yohimbe: decreased effect

Drug/food
Grapefruit juice, grapefruit: increased hypotensive effect
High-fat foods: Decreased absorption

Drug/lab test
Increased: LFTs
Decreased: potassium (IV), phosphate, platelets

NURSING CONSIDERATIONS
Assessment
• **Monitor for HF:** weight gain, crackles, peripheral edema, jugular venous distention, dyspnea
• Assess fluid volume status (I&O ratio) and record weight, color, quality, and specific gravity of urine, skin turgor, adequacy of pulses, moist mucous membranes, bilateral lung sounds, peripheral pitting edema; dehydration symptoms of decreasing output, thirst, hypotension, dry mouth, and mucous membranes should be reported
• **Allergic reactions (Stevens-Johnson syndrome):** If rash is severe with and accompanied by joint aches, mouth lesions, discontinue immediately
• **Hypertension:** assess for decreasing B/P; salt in diet, smoking, exercise, diet, weight, monitor B/P baseline and often
• **Assess anginal pain:** intensity, location, duration, alleviating factors
• Monitor potassium, renal/liver function tests, baseline and periodically if on long-term treatment

Patient problem
Impaired cardiac output (uses)
Pain (uses)
Risk for injury (adverse reactions)

Implementation
PO route
• Give without regard to meals
• To start PO give 1 hr before discontinuing IV nicardipine
• Avoid use with grapefruit, grapefruit juice
• Store in airtight container at room temperature

Continuous IV infusion route
• To convert/substitute PO to IV for adults, if PO 20 mg q8hr, start infusion at 0.5 mg/hr; if PO 30 mg q8hr, start infusion at 1.2 mg/hr; if PO 40 mg q8hr, start infusion at 2.2 mg/hr
• Dilute each 25 mg/240 ml of compatible sol (0.1 mg/ml), give slowly, titrate to patient's response, stable for 24 hr at room temperature, change IV site q12 hrs

Solution compatibilities: D₅W, D₅/0.45% NaCl, D₅/0.9% NaCl

Y-site compatibilities: Alemtuzumab, amikacin, aminophylline, aztreonam, bivalirudin, butorphanol, calcium gluconate, CARBOplatin, caspofungin, ceFAZolin, ceftizoxime, chloramphenicol, cimetidine, CISplatin, clindamycin, cytarabine, DAPTOmycin, dexmedetomidine, diltiazem, DOBUTamine, DOCEtaxel, DOPamine, DOXOrubicin hydrochloride, enalaprilat, EPINEPHrine, epirubicin, erythromycin, esmolol, famotidine, fenoldopam, fentaNYL, gentamicin, hydrocortisone, HYDROmorphone, labetalol, lidocaine, linezolid, LORazepam, magnesium sulfate, mechlorethamine, methylPREDNISolone, metroNIDAZOLE, midazolam, milrinone, morphine, nafcillin, nesiritide, nitroglycerin, nitroprusside, norepinephrine, octreotide, oxaliplatin, oxytocin, palonosetron, penicillin G potassium, potassium chloride/phosphate, quinupristin-dalfopristin, ranitidine, rocuronium, tacrolimus, tirofiban, tobramycin, trimethoprim/sulfamethoxazole, vancomycin, vasopressin, vecuronium, vinCRIStine, voriconazole, zoledronic acid

Patient/family education

• Advise patient to avoid hazardous activities until stabilized on product and dizziness is no longer a problem
• Instruct patient to limit caffeine consumption; to avoid alcohol and OTC products unless directed by a prescriber, to take without regard to food, avoid high-fat foods, to swallow sus rel product whole
• **Hypertension:** instruct patient to comply with all areas of medical regimen: diet, exercise, stress reduction, product therapy
• Instruct patient to notify prescriber of irregular heartbeat, shortness of breath, swelling of feet and hands, pronounced dizziness, constipation, nausea, hypotension, change in severity/pattern/incidence of angina
• Teach patient to use medication as directed even if feeling better; may be taken with other cardiovascular products (nitrates, β-blockers), to taper when discontinuing
• Advise patient to contact prescriber if anginal attacks continue or become worse
• Teach patient how to take pulse and when to contact health care professional
• Advise patient to avoid grapefruit/grapefruit juice
• Advise patient to rise from sitting or lying slowly to prevent orthostatic hypotension
• **Pregnancy/breastfeeding:** Identify if pregnancy is planned or suspected or if breastfeeding

Evaluation

Positive therapeutic outcome
• Decreased angina attacks
• Decreased B/P

TREATMENT OF OVERDOSE: Defibrillation, atropine for AV block, vasopressor for hypotension

---

nicotinamide
See niacin

---

nicotine
(nik'o-teen)
nicotine chewing gum
Nicorette, Thrive
nicotine inhaler (OTC, Rx)
Nicotrol Inhaler
nicotine lozenge (OTC)
Commit, Nicorette
nicotine nasal spray (Rx)
Nicotrol NS
nicotine transdermal (OTC, Rx)
Nicoderm CQ
Func. class.: Smoking deterrent
Chem. class.: Ganglionic cholinergic agonist

ACTION: Agonist at nicotinic receptors in the peripheral and central nervous systems; acts at sympathetic ganglia, on chemoreceptors of the aorta and carotid bodies; also affects adrenaline-releasing catecholamines

Therapeutic outcome: Decreased withdrawal effects when smoking cessation is attempted

USES: Deter cigarette smoking

Pharmacokinetics

Absorption	Slowly absorbed, buccal cavity
Distribution	Unknown
Metabolism	Liver; some by lungs, kidneys
Excretion	Kidneys, unchanged (20%); breast milk
Half-life	1-2 hr

Pharmacodynamics

Onset	Rapid
Peak	½ hr
Duration	Unknown

N

CONTRAINDICATIONS

Pregnancy (transdermal, inhaler), hypersensitivity, immediate post-MI recovery period, severe angina pectoris

Precautions: Pregnancy (gum), breastfeeding, vasospastic disease, dysrhythmias, diabetes mellitus, hyperthyroidism, pheochromocytoma, coronary disease, esophagitis, peptic ulcer, renal/hepatic disease; MRI (patch); soy hypersensitivity (mint lozenge)

DOSAGE AND ROUTES

Nicotine chewing gum

Adult: If patient smokes ≤25 cigarettes/day, start with 2 mg gum; if >25 cigarettes/day, start with 4 mg gum; then 1 piece of gum q1-2hr × 6 wk, then 1 piece of gum q2-4hr × 2 wk, then 1 piece of gum q4-8hr × 2 wk, then discontinue; max 24/day

Nicotine inhaler

Adult: Inhale 6 cartridges/day (24-64 mg) for up to 12 wk, then gradual reduction over 12 wk

Nicotine lozenge

Adult: If cigarette is desired >30 min after awakening, start with 1-2–mg lozenge; if <30 min after awakening, start with 4-mg lozenge; then 1 q1-2hr, max 20 lozenges/day or 5 lozenges/6 hr × 6 wk, then 1 lozenge q2-4hr × 2 wk, then 1 lozenge q4-8hr × 2 wk, then discontinue

Nicotine nasal spray

Adult: 1 spray in each nostril 1-2 ×/hr, max 5 ×/hr or 40 ×/day, max 3 mo

Nicotine transdermal/inhaler system

NicoDerm

Adult: 21 mg/day × 4-8 wk; 14 mg/day × 2-4 wk; 7 mg/day × 2-4 wk

Nicotrol

Adult: 15 mg/day × 12 wk; 10 mg/day × 2 wk; 5 mg/day × 2 wk

Nicotrol inhaler

Adult: Delivers 30% of what a smoker receives from an actual cigarette

Available forms: Gum: 2, 4 mg/piece; nicotine transdermal system (NicoDerm, Nicotine Transdermal System); 7, 14, 21 mg/day delivered; (NicoDerm) 5, 10, 15 mg/day; nicotine inhaler: 4 mg delivered; nasal spray: 0.5 mg of nicotine/actuation; lozenge: 2 mg, 4 mg

ADVERSE EFFECTS

CNS: Dizziness, vertigo, insomnia, headache, confusion, seizures, numbness, tinnitus, strange dreams

CV: Dysrhythmias, tachycardia, palpitations, edema, flushing, hypertension

EENT: Jaw ache, irritation in buccal cavity

GI: *Nausea, vomiting, anorexia, indigestion,* diarrhea, abdominal pain, constipation, eructation, irritation

RESP: Breathing difficulty, cough, hoarseness, sneezing, wheezing, bronchial spasm

INTERACTIONS

Individual drugs

Bromocriptine, cabergoline: increased vasoconstriction

Adenosine: increased effects

BuPROPion: increased B/P

Insulin: decreased effect

Cimetidine: decreased nicotine clearance

Drug classifications

Adrenergic antagonists, beta blockers: increased effect after smoking discontinuation

Ergots: increased vasoconstriction

Drug/food

Acidic foods (colas, coffee): avoid use of gum with and for 15 min after

NURSING CONSIDERATIONS

Assessment

• **Assess for adverse reaction to gum:** irritation of buccal cavity, dislike of taste, jaw ache; gum should not be used if temporomandibular condition exists

• **Assess for withdrawal symptoms:** headache, fatigue, drowsiness, restlessness, irritability, severe cravings for nicotine products before, during, and after treatment

• **Smoking:** obtain a nicotine assessment: brand of cigarettes, chewing tobacco, cigars, number of each used per day; what increases need or activities performed when each is used

• **Toxicity:** Assess for nausea, vomiting, diarrhea, headache, dizziness, dyspnea, hypotension

• **Assess for nicotine toxicity:** GI symptoms (nausea, vomiting, diarrhea), cardiopulmonary symptoms (decreased B/P, dyspnea, change in pulse), weakness, abdominal cramping, headache, blurred vision, tinnitus; product should be discontinued

• **Pregnancy/breastfeeding:** Whenever possible, avoid in pregnancy, cautious use in breastfeeding

Patient problem

Lack of knowledge of medication (teaching)

Implementation

• Give only prescribed amount, or toxicity may occur

• **Gum:** chew gum slowly for 30 min to promote buccal absorption of the product; do not chew > 45 min

• Begin product withdrawal after 3 mo of use; do not exceed 6 mo
• Do not expose to light, gum will turn color
• **Transdermal patch:** apply once a day to a nonhairy, clean, dry area of skin on upper body or upper outer arm; rotate sites to prevent skin irritation, can remove before bed if patient has strange dreams
• **Nasal spray/Inhaler:** puffing on mouthpiece delivers nicotine through the mouth
• **Lozenge:** Allow to dissolve slowly

Patient/family education

• **Toxicity:** Teach patient signs of toxicity: nausea, vomiting, diarrhea, headache, dizziness, dyspnea, hypotension
• Advise patient to begin product withdrawal after 3 mo use; max 6 mo
• Teach patient all aspects of product; give package insert to patient and explain; caution patient not to exceed prescribed dose
• Caution patient not to use during pregnancy; birth defects may occur
• Discontinue if patient is unable to stop smoking after fourth week of therapy

Gum

• Advise patient to chew gum slowly for 30 min to promote buccal absorption of the product; do not chew over 45 min
• Inform patient that gum will not stick to dentures, dental appliances
• Caution patient that gum is as toxic as cigarettes; it is to be used only to deter smoking

Transdermal patch

• Caution patient that patch is as toxic as cigarettes; to be used only to deter smoking
• Caution patient not to use during pregnancy; birth defects may occur
• Instruct patient to keep used and unused system out of reach of children and pets
• Instruct patient to apply once a day to a nonhairy, clean, dry area of skin on upper body or upper outer arm; to rotate sites to prevent skin irritation
• Instruct patient to stop smoking immediately when beginning patch treatment
• Teach patient to apply promptly after removing from protective pouch; system may lose strength
• **Nasal spray:** tilt head back, do not swallow, do not chew or inhale during administration; after smoking is stopped, use spray up to 8 wk, then discontinue over 6 wk by tapering
• **Lozenges:** allow to dissolve, avoid swallowing
• **Inhalation:** use the inhaler for 20 min by frequent puffs
• Advise patient that puffing on mouthpiece delivers nicotine through the mouth lining

• **Pregnancy/breastfeeding:** Identify if pregnancy is planned or suspected or if breastfeeding

Evaluation

Positive therapeutic outcome
• Decrease in urge to smoke
• Decreased need for gum after 3-6 mo

NIFEdipine (Rx)

(nye-fed'i-peen)
Adalat CC, Adalat XL ❖, Afeditab CR, Procardia, Procardia XL
Func. class.: Calcium channel blocker, antianginal, antihypertensive
Chem. class.: Dihydropyridine

Do not confuse: NIFEdipine/niCARdipine/ niMODipine **Procardia XL**/Protain XL

ACTION: Inhibits calcium ion influx across cell membrane during cardiac depolarization, produces relaxation of coronary vascular smooth muscle, dilates coronary vascular arteries, increases myocardial oxygen delivery in patients with vasospastic angina, dilates peripheral arteries

Therapeutic outcome: Decreased angina pectoris, decreased B/P in hypertension

USES: Chronic stable angina pectoris, variant angina, hypertension, migraine prophylaxis

Unlabeled uses: Prevention of migraines, cardiopathy, heart failure

Pharmacokinetics

Absorption	Well absorbed (PO)
Distribution	Protein binding 92%
Metabolism	Liver, extensively
Excretion	Unknown
Half-life	2-5 hr

Pharmacodynamics

	PO	PO EXT REL
Onset	20 min	Unknown
Peak	30 min-1 hr	6 hr
Duration	6-8 hr	24 hr

CONTRAINDICATIONS
Hypersensitivity to this product or dihydropyridine, cardiogenic shock

Precautions: Pregnancy, breastfeeding, children, hypotension, sick sinus syndrome, 2nd- or 3rd-degree heart block, hypotension less than 90 mm Hg systolic, hepatic injury, renal disease, acute MI, aortic stenosis, GERD, heart failure

---

DOSAGE AND ROUTES
Adult: PO immediate release, 10 mg tid; increase in 10-mg increments q7-14day, max 180 mg/24 hr or single dose of 30 mg; sus rel 30-60 mg/day; may increase q7-14day; doses >120 mg not recommended

Hypertension
Adult: PO ext rel 30-60 mg qd, titrate upward as needed; max 90 mg/day (Adalat CC); 120 mg/day (Procardia XL)
Adolescent/child (unlabeled): PO ext rel 0.25-0.5 mg/kg/day, max 3 mg/kg/day

Available forms: Caps 10, 20 mg; ext rel tabs (CC, XL) 30, 60, 90 mg

ADVERSE EFFECTS
CNS: *Headache,* fatigue, drowsiness, *dizziness,* anxiety, depression, weakness, insomnia, *light-headedness,* paresthesia, tinnitus, blurred vision, nervousness, tremor, flushing
CV: Dysrhythmias, edema, hypotension, palpitations, tachycardia
GI: *Nausea,* vomiting, diarrhea, gastric upset, constipation, increased LFTs, dry mouth, flatulence, gingival hyperplasia
GU: Nocturia, polyuria
HEMA: Bruising, bleeding, petechiae
INTEG: Rash, pruritus, *flushing,* hair loss, Stevens-Johnson syndrome, toxic epidermal necrolysis, exfoliative dermatitis
MISC: Sexual difficulties, cough, fever, chills

INTERACTIONS
Individual drugs
Cimetidine, ranitidine: increased risk of toxicity
CarBAMazepine, cycloSPORINE, phenytoin, prazosin, digoxin: increased levels of each product
QuiNIDine: decreased effects
Smoking: decreased NIFEdipine level

Drug classifications
Strong CYP3A4 inducers: use is contraindicated
Antihypertensives, β-adrenergic blockers: increased effects
NSAIDs: decreased antihypertensive effect

Drug/herb
Ginkgo biloba, ginseng, hawthorn: increased effect
Ephedra, melatonin, St. John's wort, yohimbe: decreased effect

Drug/food
Grapefruit juice: increased NIFEdipine level

Drug/lab test
Positive: ANA titer, direct Coombs' test
Increased: CPK, LDH, AST

NURSING CONSIDERATIONS
Assessment
• **Assess anginal pain:** location, intensity, duration, character, alleviating, aggravating factors
• **HF:** Peripheral edema, dyspnea, weight gain >5 lb, jugular venous distention, rales; monitor I&O ratios, daily weight
• Assess for bruising, petechiae, bleeding
• Monitor potassium, renal/liver function tests periodically during treatment; in those taking antihypertensives, beta blockers, monitor B/P often
• **Serious skin disorders:** rash starts suddenly, assess for fever, cutaneous lesions, may have pustules; discontinue product if rash present or if rash is severe, fatigue
• Assess fluid volume status (I&O ratio) and record weight, distended red veins, crackles in lung, color, quality, and specific gravity of urine, skin turgor, adequacy of pulses, moist mucous membranes, bilateral lung sounds, peripheral pitting edema; dehydration symptoms of decreasing output, thirst, hypotension, dry mouth, and mucous membranes should be reported
• Monitor cardiac status: B/P, pulse, respirations, ECG
• **GI obstruction:** ext rel products have been associated with rare reports of obstruction in those with strictures, and no known GI disease
• **Beers:** Avoid in older adults, potential for hypotension, myocardial ischemia

Patient problem
Impaired cardiac output (uses)
Pain (Uses)
Risk for injury (adverse reactions)

Implementation
PO route
• Do not use immediate release caps within 7 days of MI, coronary syndrome; do not use SL caps to reduce severe hypertension, may cause death
• Give without regard to meals
• Store in airtight container at room temperature
• Protect caps from direct light, keep in dry area, do not freeze
• **Sublingual route**
• Using a sterile needle, puncture the cap and squeeze medication in buccal/sublingual area (not an FDA-approved use), do not use in severe hypertension, may be fatal

Patient/family education
• Advise patient to avoid hazardous activities until stabilized on product and dizziness is no longer a problem

---

- Instruct patient to limit caffeine consumption; to avoid alcohol and OTC products unless directed by prescriber
- Advise patient that empty tab shells may appear in stools and are not significant
- Give without regard to meals (exception: Adelat CC should be taken on empty stomach)
- **Hypertension:** instruct patient to comply in all areas of medical regimen: diet, exercise, stress reduction, product therapy
- Tell patient to notify prescriber of irregular heartbeat, SOB, swelling of feet and hands, pronounced dizziness, constipation, nausea, hypotension, severe rash, changes in pattern/frequency/severity of angina
- Teach patient to use as directed even if feeling better; may be taken with other cardiovascular products (nitrates, β-blockers)
- Advise patient to increase fluid intake to prevent constipation
- Teach patient to check for gingival hyperplasia and report promptly
- Teach patient not to discontinue abruptly; gradually taper
- **Pregnancy/breastfeeding:** Identify if pregnancy is planned or suspected or if breastfeeding

Evaluation
Positive therapeutic outcome
- Decreased angina attacks
- Decreased B/P

TREATMENT OF OVERDOSE:
Defibrillation, atropine for AV block, vasopressor for hypotension

⚠ HIGH ALERT

nilotinib (Rx)
(nye-loe′ti-nib)
Tasigna
Func. class.: Antineoplastic—miscellaneous
Chem. class.: Protein-tyrosine kinase inhibitor

ACTION: Inhibits BCR-ABL tyrosine kinase created in chronic myeloid leukemia (CML)

Therapeutic outcome: Decrease in progression of disease

USES: Chronic phase/accelerated phase Philadelphia chromosome–positive chronic myelogenous leukemia that is resistant/intolerant to imatinib

Absorption	Unknown
Distribution	Protein binding 98%, plasma levels 3 hr
Metabolism	By CYP3A4
Excretion	Unknown
Half-life	Elimination 17 hr

Pharmacodynamics

Onset	Unknown
Peak	3 hr
Duration	Up to 12 hr

CONTRAINDICATIONS
Pregnancy, breastfeeding, hypersensitivity

BLACK BOX WARNING: Hypokalemia, hypomagnesemia, QT prolongation

Precautions: Children, women, geriatric patients, active infections, anemia, cardiac disease, bone marrow suppression, cholestasis, diabetes, gelatin hypersensitivity, infertility, galactose-free diet, lactase deficiency, neutropenia, pancreatitis, thrombocytopenia alcoholism, angina, ascites, tumor lysis syndrome, hepatic disease

DOSAGE AND ROUTES
Philadelphia chromosome–positive chronic myelogenous leukemia, accelerated phase, resistant/intolerant to prior therapy
Adult: PO 400 mg q12h; continue until disease progression or unacceptable toxicity

Philadelphia chromosome–positive chronic myelogenous leukemia, chronic phase, newly diagnosed
Adult: PO 300 mg q12hr, continue until disease progression or unacceptable toxicity

Escalation regimen for those taking a strong CYP3A4 inducer
Adult: PO increase dose as required

Adjustment following discontinuation of a strong CYP3A4 inducer
Adult: PO reduce to 400 mg/bid

Use with a strong CYP3A4 inhibitor
Adult: PO reduce dose to 400 mg/day

QT prolongation
QTcF >480 msec: Withhold dose

Myelosuppression
ANC 1 × 10⁹/L or platelets <50 × 10⁹/L: Withhold dose

Hepatic Dose
Adult: PO (Child-Pugh classes A-C): newly diagnosed CML 200 mg bid, then escalation to 300 mg bid initially

Available forms: Caps 150, 200 mg

ADVERSE EFFECTS
CNS: Headache, dizziness, fatigue, fever, flushing, paresthesia

CV: QT prolongation, palpitations, torsades de pointes, AV block

GI: *Nausea*, hepatotoxicity, vomiting, dyspepsia, *anorexia*, *abdominal pain*, constipation, pancreatitis, diarrhea, xerostomia

HEMA: Neutropenia, thrombocytopenia, anemia, pancytopenia

INTEG: *Rash*, alopecia, erythema

META: Hyperamylasemia, hyperbilirubinemia, hyperglycemia, hyperkalemia, hypocalcemia, hyponatremia, hypomagnesemia

MISC: Diaphoresis, anxiety

MS: Arthralgia, myalgia, back/bone pain, muscle cramps

RESP: Cough, dyspnea

SYST: Bleeding, tumor lysis syndrome

INTERACTIONS
Individual drugs
• Product interactions are numerous

Acetaminophen: increased hepatotoxicity

CarBAMazepine, dexamethasone, PHENobarbital, phenytoin, rifampin: decreased concentrations

Clarithromycin, erythromycin, itraconazole, ketoconazole: increased concentrations

Haloperidol, chloroquine, droperidol, pentamidine, arsenic trioxide, levomethadyl: increased QT prolongation

Pimozide, ziprasidone: do not use concurrently

Simvastatin: increased plasma concentrations

Warfarin: increased plasma concentration; avoid use with warfarin, use low-molecular-weight anticoagulants instead

Drug classifications
Class IA/III antidysrhythmics, some phenothiazines, β-agonists, local anesthetics, tricyclics, CYP3A4 inhibitors (amiodarone, clarithromycin, erythromycin, telithromycin, troleandomycin), CYP3A4 substrates (methadone, pimozide, QUEtiapine, quiNIDine, risperiDONE, ziprasidone): increased QT prolongation

Calcium channel blockers: increased plasma concentrations

Phenothiazines: do not use concurrently

Drug/herb
St. John's wort: decreased concentration

Drug/food
Grapefruit juice: increased plasma concentrations

NURSING CONSIDERATIONS
Assessment
• Assess ANC and platelets; if ANC $<1 \times 10^9$/L and/or platelets $<50 \times 10^9$/L, stop until ANC $>1.5 \times 10^9$/L and platelets $>75 \times 10^9$/L

• **Monitor CV status:** hypertension, QT prolongation can occur; monitor left ventricular ejection fraction (LVEF) baseline periodically

• **Assess for renal toxicity:** if bilirubin $>3 \times$ IULN, withhold until bilirubin levels return to $<1.5 \times$ IULN

• **Assess for hepatotoxicity:** monitor hepatic function tests, before treatment and qmo; if liver transaminases $>5 \times$ IULN, withhold until transaminase levels return to $<2.5 \times$ IULN

• **Myelosuppression:** Monitor CBC $\times 2$ mo and then monthly; differential, platelet count weekly; withhold product if WBC is <3500/mm³ or platelet count $<100,000$/mm³; notify prescriber of these results; product should be discontinued

• Monitor for bleeding: epistaxis, rectal, gingival, upper GI, genital, and wound bleeding; tumor-related hemorrhage may occur rapidly

• **Tumor lysis syndrome:** maintain hydration, correct uric acid prior to use of this product

• **Monitor electrolytes:** calcium, potassium, magnesium, sodium; lipase, phosphate; hypokalemia, hypomagnesemia should be corrected prior to use

• AST/ALT/bilirubin/lipase/amylase if increased to grade 3, withhold product; resume at 400 mg qd when levels return to grade 1 or below

• **QT prolongation:** ECG for QT prolongation, ejection fraction; assess for chest pain, palpitations, dyspnea

Patient problem
Risk of infection (uses)
Lack of knowledge of medication (teaching)

Implementation
• Do not break, crush, or chew caps; if a whole capsule cannot be swallowed, disperse capsule contents in 1 tsp of applesauce

• Give on empty stomach; separate doses by 12 hr; a make-up dose should not be taken if a dose is missed

• Store at 15°-30° C (59°-86° F)

Patient/family education
• **Infection:** Teach patient to report immediately cough, fever, chills

• Instruct patient to report bleeding, bleeding gums, blood in stools, urine, emesis

- Instruct patient to report adverse reactions immediately: SOB, bleeding
- Inform patient reason for treatment, expected result
- Advise patient that many adverse reactions may occur
- Teach patient to avoid persons with known upper respiratory infections; immunosuppression is common
- Instruct in signs/symptoms of low potassium or magnesium
- Teach patient to notify prescriber of all OTC, Rx, herbal products used; not to receive vaccinations without prescriber's approval
- **Pregnancy:** Identify if pregnancy is planned or suspected or if breastfeeding; Use contraception during treatment, do not breastfeed

Evaluation
Positive therapeutic outcome
- Decrease in progression of disease

niMODipine (Rx)
(ni-moe′dip-een)
Nimotop ✣, **Nymalize**
Func. class.: Calcium channel blocker
Chem. class.: Dihydropyridine

ACTION: Unknown, may have greater effect on cerebral arteries

Therapeutic outcome: Prevention of vascular spasm (subarachnoid hemorrhage)

USES: Prevention of cerebrovascular spasm in subarachnoid hemorrhage

Pharmacokinetics

Absorption	Well absorbed, poor bio-availability
Distribution	Crosses blood-brain barrier
Metabolism	Liver, extensively
Excretion	Kidneys
Half-life	1-2 hr

Pharmacodynamics

Onset	Unknown
Peak	1 hr
Duration	Unknown

CONTRAINDICATIONS
Sick sinus syndrome, 2nd- or 3rd-degree heart block, hypotension less than 90 mm Hg systolic, hypersensitivity

Precautions: Pregnancy, breastfeeding, children, geriatric, HF, hypotension, hepatic injury, renal disease

DOSAGE AND ROUTES
Adult: PO begin therapy within 96 hr, 60 mg q4hr × 21 days

Available forms: Caps 30 mg

ADVERSE EFFECTS
CNS: Headache, fatigue, drowsiness, dizziness, anxiety, depression, weakness, insomnia, confusion, paresthesia, somnolence
CV: Dysrhythmia, edema, HF, bradycardia, hypotension, palpitations, MI, pulmonary edema
GI: Nausea, vomiting, diarrhea, gastric upset, constipation, hepatitis, abdominal cramps
GU: Nocturia, polyuria, acute renal failure
INTEG: Rash, pruritus, urticaria, photosensitivity, hair loss
MISC: Blurred vision, flushing, nasal congestion, sweating, shortness of breath, gynecomastia, hyperglycemia, sexual difficulties

INTERACTIONS
Individual drugs
Alcohol: increased hypotension
Digoxin: increased digoxin levels, bradycardia
PHENobarbital, phenytoin: decreased effectiveness
Propranolol: increased toxicity

Drug classifications
Antihypertensives: increased hypotension
β-Adrenergic blockers: increased bradycardia
Nitrates: increased nitrates

Drug/herb
Barberry, betel palm, burdock, goldenseal, khat, khella, lily of the valley, plantain: increased effect
Yohimbe: decreased effect

NURSING CONSIDERATIONS
Assessment
- Assess fluid volume status (I&O ratio) and record weight; distended red veins; crackles in lung; color, quality, and specific gravity of urine; skin turgor; adequacy of pulses; moist mucous membranes; bilateral lung sounds; peripheral pitting edema; dehydration symptoms of decreasing output, thirst, hypotension, dry mouth and mucous membranes should be reported
- Monitor B/P and pulse; if B/P drops 30 mm Hg, call prescriber
- Monitor ALT, AST, bilirubin daily; if these are elevated, hepatotoxicity is suspected

Patient problem
Ineffective tissue perfusion (uses)
Risk of injury (adverse reactions)

N

✣ Canada only   ✗✪✪ Genetic Warning   Adverse effects: *italics* = common; red = life-threatening

Implementation
- May puncture cap and dilute in water and give through nasogastric tube; flush tube with 0.9% NaCl
- Store in airtight container at room temperature

Patient/family education
- Advise patient to avoid hazardous activities until stabilized on product and dizziness is no longer a problem
- Instruct patient to limit caffeine consumption; to avoid alcohol and OTC products unless directed by prescriber
- Advise patient that empty tab shells may appear in stools and are not significant
- Give without regard to meals (exception: Adelat CC should be taken on empty stomach)
- **Hypertension:** instruct patient to comply in all areas of medical regimen: diet, exercise, stress reduction, product therapy
- Tell patient to notify prescriber of irregular heartbeat, SOB, swelling of feet and hands, pronounced dizziness, constipation, nausea, hypotension, severe rash, changes in pattern/frequency/severity of angina
- Teach patient to use as directed even if feeling better; may be taken with other cardiovascular products (nitrates, β-blockers)
- Advise patient to increase fluid intake to prevent constipation
- Teach patient to check for gingival hyperplasia and report promptly
- Teach patient not to discontinue abruptly; gradually taper
- **Pregnancy/breastfeeding:** Identify if pregnancy is planned or suspected or if breastfeeding

Evaluation
Positive therapeutic outcome
- Prevention of neurologic damage from subarachnoid hemorrhage

---

⚠ HIGH ALERT
RARELY USED

niraparib
(nye-rap′-a-rib)
Zejula
Func. class.: Antineoplastic

USES: For the treatment of recurrent epithelial ovarian, fallopian tube, or primary peritoneal cancer

DOSAGE AND ROUTES
Adult: **PO** 300 mg qday until disease progression or unacceptable toxicity. Begin therapy no later than 8 wk after the last platinum-containing regimen

---

nitrofurantoin (Rx)
(nye-troe-fyoor′an-toyn)
Furadantin, Macrobid, Macrodantin, Novo-Furantoin ✦
Func. class.: Urinary tract antiinfective
Chem. class.: Synthetic nitrofuran derivative

ACTION: Inhibits bacterial acetyl-CoA from interfering with carbohydrate metabolism

Therapeutic outcome: Resolution of infection

USES: Urinary tract infections caused by *Escherichia coli, Klebsiella, Pseudomonas, Proteus vulgaris, Proteus morganii, Serratia, Citrobacter, Staphylococcus aureus, Staphylococcus epidermidis, Enterococcus, Salmonella, Shigella*

Pharmacokinetics
Absorption	Readily absorbed
Distribution	Crosses placenta, excreted in breast milk
Metabolism	Liver, partially
Excretion	Kidneys, 30%-50% unchanged
Half-life	20-60 min

Pharmacodynamics
Onset	Unknown
Peak	30 min
Duration	6-12 hr

CONTRAINDICATIONS
Infants <1 mo, hypersensitivity, anuria, severe renal disease, CCr <60 ml/min, at term pregnancy (38-42 wk), labor, delivery, cholestatic jaundice due to nitrofurantoin therapy

Precautions: Pregnancy, breastfeeding, geriatric, ✡ G6PD deficiency, GI disease, diabetes

DOSAGE AND ROUTES
Active infections
Adult: PO 50-100 mg qid after meals or 50-100 mg at bedtime for long-term treatment
Child: PO 5-7 mg/kg/day in 4 divided doses; 1-2 mg/kg/day for long-term treatment; max 7 mg/kg/day

Chronic suppression
Adult: PO 50-100 mg qPM
Child: PO 2 mg/kg/day qPM or 0.5-1 mg/kg q12hr if dose is not well tolerated

Available forms: Caps 25, 50, 100 mg; susp 25 mg/ml; macrocrystal caps (Macrodantin) 25, 50, 100 mg; cap (Macrobid) 100 mg (25 macrocrystals, 75 monohydrate)

ADVERSE EFFECTS

CNS: *Dizziness, headache,* drowsiness, peripheral neuropathy, chills, confusion, vertigo
CV: Bundle branch block, chest pain
GI: *Nausea, vomiting, abdominal pain, diarrhea,* cholestatic jaundice, loss of appetite, *Clostridium difficile*–associated diarrhea, hepatitis, pancreatitis
HEMA: Anemia, agranulocytosis, hemolytic anemia, leukopenia, thrombocytopenia
INTEG: Pruritus, rash, urticaria, angioedema, alopecia, tooth staining, exfoliative dermatitis
MS: Arthralgia, myalgia, numbness, peripheral neuropathy
RESP: Cough, dyspnea, pneumonitis, pulmonary fibrosis/infiltrate
SYST: Stevens-Johnson syndrome, superinfection, SLE-like syndrome

INTERACTIONS
Individual products
Magnesium trisilicate: decreased absorption
Norfloxacin: antagonist effect
Probenecid: increased nitrofurantoin levels

Drug/lab test
Increased: BUN, alkaline phosphatase, bilirubin, creatinine, blood glucose

NURSING CONSIDERATIONS
Assessment
• **Urinary tract infection:** assess for burning, pain on urination, fever; cloudy, foul-smelling urine; I&O ratio; C&S before treatment, after completion; serum creatinine, BUN
• Monitor blood count during chronic therapy
• Assess CNS symptoms: insomnia, vertigo, headache, drowsiness, seizures
• Assess allergy: fever, flushing, rash, urticaria, pruritus
• **Hepatotoxicity:** assess for yellowing of skin, eyes, dark urine, clay-colored stools; monitor AST, ALT
• **Pulmonary fibrosis, pneumonitis:** assess for dyspnea, tachypnea, persistent cough
• **Serious skin disorders:** assess for fever, flushing, rash, urticaria, pruritus

• **Peripheral neuropathy:** assess for paresthesias (more common in diabetes mellitus, electrolyte imbalances, vit B deficiency, debilitated patients)
• **CDAD:** assess for diarrhea, abdominal pain, fever, fatigue, anorexia; possible anemia, elevated WBC and low serum albumin; stop product and usually give either vancomycin or IV metroNIDAZOLE
• **Beers:** Avoid in older adults, potential for pulmonary, hepatic toxicity, peripheral neuropathy

Patient problem
Infection (uses)
Diarrhea (adverse reactions)

Implementation
• Give with meals
• Do not break, crush, chew, or open tabs, caps; store in original container
• Give after clean-catch urine for C&S
• Give two daily doses if urine output is high or if patient has diabetes

Patient/family education
• Teach patient to take with food or milk; avoid alcohol
• Teach patient to protect susp from freezing and shake well before taking
• Teach patient that product may cause drowsiness; instruct client to seek aid in walking and other activities; advise patient not to drive or operate machinery while on medication
• Teach patient that diabetics should monitor blood glucose level
• Teach patient that product may turn urine rust-yellow to brown
• **Teach patient to notify prescriber of symptoms of CDAD:** fever, diarrhea with mucous, pus, or blood; report immediately
• **Pregnancy/breastfeeding:** Identify if pregnancy is planned or suspected or if breastfeeding

Evaluation
Positive therapeutic outcome
• Decreased dysuria, fever; negative C&S

⚠ HIGH ALERT

nitroglycerin (Rx)
(nye-troe-gli′ser-in)
Intravenous (Rx)
Nitrojet ✳, Nitronel
extended release caps (Rx)
Nitrogard SR ✳, Nitro-Time
translingual spray (Rx)
Nitrolingual, Nitromist, Rho-Nitro ✳
sublingual (Rx)
Nitrostat
nitroglycerin sublingual powder
GoNitro
rectal ointment
Rectiv
topical ointment (Rx)
Nitro-Bid, Nitrol ✳, Rho-Nitro ✳
transdermal (Rx)
Minitran, Nitro-Dur Trinipatch ✳
Func. class.: Coronary vasodilator, antianginal
Chem. class.: Nitrate

ACTION: Decreases preload and afterload, which thus decreases left ventricular end-diastolic pressure and systemic vascular resistance; dilates coronary arteries and improves blood flow through coronary vasculature, dilates arterial, venous beds systemically

Therapeutic outcome: Prevention of anginal attack

USES: Chronic stable angina pectoris, prophylaxis of angina pain, HF associated with acute MI, controlled hypotension in surgical procedures, anal fissures

Pharmacokinetics

Absorption	Well absorbed (PO, buccal, SL)
Distribution	Unknown
Metabolism	Liver, extensively
Excretion	Kidney
Half-life	1-4 min

CONTRAINDICATIONS
Hypersensitivity to this product or nitrites, severe anemia, increased ICP, cerebral hemorrhage, closed-angle glaucoma, cardiac tamponade, cardiomyopathy, constrictive pericarditis

Precautions: Pregnancy, breastfeeding, children, postural hypotension, severe renal/hepatic disease, acute MI, abrupt discontinuation, hyperthyroidism

DOSAGE AND ROUTES
Adult: **SL** dissolve tab under tongue when pain begins; may repeat q5min until relief occurs; take no more than 3 tab/15 min; use 1 tab prophylactically 5-10 min before activities; **SUS REL** cap q6-12hr on empty stomach; **TOP** 1-2 inches q8hr; increase to 4 in q4hr as needed; **IV** 5 mcg/min, then increase by 5 mcg/min q3-5min; if no response after 20 mcg/min, increase by 10-20 mcg/min until desired response; **transdermal** apply a patch daily to a site free from hair; remove patch at bedtime to provide 10-12 hr nitrate-free interval to avoid tolerance
Child: **IV** initial 0.25-0.5 mcg/kg/min, titrate to patient response, usual dose 1-3 mcg/kg/min transmucosal

Anal fissures (Rectiv)
Adult: rectal apply 1 in of 0.4% ointment q12hr × 3 wk

Available forms: Translingual aerosol 0.4 mg/m spray; sus rel tabs 2.5, 6.5, 9 mg; SL tabs 0.3, 0.4, 0.6 mg; SL powder; topical oint 2%; trans syst 0.1, 0.2, 0.3, 0.4, 0.6, 0.8 mg/hr; inj 25 mg/250 ml, 50 mg/250 ml, 100 mg/250 ml, 50 mg/500 ml, 100 mg/500 ml, 200 mg/500 ml; rectal ointment 0.4% (Rectiv)

ADVERSE EFFECTS
CNS: *Headache, flushing, dizziness*
CV: *Postural hypotension,* tachycardia, collapse, syncope, palpitations
GI: Nausea, vomiting
INTEG: Pallor, sweating, rash

INTERACTIONS
Individual drugs
Alcohol: increased hypotension, CV collapse
Aspirin: increased nitrate level

Pharmacodynamics

	SUS REL	SL	TD	IV	TRANS-MUCOSAL	AEROSOL	TOPICAL OINT
Onset	20-45 min	1-3 min	½-1 hr	1-2 min	1-2 min	2 min	½-1 hr
Peak	Unknown	Unknown	Unknown	Unknown	Unknown	Unknown	Unknown
Duration	3-8 hr	½ hr	12-24 hr	3-5 min	3-5 hr	½-1 hr	2-12 hr

Heparin: decreased effects (with IV nitroglycerin)

Avanafil, sildenafil, tadalafil, vardenafil: increased fatal hypotension, do not use together

Drug classifications

Antihypertensives, β-adrenergic blockers, calcium channel blockers, diuretics: increased hypotension

Drug/lab test

Increased: urine catecholamine, urine VMA
False increase: cholesterol

NURSING CONSIDERATIONS

Assessment

• Monitor orthostatic B/P, pulse
• **Assess pain:** duration, time started, activity being performed, character; check for tolerance if taken over long period
• Monitor for headache, light-headedness, decreased B/P; may indicate a need for decreased dosage

Patient problem

Pain (uses)
Ineffective tissue perfusion (uses)
Risk of injury (uses, adverse reactions)

Implementation

PO route

• Swallow sus rel tabs whole; do not break, crush, or chew sus rel tabs
• Give 1 hr before or 2 hr after meals with 8 oz of water

SL route

• Should be dissolved under tongue or placed between gum and cheek, not swallowed
• Keep tab in original container
• If 3 SL tab in 15 min do not relieve pain, consider diagnosis of MI

Aerosol route

• Sprayed under tongue (nitrolingual); not inhaled, prime before 1st-time use or if product has not been used in > 6 wk; press valve head with forefinger

Transmucosal route

• Tab should be placed between cheek and gum line
• Do not take anything PO when tab is in place

Topical ointment route

• Apply ointment using dose-measuring papers supplied; apply to an area without hair; ointment should cover 2-3–inch area; may apply an occlusive dressing as directed

Transdermal route

• Apply transdermal patches to area without hair; press hard to adhere; if patch becomes dislodged, apply a new one

• SL tab should be held under tongue or between gum and cheek until dissolved (a few min); do not take anything by mouth when SL tab is in place

Rectal route

• Cover finger with plastic wrap, disposable glove, or finger cot, lay finger alongside 1 inch dosing line on carton, squeeze tube until equal to 1 inch dosing line, insert covered finger no further than 1st finger joint gently into anal canal and on sides, wash hands thoroughly, if too painful, apply directly to outside of anus

Continuous IV infusion route

• Diluted in D_5, D_5W, 0.9% NaCl for inf to 200-400 mcg/ml depending on patient's fluid status, common dilution is 50 mg/250 ml, use controlled inf device; use glass inf bottles, non–polyvinyl chloride inf tubing; titrate to patient response; do not use filters

Y-site compatibilities: Acyclovir, alfentanil, amikacin, aminocaproic acid, aminophylline, amiodarone, amphotericin B lipid complex, amphotericin B liposome, anidulafungin, argatroban, ascorbic acid, atenolol, atracurium, atropine, azaTHIOprine, aztreonam, benztropine, bivalirudin, bleomycin, bumetanide, buprenorphine, butorphanol, calcium chloride/gluconate, CARBOplatin, caspofungin, cefamandole, ceFAZolin, cefmetazole, cefonicid, cefoperazone, cefotaxime, cefoTEtan, cefOXitin, cefTAZidime, ceftizoxime, cefTRIAXone, cefuroxime, cephalothin, cephapirin, chloramphenicol, chlorproMAZINE, cimetidine, cisatracurium, CISplatin, clindamycin, cloNIDine, cyanocobalamin, cyclophosphamide, cycloSPORINE, cytarabine, DACTINomycin, dexamethasone, digoxin, diltiazem, diphenhydrAMINE, DOBUTamine, DOCEtaxel, DOPamine, doxacurium, DOXOrubicin, doxycycline, drotrecogin alfa, enalaprilat, ePHEDrine, EPINEPHrine, epirubicin, epoetin alfa, eptifibatide, ertapenem, erythromycin, esmolol, etoposide, famotidine, fenoldopam, fentaNYL, fluconazole, fludarabine, fluorouracil, folic acid, ganciclovir, gatifloxacin, gemcitabine, gemtuzumab, gentamicin, glycopyrrolate, granisetron, heparin, hydrocortisone, HYDROmorphone, hydrOXYzine, IDArubicin, ifosfamide, imipenemcilastatin, indomethacin, insulin (regular), irinotecan, isoproterenol, ketorolac, labetalol, lidocaine, linezolid, LORazepam, magnesium sulfate, mannitol, mechlorethamine, meperidine, metaraminol, methicillin, methotrexate, methoxamine, methyldopa, methylPREDNISolone, metoclopramide, metroNIDAZOLE, mezlocillin, micafungin, miconazole, midazolam, milrinone, minocycline, mitoXANtrone, morphine, moxalactam, mycophenolate, nafcillin, nalbuphine, naloxone, nesiritide, netilmicin, niCARdipine, nitroprusside, norepinephrine, octreotide, ondansetron, oxacillin, oxaliplatin, oxytocin, PACLitaxel, palonosetron, pamidronate, pancuronium, pantoprazole, papaverine, PEMEtrexed, penicillin G potassium/sodium, pentamidine, pentazocine, PENTobarbital, PHENobarbital, phentolamine, phenylephrine, phytonadione, piperacillin, piperacillin-tazobactam, polymyxin B, potassium chloride, procainamide, prochlorperazine, promethazine, propofol, propranolol, protamine, pyridoxine, quiNIDine, quinupristin-dalfopristin, ranitidine, remifentanil, ritodrine, rocuronium, sodium bicarbonate, succinylcholine, SUFentanil, tacrolimus, teniposide, theophylline, thiamine, thiopental, thiotepa, ticarcillin, ticarcillin-clavulanate, tigecycline, tirofiban, tobramycin, tolazoline, trimetaphan, urokinase, vancomycin, vasopressin, vecuronium, verapamil, vinCRIStine, vinorelbine, voriconazole, warfarin, zoledronic acid

Patient/family education
- Instruct patient to avoid alcohol
- Advise patient that product may cause headache; tolerance usually develops; use nonopioid analgesic
- Teach patient that product may be taken before stressful activity, exercise, sexual activity
- Inform patient that SL tab may sting when product comes in contact with mucous membranes
- Caution patient to avoid hazardous activities if dizziness occurs
- Instruct patient to comply with complete medical regimen
- Advise patient to make position changes slowly to prevent fainting
- Advise patient to never use erectile dysfunction products (sildenafil, tadalafil, vardenafil); may cause severe hypotension, death
- **Pregnancy/breastfeeding:** Identify if pregnancy is planned or suspected or if breastfeeding

Evaluation

Positive therapeutic outcome
- Decreased, prevention of anginal pain

⚠ HIGH ALERT

nitroprusside (Rx)
(nye-troe-pruss´ide)
Nitropress
Func. class.: Antihypertensive, vasodilator

ACTION: Directly relaxes arteriolar, venous smooth muscle, resulting in reduction in cardiac preload, afterload

Therapeutic outcome: Decreased B/P in hypertensive crisis, decreased preload, afterload

USES: Hypertensive crisis/urgency/induction, to decrease bleeding by creating hypotension during surgery, acute HF

Pharmacokinetics
Absorption	Complete bioavailability
Distribution	Not known
Metabolism	RBCs, tissues
Excretion	Kidneys
Half-life	2 min

Pharmacodynamics
Onset	1-2 min
Peak	Rapid
Duration	1-10 min

CONTRAINDICATIONS
Hypersensitivity, hypertension (compensatory) due to aortic coarctation or AV shunting, acute HF associated with reduced peripheral vascular resistance, toxic amblyopia, hypothyroidism

> **BLACK BOX WARNING:** Cyanide toxicity

Precautions: Pregnancy, breastfeeding, children, geriatric, fluid, electrolyte imbalances, renal/hepatic disease, hypothyroidism, anemia, increased intracranial pressure, hypovolemia

> **BLACK BOX WARNING:** Hypotension

DOSAGE AND ROUTES
Adult and child: IV INF 0.25-1.0 mcg/kg/min; max 10 mcg/kg/min

Renal dose
Adult: IV INF CCr <60 ml/min maintain doses <3 mcg/kg/min to reduce thiocyanate accumulation

Available forms: Inj 50 mg 12 ml

ADVERSE EFFECTS
CNS: *Dizziness, headache,* agitation, twitching, decreased reflexes, *restlessness*

CV: *Bradycardia,* ECG changes, tachycardia, *hypotension*
GI: Nausea, vomiting, abdominal pain
INTEG: Pain, irritation at inj site, sweating
MISC: Cyanide, thiocyanate toxicity, flushing, hypothyroidism

INTERACTIONS
Individual drugs
Enflurane, halothane; severe hypotension

Drug classifications
Circulatory depressants, ganglionic blockers, volatile liquid anesthetics: severe hypotension

Drug/herb
Hawthorn: increased antihypertensive effect

NURSING CONSIDERATIONS
Assessment

> **BLACK BOX WARNING: Hypotension:** monitor B/P q5min × 2 hr, then qhr × 2 hr; monitor pulse q4hr; monitor jugular venous distention q4hr; ECG should be monitored continuously; monitor PCWP; rebound hypertension may occur after nitroprusside is discontinued, give only with emergency equipment nearby, rapid decrease in B/P may occur

• Monitor electrolytes, blood studies: potassium, sodium, chloride, CO_2, CBC, serum glucose, serum methemoglobin if pulmonary oxygen levels are decreased, ABGs
• Check weight, I&O, edema in feet and legs daily; assess skin turgor, dryness of mucous membranes for hydration status
• Assess for signs of HF: dyspnea, edema, wet crackles
• Monitor for increased lactate, cyanide, thiocyanate levels if on long-term treatment; thiocyanate toxicity occurs at plasma levels of ≥50 mcg/ml
• Monitor for decrease in bicarbonate, $PaCO_2$, and blood pH; acidosis may occur with this product

Patient problem
Ineffective tissue perfusion (uses)
Risk for injury (uses, adverse reactions)

Implementation
Continuous IV infusion route
• Depending on B/P reading q15min
• Reconstitute 50 mg/2-3 ml of D_5W, further dilute in 250, 500, or 1000 ml of D_5W to 200, 100, 50 mcg/ml respectively; use an infusion pump only; wrap bottle with aluminum foil to protect from light; observe for color change in the inf; discard if highly discolored (blue, green,

dark red); titrate to patient response, protect from light
• Do not exceed max dose, cyanide may accumulate

Y-site compatibilities: Alfentanil, alprostadil, amikacin, aminocaproic acid, aminophylline, amphotericin B lipid complex, amphotericin B liposome, anidulafungin, argatroban, atenolol, atropine, aztreonam, benztropine, bivalirudin, bleomycin, bumetanide, buprenorphine, butorphanol, calcium chloride/gluconate, CARBOplatin, cefamandole, ceFAZolin, cefmetazole, cefonicid, cefoperazone, cefotaxime, cefoTEtan, cefOXitin, cefTAZidime, ceftizoxime, cefTRIAXone, cefuroxime, cephalothin, chloramphenicol, cimetidine, CISplatin, clindamycin, cyanocobalamin, cyclophosphamide, cycloSPORINE, cytarabine, DACTINomycin, DAPTOmycin, dexamethasone, digoxin, diltiazem, DOCEtaxel, DOPamine, doxacurium, DOXOrubicin, doxycycline, enalaprilat, ePHEDrine, EPINEPHrine, epirubicin, epoetin alfa, eptifibatide, ertapenem, esmolol, etoposide, famotidine, fenoldopam, fentaNYL, fluconazole, fludarabine, fluorouracil, folic acid, furosemide, ganciclovir, gatifloxacin, gemcitabine, gemtuzumab, gentamicin, glycopyrrolate, granisetron, heparin, hydrocortisone, HYDROmorphone, IDArubicin, ifosfamide, inamrinone, indomethacin, insulin (regular), isoproterenol, ketorolac, labetalol, lidocaine, linezolid, LORazepam, magnesium sulfate, mannitol, mechlorethamine, meperidine, metaraminol, methicillin, methoxamine, methyldopate, methylPREDNISolone, metoclopramide, metoprolol, metroNIDAZOLE, mezlocillin, micafungin, miconazole, midazolam, milrinone, minocycline, morphine, moxalactam, multiple vitamins injection, nafcillin, nalbuphine, naloxone, nesiritide, netilmicin, niCARdipine, nitroglycerin, norepinephrine, octreotide, ondansetron, oxacillin, oxaliplatin, oxytocin, PACLitaxel, palonosetron, pamidronate, pancuronium, pantoprazole, penicillin G potassium/sodium, pentamidine, PENTobarbital, PHENobarbital, phentolamine, phenylephrine, phytonadione, piperacillin, piperacillin-tazobactam, polymyxin B, potassium chloride/phosphates, procainamide, propofol, propranolol, protamine, pyridoxine, ranitidine, ritodrine, rocuronium, sodium acetate/bicarbonate, succinylcholine, SUFentanil, tacrolimus, teniposide, theophylline, thiamine, ticarcillin, ticarcillin-clavulanate, tigecycline, tirofiban, tobramycin, tolazoline, trimetaphan, urokinase, vancomycin, vasopressin, vecuronium, verapamil, vinCRIStine, zoledronic acid

Patient/family education
• Teach patient to report headache, dizziness, loss of hearing, blurred vision, dyspnea, faintness; may indicate adverse reactions, pain at IV site

• **Pregnancy/breastfeeding:** Identify if pregnancy is planned or suspected or if breastfeeding

Evaluation

Positive therapeutic outcome
• Decreased B/P in hypertension
• Absence of bleeding in surgery

TREATMENT OF OVERDOSE:
Administer amyl nitrate inh until 3% sodium nitrate sol can be prepared for **IV** administration, then inject sodium thiosulfate **IV**; correct drop in B/P with vasopressor

---

> **▲ HIGH ALERT**
> **RARELY USED**
>
> # nivolumab
> (nye-volue-mab)
> **Opdivo**
> *Func. class.:* Antineoplastic, monoclonal antibody

USES: Treatment of BRAF V600 mutation–positive unresectable/metastatic melanoma, Hodgkin's disease, non–small-cell lung cancer (NSCLC), renal cell cancer

CONTRAINDICATIONS
Hypersensitivity

DOSAGE AND ROUTES
Adult: IV INF 240 mg over 60 min q2wk until disease progression or unacceptable toxicity

Available forms: Injection 10 mg/ml

> **▲ HIGH ALERT**
>
> # norepinephrine
> (nor-ep-i-nef'rin)
> **Levophed**
> *Func. class.:* Adrenergic
> *Chem. class.:* Catecholamine

Do not confuse: norepinephrine/ EPINEPHrine

ACTION: Causes increased contractility and heart rate by acting on β-receptors in heart; also acts on a-receptors, thereby causing vasoconstriction in blood vessels; B/P is elevated, coronary blood flow improves, and cardiac output increases

Therapeutic outcome: Increased B/P with stabilization; adequate tissue perfusion

USES: Acute hypotension, shock

Absorption	Complete
Distribution	Crosses placenta
Metabolism	Liver
Excretion	Urine

Pharmacodynamics

Onset	Immediate
Peak	Rapid
Duration	1 min

CONTRAINDICATIONS
Hypersensitivity to this product or cyclopropane/ halothane anesthesia; ventricular fibrillation, tachydysrhythmias, hypovolemia

> **BLACK BOX WARNING:** Extravasation

Precautions: Pregnancy, breastfeeding, geriatric patients, arterial embolism, peripheral vascular disease, hypertension, hyperthyroidism, cardiac disease, ventricular fibrillation, tachydysrhythmias, pheochromocytoma, hypotension

DOSAGE AND ROUTES
Adult: IV INF 0.5-1 mcg/min titrated to B/P; maintenance 2-4 mcg/min; max 30 mcg/min
Child: IV INF 0.1 mcg/kg/min titrated to B/P; max 2 mcg/kg/min

Available forms: Inj 1 mg/ml

ADVERSE EFFECTS
CNS: *Headache,* anxiety, dizziness, insomnia, restlessness, tremor, cerebral hemorrhage
CV: *Palpitations, tachycardia, hypertension, ectopic beats, angina*
GI: *Nausea, vomiting*
GU: Decreased urine output
INTEG: Necrosis, tissue sloughing with extravasation, gangrene
RESP: Dyspnea
SYST: Anaphylaxis

INTERACTIONS
Individual drugs
Methyldopa: do not use norepinephrine within 2 wk of using these drugs because hypertensive crisis may result

Drug classifications
α-blockers: decreased norepinephrine action
Antihistamines, ergots, MAOIs, oxytocics, tricyclics: do not use norepinephrine within 2 wk of using these drugs because hypertensive crisis may result
Oxytocics: Increased B/P
MAOIs, tricyclics: increased pressor effect

NURSING CONSIDERATIONS
Assessment
• Assess I&O ratio; notify prescriber if output <30 ml/hr
• Assess B/P, pulse q2-3min after parenteral route, ECG during administration continuously; if B/P increases, product is decreased, CVP or PWP during inf if possible
• Assess paresthesias and coldness of extremities; peripheral blood flow may decrease

> **BLACK BOX WARNING: Extravasation:** inj site: tissue sloughing, change injection sites if blanching or vasoconstriction occurs

• Assess for sulfite sensitivity, which may be life-threatening

Patient problems
Impaired cardiac output (uses)
Ineffective tissue perfusion (uses)
Risk for injury (uses, adverse reactions)

Implementation
• Plasma expanders for hypervolemia, correct volume depletion before starting treatment

CONT IV INF route
• Dilute with 500-1000 ml D₅W or D₅/0.9% NaCl; average dilution 4 mg/1000 ml diluent (4 mcg base/ml); give as inf 2-3 ml/min; titrate to response, discontinue gradually
• Store reconstituted sol in refrigerator <24 hr, protect from light, store unopened product at room temp, do not use discolored sol

Y-site compatibilities: Alemtuzumab, alfentanil, amikacin, amiodarone, anidulafungin, argatroban, ascorbic acid, atenolol, atracurium, atropine, aztreonam, benztropine, bivalirudin, bleomycin, bumetanide, buprenorphine, butorphanol, calcium chloride/gluconate, CARBOplatin, caspofungin, cefamandole, ceFAZolin, cefmetazole, cefonicid, cefoperazone, cefotaxime, cefoTEtan, cefOXitin, cefTAZidime, ceftizoxime, ceftobiprole, cefTRIAXone, cefuroxime, cephalothin, chloramphenicol, chlorproMAZINE, cimetidine, cisatracurium, CISplatin, clindamycin, cloNIDine, cyanocobalamin, cyclophosphamide, cycloSPORINE, cytarabine, DAPTOmycin, dexamethasone, digoxin, diltiazem, diphenhydrAMINE, DOBUTamine, DOCEtaxel, DOPamine, doripenem, doxycycline, enalaprilat, ePHEDrine, EPINEPHrine, epirubicin, epoetin alfa, ertapenem, erythromycin, esmolol, etoposide, famotidine, fenoldopam, fentaNYL, fluconazole, fludarabine, gatifloxacin, gemcitabine, gentamicin, glycopyrrolate, granisetron, heparin, hydrocortisone, HYDROmorphone, hydrOXYzine, IDArubicin, ifosfamide, imipenem-cilastatin, irinotecan, isoproterenol, ketorolac, labetalol, lidocaine, linezolid, LORazepam, magnesium sulfate, mannitol, mechlorethamine, meperidine, meropenem, metaraminol, methicillin, methotrexate, methoxamine, methyldopate, methylPREDNISolone, metoclopramide, metoprolol, metroNIDAZOLE, mezlocillin, micafungin, miconazole, midazolam, milrinone, minocycline, mitoXANtrone, morphine, moxalactam, multiple vitamins injection, mycophenolate, nafcillin, nalbuphine, naloxone, netilmicin, niCARdipine, nitroglycerin, nitroprusside, octreotide, ondansetron, oxacillin, oxaliplatin, oxytocin, PACLitaxel, palonosetron, pamidronate, pancuronium, papaverine, PEMEtrexed, penicillin G potassium/sodium, pentamidine, pentazocine, phenylephrine, phytonadione, piperacillin, piperacillin-tazobactam, polymyxin B, potassium chloride, procainamide, prochlorperazine, promethazine, propofol, propranolol, protamine, pyridoxine, quiNIDine, ranitidine, remifentanil, ritodrine, succinylcholine, SUFentanil, tacrolimus, teniposide, theophylline, thiamine, thiotepa, ticarcillin, ticarcillin-clavulanate, tigecycline, tirofiban, tobramycin, tolazoline, trimetaphan, urokinase, vancomycin, vasopressin, vecuronium, verapamil, vinCRIStine, vinorelbine, vitamin B complex with C, voriconazole, zoledronic acid

Patient/family education
• Teach patient about the reason for product administration
• Advise family to report dyspnea, dizziness, chest pain
• **Pregnancy/breastfeeding:** Identify if pregnancy is planned or suspected or if breastfeeding

Evaluation
Positive therapeutic outcome
• Increased B/P with stabilization
• Adequate tissue perfusion

TREATMENT OF OVERDOSE:
Administer fluids, electrolyte replacement

N

nortriptyline (Rx)
(nor-trip'ti-leen)
Aventyl ✦, Norventyl ✦, Pamelor
Func. class.: Antidepressant, tricyclic
Chem. class.: Dibenzocycloheptene, secondary amine

Do not confuse: nortriptyline/ amitriptyline, Pamelor/Panlor DC/Tambocor

ACTION: Blocks reuptake of norepinephrine, serotonin into nerve endings, increasing action of norepinephrine, serotonin in nerve cells; has anticholinergic effects

Therapeutic outcome: Decreased symptoms of depression after 2-3 wk

USES: Major depression

Unlabeled uses: Chronic pain management

Pharmacokinetics

Absorption	Well absorbed
Distribution	Widely distributed; crosses placenta
Metabolism	Liver, extensively ✎ CYP2D6 by genetic polymorphism ($\geq$ 7% are poor metabolizers)
Excretion	Kidneys, breast milk
Half-life	18-28 hr; steady state 4-19 days

Pharmacodynamics
Unknown

CONTRAINDICATIONS
Hypersensitivity to tricyclics, carBAMazepine, recovery phase of MI

Precautions: Breastfeeding, suicidal ideation, severe depression, increased intraocular pressure, closed-angle glaucoma, urinary retention, cardiac/hepatic disease, hyperthyroidism, electroshock therapy, elective surgery, pregnancy, seizure disorders, prostatic hypertrophy

> **BLACK BOX WARNING:** Children, suicidal ideation

DOSAGE AND ROUTES
Adult: PO 25 mg tid or qid; may increase to 150 mg/day; may give daily dose at bedtime
Adolescent: PO 1-3 mg/kg/day in 3-4 divided doses or qd at bedtime; max 150 mg/day
Geriatric: PO 10-25 mg nightly, increase by 10-25 mg at weekly intervals to desired dose; usual maintenance 75 mg/day, max 150 mg/day

Available forms: Caps 10, 25, 50, 75 mg; sol 10 mg/5 ml

ADVERSE EFFECTS
CNS: *Dizziness, drowsiness,* confusion, headache, anxiety, tremors, stimulation, weakness, insomnia, nightmares, EPS (geriatric), increased psychiatric symptoms, seizures
CV: *Orthostatic hypotension,* ECG changes, *tachycardia,* hypertension, palpitations, dysrhythmias
EENT: Blurred vision, tinnitus, mydriasis, dry eyes
ENDO: SIADH, hyponatremia, hypothyroidism
GI: *Constipation, dry mouth,* nausea, vomiting, paralytic ileus, increased appetite, cramps, epigastric distress, jaundice, hepatitis, stomatitis, weight gain
GU: *Retention,* acute renal failure, sexual dysfunction
HEMA: Agranulocytosis, thrombocytopenia, eosinophilia, leukopenia
INTEG: Rash, urticaria, sweating, pruritus, photosensitivity
SYST: Serotonin syndrome

INTERACTIONS
Individual drugs
Alcohol: increased CNS depression
CloNIDine, guanethidine: decreased effects
Smoking (heavy): decreased product effect
Haloperidol, chloroquine, droperidol, pentamidine, arsenic trioxide, levomethadyl: increased QT prolongation

Drug classifications
Barbiturates, benzodiazepines, CNS depressants: increased effects
MAOIs: hypertensive episode, hyperpyretic crisis, seizures
SSRIs, SNRIs, serotonin-receptor agonists: increased serotonin syndrome, neuroleptic malignant syndrome
Class IA/III antidysrhythmics, some phenothiazines, β-agonists, local anesthetics, tricyclics, CYP3A4 inhibitors (amiodarone, clarithromycin, erythromycin, telithromycin, troleandomycin), CYP3A4 substrates (methadone, pimozide, QUEtiapine, quiNIDine, risperiDONE, ziprasidone): increased QT prolongation
Sympathomimetics (direct-acting), products increasing QT interval: increased effects
Sympathomimetics (indirect-acting): decreased effects

Drug/herb
Kava, valerian: increased CNS effect
St. John's wort: decreased nortriptyline level

Drug/lab test

Increased: serum bilirubin, blood glucose, alkaline phosphatase

Decreased: VMA, 5-HIAA

False increase: urinary catecholamines

NURSING CONSIDERATIONS
Assessment

> **BLACK BOX WARNING: Suicidal thoughts/ behaviors in children/young adults:** not approved for children; monitor for suicidal ideation in depression, adolescents, young adults

- Monitor B/P (with patient lying, standing), pulse q4hr; if systolic B/P drops 20 mm Hg, hold product, notify prescriber; take VS q4hr of patients with CV disease
- Monitor blood studies: thyroid function tests, LFTs, serum nortriptyline level/target 50-150 ng/ml if patient is receiving long-term therapy
- Monitor liver function tests: AST, ALT, bilirubin
- Check weight weekly; appetite may increase
- **QT prolongation:** assess for chest pain, palpitations, dyspnea
- Assess ECG for flattening of T-wave, bundle branch block, AV block, dysrhythmias in cardiac patients
- Assess for EPS primarily in geriatric: rigidity, dystonia, akathisia
- Assess mental status: mood, sensorium, affect, suicidal tendencies; increase in psychiatric symptoms: depression, panic
- Monitor urinary retention, constipation; constipation is more likely to occur in children or geriatric
- **Assess for withdrawal symptoms:** headache, nausea, vomiting, muscle pain, weakness; do not usually occur unless product was discontinued abruptly
- Monitor for glaucoma exacerbation and paralytic ileus
- Identify alcohol consumption; if alcohol is consumed, hold dose until AM
- **Serotonin syndrome, neuroleptic malignant syndrome:** assess for increased heart rate, shivering, sweating, dilated pupils, tremors, high B/P, hyperthermia, headache, confusion; if these occur, stop product, administer a serotonin antagonist if needed (rare)
- **Beers:** Avoid in older adults, highly anticholinergic, sedating, and causes orthostatic hypotension

Patient problem

Depression (uses)

Impaired sexual functioning (adverse reactions)

Risk for injury (adverse reactions)

Implementation

- Give with food or milk to decrease GI symptoms; mix conc with water, milk, fruit juice to disguise taste
- Give dose at bedtime if oversedation occurs during day; may take entire dose at bedtime; geriatric may not tolerate once/day dosing
- Store in tight, light-resistant container at room temp; do not freeze

Patient/family education

- Teach patient that therapeutic effects may take 2-3 wk
- Teach patient to use caution in driving and other activities requiring alertness because of drowsiness, dizziness, blurred vision; to avoid rising quickly from sitting to standing, especially geriatric
- Teach patient to avoid alcohol ingestion, MAOIs within 14 days, other CNS depressants; teach patient not to discontinue medication quickly after long-term use; may cause nausea, headache, malaise
- Teach patient to wear sunscreen or large hat to avoid burns, because photosensitivity occurs
- Teach patient to increase fluids, bulk in diet if constipation, urinary retention occur, especially geriatric, worsening depression, suicidal thoughts/behavior
- Teach patient to take gum, hard sugarless candy, or frequent sips of water for dry mouth
- **Pregnancy/breastfeeding:** Identify if pregnancy is planned or suspected or if breastfeeding

Evaluation

Positive therapeutic outcome
- Decrease in depression
- Absence of suicidal thoughts

TREATMENT OF OVERDOSE:
ECG monitoring, lavage, administer anticonvulsant

nusinersen
(neu-si-ner′sen)
Spinraza
Func. class.: Miscellaneous CNS agent-muscular dystrophy
Chem. class.: Antisense oligonucleotide

Do not confuse: Nusinersen/Neurontin, Nucynta, Spinraza/Spriva

ACTION: Increases exon 7 inclusion in SMN2 messenger ribonucleic acid (mRNA) transcripts and production of full-length SMN protein

Therapeutic outcome: Increasing muscle strength and movement

USES: Spinal muscular atrophy

Pharmacokinetics

Absorption	Unknown
Distribution	Unknown
Metabolism	Unknown
Excretion	Unknown
Half-life	133-177 days CSF, 63-87 days plasma

Pharmacodynamics

Onset	Unknown
Peak	1.7-6 hr
Duration	Unknown

CONTRAINDICATIONS: Hypersensitivity

PRECAUTIONS: Pregnancy, breastfeeding, bleeding, nephrotoxicity, requires a specialized care setting and clinician, thrombocytopenia

DOSAGE AND ROUTES
Adult/child: Intrathecal 12 mg q14 days × 3 doses, then 12 mg q30 days after third dose; maintenance 12 mg q4 months thereafter

Available forms: Injection 12 mg/5 ml single use vials

ADVERSE EFFECTS
CNS: *Headache, fever*
GI: *Constipation*, feeding difficulties, *vomiting*
GU: Renal toxicity
HEMA: *Thrombocytopenia,* coagulation changes
RESP: URI, aspiration, atelectasis
EENT: Ear infection, teething, dysphagia
MS: Back pain, scoliosis, post-lumbar puncture syndrome
MISC: *Infection,* growth inhibition

INTERACTIONS
Drug classifications: None known
Drug/lab test
Increase: PT, PTT
Decrease: Platelets

NURSING CONSIDERATIONS
Assessment
• **Coagulation studies:** Obtain platelets and PT, aPTT baseline and before each dose; monitor for bleeding
• **Nephrotoxicity:** Quantitative spot urine protein testing is required at baseline and prior to each dose; for a urinary protein concentration more than 0.2 grams/L, consider repeat testing and further evaluation; monitor for changes in urinary patterns, blood in urine

Patient problem
Impaired mobility (uses)

Implementation
Intrathecal Route
Preparation
• Allow the vial to warm to room temperature (25° C or 77° F) prior to use; do not use external heat sources to warm
• Do not administer if visible particulates are observed or if the liquid in the vial is discolored; product should be clear and colorless; a filter is not required
• Use aseptic technique; each vial is for single-use only
• Withdraw 12 mg (5 ml) from the vial into a syringe; discard unused contents
• Give within 4 hr of removal from the vial
Intrathecal administration
• Administered by, or under the direction of, healthcare professionals experienced in performing lumbar punctures
• Consider sedation as indicated by the clinical condition of the patient
• Consider ultrasound or other imaging techniques to guide intrathecal administration, particularly in younger patients
• Prior to use, remove 5 ml of cerebrospinal fluid (CSF)
• Give as an intrathecal bolus injection over 1 to 3 min using a spinal anesthesia needle. Do not administer in areas of the skin where there are signs of infection or inflammation

Patient/family education
• Reason for medication and expected results
• **Pregnancy/breastfeeding:** To notify healthcare professional if pregnancy is planned or suspected or if breastfeeding
• That continuing blood and lab tests will be required
• To report bleeding or bruising
• **Renal toxicity**: Change in urinary patterns, blood in urine

Evaluation
• Increasing muscle strength and movement

nystatin (Rx, OTC)
(nis′ta-tin)
Mycostatin, Nadostine ✹, Nilstat, Pedi-Dri, PMS-Nystatin ✹
Func. class.: Antifungal
Chem. class.: Amphoteric polyene

ACTION: Interferes with fungal DNA replication; binds sterols in fungal cell membrane, which increases permeability, resulting in leaking of cell nutrients

Therapeutic outcome: Fungistatic/fungicidal against *Candida* organisms

USES: *Candida* species causing oral, intestinal infections

Pharmacokinetics

Absorption	Poorly absorbed
Distribution	Unknown
Metabolism	Not metabolized
Excretion	Feces, unchanged
Half-life	Unknown

Pharmacodynamics

Onset	Rapid
Peak	Unknown
Duration	6-12 hr

CONTRAINDICATIONS
Hypersensitivity

Precautions: Pregnancy

DOSAGE AND ROUTES
Oral infection
Adult/adolescent/child: SUSP 400,000-600,000 units qid, use ½ dose in each side of mouth, swish and swallow, use for at least 48 hr after symptoms are resolved
Infant: SUSP 200,000 units qid (100,000 units in each side of mouth)
Newborn and premature infant: SUSP 100,000 units qid
Adult and child: Troches 200,000-400,000 units qid × up to 2 wk

GI infection
Adult: PO 500,000-1,000,000 units tid

Cutaneous candidiasis
Adult/child:
Top cream/ointment
Apply to affected area bid
Powder
Apply to affected area bid-tid

Available forms: Tabs 500,000 units; oral caps 500,000, 1,000,000 units, bulk powder; susp 1,000,000 unit/ml

ADVERSE EFFECTS
GI: Nausea, vomiting, anorexia, diarrhea, cramps
INTEG: Rash, urticaria (rare)

NURSING CONSIDERATIONS
Assessment
• **Assess for allergic reaction:** rash, urticaria; product may have to be discontinued
• Assess for predisposing factors for candidal infection: antibiotic therapy, pregnancy, diabetes mellitus, sexual partner infection (vag infections), AIDS
• Obtain culture and histologic tests to confirm organism

Patient problem
Infection (uses)

Implementation
• Store oral susp at room temp; store tabs in tight, light-resistant containers at room temp
PO route
• Give oral susp dose by placing ½ in each cheek, swish for several min, then swallow; shake susp before use
• Store oral susp at room temp, tab in airtight, light-resistant containers at room temp
Topical route
• Administer by moistening lesions with a swab coated with cream or ointment; use enough medication to cover lesions completely; give after cleansing with soap, water before each application; dry well; very moist lesions are best treated with topical powder

Patient/family education
• Instruct patient that long-term therapy may be needed to clear infection; to complete entire course of medication
• Teach patient proper hygiene: use no commercial mouthwashes for mouth infection
• Advise patient to avoid getting preparation on hands
• Instruct patient to notify prescriber if irritation occurs; product may have to be discontinued
• Inform patient that relief from itching may occur after 24-72 hr
Topical route
• Advise patient to discontinue use and notify prescriber if irritation occurs
• Teach patient to apply with glove to prevent further infection; product may stain
• Caution patient not to use occlusive dressings; to avoid use of OTC creams, ointments, lotions unless directed by prescriber
• **Pregnancy/breastfeeding:** Identify if pregnancy is planned or suspected or if breastfeeding

Evaluation

Positive therapeutic outcome
• Culture negative for *Candida*
• Decrease in size, number of lesions

nystatin topical
See Appendix B

N

ocrelizumab (Rx)
(oc"-re-liz'-ue-mab)
Ocrevus
Func. class.: Multiple sclerosis agent
Chem. class.: Monoclonal antibody

ACTION: Likely binds to CD20, a cell surface antigen present on pre-B and mature B lymphocytes. Following binding, antibody-dependent cellular cytolysis and complement-mediated lysis occur

USES: For the treatment of relapsing multiple sclerosis

Pharmacokinetics

Absorption	Complete
Distribution	Binds to lymphocytes (CD20)
Metabolism	Unknown
Excretion	Unknown
Half-life	26 days

Pharmacodynamics

Onset	Unknown
Peak	Unknown
Duration	Unknown

CONTRAINDICATIONS: Hypersensitivity, active hepatitis B infection

Precautions: Immunocompromised, pregnancy, breastfeeding, infusion-site reactions, infections, breast cancer, progressive multifocal leukoencephalopathy

DOSAGE AND ROUTES
Adult: **IV INFUSION** 300 mg as a single dose, followed by a second 300 mg 2 wk later

Subsequent infusions of 600 mg are given q6mo. The first 600 mg dose is due 6 mo after infusion one of the initial dose

Available forms: Solution for injection 30 mg/ml

SIDE EFFECTS
CNS: Progressive multifocal leukoencephalopathy
GI: Nausea, diarrhea
MS: Back pain
RESP: Cough
HEMA: Neutropenia
INTEG: Rash, itching, hypersensitivity reactions
MISC: Infection

INTERACTIONS
None significant

NURSING CONSIDERATIONS
Assessment:
• **Multiple sclerosis:** Assess for symptoms of multiple sclerosis baseline and periodically during treatment
• **Infection:** Assess for increased temperature, other flu-like symptoms; if present do not use infusion, wait until infection has been treated
• **Infusion-related reactions:** Rate of infusion modifications in response to infusion reactions depend on reaction severity:
• **Life-threatening or disabling infusion reactions:** Immediately discontinue the infusion and provide appropriate supportive treatment. Permanently discontinue
• **Severe infusion reactions:** Immediately interrupt the infusion and provide appropriate supportive treatment. Wait until all symptoms have resolved before resuming infusion. When restarting, begin at one-half of the infusion rate at the time of infusion reaction onset. If this rate is tolerated, it may be increased according to recommended infusion rate titration guidelines. The rate modifications do not change the dose administered but do increase the duration of infusion time.
• **Mild or moderate infusion reactions:** Reduce the infusion rate to one-half of the rate at the onset of the infusion reaction and maintain the reduced rate for a minimum of 30 minutes. If this rate is tolerated, it may be increased according to recommended infusion rate titration guidelines. The rate modifications do not change the dose administered but do increase the duration of infusion time.
• **Progressive multifocal leukoencephalopathy:** Assess for weakness, blurred vision, confusion, lability; if these occur, stop infusion, confirm diagnosis with MRI

Patient problems
Impaired mobility (uses)
Risk for infection (adverse reactions)

Implementation
Intermittent IV infusion route
• Visually inspect for particulate matter and discoloration; prior to use the solution is clear or slightly opalescent and colorless to pale brown
• Do not shake vial
• Vials are preservative-free and are intended for single-use only. Discard unused portion
• Withdraw dose and dilute into an infusion bag of 0.9% Sodium Chloride Injection to a final

concentration of approximately 1.2 mg/ml; do not use other diluents, as their use has not been tested
• Withdraw 10 ml (300 mg) and inject into 250 ml 0.9% Sodium Chloride Injection
• Withdraw 20 ml (600 mg) and inject into 500 ml 0.9% Sodium Chloride Injection
• No incompatibilities with polyvinyl chloride (PVC) or polyolefin (PO) bags and IV administration sets have been observed
• Use the prepared solution immediately
• *Storage*: If the solution is not used immediately, it may be refrigerated for up to 24 hr at 2° to 8° C (36° to 46° F) and 8 hr at room temperature up to 25° C (77° F), which includes infusion time. If the infusion cannot be completed within the same day, discard the remaining solution

Administration:
• Administration can cause serious infusion-related reactions. Monitor the patient during each infusion and for at least 1 hr following the completion of each infusion.
• Administration needs to be by a health care professional with appropriate medical support to manage severe infusion reactions.
• Premedication: Premedicate 30 min prior to infusion with methylprednisolone 100 mg IV (or an equivalent corticosteroid) and 30 to 60 min prior to infusion with an antihistamine (diphenhydramine) to reduce the frequency and severity of infusion reactions. An antipyretic (acetaminophen) may also be used.
• The content of the infusion bag must be at room temperature prior to infusion.
• Administer through a dedicated line using an infusion set with a 0.2 or 0.22 micron in-line filter.
• *First 2 (300 mg) infusions:* Give at an initial rate of 30 ml/hr. Increase by 30 ml/hr q30 min to a max rate of 180 ml/hr with a total infusion duration of 2.5 hr or longer.
• *Subsequent infusions (600 mg):* Give at an initial rate of 40 ml/hr. Increase by 40 ml/hr q30 min to a max rate of 200 ml/hr with a total infusion duration of 3.5 hr or longer.
• **Missed doses:** If a planned infusion is missed, give ocrelizumab as soon as possible; do not wait until the next scheduled dose. Reset the dose schedule to give the next sequential dose 6 months after the missed dose. Doses must be separated by at least 5 months.

Patient/family education
• Explain reason for product and expected result
• Explain to caregiver how to apply cream and how long to leave on the area

Evaluation
Positive therapeutic outcome
• Decreasing symptoms of multiple sclerosis

octreotide (Rx)
(ok-tree′o-tide)
SandoSTATIN, Sandostatin LAR Depot
Func. class.: Growth hormone, antidiarrheal
Chem. class.: Synthetic analog of somatostatin

Do not confuse: SandoSTATIN/SandIMMUNE

ACTION: A potent growth hormone similar to somatostatin

Therapeutic outcome: Decreased diarrhea; decreased symptoms of acromegaly, carcinoid tumors, vasoactive intestinal peptide tumors (VIPomas)

USES: Sandostatin: acromegaly, carcinoid tumors, VIPomas; **LAR Depot:** long-term maintenance of acromegaly, carcinoid tumors, VIPomas, short bowel syndrome, insulinoma, hepatorenal syndrome

Unlabeled uses: GI fistula, variceal bleeding, diarrheal conditions, pancreatic fistula, IBS, dumping syndrome

Pharmacokinetics

Absorption	Rapidly, completely absorbed
Distribution	Unknown, protein binding 65%
Metabolism	Little
Excretion	Urine, unchanged 32%
Half-life	1.7 hr

Pharmacodynamics

	Subcut/IV	IM
Onset	Unknown	Unknown
Peak	½ hr	2-4 wk
Duration	12 hr	Unknown

CONTRAINDICATIONS
Hypersensitivity

Precautions: Pregnancy, breastfeeding, children, geriatric, diabetes mellitus, hypothyroidism, renal disease

DOSAGE AND ROUTES
Acromegaly
Adult: SUBCUT/**IV** 50-100 mcg bid-tid, adjust q2wk based on growth hormone levels (Sandostatin) or IM 20 mg q4wk × 3 mo, adjust by growth hormone levels (Sandostatin LAR)

VIPomas

Adult: SUBCUT/**IV** 200-300 mcg/day in 2-4 doses for 2 wk, max 450 mcg/day; (Sandostatin) or IM 20 mg q2wk × 2 mo, adjust dose (Sandostatin LAR)

Flushing/diarrhea in carcinoid tumors

Adult: SUBCUT/**IV** 100-600 mcg/day in 2-4 doses for 2 wk, titrated to patient response (Sandostatin) or IM 20 mg q4wk × 2 mo, adjust dose (Sandostatin LAR)

GI fistula

Adult: SUBCUT 50-200 mcg q8hr

Antidiarrheal in AIDS patients (unlabeled)

Adult: SUBCUT 50 mcg q8hr PRN, increase to 500 mcg q8hr

Irritable bowel syndrome (unlabeled)

Adult: SUBCUT 100 mcg single dose to 125 mcg bid

Dumping syndrome (unlabeled)

Adult: SUBCUT 50-150 mcg/day

Variceal bleeding (unlabeled)

Adult: IV bolus **50 mcg then;** 25-50 mcg/hr CONT **IV** INF for 18 hr-5 days

Available forms: Sandostatin: inj 0.05, 0.1, 0.2, 0.5, 1 mg/ml; LAR Depot: inj powder for susp 10 mg, 20, 30 mg/5 ml

ADVERSE EFFECTS

CNS: *Headache, dizziness, fatigue, weakness,* depression, anxiety, tremors, seizures, paranoia
CV: *Sinus bradycardia, conduction abnormalities,* dysrhythmias, chest pain, shortness of breath, thrombophlebitis, ischemia, HF, hypertension, palpitations, QT prolongation
ENDO: *Hypo/hyperglycemia, ketosis, hypothyroidism,* galactorrhea, diabetes insipidus
GI: *Diarrhea, nausea, abdominal pain, vomiting, flatulence, distention, constipation,* elevated liver function tests, cholelithiasis, ileus
HEMA: Hematoma of inj site, bruise
INTEG: Rash, urticaria, pain, inflammation at inj site

INTERACTIONS

Individual drugs

Bromocriptine: decreased: effect of bromocriptine
CycloSPORINE: decreased effect of cycloSPORINE

Drug classifications

Class IA/III antidysrhythmics, some phenothiazines, β-agonists, local anesthetics, tricyclics, CYP3A4 inhibitors (amiodarone, clarithromycin, erythromycin, telithromycin, troleandomycin), CYP3A4 substrates (methadone, pimozide, QUEtiapine, quiNIDine, risperiDONE, ziprasidone): increased QT prolongation
Oral antidiabetics: decreased: effect of the oral antidiabetics; monitor blood glucose

Drug/food

Decreased: absorption of dietary fat, vit B_{12} levels

Drug/lab test

Increased: glucose
Decreased: T_4, thyroid function tests, vit B_{12}, glucose

NURSING CONSIDERATIONS

Assessment

• Identify growth hormone antibodies, IGF-1, 1-4 hr intervals for 8-12 hr after dose in acromegaly; 5-HIAA; blood glucose, serotonin levels (carcinoid tumors), plasma substance P, plasma vasoactive intestinal peptide (VIP) (VIPomas)
• Monitor for fecal fat, serum carotene, somatomedin-C q14 days, glucose; plasma serotonin levels (carcinoid tumors); plasma vasoactive intestinal peptide levels (VIPoma); serum growth hormone, serum IGF-1 baseline and periodically, diabetes to monitor blood glucose
• Monitor thyroid function tests: T_3, T_4, T_7, TSH to identify hypothyroidism
• Monitor for vital sign, B/P, pulse; hydration status
• **Assess for cardiac status:** bradycardia, conduction abnormalities, dysrhythmias; monitor ECG for QT prolongation, baseline and periodically
• **Allergic reaction:** assess for rash, itching, fever, nausea, wheezing
• Gallbladder disease, monitor for nausea, abdominal pain; monitor ultrasound of gallbladder baseline and periodically
• **Ileus:** Assess character of stools, bowel sounds baseline and throughout treatment

Patient problems

Diarrhea (uses)

Implementation

• Store in refrigerator for unopened amps, vials, or at room temp for 2 wk; protect from light; do not use discolored or cloudy sol
• Do not use if discolored or if particulates are present

IM route

• Reconstitute with diluent provided; give into gluteal immediately after reconstitution, rotate injection sites

---

SUBCUT route
• Rotate inj sites; use hip, thigh, abdomen
• Avoid using medication that is cold; allow to reach room temperature; do not use LAR Depot, do not use if discolored or if particulates are present

Direct IV route
• Give over 3 min; in an emergency carcinoid crisis, give rapid bolus, may give undiluted

Intermittent IV INF route
• Dilute in 50-200 ml D$_5$W, 0.9% NaCl; give over 15-30 min
• Solution is stable for 24 hr

Y-site compatibilities: Acyclovir, alfentanil, allopurinol, amifostine, amikacin, aminocaproic acid, aminophylline, amiodarone, amphotericin B colloidal, amphotericin B lipid complex, amphotericin B liposome, ampicillin, ampicillin-sulbactam, anidulafungin, argatroban, arsenic trioxide, atenolol, atracurium, azithromycin, aztreonam, bivalirudin, bleomycin, bumetanide, buprenorphine, busulfan, butorphanol, calcium chloride/gluconate, capreomycin, CARBOplatin, carmustine, caspofungin, ceFAZolin, cefepime, cefotaxime, cefoTEtan, cefOXitin, cefTAZidime, ceftizoxime, cefTRIAXone, cefuroxime, chloramphenicol, chlorproMAZINE, cimetidine, ciprofloxacin, cisatracurium, CISplatin, clindamycin, cyclophosphamide, cycloSPORINE, cytarabine, dacarbazine, DACTINomycin, DAPTOmycin, DAUNOrubicin, DAUNOrubicin liposome, dexamethasone, digoxin, diltiazem, diphenhydrAMINE, DOBUTamine, DOCEtaxel, dolasetron, DOPamine, DOXOrubicin, DOXOrubicin liposomal, doxycycline, droperidol, enalaprilat, ePHEDrine, EPINEPHrine, epirubicin, eptifibatide, ertapenem, erythromycin, esmolol, etoposide, famotidine, fenoldopam, fentaNYL, fluconazole, fludarabine, fluorouracil, foscarnet, fosphenytoin, furosemide, gallium nitrate, ganciclovir, gatifloxacin, gemcitabine, gentamicin, glycopyrrolate, granisetron, haloperidol, heparin, hydrALAZINE, hydrocortisone, HYDROmorphone, hydrOXYzine, IDArubicin, ifosfamide, imipenem-cilastatin, insulin (regular), irinotecan, isoproterenol, ketorolac, labetalol, lansoprazole, leucovorin, levofloxacin, lidocaine, linezolid, LORazepam, magnesium sulfate, mannitol, mechlorethamine, melphalan, meperidine, meropenem, mesna, methohexital, methotrexate, methyldopate, methylPREDNISolone, metoclopramide, metoprolol, metroNIDAZOLE, midazolam, milrinone, minocycline, mitoMYcin, mitoXANtrone, mivacurium, morphine, moxifloxacin, mycophenolate, nafcillin, nalbuphine, naloxone, nesiritide, niCARdipine, nitroglycerin, nitroprusside, norepinephrine, ondansetron, oxaliplatin, PACLitaxel, palonosetron, pamidronate, pancuronium, PEMEtrexed, pentamidine, pentazocine, PENTobarbital, PHENobarbital, phenylephrine, piperacillin, piperacillin-tazobactam, polymyxin B, potassium acetate/chloride/phosphates, procainamide, prochlorperazine, promethazine, propranolol, quiNIDine, quinupristin-dalfopristin, ranitidine, remifentanil, rocuronium, sodium acetate/bicarbonate/phosphates, streptozocin, succinylcholine, SUFentanil, sulfamethoxazole-trimethoprim, tacrolimus, teniposide, thiopental, thiotepa, ticarcillin, ticarcillin-clavulanate, tigecycline, tirofiban, tobramycin, topotecan, vancomycin, vasopressin, vecuronium, verapamil, vinBLAStine, vinCRIStine, vinorelbine, voriconazole, zidovudine, zoledronic acid

Patient/family education
• Explain reason for medication and expected results
• Advise patient that routine follow-up is needed
• Instruct parents on procedure for medication preparation and inj use; request demonstration, return demonstration; provide written instructions
• Advise patient that dizziness, drowsiness, weakness may occur; to avoid hazardous activities if these occur; to report abdominal pain immediately
• Teach diabetic patients to monitor glucose regularly
• **Pregnancy/breastfeeding:** Identify if pregnancy is planned or suspected or if breastfeeding; each patient that pregnancy may occur in acromegaly, since fertility may be restored

Evaluation
Positive therapeutic outcome
• Decreased symptoms of acromegaly, carcinoid, VIPoma
• Decreased diarrhea in AIDS

ofloxacin ophthalmic
See Appendix B

OLANZapine (Rx) REMS
(oh-lanz'a-peen)
ZyPREXA, Zyprexa Intramuscular, Zyprexa Relprevv, Zyprexa Zydis
Func. class.: Antipsychotic (first generation)/neuroleptic
Chem. class.: Thienobenzodiazepine

Do not confuse: OLANZapine/olsalazine, Zyprexa/Celexa/Zyrtec

ACTION: May mediate antipsychotic activity by both DOPamine and serotonin type 2 (5-HT$_2$)

antagonism; also, may antagonize muscarinic, histaminic (H_1), and α-adrenergic receptors

Therapeutic outcome: Decreased psychotic symptoms

USES: Schizophrenia, acute manic episodes in bipolar disorder, acute agitation

Unlabeled uses: Chemotherapy breakthrough nausea, vomiting

Pharmacokinetics

Absorption	Well absorbed
Distribution	93% plasma protein binding
Metabolism	Liver
Excretion	Kidneys
Half-life	Unknown

Pharmacodynamics

Onset	Unknown
Peak	PO 6 hr, IM 15-45 min
Duration	Unknown

CONTRAINDICATIONS
Hypersensitivity

Precautions: Pregnancy, breastfeeding, geriatric, hypertension, cardiac/renal/hepatic disease, diabetes, agranulocytosis, abrupt discontinuation, ✖ Asian patients, closed-angle glaucoma, coma, leukopenia, QT prolongation, tardive dyskinesia, torsades de pointes, suicidal ideation, stroke history, TIA

> **BLACK BOX WARNING:** Dementia, postinjection delirium/sedation syndrome

DOSAGE AND ROUTES
Schizophrenia
Adult: PO 5-10 mg/day initially, may increase dosage by 5 mg at ≥1 wk intervals; orally disintegrating tabs: open blister pack, place tab on tongue, let disintegrate, swallow; max 20 mg/day; ext rel inj (Zyprexa Relprevv) IM 150-300 mg q2wk or 405 mg q4wk
Geriatric/debilitated: PO 5 mg, may increase cautiously at 1 wk intervals, max 20 mg/day
Adolescent: PO 2.5 mg or 5 mg/day, target 10 mg/day

Acute mania or mixed episodes associated with bipolar 1 disorder
Adult: PO 10-15 mg/day, may increase dose after 24 hr by 5 mg, max 20 mg/day
Adolescent: PO 2.5 or 5 mg/day, target 10 mg/day

Acute agitation associated with schizophrenia, bipolar I mania
Adult: IM (reg rel) 10 mg once
Geriatric: IM (reg rel) 2.5-5 mg once

Available forms: Tabs 2.5, 5, 7.5, 10, 15, 20 mg; **orally disintegrating tabs** 5, 10, 15, 20 mg (Zyprexa Zydis); **powder for injection** 10 mg

ADVERSE EFFECTS
CNS: EPS (pseudoparkinsonism, akathisia, dystonia, tardive dyskinesia), seizures, headache, neuroleptic malignant syndrome (rare), *agitation*, nervousness, hostility, dizziness, hypertonia, tremor, euphoria, confusion, *drowsiness*, fatigue, *abnormal gait, insomnia, fever*, suicidal thoughts
CV: Hypotension, tachycardia, chest pain, heart failure, sudden death (geriatric, IM), orthostatic hypotension, peripheral edema
ENDO: Increased prolactin levels, hyperglycemia, hypoglycemia
GI: Dry mouth, nausea, vomiting, anorexia, constipation, abdominal pain, weight gain, appetite, dyspepsia, jaundice, hepatitis
GU: Urinary retention, urinary frequency, enuresis, impotence, amenorrhea, gynecomastia, breast engorgement, premenstrual syndrome
HEMA: Neutropenia, agranulocytosis, leukopenia
INTEG: Rash
MISC: Peripheral edema, accidental injury, hypertonia, hyperlipidemia
MS: Joint pain, twitching
RESP: *Cough, pharyngitis*, fatal pneumonia (geriatric, IM)

INTERACTIONS
Individual drugs
Alcohol: increased sedation, hypotension, CNS effects
Bromocriptine, levodopa: decreased antiparkinson activity
CarBAMazepine, omeprazole, rifampin: decreased levels of OLANZapine
Diazepam: increased hypotension, CNS effects
FluvoxaMINE: increased OLANZapine levels

Drug classifications
Anesthetics (barbiturates), antidepressants, antihistamines, CNS depressants, sedative/hypnotics: increased sedation
Anticholinergics: increased anticholinergic effects
Antihypertensives: increased hypotension
DOPamine agonists: decreased antiparkinson activity

> **BLACK BOX WARNING:** Opioids: increased respiratory depression

Drug/herb
Kava kava: Increase: toxicity
St. John's wort: Decrease: OLANZapine effect, avoid concurrent use

Drug/lab test
Increased: liver function tests, prolactin, CPK

NURSING CONSIDERATIONS
Assessment

> **BLACK BOX WARNING: Postinjection delirium/sedation syndrome (Zyprexa Relprevv):** monitor continuously for >3 hr after injection; this patient must be accompanied when leaving: assess for sedation, coma, delirium, EPS, slurred speech, altered gait, aggression, dizziness, weakness, hypertension, seizures; before leaving, confirm the patient is alert, oriented, and free of any other symptoms

• Assess mental status, assess orientation, mood, behavior, presence of hallucinations and type before initial administration and monthly, suicidal thoughts, behaviors more common in young adults
• **Renal status:** Monitor I&O ratio; palpate bladder if low urinary output occurs, especially in geriatric
• Monitor bilirubin, CBC
• Monitor urinalysis; recommended before, during prolonged therapy
• Assess affect, orientation, LOC, reflexes, gait, coordination, sleep pattern disturbances
• Monitor B/P sitting, standing, lying; take pulse and respirations q4hr during initial treatment; establish baseline before starting treatment; report drops of 30 mm Hg; obtain baseline ECG
• Assess dizziness, faintness, palpitations, tachycardia on rising
• **Assess for neuroleptic malignant syndrome:** Assess for hyperpyrexia, muscle rigidity, increased CPK, altered mental status, for acute dystonia (cheek chewing, swallowing, eyes, pill rolling), stop drug immediately
• **EPS** including akathisia (inability to sit still, no pattern to movements), tardive dyskinesia (bizarre movements of the jaw, mouth, tongue, extremities), pseudoparkinsonism (rigidity, tremors, pill rolling, shuffling gait), suicidal thoughts, behaviors
• Monitor constipation, urinary retention daily; increase bulk, water in diet
• **Beers:** Avoid in older adults except for schizophrenia, bipolar disorder, or short-term use as an antiemetic during chemotherapy, increased risk of stroke
• **Hyperglycemia:** Assess for increased hyperglycemia in diabetic patient; monitor fasting blood sugar baseline and periodically
• **Metabolic syndrome:** Assess for large weight gain; increased B/P; increased FBS, cholesterol, and triglycerides

• **DRESS:** May be fatal; fever, hepatitis, cutaneus reactions, eosinophilia, nephritis, pneumonia, discontinue immediately

Patient problem
Distorted thinking process (uses)
Impaired sexual functioning (adverse reactions)
Risk for injury (adverse reactions)

Implementation
• Give antiparkinsonian agent for EPS
• Give decreased dose in geriatric
PO route
• Give with full glass of water/milk or with food to decrease GI upset, may give without regard to food
• **Orally disintegrating tabs:** open blister pack; place tab on tongue until dissolved; swallow; no water needed; do not break, crush, chew
• Store in tight, light-resistant container
IM route (Zyprexa Intramuscular)
• Inspect for particulate, discoloration before use, if present, do not use
• Dissolve contents of vials with 2.1 ml sterile water for injection (5 mg/ml), use immediately
• Do not use IV or SUBCUT
• Inject slowly, deep into muscle mass
IM route (Zyprexa Relprevv)

> **BLACK BOX WARNING:** Available only through restricted distribution program (Zyprexa Relprevv Patient Care program 877-772-9390) due to postinjection delirium/sedation syndrome; give at a facility with emergency services, monitor for 3 hr after injection

• Use gloves to prepare, irritating to skin
• Use deep IM gluteal inj only
• Use only diluent provided in kit; give q2-4wk using 19G 1.5-inch needle in kit, in obesity use 19G 2-inch or larger needle
• Provide supervised ambulation until stabilized on medication; do not involve in strenuous exercise program because fainting is possible; patients should not stand still for long periods
• Give increased fluids to prevent constipation
• Give sips of water, candy, gum for dry mouth
• Store in airtight, light-resistant container
• Give orally disintegrating tabs: open blister pack, place tab on tongue until dissolved, swallow; no water needed

Patient/family education

> **BLACK BOX WARNING:** Teach patient about postinjection delirium/sedation syndrome; teach about all symptoms

• **Suicidal thoughts, behaviors:** Advise patient and caregiver to report immediately suicidal thoughts or behaviors

---

• Teach patient to use good oral hygiene; frequent rinsing of mouth, candy, ice chips, sugarless gum for dry mouth
• Advise patient to avoid hazardous activities until product response is determined
• Advise patient that orthostatic hypotension occurs often and to rise from sitting or lying position gradually
• Advise patient to avoid hot tubs, hot showers, tub baths, since hypotension may occur
• Advise patient to avoid abrupt withdrawal of this product, or EPS may result; product should be withdrawn slowly
• Advise patient to avoid OTC preparations (cough, hay fever, cold) unless approved by prescriber, since serious product interactions may occur; avoid use with alcohol, CNS depressants, opioids, increased drowsiness may occur
• Advise patient that in hot weather, heat stroke may occur; take extra precautions to stay cool
• **Pregnancy/breastfeeding:** Identify if pregnancy is planned or suspected or if breastfeeding, may cause EPS in infant if used in third trimester, those pregnant should enroll in the National Pregnancy Registry for Atypical Antipsychotics 866-961-2388, excreted in breast milk, avoid breastfeeding

Evaluation
Positive therapeutic outcome
• Decrease in emotional excitement; hallucinations; delusions; paranoia; reorganization of patterns of thought, speech
• Teach patient to notify prescriber if pregnancy is planned or suspected, not to breastfeed
• Teach patient to take PO without regard to food

TREATMENT OF OVERDOSE:
Lavage if orally ingested; provide airway; do not induce vomiting or use epinephrine

⚠ HIGH ALERT
olaparib
(oh-lap′a-rib)
Lynparza
Func. class.: Antineoplastic-PARP
Chem. class.: Enzyme inhibitor

USES: Treatment of deleterious or suspected deleterious germline BRCA-mutated advanced ovarian cancer in patients who have not responded successfully to ≥3 prior courses of chemotherapy, as monotherapy

CONTRAINDICATIONS: Hypersensitivity, pregnancy

DOSAGE AND ROUTES
Adult female: PO 400 mg bid (tablets), 300 mg bid (capsules) until disease progression or unacceptable toxicity. Avoid use of concomitant strong and moderate CYP3A4 inhibitors if possible.

olmesartan (Rx)
(ol-meh-sar′tan)
Benicar, Olmetec ✦
Func. class.: Antihypertensive
Chem. class.: Angiotensin II receptor (type AT₁) antagonist

Do not confuse: Benicar/Mevacor

ACTION: Blocks the vasoconstrictor and aldosterone-secreting effects of angiotensin II; selectively blocks the binding of angiotensin II to the AT_1 receptor found in tissues

Therapeutic outcome: Decreased B/P

USES: Hypertension, alone or in combination with other antihypertensives

Pharmacokinetics
Absorption	Unknown
Distribution	Protein binding 90%
Metabolism	Unknown
Excretion	Urine (50% unchanged), feces
Half-life	Unknown

Pharmacodynamics
Onset	Unknown
Peak	1-2 hr
Duration	Unknown

CONTRAINDICATIONS
Hypersensitivity

BLACK BOX WARNING: Pregnancy

Precautions: Breastfeeding, children, geriatric, hepatic disease, HF, renal artery stenosis, ✦ African descent, hyperkalemia

DOSAGE AND ROUTES
Adult: PO single agent 20 mg/day initially in patients who are not volume depleted; may be increased to 40 mg/day if needed after 2 wk
Adolescent ≤16 yr/child ≥6 yr weighing ≥35 kg: PO 20 mg/day, may increase to max 40 mg/day after 2 wk
Adolescent ≤16 yr/child ≥6 yr weighing 20-35 kg: PO 10 mg/day, may increase to max 20 mg/day after 2 wk

Volume depletion
Adult: PO start with lower dose

Available forms: Tabs 5, 20, 40 mg

ADVERSE EFFECTS
CNS: *Dizziness,* fatigue, insomnia, syncope
CV: Chest pain, peripheral edema, tachycardia, *hypotension*
EENT: Sinusitis, rhinitis, pharyngitis
GI: *Diarrhea,* abdominal pain
META: Hyperkalemia
MS: Arthralgia, pain, rhabdomyolysis
RESP: *Upper respiratory infection,* bronchitis
SYST: Angioedema

INTERACTIONS
Individual drugs
Colesevelam: Decreased antihypertensive effect
Lithium: increased effect

Drug classifications
Antihypertensives (other), diuretics: increased antihypertensive effects
COX-2 inhibitors, NSAIDs: decreased antihypertensive effect
Antioxidants: increased effects
ACE inhibitors, Potassium supplements, potassium-sparing diuretics: increased hyperkalemia

Drug/herb
Aconite: increased toxicity, death
Astragalus, cola tree: increased or decreased antihypertensive effect
Garlic, Hawthorn: increased antihypertensive effect
Black licorice, Ephedra: decreased antihypertensive effect

NURSING CONSIDERATIONS
Assessment
• **Volume depletion:** Correct volume depletion before starting therapy
• **Hypertension:** Monitor B/P, pulse; note rate, rhythm, quality; electrolytes: sodium, potassium, chloride; baselines in renal, liver function tests before therapy begins; may use antihypertensives to control B/P if needed
• **Hypotension:** Place supine; may occur with hyponatremia or in those with volume depletion; more common in those also taking a diuretic
• **Heart failure:** Monitor for edema, weight daily, jugular vein distention, dyspnea

> **BLACK BOX WARNING: Assess for pregnancy;** this product can cause fetal death when given in pregnancy, assess for pregnancy before starting therapy, do not breastfeed

Patient problem
Risk for injury (adverse reactions)
Nonadherence (teaching)

Implementation
• Give without regard to meals
• Compounded suspension may be made in the pharmacy; refrigerate up to 1 mo; shake well before use

Patient/family education
• Advise to comply with dosage schedule, even if feeling better; not to double or skip doses; if a dose is missed take when remembered if not close to next dose
• Advise patient to notify prescriber of mouth sores, fever, swelling of hands or feet, irregular heartbeat, chest pain, severe chronic diarrhea, severe weight loss
• Teach that excessive perspiration, dehydration, vomiting, diarrhea may lead to fall in B/P; to consult prescriber if these occur, maintain adequate hydration
• Teach that product may cause dizziness, fainting; light-headedness may occur, avoid hazardous activities
• Advise to rise slowly to sitting or standing position to minimize orthostatic hypotension
• Advise to avoid all OTC medications, unless approved by prescriber, severe chronic diarrhea, severe weight loss
• Teach patient that blood glucose may increase and antidiabetic product may need dosage change
• Advise to inform all health care providers of medication use
• Advise to use proper technique for obtaining B/P and acceptable parameters
• Advise patient to notify health care professional immediately of swelling of the face, lips, tongue, or trouble breathing
• Inform patient that follow-up exams will be needed

> **BLACK BOX WARNING: Pregnancy/breastfeeding:** Identify if pregnancy is planned or suspected or if breastfeeding; not to be used in pregnancy or breastfeeding

Evaluation
Positive therapeutic outcome
• Decreased B/P

olopatadine ophthalmic
See Appendix B

olsalazine (Rx)
(ohl-sal'ah-zeen)
Dipentum
Func. class.: GI Antiinflammatory
Chem. class.: Salicylate derivative

Do not confuse: olsalazine/OLANZapine

ACTION: Bioconverted to 5-aminosalicylic acid, which decreases inflammation

Therapeutic outcome: Lessening of loose diarrhea stools and cramping

USES: Maintenance of remission of ulcerative colitis in patients intolerant to sulfasalazine

Pharmacokinetics

Absorption	Colon 99% converted to mesalamine
Distribution	Colon
Metabolism	Liver
Excretion	Feces
Half-life	0.9 hr

Pharmacodynamics

Onset	Unknown
Peak	1 hr
Duration	12 hr

CONTRAINDICATIONS
Hypersensitivity to this product or salicylates

Precautions: Pregnancy, breastfeeding, children <14 yr, impaired renal/hepatic function, severe allergy, bronchial asthma

DOSAGE AND ROUTES
Adult: PO 500 mg bid, max 3 g/day

Available forms: Caps 250 mg

ADVERSE EFFECTS
CNS: Headache, hallucinations, depression, vertigo, fatigue, dizziness
GI: Nausea, vomiting, abdominal pain, diarrhea, bloating, pancreatitis
INTEG: Rash, dermatitis, urticaria

INTERACTIONS
Individual drugs
AzaTHIOprine: increased toxicity
Mercaptopurine, thioguanine: increased myelosuppression
Low Molecular-weight heparins, discontinue before using this product: Increase bleeding risk: low
Varicella vaccine, do not use within 6 wk of olsalazine: Increase Reye's syndrome development
Warfarin: increased pro-time, INR

Drug/lab test
Increased: AST, ALT

NURSING CONSIDERATIONS
Assessment
• **Assess for allergic reaction:** rash, dermatitis, urticaria, pruritus, dyspnea, bronchospasm, sulfonamides
• **Colitis:** assess bowel pattern, number of stools, consistency, frequency, pain, mucus, abdominal pain before treatment and periodically

Patient problem
Pain (uses)
Diarrhea (uses)

Implementation
• Give total daily dose evenly spaced to minimize GI intolerance, give with food
• Store in tight, light-resistant container at room temperature

Patient/family education
• Teach patient that lab work and exams will be needed during treatment
• Advise patient to take as prescribed, take missed dose as soon as remembered
• Inform patient not to operate machinery or drive until effects are known, may cause dizziness
• Advise patient to notify prescriber if symptoms do not improve or if allergic reaction or sore throat occurs
• Teach patient to report diarrhea, rash, bleeding, bruising, fever, hallucinations or if symptoms do not improve after 2 mo of therapy

Evaluation
Positive therapeutic outcome
• Absence of fever, mucus in stools, diarrhea, abdominal pain

omeprazole (Rx, OTC)
(oh-mep'ra-zole)
Losec ✦, Olex ✦, PriLOSEC, PriLOSEC OTC
Func. class.: Antiulcer, proton pump inhibitor
Chem. class.: Benzimidazole

Do not confuse: PriLOSEC/Prinivil/omeprazole/fomepizole predniSONE/PROzac/Pristiq

ACTION: Suppresses gastric secretion by inhibiting hydrogen/potassium ATPase enzyme system in the gastric parietal cell; characterized as a gastric acid pump inhibitor, since it blocks the final step of acid production

Therapeutic outcome: Absence of duodenal ulcers; decreased gastroesophageal reflux

USES: Gastroesophageal reflux disease (GERD), severe erosive esophagitis, poorly responsive systemic GERD, pathologic hypersecretory conditions (Zollinger-Ellison syndrome, systemic mastocytosis, multiple endocrine adenomas); possibly effective for treatment of duodenal ulcers with or without antiinfectives for *Helicobacter pylori*

Pharmacokinetics

Absorption	Rapidly absorbed
Distribution	Protein binding (95%); gastric parietal cells
Metabolism	Liver, extensively; by CYP2C19 🖉 some Asians, Blacks, Caucasians are poor metabolizers
Excretion	Kidneys, feces
Half-life	½-1 hr; increased in the geriatric, hepatic disease

Pharmacodynamics

Onset	1 hr
Peak	½-3½ hr
Duration	3-4 days

CONTRAINDICATIONS
Hypersensitivity to this product or benzimidazoles

Precautions: Pregnancy, breastfeeding, children; Asian, Black patients, hepatic disease

DOSAGE AND ROUTES
Active duodenal ulcers
Adult: PO 20 mg/day × 4-8 wk; associated with *H. pylori* 40 mg qAM and clarithromycin 500 mg tid on days 1-14, then 20 mg/day days 15-28

Severe erosive esophagitis/poorly responsive GERD
Adult: PO (DEL REL cap/SUSP) 20 mg/day × 4-8 wk

Pathologic hypersecretory conditions
Adult: PO 60 mg/day; may increase to 120 mg tid; daily doses >80 mg should be divided

Gastric ulcer
Adult: PO 40 mg/day × 4-8 wk
Geriatric: PO max 20 mg/day

Heartburn (OTC)
Adult: PO 1 DEL REL tab (20 mg) daily before AM meal with glass of water

Available forms: Del rel caps 10, 20, 40 mg; del rel tabs (PriLOSEC OTC) 20 mg; granules for oral susp 2.5, 10 mg (del rel)

ADVERSE EFFECTS
CNS: *Headache, dizziness, asthenia*
GI: *Diarrhea, abdominal pain, vomiting, nausea, constipation, flatulence, acid regurgitation,* abdominal swelling, anorexia, irritable colon, esophageal candidiasis, dry mouth, hepatic failure, CDAD
INTEG: Rash, dry skin, urticaria, pruritus, alopecia
MISC: *Back pain,* fever, fatigue, malaise
RESP: *Upper respiratory tract infections, cough,* epistaxis, pneumonia

INTERACTIONS
Individual drugs
Ampicillin: decreased effect of ampicillin
Calcium carbonate: decreased absorption of calcium carbonate
Cyanocobalamin: decreased absorption of cyanocobalamin
CycloSPORINE: increased cycloSPORINE levels
Diazepam: increased serum levels of diazepam
Digoxin: increased serum levels, delayed absorption of digoxin
Disulfiram: increased disulfiram levels
Flurazepam: increased flurazepam level
Gefitinib: decreased effect of gefitinib
Indinavir: decreased effect of indinavir
Iron salts: decreased absorption
Ketoconazole: decreased absorption of ketoconazole
Phenytoin: increased serum levels of phenytoin
Triazolam: increased triazolam level
Warfarin: increased bleeding tendencies

Drug classifications
Iron products: decreased absorption of iron

Drug/lab test
Increased: alkaline phosphatase, AST, ALT, bilirubin, gastrin

NURSING CONSIDERATIONS
Assessment
• Assess GI system: bowel sounds, abdomen for pain and swelling, anorexia, diarrhea, blood in stools, emesis
• ***Clostridium difficile*-associated diarrhea (CDAD):** Assess for fever, abdominal pain, bloody stool, report to prescriber immediately, may occur up to several weeks after conclusion of therapy
• **Electrolyte imbalances:** hyponatremia, hypomagnesemia in those using this product 3 mo-1 yr; if hypomagnesemia occurs, use of magnesium supplement may be sufficient; if severe, discontinue use
• **Monitor hepatic enzymes:** AST, ALT, increased alkaline phosphatase during treatment; blood studies; CBC, differential during

treatment, blood dyscrasias may occur; vitamin B_{12} in long-term treatment
• **Beers:** Avoid scheduled use >8 wk in those with hypersecretory condition, esophagitis, risk of *Clostridium difficile*, and fractures

Patient problem
Pain (uses)
Diarrhea (adverse reactions)

Implementation
• Swallow sus rel caps whole; do not break, crush, chew, or open
• Give before patient eats; may give with antacids
• **Oral suspension:** Give on empty stomach at least 1 hr before food; mix 2.5 mg packet/5 ml water or 10 mg packet/15 ml water, stir and drink; swish container with water and drink if contents remain; may be used with NG tube

Patient/family education
• Advise patient to report severe diarrhea; black, tarry stools; abdominal cramps/pain, continuing headache; product may have to be discontinued
• Teach patient not to use OTC, Rx, or herbs without prescriber consent to take as prescribed, not to double or skip doses
• Teach patient to take as directed, even if feeling better; to take missed dose as soon as remembered; not to double; PriLOSEC OTC can take up to 4 days for full effect
• Caution patient to avoid driving and other hazardous activities until response to product is known, dizziness may occur
• Caution patient to avoid alcohol, salicylates, ibuprofen; may cause GI irritation
• **Pregnancy/breastfeeding:** Identify if pregnancy is planned or suspected or if breastfeeding

Evaluation
Positive therapeutic outcome
• Absence of epigastric pain, swelling, fullness

---

ondansetron (Rx)
(on-dan′sa-tron)
Ondissolve ❦, **Zofran, Zofran ODT, Zuplenz**
Func. class.: Antiemetic
Chem. class.: 5-HT receptor antagonist

Do not confuse: Zofran/Zantac

ACTION: Prevents nausea, vomiting by blocking serotonin (5-HT) peripherally, centrally, and in the small intestine

Therapeutic outcome: Control of nausea, vomiting

USES: Prevention of nausea, vomiting associated with cancer chemotherapy, radiotherapy, and prevention of postoperative nausea, vomiting

Pharmacokinetics

Absorption	Completely absorbed (**IV**)
Distribution	Unknown
Metabolism	Liver, extensively
Excretion	Kidneys
Half-life	3.5-4.7 hr

Pharmacodynamics
Unknown

CONTRAINDICATIONS
Hypersensitivity; phenylketonuric hypersensitivity (oral disintegrating tab), torsades de pointes

Precautions: Pregnancy, breastfeeding, children, geriatric, granisetron hypersensitivity, QT prolongation, torsades de pointes

DOSAGE AND ROUTES
Prevention of nausea/vomiting (cancer chemotherapy)
Adult and child 4-18 yr: **IV** 0.15 mg/kg infused over 15 min, 30 min before start of cancer chemotherapy, max 16 mg/dose; 0.15 mg/kg is given 4 hr and 8 hr after first dose or 16 mg as a single dose; dilute in 50 ml of D_5 or 0.9% NaCl before giving; **oral dissolving film** 24 mg dissolved on tongue 30 min prior to single day chemotherapy; **rect (unlabeled)** 16 mg daily 2 hr before chemotherapy; PO 8 mg ½ hr prior to chemotherapy, repeat 4, 8 hr after 1st dose
Child ≥4 yr: PO 4 mg ½ hr prior to chemotherapy

Prevention of nausea/vomiting (radiotherapy)
Adult: PO 8 mg tid, may repeat q8hr

Prevention of postoperative nausea/vomiting
Adult: **IV**/IM 4 mg undiluted over >30 sec prior to induction of anesthesia
Child 2-12 yr: **IV** 0.1 mg/kg (≤40 kg); 4 mg (≥40 kg), give ≥30 sec

Hepatic dose
Adult: PO/IM/IV max dose 8 mg daily

Available forms: Inj 2 mg/ml, 32 mg/50 ml (premixed); tabs 4, 8 mg; oral sol 4 mg/5 ml; oral disintegrating tabs 4, 8 mg; oral dissolving film 4.8 mg

---

ADVERSE EFFECTS

CNS: *Headache,* dizziness, drowsiness, fatigue, EPS

GI: *Diarrhea, constipation, abdominal pain,* dry mouth

MISC: Rash, bronchospasm (rare), *musculoskeletal pain, wound problems, shivering, fever, hypoxia, urinary retention*

INTERACTIONS

Individual drugs

Apomorphine: increased unconsciousness, hypotension: do not use together

CarBAMazepine, phenytoin, rifampin: decreased ondansetron effect

Drug classifications

Increased QT prolongation with other products that prolong QT

Drug/lab test

Increased: LFTs

NURSING CONSIDERATIONS

Assessment

• Assess for absence of nausea, vomiting during chemotherapy

• Assess for hypersensitivity reaction: rash, bronchospasm

• **Assess for EPS** shuffling gait, tremors, grimacing, rigidity

• **QT prolongation:** monitor ECG in those with hypokalemia, hypomagnesemia, cardiac disease and those receiving other products that increase QT

• **Serotonin syndrome:** occurs when other products are given that increase CNS or peripheral serotonin levels; agitation, confusion, dizziness, diaphoresis, flushing, tremor, seizures, nausea, vomiting, diarrhea, product should be discontinued

Patient problem

Nausea (uses)
Diarrhea (adverse reactions)
Constipation (adverse reactions)

Implementation

PO route

• Regular tab; protect from light (4-mg tab)

• **Oral disintegrating tab:** do not push through foil; gently remove and immediately place on tongue to dissolve, swallow with saliva

• **Oral dissolving film:** fold pouch along dotted line to expose near notch; while folded, tear and remove film, place film on tongue until dissolved, swallow after dissolved; to reach desired dose, administer successive films, allowing each to dissolve before using another

• Check for discoloration or particulate; if particulate is present, shake to dissolve

Oral solution

• Protect from light

• Measure in calibrated oral syringe or other calibrated device

IM route

• Visually inspect for particulate or discoloration

• May give 4 mg undiluted IM; inject deeply in large muscle mass, aspirate

Direct IV route

• Give undiluted 2 mg/ml immediately preceding anesthesia induction

Intermittent IV infusion

• Give **IV** after diluting a single dose in 50 ml of 0.9% NaCl or D₅W, 0.45% NaCl; give over 15 min

• Store at room temperature for 48 hr after dilution

• Do not use IV 32-mg dose in chemotherapy; nausea/vomiting due to QT prolongation, max 16 mg/dose (adult)

Y-site compatibilities: Aldesleukin, amifostine, amikacin, aztreonam, bleomycin, CARBOplatin, carmustine, ceFAZolin, ceforanide, cefotaxme, cefOXitin, cefTAZidime, ceftizoxime, cefuroxime, chlorproMAZINE, cimetidine, cisatracurium, CISplatin, cladribine, clindamycin, cyclophosphamide, cytarabine, dacarbazine, DACTINomycin, DAUNOrubicin, dexamethasone, diphenhydrAMINE, DOXOrubicin, DOXOrubicin liposome, doxycycline, droperidol, etoposide, famotidine, filgrastim, floxuridine, fluconazole, fludarabine, gentamicin, haloperidol, heparin, hydrocortisone, HYDROmorphone, hydrOXYzine, ifosfamide, imipenem/cilastatin, magnesium sulfate, mannitol, mechlorethamine, melphalan, meperidine, mesna, methotrexate, metoclopramide, miconazole, mitoMYcin, mitoXANtrone, morphine, PACLitaxel, pentostatin, potassium chloride, prochlorperazine, ranitidine, remifentanil, streptozocin, teniposide, thiotepa, ticarcillin, ticarcillin/clavulanate, vancomycin, vinBLAStine, vinCRIStine, vinorelbine, zidovudine

Patient/family education

• Instruct patient to report diarrhea, constipation, rash, changes in respirations, or discomfort at insertion site, serotonin syndrome, EPS symptoms

• Teach patient reason for medication and expected results

• Drink with full glass of water (PO)

• **Oral disintegrating tab:** Remove strip from pouch, place on tongue, and allow to dissolve, drink water

Evaluation

Positive therapeutic outcome

• Absence of nausea, vomiting of chemotherapy, or surgery

oritavancin
(or-it′a-van′sin)
Orbactiv
Func. class.: Antiinfective agent
Chem. class.: Glycopeptide

ACTION: Inhibits bacterial cell-wall biosynthesis by preventing transglycosylation (polymerization) by binding to precursors, as well as by preventing cross-linking by binding to the peptide bridging segments of the cell wall; also disrupts the bacterial cell membrane integrity, resulting in depolarization, increased permeability, and eventual cell death

Therapeutic outcome: Resolution of infection

USES: *Enterococcus faecalis, Enterococcus faecium, Staphylococcus aureus* (MRSA), *Staphylococcus aureus* (MSSA), *Streptococcus agalactiae* (group B streptococci), *Streptococcus anginosus, Streptococcus constellatus, Streptococcus dysgalactiae, Streptococcus intermedius, Streptococcus pyogenes* (group A β-hemolytic streptococci); treatment of acute bacterial skin and skin structure infections due to gram-positive organisms, including cellulitis/erysipelas, major cutaneous abscesses, and wound infections

Pharmacokinetics

Absorption	Complete
Distribution	85% protein binding
Metabolism	Unknown
Excretion	Urine, unchanged
Half-life	245 hr

Pharmacodynamics

Onset	Unknown
Peak	Infusion's end
Duration	Unknown

CONTRAINDICATIONS: Hypersensitivity

Precautions: Anticoagulant therapy, antimicrobial resistance, breastfeeding, colitis, diarrhea, inflammatory bowel disease, infusion reactions, pregnancy, *Clostridium difficile* diarrhea, vancomycin hypersensitivity, viral infection

DOSAGE AND ROUTES
Adult: IV 1200 mg as a single dose

Available forms: Powder for injection: 400 mg

ADVERSE EFFECTS
CNS: Dizziness, flushing, headache
CV: Sinus tachycardia, phlebitis
GI: Nausea, vomiting, diarrhea, CDAD
HEMA: Anemia, eosinophilia
INTEG: Rash, vasculitis, pruritus, angioedema, infusion-related reaction
MISC: Wheezing, bronchospasm
MS: Myalgia, osteomyelitis

INTERACTIONS
Drug classifications
Products metabolized by CYP2D6 and CYP3A4: increased toxicity
Increase: bleeding risk: warfarin, avoid concurrent use

Drug/lab test
Increased: LFTs, uric acid, INR, aPTT

NURSING CONSIDERATIONS
Assessment
• **Infection:** Assess wounds, temperature, sputum, urine; monitor WBC baseline and periodically, report changes
• Monitor CBC and differential
• Infusion-related reactions, symptoms of red man's syndrome (flushing, urticaria, pruritus), slow or stop infusion
• Avoid heparin for 5 days after use of this product, a false elevated aPTT and coagulation studies occur
• Assess for fever; report to health care professional, may be *Clostridium difficile*-associated diarrhea (CDAD), may start up to 8 wk after completion of treatment
• C&S before therapy, may give product before receiving results

Patient problem
Infection (uses)
Diarrhea (adverse reactions)

Implementation
• Visually inspect for particulate matter and discoloration beforehand; the reconstituted solution is clear, colorless to pale yellow
• **Reconstitution:** Reconstitute each 400-mg vial with 40 ml sterile water for injection. Three vials are necessary for a single dose; gently swirl until dissolved.
• **Dilution:** Withdraw and discard 120 ml from a 1000-ml intravenous bag of D_5W, transfer 40 ml solution from each of the 3 reconstituted vials to the D_5W IV bag (1.2 mg/ml)
• **Storage:** Refrigerate or store at room temperature. The combined storage time (from reconstitution to dilution) and 3-hour infusion time should not exceed 6 hr at room temperature or 12 hr if refrigerated.

Intermittent IV INF
• Infuse over 3 hr, do not infuse with other medications or electrolytes, do not use saline-based solution

Patient/family education
• Teach patient reason for product, expected result
• Advise patient product is used only once to resolve infection
• **Bowel function:** To notify health care professional of diarrhea, bloody stools, cramping, fever, do not self-treat
• Teach patient to notify prescriber of rash, facial swelling, dyspnea
• Teach patient to avoid use of all OTC, herbs, supplements unless approved by prescriber
• **Pregnancy/breastfeeding:** Teach patient to notify prescriber if pregnancy is planned or suspected

Evaluation
Positive therapeutic outcome
• Resolution of infection

---

oseltamivir (Rx)
(oh-sell-tam'ih-ver)
Tamiflu
Func. class.: Antiviral
Chem. class.: Neuraminidase inhibitor

ACTION: Inhibits influenza virus neuraminidase with possible alteration of virus particle aggregation and release

Therapeutic outcome: Decreased symptoms of influenza type A

USES: Prevention/treatment of influenza type A or B

Pharmacokinetics

Absorption	Rapidly absorbed
Distribution	Protein binding 3%
Metabolism	Converted to oseltamivir carboxylate (active form)
Excretion	Eliminated by conversion, urine 99%
Half-life	1-3 hr (active form)

Pharmacodynamics

Onset	Unknown
Peak	Unknown
Duration	Up to 12 hr

CONTRAINDICATIONS
Hypersensitivity

Precautions: Pregnancy, geriatric, renal/hepatic/pulmonary/cardiac disease, infants, children, neonates, psychosis, viral infection, breastfeeding

DOSAGE AND ROUTES
Treatment
Adult and child >40 kg: PO 75 bid mg × 5 days, begin treatment within 2 days of onset of symptoms
Child 23-40 kg and ≥1 yr: PO 60 mg bid × 5 days
Child 15-23 kg and ≥1 yr: PO 45 mg bid × 5 days
Child ≤15 kg and ≥1 yr: PO 30 mg bid × 5 days

Prevention
Adult and child ≥13 yr: PO 75 mg/day × ≥10 days; begin treatment within 2 days of contact, max use 6 wk

Renal dose
Adult: PO CCr 10-30 ml/min 75 mg/day × 5 days (treatment); 75 mg every other day or 30 mg/day (prophylaxis)

Available forms: Caps 30, 45, 75 mg; powder for oral susp 6 mg/ml

ADVERSE EFFECTS
CNS: Headache, fatigue, insomnia, dizziness, seizures, delirium, self-injury (children)
GI: *Nausea, vomiting*
INTEG: Toxic epidermal necrolysis, Stevens-Johnson syndrome, erythema multiforme
RESP: Cough

INTERACTIONS
Influenza virus vaccine: Decreased effect, avoid prior to use (2 days) or after (14 days)

NURSING CONSIDERATIONS
Assessment
• **Influenza:** assess for symptoms of influenza A: increased temperature, malaise, aches and pains
• **Behavioral symptoms:** Assess for hallucinations, abnormal behaviors, delirium (rare)

Patient problem
Infection (uses)
Risk for infection (uses)

Implementation
• Give within 2 days of symptoms of influenza; continue for 5 days
• Give at least 4 hr before bedtime to prevent insomnia
• 12 mg/ml concentration will be available for a limited time, new product is 6 mg/ml concentration, take care to give correct dose
• Give without regard to food, give with food for GI upset, take with full glass of water

• **Oral susp:** loosen powder from side of bottle 55 ml; shake well (6 mg/ml); remove child-resistant cap and push bottle adapter into neck of bottle, close tightly with child-resistant cap to ensure sealing; use within 17 days of preparation when refrigerated or 10 days at room temperature, write expiration date on bottle, shake well before use, use oral syringe provided but only with markings for 30, 45, 60 ml; confirm dosing instructions are in same units as syringe provided
• Store in airtight, dry container

Patient/family education
• Teach patient about all aspects of product therapy
• Teach patient to avoid hazardous activities if dizziness occurs
• Advise patient to take as soon as symptoms appear, to take full course, even if feeling better
• Advise patient to take missed dose as soon as remembered if within 2 hr of next dose
• Teach patient to stop product immediately and report to prescriber skin rash, delirium, psychosis, hallucinations (child)
• Advise patient that product is not a substitute for a flu shot
• Inform patient to avoid other products without approval of prescriber
• **Pregnancy/breastfeeding:** Identify if pregnancy is planned or suspected or if breastfeeding

Evaluation
Positive therapeutic outcome
• Absence of fever, malaise, cough, dyspnea in influenza A

RARELY USED

osimertinib
(oh-si-mer′ ti-nib)
Tagrisso
Func. class.: Antineoplastic, epidermal growth factor receptor inhibitor

---

USES: Metastatic epidermal growth factor receptor T790M mutation positive non–small cell lung cancer after other treatment with EGFR tyrosine kinase inhibitor

CONTRAINDICATIONS: Hypersensitivity, pregnancy, breastfeeding, strong CYP3A4 inhibitors or inducers

DOSAGE AND ROUTES
Adult: PO 80 mg qday until disease progression or unacceptable toxicity

---

RARELY USED

ospemifene
(os-pem′ i-feen)
Osphena
Func. class.: Hormone, estrogen agonist, antagonist

USES: Severe dyspareunia due to menopausal vaginal atropy

CONTRAINIDCATIONS: Hypersensitivity, abnormal genital bleeding, estrogen-dependent cancers, thrombosis, pregnancy, breastfeeding

DOSAGE AND ROUTES
Adult: PO 60 mg qday

RARELY USED

oxacillin
(ox-a-sill′in)
Func. class: Anti-infective, penicillinase-resistant penicillin

---

USES: Bone, joint infections, UTI, endocarditis, septicemia, meningitis

CONTRAINDICATIONS: Hypersensitivity to this product or penicillins or cephalosporins (cross-sensitivity)

DOSAGE AND ROUTES
Adult and child ≥40 kg: IM/IV 250-2000 mg q4-6 hr, max 12 g/day
Child <40 kg IM/IV 100-200 mg/kg/day divided q4-6 hr, max 12 g/day

---

⚠ HIGH ALERT

oxaliplatin (Rx)
(ox-al-i′plat-in)
Eloxatin
Func. class.: Antineoplastic
Chem. class.: 3rd-generation platinum analog, alkylating agent

---

ACTION: Forms cross links, inhibiting DNA replication and transcription, cell-cycle nonspecific

Therapeutic outcome: Decreased size of tumor, spread of malignancy

---

USES: Metastatic carcinoma of the colon or rectum in combination with 5-FU/leucovorin

Unlabeled uses: Relapsed or refractory non-Hodgkin's lymphoma, advanced ovarian cancer

Pharmacokinetics

Absorption	Complete
Distribution	15% of platinum in systemic circulation; 85% is either in tissues or being eliminated in urine, protein binding 90%
Metabolism	Liver
Excretion	Urine
Half-life	40 days

Pharmacodynamics

Unknown

CONTRAINDICATIONS

Pregnancy, breastfeeding, radiation therapy or chemotherapy within 1 mo, thrombocytopenia, smallpox vaccination

> **BLACK BOX WARNING:** Hypersensitivity to this product or other platinum products

Precautions: Children, geriatric, pneumococcus vaccination, renal disease

DOSAGE AND ROUTES

Dosage protocols may vary

Adult: IV INF *Day 1:* oxaliplatin 85 mg/m² in 250-500 ml D₅W and leucovorin 200 mg/m² in D₅W, give both over 2 hr at the same time in separate bags using a Y-line, followed by 5-FU 400 mg/m² **IV** BOL over 2-4 min, then 5-FU 600 mg/m² **IV** INF in 500 ml D₅W as a 22-hr CONT INF; *Day 2:* leucovorin 200 mg/m² **IV** INF over 2 hr, then 5-FU 400 mg/m² **IV** BOL over 2-4 min, then 5-FU 600 mg/m² **IV** INF in 500 ml D₅W as a 22-hr CONT INF; repeat cycle q2wk

With 5-FU/LV for adjuvant treatment of stage III colon cancer in those who have had complete resection of the primary tumor

Renal dose

Adult: IV CCr <30 ml/min: reduce starting dose to 65 mg/m²

Available forms: Powder for inj 50, 100 mg single-use vials (5 mg/ml); solution for inj 50 mg/10 ml, 100 mg/20 ml, 200 mg/40 ml

ADVERSE EFFECTS

CNS: Peripheral neuropathy, fatigue, headache, dizziness, insomnia, reversible posterior leukoencephalopathy syndrome
CV: Cardiac abnormalities, thromboembolism
EENT: *Decreased visual acuity, tinnitus, hearing loss*
GI: *Severe nausea, vomiting, diarrhea, weight loss,* stomatitis, anorexia, gastroesophageal reflux, constipation, dyspepsia, mucositis, flatulence
GU: Hematuria, dysuria, creatinine
HEMA: Thrombocytopenia, leukopenia, pancytopenia, neutropenia, anemia, hemolytic uremic syndrome
INTEG: *Alopecia,* rash, flushing, extravasation, redness, swelling, pain at inj site
META: Hypokalemia
RESP: Fibrosis, dyspnea, cough, rhinitis, URI, pharyngitis
SYST: Anaphylaxis, angioedema

INTERACTIONS

Drug classifications

Class Ia/III antidysrythmics: Increased QT prolongation
Live virus vaccines: decreased antibody response
Myelosuppressives: increased myelosuppression
Taxanes: increased oxaliplatin toxicity
Nephrotoxics: Increased nephrotoxicity

Drug/lab test

Increased: ALT, AST, bilirubin, creatinine
Decreased: potassium, neutrophils, WBC, platelets

NURSING CONSIDERATIONS

Assessment

• **Bone marrow depression:** monitor CBC, differential, platelet count weekly; withhold product if WBC is <4000 or platelet count is <100,000; notify prescriber of results
• Monitor renal function tests: BUN, creatinine, serum uric acid, urine CCr before, electrolytes during therapy; dose should not be given if BUN >19 mg/dl; creatinine <1.5 mg/dl; I&O ratio; report fall in urine output of <30 ml/hr

> **BLACK BOX WARNING: Assess for anaphylaxis:** wheezing, tachycardia, facial swelling, fainting, rash, dyspnea, hives; discontinue product and report to prescriber; resuscitation equipment should be nearby with EPINEPHrine, corticosteroids

• **Reversible posterior leukoencephalopathy syndrome:** Assess for diarrhea, infection, fever; notify health care professional immediately
• Monitor temp (may indicate beginning infection)
• Monitor liver function tests before, during therapy (bilirubin, AST, ALT, LDH) as needed or monthly
• **Assess for bleeding:** hematuria, guaiac, bruising or petechiae, mucosa or orifices; obtain prescription for viscous lidocaine (Xylocaine)

• **Peripheral neuropathy:** usually occurs 1-2 days of use; may diminish in 2 wk; some may be permanent; avoid use of cold or ice that will make condition worse
• **Pulmonary fibrosis:** assess for cough, crackles, dyspnea, pulmonary infiltrate; discontinue immediately; may be fatal

Patient problem

Nausea (adverse reactions)
Risk for injury (adverse reactions)
Risk for infection (adverse reactions)

Implementation

Intermittent IV INF route

• Premedicate with antiemetics including 5-HT₃ blockers, with or without dexamethasone, prehydration is not needed
• Do not reconstitute or dilute with sodium chloride or any chloride-containing solutions, do not use aluminum equipment during any preparation or administration, will degrade platinum; do not refrigerate unopened powder or solution; do not freeze; protect from light
• Use cytotoxic handling procedures; prepare in biological cabinet using gown, gloves, mask; do not allow product to come in contact with skin; use soap and water if contact occurs
• EPINEPHrine, antihistamines, corticosteroids for hypersensitivity reaction
• **Lyophilized powder:** reconstitute vial 50 mg/10 ml, or 100 mg/20 ml sterile water for inj or D₅W, after reconstitution, solution may be stored for ≤24 hr in refrigerator, after dilution in 250-500 ml D₅W, may store ≤24 hr in refrigerator or 6 hr at room temp, infuse over 2 hr
• **Aqueous solution:** dilute in 250-500 ml of D₅W, after dilution may store ≤24 hr refrigerator, 6 hr at room temp, infuse over 2 hr

Y-site compatibilities: Alfentanil, amifostine, amikacin, aminocaproic acid, amiodarone, amphotericin B colloidal, amphotericin B lipid complex, amphotericin B liposome, ampicillin, ampicillin-sulbactam, anidulafungin, atenolol, atracurium, azithromycin, aztreonam, bivalirudin, bleomycin, bumetanide, buprenorphine, butorphanol, calcium chloride/gluconate, CARBOplatin, caspofungin, ceFAZolin, cefotaxime, cefoTEtan, cefOXitin, cefTAZidime, ceftizoxime, cefTRIAXone, cefuroxime, chloramphenicol, chlorproMAZINE, cimetidine, ciprofloxacin, cisatracurium, CISplatin, clindamycin, cyclophosphamide, cycloSPORINE, cytarabine, dacarbazine, DACTINomycin, DAPTOmycin, DAUNOrubicin, dexamethasone, digoxin, diltiazem, diphenhydrAMINE, DOBUTamine, DOCEtaxel, dolasetron, DOPamine, doxacurium, DOXOrubicin, doxycycline, droperidol, enalaprilat, ePHEDrine, EPINEPHrine,

epirubicin, ertapenem, erythromycin, esmolol, etoposide, famotidine, fenoldopam, fentaNYL, fluconazole, fludarabine, foscarnet, fosphenytoin, furosemide, gatifloxacin, gemcitabine, gemtuzumab, gentamicin, glycopyrrolate, granisetron, haloperidol, heparin, hydrALAZINE, hydrocortisone, HYDROmorphone, hydrOXYzine, IDArubicin, ifosfamide, imipenem-cilastatin, inamrinone, insulin (regular), irinotecan, isoproterenol, ketorolac, labetalol, leucovorin, levofloxacin, levorphanol, lidocaine, linezolid, LORazepam, magnesium sulfate, mannitol, meperidine, meropenem, mesna, metaraminol, methyldopate, methylPREDNISolone, metoclopramide, metoprolol, metroNIDAZOLE, midazolam, milrinone, minocycline, mitoMYcin, mitoXANtrone, mivacurium, morphine, nafcillin, nalbuphine, naloxone, nesiritide, niCARdipine, nitroglycerin, nitroprusside, norepinephrine, octreotide, ondansetron, PACLitaxel, palonosetron, pancuronium, PEMEtrexed, pentamidine, pentazocine, phenylephrine, piperacillin, polymyxin B, potassium chloride/phosphates, procainamide, prochlorperazine, promethazine, propranolol, quiNIDine, quinupristin-dalfopristin, ranitidine, rocuronium, sodium acetate/phosphates, succinylcholine, SUFentanil, sulfamethoxazole-trimethoprim, tacrolimus, teniposide, theophylline, thiotepa, ticarcillin, ticarcillin-clavulanate, tigecycline, tirofiban, tobramycin, tolazoline, topotecan, trimethobenzamide, vancomycin, vasopressin, vecuronium, verapamil, vinBLAStine, vinCRIStine, vinorelbine, voriconazole, zidovudine, zoledronic acid

Patient/family education

• **Advise patient to report signs of infection:** increased temp, sore throat, flulike symptoms
• **Advise patient to report signs of anemia:** fatigue, headache, faintness, shortness of breath, irritability
• **Advise patient to report bleeding;** avoid use of razors, commercial mouthwash
• Advise patient to avoid aspirin, ibuprofen, NSAIDs, alcohol; may cause GI bleeding
• Advise patient to report any changes in breathing, coughing
• Advise patient to report numbness, tingling in face or extremities, poor hearing or joint pain, swelling
• Advise patient not to receive vaccines during treatment
• **Pregnancy/breastfeeding:** Identify if pregnancy is planned or suspected or if breastfeeding;
• Advise patient to use contraception during treatment and 4 mo after; this product may cause infertility
• Teach patient to avoid contact with cold (air, ice, liquid); causes acute dysesthesias

---

Evaluation
Positive therapeutic outcome
• Decreased tumor size, spread of malignancy

⚠ HIGH ALERT

oxazepam (Rx)
(ox-az'e-pam)
Novoxapan ✳, **Oxpam** ✳, **Serax** ✳,
Zopex ✳
Func. class.: Sedative-hypnotic;
antianxiety
Chem. class.: Benzodiazepine,
short-acting
Controlled substance schedule IV

ACTION: Depresses subcortical levels of CNS, including limbic system, reticular formation; potentiates GABA

Therapeutic outcome: Decreased anxiety, successful alcohol withdrawal, relaxation

USES: Anxiety, alcohol withdrawal

Pharmacokinetics

Absorption	Well absorbed
Distribution	Widely distributed; crosses placenta, blood-brain barrier, protein binding 95%
Metabolism	Liver
Excretion	Kidneys, breast milk
Half-life	5-15 hr

Pharmacodynamics

Onset	½-1½ hr
Peak	Unknown
Duration	6-12 hr

CONTRAINDICATIONS
Pregnancy, breastfeeding, children <6 yr, hypersensitivity to benzodiazepines, closed-angle glaucoma, psychosis

Precautions: Geriatric, debilitated, renal/hepatic disease, depression, suicidal ideation, dementia, sleep apnea, seizure disorder

BLACK BOX WARNING: Depressants, respiratory depression

DOSAGE AND ROUTES
Anxiety
Adult: PO 15-30 mg tid-qid, max 120 mg/day
Geriatric: PO 10 mg daily bid-tid, max 60 mg/day

Alcohol withdrawal
Adult: PO 15-30 mg tid-qid

Severe anxiety syndrome; agitation; anxiety with depression
Adult and child >12 yr: PO 15-30 mg tid-qid

Available forms: Caps 10, 15, 30 mg

ADVERSE EFFECTS
CNS: *Dizziness, drowsiness,* confusion, headache, anxiety, tremors, fatigue, depression, insomnia, hallucinations, paradoxical excitement, transient amnesia
CV: *Orthostatic hypotension,* ECG changes, tachycardia, hypotension
EENT: *Blurred vision,* tinnitus, mydriasis
GI: Nausea, vomiting, anorexia, drug-induced hepatitis
HEMA: Leukopenia
INTEG: Rash, dermatitis, itching
SYST: Dependence

INTERACTIONS
Individual drugs
Alcohol: increased CNS depression
Disulfiram: increased oxazepam effects
Levodopa: decreased effects of levodopa
Phenytoin, theophylline, valproic acid: decreased oxazepam effects

Drug classifications

BLACK BOX WARNING: CNS depressants: increased oxazepam effects, respiratory depression

BLACK BOX WARNING: Oral contraceptives: increased or decreased oxazepam effect

Drug/herb
Kava, melatonin, valerian: increased CNS depression

Drug/lab test
Increased: AST, ALT, serum bilirubin
Decreased: WBC

NURSING CONSIDERATIONS
Assessment

BLACK BOX WARNING: Respiratory depression: Not to be used in preexisting respiratory depression, use cautiously in severe pulmonary disease, monitor respirations

• Monitor CBC and LFTs, periodically
• **Assess mental status:** mood, sensorium, anxiety, affect, sleeping pattern, drowsiness,

---

dizziness, suicidal thoughts, behavior; physical dependency, withdrawal symptoms: anxiety, panic attacks, agitation, seizures, headache, nausea, vomiting, muscle pain, weakness, sedation suicidal thoughts, behavior; indications of increasing tolerance and abuse

• Monitor B/P with patient lying, standing; pulse; if systolic B/P drops 20 mm Hg, hold product, notify prescriber

• **Beers:** Avoid in older adults, delirium, cognitive impairment may occur

Patient problem
Anxiety (uses)
Risk for injury (adverse reactions)

Implementation
• Give with food or milk for GI symptoms; tab may be crushed if patient is unable to swallow medication whole
• Taper product (0.5 mg q3day) before discontinuing

Patient/family education
• Teach patient that product may be taken without regard to food or fluids; tab may be crushed or swallowed whole
• Caution patient not to use for everyday stress or longer than 4 mo unless directed by prescriber; not to take more than prescribed amount; not to double doses or skip doses
• Advise patient to avoid OTC preparations, herbals, supplements unless approved by prescriber; alcohol and CNS depressants will increase CNS depression
• Caution patient to avoid driving and activities that require alertness, since drowsiness may occur; to avoid alcohol and other psychotropic medications; to rise slowly or fainting may occur, especially geriatric; that drowsiness may worsen at beginning of treatment
• Caution patient not to discontinue medication abruptly after long-term use; withdrawal symptoms include vomiting, cramping, tremors, seizures
• Advise patient to use sugarless gum, hard candy, frequent sips of water for dry mouth
• Teach patient that drowsiness may worsen at beginning of treatment
• **Pregnancy/breastfeeding:** Teach patient to notify prescriber if pregnancy is planned or suspected

Evaluation
Positive therapeutic outcome
• Decreased anxiety, restlessness, sleeplessness (short-term treatment only)

TREATMENT OF OVERDOSE:
Lavage, VS, supportive care

OXcarbazepine (Rx)
(ox'kar-baz'uh-peen)
Oxtellar XR, Trileptal
Func. class.: Anticonvulsant

Do not confuse: OXcarbazepine/carBAMazepine

ACTION: May inhibit nerve impulses by limiting influx of sodium ions across cell membrane in motor cortex

Therapeutic outcome: Absence of seizures

USES: Partial seizures

Unlabeled uses: Trigeminal neuralgia

Pharmacokinetics

Absorption	Unknown
Distribution	Unknown
Metabolism	Liver; 95% renal extraction
Excretion	Unknown
Half-life	Unknown

Pharmacodynamics

Onset	Unknown
Peak	4-6 hr
Duration	Unknown

CONTRAINDICATIONS
Hypersensitivity

Precautions: Pregnancy, breastfeeding, children <4 yr, hypersensitivity to carbamazepine, renal disease, fluid restriction, hyponatremia, abrupt discontinuation, suicidal ideation, ✪ positive for HLA-B 1502 allele

DOSAGE AND ROUTES
Seizures adjunctive therapy
Adult: PO 300 mg bid, may be increased by 600 mg/day in divided doses bid at weekly intervals; maintenance 1200 mg/day; **ext rel** 600 mg/day × 1 wk, increase weekly in 600 mg/day increments to 1200-2400 mg/day

Child 4-16 yr: PO 8-10 mg/kg/day divided bid, dose is determined by weight, increase by 5 mg/kg/day q3 days, max doses are weight dependent

Child 2≤4 yr: PO 8-10 mg/kg daily in two divided doses, max 600 mg daily

Conversion to monotherapy in partial seizures
Adult: PO 300 mg bid with reduction in other anticonvulsants, increase OXcarbazepine by 600 mg/day qwk over 2-4 wk; withdraw other anticonvulsants over 3-6 wk, max 2400 mg/day

Initiation of monotherapy in partial seizures
Adult: PO 300 mg bid, increase by 300 mg/day q3day to 1200 mg divided bid, max 2400 mg/day

Renal dose
Adult: PO CCr <30 ml/min 150 mg bid and increase slowly

Available forms: Film-coated tabs 150, 300, 600 mg; oral susp 300 mg/5 ml; ext rel tab 150, 300, 600 mg

ADVERSE EFFECTS
CNS: *Headache, dizziness, confusion, fatigue,* feeling abnormal, ataxia, abnormal gait, tremors, anxiety, agitation, worsening of seizures, suicidal ideation/behavior
CV: *Hypotension,* chest pain, edema, bradycardia, syncope
EENT: *Blurred vision, diplopia, nystagmus,* rhinitis, sinusitis
ENDO: Hypothyroidism, hot flashes
GI: *Nausea, constipation, diarrhea,* anorexia, vomiting, abdominal pain, gastritis
GU: Urinary frequency, hematuria, menses change
INTEG: Purpura, rash, acne
META: Hyponatremia
RESP: Flulike symptoms
SYST: Angioedema, anaphylaxis, Stevens-Johnson syndrome, toxic epidermal necrolysis, drug reaction with eosinophilia and systemic symptoms (DRESS)

INTERACTIONS
Individual products
Alcohol: increased CNS depression
CarBAMazepine: decreased carBAMazepine level, decreased OXcarbazepine levels
Felodipine: decreased effects of felodipine
PHENobarbital, valproic acid, verapamil: decreased OXcarbazepine level
Phenytoin: decreased OXcarbazepine level

Drug classifications
Contraceptives (oral): decreased oral contraceptive level
CYP3A4 substrates (cyclosporine, itraconazole, rivaroxaban): decreased effect of substrates

Drug/herb
Ginkgo: increased anticonvulsant effect
Ginseng, santonica: decreased anticonvulsant effect

Drug/lab test
Decreased: sodium

NURSING CONSIDERATIONS
Assessment
• **Assess seizure activity,** including frequency, duration, and aura; provide seizure precautions

• Assess mental status including mood, sensorium, affect, behavioral changes, suicidal thoughts, behavior; if mental status changes, notify prescriber; usually occurs within the first 3 mo of treatment, but may occur ≤1 yr; if this product is being used with other products that decrease sodium, monitor sodium levels
• **Assess for serious skin reactions:** angioedema, anaphylaxis, Stevens-Johnson syndrome
• **Pregnancy:** pregnant patients should enroll in Antiepileptic Drug Pregnancy Registry 888-233-2334, do not breastfeed, excreted in breast milk
• **Beers:** Avoid in older adults unless safer alternatives are not available, ataxia, impaired psychomotor function may occur

Patient problem
Risk for injury (uses, adverse reactions)

Implementation
• Store product at room temperature
• Provide assistance with ambulation during early part of treatment; dizziness may occur
• Give product with food, milk to decrease GI symptoms
• **Oral susp:** shake well, use calibrated oral syringe provided, use or discard within 7 days of opening
• **Ext rel:** do not crush, break, or chew

Patient/family education
• Caution patient to avoid driving, other activities that require alertness
• Instruct patient to take twice a day at same intervals (immediate release)
• Advise patient not to discontinue medication quickly after long-term use, seizures may increase
• Instruct patient to avoid use of alcohol while taking this medication
• Instruct patient to use alternative contraception if using hormonal method, to report if pregnancy is planned or suspected, pregnancy
• Teach patient caregivers to report skin rashes immediately; serious skin reactions can occur
• Instruct patient to inform prescriber if allergic to carBAMazepine; multisystem hypersensitivity may occur, to report fever, other allergic symptoms
• Instruct patient to report suicidal thoughts/behavior immediately

Evaluation
Positive therapeutic outcome
- Decreased seizure activity

TREATMENT OF OVERDOSE:
Give 0.9% NaCl (hypotensive state), atropine (bradycardia); use benzodiazepines, barbiturates for seizures

oxybutynin (Rx, OTC)
(ox-i-byoo'ti-nin)
Ditropan XL, Oxytrol ✤

Oxybutynin gel
Gelnique

Oxybutynin, Transdermal
Oxytrol, Oxytrol for Women
Func. class.: Anticholinergic, urinary antispasmatic
Chem. class.: Synthetic tertiary amine

Do not confuse: Ditropan/diazepam/diprivan

ACTION: Relaxes smooth muscles in urinary tract by inhibiting acetylcholine at postganglionic sites

Therapeutic outcome: Decreased symptoms of urgency, nocturia, incontinence

USES: Antispasmodic for neurogenic bladder, overactive bladder in females (OTC)

Pharmacokinetics

Absorption	Rapidly absorbed
Distribution	Unknown
Metabolism	Liver
Excretion	Unknown
Half-life	Unknown

Pharmacodynamics

Onset	½-1 hr
Peak	3-4 hr
Duration	6-10 hr

CONTRAINDICATIONS
Hypersensitivity, GI obstruction, urinary retention, glaucoma, severe colitis, myasthenia gravis, unstable CV, infants

Precautions: Pregnancy, breastfeeding, children <12 yr, geriatric, suspected glaucoma, cardiac disease, dementia

DOSAGE AND ROUTES
Adult: PO 5 mg bid-tid, max 5 mg qid; ext rel tabs 5-10 mg/day, may increase by 5 mg, max 30 mg/day; transdermal apply one patch to abdomen, hip, buttock 2 ×/wk (q3-4day); GEL apply contents of 1 packet to abdomen, upper arms, shoulders, thighs daily
Geriatric: PO 2.5-5 mg bid-tid, increase by 2.5 mg q several days
Child ≥6 yr: PO 5 mg bid, not to exceed 5 mg tid; ext rel 5 mg/day, max 20 mg/day
Child 1-5 yr: PO 0.2 mg/kg/dose 2-3 ×/day

Available forms: Syr 5 mg/5 ml; tabs 5 mg; ext rel tabs 5, 10, 15 mg; transdermal 3.9 mg/day; top gel 10% (Gelnique)

ADVERSE EFFECTS
CNS: *Anxiety, restlessness, dizziness,* somnolence, insomnia, nervousness, seizures, headache, drowsiness, confusion
CV: *Palpitations, sinus tachycardia,* hypertension, peripheral edema, QT prolongation
EENT: Blurred vision, increased intraocular tension; dry mouth, throat, dry eyes
GI: *Nausea, vomiting, anorexia,* abdominal pain, constipation, *dyspepsia,* diarrhea, taste perversion, GERD
GU: Dysuria, impotence, retention, hesitancy
MISC: Hyperthermia, anaphylaxis, angioedema

INTERACTIONS
Individual drugs
Acetaminophen: decreased levels of acetaminophen
Amantadine: increased anticholinergic effects
Atenolol: increased levels of atenolol
Digoxin: increased levels of digoxin
Haloperidol, chloroquine, droperidol, pentamidine, arsenic trioxide, levomethadyl: increased QT prolongation
Levodopa: decreased levels of levodopa
Nitrofurantoin: increased levels of nitrofurantoin

Drug classifications
Antihistamines, other anticholinergics: increased anticholinergic effects
Benzodiazepines, sedatives, hypnotics, opioids: increased CNS depression
Class IA/III antidysrhythmics, some phenothiazines, β-agonists, local anesthetics, tricyclics, CYP3A4 inhibitors (amiodarone, clarithromycin, erythromycin, telithromycin, troleandomycin), CYP3A4 substrates (methadone, pimozide, QUEtiapine, quiNIDine, risperiDONE, ziprasidone): increased QT prolongation

---

NURSING CONSIDERATIONS
Assessment
• **Assess for allergic reactions:** rash, urticaria; if these occur, product should be discontinued; swelling of face, tongue, throat
• **Assess urinary patterns:** distention, nocturia, frequency, urgency, incontinence; catheterization may be required to remove residual urine; urinary tract infections should be treated
• **QT prolongation:** assess ECG for QT prolongation, ejection fraction; assess for chest pain, palpitations, dyspnea
• **Beers:** Avoid in older adults, delirium risk is increased

Patient problem
Impaired urination (uses)
Pain (uses)

Implementation
PO route
• Do not break, crush, or chew ext rel tabs
• May be given with meals or fluids or on an empty stomach
Topical route
• Wash hands, apply to clean, dry, intact skin on abdomen, upper arms/shoulders, thighs, avoid navel, rotate sites
• Squeeze contents in palm of hand or directly on this site, rub gently
• Do not bathe, exercise, swim for 1 hr after application
• Allow to dry before putting on clothing
• Do not be near flame, fire, or smoke until gel has dried
• Delivers 100 mg
Transdermal route
• Apply to clean, dry, intact skin on the abdomen, hip, buttock, use firm pressure, not affected by showering/bathing; rotate sites
• Delivers 3.9 mg/day

Patient/family education
• Advise patient to avoid hazardous activities until response to product is known; dizziness, blurred vision may occur
• Caution patient to avoid OTC medication with alcohol or other CNS depressants
• Teach patient to use frequent rinsing of mouth, sips of water for dry mouth
• Teach patient to stay cool; avoid hot weather, strenuous activity since overheating may occur; product decreases perspiration
• Advise patient to report CNS effects: confusion, anxiety, anticholinergic effect in the geriatric
• **Pregnancy/breastfeeding:** Identify if pregnancy is planned or suspected or if breastfeeding

Transdermal
• Instruct patient to change patch 2×/wk and not to use same site within 7 days
• Instruct patient to use container that is not accessible to pets/children and to dispose of container after use
• Instruct patient to open patch immediately before using
• Instruct patient to remove patch during MRI
Topical gel
• **Instruct patient to rotate sites**
• Instruct patient to apply to clean, dry skin on abdomen, upper arm/shoulders/thighs
• Teach patient that gel is flammable

Evaluation
Positive therapeutic outcome
• Absence of dysuria, frequency, nocturia, incontinence

⚠ HIGH ALERT

oxyCODONE (Rx)
(ox-i-koe′done)
Oyado, OxyCONTIN, Oxy IR ✦, Supeudol, Xampza
oxyCODONE/ acetaminophen (Rx)
Endocet, Nalocet, Percocet, Primlev, Roxicet, Xartemis XR
oxyCODONE/aspirin (Rx)
Endodan, Percodan
oxyCODONE/ibuprofen (Rx)
Func. class.: Opiate analgesic
Chem. class.: Semisynthetic derivative
Controlled substance schedule II

Do not confuse: oxyCODONE/ HYDROcodone/OxyCONTIN

ACTION: Inhibits ascending pain pathways in CNS, increases pain threshold, alters pain perception

Therapeutic outcome: Decreased pain

USES: Moderate to severe pain

Unlabeled uses: Postherpetic neuralgia (cont rel)

Pharmacokinetics
Absorption	Well absorbed
Distribution	Widely distributed; crosses placenta, protein binding 45%
Metabolism	Liver, extensively
Excretion	Kidneys, breast milk
Half-life	3-5 hr

Pharmacodynamics

	PO	RECT
Onset	15-30 min	Unknown
Peak	½-1 hr	Unknown
Duration	Reg rel 2-6 hr, cont rel 12 hr	4-6 hr

CONTRAINDICATIONS

Hypersensitivity, addiction (opiate), asthma, ileus

> **BLACK BOX WARNING:** Respiratory depression

Precautions: Pregnancy, breastfeeding, children <18 yr, addictive personality, increased ICP, MI (acute), severe heart disease, renal/hepatic disease, bowel impaction

> **BLACK BOX WARNING:** Opioid-naïve patients, substance abuse, accidental exposure, potential for overdose/poisoning, status asthmaticus

DOSAGE AND ROUTES
Severe pain

Adult: PO 10-30 mg q4hr (5-15 mg q4-6hr for opiate naïve patients); CONC SOL is extremely concentrated, do not use interchangeably; CONT REL 10 mg q12hr in opiate-naïve patients

Child >5 yr and adolescent (unlabeled): PO 0.2 mg/kg given 30 min before procedure

Available forms: **OxyCODONE:** cont rel tabs (OxyCONTIN) 10, 15, 20, 30, 40, 80, 160 mg; immediate rel tabs 5, 7.5, 10, 15, 20, 30 mg; immediate rel caps 5 mg; oral sol 5 mg/5 ml, 20 mg/ml; Ext rel cap 13.5, 18, 27, 36 mg **oxyCODONE with acetaminophen:** 2.5 mg/325 mg, 5 mg/325 mg; 7.5 mg/325 mg, 7.5 mg/500 mg, 10 mg/325 mg; oral sol 5 mg/325 mg/5 ml; **oxyCODONE with aspirin:** 4.835 mg/325 mg; **oxyCODONE with ibuprofen:** 5 mg/400 mg

ADVERSE EFFECTS

CNS: *Drowsiness, dizziness, confusion, headache, sedation, euphoria,* fatigue, abnormal dreams, thoughts, hallucinations
CV: Palpitations, bradycardia, change in B/P
EENT: Tinnitus, blurred vision, miosis, diplopia
GI: *Nausea, vomiting, anorexia, constipation, cramps,* gastritis, dyspepsia, biliary spasms
GU: Increased urinary output, dysuria, urinary retention
INTEG: *Rash,* urticaria, bruising, flushing, diaphoresis, pruritus
RESP: Respiratory depression

INTERACTIONS
Individual drugs

Alcohol: increased respiratory depression, hypotension, sedation
Cimetidine: increased toxicity

Drug classifications

Antipsychotics, CNS depressants, opioids, sedative/hypnotics, skeletal muscle relaxants: increased respiratory depression, hypotension
CYP3A4 inhibitors: increased oxyCODONE level
MAOIs: increased toxicity

Drug/herb

St. John's wort, valerian: increased sedative effect

Drug/lab test

Increased: amylase, lipase

NURSING CONSIDERATIONS
Assessment

• **Pain:** assess intensity, location, type, characteristics; need for pain medication by pain/sedation scoring; physical dependence
• Monitor I&O ratio; check for decreasing output; may indicate urinary retention
• **CNS changes:** assess for dizziness, drowsiness, hallucinations, euphoria, LOC, pupil reaction
• **Allergic reactions:** assess for rash, urticaria

> **BLACK BOX WARNING: Respiratory dysfunction:** assess for respiratory depression, character, rate, rhythm; notify prescriber if respirations are <10/min; also B/P, pulse take baseline and periodically

• **Bowel status:** assess for constipation; stimulate laxative may be needed with fluids, fiber
• Monitor VS after parenteral route; note muscle rigidity, product history, renal, liver function tests, respiratory dysfunction: respiratory depression, character, rate, rhythm; notify prescriber if respirations are <10/min

> **BLACK BOX WARNING: Substance abuse:** assess for substance abuse in patient/family/friends before prescribing; monitor for abuse; may crush, chew, snort, or inject ex rel product; may be fatal

> **BLACK BOX WARNING: Accidental exposure:** dispose of properly away from pets, children

> **BLACK BOX WARNING: Pregnancy/breastfeeding:** Use only if benefits outweigh fetal risk, neonatal opioid withdrawal syndrome may occur with extended user, avoid breastfeeding, excreted in breast milk

---

• **Beers:** Avoid in older adults, ataxia, impaired psychomotor function may occur

Patient problem
Pain (uses)
Constipation (adverse reactions)
Impaired breathing (adverse reactions)

Implementation
• Clarify all orders, fatalities have occurred
• Regular administration is more effective than PRN, give before pain becomes severe
• Discontinue gradually after long-term use
• OxyCODONE should be titrated from the initial recommended dosage to the dose required to relieve pain
• There is no maximum dose of oxyCODONE; however, careful titration is required until tolerance develops to some of the side effects (drowsiness and respiratory depression)
• Store in light-resistant area at room temp
Immediate-release tablets
• May be administered with food or milk to minimize GI irritation
Oxycodone extended-release caps (Xtampza ER) administration
• Take with food and with approximately the same amount of food in order to ensure consistent plasma concentrations
• The capsule contents may be sprinkled onto soft foods (applesauce, pudding, yogurt, ice cream, or jam) or into a cup and then given directly into the mouth; swallow immediately and rinse mouth to ensure all contents have been swallowed. Discard capsule shells after administration
• The capsule contents may be given through an NG or gastrostomy tube. Flush the tube with water. Open a capsule and pour the contents directly into the tube. Do not premix capsule contents with the liquid that will be used to flush the tube. Draw up 15 ml of water into a syringe, insert the syringe into the tube, and flush the contents through the tube. Repeat flushing twice using 10 ml of water with each flush. Milk or liquid nutritional supplement may be used as an alternative to water when flushing capsule contents through the tube
• Extended-release 36-mg capsules are for use ONLY in opioid-tolerant patients
• Monitor patients closely for respiratory depression, particularly within the first 24 to 72 hr after initiation or dose escalation

Controlled-release tablets (OxyCONTIN)
• Administer whole; do not crush, chew, or break in half. Taking chewed, broken, or crushed controlled-release tabs could lead to the rapid release and absorption of a potentially toxic dose of oxyCODONE
• OxyCONTIN brand tablets: Due to hydrogelling nature of the 2010 reformulation, do not presoak, lick, or otherwise wet tab prior to dose administration. Administer 1 tab at a time; allow patient to swallow each tab separately with sufficient liquid to ensure prompt and complete transit through the esophagus
• OxyCODONE controlled-release (OxyCONTIN) 60 mg and 80 mg tablets are for use ONLY in opioid-tolerant patients
• May be administered with or without food
Oral concentrate solution route
• A highly concentrated solution (20 mg oxyCODONE/ml), care should be taken in dispensing and administering this medication. The solution may be added to 30 ml of a liquid or semisolid food. If the medication is placed in liquid or food, consume immediately; do not store diluted oxyCODONE for future use
PO route
• Do not break, crush, or chew cont rel tabs; give q12hr, no more frequently
• May be given with food or milk to lessen GI upset
• Use 80-, 160-mg cont rel tabs (oxyCONTIN) only in opioid-tolerant patients

Patient/family education
• Advise patients to avoid CNS depressants: alcohol, sedative/hypnotics
• Discuss with patient that dizziness, drowsiness, and confusion are common; to avoid getting up without assistance
• Discuss in detail all aspects of the product, including purpose and what to expect
• Advise patient to make position changes slowly to lessen orthostatic hypotension
• Advise patient to avoid CNS depressants, alcohol
• Advise patient to avoid operating machinery, driving if drowsiness occurs
• Teach patient that withdrawal symptoms may occur after long-term use: nausea, vomiting, cramps, fever, faintness, anorexia

Evaluation
Positive therapeutic outcome
• Decreased pain

TREATMENT OF OVERDOSE:
Naloxone 0.2-0.8 **IV**, O₂, **IV** fluids, vasopressors; caution with patients physically dependent on opioids

oxymetazoline nasal agent
See Appendix B

oxymetazoline ophthalmic
See Appendix B

⚠ HIGH ALERT

oxytocin (Rx)
(ox-i-toe′sin)
Pitocin
Func. class.: Oxytocic hormone

ACTION: Acts directly on myofibrils, producing uterine contraction; stimulates breast milk letdown, vasoactive antidiuretic effect

Therapeutic outcome: Stimulation of labor, control of bleeding; stimulation of milk letdown

USES: Stimulation, induction of labor; missed or incomplete abortion; postpartum bleeding

Pharmacokinetics

Absorption	Well absorbed (nasal); completely absorbed (**IV**)
Distribution	Widely distributed (extracellular fluid)
Metabolism	Liver, rapidly
Excretion	Kidneys
Half-life	3-12 min

Pharmacodynamics

	Nasal	IV	IM
Onset	5 min	Rapid	3-7 min
Peak	Unknown	Unknown	Unknown
Duration	20 min	1 hr	1 hr

CONTRAINDICATIONS
Hypersensitivity, serum toxemia, cephalopelvic disproportion, fetal distress, hypertonic uterus, prolapsed umbilical cord, active genital herpes

Precautions: Cervical/uterine surgery, uterine sepsis, primipara >35 yr, 1st/2nd stage of labor

BLACK BOX WARNING: Elective induction of labor

DOSAGE AND ROUTES
Labor induction
Adult: IV 1-2 milliunit/min, increase by 1-2 milliunit q15-60min until regular contractions occur, then decrease dosage

Postpartum hemorrhage
Adult: IV 10-40 units in 1000 ml nonhydrating diluent infused at 20-40 milliunit/min
Adult: IM 3-10 units after placenta delivery

Incomplete abortion
Adult: IV INF 10 units/500 ml D₅W or 0.9% NaCl run at 10-20 milliunit/min; max 30 units/12 hr

Fetal stress test
Adult: IV 0.5 milliunit/min; increase q20min until 3 contractions occur at 10 min

Available forms: Inj 10 units/ml

ADVERSE EFFECTS
CNS: Seizures, tetanic contractions
CV: Hypo/hypertension, dysrhythmias, increased pulse, bradycardia, tachycardia, premature ventricular contractions
FETUS: Dysrhythmias, jaundice, hypoxia, intracranial hemorrhage
GI: Anorexia, nausea, vomiting, constipation
GU: Abruptio placentae, decreased uterine blood flow
HEMA: Increased hyperbilirubinemia
INTEG: Rash
RESP: Asphyxia
SYST: Water intoxication of mother

INTERACTIONS
Drug classifications
Vasopressors: Increase: increased hypertension

Drug/herb
Ephedra: Increase: hypertension

NURSING CONSIDERATIONS
Assessment
• **Assess labor contractions:** fetal heart tones, frequency, duration, intensity of contractions; if fetal heart tones increase or decrease significantly or if contractions are longer than 1 min, notify prescriber; turn patient on left side to increase oxygen to fetus
• **Assess for water intoxication:** confusion, anuria, drowsiness, headache; monitor I&O; notify prescriber
• Watch for fetal distress, acceleration, deceleration, fetal presentation, pelvic dimensions
• Monitor B/P, pulse, respiratory rate, rhythm, depth

- Assess for fetal presentation, pelvic dimensions before use
- Provide an environment conducive to letdown reflex
- Monitor continuously, discontinue immediately if fetal distress occurs or uterine hyperactivity occurs

Patient problem
Lack of knowledge of medication (teaching)

Implementation

Oxytocin administration
- Give by IV infusion or IM
- Before use, an IV infusion of NS should be already running for use in case of adverse reactions. Magnesium sulfate should be readily available if relaxation of the myometrium is needed
- Visually inspect parenteral product for particulate matter and discoloration before use

IV infusion route
- *Induction of labor:* Dilute 1 ml (10 units) in 1000 ml of a compatible IV infusion solution. Rotate infusion bottle for thorough mixing. The resultant infusion should contain 10 milliunits/ml
- *Control of postpartum uterine bleeding:* Dilute 10-40 units in a compatible IV solution or to an already infusing solution. The maximum concentration is 40 units in 1000 ml of solution
- *Incomplete, inevitable, or elective abortion:* Dilute 10 units in 500 ml of a compatible IV solution
- Administer using an infusion pump to ensure accurate dosing

IM route
- Inject into a large muscle mass, aspirate before injection to avoid injection into a blood vessel

Y-site compatibilities: acyclovir, alfentanil, allopurinol, amikacin, aminocaproic acid, aminophylline, amphotericin B liposome (AmBisome), anidulafungin, argatroban, ascorbic acid injection, atenolol, atracurium, atropine, azaTHIOprine, azithromycin, aztreonam, benztropine, bivalirudin, bumetanide, buprenorphine, butorphanol, calcium chloride/gluconate, capreomycin, caspofungin, cefamandole, ceFAZolin, cefepime, cefoperazone, cefotaxime, cefotetan, cefoxitin, cefTAZidime, ceftizoxime, cefTRIAXone, cefuroxime, chloramphenicol, chlorothiazide, chlorpheniramine, cimetidine, ciprofloxacin, cisatracurium, clindamycin, cloxacillin, colistimethate, cyanocobalamin, cyclophosphamide, cycloSPORINE, DAPTOmycin, dexamethasone, dexmedetomidine, digoxin, dilTIAZem, diphenhydramine, dobutamine, dolasetron, dopamine, doxycycline, droperidol, edetate calcium disodium, enalaprilat, ePHEDrine,

EPINEPHrine, epoetin alfa, eptifibatide, ergonovine, ertapenem, erythromycin, esmolol, famotidine, fenoldopam, fentaNYL, fluconazole, folic acid (as sodium salt), foscarnet, fosphenytoin, furosemide, gallamine, ganciclovir, gatifloxacin, gentamicin, glycopyrrolate, granisetron, heparin, hydrocortisone sodium succinate, HYDROmorphone, hydrOXYzine, imipenem-cilastatin, isoproterenol, kanamycin, ketamine, ketorolac, labetalol, lactated Ringer's injection, lansoprazole, lepirudin, leucovorin, levoFLOXacin, lidocaine, lincomycin, linezolid, lorazepam, magnesium sulfate, mannitol, mechlorethamine, meperidine, mephentermine, meropenem, metaraminol, methyldopate, methylPREDNISolone, metoclopramide, metoprolol, metronidazole, midazolam, milrinone, minocycline, morphine, moxifloxacin, multiple vitamins injection, mycophenolate mofetil, Nafcillin, nalbuphine, nalorphine, naloxone, nesiritide, netilmicin, niCARdipine, nitroglycerin, nitroprusside, norepinephrine, ondansetron, oxacillin, palonosetron, pamidronate, papaverine, penicillin G potassium/sodium, pentamidine, pentazocine, PENTobarbital, PHENobarbital, phentolamine, phenylephrine, phytonadione, piperacillin sodium, piperacillin-tazobactam, polymyxin B, potassium acetate/chloride/phosphates, procainamide, prochlorperazine, prochlorperazine, promazine, promethazine, propranolol, protamine, pyridoxine, quinupristin-dalfopristin, raNITIdine, Ringer's injection, sodium acetate/bicarbonate/phosphates, streptomycin, succinylcholine, SUFentanil, tacrolimus, theophylline, thiamine hydrochloride, ticarcillin disodium, ticarcillin disodium-clavulanate potassium, tigecycline, tirofiban hydrochloride, tobramycin sulfate, tolazoline, trimetaphan, tubocurarine, urokinase, vancomycin, vasopressin, verapamil, vitamin B complex with C, voriconazole, warfarin, zidovudine, zoledronic acid

Patient/family education
- Teach patient to report increased blood loss, abdominal cramps, increased temp or foul-smelling lochia, nausea, blurred vision, itching, swelling
- Advise patient that contractions will be similar to menstrual cramps, gradually increasing in intensity

BLACK BOX WARNING: Elective induction of labor; use only for induction when medically necessary

Evaluation
Positive therapeutic outcome
- Stimulation of milk letdown (nasal)
- Induction of labor
- Decreased postpartum bleeding

⚠ HIGH ALERT

pACLitaxel (Rx)
(pa-kli-tax'el)
pACLitaxel protein-bound particles (Rx)
Abraxane
Func. class.: Antineoplastic—miscellaneous
Chem. class.: Taxane

Do not confuse: PACLitaxel/PARoxetine/Paxil

ACTION: Inhibits the reorganization of the microtubule network needed for interphase and mitotic cellular functions; also causes abnormal bundles of microtubules during cell cycle and multiple esters of microtubules during mitosis

Therapeutic outcome: Prevention of rapidly growing malignant cells

USES: PACLitaxel metastatic carcinoma of the ovary, breast carcinoma, AIDS-related Kaposi's sarcoma (second line), non–small cell lung cancer (first line), adjuvant treatment for node-positive breast cancer, prostate, esophageal cancer, melanoma paclitaxel protein-bound particles: Metastatic breast cancer after failure or relapse, metastatic pancreatic adenocarcinoma

Pharmacokinetics

Absorption	Completely absorbed
Distribution	89%-98% protein binding
Metabolism	Liver, extensively
Excretion	Unknown
Half-life	5-17 hr

Pharmacodynamics

Onset	Unknown
Peak	1-2 wk
Duration	3 wk

CONTRAINDICATIONS

Pregnancy, hypersensitivity to paclitaxel or other products with polyoxyethylated castor oil, albumin

BLACK BOX WARNING: Neutropenia (neutrophils <1500/mm³)

Precautions: Breastfeeding, children, CV/hepatic disease, CNS disorder, renal disease, bone marrow suppression, dental disease/work, extravasation, females, geriatric patients, herpes, infection, infertility, jaundice, ocular exposure, radiation therapy, thrombocytopenia, vaccination

BLACK BOX WARNING: Taxane hypersensitivity, requires a specialized care setting and an experienced clinician, bone marrow supression

DOSAGE AND ROUTES
≫ PACLitaxel
Ovarian carcinoma
Adult: IV INF 135 mg/m² given over 24 hr q3wk, then CISplatin 75 mg/m² or 175 mg/m² over 3 hr q3wk (refractory or metastatic) or 175 mg/m² over 3 hr

Advanced ovarian carcinoma (node positive)
Adult: IV INF 175 mg/m² with CISplatin 75 mg/m² over 3 hr q3wk with doxorubicin

Breast carcinoma-node positive
Adult: IV INF 175 mg/m² over 3 hr q3wk × 4 courses with doxorubicin

AIDS-related Kaposi's sarcoma
Adult: IV INF 135 mg/m² over 3 hr q3wk or 100 mg/m² over 3 hr q2wk

1st line non–small cell lung cancer
Adult: IV INF 135 mg/m²/24 hr with CISplatin 75 mg/m² × 3 wk

≫ PACLitaxel protein-bound particles
Breast cancer
Adult: IV 260 mg/m² q3wk
Pancreatic cancer
Adult: IV 125 mg/m2 over 30-40 min on Day 1, 8, 15 of each 28-day cycle

Hepatic dose
Adult, for dose reduction 135 mg/m² 24 hr IV inf: AST/ALT 2-10 × ULN, total bilirubin ≤1.5 mg/dl: give 100 mg/m²; AST/ALT <10 × ULN, total bilirubin 1.6-7.5 mg/dl: give 50 mg/m²; AST/ALT ≥10 × ULN or total bilirubin >7.5 mg/dl: avoid use
Adult, for dose reduction 175 mg/m² 3 hr IV inf: AST/ALT <10 × ULN, total bilirubin 1.26-2 × ULN: 135 mg/m²; AST/ALT <10 × ULN, total bilirubin 2.01-5 × ULN: give 90 mg/m²; AST/ALT ≥10 × ULN or total bilirubin >5 × ULN: avoid use

Available forms: Inj 6 mg/5 ml, powder for inj, lyophilized 100 mg in single-use vials (Abraxane)

ADVERSE EFFECTS
CNS: Peripheral neuropathy, dizziness, seizures, headache
CV: *Bradycardia, hypotension, abnormal ECG*
GI: *Nausea, vomiting, diarrhea, mucositis,* pancreatitis
GU: Renal failure

HEMA: Neutropenia, leukopenia, thrombocytopenia, anemia
INTEG: Alopecia, tissue necrosis, generalized urticaria, flushing
MS: *Arthralgia, myalgia*
RESP: Pulmonary embolism, dyspnea, cough
SYST: *Hypersensitivity reactions,* anaphylaxis, Stevens-Johnson syndrome, toxic epidermal necrolysis, angioedema

INTERACTIONS
Individual drugs
DOXOrubicin: increased levels of DOXOrubicin
Cisplatin: Increased myelosuppression
Gemibibrozil: Increased toxicity
Radiation: increased myelosuppression

Drug classifications
CYP3A4 inhibitors (clarithromycin, indinavir, ketoconazole, ritonavir, saquinavir):
  Increased effect, toxicity
  CYP3A4 inducers: (carbamazepine, phenytoin, rifampin):
  Decreased effect, failure of treatment
Antineoplastics: increased myelosuppression
CYP2C8, CYP2C9 inducers: decreased PACLitaxel level
Vaccines (live virus): decreased immune response

Drug/lab test
Increased: AST/ALT, alk phos, triglycerides
Decreased: neutrophils, platelets, WBCs, Hgb

NURSING CONSIDERATIONS
Assessment
• Assess CNS changes: confusion, paresthesias, psychosis, tremors, seizures, neuropathies; product should be discontinued
• Check buccal cavity for dryness, sores or ulceration, white patches, oral pain, bleeding, dysphagia; obtain prescription for viscous lidocaine (Xylocaine) to use in mouth

> **BLACK BOX WARNING:** Requires a specialized care setting such as a hospital or facility capable of managing complications; should be used by a clinician experienced in cytotoxic agents

• **Cardiovascular status:** monitor ECG continuously in CV conditions; monitor for hypotension, sinus bradycardia/tachycardia
• **Peripheral neuropathy:** assess for paresthesias, numbness; during inf use ice packs on extremities to lessen continued neuropathy; use ice on extremities when infusing
• Stevens Johnson syndrome: Assess for rash, fever, fatigue, blisters, discontinue if these occur

• Paclitaxel: Monitor CBC and differential baseline and periodically, leukocytes < 1500/mm3, platelets < 100,000/mm3 hold and notify health care professional, Nadir is 11 days (leukopenia) recovery 15-21 days
• Paclitaxel Protein Bound Particles: Monitor CBC and differential baseline and on days 1, 8, 15. Hold if neutrophils < 1500/mm3 × 1 wk reduce all doses
• **Arthralgia, myalgia:** may begin 2-3 days after infusion and continue for 4-5 days, may use analgesics
• **Nausea, vomiting:** premedicate with antiemetics, nausea and vomiting occur often
• Monitor renal function tests: BUN, creatinine, serum uric acid, urine CCr before, during therapy; check I&O ratio; report fall in urine output to <30 ml/hr
• Assess effects of alopecia on body image; discuss feelings about body changes
• VS during 1st hr of inf, check IV site for signs of infiltration

> **BLACK BOX WARNING:** Hypersensitivity reactions, anaphylaxis, hypotension, dyspnea, angioedema, generalized urticaria: discontinue inf immediately; keep emergency equipment available, monitor continuously during first 30-60 min, then periodically, usually occur in first few minutes, pretreat with dexamethasone, diphenhydramine

• **Flush:** for mild to moderate flush, may continue diphenhydrAMINE for up to 48 hr (not required in paclitaxel protein bound)
• Effects of alopecia on body image; discuss feelings about body changes
• **Pregnancy/breastfeeding:** Do not use in pregnancy, breastfeeding

Patient problem
Risk for infection (adverse reactions)

Implementation

> **BLACK BOX WARNING: Bone marrow suppression** Monitor CBC, differential, platelet count weekly; withhold product if WBC is <1500/mm³ or platelet count is <100,000/mm³, notify prescriber of results

• If CISplatin is given, use after taxane

>> PACLitaxel

Paclitaxel Continuous IV INF route
• After premedicating with dexamethasone 20 mg PO 12 hr and 6 hr before paclitaxel, diphenhydrAMINE 50 mg IV 0.5-1 hr before PACLitaxel and cimetidine 300 mg or ranitidine 50 mg IV 0.5-1 hr before PACLitaxel

- For extravasation if given by regular IV, not port
- Dilute 30 mg vial in 5 mL of 0.9% NaCl, D$_5$, D$_5$W and 0.9% NaCl, D$_5$LR (0.3-1.2 mg/ml), use in-line filter ≤0.22 micron, give as 3 hr (breast cancer, febrile sarcoma) or 24 hr inf (ovarian cancer)
- Use only glass bottles, polypropylene, polyolefin bags and administration sets; do not use PVC inf bags or sets

Y-site compatibilities: Acyclovir, amikacin, aminophylline, ampicillin/sulbactam, bleomycin, butorphanol, calcium chloride, CARBOplatin, cefepime, cefoTEtan, cefTAZidime, cefTRIAXone, cimetidine, CISplatin, cladribine, cyclophosphamide, cytarabine, dacarbazine, dexamethasone, diphenhydrAMINE, DOXOrubicin, droperidol, etoposide, famotidine, floxuridine, fluconazole, fluorouracil, furosemide, ganciclovir, gentamicin, granisetron, haloperidol, heparin, hydrocortisone, HYDROmorphone, ifosfamide, LORazepam, magnesium sulfate, mannitol, meperidine, mesna, methotrexate, metoclopramide, morphine, nalbuphine, ondansetron, pentostatin, potassium chloride, prochlorperazine, propofol, ranitidine, sodium bicarbonate, thiotepa, vancomycin, vinBLAStine, vinCRIStine, zidovudine

>> Paclitaxel Protein-Bound Particles

Intermittent IV INF route
- No pref medication for allergic reactions is needed
- Reconstitute vial by injecting 20 ml of 0.9% NaCl; slowly inject the 20 ml of 0.9% NaCl over at least 1 min to direct the sol flow on wall of vial (5mg/mL); do not inject 0.9% NaCl directly onto lyophilized cake (foaming will occur); allow vial to sit for at least 15 min to ensure proper wetting of lyophilized cake; gently swirl or invert vial slowly for at least 2 min until completely dissolved, should look milky
- Use PVC IV bag, do not use a filter
- Solution is stable for 8 hr, refrigerated
- Give over 30 min

Patient/family education
- Teach patient to notify prescriber if pregnancy is planned or suspected, do not breastfeed
- Teach patient to avoid use of products containing aspirin or ibuprofen, razors, commercial mouthwash, since bleeding may occur; to report symptoms of bleeding (hematuria, tarry stools)
- Instruct patient to report signs of anemia (fatigue, headache, irritability, faintness, shortness of breath) and CNS reactions (confusion, psychosis, nightmares, seizures, severe headaches)

- Teach patient to rinse mouth tid-qid with water, club soda; brush teeth bid-qid with soft brush or cotton-tipped applicators for stomatitis; use unwaxed dental floss
- Inform patient that hair may be lost during treatment; a wig or hairpiece may make patient feel better; new hair may be different in color, texture
- Inform patient that receiving vaccinations during therapy may cause serious reactions

Evaluation

Positive therapeutic outcome
- Prevention of rapid division of malignant cells

⚠ HIGH ALERT

palbociclib
(pal-boe-sye′klib)
Ibrance
Func. class.: Antineoplastic
Chem. class.: Signal transduction inhibitor, Kinase inhibitor

ACTION: Inhibits progression of the cell cycle from G$_1$ into S phase, decreased proliferation of ER-positive breast cancer cell lines. When combined with antiestrogen therapy (letrozole), decreases retinoblastoma protein (Rb) phosphorylation, reducing E2F expression and signaling, and increasing growth arrest

Therapeutic outcome: Decreased progression, spread of cancer

USES: Treatment of estrogen receptor (ER)–positive, HER2-negative advanced breast cancer in postmenopausal women, in combination with letrozole as initial endocrine-based therapy

Pharmacokinetics

Absorption	Unknown
Distribution	85% protein bound
Metabolism	Metabolized by CYP3A
Excretion	Unknown
Half-life	Elimination half-life was 24-34 hr

Pharmacodynamics

Onset	Unknown
Peak	Peak 6-12 hr
Duration	Unknown

CONTRAINDICATIONS: Hypersensitivity, pregnancy, lactation

Precautions: Children, fungal/viral infection, infants, infertility, neutropenia, testicular failure, thromboembolic disease

DOSAGE AND ROUTES
Hormone receptor (HR)-positive, HER2-negative advanced or metastatic breast cancer
Adult: females PO 125 mg qday with food for 21 days then 7 days rest; with strong CYP3A4 inhibitors 75 mg q day × 21 days, then 7 day rest

Available forms: Caps 75, 100, 125 mg

ADVERSE EFFECTS
CNS: Weakness, fever, fatigue
EENT: Stomatitis, pharyngitis, sinusitis, epistaxis
GI: Vomiting, nausea, anorexia, diarrhea
HEMA: Thrombocytopenia, neutropenia, leukopenia, lymphopenia, anemia
MISC: Peripheral neuropathy, alopecia, infection, pulmonary embolism, thromboembolism

INTERACTIONS
Individual cyclosporine, ergotamine, everolimus, fentanyl, pimozide, quinidine, sirolimus, tacrolimus: Increased effect, toxicity, dosage reduction may be needed

Drug classifications
CYP3A inhibitors (clarithromycin, itraconazole, nefazodone, ritonavir, saquinivir, verapamil): Increased effect, toxicity, avoid using together
CYP3A inducers (carbamazepine, phenytoin, rifampin): Decreased effect, avoid using together

Drug/herb
St. John's wort: Avoid concurrent use

Drug/food
Avoid use with grapefruit juice

NURSING CONSIDERATIONS
Assessment
• **Pulmonary embolism/thromboembolic events:** Assess for dyspnea/shortness of breath, chest pain, arm or leg swelling, sudden numbness or weakness, severe headache or confusion, or problems with vision, speech, or balance
• **Bone marrow suppression:** Monitor CBC/ differential baseline and on day 15 of 2 cycles, 15 day is expected until neutrophils decrease, felomine neutropenia may occur

Patient problem
Risk for infection (adverse reactions)
Risk for injury (adverse reactions)

Implementation
• Give at same time of day with food and letrozole, capsules should be swallowed whole, do not cut, open, chew, do not use if capsule is not intact
Treatment-related hepatotoxicity:
• **Grade 1 or 2 hepatotoxicity:** No dosage change
• **Grade ≥3 hepatotoxicity (AST or ALT >5 × ULN or total bilirubin >3 × ULN) that persists despite medical treatment:** Hold until toxicity resolves to grade ≤2 (AST or ALT ≤5 × ULN or total bilirubin ≤3 × ULN), resume treatment at the next lower dose level if not considered a safety risk for the patient; discontinue if grade ≥3 toxicity occurs at a dose of 75 mg/day
Treatment-related nephrotoxicity:
• **Grade 1 or 2 nephrotoxicity:** No change
• **Grade ≥3 nephrotoxicity (CCr >3 × baseline or >4 mg/dl, or requiring hospitalization or dialysis) that persists despite medical treatment:** Hold therapy. When toxicity resolves to grade ≤2 (CCr <3 × baseline or <4 mg/dl), resume at the next lower dose level if not considered a safety risk for the patient, discontinue if grade ≥3 toxicity occurs at a dose of 75 mg/day.

Patient/family education
• Identify if pregnancy is planned or suspected. Discuss the need for contraception due to possible fetal harm; avoid breastfeeding
• Advise patient laboratory testing will be needed during treatment
• Advise patient to take as prescribed, not to skip or double doses, review " Patient Information " sheet
• Teach patient to notify provider of infection
• Advise patient to discuss OTC, Rx, herbals, supplements with health care professional
• **Pulmonary/thromboembolic events:** Instruct patient to seek medical attention if dyspnea/shortness of breath, chest pain, arm or leg swelling, sudden numbness or weakness, severe headache or confusion, or problems with vision, speech, or balance develop
• Teach patient to not take with grapefruit juice
• **Pregnancy:** Product can cause fetal harm; identify if the patient is pregnant or if pregnancy is planned

Evaluation
Positive therapeutic outcome
• Decreased progression of breast cancer

paliperidone (Rx)
(pal-ee-per'i-done)
Invega, Invega Sustenna, Invega Trinza
Func. class.: Antipsychotic (2nd generation)
Chem. class.: Benzisoxazole derivative

Do not confuse: Invega/Iveegam,
paliperidone/risperidone

ACTION: Mediated through both dopamine type 2 (D_2) and serotonin type 2 (5-HT_2) antagonism

Therapeutic outcome: Decrease in emotional excitement, hallucinations, delusions, paranoia; reorganization of patterns of thought, speech

USES: Schizophrenia, schizoaffective disorder

Pharmacokinetics

Absorption	Unknown
Distribution	Unknown, protein binding >74%
Metabolism	Unknown
Excretion	80% urine, 11% feces
Half-life	Elimination 23 hr

Pharmacodynamics

Onset	Unknown
Peak	24 hr
Duration	Unknown

CONTRAINDICATIONS
Breastfeeding, seizure disorders, AV block, geriatric, QT prolongation, torsades de pointes, hypersensitivity to this product or risperidone

Precautions: Pregnancy, children, renal/hepatic disease, obesity, Parkinson's disease, suicidal ideation, diabetes mellitus, hematologic disease

BLACK BOX WARNING: Mortality-related psychosis in dementia

DOSAGE AND ROUTES
Adult: PO 6 mg/day; max 12 mg/day; IM 234 mg on day 1, then 156 mg 1 wk later; after 2nd dose, give 117 mg qmo, range 39-234 mg
Child/adolescent ≥12 yr and ≥51 kg: PO 3 mg/day, may increase if needed by 3 mg/day in intervals >5 days up to max 12 mg/day; <51 kg max 6 mg/day

Renal dose
Adult: PO CCr 50-79 ml/min, 3 mg/day, max 6 mg/day; ext rel/IM 156 mg on day 1, 117 mg 1 wk later, then 78 mg each mo CCr 10-49 ml/min, 1.5 mg/day, max 3 mg/day; IM not recommended

Available forms: Ext rel tabs 1.5, 3, 6, 9 mg; ext rel susp for inj 39 mg/0.25 ml, 78 mg/0.5 ml, 117 mg/0.75 ml, 156 mg/1 ml, 234 mg/1.5 ml; Invega Trinza extended-release suspension 273, 410, 546, 819 mg

ADVERSE EFFECTS
CNS: *EPS, pseudoparkinsonism, akathisia, dystonia, tardive dyskinesia; drowsiness, insomnia, agitation, anxiety, headache,* seizures, neuroleptic malignant syndrome, dizziness, suicidal thoughts/behaviors
CV: Orthostatic hypotension, tachycardia, heart failure, QT prolongation, dysrhythmias
EENT: Blurred vision, cough
ENDO: Insulin increase, hyperinsulinemia, weight gain, hyperglycemia, dyslipidemia
GI: *Nausea,* vomiting, *anorexia, constipation,* weight gain in adolescents, xerostomia
GU: Menstrual irregularities, impotence, priapism
MS: Arthralgia
MISC: Amgioedema, anaphylaxis
HEMA: Agranulocytosis, leukopenia, neutropenia

INTERACTIONS
Individual drugs
Abarelix, alfuzosin, amoxapine, apomorphine, chloroquine, dasatinib, dolasetron, droperidol, flecainide, pimozide: increased QT prolongation
Alcohol: increased sedation
Carbamazepine: decreased levels, increase dose of paliperidone may be needed
Levodopa: decreased levodopa effect
Lithium: increased neurotoxicity
Valproic acid: increased effect, dose decrease of periperidone may be needed

Drug classifications
Antihypertensives, nitrates: Increased orthostatic hypotension
Azole antifungals; β-blockers; class IA, III antidysrhythmics; halogenated anesthetics; some antipsychotics; some phenothiazines; tricyclics (high doses): increased QT prolongation
SSRIs, SNRIs: increased serotonin syndrome, increased neuroleptic malignant syndrome
Other CNS depressants, sedatives/hypnotics, opiates: increased sedation

---

⚠ Nurse Alert　　　　✴ Key NCLEX® Drug　　　　>> Drug Specifics

Drug/herb
Betel palm, kava: increased EPS
Cola tree, hops, nettle, nutmeg: increased action
Kava: increased CNS depression

Drug/lab test
Increased: prolactin levels

NURSING CONSIDERATIONS
Assessment

> **BLACK BOX WARNING: Assess mental status;** mood, behavior, confusion, orientation, suicidal thoughts/behaviors; dementia especially in geriatric patients before initial administration and periodically

• **QT prolongation:** monitor ECG for QT prolongation, ejection fraction; assess for chest pain, palpitations, dyspnea
• Assess AIMS assessment, blood glucose, CBC, glycosylated hemoglobulin A1C (HbA1C), LFTs, neurologic function, pregnancy testing, serum creatinine/electrolytes/lipid profile/prolactin, thyroid function tests, weight
• Monitor for swallowing of PO medication; check for hoarding or giving of medication to other patients
• Monitor I&O ratio; palpate bladder if urinary output is low
• Assess affect, orientation, LOC, reflexes, gait, coordination, sleep pattern disturbances
• Monitor B/P standing and lying; also pulse, respirations; take these during initial treatment; establish baseline before starting treatment; report drops of 30 mm Hg; watch for ECG changes
• Assess for dizziness, faintness, palpitations, tachycardia on rising
• **Hyperprolactinemia:** assess for sexual dysfunction, decreased menstruation, breast pain
• **Assess for EPS,** including akathisia, tardive dyskinesia (bizarre movements of the jaw, mouth, tongue, extremities), pseudoparkinsonism (rigidity, tremors, pill rolling, shuffling gait)
• **Serotonin syndrome, neuroleptic malignant syndrome:** assess for increased heart rate, shivering, sweating, dilated pupils, tremors, high B/P, monitor for hyperthermia, headache, confusion; if these occur, stop product, administer a serotonin antagonist if needed
• Assess for constipation, urinary retention daily; if these occur, increase bulk and water in diet; monitor for weight gain in adolescents
• **Beers:** Avoid in older adults except for schizophrenia, bipolar disorder, or short-term use as an antiemetic in chemotherapy, increases stroke risk
• **Pregnancy/breastfeeding:** Use only if benefits outweigh fetal risk, EPS may result in neonate EPS, pregnant patients should enroll in the National Registry for Atypical Antipsychotics (866-961-2388), do not breastfeed

Patient problem
Distorted thinking process (uses)
Risk for injury (uses, adverse reactions)

Implementation
PO route
• Do not break, crush, or chew ext rel tabs, use plenty of water
• Give without regard for food
• Give a reduced dose to the geriatric patient
• Give antiparkinsonian agent on order from prescriber; to be used for EPS
• Avoid use with CNS depressants
• Supervise ambulation until patient is stabilized on medication; do not involve in strenuous exercise program, because fainting is possible; patient should not stand still for a long time
• Increase fluids to prevent constipation
• Provide sips of water, candy, gum for dry mouth
• Store in airtight, light-resistant container
IM route
• Use for IM only, do not use IV or SUBCUT, injection kits contain a prefilled syringe and 2 safety needles, for single use only, shake for 10 secs
• **Deltoid injection:** ≥ 90 kg use 1.5 inch, 22 G needle; < 90 kg use 1 inch, 23 G needle, alternate injections between deltoid muscles
• **Gluteal injection:** use 1.5 inch, 22 G needle; attach needle to luer connection in clockwise motion, pull needle sheath away using straight pull, bring syringe with attached needle upright to de-aerate, de-aerate, inject; after injection, use finger, thumb or flat surface to activate needle protection system, until click heard, use deltoid × 2 dosages

Patient/family education
• Advise patient that orthostatic hypotension may occur and to rise from sitting or lying position gradually
• Advise patient to avoid hot tubs, hot showers, tub baths; hypotension may occur
• Caution patient to avoid abrupt withdrawal of this product; EPS may result; product should be withdrawn slowly
• Teach patient to avoid OTC preparations (cough, hay fever, cold) unless approved by prescriber; serious product interactions may occur; avoid use of alcohol; increased drowsiness may occur
• Advise patient to avoid hazardous activities if drowsy or dizzy
• Teach patient compliance with product regimen; non-absorbable tab shell is expelled in stool
• Teach patient to avoid abrupt withdrawal of this product, EPS may result; that product should be withdrawn slowly

• Teach patient to report impaired vision, tremors, muscle twitching
• Caution patient that heat stroke may occur in hot weather; take extra precautions to stay cool
• Teach patient to use contraception, inform prescriber if pregnancy is planned or suspected

> **BLACK BOX WARNING: Suicidal thoughts/ behaviors:** Teach patient/family to notify prescriber of suicidal thoughts, behaviors, or other changes in behavior; identify dementia in the elderly

Evaluation
Positive therapeutic outcome
• Decrease in emotional excitement, hallucinations, delusions, paranoia; reorganization of patterns of thought, speech

TREATMENT OF OVERDOSE:
Lavage if orally ingested; provide airway; *do not induce vomiting*

palonosetron (Rx)
(pa-lone-o'se-tron)
Aloxi
Func. class.: Antiemetic
Chem. class.: 5-HT₃ receptor antagonist

ACTION: Prevents nausea, vomiting by blocking serotonin peripherally, centrally, and in the small intestine at the 5-HT$_3$ receptor

Therapeutic outcome: Decreased nausea, vomiting during chemotherapy

USES: Prevention of nausea, vomiting associated with cancer chemotherapy; postoperative nausea/vomiting

Pharmacokinetics

Absorption	Unknown
Distribution	62% protein bound
Metabolism	Liver
Excretion	Unchanged product and metabolites excreted by kidney
Half-life	40 hr

Pharmacodynamics
Unknown

CONTRAINDICATIONS
Hypersensitivity

Precautions: Pregnancy, breastfeeding, children, geriatric, with hypokalemia, hypomagnesemia, patients taking diuretics

DOSAGE AND ROUTES
Prevention of Chemotherapy induced nausea/vomiting
Adult: **IV** 0.25 mg as a single dose over 30 sec, 30 min prior to chemotherapy, max 0.25 mg **IV**
Child 1 mon–< 17 yr **IV** 20 mcg/kg, max 1.5 mg given 30 min prior to chemotherapy

Postoperative nausea/vomiting prophylaxis for up to 24 hr after surgery
Adult: **IV** 0.075 mg given over 10 sec immediately before induction

Available forms: Inj 0.075 mg/1.5 mL, 0.25 mg/5 ml, single use

ADVERSE EFFECTS
CNS: *Headache, dizziness, drowsiness*
GI: *Diarrhea, constipation*
MISC: Serotonin Syndrome

INTERACTIONS
Individual drugs
Buspirone, fentanyl, lithium, methylene blue, tramadol: Increased serotonin syndrome

Drug classifications
Class 1A antidysrhythmics (disopyramide, procainamide, quiNIDine), class III antidysrhythmics (amiodarone, dofetilide, ibutilide), diuretics (except potassium sparing), some phenothiazines: possible QT prolongation
SSRIs, SNRIs, MAOIs, tricyclic antidepressants, triptans: Increased serotonin syndrome

Drug/lab test
Increase: potassium

NURSING CONSIDERATIONS
Assessment
• Monitor for absence of nausea, vomiting during chemotherapy
• **Assess hypersensitivity reaction:** rash, bronchospasm
• Assess for agents that cause QT prolongation, avoid using those products

Patient problem
Nausea (uses)
Diarrhea (adverse reactions)
Constipation (adverse reactions)

Implementation

> **Direct IV route**
> • Give 30 mins prior to chemotherapy or immediately before anesthesia
> • Give over 30 secs (Adult) 15 secs (Child) for chemotherapy, 10 secs for anesthesia

---

- Do not mix with other products; flush **IV** line with 0.9% NaCl before, after administration
- Store at room temperature
- **Chemotherapy nausea/vomiting:** give as a single dose over 30 seconds
- **Postoperative nausea/vomiting:** give over 10 seconds immediately prior to anesthesia induction

Y-site compatibilities: Alemtuzumab, alfentanil, amikacin, aminocaproic acid, aminophylline, amiodarone, amphotericin B liposome, ampicillin, ampicillin/sulbactam, atracurium, atropine, azithromycin, aztreonam, bivalirudin, bleomycin, bumetanide, buprenorphine, busulfan, butorphanol, calcium acetate/chloride/gluconate, CARBOplatin, carmustine, caspofungin, ceFAZolin, cefepime, cefotaxime, cefoTEtan, cefOXitin, cefTAZidime, ceftizoxime, cefTRIAXone, cefuroxime, chloramphenicol, chlorproMAZINE, cimetidine, ciprofloxacin, cisatracurium, CISplatin, clindamycin, cyclophosphamide, cycloSPORINE, cytarabine, dacarbazine, DACTINomycin, dantrolene, DAPTOmycin, DAUNOrubicin, dexamethasone, dexmedetomidine, dexrazoxane, digoxin, diltiazem, diphenhydrAMINE, DOBUTamine, DOCEtaxel, DOPamine, doxacurium, DOXOrubicin hydrochloride, droperidol, enalaprilat, ePHEDrine, EPINEPHrine, epirubicin, eptifibatide, erythromycin, esmolol, etoposide, etoposide phosphate, famotidine, fenoldopam, fentaNYL, fluconazole, fludarabine, fluorouracil, foscarnet, fosphenytoin, furosemide, gemcitabine, gentamicin, glycopyrrolate, haloperidol, heparin, hydrALAZINE, hydrocortisone, HYDROmorphone, IDArubicin, ifosfamide, inamrinone, insulin, irinotecan, isoproterenol, ketorolac, labetalol, leucovorin, levofloxacin, lidocaine, linezolid, LORazepam, magnesium sulfate, mannitol, mechlorethamine, melphalan, meperidine, meropenem, mesna, metaraminol, methotrexate, methyldopate, metoclopramide, metoprolol, metroNIDAZOLE, midazolam, milrinone, mitoMYcin, mitoXANtrone, mivacurium, morphine, nalbuphine, naloxone, neostigmine, nesiritide, niCARdipine, nitroglycerin, nitroprusside, norepinephrine, octreotide, oxaliplatin, oxytocin, PACLitaxel, pamidronate, pancuronium, pentazocine, PHENobarbital, phentolamine, phenylephrine, piperacillin/tazobactam, potassium acetate/chloride/phosphates, procainamide, prochlorperazine, promethazine, propranolol, quinupristin/dalfopristin, ranitidine, remifentanil, rocuronium, sodium acetate/bicarbonate/phosphates, streptozocin, succinylcholine, SUFentanil, tacrolimus, teniposide, theophylline, thiotepa, ticarcillin/clavulanate, tigecycline, tirofiban, tobramycin, topotecan, trimethobenzamide, trimethoprim/sulfamethoxazole, vancomycin, vasopressin, vecuronium, verapamil, vinBLAStine, vinCRIStine, vinorelbine, zidovudine

Patient/family education

- Teach to report diarrhea, constipation, rash, or changes in respirations or discomfort at insertion site
- Teach patient reason for product, expected results

Evaluation

Positive therapeutic outcome

- Absence of nausea, vomiting during cancer chemotherapy

pamidronate (Rx)

(pam-i-drone´ate)

Aredia ✦

Func. class.: Bone resorption inhibitor, electrolyte modifier

Chem. class.: Bisphosphonate

Do not confuse: Aredia/Adriamycin

ACTION: Inhibits bone resorption, apparently without inhibiting bone formation and mineralization; absorbs calcium phosphate crystals in bone and may directly block dissolution of hydroxyapatite crystals of bone

Therapeutic outcome: Serum calcium at normal level

USES: Moderate to severe Paget's disease, hypercalcemia, osteolytic bone metastases in breast cancer patients, multiple myeloma

Unlabeled uses: Postmenopausal osteoporosis, hyperparathyroidism

Pharmacokinetics

Absorption	Rapidly cleared from circulation
Distribution	Mainly to bones, primarily in areas of high bone turnover
Metabolism	Unknown
Excretion	Kidneys, unchanged (50%)
Half-life	Biphasic 27 hr; from bone to 300 days

Pharmacodynamics

Onset	1 day
Peak	1 wk
Duration	Unknown

CONTRAINDICATIONS

Pregnancy, hypersensitivity to bisphosphonates

Precautions: Children, nursing mothers, renal dysfunction, poor dentition

DOSAGE AND ROUTES
Hypercalcemia of malignancy

Adult: IV INF 60-90 mg as a single dose in moderate hypercalcemia, 90 mg in severe hypercalcemia given over 2-24 hr; dose should be diluted in 1000 ml 0.45% NaCl, 0.9% NaCl, or D_5W; wait 7 days before 2nd course

Osteolytic lesions

Adult: IV 90 mg/500 ml of D_5W, 0.45% NaCl, or 0.9% NaCl given over 4 hr on a monthly basis (multiple myeloma) or over 2 hr q3-4wk (breast carcinoma)

Paget's disease

Adult: IV INF 30 mg/day given over 4 hr × 3 days

Available forms: Powder for inj 30, 90 mg/vial; inj 3, 6, 9 mg/ml in 10 mL vials

ADVERSE EFFECTS

CNS: Fatigue, *fever*
CV: *Hypertension,* atrial fibrillation
EENT: Ocular pain, inflammation, vision impairment
GI: *Abdominal pain, anorexia, constipation, nausea, vomiting,* dyspepsia
GU: Renal failure
HEMA: Thrombocytopenia, anemia, leukopenia
INTEG: Redness, swelling, induration, pain on palpation at site of catheter insertion
META: Hypokalemia, hypomagnesemia, hypophosphatemia, hypocalcemia, hypothyroidism
MS: *Severe bone pain,* myalgia, osteonecrosis of the jaw
RESP: Coughing, dyspnea, URI
SYST: Angioedema, anaphylaxis

INTERACTIONS

None significant

Drug/lab test

Increased: creatinine
Decreased: potassium, magnesium, phosphate, calcium, WBC, platelets

NURSING CONSIDERATIONS
Assessment

• **Dental health:** Optimal dental health should be obtained before treatment with this product; give antiinfectives for dental extractions
• Monitor WBCs, platelets, electrolytes, creatinine, BUN, Hgb/Hct prior to beginning treatment

• Temperature may be elevated during the first 3 days after a dose; risk of fever increases as dose increases
• **Renal disease:** max 90 mg single dose, longer infusions >2 hr may increase risk for renal toxicity
• **Hypocalcemia:** assess for nausea, vomiting, constipation, thirst, dysrhythmias, hypocalcemia, paresthesia, twitching, laryngospasm, Chvostek's, Trousseau's signs; **hypercalcemia:** thirst, nausea, vomiting, dysrhythmias
• **Dehydration/hypovolemia:** should be corrected during treatment of hypercalcemia, prior to therapy; maintain adequate urine output
• **Pregnancy/breastfeeding:** Do not use in pregnancy/breastfeeding, use contraception
• Assess for atrial fibrillation
• Assess fluid volume status: check I&O ratio and record, assess for distended red veins, crackles in lung, color, quality, and specific gravity of urine, skin turgor, adequacy of pulses, moist mucous membranes, bilateral lung sounds, peripheral pitting edema
• Monitor electrolytes: phosphorus, potassium, sodium, calcium, magnesium; also include BUN, creatinine, CBC, platelets, hemoglobin, electrolytes (calcium, potassium, magnesium)
• Assess B/P before, during therapy
• Assess for pain: in joints or on exertion, duration and characteristics; analgesics may be ordered
• Assess for phlebitis at **IV** site: swelling, redness, pain, warmth

Patient problem

Pain (uses)
Risk for injury (adverse reactions)

Implementation

IV route
• Use saline hydration to produce 2000 mL/24 hr of urine output
• Avoid diuretics prior to treatment
• After reconstituting by adding 10 ml of sterile water for inj to each vial (30 mg/10 ml or 90 mg/10 ml depending on vial used): add to 1000 ml of sterile 0.45%, 0.9% NaCl, D_5W, run over 2-24 hr **(hypercalcemia);** dilute reconstituted sol in 500 ml of 0.9% NaCl, 0.45% NaCl, or D_5W, give over 4 hr **(multiple myeloma, Paget's disease);** dilute reconstituted sol in 250 ml of 0.9% NaCl, 0.45% NaCl or D_5W, give over 2 hr **(osteolytic bone metastases of breast cancer)**
• Store inf sol for up to 24 hr at room temperature
• Monitor IV site for pain, redness
• Reconstituted sol with sterile water may be stored under refrigeration for up to 24 hr
• Do not mix with calcium-containing inf sol such as Ringer's sol

---

Y-site compatibilities: Acyclovir, alfentanil, allopurinol, amifostine, amikacin, aminocaproic acid, aminophylline, amphotericin B lipid complex, amphotericin B liposome, ampicillin, anidulafungin, atenolol, atracurium, azithromycin, aztreonam, bivalirudin, bleomycin, bumetanide, buprenorphine, butorphanol, CARBOplatin, carmustine, ceFAZolin, cefepime, cefoperazone, cefotaxime, cefoTEtan, cefOXitin, cefTAZidime, ceftizoxime, cefTRIAXone, cefuroxime, chloramphenicol, chlorproMAZINE, cimetidine, ciprofloxacin, cisatracurium, CISplatin, clindamycin, cyclophosphamide, cycloSPORINE, cytarabine, dacarbazine, DAPTOmycin, dexamethasone, dexmedetomidine, dexrazoxane, digoxin, diltiazem, diphenhydrAMINE, DOBUTamine, DOCEtaxel, dolasetron, DOPamine, doxacurium, DOXOrubicin, doxycycline, droperidol, enalaprilat, ePHEDrine, EPINEPHrine, epirubicin, ertapenem, erythromycin, esmolol, etoposide, famotidine, fenoldopam, fentaNYL, fluconazole, fludarabine, fluorouracil, foscarnet, fosphenytoin, furosemide, gallium, ganciclovir, gatifloxacin, gemcitabine, gentamicin, glycopyrrolate, granisetron, haloperidol, heparin, hetastarch 6%, hydrALAZINE, hydrocortisone, HYDROmorphone, hydrOXYzine, ifosfamide, imipenem-cilastatin, inamrinone, insulin (regular), isoproterenol, ketorolac, labetalol, levofloxacin, levorphanol, lidocaine, linezolid, LORazepam, magnesium sulfate, mannitol, mechlorethamine, melphalan, meperidine, meropenem, mesna, metaraminol, methotrexate, methyldopate, methylPREDNISolone, metoclopramide, metoprolol, metroNIDAZOLE, midazolam, milrinone, minocycline, mitoXANtrone, mivacurium, morphine, mycophenolate, nafcillin, nalbuphine, naloxone, nesiritide, niCARDipine, nitroglycerin, nitroprusside, norepinephrine, octreotide, ondansetron, oxytocin, PACLitaxel, palonosetron, pancuronium, PEMEtrexed, pentamidine, pentazocine, PENTobarbital, PHENobarbital, phenylephrine, piperacillin, polymyxin B, potassium chloride/phosphates, procainamide, prochlorperazine, promethazine, propranolol, quiNIDine, quinupristin-dalfopristin, ranitidine, remifentanil, rocuronium, sodium acetate/bicarbonate/phosphates, succinylcholine, SUFentanil, sulfamethoxazole-trimethoprim, teniposide, theophylline, thiopental, thiotepa, ticarcillin, ticarcillin-clavulanate, tigecycline, tirofiban, tobramycin, tolazoline, topotecan, trimethobenzamide, vancomycin, vasopressin, vecuronium, verapamil, vinBLAStine, vinCRIStine, vinorelbine, voriconazole, zidovudine

Patient/family education

• Advise patient to report hypercalcemic relapse: nausea, vomiting, bone pain, thirst; unusual muscle twitching, muscle spasms, severe diarrhea, constipation, ocular symptoms
• Advise patient to continue with dietary recommendations, including calcium and vit D
• To obtain an analgesic from provider for bone pain
• Advise patient that small, frequent meals may help nausea/vomiting
• Advise patient to maintain good oral hygiene, have regular dental check-ups
• Teach patient to report dental or jaw pain to prescriber immediately
• Teach patient to notify prescriber if pregnancy is planned or suspected, to use contraception

Evaluation

Positive therapeutic outcome
• Decreased calcium levels to normal

pancrelipase (Rx)

(pan-kre-li′pase)
Creon ✱, Cotazym ✱ Pancrease ✱, Pancreaze, Pertyze, Ultrase, VioKase, Zenpep
Func. class.: Digestant
Chem. class.: Pancreatic enzyme (bovine/porcine)

ACTION: Pancreatic enzyme needed for breakdown of substances released from the pancreas

Therapeutic outcome: Increases protein, fat, carbohydrate digestion

USES: Exocrine pancreatic secretion insufficiency, cystic fibrosis (digestive aid), steatorrhea, pancreatic enzyme deficiency

Pharmacokinetics
Unknown

Pharmacodynamics
Unknown

CONTRAINDICATIONS
Allergy to pork

Precautions: Pregnancy, ileus, pancreatitis, Crohn's disease, diabetes mellitus

DOSAGE AND ROUTES
Many products listed above are not interchangeable

P

Del rel caps—Creon caps, Zenpep caps, Pancreaze caps

Adult/adolescent/child ≥4 yr: PO 500 lipase units/kg/meal, titrate based on response, max 2500 lipase units/kg/meal

Child 1<4 yr: PO 1000 lipase units/kg/meal, titrate based on response, max 2500 lipase units/kg/meal

Available forms: Tabs (VioKase) 10, 20 units; cap, del rel 4, 8, 16 units (Pancrecarb MS), 12, 18, 20 units (Ultrase MT), Ultrase: cap 3000, 4200, 5000, 6000, 8000, 10,500, 12,000, 15,000, 16,000, 16,800, 24,000, 25,000 units

ADVERSE EFFECTS

ENDO: Hyperglycemia, hypoglycemia
GI: Anorexia, nausea, vomiting, diarrhea, cramping, bloating
GU: Hyperuricuria, hyperuricemia

INTERACTIONS
Individual drugs

Acarbose, miglitol: decreased effects of each specific drug
Cimetidine, iron (oral): decreased absorption of pancrelipase

Drug classifications

Antacids: decreased absorption of pancrelipase

NURSING CONSIDERATIONS
Assessment

• Monitor I&O ratio; watch for increasing urinary output
• Monitor fecal fat, nitrogen, pro-time during treatment
• Monitor for polyuria, polydipsia, polyphagia (may indicate diabetes mellitus); monitor glucose level more frequently
• Assess for allergy to pork; patient may also be sensitive to this product
• Assess for appropriate weight, height, development; there may be a developmental lag
• Check stools for steatorrhea, which signifies undigested fat content
• **Pregnancy/breastfeeding:** Use only if clearly needed, can be used in breastfeeding

Patient problem

Diarrhea (adverse reactions)

Implementation

• Give after antacid or cimetidine; decreased pH inactivates product
• Administer low-fat diet to decrease GI symptoms
• Provide adequate hydration
• Store in airtight container at room temperature
• Do not crush, chew del rel products, caps

Patient/family education

• Teach patient to always take with food, not to crush, chew del rel product, caps
• Instruct patient to store at room temperature, away from moisture
• Teach patient to take tab with 8 oz or more water, not to let tab sit in mouth; have patient take tab sitting up only
• Advise patient to notify prescriber of allergic reactions, abdominal pain, cramping, or hematuria

Evaluation
Positive therapeutic outcome

• Absence of steatorrhea
• Improved digestion of carbohydrates, proteins, fat

⚠ HIGH ALERT

pancuronium (Rx)

(pan-cure-oh′nee-yum)
Func. class.: Neuromuscular blocker (nondepolarizing)
Chem. class.: Synthetic curariform

ACTION: Inhibits transmission of nerve impulses by binding with cholinergic receptor sites, antagonizing action of acetylcholine

Therapeutic outcome: Paralysis of all skeletal muscles

USES: Facilitation of endotracheal intubation, skeletal muscle relaxation during mechanical ventilation, surgery, or general anesthesia

Pharmacokinetics

Absorption	Complete bioavailability
Distribution	Extracellular space; crosses placenta
Metabolism	Plasma
Excretion	Kidneys, unchanged
Half-life	2 hr

Pharmacodynamics

Onset	3-5 min, dose dependent
Peak	3-5 min
Duration	35-40 min

CONTRAINDICATIONS

Hypersensitivity to bromide ion

Precautions: Pregnancy, breastfeeding, children <2 yr, renal/hepatic/cardiac/neuromuscular disease, electrolyte imbalances, dehydration, previous anaphylactic reactions (other neuromuscular blockers), respiratory insufficiency

---

DOSAGE AND ROUTES

Adult/child/infant >1 mo: IV 0.04-0.1 mg/kg initially or 0.05 mg/kg after initial dose of succinylcholine; maintenance 0.01 mg/kg 60-100 min after initial dose, then 0.01 mg/kg q25-60min as needed; in obese patients, use ideal body weight

Neonate <1 mo: IV test dose 0.02 mg/kg, then 0.03 mg/kg/dose initially, repeat 2 × as needed at 5-10 min intervals; maintenance 0.03-0.09 mg/kg/dose q30min-4hr as needed

Available forms: Inj 1, 2 mg/ml

ADVERSE EFFECTS

CV: Bradycardia, tachycardia; increased, decreased B/P, ventricular extrasystoles, edema, hypotension
EENT: Increased secretions
INTEG: Rash, flushing, pruritus, urticaria, sweating, salivation
MS: Weakness to prolonged skeletal muscle relaxation
RESP: Prolonged apnea, bronchospasm, cyanosis, respiratory depression, dyspnea
SYST: Anaphylaxis

INTERACTIONS
Individual products
Clindamycin, enflurane, isoflurane, lincomycin, lithium, quiNIDine: increased neuromuscular blockade
Theophylline: dysrhythmias

Drug classifications
Aminoglycosides, anesthetics (local), analgesics (opioid), polymyxin antiinfectives, thiazides: increased neuromuscular blockade

Drug/lab test
Decreased: cholinesterase

NURSING CONSIDERATIONS
Assessment
• Monitor vital signs (B/P, pulse, respirations, airway) until fully recovered; note rate, depth, pattern of respirations, strength of hand grip; patient should be intubated before use
• Monitor for electrolyte imbalances (potassium, magnesium) before product is used; electrolyte imbalances may lead to increased action of this product
• **Monitor for recovery:** decreased paralysis of face, diaphragm, leg, arm, rest of body; residual weakness and respiratory problems may occur during recovery period
• **Assess for hypersensitive reactions, anaphylaxis:** rash, fever, respiratory distress, pruritus; product should be discontinued

• **Pregnancy/breastfeeding:** Use only if benefits outweigh fetal risk, breast milk excretion unknown

Patient problem
Impaired breathing (uses)
Risk for injury (adverse reactions)

Implementation
• Use peripheral nerve stimulator (anesthesiologist) to determine neuromuscular blockade; deep tendon reflexes should be monitored during extended periods

Direct IV route
• Give undiluted over 1-2 min (1 mg/ml [10 ml vial], 2 mg/ml [2, 5 ml vial])
Intermittent IV infusion route
• Add 100 mg of product to 250 ml D₅W, 0.9% NaCl, or LR (0.4 mg/ml)
• Store in light-resistant area
• Give anticholinesterase to reverse neuromuscular blockade

Y-site compatibilities: Aminophylline, ceFAZolin, cefuroxime, cimetidine, DOBUTamine, DOPamine, EPINEPHrine, esmolol, fentaNYL, fluconazole, gentamicin, heparin, hydrocortisone, isoproterenol, LORazepam, midazolam, morphine, nitroglycerin, nitroprusside, ranitidine, sulfamethoxazole/trimethoprim, vancomycin

Patient/family education
• Provide reassurance if communication is difficult during recovery from neuromuscular blockade
• Provide explanation to patients regarding all procedures or treatments; patient will remain conscious if anesthesia is not given also

Evaluation
Positive therapeutic outcome
• Paralysis of jaw, eyelid, head, neck, rest of body as evaluated by peripheral nerve stimulator

TREATMENT OF OVERDOSE:
Neostigmine, atropine; monitor VS; may require mechanical ventilation

⚠ HIGH ALERT

panitumumab (Rx)
(pan-i-tue′moo-mab)
Vectibix
Func. class.: Antineoplastic—miscellaneous
Chem. class.: Multikinase inhibitor, signal transduction inhibitor

ACTION: Decreases growth and survival of cancer cells by competitive inhibition of EGFR receptor

Therapeutic outcome: Decrease in colon carcinoma progression

USES: EGFR expressing metastatic colorectal cancer, not beneficial in *KRAS* mutations in codon 12 or 13

Pharmacokinetics

Absorption	38%-49%, high-fat meal decreases absorption
Distribution	Protein binding 99.5%
Metabolism	Liver, oxidative metabolism by CYP3A4, glucuronidation by UGT1A9, some Asian patients (15%-20%) are poor metabolizers
Excretion	Feces 77%
Half-life	Elimination 7.5 day

Pharmacodynamics

Onset	Unknown
Peak	3 hr
Duration	Unknown

CONTRAINDICATIONS
Hypersensitivity

Precautions: Pregnancy, breastfeeding, children, hepatic disease, acute bronchospasm, diarrhea, hamster protein allergy, hypomagnesemia, hypotension, pulmonary fibrosis, sepsis, *KRAS* mutations, soft-tissue toxicities infusion-related reactions

> **BLACK BOX WARNING:** Exfoliative dermatitis

DOSAGE AND ROUTES
Adult: IV INF 6 mg/kg over 60 min q2wk; doses > 1000 mg over 90 min

Available forms: Sol for inj 20 mg/ml (100 mg/5 ml, 400 mg/20 ml)

ADVERSE EFFECTS
CNS: Fatigue
CV: Peripheral edema
EENT: Ocular irritation, ocular toxicity
GI: *Nausea, diarrhea, vomiting,* anorexia, mouth ulceration, abdominal pain, constipation
HEMA: Thrombophlebitis
INTEG: *Rash,* pruritus, exfoliative dermatitis, skin fissure, angioedema, severe/fatal infusion reactions
META: Hypocalcemia, hypomagnesemia, antibody formation
RESP: Bronchospasm, cough, dyspnea, hypoxia, pulmonary fibrosis/embolism, pneumonitis, wheezing, interstitial lung disease

INTERACTIONS
Drug classifications
Antineoplastics, other: do not use with other products

NURSING CONSIDERATIONS
Assessment
• **Pulmonary fibrosis:** assess for dyspnea, cough, wheezing, may need to discontinue

> **BLACK BOX WARNING: Serious skin disorders:** assess for fever, sore throat, fatigue, then lesions in mouth, lips; withhold product, notify prescriber

• Monitor serum electrolytes periodically (calcium, magnesium)
• Assess for signs of infection: increased temperature
• Assess for diarrhea
• **Assess for signs of infusion reactions:** bronchospasm, fever, chills, hypotension; may require discontinuation; have emergency equipment available
• **Assess for signs of ocular toxicity:** ocular irritation, hyperemia
• **Pregnancy/breastfeeding:** Do not use in pregnancy, breastfeeding

Patient problem
Impaired gas exchange (adverse reactions)
Risk for infection (adverse reactions)

Implementation
• Assess for KRAS prior to use

Intermittent IV infusion route
• Give in hospital or clinic setting with full resuscitation equipment
• Give only as IV inf using controlled IV inf pump; do not give **IV** push or bolus; use low-protein binding 0.2 or 0.22 micron in-line filter; flush line with 0.9% NaCl before, after administration
• Give over 60 min through a peripheral line or in-dwelling catheter; inf doses of >1000 mg over 90 min
• Dilute in 100 ml of 0.9% NaCl; dilute doses >1000 mg in 150 ml of 0.9% NaCl; mix by inverting; max 10 mg/ml; use within 6 hr if stored at room temperature; can be stored between 2°-8° C for up to 24 hr
• Store unopened vials in refrigerator; do not shake; protect from direct sunlight; do not freeze
Dosage adjustment for infusion/dermatologic reaction
• **Grade 1/2:** reduce infusion by 50%; Grade 3/4: terminate, permanently discontinue depending on severity/resistance

Patient/family education
• **Instruct patient to report adverse reactions immediately:** difficulty breathing, mouth sores, skin rash, ocular toxicity
• Teach patient reason for treatment, expected results, adverse reactions

---

• Teach males/females to use contraception while taking this product and for 6 mo after treatment; do not breastfeed for at least 2 mo after treatment, enroll in Amgen's Pregnancy Surveillance Program (800-772-6436)

• Advise to use sunscreen while taking, 2 mo after

Evaluation
Positive therapeutic outcome
• Decrease in colon carcinoma progression

---

pantoprazole (Rx)
(pan-toe-pray′zole)
Panto IV ✤, Pantoloc ✤, Protonix, Protonix IV, Tecta ✤
Func. class.: Proton pump inhibitor
Chem. class.: Benzimidazole

Do not confuse: Protonix/Lotronex/Protamine

ACTION: Suppresses gastric secretion by inhibiting hydrogen/potassium ATPase enzyme system in gastric parietal cell; characterized as gastric acid pump inhibitor, since it blocks final step of acid production

Therapeutic outcome: Absence of epigastric fullness, pain, swelling

USES: Gastroesophageal reflux disease (GERD), severe erosive esophagitis, maintenance, long-term pathological hypersecretory conditions including Zollinger-Ellison syndrome

Pharmacokinetics
Absorption	Unknown
Distribution	Protein binding 97%
Metabolism	Unknown
Excretion	Urine-metabolites, feces, decreased rate in geriatric patients; ✒ some Asian patients (15%-20%) may be poor metabolizers
Half-life	1½ hr

Pharmacodynamics
Onset	Unknown
Peak	2.4 hr
Duration	>24 hr

CONTRAINDICATIONS
Hypersensitivity to this product or benzimidazole

Precautions: Pregnancy, breastfeeding, children, proton pump hypersensitivity

DOSAGE AND ROUTES
GERD
Adult: PO 40 mg/day × 8 wk, may repeat course

Erosive esophagitis
Adult: IV 40 mg/day × 7-10 days; PO 40 mg/day × 8 wk; may repeat PO course
Child ≥ 5 yr and ≥ 40 Kg PO 40 mg q day for up to 8 wk, 15-39 Kg 20 mg q day for up to 8 wk

Pathologic hypersecretory conditions
Adult: PO 40 mg bid; **IV** 80 mg q12hr; max 240 mg/day

Available forms: Del rel tabs 20, 40 mg; powder for inj 40 mg/vial; del rel granules for susp 40 mg

ADVERSE EFFECTS
CNS: *Headache,* insomnia, asthenia, fatigue, malaise, insomnia, somnolence
GI: *Diarrhea, abdominal pain,* flatulence, pancreatitis, weight changes, CDAD
INTEG: *Rash*
META: Hyperglycemia, weight gain/loss, hyponatremia, hypomagnesemia, vitamin B_{12} deficiency
MS: Myalgia

INTERACTIONS
Individual drugs
Calcium carbonate, sucralfate, vit B_{12}, ketoconazole, itraconazole, atazanavir, ampicillin, iron salts: decreased absorption of these products, separate doses
Warfarin: increased risk of bleeding

Drug Classifications
Protease inhibitors (atazanavir, indinavir, nelfinavir): Decreased effect of each of these drugs

Drug/herb
St. John's wort: decreased effect of pantoprazole

NURSING CONSIDERATIONS
Assessment
• CDAD: Assess GI system: bowel sounds, abdomen for pain, swelling, anorexia, diarrhea with blood, mucus
• Monitor hepatic enzymes: AST, ALT, alkaline phosphatase during treatment
• **Electrolyte imbalances:** hyponatremia; hypomagnesemia in those using this product (3 mo-1 yr); if hypomagnesemia occurs, use of magnesium supplements may be sufficient; if severe, discontinuation of this product may be required
• **Beers:** Avoid in older adults for >8 wk unless for high-risk patients, risk of *Clostridium difficile,* fractures

---

Patient problem
Pain (uses)

Implementation
- Swallow del rel tabs whole; do not break, crush, or chew
- May take with or without food
- **Suspension:** give in apple juice 30 min before a meal or sprinkled on 1 tbsp of applesauce

IV route
- **Use of Protonix IV vials with spiked IV system adaptors is not recommended**
- Visually inspect for particulate matter and discoloration prior to use
- Give as an IV infusion over 15 min either through a dedicated line or a Y-site; a 2-min slow injection regimen is also approved; do not give fast IV push
- When using a Y-site, immediately stop use if a precipitation or discoloration occurs
Reconstitution of vial:
- Use 40 mg vial/10 ml NS; do not freeze
2-minute slow intravenous (IV) infusion injection:
- Dilute one or two 40-mg vials with 10 ml NS per vial to 4 mg/ml, store up to 24 hr at room temperature prior to use; infuse slowly over at least 2 min; do not give with other IV fluids or medications; flush line with D₅W, NS, or LR before and after each dose
15-minute intravenous (IV) infusion:
- Dilute each 40 mg dose with 10 ml NS; the reconstituted vial should be further admixed with 100 ml (for one vial) or 80 ml (for 2 vials) of D₅W, NS, or LR (to 0.4 mg/ml or 0.8 mg/ml, respectively), store up to 6 hr at room temperature prior to further dilution; the admixed solution (0.4 mg/ml or 0.8 mg/ml) may be stored at room temperature and must be used within 24 hr from the time of initial reconstitution; infuse over 15 min at 7 ml/min; do not administer with other IV fluids or medications; flush the IV line with D₅W, NS, or LR before and after each dose

Patient/family education
- Advise patient to report severe diarrhea; product may have to be discontinued (CDAD)
- Advise patient with diabetes that hyperglycemia may occur
- Advise patient to avoid hazardous activities; dizziness may occur
- Advise patient to avoid alcohol, salicylates, ibuprofen; may cause GI irritation
- Inform patient to take as directed not to skip or double doses
- Pregnancy/breastfeeding: Identify if pregnancy is planned or suspected or if breastfeeding

Evaluation
Positive therapeutic outcome
- Absence of epigastric pain, swelling, fullness

PARoxetine hydrochloride (Rx)
Paxil, Paxil CR
Paroxetine mesylate
(par-ox'e-teen)
Brisdelle, Pexeva
Func. class.: Antidepressant, selective serotonin reuptake inhibitor (SSRI)
Chem. class.: Phenylpiperidine derivative

Do not confuse: PARoxetine/FLUoxetine/PACLitaxel, Piroxicam **Paxil**/PACLitaxel/Doxil/Plavix/Lexiva

ACTION: Inhibits CNS neuron reuptake of serotonin but not of norepinephrine or DOPamine

Therapeutic outcome: Relief of depression

USES: Major depressive disorder, obsessive-compulsive disorder, panic disorder, generalized anxiety disorder, posttraumatic stress disorder, premenstrual disorders, social anxiety disorder

Unlabeled uses: Premature ejaculation

Pharmacokinetics

Absorption	Well absorbed
Distribution	Widely distributed; crosses blood-brain barrier, protein-binding 95%
Metabolism	Liver, mostly by CYP2D6 enzyme system ♥ℴⓧ, 7% may be poor metabolizers
Excretion	Kidneys, unchanged (2%); breast milk
Half-life	21 hr (reg rel); 15-20 hr (cont rel)

Pharmacodynamics

Onset	Unknown
Peak	5.2 hr
Duration	Unknown

CONTRAINDICATIONS
Pregnancy, hypersensitivity, MAOI use, alcohol use

Precautions: Breastfeeding, geriatric, seizure history, patients with history of mania, renal/hepatic disease

BLACK BOX WARNING: Children, suicidal ideation

DOSAGE AND ROUTES
Depression
Adult: PO 20 mg/day in AM; after 4 wk if no clinical improvement is noted, dosage may be increased by 10 mg/day weekly to desired response; max 50 mg/day; or CONT REL 25 mg/day, may increase by 12.5 mg/day weekly up to 62.5 mg/day

Geriatric: PO 10 mg/day, increase by 10 mg to desired dose, max 40 mg/day

Obsessive-compulsive disorder
Adult: PO 40 mg/day in AM; start with 20 mg/day, increase 10 mg/day increments, max 60 mg/day

Panic disorder
Adult: Start with 10 mg/day and increase in 10 mg/day increments to 40 mg/day, max 60 mg/day; or CONT REL 12.5 mg/day max 75 mg/day

Generalized anxiety disorder
Adult: PO 20 mg/day in AM, range 20-50 mg/day

Posttraumatic stress disorder
Adult: PO 20 mg/day, range 20-60 mg/day

Premenstrual disorders
Adult: CONT REL 12.5 mg/day in AM

Renal dose
Adult: PO CCr 30-60 ml/min lower doses may be needed, CCr <30 ml/min 10 mg/day in AM, may increase to 10 mg/day qwk, max 40 mg/day; or CONT REL 12.5 mg/day max 50 mg/day

Hepatic dose
Adult: PO 10 mg/day initially, max 40 mg regular release, CONT REL 12.5 mg/day initially, max 50 mg/day

Available forms: Tabs 10, 20, 30, 40 mg; oral susp 10 mg/5 ml; cont rel 12.5, 25, 37.5 mg, cap 7.5 mg

ADVERSE EFFECTS
CNS: *Headache, nervousness, insomnia, drowsiness, anxiety, tremor, dizziness, fatigue, sedation,* abnormal dreams, agitation, apathy, euphoria, hallucinations, delusions, psychosis, seizures
CV: Vasodilatation, postural hypotension, palpitations, bleeding, chest pain
EENT: Visual changes
GI: *Nausea, diarrhea, constipation, dry mouth, anorexia,* dyspepsia, vomiting, taste changes, flatulence, decreased appetite, cramps
GU: Dysmenorrhea, decreased libido, urinary frequency, UTI, amenorrhea, cystitis, impotence, decreased sperm quality, decreased fertility, *abnormal ejaculation* (male)
INTEG: *Sweating,* rash, photosensitivity
MS: Pain, arthritis, myalgia, myopathy

RESP: Infection, pharyngitis, nasal congestion, sinus headache, sinusitis, cough, dyspnea, yawning
SYST: Fever, abrupt withdrawal syndrome, Stevens Johnson Syndrome, Serotonin syndrome, neuroleptic syndrome, suicidal thoughts/behaviors

INTERACTIONS
Individual drugs
Bupropion, cyclobenzeprine, limeolid, trazadone, tramadol: Increased serotonin syndrome
Cimetidine: increased PARoxetine levels
Digoxin: decreased effect of digoxin
L-tryptophan: increased agitation
PHENobarbital: decreased PARoxetine levels
Phenytoin: decreased effect of PARoxetine
Pimozide: potentially fatal reactions
Theophylline: increased theophylline levels
Thioridazine: do not use with PARoxetine; hypertensive crisis, seizures, potentially fatal reactions can occur
Warfarin: increased bleeding

Drug classifications
CYP2D6 inhibitors (aprepitant, dclavirdine, imatinib, nefazodone): increased toxicity
Highly protein-bound products: increased side effects
MAOIs: hypertensive crisis, seizures; do not use together; potentially fatal reactions can occur
SSRIs, SNRIs, atypical antipsychotics, serotonin-receptor agonists, tricyclics, amphetamines: increased serotonin syndrome
NSAIDs, thrombolytics, salicylates, platelet inhibitors, anticoagulants: increased bleeding

Drug/herb
SAMe, St. John's wort, tryptophan: possible serotonin syndrome, avoid use

NURSING CONSIDERATIONS
Assessment

> **BLACK BOX WARNING: Depression/OCD/anxiety/panic attacks:** assess mental status: mood, sensorium, affect, suicidal tendencies (especially in child/young adult), increase in psychiatric symptoms, increasing obsessive thoughts, compulsive behaviors, restrict amount available

• **Postural hypotension:** monitor B/P (lying/standing), pulse q4hr; if systolic B/P drops 20 mm Hg, hold product, notify prescriber; take vital signs q4hr in patients with CV disease
• **Renal status:** monitor BUN, creatinine, urinary retention

• **Withdrawal symptoms:** assess for headache, nausea, vomiting, muscle pain, weakness; not usual unless product discontinued abruptly, taper over 1-2 wk
• **Serotonin, neuroleptic malignant syndrome:** assess for hallucinations, coma, headache, agitation, shivering/sweating, tachycardia, diarrhea, tremor, hypertension, hyperthermia, rigidity, delirium, coma, myoclonus, agitation, nausea, vomiting
• Monitor blood studies: CBC, leukocytes, differential, cardiac enzymes if patient is receiving long-term therapy
• Monitor hepatic studies: AST, ALT, bilirubin
• Check weight weekly; appetite may increase with product
• Monitor urinary retention, constipation; constipation is more likely to occur in children or geriatric
• Identify alcohol consumption; if alcohol is consumed, hold dose until AM
• **Pregnancy/breastfeeding:** Do not use in pregnancy/breastfeeding

Patient problem
Depression (uses)
Risk for Injury (adverse reactions)

Implementation
• Give with food or milk for GI symptoms; store at room temperature; do not freeze
• Give crushed if patient is unable to swallow whole, regular release only
• Use gum, hard candy, frequent sips of water for dry mouth
• Avoid use with other CNS depressants
• **Oral susp:** shake, measure with oral syringe or calibrated measuring device
• **Cont rel tab:** do not cut, chew, crush; do not give concurrently with antacids

Patient/family education
• Advise patient that therapeutic effects may take 1-4 wk
• Teach patient to use caution in driving and other activities requiring alertness because of drowsiness, dizziness, blurred vision; to avoid rising quickly from sitting to standing, especially geriatric
• Caution patient to avoid alcohol ingestion, other CNS depressants, and OTC medication unless prescribed
• Caution patient not to discontinue medication quickly after long-term use; may cause nausea, anxiety, headache, malaise; do not double doses if one is missed
• Advise patient to use gum, hard sugarless candy, or frequent sips of water for dry mouth; if dry mouth continues an artificial saliva product may be used

> **BLACK BOX WARNING:** Advise patient that depression may worsen, suicidal thoughts/behavior may occur (especially in child/young adult), to notify prescriber immediately

• Advise patient to discuss sexual side effects: impotence, possible male infertility while taking this product

Evaluation
Positive therapeutic outcome
• Decrease in depression
• Absence of suicidal thoughts

TREATMENT OF OVERDOSE:
Gastric lavage, maintain airway; for seizures give diazepam, symptomatic treatment

---

RARELY USED

patiromer
(pa-tir′ oh-mer)
Veltassa
Func. class.: Electrolyte modifier

USES: Hyperkalemia

CONTRAINDICATIONS: Hypersensitivity, bowel impaction, GI obstruction, severe constipation

DOSAGE AND ROUTES
Adult: PO 8.4 g q day titrate at 1 wk interval to achieve potassium levels WNL

⚠ HIGH ALERT

pazopanib
(paz-oh′pa-nib)
Votrient
Func. class.: Antineoplastic biologic response modifier/multikinase angiogenesis inhibitor
Chem. class.: Kinase inhibitor

Do not confuse: pazopanib/ponatinib

ACTION: Targets vascular endothelial growth factor receptors; a multikinase angiogenesis inhibitor

Therapeutic outcome: Decrease in size, spread of tumor

USES: Advanced renal cell carcinoma; soft-tissue sarcoma patients who have received prior chemotherapy

---

Pharmacokinetics

Absorption	Unknown
Distribution	Protein binding 99%
Metabolism	Unknown
Excretion	Unknown
Half-life	31 hr

Pharmacodynamics

Onset	Unknown
Peak	2-4 hr
Duration	24 hr

CONTRAINDICATIONS

Pregnancy, hypothyroidism, QT prolongation, MI, wound dehiscence, hypertension

Precautions: Breastfeeding, children, cardiac/renal/hepatic/dental disease, GI bleeding

> **BLACK BOX WARNING:** Hepatic disease

DOSAGE AND ROUTES

Adult: **PO** 800 mg/day without food (1 hr before, 2 hr after a meal), may decrease to 400 mg/day if not tolerated (renal cell cancer); or adjust in 200-mg increments based on toxicity (soft-tissue sarcoma); **use with strong CYP3A4 inhibitors 400 mg q d**

Hepatic dose
Adult: PO 200 mg q day (moderate hepatic disease)

Available forms: Tabs 200 mg

ADVERSE EFFECTS

CNS: Intracranial bleeding, headache
CV: Heart failure, hypertension, hypertensive crisis, chest pain, MI, QT prolongation, torsades de pointes
GI: Nausea, hepatotoxicity, vomiting, dyspepsia, GI hemorrhage, anorexia, abdominal pain, GI perforation, pancreatitis, diarrhea; hepatotoxicity (geriatric)
HEMA: Neutropenia, thrombocytopenia, bleeding
INTEG: Rash, alopecia
MISC: Fatigue, epistaxis, pyrexia, hot sweats, increased weight, flulike symptoms, hypothyroidism, hand–foot syndrome, retinal tear/detachment

INTERACTIONS
Individual drugs

Arsenic trioxide, levomethadyl, haloperidol, chloroquine, droperidol, pentamidine: increased QT prolongation, pazopanib concentrations
Simvastatin: increased plasma concentrations of this agent

Warfarin: avoid use with warfarin; use low-molecular-weight anticoagulants instead; increased plasma concentration of warfarin

Drug classifications

Class IA/III antidysrhythmics, some phenothiazines, beta-agonists, local anesthetics, tricyclics; CYP3A4 inhibitors (amiodarone, clarithromycin, erythromyoin, telithromycin, ketoconazole, troleandomycin); CYP3A4 substrates (methadone, pimozide, QUEtiapine, quiNIDine, risperiDONE, ziprasidone): increased QT prolongation, increased pazopanib concentrations
Calcium-channel blockers, ergots: increased plasma concentrations of these agents
CYP3A4 inhibitors (clarithromycin, ketoconazole, ritonavir): Increased levels, avoid using together
CYP3A4 inducers (dexamethasone, phenytoin, carBAMazepine, rifampin, PHENobarbital): decreased pazopanib concentrations

Drug/food
Grapefruit juice: avoid use; increased pazopanib effect

Drug/herb
St. John's wort: decreased pazopanib concentration

NURSING CONSIDERATIONS
Assessment

> **BLACK BOX WARNING: Hepatic disease:** fatal hepatotoxicity can occur; obtain LFTs baseline and at least every 2 wk × 2 mo, then monthly

Fatal bleeding: from GI, respiratory, GU tracts, permanently discontinue in those with severe bleeding
• **Palmar-plantar erythrodysesthesia (hand–foot syndrome):** more common in those previously treated; assess for swelling, numbness, desquamation on palms and soles
• **GI perforation/fistula:** discontinue if this occurs, assess for pain in epigastric area, dyspepsia, flatulence, fever, chills
• **Hypertension/hypertensive crisis:** hypertension usually occurs in the first cycle; in those with preexisting hypertension, do not start treatment until B/P is controlled; monitor B/P every wk × 6 wk, then at start of each cycle or more often if needed, temporarily or permanently discontinue for severe uncontrolled hypertension

- Monitor LFTs prior to and at 3, 5, 7, 9 wks, then 3 mon, 4 mon if symptoms are present; thyroid function test
- **Hepatotoxicity:** Notify healthcare provider immediately of yellow skin, eyes, clay-colored stools, dark urine
- **Bleeding:** Teach patient to notify provider of bruising, bleeding from any orifice
- **Blood Clots:** Notify provider immediately of Pain in legs, trouble breathing, chest pain, swelling in legs, arms; notify provider immediately
- **Pregnancy/breastfeeding:** Do not use in pregnancy, breastfeeding

Patient problem
Risk of Injury (adverse reactions)
Lack of Knowledge of medication (teaching)

Implementation
- Give on an empty stomach (1 hr before or 2 hr after a meal); separate doses by 24 hr
- Do not crush tablets, can lead to an increased rate of absorption, which can affect systemic exposure; only intact, whole tablets should be used
- If a dose is missed, it should not be taken if it is ≤12 hr until the next dose
- Store at 77°F (25°C)

Patient/family education
- Advise patient to report adverse reactions immediately: heart attack, stroke
- Teach patient about reason for treatment, expected results
- Inform patient that effect on male fertility is unknown
- Do not crush or chew tabs, take on empty stomach 1 hr before or 2 hr after meals, avoid grapefruit juice, provide "Medication Guide"

Evaluation

Positive therapeutic outcome
- Decrease in size, spread of tumor

---

pegaspargase (Rx)
(peg-as'-per-gase)
Oncaspar
Func. class.: Antineoplastic
Chem. class.: Escherichia coli enzyme

ACTION: Indirectly inhibits protein synthesis in tumor cells; without amino acid, DNA, RNA synthesis is halted; asparagine, protein synthesis is halted; G1 phase of cell cycle specific; a nonvesicant; a modified version of L-asparaginase

Therapeutic outcome: Prevention of rapidly growing malignant cells

USES: Acute lymphocytic leukemia unresponsive to other agents in combination with other antineoplastics

Pharmacokinetics

Absorption	Complete bioavailability
Distribution	Intravascular spaces
Metabolism	Unknown
Excretion	Reticuloendothelial system
Half-life	5 1/2 days

Pharmacodynamics

Onset	Rapid
Peak	Unknown
Duration	2 wk

CONTRAINDICATIONS: Breastfeeding, infants, hypersensitivity, pancreatitis, acute bronchospasm, bleeding, coagulopathy, coronary thrombosis, DIC, hypotension

Precautions: Pregnancy, renal/hepatic/CNS disease, *E. coli* protein hypersensitivity, hemophilia, tumor lysis syndrome, infection

DOSAGE AND ROUTES
In combination
Adult and child: IV/IM 2500 international units/m2 q14day, run **IV** over 1-2 hr in 100 ml of 0.9% NaCl or D5W through a running **IV**; IM should be no more than 2 ml in one inj site used in combination with other chemotherapeutics

Available forms: Inj 750 international units/ml in a phosphate-buffered saline sol

ADVERSE EFFECTS
CNS: Neuritis, dizziness, headache, coma, depression, fatigue, confusion, hallucinations, seizures, intracranial bleeding
CV: Chest pain, hypotension
ENDO: Hyperglycemia
GI: *Nausea, vomiting, anorexia, cramps, stomatitis*, hepatotoxicity, pancreatitis, *diarrhea*
GU: Urinary retention, renal failure, glycosuria, polyuria, azotemia, uric acid neuropathy
HEMA: Thrombocytopenia, leukopenia, myelosuppression, anemia, decreased clotting factors, pancytopenia, DIC
INTEG: *Rash*, urticaria, chills, fever
RESP: Fibrosis, pulmonary infiltrate, severe bronchospasm
SYST: Anaphylaxis, hypersensitivity, angioedema

INTERACTIONS
Individual drugs
Aspirin, heparin, warfarin: coagulation factor imbalances
Methotrexate: decreased action of methotrexate

Drug classifications

Corticosteroids: increased hypoglycemia

NSAIDs, salicylates, platelet inhibitors, thrombolytics: increased bleeding risk

Live virus vaccines: decreased immune responses

NURSING CONSIDERATIONS
Assessment

• Assess for signs and symptoms of pancreatitis (nausea, vomiting, severe abdominal
pain), anaphylaxis (bronchospasm, dyspnea),
cyanosis; monitor amylase, glucose

• Assess symptoms indicating severe
allergic reaction: rash, pruritus, urticaria,
purpuric skin lesions, itching, flushing; monitor for joint pain, bronchospasm, hypotension; epinephrine and crash carts should be
nearby

• Monitor for frequency of stools, characteristics: cramping, acidosis; signs of dehydration:
rapid respirations, poor skin turgor, decreased
urine output, dry skin, restlessness, weakness

• Monitor CBC, differential, platelet count
weekly; withhold product if WBC is <4000/
mm^3 or platelet count is <100,000/mm^3; notify
physician of results; also assess pro-time, PTT,
and thrombin time, which may be increased

• Monitor renal function tests: BUN, creatinine,
serum uric acid, urine CCr before, during
therapy; check I&O ratio; report fall in urine
output to <30 ml/hr; patient should be well hydrated with 2-3 L/day to prevent urate deposits

• Monitor temp q4hr (may indicate beginning
of infection)

• Monitor liver function tests before, during
therapy (bilirubin, AST, ALT, LDH) as needed or
monthly; check for jaundice of skin and sclera,
dark urine, clay-colored stools, itchy skin,
abdominal pain, fever, diarrhea; also monitor
cholesterol, alkaline phosphatase

• Assess for bleeding: hematuria, stool guaiac,
bruising or petechiae, mucosa or orifices q8hr;
check for inflammation of mucosa, breaks in
skin

• Identify edema in feet, joint pain, stomach
pain, shaking

Patient problems

• Risk for infection (adverse reactions)
• Risk for injury (adverse reactions)
• Lack of knowledge of medication (teaching)

Implementation

• Preparation by trained personnel is required
in controlled environment

• Provide antiemetic 30-60 min before giving
product and prn to prevent vomiting; administer
antibiotics for prophylaxis of infection

• Provide a liquid diet: carbonated beverages;
gelatin may be added if patient is not nauseated
or vomiting

IM route

• No dilution needed; inject in large muscle; do
not give more than 2 ml in one injection site,
aspirate; preferred route

Intermittent IV infusion route

• Dilute contents of vial 1100 ml 0.9% NaCl or
D5W; give over 1-2 hr through freely running IV
solution; keep refrigerated, do not freeze

• Provide allopurinol or sodium bicarbonate
to reduce uric acid levels, alkalinization of
urine

Patient/family education

• Advise patient that contraceptive measures
are recommended during therapy; product is
teratogenic

• Teach patient to avoid use of products containing aspirin or NSAIDs, razors, commercial
mouthwash because bleeding may occur; to
report symptoms of bleeding (hematuria, tarry
stools)

• Teach patient to report signs of anemia (fatigue, headache, irritability, faintness, shortness
of breath)

• Tell patient to avoid crowds and persons with
respiratory tract infections to prevent patient
infection

• Advise patient to avoid vaccinations; serious
reactions can occur

• Teach patient to report nausea, vomiting,
bruising, bleeding, stomatitis, severe diarrhea,
jaundice, chest pain, abdominal pain, trouble
breathing, rash

Evaluation
Positive therapeutic outcome

• Prevention of rapid division of malignant cells

⚠ HIGH ALERT

pegfilgrastim (Rx)

(peg-fill-grass′stim)

Neulasta, Neulasta Onpro Kit

Func. class.: Hematopoietic agent

ACTION: Stimulates proliferation and differentiation of neutrophils

Therapeutic outcome: Absence of infection

USES: To decrease infection in patients receiving antineoplastics that are myelosuppressive;
to increase WBC in patients with product-induced
neutropenia

Pharmacokinetics

Absorption	Unknown
Distribution	Unknown
Metabolism	Unknown
Excretion	Unknown
Half-life	15-80 hr; 20-38 hr (child)

Pharmacodynamics

Unknown

CONTRAINDICATIONS
Hypersensitivity to proteins of *E. coli,* filgrastim

Precautions: Pregnancy, breastfeeding, child <45 kg, adolescents, myeloid malignancies, sickle cell disease, leukocytosis, splenic rupture, allergic-type reactions, ARDS, peripheral blood stem cell mobilization (PBSC)

DOSAGE AND ROUTES
Adult/Child > 45 kg: SUBCUT 6 mg per chemotherapy cycle

Available forms: Sol for inj 6 mg/0.6 ml

ADVERSE EFFECTS
CNS: Fever, fatigue, headache, dizziness, insomnia, peripheral edema
GI: Splenic rupture
GU: glomerulonephritis
HEMA: Sickle cell crisis
INTEG: Alopecia, Capillary leak Syndrome
MISC: Chest pain, hyperuricemia, anaphylaxis, flulike syndrome, angioedema, antibody formation
MS: Skeletal pain
RESP: Respiratory distress syndrome

INTERACTIONS
Individual drug
Lithium: increased release of neutrophils

Drug classifications
Cytotoxic chemotherapy agents: do not use this product concomitantly or 2 wk before or 24 hr after administration of cytotoxics

Drug/lab test
Increased: uric acid, LDH, alkaline phosphatase

NURSING CONSIDERATIONS
Assessment
• **Assess for allergic reactions, anaphylaxis:** rash, urticaria; discontinue this product, have emergency equipment nearby
• Monitor blood studies: CBC, platelet count before treatment and twice weekly; neutrophil counts may be increased for 2 days after therapy

• **ARDS:** assess for dyspnea, fever, tachypnea, occasional confusion; obtain ABGs, chest x-ray, product may need to be discontinued
• Monitor B/P, respirations, pulse before, during therapy
• **Assess for bone pain,** give mild analgesics
• **Pregnancy/breastfeeding:** Pregnant patient should enroll in Amgen's Pregnancy Surveillance Program (800-772-6436), cautious use in breastfeeding, excretion unknown

Patient problem
Risk for infection (uses)
Immunologic impairment (uses)
Pain (adverse reactions)

Implementation
SUBCUT route
• Give using single-use vials; after dose is withdrawn, do not reenter vial
• Do not use 6-mg fixed dose in infants, children, or others <45 kg
• Inspect sol for discoloration, particulates; if present, do not use
• Do not administer in the period 14 days before and 24 hr after cytotoxic chemotherapy
• Store in refrigerator; do not freeze; may store at room temp up to 6 hr, avoid shaking, protect from light

Patient/family education
• Teach the technique for self-administration: dose, side effects, disposal of containers and needles; provide instruction sheet; that injection site pain may occur
• Teach patient to notify prescriber immediately of allergic reaction, trouble breathing, abdominal pain

Evaluation

Positive therapeutic outcome
• Absence of infection

RARELY USED

peginterferon beta 1a
(peg-in-ter-feer'on bay-ta)
Plegridy
Func. class.: Immune modifier

USES: Relapsing multiple sclerosis

CONTRAINDICATIONS: Hypersensitivity to this product or peginterferon

DOSAGE AND ROUTES
Adult: SUBCUT 63 mcg initially, then 94 mcg on day 15, and then 125 mcg q 14 days

---

pegloticase (Rx)

(peg-loe′ti-kase)

Krystexxa

Func. class.: Antigout agent
Chem. class.: Pegylated, recombinant, mammalian urate oxidase enzyme

ACTION: Lowers plasma uric acid concentration by converting uric acid to allantoin, which is readily excreted by the kidneys

USES: Chronic gout in patients experiencing treatment failure

Pharmacokinetics

Absorption	Complete
Distribution	Unknown, remains primarily in intravascular space
Metabolism	Unknown
Excretion	Unknown
Half-life	2 wk, mean nadir uric acid concentration 24-72 hr

Pharmacodynamics

Onset	Unknown
Peak	24-72 hr
Duration	Unknown

CONTRAINDICATIONS:

BLACK BOX WARNING: Hypersensitivity, G6PD deficiency

Precautions: Pregnancy, breastfeeding, children/infants/neonates, ✖ African-American patients, heart failure

BLACK BOX WARNING: Requires specialized setting, experienced clinician; serious hypersensitivity; **methemoglobinemia**

DOSAGE AND ROUTES

Adult: IV INFUSION 8 mg over 2 hr q2wk

Available forms: Sol for inj 8 mg/mL

SIDE EFFECTS

CNS: Dizziness, fatigue, fever
CV: *Chest pain,* heart failure, hypotension
GI: *Nausea,* vomiting, diarrhea, constipation
GU: Nephrolithiasis
HEMA: Anemia
INTEG: Ecchymosis, *erythema, pruritus, urticaria*
MS: Back pain, arthralgia, muscle spasm
SYST: Antibody formation, infection, anaphylaxis, infusion-related reactions
RESP: *Dyspnea,* upper respiratory infection

INTERACTIONS

Do not use with urate-lowering agents (allopurinol, probenecid, febuxostat, sulfinpyrazone)

NURSING CONSIDERATIONS

Assessment:

• **Gout:** Assess for pain in big toe, feet, knees, redness, swelling, tenderness lasting a few days to weeks; intake of alcohol, purines, if patient is overweight or taking diuretics
• Obtain uric acid levels at baseline, before administration; two consecutive uric acid levels of >6 mg/dL may indicate therapy failure; greater chance of anaphylaxis; infection-related reactions

BLACK BOX WARNING: Specialized care setting: use only in facility where emergency equipment is available, anaphylaxis may occur

BLACK BOX WARNING: Infusion reactions: monitor for reactions for ≥1 hr after use

BLACK BOX WARNING: Assess for G6PD deficiency, methemoglobinemia

• **Pregnancy/breastfeeding:** Use only if benefits outweigh fetal risk; avoid breastfeeding, excretion unknown

Patient problem

Pain (uses)
Impaired mobility (uses)

Implementation:
Intermittent IV INFUSION route

• **Reconstitute:** Visually inspect for particulate matter, discoloration whenever sol/container permits; use aseptic technique; withdraw 8 mg (1 mL) of product/250 mL 0.9% NaCl or 0.45% NaCl; invert several times to mix, do not shake; discard remaining product in vial
• **Premedicate:** With antihistamines and corticosteroids in all patients and acetaminophen if deemed necessary to prevent anaphylaxis, infusion site reactions
• **Infusion:** If refrigerated, allow to come to room temperature; do not warm artificially; give over 120 min; do not give IV push or bolus; use infusion by gravity feed, syringe-type pump, or infusion pump; given in a specialized setting by those who can manage anaphylaxis or inj-site reactions; monitor during and for 1 hr after infusion; if reaction occurs, slow or stop infusion, may be restarted at a slower rate; do not admix
• Store diluted product in refrigerator or at room temperature for up to 4 hr; refrigerator is preferred; protect from light; do not freeze; use within 4 hr of preparation

Patient/family education:
• Teach patient about reason for infusion, expected results
• Advise patient to notify prescriber during infusion of allergic reactions or redness, swelling, pain at infusion site
• Teach patient that continuing follow-up exams and uric acid levels will be needed

Evaluation
• Positive therapeutic outcome: Decreased uric acid levels; relief of pain, swelling, redness in toes, feet, knees

---

⚠ HIGH ALERT

pembrolizumab

(pem'broe-liz'ue-mab)
Keytruda
Func. class.: Antineoplastic, biologic response modifier
Chem. class.: Monoclonal antibody

ACTION: A human monoclonal antibody that binds to the programmed death receptor-1 (PD-1) found on T cells and blocks the interaction of PD-1 with its ligands, PD-L1 and PD-L2, on the tumor cell

Therapeutic outcome: Decreased progression of multiple myeloma

USES: Unresectable or metastatic malignant melanoma in those who have disease progression after ipilimumab or in BRAF V600 mutation–positive patients who have disease progression after ipilimumab and a BRAF inhibitor. Metastatic non-small lung cancer with high PD-L1 expression lacking EGFR or ALK, recurrent head and neck squamous cell carcinoma, Hodgkin lymphoma

Pharmacokinetics

Absorption	complete
Distribution	Unknown
Metabolism	Unknown
Excretion	Unknown
Half-life	22-26 days

Pharmacodynamics

Onset	Unknown
Peak	Unknown
Duration	Unknown

CONTRAINDICATIONS: Hypersensitivity, pregnancy, breastfeeding

Precautions: Immune-mediated colitis, immune-mediated hepatitis, immune-mediated hyperthyroidism/hypothyroidism; immune-mediated nephritis, acute interstitial nephritis, and renal failure; immune-mediated pneumonitis, adrenocortical insufficiency, arthritis, exfoliative dermatitis, hemolytic anemia, hypophysitis, myasthenia syndrome, myositis, optic neuritis, pancreatitis, partial seizures after inflammatory foci identified in brain parenchyma, rhabdomyolysis, uveitis, incidence of abortion/stillbirths

DOSAGE AND ROUTES
Adult: IV INF: 200mg over 30 min q3wk until disease progression, up to 24 months in some

Available forms: Powder for injection 50 mg/vial; solution for injection 25 mg/mL

ADVERSE EFFECTS
CNS: Seizures, myasthenia gravis, headache, fever, insomnia, chills, dizziness, fatigue
EENT: Optic neuritis
ENDO: Hyponatremia, hypothyroidism/hyperthyroidism, hyperglycemia, hypocalcemia, immune-mediated hypophysitis
GI: Nausea, vomiting, abdominal pain, pancreatitis, colitis, diarrhea, hepatitis, constipation
GU: Interstitial nephritis, renal failure
INTEG: Rash, pruritus, skin discoloration
MS: Myalgia, immune-mediated rhabdomyolysis
RESP: Cough, dyspnea, pneumonitis
SYST: Exfoliative dermatitis

INTERACTIONS
Drug/lab test
Increased: LFTs, renal function studies

NURSING CONSIDERATIONS
Assessment
• **Hyperglycemia:** May cause diabetes mellitus type 1 or diabetic ketoacidosis
• For hyperthyroidism/hypothyroidism, assess for renal function studies baseline, periodically during therapy, CCr, BUN, monitor for nephritis
• For pneumonitis, assess for new or worsening cough, chest pain, shortness of breath, confirm with x-ray; give corticosteroids ≥ grade 2, withhold in grade 2, resume in grade 1
• **Immune-mediated hepatitis:** Liver function tests and hepatitis (jaundice, severe nausea/vomiting, easy bleeding or bruising; withhold and give corticosteroids if grade 2 hepatitis (AST or ALT >3-5 × ULN or total bilirubin >1.5-3 × ULN)

Patient problem
Risk of infection (adverse reactions)
Diarrhea (adverse reactions)
Lack of knowledge of medication (teaching)

Implementation
Intermittent IV INF route
• Add 2.3 ml of sterile water for injection, 50-mg vial (25 mg/ml); inject sterile water along the walls of the vial and not directly on the powder
• Gently swirl and allow up to 5 min for bubbles to clear, do not shake; solution will be clear to slightly opalescent, colorless to slightly yellow
• Add the required amount of product to a bag of normal saline (0.9% sodium chloride injection) to a final diluted concentration between 1 and 10 mg/ml; mix by gentle inversion
• Discard any unused solution left in the vial
• Storage after reconstitution and dilution: Store at room temperature up to 4 hr or refrigerate up to 24 hr (includes reconstitution, dilution, and administration time). If refrigerated, allow the diluted solution to warm to room temperature before use, give over 30 min.
• Use a sterile, nonpyrogenic, low-protein binding 0.2- to 5-micron in-line or add-on filter
• Do not use with other drugs through the same infusion line
• **Grade 2 or 3 toxicity:** Withhold and give corticosteroids; resume when the adverse event recovers to grade ≤1. Permanently discontinue if there is no recovery within 12 wk, if the corticosteroid dose cannot be reduced to ≤10 mg/day of predniSONE (or equivalent) within 12 wk, or for recurrent severe or grade 3 colitis.
• **Grade 4 toxicity:** Permanently discontinue, give corticosteroids
Hepatitis:
• **Grade 2 toxicity (AST or ALT >3-5 × upper limit of normal [ULN] or total bilirubin ≤1.5-3 × ULN):** Withhold and give corticosteroids; resume when adverse event recovers to grade 1 or less. Permanently discontinue if there is no recovery within 12 wks or if the corticosteroid dose cannot be reduced to ≤10 mg/day of predniSONE (or equivalent) within 12 wks.
• **Grade 3 or 4 toxicity (AST or ALT >5 × ULN or total bilirubin >3 × ULN):** Permanently discontinue, give corticosteroids
• **Liver metastases and grade 2 elevated transaminase levels at baseline:** Permanently discontinue if AST/ALT levels increase by ≥50% over baseline and transaminase level elevations persist for at least 1 wk

Patient/family education
• **Pregnancy:** Assess if pregnancy is planned or suspected; if breastfeeding, instruct patient to use highly effective contraceptive methods during and for 4 months after treatment, to contact their health care provider if pregnancy is suspected or confirmed
• Teach patient to notify prescriber immediately of signs of colitis, pneumonitis, hepatitis, hypophysitis
• **Hyperglycemia:** Teach about signs and symptoms of hyperglycemia, diabetes, ensure right glucose control, report
• Teach patient that prophylactic folic acid and B$_{12}$ injections may be necessary 1 wk before therapy to prevent bone marrow suppression and GI symptoms
• **Immune-mediated hypophysitis:** Headache, weakness, fainting, dizziness, blurred vision, use corticosteroid if >grade 2, discontinue if >grade 3

Evaluation
Positive therapeutic outcome
• Decreased progression of multiple myeloma

⚠ HIGH ALERT

PEMEtrexed (Rx)
(pem-ah-trex′ed)
Alimta
Func. class.: Antineoplastic-antimetabolite
Chem. class.: Folic acid antagonist

Do not confuse: pemetrexed/pralatrexate

ACTION: Inhibits multiple enzymes that reduce folic acid, which is needed for cell replication

Therapeutic outcome: Decreased spread of mesothelioma, decreased tumor size

USES: Malignant pleural mesothelioma in combination with CISplatin; non–small cell lung cancer as a single agent; non-squamous non–small cell lung cancer (first-line treatment)

Pharmacokinetics
Absorption	Unknown
Distribution	81% protein binding
Metabolism	Not metabolized
Excretion	Excreted in urine (unchanged 70%-90%) Not known if it is excreted in breast milk
Half-life	3.5 hr

Pharmacodynamics

Unknown

CONTRAINDICATIONS

Pregnancy, hypersensitivity, ANC <1500 cells/mm^3, CCr <45 ml/min, thrombocytopenia (<100,000/mm^3), anemia

Precautions: Breastfeeding, children, renal/hepatic disease

DOSAGE AND ROUTES

Adult: IV INF 500-600 mg/m^2 given over 10 min on day 1 of a 21-day cycle with CISplatin 75 mg/m^2 INF over 2 hr beginning ½ hr after end of PEMEtrexed INF

Renal dose

Adult: IV infusion CCr <45 ml/min, not recommended

Available forms: Inj, single-use vials, 100, 500 mg

ADVERSE EFFECTS

CNS: *Fatigue, fever, mood alteration, neuropathy*

CV: Thrombosis/embolism, *chest pain*, arrhythmia exacerbation

GI: *Nausea, vomiting, anorexia, diarrhea, ulcerative stomatitis, constipation, dehydration*

GU: Renal failure, *creatinine elevation*

HEMA: Neutropenia, leukopenia, thrombocytopenia, myelosuppression, anemia

INTEG: *Rash, desquamation*

RESP: *Dyspnea*

SYST: Infection with/without neutropenia, radiation recall reaction

INTERACTIONS

Individual Drugs

Probenecid: Increased effect of premetrexel

Drug classifications

Nephrotoxic products (NSAIDs): decreased PEMEtrexed clearance, avoid NSAIDs for 2-5 days prior to use

NURSING CONSIDERATIONS

Assessment

• **Bone marrow depression:** monitor CBC, differential, platelet count; monitor for nadir and recovery on days 8, 15 of the cycle; a new cycle should not begin if ANC < 1500 cells/mm^3, platelets are < 100,000 cells/mm^3, creatinine clearance < 45 ml/min, if platelet nadir is < 50,000/mm^3, decreased both products by 50%

• Neurotoxicity: Monitor renal tests: BUN, serum uric acid, urine CCr, electrolytes before, during therapy

• For previous radiation treatments; radiation recall reactions have occurred (erythema, exfoliative dermatitis, pain, burning)

• Monitor I&O ratio; report fall in urine output to <30 ml/hr

• Monitor temp q4hr; fever may indicate beginning infection; no rectal temps

• Assess bleeding time, coagulation time during treatment; bleeding: hematuria, guaiac, bruising or petechiae, mucosa or orifices q8hr

• Assess buccal cavity q8hr for dryness, sores, ulceration, white patches, oral pain, bleeding, dysphagia

• **Assess for symptoms indicating severe allergic reaction/toxic epidermal necrolysis:** rash, urticaria, itching, flushing

• **Pregnancy/breastfeeding:** Do not use in pregnancy, breastfeeding

Patient problem

Risk of infection (adverse reactions)

Risk of injury (adverse reactions)

Implementation

• Administer vit B$_{12}$ and low-dose folic acid as a prophylactic measure to treat related hematologic, GI toxicity; at least folic acid (1 mg) must be taken in the 7 days preceding first dose and for 21 days after discontinuing

• Premedicate with a corticosteroid (dexamethasone) given PO bid the day before, day of, and day after administration of PEMEtrexed

• **Bleeding:** assess for bleeding time, coagulation time during treatment; bleeding; hematuria, guaiac, bruising or petechiae, mucosa or orifices q8hr

• Use a liquid diet: carbonated beverage, gelatin; dry toast, crackers may be added when patient is not nauseated or vomiting

• Assist patient with rinsing of mouth tid-qid with water, club soda; brushing of teeth bid-tid with soft brush or cotton-tipped applicators for stomatitis; use unwaxed dental floss

IV route

• Use cytotoxic handling procedures

• Reconstitute 500-mg vial/20 ml 0.9% NaCl inj (preservative free) = 25 mg/ml, swirl until dissolved, further dilute with 100 ml 0.9% NaCl inj (preservative free), give as IV inf over 10 min

• Use only 0.9% NaCl inj (preservative free) for reconstitution, dilution

---

• Store at 77° F, excursions permitted 59°-86°F, not light sensitive, discard unused portions

Dosage adjustments

Do not begin a new cycle unless neutrophils (ANC) $\geq$1500 cells/mm³, platelets $\geq$100,000 cells/mm³, CCr is $\geq$45 ml/min

• **Platelet nadir <50,000/mm³ regardless of the ANC:** If necessary, delay until platelet count recovery, reduce PEMEtrexed and CISplatin by 50%; if grade 3/4 toxicity occurs after 2 reductions, discontinue both products

• **ANC nadir <500/mm³ when platelet nadir is $\geq$50,000/mm³:** If necessary, delay until ANC recovery, reduce PEMEtrexed and CISplatin by 75%; if grade 3/4 toxicity occurs after 2 reductions, discontinue both products

• **CTC Grade 3/4 nonhematologic toxicity including diarrhea requiring hospitalization and excluding neurotoxicity, mucositis, and grade 3 transaminase elevations:** Withhold therapy until pre-therapy value or condition, reduce by 75% both products, if grade 3 or 4 toxicity occurs after 2 reductions, discontinue both products

• **CTC grade 3/4 mucositis:** Withhold therapy until pre-therapy value or condition, reduce 50% of PEMEtrexed; if grade 3 or 4 mucositis occurs after 2 dosage reductions, discontinue both products

• **CTC grade 2 neurotoxicity:** Withhold therapy until pre-therapy value or condition, reduce dose of CISplatin by 50%

• **CTC grade 3/4 neurotoxicity:** discontinue both products

Y-site compatibilities: Acyclovir sodium, alfentanil, allopurinol, amifostine, amikacin, aminocaproic acid, aminophylline, amiodarone, amphotericin B lipid complex, amphotericin B liposome, ampicillin, ampicillin-sulbactam, atenolol, atracurium, azithromycin, aztreonam, bivalirudin, bleomycin, bumetanide, buprenorphine, butorphanol, CARBOplatin, carmustine, ceftizoxime, cefTRIAXone, cefuroxime, cimetidine, cisatracurium, CISplatin, clindamycin, cyclophosphamide, cycloSPORINE, cytarabine, DACTINomycin, DAPTOmycin, dexamethasone, digoxin, diltiazem, diphenhydrAMINE, DOCEtaxel, dolasetron, DOPamine, doxacurium, enalaprilat, ePHEDrine, EPINEPHrine, eptifibatide, ertapenem, esmolol, etoposide, famotidine, fenoldopam, fentaNYL, fluconazole, fludarabine, fluorouracil, foscarnet, fosphenytoin, furosemide, ganciclovir, gatifloxacin, glycopyrrolate, granisetron, haloperidol, heparin, hydrocortisone, HYDROmorphone, hydrOXYzine, ifosfamide, imipenem-cilastatin, insulin (regular), isoproterenol, ketorolac, labetalol, leucovorin, levofloxacin, lidocaine, linezolid, LORazepam, magnesium, mannitol, meperidine, meropenem, mesna, methyldopate, methylPREDNISolone, metoclopramide, metoprolol, midazolam, milrinone, mitoMYcin, mivacurium, morphine, moxifloxacin, nafcillin, naloxone, nesiritide, nitroglycerin, norepinephrine, octreotide, oxaliplatin, PACLitaxel, pamidronate, pancuronium, PENTobarbital, PHENobarbital, piperacillin-tazobactam, polymyxin B, potassium chloride/phosphates, procainamide, promethazine, propranolol, ranitidine, remifentanil, rocuronium, sodium acetate/bicarbonate/phosphates, succinylcholine, SUFentanil, sulfamethoxazole-trimethoprim, tacrolimus, theophylline, thiopental, thiotepa, ticarcillin, ticarcillin-clavulanate, tigecycline, tirofiban, trimethobenzamide, vancomycin, vecuronium, verapamil, vinBLAStine, vinCRIStine, vinorelbine, zidovudine, zoledronic acid

Patient/family education

• Instruct patient to report any complaints, side effects to nurse or prescriber: black tarry stools, chills, fever, sore throat, bleeding, bruising, cough, shortness of breath, dark or bloody urine

• Instruct patient to avoid foods with citric acid, hot or rough texture if stomatitis is present

• Instruct patient to report stomatitis: any bleeding, white spots, ulcerations in mouth to prescriber; tell patient to examine mouth daily, report symptoms to nurse, use good oral hygiene

• Advise patient to discuss with healthcare professional OTC, Rx, herbals, supplements taken, to avoid alcohol

• Advise patient to avoid use of razors, commercial mouthwash

• Teach to eat foods high in folic acid and take supplements as prescribed

• **Pregnancy/breastfeeding:** Advise patient that contraceptive measures are recommended during therapy and for at least 8 wk following cessation of therapy, to discontinue breastfeeding; toxicity to infant may occur

Evaluation

Positive therapeutic outcome

• Decreased spread of malignancy

penciclovir topical
See Appendix B

PENICILLINS

penicillin G benzathine (Rx)
(pen-i-sill′in)
Bicillin L-A
penicillin G Potassium (Rx)
Pfizerpen
penicillin G procaine (Rx)
penicillin G Sodium (Rx)
Crystapen ✦
penicillin V (Rx)
Apo-Pen-VK ✦, **Novo-Pen-VK** ✦,
Pen-VK ✦, **Penicillin VK**
Func. class.: Broad-spectrum antiinfective
Chem. class.: Natural penicillin

ACTION: Interferes with cell wall replication of susceptible organisms; osmotically unstable cell wall swells and bursts from osmotic pressure, resulting in cell death

Therapeutic outcome: Bactericidal effects on the gram-positive cocci *Staphylococcus, Streptococcus pyogenes, Streptococcus viridans, Streptococcus faecalis, Streptococcus bovis, Streptococcus pneumoniae;* gram-negative cocci *Neisseria gonorrhoeae;* gram-positive bacilli *Actinomyces, Bacillus anthracis, Clostridium perfringens, Clostridium tetani, Corynebacterium diphtheriae, Listeria monocytogenes;* gram-negative bacilli *Escherichia coli, Proteus mirabilis, Salmonella, Shigella, Enterobacter, Streptobacillus moniliformis;* spirochete *Treponema pallidum*

USES: Respiratory tract infections, scarlet fever, erysipelas, otitis media, pneumonia, skin and soft tissue infections, gonorrhea

>> Penicillin G benzathine
Pharmacokinetics

Absorption	Delayed; prolonged drug levels
Distribution	Widely distributed; crosses placenta
Metabolism	Liver, minimally
Excretion	Kidneys, unchanged; breast milk
Half-life	½-1 hr

Pharmacodynamics

Onset	Slow
Peak	12-24 hr
Duration	1-4 wk

>> Penicillin G
Pharmacokinetics

Absorption	Variably absorbed (PO); well absorbed (IM)
Distribution	Widely distributed; crosses placenta
Metabolism	Liver, minimally
Excretion	Kidneys, unchanged; breast milk
Half-life	½-1 hr

Pharmacodynamics

	PO	IM	IV
Onset	Rapid	Rapid	Rapid
Peak	1 hr	¼-½ hr	Immediate
Duration	Unknown	Unknown	Unknown

>> Penicillin G procaine
Pharmacokinetics

Absorption	Delayed; prolonged drug levels
Distribution	Widely distributed; crosses placenta
Metabolism	Liver, minimally
Excretion	Kidneys, unchanged; breast milk
Half-life	½-1 hr

Pharmacodynamics

Onset	Slow
Peak	1-4 hr
Duration	15 hr

>> Penicillin V
Pharmacokinetics

Absorption	Widely absorbed
Distribution	Widely distributed; crosses placenta
Metabolism	Liver, minimally
Excretion	Kidneys, unchanged; breast milk
Half-life	½-1 hr

Pharmacodynamics

Onset	Rapid
Peak	½ hr
Duration	Unknown

CONTRAINDICATIONS
Hypersensitivity to penicillins, corn

Precautions: Pregnancy, breastfeeding, hypersensitivity to cephalosporins/carbapenem/sulfite, severe renal disease, GI disease, asthma

> **BLACK BOX WARNING:** Penicillin G benzathine: IV use

DOSAGE AND ROUTES
>> **Penicillin G benzathine**
Early syphilis
Adult: IM 2.4 million units in single dose
Congenital syphilis
Child <2 yr: IM 50,000 units/kg in single dose, max 2.4 million units as a single inj
Prophylaxis of rheumatic fever, glomerulonephritis
Adult and child: IM 1.2 million units q mon or 600,000 units q 2 wks
Upper respiratory tract infections (group A streptococcal)
Adult: IM 1.2 million units in single dose
Child >27 kg: IM 900,000 units in single dose
Child <27 kg: IM 300,000-600,000 units in single dose

Available forms: Inj 300,000 units/ml; 600,000 units/ml

>> **Penicillin G potassium**
Pneumococcal/streptococcal infections (serious)
Adult: IM/IV 5-24 million units in divided doses q4-6hr
Child <12 yr: IV 150,000-300,000 units/kg/day in 4-6 divided doses; max 24 million units/day
Most infections
Adult: IM/IV 1-5 million units q 4-6 hr
Child: IM/IV 8333-16,667 units/kg q 4 hr; 12,550-25,000 units/kg q 4 hr; up to 250,000 units/kg q day in divided doses, if more serious 300,000 units/kg q day
Infants< 7 day: IV 25,000 units/kg q 12 hr, meningitis 100,000-150,000 units/kg q day in divided doses
Renal dose
CCr >10 ml/min, give full loading dose, then ½ of loading dose q8-10hr

Available forms: Inj 1, 2, 3 million units/50 ml; powder for inj 1, 5, 20 million units/vial

>> **Penicillin G procaine**
Moderate to severe pneumococcal infections
Adult: IM 600,000-1.2 million units in 1 or 2 doses/day for 10 days to 2 wk
Child IM: 50,000 units/kg q day × 10-14 days (congenital syphilis)

Available forms: Inj 600,000 units/ml

>> **Penicillin V**
Most Infections
Adult/Child ≥ 12 yr: PO 125-500 mg q6-8 hr
Child <12: 125 mg q 12 hr (Streptococcus pneumonia, sickle cell); 12.5 mg/kg q 6 hr (Lyme disease unlabeled)

Prevention of Rheumatic fever/chorea
Adult: PO 125-250 mg bid continuously

Available forms: Tabs 250, 500 mg; powder for oral sol 125, 250 mg/5 ml

ADVERSE EFFECTS
CNS: Lethargy, hallucinations, anxiety, depression, twitching, coma, seizures, hyperreflexia
GI: *Nausea, vomiting, diarrhea,* increased AST, ALT, abdominal pain, glossitis, colitis, CDAD
GU: Oliguria, proteinuria, hematuria, *vaginitis, moniliasis,* glomerulonephritis, renal tubular damage
HEMA: Anemia, increased bleeding time, bone marrow depression, granulocytopenia, hemolytic anemia
META: Hyperkalemia, hypokalemia, alkalosis, hypernatremia
MISC: Local pain, tenderness and fever with IM inj, anaphylaxis serum sickness, Stevens-Johnson syndrome

INTERACTIONS
Individual drugs
Aspirin, probenecid: increased penicillin levels
Heparin: increased effect of heparin
Methotrexate: increased effect of methotrexate
Typhoid vaccine: decreased effect of vaccine

Drug classifications
Contraceptives (oral): decreased contraceptive effectiveness
Tetracyclines: decreased antimicrobial effectiveness of penicillin

Drug/lab test
False positive: urine glucose, urine protein

NURSING CONSIDERATIONS
Assessment
• Assess patient for previous sensitivity reaction to penicillins or cephalosporins; cross-sensitivity

between penicillins and cephalosporins is common

• **Assess patient for signs and symptoms of infection** including characteristics of wounds, sputum, urine, stool, WBC >10,000/mm³, earache, fever; obtain information baseline, during treatment

• Obtain C&S before beginning drug therapy to identify if correct treatment has been initiated

• **Assess for allergic reactions:** rash, urticaria, pruritus, chills, fever, joint pain; angioedema may occur a few days after therapy begins; EPINEPHrine, resuscitation equipment should be available for anaphylactic reaction

• **CDAD:** Assess for diarrhea, abdominal pain, fever, fatigue, anorexia; possible anemia, elevated WBC and low serum albumin; stop product and usually give either vancomycin or IV metroNIDAZOLE

• Identify urine output; if decreasing, notify prescriber (may indicate nephrotoxicity); also check for increased BUN, creatinine

• Monitor blood studies: AST, ALT, CBC, Hct, bilirubin, LDH, alkaline phosphatase, Coombs' test monthly if patient is on long-term therapy

• Monitor electrolytes: potassium, sodium, chloride monthly if patient is on long-term therapy

• Assess bowel pattern daily; if severe diarrhea occurs, product should be discontinued; may indicate CDAD

• Monitor for bleeding: ecchymosis, bleeding gums, hematuria, stool guaiac daily if on long-term therapy

• **Assess for overgrowth of infection:** perineal itching, fever, malaise, redness, pain, swelling, drainage, rash, diarrhea, change in cough, sputum

Patient problem

Infection (uses)
Diarrhea (adverse reactions)

Implementation
>> Penicillin G benzathine
IM route
• No dilution needed, shake well, give deeply IM in large muscle mass, avoid intravascular inj; aspirate; do not give **IV**

>> Penicillin G
• Penicillin G sodium or potassium can be given IM or IV, vials containing 10 or 20 million units are not for IM use

Intermittent IV infusion route
• **Vials/bulk packages;** dilute according to manufacturer's directions
• **Frozen bags:** thaw at room temp, do not force thaw, no reconstitution needed
• Final conc (100,000-500,000 units/ml, adults; 50,000 units/ml, neonate/infant)
• Total daily dose divided q4-6hr and given over 1-2 hr (adult), 15 min (infant/neonate)

>> Penicillin G potassium
Y-site compatibilities: Acyclovir, amiodarone, aztreonam, atropine, benztropine, bumetanide, buprenorphine, butorphanol, calcium chloride/gluconate, ceFAZolin, cefTRIAXone, cefuroxime, chloramphenicol, clindamycin, cyclophosphamide, diltiazem, enalaprilat, esmolol, fluconazole, foscarnet, heparin, HYDROmorphone, labetalol, magnesium sulfate, meperidine, morphine, perphenazine, potassium chloride, tacrolimus, theophylline, vit B/C

>> Penicillin G procaine
• No dilution needed, give deep IM inj; avoid intravascular inj; aspirate; do not give IV
• Reconstitute with 0.9% NaCl, sterile water for inj, D₅W; refrigerate unused portion
• Shake medication before administering
• IM route may include procaine reactions: fear of death, depression, seizures, anxiety, confusion, hallucinations

>> Penicillin V
• Orally on empty stomach for best absorption
• **Oral susp:** tap bottle to loosen, add ½ total amount of water, shake, add remaining water, shake; final conc (125 or 250); store in refrigerator after reconstitution, discard after 14 days
• Give in even doses around the clock; if GI upset occurs, give with food; product must be given for 10-14 days to ensure organism death and prevent superinfection; store in tight container
• Shake susp; store in refrigerator for 2 wk or for 1 wk at room temperature

Patient/family education
• Teach patient to report sore throat, bruising, bleeding, joint pain; may indicate **blood dyscrasias (rare)**; CNS effects: depression, hallucinations, seizures
• Advise patient to contact prescriber if vaginal itching, loose foul-smelling stools, furry tongue occur; may indicate **superinfection**
• Instruct patient to take all medication prescribed for the length of time ordered
• Advise patient to notify prescriber of diarrhea with blood or pus, which may indicate CDAD

- **Sexually transmitted infection:** All partners must be notified and treated
- **Suspension:** Teach patient to shake suspension well before each dose, store in refrigerator for up to 2 wk
- **Pregnancy:** Identify if pregnancy is planned or suspected or if breastfeeding

Evaluation

Positive therapeutic outcome
- Absence of signs/symptoms of infection (WBC <10,000/mm^3, temp WNL, absence of red, draining wounds, earache)
- Reported improvement in symptoms of infection

TREATMENT OF ANAPHYLAXIS:
Withdraw product, maintain airway, administer EPINEPHrine, SUBCUT × 3 doses, followed by an epinephrine drip, O$_2$, **IV** corticosteroids, inhaled bronchodilator

pentamidine (Rx)
(pen-tam'i-deen)
Nebupent, Pentam 300
Func. class.: Antiprotozoal
Chem. class.: Aromatic diamide derivative

ACTION: Interferes with DNA/RNA synthesis in protozoa; has direct effect on islet cells in the pancreas

Therapeutic outcome: Protozoa death

USES: Treatment/prevention of *Pneumocystis jiroveci* infections

Unlabeled uses: PJP (Inhalation)

Pharmacokinetics

Absorption	Well absorbed (IM); minimally absorbed (INH); completely absorbed (**IV**)
Distribution	Widely distributed; does not appear in CSF
Metabolism	Not known
Excretion	Kidneys, unchanged (up to 30%)
Half-life	9-13 hr; increased in renal disease

Pharmacodynamics

	IM	IV	INH
Onset	Unknown	Unknown	Unknown
Peak	0.5-1 hr	Inf end	Unknown
Duration	Unknown	Unknown	Unknown

CONTRAINDICATIONS
Hypersensitivity

Precautions: Pregnancy, breastfeeding, children, blood dyscrasias, cardiac/renal/hepatic disease, diabetes mellitus, hypocalcemia, hyper/hypotension, anemia

DOSAGE AND ROUTES
Adult and child ≥4 mo: IV/IM 4 mg/kg/day × 2-3 wk; NEB 150 mg q 2 wk or 300 mg via Respirgard II jet nebulizer given q4wk for prevention (Nebupent)

Available forms: Inj; aerosol 300 mg/vial; sol for aerosol 300 mg ✦

ADVERSE EFFECTS
CNS: Disorientation, hallucinations, confusion
CV: Hypotension, chest pain
GI: *Nausea*, diarrhea, metallic taste
HEMA: Anemia, leukopenia, thrombocytopenia
INTEG: Sterile abscess, pain at inj site, pruritus, urticaria, rash
META: *Hypoglycemia*
MISC: Night sweats, anaphylaxis, Stevens-Johnson syndrome
RESP: Cough, shortness of breath, bronchospasm (with aerosol), sore throat

INTERACTIONS
Individual drugs
Amphotericin B, CISplatin, vancomycin: increased nephrotoxicity
Erythromycin IV: fatal dysrhythmias
Haloperidol, chloroquine, droperidol, pentamidine; arsenic trioxide, levomethadyl: increased QT prolongation
Radiation: bone marrow suppression

Drug classifications
Aminoglycosides NSAIDs: increased nephrotoxicity
Antineoplastics: increased bone marrow depression, monitor blood studies
Class IA/III antidysrhythmics, some phenothiazines, β-agonists, local anesthetics, tricyclics, CYP3A4 inhibitors (amiodarone, clarithromycin, erythromycin, telithromycin, troleandomycin), CYP3A4 substrates (methadone, pimozide, QUEtiapine, quiNIDine, risperiDONE, ziprasidone): increased QT prolongation

Drug/lab test
Decrease: WBC, platelets, Hbg, Hct, calcium, magnesium, bilirubin, alkaline phosphatase
Increase: BUN, creatinine potassium, LFTs

P

NURSING CONSIDERATIONS
Assessment
- **Assess any patient with compromised renal system:** product is excreted slowly in poor renal system function; toxicity may occur rapidly
- **QT prolongation:** ECG for QT prolongation, ejection fraction; assess for chest pain, palpitations, dyspnea
- **Assess patient for infection,** including increased temp, thick sputum, WBC >10,000/mm³; monitor these signs of infection throughout treatment; obtain C&S before beginning therapy; treatment may begin after culture is obtained
- Assess respiratory system including rate, rhythm, bilateral lung sounds, SOB, wheezing, dyspnea
- **Serious skin reactions:** Assess for rash, fever, fatigue, muscle/joint aches, oral lesions, blisters, discontinue product immediately if these occur
- **Pancreatitis:** Assess for nausea, vomiting, severe abdominal pain, monitor the lab values of lipase/amylase that will be elevated, if these occur product may need to be discontinued
- Monitor ECG for cardiac dysrhythmias in cardiac patients; ECG and pulse should be checked frequently during treatment, since cardiotoxicity can occur
- Assess for hypoglycemia including nausea, tremors, anxiety, chills, diaphoresis, headache, hunger, cold, pale skin; this side effect can last for several mo after treatment is completed
- Monitor renal function tests including BUN, urinalysis, creatinine; obtain at baseline and frequently during treatment; nephrotoxicity may occur; check I&O, report hematuria, oliguria
- Monitor blood studies including blood glucose, CBC, platelets; blood glucose fluctuations are common; anemia, leukopenia, thrombocytopenia can occur
- Monitor liver function studies including AST, ALT, alkaline phosphatase, bilirubin before beginning treatment and every 3 days during therapy
- Monitor calcium and magnesium before beginning treatment and every 3 days during therapy; hypocalcemia may occur

Patient problem
Infection (uses)
Risk of infection (uses)

Implementation
Inhalation route
- Through nebulizer, using Respirgard II jet nebulizer; mix contents in 6 ml of sterile water; do not use low pressure (<20 psi); flow rate should be 5-7 L/min (40-50 psi) air or O_2 source over 30-45 min until chamber is empty
IM route
- 300 mg diluted in 3 ml sterile water (100 mg/mL); give deep IM by Z-track; painful by this route, rotate inj site

Intermittent IV infusion route
- 300 mg/3-5 ml of sterile water for inj, D_5W; withdraw dose and further dilute in 50-250 ml of D_5W; diluted sol is stable for 48 hr; discard unused sol; give over 1 hr or more
- Assess IV site frequently, has vesicant properties

Y-site compatibilities: alemtuzumab, alfentanil, aminocaproic acid, anidulafungin, argatroban, atracurium, atropine, benztropine, buprenorphine, calcium gluconate, CARBOplatin, caspofungin, chlorpromazine, cimetidine, CISplatin, cyclophosphamide, cycloSPORINE, cytarabine, DACTINomycin, diltiazem, gatifloxacin, zidovudine

Patient/family education
- Teach patient to report sore throat, fever, fatigue; could indicate superinfection
- Teach patient to make position changes slowly to prevent orthostatic hypotension
- Advise patient to maintain adequate fluid intake
- Teach patient to complete entire course of medication
- **Pancreatitis:** Advise patient to report to provider immediately nausea, vomiting, severe abdominal pain
- Pregnancy/breastfeeding: Identify if pregnancy is planned or suspected or if breastfeeding
- Advise patient to report immediately rash, fever, sore throat, or flu like symptoms, to avoid crowds, persons with known infections

Evaluation
Positive therapeutic outcome
- Decreased signs and symptoms of protozoan infections
- Decreased signs and symptoms of *P. jiroveci* pneumonia in HIV infections

---

RARELY USED

perampanel
(per-am'pa-nel)
Fycompa
Func. class.: Anticonvulsant, glutamate receptor antagonist
Schedule III

USES: Adjunctive treatment of partial onset seizures, generalized tonic-clonic seizures in combination with other anticonvulsants

CONTRAINDICATIONS: Hypersensitivity, severe hepatic disease

> **BLACK BOX WARNING:** Behavioral changes

DOSAGE AND ROUTES
Adult/child ≥12 yr: **PO 2** mg q day at bedtime, may increase by 2 mg/day weekly up to 4-12 mg/day (partial onset seizures) 8-12 mg/day (tonic-clonic seizures)

perindopril (Rx)
(per-in-doe-pril)
Aceon, Coversyl
Func. class.: Antihypertensive
Chem. class.: Angiotensin-converting enzyme (ACE) inhibitor

ACTION: Selectively suppresses renin angiotensin-aldosterone system; inhibits ACE; prevents conversion of angiotensin I to angiotensin II, resulting in dilatation of arterial and venous vessels

Therapeutic outcome: Decreased B/P in hypertension

USES: Hypertension alone or in combination, stable artery disease

Pharmacokinetics

Absorption	Well absorbed
Distribution	Unknown
Metabolism	Liver
Excretion	Kidneys
Half-life	Unknown

Pharmacodynamics

Onset	Unknown
Peak	Unknown
Duration	Unknown

CONTRAINDICATIONS: Hypersensitivity, history of angioedema

> **BLACK BOX WARNING:** Pregnancy

Precautions: Breastfeeding, renal disease, hyperkalemia, hepatic failure, dehydration, bilateral renal artery stenosis, cough, angioedema, severe HF

DOSAGE AND ROUTES
Hypertension
Adult: PO 4 mg/day, may increase or decrease to desired response; range 4-8 mg/day, may give in two divided doses or as a single dose; max 16 mg/day

Patients taking diuretics
Adult: PO 2-4 mg/day in 1-2 divided doses, range 4-8 mg/day

Stable CAD
Adult: PO 4 mg/day 2 wk, then increase as tolerated to 8 mg/day

Renal dose
Adult: PO CCr 16-29 ml/min, 2 mg every other day; CCr 30-59 ml/min 2 mg/day

Available forms: Tabs, scored 2, 4, 8 mg

ADVERSE EFFECTS
CNS: *Insomnia, dizziness,* paresthesias, headache, fatigue, anxiety, depression
CV: *Hypotension,* chest pain, tachycardia, dysrhythmias, syncope
EENT: *Tinnitus,* visual changes, sore throat, double vision, dry burning eyes
GI: Nausea, vomiting, colitis, cramps, diarrhea, constipation, flatulence, dry mouth, loss of taste
GU: Proteinuria, renal failure, increased frequency of polyuria or oliguria
HEMA: Agranulocytosis, neutropenia
INTEG: Rash, purpura, alopecia, hyperhidrosis
META: Hyperkalemia
RESP: Dyspnea, dry cough, crackles
SYST: Angioedema

INTERACTIONS
Individual drugs
Allopurinol: increased hypersensitivity
Lithium: increased serum levels

Drug classifications
Antihypertensives, diuretics: increased hypotension
Antihypertensives, neuromuscular blocking agents: increased effects
Diuretics (potassium-sparing), potassium supplements, salt substitutes: hyperkalemia
NSAIDs: decreased effects
NSAIDs, salicylates: decreased antihypertensive effect

P

Drug/herb
Hawthorn: increased antihypertensive effect
Ephedra: decreased antihypertensive effect

Drug/lab test
Interference: glucose/insulin tolerance tests

NURSING CONSIDERATIONS
Assessment
• **Hypertension:** monitor B/P, orthostatic hypotension, syncope; if changes occur dosage change may be required
• Monitor blood studies: neutrophils, decreased platelets
• **HF:** Check for edema in feet, legs daily
• Monitor renal studies: protein, BUN, creatinine; increased levels may indicate nephrotic syndrome and renal failure
• Monitor renal symptoms: polyuria, oliguria, frequency, dysuria
• Establish baselines in renal, liver function tests before therapy begins
• Check potassium levels throughout treatment, although hyperkalemia rarely occurs
• **Assess for allergic reactions:** rash, fever, pruritus, urticaria; product should be discontinued if antihistamines fail to help; angioedema: facial swelling, urticaria, product should be discontinued; may be more common in African-Americans

Patient problems
• Impaired cardiac output (uses)
• Risk for injury (adverse reactions)
• Lack of knowledge of medication (teaching)
• Nonadherence (teaching)

Implementation
• Store in airtight container at 86° F (30° C) or less
• Severe hypotension may occur after first dose of this medication; decreased hypotension may be prevented by reducing or discontinuing diuretic therapy 3 days before beginning perindopril therapy
• Give by **IV** inf of 0.9% NaCl (as ordered) to expand fluid volume if severe hypotension occurs

Patient/family education
• Advise patient not to discontinue product abruptly; advise patient to tell all persons associated with health care about product taken
• Teach patient not to use OTC products (cough, cold, allergy medications) unless directed by physician; serious side effects can occur; xanthines, such as coffee, tea, chocolate, cola, can prevent action of product

• Instruct patient on the importance of complying with dosage schedule, even if feeling better; to continue with medical regimen to decrease B/P: exercise, cessation of smoking, decreasing stress, diet modifications
• Emphasize the need to rise slowly to sitting or standing position to minimize orthostatic hypotension; not to exercise in hot weather, which can cause increased hypotension
• Advise patient to notify prescriber of mouth sores, sore throat, fever, swelling of hands or feet, irregular heartbeat, chest pain, coughing, shortness of breath
• Caution patient to report excessive perspiration, dehydration, vomiting, diarrhea; may lead to fall in B/P
• Caution patient that product may cause dizziness, fainting, light-headedness; may occur during first few days of therapy; to avoid activities that may be hazardous
• Teach patient how to take B/P, normal readings for age group

> **BLACK BOX WARNING:** Notify prescriber if pregnancy is planned or suspected

Evaluation
Positive therapeutic outcome
• Decreased B/P in hypertension

TREATMENT OF OVERDOSE:
Lavage, **IV** atropine for bradycardia, **IV** theophylline for bronchospasm, digoxin, O^2; diuretic for cardiac failure, hemodialysis

---

RARELY USED

permethrin
(per-meth'rin)
Elimite
Func. class.: Pediculocides

USES: Scabies

CONTRAINDICATIONS: Hypersensitivity

DOSAGE AND ROUTES
Adults, Adolescents, Children, and Infants ≥2 months: Topical massage 5% cream into the skin from the head to the soles of the feet. Usually 30 g is sufficient for the average adult. Wash cream off after 8 to 14 hr. One application is generally curative.

---

pertuzumab
(per-too'zoo-mab)
Perjeta
Func. class.: Antineoplastic
Chem. class.: HER2/ new antagonist

ACTION: Blocks liquid-dependent action of ᴳᴱᴺ human epidermal growth factor-2 (HER2), inhibiting signal pathways

Therapeutic outcome: Decreased size, spread of tumor

USES: First-line treatment of (HER2) positive metastatic breast cancer with trastuzumab and DOCEtaxel

Pharmacokinetics

Absorption	Complete
Distribution	Unknown
Metabolism	Unknown
Excretion	Unknown
Half-life	18 days

Pharmacodynamics

Onset	Unknown
Peak	Unknown
Duration	Unknown

CONTRAINDICATIONS
Hypersensitivity

BLACK BOX WARNING: Pregnancy

Precautions: Breastfeeding, children, infants, neonates, cardiac arrhythmias, MI, cardiac disease, heart failure, hypertension, infusion-related reactions, ᴳᴱᴺ Asian patients

BLACK BOX WARNING: Heart failure, ventricular dysfunction

DOSAGE AND ROUTES
Adult: IV 840 mg over 60 min, then after 3 wk 420 mg over 30–60 min every 3 wk; give with trastuzumab 8 mg/kg IV over 90 min, then after 3 wk 6 mg/kg over 30–90 min every 3 wk and DOCEtaxel 75 mg/m 2 IV every 3 wk; dosage may be escalated to 100 mg/m²

Available forms: Solution for inj 420 mg/ 14 ml (single-use vials) 30 mg/mL

ADVERSE EFFECTS
CNS: Headache, fever, peripheral neuropathy, chills, fatigue, asthenia, dizziness
CV: Heart failure
EENT: Lacrimation, stomatitis
GI: Nausea, vomiting, diarrhea, dysgeusia, anorexia, constipation
HEMA: Anemia, neutropenia, arthralgia
RESP. Upper respiratory infection, cough
SYST: Anaphylaxis, antibody formation
INTEG: *Alopecia*

NURSING CONSIDERATIONS
Assessment
• **HER2 overexpression**: Testing should be done to identify HER2 overexpression before using this product
• **Decreased left ventricular ejection fraction (LVEF):** Can occur and is increased in those with a history of prior anthracycline use or radiotherapy to the chest; evaluate LVEF at baseline and every 3 mo; withhold therapy × 3 wk if LVEF is <40% or LVEF is 40%–45% with a 10% or greater absolute decrease from baseline; resume therapy if the LVEF is recovered to >45% or to 40%–45% with <10% absolute decrease at reassessment; if the LVEF has not improved or has declined further, consider permanently discontinuing pertuzumab and trastuzumab after a risk/benefit assessment
• **Infusion-related reactions/hypersensitivity:** Assess anaphylactoid reaction, acute infusion reaction, cytokine-release syndrome 60 min after the first infusion, 30 min after other infusions; monitor for pyrexia, chills, fatigue, headache, asthenia, hypersensitivity, and vomiting; if a significant reaction occurs, slow or interrupt the infusion; permanent discontinuation may be needed in severe reactions
• **Neutropenia:** Can occur, but occurs more commonly when trastuzumab is also used and in ᴳᴱᴺ Asian patients, monitor CBC with differential baseline and periodically
• Upper respiratory infection: Monitor for dyspnea, shortness of breath, fever

BLACK BOX WARNING: Pregnancy: Determine if pregnancy is planned or suspected; patients who become pregnant during therapy should report exposure to the Genentech Adverse Event line at 888-835-2555 and enroll in the MOTHER pregnancy registry at 800-690-6720

P

Patient problem
Impaired cardiac output (adverse reactions)
Risk for injury (adverse reactions)

Implementation
• Visually inspect for particulate matter and discoloration

Dilution and preparation
• Withdraw the calculated dose from the vial and add to a 250 ml 0.9% sodium chloride to PVC or non-PVC polyolefin infusion bag; do not dilute with dextrose 5% solution
• Dilute in normal saline only; do not mix or dilute with other drugs or dextrose solutions
• Mix the diluted solution by gentle inversion; do not shake

IV infusion
• Administer the diluted solution immediately
• Do not administer as an IV push or bolus
• Give the first dose of 840 mg over 60 min and subsequent 420-mg doses over 30–60 min
• If the diluted solution is not used immediately, store at 2°–8° C for up to 24 hr

Delayed or missed doses
• If time since previous dose is 6 wk, give 420 mg IV (do not wait for next scheduled dose)
• If time since previous dose is 6 wk, give 840 mg IV over 60 min, followed 3 wk later by 420 mg IV over 30–60 min repeated every 3 wk
• If DOCEtaxel is discontinued, this product and trastuzumab may continue

Patient/family education
• Teach patient to notify prescriber immediately of infection: cough, fever, chills, sore throat
• Teach patient to avoid all OTC, Rx, herbals, supplements unless approved by prescriber, not to use aspirin, NSAIDs, alcohol
• Teach patient to notify prescriber of peripheral neuropathy
• Hair loss is common

> **BLACK BOX WARNING:** Counsel women of childbearing age on the need for contraception during and for 6 mo after therapy; advise patients who suspect pregnancy to contact their health care provider immediately; discontinue breastfeeding

Evaluation

Positive therapeutic outcome
• Decreased size, spread of tumor

---

phenazopyridine (Rx, OTC)
(fen-az-o-peer′-i-deen)
Baridium, Phenazo ✦, Pyridium, Pyridium Plus
Func. class.: Nonopioid analgesic, urinary
Chem. class.: Azodye

ACTION: Exerts analgesic, anesthetic action on the urinary tract mucosa

Therapeutic outcome: Decreased pain, burning when urinating

USES: Urinary tract irritation, infection (for symptoms only of pain, burning, itching) used with urinary antiinfectives

Pharmacokinetics

Absorption	Well absorbed
Distribution	Unknown; crosses placenta
Metabolism	Unknown
Excretion	Kidneys, unchanged
Half-life	Unknown

Pharmacodynamics

Onset	Unknown
Peak	5-6 hr
Duration	8 hr

CONTRAINDICATIONS: Hypersensitivity, renal insufficiency, hepatic disease, uremia

Precautions: Pregnancy, breastfeeding, children <12 yr, geriatric patient, contact lens use

DOSAGE AND ROUTES
Adult: PO 200 mg tid ×2 days or less when used with antibacterial for UTI
Child 6-12 yr: PO 4 mg/kg tid ×2 days

Renal dose
Adult: PO CCr 50-80 ml/min give dose 8-16 hr; CCr <50 ml/min do not use

Available forms: Tabs 95, 97.2, 100, 200 mg

ADVERSE EFFECTS
CNS: Headache, aseptic meningitis
GI: *Nausea*, hepatic toxicity
GU: Renal toxicity, *orange-red urine*
HEMA: Methemoglobinemia
INTEG: Rash, pruritus, skin pigmentation
SYST: Anaphylaxis

INTERACTIONS

Drug/lab test
Interference: urinalysis

NURSING CONSIDERATIONS
Assessment
- Assess urinary status: burning, pain, itching, urgency, frequency; hematuria before, during, after completion of product therapy
- Monitor liver function tests: AST, ALT, bilirubin if patient is on long-term therapy

Assess for hepatotoxicity: dark urine, clay-colored stools, yellowing of skin and sclera, itching, abdominal pain, fever, diarrhea if patient is on long-term therapy
- **Assess for allergic reactions:** rash, urticaria; if these occur, product may have to be discontinued

Patient problems
Lack of knowledge of medication (teaching)
Pain (uses)
Impaired urination (uses)

Implementation
- Give to patient crushed or whole; chew tab should be chewed
- Give with food or milk to decrease gastric symptoms

Patient/family education
- Advise patient to report any symptoms of hepatotoxicity
- Caution patient not to exceed recommended dosage and to take with meals; to read label on other OTC products
- Teach patient not to discontinue after pain is relieved but continue to take concurrent prescribed antiinfective until finished
- Inform patient urine may turn red-orange; body fluids may stain clothing or contact lenses

Evaluation
Positive therapeutic outcome
- Decrease in pain, burning, itching when urinating

TREATMENT OF OVERDOSE:
Methylene blue 1-2 mg/kg **IV** or vit C 100-200 mg PO

⚠ HIGH ALERT

PHENobarbital (Rx)
(fee-noe-bar′-bit-tal)
Luminal, PMS-PHENobarbital
Func. class.: Anticonvulsant
Chem. class.: Barbiturate
Controlled substance schedule IV

Do not confuse: PHENobarbital/PENTobarbital

ACTION: Decreases impulse transmission; increases seizure threshold at cerebral cortex level

Therapeutic outcome: Sedation, anticonvulsant, improved energy

USES: All forms of epilepsy, status epilepticus, febrile seizures in children, sedation, insomnia

Pharmacokinetics

Absorption	Slow (70%-90%) (PO/IM/IV)
Distribution	Not known; crosses placenta
Metabolism	Liver (75%)
Excretion	Kidneys (25% unchanged)
Half-life	2-6 days

Pharmacodynamics

	PO	IM	IV
Onset	30-60 min	10-30 min	5 min
Peak	Unknown	Unknown	30 min
Duration	6-8 hr	4-6 hr	4-6 hr

CONTRAINDICATIONS: Pregnancy, breastfeeding, geriatric, hypersensitivity to barbiturates, porphyria, hepatic/respiratory disease, nephritis, hyperthyroidism, diabetes mellitus

Precautions: Anemia, renal disease

DOSAGE AND ROUTES
Seizures
Adult: PO 1-3 mg/kg/day in divided doses bid, tid, or total dose at bedtime
Child 5-12 yr: PO 3-6 mg/kg/day in 1-2 divided doses
Child 1-5 yr: PO 6-8 mg/kg/day in 1-2 divided doses
Infant: PO 5-6 mg/kg/day in 1-2 divided doses
Neonate: PO 3-4 mg/kg/day as a single dose

Status epilepticus
Adult: IV INF 10 mg/kg; run no faster than 50 mg/min; may give up to 30 mg/kg
Child: IV INF 5-10 mg/kg; may repeat q10-15min up to 20 mg/kg; run no faster than 50 mg/min

Insomnia
Adult: PO/IM/SUBCUT 100-200 mg
Child (unlabeled): PO/IM/SUBCUT 3-5 mg/kg

Sedation
Adult: PO 30-120 mg/day in 2-3 divided doses
Child: PO 3-5 mg/kg/day in 3 divided doses

Preoperative sedation
Adult: IM 100-200 mg 1-1 1/2 hr before surgery
Child: PO/IM/IV 1-3 mg/kg 1-1 1/2 hr before surgery

P

Available forms: Caps 15 mg; elix 20 mg/5 ml; tabs 15, 30, 32, 60, 65, 100 mg; inj 30, 60, 65, 130 mg/ml

ADVERSE EFFECTS

CNS: Paradoxical excitement (geriatric), drowsiness, lethargy, *hangover headache,* flushing, hallucinations, coma
GI: Nausea, vomiting, diarrhea, constipation
HEMA: Agranulocytosis, megaloblastic anemia, thrombocytopenia, thrombophlebitis
INTEG: Rash, urticaria, Stevens-Johnson syndrome, angioedema, local pain, swelling, necrosis, scaling eczema

INTERACTIONS

Individual drugs
Alcohol: increased CNS depression
Chloramphenicol, disulfiram: increased effects
Doxycycline, metroNIDAZOLE, quiNIDine, theophylline: decreased effectiveness
Furosemide: increased orthostatic hypotension
Valproic acid: increased sedation

Drug classifications
Anticoagulants, glucocorticoids, estrogens, hormonal contraceptives: decreased effectiveness
CNS depressants: increased effects
MAOIs, skeletal muscle relaxants (nondepolarizing), sulfonamides: increased effects

Drug/herb
Chamomile, eucalyptus, hops, kava, valerian: increased CNS depression
St. John's wort: decreased barbiturate effect

NURSING CONSIDERATIONS

Assessment
• Assess mental status: mood, sensorium, affect, memory (long, short), especially geriatric; if using as a hypnotic, assess sleep patterns during therapy; product suppresses REM sleep with dreaming
• Withdrawal insomnia may occur after short-term use; do not start using product again; insomnia improves in 1-3 nights; may experience increased dreaming
• Assess respiratory dysfunction: respiratory depression, character, rate, rhythm when using IV; hold product if respirations are <10/min or if pupils are dilated; also check VS q30min after parenteral route for 2 hr
• **Assess for barbiturate toxicity:** hypotension; pulmonary constriction; cold, clammy skin; cyanosis of lips; CNS depression; nausea; vomiting; hallucinations; delirium; weakness; coma; pupillary constriction; mild symptoms occur in 8-12 hr without product

• **Assess for pain** in post-op patients; pain threshold is lowered in patients taking this medication
• **Assess for blood dyscrasias:** fever, sore throat, bruising, rash, jaundice, epistaxis (long-term treatment only)
• **Assess seizure activity,** including type, location, duration, character; provide seizure precaution

Patient problems
• Risk for injury (adverse reactions)
• Lack of knowledge of medication (teaching)
• Impaired sleep (uses)

Implementation
• Give medication after removal of cigarettes to prevent fires
• Give medication after trying conservative measures for insomnia
PO route
• Tab may be crushed and mixed with food if swallowing is difficult; also may be mixed with other fluids 30-60 min before bedtime for expected sleeplessness; on empty stomach for best absorption
• Oral sol: use undiluted or mixed with water or other fluids; use calibrated measuring device
IM route
• Give inj in deep muscle mass (gluteal) to minimize irritation to tissues
• Split inj of >5 ml into two, since irritation to tissues may occur
Direct IV route
• Use large vein to prevent extravasation; if extravasation occurs, use moist heat to the area and 5% procaine sol injected into area; give at 65 mg or less/min; titrate to patient's response

Y-site compatibilities: Doxapram, enalaprilat, fentaNYL, fosphenytoin, levofloxacin, meropenem, methadone, morphine, propofol, SUFentanil

Patient/family education
• Teach patient that hangover is common
• Instruct patient that product is indicated only for short-term treatment of insomnia and is probably ineffective after 2 wk
• Inform patient that physical dependency may result when used for extended time (45-90 days depending on dosage)
• Teach patient to avoid driving and other activities requiring alertness
• Caution patient to avoid alcohol ingestion and CNS depressants; serious CNS depression may result
• Instruct patient not to discontinue medication quickly after long-term use; may cause seizures; product should be tapered over 1 wk; take exactly as prescribed

---

⚠ Nurse Alert   ✦ Key NCLEX® Drug   >> Drug Specifics

- Emphasize the need to tell all prescribers that a barbiturate is being taken
- Teach the patient to make position changes slowly; orthostatic hypotension may occur
- Teach patient that response may take 4 days to 2 wk
- Instruct patient to notify prescriber immediately if bruising, bleeding occur, which may indicate blood dyscrasias

Evaluation
Positive therapeutic outcome
- Improved sleeping patterns
- Decreased seizure activity
- Sedative preoperatively

TREATMENT OF OVERDOSE:
Lavage, activated charcoal, warming blanket, VS, hemodialysis, alkalinize urine, give **IV** volume expanders, **IV** fluids

phenylephrine (Rx)
(fen-ill-ef ′rin)
Neo-Synephrine 🍁, **Vazculep**
Func. class.: Adrenergic, direct acting
Chem. class.: Direct sympathomimetic amine (beta-agonist)

ACTION: Powerful and selective receptor agonist causing contraction of blood vessels, vasoconstriction of eye arterioles; decreases eye engorgement by stimulation of beta-adrenergic receptors

Therapeutic outcome: Increased B/P, decreased nasal congestion, decreased eye irritation

USES: Hypotension, paroxysmal supraventricular tachycardia, shock, B/P maintenance during spinal anesthesia, topical ocular vasoconstrictor in uveitis, open-angle glaucoma; preoperative, diagnostic procedures, refraction without cycloplegia; nasal congestion

Pharmacokinetics

Absorption	Well absorbed (IM); completely absorbed (IV); minimally absorbed (nasal, ophth)
Distribution	Unknown
Metabolism	Liver
Excretion	Unknown
Half-life	Unknown

Pharmacodynamics

	SUBCUT/IM	IV
Onset	15 min	Rapid
Peak	Unknown	Unknown
Duration	45-60 min	20-30 min

CONTRAINDICATIONS
Hypersensitivity, closed angle glaucoma, ventricular fibrillation, tachydysrhythmias, pheochromocytoma, severe hypertension

Precautions: Pregnancy, breastfeeding, geriatric, hyperthyroidism, severe arteriosclerosis, arterial embolism, peripheral vascular disease, bradycardia, myocardial disease, partial heart block

> **BLACK BOX WARNING:** Cardiac disease, extravasation

DOSAGE AND ROUTES
Hypotension
Adult: SUBCUT/IM 2-5 mg; may repeat q10-15min if needed, do not exceed initial dose; IV 0.1-0.5 mg, may repeat q10-15 min if needed, do not exceed initial dose
Child: IM/SUBCUT 0.1 mg/kg/dose q1-2hr prn

Supraventricular tachycardia
Adult: **IV** max 0.5 mg given rapidly, max single dose 1 mg

Shock
Adult: **IV** INF 10 mg/500 ml of D5W given 100-180 mcg/min (if 20 gtt/ml device is used), then maintenance of 40-60 mcg/min (if 20 gtt/ml device is used); use inf pump
Child: **IV** BOL 5-20 mcg/kg/dose q10-15min; **IV** INF 0.1-0.5 mcg/kg/min

Available forms: Inj 1% (10 mg/ml)

ADVERSE EFFECTS
CNS: *Headache, dizziness, anxiety, tremor, insomnia*
CV: Reflex bradycardia, dysrhythmias, *hypertension*, tachycardia, palpitations, ectopic beats, angina
GI: *Nausea, vomiting*
INTEG: Necrosis, tissue sloughing with extravasation, gangrene
MISC: Anaphylaxis

INTERACTIONS
Individual drugs
Digoxin: increased dysrhythmias

P

Drug classifications
Alpha-blockers: decreased phenylephrine action
Antidepressants (tricyclics), H1 antihistamines: increased pressor effect
General anesthetics: increased dysrhythmias
MAOIs: do not use within 2 wk, hypertensive crisis may result
Oxytocics: increased B/P

NURSING CONSIDERATIONS

Assessment
• Monitor I&O ratio; notify prescriber if output <30 ml/hr
• Monitor ECG during administration continuously; if B/P increases, product is decreased
• Monitor B/P and pulse q5min after parenteral route; CVP or PWP during inf if possible
• Assess for paresthesias and coldness of extremities; peripheral blood flow may decrease

Patient problems
• Impaired cardiac output (uses)
• Lack of knowledge of medication (teaching)
• Ineffective tissue perfusion (uses)

Implementation
IV route
• Give plasma expanders for hypovolemia
• Give **IV** after diluting 1 mg/9 ml of sterile water for inj; give dose over 30-60 sec; may be diluted 10 mg/500 ml of D5W or 0.9% NaCl; titrate to patient's response; low normal B/P; check for extravasation; check site for infiltration; use inf pump
• Store reconstituted sol in refrigerator for no longer than 24 hr
• Do not use discolored sol

Y-site compatibilities: Famotidine, haloperidol, inamrinone, zidovudine

Patient/family education
• Inform patient of reason for product administration and expected result
• Advise patient to report pain at inf site immediately
• Instruct patient to report change in vision, blurring, loss of sight; breathing trouble, sweating, flushing

Evaluation
Positive therapeutic outcome
• Increased B/P with stabilization

phenylephrine nasal agent
See Appendix B

phenylephrine ophthalmic
See Appendix B

phenytoin (Rx)
(fen′i-toyn)
Dilantin, ❋, Phenytek, Tremytoine ❋
Func. class.: Anticonvulsant/antidysrhythmic (class IB)
Chem. class.: Hydantoin

ACTION: Inhibits spread of seizure activity in motor cortex by altering ion transport; increases AV conduction to decrease dysrhythmias

Therapeutic outcome: Decreased seizures, absence of dysrhythmias

USES: Generalized tonic-clonic seizures, status epilepticus, nonepileptic seizures associated with Reye's syndrome or after head trauma, complex/partial seizures

Pharmacokinetics

Absorption	Slowly absorbed from GI tract; erratic (IM)
Distribution	Crosses placenta, 90%-95% protein binding
Metabolism	Liver, extensively
Excretion	Kidneys, minimally; enters breast milk
Half-life	7-42 hr, dose dependent

Pharmacodynamics

	PO	PO-EXT REL	IM	IV
Onset	2-24 hr	2-24 hr	Erratic	1-2 hr
Peak	1½-3 hr	4-12 hr	Erratic	Unknown
Duration	6-12 hr	12-36 hr	12-24 hr	12-24 hr

CONTRAINDICATIONS
Pregnancy, hypersensitivity, psychiatric condition, bradycardia, SA and AV block, Stokes-Adams syndrome

Precautions: Geriatric, allergies, renal/hepatic disease, petit mal seizures, hypotension, myocardial insufficiency, ᴺᴼᴱ Asian patients positive for HLA-B 1502, hepatic failure, acute intermittent porphyria

DOSAGE AND ROUTES
Seizures
Adult: PO 15-20 mg/kg (EXT REL) in 3-4 divided doses given q2hr or 400 mg, then 300 mg q2hr × 2 doses, maintenance 4-7 mg/kg/day; max 600 mg/day; **IV** 15-20 mg/kg, max 25-50 mg/min then 100 mg q6-8hr

Child: PO 5 mg/kg/day in 2-3 divided doses, maintenance 4-8 mg/kg/day in 2-3 divided doses, max 300 mg/day; **IV** 15-20 mg/kg at 1-3 mg/kg/min

Status epilepticus
Adult: **IV** 15-20 mg/kg, max 25-50 mg/min; may give 100 mg q6-8hr thereafter

Child: **IV** 15-20 mg/kg, max in divided doses 1-3 mg/kg/min

Ventricular dysrhythmias
Adult: PO loading dose 1 g divided over 24 hr, then 500 mg/day × 2 days; **IV** 250 mg given over 5 min until dysrhythmias subside or 1 g is given, or 100 mg q15min until dysrhythmias subside or 1 g is given

Child: PO 3-8 mg/kg or 250 mg/m²/day as single dose or divided in 2 doses; **IV** 3-8 mg/kg given over several min, or 250 mg/m²/day as single dose or divided in 2 doses

Renal dose
Adult: Do not use loading dose if CCr <10 ml/min or hepatic failure

Available forms: Susp 25 mg/5 ml; chew tabs 50 mg; inj 50 mg/ml; ext rel caps 100, 200, 300 mg; prompt rel caps 100 mg

ADVERSE EFFECTS
CNS: Dizziness, insomnia, paresthesias, depression, suicidal tendencies, aggression, headache, confusion, slurred speech, peripheral neuropathy

CV: Hypotension, ventricular fibrillation, bradycardia, cardiac arrest

EENT: Nystagmus, diplopia, blurred vision

ENDO: Diabetes insipidus

GI: Nausea, vomiting, constipation, anorexia, weight loss, hepatitis, jaundice, gingival hyperplasia, abdominal pain

GU: Nephritis, urine discoloration, sexual dysfunction

HEMA: Agranulocytosis, leukopenia, aplastic anemia, thrombocytopenia, megaloblastic anemia

INTEG: Rash, lupus erythematosus, Stevens-Johnson syndrome, hirsutism, toxic epidermal necrolysis

SYST: Hypocalcemia, purple glove syndrome (IV), exacerbation of myasthenia gravis

INTERACTIONS
Individual drugs
Alcohol (chronic use), calcium (high dose), carBAMazepine, folic acid, rifampin: decreased effects of phenytoin

Chloramphenicol, cimetidine, cycloSERINE, disulfiram, alcohol, amiodarone, FLUoxetine, gabapentin, methylphenidate, felbamate, traZODone, diazepam, valproate: increased phenytoin effect

Delavirdine: decreased response, resistance, do not use together

Drug classifications
Antacids, barbiturates: decreased effect of phenytoin

Antidepressants (tricyclics), benzodiazepines, sulfonamides, H_2 antagonists, azole antifungals, estrogens, succinimides, phenothiazines, salicylates: increased phenytoin level

Drug/food
Enteral tube feeding: may decrease absorption of oral product, do not use enteral feedings 2 hr before and after dose

Drug/lab test
Increased: glucose, alkaline phosphatase, BSP

Decreased: dexamethasone, metyrapone test serum, urinary steroids

NURSING CONSIDERATIONS
Assessment
• Assess product level: toxic level 30-50 mcg/ml; therapeutic level 7.5-20 mcg/ml, wait ≥1 wk to determine level

• **Assess mental status:** mood, sensorium, affect, memory (long, short), especially geriatric; suicidal thoughts/behaviors

• **Phenytoin hypersensitivity syndrome:** assess 3-12 wk after start of treatment: rash, temp, lymphadenopathy; may cause hepatotoxicity, renal failure, rhabdomyolysis

• **Serious skin disorders:** assess for beginning rash that may lead to Stevens-Johnson syndrome or toxic epidermal necrolysis; phenytoin should not be used again, may occur more often in Asian patients with HLA-B 1502

• **Purple glove syndrome:** with IV use

• **Phenytoin level:** toxic level 30-50 mcg/ml, therapeutic level: 7.5-20 mcg/ml, wait ≥1 wk to draw levels

• **Seizures:** assess for duration, type, intensity, precipitating factors, obtain EEG periodically, monitor therapeutic level

• Blood studies: CBC, platelets q2wk until stabilized, then qmo × 12, then q3mo; discontinue

product if neutrophils <1600/m³; renal function: albumin conc; folic acid levels, LFTs
- **Blood dyscrasias:** assess fever, sore throat, bruising, rash, jaundice, epistaxis (long-term treatment only)
- Assess renal studies: urinalysis, BUN, urine creatinine
- Monitor blood studies: RBC, Hct, Hgb, reticulocyte counts weekly for 4 wk then monthly; also check thyroid function tests, serum calcium
- Monitor ECG, B/P, respiratory function during IV loading dose; verify patency of IV access port prior to IV infusion
- Monitor EEG function and serum levels periodically
- Monitor liver function tests for renal failure: ALT, AST, bilirubin, creatinine
- Assess for signs of physical withdrawal if medication suddenly discontinued
- Assess eye problems: need for ophth exam before, during, after treatment (slit lamp, funduscopy, tonometry)
- **Monitor for toxicity:** bone marrow depression, nausea, vomiting, ataxia, diplopia, CV collapse, slurred speech, confusion
- **Beers:** Avoid use in older adults unless safer alternatives are not available, ataxia, impaired psychomotor function may occur
- **Pregnancy/breastfeeding:** Pregnant patient should enroll in the Antiepileptic Drug Pregnancy Registry (888-233-2334), may cause fetal malformations, use other options when possible, breastfeeding is not recommended

Patient problem
Risk for injury (uses, adverse reactions)

Implementation
PO route
- Do not interchange chewable product with caps, not equivalent; only ext rel caps are to be used for once-a-day dosing
- Give with meals to decrease GI upset
- Chew tab can be crushed or chewed; cap can be opened and mixed with foods or fluids; cap and tab are not interchangeable, only ext rel cap is to be used for once-a-day dosing
- Do not take antacids or antidiarrheals within 2-3 hr of taking phenytoin
- **Oral suspension:** shake well before each dose G tube/NG tube; dilute susp prior to administration; flush tube with 20 ml water after dose; hold tube feedings 1 hr before and 1 hr after dose
- Allow 7-10 days between dosage changes
- Divided PO doses with or after meals to decrease adverse effects
- 2 hr before or after antacid, enteral feeding

- Shake oral susp well; use measuring device for correct dose

Direct IV route

> **BLACK BOX WARNING:** Give undiluted at ≤50 mg/min (adult) 1-3 mg/kg/min (neonates); 0.5-1 mg/kg/min

Intermittent IV INF route

> **BLACK BOX WARNING:** Dilute dose in NS to ≤6.7 mg/ml, complete inf within 1 hr of preparation, use 0.22 or 0.55 micron in-line particulate final filter between **IV** catheter and tubing, flush the **IV** line or catheter with NS before and after use, give at ≤50 mg/min (adult), 0.5-1 mg/kg/min (child, infant, neonate)

Patient/family education
- Teach patient to carry/wear emergency ID stating name, products taken, condition, prescriber's name and phone number
- Advise patient to avoid driving and other activities that require alertness until product response is known; dizziness, drowsiness can occur
- Advise patient to avoid alcohol ingestion and CNS depressants unless approved by prescriber; increased sedation may occur
- Teach patient not to discontinue medication quickly after long-term use; taper off over several wk
- Advise patient that urine may turn pink, red, or brown
- Caution patient to avoid antacids or antidiarrheals within 2-3 hr of taking phenytoin
- Instruct patient in proper oral hygiene to prevent gingival hyperplasia; to visit dentist routinely
- Teach patient to notify prescriber of unusual bleeding, bruising, petechiae (bleeding), clay-colored stools, abdominal pain, dark urine, yellowing of skin/eyes (hepatotoxicity); slurred speech, headache, drowsiness
- Teach patient to report suicidal thoughts/ behaviors immediately
- Teach patient to use nonhormonal contraception, to notify prescriber if pregnancy is planned or suspected

Evaluation
Positive therapeutic outcome
- Decreased seizure activity
- Decreased dysrhythmias
- Relief of pain

---

phosphate/bisphosphate

(foss'fate/bye-foss'fate)

Fleet Enema, OsmoPrep

Func. class.: Saline laxative

USES: Chronic constipation; prep for colonoscopy (OsmoPrep)

CONTRAINDICATIONS: Hypersensitivity, GI obstruction, abdominal pain, severe renal/CV disease, pregnancy (at term)

DOSAGE AND ROUTES

Constipation

Adult: PO 15 ml as a single dose

Child 5-9 yr: PO 7.5 ml as a single dose

Adult/child >12 yr: Rectal 118 mL (Fleet Enema)

Child >2 to 11 yr: Rectal 1/2 of adult dose

Bowel cleansing (OsmoPrep)

Adult: PO PM before colonoscopy 4 tablets q15min with 8 oz of water (20 tablets); morning of colonoscopy 4 tablets q15min with 8 oz of water 3-5 hr prior to exam (12 tablets)

physostigmine ophthalmic

See Appendix B

phytonadione (vit K₁) (Rx)

(fye-toe-na-dye'one)

Mephyton

Func. class.: Vitamin K₁, fat-soluble vitamin

Do not confuse: Mephyton/methadone

ACTION: Needed for adequate blood clotting (factors II, VII, IX, X)

Therapeutic outcome: Prevention of bleeding

USES: Vitamin K malabsorption, hypoprothrombinemia, prevention of hypoprothrombinemia caused by oral anticoagulants, prevention of hemorrhagic disease of the newborn

Pharmacokinetics

Absorption	Well absorbed (PO, IM, SUBCUT)
Distribution	Crosses placenta
Metabolism	Liver, rapidly
Excretion	Breast milk
Half-life	Unknown

Pharmacodynamics

	PO	SUBCUT/IM
Onset	6-12 hr	1-2 hr
Peak	Unknown	6 hr
Duration	Unknown	14 hr

CONTRAINDICATIONS

Hypersensitivity, severe hepatic disease, last few wk of pregnancy

Precautions: Pregnancy, neonates, hepatic disease, IV use

> **BLACK BOX WARNING:** Risk of anaphylaxis

DOSAGE AND ROUTES

Hypoprothrombinemia caused by vitamin K malabsorption

Adult: PO/IM 2.5-25 mg; may repeat or increase to 50 mg

Child: PO 2.5-5 mg

Infant: PO/IM 2 mg

Prevention of hemorrhagic disease of the newborn

Neonate: IM 0.5-1 mg within 1 hr after birth; repeat in 2-3 wk if required

Hypoprothrombinemia caused by oral anticoagulants

Adult and child: PO/SUBCUT/IM 1-10 mg, may repeat 12-48 hr after PO dose or 6-8 hr after SUBCUT/IM dose, based on INR

Available forms: Tabs 5 mg; inj 10 mg/ml, 1 mg/0.5 ml

ADVERSE EFFECTS

CNS: Headache, brain damage (large doses)

GI: Nausea, decreased liver function tests

HEMA: Hemolytic anemia, hemoglobinuria, hyperbilirubinemia

INTEG: Rash, urticaria

RESP: Bronchospasm, dyspnea, chest constriction, respiratory arrest

INTERACTIONS

Individual drugs

Sucralfate, mineral oil: decreased action of phytonadione

Warfarin: decreased action of warfarin (large dose of this product)

Drug classifications

Oral anticoagulants: decreased anticoagulant effect

Bile acid sequestrants, antiinfectives, salicylates: decreased action of phytonadione

P

Drug/food
Olestra: decreased vit K levels

NURSING CONSIDERATIONS
Assessment
• Monitor pro-time during treatment (2-sec deviation from control time, bleeding time, and clotting time), INR
• Monitor for bleeding, INR pulse, and B/P
• Assess nutritional status: liver (beef), spinach, tomatoes, coffee, asparagus, broccoli, cabbage, lettuce, greens
• Assess for bleeding or bruising: hematuria, black tarry stools, hematemesis
• **Pregnancy/breastfeeding:** Usually not needed in pregnancy, may breastfeed

Patient problem
Ineffective tissue perfusion (uses)
Nausea (adverse reactions)

Implementation
IM route
• Only use when other routes are not possible (deaths have occurred from allergic reactions)

Intermittent IV infusion route
• Give **IV** after diluting with D_5 NS 10 ml or more; give max 1 mg/min
• Give **IV** only when other routes not possible (deaths have occurred)
• Store in airtight, light-resistant container

Y-site compatibilities: Alfentanil, amikacin, aminophylline, ascorbic acid, atracurium, atropine, azaTHIOprine, aztreonam, bumetanide, buprenorphine, butorphanol, calcium chloride/gluconate, ceFAZolin, cefonicid, cefoperazone, cefotaxime, cefoTEtan, cefOXitin, cefTAZidime, ceftizoxime, cefTRIAXone, cefuroxime, chloramphenicol, chlorproMAZINE, cimetidine, clindamycin, cyanocobalamin, cycloSPORINE, dexamethasone, digoxin, diphenhydrAMINE, DOPamine, doxycycline, enalaprilat, ePHEDrine, EPINEPHrine, epoetin alfa, erythromycin, esmolol, famotidine, fentaNYL, fluconazole, folic acid, furosemide, ganciclovir, gentamicin, glycopyrrolate, heparin, hydrocortisone, imipenem-cilastatin, indomethacin, insulin, isoproterenol, ketorolac, labetalol, lidocaine, mannitol, meperidine, metaraminol, methoxamine, methyldopa, metoclopramide, metoprolol, metroNIDAZOLE, midazolam, morphine, multivitamins, nafcillin, nalbuphine, naloxone, nitroglycerin, nitroprusside, norepinephrine, ondansetron, oxacillin, oxytocin, papaverine, penicillin G potassium, pentamidine, pentazocine, PENTobarbital, PHENobarbital, phentolamine, phenylephrine, potassium chloride, procainamide, prochlorperazine, propranolol, pyridoxine, ranitidine, sodium bicarbonate, succinylcholine, SUFentanil, theophylline, thiamine, ticarcillin/clavulanate, tobramycin, tolazoline, trimethaphan, urokinase, vancomycin, vasopressin, verapamil, vitamin B with C

Patient/family education
• Teach patient not to take other supplements unless directed by prescriber; to take this medication as directed
• Teach patient necessary foods high in vit K to be included in diet
• Advise patient to avoid IM inj, hard toothbrush, flossing; use electric razor until treatment is terminated
• Instruct patient to report symptoms of bleeding: bruising, nosebleeds, blood in urine, heavy menstruation, black tarry stools
• Caution patient not to use OTC medications unless approved by prescriber
• Stress the need for periodic lab tests to monitor coagulation levels
• Stress the need for patient to carry/wear emergency ID with condition, treatment, and medications taken

Evaluation
Positive therapeutic outcome
• Decreased bleeding tendencies
• Decreased pro-time
• Decreased clotting time

pilocarpine ophthalmic
See Appendix B

RARELY USED
pilocarpine (oral)
(pye-loe-kar′peen)
Salagen
Func. class.: Cholinergic

USES: Xerostomia from radiation treatment

CONTRAINDICATIONS: Hypersensitivity, asthma, closed-angle glaucoma

DOSAGE AND ROUTES
Adult: PO 5 mg tid, then titrate to response

pimavanserin
(pim-a-vans'er-in)
Nuplazid
Func. class.: Atypical antipsychotic

ACTION: The exact mechanism of action is unknown; may be mediated through inverse agonist and antagonist activity at serotonin 5-HT2A receptors, and to a lesser extent at 5-HT2C receptors

Therapeutic outcome: Decrease in hallucinations, delusions, paranoia; reorganization of patterns of thought and speech

USES: The treatment of hallucinations and delusions associated with Parkinson's disease psychosis

Pharmacokinetics

Absorption	Unknown
Distribution	Protein binding
Metabolism	Hepatic metabolism occurs through CYP3A4 and CYP3A5, and to a lesser extent CYP2J2, CYP2D6 with a major active metabolite
Excretion	0.55% eliminated unchanged in the urine and 1.53% was eliminated in feces after 10 days
Half-life	Plasma half-lives of drug and metabolite are 57 hr and 200 hr, respectively

Pharmacodynamics

Onset	Unknown
Peak	6 hr
Duration	Unknown

CONTRAINDICATIONS
Hypersensitivity

Precautions: Alcoholism, bradycardia, breastfeeding, cardiac arrhythmias, cardiac disease, children, coronary artery disease, diabetes mellitus, females, geriatric patients, heart failure, hepatic disease, hypertension, hypocalcemia, hypokalemia, hypomagnesemia, long QT syndrome, malnutrition, myocardial infarction, pregnancy, QT prolongation, renal failure, renal impairment, stroke, thyroid disease

BLACK BOX WARNING: Dementia-related psychosis

DOSAGE AND ROUTES
Adult: PO 34 mg (taken as two 17-mg tablets) qday, without titration

Hepatic dose
Adult: PO Not recommended

Renal dose
Adult: PO CCr 30 ml/min or more: No dosage adjustment needed; CCr <30 ml/min: Not recommended

Other dosage adjustments
• **Patients receiving a strong CYP3A4 inhibitor:** 17 mg qday
• **Patients receiving a strong CYP3A4 inducer:** Monitor for reduced effect, increase dose if needed

Available forms: Tab 17 mg

ADVERSE EFFECTS

CNS: Confusion, hallucinations, fatigue, stroke, dizziness

GI: Nausea, constipation

MISC: Peripheral edema, infection, QT prolongation

INTERACTIONS
Drug classifications
CYP2D6 inhibitors (fluoxetine, paroxetine, quinidine), CYP3A4 inhibitors (erythromycin, ketoconazole); reduce dose of pimavanserin: increased effects of pimavanserin
Other CNS depressants: increased sedation
Products that cause QT prolongation:
Increase: QT prolongation, CYP3A4 inducers (carbamazepine): decreased pimavanserin effects

Drug/herb
St. John's wort: decreased pimavanserin effect

NURSING CONSIDERATIONS
Assessment

BLACK BOX WARNING: Dementia-related psychosis: At increased risk of death, avoid using

• Swallowing of medication, check for hoarding, giving product to other patients
• AIMS assessment, neurologic function, LFTs, serum electrolytes, creatinine monthly
• Constipation daily, if this occurs, increase bulk, water in diet, stool softeners, laxatives may be needed
• **QT prolongation:** Avoid in those with cardiac disease or other risk factors for QT prolongation, torsades de pointes (TdP), and/or sudden death such as cardiac arrhythmias, congenital long QT syndrome, heart failure, bradycardia, myocardial infarction, hypertension, coronary artery

disease, hypomagnesemia, hypokalemia, hypocalcemia, or in patients receiving medications known to prolong the QT interval. Females, elderly patients, patients with diabetes mellitus, thyroid disease, malnutrition, alcoholism, or hepatic impairment may also be at increased risk for QT prolongation
• **Renal disease:** Product is not recommended for patients with severe renal impairment (CCr <30 ml/min)
• **Hepatic disease:** Product is extensively metabolized in the liver, use is not recommended in patients with mild, moderate, or severe hepatic disease
• **Stroke:** Avoid antipsychotics to treat delirium or dementia-related behavioral problems unless nonpharmacologic options have failed or are not possible and the patient is a substantial threat to self or others, avoid use in those with a history of falls or fractures
• **Hyponatremia:** Product can cause hyponatremia and SIADH, and the elderly are at increased risk of developing these conditions, sodium levels should be closely monitored when starting or changing dosages of antipsychotics in older adults

Patient problem
Distorted thinking process (uses)

Implementation:
• Give without regard to food

PATIENT/FAMILY EDUCATION
• Teach patient to avoid hazardous activities until response is known, dizziness may occur
• Teach patient that compliance with dose is needed
• Teach patient to avoid OTC products unless approved by prescriber

Evaluation: Decrease in hallucinations, delusions, paranoia; reorganization of patterns of thought and speech

pimecrolimus topical
See Appendix B

⚠ HIGH ALERT

pioglitazone (Rx)
(pie-oh-glye′ta-zone)
Actos
Func. class.: Antidiabetic, oral
Chem. class.: Thiazolidinedione

Do not confuse: Actos/Actonel

ACTION: Specifically targets insulin resistance, an insulin sensitizer; regulates the transcription of a number of insulin-responsive genes

Therapeutic outcome: Decreased symptoms of diabetes mellitus

USES: Type 2 diabetes mellitus

Pharmacokinetics
Absorption	Unknown
Distribution	Protein binding >99%
Metabolism	Unknown
Excretion	Kidneys
Half-life	3-7 hr, terminal 16-24 hr

Pharmacodynamics
Onset	Unknown
Peak	6-12 wk
Duration	Unknown

CONTRAINDICATIONS
Breastfeeding, children, hypersensitivity to thiazolidinediones, diabetic ketoacidosis

> **BLACK BOX WARNING:** NYHA Class III/IV heart failure

Precautions: Pregnancy, thyroid/renal/hepatic disease, edema, geriatric patients with CV disease, polycystic ovary syndrome, bladder cancer, osteoporosis, pulmonary disease, secondary malignancy

DOSAGE AND ROUTES
Monotherapy
Adult: PO 15-30 mg/day, may increase to 45 mg/day; with strong CYP2C8 max 15 mg/day; those with NYHA class I/II heart failure max 15 mg/day

Combination therapy
Adult: PO 15-30 mg/day with a sulfonylurea, metformin, or insulin; decrease sulfonylurea dose if hypoglycemia occurs; decrease insulin dose by 10%-25% if hypoglycemia occurs or if plasma glucose is <100 mg/dl; max 45 mg/day

Hepatic dose
Do not use in active liver disease or if ALT >2.5 × ULN

Available forms: Tabs 15, 30, 45 mg

ADVERSE EFFECTS
CNS: *Headache*
CV: MI, heart failure, death (geriatric patients)
ENDO: Hyper/hypoglycemia
MISC: *Myalgia, sinusitis, upper respiratory tract infection, pharyngitis,* hepatotoxicity, edema, weight gain, anemia, macular edema; risk of bladder cancer (use >1 yr), peripheral/pulmonary edema
MS: Fractures (females), rhabdomyolysis, myalgia

INTERACTIONS
Individual drugs
Atorvastatin: decreased effect of this product
Fluconazole, itraconazole, ketoconazole, miconazole, voriconazole: decreased pioglitazone effect

Drug classifications
CYP2C8 inducers: decreased pioglitazone effect
Oral contraceptives: decreased effect, use an alternative contraceptive method

Drug/herb
Garlic, green tea, horse chestnut: increased hypoglycemia

Drug/lab test
Increased: CPK, LFTs, HDL, cholesterol
Decreased: glucose, Hct/Hgb

NURSING CONSIDERATIONS
Assessment

> **BLACK BOX WARNING: Heart failure:** do not use in NYHA Class III/IV; excessive/rapid weight gain > 5 lb, dyspnea, edema; may need to be reduced or discontinued, monitor daily weights

• **Hypoglycemic reactions:** assess for hypoglycemic reactions (sweating, weakness, dizziness, anxiety, tremors, hunger), hyperglycemic reactions soon after meals (rare)
• **Bladder cancer:** Avoid use in patients with history of bladder cancer; use of pioglitazone >1 yr has been correlated with an increase in bladder cancer; may occur more often with insulin or other antidiabetics
• **Hepatic disease:** check LFTs periodically: AST, LDH; do not start treatment in active heart disease or if ALT >2.5× upper limit of normal; if treatment has already begun, follow closely with continuing ALT levels; if ALT increases to >3× upper limit of normal, recheck ALT as soon as possible, if ALT remains >3× upper limit of normal, discontinue
• Monitor FBS, glycosylated HbA1c, plasma lipids/lipoproteins, B/P, body weight during treatment
• Monitor CBC with differential prior to and during therapy, more necessary in those with anemia, Hct/Hgb (may be decreased in first few months of treatment)
• **Beers:** Avoid use in older adults, may promote fluid retention and/or exacerbate heart failure

Patient/family education
• Teach patient to self-monitor using a blood glucose meter
• Teach patient symptoms of hypo/hyperglycemia, what to do about each (rare)
• Advise patient that product must be continued on daily basis; explain consequence of discontinuing product abruptly
• Advise patient to avoid OTC medications or herbal preparations unless approved by prescriber; to report weight gain, edema
• Advise patient that diabetes is lifelong illness; that this product is not a cure, only controls symptoms
• Teach patient not to use if breastfeeding
• Teach patient that lab work, eye exams will be needed periodically
• Pregnancy/breastfeeding: Instruct patient to notify prescriber if oral contraceptives are used, effect may be decreased

Patient problem
Excess food intake (uses)
Nonadherence (teaching)

Implementation
• Convert from other oral hypoglycemic agents; change may be made with gradual dosage change; monitor serum glucose during conversion
• Give once a day without regard to meals
• Give tabs crushed and mixed with meal or fluids for patients with difficulty swallowing
• Store in airtight container in cool environment

Evaluation
Positive therapeutic outcome
• Decrease in polyuria, polydipsia, polyphagia; clear sensorium; absence of dizziness; stable gait; blood glucose, A1c improvement

piperacillin/tazobactam (Rx)
(pip'er-ah-sill'in/ta-zoe-bak'tam)
Tazocin ✦, Zosyn
Func. class.: Broad-spectrum antiinfective
Chem. class.: Extended-spectrum penicillin

ACTION: Interferes with cell wall replication of susceptible organisms; tazobactam is a β-lactamase inhibitor, protects piperacillin from enzymatic degradation

Therapeutic outcome: Bactericidal effects for piperacillin-resistant β-lactamase, *Escherichia coli, Staphylococcus aureus, Bacteroides fragilis, Bacteroides ovatus, Bacteroides thetaiotaomicron, Bacteroides vulgatus, Haemophilus influenzae*

USES: Moderate to severe infections: piperacillin-resistant, β-lactamase strains causing infections in respiratory tract, skin, skin structure, urinary tract, bone, and joint; gonorrhea, pneumonia, infections from penicillinase-producing staphylococci, streptococci

Pharmacokinetics

Absorption	Well absorbed (80%)
Distribution	Widely distributed; crosses placenta
Metabolism	Not metabolized
Excretion	Kidneys, unchanged (90%); bile (10%); breast milk
Half-life	0.7-1.3 hr

Pharmacodynamics

Onset	Rapid
Peak	Inf end
Duration	Unknown

CONTRAINDICATIONS
Hypersensitivity to penicillins; neonates, carbapenem allergy

Precautions: Pregnancy, breastfeeding, HF, seizures, hypersensitivity to cephalosporins, renal insufficiency in neonates, GI disease, electrolyte imbalances, biliary obstruction

DOSAGE AND ROUTES
Nosocomial pneumonia
Adult: IV 4.5 g q6hr or 3.375 g q4hr with an aminoglycoside or antipseudomonal fluoroquinolone × 1-2 wk

Appendicitis/peritonitis
Child ≥40 kg (88 lb): IV 3.375 g q6hr × 7-10 days
Child ≥9 mo and <40 g: IV 100 mg (piperacillin)/q8hr × 7-10 days
Infant 2 mo to <9 mo: IV 80 mg/kg (piperacillin) q8hr × 7-10 days

Renal dose
Adult: IV CCr 20-40 ml/min give 3.375 g q6hr (nosocomial pneumonia); give 2.25 g q6hr (all other indications); CCr <20 ml/min, give 2.25 g q6hr (nosocomial pneumonia); give 2.25 g q8hr (all other indications)

Available forms: Powder for inj 2 g piperacillin/0.25 g tazobactam, 3 g piperacillin/0.375 g tazobactam, 4 g piperacillin/0.5 g tazobactam, 36 g piperacillin/4.5 g tazobactam

ADVERSE EFFECTS
CNS: Headache, insomnia, dizziness, fever, lethargy, hallucinations, anxiety, depression, twitching, seizures, vertigo
CV: Cardiac toxicity, edema
GI: *Nausea, vomiting, diarrhea,* increased AST, ALT, abdominal pain, glossitis, constipation, pseudomembranous colitis, pancreatitis
GU: Oliguria, proteinuria, hematuria, *vaginitis, moniliasis,* glomerulonephritis, renal failure

HEMA: Anemia, increased bleeding time, bone marrow depression, agranulocytosis, hemolytic anemia
INTEG: Rash, pruritus, exfoliative dermatitis
META: Hypokalemia, hypernatremia
SYST: Serum sickness, anaphylaxis, Stevens-Johnson syndrome

INTERACTIONS
Individual drugs
Aspirin, probenecid: increased piperacillin levels
Methotrexate: increased effect of methotrexate

Drug classifications
Aminoglycosides (**IV**): decreased piperacillin effect
Anticoagulants (oral): increased effect of anticoagulants
Contraceptives (oral): decreased contraceptive effectiveness
Neuromuscular blockers: increased effects
Tetracyclines: decreased antimicrobial effectiveness of piperacillin

Drug/lab test
Increased: eosinophilia, neutropenia, leucopenia, serum creatinine, PTT, AST, ALT, alkaline phosphatase, bilirubin, BUN, electrolytes
Decreased: Hct, Hgb, electrolytes
False positive: urine glucose, urine protein, Coombs' test

NURSING CONSIDERATIONS
Assessment
• Assess patient for previous sensitivity reaction to penicillins or other cephalosporins; cross-sensitivity between penicillins and cephalosporins is common
• Assess patient for signs and symptoms of infection, including characteristics of wounds, sputum, urine, stool, WBC >10,000/mm^3, fever; obtain information baseline, during treatment
• Obtain C&S before beginning product therapy to identify if correct treatment has been initiated
• **Assess for allergic reactions:** rash, urticaria, pruritus, chills, fever, joint pain; angioedema may occur a few days after therapy begins; EPINEPHrine, resuscitation equipment should be available for anaphylactic reaction
• Identify urine output; if decreasing, notify prescriber (may indicate nephrotoxicity); also check for increased BUN, creatinine
• Monitor blood studies: AST, ALT, CBC, Hct, bilirubin, LDH, alkaline phosphatase, Coombs' test monthly if patient is on long-term therapy
• Monitor electrolytes: potassium, sodium, chloride monthly if patient is on long-term therapy

- **CDAD:** assess for diarrhea, abdominal pain, fever, fatigue, anorexia; possible anemia, elevated WBC and low serum albumin; stop product and usually give either vancomycin or IV metroNIDAZOLE
- Monitor for bleeding: ecchymosis, bleeding gums, hematuria, stool guaiac daily if on long-term therapy
- **Assess for overgrowth of infection.** perineal itching, fever, malaise, redness, pain, swelling, drainage, rash, diarrhea, change in cough, sputum
- **Pregnancy/breastfeeding:** Use only if clearly needed, cautious use in breastfeeding

Patient problem
Infection (uses)
Risk for injury (adverse reactions)

Implementation
- Separate aminoglycoside from piperacillin to avoid inactivation

Intermittent IV infusion route
- Reconstitute each 1 g of product/5 ml 0.9% NaCl for inj or sterile water for inj, dextrose 5%; shake well; further dilute in at least 50 ml compatible IV sol and run as int inf over at least 30 min

ADD-Vantage IV solution: reconstitution
- Reconstitute with 0.9% NaCl or D₅W in the appropriate flexible diluent container provided; for 500 mg vials, use at least a 100 ml diluent container and for 750 mg and 1 g vials, use only the 250 ml diluent container
- Remove the protective covers from the top of the vial and vial port. Remove vial cap (do not access with a syringe) and vial port cover. Screw the vial into the vial port until it will go no further to assure a seal. Once vial is sealed to the port, do not remove. To activate the contents of the vial, squeeze the bottom of the diluent container gently to inflate the portion of the container surrounding the end of the drug vial. With the other hand, push the drug vial down into the container telescoping walls of the container and grasp the inner cap of the vial through the walls of the container. Pull the inner cap from the drug vial. Verify the rubber stopper has been pulled out, allowing the drug and diluent to mix. Mix the container contents thoroughly
- *Storage after reconstitution:* The admixture solution may be stored for up to 24 hr at room temperature. Do not refrigerate or freeze after reconstitution
- Do not use in series connections with flexible containers

Pre-mixed Galaxy IV solution
- Thaw frozen containers at room temperature (20-25° C or 68-77° F) or under refrigeration (2-8° C or 36-46° F). Do not force thaw by immersion in water baths or by microwaving. Check for leaks by squeezing bag firmly
- Do not admix
- Contents of the solution may precipitate in the frozen state and should dissolve with little or no agitation once the solution has reached room temperature
- *Storage:* The thawed solution is stable for 24 hours at room temperature or for 14 days under refrigeration. Do not refreeze thawed product
- Do not use plastic containers in series connections as this could result in an embolism due to residual air being drawn from the primary container before administration of the fluid from the secondary container is complete

IV infusion
- Infuse IV over at least 30 min. Ambulatory intravenous infusion pumps can be used; the solution is stable for up to 12 hr at room temperature

Y-site compatibilities: Alfentanil, allopurinol, amifostine, amikacin, aminocaproic acid, aminophylline, amphotericin B lipid complex, amphotericin B liposome, anidulafungin, argatroban, atenolol, aztreonam, bivalirudin, bleomycin, bumetanide, buprenorphine, busulfan, butorphanol, calcium acetate/chloride/gluconate, CARBOplatin, carmustine, cefepime, chloramphenicol, cimetidine, clindamycin, cyclophosphamide, cycloSPORINE, cytarabine, DACTINomycin, DAPTOmycin, dexamethasone, dexrazoxane, diazepam, digoxin, diphenhydrAMINE, DOCEtaxel, DOPamine, doxacurium, enalaprilat, ePHEDrine, EPINEPHrine, eptifibatide, erythromycin, esmolol, etoposide, fenoldopam, fentaNYL, floxuridine, fluconazole, fludarabine, fluorouracil, foscarnet, fosphenytoin, furosemide, gallium, granisetron, heparin, hydrocortisone, HYDROmorphone, ifosfamide, isoproterenol, ketorolac, lansoprazole, lepirudin, leucovorin, lidocaine, linezolid, LORazepam, magnesium sulfate, mannitol, mechlorethamine, melphalan, meperidine, mesna, metaraminol, methotrexate, methylPREDNISolone, metoclopramide, metoprolol, metroNIDAZOLE, milrinone, morphine, naloxone, nitroglycerin, nitroprusside, norepinephrine, octreotide, ondansetron, oxytocin, PACLitaxel, palonosetron, pamidronate, pancuronium, PEMEtrexed, PENTobarbital, PHENobarbital, phentolamine, phenylephrine, plicamycin, potassium chloride/phosphates, procainamide, ranitidine, remifentanil,

P

riTUXimab, sargramostim, sodium acetate/bicarbonate/phosphates, succinylcholine, SUFentanil, sulfamethoxazole-trimethoprim, tacrolimus, telavancin, teniposide, theophylline, thiotepa, tigecycline, tirofiban, trimethobenzamide, vasopressin, vinBLAStine, vinCRIStine, voriconazole, zidovudine, zoledronic acid

Patient/family education
• Teach patient to report sore throat, bruising, bleeding, joint pain; may indicate blood dyscrasias (rare)
• Advise patient to contact prescriber if vaginal itching, loose foul-smelling stools, furry tongue occur; may indicate **superinfection**
• Advise patient to notify prescriber of diarrhea with blood or pus, which may indicate CDAD

Evaluation
Positive therapeutic outcome
• Absence of signs/symptoms of infection (WBC <10,000/mm³, temp WNL, absence of red, draining wounds)
• Reported improvement in symptoms of infection

TREATMENT OF ANAPHYLAXIS: Withdraw product, maintain airway, administer EPINEPHrine, aminophylline, O₂, **IV** corticosteroids

---

pitavastatin (Rx)
(pit′a-va-stat′in)
Livalo
Func. class.: Antilipidemic
Chem. class.: HMG-CoA reductase inhibitor

Do not confuse: pitavastatin/pravastatin

ACTION: Inhibits HMG-CoA reductase enzyme, which reduces cholesterol synthesis, high doses lead to plaque regression

Therapeutic outcome: Decreased cholesterol levels and LDLs, increased HDLs

USES: As an adjunct in primary hypercholesterolemia (types Ia, Ib), dysbetalipoproteinemia, elevated triglyceride levels; prevention of cardiovascular disease by reduction of heart risk in those with mildly elevated cholesterol

Pharmacokinetics

Absorption	Unknown
Distribution	Concentrations are lower in healthy African Americans
Metabolism	Liver
Excretion	Urine, feces
Half-life	12 hr

Pharmacodynamics
Unknown

CONTRAINDICATIONS
Pregnancy, breastfeeding, hypersensitivity, active liver disease, cholestasis

Precautions: Past liver disease, alcoholism, severe acute infections, trauma, severe metabolic disorders, electrolyte imbalance, seizures, surgery, organ transplant, endocrine disease, females, hypotension, renal disease

DOSAGE AND ROUTES
Adult: PO 2 mg/day, usual range 1-4, max 4 mg/day

Renal dose
Adult: PO CCr 30-60 ml/min 1 mg qd, max 2 mg qd; CCr <30 ml/min on hemodialysis 1 mg qd, max 2 mg qd; CCr <30 ml/min not on hemodialysis—not recommended

Available forms: Tabs 1, 2, 4 mg

ADVERSE EFFECTS
CNS: Headache
GI: Constipation, diarrhea
INTEG: Rash, pruritus, alopecia
MS: Myalgia, rhabdomyolysis, arthralgia
RESP: Pharyngitis

INTERACTIONS
Individual drugs
Clofibrate, cycloSPORINE, erythromycin, gemfibrozil, niacin: increased risk of rhabdomyolysis
Colestipol: decreased action of atorvastatin
Erythromycin: increased levels of atorvastatin

Drug classifications
Antifungals (azole): possible rhabdomyolysis

Drug/herb
Red yeast rice: increased pitavastatin effect

Drug/lab test
Increased: bilirubin, alkaline phosphatase, ALT, AST
Interference: thyroid function tests

NURSING CONSIDERATIONS
Assessment
• Assess nutrition: fat, protein, carbohydrates; nutritional analysis should be completed by dietitian before treatment
• **Rhabdomyolysis:** assess for muscle pain, tenderness; obtain CPK if these occur; product may need to be discontinued
• Monitor bowel pattern daily; diarrhea may be a problem

- Monitor triglycerides, cholesterol at baseline, throughout treatment; LDL and VLDL should be watched closely; if increased, product should be discontinued
- Monitor liver function studies q1-2mo during the first 1½ yr of treatment; AST, ALT, liver function tests may be increased
- Monitor renal studies in patients with compromised renal system; BUN, I&O ratio, creatinine
- Assess eyes via ophthalmic exam 1 mo after treatment begins, annually
- **Pregnancy/breastfeeding:** Do not use in pregnancy, breastfeeding

Patient problem
Nonadherence (teaching)

Implementation
- Administer total daily dose at any time of day
- Store in cool environment in tight container protected from light

Patient/family education
- Inform patient that compliance is needed for positive results to occur, not to double doses
- Teach patient that risk factors should be decreased: high-fat diet, smoking, alcohol consumption, absence of exercise
- Advise patient to notify prescriber if the GI symptoms of diarrhea, abdominal or epigastric pain, nausea, vomiting; chills, fever, sore throat; muscle pain, weakness occur
- Advise patient that treatment will take several years
- Advise patient that blood work will be necessary during treatment
- Teach patient that product may increase blood glucose level
- Advise patient not to take if pregnant, avoid breastfeeding

Evaluation

Positive therapeutic outcome
- Decreased cholesterol levels, serum triglyceride
- Improved ratio of HDLs

plazomicin
(pla-zoe-mye' sin)
Zemdri
Func. class.: Anti-infective aminoglycoside

ACTION: Bactericidal; inhibits bacterial protein synthesis through irreversible binding to the 30 S ribosomal subunit of susceptible bacteria

Therapeutic outcome: Absence of fever, draining wounds, negative C&S after treatment

USES: Treatment of complicated urinary tract infection (UTI), including pyelonephritis

Pharmacokinetics

Absorption	Unknown
Distribution	Protein binding 20%
Metabolism	Not metabolized
Excretion	Kidneys
Half-life	Unknown

Pharmacodynamics

Onset	Unknown
Peak	Unknown
Duration	Unknown

CONTRAINDICATIONS: Aminoglycoside hypersensitivity, pregnancy

PRECAUTIONS: Breastfeeding, colitis, diarrhea, geriatrics, GI disease, hearing impairment, myasthenia gravis, pseudomembranous colitis, renal disease

> **BLACK BOX WARNING:** Nephrotoxicity, neuromuscular blockade, ototoxicity, pregnancy

DOSAGE AND ROUTES
Adult: IV 15 mg/kg q24 hr for 4 to 7 days

Available forms: Solution for injection 500 mg/10 ml, single dose

ADVERSE EFFECTS
GI: Nausea, vomiting, diarrhea
GU: Decreased renal function, nephrotoxicity
CNS: Headache
CV: Hypo-hypertension
MISC: Ototoxicity

INTERACTIONS
Drug classifications

> **BLACK BOX WARNING:** Cephalosporins, acyclovir, vancomycin, amphotericin B, cyclosporine, loop diuretics, cidofovir; increase: nephrotoxicity

> **BLACK BOX WARNING:** IV loop diuretics; increase: ototoxicity

> **BLACK BOX WARNING:** Anesthetics, nondepolarizing neuromuscular blockers; increase: neuromuscular blockade, respiratory depression

P

Drug/lab test
Increase: BUN, creatinine

NURSING CONSIDERATIONS
Assessment
• Assess weight before treatment; calculation of dosage is usually based on ideal body weight but may be calculated on actual body weight
• Monitor vital signs during infusion; watch for hypotension, change in pulse
• Check IV site for thrombophlebitis (pain, swelling, redness); change site if needed; apply warm compress to discontinued site

> **BLACK BOX WARNING: Nephrotoxicity**: Is greater in those with impaired renal function, the elderly, and in those receiving other nephrotoxic medications; monitor creatinine clearance in all patients prior to starting therapy and daily; therapeutic drug monitoring (TDM) is recommended for complicated urinary tract infection patients with CCr <90 ml/min to avoid potentially toxic levels; I&O ratio; urinalysis daily for casts, protein; report sudden drop in urinary output

> **BLACK BOX WARNING: Ototoxicity:** Assess for hearing loss, tinnitus, and/or vertigo; assess hearing baseline and throughout treatment; may be irreversible and may not become evident until after completion of therapy, usually in patients with a family history of hearing loss, with renal impairment, and in those receiving higher doses and/or longer durations of therapy than recommended

> **BLACK BOX WARNING: Neuromuscular blockade:** In those with neuromuscular disorders (myasthenia gravis) or in those receiving neuromuscular blocking agents; respiratory paralysis may occur

• **Pregnancy/breastfeeding**: Can cause fetal harm when administered to a pregnant woman, do not use in pregnancy; considered compatible with breastfeeding
• For dehydration, provide adequate hydration 1500-2000 ml/day

Patient problem
Infection (uses)

Implementation
Intermittent IV Infusion Route
• Obtain C&S before treatment; begin treatment before results
• Visually inspect for particulate matter and discoloration prior to use; product should be clear, colorless to yellow solution

Dilution
• Withdraw needed volume of solution (50 mg/ml) for the required dose
• Dilute in 0.9% sodium chloride injection or Lactated Ringer's Injection to achieve a final volume of 50 ml
• *Storage:* Discard any unused portion of vial; dilution may be stored at room temperature for 24 hr at concentrations of 2.5 to 45 mg/ml

Infuse
• Over 30 min

Patient/family education

> **BLACK BOX WARNING: Ototoxicity**: Teach patient to report hearing loss, ringing, roaring in ears, and feeling of fullness in the head

• Advise patient to report headache, dizziness, symptoms of overgrowth of infection, renal impairment, symptoms of nephrotoxicity
• Teach patient to report redness, swelling at infusion site
• Advise patient to drink plenty of fluids each day
• **Pregnancy/breastfeeding:** Teach patient to notify healthcare provider if pregnancy is planned or suspected or if breastfeeding

Evaluation
• Absence of fever, draining wounds, negative C&S after treatment

plecanatide
(ple-kan'-a-tide)
Trulance
Func. class.: Laxative
Chem. class.: Guanylate cyclase-C agonist

ACTION: Binds to GC-C and acts locally on the luminal surface of the intestinal epithelium. Activation of GC-C results in an increase in both intracellular and extracellular concentrations of cyclic guanosine monophosphate (cGMP); this action results in increased intestinal fluid and accelerated gastrointestinal (GI) transit

USES: Chronic idiopathic constipation, IBS-C

Pharmacokinetics

Absorption	Minimal
Distribution	GI tract
Metabolism	Active metabolite, in intestine
Excretion	Unknown
Half-life	Unknown

Pharmacodynamics

Onset	1 wk
Peak	Up to 12 wk
Duration	2 wk after last dose

CONTRAINDICATIONS: Hypersensitivity, GI obstruction

> **BLACK BOX WARNING.** Child <6 yr

Precautions: Pregnancy, breastfeeding

DOSAGE AND ROUTES
Adult: PO 3 mg daily

Available forms: Tabs 3 mg

SIDE EFFECTS
CNS: Dizziness
GI: Diarrhea, flatulence, abdominal distention, abdominal tenderness, nausea
GU: UTI
RESP: Sinusitis, upper respiratory tract infection

INTERACTIONS
Drug/lab test
Increase: AST/ALT

NURSING CONSIDERATIONS

Assessment: Bowel pattern: Assess frequency, consistency, baseline and periodically; provide adequate hydration if diarrhea occurs

Patient problems
Constipation (uses)
Diarrhea (adverse reactions)

Implementation
• Give without regard to food
• Swallow whole; tablets may be crushed and given with applesauce or in water, may be given orally or via NG tube

Patient/family education:
• **Pregnancy/breastfeeding:** Teach patient to notify health care professional if pregnancy is planned or suspected or if breastfeeding
• Teach patient to notify health care professionals of all OTC, Rx, herbals, or supplements taken
• Teach patient to take as directed, not to double or skip doses; that if dose is missed, to take next regularly scheduled dose when due

Evaluation:
• Positive therapeutic outcome
  • Complete bowel movements

> **RARELY USED**
> ## polyethylene glycol
> (po-lee-eth'e-leen glye'kole)
> **ClearLax ✦, GlycoLax, Lax-a Day ✦, MiraLax, PegaLax ✦, PolyLax ✦, Relaxa ✦, RestorLax ✦**
> *Func. class.:* Osmotic laxative

USES: Constipation

CONTRAINDICATION: Hypersensitivity, GI obstruction, megacolon, GI perforation

DOSAGE AND ROUTES
Adult: PO 17 g (a heaping tablespoon) in 8 oz of water
Child >6 mo: PO 0.5-1.5 g/kg/day, titrate to max 17 g if needed

> ## posaconazole (Rx)
> (poe'sa-kon'a-zole)
> **Noxafil, Posanol ✦**
> *Func. class.:* Antifungal, systemic
> *Chem. class.:* Triazole derivative

ACTION: Inhibits a portion of cell wall synthesis; alters cell membranes and inhibits several fungal enzymes

Therapeutic outcome: Decreased fever, malaise, rash; negative C&S for infecting organism

USES: Prevention of aspergillus, candida infection, oropharyngeal candidiasis in the immunocompromised, chemotherapy-induced neutropenia, mucocutaneous candidiasis

Pharmacokinetics

Absorption	Well absorbed, enhanced by food
Distribution	Protein binding 98%-99%
Metabolism	Liver
Excretion	Feces, 77% unchanged
Half-life	19-35 hr

Pharmacodynamics

Onset	Unknown
Peak	3-5 hr
Duration	Unknown

CONTRAINDICATIONS
Hypersensitivity to this product or other systemic antifungal or azoles, fungal meningitis, onchomycosis or dermatomycosis in cardiac dysfunction, use with ergots, sirolimus, CYP3A4 substrates

P

Precautions: Pregnancy, breastfeeding, children, hepatic/cardiac/renal disease

DOSAGE AND ROUTES

Adult/adolescent: PO 600 mg/day in 2-4 divided doses

Oropharyngeal candidiasis

Adult: PO 100 mg bid × 1 day, then 100 mg/day × 13 days

Oropharyngeal candidiasis resistant to fluconazole or itraconazole

Adult/Child ≥13 yr: PO 400 mg bid

Available forms: Oral susp 200 mg/5 ml; delayed release tab 100 mg; solution for injection 300 mg/16.7 ml

ADVERSE EFFECTS

CNS: *Headache, dizziness,* insomnia, fever, rigors, weakness, anxiety

CV: Hypo/hypertension, tachycardia, anemia, QT prolongation, torsades de pointes

GI: *Nausea, vomiting, anorexia, diarrhea,* cramps, abdominal pain, flatulence, GI bleeding, hepatotoxicity

GU: Gynecomastia, impotence, decreased libido

INTEG: *Pruritus,* fever, *rash,* toxic epidermal necrolysis

MISC: *Edema, fatigue,* malaise, hypokalemia, tinnitus, rhabdomyolysis

INTERACTIONS

Individual drugs

Atorvastatin, lovastatin: do not use concurrently

BusPIRone, busulfan, clarithromycin, cycloSPORINE, diazepam, digoxin, felodipine, indinavir, isradipine, midazolam, niCARdipine, NIFEdipine, niMODipine, phenytoin, quiNIDine, ritonavir, saquinavir, tacrolimus, warfarin: increased levels, toxicity

Haloperidol, chloroquine, droperidol, pentamidine; arsenic trioxide, levomethadyl: increased QT prolongation

Cimetidine, phenytoin: decreased posaconazole level

Didanosine, rifamycin: decreased posaconazole action

Dofetilide, pimozide, quiNIDine, halofantrine: life-threatening reactions, increased QT prolongation

Midazolam (oral), triazolam: increased sedation

QuiNIDine: increased tinnitus, hearing loss

Drug classifications

Antacids, H₂-receptor antagonists, rifamycins: decreased posaconazole action

Class IA/III antidysrhythmics, some phenothiazines, beta agonists, local anesthetics, tricyclics, CYP3A4 inhibitors (amiodarone, clarithromycin, erythromycin, telithromycin, troleandomycin), CYP3A4 substrates (methadone, pimozide, QUEtiapine, quiNIDine, risperiDONE, ziprasidone): increased QT prolongation

Ergots: life-threatening reactions, increased QT prolongation

Other hepatotoxic products: increased hepatotoxicity

Calcium channel blockers, HMG-CoA reductase inhibitors, vinca alkaloids: increased levels, toxicity

Oral hypoglycemics: increased severe hypoglycemia

Drug/food

Food: increased absorption

NURSING CONSIDERATIONS

Assessment

- **Rhabdomyolysis:** assess for muscle pain, increased CPK, weakness, swelling of affected muscles; if these occur and if confirmed by CPK, product should be discontinued
- **QT prolongation:** monitor ECG for QT prolongation, ejection fraction; assess for chest pain, palpitations, dyspnea
- Assess for type of infection; may begin treatment before obtaining results
- Assess for infection: temp, WBC, sputum, baseline, periodically, breakthrough infections may occur when used with fosamprenavir
- Monitor I&O ratio, potassium levels
- Monitor liver function tests (ALT, AST, bilirubin) if on long-term therapy
- Assess for allergic reaction: rash, photosensitivity, urticaria, dermatitis
- **Assess for hepatotoxicity:** nausea, vomiting, jaundice, clay-colored stools, fatigue
- **Pregnancy/breastfeeding:** Use only if benefits outweigh fetal risk, may cause malformations, breastfeeding isn't recommended

Patient problem

Infection (uses)
Diarrhea (adverse reactions)

Implementation

PO route

- **Oral susp:** give after shaking well; use calibrated measuring device; take only with a full meal or liquid nutritional supplements such as Ensure; rinse measuring device after each use

- Store in a tight container in refrigerator; do not freeze
- **Delayed-release tab:** Do not divide, chew, or crush; give with food

IV route

Intermittent IV infusion:
- Use 0.22 micron PES or PVDF filter, give slowly over 90 min through central line; if central line is not available, may give a single dose through a peripheral line over 30 min; do not give multiple doses by this method

Dilution:
- Bring to room temperature, transfer 16.7 ml of posaconazole to IV solution that is sufficient for final concentration of 1-2 mg/ml, use immediately (diluted solution)
- Store up to 2 hr refrigerated

Patient/family education
- Teach patient that long-term therapy may be needed to clear infection (1 wk-6 mo depending on infection)
- Advise patient to avoid hazardous activities if dizziness occurs
- Advise patient to take 2 hr before administration of other products that increase gastric pH (antacids, H_2-blockers, omeprazole, sucralfate, anticholinergics); to notify health care provider of all medications taken (many interactions)
- Teach the patient the importance of compliance with product regimen; to use alternative method of contraception
- Teach patient to notify prescriber of GI symptoms, signs of hepatic dysfunction (fatigue, nausea, anorexia, vomiting, dark urine, pale stools)
- Teach patient to take during meal or within 20 min of eating

Evaluation

Positive therapeutic outcome
- Decreased fever, malaise, rash, negative C&S for infecting organism

---

RARELY USED

potassium/sodium phosphates
(po-tas´e-um/soe´dee-um-foss´fates)
K-Phos M, F, K-Phos Neutral, K-Phos No. 2, Neutra-Phos, Uro-KP Neutral
Func. class.: Mineral/electrolyte replacement

USES: Phosphate depletion, prevention of kidney stones (calcium)

CONTRAINDICATIONS: Hyperkalemia, hypocalcemia, severe renal disease, hyperphosphatemia

---

DOSAGE AND ROUTES

Urinary acidification
Adult: PO 2 tablets QID

Phosphorus maintenance
Adult: PO 50-150 mmol/day in divided doses
Child: PO 2-3 mmol/kg/day in divided doses

Phosphorous supplement
Adult/child >4 yr: PO 250-500 mg qid
Child <4 yr: PO 250 mg qid

---

potassium acetate/ potassium bicarbonate (Rx, OTC)
K-Effervescent, Klor-Con EF, K-Vescent
potassium bicarbonate potassium chloride (Rx, OTC)
potassium bicarbonate/ potassium citrate (Rx, OTC)

⚠ HIGH ALERT

potassium chloride (Rx, OTC)
Micro-K-10, Klor-Con, K-Tab, Micro-K
potassium gluconate (Rx, OTC)
Func. class.: Electrolyte, mineral replacement
Chem. class.: Potassium

ACTION: Needed for adequate transmission of nerve impulses and cardiac contraction, renal function, intracellular ion maintenance

Therapeutic outcome: Potassium level 3.0-5.0 mg/dl

USES: Prevention and treatment of hypokalemia

Pharmacokinetics

Absorption	Unknown
Distribution	Unknown
Metabolism	Unknown
Excretion	Kidneys, feces
Half-life	Unknown

Pharmacodynamics

	PO	IV
Onset	30 min	Immediate
Peak	Unknown	Unknown
Duration	Unknown	Unknown

CONTRAINDICATIONS
Renal disease (severe), severe hemolytic disease, Addison's disease, hyperkalemia, acute dehydration, extensive tissue breakdown

Precautions: Pregnancy, cardiac disease, potassium-sparing diuretic therapy, systemic acidosis

DOSAGE AND ROUTES
Hypokalemia (prevention) (bicarbonate, chloride, gluconate)
Adult: PO 20 mEq/day in 1-2 divided doses
Child: PO 1-2 mEq/day in 1-2 divided doses

Hypokalemia, digoxin toxicity (acetate, chloride)
Adult: serum potassium conc > 2.5 mEq/L: IV max 10 mEq/l hr, with 24 hr dose max 200 mEq, initial dose of 20-40 mEq has been recommended; PO 40-100 mEq/day in 2-4 divided doses
Child: IV 0.25-0.5 mEq/g/dose, at 0.25-0.5 mEq/kg/hr; PO 2-5 mEq/day in divided doses

Available forms: Tabs for sol 6.5, 25 mEq; ext rel caps 8, 10 mEq; powder for sol 3.3, 5, 6.7, 10, 13.3 mEq/5 ml; tabs 2, 4, 5, 13.4 mEq; ext rel tabs 6.7, 8, 10 mEq; elix 6.7 mEq/5 ml; oral sol 2.375 mEq/5 ml; inj for prep of IV 1.5, 2, 2.4, 3, 3.2, 4.4, 4.7 mEq/ml

ADVERSE EFFECTS
CNS: Confusion
CV: Bradycardia, *cardiac depression*, dysrhythmias, arrest, peaking T waves, lowered R and depressed RST, prolonged P–R interval, widened QRS complex
GI: *Nausea, vomiting, cramps,* pain, *diarrhea,* ulceration of small bowel
GU: Oliguria
INTEG: Cold extremities, rash

INTERACTIONS
Drug classifications
Angiotensin-converting enzyme inhibitors, calcium, diuretics (potassium-sparing), magnesium, potassium phosphate, IV, other potassium products: increased hyperkalemia

NURSING CONSIDERATIONS
Assessment
• **Hyperkalemia:** Assess ECG for peaking T-waves, lowered R, depressed RST, prolonged PR interval, widening QRS complex, hyperkalemia; product should be reduced or discontinued; monitor potassium level during treatment (3.5-5.0 mg/dl is normal level)
• Monitor hydration status, I&O ratio; watch for decreased urinary output; notify prescriber immediately; check urinary pH in patients receiving the product as a urinary acidifier
• Assess cardiac status: rate, rhythm, CVP, PWP, PAWP if being monitored directly

Patient problem
Risk of injury (uses, adverse reactions)

Implementation
PO route
• Do not break, crush, or chew ext rel tabs/caps or enteric-coated products
• Give with meal or after meal; take cap with full glass of liquid; dissolve effervescent tab, powder in 8 oz of cold water or juice; do not give IM, SUBCUT
• Store at room temperature

IV route
• Give through large-bore needle to decrease vein inflammation; check for extravasation; administer in large vein, avoiding scalp vein in child
• After diluting in large volume of IV sol give as an IV inf slowly to prevent toxicity; never give IV bol or IM

>> Potassium Chloride
• Must be diluted, concentrated potassium infections are fatal

Continuous IV infusion route
• Conc max 80 mEq/L for peripheral line, 120 mEq/L central line
• Dehydrated patients should receive 1 L of potassium-free hydration sol; then infuse 10 mEq/hr; in severe hypokalemia rate may be 40 mEq/hr

Y-site compatibilities: Acyclovir, aldesleukin, allopurinol, amifostine, aminophylline, amiodarone, ampicillin, atropine, aztreonam, betamethasone, calcium gluconate, cefmetazole, cephalothin, cephapirin, chlordiazePOXIDE, chlorproMAZINE, ciprofloxacin, cladribine, cyanocobalamin, dexamethasone, digoxin, diltiazem, diphenhydrAMINE, DOBUTamine, DOPamine, droperidol, edrophonium, enalaprilat, EPINEPHrine, esmolol, estrogens, ethacrynate, famotidine, fentaNYL, filgrastim, fludarabine, fluorouracil, furosemide, gallium, granisetron, heparin, hydrALAZINE, IDArubicin, indomethacin, inamrinone, regular insulin, isoproterenol, kanamycin, labetalol, lidocaine, LORazepam, magnesium sulfate, melphalan, meperidine, methicillin, methoxamine, methylergonovine, midazolam, minocycline, morphine, neostigmine, norepinephrine, ondansetron, oxacillin, oxytocin, PACLitaxel, penicillin G potassium,

---

pentazocine, phytonadione, piperacillin/tazobactam, predniSOLONE, procainamide, prochlorperazine, propofol, propranolol, pyridostigmine, sargramostim, scopolamine, sodium bicarbonate, succinylcholine, tacrolimus, teniposide, theophylline, thiotepa, trimethaphan, trimethobenzamide, vinorelbine, zidovudine

Patient/family education
• Teach patient to eat foods rich in potassium after medication is discontinued
• Advise patient to avoid OTC products: antacids, salt substitutes, analgesics, vit preparations, unless specifically directed by prescriber; avoid licorice in large amounts, may cause hypokalemia, sodium retention
• Advise patient to report hyperkalemia symptoms or continued hypokalemia symptoms
• Tell patient to take cap with full glass of liquid; to dissolve powder or tab completely in at least 120 ml of water or juice; not to crush, chew caps or tabs
• Emphasize importance of regular follow-up and periodic potassium levels

Evaluation

Positive therapeutic outcome
• Absence of fatigue, muscle weakness, and decreased thirst and urinary output, cardiac changes
• Potassium level normal

pramipexole (Rx)
(pra-mi-pex'ol)
Mirapex, Mirapex ER
Func. class.: Antiparkinsonian agent
Chem. class.: Dopamine receptor agonist, nonergot

ACTION: Selective agonist for D_2 receptors (presynaptic/postsynaptic sites); binding at D_3 receptor contributes to antiparkinson effects

Therapeutic outcome: Decreased symptoms of Parkinson's disease (involuntary movements)

USES: Idiopathic Parkinson's disease, restless leg syndrome

Pharmacokinetics

Absorption	Well absorbed
Distribution	Widely distributed
Metabolism	Liver, minimally
Excretion	Kidneys, unchanged
Half-life	8 hr; 12 hr in geriatric

Pharmacodynamics

Onset	Unknown
Peak	2 hr
Duration	Unknown

CONTRAINDICATIONS
Hypersensitivity

Precautions: Pregnancy renal/cardiac disease, MI with dysrhythmias, affective disorders, psychosis, preexisting dyskinesias, history of falling asleep during daily activities, rapid dose reduction

DOSAGE AND ROUTES
Initial treatment
Adult: PO from a starting dose of 0.375 mg/day given in 3 divided doses, increase gradually by 0.125 mg/dose at 5-7–day intervals until total daily dose of 4.5 mg is reached; ER 0.375 mg qd, may increase up to 0.75 mg/day, then increments of 0.75 mg/day ≤5-7 days, max 4.5 mg/day

Restless leg syndrome
Adult: PO 0.125 mg 2-3 hr before bedtime, increase gradually, max 0.5 mg/day

Renal dose
Adult: PO CCr 35-59 ml/min 0.125 mg bid, may increase q5-7day to 1.5 mg bid; CCr 15-34 ml/min 0.125 mg/day, may increase q5-7day to 1.5 mg/day

Available forms: Tabs 0.125, 0.25, 0.5, 0.75, 1, 1.5 mg; cap ER 0.375, 0.75, 1.5, 2.25, 3.0, 3.75, 4.5 mg

ADVERSE EFFECTS
CNS: *Agitation, insomnia,* psychosis, hallucinations, depression, dizziness, headache, confusion, amnesia, dream disorder, asthenia, dyskinesia, hypersomnolence, sudden sleep onset, impulse-control disorders
CV: *Orthostatic hypotension,* edema, syncope, tachycardia, increased B/P, heart rate
EENT: Blurred vision
ENDO: Antidiuretic hormone secretion (SIADH)
GI: *Nausea, anorexia,* constipation, dysphagia, dry mouth
GU: Impotence, urinary frequency
HEMA: Hemolytic anemia, leukopenia, agranulocytosis
INTEG: Pruritus

INTERACTIONS
Individual drugs
Cimetidine, diltiazem, levodopa, quiNIDine, ranitidine, triamterene, verapamil: increased pramipexole levels
Metoclopramide: decreased pramipexole levels

Drug classifications

Butyrophenones, DOPamine agonists, phenothiazines: decreased pramipexole effect

NURSING CONSIDERATIONS

Assessment

• Monitor B/P, ECG, respiration during initial treatment; hypo/hypertension should be reported

• Assess mental status: affect, mood, behavioral changes, depression; complete suicide assessment

• Assess for involuntary movements in parkinsonism: akinesia, tremors, staggering gait, muscle rigidity, drooling; these symptoms should improve with therapy

• **Assess for sleep attacks:** may fall asleep during activities, without warning; may need to discontinue medication

Patient problem

Impaired mobility (uses)
Risk for injury (uses, adverse reactions)
Impaired sleep (adverse reactions)

Implementation

• Adjust dosage to patient's response
• Give with meals to decrease GI upset

Patient/family education

• Advise patient that therapeutic effects may take several wk to a few mo

• Caution patient to change positions slowly to prevent orthostatic hypotension

• Instruct patient to use product exactly as prescribed; if product is discontinued abruptly, parkinsonian crisis may occur; if treatment is to be discontinued, taper over 1 wk; avoid alcohol, OTC sleeping products

• Teach patient to notify prescriber of impulse control disorders: shopping

• Advise patient to notify prescriber if pregnancy is planned or suspected, or if breastfeeding

Evaluation

Positive therapeutic outcome

• Decreased akathisia, other involuntary movements
• Improved mood

pramoxine topical

See Appendix B

⚠ HIGH ALERT

prasugrel (Rx)

(pra′soo-grel)

Effient

Func. class.: Platelet aggregation inhibitor
Chem. class.: ADP receptor antagonist

ACTION: Inhibits ADP-induced platelet aggregation

Therapeutic outcome: Absence of MI, stroke

USES: Reducing the risk of stroke, MI, vascular death, peripheral arterial disease in high-risk patients

Pharmacokinetics

Absorption	Rapidly absorbed
Distribution	Unknown
Metabolism	Liver CYP3A4, CYP2B6
Excretion	Urine, feces
Half-life	7-8 hr

Pharmacodynamics

Onset	Unknown
Peak	30 min
Duration	Unknown

CONTRAINDICATIONS

Hypersensitivity, stroke, TIA

BLACK BOX WARNING: Active bleeding

Precautions: Pregnancy, breastfeeding, children, hepatic disease, increased bleeding risk, neutropenia, agranulocytosis, renal disease, surgery, trauma, thrombotic thrombocytopenia purpura, Asian patients, weight <60 kg, CABG, geriatric, abrupt discontinuation

DOSAGE AND ROUTES

Adult/geriatric <75 yr and ≥60 kg: PO 60 mg loading dose, then 10 mg qd with aspirin (75-325 mg/day)

Adult/geriatric <75 yr and <60 kg: PO 60 mg loading dose, then 5 mg qd

Geriatric >75 yr: Not recommended

Available forms: Tabs 5, 10 mg

ADVERSE EFFECTS

CNS: Headache, dizziness

CV: Edema, atrial fibrillation, bradycardia, chest pain, hyper/hypotension

GI: Nausea, vomiting, diarrhea

HEMA: Epistaxis, leukopenia, thrombocytopenia, neutropenia, anaphylaxis, angioedema, anemia
INTEG: Rash, hypercholesterolemia
MISC: Fatigue, intracranial hemorrhage, secondary malignancy, angioedema
MS: Back pain

INTERACTIONS
Individual drugs
Abciximab, aspirin, eptifibatide, rifampin, tirofiban, ticlopidine, treprostinil: increased bleeding risk

Drug classifications
Anticoagulants, thrombolytics, NSAIDs, SSRIs: increased bleeding risk

NURSING CONSIDERATIONS
Assessment
• **Assess for thrombotic/thrombocytic purpura:** fever, thrombocytopenia, neurolytic anemia
• Monitor hepatic studies: AST, ALT, bilirubin, creatinine (long-term therapy)
• Monitor blood studies: CBC, differential, Hct, Hgb, PT, cholesterol (long-term therapy)

> **BLACK BOX WARNING: Bleeding:** may be fatal, decreased B/P in those who have had CABG may be the first indication; bleeding should be controlled while continuing product; may use transfusion; do not use within 1 wk of CABG; may use lower doses in those <60 kg

• **Beers:** Avoid use in those ≥ 75 yr old, increased bleeding risk

Patient problem
Risk of injury (adverse reactions)
Lack of knowledge of medication (teaching)

Implementation
• Give with food to decrease gastric symptoms
• Do not break tablets, tablet may be crushed and mixed in food, fluids
• Do not discontinue therapy abruptly

Patient/family education
• Advise that blood work will be necessary during treatment
• Teach to report any unusual bruising, bleeding to prescriber; that it may take longer to stop bleeding
• Advise to take with food or just after eating to minimize GI discomfort
• Advise to report diarrhea, skin rashes, subcutaneous bleeding, chills, fever, sore throat
• Teach to tell all health care providers that prasugrel is used; may be withheld before surgery
• **Pregnancy/breastfeeding:** Identify if pregnancy is planned or suspected

Evaluation
Positive therapeutic outcome
• Absence of stroke, MI

pravastatin (Rx)
(pra′va-sta-tin)
Pravachol, PravASA ♣
Func. class.: Antilipidemic

Do not confuse: Pravachol/Prevacid

ACTION: Inhibits biosynthesis of VLDL, LDL, which are responsible for cholesterol development, by inhibiting the enzyme HMG-CoA reductase

Therapeutic outcome: Decreasing cholesterol levels and LDL, increased HDL

USES: As an adjunct in primary hypercholesterolemia types IIa, IIb, III, IV, atherosclerosis; to reduce the risk of recurrent MI, primary/secondary CV events; reduce stroke, TIAs

Pharmacokinetics
Absorption	Poorly absorbed, erratic
Distribution	Protein binding 80%
Metabolism	Liver, extensively
Excretion	Feces (70%-75%); kidneys, unchanged (20%); breast milk (minimal)
Half-life	2 hr

Pharmacodynamics
Onset	Unknown
Peak	1-1½ hr
Duration	Unknown

CONTRAINDICATIONS
Pregnancy, breastfeeding, hypersensitivity, active liver disease

Precautions: Past liver disease, alcoholism, severe acute infections, trauma, severe metabolic disorders, electrolyte imbalances, renal disease

DOSAGE AND ROUTES
Adult: PO 40-80 mg/day at bedtime (range 20-80 mg/day), start at 10 mg/day if also on immunosuppressants
Adolescent 14-18 yr: PO 40 mg/day
Child 8-13 yr: PO 20 mg/day
Geriatric: PO 10 mg/day, initially

Renal dose
Adult: PO 10-20 mg daily at bedtime, increase at 4-wk intervals

Available forms: Tabs 10, 20, 40, 80 mg

ADVERSE EFFECTS

CNS: Headache, dizziness, fatigue, confusion
CV: Chest pain
EENT: Lens opacities
GI: Nausea, constipation, diarrhea, flatus, abdominal pain, heartburn, liver dysfunction, pancreatitis, hepatitis
GU: Renal failure (myoglobinuria)
INTEG: Rash, pruritus
MS: Muscle cramps, myalgia, myositis, rhabdomyolysis
RESP: Common cold, rhinitis, cough

INTERACTIONS
Individual drugs
Clarithromycin, clofibrate, cycloSPORINE, erythromycin, gemfibrozil, itraconazole, niacin: increased risk for myopathy

Drug classifications
Bile acid sequestrants: decreased pravastatin bioavailability
Protease inhibitors: increased risk of myopathy

Drug/herb
St. John's wort: decreased effect
Red yeast rice: increased adverse reactions
Eucalyptus: increased hepatotoxicity

Drug/lab test
Increased: CPK, liver function tests
Altered: thyroid function tests

NURSING CONSIDERATIONS
Assessment
• Assess nutrition: fat, protein, carbohydrates; nutritional analysis should be completed by dietitian before treatment
• Monitor triglycerides, esterol, cholesterol at baseline, throughout treatment; LDL and HDL should be watched closely; if increased, product should be discontinued
• Rhabdomyolysis: assess for muscle tenderness, pain; obtain CPK; therapy should be discontinued
• Monitor ophth status yearly
• **Pregnancy/breastfeeding:** Do not use in pregnancy, breastfeeding

Patient problem
Nonadherence (teaching)

Implementation
• Give at bedtime only; give 1 hr before or 2 hr after bile acid sequestrants
• Store in cool environment in airtight, light-resistant container

Patient/family education
• Inform patient that compliance is needed for positive results to occur; not to double doses or skip doses
• Teach patient that risk factors should be decreased: high-fat diet, smoking, alcohol consumption, absence of exercise
• Advise patient to notify prescriber of weakness, tenderness, or limited mobility, blurred vision, severe GI symptoms, dizziness, headache, muscle pain, fever
• **Pregnancy/breastfeeding:** Explain to patient that contraception is necessary, since product produces teratogenic effects, not to breastfeed
• Advise patient to use sunscreen, protective clothing to prevent burns
• **Hepatic disease:** Instruct patient to notify prescriber of lack of appetite, yellow sclera and skin, dark urine, abdominal pain, weakness

Evaluation
Positive therapeutic outcome
• Decreased cholesterol, serum triglyceride levels and improved ratio with HDL

prazosin (Rx)
(pra′zoe-sin)
Minipress
Func. class.: Antihypertensive
Chem. class.: α_1-Adrenergic blocker, peripheral

ACTION: Blocks α-mediated vasoconstriction of adrenergic receptors, inducing peripheral vasodilatation

Therapeutic outcome: Decreased B/P in hypertension; decreased cardiac preload, afterload

USES: Hypertension, benign prostatic hypertrophy to decrease urine outflow obstruction

Unlabeled uses: Posttraumatic stress disorder (PTSD)

Pharmacokinetics

Absorption	60%
Distribution	Widely distributed
Metabolism	Liver, extensively; protein binding 97%
Excretion	Kidneys, unchanged (10%); bile (90%)
Half-life	2-3 hr

Pharmacodynamics

Onset	2 hr
Peak	1-3 hr
Duration	6-12 hr

CONTRAINDICATIONS

Hypersensitivity

Precautions: Pregnancy, breastfeeding, children, geriatric patients, prostate cancer, ocular surgery, orthostatic hypotension

DOSAGE AND ROUTES
Hypertension

Adult: PO 1 mg bid or tid, increasing to 20 mg/day in divided doses if required, usual range 6-15 mg/day; max 1 mg initially, max 20-40 mg/day
Child: PO 5 mcg/kg q6hr; max 400 mcg/kg/day or 15 mg/day

Benign prostatic hyperplasia
Adult: PO 2 mg bid

Post-traumatic stress disorder (unlabeled)
Adult PO: 1 mg/day at bedtime, titrate over 10 days to max 15 mg/day

Available forms: Caps 1, 2, 5 mg

ADVERSE EFFECTS

CNS: *Dizziness, headache, drowsiness,* anxiety, depression, vertigo, *weakness,* fatigue, syncope
CV: *Palpitations, orthostatic hypotension,* tachycardia, edema, rebound hypertension
EENT: Blurred vision, epistaxis, tinnitus, dry mouth, red sclera
GI: *Nausea,* vomiting, diarrhea, constipation, abdominal pain, pancreatitis
GU: Urinary frequency, incontinence, impotence, priapism, water and sodium retention

INTERACTIONS
Individual drugs

Alcohol, nitroglycerin: increased hypotension
CloNIDine: decreased antihypertensive effect

Drug classifications

Antihypertensives, β-adrenergic blockers, phosphodiesterase inhibitors (vardenafil, tadalafil, sildenafil), diuretics, MAOIs: increased hypotension
NSAIDs: decreased antihypertensive effect

Drug/herb

Hawthorn: increased antihypertensive effect

Drug/lab test

Increased: urinary norepinephrine, BUN, uric acid, LFTs
Positive: ANA titer

NURSING CONSIDERATIONS
Assessment

• **Hypertension/HF:** Monitor B/P, orthostatic hypotension usually occurs on first dose, syncope; check for edema in feet, legs daily; monitor I&O, weight daily; notify prescriber of changes
• Assess for allergic reactions: rash, fever, pruritus, urticaria; product should be discontinued if antihistamines fail to help
• **Beers:** Avoid use as an antihypertensive in older adults, high risk of orthostatic hypotension

Patient problems

Nonadherence (teaching)

Implementation

• Severe hypotension may occur after first dose of this medication; hypotension may be prevented by reducing or discontinuing diuretic therapy 3 days before beginning prazosin therapy
• Give same time each day
• Store in airtight container at 86° F (30° C) or less
• Give without regard to meals
• Store at room temperature

Patient/family education

• Instruct patient not to discontinue product abruptly; stress the importance of complying with dosage schedule, even if feeling better; if dose is missed, take as soon as remembered; take at same time each day
• Advise patient not to use OTC products (cough, cold, allergy) unless directed by prescriber; also to avoid large amounts of caffeine, alcohol; do not crush, chew caps
• Emphasize the need to rise slowly to sitting or standing position to minimize orthostatic hypotension
• Teach patient not to notify prescriber of mouth sores, sore throat, fever, swelling of hands or feet, irregular heartbeat, chest pain
• Caution patient to report excessive perspiration, dehydration, vomiting, diarrhea; may lead to fall in B/P
• Caution patient that product may cause dizziness, fainting, light-headedness; may occur during 1st few days of therapy; to avoid hazardous activities
• Teach patient how to take B/P and normal readings for age group; instruct to take B/P q7day

Evaluation

Positive therapeutic outcome
• Decreased B/P in hypertension

TREATMENT OF OVERDOSE:

Administer volume expanders or vasopressors, discontinue product, place patient in supine position

prednisoLONE (Rx)
(pred-niss'oh-lone)
Orapred, Orapred ODT, Pediapred Prelone
Func. class.: Corticosteroid, synthetic
Chem. class.: Intermediate-acting gluco-corticoid

Do not confuse: prednisoLONE/
predniSONE

ACTION: Decreases inflammation by suppressing migration of polymorphonuclear leukocytes, fibroblasts; reversal to increase capillary permeability and lysosomal stabilization

Therapeutic outcome: Decreased inflammation, decreased adrenal insufficiency

USES: Severe inflammation, immunosuppression, neoplasms, asthma

Pharmacokinetics

Absorption	Well absorbed (PO, IM), completely absorbed (**IV**)
Distribution	Widely distributed, crosses placenta
Metabolism	Liver, extensively
Excretion	Kidney, breast milk
Half-life	2-4 hr

Pharmacodynamics

	PO	IM (phos-phate)	IV	IA/IL
Onset	1 hr	Rapid	Rapid	Slow
Peak	2 hr	1 hr	Un-known	Un-known
Duration	1½ days	Un-known	Un-known	Up to 1 mo

CONTRAINDICATIONS
Hypersensitivity, fungal infections, varicella, viral infection

Precautions: Pregnancy, breastfeeding, children, diabetes mellitus, glaucoma, osteoporosis, seizure disorders, ulcerative colitis, HF, myasthenia gravis, thromboembolism, peptic ulcer disease, renal disease, Cushing syndrome, abrupt discontinuation, children, acute MI, GI ulcers, hypertension, hepatitis, psychosis

DOSAGE AND ROUTES
Most conditions
Adult: PO 5-60 mg/day as a single dose or in divided doses

Adolescent/child/infant: PO 0.14-2 mg/kg or 4-60 mg/m²/day in 3-4 divided doses

Multiple Sclerosis
Adult: PO 200 mg/day x 7 day, then 80 mg every other day × 1 mo
Adolescent/child/infant: PO 0.14-2 mg/kg or 4-60 mg/m²/day in 3-4 divided doses

Antiinflammatory
Adult: PO 5-60 mg/day as a single dose or in divided doses
Adolescent/child/infant: PO 0.14-2 mg/kg or 4-60 mg/m²/day in 3-4 divided doses

Acute asthma exacerbation
Adult/adolescent: PO 40-60 mg/day as a single dose or in 2 divided doses for 3-10 days
Child 5-12 yr: PO 1-2 mg/day (up to 60 mg) in 2 divided doses for 3-10 days
Infant/child ≤4 yr: PO 1-2 mg/kg/day (up to 30 mg) in 2 divided doses for 3-10 days

Available forms: Tabs 5 mg; oral sol 5 mg/5 ml, 10 mg/5 ml, 15 mg/5 ml, 25 mg/5 ml; oral suspension 5 mg/mL; oral disintegrating tab 10, 15, 30 mg

ADVERSE EFFECTS
CNS: *Depression,* flushing, sweating, headache, mood changes
CV: *Hypertension,* circulatory collapse, thrombophlebitis, embolism, tachycardia
EENT: Fungal infections, increased intraocular pressure, blurred vision
GI: *Diarrhea, nausea, abdominal distention,* GI hemorrhage, increased appetite, pancreatitis
INTEG: Acne, poor wound healing, ecchymosis, petechiae
MS: Fractures, osteoporosis, weakness, arthralgia, myopathy, tendon rupture
MISC: Hyperglycemia

INTERACTIONS
Individual drugs
Alcohol, amphotericin B, cycloSPORINE, digitalis, indomethacin, NSAIDs: increased side effects
Ambenonium, isoniazid, neostigmine, somatrem: decreased effects of each specific product
Cholestyramine, colestipol, ePHEDrine, phenytoin, rifampin, theophylline: decreased action of prednisoLONE
Indomethacin, ketoconazole: increased action of prednisoLONE

Drug classifications
Antibiotics (macrolide), contraceptives (oral), estrogens, salicylates: increased action of prednisoLONE

Anticholinesterases, anticoagulants, anticonvulsants, antidiabetics, salicylates, toxoids, vaccines: decreased effects of each specific product

Azole antifungals, cycloSPORINE: increased toxicity

Barbiturates: decreased action of prednisoLONE

CYP3A4 inducers: decreased prednisoLONE effect

CYP3A4 inhibitors: increased prednisoLONE effect

Diuretics, salicylates: increased side effects

Quinolones: increased tendon rupture

Drug/lab test

Increased: cholesterol, sodium, blood glucose, uric acid, calcium, urine glucose

Decreased: calcium, potassium, T_4, T_3, thyroid ^{131}I uptake test, urine 17-OHCS, 17-KS, PBI

False negative: skin allergy tests

NURSING CONSIDERATIONS
Assessment

• Monitor potassium, blood glucose, urine glucose while patient is on long-term therapy; hypokalemia and hyperglycemia may occur

• Monitor weight daily; notify prescriber of weekly gain >5 lb; monitor I&O ratio; be alert for decreasing urinary output and increasing edema

• Monitor B/P, pulse; notify prescriber if chest pain occurs

• Monitor plasma cortisol levels during long-term therapy (normal level 138-635 nmol/L [SI units] when measured at 8 AM)

• **Assess infection:** increased temp, WBC even after withdrawal of medication; product masks infection symptoms

• **Assess for potassium depletion:** paresthesias, fatigue, nausea, vomiting, depression, polyuria, dysrhythmias, weakness, edema, hypertension, cardiac symptoms

• **Adrenal insufficiency:** assess for nausea, vomiting, lethargy, restlessness, confusion, baseline and periodically

• Assess mental status: affect, mood, behavioral changes, aggression

• Monitor temp; if fever develops, product should be discontinued

• **Beers:** Avoid in older adults with or at high risk of delirium

Patient problem

Risk for infection (adverse reactions)
Risk for injury (adverse reactions)
Nonadherence (teaching)

Implementation

• **Oral sol:** use calibrated measuring devices

• **Orally disintegrating tabs:** place on tongue, allow to dissolve, swallow; or swallow whole; do not cut, split

Patient/family education

• Advise patient to carry/wear emergency ID as steroid user

• Advise patient to notify prescriber if therapeutic response decreases; dosage adjustment may be needed

• Caution patient not to discontinue abruptly; adrenal crisis can result; take exactly as prescribed

• Caution patient to avoid OTC products: salicylates, cough products with alcohol, cold preparations unless directed by prescriber

• Teach patient all aspects of product usage including cushingoid symptoms (moon face, buffalo hump, rapid weight gain, excessive sweating, stretch marks)

• **Teach patient symptoms of adrenal insufficiency:** nausea, anorexia, fatigue, dizziness, dyspnea, weakness, joint pain and why to notify provider

• Advise patient that long-term therapy may be needed to clear infection (1-2 mo depending on type of infection)

• **Pregnancy/breastfeeding:** Not recommended in pregnancy, cautious use in breastfeeding. Identify if pregnancy is planned or suspected or if breastfeeding

Evaluation

Positive therapeutic outcome
• Decreased inflammation

prednisoLONE ophthalmic
See Appendix B

predniSONE (Rx)
(pred′ni-sone)
Winipred ✚
Func. class.: Corticosteroid
Chem. class.: Intermediate-acting glucocorticoid

Do not confuse: predniSONE/
methylPREDNISolone/prednisoLONE/PriLOSEC

ACTION: Decreases inflammation by increasing capillary permeability and lysosomal stabilization, minimal mineralocorticoid activity

Therapeutic outcome: Decreased inflammation, decreased adrenal insufficiency

USES: Severe inflammation, neoplasms, multiple sclerosis, collagen disorders, dermatologic disorders

Pharmacokinetics

Absorption	Well absorbed
Distribution	Widely distributed, crosses placenta
Metabolism	Liver, extensively
Excretion	Kidney, breast milk
Half-life	3-4 hr

Pharmacodynamics

Onset	Unknown
Peak	1-2 hr; del rel 6-6½ hr
Duration	1½ days

CONTRAINDICATIONS
Hypersensitivity

Precautions: Pregnancy, diabetes mellitus, glaucoma, osteoporosis, seizure disorders, ulcerative colitis, HF, myasthenia gravis, renal disease, esophagitis, peptic ulcer, cataracts, coagulopathy, abrupt discontinuation, children, corticosteroid hypersensitivity, Cushing syndrome, thromboembolism, geriatrics, acute MI

DOSAGE AND ROUTES
Most Uses
Adult: PO 5-60 mg/day or divided bid-qid
Child: PO 0.05-2 mg/kg/day divided 1-4 ×/day

Nephrotic syndrome
Child: PO 2 mg/kg/day in divided doses until urine is protein-free for 3 consecutive days, then 1-1.5 mg/kg/day every other day × 4 wk

Multiple sclerosis
Adult: PO 200 mg/day × 1 wk, then 80 mg every other day × 1 mo

Asthma
Adult/adolescent: PO 40-80 mg/day in 1-2 divided doses until PEF is 70% of predicted or personal best
Child: PO 1 mg/kg (max 60 mg)/day in 2 divided doses until PEF is 70% of predicted or personal best

Available forms: Tabs 1, 2.5, 5, 10, 20, 50 mg; oral sol 5 mg/5 ml; del rel tab 1, 2, 5 mg

ADVERSE EFFECTS
CNS: Depression, flushing, sweating, headache, mood changes
CV: Hypertension, thrombophlebitis, embolism, tachycardia, fluid retention
EENT: Fungal infections, increased intraocular pressure, blurred vision
GI: Diarrhea, nausea, abdominal distention, GI hemorrhage, increased appetite, pancreatitis
INTEG: Acne, poor wound healing, ecchymosis, petechiae

META: Hyperglycemia
MS: Fractures, osteoporosis, weakness

INTERACTIONS
Individual drugs
Alcohol, amphotericin B, cycloSPORINE, digoxin: increased side effects
Isoniazid, neostigmine, somatrem: decreased effects of each specific product
Cholestyramine, colestipol, phenytoin, rifampin, theophylline: decreased action of predniSONE
Ketoconazole: increased action of predniSONE

Drug classifications
Anticholinesterases, anticoagulants, anticonvulsants, antidiabetics, toxoids, vaccines: decreased effects of each specific product
Antiinfectives (macrolide), contraceptives (oral), estrogens: increased action of predniSONE
Barbiturates: decreased action of predniSONE
CYP3A4 inducers: decreased predniSONE effect
CYP3A4 inhibitors: increased predniSONE effect
Diuretics: increased side effects
NSAIDs: increased side effects, increased action of predniSONE
Quinolones: increased tendon rupture
Salicylates: increased side effects, increased action of predniSONE, decreased effects of salicylates

Drug/herb
Ephedra (ma huang): decreased predniSONE effect

Drug/lab test
Increased: cholesterol, sodium, blood glucose, uric acid, calcium, urine glucose
Decreased: calcium, potassium, T_4, T_3, thyroid ^{131}I uptake test, urine 17-OHCS, 17-KS, PBI
False negative: skin allergy tests

NURSING CONSIDERATIONS
Assessment
• **Adrenal insufficiency:** assess for nausea, vomiting, anorexia, confusion, hypotension, weight loss before and during treatment; HPA suppression may be precipitated by abrupt withdrawal
• Monitor potassium, blood glucose, urine glucose while on long-term therapy; hypokalemia and hyperglycemia may occur
• Monitor weight daily; notify prescriber of weekly gain >5 lb; monitor I&O ratio; be alert for decreasing urinary output and increasing edema, rales/crackles, notify provider if present
• Monitor B/P, pulse; notify prescriber if chest pain occurs

• Monitor plasma cortisol levels during long-term therapy (normal level 138-635 nmol/L when measured at 8 AM)
• Assess adrenal function periodically for hypothalamic-pituitary-adrenal axis suppression
• Assess infection: increased temp, WBC even after withdrawal of medication; product masks infection symptoms
• **Assess for potassium depletion:** paresthesias, fatigue, nausea, vomiting, depression, polyuria, dysrhythmias, weakness, edema, hypertension, cardiac symptoms
• Assess mental status: affect, mood, behavioral changes, aggression
• Monitor temp; if fever develops, product should be discontinued
• Assess for systemic absorption: increased temp, inflammation, irritation (topical)
• **Beers:** Avoid in older adults with a high risk of delirium

Patient problem

Risk for infection (adverse reactions)
Risk for injury (adverse reactions)
Nonadherence (teaching)

Implementation

• Regular tabs may be crushed and given with food or fluids
• **Oral Solution:** Use calibrated measuring device to measure
• Give with food or milk to decrease GI symptoms; use measuring device for liquid route
• For long-term use, alternative product therapy is recommended, to decrease adverse reactions
• **Del rel tab:** swallow whole, do not break, crush, or chew; give once daily

Patient/family education

• Advise patient that emergency ID as corticosteroid user should be carried or worn
• Advise patient to notify prescriber if therapeutic response decreases; dosage adjustment may be needed
• Caution patient not to discontinue abruptly; adrenal crisis can result
• Caution patient to avoid OTC products: salicylates, cough products with alcohol, cold preparations unless directed by prescriber
• Teach patient all aspects of product use including cushingoid symptoms
• Teach patient symptoms of adrenal insufficiency: nausea, anorexia, fatigue, dizziness, dyspnea, weakness, joint pain
• Teach patient to notify provider before surgery
• Inform patient that continuing blood work and follow ups will be needed

• Advise patient that long-term therapy may be needed to clear infection (1-2 mo depending on type of infection)
• Teach patient with diabetes that antidiabetic agents may need adjustment, blood glucose may increase
• **Pregnancy:** Teach patient to notify prescriber if pregnancy is planned or suspected; cleft palate, stillbirth, abortion reported

Evaluation

Positive therapeutic outcome
• Decreased inflammation

pregabalin (Rx)
(pre-gab'a-lin)
Lyrica
Func. class.: Anticonvulsant
Chem class.: gamma amminobytyric acid (GABA) analogue
Controlled substance schedule V

Do not confuse: Lyrica/Lapressor

ACTION: Binds to high-voltage–gated calcium channels in CNS tissues; this may lead to anticonvulsant action, similar to the inhibitory neurotransmitter GABA; anxiolytic, analgesic, and antiepileptic properties

Therapeutic outcome: Decreased seizure activity, decreased neuropathic pain

USES: Neuropathic pain associated with spinal cord injury, diabetic peripheral neuropathy, partial-onset seizures, postherpetic neuralgia, fibromyalgia

Pharmacokinetics

Absorption	Well absorbed
Distribution	Not bound to plasma proteins
Metabolism	Negligible
Excretion	90% unchanged, urine
Half-life	6 hr

Pharmacodynamics

Onset	Unknown
Peak	1.5 hr
Duration	Unknown

CONTRAINDICATIONS

Hypersensitivity to this product or gabapentin, abrupt discontinuation

Precautions: Pregnancy, breastfeeding, children <12 yr, geriatric, renal disease, PR interval prolongation, creatine kinase elevations, HF (class III, IV), decreased platelets, drug abuse, dependence, glaucoma, myopathy, angioedema history, suicidal behavior

DOSAGE AND ROUTES
Diabetic peripheral neuropathic pain
Adult: PO/oral sol 50 mg tid, may increase to 300 mg/day (max) within 1 wk, adjust in renal disease

Partial onset seizures
Adult: PO/oral sol 75 mg bid or 50 mg tid; may increase to 600 mg/day (max)

Postherpetic neuralgia
Adult: PO/oral sol 150 mg/day in 2-3 doses, may increase to 300 mg/day in 2-3 divided doses, if higher dose is needed in 2-4 wk, may increase to 600 mg/day in 2-3 divided doses

Fibromyalgia, spinal cord injury/pain
Adult: PO/oral sol 75 mg bid, may increase to 150 mg bid within 1 wk and 225 mg bid after 1 wk

Renal dose
PO CCr 30-60 ml/min 75-300 mg/day in 2-3 divided doses; CCr 15-30 ml/min 25-150 mg/day in 1-2 divided doses, CCr <15 ml/min 25-75 mg/day in a single dose

Available forms: Caps 25, 50, 75, 100, 150, 200, 225, 300 mg; oral sol 20 mg/ml

ADVERSE EFFECTS
CNS: *Drowsiness, dizziness,* abnormal thinking
EENT: *Dry mouth,* blurred vision, sinusitis
GI: Constipation, abdominal pain, weight gain, nausea, vomiting, increased appetite
HEMA: thrombocytopenia
MS: Back pain, rhabdomyolysis, myopathy
MISC: Pruritus, *peripheral edema,* angioedema, suicidal ideation, drowsiness

INTERACTIONS
Individual drugs
Alcohol: increased CNS depression
Pioglitazone, rosiglitazone: Increased fluid retention and weight gain

Drug classifications
ACE inhibitors: Increased risk of angioedema
Anxiolytics, barbiturates, general anesthetics, hypnotics, opiate agonists, phenothiazines, sedating H_1 blockers, sedatives, thiazolidinediones, tricyclics: increased CNS depression

Drug/lab test
Increased: creatine kinase
Decreased: platelets

NURSING CONSIDERATIONS
Assessment
• **Assess for seizures:** aura, location, duration, activity at onset, use seizure precaution
• **Assess for pain:** location, duration, characteristics if using for diabetic neuropathy, spinal cord injury, neuralgia
• Monitor renal function tests: urinalysis, BUN, urine creatinine q3mo, creatine kinase; if markedly increased, discontinue
• **Assess mental status:** mood, sensorium, affect, behavioral changes, suicidal thoughts, behavior; if mental status changes, notify prescriber
• **Angioedema/hypersensitivity:** monitor for blisters, hives, rash, dyspnea, wheezing; angioedema; if these occur, discontinue: cross-hypersensitivity with this product and gabapentin may occur
• **Rhabdomyolysis and creatinine kinase elevations (rare):** monitor for muscle pain, tenderness, weakness accompanied by malaise or fever; product should be discontinued
• Hemolytic anemia may be severe in Asian, Mediterranean individuals
• **Beers:** Avoid in older adults unless safer alternative is not available, may cause ataxia, impaired psychomotor function
• **Pregnancy/breastfeeding:** Use only if benefits outweigh fetal risk, may cause fetal toxicity; pregnant patients should enroll in the Antiepileptic Drug Pregnancy Registry (888-233-2334), do not breastfeed

Patient problem
Risk for Injury (uses, adverse reactions)
Pain (uses)

Implementation
• Do not crush or chew caps; caps may be opened and contents put in applesauce or dissolved in juice
• Give without regard to meals
• Gradually withdraw over 7 days; abrupt withdrawal may precipitate seizures
• Store at room temperature away from heat and light
• Give hard candy, frequent rinsing of mouth, gum for dry mouth
• Provide assistance with ambulation during early part of treatment; dizziness occurs
• Provide seizure precautions: padded side rails; move objects that may harm patient
• Provide increased fluids, bulk in diet for constipation
• **Oral sol:** should be written in mg and calculated to mL

Patient/family education
• Advise patient to carry emergency ID stating patient's name, products taken, condition, prescriber's name and phone number
• Advise patient to avoid driving, other activities that require alertness: dizziness, drowsiness may occur, those with seizures should obtain written notice that driving is acceptable
• Teach patient not to discontinue medication quickly after long-term use, taper over ≥1 wk; withdrawal-precipitated seizures may occur, not to double doses if dose is missed, take if 2 hr or more before next dose
• Teach patient to report muscle pain, tenderness, weakness, when accompanied by fever, malaise
• Advise patient to avoid alcohol, live virus vaccines
• Teach patient to notify prescriber if pregnancy is planned or suspected; avoid breastfeeding

Evaluation

Positive therapeutic outcome
• Decreased seizure activity; decrease in neuropathic pain

TREATMENT OF OVERDOSE:
Lavage, VS, hemodialysis

prochlorperazine (Rx)
(proe-klor-pair'a-zeen)
Compro, Prochlorazine ✽
Func. class.: Antiemetic/antipsychotic
Chem. class.: Phenothiazine, piperazine derivative

Do not confuse: prochlorperazine/chlorproMAZINE

ACTION: Decreases DOPamine neurotransmission by increasing DOPamine turnover through blockade of the D_2 somatodendritic autoreceptor in the meso-limbic system

Therapeutic outcome: Decreased nausea, vomiting, decreased signs and symptoms of psychosis

USES: Nausea, vomiting, psychosis

Pharmacokinetics

Absorption	Variably absorbed (PO); well absorbed (IM)
Distribution	Widely distributed, high concentration in CNS, crosses placenta
Metabolism	Liver, extensively; GI mucosa
Excretion	Kidneys, breast milk
Half-life	Unknown

Pharmacodynamics

	PO	PO-SUS REL	RECT	IM	IV
Onset	½ hr	Unkn	1 hr	10-20 min	4-5 min
Peak	Unkn	Unkn	Unkn	Unkn	Unkn
Duration	3-4 hr	10-12 hr	3-4 hr	4-6 hr; children: 12 hr	3-4 hr

CONTRAINDICATIONS
Hypersensitivity to phenothiazines, coma, infants/neonates/child <2 yr or <20 lb, surgery

Precautions: Pregnancy, breastfeeding, geriatric, seizure, encephalopathy, glaucoma, hepatic disease, Parkinson's disease, BPH

> **BLACK BOX WARNING:** Increased mortality in elderly patients with dementia-related psychosis

DOSAGE AND ROUTES
Postoperative nausea/vomiting
Adult: IM 5-10 mg 1-2 hr before anesthesia; may repeat in 30 min; **IV** 5-10 mg 15-30 min before anesthesia; **IV INF** 20 mg/L D_5W or 0.9% NaCl 15-30 min before anesthesia, max 40 mg/day

Severe nausea/vomiting
Adult: PO 5-10 mg tid-qid; SUS REL 15 mg/day in AM or 10 mg q12hr; RECT 25 mg/bid; IM 5-10 mg; may repeat q3-4hr prn, max 40 mg/day
Child 18-39 kg: PO 2.5 mg tid or 5 mg bid; IM 0.132 mg/kg, q3-4hr prn, max 15 mg/day
Child 14-17 kg: PO/RECT 2.5 mg bid-tid; IM 0.132 mg/kg, q3-4hr prn, max 10 mg/day
Child 9-13 kg: PO/RECT 2.5 mg daily-bid; IM 0.132 mg/kg, q3-4hr prn, max 7.5 mg/day

Antipsychotic
Adult and child ≥12 yr: PO 5-10 mg tid-qid; may increase q2-3day, max 150 mg/day; IM 10-20 mg q2-4hr up to 4 doses, then 10-20 mg q4-6hr, max 200 mg/day; RECT 10 mg tid-qid, may increase by 5-10 mg q2-3day as needed
Child 2-12 yr: PO 2.5 mg bid-tid; IM 0.132 mg/kg, change to oral ASAP

Antianxiety
Adult and child ≥12 yr: PO 5 mg tid-qid, max 20 mg/day or >12 wk; IM 5-10 mg q3-4hr, max 40 mg/day; **IV** 2.5-10 mg; max 40 mg/day
Child 2-12 yr: IM 0.132 mg/kg, change to oral ASAP

Available forms: tabs 5, 10 mg; supp 10 ✽, 25 mg; solution for injection 5 mg/ml

ADVERSE EFFECTS

CNS: Tardive dyskinesia, *euphoria,* depression, EPS, restlessness, tremor, dizziness, neuroleptic malignant syndrome, drowsiness, headache
CV: Tachycardia, hypotension, ECG changes
EENT: Blurred vision, dry eyes
GI: Nausea, vomiting, anorexia, dry mouth, diarrhea, constipation, weight loss, metallic taste, cramps
HEMA: Agranulocytosis
MISC: Impotence, color change of urine
RESP: Respiratory depression

INTERACTIONS
Individual drugs
Lithium: decreased prochlorperazine effect

Drug classifications
Antacids, barbiturates: decreased prochlorperazine effect
Anticholinergics, antidepressants, antiparkinson products: increased anticholinergic effects
SSRIs, SNRIs: increased serotonin syndrome, increased neuroleptic malignant syndrome
CNS depressants: increased CNS depression

Drug/herb
Chamomile, valerian, hops, kava: Increased CNS depressants
Dong quai: avoid use

Drug/lab test
Increased: liver function tests, cardiac enzymes, cholesterol, blood glucose, prolactin, bilirubin, PBI, ^{131}I, alkaline phosphatase, leukocytes, granulocytes, platelets
Decreased: hormones (blood and urine)
False positive: pregnancy tests, urine bilirubin
False negative: urinary steroids, 17-OHCS, pregnancy tests

NURSING CONSIDERATIONS
Assessment
• Assess mental status: orientation, mood, behavior, presence and type of hallucinations before initial administration and monthly; this product should significantly reduce psychotic behavior
• Check for swallowing of PO medication; check for hoarding or giving of medication to other patients
• Monitor I&O ratio; palpate bladder if low urinary output occurs, especially in geriatric; urinalysis recommended before, during prolonged therapy
• Monitor bilirubin, CBC, liver function tests monthly; blood dyscrasias, hepatotoxicity may occur

• Assess affect, orientation, LOC, reflexes, gait, coordination, sleep pattern disturbances
• Monitor B/P with patient sitting, standing, and lying; take pulse and respirations q4hr during initial treatment; establish baseline before starting treatment; report drops of 30 mm Hg; obtain baseline ECG, Q-wave and T-wave changes
• Check for dizziness, faintness, palpitations, tachycardia on rising; severe orthostatic hypotension is common
• **Identify neuroleptic malignant syndrome:** hyperpyrexia, muscle rigidity, increased CPK, altered mental status, seizures, fever, tachycardia, dyspnea, fatigue, loss of bladder control; notify prescriber immediately; product should be discontinued
• Assess for EPS including akathisia (inability to sit still, no pattern to movements), tardive dyskinesia (bizarre movements of the jaw, mouth, tongue, extremities), pseudoparkinsonism (ragged tremors, pill rolling, shuffling gait); an antiparkinsonism product should be prescribed
• Assess for constipation, urinary retention daily; if these occur, increase bulk, water in diet
• **Pregnancy/breastfeeding:** Use only if benefits outweigh fetal risk, EPS may result, cautious use in breastfeeding, excreted in breast milk
• **Beers:** Avoid in older adults with a high risk of delirium

Patient problem
Distorted thinking process (use)
Nausea (uses)

Implementation
IM route
• Inject slowly in deep muscle mass; do not give SUBCUT; aspirate to avoid **IV** administration; do not administer sol with a precipitate; have patient lie down afterward for at least 30 min

Direct IV route
• May give undiluted or dilution by slow IV, do not give as bolus
Intermittent IV infusion route
• May dilute 20 mg/L NaCl and give as inf 15-30 min prior to anesthesia induction
Continuous IV Infusion
• May give using 20 mg/L of compatible solution

Y-site compatibilities: Amsacrine, calcium gluconate, CISplatin, cladribine, cyclophosphamide, cytarabine, DOXOrubicin, fluconazole, granisetron, heparin, hydrocortisone, melphalan, methotrexate, ondansetron, PACLitaxel, potassium chloride, propofol, sargramostim, SUFentanil, teniposide, thiotepa, vinorelbine, vit B/C

Patient/family education
- Teach patient to use good oral hygiene; frequent rinsing of mouth, sugarless gum for dry mouth since oral candidiasis may occur
- Caution patient to avoid hazardous activities until product response is determined; dizziness, blurred vision may occur
- Inform patient that orthostatic hypotension occurs often and to rise from sitting or lying position gradually; to remain lying down after IM inj for at least 30 min; tell patient to avoid hot tubs, hot showers, tub baths, since hypotension may occur; tell patient that in hot weather heat stroke may occur; take extra precautions to stay cool
- Advise patient to avoid abrupt withdrawal of this product, or EPS may result; product should be withdrawn slowly
- Teach patient to avoid OTC preparations (cough, hay fever, cold) unless approved by prescriber, since serious product interactions may occur; avoid use with alcohol, CNS depressants; increased drowsiness may occur; avoid activities requiring mental alertness
- Instruct patient to avoid sun or use sunscreen, sunglasses, and protective clothing to prevent burns
- Advise patient to take antacids 2 hr before or after taking this product
- Advise patient to report sore throat, malaise, fever, bleeding, mouth sores; if these occur, CBC should be done and product discontinued
- Teach patient not to double or skip doses
- Inform patient that urine may turn pink to reddish brown
- Instruct patient to report dark urine, clay-colored stools, bleeding, bruising, rash, blurred vision
- Advise patient that suppositories may contain coconut/palm oil

Evaluation

Positive therapeutic outcome
- Relief of nausea and vomiting
- Decrease in emotional excitement, hallucinations, delusions, paranoia
- Reorganization of patterns of thought, speech

TREATMENT OF OVERDOSE:
Lavage if orally ingested; provide airway; *do not induce vomiting or use EPINEPHrine*

progesterone (Rx)
(proe-jess'ter-one)
Crinone, Endometrin, Prometrium, Utrogestran ✤
Func. class.: Hormone, Progestogen
Chem. class.: Progesterone derivative

ACTION. Inhibits secretion of pituitary gonadotropins, which prevents follicular maturation, ovulation; stimulates growth of mammary tissue; antineoplastic action against endometrial cancer

Therapeutic outcome: Decreased abnormal uterine bleeding, absence of amenorrhea

USES: Contraception, amenorrhea, premenstrual syndrome, abnormal uterine bleeding, endometrial hyperplasia prevention, assisted reproductive technology (ART) gel

Unlabeled uses: Corpus luteum insufficiency

Pharmacokinetics
Absorption	Unknown
Distribution	(protein binding 90%)
Metabolism	Liver 50%
Excretion	Breast milk kidneys
Half-life	A few minutes

Pharmacodynamics
	IM	RECT	VAG
Onset	Unknown	Unknown	Unknown
Peak	Unknown	Unknown	Unknown
Duration	24 hr	24 hr	24 hr

CONTRAINDICATIONS
Pregnancy, thromboembolic disorders, reproductive cancer, genital bleeding (abnormal, undiagnosed), cerebral hemorrhage, ectopic pregnancy, PID, STDs, thrombophlebitis, hypersensitivity to this product, peanuts, or peanut oil

BLACK BOX WARNING: Breast cancer

Precautions: Breastfeeding, hypertension, asthma, blood dyscrasias, gallbladder disease, HF, diabetes mellitus, bone disease, depression, migraine headache, seizure disorders, renal/hepatic disease, family history of breast or reproductive tract cancer

BLACK BOX WARNING: Cardiac disease, dementia

DOSAGE AND ROUTES
Secondary Amennorhea
Adult: PO 400 mg q day in PM × 10 days; Vaginal 45 mg (1 applicator 4% gel) every other day up to 6 days, may increase to 90 mg (1 applicator 8% gel every other day up to 6 days

Infertility
Adult: Vag 90 mg/day (micronized gel); 100 mg 2-3 times/day, starting day after oocyte retrieval and up to 10 wk total

Amenorrhea/functional uterine bleeding
Adult: IM 5-10 mg/day × 6-8 doses

Endometrial hyperplasia prevention
Adult: PO 200 mg/day × 14 days on days 8-21 (28 day cycle) or on days 12-25 (30 day cycle)

Assisted reproductive technology
Adult: GEL 90 mg (8%) vaginally daily, for supplementation; 90 mg (8%) vaginally bid for replacement; if pregnancy occurs, continue × 10-12 wk

Corpus luteum insufficiency (unlabeled)
Adult: VAG insert 90-100 mg bid-tid starting at oocyte retrieval and continuing up to 10-12 wk of gestation

Available forms: Caps 100, 200 mg; inj 50 mg/ml; powder micronized; vag gel 4%, 8%; vag insert 100 mg; supp 25, 100, 200, 500 mg, compounding kit 25, 50, 100, 200, 400 mg; oil for IM injection 50 mg/mL

ADVERSE EFFECTS
CNS: *Dizziness, headache,* depression, *fatigue,* mood swings
CV: Thrombophlebitis, thromboembolism, stroke, pulmonary embolism
EENT: Diplopia, retinal thrombosis
GI: *Nausea,* vomiting, anorexia, cramps, increased weight, cholestatic jaundice, *constipation,* abdominal pain
GU: Amenorrhea, cervical erosion, breakthrough bleeding, dysmenorrhea, nocturia, breast changes, *gynecomastia,* endometriosis, spontaneous abortion, breast pain, ectopic pregnancy
INTEG: Rash, urticaria, acne, hirsutism, alopecia, photosensitivity
META: Hyperglycemia
SYST: Angioedema, anaphylaxis

INTERACTIONS
Individual Drugs
Bromocriptine: Decreased effect

Drug/lab test
Increased: alkaline phosphatase, nitrogen (urine), pregnanediol, amino acids, factors VII, VIII, IX, X
Decreased: GTT, HDL

NURSING CONSIDERATIONS
Assessment
• Monitor B/P at beginning of treatment and periodically; check weight daily; notify prescriber of weekly weight gain >5 lb
• Monitor I&O ratio: be alert for decreasing urinary output, increasing edema, hypertension
• Assess liver function tests: ALT, AST, bilirubin baseline and periodically during long-term therapy
• Assess edema, hypertension, cardiac symptoms, jaundice
• **Amenorrhea:** Assess current and past menstrual history, use approximately 8 days before normal menstruation
• **Bleeding, dysfunctional:** Monitor pad count
• Assess mental status: affect, mood, behavioral changes, depression
• **Pregnancy/breastfeeding:** Do not use in pregnancy, breastfeeding

Patient problem
Impaired sexual functioning (uses)
Risk for Injury (adverse reactions)

Implementation
PO route
• Do not crush, break, chew caps, give one dose in AM
• With food or milk to decrease GI symptoms
• Start progesterone 14 days after estrogen dose, if given concomitantly
Vaginal route
• Wait at least 6 hr after any vaginal treatment before using vaginal gel, use applicator provided
IM route
• Give titrated dose; use lowest effective dosage; give oil sol deep in large muscle mass; rotate sites
• Check for particulate matter and discoloration prior to injecting

Patient/family education
• Teach patient to avoid activities requiring mental alertness until effects are realized; can cause dizziness
• Teach patient to report breast lumps, vaginal bleeding, edema, jaundice, dark urine, clay-colored stools, dyspnea, headache, blurred vision, abdominal pain, numbness or stiffness in legs, chest pain
• Inform patient follow up and testing will be needed

⚠ Nurse Alert   ✴ Key NCLEX® Drug   >> Drug Specifics

- Advise patient to notify providers of use of product
- Teach patient to use sunscreen, protective clothing to prevent photosensitivity
- Teach patient to report suspected pregnancy
- Teach patient to avoid gel with other vaginal products; if to be used together, to separate by 6 hr; for vaginal route, teach patient proper insertion technique

Evaluation

Positive therapeutic outcome
- Decreased abnormal uterine bleeding
- Absence of amenorrhea
- Prevented pregnancy

⚠ HIGH ALERT

promethazine (Rx)

(proe-meth′a-zeen)
Histamil ✱
Func. class.: Antihistamine, H₁-receptor antagonist; antiemetic; sedative/hypnotic
Chem. class.: Phenothiazine derivative

ACTION: Acts on blood vessels, GI, respiratory system by competing with histamine for H₁-receptor site; decreases allergic response by blocking histamine

Therapeutic outcome: Absence of allergy symptoms and rhinitis, absence of nausea/vomiting, sedation

USES: Motion sickness, rhinitis, allergy symptoms, sedation, nausea, preoperative and postoperative sedation

Pharmacokinetics

Absorption	Well absorbed (PO, IM); erratically absorbed (RECT)
Distribution	Widely distributed; crosses the blood-brain barrier, placenta
Metabolism	Liver
Excretion	Kidneys, breast milk
Half-life	10-16 hr

Pharmacodynamics

	PO/IM/RECT	IV
Onset	20 min	3-5 min
Peak	Unknown	Unknown
Duration	4-12 hr	4-6 hr

CONTRAINDICATIONS

Hypersensitivity to H₁-receptor antagonist, agranulocytosis, bone marrow suppression, breastfeeding, coma, jaundice, Reye's syndrome

BLACK BOX WARNING: Infants, intraarterial/SUBCUT use, neonates, children, extravasation

Precautions: Pregnancy, renal/cardiac/hepatic disease, asthma, seizure disorder, prostatic hypertrophy, bladder obstruction, glaucoma, COPD, GI obstruction, ileus, CNS depression, diabetes, sleep apnea, urinary retention

BLACK BOX WARNING: IV use, tissue necrosis

DOSAGE AND ROUTES
Nausea/vomiting
Adult: PO/IM/**IV**/RECT 12.5-25 mg; q4-6hr prn
Child >2 yr: PO/IM/**IV**/RECT 0.25-0.5 mg/kg q4-6hr prn

Motion sickness
Adult: PO 25 mg bid; give 30-60 min before departure and q8-12hr prn
Child >2 yr: PO/IM/RECT 12.5-25 mg bid; give 30-60 min before departure and q8-12hr prn

Allergy/rhinitis (unlabeled)
Adult: PO 12.5 mg qid, or 25 mg at bedtime
Child ≥2 yr: PO 6.25-12.5 mg tid or 25 mg at bedtime

Sedation
Adult: PO/IM 25-50 mg at bedtime
Child ≥2 yr: PO/IM/RECT 12.5-25 mg at bedtime

Sedation (preoperative/ postoperative)
Adult: PO/IM/**IV** 25-50 mg
Child ≥2 yr: PO/IM/**IV** 0.5-1.1 mg/kg

Available forms: Tabs 12.5, 25, 50 mg; supp 12.5, 25, 50 mg; inj 25, 50 mg/ml; oral solution 6.25, 10 mg/5mL

ADVERSE EFFECTS
CNS: *Dizziness, drowsiness,* poor coordination, fatigue, anxiety, euphoria, confusion, paresthesia, neuritis, EPS, neuroleptic malignant syndrome
CV: Hyper/hypotension, palpitations, tachycardia, orthostatic hypotension
EENT: Blurred vision, dilated pupils, tinnitus, nasal stuffiness, dry nose, throat, mouth, photosensitivity
GI: *Constipation,* dry mouth, nausea, vomiting, anorexia, diarrhea
GU: *Retention,* frequency
INTEG: Rash, urticaria, photosensitivity, tissue necrosis (infiltration IV site)

P

✱ Canada only　　　🏵 Genetic Warning　　　Adverse effects: *italics* = common; red = life-threatening

INTERACTIONS
Individual drugs
Alcohol: increased CNS depression
Heparin: decreased oral anticoagulants effect

Drug classifications
Antidepressants (tricyclics), barbiturates, CNS
depressants, opiates, sedative/hypnotics:
increased CNS depression
MAOIs: increased promethazine effect

Drug/lab test
Increase: glucose
False negative: skin allergy tests (discontinue
antihistamines 3 days before testing), urine
pregnancy test
False positive: urine pregnancy test
Interference: blood grouping (ABO), GTT

NURSING CONSIDERATIONS
Assessment

> **BLACK BOX WARNING: Child:** Not to be used
> in children <2 yr: fatal respiratory depression
> may occur; use cautiously in children >2 yr:
> seizures, paradoxical CNS stimulation may
> occur

- **Neuroleptic malignant syndrome:** assess
for fever, confusion, diaphoresis, rigid
muscles, elevated CPK, encephalopathy,
discontinue product, notify prescriber
- Monitor CBC during long-term therapy;
blood dyscrasias may occur but are rare
- **Respiratory depression/sedation:** Monitor for degree of sedation, respiratory rate, CNS
depressants may cause increased sedation
- **EPS:** Assess for pseudoparkinsonism, dystonia, akathisia, may be worse in geriatric patients
- **Anticholinergic effects:** monitor for dry
mouth, confusion, urinary retention, more common in geriatric patients
- Monitor cardiac status: VS, palpitations,
increased pulse, hypo/hypertension
- **Pregnancy/breastfeeding:** Use only if
benefits outweigh fetal risk, do not breastfeed

Patient problem
Nausea (uses)
Risk for injury (adverse reactions)

Implementation
PO route
- With meals for GI symptoms; absorption may
slightly decrease
- When used for motion sickness, 30 min-1 hr
before travel
IM route
- IM inj in deep in large muscle; rotate site,
necrosis may occur from Subcut injection, give
only IM

Direct IV route

> **BLACK BOX WARNING:** Check for extravasa-
> tion: burning, pain, swelling at **IV** site, can
> cause tissue necrosis

- Do not use if precipitate is present
- Rapid administration may cause transient
decrease in B/P
- After diluting each 25-50 mg/9 ml of NaCl for
inj; give 25 mg or less/2 min

Y-site compatibilities: alfentanil, amifostine, amikacin, aminocaproic acid, amsacrine,
anidulafungin, ascorbic acid, atenolol, atracurium, atropine, aztreonam, benztropine, bivalirudin, bleomycin, bumetanide, buprenorphine,
butorphanol, calcium chloride/gluconate, CAR-
BOplatin, caspofungin, chlorproMAZINE, cimetidine, ciprofloxacin, cisatracurium, CISplatin,
cladribine, codeine, cyanocobalamin, cyclophosphamide, cycloSPORINE, cytarabine,
DACTINomycin, DAPTOmycin, dexmedetomidine, digoxin, diltiazem, diphenhydrAMINE, DO-
BUTamine, DOCEtaxel, DOPamine, doxacurium,
DOXOrubicin, doxycycline, enalaprilat, ePHED-
rine, EPINEPHrine, epirubicin, epoetin, eptifibatide, erythromycin, esmolol, etoposide, famotidine, fenoldopam, fentaNYL, filgrastim,
fluconazole, fludarabine, gemcitabine, gentamicin, glycopyrrolate, granisetron, HYDROmorphone, hydrOXYzine, IDArubicin, ifosfamide, insulin (regular), irinotecan, isoproterenol,
labetalol, levofloxacin, lidocaine, linezolid, LORazepam, LR, magnesium sulfate, mannitol, mechlorethamine, melphalan, meperidine, metaraminol,
methoxamine, methyldopa, metoclopramide,
metoprolol, metroNIDAZOLE, miconazole, midazolam, milrinone, mitoXANtrone, morphine, mycophenolate, nalbuphine, naloxone, netilmicin,
nitroglycerin, norepinephrine, octreotide, ondansetron, oxaliplatin, oxytocin, PACLitaxel, palonosetron, pamidronate, pancuronium, PEMEtrexed,
pentamidine, pentazocine, phenylephrine, polymyxin B, procainamide, prochlorperazine, propranolol, protamine, pyridoxine, quiNIDine, quinupristin-dalfopristin, ranitidine, remifentanil,
Ringer's, ritodrine, riTUXimab, rocuronium, sargramostim, sodium acetate, succinylcholine, SUF-
entanil, tacrolimus, teniposide, theophylline, thiamine, thiotepa, tigecycline, tirofiban, TNA,
tobramycin, tolazoline, trastuzumab, trimethaphan,
vancomycin, vasopressin, vecuronium, verapamil,
vinCRIStine, vinorelbine, voriconazole

Patient/family education
- Inform patient that a false-negative result may
occur with skin testing; these procedures should
not be scheduled until 3 days after discontinuing
use

- Advise patient to take 30 min before departure to prevent motion sickness
- Caution patient to avoid hazardous activities, activities requiring alertness, since dizziness may occur; instruct patient to request assistance with ambulation
- Advise patient to use frequent sips of water, sugarless gum to minimize dry mouth
- Inform patient to change positions slowly to minimize orthostatic hypotension
- Advise patient to use sunscreen, protective clothing to prevent sun burns
- Teach patient to avoid driving, hazardous activities until reaction is known, dizziness may occur
- Advise patient to avoid alcohol, other depressants; serious CNS depression may occur
- Teach patient all aspects of product use; to notify prescriber if confusion, sedation, hypotension, jaundice, fever occur; to avoid driving and other hazardous activity if drowsiness occurs
- Advise patient to take 1 hr before or 2 hr after meals to facilitate absorption
- Caution patient not to exceed recommended dosage; dysrhythmias may occur
- Inform patient hard candy, gum, frequent rinsing of mouth may be used for dryness

Evaluation

Positive therapeutic outcome
- Absence of motion sickness
- Absence of nausea, vomiting

proparacaine ophthalmic
See Appendix B

A HIGH ALERT

propofol (Rx)
(pro'poh-fole)
Diprivan
Func. class.: General anesthetic

Do not confuse: Diprivan/Diflucan/Ditropan

ACTION: Produces dose-dependent CNS depression by activation of GABA receptor, hypnotic

Therapeutic outcome: Induction of anesthesia

USES: Induction or maintenance of anesthesia as part of balanced anesthetic technique; sedation in mechanically ventilated patients

Pharmacokinetics

Absorption	Completely absorbed
Distribution	Rapid
Metabolism	Liver, conjugation to active metabolites; 95%-99% protein binding, crosses placenta, enters breast milk, crosses blood brain barrier
Excretion	Urine
Half-life	3-12 hr

Pharmacodynamics

Onset	15-30 sec
Peak	Unknown
Duration	Unknown

CONTRAINDICATIONS
Hypersensitivity to product or soybean oil, egg, benzyl alcohol (some products)

Precautions: Pregnancy, breastfeeding, children, geriatric, respiratory depression, severe respiratory disorders, cardiac dysrhythmias, labor and delivery, renal disease, hyperlipidemia

DOSAGE AND ROUTES
General Anesthesia
Adult <55 yr: IV 40 mg q10sec until induction onset; **maintenance:** 100-200 mcg/kg/min or **IV BOL** 20-50 mg prn, allow 3-5 min between adjustments
Child ≥3 yr: IV Induction: 2.5-3.5 mg/kg over 20-30 sec when not premedicated or lightly premedicated
Child 2 mo-16 yr maintenance: IV 125-300 mcg/kg/min, lower dose for ASA III or IV

Monitored Anesthesia Care (MAC) sedation
Adult < 55 yr: IV 100-150 mcg/kg infusion or 0.5 mg/kg by slow infusion; maintenance 25-75 mcg/kg/min infusion or boluses of 10-20 mg; Geriatric, debilitated; ASA IA/IV: IV initial use slower rates; maintenance use 20% less than adult dose

ICU sedation
Adult: IV 5 mcg/kg/min over 5 min; may increase by 5-10 mcg/kg/min over 5-10 min until desired response (Diprivan or generic)

Available forms: Inj 10 mg/ml in 20 ml ampule, vials, syringes

ADVERSE EFFECTS

CNS: Involuntary movement, headache, fever, dizziness, shivering, euphoria, fatigue
CV: *Bradycardia, hypotension,* hypertension
GI: *Nausea, vomiting,* dry mouth, swallowing
GU: Urine retention, green urine
INTEG: *Flushing, phlebitis, hives, burning/ stinging at inj site,* rash
RESP: Apnea, *cough, hiccups*
SYST: Propofol infusion syndrome

INTERACTIONS
Individual drugs
Alcohol: increased CNS depression

Drug classifications
Antipsychotics, CNS depressants (sedative-hypnotics, opioid analgesics), inhalational anesthetics, skeletal muscle relaxants: increased CNS depression

Drug/herb
St. John's wort: increased propofol effect

NURSING CONSIDERATIONS
Assessment
• Assess inj site: phlebitis, burning, stinging
• **Monitor ECG for changes:** PVC, PAC, ST segment changes; monitor VS (B/P, pulse, respirations)
• Assess CNS changes: movement, jerking, tremors, dizziness, LOC, pupil reaction
• Avoid general anesthetic use in child <3 yr, may negatively affect the brain
• Assess allergic reactions: hives
• **Assess respiratory dysfunction:** respiratory depression, character, rate, rhythm; notify prescriber if respirations are <10/min, apnea may occur ≥ 1 min, check airway ventilation, determine level of sedation
• **ICU Sedation:** Test wake up on daily basis to determine needed dose for sedation; do not discontinue abruptly during test
• **Propofol infusion syndrome:** assess for rhabdomyolysis, renal failure, hyperkalemia, metabolic acidosis, cardiac dysrhythmias, heart failure, usually between 35 and 93 hr after inf began, at >5 mg/kg/hr for >58 hr

Patient problem
Impaired breathing (adverse reactions)
Risk of Injury (adverse reactions)

Implementation
IV route
• Shake well before use; dilution is not necessary but if diluted, use only D_5W to ≥2 mg/ml; give over 3-5 min, titrate to needed level of sedation; use only glass containers when mixing, not stable in plastic; use aseptic technique when transferring from original container
• Only with resuscitative equipment available, only by qualified persons trained in anesthesia

Y-site compatibilities: Acyclovir, alfentanil, aminophylline, ampicillin, aztreonam, bumetanide, buprenorphine, butorphanol, calcium gluconate, CARBOplatin, ceFAZolin, cefoperazone, cefotaxime, cefoTEtan, cefOXitin, ceftizoxime, cefTRIAXone, cefuroxime, chlorproMAZINE, cimetidine, CISplatin, clindamycin, cyclophosphamide, cycloSPORINE, cytarabine, dexamethasone, diphenhydrAMINE, DOBUTamine, DOPamine, doxycycline, droperidol, enalaprilat, ePHEDrine, EPINEPHrine, esmolol, famotidine, fentaNYL, fluconazole, fluorouracil, furosemide, ganciclovir, glycopyrrolate, granisetron, haloperidol, heparin, hydrocortisone, HYDROmorphone, hydrOXYzine, ifosfamide, imipenem/cilastatin, inamrinone, regular insulin, isoproterenol, ketamine, labetalol, levorphanol, lidocaine, LORazepam, magnesium sulfate, mannitol, meperidine, mezlocillin, miconazole, morphine, nafcillin, nalbuphine, naloxone, nitroglycerin, norepinephrine, ofloxacin, PACLitaxel, PENTobarbital, PHENobarbital, piperacillin, potassium chloride, prochlorperazine, propranolol, ranitidine, scopolamine, sodium bicarbonate, sodium nitroprusside, succinylcholine, SUFentanil, thiopental, ticarcillin, ticarcillin/clavulanate, vecuronium, verapamil

Solution compatibilities: (If given together via Y-site) D_5W, D_5LR, LR, D_5/0.45% NaCl, D_5/0.2% NaCl

Patient/family education
• Teach patient that this medication will cause dizziness, drowsiness, sedation; to avoid hazardous activities until drug effect wears off, may cause burning sensation during administration
• Advise patient to avoid CNS depressants following use and for 24 hrs

Evaluation
Positive therapeutic outcome
• Induction of anesthesia
• Sedation in ICU

TREATMENT OF OVERDOSE:
Discontinue product; administer vasopressor agents or anticholinergics, artificial ventilation

⚠ HIGH ALERT

propranolol (Rx)

(proe-pran´oh-lole)

Hemanegeol, Inderal LA, InnoPran XL

Func. class.: Antihypertensive, antianginal, antidysrhythmic (class III)

Chem. class.: β-Adrenergic blocker

Do not confuse: propranolol/Pravachol

ACTION: Nonselective β-blocker with negative inotropic, chronotropic, dromotropic properties

Therapeutic outcome: Decreased B/P, heart rate

USES: Chronic stable angina pectoris, hypertension, supraventricular dysrhythmias, migraine prophylaxis, pheochromocytoma, cyanotic spells related to hypertrophic subaortic stenosis, essential tremor, acute MI, vascular headache prophylaxis

Unlabeled uses: Prevention of variceal bleeding caused by portal hypertension, akathisia induced by antipsychotics, lithium-induced tremor, attenuation of hypermetabolism in severe burns

Pharmacokinetics

Absorption	Well absorbed (PO); slowly absorbed (ext rel); completely absorbed (**IV**)
Distribution	Widely distributed, crosses blood-brain barrier, protein binding 90%
Metabolism	Liver, extensively by CYP2D6 enzyme system, ⟋⟍ 7% of population are poor metabolizers
Excretion	Kidneys
Half-life	3-8 hr; ext rel 8-11 hr

Pharmacodynamics

	PO	PO-EXT REL	IV
Onset	½ hr	Unknown	Rapid
Peak	1-1½ hr	6 hr	1 min
Duration	6-12 hr	24 hr	2-4 hr

CONTRAINDICATIONS

Hypersensitivity to this product, cardiogenic shock, AV heart block, bronchospastic disease, sinus bradycardia, bronchospasm, asthma

Precautions: Pregnancy, breastfeeding, children, diabetes mellitus, renal/hepatic disease, hyperthyroidism, COPD, myasthenia gravis, peripheral vascular disease, hypotension, cardiac failure, Raynaud's disease, sick sinus syndrome, vasospastic angina, smoking, Wolff-Parkinson-White syndrome, thyrotoxicosis

BLACK BOX WARNING: Abrupt discontinuation

DOSAGE AND ROUTES

Dysrhythmias

Adult: PO 10-30 mg tid-qid; **IV** BOL 1-3 mg given 1 mg/min; may repeat in 2 min; may repeat q4hr thereafter

Child: PO 1 mg/kg/day divided in 2 doses, **IV** 0.01-0.1 mg/kg over 5 min

Hypertension

Adult: PO 40 mg bid or 80 mg/day (EXT REL) initially; usual dosage 120-240 mg/day bid-tid or 120-160 mg/day (EXT REL)

Child: PO 0.5-1 mg/kg/day divided q6-12hr

Angina

Adult: PO 10-20 mg bid-qid, increase at 3-7 day intervals up to 160-320 mg/day, or ext rel 80 mg/day, increase at 3-7 day intervals up to 160-320 mg/day

MI prophylaxis

Adult: PO 180-240 mg/day tid-qid starting 5 days to 2 wk after MI

Pheochromocytoma

Adult: PO 60 mg/day × 3 days preoperatively in divided doses or 30 mg/day in divided doses (inoperable tumor)

Migraine

Adult: PO 80 mg/day (EXT REL) or in divided doses; may increase to 160-240 mg/day in divided doses

Child: PO 0.6-1.5 mg/kg/day divided q8hr

Child ≤35 kg (unlabeled): PO 10-20 mg tid

Essential tremor

Adult: PO 40 mg bid; usual dosage 120 mg/day

Available forms: Ext rel caps 60, 80, 120, 160 mg; tabs 10, 20, 40, 60, 80 mg; inj 1 mg/ml; oral solution 20 mg, 40 mg/5 mL; oral solution (Hemanegeol) 4.28 mg/mL

ADVERSE EFFECTS

CNS: Depression, hallucinations, *dizziness, fatigue,* lethargy, paresthesia, bizarre dreams, disorientation

CV: Bradycardia, *hypotension,* HF, palpitations, AV block, peripheral vascular insufficiency, vasodilatation, pulmonary edema, dysrhythmias, cold extremities

P

EENT: Sore throat, laryngospasm, blurred vision, dry eyes

GI: Nausea, vomiting, diarrhea, colitis, constipation, cramps, dry mouth, hepatomegaly, gastric pain, acute pancreatitis

GU: Impotence, decreased libido, UTIs

HEMA: Agranulocytosis, thrombocytopenia

INTEG: Rash, pruritus, fever, Stevens-Johnson syndrome, toxic epidermal necrolysis

META: Hyperglycemia, hypoglycemia

MISC: Facial swelling, weight change, Raynaud's phenomenon

MS: Joint pain, arthralgia, muscle cramps, pain

RESP: Dyspnea, respiratory dysfunction, bronchospasm, cough

INTERACTIONS
Individual drugs
Cimetidine: increased β-blocking effect

Disopyramide: increased negative inotropic effects

Haloperidol, prazosin, quiNIDine: increased hypotension

Propafenone: increased propranolol levels

Smoking: decreased propranolol levels

Drug classifications
Barbiturates: decreased β-blocking effect

Calcium channel blockers, neuromuscular blockers: increased effects

Phenothiazines: increased toxicity

Drug/herb
Hawthorn: increased antihypertensive effect

Avoid use with feverfew, ma huang: decreased antihypertensive effect

Drug/lab test
Increased: serum potassium, serum uric acid, AST, ALT, alkaline phosphatase, LDH

Decreased: blood glucose

Interference: glaucoma testing

NURSING CONSIDERATIONS
Assessment
• Monitor B/P during beginning treatment, periodically thereafter; pulse; note rate, rhythm, quality; check apical/radial pulse before administration; notify prescriber of any significant changes (pulse <50 bpm or systolic B/P <90 mm Hg)

> **BLACK BOX WARNING: Abrupt withdrawal:** taper over 1-2 weeks; do not discontinue abruptly; dysrhythmias, angina, myocardial ischemia, or MI may recur

• Monitor ECG continuously if using an antidysrhythmic IV, PCWP (pulmonary capillary wedge pressure), CVP (central venous pressure)

• Assess for edema in feet, legs daily; monitor; check for jugular vein distention, crackles bilaterally; dyspnea (HF)

• Monitor skin turgor, dryness of mucous membranes for hydration status, especially geriatric

• Assess for headache, light-headedness, decreased B/P; may indicate need for decreased dose; may aggravate symptoms of arterial insufficiency

• **Headache:** Assess for frequency, characteristics, aggravating factors

• **Stevens Johnson Syndrome:** Monitor for rash, fever, blisters, fatigue, report to health care professional immediately

• Monitor hepatic enzymes: AST, ALT, bilirubin; blood glucose (diabetes mellitus)

• **Angina pain:** Assess duration, time started, activity being performed, character

• Assess for tolerance with long-term use

• Fluid overload: Monitor weight daily; report gain of >5 lb

• Monitor I&O ratio, CCr if kidney damage is diagnosed; fatigue, weight gain, jugular distention, dyspnea, peripheral edema, crackles

• **Pregnancy/breastfeeding:** Use only if benefits outweigh fetal risk, cautious use in breastfeeding

Patient problem
Impaired cardiac output (adverse reactions)

Risk for injury (adverse reactions)

Nonadherence (teaching)

Implementation
PO route
• Do not break, crush, chew, or open ext rel cap

• Do not use ext rel cap for essential tremor, MI, cardiac dysrhythmias; do not use InnoPran XL in hypertropic subaortic stenosis, migraine, angina pectoris

• Ext rel caps should be taken daily; InnoPran XL should be taken at bedtime

• May mix oral sol with liquid or semisolid food; rinse container to get entire dose

• Give with 8 oz water with food; food enhances bioavailability

• Do not give with aluminum-containing antacid; may decrease GI absorption

Direct IV route
• IV undiluted or diluted 10 ml D₅W for inj; give 0.5 mg or less/min (adult); give over 10 min (child)

Intermittent IV infusion route
• May be diluted in 50 ml NaCl and run 1 mg over 10-15 min

Y-site compatibilities: Acyclovir, alfentanil, alteplase, amikacin, aminocaproic acid, aminophylline, anidulafungin, ascorbic acid, atracurium, atropine, azaTHIOprine, aztreonam, benztropine, bivalirudin, bleomycin, bumetanide, buprenorphine, butorphanol, calcium chloride/gluconate, CARBOplatin, caspofungin, cefamandole, ceFAZolin, cefmetazole, cefonicid, cefoperazone, cefotaxime, cefoTEtan, cefOXitin, cefTAZidime, ceftizoxime, cefTRIAXone, cefuroxime, cephalothin, cephapirin, chloramphenicol, chlorproMAZINE, cimetidine, CISplatin, clindamycin, cyanocobalamin, cyclophosphamide, cycloSPORINE, cytarabine, DACTINomycin, DAPTOmycin, dexamethasone, digoxin, diltiazem, diphenhydrAMINE, DOBUTamine, DOCEtaxel, DOPamine, doxacurium, DOXOrubicin, doxycycline, enalaprilat, ePHEDrine, EPINEPHrine, epirubicin, epoetin alfa, eptifibatide, ertapenem, erythromycin, esmolol, etoposide, etoposide phosphate, famotidine, fenoldopam, fentaNYL, fluconazole, fludarabine, fluorouracil, folic acid, furosemide, ganciclovir, gatifloxacin, gemcitabine, gemtuzumab, gentamicin, glycopyrrolate, granisetron, heparin, hydrocortisone, HYDROmorphone, hydrOXYzine, IDArubicin, ifosfamide, imipenem-cilastatin, inamrinone, irinotecan, isoproterenol, ketorolac, labetalol, levofloxacin, lidocaine, linezolid, LORazepam, magnesium, mannitol, mechlorethamine, meperidine, metaraminol, methicillin, methotrexate, methoxamine, methyldopate, methylPREDNISolone, metoclopramide, metoprolol, metroNIDAZOLE, mezlocillin, miconazole, midazolam, milrinone, minocycline, mitoXANtrone, morphine, moxalactam, multiple vitamins, mycophenolate, nafcillin, nalbuphine, naloxone, nesiritide, netilmicin, nitroglycerin, nitroprusside, norepinephrine, octreotide, ondansetron, oxacillin, oxaliplatin, oxytocin, palonosetron, pamidronate, pancuronium, papaverine, PEMEtrexed, penicillin G potassium/sodium, pentamidine, pentazocine, PENTobarbital, PHENobarbital, phenylephrine, phytonadione, piperacillin, polymyxin B, potassium chloride, procainamide, prochlorperazine, promethazine, propofol, protamine, pyridoxine, quiNIDine, quinupristin-dalfopristin, ranitidine, ritodrine, rocuronium, sodium acetate/bicarbonate, succinylcholine, SUFentanil, tacrolimus, teniposide, theophylline, thiamine, thiotepa, ticarcillin, ticarcillin-clavulanate, tigecycline, tirofiban, tobramycin, tolazoline, trimetaphan, urokinase, vancomycin, vasopressin, vecuronium, verapamil, vinCRIStine, vinorelbine, vitamin B complex/C, voriconazole, zoledronic acid

Patient/family education

• Teach patient not to discontinue product abruptly (life-threatening dysrhythmias, exacerbation of angina, MI); to take at same time of day either with or without food consistently; taper over at least a few wk
• Teach patient not to use OTC products containing α-adrenergic stimulants (such as nasal decongestants, cold preparations); to avoid alcohol, smoking and to limit sodium intake as prescribed; blood glucose (diabetes mellitus)
• **Diabetes:** Teach patient to monitor glucose closely; glucose levels may be increased or decreased to monitor for hypo/hyperglycemic reactions
• Instruct patient to comply with weight control, dietary adjustments, modified exercise program
• Instruct patient to carry/wear emergency ID to identify product being taken, allergies; tell patient product controls symptoms but does not cure
• Caution patient to avoid hazardous activities if dizziness, drowsiness are present
• **Teach patient to report symptoms of HF:** difficulty breathing, especially on exertion or when lying down, night cough, swelling of extremities or bradycardia, dizziness, confusion, depression, fever
• Advise patient that sensitivity to cold may occur
• Teach patient to monitor blood glucose; may mask symptoms of hypoglycemia
• Teach patient how to take pulse, B/P; withhold if <50 bpm or systolic B/P <90 mm Hg
• Teach patient to rise slowly to prevent orthostatic hypotension

Evaluation

Positive therapeutic outcome
• Decreased B/P in hypertension (after 1-2 wk)
• Decreased tremors
• Absence of dysrhythmias
• Decreased migraine headaches

TREATMENT OF OVERDOSE:
Lavage, **IV** atropine for bradycardia, **IV** theophylline for bronchospasm, digoxin, O_2, diuretic for cardiac failure, hemodialysis, **IV** glucose for hyperglycemia, **IV** diazepam (or phenytoin) for seizures

⚠ HIGH ALERT

propylthiouracil (Rx)

(proe-pill-thye-oh-yoor′a-sill)

Propyl-Thyracil ✤

Func. class.: Thyroid hormone antagonist (antithyroid)

Chem. class.: Thioamide

Do not confuse: propylthioracil/thiouracil

ACTION: Blocks synthesis peripherally of T_3, T_4, inhibits organification of iodine

Therapeutic outcome: Decreased T_3, T_4 levels, hyperthyroid symptoms

USES: Preparation for thyroidectomy, thyrotoxic crisis, hyperthyroidism, thyroid storm

Pharmacokinetics

Absorption	Rapidly absorbed
Distribution	Crosses placenta, concentration in thyroid gland
Metabolism	Liver
Excretion	Urine, bile, breast milk
Half-life	1-2 hr

Pharmacodynamics

Onset	30-40 min
Peak	Unknown
Duration	2-4 hr

CONTRAINDICATIONS

Pregnancy, breastfeeding, hypersensitivity

Precautions: Infection, bone marrow depression, hepatic disease, fever, agranulocytosis, hepatitis, jaundice

BLACK BOX WARNING: Hepatic disease

DOSAGE AND ROUTES

Thyrotoxic crisis

Adult and child: PO 200-400 mg q4h for 1st 24 hr

Preparation for thyroidectomy

Adult: PO 600-1200 mg/day

Child: PO 10 mg/kg/day in divided doses

Hyperthyroidism

Adult: PO 100 mg tid increasing to 300 mg q8hr if condition is severe; continue to euthyroid state, then 100 mg daily-tid

Child >6 yr: PO 50 mg/day divided doses q8hr, titrate based on TSH/free T_4 levels

Neonate (unlabeled): PO 10 mg/kg/day in divided doses

Available forms: Tabs 50, 100 ✤ mg

ADVERSE EFFECTS

CNS: *Drowsiness, headache, vertigo, fever,* paresthesias, neuritis

GI: *Nausea, diarrhea, vomiting,* jaundice, hepatitis, loss of taste, liver failure, death

GU: Nephritis

HEMA: Agranulocytosis, leukopenia, thrombocytopenia, hypothrombinemia, lymphadenopathy, bleeding, vasculitis, periarteritis

INTEG: *Rash, urticaria, pruritus, alopecia, hyperpigmentation,* lupuslike syndrome

MS: Myalgia, arthralgia, nocturnal muscle cramps, osteoporosis

INTERACTIONS

Individual drugs

Heparin: decreased anticoagulant effect

Lithium: increased antithyroid effect

Potassium/sodium iodide: increased effects

Radiation: increased bone marrow depression

Drug classifications

Anticoagulants (oral): decreased anticoagulant effect

Antineoplastics: increased bone marrow depression

Phenothiazines: increased agranulocytosis

Drug/lab test

Increased: pro-time, AST, ALT, alkaline phosphatase

NURSING CONSIDERATIONS

Assessment

• Monitor pulse, B/P, temp; I&O ratio; check for edema (puffy hands, feet, periorbits); indicates hypothyroidism

• Check weight daily with same clothing, scale, time of day

• **Hyperthyroidism:** monitor for weight loss, nervousness, insomnia, fever, diaphoresis, tremors; monitor clinical response: after 3 wk should include increased weight, decreased pulse, decreased T_4

• **Hypothyroidism:** monitor for constipation, dry skin, weakness, headache

• Monitor T_3, T_4, which are increased; check serum TSH, which is decreased; assess free thyroxine index, which is increased if dosage is too low; discontinue product 3-4 wk before radioactive iodine uptake test

• **Blood dyscrasias:** Monitor CBC with differential; leukopenia, thrombocytopenia, agranulocytosis, monitor periodically; agranulocytosis may develop in first 2 mo of treatment, discontinue treatment

• **Overdose:** Assess for peripheral edema, heat intolerance, diaphoresis, palpitations, dysrhythmias, severe tachycardia, increased temp, delirium, CNS irritability

- **Hypersensitivity:** Assess for rash, enlarged cervical lymph nodes; product may have to be discontinued
- **Hypoprothrombinemia:** assess for bleeding, petechiae, ecchymosis
- **Bone marrow depression:** assess for sore throat, fever, fatigue

> **BLACK BOX WARNING: Hepatotoxicity:** monitor LFTs before and during treatment; jaundice, nausea, vomiting, abdominal pain, anorexia, diarrhea, fatigue

- **Pregnancy/benefits:** Do not use in pregnancy, breastfeeding

Patient problem
Risk of Injury (uses)
Nonadherence (teaching)
Lack of knowledge of medication (teaching)

Implementation
- Give with meals to decrease GI upset
- Give at same time each day to maintain product level
- Give lowest dosage that relieves symptoms
- Store in light-resistant container

Patient/family education
- Teach patient to take pulse daily and to keep graph of weight, pulse, mood
- Advise patient to report redness, swelling, sore throat, mouth lesions, which indicate blood dyscrasias (yellow skin/eyes, clay-colored stools, dark urine)
- Caution patient to avoid OTC products that contain iodine; that seafood, other iodine-containing foods may be restricted by prescriber
- Teach patient that response may take several mo if thyroid is large
- **Teach patient symptoms/signs of overdose:** periorbital edema, cold intolerance, mental depression; notify prescriber at once
- Teach patient symptoms of inadequate dose: tachycardia, diarrhea, fever, irritability; prescriber should be notified to adjust dosage
- Teach patient follow ups and lab work will be needed
- Teach patient to take medication exactly as prescribed, not to skip or double doses; missed doses should be taken when remembered up to 1 hr before next dose
- Instruct patient to carry/wear emergency identification indicating medication taken and condition being treated
- **Pregnancy:** Notify prescriber immediately if pregnancy is planned or suspected, do not breastfeed

Evaluation
Positive therapeutic outcome
- Weight gain
- Decreased pulse
- Decreased T$_4$
- Decreased B/P

protamine (Rx)
(proe′ta-meen)
Func. class.: Heparin antagonist
Chem. class.: Low-molecular-weight protein

Do not confuse: Protamine/Protonix

ACTION: Binds heparin, making it ineffective

Therapeutic outcome: Prevention of heparin overdose

USES: Heparin overdose; neutralizes heparin in procedures, hemorrhage

Pharmacokinetics
Absorption	Completely absorbed
Distribution	Unknown
Metabolism	Degrades
Excretion	Unknown
Half-life	Unknown

Pharmacodynamics
Onset	1 min
Peak	Unknown
Duration	2 hr

CONTRAINDICATION
> **BLACK BOX WARNING:** Hypersensitivity

Precautions: Pregnancy, breastfeeding, fish allergy, diabetes, previous exposure to protamine, insulins, heparin rebound or bleeding

> **BLACK BOX WARNING:** Requires a specialized care setting

DOSAGE AND ROUTES
Heparin overdose
Adult and child: IV 1 mg of protamine/100 units of heparin given; administer slowly over 1-3 min; max 50 mg/10 min

Enoxaparin overdose
Adult: IV 1 mg of protamine/1 mg enoxaparin

Dalteparin/overdose
Adult: IV 1 mg of protamine/100 anti-Xa unit

Available forms: Inj 10 mg/ml

ADVERSE EFFECTS

CV: Hypotension, bradycardia, circulatory collapse, capillary leak
GI: Nausea, vomiting
HEMA: Bleeding
INTEG: *Rash,* dermatitis, urticaria
RESP: Dyspnea, pulmonary edema, severe respiratory distress, bronchospasm
SYST: Anaphylaxis, angioedema

NURSING CONSIDERATIONS
Assessment
• Monitor blood studies (Hct, platelets, occult blood stools) q3mo
• Monitor coagulation tests (aPTT, ACT) 15 min after dose, then in several hr
• Monitor VS, B/P, pulse q30min, plus 3 hr after dose
• **Bleeding:** Assess for bleeding 30 min-18 hrs after dose in cardiac surgery

> **BLACK BOX WARNING: Assess for hypersensitivity:** skin rash, urticaria, dermatitis, cough, wheezing, have emergency equipment nearby; men who have had a vasectomy may be more prone to hypersensitivity, fish hypersensitivity, also in higher doses

• Assess for allergy to salmon; use with caution in these patients

Patient problem
Ineffective tissue perfusion (uses)
Risk for injury (adverse reactions)

Implementation
Direct IV route
• May give undiluted or diluted
• After reconstituting 50 mg/5 ml sterile bacteriostatic water for inj, shake; give 20 mg or less over 1-3 min, do not give rapidly

Y-site compatibilities: Alfentanil, amikacin, aminophylline, ascorbic acid, atracurium, atropine, azaTHIOprine, aztreonam, benztropine, bumetanide, buprenorphine, butorphanol, calcium chloride/gluconate, ceftazidime, chlorproMAZINE, cimetidine, clindamycin, cyanocobalamin, cycloSPORINE, digoxin, diphenhydrAMINE, DOBUTamine, DOPamine, doxycycline, enalaprilat, ePHEDrine, EPINEPHrine, epoetin alfa, erythromycin, esmolol, famotidine, fentaNYL, fluconazole, ganciclovir, gentamicin, glycopyrrolate, hydrOXYzine, imipenem-cilastatin, inamrinone, iohexol, iopamidol, iothalamate, isoproterenol, labetalol, lidocaine, magnesium, mannitol, meperidine, metaraminol, methoxamine, methyldopate, metoclopramide, metoprolol, miconazole, midazolam, minocycline, morphine, multiple vitamins, nalbuphine, naloxone, netilmicin, nitroglycerin, nitroprusside, norepinephrine, ondansetron, oxytocin, papaverine, pentazocine, phenylephrine, polymyxin B, potassium chloride, procainamide, prochlorperazine, promethazine, propranolol, pyridoxine, quiNIDine, ranitidine, Ringer's, ritodrine, sodium bicarbonate, succinylcholine, SUFentanil, theophylline, thiamine, tobramycin, tolazoline, trimetaphan, urokinase, vancomycin, vasopressin, verapamil

Patient/family education
• Explain reason for medication and expected results; not to take if allergic to fish
• Caution patient to avoid contact activities that may result in bleeding
• Inform the patient about the purpose of product, expected result
• Teach patient to avoid activities where bleeding may occur such as shaving, use of hard bristle toothbrush, injections, rectal temperatures, until risk of bleeding has past

Evaluation
Positive therapeutic outcome
• Reversal of heparin overdose

pseudoephedrine (OTC)
(soo-doe-e-fed'rin)
Eltor ✦, Nasofed, Sudafed, Sudafed 24 hour, Sudogest
Func. class.: Adrenergic
Chem. class.: Substituted phenylethylamine
Controlled Substance V

Do not confuse: Sudafed/Sotalol

ACTION: Primary activity through α-adrenergic effects on respiratory mucosal membranes reducing congestion, hyperemia, edema; minimal bronchodilatation secondary to β-adrenergic effects

Therapeutic outcome: Decreased nasal congestion, swelling

USES: Nasal decongestant, otitis media adjunct, adjunct with antihistamines

Pharmacokinetics
Absorption	Well absorbed
Distribution	Enters CSF, crosses placenta
Metabolism	Liver, partially
Excretion	Kidneys, unchanged (75%); breast milk
Half-life	7 hr (adult), 3 hr (child)

Pharmacodynamics		
	PO	**PO-EXT REL**
Onset	15-30 min	1 hr
Peak	Unknown	Unknown
Duration	4-6 hr	12 hr

CONTRAINDICATIONS
Hypersensitivity to sympathomimetics, closed-angle glaucoma

Precautions: Pregnancy, breastfeeding, cardiac disorders, hyperthyroidism, diabetes mellitus, prostatic hypertrophy, hypertension, child < 4 yr

DOSAGE AND ROUTES
Adult and child >12 yr: PO 60 mg q6hr; EXT REL 120 mg q12hr or 240 mg q24hr
Geriatric: PO 30-60 mg q6hr prn
Child 6-12 yr: PO 30 mg q6hr, max 120 mg/day
Child 4-6 yr: PO 15 mg q6hr, max 60 mg/day

Available forms: Ext rel caps 120, 240 mg; oral sol 15 mg, 30 mg/5 ml; tabs 30, 60 mg; ext rel tabs 120, 240 mg

ADVERSE EFFECTS
CNS: *Tremors, anxiety,* stimulation, insomnia, headache, dizziness, hallucinations, seizures (geriatric)
CV: Palpitations, tachycardia, hypertension, chest pain, dysrhythmias, CV collapse
EENT: Dry nose, irritation of nose and throat
GI: *Anorexia, nausea, vomiting,* dry mouth, ischemic colitis
GU: Dysuria

INTERACTIONS
Drug classifications
Antidepressants (tricyclics), MAOIs: hypertensive crisis, do not use together
Urinary acidifiers: decreased effect of pseudoephedrine
Urinary alkalizers, adrenergics, β-blockers, phenothiazines, tricyclics: increased effect of pseudoephedrine

NURSING CONSIDERATIONS
Assessment
• Monitor for nasal congestion; auscultate lung sounds; check for tenacious bronchial secretions; children with otitis media should be assessed for eustachian tube congestion
• Monitor B/P and pulse baseline and throughout treatment
• **Beers:** Avoid in older adults, CNS stimulant effects, seizures, hallucinations, excitation

Patient problem
Impaired airway clearance (uses)

Implementation
• Swallow tab and ext rel cap whole; do not break, crush, or chew
• Avoid taking at or near bedtime if insomnia occurs
• Store at room temperature
• OTC preparations require an ID, tracked, Schedule V

Patient/family education
• Teach patient reason for product administration and expected results
• Instruct patient not to use continuously or for longer then 7 days if symptoms do not improve or fever occurs, or more than recommended dose; rebound congestion may occur
• Advise patient to check with prescriber before using other products, as product interactions may occur
• Advise patient to avoid taking near bedtime; stimulation can occur
• Caution patient not to use if stimulation, restlessness, tremors occur
• Notify parents of possible excessive agitation in children, not to use in child < 4 yr
• Advise patient to notify prescriber of anxiety, slow or fast heart rate, dyspnea, seizures
• Ext rel: do not divide, crush, chew, or dissolve
• Do not use within 14 days of MAOIs

Evaluation
Positive therapeutic outcome
• Decreased nasal, eustachian tube congestion

---

pyrazinamide (Rx)
(peer-a-zin´-a-mide)
Tebrazid
Func. class.: Antitubercular agent
Chem. class.: Pyrazinoic acid amine/nicoturimide analog

ACTION: Bactericidal interference with lipid; nucleic acid biosynthesis is possible

Therapeutic outcome: Bactericidal for *Mycobacterium* species

USES: Tuberculosis, as an adjunct when other products are not feasible

Pharmacokinetics	
Absorption	Well absorbed
Distribution	Widely distributed
Metabolism	Liver, extensively
Excretion	Kidneys, breast milk
Half-life	9-10 hr

Pharmacodynamics

Onset	Unknown
Peak	2 hr
Duration	9 1/2 hr; metabolites 12 hr

CONTRAINDICATIONS: Hypersensitivity, severe hepatic damage, acute gout

Precautions: Pregnancy, child <13 yr, renal failure, diabetes, porphyria, chronic gout

DOSAGE AND ROUTES
HIV negative
Adult/adolescent: PO 15-30 mg/kg/day, max 30 mg/kg/day or 3 g/day; CDC max 50 mg/kg/dose or 4 g max

Renal dose
Adult: PO CCr 10-50 ml/min, give dose q48-72hr; CCr <10 ml/min give dose q72hr

Available forms: Tabs 500 mg

ADVERSE EFFECTS
CNS: Headache
GI: Hepatotoxicity, abnormal liver function tests, peptic ulcer, nausea, vomiting, anorexia, cramps, diarrhea
GU: Urinary difficulty, increased uric acid
HEMA: Hemolytic anemia
INTEG: Photosensitivity, urticaria

INTERACTIONS
Drug/lab test
Increased: PBI
Decreased: 17-KS

NURSING CONSIDERATIONS
Assessment
• C&S studies should be done before treatment begins and periodically during treatment
• Monitor serum uric acid, which may be elevated and cause gout symptoms
• **Hepatotoxicity:** monitor liver function tests weekly: ALT, AST, bilirubin; hepatic status: decreased appetite, jaundice, dark urine, fatigue
• Monitor renal status before treatment, monthly thereafter: BUN, creatinine, output, specific gravity, urinalysis, uric acid
• Monitor mental status often: affect, mood, behavioral changes; psychosis may occur

Patient problem
• Diarrhea (adverse reactions)
• Infection (uses)
• Risk for injury (adverse reactions)
• Lack of knowledge of medication (teaching)
• Nonadherence (teaching)

Implementation
• Give with meals to decrease GI symptoms
• Give antiemetic if vomiting occurs
• May be given with other antitubercular products

Patient/family education
• Instruct patient that compliance with dosage schedule, duration is necessary and that scheduled appointments must be kept or relapse may occur

pyridostigmine (Rx)
(peer-id-oh-stig'meen)
Mestinon, Mestinon SR ✹, Mestinon Timespan, Regonol
Func. class.: Cholinergic, anticholinesterase
Chem. class.: Tertiary amine carbamate

ACTION: Inhibits destruction of acetylcholine, which increases concentration at sites where acetylcholine is released; this facilitates transmission of impulses across myoneural junction

Therapeutic outcome: Decreased action of nondepolarizing muscle relaxant; increased muscle strength in myasthenia gravis

USES: Nondepolarizing muscle relaxant antagonist, myasthenia gravis, pretreatment in nerve gas exposure (military only)

Pharmacokinetics

Absorption	Poorly absorbed (PO)
Distribution	Widely distributed, crosses placenta
Metabolism	Liver, plasma cholinesterase
Excretion	Kidneys
Half-life	2 hr (**IV**); 4 hr (PO)

Pharmacodynamics

	PO	PO-EXT REL	IM/IV
Onset	20-30 min	½-1 hr	2-15 min
Peak	Unknown	Unknown	Unknown
Duration	3-6 hr	3-6 hr	2-4 hr

CONTRAINDICATIONS
Bradycardia, hypotension, obstruction of intestine, renal system, bromide, benzyl alcohol sensitivity, cholinesterase inhibitor toxicity

Precautions: Pregnancy seizure disorders, bronchial asthma, coronary occlusion, hyperthyroidism, dysrhythmias, peptic ulcer, megacolon, poor GI motility

---

⚠ Nurse Alert   ✹ Key NCLEX® Drug   >> Drug Specifics

DOSAGE AND ROUTES
Myasthenia gravis
Adult: PO 600 mg/day in 5-6 divided doses, max 1.5 g/day; IM/IV 2 mg; SUS REL 180-540 mg/day or bid at intervals of at least 6 hr
Child: PO 7 mg/kg/day in 5-6 divided doses; IM/IV 0.05-0.15 mg/kg/dose

Nondepolarizing neuromuscular blocker antagonist
Adult: 0.6-1.2 mg IV atropine, then 0.1-0.25 mg/kg/dose
Child: IV 0.1-0.25 mg/kg/dose

Nerve gas exposure prophylaxis (military)
Adult: PO 30 mg q8hr if threat of exposure to Soman gas is anticipated, start several hours before exposure and discontinue upon exposure; after this product is discontinued, give antidotes (atropine, pralidoxime)

Available forms: Tabs 60 mg; ext rel tabs 180 mg; syr 60 mg/5 ml; inj 5 mg/ml

ADVERSE EFFECTS
CNS: Dizziness, headache, sweating, weakness, seizures, uncoordination, paralysis, drowsiness, LOC
CV: Tachycardia, dysrhythmias, bradycardia, AV block, hypotension, ECG changes, cardiac arrest, syncope
EENT: Miosis, blurred vision, lacrimation, vision changes
GI: *Nausea, diarrhea, vomiting, cramps, increased salivary and gastric secretions, peristalsis*
GU: Frequency, incontinence, urgency
INTEG: Rash, urticaria, flushing
RESP: Respiratory depression, bronchospasm, constriction, laryngospasm, respiratory arrest
SYST: Cholinergic crisis

INTERACTIONS
Individual drugs
Atropine, gallamine, metocurine, pancuronium, tubocurarine: decreased action
Succinylcholine: increased action of pyridostigmine
Magnesium, mecamylamine, polymyxin, procainamide, quiNIDine: decreased action of pyridostigmine

Drug classifications
Aminoglycosides, anesthetics, antidysrhythmics, corticosteroids, quinolones: decreased action of pyridostigmine

NURSING CONSIDERATIONS
Assessment
• **Myasthenia gravis:** assess for fatigue, ptosis, diplopia, difficulty swallowing, SOB, hand/gait

before and after product, improvement should be seen after 1 hr
• Monitor I&O ratio; check for urinary retention or incontinence
• **Toxicity:** assess for bradycardia, hypotension, bronchospasm, headache, dizziness, seizures, respiratory depression; product should be discontinued if toxicity occurs
• Monitor VS, respiration; increased B/P during test and at baseline
• Monitor diabetic patient carefully, since this product lowers blood glucose

Patient problem
Impaired breathing (uses)
Impaired mobility (uses)
Risk for Injury (uses, adverse reactions)

Implementation
• Only with atropine sulfate available for cholinergic crisis
• Only after all other cholinergics have been discontinued
• Increased doses for tolerance, as ordered
• Larger doses after exercise or fatigue, as ordered
• Do not break, crush, or chew sus rel tabs
PO route
• On empty stomach for better absorption

IV route
• Undiluted (5 mg/ml), give through Y-tube or 3-way stopcock, give 0.5 mg or less/min (myasthenia gravis); 5 mg/min (reversal of nondepolarizing neuromuscular blockers)

Y-site compatibilities: Heparin, hydrocortisone, potassium chloride, vit B/C
• Storage at room temperature

Patient/family education
• Advise patient to carry/wear emergency ID specifying myasthenia gravis, products taken
• Teach patient that product doesn't cure but relieves symptoms
• Teach patient to avoid driving, other hazardous activities until effect is known
• Advise patient not to drink alcohol
• Advise patient to take with food to decrease gastric side effects
• Teach patient to report weakness (cholinergic crisis, or overdose), bradycardia

Evaluation
Positive therapeutic outcome
• Increased muscle strength, hand grasp, improved gait, absence of labored breathing (if severe); reversal of nondepolarizing neuromuscular blockers; prevention of nerve gas toxicity

TREATMENT OF OVERDOSE:
Discontinue product, atropine 1-4 mg IV

pyridoxine (vitamin B₆) (OTC, Rx)
(peer-i-dox'een)
Neuro-K, Pyri 500
Func. class.: Vitamin B₆, water soluble

ACTION: Needed for fat, protein, carbohydrate metabolism; enhances glycogen release from liver and muscle tissue; needed as coenzyme for metabolic transformations of a variety of amino acids

Therapeutic outcome: Absence of vit B₆ deficiency

USES: Vitamin B₆ deficiency associated with the following: inborn errors of metabolism, seizures, isoniazid therapy, oral contraceptives, alcoholism, polyneuritis

Pharmacokinetics

Absorption	Well absorbed (PO)
Distribution	Stored in liver, muscle, brain; crosses placenta
Metabolism	Unknown
Excretion	Kidneys, unchanged (not used)
Half-life	15-20 days

Pharmacodynamics

Unknown

CONTRAINDICATION
Hypersensitivity

Precautions: Pregnancy, breastfeeding, children, Parkinson's disease, patients taking levodopa should avoid supplemental vitamins with >5 mg pyridoxine

DOSAGE AND ROUTES
RDA
Adult: PO (male) 1.7-2 mg; (female) 1.4-1.6 mg
Child 9-13 yr: PO 1 mg/day
Child 4-8 yr: PO 0.6 mg/day
Child 1-3 yr: PO 0.5 mg/day
Infant 7-12 mo: PO 0.3 mg/day

Vitamin B₆ deficiency
Adult: PO 5-25 mg/day × 3 wk
Child: PO 10 mg until desired response

Pyridoxine deficiency neuritis/seizure (not drug induced)
Adult: PO without neuritis 2.5-10 mg/day, after corrected 2-5 mg/day; with neuritis 100-200 mg/day × 3 wk, then 2-5 mg/day
Child: PO without neuritis 5-25 mg/day × 3 wk, then 1.5-2.5 mg/day in a multivitamin; with neuritis 10-50 mg/day × 3 wk, then 1-2 mg/day
Neonate with seizures: IM/IV 50-100 mg as a single dose

Deficiency caused by isoniazid, cycloSERINE, hydrALAZINE, penicillamine
Adult: PO 100-300 mg/day
Child: PO 10-50 mg/day

Prevention of deficiency caused by isoniazid, cycloSERINE, hydrALAZINE, penicillamine
Adult: PO 25-100 mg/day
Child: PO 1.2 mg/kg/day

Available forms: Capsules 250 mg; Tabs 25, 50, 100, 250, 500 mg; ext rel tabs 200, 500 mg; inj 100 mg/ml; ext rel caps 200, 500 mg

ADVERSE EFFECTS
CNS: Paresthesia, flushing, warmth, lethargy (rare with normal renal function)
INTEG: Pain at inj site

INTERACTIONS
Individual drugs
Chloramphenicol, cycloSERINE, hydrALAZINE, isoniazid, penicillamine: decreased effects of pyridoxine
Levodopa: decreased effects of levodopa

Drug classifications
Contraceptives (oral), immunosuppressants: decreased effects of pyridoxine

NURSING CONSIDERATIONS
Assessment
• Monitor pyridoxine levels throughout treatment
• Assess nutritional status: yeast, liver, legumes, bananas, green vegetables, whole grains
• Assess for pyridoxine (B₆) deficiency: nausea, vomiting, dermatitis, cheilosis, seizures, irritability, dermatitis before, during treatment
• Assess neurological status: paresthesia, lethargy
• Monitor blood tests: Hct, Hgb
• **Malabsorption:** Assess for malabsorption, may require injection if abnormal GI motility or absorption is present
• **Pregnancy/breastfeeding:** Safe in pregnancy, breastfeeding

Patient problem
Impaired nutritional intake (uses)

Implementation
PO route
• Swallow ext rel cap and ext rel tabs whole; do not break, crush, or chew
IM route
• Rotate sites to avoid pain; burning or stinging at site may occur; give by Z-track to minimize pain
• Store in airtight, light-resistant container
IV route
• Give **IV** undiluted or added to most **IV** sol; give 50 mg or less/1 min if undiluted

---

Syringe compatibilities: Doxapram

Additive incompatibilities: Erythromycin, iron salts, kanamycin, riboflavin, streptomycin

Patient/family education

• Teach patient to avoid other vitamin supplements unless directed by prescriber
• Advise patient to increase meat, bananas, potatoos, lima beans, whole grain cereals in diet which are high in vit B_6
• Caution patient not to increase dosage, since serious reactions may occur
• Teach patient to take as prescribed, not to skip, double doses, if dose is missed, skip
• **Pregnancy/breastfeeding:** Identify if pregnancy is planned or suspected or if breastfeeding

Evaluation

Positive therapeutic outcome

• Absence of nausea, vomiting, anorexia, skin lesions, glossitis, stomatitis, edema, seizures, restlessness, paresthesia

QUEtiapine (Rx)

(kwe-tie'a-peen)
SEROquel, Seroquel XR
Func. class.: Antipsychotic
Chem. class.: Dibenzodiazepine

Do not confuse: QUEtiapine/OLANZapine
SEROquel/Serzone/SINEquan

ACTION: Functions as an antagonist at multiple neurotransmitter receptors in the brain including $5-HT_{1A}$, $5-HT_2$, DOPamine D_1, D_2, H_1, adrenergic α_1, α_2 receptors

Therapeutic outcome: Decreased hallucinations and disorganized thought

USES: Bipolar disorder, bipolar I disorder, depression, mania, schizophrenia

Pharmacokinetics

Absorption	Rapidly
Distribution	Widely
Metabolism	Liver, extensively; inhibits P450 CYP3A4 enzyme system; 83% protein
Excretion	Excretion <1% unchanged urine
Half-life	≥6 hr

Pharmacodynamics

Onset	Unknown
Peak	1.5 hr
Duration	Up to 12 hr

CONTRAINDICATIONS

Hypersensitivity, breastfeeding

Precautions: Pregnancy, geriatric, long-term use, seizures, hepatic disease, breast cancer, QT prolongation, CV disease, Parkinson's, brain tumor, hematological disease, torsades de pointes, cataracts, dehydration

> **BLACK BOX WARNING:** Children, suicide, dementia

DOSAGE AND ROUTES
Schizophrenia

Adult: PO (not at risk for hypotension) 25 mg bid on day 1, increase by 25-50 mg divided two to three times on day 2 and day 3 to a target of 300-400 mg/day in divided doses on day 4; make further dosage adjustments in 25-50 mg bid increments, max 800 mg/day; **ext rel** 300 mg q day, increase by 300 mg/day, max 800 mg/day
Adolescents 13-17 yr: PO 25 mg bid on day 1, 50 mg bid on day 2, 100 mg bid on day 3,

150 mg bid on day 4, 200 bid mg on day 5; ext rel 50 mg on day 1, then 100 mg on day 2 , 200 mg on day 3, 300 mg on day 4, 400 mg on day 5
Geriatric: PO ext rel 50 mg/day; may increase in 50 mg/day increments

Bipolar I disorder

Adult: PO (monotherapy or as adjunct to lithium or divalproex) 50 mg bid on day 1, 100 mg on day 2 in 2 divided doses as tolerated to 400 mg on day 4; range 400-800 mg/day; **ext rel** give in evening 300 mg qday day 1, then 600 mg qday day 2, then adjusted as tolerated
Adolescents 10-17 yr: PO 25 mg bid (day 1), then 50 mg bid (day 2), then 100 mg bid (day 3), then 150 mg (day 4), then 200 mg bid (day 5), then ≤100 mg/day increase, max 600 mg/day

Psychotic disorders

Adult: PO 25 mg bid, titrate upward; XR: 300 mg/day in PM, range 400-800 mg/day

Depressive disorder

Adult: PO EXT REL 50 mg/day in the PM on day 1, 2; on day 3 give 150 mg in the PM, max 600 mg/day
Geriatric: PO EXT REL 50 mg; may increase by 50 mg/day based on response; ext rel 50 mg in evening, max 800 mg/day

Available forms: Tabs 25, 50, 100, 200, 300, 400 mg; ext rel tab 50, 150, 200, 300, 400 mg

ADVERSE EFFECTS

CNS: EPS, pseudoparkinsonism, akathisia, dystonia, tardive dyskinesia, drowsiness, insomnia, agitation, anxiety, *headache,* seizures, neuroleptic malignant syndrome, dizziness, dystonia, restless legs syndrome
CV: Orthostatic hypotension, tachycardia, QT prolongation, CV disease, Parkinson's disease, cardiomyopathy, myocarditis
ENDO: SIADH, hyperglycemia
GI: Nausea, anorexia, constipation, abdominal pain, dry mouth, pancreatitis
HEMA: Leukopenia, agranulocytosis
INTEG: Rash DRESS
META: Hyponatremia
MISC: Asthenia, back pain, fever, ear pain
MS: Rhabdomyolysis
RESP: Rhinitis
SYST: Stevens-Johnson syndrome, anaphylaxis

INTERACTIONS
Individual drugs

Alcohol: increased CNS depression
CarBAMazepine, phenytoin, rifampin, thioridazine: increased QUEtiapine clearance
Chloroquine, clarithromycin, droperidol, erythromycin, haloperidol, methadone, pentamidine: increased QT prolongation

---

Cimetidine: decreased QUEtiapine clearance

Erythromycin: increased effects of erythromycin

Fluconazole, itraconazole, ketoconazole: increased action of QUEtiapine

Levodopa: decreased effect of levodopa

Lithium: increased neurotoxicity

LORazepam: decreased effect of LORazepam

Drug classifications

Analgesics (opioid), antihistamines, sedatives-hypnotics: increased CNS depression

Antihypertensives: increased hypotension

Barbiturates, glucocorticoids: increased clearance of quetiapine, decreased quetiapine effect

β-agonists, class IA/III antidysrhythmics, local anesthetics, macrolide antiinfectives (clarithromycin), phenothiazines (some), tricyclics: increased QT prolongation

DOPamine agonists: decreased effects of DOPamine agonists

NURSING CONSIDERATIONS
Assessment

• Assess CV status: QT prolongation, tachycardia, orthostatic B/P

> **BLACK BOX WARNING:** Mental status before initial administration, AIMS assessment; affect, orientation, LOC, reflexes, gait, coordination, sleep pattern disturbances; suicidal thoughts/behavior (child/young adult); dementia (geriatric patients)

> **BLACK BOX WARNING:** Not to be used in child <10 yr (immediate release) or <18 yr (extended release)

> **BLACK BOX WARNING: Suicide:** restrict amount of product given, usually suicidal thoughts, behavior occur early in treatment and in children/adolescents/young adults

• Check that patient swallows all PO medication; check for hoarding or giving of medication to other patients

• Obtain baselines in blood glucose, liver function tests, neurologic status, ophthalmologic exam, weight, thyroid function tests, serum electrolytes/creatinine/lipid profile/prolactin

• Monitor B/P with patient in sitting, standing, and lying positions; take pulse and respirations q4hr during initial treatment; establish baseline before starting treatment; report drops of 30 mm Hg; obtain baseline ECG and monitor Q- and T-wave changes

• Check for dizziness, faintness, palpitations, tachycardia on rising; severe orthostatic hypotension is common

• **Serious rash:** Stevens-Johnson syndrome, discontinue product, may cause rash, fever, joint pain, lesions

• **Pancreatitis:** Assess for nausea, vomiting, severe abdominal pain

• **Identify for neuroleptic malignant syndrome:** hyperpyrexia, muscle rigidity, increased CPK, altered mental status, seizures, tachycardia, diaphoresis, hyper/hypotension, fatigue; product should be discontinued and prescriber notified immediately

• **Assess for EPS** including akathisia (inability to sit still, no pattern to movements), tardive dyskinesia (bizarre movements of the jaw, mouth, tongue, extremities), pseudoparkinsonism (rigidity, tremors, pill rolling, shuffling gait); an antiparkinson product should be prescribed

• **DRESS:** Assess for fever, hepatitis, swelling of face, myositis; monitor eosinophils that may be elevated; discontinue

• **Hyperprolactinemia:** Assess for sexual dysfunction, menstrual changes

• **Pregnancy/breastfeeding:** Use only if benefits outweigh fetal risk, pregnant patients should enroll in the National Pregnancy Registry for Atypical Antipsychotics 1-866-961-2388, EPS may develop in the infant, breastfeeding isn't recommended, excreted in breast milk

• **Beers:** Avoid in older adults except for schizophrenia, bipolar disorder, or short-term use as an antiemetic for chemotherapy, increased risk of stroke

Patient problem

Distorted thinking process (uses)
Depression (uses)

Implementation

• Give reduced dosage in geriatric patients

• Avoid use of CNS depressants

• Give **immediate release** without regard to meals

• Give **extended release** without food or with light meal, swallow whole, do not split, crush, chew

• Supervise ambulation until patient is stabilized on medication; do not involve in strenuous exercise program because fainting is possible; patient should not stand still for a long time

• If there is a week of absence of therapy, initiate at beginning dose

• Provide sips of water, sugarless candy, gum for dry mouth

• Store in airtight, light-resistant container

Patient/family education
• Teach patient to use good oral hygiene; frequent rinsing of mouth, sugarless gum for dry mouth
• Caution patient to avoid hazardous activities until product response is determined; dizziness, blurred vision may occur
• Inform patient that orthostatic hypotension occurs often; patient should rise from sitting or lying position gradually; avoid hot tubs, hot showers, and tub baths because hypotension may occur; inform patient that heat stroke may occur in hot weather, to take extra precautions to stay cool, drink plenty of fluids
• Advise patient to avoid abrupt withdrawal of this product or EPS may result; product should be withdrawn slowly
• Teach patient to avoid OTC preparations (cough, hayfever, cold), herbals, supplements unless approved by prescriber; serious product interactions may occur; avoid use with alcohol, CNS depressants because increased drowsiness may occur
• Advise patient to take medication only as prescribed, not to use other products unless approved by prescriber; not to stop abruptly
• Advise patient that follow-up is necessary including LFTs, blood glucose, neurologic/ophthalmic function, cholesterol profile, weight
• If drowsiness occurs, avoid hazardous activities such as driving
• Advise patient to notify prescriber if pregnancy is planned, suspected; do not breastfeed
• Teach patient to notify health care professionals of use before surgery
• Advise patient to notify prescriber immediately of fever, difficulty breathing, fatigue, sore throat, rash, bleeding

> **BLACK BOX WARNING: Suicide:** To notify provider of thoughts, behavior, primarily in children/adolescents/young adults or worsening depression, severe anxiety, panic attacks, insomnia

• **Pregnancy/breastfeeding:** Advise patient to notify prescriber if pregnancy is planned, suspected; do not breastfeed

Evaluation
Positive therapeutic outcome
• Decrease in emotional excitement, hallucinations, delusions, paranoia
• Reorganization of patterns of thought, speech

TREATMENT OF OVERDOSE:
Lavage, provide airway

quinapril (Rx)
(kwin′a-pril)
Accupril
Func. class.: Antihypertensive
Chem. class.: Angiotensin-converting enzyme (ACE) inhibitor

Do not confuse: Accupril/Aciphex

ACTION: Selectively suppresses renin-angiotensin-aldosterone system; inhibits ACE, prevents conversion of angiotensin I to angiotensin II; results in dilatation of arterial, venous vessels

Therapeutic outcome: Decreased B/P in hypertension

USES: Hypertension, alone or in combination with thiazide diuretics, systolic HF

Pharmacokinetics
Absorption	≥60%
Distribution	Protein binding 97%, crosses placenta
Metabolism	Liver (active metabolites quinaprilat)
Excretion	Metabolites urine (60%), feces (37%)
Half-life	2 hr

Pharmacodynamics
Onset	½-1 hr
Peak	1-2 hr
Duration	24 hr

CONTRAINDICATIONS
Children, hypersensitivity to ACE inhibitors, angioedema

> **BLACK BOX WARNING:** Pregnancy

Precautions: Breastfeeding, geriatric, impaired renal/liver function, dialysis patients, hypovolemia, blood dyscrasias, bilateral renal stenosis, cough, pregnancy 1st trimester, hyperkalemia, aortic stenosis, ✒ African descent

DOSAGE AND ROUTES
Hypertension
Adult: PO 10-20 mg/day initially, then 20-80 mg/day divided bid or daily (monotherapy), start at 5 mg/day (with diuretics), titrate up to 80 mg/day
Geriatric: PO 10 mg/day, titrate to desired response (monotherapy), start at 2.5 mg/day (with diuretics), titrate ≥ 2 wk

Heart failure
Adult: PO 5 mg bid, may increase qwk until 20-40 mg/day in 2 divided doses

Renal dose
Adult: PO CCr 61-89 ml/min start or 10 mg/day (hypertension), 5 mg bid (heart failure); CCr 30-60 ml/min 5 mg/day initially; CCr 10-29 ml/min 2.5 mg/day initially

Available forms: Tabs 5, 10, 20, 40 mg

ADVERSE EFFECTS

CNS: Headache, dizziness, fatigue, somnolence, depression, malaise, nervousness, vertigo, syncope

CV: Hypotension, postural hypotension, syncope, palpitations, *angina pectoris,* MI, tachycardia, vasodilatation, chest pain

GI: Nausea, diarrhea, constipation, vomiting, gastritis, GI hemorrhage, dry mouth

GU: Increased BUN, creatinine, decreased libido, impotence

INTEG: Angioedema, rash, sweating, photosensitivity, pruritus

META: Hyperkalemia

MISC: Back pain, amblyopia

MS: Myalgia

RESP: *Cough,* pharyngitis, dyspnea

INTERACTIONS
Individual drugs
Aliskiren (diabetic patients): increased hyperkalemia
Alcohol: increased hypotension (large amounts)
Lithium: increased toxicity
HydrALAZINE, prazosin: use caution
Tetracycline: decreased absorption of tetracycline

Drug classifications
Adrenergic blockers, antihypertensives, diuretics, ganglionic blockers, nitrates, phenothiazines: increased hypotension
Diuretics (potassium sparing), potassium supplements, sympathomimetics, ACE/angiotensin II receptor antagonists, vasodilators: use caution
NSAIDs: decreased hypotensive effect of quinapril

Drug/herb
Cough: capsaicin
Decrease antihypertensive effect: ma huang

Drug/food
Hyperkalemia: do not use with potassium-containing salt substitutes; read label carefully

Drug/lab test
Increased: Potassium, creatinine, BUN, LFTs

NURSING CONSIDERATIONS
Assessment
• **Hypertension:** monitor B/P, check for orthostatic hypotension, syncope; if changes occur, dosage change may be required
• **HF:** check for edema in feet, legs daily, weight daily
• **Collagen vascular disease:** monitor blood studies: neutrophils, decreased platelets; WBC with differential baseline, periodically q3mo; if neutrophils <1000/mm³ discontinue treatment
• Monitor renal function tests (protein, BUN, creatinine) and periodically liver function tests, uric acid; glucose may be elevated; watch for increased levels that may indicate nephrotic syndrome and renal failure; monitor renal symptoms: polyuria, oliguria, frequency, dysuria
• Check potassium levels throughout treatment, although hyperkalemia rarely occurs
• **Allergic reactions:** Angioedema, rash, fever, pruritus, swelling of eyes/face/neck/throat, difficulty breathing; product should be discontinued, angioedema is more common in Black patients

> **BLACK BOX WARNING:** Assess for pregnancy; pregnancy; if pregnancy is suspected, discontinue product

Patient problem
Risk for injury (adverse reactions)
Nonadherence (teaching)

Implementation
• Tabs may be crushed if necessary, without regard to food
• Store in airtight container at 86° F (30° C) or less
• Do not use with high-fat meal, decreases absorption
• Severe hypotension may occur after 1st dose of this medication; may be prevented by reducing or discontinuing diuretic therapy 3 days before beginning quinapril therapy

Patient/family education
• Advise patient not to discontinue product abruptly; advise patient to tell all persons associated with care
• Teach patient not to use OTC products (cough, cold, allergy) unless directed by physician; serious side effects can occur; avoid high-fat meal at time of dose
• Inform patient that xanthines such as coffee, tea, chocolate, cola can prevent action of product

• Caution patient on the importance of complying with dosage schedule, even if feeling better; to continue with medical regimen to decrease B/P: exercise, cessation of smoking, decreasing stress, diet modifications

• Emphasize the need to rise slowly to sitting or standing position to minimize orthostatic hypotension; not to exercise in hot weather or increased hypotension can occur

• **Allergic reactions:** assess for allergic reactions: rash, fever, pruritus, urticaria; product should be discontinued if antihistamines fail to help

• Teach patient to notify prescriber of mouth sores, sore throat, fever, swelling of hands or feet, irregular heartbeat, chest pain, coughing, shortness of breath

• Caution patient to report excessive perspiration, dehydration, vomiting, diarrhea; may lead to fall in B/P, maintain adequate hydration

• Caution patient that product may cause dizziness, fainting, light-headedness; may occur during 1st few days of therapy; to avoid activities that may be hazardous

• Teach patient how to take B/P, and normal readings for age group

• Teach patient product may cause skin rash or impaired taste perception

BLACK BOX WARNING: Pregnancy, to report if pregnancy is planned or suspected, do not use in pregnancy, breastfeeding, do not breastfeed

Evaluation
Positive therapeutic outcome
• Decreased B/P in hypertension

TREATMENT OF OVERDOSE:
0.9% NaCl **IV** inf, hemodialysis

RARELY USED

quinupristin/dalfopristin
(kwin-oo-pris'tin/dal-foe-pris'tin)
Synercid
Func. class.: Antiinfective, streptogramins

USES: Complicated skin, skin structure infections (*Staphylococcus aureus* methicillin susceptible, *Streptococcus pyogenes*)

CONTRAINDICATION: Hypersensitivity

DOSAGE AND ROUTES
Adult/child 12-17 yr: IV 7.5mg/kg q12hr × ≥7 days

RABEprazole (Rx)

(rab-ee-pray'zole)

Aciphex, Aciphex Sprinkle, Pariet ✦

Func. class.: Proton pump inhibitor
Chem. class.: Benzimidazole

Do not confuse: Aciphex/Aricept/Accupril
RABEprazole/ARIPiprazole

ACTION: Suppresses gastric secretion by inhibiting hydrogen/potassium ATPase enzyme system in the gastric parietal cell; characterized as a gastric acid pump inhibitor, since it blocks the final step of acid production

Therapeutic outcome: Absence of duodenal ulcers; decreased gastroesophageal reflux

USES: Gastroesophageal reflux disease (GERD), severe erosive esophagitis, poorly responsive systemic GERD, pathologic hypersecretory conditions (Zollinger-Ellison syndrome, systemic mastocytosis, multiple endocrine adenomas); treatment of duodenal ulcers with or without antiinfectives for *Helicobacter pylori;* daytime, nighttime heartburn

Pharmacokinetics

Absorption	50%
Distribution	Protein binding 96.3%
Metabolism	Liver, extensively by CYP2C19 🗲Ⓖⓧ
Excretion	Kidneys, feces, metabolites
Half-life	1-2 hr

Pharmacodynamics

Unknown

CONTRAINDICATIONS

Hypersensitivity to this product or proton pump inhibitors (PPIs)

Precautions: Pregnancy, breastfeeding, children, 🗲Ⓖⓧ Asian patients, diarrhea, geriatric patients, gastric cancer, hepatic/GI disease, IBS, osteoporosis, pseudomembranous colitis, ulcerative colitis, vit B_{12} deficiency

DOSAGE AND ROUTES
Healing of duodenal ulcers

Adult: PO 20 mg/day × ≤4 wk, to be taken after breakfast

Erosive esophagitis/GERD

Adult: PO Delayed release tabs 20 mg/day × 4-8 wk

Adolescent and child ≥12 yr: PO Delayed release tabs 20 mg/day up to 8 wk, may use an additional course

Child 1-11 yr (≥15 kg): PO (sprinkle) 10 mg qday up to 12 wk; (<15 kg) 5 mg qday up to 12 wk; may increase to 10 mg qday if needed

H. pylori eradication

Adult: PO 20 mg bid × 7 days with amoxicillin 1 g bid × 7 days with clarithromycin 500 mg bid × 7 days

Available forms: Del rel tabs 20 mg; delayed release caps 5, 10 mg

ADVERSE EFFECTS

CNS: *Headache, dizziness*
EENT: Tinnitus, taste perversion
GI: *Diarrhea, abdominal pain, vomiting, nausea, constipation, flatulence, acid regurgitation,* abdominal swelling, anorexia, *Clostridium difficile*–associated diarrhea, hepatitis, hepatic encephalopathy
MISC: *Back pain,* infection, arthralgia, myalgia, osteoporosis, fractures, Stevens-Johnson syndrome

INTERACTIONS
Individual drugs

Digoxin, methotrexate, nelfinavir/omeprazole: increased levels of each of these products
Ketoconazole, itraconazole, iron salts, atazanavir/ritonavir, ampicillin, cycloSPORINE: decreased levels of each of these products
Calcium carbonate, sucralfate, vitamin B_{12}: decreased rabeprazole levels
Clarithromycin, phenytoin: increased levels of rabeprazole
Warfarin, clopidogrel: increased bleeding risk, monitor PT, INR

Drug classifications

Benzodiazepines, antacids, other proton pump inhibitors, H_2 blockers: increased levels of rabeprazole
Protease inhibitors: Decreased level of protease inhibitors

Drug/herb

St. John's wort: decreased levels of rabeprazole

Drug/lab test

Decreased: magnesium

NURSING CONSIDERATIONS
Assessment

• Assess GI system: bowel sounds q8hr, abdomen for pain and swelling, anorexia
• **CDAD** may occur with most antibiotic therapy; assess for watery diarrhea, abdominal pain, fever, may occur several weeks after treatment concludes
• **Vitamin B_{12} deficiency/cyanocobalamin/ hypomagnesemia:** may occur several weeks after treatment concludes; use magnesium,

vit B_{12}, cyanocobalamin supplement; if severe, discontinuing of product may be needed

• Monitor hepatic enzymes: AST, ALT, increased alkaline phosphatase during treatment

• Assess for low magnesium level: tremors, muscle soreness, spasms, anxiety, change in heart rate, palpitations, obtain magnesium level

• Obtain susceptibility testing if *H. pylori* treatment is ineffective; another antiinfective may be needed

• **Osteoporosis/fractures:** May occur with prolonged high-dose use, usually in those 50 yr, make sure adequate vitamin D and calcium are taken

• **Beers:** Avoid scheduled use >8 wk in older adults unless for high-risk patients

Patient problem
Pain (uses)

Implementation
PO route

• Do not break, crush, or chew del rel tab

• Give after breakfast daily with a full glass of water, without regard to food

• **Delayed-release capsule:** Open, use on a spoonful of applesauce or liquid, give immediately, (within 15 min) 2h before a meal; do not crush, chew delayed-release product

Patient/family education

• **CDAD:** Advise patient to report severe diarrhea; product may have to be discontinued

• Inform diabetic patient that hypoglycemia can occur; monitor blood glucose closely

• Caution patient to avoid driving and other hazardous activities until response to product is known, take delayed release tab whole, do not cut, break; that cap should be opened and sprinkled on food (applesauce), to take within 15 min and 30 min before a meal

• Caution patient to avoid alcohol, salicylates, NSAIDs; may cause GI irritation

• Advise patient to wear sunscreen, protective clothing to prevent burns

• Advise patient to notify prescriber if pregnancy is planned or suspected

• Advise patient that fractures may occur with use > 1 yr

Evaluation
Positive therapeutic outcome

• Absence of epigastric pain, swelling, fullness; decreased symptoms of GERD after 4-8 wk

raloxifene (Rx)
(ral-ox'ih-feen)
Evista
Func. class.: Bone resorption inhibitor
Chem. class.: Hormone modifier, selective estrogen receptor modulator (SERM)

ACTION: Tissue-selective estrogen agonist/antagonist; agonist activity in bone and lipid metabolism, antagonistic activity on breast and uterus, reduces resorption of bone and decreases bone turnover

Therapeutic outcome: Absence or decrease of osteoporosis in postmenopausal women

USES: Prevention, treatment of osteoporosis in postmenopausal women, breast cancer prophylaxis in postmenopausal women with osteoporosis or in postmenopausal women at high risk for developing the disease, invasive breast cancer risk reduction

Pharmacokinetics
Absorption	Unknown
Distribution	Highly protein bound
Metabolism	Liver, extensively
Excretion	Feces, breast milk
Half-life	28-32 hr

Pharmacodynamics
Onset	Unknown
Peak	Unknown
Duration	24 hr

CONTRAINDICATIONS
Pregnancy, breastfeeding, hypersensitivity

> **BLACK BOX WARNING:** Women with active or history of venous thromboembolic events

Precautions: Hepatic/CV disease, cervical/uterine cancer, elevated triglycerides, pulmonary embolism

> **BLACK BOX WARNING:** Stroke

DOSAGE AND ROUTES
Postmenopausal women: PO 60 mg/day, max 60 mg/day

Available forms: Tabs 60 mg

ADVERSE EFFECTS

CNS: Insomnia, depression, migraines, fever
CV: Hot flashes, peripheral edema, thromboembolism, stroke, chest pain
EENT: Pharyngitis, sinusitis, laryngitis
GI: *Nausea*, vomiting, diarrhea, dyspepsia, abdominal pain
GU: Vaginitis, leukorrhea, *hot flashes*, cystitis, vaginal bleeding
INTEG: Rash, sweating
META: Weight gain, peripheral edema
MS: Arthralgia, myalgia, *leg cramps*, arthritis
RESP: Increased cough, pneumonia

INTERACTIONS
Individual drugs
Ampicillin, cholestyramine: decreased action of raloxifene
Levothyroxine, liotrix: decreased action

Drug classifications
Anticoagulants: decreased action of anticoagulants
Bile acid sequestrants: decreased action of raloxifene
Highly protein-bound products (naproxen, ibuprofen, diazoxide), administer cautiously

Drug/food
Soy: decreased effect of raloxifene

Drug/lab test
Increased: triglycerides

NURSING CONSIDERATIONS
Assessment

> **BLACK BOX WARNING:** For history of stroke, TIA, thrombosis, atrial fibrillation, hypertension, smoking; venous thrombosis may occur; avoid prolonged sitting, discontinue 3 days before surgery or other immobilization

• Obtain bone density test baseline, periodically throughout treatment; bone-specific alkaline phosphatase; osteocalcin, collagen breakdown baseline and periodically
• Monitor B/P, watch for increase caused by H_2O and sodium retention

Patient problem
Risk for injury (uses, adverse reactions)

Implementation
• Administer without regard to meals
• Add calcium supplement, vit D if lacking
• Do not use during prolonged bed rest

Patient/family education

> **BLACK BOX WARNING:** Teach patients to discontinue product 72 hr before prolonged bedrest, to report possible blood clots immediately, usually during first few months of therapy

• Advise patient to avoid maintaining one position for long periods
• Advise patient to take calcium supplements, vit D if intake is inadequate
• Advise patient to increase exercise using weights
• Advise patient to stop smoking and to decrease alcohol consumption
• Inform patient that this product does not help control hot flashes
• Instruct patient to report fever, acute migraine, insomnia, emotional distress, UTI, or vaginal itching, uterine bleeding (abnormal), breast lumps

> **BLACK BOX WARNING:** Teach patient to report swelling, warmth, or pain in calves, may indicate clot

• **Pregnancy:** Advise patient to notify prescriber if pregnancy is planned or suspected, not to use in pregnancy or breastfeeding
• Provide product package insert and discuss with patient

Evaluation
Positive therapeutic outcome
• Prevention, treatment of osteoporosis

raltegravir (Rx)
(ral-teg'ra-vir)
Isentress, Isentress HD
Func. class.: Antiretroviral
Chem. class.: HIV integrase strand transfer inhibitor (ISTIs)

ACTION: Inhibits catalytic activity of HIV integrase, which is an HIV-encoded enzyme needed for replication

Therapeutic outcome: Improvement in CD4, T-cell counts

USES: HIV in combination with other antiretrovirals

Pharmacokinetics

Absorption	Unknown
Distribution	Unknown
Metabolism	Liver by uridine diphosphate glucuronosyltransferase (✿ UGT1A1 enzyme system)
Excretion	51% feces, 32% urine
Half-life	9 hr

Pharmacodynamics

Onset	Unknown
Peak	3 hr
Duration	Up to 12 hr

CONTRAINDICATIONS
Hypersensitivity, breastfeeding

Precautions: Pregnancy, children, geriatric, hepatic disease, immune reconstitution syndrome, hepatitis, antimicrobial resistance, lactase deficiency

DOSAGE AND ROUTES
Adult and adolescent ≥16 yr: PO 400 mg bid, if using with rifampin give 800 mg bid

Child ≥40 kg treatment naive or immunosuppressed (initial 400 mg bid): PO tab 1200 mg qday 400 mg bid, chew tab 300 mg qday

Child ≥4 wk and ≥25 kg: PO tab 400 mg bid, chew tab (25-28 kg) 150 mg bid, (28-39.9 kg) 200 mg bid, ≥40 kg 300 mg bid

Child ≥4 wk and <25 kg: chew tab 150 mg bid

Child ≥4 wk and 14–<20 kg: susp 100 mg bid, chew tab 100 mg bid

Child ≥4 wk and 11–<14 kg: susp 80 mg bid, chew tab 75 mg bid

Child ≥4 wk and 8–<11 kg: susp 60 mg bid

Child ≥4 wk and 6–<8 kg: susp 40 mg bid

Child ≥4 wk and 4–<6 kg: susp 30 mg bid

Child ≥4 wk and 3–<4 kg: susp 20 mg bid

Available forms: Tabs 400, 600 mg; chew tabs 25, 100 mg; granules for oral suspension 100/packet mg

ADVERSE EFFECTS
CNS: *Fatigue,* fever, *dizziness, headache,* asthenia, suicidal ideation, insomnia
CV: MI
GI: *Nausea,* vomiting, *diarrhea,* abdominal pain, gastritis, hepatitis
GU: Acute renal failure
HEMA: Anemia, neutropenia
INTEG: Rash, urticaria, pruritus, pain or phlebitis at IV site, unusual sweating, alopecia, Stevens-Johnson syndrome, toxic epidermal necrolysis
META: Hyperamylasemia, hyperglycemia, lipodystrophy
MS: Myopathy, rhabdomyolysis
SYST: Immune reconstitution syndrome

INTERACTIONS
Individual drugs
Rifampin, efavirenz, tenofovir, tipranavir/ritonavir: decreased raltegravir levels

Drug classifications
Fibric acid derivatives, HMG-CoA reductase inhibitors: increased rhabdomyolysis, myopathy, elevated CPK

H_2 blockers, protein pump inhibitors, UGT1A1 inhibitors (atazanavir): increased raltegravir effect

Drug/lab test
Increased: total/HDL/LDL cholesterol

NURSING CONSIDERATIONS
Assessment
• **HIV infection:** monitor CD4, T-cell count, plasma HIV RNA, viral load; resistance testing prior to therapy and at treatment failure
• **Rhabdomyolysis:** Assess for muscle pain, dark urine, increased; product should be discontinued
• **Suicidal thoughts, behavior:** monitor for depression, more common in those with mental illness
• **Immune reconstitution syndrome:** usually during initial phase of treatment, may give antiinfective before starting, opportunistic infections or autoimmune disorders may occur
• Monitor total HDL/LDL cholesterol baseline and periodically; all may be elevated; pregnancy test, CBC with differential, hepatitis B serology, plasma hepatitis C RNA, urinalysis, blood glucose, LFTs serum bilirubin (total and direct), baseline and periodically
• Assess skin eruptions: rash, urticaria, itching may indicate Stevens-Johnson syndrome
• **Pregnancy/breastfeeding:** Pregnant patients need to enroll in the Antiretroviral Pregnancy Registry 800-258-4263, do not breastfeed

Patient problem
Infection (uses)
Nonadherence (teaching)

Implementation
PO route
• Tablets and chew tablets are not interchangeable
• Chew tabs should be chewed or swallowed whole
• Do not break, crush, or chew tabs
• May give without regard to meals, with 8 oz of water
• Store at room temperature
Oral suspension
• Open foil; use 5 ml of water in provided measuring cup; close, then swirl; don't turn upside down; use oral syringe to administer; use within 30 min; discard any remaining suspension

---

Patient/family education
• Teach patient to take as prescribed; if dose is missed, take as soon as remembered up to 1 hr before next dose; do not double dose, do not share with others
• Teach patient to report rash, muscle pain
• Teach patient that sexual partners need to be told that patient has HIV
• Advise patient that product does not cure infection, just controls symptoms, does not prevent infecting others
• Teach patient to report sore throat, fever, fatigue (may indicate immune reconstitution syndrome)
• Advise patient that product must be taken in equal intervals 2×/day to maintain blood levels for duration of therapy
• Advise patient that regular exams and blood work will be needed
• Advise patient to notify prescriber immediately of suicidal thoughts, behavior
• **Pregnancy:** Advise patient to notify prescriber if pregnancy is planned or suspected, not to breastfeed

Evaluation
Positive therapeutic outcome
• Improvement in CD4, T-cell counts, viral load
• Decreased progression of AIDS, HIV

⚠ HIGH ALERT

ramelteon (Rx)
(rah-mel'tee-on)
Rozerem
Func. class.: Sedative-hypnotic, anti-anxiety
Chem. class.: Melatonin receptor agonist

Do not confuse: Rozerem/Razadyne

ACTION: Binds selectively to melatonin receptors (MT_1, MT_2); thought to be involved in circadian rhythm and the normal sleep-wake cycle

Therapeutic outcome: Ability to fall asleep easily and decrease early-morning awakenings

USES: Insomnia (difficulty with sleep onset)

Pharmacokinetics

Absorption	Well
Distribution	Protein binding 82%, to tissue
Metabolism	Rapid first-pass metabolism, liver by CYP1A2
Excretion	84% urine, 4% feces
Half-life	2-5 hr metabolite

Pharmacodynamics

Onset	Unknown
Peak	½-1½ hr
Duration	Unknown

CONTRAINDICATIONS
Breastfeeding, infants, children, hypersensitivity

Precautions: Pregnancy, hepatic disease, alcoholism, seizure disorder, sleep apnea, suicidal ideation, angioedema, depression, sleep-related behavior (sleepwalking), schizophrenia, bipolar disorder, alcohol intoxication, hepatic encephalopathy, aortic stenosis

DOSAGE AND ROUTES
Adult: PO 8 mg within 30 min of bedtime

Hepatic dose
Do not use in severe hepatic disease; use with caution in mild to moderate hepatic disease

Available forms: Tabs 8 mg

ADVERSE EFFECTS
CNS: Dizziness, somnolence, fatigue, headache, worsening insomnia, depression
GI: Nausea
SYST: Severe allergic reactions, angioedema

INTERACTIONS
Individual drugs
Alcohol, ciprofloxacin, fluconazole, fluvoxaMINE, ketoconazole: increased ramelteon effect, toxicity

Drug classifications
Antiretroviral protease inhibitors: possible toxicity
Anxiolytics, azole antifungals, barbiturates, CNS depressants, opioids, CYP1A2 inhibitors, strong CYP2C9 inhibitors, strong CYP3A4 inhibitors, hypnotics, sedatives: increased ramelteon effect, toxicity
Strong CYP inducers (rifampin): decreased ramelteon effect

Drug/food
High-fat/heavy meal: prolonged absorption, sleep onset reduced

Drug/lab test
Increased: protein level
Decreased: testosterone level

NURSING CONSIDERATIONS
Assessment
• **Sleep characteristics:** assess type of sleep problem: falling asleep, staying asleep; complex sleep disorders (sleep walking/driving/eating) after taking product
• Assess mental status: mood, sensorium, affect, memory (long, short), suicidal thoughts/behaviors

R

• **Severe hypersensitivity reactions:** Assess for angioedema (facial swelling); discontinue product; notify prescriber immediately
• **LFTS:** Before treatment, periodically
• **Beers:** Avoid in older adults with a high risk of delirium, delirium might be induced or worsened
• **Pregnancy/breastfeeding:** Use only if benefits outweigh fetal risk, may be toxic to fetus, cautious use in breastfeeding, excretion is unknown

Patient problem
Impaired sleep (uses)

Implementation
• Give within 30 min of bedtime for sleeplessness, give on empty stomach for fast onset, do not give within 1 hr of high-fat foods
• Store in tight container in cool environment
• Do not break, chew, crush tabs; swallow whole

Patient/family education
• Advise patient to avoid driving or other activities requiring alertness until product is stabilized; drowsiness may continue the next day
• Advise patient to avoid alcohol ingestion or CNS depressants, opioids
• Advise patient to immediately report swelling of face, tongue; trouble breathing
• Teach patient alternative measures to improve sleep: reading, exercise several hr before bedtime, warm bath, warm milk, TV, self-hypnosis, deep breathing
• Advise patient to take within 30 min before going to bed
• Advise patient not to ingest a high-fat/heavy meal before taking
• Med guide should be given to patient and reviewed
• Teach patient to report if pregnancy is planned or suspected, avoid breastfeeding

Evaluation

Positive therapeutic outcome
• Ability to sleep at night, decreased amount of early-morning awakening

---

ramipril (Rx)
(ra-mi′pril)
Altace
Func. class.: Antihypertensive
Chem. class.: Angiotensin-converting enzyme (ACE) inhibitor

Do not confuse: ramipril/enalapril, Altace/alteplase

ACTION: Selectively suppresses renin-angiotensin-aldosterone system; inhibits ACE; prevents conversion of angiotensin I to angiotensin II; results in dilatation of arterial, venous vessels

Therapeutic outcome: Decreased B/P in hypertension

USES: Hypertension, alone or in combination with thiazide diuretics; HF (after MI), reduction in risk of MI, stroke, death from CV disorders

Pharmacokinetics

Absorption	Well absorbed
Distribution	Not known, crosses placenta
Metabolism	Liver, extensively; protein binding 73%
Excretion	Urine
Half-life	Ramipril (5 hr), ramiprilat (13-17 hr)

Pharmacodynamics

Onset	½-1 hr
Peak	1-3 hr
Duration	24-72 hr

CONTRAINDICATIONS
Breastfeeding, children, hypersensitivity to ACE inhibitors, history of ACE inhibitor–induced angioedema

> **BLACK BOX WARNING:** Pregnancy

Precautions: Impaired renal/liver function, dialysis patients, hypovolemia, blood dyscrasias, COPD, HF, asthma, geriatric, renal artery stenosis, cough, ⦿ African descent

DOSAGE AND ROUTES
Hypertension
Adult: PO 2.5 mg/day initially, then 2.5-20 mg/day divided bid or daily

HF/Post MI
Adult: PO 1.25-2.5 mg bid, may increase to 5 mg bid

Reduction in risk of MI, stroke, death
Adult: PO 2.5 mg/day × 7 days, then 5 mg/day × 21 days, then may increase to 10 mg/day

Renal impairment
Adult: PO CCr <40 ml/min; reduce by 50%, titrate upward to max 5 mg/day

Available forms: Caps 1.25, 2.5, 5, 10 mg

ADVERSE EFFECTS
CNS: *Headache, dizziness,* anxiety, insomnia, paresthesia, fatigue, depression, malaise, vertigo
CV: *Hypotension,* chest pain, palpitations, angina, syncope, dysrhythmia, heart failure, MI

GI: Nausea, constipation, vomiting, anorexia, diarrhea, abdominal pain
GU: Proteinuria, increased BUN, creatinine, impotence
INTEG: Rash, sweating, photosensitivity, pruritus
META: *Hyperkalemia,* hyperglycemia
MS: Arthralgia, arthritis, myalgia
RESP: Cough, dyspnea

INTERACTIONS
Individual drugs
Do not use with aliskiren in moderate-severe renal disease
Alcohol: increased hypotension (large amounts)
Lithium: increased serum levels
HydrALAZINE, prazosin: increased toxicity
Indomethacin: decreased antihypertensive effect

Drug classifications
Adrenergic blockers, antihypertensives, diuretics, ganglionic blockers, nitrates: increased hypotension
Antacids: decreased absorption
Diuretics (potassium sparing), potassium supplements, sympathomimetics, vasodilators: increased toxicity
NSAIDs, salicylates: decreased antihypertensive effect

Drug/food
Potassium salt substitutes: increased hyperkalemia, avoid use

Drug/herb
Hawthorn: increased antihypertensive effect
Ephedra: decreased antihypertensive effect

Drug/lab test
Increased: LFTs, BUN, creatinine, glucose, potassium
Decreased: RBC, Hgb, platelets

NURSING CONSIDERATIONS
Assessment
• **HF:** Check for edema in feet, legs daily, weight daily
• **Hypertension:** Monitor B/P baseline and regularly, check for orthostatic hypotension, syncope; if changes occur, dosage may need to be changed
• **Monitor blood tests:** neutrophils, decreased platelets; WBC with differential baseline, periodically q3mo; if neutrophils are <1000/mm³, discontinue treatment
• **Renal disease:** Monitor renal function tests: protein, BUN, creatinine, potassium, sodium; watch for increased levels that may indicate nephrotic syndrome and renal failure; monitor renal symptoms: polyuria, oliguria, frequency, dysuria; establish baselines in renal, liver

function tests before therapy begins and monitor periodically; liver function tests, uric acid, and glucose may be increased
• Check potassium levels throughout treatment, hyperkalemia occurs
• **Allergic reactions: angioedema, Stevens-Johnson syndrome;** assess for rash, fever, pruritus, urticaria; product should be discontinued if antihistamines fail to help
• Monitor electrolytes baseline and periodically, potassium may be increased

Patient problem
Risk for injury (adverse reactions)

Implementation
• Caps may be opened and added to food, mixture is stable for 24 hr at room temperature, 48 hr refrigerated
• Swallow cap or tablets whole; do not chew, crush
• Store in airtight container at 86° F (30° C) or less

Patient/family education
• Caution patient not to discontinue product abruptly; advise patient to tell all persons associated with care
• Teach patient not to use OTC products (cough, cold, allergy), herbals, supplements unless directed by prescriber; serious side effects can occur; xanthines such as coffee, tea, chocolate, cola can prevent action of product
• Instruct patient on the importance of complying with dosage schedule, even if feeling better; to continue with medical regimen to decrease B/P: exercise, cessation of smoking, decreasing stress, diet modifications
• Emphasize the need to rise slowly to sitting or standing position to minimize orthostatic hypotension; not to exercise in hot weather because increased hypotension can occur
• Teach patient to notify prescriber of mouth sores, sore throat, fever, swelling of hands or feet, irregular heartbeat, chest pain, coughing, shortness of breath
• Caution patient to report excessive perspiration, dehydration, vomiting, diarrhea; may lead to fall in B/P, maintain hydration
• Caution patient that product may cause dizziness, fainting, light-headedness; may occur during 1st few days of therapy; to avoid activities that may be hazardous
• Teach patient how to take B/P, and normal readings for age group

BLACK BOX WARNING: Inform prescriber if pregnancy is planned, do not use in pregnancy, breastfeeding

R

Evaluation
Positive therapeutic outcome
- Decreased B/P in hypertension

TREATMENT OF OVERDOSE:
0.9% NaCl **IV** inf, hemodialysis

ranitidine (Rx)
(ra-nit'i-deen)
Acid Reducer ✤, Zantac, Zantac 75, Zantac 150, Zantac 300 ✤, Zantac EFFER-dose
Func. class.: H₂ histamine receptor antagonist

Do not confuse: ranitidine/amantadine/ rimantadine, **Zantac**/Xanax/Zofran/ZyrTEC

ACTION: Inhibits histamine at H₂ receptor site in the gastric parietal cells, which inhibits gastric acid secretion

Therapeutic outcome: Healing of duodenal ulcers or gastric ulcers; prevention of duodenal ulcers; decreased symptoms of gastroesophageal reflux disease (GERD), Zollinger-Ellison syndrome, or heartburn

USES: Short-term treatment of duodenal and gastric ulcers and maintenance; management of GERD, Zollinger-Ellison syndrome, active duodenal ulcers with *Helicobacter pylori* in combination with clarithromycin, hypersecretory conditions, stress ulcers, erosive esophagitis (maintenance), systemic mastocytosis, multiple endocrine adenoma syndrome, heartburn

Pharmacokinetics

Absorption	Well absorbed (PO, IM), completely absorbed (**IV**)
Distribution	Widely distributed, crosses placenta
Metabolism	Liver (30%)
Excretion	Kidneys unchanged (70%)
Half-life	2-3 hr, increased renal disease

Pharmacodynamics

	PO	IM/IV
Onset	Unknown	Unknown
Peak	2-3 hr	15 min
Duration	8-12 hr	8-12 hr

CONTRAINDICATIONS
Hypersensitivity

Precautions: Pregnancy, breastfeeding, child <12 yr, renal/hepatic disease

DOSAGE AND ROUTES
Erosive esophagitis
Adult: PO 150 mg qid for up to 12 wk
Child ≥1 mo: PO 5-10 mg/kg/day in 2-3 divided doses

Duodenal ulcer
Adult: PO 150 mg bid or 300 mg/day after PM meal or at bedtime, maintenance 150 mg at bedtime
Infant and child: PO 2-4 mg/kg bid, max 300 mg/day

Zollinger-Ellison syndrome
Adult: PO 150 mg bid, may increase if needed

Gastric ulcer
Adult: PO 150 mg bid × 6 wk, then 150 mg at bedtime
Infant/child: PO 2-4 mg/kg bid, max 300 mg/day

GERD
Adult: PO 150 mg bid

Renal dose
Adult: CCr <50 ml/min give 50% of dose or extend dosing interval

Available forms: Tab 75, 150, 300 mg; sol for inj 25 mg/ml; caps 150, 300 mg; syrup 15 mg/ml

ADVERSE EFFECTS
CNS: Headache, dizziness, hallucinations (geriatric)
EENT: Blurred vision
GI: Constipation, abdominal pain, diarrhea, nausea, vomiting, hepatotoxicity
INTEG: Anaphylaxis, angioedema, burning at inj site

INTERACTIONS
Individual drugs
Atazanavir, delavirdine: Decreased absorption of each product
Ketoconazole: decreased effect of ketoconazole, give 2 hr before ranitidine
Procainamide: increased absorption, toxicity
Warfarin: decreased warfarin clearance

Drug classifications
Iron salts: decreased effects of iron salts

Drug/lab test
Increased: AST, creatinine, ALT
False positive: urine protein (multistix)

NURSING CONSIDERATIONS
Assessment
- **GI complaints:** assess patient with ulcers or suspected ulcers: epigastric or abdominal pain, hematemesis, occult blood in stools, blood in gastric aspirate before, throughout treatment

• Monitor I&O ratio, BUN, creatinine, CBC with differential monthly
• **Beers:** Avoid in older adults with or at high risk of delirium, may induce or make delirium worse, report confusion

Patient problem
Pain (uses)

Implementation
• Store at room temp
• Give qday dose at bedtime
PO route
• May be given with or without meals
• Give antacids 1 hr before or 1 hr after this product
IM route
• No dilution needed; inject in large muscle mass, aspirate

IV direct route
• Dilute to max 2.5 mg/ml (50 mg/20 ml) using 0.9% NaCl (nonpreserved) or D₅W, give dose over ≥5 min (max 4 mg/ml)
Intermittent IV INF route
• Dilute to max 0.5 mg/ml with D₅W, 0.9% NaCl, give over 15-20 min (5-7 ml/min); premixed ready-to-use bags as 1 mg/ml (50 mg/50 ml), inf over 15-20 min
Continuous 24 hr IV INF route
• **Adult:** dilute 150 mg/250 ml of D₅W or 0.9% NaCl, run over 24 hr (6.25 mg/hr or as directed); use inf device and use within 48 hr; *Zollinger-Ellison:* dilute in D₅W or 0.9% NaCl, max concentration 2.5 mg/ml, use inf device

Y-site compatibilities: Acyclovir, aldesleukin, alemtuzumab, alfentanil, allopurinol, amifostine, amikacin, aminophylline, amphotericin B liposome, amsacrine, anakinra, anidulafungin, ascorbic acid, atracurium, atropine, aztreonam, bivalirudin, bumetanide, buprenorphine, butorphanol, calcium chloride/gluconate, CARBOplatin, ceFAZolin, cefepime, cefonicid, cefoperazone, cefotaxime, cefoTEtan, cefOXitin, cefTAZidime, ceftizoxime, cefTRIAXone, cefuroxime, chloramphenicol, chlorproMAZINE, cimetidine, ciprofloxacin, cisatracurium, CISplatin, clindamycin, cyanocobalamin, cyclophosphamide, cycloSPORINE, cytarabine, DACTINomycin, DAPTOmycin, dexamethasone, dexmedetomidine, digoxin, diltiazem, DOBUTamine, DOCEtaxel, DOPamine, doripenem, doxacurium, doxapram, DOXOrubicin, DOXOrubicin liposome, doxycycline, enalaprilat, ePHEDrine, EPINEPHrine, epirubicin, epoetin alfa, ertapenem, erythromycin, esmolol, etoposide, etoposide phosphate, famotidine, fenoldopam, fentaNYL, filgrastim,

fluconazole, fludarabine, fluorouracil, folic acid, foscarnet, furosemide, ganciclovir, gemcitabine, gentamicin, glycopyrrolate, granisetron, heparin, hydrocortisone, HYDROmorphone, IDArubicin, ifosfamide, imipenem/cilastatin, inamrinone, indomethacin, isoproterenol, ketorolac, labetalol, levofloxacin, lidocaine, linezolid, LORazepam, magnesium sulfate, mannitol, mechlorethamine, melphalan, meperidine, metaraminol, methotrexate, methoxamine, methyldopate, methylPREDNISolone, metoclopramide, metoprolol, metroNIDAZOLE, midazolam, milrinone, mitoXANtrone, morphine, nalbuphine, naloxone, nesiritide, niCARdipine, nitroglycerin, nitroprusside, norepinephrine, octreotide, ondansetron, oxacillin, oxaliplatin, oxytocin, PACLitaxel, palonosetron, pancuronium, papaverine, PEMEtrexed, penicillin G, pentamidine, pentazocine, PENTobarbital, PHENobarbital, phentolamine, phenylephrine, phytonadione, piperacillin/tazobactam, potassium chloride, procainamide, prochlorperazine, promethazine, propofol, propranolol, protamine, pyridoxine, remifentanil, riTUXimab, rocuronium, sargramostim, sodium acetate/bicarbonate, succinylcholine, SUFentanil, tacrolimus, teniposide, theophylline, thiamine, thiopental, thiotepa, ticarcillin/clavulanate, tigecycline, tirofiban, tobramycin, tolazoline, trastuzumab, trimetaphan, urokinase, vancomycin, vecuronium, vinCRIStine, vinorelbine, warfarin, zidovudine, zoledronic acid

Patient/family education
• Advise patient to avoid driving, other hazardous activities until stabilized on this medication; drowsiness or dizziness may occur
• Inform patient that smoking decreases the effectiveness of the product; that smoking cessation should be considered, to avoid alcohol
• Instruct patient that product must be continued for prescribed time to be effective and taken exactly as prescribed; doses should not be doubled; a missed dose should be taken when remembered up to 1 hr before next dose
• Inform patient to report diarrhea, black tarry stools, sore throat, rash, dizziness, confusion, or delirium to prescriber immediately
• Teach patient to report immediately coffee-grounds emesis, abdominal pain, cramping
• **Pregnancy/breastfeeding:** Identify if pregnancy is planned or suspected or if breastfeeding

R

Evaluation
Positive therapeutic outcome
- Decreased pain in abdomen, heartburn
- Healing of ulcers
- Absence of gastroesophageal reflux

ranolazine (Rx)
(ruh-no'luh-zeen)
Ranexa
Func. class.: Antianginal
Chem. class.: Piperazine derivative

ACTION: Antianginal, antiischemic; unknown, may work by inhibiting portal fatty-acid oxidation

Therapeutic outcome: Decreased anginal pain and number of episodes

USES: Chronic stable angina pectoris; use in those that have not responded to other treatment options; should be used in combination with other antianginals such as amlodipine, β-blockers, or nitrates

Pharmacokinetics

Absorption	Varied absorption
Distribution	Protein binding 62%
Metabolism	Liver, extensively by CYP3A, CYP2D6 (lesser)
Excretion	Urine 75%, feces 25%
Half-life	7 hr

Pharmacodynamics

Onset	Unknown
Peak	2-5 hr
Duration	Unknown

CONTRAINDICATIONS
Preexisting QT prolongation, hepatic disease (Child-Pugh class A, B, C), hypersensitivity, hypokalemia, renal failure, torsades de pointes, ventricular dysrhythmia, ventricular tachycardia, hepatic cirrhosis

Precautions: Pregnancy, breastfeeding, children, geriatric, renal disease, hypotension, females at risk for torsades de pointes

DOSAGE AND ROUTES
Chronic angina
Adult: PO 500 mg bid and increased to 1000 mg bid based on response; max 1000 mg bid, limit to 500 mg bid in those taking moderate CYP3A4 inhibitors

Available forms: Ext rel tabs 500, 1000 mg

ADVERSE EFFECTS
CNS: *Headache, dizziness,* hallucinations

CV: Palpitations, QT prolongation, orthostatic hypotension
EENT: Tinnitus
GI: Nausea, vomiting, constipation, dry mouth
MISC: Peripheral edema
RESP: Dyspnea

INTERACTIONS
Individual drugs
Haloperidol, chloroquine, droperidol, pentamidine, arsenic trioxide, levomethadyl; CYP3A4 substrates (methadone, pimozide, QUEtiapine, quiNIDine, risperiDONE, ziprasidone): increased QT prolongation

Digoxin, simvastatin: increased action of digoxin, simvastatin

Diltiazem, dofetilide, ketoconazole, PARoxetine, quiNIDine, sotalol, thioridazine, verapamil, ziprasidone: increased ranolazine action, avoid using together

Drug classifications
Anti-retroviral protease inhibitors: increased ranolazine absorption, toxicity

Class IA/III antidysrhythmics, some phenothiazines, β-agonists, local anesthetics, tricyclics; CYP3A4 inhibitors (amiodarone, clarithromycin, erythromycin, telithromycin, troleandomycin); CYP3A4 substrates (methadone, pimozide, QUEtiapine, quiNIDine, risperiDONE, ziprasidone): increased QT prolongation; macrolides (clarithromycin, erythromycin, troleandomycin): increased QTc interval

Drug/herb
St. John's wort: decreased ranolazine level, do not use together

Drug/food
Do not use with grapefruit or grapefruit juice

NURSING CONSIDERATIONS
Assessment
- **Angina:** characteristics of pain (intensity, location, duration, alleviating/precipitating factors)
- Assess cardiac status: B/P, pulse, respiration
- **QT prolongation:** ECG for QT prolongation, ejection fraction; assess for chest pain, palpitations, dyspnea, torsades de pointes may occur
- Renal function: Assess serum creatinine, BUN, renal impairment may occur rapidly

Patient problem
Ineffective tissue perfusion
Risk for injury (uses, adverse reactions)

Implementation
- Use in combination with H2 blockers, metroNIDAZOLE, proton pump inhibitor, and clarithromycin for *H. pylori*

• **Ext rel tabs:** Do not break, crush, or chew tabs; give products as prescribed; do not double or skip dose
• Give bid, without regard to meals
• Do not use with grapefruit juice or grapefruit

Patient/family education
• Teach patient to avoid hazardous activities until stabilized on product, dizziness is no longer a problem
• Advise patient to avoid OTC drugs, grapefruit juice, drugs prolonging QTc (quiNIDine, dofetilide, sotalol, erythromycin, thioridazine, ziprasidone or protease inhibitors, diltiazem, ketoconazole, macrolide antibiotics, verapamil) unless directed by prescriber
• Advise patient to comply in all areas of medical regimen
• Teach patient to notify all health care providers of this product use
• Teach patient not to chew or crush
• Advise patient to notify prescriber of palpitations, dizziness, fainting, edema, dyspnea
• For acute angina take other products prescribed; this product doesn't decrease acute attack
• **Pregnancy/breastfeeding:** Identify if pregnancy is planned or suspected or if breastfeeding

Evaluation
Positive therapeutic outcome
• Decreased anginal pain, attacks and number of episodes

rasagiline (Rx)
(ra-sa'ji-leen)
Azilect
Func. class.: Antiparkinson agent
Chem. class.: MAOI, type B

ACTION: Inhibits MAO type B at recommended doses; may increase DOPamine levels

Therapeutic outcome: Improved symptoms in those with Parkinson's disease

USES: Idiopathic Parkinson's disease monotherapy or with levodopa

Pharmacokinetics

Absorption	35%-40%
Distribution	Protein binding >88%-94%
Metabolism	Liver, CYP1A2
Excretion	Kidneys, <1%
Half-life	1.3

Pharmacodynamics

Onset	Varies
Peak	1 hr
Duration	1 wk

CONTRAINDICATIONS
Breastfeeding, hypersensitivity to this product or MAOIs, pheochromocytoma

Precautions: Pregnancy, children, psychiatric disorders, severe hepatic disorders

DOSAGE AND ROUTES
Parkinson's disease
Monotherapy
Adult: PO 1 mg/day

Adjunctive therapy
Adult: PO 0.5 mg/day, may be increased to 1 mg/day; change of levodopa dose in adjunct therapy; reduced levodopa dose may be needed

Hepatic dose
Adult: PO 0.5 mg in mild hepatic disease

Concomitant ciprofloxacin, other CYP1A2 inhibitors
Adult: PO 0.5 mg; plasma concentrations of rasagiline may double

Available forms: Tabs 0.5, 1 mg

ADVERSE EFFECTS
Monotherapy
CNS: Drowsiness, hallucinations, depression, headache, malaise, paresthesia, vertigo, syncope
CV: Angina, hypertensive crisis (ingestion of tyramine products), orthostatic hypotension
GI: *Nausea*, diarrhea, dry mouth, dyspepsia
GU: Impotence, decreased libido
HEMA: Leukopenia
INTEG: Alopecia, skin cancers
MISC: Conjunctivitis, fever, flu syndrome, neck pain, allergic reaction, alopecia
MS: Arthralgia, arthritis, dyskinesia, falls
RESP: Rhinitis

INTERACTIONS
Individual drugs
Ciprofloxacin: increased levels of rasagiline up to twofold
Meperidine: do not give together; serious reaction

Drug classifications
Sympathomimetics: do not give; serious reaction including coma and death may occur

R

Antidepressants (tricyclics, SSRIs, SNRIs, mirtazapine, cyclobenzaprine): increased severe CNS toxicity, serotonin syndrome

CYP1A2 inhibitors (atazanavir, mexiletine, taurine): increased levels of rasagiline up to twofold

MAOIs: increased hypertensive crisis

Drug/herb
St. John's wort, yohimbe: do not use together

Drug/food
Do not use with food/liquids that contain large amounts of tyramine (cured meats, cheeses, pickled products)

Drug/lab test
Increased: LFTs
Decreased: WBCs

NURSING CONSIDERATIONS
Assessment
• **Assess for Parkinson's symptoms:** tremor, ataxia, muscle weakness and rigidity; baseline, periodically; assess for increased dyskinesia and postural hypotension if used in combination with levodopa

• Assess mental status: hallucinations, confusion, notify prescriber of significant reactions

• **Serotonin syndrome:** Assess for Agitation, coma, tachycardia, hyperreflexia, nausea, vomiting, may be precipitated in those taking SSRIs, SNRIs

• **Assess for hypertensive crisis:** severe headache, blurred vision, seizures, chest pain, difficulty thinking, nausea/vomiting, signs of stroke; any unexplained severe headache should be considered to be hypertensive crisis

• Monitor cardiac status: B/P, periodically, orthostatic hypotension during first 2 months of treatment

• **Tyramine products:** assess for foods, other medications, may lead to hypertensive crisis (tachycardia, bradycardia, chest pain, nausea, vomiting, sweating, dilated pupils)

Patient problem
Risk for injury (uses, adverse reactions)
Impaired mobility (uses)

Implementation
• Give with meals to prevent nausea; continuing therapy usually reduces or eliminates nausea; do not give with foods/liquids containing large amounts of tyramine

• Give reduced dose of carbidopa/levodopa cautiously

• **Renal failure:** in dialysis, increase dose slowly

Patient/family education
• Advise patient to change position slowly to prevent orthostatic hypotension

• Instruct patient to avoid hazardous activities until stabilized; dizziness can occur

• Advise patient to rinse mouth frequently, use sugarless gum to alleviate dry mouth

• Teach patient to take as prescribed, not to miss dose or double doses; take missed dose as soon as remembered if several hours before next dose

• Teach patient to prevent hypertensive crisis by avoiding tyramine foods >150 mg, give list to patient

• Teach patient to avoid CNS depressants, alcohol

• If drowsiness, daytime sleepiness, or falling asleep occurs, product may need to be discontinued

• Skin should be checked periodically for possible skin cancer, higher incidence in Parkinson's disease

• **Pregnancy/breastfeeding:** Identify if pregnancy is planned or suspected or if breastfeeding

Evaluation
Positive therapeutic outcome
• Improved symptoms in those with Parkinson's disease (decreasing tremors, ataxia, muscle weakness/rigidity)

⚠ HIGH ALERT

rasburicase (Rx)
(rass-burr'i-case)
Elitek, Fasturtec ✦
Func. class.: Enzyme
Chem. class.: Recombinant urate-oxidase enzyme

ACTION: Catalyzes enzymatic oxidation of uric acid into an inactive and a soluble metabolite (allantoin)

Therapeutic outcome: Decreased uric acid levels

USES: To reduce uric acid levels in leukemia, lymphoma, solid tumor malignancies who are receiving chemotherapy

Pharmacokinetics

Absorption	Complete
Distribution	Unknown
Metabolism	Unknown
Excretion	Unknown
Half-life	16-24 hr

Pharmacodynamics

Onset	Unknown
Peak	Unknown
Duration	Up to 12 hr

CONTRAINDICATIONS

Hypersensitivity

> **BLACK BOX WARNING:** ⚕ G6PD deficiency (Mediterranean, African descent), hemolytic reactions, or methemoglobinemia reactions to this product

Precautions: Pregnancy, breastfeeding, children <2 yr, anemia, acute bronchospasm, angina, patients of African or Mediterranean ancestry ⚕, hypotension

> **BLACK BOX WARNING:** Anaphylaxis, interference with uric acid measurements

DOSAGE AND ROUTES

Adult/adolescent/child/infant: IV INF 0.2 mg/kg as a single daily dose × 5 days

Available forms: Powder for inj 1.5, 7.5 mg/vial

ADVERSE EFFECTS

CNS: *Headache,* fever
CV: Chest pain, hypotension
GI: *Nausea, vomiting, anorexia, diarrhea, abdominal pain, constipation, dyspepsia, mucositis*
HEMA: Neutropenia with fever, hemolysis, methemoglobinemia
INTEG: *Rash*
MISC: Edema
SYST: Anaphylaxis, hemolysis, sepsis

INTERACTIONS

Individual drugs
Drug/lab

> **BLACK BOX WARNING:** Interference: uric acid

NURSING CONSIDERATIONS
Assessment

> **BLACK BOX WARNING:** Assess for anaphylaxis (dyspnea, urticaria, flushing, wheezing, swelling of lips, tongue, throat); have emergency equipment nearby

• Monitor blood studies: BUN, serum uric acid, urine CCr, electrolytes, CBC with differential before, during therapy
• Monitor temp; fever may indicate beginning infection; no rectal temp
• Assess for ⚕ G6PD deficiency, hemolytic reactions, methemoglobinemia; these patients should not be given this agent, screen patients who are higher risk for these disorders
• Assess GI symptoms: frequency of stools, cramping; if severe diarrhea occurs, fluid and electrolytes may need to be given

Patient problem

Diarrhea (adverse reactions)
Lack of knowledge of medication (teaching)

Implementation

Intermittent IV INF route

• Number of vials that are needed are based on weight and concentration required
• Reconstitute with diluent provided, add 1 ml of diluent/vial, swirl, withdraw amount needed and mix with 0.9% NaCl to final volume of 50 ml, use within 24 hr, give over 30 min, do not use filter, use different line, if not possible flush with ≥15 ml of NaCl before and after use
• Chemotherapy is started 4-24 hr after 1st dose

Patient/family education

• Advise of reason for therapy, expected results
• **Pregnancy/breastfeeding:** Identify if pregnancy is planned or suspected or if breastfeeding

Evaluation

Positive therapeutic outcome

• Decreased uric acid levels in children when antineoplastics causing high uric acid levels are used

---

> ⚠ **HIGH ALERT**
>
> ## regorafenib
> (re'goe-raf'e-nib)
> **Stivarga**
> *Func. class.:* Antineoplastic multikinase inhibitor
> *Chem. class.:* Signal transduction inhibitor (STI)

ACTION: Inhibits tyrosine kinase in patients with colorectal cancer

Therapeutic outcome: Decrease in spread or size of tumor

USES: Metastatic colorectal cancer in those who have received fluoropyrimidine, oxaliplatin, irinotecan-based chemotherapy, an ⚕ anti-VEGF therapy; and an anti-EGFR therapy if *KRAS* wild type

Pharmacokinetics

Absorption	Well
Distribution	Protein binding 99%
Metabolism	by CYP3A4, UGT1A0
Half-life	14–58 hr

Pharmacodynamics

Onset	Unknown
Peak	Unknown
Duration	Unknown

CONTRAINDICATIONS
Pregnancy

Precautions: Breastfeeding, children, geriatric patients, cardiac/renal/hepatic/dental disease, fistula, GI bleeding or perforation, bone marrow suppression, infection, wound dehiscence, thrombocytopenia, neutropenia, immunosuppression

> **BLACK BOX WARNING:** Hepatic disease

DOSAGE AND ROUTES
Adult: PO 160 mg/day with a low-fat breakfast × 21 days of a 28-day cycle, cycles may be repeated

Hepatic dose
Baseline mild (Child-Pugh class A) or moderate (Child-Pugh class B): No change; baseline severe hepatic impairment (Child-Pugh class C): use not recommended

Available forms: Tabs 40 mg

ADVERSE EFFECTS
CNS: Headache, tremor
CV: Hypertensive crisis, MI
EENT: Blurred vision, conjunctivitis
GI: Hepatotoxicity, GI hemorrhage, diarrhea, GI perforation, xerostomia
HEMA: Neutropenia, thrombocytopenia, bleeding
INTEG: Rash, alopecia
META: Hypokalemia
MISC: Fatigue, decreased weight, hand–foot syndrome, hypothyroidism

INTERACTIONS
Individual drugs
Simvastatin: Increased plasma concentrations of simvastatin
Warfarin: Increased plasma concentration of warfarin; avoid use; use low-molecular-weight anticoagulants instead

Drug classifications
CYP3A4 inhibitors (ketoconazole, itraconazole, erythromycin, clarithromycin): Increase: regorafenib concentrations
Calcium-channel blockers, ergots: Increased plasma concentrations of each product
CYP3A4 inducers (dexamethasone, phenytoin, carBAMazepine, rifampin, PHENobarbital): Decrease: regorafenib concentrations

Drug/food
Grapefruit juice; avoid use while taking product: Increased regorafenib effect

Drug/herb
St. John's wort: Decreased imatinib concentration

NURSING CONSIDERATIONS
Assessment

> **BLACK BOX WARNING: Hepatic disease:** fatal hepatotoxicity can occur; obtain LFTs baseline and at least every 2 wk × 2 mo, then monthly

- **Fatal bleeding:** Assess from GI, respiratory, GU tracts; permanently discontinue in those with severe bleeding
- Assess any wounds for healing, report wound dehiscence, stop medication, notify prescriber
- **Palmar–plantar erythrodysesthesia (hand–foot syndrome):** More common in those previously treated; assess for reddening, swelling, numbness, desquamation on palms, soles
- **GI perforation/fistula:** Discontinue if this occurs, assess for pain in epigastric area, dyspepsia, flatulence, fever, chills
- **Hypertension/hypertensive crisis:** Hypertension usually occurs in the first cycle in those with preexisting hypertension, do not start treatment until B/P is controlled; monitor B/P every wk × 6 wk, then at start of each cycle or more often if needed, temporarily or permanently discontinue for severe uncontrolled hypertension
- **Pregnancy:** To identify if patient is pregnant or if pregnancy is planned, identify contraception type in both men and women, do not use in pregnancy, breastfeeding

Patient problem
Risk of infection (adverse reactions)
Lack of knowledge of medication (teaching)

Implementation
- Store at 77°F (25°C)
- Give at the same time each day with a low-fat breakfast that contains less than 30% fat such as 2 slices of white toast with 1 TBSP of low-fat margarine and 1 TBSP of jelly, and 8 oz of skim milk; or 1 cup of cereal, 8 oz of skim milk, 1 slice of toast with jam, apple juice, and 1 cup of coffee or tea
- Swallow tablets whole
- If a dose is missed, take as soon as possible that day; do not take 2 doses on the same day
- **Hand–foot skin reaction:** Reduce to 120 mg (grade 2 palmar–plantar erythrodysesthesia); hold if grade 2 toxicity does

not improve in 7 days or recurs; hold for 7 days in grade 3 toxicity; reduce to 80 mg for recurrent grade 2 toxicity; discontinue if 80 mg is not tolerated
• **Hypertension:** Hold in grade 2 hypertension
• **Other severe toxicity (except hepatotoxicity):** Hold until toxicity resolves in grade 3 or 4 toxicity; consider the risk/benefits of continuing therapy in grade 4 toxicity, reduce dosage to 120 mg; if grade 3 or 4 toxicity recurs, hold until toxicity resolves, then reduce to 80 mg; discontinue in those who do not tolerate 80-mg dose

AST/ALT elevations during therapy:
For grade 3 AST/AST level elevations, hold dose; if therapy is continued, reduce to 120 mg after levels recover; discontinue in those with AST/ALT $>20 \times$ ULN; AST/ALT $>3 \times$ ULN and bilirubin $>2 \times$ ULN; recurrence of AST/ALT $>5 \times$ ULN despite a reduction to 120 mg

Patient/family education
• Teach patient to report adverse reactions immediately: bleeding, rash
• Teach patient the reason for treatment, expected results
• Advise patient that effect on male fertility is unknown
• Teach patient to take at same time of day with low-fat food, do not use grapefruit juice, take missed dose on same day, do not take multiple doses on the same day, keep in original container
• Teach patient to report immediately hepatic effects (yellowing skin, eyes, nausea, vomiting, dark urine), increase B/P, (severe headache); GI perforation/fistula (dyspepsia, flatulence, fever, chills, epigastric pain)
• **Pregnancy:** Not to use in pregnancy if suspected or if breastfeeding, men and women to use contraception during and for 2 mo after termination of treatment

Evaluation
Positive therapeutic outcome
• Decrease in spread or size of tumor

RARELY USED

reteplase
(re′te-plase)
Retavase
Func. class: Thrombolytic, plasminogen activator

USES: Acute MI

CONTRAINDICATIONS: Hypersensitivity, active internal bleeding, CVA, severe uncontrolled hypertension, intracranial/spinal trauma, aneurysm

DOSAGE AND ROUTES
Adult: IV 10 units, then 10 more units 30 min later

retapamulin topical
See Appendix B

retinoic acid
See tretinoin

revefenacin
(rev′ e-fen′ a-sin)
Yupelri
Func. class.: Respiratory muscarinic antagonists—long acting

ACTION: In the airways, it exhibits pharmacological effects through inhibition of the M3 receptor at the smooth muscle leading to bronchodilation

Therapeutic outcome: Prevention or relief of the symptoms of COPD

USES: Maintenance treatment of those with COPD

Pharmacokinetics

Absorption	Unknown
Distribution	Extensively distributed to tissues
Metabolism	Via hydrolysis to a metabolite
Excretion	Excreted 54% feces, 27% urine
Half-life	Of active metabolite 22-70 hr

Pharmacodynamics

Onset	Unknown
Peak	Unknown
Duration	Unknown

CONTRAINDICATIONS:
Hypersensitivity

PRECAUTIONS: Acute/paradoxical bronchospasm, acutely deteriorating COPD, acute symptoms, other anticholinergics, breastfeeding, cardiac disease, children, closed-angle glaucoma, dementia, driving or hazardous tasks, geriatrics, hepatic disease, ocular exposure, pregnancy, prostatic hypertrophy, urinary retention/obstruction

R

DOSAGE AND ROUTES
Adult: **INH** One 175 mcg vial (3 ml) once daily, by oral inhalation only

Available forms: 175 mcg/3 ml solution for inhalation

ADVERSE EFFECTS
CNS: Headache
Resp: Cough, nasopharyngitis, upper respiratory tract infection
MS: Back pain

INTERACTIONS
Drug classifications
Other anticholinergics: Increased: anticholinergic effect, avoid coadministration
OATP1B1, OATP1B3 inhibitors (rifampicin, cyclosporine): Increased revefenacin effect; avoid coadministration

NURSING CONSIDERATIONS
Assessment
• **Respiratory status:** Monitor lung sounds, pulse, B/P prior to and after product is given; note wheezing, shortness of breath, cough; monitor pulmonary function tests at baseline and periodically
• **Pregnancy/breastfeeding:** There are no well-controlled studies; animal studies showed no evidence of fetal harm; anticholinergics suppress lactation

Potential problem
Impaired gas exchange (uses)

Implementation
Oral inhalation route
• Give by oral inhalation via nebulizer only; do not swallow; no dilution necessary; single-dose vials are ready-to-use
• Only remove the unit-dose vial from the foil pouch immediately before use; product should be colorless; discard if the solution is not colorless
• Do not mix with other drugs
• Give the inhalation solution via a standard jet nebulizer connected to an air compressor, give over 8 min
• Discard the vial and any residual solution after use

Patient/family education
• Teach patient to contact healthcare provider if symptoms are not relieved or if shortness of breath continues or if bronchospasm occurs
• Teach patient to notify healthcare provider of all OTC Rx, herbals, and supplements taken; not to start or stop products without approval of provider
• Advise patient not to swallow during nebulization

• Inform patient that pulmonary function tests will be monitored periodically
• **Pregnancy/breastfeeding:** Teach patient to inform healthcare provider if pregnancy is planned or suspected or if breastfeeding

Evaluation
• Prevention or relief of the symptoms of COPD

Rh_o (D) immune globulin, standard dose IM
HyperRHO Full Dose, Rho Gam Ultra Filtered Plus
Rh_o (D) immune globulin microdose IM
HyperRHO S/D mini-Dose, MICRhoGAM, Mini-Gamulin R
Rh_o (D) immune globulin microdose (IM, IV)
Rhophylac, WinRho SDF
Rh_o (D) immune globulin IV

Func. class.: Immune globulins

ACTION: Suppresses immune nonsensitized Rh_o (D or D^u)-negative patients who are exposed to Rh_o (D or D^u)-positive blood

Therapeutic outcome: Absence of Rh factor and transfusion error

USES: Prevention of isoimmunization in Rh-negative women exposed to Rh-positive blood given after abortions, miscarriages, amniocentesis, chronic idiopathic thrombocytopenic purpura (Rhophylac)

Pharmacokinetics
Absorption	Complete (IV), Well (IM)
Distribution	Unknown
Metabolism	Unknown
Excretion	Unknown
Half-life	30 days

Pharmacodynamics
Onset	Rapid
Peak	Unknown
Duration	Unknown

CONTRAINDICATIONS
Previous immunization with this product, Rh_o (D)-positive/D^u-positive patient

BLACK BOX WARNING: Hemolysis

Precautions: Pregnancy

> **BLACK BOX WARNING:** Requires a specialized setting

DOSAGE AND ROUTES
RhoD immune globulin (IM only)
Adult and adolescent ≥16 yr: IM ([Hyper-RHO S/D] [full dose only]) 300 mcg at 28 wk gestation, repeat within 72 hr of delivery of confirmed Rho(D)-positive infant; IM/IV (WinRho SDF only) 300 mcg (1500 international units) at 28 wk gestation; if given earlier in pregnancy, give at 12-wk intervals during pregnancy, a 120-mcg (600 international units) dose; IM/IV should be given as soon as possible and preferably within 72 hr of delivery of a confirmed Rho(D)-positive infant

Massive fetomaternal hemorrhage (>15 ml)
Adult and adolescent ≥16 yr: IM (Rho-Gam) 20 mcg/ml of Rho(D)-positive fetal RBCs 300 mcg (1500 units) per every 15 ml of fetal blood cells or 30 ml of whole blood, multiple syringes may be injected IM at the same time in different sites, give within 72 hr of exposure, repeat dose within 72 hr of delivery; IM/IV (WinRho SDF only) if large fetomaternal hemorrhage is suspected, give IV 9 mcg (45 units) or IM 12 mcg (60 units) for every ml of fetal whole blood, give IV 600 mcg (3000 units) q8hr or IM 1200 mcg (6000 units) q12hr until total dose is given, total dose should be given within 72 hr of exposure

Threatened abortion at any stage of pregnancy
Adult and adolescent ≥16 yr: IM ([Hyper-RHO S/D] [full dose only]) 300 mcg (1500 units) as soon as possible; if given 13-18 wk gestation, give another 300 mcg (1500 units) at 26-28 wk gestation; repeat dose within 72 hr of delivery; IM (RhoGam only) 300 mcg (1500 units) as soon as possible and within 72 hr; IM/IV (Rhophylac only) 300 mcg (1500 units) as soon as possible and within 72 hr; IM/IV (WinRho SDF only) 300 mcg (1500 units) as soon as possible and within 72 hr, repeat dose at 12-wk intervals during pregnancy and 120 mcg (600 units) as soon as possible after delivery and within 72 hr

Termination of pregnancy, or ectopic pregnancy that occurs ≤12 wk gestation
Adult and adolescent ≥16 yr: IM (Minidose, HYperRHO Minidose, MICRORhoGAM only) 50 mcg (250 units) as soon as possible, give within 3 hr of spontaneous or surgical removal, if possible within 72 hr

Termination of pregnancy, or ruptured tubal pregnancy that occurs ≥13 wk
Adult and adolescent ≥16 yr: IM (full dose [HyperRHO S/D] RhoGAM only) 300 mcg (1500 units) as soon as possible and within 72 hr of event

Amniocentesis, chorionic villus sampling, abdominal trauma, ruptured tubal pregnancy up to 34 wk gestation
Adult and adolescent ≥16 wk: IM/IV (WinRho SDF only) 300 mcg (1500 units) within 72 hr, repeat at 12-wk intervals during pregnancy, give 120 mcg (600 units) as soon as possible and preferably within 72 hr of delivery

Available forms: Hyper RHO S/D solution for injection 1500 IU/prefilled syringe; MICRRho-GAM Ultra Filtered Plus Solution for inj 50 mcg/ml; RhoGam Ultra Filtered Plus Solution for inj 50 mcg; Rhophylac Pre-Filled Syringes Solution for inj 300 mcg/2 ml; WinRho SDF Liquid for inj

ADVERSE EFFECTS
CNS: Lethargy, dizziness, headache
CV: Hypo/hypertension
HEMA: Anemia, disseminated intravascular coagulation, intravascular hemolysis
INTEG: Irritation at inj site, fever
MISC: Infection, ARDS, anaphylaxis, pulmonary edema, DIC
MS: Myalgia

INTERACTIONS
Drug classifications
Live virus vaccines (measles, mumps, rubella): decreased antibody response to vaccine

NURSING CONSIDERATIONS
Assessment
• Assess for allergies, reactions to immunizations; previous immunization with this product
• **Intravascular hemolysis:** assess for back pain, chills, hemoglobinuria, renal insufficiency; usually when WinRho SDF is given in those with immune thrombocytopenia purpura
• Obtain type and cross-match of mother's blood and of neonate's cord blood; neonate must be Rh₀(D)-positive, mother must be Rh₀(D)-negative and (Dᵘ)-negative, medication should be given if there is a doubt

Patient problem
Lack of knowledge of medication (teaching)
Risk of injury (uses)

Implementation
• HyperRHO S/D, MICRRhoGAM, RhoGAM are given by IM only; do not give IV

- Rhophylac may be given IM or **IV**
- Inspect for particulate matter; do not use if particulate matter is present
- Do not confuse different types
- Reconstitution/dilution: no reconstitution or dilution is needed for (HyperRHO S/D), Rhophylac, MICRoGAM, RhoGAM, or the liquid formulation of WinRho SDF

IM route
- Use aseptic technique, observe for 20 min after administration
- Bring Rhophylac to room temperature before using
- Inject into the deltoid muscle of upper arm or anterolateral portion of the upper thigh; do not inject into gluteal muscle
- If dose calculated will need multiple vials or syringes, use different sites at the same time

IV route
- Use aseptic technique
- WinRhoSDF: remove entire contents of vial to obtain calculated dose; if partial vial contents are required for dosage calculation, withdraw the entire vial contents to ensure correct calculation; inf correct calculated dose over 3-5 min; do not inf with other fluids or products
- Rhophylac: bring to room temperature; inf by slow **IV**; observe for 20 min

Patient/family education
- Teach patient how product works; that product must be given after subsequent deliveries if subsequent babies are Rh-positive
- **Intravascular hemolysis:** Teach patient to report immediately: shaking, fever, chills, dark urine, swelling of hand or feet, back pain, SOB

Evaluation

Positive therapeutic outcome
- Prevention of $Rh_o(D)$ sensitization in transfusion error
- Prevention of erythroblastosis fetalis in subsequent $Rh_o(D)$-positive neonates

---

ribociclib
(rye-boe-sye′-klib)
Kisqali
Func. class.: Antineoplastic
Chem. class.: Protein kinase inhibitors

ACTION: A cyclin-dependent kinase (CDK) 4 and 6 inhibitor. Regulates cell cycle progression through phosphorylation of the retinoblastoma protein. The combination of ribociclib and an antiestrogen such as letrozole inhibited tumor growth more than either agent alone. It is a protein kinase inhibitor

USES: For the initial endocrine-based treatment of hormone receptor (HR)-positive, HER2-negative advanced or metastatic breast cancer in combination with an aromatase inhibitor in postmenopausal women

Absorption	Unknown
Distribution	Protein binding 70%
Metabolism	Extensively metabolized (CYP3A4)
Excretion	Unchanged drug 17% and 12% in feces and urine, respectively,
Half-life	29.7-54.7 hr/fecal excretion 97.1%

Pharmacodynamics

Onset	Unknown
Peak	1-4 hr
Duration	Unknown

CONTRAINDICATIONS
Hypersensitivity

Precautions: Breastfeeding, contraception requirements, hepatic disease, hepatotoxicity, infertility, neutropenia, pregnancy, pregnancy testing, reproductive risk, thromboembolic disease

DOSAGE AND ROUTES
Hormone receptor (HR)-positive, HER2-negative advanced or metastatic breast cancer
Adult: 600 mg qday on days 1 to 21, followed by 7 days of rest, in combination with letrozole (2.5 mg daily) or another aromatase inhibitor on days 1 to 28; repeat cycle q28days

Available forms: Tablets 200, 400, 600 mg

Therapeutic drug monitoring
Neutropenia:
- *ANC ≥ 1000 cells/mm³ (grade 2 or less):* No change
- *ANC 500 cells/mm³ to 999 cells/mm³ (grade 3):* Hold. For the first occurrence of grade 3 neutropenia, resume at the original dose level when the ANC returns to ≥ 1000 cells/mm³ (grade 2 or less); for recurrent grade 3 neutropenia, resume at the next lower dose level (reduce 600 mg to 400 mg; reduce 400 mg to 200 mg). If further dose reduction below 200 mg per day is required, discontinue
- *ANC <500 cells/mm³ (grade 4):* Hold. Resume at the next lower dose level when the ANC returns to ≥1000 cells/mm³ (grade 2 or

less) (reduce 600 mg to 400 mg; reduce 400 mg to 200 mg). If further dose reduction below 200 mg per day is required, discontinue

Neutropenic fever

• *ANC 500 cells/mm³ to 999 cells/mm³ (grade 3 neutropenia) with single episode of fever >38.3°C (or) above 38°C for more than 1 hr and/or concurrent infection:* Hold, resume at the next lower dose level when the ANC returns to ≥1000 cells/mm³ (grade 2 or less) (reduce 600 mg to 400 mg; reduce 400 mg to 200 mg). If further dose reduction below 200 mg per day is required, discontinue

QT prolongation

• *QTcF 481 to 500 msec and no serious arrhythmia:* Hold, monitor ECG frequently. For the first occurrence, resume at the same dose when QTcF prolongation resolves to ≤480 msec; for a recurrence of QTcF >480 msec, resume at the next lower dose level (reduce 600 mg to 400 mg; reduce 400 mg to 200 mg). If further dose reduction below 200 mg per day is required, discontinue

• *QTcF greater than 500 msec and no serious arrhythmia:* Repeat ECG. If the QTcF >500 msec on at least 2 separate ECGs at the same visit, hold; monitor ECG more frequently. Resume at the next lower dose level (reduce 600 mg to 400 mg; reduce 400 mg to 200 mg) when QTcF prolongation resolves to ≤480 msec. If further dose reduction below 200 mg per day is required, discontinue

• *QTcF >500 msec OR >60 msec change from baseline AND associated with torsades de pointes, polymorphic ventricular tachycardia, unexplained syncope, or signs/symptoms of serious arrhythmia:*

Hepatic dose

• *Mild hepatic impairment (Child-Pugh class A):* No change; *moderate to severe hepatic impairment (Child-Pugh class B or C):* Reduce the starting dose to 400 mg qday

• *AST/ALT greater than ULN to 3 times ULN (grade 1); total bilirubin less than 2 times ULN:* No change

• *AST/ALT 3.01 to 5 times ULN (grade 2); total bilirubin less than 2 times ULN:* If baseline hepatic impairment was grade 2, continue; monitor LFTs more frequently. If baseline was grade 0 or 1, hold. For the first occurrence of grade 2 hepatotoxicity, resume treatment at original dose, when AST/ALT resolve ≤ to baseline. For recurrent grade 2 hepatotoxicity, resume at the next lower dose level (reduce 600 mg to 400 mg; reduce 400 mg to 200 mg), monitor LFTs

more frequently. If further dose reduction below 200 mg/day is required, discontinue

• *AST/ALT greater than 3 times ULN (greater than grade 2); total bilirubin GREATER than 2 times ULN (irrespective of baseline; in the absence of cholestasis):* Discontinue AST/ALT 5.01 to 20 times ULN; (grade 3); total bilirubin less than 2 times ULN: Hold. For the first occurrence of grade 3 hepatotoxicity, resume at the next lower dose level when AST/ALT recover to ≤ baseline grade (reduce 600 mg to 400 mg; reduce 400 mg to 200 mg). monitor LFTs more frequently. If further dose reduction below 200 mg per day is required, discontinue. Discontinue for recurrent grade 3 hepatotoxicity

• *AST/ALT greater than 20 times ULN (grade 4); total bilirubin less than 2 times ULN:* Discontinue

Nephrotoxicity dosage adjustments

Serum creatinine (SCr) less than or equal to 3 times the upper limit of normal (ULN) or glomerular filtration rate (GFR) greater than or equal to 25% of the lower limit of normal (LLN) (grade 1 or 2): No change

SCr 3.01 to 6 times ULN or GFR less than 25% of LLN (chronic dialysis not indicated) (grade 3): Hold. For the first occurrence of a grade 3, resume at the original dose ≤ grade 1; for a recurrent grade 3, resume at the next lower dose level (reduce 600 mg to 400 mg; reduce 400 mg to 200 mg). If further dose reduction below 200 mg per day is required, discontinue

SCr greater than 6 times ULN or requiring chronic dialysis or renal transplant (grade 4): Discontinue

ADVERSE EFFECTS

CV: QT prolongation, peripheral edema
GI: Diarrhea, abdominal pain, anorexia, nausea, vomiting, constipation, stomatitis, weight loss
CNS: Fatigue, headache, insomnia
MS: Back pain
Dermatologic: *Alopecia, skin rash, pruritus*
HEMA: Leukemia, neutropenia
MISC: Infection

INTERACTIONS

Drugs known to prolong QT interval: Increased QT prolongation, avoid concomitant use
Strong or moderate CYP3A4 inhibitors- Increased ribociclib effect, avoid concomitant use, if cannot be avoided, reduce dose
Strong or moderate CYP3A4 inducers: Decreased ribociclib effect, avoid concomitant use

Drug/lab test
Increase: LFTs

Drug/food
To avoid pomegranate/pomegranate juice, and grapefruit/grapefruit juice

NURSING CONSIDERATIONS
Assessment
• **Hepatotoxicity:** Including elevated transaminases with or without an elevation in total bilirubin, may occur in combination therapy with ribociclib plus letrozole. Monitor LFTs baseline, q2wk for the first 2 cycles, before the next 4 cycles, and then as needed. A dose interruption, reduction, or discontinuation of therapy may be necessary. Use with caution in those with baseline hepatic disease; reduce dose in Child-Pugh class B or C hepatic disease
• **Bone marrow suppression:** Neutropenia is the most frequent. The median time to onset of grade 2 or higher neutropenia was 16 days, with the median time to resolution (to normalization or grade <3) of 15 days. Monitor a CBC baseline, q2wk for the first 2 cycles, before the next 4 cycles, and then as needed. A dose interruption, reduction, or discontinuation of therapy may be needed in those with an absolute neutrophil count (ANC) <1000 cells/mm³
• **Long QT syndrome:** Avoid the use in long QT syndrome, uncontrolled or significant cardiac disease (cardiac arrhythmias, recent MI, heart failure, unstable angina, bradycardia or bradyarrhythmias), electrolyte imbalance (hypomagnesemia, hypokalemia, hypocalcemia), with products causing prolonged QT interval or strongly inhibit CYP3A4, as this may lead to prolongation of the QTcF interval. Use with caution in conditions that increase the risk of QT prolongation (hypertension, CAD). Females, geriatric patients, diabetes mellitus, thyroid disease, malnutrition, alcoholism, or hepatic disease may also be at increased risk for QT prolongation. Assess ECG before starting therapy; do not start product if QTcF >450 msec. Repeat ECG at day 14 of the first cycle, at the beginning of the second cycle, and then as needed; prolongation of the QTcF interval may require interruption of therapy, dose reduction, or discontinuation of therapy. Monitor serum electrolytes (potassium, calcium, phosphorous and magnesium) baseline, at the beginning of the first 6 cycles, and as needed; correct electrolyte imbalances before starting product
• **Pregnancy/breastfeeding:** Avoid by females of reproductive potential during treatment and for at least 3 wk after the last dose, can cause fetal harm or death when used during pregnancy; discontinue breastfeeding during treatment and for 3 wk after the final dose. It is not known whether present in breast milk. Obtain a pregnancy test before starting treatment

Patient problem
Risk of injury (adverse reactions)

Implementation
• Take ribociclib and letrozole at the same time every day, preferably in the morning
• Swallow tablets whole; do not chew, crush, or split. Not to take if broken, cracked
• If a dose is missed, or if the patient vomits, do not replace the missed dose. Resume with the next scheduled daily dose

Patient/family education
• **Pregnancy/breastfeeding:** Teach patient not to use in pregnancy, breastfeeding, contraception should be used during and for at least 3 wk after last dose
• **Hepatotoxicity:** Teach patient should report immediately yellowing of skin or eyes, dark urine
• **QT Prolongation:** Teach patient the signs and symptoms of QT prolongation (irregular or rapid heartbeat, fainting). Advise to contact their health care provider immediately if any of these occur
• **Neutropenia:** Teach patient to immediately contact their health care provider if a fever occurs, usually may occur with an infection
• **Drug Interactions:** Teach patient to avoid pomegranate/pomegranate juice, and grapefruit/grapefruit juice; to avoid strong CYP3A inhibitors, strong CYP3A inducers, and drugs known to prolong the QT interval; all OTC/RX and herbals, supplements should be approved by provider

Evaluation
Positive therapeutic outcome
• Decrease in size of cancerous tumor

---

riboflavin (vitamin B₂) (OTC)
(rye'bo-flay-vin)
Func. class.: Vitamin B₂, water soluble

ACTION: Needed for respiratory reactions (catalyzes proteins) and for normal vision

Therapeutic outcome: Prevention or treatment of riboflavin deficiency

USES: Vitamin B₂ deficiency or polyneuritis; cheilosis adjunct with thiamine

Precautions: Pregnancy

Pharmacokinetics

Absorption	Well absorbed (by active transport)
Distribution	60% protein bound, widely distributed, crosses placenta
Metabolism	Unknown
Excretion	Kidneys (unchanged), excess amounts
Half-life	1-1½ hr

Pharmacodynamics

Unknown

DOSAGE AND ROUTES
Deficiency
Adult: PO 5-30 mg/day
Child ≥12 yr: PO 3-10 mg/day, then 0.6 mg/1000 cal ingested

RDA
Adult: PO (Males) 1.3 mg; (females) 1.1 mg

Available forms: Tabs 5, 10, 25, 50, 100, 250 mg

ADVERSE EFFECTS
GU: Yellow discoloration of urine (large doses)

INTERACTIONS
Individual drugs
Alcohol, probenecid: increased riboflavin need
Tetracycline: decreased action of tetracycline

Drug classifications
Antidepressants (tricyclics), phenothiazines: increased riboflavin need

Drug/lab test
False increase: urinary catecholamines

NURSING CONSIDERATIONS
Assessment
• Assess patient's nutritional status: liver, eggs, dairy products, yeast, whole grain, green vegetables
• Assess for vit B$_2$ deficiency: photophobia, cheilosis, stomatitis, ocular swelling
• **Pregnancy/breastfeeding:** Considered safe in pregnancy, breastfeeding at recommended dietary levels

Patient problem
Lack of knowledge of medication (teaching)

Implementation
• Give with food for better absorption
• Store in airtight, light-resistant container

Patient/family education
• Inform patient that urine may turn bright yellow

• Instruct patient about needed addition of foods that are rich in riboflavin

Evaluation
Positive therapeutic outcome
• Absence of headache; GI problems; cheilosis; skin lesions; depression; burning, itchy eyes; anemia

rifabutin (Rx)
(riff'a-byoo-tin)
Mycobutin
Func. class.: Antimycobacterial
Chem. class.: Rifamycin S derivative

Do not confuse: rifabutin/rifampin/rifapentine

ACTION: Inhibits DNA-dependent RNA polymerase in susceptible strains

Therapeutic outcome: Antimycobacterial death of *Escherichia coli, Bacillus subtilis;* mechanism of action against *Mycobacterium avium* unknown

USES: Prevention of *M. avium* complex (MAC) in patients with advanced HIV infection

Pharmacokinetics

Absorption	Well absorbed
Distribution	Widely distributed
Metabolism	Liver
Excretion	Kidney
Half-life	45 hr

Pharmacodynamics

Onset	Unknown
Peak	2-3 hr
Duration	Unknown

CONTRAINDICATIONS
Hypersensitivity, active TB, WBC <1000/mm^3, platelets <50,000/mm^3

Precautions: Pregnancy, breastfeeding, children, hepatic disease, blood dyscrasias

DOSAGE AND ROUTES
Adult: PO 300 mg/day (may take as 150 mg bid); max 600 mg/day

Renal dose
Adult: PO CCr <30 ml/min reduce dose by 50%

Available forms: Caps 150 mg

R

ADVERSE EFFECTS

CNS: *Headache,* fatigue, anxiety, confusion, insomnia
GI: *Nausea, vomiting, anorexia, diarrhea,* heartburn, hepatitis, discolored saliva, *Clostridium difficile*–associated diarrhea (CDAD)
GU: Discolored urine
HEMA: Hemolytic anemia, eosinophilia, thrombocytopenia, leukopenia
INTEG: *Rash*
MISC: Flulike syndrome, shortness of breath, chest pressure
MS: Asthenia, arthralgia, myalgia

INTERACTIONS
Individual drugs
Amprenavir, busPIRone, clofibrate, cycloSPORINE, dapsone, delavirdine, disopyramide, doxycycline, efavirenz, fluconazole, indinavir, ketoconazole, losartan, nelfinavir, nevirapine, phenytoin, quiNIDine, saquinavir, theophylline, zidovudine, zolpidem: decreased action of each specific product
Ritonavir: increased rifabutin level

Drug classifications
Anticoagulants, antidepressants (tricyclics), barbiturates, β-blockers, contraceptives (oral), corticosteroids, estrogens, sulfonylureas: decreased action of each specific product

Drug/food
High-fat foods: decreased absorption

Drug/lab test
Interference: folate level, vit B_{12}, BSP, gallbladder tests

NURSING CONSIDERATIONS
Assessment
• **Assess for active TB:** chest x-ray, sputum culture, blood culture, biopsy of lymph nodes, obtain PPD test; product should be given only for MAC and never for TB
• Monitor CBC for neutropenia, thrombocytopenia, eosinophilia
• **CDAD:** assess for diarrhea, abdominal pain, fever, fatigue, anorexia; possible anemia, elevated WBC and low serum albumin; stop product and usually give either vancomycin or IV metroNIDAZOLE, report immediately, may occur several weeks after discontinuing treatment

Patient problem
Infection (uses)
Nonadherence (teaching)

Implementation
• Give with meals to decrease GI symptoms; better to take on empty stomach 1 hr before or 2 hr after meals; high-fat food slows absorption, may take in 2 divided doses, may open capsule and mix with applesauce if unable to swallow whole
• Give antiemetic if vomiting occurs

Patient/family education
• Caution patient that compliance with dosage schedule and duration is necessary
• Instruct patient that scheduled appointments must be kept or relapse may occur
• Instruct patient to notify prescriber if hepatitis, neutropenia, or thrombocytopenia occurs: sore throat, fever, bleeding, bruising, yellow sclera, anorexia, nausea, vomiting, fatigue, weakness; myositis: muscle or bone pain
• **Hepatotoxicity:** Teach patient that decreased appetite, jaundice, dark urine, fatigue may occur to report immediately
• Advise patient that urine, feces, saliva, sputum, sweat, tears may be colored red-orange; soft contact lenses may become permanently stained
• **Pregnancy/breastfeeding:** Caution patients using oral contraceptives to use a nonhormonal method of birth control because rifabutin may decrease efficiency of oral contraceptives; to notify prescriber if pregnancy is planned or suspected, do not use in pregnancy, breastfeeding

Evaluation
Positive therapeutic outcome
• Decreased symptoms of *M. avium* in patients with HIV

---

rifampin (Rx)
(rif′am-pin)
Rifadin, Rofact ✽
Func. class.: Antitubercular
Chem. class.: Rifamycin B derivative

Do not confuse: rifampin/rifabutin/rifaximin

ACTION: Inhibits DNA-dependent polymerase, decreases tubercle bacilli replication

Therapeutic outcome: Bactericidal against the following organisms: mycobacteria, *Staphylococcus aureus, Haemophilus influenzae, Neisseria meningitidis, Legionella pneumophila*

USES: Pulmonary TB, meningococcal carriers (prevention)

Unlabeled uses: *Haemophilus influenzae* type B prevention in close contacts

---

Pharmacokinetics

Absorption	Well absorbed (PO), completely absorbed (**IV**)
Distribution	Widely distributed, crosses placenta
Metabolism	Liver—extensively
Excretion	Feces
Half-life	1-5 hr

Pharmacodynamics

	PO	IV
Onset	Rapid	Rapid
Peak	2-3 hr	Inf end
Duration	Unknown	Unknown

CONTRAINDICATIONS

Hypersensitivity to this product or rifamycins, active *Neisseria meningitidis* infection

Precautions: Pregnancy, breastfeeding, children <5 yr, hepatic disease, blood dyscrasias

DOSAGE AND ROUTES
Tuberculosis

Adult: PO/**IV** max 600 mg/day as single dose 1 hr before or 2 hr after meals, or 10 mg/kg/day 5 days/wk or 2-3 ×/wk

Child >5 yr: PO/**IV** 10-20 mg/kg/day as single dose 1 hr before or 2 hr after meals, max 600 mg/day, with other antitubercular products

6-mo regimen: 2-mo treatment of isoniazid, rifampin, pyrazinamide, and possibly streptomycin or ethambutol; then rifampin and isoniazid × 4 mo

9-mo regimen: Rifampin and isoniazid supplemented with pyrazinamide or streptomycin or ethambutol

Meningococcal carriers

Adult: PO/**IV** 600 mg bid × 2 days, max 600 mg/dose

Child >5 yr: PO/**IV** 10-20 mg/kg bid × 2 days, max 600 mg/dose

Infant 3 mo-1 yr: PO 5 mg/kg bid for 2 days

H. influenzae prophylaxis (unlabeled)

Adult: PO 600 mg/day × 4 days
Child: PO 20 mg/kg/day × 4 days
Neonates: PO 10 mg/kg/day × 4 days

Available forms: Caps 150, 300 mg; powder for inj 600 mg/vial

ADVERSE EFFECTS

CNS: Headache, fatigue, anxiety, drowsiness, confusion
EENT: Visual disturbances
GI: *Nausea, vomiting, anorexia, diarrhea,* Clostridium difficile–associated diarrhea (CDAD), *heartburn,* sore mouth and tongue, pancreatitis, elevated liver function tests
GU: Hematuria, acute renal failure, hemoglobinuria
HEMA: Hemolytic anemia, eosinophilia, thrombocytopenia, leukopenia
INTEG: Rash, pruritus, urticaria
MISC: Flulike syndrome, menstrual disturbances, edema, SOB, Stevens-Johnson syndrome, toxic epidermal necrolysis, angioedema, anaphylaxis, DRESS
MS: Ataxia, weakness
MISC: Staining of teeth, contact lens; coloring to urine, sweat, tears, sputum

INTERACTIONS
Individual drugs

Acetaminophen, alcohol, chloramphenicol, clofibrate, cycloSPORINE, dapsone, digoxin, diltiazem, doxycycline, haloperidol, NIFEdipine, phenytoin, theophylline, verapamil, zidovudine: decreased effect of specific product
Isoniazid: increased hepatotoxicity, alcohol, ketoconazole, pyrazinamide

Drug classifications

Anticoagulants, antidiabetics, barbiturates, benzodiazepines, β-blockers, contraceptives (oral), glucocorticoids, hormones, imidazole antifungals: decreased effect of each product
Protease inhibitors: do not use together

Drug/lab test

Increased: alk phosphatase, ALT, AST, uric acid, bilirubin, eosinophils
Increased: LFTs
Decreased: Hgb
Interference: folate level, vit B_{12}

NURSING CONSIDERATIONS
Assessment

• **Infection:** assess sputum culture, lung sounds, susceptibility tests baseline and periodically to determine effectiveness and resistance
• C&S should be performed before beginning treatment, during, and after therapy is completed
• Monitor liver function tests qmo: ALT, AST, bilirubin, decreased appetite, jaundice, dark urine, fatigue
• Monitor renal status: before, qmo: BUN, creatinine, output, specific gravity, urinalysis
• **CDAD:** assess for diarrhea, abdominal pain, fever, fatigue, anorexia; possible anemia, elevated WBC and low serum albumin; stop product and usually give either vancomycin or IV metroNIDAZOLE

• Monitor mental status often: affect, mood, behavioral changes; psychosis may occur
• **Serious skin reactions:** assess for fever, sore throat, fatigue, ulcers, lesions in mouth, lips, rash; can be fatal
• DRESS: Assess for rash, fever, large lymph nodes; discontinue product if these occur

Patient problem
Infection (uses)
Nonadherence (teaching)

Implementation
• Do not give IM or SUBCUT
PO route
• On empty stomach, 1 hr before or 2 hr after meals with a full glass of water; give with other products for TB
• Antiemetic if vomiting occurs
• Capsules may be opened and mixed with applesauce or gelatin

Intermittent IV INF route
• After diluting each 600 mg/10 ml of sterile water for inj (60 mg/ml), swirl, withdraw dose, and dilute in 100 ml or 500 ml of D₅W given as an inf over 3 hr, or if diluted in 100 ml, give over ½ hr; do not admix with other sol or medications

Y-site compatibilities: Amiodarone, bumetanide, midazolam, pantoprazole, vancomycin

Patient/family education
• Instruct patient that compliance with dosage schedule, duration is necessary, take on an empty stomach 1 hr before or 2 hr after food
• Instruct patient that scheduled appointments must be kept or relapse may occur
• Instruct patient to notify prescriber if hepatitis, neutropenia, or thrombocytopenia occurs: sore throat, fever, bleeding, bruising, yellow sclera, anorexia, nausea, vomiting, fatigue, weakness, diarrhea with pus, mucus, blood
• Advise patient that urine, feces, saliva, sputum, sweat, tears may be colored red-orange; soft contact lenses may be permanently stained
• **Pregnancy/breastfeeding:** Caution patients using oral contraceptives to use a nonhormonal method of birth control because rifabutin may decrease the efficiency of oral contraceptives, to notify prescriber if pregnancy is planned or suspected
• Advise patient to avoid alcohol; hepatotoxicity may occur

Evaluation

Positive therapeutic outcome
• Decreased symptoms of TB

rifaximin (Rx)
(rif-ax'i-min)
Xifaxan, Zaxine ✸
Func. class.: Misc. antiinfective
Chem. class.: Analog of rifampin

Do not confuse: rifaximin/rifampin

ACTION: Binds to bacterial DNA dependent RNA polymerase, thereby inhibiting bacterial RNA synthesis

Therapeutic outcome: Bacterial action against *E. coli*

USES: Traveler's diarrhea in those ≥12 yr old, caused by *E. coli*, hepatic encephalopathy, irritable bowel syndrome

Pharmacokinetics
Absorption	Low, systemic
Distribution	To GI tract
Metabolism	Induces CYP3A4
Excretion	Feces
Half-life	6 hr

Pharmacodynamics
Onset	Unknown
Peak	1-4 hr
Duration	Unknown

CONTRAINDICATIONS
Hypersensitivity to this product or rifamycins, diarrhea with fever, blood in stool

Precautions: Pregnancy, breastfeeding, children, geriatric patients

DOSAGE AND ROUTES
Traveler's diarrhea
Adult and child ≥12 yr: PO 200 mg tid × 3 days without regard to meals

Hepatic encephalopathy
Adult: PO 550 mg bid

IBS
Adults: PO 550 mg tid × 14 days, may give another two courses if recurrence

Available forms: Tabs 200, 550 mg

ADVERSE EFFECTS
CNS: Abnormal dreams, dizziness, insomnia, *headache*, fatigue, depression
CV: Hypotension, chest pain, peripheral edema, ascites

GI: *Abdominal pain, constipation, defecation urgency, flatulence, nausea, rectal tenesmus,* vomiting, ascites, *Clostridium difficile*–associated diarrhea (CDAD)

GU: Proteinuria, polyuria, increased urinary frequency

MISC: *Pyrexia,* motion sickness, tinnitus, rash, photosensitivity, exfoliative dermatitis

MC: Arthralgia, muscle pain, myalgia

RESP: Dyspnea, cough, pharyngitis

INTERACTIONS
Individual drugs
Afatinib: increased effect of afatinib

Drug classifications
P-glycoprotein inhibitors: Increased levels

Drug/lab test
Increased: LFTs, potassium
Decreased: blood glucose, sodium

NURSING CONSIDERATIONS
Assessment
• Assess for GI symptoms: amount and character of diarrhea, abdominal pain, nausea, vomiting; do not use in those with blood in stool, increased temperature with diarrhea
• Assess for overgrowth of infection and CDAD
• **Pregnancy/breastfeeding:** Do not use in first trimester, use only if benefits outweigh fetal risk, do not breastfeed, excretion unknown

Patient problem
Infection (uses)
Diarrhea (uses)

Implementation
• May be administered without regard to food

Patient/family education
• Instruct patient to discontinue rifaximin and notify prescriber if diarrhea persists for more than 24-48 hr, if diarrhea worsens, or if blood is in stools and fever is present
• Advise patient to avoid hazardous activities if dizziness occurs
• Teach patient to take without regard to food
• Teach patient to take as directed, to consume all of the product prescribed

Evaluation

Positive therapeutic outcome
• Absence of infection

rilpivirine
(ril-pi-vir′ine)
Edurant
Func. class.: Antiretroviral
Chem. class.: Non-nucleoside transcriptase inhibitors (NNTIs)

ACTION. Inhibits HIV-1 reverse transcriptase; unlike nucleoside reverse transcriptase inhibitors (NRTIs), it does not compete for binding nor does it require phosphorylation to be active. Binds directly to a site on reverse transcriptase; causing disruption of the enzyme's active site thereby blocking RNA-dependent and DNA-dependent DNA polymerase activities

Uses: HIV in combination with other antiretrovirals

Pharmacokinetics

Absorption	Increased effect 40% (food), decreased effect 50% (high protein drink)
Distribution	Protein binding (99.7%) to albumin
Metabolism	Via oxidation CYP3A system
Excretion	Feces 25% excreted unchanged (85%); urine (6.1%)
Half-life	Terminal elimination 50 hr

Pharmacodynamics

Onset	Unknown
Peak	4-5 hr
Duration	Unknown

CONTRAINDICATIONS
Hypersensitivity

Precautions: Pregnancy, breastfeeding, immune reconstitution syndrome, antimicrobial resistance, pancreatitis, depression, suicidal ideation, neonates, infants, children, adolescents <18 yr, QT prolongation, torsades de pointes, hyperlipidemia, hypertriglyceridemia, hypercholesterolemia

DOSAGE AND ROUTES
Human immunodeficiency virus (HIV) in combination with other antiretroviral agents
Adult/child ≥12 yr and ≥35 kg: PO 25 mg/day with a meal, if using with rifabutin also, increase rilpivirine dose to 50 mg qday; give with other antiretroviral agents.

Available forms: Tab 25 mg

ADVERSE EFFECTS
CNS: Depressed mood, dizziness, drowsiness, insomnia
GI: Hepatotoxicity
INTEG: Drug reaction with eosinophilia and systemic symptoms (DRESS)
MISC: Immune reconstitution syndrome

INTERACTIONS
Individual drugs
Aminoglutethimide, bexarotene, bosentan, efavirenz, flutamide, griseofulvin, metyrapone, modafinil, nafcillin, nevirapine, pioglitazone, primidone, ritonavir, topiramate: Decreased rilpivirine effect, treatment failure

Abarelix, alfuzosin, amiodarone, amoxapine, apomorphine, artemether, asenapine, chloroquine, ciprofloxacin, citalopram, cloZAPine, cyclobenzaprine, dasatinib, dolasetron, dronedarone, droperidol, eribulin, flecainide, fluconazole, gatifloxacin, gemifloxacin, haloperidol, iloperidone, lapatinib, levofloxacin, lopinavir, lumefantrine, maprotiline, mefloquine, moxifloxacin, nilotinib, norfloxacin, octreotide, ofloxacin, OLANZapine, ondansetron, paliperidone, palonosetron, pentamidine, posaconazole, QUEtiapine, ranolazine, saquinavir: Increased QT prolongation

Fluconazole, voriconazole: Increased rilpivirine adverse reactions, fungal infections

Drug classifications
CYP3A4 inducers (phenytoin, fosphenytoin, barbiturates, OXcarbazepine, carBAMazepine, rifabutin, rifampin, rifapentine, dexamethasone), proton pump inhibitors (PPIs): Decreased rilpivirine effect, treatment failure

H$_2$ receptor antagonists (cimetidine, famotidine, nizatidine, ranitidine): Decreased rilpivirine effect, treatment failure; give 12 hr before or 4 hr after rilpivirine

Antacids: Decreased rilpivirine effect; use 2 hr or more before, or 4 hr after rilpivirine

CYP3A4 inhibitors (aldesleukin, amiodarone, aprepitant, atazanavir, basiliximab, boceprevir, bromocriptine, chloramphenicol, clarithromycin, conivaptan, dalfopristin, danazol, darunavir, dasatinib, delavirdine, diltiazem, dronedarone, efavirenz, erythromycin, ethinyl estradiol, fluconazole, FLUoxetine, fluvoxaMINE, fosamprenavir, fosaprepitant, IL-2, imatinib, indinavir, isoniazid, itraconazole, ketoconazole, lanreotide, lapatinib, miconazole, nefazodone, nelfinavir, niCARdipine, octreotide, posaconazole, quiNINE, ranolazine, rifaximin, tamoxifen, telaprevir, telithromycin, tipranavir, troleandomycin, verapamil, voriconazole, zafirlukast): Increased rilpivirine effect

Class IA/III antidysrhythmics, some phenothiazines, beta agonists, local anesthetics, tricyclics, CYP3A4 inhibitors (amiodarone, arsenic trioxide, clarithromycin, erythromycin, levomethadyl, telithromycin, troleandomycin); CYP3A4 substrates (methadone, pimozide, QUEtiapine, quiNIDine, risperiDONE, ziprasidone), halogenated anesthetics: Increased QT prolongation

Drug/herb
St. John's wort: Decreased effect; do not use together

Drug/food
Increased adverse reactions: grapefruit juice

NURSING CONSIDERATIONS
Assessment
• **HIV:** Assess symptoms of HIV, including opportunistic infections before and during treatment; some may be life-threatening; monitor plasma HIV RNA, CD4+, CD8+ cell counts, serum β-2 microglobulin, serum ICD+24 antigen levels; treatment failures occur more frequently in those with baseline HIV-1 RNA concs >100,000 copies/ml than in patients with concs <100,000 copies/ml; monitor serum cholesterol, lipid panel, assess for redistribution of body fat

• Antiretroviral drug resistance testing before initiation of therapy in antiretroviral treatment-naive patients

• For adults and adolescents, initiation of antiretroviral therapy is recommended in any patient with a history of an AIDS-defining infection; with a CD4 ≤500/mm^3; who is pregnant; who has HIV-associated nephropathy; or who is being treated for hepatitis B (HBV) infection

• **DRESS:** May occur 2-8 wk, skin eruptions, eosinophilia, lymphadenopathy, fever, inflammation of internal organs, if these occur, report immediately, usually systemic steroids are given

• **Hepatic disease:** monitor for elevated hepatic enzymes (>2.5 × ULN); grade 3 and 4 may be higher in patients co-infected with hepatitis B or C

• **Pregnancy/breastfeeding:** Enroll pregnant patient in the Antiretroviral Pregnancy Registry 800-258-4263, do not breastfeed, excretion unknown, use nonhormonal contraceptive

Patient problem
Infection (uses)
Nonadherence (teaching)

Implementation
• Store at room temperature away from heat and moisture

Patient/family education
• Teach patient that product is not a cure but controls symptoms, that continuing use is required
• Teach patient that product must be taken in combination with other prescribed products, that if dose is missed, not to take if next dose is within 12 hr, to discuss all products taken including OTC, Rx, herbals, supplements, as there are many interactions
• Advise patient that dizziness may occur, not to drive until response is known
• Teach patient to report hypersensitivity reactions
• Teach patient to report if pregnancy is suspected immediately, do not breastfeed

Evaluation

Positive therapeutic outcome
• Control of HIV-related symptoms

risedronate (Rx)
(rih-sed′roh-nate)
Actonel, Actonel DR ✽, Atelvia
Func. class.: Bone resorption inhibitor
Chem. class.: Bisphosphonate

Do not confuse: Actonel/Actos

ACTION: Inhibits bone resorption; absorbs calcium phosphate crystal in bone and may directly block dissolution of hydroxyapatite crystals of bone

Therapeutic outcome: Increased bone mass, activity without fractures

USES: Paget's disease; prevention, treatment of osteoporosis in postmenopausal women; glucocorticoid-induced osteoporosis; osteoporosis in men

Pharmacokinetics

Absorption	Poor
Distribution	To bones (50%)
Metabolism	Unknown
Excretion	Kidneys, feces
Half-life	PO 23 hr, delayed release 56 hr ⅗ determined by poor metabolizers or average metabolizers

Pharmacodynamics

	PO	Del Rel
Onset	1 hr	Unknown
Peak	1 hr	3 hr
Duration	Unknown	Unknown

CONTRAINDICATIONS
Hypersensitivity to bisphosphonates, inability to stand or sit upright for ≥30 min, esophageal stricture, achalasia, hypocalcemia

Precautions: Pregnancy, breastfeeding, children, renal disease, active upper GI disorders, dental disease, hyperparathyroidism, infection, vitamin D deficiency, coagulopathy, chemotherapy, asthma

DOSAGE AND ROUTES
Paget's disease (Actonel)
Adult: PO 30 mg/day × 2 mo; give calcium and vit D if dietary intake is lacking; if relapse occurs, retreatment is advised

Treatment/prevention of postmenopausal osteoporosis
Adult: PO 5 mg/day or 35 mg qwk or 75 mg/day × 2 consecutive days 2 × mo or 150 mg qmo

Glucocorticoid osteoporosis
Adult: PO 5 mg/day

Osteoporosis in men
Adult: PO 35 mg qwk

Renal dose
Adult: PO CCr <30 mg/min, avoid use

Available forms: Tabs 5, 30, 35, 75, 150 mg; tab, weekly 35 mg

ADVERSE EFFECTS
CNS: Dizziness, headache, depression, *asthenia, dizziness, insomnia, weakness*
CV: Chest pain, hypertension, atrial fibrillation
GI: *Abdominal pain,* diarrhea, *nausea,* constipation, esophagitis
MS: *Severe muscle/joint/bone pain,* osteonecrosis of the jaw, fractures
MISC: Rash, UTI, pharyngitis, hypocalcemia, hypophosphatemia, increased PTH
SYST: Angioedema

INTERACTIONS
Drug classifications
Aluminum, antacids, calcium, iron, magnesium salts: decreased absorption of risedronate
NSAIDs, salicylates: increased GI irritation
H₂ antagonists, proton pump inhibitors: decreases absorption of delayed release risedronate; do not use together

R

✽ Canada only   ⅗ Genetic Warning   Adverse effects: *italics* = common; red = life-threatening

Drug/food
Food: decreased bioavailability; take ½ hr before food or drinks other than water

Drug/lab test
Decreased: calcium, phosphorus

NURSING CONSIDERATIONS
Assessment
• **Paget's disease:** assess for headache, bone pain, increased head circumference
• **Osteoporosis:** in men or postmenopausal women; bone density study prior to and periodically during treatment
• **Hypocalcemia:** assess for paresthesia, twitching, laryngospasm, Chvostek's/Trousseau's signs
• **Serious skin reactions:** assess for angioedema
• Assess for atrial fibrillation
• Monitor phosphate, alkaline phosphatase, calcium; creatinine, BUN (renal disease)
• **Hypercalcemia:** assess for paresthesia, twitching, laryngospasm, Chvostek's/Trousseau's signs
• Assess dental health, cover with antiinfectives prior to dental extraction
• **Beers:** Avoid use in older adults except for schizophrenia, bipolar disorder, or as a short-term antiemetic in chemotherapy

Patient problem
Risk for injury (uses)

Implementation
• Give PO for 2 mo to be effective in Paget's disease
• Give with a full glass of water; patient should be in upright position, give delayed release tablet in AM after breakfast, only use with food (delayed release)
• Administer supplemental calcium and vit D in Paget's disease
• Give daily ≥30 min before meals
• Store in cool environment out of direct sunlight

Patient/family education
• Advise patient to sit upright for ½ hr after dose to prevent irritation
• Teach patient to notify prescriber immediately if difficulty swallowing, severe heartburn, or pain in chest
• Instruct patient to comply with dietary restrictions, maintain good oral hygiene, exercise regimen
• Advise patient to notify prescriber if pregnancy is planned or suspected

Evaluation
Positive therapeutic outcome
• Increased bone mass, absence of fractures

risperiDONE (Rx)
(res-pare′a-done)
RisperDAL, Risperdal Consta, Risperdal M-TAB
Func. class.: Antipsychotic
Chem. class.: Benzisoxazole derivative

Do not confuse: RisperDAL/reserpine

ACTION: Unknown; may be mediated through both DOPamine type 2 (D_2) and serotonin type 2 (5-HT_2) antagonism

Therapeutic outcome: Decreased hallucinations and disorganized thought

USES: Irritability associated with autism, bipolar disorder, mania, schizophrenia

Pharmacokinetics
Absorption	Unknown
Distribution	Unknown
Metabolism	Liver, extensively
Excretion	Urine 90%
Half-life	3-24 hr

Pharmacodynamics
Onset	Unknown
Peak	1-2 hr
Duration	Up to 12 hr

CONTRAINDICATIONS
Hypersensitivity, seizure

Precautions: Pregnancy, children, geriatric, cardiac/renal/hepatic disease, breast cancer, Parkinson's disease, CNS depression, brain tumor, dehydration, diabetes, hematologic disease, seizure disorders, breastfeeding, abrupt discontinuation, suicidal ideation, phenylketonuria

> **BLACK BOX WARNING:** Increased mortality in elderly patients with dementia-related psychosis

DOSAGE AND ROUTES
Adult: PO 2 mg/day as a single dose or 2 divided doses, adjust dose at intervals of ≥24 hr and 1-2 mg/day as tolerated to 4-8 mg/day; IM establish dosing with PO prior to IM 25 mg q2wk, may increase to max 50 mg q2wk
Adolescent: PO 0.5 mg/day in AM or PM, adjust dose at intervals of ≥24 hr and 0.5-1 mg/day as tolerated to 3 mg/day
Geriatric: PO 0.5 mg daily-bid, increase by 1 mg qwk; IM 25 mg q2wk

---

Hepatic dose/renal dose
Adult: PO 0.5 mg, increase by 0.5 mg bid, then increase to 1.5 mg bid at intervals ≥1 wk

Available forms: Tabs 0.25, 0.5, 1, 2, 3, 4 mg; oral sol 1 mg/ml; orally disintegrating tabs 0.25, 0.5, 1, 2, 3, 4 mg; long-acting inj kit (Risperdal Consta) 12.5, 25, 37.5, 50 mg

ADVERSE EFFECTS
CNS: *EPS (pseudoparkinsonism, akathisia, dystonia, tardive dyskinesia), drowsiness, insomnia, agitation, anxiety, headache,* neuroleptic malignant syndrome, dizziness, seizures, suicidal ideation, head titubation (shaking)
CV: Orthostatic hypotension, tachycardia, heart failure, sudden death (geriatric), AV block
EENT: Blurred vision, tinnitus
GI: *Nausea,* vomiting, *anorexia, constipation,* jaundice, weight gain
GU: Hyperprolactinemia, gynecomastia, dysuria
HEMA: Neutropenia, granulocytopenia
MS: Rhabdomyolysis
MISC: Renal artery disease; weight gain, hyperprolactinemia (child)
RESP: Rhinitis, sinusitis, upper respiratory infection, cough

INTERACTIONS
Individual drugs
Alcohol: increased sedation
• Chloroquine, clarithromycin, droperidol, erythromycin, haloperidol, methadone, pentamidine, thioridazine, ziprasidone: increased QT prolongation
CarBAMazepine: increased risperiDONE excretion
Furosemide: increased risk of death in dementia-related psychosis
Levodopa: decreased levodopa effect
TraMADol: increased seizures
Valproic acid, verapamil: increased risperiDONE levels

Drug classifications
Acetylcholinesterase inhibitors, CYP2D6 inhibitors, SSRIs: increased risperiDONE levels
Antipsychotics: increased EPS
β-agonists, class IA/III antidysrhythmics, local anesthetics, some phenothiazines, tricyclics: increased QT prolongation
CNS depressants: increased sedation
CYP2D6 inducers (carBAMazepine, barbiturates, phenytoin, rifampin): decreased risperiDONE action
CYP2D6 inhibitors (selective serotonin reuptake inhibitors): serotonin syndrome, neuroleptic malignant syndrome

Drug/herb
Echinacea: decreased risperiDONE effect

Drug/lab test
Increased: prolactin levels, blood glucose, lipids

NURSING CONSIDERATIONS
Assessment
• Suicidal thoughts, behaviors often occur when depression is lessened; assess mental status: orientation, mood, behavior, presence and type of hallucinations before initial administration, monthly; this product should significantly reduce psychotic behavior
• Monitor thyroid function test, blood glucose, serum electrolytes/prolactin/lipid profile, bilirubin, creatinine, weight, pregnancy test, CBC, LFTs, AIMS assessment, and weight baseline periodically
• Assess affect, orientation, LOC, reflexes, gait, coordination, sleep pattern disturbances
• **QT prolongation:** Monitor B/P with patient in sitting, standing, and lying positions; take pulse and respirations q4hr during initial treatment; establish baseline before starting treatment; report drops of 30 mm Hg; obtain baseline ECG and monitor Q- and T-wave changes
• Check for dizziness, faintness, palpitations, tachycardia on rising; severe orthostatic hypotension is common
• **Assess for neuroleptic malignant syndrome:** hyperpyrexia, muscle rigidity, increased CPK, altered mental status; product should be discontinued
• **EPS:** Assess for akathisia (inability to sit still, no pattern to movements), tardive dyskinesia (bizarre movements of the jaw, mouth, tongue, extremities), pseudoparkinsonism (rigidity, tremors, pill rolling, shuffling gait); an antiparkinsonian product should be prescribed
• Assess for constipation, urinary retention daily; if these occur, increase bulk, water in diet
• Assess for weight gain, hyperglycemia, metabolic changes in diabetes, increased lipids
• **Pregnancy/breastfeeding:** EPS may occur in the neonate, enroll pregnant patient in the National Pregnancy Registry for Atypical Antipsychotics 866-961-2388, do not breastfeed, excreted in breast milk
• **Beers:** Avoid use in older adults except for schizophrenia, bipolar disorder, or as a short-term antiemetic in chemotherapy

Patient problem
Distorted thinking process (uses)
Risk for injury (adverse reactions)

Implementation
PO route
- Reduced dosage in geriatric patients
- Anticholinergic agent on order from prescriber, to be used for EPS
- Avoid use with CNS depressants
- Conventional tabs: give without regard to meals
- **Oral disintegrating tab** (Risperdal M-Tab): do not open blister pack until ready to use; tear 1 of the 4 units apart at perforation; peel back foil; do not push tab through foil; remove from pack and place on tongue; tab disintegrates in seconds and can be swallowed with or without liquids, do not split or chew
- **Oral solution:** may dilute 3-4 oz of a beverage, measure dose using calibrated pipette, not compatible with tea, cola; compatible with water, coffee, orange juice, low-fat milk

IM route
- Only use the diluent and needle provided; prior to admixing, allow to come to room temperature for 30 minutes prior to reconstitution
- Remove colored cap from the vial without removing rubber stopper. Wipe top of the grey stopper with an alcohol wipe
- Peel back the blister pouch and remove the Vial Access Device by holding between the white luer cap and the skirt. Do not touch the spike tip at any time
- Place the vial on a hard surface and hold the base. Orient the Vial Access Device vertically over the vial so that the spike tip is at the center of the vial's rubber stopper
- With a straight downward push, press the spike tip of the Vial Access Device through the center of the vial's rubber stopper until the device securely snaps onto the vial top
- Hold the base of the vial and swab the syringe connection point (blue circle) of the Vial Access Device with an alcohol wipe and allow to dry prior to attaching the syringe
- While holding the white collar of the syringe, insert and press the syringe tip into the blue circle of the Vial Access Device and twist.
- Inject the entire contents of the syringe containing the diluent into the vial
- Shake the vial vigorously while holding the plunger rod down with the thumb. Mixing is complete when the suspension appears uniform, thick, and milky colored, and all the powder is dispersed in liquid. The microspheres will be visible in liquid, but no dry microspheres remain
- Invert the vial and withdraw the entire content of the suspension from the vial into the syringe. Tear the section of the vial label at the perforation and apply the detached label to the syringe for ID
- While holding the white collar of the syringe, unscrew the syringe from the Vial Access Device, then discard both the vial and the Vial Access Device
- Select the appropriate color-coded needle provided with the kit. Two distinct needles are provided. The needle with the yellow colored hub and print is for injection into the gluteal (2-inch needle) and the needle with the green colored hub and print is for deltoid (1-inch needle). They are not interchangeable; do not use the needle intended for gluteal injection for deltoid injection, and vice versa
- Peel the blister pouch of the Needle-Pro safety device open halfway. Grasp the transparent needle sheath using the plastic peel pouch. To prevent contamination, do not touch the orange Needle-Pro safety device's luer connector. While holding the white collar of the syringe, attach the luer connection of the orange Needle-Pro safety device to the syringe with an easy clockwise twisting motion
- While holding the white collar of the syringe, grasp the transparent needle sheath and seat the needle firmly on the orange Needle-Pro safety device with a push and a clockwise twist. Seating the needle will secure the connection between the needle and the orange Needle-Pro safety device
- Re-suspend the microspheres in the syringe by shaking vigorously

Patient/family education
- Teach patient to use good oral hygiene; frequent rinsing of mouth, sugarless gum for dry mouth
- Caution patient to avoid hazardous activities until product response is determined; dizziness, blurred vision may occur
- Inform patient that orthostatic hypotension occurs often; patient should rise from sitting or lying position gradually and remain lying down for at least 30 min after IM inj
- Instruct patient to avoid hot tubs, hot showers, tub baths; hypotension may occur
- Inform patient that heat stroke may occur in hot weather and to take extra precautions to stay cool
- Advise patient to avoid abrupt withdrawal of this product, or EPS may result; product should be withdrawn slowly
- Teach patient to avoid OTC preparations (cough, hay fever, cold) unless approved by prescriber; serious product interactions may occur; avoid use with alcohol, CNS depressants because increased drowsiness may occur

---

- Teach patient to notify provider of suicidal thoughts/behaviors
- Advise patient to use contraception, to inform prescriber if pregnancy is planned or suspected

Evaluation
Positive therapeutic outcome
- Decrease in emotional excitement, hallucinations, delusions, paranoia
- Reorganization of patterns of thought, speech

TREATMENT OF OVERDOSE:
Lavage, provide airway

ritonavir (Rx)
(ri-toe′na-veer)

Norvir

Func. class.: Antiretroviral
Chem. class.: Protease inhibitor

Do not confuse: ritonavir/retrovir

ACTION: Inhibits HIV-1 protease and prevents maturation of the infectious virus

Therapeutic outcome: Improvement of HIV-1 infection

USES: HIV-1 in combination with at least 2 other antiretrovirals

Pharmacokinetics

Absorption	Well
Distribution	Unknown
Metabolism	98% protein binding, liver
Excretion	Unknown
Half-life	3-5 hr

Pharmacodynamics

Onset	Unknown
Peak	2-4 hr
Duration	Unknown

CONTRAINDICATIONS
Hypersensitivity

BLACK BOX WARNING: Coadministration with other drugs

Precautions: Pregnancy, breastfeeding, children, liver disease, pancreatitis, diabetes, hemophilia, AV block, hypercholesterolemia, immune reconstitution syndrome, neonates, cardiomyopathy, immune reconstitution syndrome

DOSAGE AND ROUTES
Adult/adolescent >16 yr: PO 600 mg bid; if nausea occurs, begin dose at ½ and gradually increase, max 1200 mg/day in divided doses

Adolescent ≤16 yr/child/infant: PO 400 mg/m² bid up to 1200 mg/day in divided doses; may start lower and escalate

Available forms: Caps 100 mg; oral sol 80 mg/ml, tab 100 mg

ADVERSE EFFECTS
CNS: *Paresthesia*, headache, seizures, dizziness, insomnia, fever, asthenia, intracranial bleeding
CV: QT, PR interval prolongation
GI: *Diarrhea*, buccal mucosa ulceration, *abdominal pain*, *nausea*, *taste perversion*, dry mouth, *vomiting*, *anorexia*, pancreatitis, pseudomembranous colitis, hepatitis
HEMA: leukopenia, thrombocytopenia
INTEG: Rash
MISC: Asthenia, angioedema, anaphylaxis, Stevens-Johnson syndrome, increased lipids, lipodystrophy, toxic epidermal necrolysis, immune reconstitution syndrome
MS: Pain, rhabdomyolysis, myalgia

INTERACTIONS
Individual drugs

BLACK BOX WARNING: Amiodarone, astemizole, buPROPion, cisapride, cloZAPine, desipramine, encainide, ergotamine, flecainide, meperidine, midazolam, pimozide, piroxicam, propafenone, propoxyphene, quiNIDine, ranolazine, saquinavir, terfenadine, triazolam, zolpidem: toxicity, do not use together

Atovaquone, divalproex, ethinyl estradiol, lamoTRIgine, phenytoin, sulfamethoxazole, theophylline, voriconazole, zidovudine: decreased levels of each drug
Bosentan: increased levels of bosentan
Clarithromycin: increased level of both products
ddI: increased levels of both products
Fluconazole: increased ritonavir level

BLACK BOX WARNING: Haloperidol, chloroquine, droperidol, pentamidine, arsenic trioxide, levomethadyl: increased QT prolongation

Nevirapine, phenytoin: decreased ritonavir levels

Drug classifications
Anticoagulants: decreased levels of anticoagulants
Azole antifungals, benzodiazepines, HMG-CoA reductase inhibitors, interleukins: toxicity, do not use together
Barbiturates, rifamycins: decreased ritonavir level

R

BLACK BOX WARNING: Class IA/III antidysrhythmics, some phenothiazines, β-agonists, local anesthetics, tricyclics, CYP3A4 inhibitors (amiodarone, clarithromycin, erythromycin, telithromycin, troleandomycin), CYP3A4 substrates (dasatinib, methadone, pimozide, QUEtiapine, quiNIDine, risperiDONE, ziprasidone): increased QT prolongation

CYP2D6 inhibitors: toxicity, do not use together

Drug/herb
Red yeast rice: avoid use
St. John's wort: decreased ritonavir levels, avoid concurrent use

Drug/lab test
Increased: ALT, GGT, AST, CK, cholesterol, triglycerides, uric acid
Decreased: Hct, RBC, Hgb, neutrophils, WBC

NURSING CONSIDERATIONS
Assessment
• **HIV:** Monitor viral load and CD4, blood glucose, plasma HIV RNA, serum cholesterol, lipid profile baseline, throughout therapy; resistance testing prior to starting therapy and after treatment failure
• **QT prolongation:** ECG for QT prolongation, ejection fraction; assess for chest pain, palpitations, dyspnea
• **Rhabdomyolysis:** muscle pain, increased CPK, weakness, swelling of affected muscles, dark urine; if these occur and if confirmed by CPK, product should be discontinued
• **Immune reconstitution syndrome:** may occur with combination therapy, may develop inflammatory response with opportunistic infection (MAC, Graves disease, Guillain-Barré syndrome, TB, PCP), may occur during initial treatment or months afterward
• Assess signs of infection, anemia
• Assess liver function tests: ALT, AST; in those with hepatic disease, monitor q3mo
• Monitor C&S before product therapy; product may be taken as soon as culture is done; repeat C&S after treatment; determine the presence of other STDs
• Assess bowel pattern before, during treatment; if severe abdominal pain with bleeding occurs, product should be discontinued; monitor hydration

• **Serious skin disorders:** Assess for Stevens-Johnson syndrome, angioedema; anaphylaxis, toxic epidermal necrolysis
• **Pregnancy/breastfeeding:** Enroll pregnant patient in the Antiretroviral Pregnancy Registry 800-258-4263, do not breastfeed

Patient problem
Infection (uses)
Nonadherence (teaching)

Implementation
• Oral sol: Shake oral sol well, use calibrated measuring device
• Store caps in refrigerator
• Mix liquid formulation with chocolate milk or liquid nutritional supplement to improve taste
• When switching from cap to tab, more GI symptoms may occur that will lessen over time
• Use dosage titration to minimize side effects
• Overdose: infants, children 43.2% alcohol, 26.57% propylene glycol oral solution, calculate total amount of alcohol, propylene glycol from all products given

Patient/family education
• Teach patient to take as prescribed; if dose is missed, take as soon as remembered up to 1 hr before next dose; do not double dose
• Teach patient that product must be taken in equal intervals around the clock to maintain blood levels for duration of therapy
• Teach patient that product is not a cure for HIV; opportunistic infections may continue to be acquired, and others may continue to contract HIV from the patient

BLACK BOX WARNING: Advise patient to avoid other Rx, OTC meds, herbs, supplements unless approved by prescriber, not to use St. John's wort, that it decreases this product's effect

• Inform that redistribution of body fat or accumulation of body fat may occur

Evaluation
Positive therapeutic outcome
• Decreasing symptoms of HIV
• Improving viral load and CD4 cell counts

---

750 mg/m² on day 1, vinCRIStine **IV** 1.4 mg/m² (max of 2 mg) on day 1, and predniSONE 40 mg/m²/day **PO** on days 1-5

Follicular, CD20-positive, B-cell non-Hodgkin's lymphoma (NHL) (complete or partial response)
Adult: **IV** 375 mg/m² **IV** q8wk × 12 doses as maintenance therapy starting 8 wk after the completion of induction chemotherapy with 8 doses of riTUXimab with 6-8 cycles of cyclophosphamide, vinCRIStine, and predniSONE 4-6 cycles of cyclophosphamide, DOXOrubicin, vinCRIStine, and predniSONE

As a component of the Zevalin (ibritumomab tiuxetan) regimen
Adult: **IV**; as a required component of the ibritumomab regimen; riTUXimab 250 mg/m² given within 4 hr prior to the administration of Yttrium-90 ibritumomab that may occur on day 7, 8, or 9

First-line treatment of diffuse large B-cell, non-Hodgkin's lymphoma (NHL)
Adult 18-59 yr: **IV** 375 mg/m² on day 1 of each cycle for up to 8 infusions

Low-grade, CD20-positive, B-cell non-Hodgkin's lymphoma (NHL)
Adult: **IV** 375 mg/m² qwk × 4 wk repeated q6mo × 2 years (total of 16 doses) as maintenance therapy starting 4 wk after the completion of first-line chemotherapy with 6 to 8 cycles of cyclophosphamide, vinCRIStine, and predniSONE (CVP)

Rheumatoid arthritis
Adult: **IV** infusion 1000 mg initially, then another 1000 mg in 2 wk

GPA/MPA
Adult: **IV** 375 mg/m² qwk × 4 wk

Available forms: Inj 10 mg/ml (100 mg/10 ml, 500 mg/50 ml)

ADVERSE EFFECTS
CNS: Life-threatening brain infection (progressive multifocal leukoencephalopathy)
CV: Cardiac dysrhythmias, heart failure, MI, superventricular tachycardia, hypertension, angina
GI: *Nausea, vomiting, anorexia,* GI obstruction/perforation
GU: Renal failure
HEMA: Leukopenia, neutropenia, thrombocytopenia, anemia

⚠ HIGH ALERT
riTUXimab (Rx)
(rih-tuks´ih-mab)
Rituxan
Func. class.: Antineoplastic—miscellaneous; DMARD
Chem. class.: Murine/human monoclonal antibody

ACTION: Directed against the CD20 antigen that is found on malignant B lymphocytes; CD20 regulates a portion of cell cycle initiation/differentiation

Therapeutic outcome: Decreased tumor size, prevention of spread of cancer

USES: Non-Hodgkin's lymphoma ✏ (CD20 positive, B-cell), bulky disease (tumors >10 cm), rheumatoid arthritis, Wegener's granulomatosis, microscopic polyangiitis

Pharmacokinetics

Absorption	Unknown
Distribution	Binds to CD20 sites on lymphoma cells
Metabolism	Unknown
Excretion	Unknown
Half-life	Varies

Pharmacodynamics
Unknown

CONTRAINDICATIONS
Hypersensitivity, murine proteins

Precautions: Pregnancy, breastfeeding, children, geriatric, cardiac/renal/pulmonary conditions

> **BLACK BOX WARNING:** Exfoliative dermatitis, infusion-related reactions, progressive multifocal leukoencephalopathy, hepatitis B exacerbation

DOSAGE AND ROUTES
Relapsed or refractory low-grade or follicular, CD20 positive, B-cell non-Hodgkin's lymphoma (NHL)
Adult: **IV** 375 mg/m² qwk × 4 doses, may retreat with 4 more doses of 375 mg/m² qwk

First-line treatment of follicular, CD20-positive, B-cell non-Hodgkin's lymphoma (NHL), in combination with chemotherapy
Adult: **IV** 375 mg/m² on day 1 of each cycle for up to 8; may be given with cyclophosphamide **IV**

INTEG: *Irritation at inj site, rash,* fatal mucocutaneous infections (rare)
MISC: *Fever,* chills, asthenia, *headache,* angioedema, hypotension, myalgia, bronchospasm, ARDs
SYST: Stevens-Johnson syndrome, exfoliative dermatitis, toxic epidermal necrolysis, tumor lysis syndrome
META: Hyperkalemia, hypocalcemia, hyperphosphatemia

INTERACTIONS
Individual drugs
CISplatin: increased nephrotoxicity—avoid concurrent use; if used, monitor renal status
Drug classifications
Anticoagulants, NSAIDs: increased bleeding risk
Antihypertensives: increased hypotension, separate by 12 hr

NURSING CONSIDERATIONS
Assessment

> **BLACK BOX WARNING:** Assess for signs of fatal inf reaction: hypoxia, pulmonary infiltrates, ARDS, MI, ventricular fibrillation, cardiogenic shock; most fatal inf reactions occur with first inf, discontinue product

> **BLACK BOX WARNING: Hepatitis B exacerbation or fulminant hepatitis,** hepatic failure, death may occur during or after treatment, screen all patients for HBV (HBsAg and HBc titers) before use, monitor those with current or prior HBV for signs of hepatitis or HBV reactivation for several months after therapy, if reactivation occurs, discontinue product

> **BLACK BOX WARNING:** Assess for signs of **severe mucocutaneous reactions**: Stevens-Johnson syndrome, lichenoid dermatitis, toxic epidermal lysis; signs occur 1-13 wk after product was given, discontinue treatment immediately

> **BLACK BOX WARNING:** Assess for **tumor lysis syndrome:** acute renal failure requiring hemodialysis, hyperkalemia, hypocalcemia, hyperuricemia, hyperphosphatasemia; allopurinol and adequate hydration may be needed

> **BLACK BOX WARNING: Multifocal leukoencephalopathy:** confusion, dizziness, lethargy, hemiparesis, monitor periodically

• Monitor CBC, differential, platelet count weekly; withhold product if WBC is <3500/mm³ or platelet count <100,000/mm³; notify prescriber of these results; product should be discontinued
• Monitor ECG, serum creatinine/BUN, electrolytes, uric acid; correct electrolyte imbalances before use, hyperkalemia, hypocalcemia, hyperphosphatemia occur often
• Assess GI symptoms: frequency of stools, abdominal pain, perforation/obstruction may occur
• **Infection:** assess for fever, increased temperature, flulike symptoms in those with WG and MPA, in those using DMARDs
• **Pregnancy/breastfeeding:** Contraception should be used, enroll pregnant patient in the Mother To Baby Autoimmune Diseases Study 877-311-8972 (patients with rheumatoid arthritis); do not breastfeed, excretion unknown

Patient problem
Risk for infection (uses)
Risk for injury (adverse reactions)

Implementation
Intermittent IV infusion route
• Hold antihypertensive 2 hr before administration
• Administer after diluting to a final conc of 1-4 mg/ml; use 0.9% NaCl, D₅W, gently invert bag to mix; do not mix with other products
• Increase fluid intake to 2-3 L/day to prevent dehydration, unless contraindicated
• Store vials at 36° F-40° F; protect vials from direct sunlight; inf sol is stable at 36° F-46° F for 24 hr and at room temp for another 12 hr

Y-site compatibilities: Acyclovir, amifostine, amikacin, aminophylline, ampicillin, ampicillin/sulbactam, aztreonam, bleomycin, bumetanide, buprenorphine, busulfan, butorphanol, calcium gluconate, CARBOplatin, carmustine, ceFAZolin, cefoperazone, cefotaxime, cefoTEtan, cefOXitin, cefTAZidime, ceftizoxime, cefTRIAXone, cefuroxime, chlorproMAZINE, cimetidine, CISplatin, clindamycin, cyclophosphamide, cytarabine, DACTINomycin, DAUNOrubicin hydrochloride, dexamethasone, dexrazoxane, digoxin, diphenhydrAMINE, DOBUTamine, DOCEtaxel, DOPamine, DOXOrubicin liposome, doxycycline, droperidol, enalaprilat, etoposide phosphate, famotidine, fentaNYL, filgrastim, floxuridine, fluconazole, fludarabine, fluorouracil, ganciclovir, gemcitabine, gentamicin, granisetron, haloperidol, heparin, hydrocortisone, HYDROmorphone, IDArubicin, ifosfamide, imipenem/cilastatin, irinotecan, leucovorin, levorphanol, LORazepam, magnesium sulfate, mannitol, meperidine, mesna, methotrexate, methylPREDNISolone, metoclopramide, metroNIDAZOLE, mitoMYcin, mitoXANtrone, morphine, nalbuphine, netilmicin, PACLitaxel, pentamidine, piperacillin/tazobactam, plicamycin, potassium chloride, prochlorperazine, promethazine, ranitidine, sargramostim, streptozocin, teniposide, theophylline, thiotepa, ticarcillin/clavulanate, tobramycin, trimethoprim/sulfamethoxazole, trimethobenzamide, vinBLAStine, vinCRIStine, vinorelbine, zidovudine

Additive incompatibilities: Do not admix with other products

Patient/family education
• Advise patient to report to prescriber possible infection (cough, fever, chills, sore throat), renal issues (painful urination, back/side pain), bleeding (gums, stools, bruising, urine, emesis, fatigue), chest pain
• Advise to avoid OTC products
• Avoid use with vaccines, toxoids
• Advise patient to increase fluid intake
• Teach to use contraception during and up to 12 mo after therapy

Evaluation

Positive therapeutic outcome
• Prevention of increasing cancer progression

⚠ HIGH ALERT

rivaroxaban
(ri-va-rox′a-ban)
Xarelto
Func. class.: Anticoagulant
Chem. class.: Factor Xa inhibitor

ACTION: A novel, oral anticoagulant that selectively and potently inhibits coagulation factor Xa

Therapeutic outcome: Prevention of DVT, stroke, and systemic embolism

USES: For deep venous thrombosis (DVT) prophylaxis, pulmonary embolism (PE), in patients undergoing knee or hip replacement surgery; for stroke prophylaxis and systemic embolism prophylaxis in patients with nonvalvular atrial fibrillation

Pharmacokinetics

Absorption	80%-100%
Distribution	Protein binding (92%-95%)
Metabolism	Oxidative degradation
Excretion	Urine (66%), feces (17%)
Half-life	5-9 hr; geriatric: 11-13 hr

Pharmacodynamics

Onset	Unknown
Peak	2-4 hrs
Duration	Unknown

CONTRAINDICATIONS
Severe hypersensitivity

Precautions: Moderate or severe hepatic disease (Child-Pugh Class B or C), hepatic disease associated with coagulopathy, creatinine clearance <30 ml/min for use as DVT prophylaxis and <15 ml/min for stroke and systemic embolism prophylaxis in nonvalvular atrial fibrillation, dental procedures, neonates, infants, children, adolescents, pregnancy aneurysm, diabetes retinopathy, breastfeeding, diverticulitis, endocarditis, geriatrics, GI bleeding, hypertension, obstetric delivery, peptic ulcer disease, stroke, surgery

DOSAGE AND ROUTES
Deep venous thrombosis (DVT) prophylaxis, (knee or hip replacement surgery)
Administer the initial dose at least 6–10 hr after surgery once hemostasis has been established
Adult: PO 10 mg daily for 12 days after knee replacement surgery or for 35 days after hip replacement

Stroke prophylaxis and systemic embolism prophylaxis (nonvalvular atrial fibrillation)
Adult: PO 20 mg daily with the evening meal (CrCl > 50 ml/min)

Renal dose
Adult: PO (nonvalvular atrial fibrillation) CCr 15-50 ml/min, 15 mg/day; CCr <15 ml/min, avoid use; (treatment/prophylaxis of DVT/pulmonary embolism) CCr <30 ml/min, avoid use

Hepatic dose
Adult: PO Child-Pugh class B or C: avoid use

Available forms: Tab 10, 15, 20, 50 mg

ADVERSE EFFECTS
GI: Cholestasis, *cytolytic hepatitis*, *hyperbilirubinemia*, *increased hepatic enzymes*, *jaundice*, nausea
HEMA: Adrenal bleeding, bleeding, *cerebral hemorrhage*, *epidural hematoma*, *GI bleeding*, *hemiparesis*, *intracranial bleeding*, *retinal hemorrhage*, *retroperitoneal hemorrhage*, *subdural hematoma*, *thrombocytopenia*

R

INTEG: Anaphylactic reaction, anaphylactic shock, blister, hypersensitivity, pruritus
SYST: Stevens-Johnson syndrome

> **BLACK BOX WARNING:** Active bleeding

> **BLACK BOX WARNING:** Abrupt discontinuation, epidermal/spinal anesthesia

INTERACTIONS
Individual drugs
Clarithromycin, conivaptan, erythromycin, itraconazole, ketoconazole, lopinavir/ritonavir, nicardipine: increased rivaroxaban effect, possible bleeding

CarBAMazepine, phenytoin, rifampin, ritonavir: decreased rivaroxaban effect

Amiodarone, azithromycin, darunavir, diltiazem, dronedarone, felodipine, fluconazole, lapatinib, mifepristone, nelfinavir, pantoprazole, posaconazole, quiNIDine, ranolazine, saquinavir, tamoxifen, telithromycin, verapamil: increased rivaroxaban effect in renal impairment

Drug classifications
NSAIDs, other anticoagulants, platelet inhibitors, salicylates, thrombolytics: increased rivaroxaban effect, possible bleeding

Drug/herb
St. John's wort: decreased rivaroxaban effect

Drug/food
Grapefruit juice: increased rivaroxaban effect in renal disease

Food: decreased rivaroxaban effect

NURSING CONSIDERATIONS
Assessment

> **BLACK BOX WARNING: Bleeding:** Monitor for bleeding, including bleeding during dental procedures, easy bruising, blood in urine, stools, emesis, sputum, epistaxis; there is no specific antidote

> **BLACK BOX WARNING: Abrupt discontinuation:** Avoid the abrupt discontinuation unless an alternative anticoagulant is used in those with atrial fibrillation; discontinuing puts patients at increased risk for thrombotic events; if this product must be discontinued for reasons other than pathological bleeding, consider administering another anticoagulant

> **BLACK BOX WARNING: Epidural/spinal anesthesia:** Epidural or spinal hematomas that may result in long-term/permanent paralysis may occur in patients who have received anticoagulants and are receiving neuraxial anesthesia or undergoing spinal puncture. The epidural catheter should not be removed <18 hr after the last dose of rivaroxaban; do not administer the next rivaroxaban dose <6 hr after the catheter removal; delay rivaroxaban administration for 24 hr if traumatic puncture occurs. Monitor for neuro changes

• **Hepatic/Renal disease:** Increase in effect of this product in hepatic disease (Child-Pugh Class B or C), hepatic disease with coagulopathy; renal failure/severe renal impairment (creatinine clearance <30 ml/min in DVT prophylaxis and <15 ml/min for stroke/systemic embolism prophylaxis in nonvalvular atrial fibrillation); product should be discontinued in acute renal failure; reduce dose in those with atrial fibrillation and CrCl 15-50 ml/min; monitor renal function periodically (creatinine clearance, BUN)

• **Pregnancy/breastfeeding:** Identify if pregnancy is suspected or planned; pregnancy-related hemorrhage may occur, and anticoagulation cannot be monitored with standard laboratory testing; breastfeeding should be discontinued prior to use of this product, use only if benefits outweigh fetal risk

• **Beers:** Avoid use in older adults with CCr <30 ml/min, reduce dose in CCr 30-50 ml/min

Patient problem
Ineffective tissue perfusion (uses)

Implementation
• **For DVT prophylaxis:** give daily without regard to food, give initial dose ≥6-10 hr after surgery when hemostasis has been established

• **For stroke/systemic embolism prophylaxis:** give daily with evening meal

• If dose is not given at correct time, give as soon as possible on the same day

• Unless pathological bleeding occurs, do not discontinue rivaroxaban in the absence of alternative

• Store at room temperature

• 15-, 20-mg tablets should be taken with food, for those unable to swallow whole, 15-mg and 20-mg tablets may be crushed, mixed with applesauce, immediately following administration, instruct to eat, crushed tablets are stable in applesauce for up to 4 hr

• 10-mg tablet can be taken without regard to food

Nasogastric (NG) tube or gastric feeding tube

- Confirm gastric placement of tube
- Crush 15-mg or 20-mg tablet, suspend in 50 ml of water, and administer via NG or gastric feeding tube
- To minimize reduced absorption, avoid administration distal to the stomach
- Enteral feeding should follow immediately administration of a crushed dose
- Crushed tablets are stable in water for up to 4 hours

Missed doses

- Patients receiving 15 mg twice daily should take their missed dose immediately to ensure intake of 30 mg per day. Two 15-mg tablets may be taken at once followed by the regular 15 mg twice daily dose the next day
- For patients receiving once daily dosing, take the missed dose as soon as it is remembered

Patient/family education

- Advise patient to report numbness of extremities, weakness, tingling, contact prescriber immediately (neuraxial anesthesia, spinal puncture)
- Advise patient to report if pregnancy is planned or suspected, not to breastfeed
- Teach patient to report bleeding (bruising, blood in urine, stools, sputum, emesis, heavy menstrual flow) and to use soft toothbrush, electric shaver
- Advise patient to inform all health care providers of use; report to prescriber all products used, to take all medication for duration, exactly as prescribed, to prevent clots, notify prescriber if unable to so a different anticoagulant may be used
- Advise patient to avoid abrupt discontinuation without another blood thinner
- Instruct patients, especially those with dental disease, in proper oral hygiene, including caution in use of regular toothbrushes, dental floss, and toothpicks.

Evaluation

Positive therapeutic outcome

- Prevention of DVT, stroke and systemic embolism

rivastigmine (Rx)

(riv-as-tig′mine)
Exelon, Exelon Patch
Func. class.: Anti-Alzheimer's agent
Chem. class.: Cholinesterase inhibitor

ACTION: Potent selective inhibitor of brain acetylcholinesterase (AChE) and butyrylcholinesterase (BChE)

Therapeutic outcome: Decreased signs and symptoms of Alzheimer's dementia

USES: Mild to severe Alzheimer's dementia, mild to moderate Parkinson's disease dementia (PDD)

Pharmacokinetics

Absorption	Rapidly, completely absorbed
Distribution	40% protein binding
Metabolism	To decarbamylated metabolite
Excretion	Kidney—metabolites, clearance lowered in geriatric, hepatic disease, increased nicotine use
Half-life	1½ hr

Pharmacodynamics

Onset	Unknown
Peak	1 hr
Duration	Unknown

CONTRAINDICATIONS

Hypersensitivity to this product, other carbamates

Precautions: Pregnancy, breastfeeding, children, renal/hepatic/respiratory disease, seizure disorder, asthma, urinary obstruction, peptic ulcer, increased intracranial pressure, surgery, GI bleeding, jaundice

DOSAGE AND ROUTES

Adult: PO 1.5 mg bid with food for 4 wk or more, may increase to 3 mg bid after 4 wk or more; may increase to 4.5 mg bid and thereafter 6 mg bid, max 12 mg/day; **transdermal** apply 4.6 mg/24 hr after 4 wk or more, may increase to 9.5 mg/24 hr; max 13.3 mg/24 hr; for those using 6-12 mg/day PO and switching to transdermal use one 9.5 mg/24 hr; for those using <6 mg/day PO and switching to transdermal use one 4.6 mg/24 hr

Available forms: Caps 1.5, 3, 4.5, 6 mg; transdermal patch 4.6, 9.5 mg/24 hr

ADVERSE EFFECTS

CNS: *Tremors, confusion, insomnia,* psychosis, hallucination, depression, dizziness, headache, anxiety, somnolence, fatigue, syncope, EPS, exacerbation of Parkinson's disease
CV: QT prolongation, AV block, cardiac arrest, MI, angina, palpitations, bradycardia
GI: *Nausea, vomiting, anorexia, abdominal distress, flatulence,* diarrhea, constipation, dyspepsia, colitis, eructation, fecal incontinence, GI bleeding/obstruction, GERD, gastritis, pancreatitis
MISC: UTI, asthenia, increased sweating, hypertension, flulike symptoms, weight change

R

INTERACTIONS
Individual drugs
Nicotine: increased metabolism, decreased blood level of rivastigmine

Drug classifications
Anticholinergics, phenothiazines, sedating H_1 blockers, tricyclics: decreased rivastigmine effect

Cholinergic agonists, other cholinesterase inhibitors: increased synergistic effect

NSAIDs: increased GI effects

NURSING CONSIDERATIONS
Assessment
• Monitor liver function tests: AST, ALT, alkaline phosphatase, LDH, bilirubin, CBC
• Assess for severe GI effects: nausea, vomiting, anorexia, weight loss, GI bleeding
• Monitor B/P, respiration during initial treatment; hypo/hypertension should be reported
• **Cognitive/mental status:** affect, mood, behavioral changes, depression; complete suicide assessment
• **Pregnancy/breastfeeding:** Use only if clearly needed, do not breastfeed, excretion unknown
• **Beers:** Avoid use in older adults, increased risk of orthostatic hypotension or bradycardia

Patient problem
Distorted thinking process (uses)
Risk for injury (adverse reactions)

Implementation
• Give with meals; take with AM and PM meal even though absorption may be decreased
• Provide assistance with ambulation during beginning therapy
• Discontinue treatment for several doses and restart at same or next lower dosage level if adverse reactions cause intolerance
• If treatment is interrupted for longer than several days, treatment should be initiated with the lowest daily dose and titrated as indicated above
Transdermal route
• Apply to clean, hairless, dry skin; not in an area that clothing will rub; rotate sites daily; remove liner; apply firmly; may be used during water activities; avoid saunas, avoid excess sunlight or external heat, each 5 cm^2 patch contains 9 mg base, rate of 4.6 mg/24 hr, each 10 cm^2 patch is 18 mg base, rate of 9.5 mg/24 hr

Patient/family education
• Teach patient procedure for giving **oral sol**; use instruction sheet provided; teach application of **transdermal** product, to fold in half and discard, not to get in eyes, to wash hands after

application, to not use heating pad, sauna, tanning bed
• Teach patient to notify prescriber of severe GI effects, do not discontinue abruptly
• Teach patient that product may cause dizziness, anorexia, weight loss

Evaluation
Positive therapeutic outcome
• Increased coherence, decreased symptoms of Alzheimer's disease, improved mood
• Teach patient to give with food in AM, PM
• Teach patient to report nausea, vomiting, diarrhea
• Advise to inform prescriber of all products taken

rizatriptan (Rx)
(rye-zah-trip′tan)
Maxalt, Maxalt-MLT
Func. class.: Migraine agent
Chem. class.: 5-HT$_1$-like receptor agonist

ACTION: Binds selectively to the vascular 5-HT$_{1B/1D}$ receptor subtype, exerts antimigraine effect; causes vasoconstriction in cranial arteries

Therapeutic outcome: After treatment, relief of migraine

USES: Acute treatment of migraine

Pharmacokinetics
Absorption	Unknown
Distribution	Unknown
Metabolism	Liver (metabolite)
Excretion	Urine/feces
Half-life	2-3 hr

Pharmacodynamics
Onset	10 min-2 hr
Peak	Unknown
Duration	Unknown

CONTRAINDICATIONS
Angina pectoris, history of MI, documented silent ischemia, Prinzmetal's angina, ischemic heart disease, concurrent ergotamine-containing preparations, uncontrolled hypertension, hypersensitivity, basilar or hemiplegic migraine

Precautions: Pregnancy, breastfeeding, children, postmenopausal women, men >40 yr, geriatric, risk factors for CAD, hypercholesterolemia, obesity, diabetes, impaired renal/hepatic function

---

DOSAGE AND ROUTES

Adult: **PO** 5-10 mg single dose, redosing separate by 2 hr or more; max 30 mg/24 hr, use 5 mg in patient on propanolol; max 15 mg/24 hr

Available forms: Tabs (Maxalt) 5, 10 mg; orally disintegrating tabs (Maxalt-MLT) 5, 10 mg

ADVERSE EFFECTS

CNS. *Dizziness, drowsiness, headache, fatigue,* warm/cold sensation, flushing

CV: MI, ventricular fibrillation, ventricular tachycardia, coronary artery vasospasm, peripheral vascular ischemia, ECG changes

ENDO: Hot flashes, mild increase in growth hormone

GI: *Nausea,* dry mouth, diarrhea, abdominal pain, ischemic colitis

RESP: Chest tightness, pressure, dyspnea

INTERACTIONS
Individual drugs

Cimetidine, isocarboxazid, pargyline, phenelzine, propranolol, trancyclomine: increased rizatriptan action

Ergot: increased vasospastic effects

Sibutramine: increased levels of sibutramine

Drug classifications

Contraceptives (oral), MAOIs, MAOIs (nonselective types A and B): increased rizatriptan action

Ergot derivatives, 5-HT$_1$ receptor agonists: increased vasospastic effects

Selective serotonin reuptake inhibitors: increased weakness, hyperreflexia, incoordination

Drug/herb

St. John's wort: serotonin syndrome

NURSING CONSIDERATIONS
Assessment

• Assess for stress level, activity, recreation, coping mechanisms

• Assess neurologic status: LOC, blurring vision, nausea, vomiting, tingling in extremities preceding headache

• **Ingestion of tyramine-containing foods:** Monitor for pickled products, beer, wine, aged cheese, food additives, preservatives, colorings, artificial sweeteners, chocolate, caffeine, which may precipitate these types of headaches

• **Pregnancy/breastfeeding:** Enroll in the registry 800-986-8999, cautious use in breastfeeding, excretion unknown

Patient problem

Distorted thinking process (uses)

Risk for injury (uses, adverse reactions)

Implementation

• Provide quiet, calm environment with decreased stimulation for noise, bright light, excessive talking

• Do not open blister pack until ready to use, put orally disintegrating tab on tongue to dissolve; swallow with saliva

Patient/family education

• **Teach patient use of orally disintegrating tab:** instruct patient not to open blister until use, to peel blister open with dry hands, to place tab on tongue, where it will dissolve, and to swallow with saliva (contains phenylalanine)

• Advise patient to report any side effects to prescriber

• Teach patient that product does not prevent or reduce number of migraines, main action is abortive, if first dose does not relieve pain, do not use more, notify prescriber

• Advise patient to use alternative contraception while taking product if oral contraceptives are being used

Evaluation

Positive therapeutic outcome

• Decrease in frequency, severity of headache

RARELY USED

rolapitant
(rol-ap'i-tant)
Varubi
Func. class.: Antiemetic, neurokinin antagonist

R

USES: Nausea, vomiting associated with cancer chemotherapy

CONTRAINDICATIONS
Hypersensitivity

DOSAGE AND ROUTES
Adult: **PO** 180 mg 1-2 hr prior to chemotherapy with dexamethasone and a 5-Ht$_3$ antagonist

rOPINIRole (Rx)
(roe-pin'e-role)
Requip, Requip XL
Func. class.: Antiparkinsonian agent
Chem. class.: Dopamine-receptor agonist, nonergot

Do not confuse: rOPINIRole/risperiDONE

ACTION: Selective agonist for DOPamine D$_2$ receptors (presynaptic/postsynaptic sites); binding at D$_3$ receptor contributes to antiparkinson effects

---

Therapeutic outcome: Decreased symptoms of Parkinson's disease (involuntary movements)

USES: Parkinsonism, restless legs syndrome

Pharmacokinetics

Absorption	Well absorbed
Distribution	Widely distributed
Metabolism	Liver, extensively by the liver by CYP450 CYP1A2 enzyme system
Excretion	Kidneys
Half-life	6 hr

Pharmacodynamics

Unknown

CONTRAINDICATIONS

Hypersensitivity

Precautions: Pregnancy, cardiac/renal/hepatic disease, dysrhythmias, affective disorders, psychosis

DOSAGE AND ROUTES

Parkinson's disease

Adult: PO (regular release) Initially, 0.25 mg PO tid × first wk; gradually titrate at weekly intervals; wk 2: give 0.5 mg tid; wk 3: 0.75 mg tid; wk 4; titrate to 1 mg tid; after wk 4, may increase by 1.5 mg/day wk, max 9 mg/day total dose, and then by 3 mg/day qwk, max 24 mg/day; PO (ext rel) Initially, 2 mg/day × 1-2 wk, may increase by mg/day at intervals ≥1 wk based upon response; max 24 mg/day. If significant interruption of therapy occurs, retitration may be necessary

For conversion from immediate-release to ext rel tablets

Oral dosage (ext rel tablets):

Adults currently on 0.75-2.25 mg/day: Give 2 mg/day ext rel

Adults currently on 3-4.5 mg/day: Give 4 mg/day ext rel

Adults currently on 6 mg/day: Give 6 mg/day ext rel

Adults currently on 7.5-9 mg/day: Give 8 mg/day ext rel

Adults currently on 12 mg/day: Give 12 mg/day ext rel

Adults currently on 15-18 mg/day: Give 16 mg/day ext rel

Adults currently on 21 mg/day: Give 20 mg/day ext rel

Adults currently on 24 mg/day: Give 24 mg/day ext rel

For the treatment of restless legs syndrome (RLS)

Adult: PO (reg rel) Initially, 0.25 mg/day, give 1-3 hr before bedtime; days 3-7, may increase to 0.5 mg/day; at the beginning of wk 2 (day 8) the dose may be increased to 1 mg/day × 1 wk; weeks 3-6, dose may be titrated up by 0.5 mg/wk (from 1.5-3 mg over the 5-wk period), as needed to achieve desired effect; wk 7, may increase dose to 4 mg/day; dose is titrated based on clinical response; give all doses 1-3 hr before bedtime

Available forms: Tabs 0.25, 0.5, 1, 2, 3, 4, 5 mg; ext rel tab 2, 4, 6, 8, 12 mg

ADVERSE EFFECTS

CNS: Dystonia, *agitation, insomnia,* dizziness, psychosis, hallucinations, depression, somnolence, sleep attacks, impulse-control disorders

CV: *Orthostatic hypotension,* hypotension, syncope, palpitations, tachycardia, hypertension

EENT: Blurred vision

GI: *Nausea, vomiting, anorexia, dry mouth,* constipation, dyspepsia, flatulence

GU: Impotence, urinary frequency

HEMA: Hemolytic anemia, leukopenia, agranulocytosis

INTEG: Rash, sweating

RESP: Pharyngitis, rhinitis, sinusitis, bronchitis, dyspnea

INTERACTIONS

Individual drugs

Cimetidine, ciprofloxacin, digoxin, diltiazem, enoxacin, erythromycin, fluvoxamine, levodopa, mexiletine, norfloxacin, tacrine, theophylline: increased effect of rOPINIRole

Metoclopramide: decreased rOPINIRole effect

Drug classifications

Butyrophenones, phenothiazines, thioxanthenes: decreased ropinirole effect

NURSING CONSIDERATIONS

Assessment

• Monitor B/P, respiration during initial treatment; hypotension or hypertension should be reported

• Assess mental status: affect, mood, behavioral changes, depression; complete suicide assessment

• **Parkinsonism:** assess for akinesia, tremors, staggering gait, muscle rigidity, drooling; these symptoms should improve with therapy

• **Sleep attacks:** assess for drowsiness, falling asleep without warning even during hazardous activities

• **Pregnancy/breastfeeding:** Use only if benefits outweigh fetal risk, avoid breastfeeding, excretion unknown

Patient problem
Impaired mobility (uses)
Risk for injury (uses, adverse reactions)

Implementation
• Give product until NPO before surgery
• Adjust dosage to patient's response
• Give with meals to decrease GI upset
• Test for diabetes mellitus, acromegaly if patient is receiving long-term therapy

Patient/family education
• Teach patient to notify prescriber if pregnancy is planned or suspected, pregnancy, breast-feeding
• Teach patient to take with food to prevent nausea
• Teach patient to report hallucinations, confusion (usually in geriatrics)
• Advise patient that therapeutic effects may take several wk to a few mo
• Caution patient to change positions slowly to prevent orthostatic hypotension
• Instruct patient to use product exactly as prescribed; if product is discontinued abruptly, parkinsonian crisis may occur
• Teach patient that drowsiness, sleeping attacks may occur, to avoid driving or other hazardous activities until response is known
• Teach patient to avoid alcohol and CNS depressants (cough and cold products)
• Teach patient to notify prescriber of unusual urges

Evaluation
Positive therapeutic outcome
• Decreased akathisia, other involuntary movements
• Increased mood

---

ropivacaine (Rx)
(roe-pi'va-kane)
Naropin
Func. class.: Local anesthetic
Chem. class.: Amide

ACTION: Competes with calcium for sites in nerve membrane that control sodium transport across cell membrane; decreases rise of depolarization phase of action potential

Therapeutic outcome: Maintenance of local anesthesia

USES: Peripheral nerve block, caudal anesthesia, central neural block, vaginal, epidural, spinal block

Pharmacokinetics
Absorption	Complete
Distribution	Unknown
Metabolism	Liver
Excretion	Kidneys
Half-life	Unknown

Pharmacodynamics
Onset	2-8 min
Peak	Unknown
Duration	3 hr, varies with inj site

CONTRAINDICATIONS
Children <12 yr, geriatric, hypersensitivity to amide local anesthetics, severe liver disease, severe hypotension, complete heart block

Precautions: Pregnancy, severe product allergies, hyperthyroidism, CV, hepatic/neurologic disease

DOSAGE AND ROUTES
Lumbar epidural block for C-section
Adult: 20-30 ml of 0.5% SOL, or 15-20 ml of 0.75% SOL

Thoracic epidural
Adult: 5-15 ml of 0.5%-0.75% SOL

Major nerve block
Adult: 35-50 ml of 0.5% SOL or 10-40 ml of 0.75% SOL

Labor pain epidural
Adult: 10-20 ml of 0.2% SOL, then 6-14 ml/hr

Postoperative (lumbar/thoracic epidural)
Adult: 6-14 ml/hr of 0.2% SOL

Infiltration/minor nerve block
Adult: 1-100 ml of 0.2% SOL or 1-40 ml of 0.5% SOL

Available forms: Inj 2, 5, 7.5 mg/ml

ADVERSE EFFECTS
CNS: Anxiety, restlessness, seizures, loss of consciousness, drowsiness, disorientation, tremors, shivering, paresthesia
CV: Myocardial depression, cardiac arrest, dysrhythmias, bradycardia, *hypo*/hypertension, fetal bradycardia
EENT: Blurred vision, tinnitus, pupil constriction
ENDO: Hypokalemia
GI: Nausea, vomiting
GU: Urinary retention
INTEG: Rash, urticaria, allergic reactions, edema, burning, skin discoloration at injection site, tissue necrosis
RESP: Status asthmaticus, respiratory arrest, anaphylaxis

R

INTERACTIONS
Individual drugs
Amiodarone, cimetidine, ciprofloxacin, fluvoxaMINE, imipramine, theophylline: increased effect

Chloroprocaine: decreased action of ropivacaine

Enflurane, EPINEPHrine, halothane: increased dysrhythmias

Drug classifications
Antidepressants (tricyclics), MAOIs, phenothiazines: increased hypertension

Azole antifungals: increased effect

NURSING CONSIDERATIONS
Assessment
- Assess B/P, pulse, respiration during treatment
- Assess fetal heart tones during labor
- Assess allergic reactions: rash, urticaria, itching
- Assess cardiac status: ECG for dysrhythmias, pulse, B/P during anesthesia

Patient problem
Risk of injury (adverse reactions)

Implementation
- Give only with resuscitative equipment nearby
- Give only products without preservatives for epidural or caudal anesthesia
- Use new sol; discard unused portions

Evaluation
Positive therapeutic outcome
- Anesthesia necessary for procedure

TREATMENT OF OVERDOSE:
Airway, O_2, vasopressor, **IV** fluids, anticonvulsants for seizures

---

rosuvastatin (Rx)
(roe-soo′va-sta-tin)
Crestor
Func. class.: Antilipemic
Chem. class.: HMG-CoA reductase inhibitor

ACTION: Inhibits HMG-CoA reductase, which reduces cholesterol synthesis

Therapeutic outcome: Decreasing cholesterol levels

USES: As an adjunct in primary hypercholesterolemia (types IIa, IIb), mixed dyslipidemia elevated serum triglycerides, homozygous/heterozygous familial hypercholesterolemia (FH), slowing of atherosclerosis, CV disease prophylaxis, MI, stroke prophylaxis (normal LDL)

Pharmacokinetics

Absorption	Unknown
Distribution	88% protein bound, crosses placenta
Metabolism	Minimal liver metabolism (about 10%)
Excretion	Primarily in feces (90%)
Half-life	19 hr

Pharmacodynamics

Onset	Unknown
Peak	3-5 hr
Duration	Unknown

CONTRAINDICATIONS
Pregnancy, breastfeeding, hypersensitivity, active liver disease

Precautions: Children <10 yr, geriatric, past liver disease, alcoholism, severe acute infections, trauma, hypotension, uncontrolled seizure disorders, severe metabolic disorders, electrolyte imbalances, severe renal impairment, hypothyroidism, Asian patients

DOSAGE AND ROUTES
Patient should first be placed on a cholesterol-lowering diet

Hypercholesterolemia, hyperlipoproteinemia, and/or hypertriglyceridemia
Adult: PO 10 mg q day, 5 mg q day in those requiring less aggressive LDL-reductions, patients with CrCl less than 30 ml/min, or patients at higher risk for myopathy

Homozygous familial hypercholesterolemia (HoFH)
Adult: PO 20 mg q day.
Children and Adolescents: 7 to 17 years PO 20 mg q day

Pediatric patients with heterozygous familial hypercholesterolemia (HeFH)
Children and Adolescents: 10 to 17 yrs PO 5 to 20 mg q day, Individualize based on the goals of therapy. Adjust dose q4 wk or more
Children 8 to 9 yrs: PO 5 to 10 mg qday, individualize based on the goals of therapy. Adjust dose q4wk or more

---

For slowing the progression of atherosclerosis

Adults: PO 10 mg qday. 5 mg qday may be initiated in those requiring less aggressive LDL-reductions, patients with CCr less than 30 ml/min, or patients at higher risk for myopathy.

For primary prevention of cardiovascular disease

Adults: PO 10 to 20 mg q day, with a dose range of 5 to 40 mg q day.

Renal Dose

Adult: PO CCr < 30 ml/min: Initially, 5 mg q day in those not receiving dialysis. Max 10 mg q day

Available forms: Tabs 5, 10, 20, 40 mg

ADVERSE EFFECTS

CNS: *Headache, dizziness,* insomnia, paresthesia, confusion
GI: *Nausea, constipation, abdominal pain, flatus, diarrhea, dyspepsia, heartburn,* kidney failure, liver dysfunction, vomiting
HEMA: Thrombocytopenia, hemolytic anemia, leukopenia
INTEG: *Rash, pruritus*
MS: *Asthenia, muscle cramps, arthritis, arthralgia, myalgia,* myositis, rhabdomyolysis, leg, shoulder, or localized pain
RESP: Rhinitis, sinusitis, *pharyngitis,* increased cough

INTERACTIONS
Individual drugs
Alcohol: increased hepatotoxicity
Clofibrate, cycloSPORINE, gemfibrozil, niacin: increased myalgia, myositis
Warfarin: increased bleeding

Drug classifications
Antifungals (azole), antiretroviral protease inhibitors, fibric acid derivatives: increased myalgia, myositis
Bile acid sequestrants: increased effects

Drug/herb
St. John's wort: decreased rosuvastatin effect

Drug/lab test
Increased: CPK, liver function tests

NURSING CONSIDERATIONS
Assessment
• Assess diet: obtain diet history including fat, cholesterol in diet
• Monitor fasting cholesterol, LDL, HDL, triglycerides periodically during treatment
• Liver function: monitor liver function tests q1-2mo during the first 1½ yr of treatment; AST, ALT, liver function tests may increase

• Monitor renal function in patients with compromised renal system: BUN, creatinine, I&O ratio
• Obtain ophthalmic exam before, 1 mo after treatment begins, annually; lens opacities may occur
• **Rhabdomyolysis:** Assess for muscle pain, tenderness, obtain CPK; if these occur, product may need to be discontinued; for Asian ancestry: increased blood levels, rhabdomyolysis
• **Pregnancy/breastfeeding:** Do not use in pregnancy, breastfeeding

Patient problem
Risk for injury (uses)
Nonadherence (teaching)

Implementation
• May be taken at any time of day, with or without food
• Store in cool environment in airtight, light-resistant container

Patient/family education
• Advise to report suspected pregnancy, to use contraception while taking this product, pregnancy, not to breastfeed
• Advise that blood work and ophthalmic exam will be necessary during treatment
• Teach to report blurred vision, severe GI symptoms, dizziness, headache, muscle pain, weakness
• Teach that previously prescribed regimen will continue: low-cholesterol diet, exercise program, smoking cessation; liver injury (jaundice, anorexia, abdominal pain)

Evaluation

Positive therapeutic outcome
• Cholesterol at desired level after 8 wk

⚠ HIGH ALERT

rucaparib
(roo-kap' a-rib)
Rubraca
Func. class.: Antineoplastic
Chem. class.: (PARP) Poly (ADP-ribose) polymerase inhibitor

ACTION: Inhibits poly (ADP-ribose) polymerase (PARP) enzymes; inhibition of PARP enzyme activity results in increased PARP-DNA complexes; causing DNA damage, apoptosis, and cell death

Therapeutic outcome: Decrease in growth, spread of cancer

USES: Treatment of BRCA 🐾 mutation-positive epithelial ovarian, fallopian tube, or primary peritoneal cancer in patients who have received two or more prior chemotherapy regimens as monotherapy

Pharmacokinetics

Absorption	Unknown
Distribution	70% protein binding
Metabolism	Metabolized by CYP2D6 (major) and CYP3A4, CYP1A2 (minor)
Excretion	Unknown
Half-life	17-19 hr

Pharmacodynamics

Onset	Unknown
Peak	1.9 hr
Duration	Unknown

CONTRAINDICATIONS: Hypersensitivity

PRECAUTIONS: Breastfeeding, contraceptive requirements, leukemia, myelodysplastic syndrome (MDS), pregnancy, pregnancy testing, reproductive risk

DOSAGE AND ROUTES
Adult: PO 600 mg bid continue until disease progression or severe toxicity

Available forms: Tablets 200 mg, 300 mg

ADVERSE EFFECTS
CNS: Fatigue, dizziness, fever, asthenia
GI: Nausea, vomiting, constipation, anorexia, abdominal pain, diarrhea, dysgeusia
Hema: Anemia, thrombocytopenia, neutropenia, febrile neutropenia, myelodysplastic syndrome (MDS)/acute myeloid leukemia
Resp: Dyspnea
Integ: Pruritus, rash, photosensitivity, hand-foot syndrome

INTERACTIONS
None known

Drug/lab test
Increase: AST/ALT, cholesterol
Decrease: ANC, Hb, platelets

NURSING CONSIDERATIONS
Assessment
• **Myelodysplastic syndrome (MDS)/acute myeloid leukemia (AML)**: Monitor for signs and symptoms of MDS/AML; all

patients had received prior treatment with platinum-containing chemotherapy and other DNA-damaging agents; monitor CBC baseline and monthly; do not start until prior hematologic toxicity resolves to grade 1 or less. For prolonged hematologic toxicity (greater than 4 weeks), hold therapy or reduce the dose and check a CBC every week until recovery; discontinue if a diagnosis of MDS or AML occurs
• **Pregnancy/breastfeeding:** Assess for pregnancy/breastfeeding; not to use during or for 6 months after treatment; can cause fetal harm or death; do not breastfeed during or for 2 wks after the final dose
• Monitor AST/ALT, cholesterol, creatinine; all may be elevated

Patient problem

Implementation
• May give without regard to food; approximately 12 hr apart
• If a dose is missed, the patient should take the next dose at the regularly scheduled time; do not replace doses if vomiting occurs

Patient/family education
• Inform patient to notify prescriber of all OTC, Rx, and herbal products taken, and not to start new products without prescriber approval
• **Pregnancy/breastfeeding:** Teach patient not to use during or for 6 months after treatment; can cause fetal harm or death; do not breastfeed during or for 2 wks after the final dose; pregnancy testing should be done prior to use
• **Myelodysplastic syndrome (MDS)/acute myeloid leukemia (AML):** Teach patient to report weakness, fatigue, bruising, bleeding, trouble breathing, blood in urine, stool, emesis; teach patient that continuing blood work will be needed
• **Photosensitivity:** Advise patient to wear protective clothing, sunscreen, or stay out of the sun to prevent burns

Evaluation
• Therapeutic response: Decrease in growth, spread of cancer

safinamide
(sa-fin'-a-mide)
Xadago
Func. class.: Antiparkinson's agent
Chem. class.: MAO type B inhibitor

ACTION: The precise mechanism of action of safinamide in treating "off" episodes in Parkinson's disease is unknown; however, one mechanism may be related to its MAO-B inhibitory activity, which causes an increase in dopamine levels centrally. The elevated dopamine levels and subsequent increased dopaminergic activity are likely to mediate the beneficial effects of safinamide

USES: For adjunctive treatment to levodopa-carbidopa therapy in patients with Parkinson's disease experiencing "off" episodes

Pharmacokinetics

Absorption	Unknown
Distribution	Not highly protein bound
Metabolism	Inhibits intestinal breast cancer resistance protein (BCRP)
Excretion	Excreted via kidneys 5% (unchanged), 76% recovered in the urine
Half-life	20-26 hr

Pharmacodynamics

Onset	Unknown
Peak	2-3 hr
Duration	Unknown

CONTRAINDICATIONS
Hypersensitivity, MAOI therapy

Precautions: Abrupt discontinuation, alcoholism, breastfeeding, pregnancy, cataracts, use with CNS depressants, dental work, diabetic retinopathy, hypertension, hepatic disease, impulse control problems, psychosis, schizophrenia, surgery, uveitis

DOSAGE AND ROUTES
For adjunctive treatment to levodopa-carbidopa therapy in patients with Parkinson's disease experiencing "off" episodes
Adult: PO 50 mg per day, initially. May increase after 2 wk to 100 mg qday, based on need and tolerability. Max: 100 mg/day.

Available forms: Tablet 50, 100 mg

ADVERSE EFFECTS
CNS: Drowsiness, dyskinesia, insomnia, impulse control symptoms, neuroleptic malignant syndrome, psychosis, serotonin syndrome

CV: Orthostatic hypotension

MISC: Cough, dyspepsia, cataracts

INTERACTIONS
Drug classifications
Anxiolytics, sedatives; hypnotics barbiturates: Increased severe somnolence, avoid using together
MAOIs, linezolid: Increased hypertension, hypertensive crisis, do not use within 14 days of these products
Some other opioids; SNRIs; tricyclic antidepressants and other cyclic antidepressants; triazolopyridine antidepressants; cyclobenzaprine; stimulants (methylphenidate, amphetamines): Increased serotonin syndrome, use the lowest dose
Decreased safinamide effects: Atypical antipsychotics

Individual drugs
ALPRAZolam, clonazePAM, zolpidem, zaleplon: Increased severe somnolence, avoid using together
Meperidine, dextromethorphan: Increased serotonin syndrome, use lowest dose

NURSING CONSIDERATIONS
Assessment
• **Parkinson's disease:** Assess for changes before and during treatment; tremors, pin-rolling movement, balance, anxiety, drooling, depression, delusions, hallucinations, insomnia, shuffling gait; decreasing of "off" periods
• **Mental status:** Assess for affect, depression, mood, complete suicide assessment
• **Hypertension:** May cause hypertension, exacerbate preexisting hypertension, or cause hypertensive crisis. Monitor for new-onset hypertension or hypertension that is not adequately controlled after starting product, adjust dose if elevations in B/P are sustained, do not exceed max dose; monitor for hypertension if coadministered with sympathomimetics (prescription or nonprescription nasal, oral, and ophthalmic decongestants, cold preparations)
• **Drug interactions:** Review drug interactions before use. There are many serious reactions
• **Impulse control:** Inquire periodically about new or worsening impulse control symptoms, (gambling, increased sexual urges, binge eating, intense urges to spend money, or other intense urges); if these occur dose reduction or discontinuation may be needed

S

• **Pregnancy/breastfeeding:** May cause fetal harm, use in pregnancy only if the potential benefit outweighs fetal risk; do not use in breastfeeding, serious adverse reactions may occur

• **Hepatic disease:** Monitor LFTs baseline and periodically in those with hepatic disease

• Neuroleptic malignant syndrome-like symptoms: Assess for elevated temperature, muscular rigidity, altered consciousness, and autonomic instability, may occur with rapid dose reduction

• **Serotonin syndrome**: Assess for nausea, vomiting, sedation, dizziness, diaphoresis (sweating), facial flushing, mental status changes, myoclonus, restlessness, shivering, and hypertension. If serotonin syndrome occurs, any serotonergic agents should be discontinued

Patient problem
Impaired mobility (uses)

Implementation
• Give at the same time each day; may be given with or without food
• If a dose is missed, take the next dose at the usual time on the next day
• Food and drug interactions with safinamide can be serious. Patients should avoid foods/beverages containing large amounts of tyramine

Patient/family education
• **Impulse control:** Teach patient that impulse control symptoms (gambling, increased sexual urges, binge eating, intense urges to spend money, or other intense urges) may occur, to report to provider
• **Pregnancy/breastfeeding:** Teach patient to report if pregnancy is planned or suspected or if breastfeeding
• Advise patient not to drive or engage in hazardous activities until result of product is known, drowsiness may occur
• Advise patient to change position slowly to prevent orthostatic hypotension
• Teach patient to use product as prescribed, if discontinued abruptly, neuroleptic malignant syndrome-like symptoms may occur, taper gradually
• Advise patient to use physical activity to maintain mobility, lessen spasms

Evaluation
Positive therapeutic outcome
• Decreased "off" periods in Parkinson's disease

salicylic acid topical
See Appendix B

salmeterol (Rx)
(sal-met′er-ole)
Serevent Diskhaler Disk, Serevent Diskus
Func. class.: Adrenergic β₂ agonist, (long acting) bronchodilator

ACTION: Causes bronchodilatation by action on β₂ (pulmonary) receptors by increasing levels of cyclic AMP, which relaxes smooth muscle; with very little effect on heart rate

Therapeutic outcome: Ease of breathing

USES: Prevention of exercise-induced asthma, bronchospasm, COPD

Pharmacokinetics
Absorption	Minimal
Distribution	Local
Metabolism	Unknown
Excretion	Unknown
Half-life	4 hr

Pharmacodynamics
Onset	5-15 min
Peak	4 hr
Duration	12 hr

CONTRAINDICATIONS
Hypersensitivity to sympathomimetics, tachydysrhythmias, severe cardiac disease, monotherapy treatment of asthma

Precautions: Pregnancy, breastfeeding, cardiac disorders, hyperthyroidism, diabetes mellitus, hypertension, prostatic hypertrophy, closed-angle glaucoma, seizures, acute asthma, as a substitute for corticosteroids, QT prolongation

> **BLACK BOX WARNING:** Asthma-related death, children <4 yr

DOSAGE AND ROUTES
Adult/child ≥4 yr: Asthma INH 50 mcg (one inhalation as dry powder); **exercise-induced bronchospasm:** 50 mcg (1 INH) ½-1 hr prior to exercise

Available forms: Inhalation powder 50 mcg/blister

ADVERSE EFFECTS
CNS: *Anxiety,* insomnia, *headache,* dizziness, fever
CV: Palpitations, tachycardia, angina

GI: Nausea, vomiting, abdominal pain
MS: Muscle cramps
RESP: Paradoxical bronchospasm, cough, asthma-related death

INTERACTIONS
Drug classifications
Antidepressants (tricyclics, MAOIs): increased salmeterol action

β-Adrenergic blockers: decreased therapeutic effect

Bronchodilators, aerosol: increased action of bronchodilator

CYP3A4 inhibitors (itraconazole, ketoconazole, nelfinavir, nefazodone, saquinavir): increased CV effects, avoid using together

Drug/herb
Betel palm, butterbur, coffee, cola nut, figwort, fumitory, guarana, hawthorn, lily of the valley, motherwort, plantain, tea (black, green), yerba maté: increased stimulation

NURSING CONSIDERATIONS
Assessment
• **Respiratory function:** assess vital capacity, FEV, ABGs, lung sounds, heart rate, rhythm (baseline), and periodically during treatment
• **Paradoxical bronchospasm:** monitor for dyspnea, wheezing, chest tightness, do not use in bronchospasm

> **BLACK BOX WARNING:** Children should not use this product as monotherapy for asthma; use only with persistent asthma in those that are not well-controlled with a long-term asthma product, after product controls asthma, use another bronchodilator

• **Hypersensitivity:** Assess for rash, urticaria, rarely leads to anaphylaxis, angioedema

> **BLACK BOX WARNING:** Asthma-related death

Patient problem
Ineffective airway clearance (uses)
Risk of injury (uses, adverse reactions)

Implementation
• Shake aerosol container, ask patient to exhale, then place mouthpiece in mouth, inhale slowly, hold breath, remove, exhale slowly
• Use this medication before other medications and allow at least 1 min between each
• Store in foil pouch; do not expose to temp >86° F (30° C); discard 6 wk after removal from foil pouch

• Use 1/2 hr prior to exercise for exercise-induced bronchospasm prevention; do not use additional doses if using bid
• Don't use spacer with this product

Patient/family education
• Caution patient not to use OTC medications unless approved by health care professional, because extra stimulation may occur
• Instruct patient to use this medication before other medications and to allow at least 1 min between each, to prevent overstimulation
• Teach patient how to use inhaler; to wash inhaler in warm water daily and dry; to avoid smoking, smoke-filled rooms, and persons with respiratory infections; review package insert with patient
• Instruct patient on administration of dose, not to use more than prescribed; serious side effects may occur
• Teach patient not to use for exercise-induced bronchospasm, never exhale into diskus, hold level, keep mouthpiece dry
• Teach patient not to use for treatment of acute exacerbation, a fast-acting β-blocker should be used instead
• Teach patient to report immediately dyspnea after use, if 1 canister or more is used in 2 mo time
• **Multidose:** Advise patient not to get canister or mouthpiece wet, not to use spacer, not to exhale into mouthpiece
• Teach patient to take other products as prescribed

> **BLACK BOX WARNING: Asthma-related death:** Teach patient to seek medical attention immediately for serious asthma attack, death may be greater in Black patients

• Advise patient to use 1/2-1 hr before exercising if using to prevent exercise-induced bronchospasm
• **Pregnancy/breastfeeding:** Advise patient to notify provider if pregnancy is planned or if breastfeeding

Evaluation
Positive therapeutic outcome
• Absence of dyspnea, wheezing
• Improved airway exchange
• Improved ABGs

TREATMENT OF OVERDOSE:
Administer a β$_2$-adrenergic blocker

S

sarilumab
(sar-il' ue-mab)
Kevzara
Func. class.: Antirheumatic, immunosuppressive
Chem. class.: Interleukin antagonist, monoclonal antibody

ACTION: Inhibits interleukin-6 (IL-6) receptors by binding to them; antiinflammatory action and a reduction in C-reactive protein

Therapeutic outcome: Slowing progression of rheumatoid arthritis

USES: Treatment of moderately to severely active rheumatoid arthritis

Pharmacokinetics

Absorption	Unknown
Distribution	Unknown
Metabolism	Unknown
Excretion	Unknown
Half-life	150 mg dose is 8 days, 200 mg dose 10 days

Pharmacodynamics

Onset	Unknown
Peak	2-4 days depending on dose
Duration	28-43 days depending on dose

CONTRAINDICATIONS: Hypersensitivity, active infections, active severe hepatic disease, ANC <2000/mm3, platelets <150,000/mm3

PRECAUTIONS: Chronic/recurrent infections, corticosteroid therapy, diabetes mellitus, TB, diverticulitis, risk of GI perforation, hepatic disease (Child-Pugh B), severe renal disease, pregnancy, lactation, children, geriatrics, HIV, neoplastic disease

> **BLACK BOX WARNING:** Infection

DOSAGE AND ROUTES
Adult: SUBCUT 200 mg q2 wk

Available forms: Solution for SUBCUT injection 150 mg/1.14 ml, 200 mg/1.14 ml single-use prefilled syringes

ADVERSE EFFECTS
GU: UTI
GI: GI perforation
HEMA: Thrombocytopenia, neutropenia, leukopenia
RESP: URI, dyspnea
INTEG: Injection site reactions, rash, pruritus

MISC: Infections (TB), hypersensitivity, immunosuppression, malignancy

INTERACTIONS
Drug classifications
CYP450 substrates (cyclosporine, atorvastatin, lovastatin, theophylline, warfarin, hormonal contraceptives); altered effect; monitor substrate levels
DMARDs, TNF antagonists, corticosteroids, live virus vaccines, increased immunosuppression, infections

NURSING CONSIDERATIONS
Assessment
• **Infection:** Assess for flulike symptoms, fever, dyspnea, inflammation of wounds; a TB test should be performed before starting treatment
• **Reactivation of viral herpes zoster:** Assess for blisters, rash; **hepatitis B:** assess for dark urine, jaundice, clay-colored stools, weakness, fatigue, anorexia, nausea, vomiting, abdominal pain; any of these symptoms should be reported immediately
• **Blood studies:** Monitor **AST/ALT** baseline and at 4 and 8 wks after starting therapy and every 3 months thereafter; **lipid levels:** monitor baseline and 4 and 8 wks after starting treatment and then every 6 months thereafter; platelets: baseline and 4 and 8 wks after string therapy and every 3 months thereafter; **neutrophils:** monitor baseline and 4 and 8 wks after starting therapy and then every 3 months thereafter

Patient problem
Pain (uses)
Impaired mobility (uses)

Implementation
SUBCUT Route
• A TB test is required prior to use; do not start on therapy if patient has latent TB, treat first
• Visually inspect for particulate matter and discoloration prior to use; product is a clear and colorless to pale yellow
• Allow to sit at room temperature for 30 min
• Inject full amount of the syringe
• Do not rub the injection site
• Dispose of the used syringe or pen properly; do not recap after use; do not reuse the pen or the syringe
• Rotate injection sites with each injection
Storage: Use within 14 days after being taken out of the refrigerator

Patient/family education
• Inform patient the reason for therapy and expected result

- **Subcut:** Teach patient family member correct injection technique and disposal of syringes; give the medication guide to patient and review it
- **Infection:** Teach patient to report immediately fever, flulike symptoms, cough, blood in emesis, urine, stools; **hypersensitivity:** rash, itching
- **Pregnancy/breastfeeding:** Teach patient to notify prescriber if pregnancy is planned or suspected or if breastfeeding; pregnant women should enroll in the pregnancy registry at 1-877-311-8972
- Teach patient to avoid live virus vaccines while taking this product; vaccinations should be brought up-to-date before treatment if needed
- Advise patient to avoid OTC herbal products or supplements without consent of prescriber; discuss with all prescribers all medications and products taken

Evaluation
- Slowing progression of rheumatoid arthritis

> **⚠ HIGH ALERT**
>
> **saxagliptin (Rx)**
> (sax-a-glip′tin)
> **Onglyza**
> *Func. class.:* Antidiabetic, oral
> *Chem. class.:* Dipeptidyl-peptidase-4 (DPP-4) inhibitor

Do not confuse: saxagliptin/sitaGLIPtin

ACTION: Slows the inactivation of incretin hormones, improves glucose homeostasis, improves glucose-dependent insulin synthesis, lowers glucagon secretions and slows gastric emptying time

Therapeutic outcome: Decrease in polyuria, polydipsia, polyphagia; clear sensorium; absence of dizziness; stable gait; blood glucose at normal level

USES: Type 2 diabetes mellitus as monotherapy or in combination with other antidiabetic agents

Pharmacokinetics

Absorption	Rapidly, well
Distribution	Unknown
Metabolism	Liver by CYP3A4/5
Excretion	Kidneys 24% unchanged, feces 22%
Half-life	2.5 hr, 3.1 hr metabolite

Pharmacodynamics

Onset	Unknown
Peak	1-4 hr
Duration	24 hr

CONTRAINDICATIONS
Hypersensitivity, angioedema, serious rash, type 1 diabetes, ketoacidosis

Precautions: Pregnancy, geriatric, GI obstruction, thyroid disease, surgery, renal/hepatic disease, trauma, diabetic ketoacidosis (DKA), type 1 diabetes mellitus, heart failure

DOSAGE AND ROUTES
Adult: PO 2.5-5 mg; may use with other antidiabetic agents (metformin, pioglitazone, rosiglitazone), if used with insulin, a lower dose is needed; max 2.5 mg with strong 3A4-5 inhibitors

Renal dose
Adult: PO CCr ≤50 ml/min 2.5 mg/day; hemodialysis: 2.5 mg qday after hemodialysis

Available forms: Tabs 2.5; 5 mg

ADVERSE EFFECTS
CNS: *Headache*
CV: Edema, HF
EENT: Sinusitis
ENDO: Hypoglycemia (renal impairment)
GI: *Nausea, vomiting,* abdominal pain, pancreatitis
INTEG: Urticaria, angioedema, anaphylaxis

INTERACTIONS
Individual drugs
Aripiprazole, cloZAPine, fosphenytoin, OLANZapine, phenytoin, QUEtiapine, risperiDONE, ziprasidone: decreased antidiabetic effect
Cimetidine, disopyramide: increased saxagliptin level
Cimetidine, FLUoxetine: increased hypoglycemia
Digoxin: increased levels of digoxin

Drug classifications
ACE inhibitors, estrogens, oral contraceptives, phenothiazines, progestins, protease inhibitors, sympathomimetics, thiazide diuretics: decreased antidiabetic effect
Androgens, β-blockers, corticosteroids, fibric acid derivatives, insulins, MAOIs, salicylates: increased hypoglycemia, dosage reduction may be needed

Drug/herb
Garlic, horse chestnut: increased antidiabetic effect

Drug/lab test
Decreased: lymphocytes, glucose

NURSING CONSIDERATIONS
Assessment
• **Hypoglycemic reactions** assess for sweating, weakness, dizziness, anxiety, tremors, hunger; monitor blood glucose (BG) as needed
• Monitor CBC (baseline, periodically) during treatment; check liver function tests periodically, AST, LDH, renal studies: BUN, creatinine during treatment; glycosylated hemoglobin HbA1C
• **Heart failure:** Assess for history of risk factors for heart failure, use cautiously in these patients
• **Pancreatitis:** Assess for abdominal pain, nausea, vomiting; discontinue product immediately, previous pancreatitis may be a contributing factor

Patient problem
Excess food intake (uses)
Nonadherence (teaching)

Implementation
PO route
• May be taken with or without food
• Conversion from other antidiabetic agents; change may be made with gradual dosage change
• Store in tight container at room temperature
• Do not break or cut tabs

Patient/family education
• Teach patient to use regular self-monitoring of blood glucose using blood glucose meter
• Teach patient the symptoms of hypo/hyperglycemia; what to do about each
• Teach patient that product must be continued on daily basis; explain consequence of discontinuing product abruptly
• Advise patient to avoid OTC medications, alcohol, digoxin, exenatide, insulins, nateglinide, repaglinide, and other products that lower blood sugar, unless approved by prescriber
• Teach patient that diabetes is a lifelong illness; that this product is not a cure, only controls symptoms
• Teach patient that all food included in diet plan must be eaten to prevent hypo/hyperglycemia
• Teach patient to carry emergency ID
• Teach patient to take product without regard to food
• Teach patient to notify prescriber when surgery, trauma, or stress occurs, as dose may need to be adjusted, or insulin used
• **Pancreatitis:** Teach patient to immediately report and stop taking product if severe abdominal pain with vomiting occurs
• **Hypersensitivity:** Advise patient to immediately seek medical assistance and stop product if itching, rash, swelling of face, tongue occur
• **Pregnancy/breastfeeding:** Advise patient if pregnancy is planned or suspected or if breastfeeding

Evaluation
Positive therapeutic outcome
• Decrease in polyuria, polydipsia, polyphagia; clear sensorium; absence of dizziness; stable gait; blood glucose at normal level

---

RARELY USED

scopolamine (Rx)
(skoe-pol′a-meen)
Transderm-Scop
Func. class.: Cholinergic blocker
Chem. class.: Belladonna alkaloid

USES: Prevention of motion sickness

CONTRAINDICATIONS
Hypersensitivity, closed-angle glaucoma, myasthenia gravis, GI/GU obstruction, hypersensitivity to belladonna, barbiturates

DOSAGE AND ROUTES
Adult: Transdermal 1 patch placed behind ear 4 hr before travel, reapply q3day

---

RARELY USED

secnidazole
Solosec
Func. class.: Antiinfective

USES: For the treatment of bacterial vaginosis

DOSAGE AND ROUTES
Adult: PO 2 g PO as a single dose

---

selegiline (Rx)
(se-le′ji-leen)
Eldepryl, Emsam, Zelapar
Func. class.: Antiparkinson agent, antidepressant
Chem. class.: MAOI, type B

Do not confuse: selegiline/Salagen
Zelapar/ZyPREXA

ACTION: Increased dopaminergic activity by inhibition of MAO type B activity; not fully understood

---

Therapeutic outcome: Decreased symptoms of Parkinson's disease, depression

USES: Adjunct management of Parkinson's disease in patients being treated with levodopa/carbidopa who have responded poorly to therapy, depression (transdermal)

Pharmacokinetics

Absorption	Well absorbed (PO)
Distribution	Widely distributed
Metabolism	Rapidly, liver
Excretion	Metabolites N-desmethyl-deprenyl, amphetamine, methamphetamine, urine (45%)
Half-life	10 hr; oral disintegrating tab 1.3 hr; transdermal 18-25 hr

Pharmacodynamics

	PO	Orally disintegrating tab	TD
Onset	Unknown	5 min	Unknown
Peak	½-2 hr	10-15 min	2 wk
Duration	Unknown	Unknown	Unknown

CONTRAINDICATIONS

Children/adolescents (suicide/hypertensive crisis), hypersensitivity, breastfeeding, MAOIs

Precautions: Pregnancy, abrupt discontinuation, alcoholism, ambient temperature increases, behavioral changes, bipolar disorders, driving or operating machinery, geriatrics, heating pad, hepatic disease, hypertension, hypotension, melanoma, phenylketonuria, psychosis, renal disease, sunlight exposure

> **BLACK BOX WARNING:** Children or adolescents (transdermal)

> **BLACK BOX WARNING:** Suicidal ideation

DOSAGE AND ROUTES

Adult: PO 5 mg bid at breakfast and lunch **oral disintegrating tab** 1.25 mg (1 tab) initially, then 2.5 (2 tabs) dissolved on tongue daily before breakfast × 6 wk or more; max 2.5 mg/day; **transdermal** (depression) 6 mg/24 hr initially, increase by 3 mg/24 hr at ≥2 wk, up to 12 mg/24 hr if needed

Available forms: Tabs 5 mg, caps 5 mg; oral disintegrating tabs 1.25 mg; transdermal 6 mg/24 hr (20 mg/20 cm²), 9 mg/24 hr (30 mg/30 cm²), 12 mg/24 hr (40 mg/40 cm²)

ADVERSE EFFECTS

CNS: Increased tremors, tardive dyskinesia, dystonic symptoms, hallucinations, dizziness, mood changes, nightmares, delusions, headache, migraine, confusion, anxiety, suicide in children/adolescents, suicidal ideation in adults, serotonin syndrome
CV: Orthostatic hypotension, hypertensive crisis (children)
EENT: Tinnitus
GI: *Nausea*, weight loss, anorexia, diarrhea, vomiting, constipation, flatulence
GU: Hesitation, retention, frequency
INTEG: Increased sweating, melanoma, acne, pruritus
RESP: Cough

INTERACTIONS
Individual drugs
Dextromethorphan: increased unusual behavior, psychosis
FLUoxetine, fluvoxaMINE, PARoxetine, sertraline: increased serotonin syndrome (confusion, seizures, fever, hypertension, agitation) discontinue 5 wk before selegiline
Levodopa/carbidopa: increased side effects
Meperidine opioids: do not use, fatal reaction

Drug/lab test
Decreased: VMA
False positive: urine ketones, urine glucose
False negative: urine glucose (glucose oxidase)
False increase: uric acid, urine protein

NURSING CONSIDERATIONS
Assessment
• **Parkinson's symptoms:** assess for rigidity, unsteady gait, weakness, tremors; these should decrease in severity
• Monitor cardiac status: tachycardia, bradycardia; B/P, respiration throughout treatment

> **BLACK BOX WARNING: Depression:** Assess mental status: affect, mood, behavioral changes, depression; perform suicide assessment, suicidal ideation may occur; report change in symptoms, worsening depression, or suicidal thoughts/behaviors; treatment may need to be changed

• Assess for opioids; if patient has received, do not give selegiline; fatal reactions have occurred
• **Orthostatic hypotension:** May occur during first few weeks of use, more frequent in those >60 yr

S

Patient problem
Impaired mobility (uses)
Depression (uses)
Transdermal risk of injury (uses, adverse reactions)

Implementation
• Do not use in children due to risk for hypertensive crisis
• Adjust dosage to patient's response
• Give with meals; limit protein taken with product
• Give at doses <10 mg/day because of risks associated with nonselective inhibition of MAO
• **Parkinson's syndrome:** reduce levodopa/carbidopa by 10%-30% after 2-3 days of selegiline
• **Oral disintegrating tab:** peel back foil, place tab on tongue, allow to dissolve, swallow with saliva, no fluids for 5 min before and after use; avoid using >2.5 mg/day, hypertensive crisis is more common

Transdermal route (depression)
• Apply to dry, intact skin on upper torso/thigh or outer surface of upper arm q24hr

> **BLACK BOX WARNING:** Do not use in children <12 yr

• When using 9 mg/24 hr or 12 mg/24 hr specific manufacturer recommendations for tyramine intake must be followed to prevent hypertensive crisis

Patient/family education
• Caution patient to change positions slowly to prevent orthostatic hypotension
• **Hypertensive crisis:** teach patient to report nausea, vomiting, sweating, agitation, change in mental status, headache, chest pain to prescriber immediately; instruct patient not to exceed recommended dose of 10 mg
• Teach patient to use during the day to prevent insomnia
• Caution patient to use product exactly as prescribed; if product is discontinued abruptly, parkinsonian crisis may occur
• Instruct patient to avoid foods high in tyramine: cheese, pickled products, wine, beer, large amounts of caffeine as per manufacturer
• **Serotonin syndrome:** teach patient to report twitching, sweating, shivering, diarrhea to prescriber immediately
• Teach patient to avoid heating pads, hot tubs when using transdermal products
• Teach patient to avoid hazardous activities until response is known
• **Pregnancy:** teach patient to report if pregnancy is planned or suspected; do not breastfeed

Evaluation
Positive therapeutic outcome
• Decreased symptoms of Parkinson's disease

TREATMENT OF OVERDOSE:
IV fluids for hypertension, **IV** dilute pressure agent for B/P titration

selenium topical
See Appendix B

RARELY USED

semaglutide
Ozempic
Func. class.: Antidiabetic

USES: For the treatment of type 2 diabetes

DOSAGE AND ROUTES
For the treatment of type 2 diabetes mellitus in combination with diet and exercise
Adult: SUBCUT Initially, 0.25 mg every 7 days (weekly), give at any time of day, with or without meals; after 4 wk increase the dose to 0.5 mg qwk

sennosides (OTC)
(sen'oh-sides)
Black Draught, Ex-Lax, Fletcher's Castoria, Maximum Relief Ex-Lax, Senna-Gen, Senokot, SenokotXTRA
Func. class.: Laxative-stimulant
Chem. class.: Anthraquinone

ACTION: Stimulates peristalsis by action on Auerbach's plexus; softens feces by increasing water and electrolytes in large intestine

Therapeutic outcome: Decreased constipation

USES: Acute constipation; bowel preparation for surgery or exam, prevention of constipation in those taking opiates long term

Pharmacokinetics

Absorption	Minimally absorbed (PO)
Distribution	Unknown
Metabolism	Not metabolized
Excretion	Kidneys, feces
Half-life	Unknown

Pharmacodynamics

	PO	Rect
Onset	6-24 hr	Unknown
Peak	Unknown	Unknown
Duration	3-4 days	Unknown

CONTRAINDICATIONS: Breast-feeding, hypersensitivity, GI bleeding, intestinal obstruction, HF, abdominal pain, nausea/vomiting, appendicitis, acute surgical abdomen

Precautions: Pregnancy

DOSAGE AND ROUTES
Adult: PO 12-50 mg qd or bid
Child 6-12 yr: PO 6-25 mg qd or bid
Child 2-6 yr: PO 3-12.5 qd or bid

Available forms: Tabs 6, 8.6, 15, 25 mg; syr 8.8 mg/5 ml; liquid 33.3 mg/ml

ADVERSE EFFECTS
GI: *Nausea, vomiting, anorexia, abdominal cramps,* diarrhea, flatulence
GU: Pink-red or brown-black discoloration of urine
META: Hypocalcemia, enteropathy, alkalosis, hypokalemia, tetany

INTERACTIONS
Individual drugs
Disulfiram: do not use together

Drug/herb
Flax, senna: increased laxative effect

NURSING CONSIDERATIONS
Assessment
• **Stool:** assess color, consistency, amount; cramping, rectal bleeding, nausea, vomiting; if these symptoms occur, product should be discontinued; identify cause of constipation; identify whether fluids, bulk, or exercise is missing from lifestyle

Nursing diagnoses
• Constipation (uses)
• Diarrhea (side effects)
• Lack of knowledge of medication (teaching)
• Nonadherence (teaching)

Patient problem
Constipation (uses)

Implementation
PO route
• Administer on empty stomach for more rapid results
• Give with a full glass of water in AM or PM (oral dose); evacuation occurs 6-12 hr later

• Dissolve granules in water or juice before administration
• Shake oral sol before giving

Patient/family education
• Discuss with patient that adequate fluid consumption is necessary
• Inform patient that normal bowel movements do not always occur daily
• Teach patient not to use in presence of abdominal pain, nausea, vomiting; tell patient to notify prescriber if constipation is unrelieved or if symptoms of electrolyte imbalance occur: muscle cramps, pain, weakness, dizziness, excessive thirst
• Teach patient to use other ways to decrease constipation: water, bulk in diet, exercise

Evaluation
Positive therapeutic outcome
• Decreased constipation in 8-10 hr

sertraline (Rx)
(ser′tra-leen)
Zoloft
Func. class.: Antidepressant
Chem. class.: Selective serotonin reuptake inhibitor (SSRI)

Do not confuse: Zoloft/Zocor

ACTION: Inhibits serotonin reuptake in CNS, thus increasing action of serotonin; does not affect DOPamine, norepinephrine

Therapeutic outcome: Relief of depression, obsessive-compulsive disorder (OCD), post-traumatic stress disorder (PTSD), panic disorder

USES: Major depression, OCD, PTSD, social anxiety disorder, panic disorder, premenstrual dysphoric disorder (PMDD), separation anxiety disorder

Unlabeled use: Generalized anxiety disorder

Pharmacokinetics

Absorption	Well absorbed
Distribution	Extensive–tissues, protein binding 99%
Metabolism	Liver, extensively
Excretion	Feces (14%)
Half-life	26 hr

Pharmacodynamics

Onset	Unknown
Peak	4.5-8.4 hr
Duration	Unknown

CONTRAINDICATIONS

Hypersensitivity to this product or selective serotonin reuptake inhibitors

Precautions: Pregnancy, breastfeeding, geriatric, renal/hepatic disease, epilepsy, recent MI, latex sensitivity (dropper of oral conc)

> **BLACK BOX WARNING:** Suicidal ideation, children

DOSAGE AND ROUTES
Major depression/OCD
Adult/geriatric: PO 25-50 mg/day; may increase to a maximum of 200 mg/day, do not change dose at intervals of <1 wk; administer daily in AM or PM

Child 6-12 yr (unlabeled): PO 25 mg/day, max 200 mg/day

Premenstrual disorders
Adult: PO 50-150 mg nightly

PTSD/Social anxiety disorder/panic disorder
Adult: PO 25 mg qday, may increase by 50 mg qday after 7 days, range 50-200 mg/day

Hepatic dose
Adult: PO; use lower dose or less frequent dosing intervals

Available forms: Tabs 25, 50, 100 mg; oral concentrate 20 mg/ml; capsules: 25, 50 ❀, 100 mg ❀

ADVERSE EFFECTS

CNS: *Insomnia, agitation, dizziness, headache, fatigue,* confusion, gait abnormality (geriatric), neuroleptic malignant syndrome–like reactions, serotonin syndrome, suicidal ideation, anxiety, drowsiness
CV: Palpitations, chest pain
EENT: Vision abnormalities, yawning, tinnitus, intraocular pressure
ENDO: Syndrome of inappropriate antidiuretic hormone (geriatric), diabetes mellitus
GI: *Diarrhea, nausea, constipation, anorexia, dry mouth,* dyspepsia, *vomiting, flatulence,* weight gain/loss
GU: *Male sexual dysfunction,* menstrual disorders, urinary frequency
INTEG: Increased sweating, rash, hot flashes
MISC: Hyponatremia, neonatal abstinence syndrome, fever

INTERACTIONS
Individual drugs

Bupropion, cyclobenzeprine, tramadol, trazedone: increased serotonin syndrome risk
Cimetidine, warfarin: increased sertraline effect

CloZAPine: increased effects of cloZAPine
Diazepam: increased diazepam effect
Disulfiram: disulfiram reaction with oral conc due to alcohol content
Lithium: altered lithium levels
Phenytoin: increased effects of phenytoin
Pimozide: sertraline is contraindicated with pimozide, fatal reactions, avoid concurrent use
Sibutramine, traZODone, busPIRone, linezolid, traMADol: increased serotonin syndrome, increased neuroleptic malignant syndrome
SUMAtriptan: increased SUMAtriptan effects
TOLBUTamide: increased effect of TOLBUTamide
Warfarin: increased warfarin effect

Drug classifications

Anticoagulants, NSAIDs, thrombolytics, platelet inhibitors, salicylates: increased bleeding risk
Antidepressants (tricyclics), benzodiazepines: increased effect
Highly protein-bound products: increased sertraline levels
SSRIs, SNRIs, serotonin-receptor agonists, tricyclics: increased serotonin syndrome, increased neuroleptic malignant syndrome, avoid concurrent use
MAOIs: fatal reactions

Drug/herb
Kava, valerian: increased CNS effect
SAM-e, St. John's wort, tryptophan: increased effect of SSRIs, serotonin syndrome; do not use together

Drug/lab test
Increased: AST, ALT
False positive: urine screen for benzodiazepines

NURSING CONSIDERATIONS
Assessment

> **BLACK BOX WARNING: Depression/OCD/PTSD:** Assess mental status: mood, sensorium, affect, suicidal tendencies (child/young adult); increase in psychiatric symptoms: depression, panic attacks, OCD, PTSD, social anxiety disorder, usually occurs in first few months of treatment

• **Premenstrual dysphoric disorder:** Assess for emotional lability, sadness, hopelessness, insomnia, anxiety, food cravings, breast pain/tenderness
• Identify alcohol consumption; if alcohol is consumed, hold dose until AM
• **Serotonin syndrome:** assess for hyperthermia, hypertension, rigidity, delirium, coma, myoclonus or neuroleptic malignant-like

syndrome (muscle cramps, fever, unstable B/P, agitation, tremors, mental changes)
• LFTs, thyroid function test, growth rate, weight baseline and periodically
• **Hypertension:** B/P (lying/standing), pulse q4hr; if systolic B/P drops 20 mm Hg, hold product, notify prescriber; VS q4hr in patients with CV disease
• Weight qwk; appetite may decrease with product
• Urinary retention, constipation, especially in geriatric patients
• **Beers:** Avoid in older adults unless safer alternatives are not available, may cause ataxia, impaired psychomotor function

Patient problem
Depression (uses)
Risk for injury (adverse reactions)

Implementation
• Administer dosage at bedtime if oversedation occurs during day; may take entire dose at bedtime
• Give with food, milk for GI symptoms
• Give tablets crushed if patient is unable to swallow medication whole
• Use sugarless gum, hard candy; frequent sips of water for dry mouth
• **Oral concentration:** dilute before use with 4 oz (½ cup) of water, orange juice, ginger ale, or lemon/lime soda; do not mix with other liquids
• Store at room temperature; do not freeze
• Dropper contains latex

Patient/family education
• Teach patient that therapeutic effects may take 1 wk or longer
• Instruct patient to use caution in driving or other activities requiring alertness because of drowsiness, dizziness, blurred vision; to avoid rising quickly from sitting to standing, especially geriatric
• Advise patient to avoid alcohol ingestion, other CNS depressants
• **Teach patient not to discontinue medication quickly after long-term use:** may cause nausea, headache, malaise
• Caution patient to wear sunscreen or large hat because photosensitivity can occur
• Teach patient to increase fluids, bulk in diet if constipation, urinary retention occur, especially geriatric
• Instruct patient to take gum, hard sugarless candy, or frequent sips of water for dry mouth
• Teach patient that medication may be taken without regard to food
• **Serotonin syndrome:** teach patient to report agitation, nausea, vomiting, diarrhea, twitching, sweating, shivering to prescriber immediately
• Advise patient that follow-up exams will be needed

> **BLACK BOX WARNING: Suicidal ideation:** Teach patient that suicidal thoughts/behavior may occur (children/adolescents)

• Instruct patient to notify prescriber if pregnant or planning to become pregnant or breastfeed

Evaluation
Positive therapeutic outcome
• Decrease in depression, OCD, PTSD, PMDD
• Absence of suicidal thoughts

TREATMENT OF OVERDOSE:
ECG monitoring, induce emesis, lavage, administer anticonvulsant

sildenafil (Rx)
(sil-den′a-fill)
Revatio, Viagra
Func. class.: Erectile agent; antihypertensive, pulmonary vasodilator
Chem. class.: Phosphodiesterase 5 inhibitor

Do not confuse: Viagra/Allegra

ACTION: Enhances the effect of nitric oxide (NO) by inhibiting phosphodiesterase type 5 (PDE5), which is necessary for degrading cyclic GMP in the corpus cavernosum

Therapeutic outcome: Ability to achieve and maintain erection

USES: Treatment of erectile dysfunction (Viagra), pulmonary hypertension; improvement in exercise ability

Pharmacokinetics

Absorption	Rapidly, bioavailability (40%)
Distribution	Unknown
Metabolism	Liver (active metabolites)
Excretion	Feces, urine
Half-life	4 hr

Pharmacodynamics

Onset	Unknown
Peak	½-1½ hr
Duration	Unknown

CONTRAINDICATIONS
Hypersensitivity to this product or nitrates

Precautions: Pregnancy, anatomical penile deformities, sickle cell anemia, leukemia, multiple myeloma, retinitis pigmentosa, bleeding disorders, active peptic ulceration, CV/renal/hepatic disease, multidrug antihypertensive regimens, geriatric patients

DOSAGE AND ROUTES
Erectile dysfunction (Viagra only)
Adult male <65 yr: PO 50 mg 1 hr before sexual activity; may be increased to 100 mg or decreased to 25 mg; max frequency once/day use with alpha blockers: space 50-100 mg dose ≥4 hr of alpha blocker
Adult ≥65 yr (male): PO 25 mg prn about 1 hr before sexual activity

Renal/hepatic dose
Adult: PO (Child-Pugh A, B) 25 mg, take 1 hr before sexual activity, do not use more than 1 ×/day; CCr <30 ml/min 25 mg starting dose

Pulmonary hypertension (Revatio only)
Adult: PO 20 mg tid, take 4-6 hr apart; **IV BOL** 10 mg tid

Available forms: Tabs (Viagra), 25, 50, 100 mg; tabs (Revatio) 25mg; sol for inj 10 mg/12.5 ml (Revatio); powder for oral suspension 10 mg/mL (Revatio)

IV push route
• Give undiluted; check for solution that is discolored or precipitate is present; give tid

ADVERSE EFFECTS
CNS: *Headache, flushing, dizziness,* transient global amnesia, seizures
CV: MI, sudden death, CV collapse, TIAs, ventricular dysrhythmias, CV hemorrhage
MISC: *Dyspepsia, nasal congestion, UTI, abnormal vision, diarrhea, rash,* NAION (nonarteritic ischemic optic neuropathy), hearing loss, priapism, sickle cell crisis

INTERACTIONS
Individual drugs
Alcohol, amLODIPine: decreased B/P
Bosentan, rifampin, carBAMazepine, dexamethasone, phenytoin, nevirapine, rifabutin, troglitazone: decreased sildenafil levels
Cimetidine, erythromycin, itraconazole, ketoconazole, tacrolimus: increased sildenafil levels
Riociguat: Fatal fall in B/P, do not use together

Drug classifications
Antacids, barbiturates, CYP450 inducers: decreased sildenafil levels

Antiretroviral protease inhibitors: increased sildenafil levels
α-Blockers, angiotensin II receptor blockers: decreased B/P
Nitrates: fatal fall in B/P; do not use together

Drug/food
Grapefruit: increased product effect
High-fat meal: decreased absorption

NURSING CONSIDERATIONS
Assessment
• For erectile dysfunction before use (Viagra), question about whether failure to achieve erection or failure to maintain intercourse, anorgasmia
• **Pulmonary hypertension:** Assess cardiac status, hemodynamic parameters, exercise tolerance in pulmonary hypertension: B/P pulse (Revatio)
• **Phosphodiesterase type 5 inhibitors with lopinavir/ritonavir (Kaletra):** assess for hypotension, visual changes, prolonged erection, syncope; give only 25 mg q48hr and monitor for adverse reactions
• Identify organic nitrates that should not be used with this product
• Assess for any severe loss of vision while taking this or any similar products; these products should not be used if vision loss has occurred
• **Assess for MI, sudden death, CV collapse:** Those with an MI within 6 mo, resting hypotension <90/50, resting hypertension >170/100, fluid depletion should use this product cautiously, may occur right after sexual activity to days afterward
• **Sickle cell crisis (vasoocclusive crisis):** when used for pulmonary hypertension, may require hospitalization

Patient problem
Impaired sexual functioning (uses)

Implementation
PO route
• **Erectile dysfunction:** give approximately 1 hr before sexual activity, do not use more than once a day, give on empty stomach for better absorption
• Tab may be split
• **Pulmonary hypertension:** Give 3×/day, 4-6 hr apart

IV push route
• Give undiluted, check for solution that is discolored or precipitate is present, give TID

Patient/family education

• Teach patient that product does not protect against STDs, including HIV
• Teach patient that product absorption is reduced with a high-fat meal, to take on empty stomach for faster absorption, to take 30 min to 4 hr before sexual activity, peak in 2 hr
• Teach patient to notify prescriber immediately and stop taking product if vision loss occurs
• Do not use more often than 100 mg in 24 hr
• Teach patient that product should not be used with nitrates in any form or soluble guanylate cyclase stimulators (pulmonary hypertension: Riociguat)
• Teach patient that tab may be split
• Teach patient to notify prescriber immediately and to stop taking product if vision/hearing loss occurs or erection lasts >4 hr
• Teach patient to use only as directed
• Advise patient that color change that is visualized may change
• **Pregnancy/breastfeeding:** Viagra not indicated for women; Revatio: identify if pregnancy is planned or suspected or if breastfeeding

Evaluation

Positive therapeutic outcome

• Ability to achieve and maintain an erection (Viagra); decreasing pulmonary hypertension (Revatio)

---

silodosin (Rx)

(si-lo'do-seen)
Rapaflo
Func. class.: Selective α_1-adrenergic blocker, BPH agent
Chem. class.: Sulfamoylphenethylamine derivative

ACTION: Binds preferentially to α_{1A}-adrenoceptor subtype located mainly in the prostate

Therapeutic outcome: Decreased symptoms of benign prostatic hyperplasia

USES: Symptoms of benign prostatic hyperplasia (BPH)

Pharmacokinetics

Absorption	Decreased with high-fat/high-calorie meal
Distribution	Extensive protein binding 97%
Metabolism	Liver extensively by CYP3A4, UGT2B7
Excretion	Urine (34%), feces (55%)
Half-life	13.3 hr; 24 hr (metabolite)

Pharmacodynamics

Onset	Rapid
Peak	Up to 24 hr
Duration	Up to 24 hr

CONTRAINDICATIONS

Hypersensitivity, renal failure, hepatic disease

Precautions: Pregnancy breastfeeding, children, renal/hepatic disease, females, hypotension, ocular surgery, orthostatic hypotension, prostate cancer, syncope, geriatric patients

DOSAGE AND ROUTES

Adult: PO 8 mg/day with a meal; max 8 mg/day

Renal dose

Adult: PO CCr 30-49 ml/min 4 mg/day; CCr <30 ml/min not recommended

Available forms: Capsules 4, 8 mg

ADVERSE EFFECTS

CNS: *Dizziness, headache,* insomnia
CV: Orthostatic hypotension
EENT: Nasal congestion
GI: Diarrhea
GU: *Abnormal ejaculation,* priapism, urinary incontinence
INTEG: Rash, pruritus, allergic reactions

INTERACTIONS

Drug classifications

CYP3A4 inhibitors (clarithromycin, itraconazole, ritonavir, anti-retroviral protease inhibitors, aprepitant, chloramphenicol, conivaptan, dalfopristin, danazol, delavirdine, efavirenz, fosaprepitant, fluconazole, fluvoxaMINE, imatinib, isoniazid, mifepristone, nefazodone, tamoxifen, telithromycin, troleandomycin, voriconazole, zileuton, zafirlukast), P-gb inhibitors: increased silodosin effect

Drug/food

Grapefruit juice: increased silodosin effect

Drug/lab test

Increased: LFTs

NURSING CONSIDERATIONS

Assessment

• **Prostatic hyperplasia:** assess for change in urinary patterns, baseline and throughout treatment, testing for prostate cancer prior to administration is recommended; monitor BUN, uric acid, urodynamic studies (urinary flow rates, residual volume), CCr, contraindicated in CCr <30 ml/min; assess I&O ratios, weight daily, edema; report weight gain or edema
• B/P, monitor for orthostatic hypotension
• **Pregnancy/breastfeeding:** Not indicated for women

S

Patient problem
Impaired urination (uses)
Risk for injury (adverse reactions)

Implementation
• Give with meal at same time of day
• May open capsule and sprinkle on food if unable to swallow cap; use water afterward
• Store at room temperature; protect from light and moisture

Patient/family education
• Caution patient not to drive or operate machinery until effect is known
• Advise patient not to use with grapefruit juice
• Teach patient to rise slowly to minimize orthostatic hypotension
• Advise patient to discuss all OTC, Rx, herbals, supplements with health care professional
• Advise patient that follow-up exams will be needed
• Teach patient to take with same meal each day, contents of capsule may be sprinkled on room-temperature applesauce if used within 5 min, follow with 8 oz of water

Evaluation

Positive therapeutic outcome
• Decreased symptoms of benign prostatic hyperplasia

silver nitrate 1% ophthalmic
See Appendix B

silver nitrate sulfacetamide sodium ophthalmic
See Appendix B

silver sulfADIAZINE topical
See Appendix B

simvastatin (Rx)
(sim-va-stat′in)
Zocor
Func. class.: Antilipidemic
Chem. class.: HMG-CoA reductase inhibitor

Do not confuse: Zocor/Zoloft

ACTION: Inhibits HMG-CoA reductase enzyme, which reduces cholesterol synthesis; this enzyme is needed for cholesterol production

Therapeutic outcome: Decreasing cholesterol levels and LDLs, increased HDLs

USES: As an adjunct in primary hypercholesterolemia (types IIa, IIb), isolated hypertriglyceridemia (Frederickson type IV) and type III hyperlipoproteinemia, CAD, heterozygous familial hypercholesterolemia; MI/stroke prophylaxis

Pharmacokinetics

Absorption	85%
Distribution	Unknown, protein binding 98%
Metabolism	Liver—extensively
Excretion	70% feces, 20% kidneys
Half-life	3 hr

Pharmacodynamics

Onset	Unknown
Peak	Up to 4 wk
Duration	Unknown

CONTRAINDICATIONS
Pregnancy, breastfeeding, hypersensitivity, active liver disease

Precautions: Past liver disease, alcoholism, severe acute infections, trauma, severe metabolic disorders, electrolyte imbalances, Chinese patients

DOSAGE AND ROUTES
Adult: PO 20-40 mg/day in PM initially, usual range 5-40 mg/day daily in PM max, 40 mg/day

With diltiazem/verapamil
Adult: PO 5-10 mg q PM
Child and adolescent ≥10 yr including girls ≥1 yr postmenarche: PO 10 mg q PM

With amiodarone, amLODIPine, ranolazine
Adult: PO 5-20 mg/day in evening, max 20 mg/day

Heterozygous familial hypercholesterolemia
Adult: PO 40 mg qday in evening; make dosage adjustments q4wk

Heterozygous familial hypercholesterolemia in boys and postmenarchal girls
Child 10-17 yr: PO 10 mg qday in the evening, max 40 mg/day

Renal dose
Adult: PO 5 mg qday in the evening (severe renal disease)

Available forms: Tabs 5, 10, 20, 40, 80 mg

ADVERSE EFFECTS
CNS: Headache, cognitive impairment
GI: Nausea, constipation, diarrhea, dyspepsia, flatus, abdominal pain, liver dysfunction, pancreatitis, hyperglycemia
INTEG: Rash, pruritus

MS: Muscle cramps, myalgia, myositis, rhabdomyolysis, myopathy
RESP: Upper respiratory tract infection

INTERACTIONS
Individual drugs
Clarithromycin, clofibrate, cycloSPORINE, erythromycin, gemfibrozil, itraconazole, ketoconazole, niacin, danazol, delavirdine, nefazodone, verapamil, diltiazem, amiodarone, azole antifungals, telithromycin: increased myalgia, myositis, rhabdomyolysis
CycloSPORINE, gemfibrozil: do not use with simvastatin
Digoxin: increased digoxin levels
Warfarin: increased risk of bleeding

Drug classifications
Macrolide antiinfectives, protease inhibitors: increased myalgia, myositis, rhabdomyolysis
Increased: simvastatin effect ATP1B1 inhibitors

Drug/herb
Red yeast rice, kava; eucalyptus: increased simvastatin effect
St. John's wort: decreased effect

Drug/food
Increased: simvastatin level: grapefruit juice (large amounts)

Drug/lab test
Increased: CPK, liver function tests, HbA1C, ALT/AST

NURSING CONSIDERATIONS
Assessment
• Assess nutrition: fat, protein, carbohydrates; nutritional analysis should be completed by dietitian before treatment is initiated
• **Rhabdomyolysis:** assess for muscle tenderness, increased CPK levels 10× ULN; therapy should be discontinued, more likely in those receiving >80 mg/day, first year of treatment, those ≥65 yr, females
• 🧬 **Chinese patients:** Avoid high doses (80 mg) if taking niacin >1 g/day, may increase myopathy
• Monitor bowel pattern daily; diarrhea may occur
• Monitor triglycerides, cholesterol baseline, throughout treatment; LDL, HDL, triglycerides and cholesterol should be watched closely at 6-8 wk and q6mo; if increased, product should be discontinued

Patient problem
Nonadherence (teaching)

Implementation
• Once a day in OM
• Store in cool environment in tight container protected from light

• Avoid grapefruit juice
• Discontinuing use before surgery is recommended in renal failure, restart afterward

Patient/family education
• Inform patient that compliance is needed for positive results to occur, not to double doses
• Advise patient to lower risk factors: high-fat diet, smoking, alcohol consumption, absence of exercise, smoking cessation
• Teach patient to take in evening
• Teach patient to report muscle pain, weakness, abdominal pain, dark urine, yellowing of skin or eyes, memory loss
• Teach patient this product may affect blood sugar levels if patient has diabetes
• Teach patient follow-up exams will be needed
• Advise patient to notify prescriber of planned or suspected pregnancy or if breastfeeding

Evaluation
Positive therapeutic outcome
• Decreased cholesterol levels, serum triglycerides and improved ratio with HDLs

---

⚠ HIGH ALERT

sirolimus (Rx)
(seer-roe'li-mus)
Rapamune
Func. class.: Immunosuppressant
Chem. class.: Macrolide

ACTION: Produces immunosuppression by inhibiting T-lymphocyte activation and proliferation

Therapeutic outcome: Prevention of rejection in organ transplant

USES: Organ transplants: to prevent rejection, recommended use is with cycloSPORINE and corticosteroids

Pharmacokinetics

Absorption	Rapidly absorbed
Distribution	To major organs, 92% protein binding
Metabolism	Liver; extensively by CYP3A4
Excretion	91% (feces)
Half-life	57-63 hr

Pharmacodynamics

Onset	Unknown
Peak	1 hr single dose, 2 hr multiple dosing
Duration	Unknown

S

CONTRAINDICATIONS

Breastfeeding, hypersensitivity to this product or to components of the product

Precautions: Pregnancy, children <13 yr, severe cardiac/renal/hepatic disease, diabetes mellitus, hyperkalemia, hyperuricemia, hypertension, interstitial lung disease, hyperlipidemia, soy lecithin hypersensitivity

> **BLACK BOX WARNING:** Lymphomas, infection, other malignancies, liver/lung transplant, requires a specialized setting, requires an experienced clinician

DOSAGE AND ROUTES

Kidney transplant
Adult/adolescent ≥40 kg: PO 2 mg daily with 6 mg loading dose
Child >13 yr <40 kg (88 lb): PO 1 mg/m^2/day, 3 mg/m^2/loading dose

Hepatic dose
Adult and child ≥13 yr <40 kg: PO reduce by 33% in maintenance dose (mild to moderate hepatic impairment); reduce by 50% in maintenance dose (severe hepatic impairment)

Lymphangioleimyomatosis
Adult: PO 2 mg q day, trough level (whole blood) after 10-20 days, titrate to 5-15 mg/mL, then monitor trough q 3 mo

Available forms: Oral sol 1 mg/ml; tabs 0.5, 1, 2 mg

ADVERSE EFFECTS

CNS: *Tremors, headache, insomnia*, paresthesia, chills, fever, progressive multifocal leukoencephalopathy (PML)
CV: Hypo/hypertension, atrial fibrillation, HF, palpitations, tachycardia, peripheral edema, thrombosis
EENT: Blurred vision, photophobia
GI: Nausea, vomiting, diarrhea, constipation, hepatotoxicity, CDAD
GU: UTI, renal failure, nephrotic syndrome, amenorrhea
HEMA: Anemia, thrombocytopenia, leukopenia
INTEG: *Rash, acne*, photosensitivity
META: Increased creatinine, edema, hypercholesterolemia, *hyperlipemia*, hypophosphatemia, weight gain, hyperglycemia, hypo/hyperkalemia, hyperuricemia, hypomagnesemia, hypertriglyceridemia
MS: Arthralgia
RESP: Pleural effusion, atelectasis, *dyspnea*, pneumonitis, pulmonary embolism/fibrosis, pulmonary hypertension, interstitial lung disease
SYST: Lymphoma, exfoliative dermatitis

INTERACTIONS
Individual drugs
Bromocriptine, cimetidine, cycloSPORINE, danazol, erythromycin, metoclopramide: increased blood level
CarBAMazepine, PHENobarbital, phenytoin, rifamycin, rifapentine: decreased blood levels

Drug classifications
ACE inhibitors, angiotensin II receptor antagonists, cephalosporins, iodine-containing radiopaque contrast media, neuromuscular blockers, NSAIDs, penicillins, salicylates, thrombolytics: increased angioedema
Antifungal agents, calcium channel blockers, HIV protease inhibitors: increased blood levels
Live virus vaccines: decreased effect of vaccines

Drug/herb
St. John's wort: decreased sirolimus effect

Drug/food
Food: alters bioavailability, use consistently with or without food
Grapefruit juice: do not use with grapefruit juice

Drug/lab test
Increased: LFTs, alk phos, lipids, triglycerides, total cholesterol, BUN, creatinine, LDH, phosphate
Decreased: platelets, sodium
Increased or decreased: magnesium, glucose, calcium

NURSING CONSIDERATIONS
Assessment
• **Wound dehiscence and anastomotic disruption:** assess wound, vascular, airway, ureteral, biliary, inhibition of growth factors; do not combine with corticosteroids, not recommended in lung or liver transplant

> **BLACK BOX WARNING: Infection:** Immunosuppression may lead to susceptibility to infection

> **BLACK BOX WARNING: Neoplastic disease:** Lymphoma, skin cancer may occur, limit UV exposure, use protective clothing, sunscreen not recommended, mortality and graft loss may occur

• **Anaphylaxis, angioedema, exfoliative dermatitis:** assess for, more common when given with ACE inhibitors; do not use if a hypersensitivity reaction occurs
• **Bone marrow suppression:** Hgb, WBC, platelets monthly during treatment; if leukocytes are <3000/mm^3 or platelets <100,000/mm^3, product should be discontinued or reduced; decreased Hgb level

---

- Monitor blood levels in those who may have altered metabolism, trough levels ≥15 ng/ml are associated with increased adverse reactions
- **Pulmonary fibrosis, pulmonary effusion, pneumonitis:** assess for dyspnea, cough, hypoxia; some fatal cases have occurred
- Monitor lipid profile: cholesterol, triglycerides; a lipid-lowering agent may be needed

> **BLACK BOX WARNING.** Creatinine/BUN, CBC, serum potassium

- **High risk:** those with Banff grade 3 acute rejection or vascular rejection prior to cycloSPORINE withdrawal, dialysis dependent, creatinine >4.5 mg/dl, 🐭 African descent, re-transplant, multiorgan transplant, high panel of reactive antibodies
- **Hepatotoxicity:** alk phos, AST, ALT, amylase, bilirubin: dark urine, jaundice, itching, light-colored stools; product should be discontinued

Patient problem
Immunologic impairment (uses)
Risk for infection (adverse reactions)

Implementation
- Administer prophylaxis for *Pneumocystis jiroveci* pneumonia for 1 yr after transplantation; prophylaxis for cytomegalovirus (CMV) is recommended for 90 days after transplantation in those at increased risk for CMV
- Use amber oral dose syringe and withdraw amount of oral sol needed; empty correct dose into plastic/glass container holding 60 ml of water/orange juice, stir vigorously and have patient drink at once, refill container with additional 120 ml of water/orange juice, stir vigorously, and have patient drink at once; if using a pouch squeeze entire contents into container and follow preceding directions
- Give all medications PO if possible; avoid IM inj because bleeding may occur
- Give for 3 days before transplant surgery; patients should be placed in protective isolation, give at same time of day, give 4 hr after cycloSPORINE oral sol or caps, do not use with grapefruit juice
- Store protected from light; refrigerate; stable for 24 months

> **BLACK BOX WARNING:** Only those experienced in immunosuppressant therapy and transplant should use this drug; must use in a specialized care setting with adequate medical equipment

Patient/family education
- Instruct patient to report fever, rash, severe diarrhea, chills, sore throat, fatigue because serious infections may occur; clay-colored stools, cramping may indicate hepatotoxicity; fever, chills, sore throat (infection)
- Caution patient to avoid crowds or persons with known infections to reduce risk of infection
- Teach patient to use sunscreen, protective clothing to prevent burns
- Teach patient that lifelong use is required to prevent rejection
- Teach patient that continuing follow-up exams and blood work will be required
- Teach patient to take at same time, consistently, with or without regard to food, avoid grapefruit juice
- Teach patient to take 4 hr after oral cycloSPORINE
- **Pregnancy/breastfeeding:** Teach patient to use contraception before, during, and 12 wk after product has been discontinued; avoid breastfeeding
- Advise patient to avoid live virus vaccines during treatment

Evaluation

Positive therapeutic outcome
- Absence of graft rejection

> **⚠ HIGH ALERT**
>
> ## sitaGLIPtin (Rx)
> (sit-a-glip′tin)
> **Januvia**
> *Func. class.:* Antidiabetic, oral
> *Chem. class.:* Dipeptidyl-peptidase-4 inhibitor (DPP-4 inhibitor)

ACTION: Slows the inactivation of incretin hormones; improves glucose homeostasis, improves glucose-dependent insulin secretion, lowers glucagon secretions and slows gastric emptying time

Therapeutic outcome: Decrease in polyuria, polydipsia, polyphagia; clear sensorium; absence of dizziness; stable gait; blood glucose at normal level

USES: Type 2 diabetes mellitus as monotherapy or in combination with other antidiabetic agents

Pharmacokinetics

Absorption	Rapidly
Distribution	Unknown
Metabolism	Unknown
Excretion	Kidneys, 79% unchanged
Half-life	12.4 hr

Pharmacodynamics

Onset	Unknown
Peak	1-4 hr
Duration	Up to 24 hr

CONTRAINDICATIONS

Angioedema, diabetic ketoacidosis (DKA)

Precautions: Pregnancy, geriatric, hypersensitivity, GI obstruction, thyroid disease, surgery, renal/hepatic disease, trauma, breastfeeding, pancreatitis, hypercortisolism, hyperglycemia, hyperthyroidism, hypoglycemia, ileus, pituitary insufficiency, surgery, type 1 diabetes mellitus, adrenal insufficiency, burns, diabetic ketoacidosis

DOSAGE AND ROUTES

Adult: PO 100 mg/day; when used with a sulfonylurea or insulin

Renal dose

Adult: PO CCr 30-50 ml/min 50 mg qd; CCr <30 ml/min 25 mg qd

Available forms: Tabs 25, 50, 100 mg

ADVERSE EFFECTS

CNS: *Headache*
ENDO: Hypoglycemia
GI: *Nausea, vomiting,* abdominal pain, diarrhea, pancreatitis, constipation
GU: Acute renal failure
MISC: Peripheral edema, upper respiratory infection
SYST: Anaphylaxis, Stevens-Johnson syndrome, angioedema

INTERACTIONS

Individual drugs
Digoxin: increased levels of digoxin

Drug classifications
Antidiabetic (insulin, glipizide, glimerpiride, glyburide): increase hypoglycemia

Drug/herb
Garlic, green tea, horse chestnut: increased antidiabetic effect

Drug/lab test
Increased: creatinine, LFTs

NURSING CONSIDERATIONS

Assessment
• **Hypoglycemic reactions:** assess for sweating, weakness, dizziness, anxiety, tremors, hunger, hyperglycemic reactions soon after meals
• Monitor CBC (baseline, q3mo) during treatment; check liver function tests periodically, AST, LDH, renal studies: BUN, creatinine during treatment; Hgb A1c

• **Serious skin reactions:** assess for swelling of face, mouth, lips, dyspnea, wheezing
• **Pancreatitis:** assess for severe abdominal pain, nausea, vomiting; discontinue product; monitor amylase, lipase
• **Renal studies:** monitor BUN, creatinine during treatment, especially in geriatrics or those with renal disease
• Monitor hemoglobin A1C; monitor blood glucose as needed

Patient problem
Excess food intake (uses)
Nonadherence (teaching)

Implementation
• May be taken with or without food
• Conversion from other antidiabetic agents; change may be made with gradual dosage change
• Store in tight container at room temperature
• Do not split, crush, chew, swallow whole

Patient/family education
• Teach patient to use regular self-monitoring of blood glucose using blood glucose meter
• Teach patient the symptoms of hypo/hyperglycemia, what to do about each
• Teach patient that product must be continued on daily basis; explain consequence of discontinuing product abruptly
• Advise patient to avoid OTC medications, alcohol, digoxin, exenatide, insulins, nateglinide, repaglinide, and other products that lower blood sugar, unless approved by prescriber
• Teach patient that diabetes is a lifelong illness; that this product is not a cure, only controls symptoms
• Teach patient that all food included in diet plan must be eaten to prevent hypo/hyperglycemia
• Teach patient to carry emergency ID
• Teach patient to notify prescriber immediately of hypersensitivity reactions (rash, swelling of face, trouble breathing)
• Advise patient to report severe joint pain immediately, may have a late onset
• Teach patient to notify prescriber if pregnancy is planned or suspected; to continue health regimen (diet, exercise)

Evaluation

Positive therapeutic outcome
• Decrease in polyuria, polydipsia, polyphagia; clear sensorium; absence of dizziness; stable gait, blood glucose, A1C improvement

sodium bicarbonate (Rx, OTC)

baking soda, Bell-Ans,
Citrocarbonate, Neut, Soda mint ♦

Func. class.: Alkalinizer; antacid
Chem. class.: NaHCO₃

ACTION: Orally neutralizes gastric acid, which forms water, NaCl, CO_2; increases plasma bicarbonate, which buffers H⁺ ion concentration; reverses acidosis IV

Therapeutic outcome: Correction of acidosis, gastric acid neutralization

USES: Acidosis (metabolic), cardiac arrest, alkalinization (systemic/urinary); antacid (PO); salicylate poisoning

Pharmacokinetics

Absorption	Unknown
Distribution	Widely distributed—extracellular fluids
Metabolism	Unknown
Excretion	Kidneys
Half-life	Unknown

Pharmacodynamics

	PO	IV
Onset	2 min	Rapid
Peak	½ hr	Rapid
Duration	1-3 hr	Unknown

CONTRAINDICATIONS

Respiratory/metabolic alkalosis, hypochloremia, hypocalcemia

Precautions: Pregnancy, HF, cirrhosis, toxemia, renal disease, hypertension, hypokalemia, breastfeeding, hypernatremia, Bartter's syndrome, Cushing's syndrome, hyperaldosteronism, children

DOSAGE AND ROUTES

Acidosis, metabolic (not associated with cardiac arrest)

Adult and child: IV INF 2-5 mEq/kg over 4-8 hr depending on CO_2, pH, ABGs

Cardiac arrest

Adult and child: IV BOL 1 mEq/kg of 7.5% or 8.4% SOL, then 0.5 mEq/kg q5-10min, then doses based on ABGs

Infant: IV 1 mEq/kg over several min (use only the 0.5 mEq/ml [4.2%] sol for inj)

Alkalinization of urine

Adult: PO 325 mg-2 g qid or 48 mEq/kg (4 g), then 12-24 mEq q4hr

Child: PO 84-840 mg/kg/day (1-10 mEq/kg), in divided doses q4-6hr

Antacid

Adult: PO 300 mg-2 g chewed, taken with water daily-qid

Available forms: Tabs 300, 325, 600, 650 mg; inj 4.2%, 5%, 7.5%, 8.4%

ADVERSE EFFECTS

CNS: Irritability, headache, confusion, stimulation, tremors, *twitching, hyperreflexia,* tetany, weakness, seizures caused by alkalosis
CV: Irregular pulse, cardiac arrest, water retention, edema, weight gain
GI: Flatulence, *belching, distention*
GU: Calculi
META: *Alkalosis*
MS: Muscular twitching, tetany, irritability

INTERACTIONS

Individual drugs

ChlorproPAMIDE, lithium: decreased effect of each specific product
Flecainide, mecamylamine, pseudoephedrine, quiNIDine, quiNINE: increased effects of each specific product

Drug classifications

Amphetamines, anorexiants, sympathomimetics: increased effects of each specific product
Barbiturates: decreased effects of barbiturates
Benzodiazepines: decreased effects of each specific product
Corticosteroids: increased sodium; decreased potassium, decreased effects of corticosteroids
Ketoconazoles: decreased effects of ketoconazoles
Salicylates: decreased effect of salicylates

Drug/herb

Oak bark: decreased action of sodium bicarbonate

Drug/lab test

Increased: sodium, lactate
Decreased: potassium

NURSING CONSIDERATIONS

Assessment

• Assess respiratory and pulse rate, rhythm, depth, lung sounds; notify prescriber of abnormalities
• Assess for CO_2 in GI tract; may lead to perforation if ulcer is severe
• **Fluid balance** (I&O ratio, weight daily, edema); notify prescriber of fluid overload, assess for edema, crackles, SOB
• Monitor electrolytes, blood pH, PO_2, HCO_3 during beginning treatment; ABGs frequently during emergencies

S

• Monitor extravasation with **IV** administration (tissue sloughing, ulceration, and necrosis)
• **Alkalosis:** irritability, confusion, twitching, hyperreflexia, stimulation, slow respirations, cyanosis, irregular pulse
• **Milk-alkali syndrome:** confusion, headache, nausea, vomiting, anorexia, urinary stones, hypercalcemia
• **Pregnancy/breastfeeding:** Use as an antacid is considered unsafe, may breastfeed

Patient problem
Impaired gas exchange (uses)
Fluid imbalance (adverse reactions)

Implementation
PO route
• Antacid tab must be chewed and taken with 8 oz of water
• Dissolve effervescent tab in water
• May be used to neutralize gastric acid in peptic ulcer disease, given 1 and 3 hr after meals and at bedtime

Direct IV route
• Use in cardiac emergencies, use ampules or prefilled syringes only, give by rapid bolus dose, flush with 0.9% NaCl before and after use
Continuous IV infusion route
• Prepared sol or diluted in an equal amount of any dextrose/saline combination; administer 2-5 mEq/kg over 4-8 hr, max 50 mEq/hr; slower rate in children

Y-site compatibilities: Acyclovir, amifostine, asparaginase, aztreonam, bivalirudin, bumetanide, cefepime, cefmetazole, cefTRIAXone, chloramphenicol, cyclophosphamide, cytarabine, DAUNOrubicin, dexamethasone, DOXOrubicin, etoposide, famotidine, fentaNYL, filgrastim, fluconazole, fludarabine, furosemide, gallium nitrate, gemcitabine, gentamicin, granisetron, heparin, hydrocortisone sodium succinate, ifosfamide, indomethacin, insulin, ketorolac, labetalol, levofloxacin, lidocaine, linezolid, LORazepam, magnesium sulfate, melphalan, mesna, meperidine, methylPREDNISolone, metoclopramide, metoprolol, metroNIDAZOLE, milrinone, morphine, nafcillin, nitroglycerin, nitroprusside, PACLitaxel, palonosetron, pantoprazole, PEMEtrexed, penicillin G potassium, phenylephrine, phytonadione, piperacillin/tazobactam, potassium chloride, procainamide, propofol, propranolol, protamine, ranitidine, remifentanil, tacrolimus, teniposide, thiotepa, ticarcillin/clavulanate, tirofiban, tobramycin, tolazoline, vasopressin, vitamin B complex with C, voriconazole

Patient/family education
• Instruct patient to chew antacid tab and drink 8 oz of water; not to take antacid with milk

because milk-alkali syndrome may result; not to use antacid for more than 2 wk
• Advise patient to notify prescriber if indigestion is accompanied by chest pain; trouble breathing; diarrhea; dark, tarry stools; vomit that looks like coffee grounds; swelling of feet/ankles
• Teach patient about sodium-restricted diet; to avoid use of baking soda for indigestion

Evaluation
Positive therapeutic outcome
• ABGs, electrolytes, blood pH, HCO_3 normal levels
• Decreased gastric pain

sodium biphosphate/ sodium phosphate (OTC)
Fleet Enema, Phospho-soda
Func. class.: Laxative, saline

ACTION: Increases water absorption in the small intestine by osmotic action; laxative effect occurs by increased peristalsis and water retention

Therapeutic outcome: Absence of constipation

USES: Constipation, bowel or rectal preparation for surgery, examination

Pharmacokinetics
Absorption	Up to 20% (rec)
Distribution	Unknown
Metabolism	Unknown
Excretion	Kidneys
Half-life	Unknown

Pharmacodynamics
	PO	Rect
Onset	½-3 hr	5 min
Peak	Unknown	Unknown
Duration	Unknown	Unknown

CONTRAINDICATIONS
Hypersensitivity, rectal fissures, abdominal pain, nausea/vomiting, appendicitis, acute surgical abdomen, ulcerated hemorrhoids, Na-restricted diets, renal failure, hyperphosphatemia, hypocalcemia, hypokalemia, hypernatremia, Addison's disease, HF, ascites, bowel perforation, megacolon, imperforate anus

BLACK BOX WARNING: GI obstruction, renal failure

Precautions: Pregnancy

BLACK BOX WARNING: Colitis, elderly, hypovolemia, renal disease

DOSAGE AND ROUTES
Adult: PO 20-30 ml (Phospho-soda)
Child: PO 5-15 ml (Phospho-soda)
Adult and child >12 yr: RECT enema (118 ml)
Child 2-12 yr: RECT ½ enema (59 ml)

Available forms: Enema 7 g/phosphate and 19 g/biphosphate/118 ml; oral sol 18 g phosphate/48 g biphosphate/100 ml

ADVERSE EFFECTS
CV: Dysrhythmias, cardiac arrest, hypotension, widening QRS complex
GI: *Nausea, cramps,* diarrhea
META: Electrolyte, fluid imbalances

NURSING CONSIDERATIONS
Assessment
• Assess stools: color, amount, consistency
• Assess for bowel pattern, bowel sounds (frequency, intensity), flatulence, distention, increased temp, dietary patterns (fluid, bulk), exercise
• Assess for cramping, rectal bleeding, nausea, vomiting; if these symptoms occur, product should be discontinued

Patient problem
Constipation (uses)

Implementation
PO route
• Give on empty stomach
• Mix oral sol in cold water
• Take alone for better absorption; do not take within 1 hr of other products

Patient/family education
• Advise patient not to use laxatives or enema for long-term therapy; bowel tone will be lost
• Teach patient that normal bowel movements do not always occur daily
• Caution patient not to use in presence of abdominal pain, nausea, vomiting
• Caution patient to notify prescriber if constipation is unrelieved or if symptoms of electrolyte imbalance occur: muscle cramps, pain, weakness, dizziness, excessive thirst
• Instruct patient to maintain adequate fluid consumption to help prevent constipation

Evaluation
Positive therapeutic outcome
• Decrease in constipation

sodium polystyrene sulfonate (Rx)
(po-lee-stye′reen)
Kalexate, Kayexalate, Kionex, SPS
Func. class.: Potassium-removing resin
Chem. class.: Cation exchange resin

ACTION: Removes potassium by exchanging sodium for potassium in body; occurs primarily in large intestine

Therapeutic outcome: Potassium levels within accepted range

USES: Hyperkalemia in conjunction with other measures

Pharmacokinetics
Absorption	None
Distribution	None
Metabolism	None
Excretion	Feces
Half-life	Unknown

Pharmacodynamics
	PO	Rect
Onset	2-12 hr	2-12 hr
Peak	Unknown	Unknown
Duration	6-24 hr	4-6 hr

CONTRAINDICATIONS
Hypersensitivity to saccharin or parabens that may be in some products; GI obstruction, neonate (reduced gut motility)

Precautions: Pregnancy, geriatric, renal failure, HF, severe edema, severe hypertension, sodium restriction, constipation, GI bleeding, hypocalcemia

DOSAGE AND ROUTES
Adult: PO 15 g daily-qid; RECT enema 30-50 q1-2hr initially prn, then q6hr prn
Child (unlabeled): PO 1 g/kg q6hr prn; RECT 1 g/kg q2-6hr prn

Available forms: Powder for susp 453.6 g, 454 g; oral susp 15 g/60 ml

ADVERSE EFFECTS
GI: *Constipation,* anorexia, nausea, vomiting, diarrhea (sorbitol), *fecal impaction,* gastric irritation
META: Hypocalcemia, hypokalemia, hypomagnesemia, sodium retention

S

INTERACTIONS
Individual drugs
Sorbitol: increased colonic necrosis, do not use concurrently

Lithium: decreased effect of lithium

Drug classifications
Diuretics (loop), cardiac glycosides: increased hypokalemia

Magnesium/calcium antacids: increased metabolic acidosis

Thyroid hormones: decreased effect of thyroid hormones

NURSING CONSIDERATIONS
Assessment
• Assess bowel function daily: amount of stool, color, characteristics

• Assess for hypotension: confusion, irritability, muscular pain, weakness

• Hyperkalemia: assess for confusion, dyspnea, weakness, dysrhythmias

• Monitor electrolytes: potassium, sodium, calcium, magnesium; I&O ratio, weight daily

• **Hypokalemia:** Monitor ECG for spiked T-waves, depressed ST segments, prolonged QT interval, and widening QRS complex

• Monitor I&O ratio, weight daily, crackles, dyspnea, jugular vein distention, edema

• Monitor for digoxin toxicity (nausea, vomiting, blurred vision, anorexia, dysrhythmia) in those receiving digoxin

Patient problem
Constipation (adverse reactions)

Implementation
PO route
• **Powdered resin:** Use orally as a suspension in water or in a syrup. Fluid ranges 20-100 ml, depending on the dose, or 3-4 ml per g of resin. Suspensions should be freshly prepared and not stored for longer than 24 hr. The powder should not be mixed with foods or liquids that contain a large amount of potassium (bananas or orange juice)

Rectal route
• Precede retention enema with a cleansing enema; Gently insert a soft, large (French 28) rubber tube into the rectum for a distance of about 20 cm; the tip should be well into the sigmoid colon. Tape the tube in place. Suspend the sodium polystyrene sulfonate powdered resin in 100 ml (water or sorbitol) warmed to body temperature. The particles should be kept suspended by stirring the suspension during administration. Alternatively, 120-180 ml of a commercially available suspension may be administered as a retention enema after the suspension has been warmed to body temperature. Following administration, flush the tube with 50-100 ml of fluid and clamp the tube and leave in place. The suspension should be retained in the colon for at least 30-60 min or for several hours, if possible

• After several hours have passed, administer a cleansing enema using a nonsodium containing solution at body temperature. Drain fluid through a Y-tube connection. Observe the drainage if sorbitol was used

Patient/family education
• Explain reason for medication and expected results

• Teach patient to avoid laxatives, antacids, electrolyte-based products unless approved by prescriber

• Teach patient to use a low-potassium diet, provide sample diet

Evaluation
Positive therapeutic outcome
• Potassium level 3.5-5 mg/dl

sofosbuvir/velpatasvir
(soe-fosbue-vir/vel-patas-vir)
Epclusa
Func. class.: Antiviral, antihepatitis agent

ACTION: Sofosbuvir: A nucleotide prodrug that prevents hepatitis C viral (HCV) replication by inhibiting the activity of HCV NS5B RNA polymerase. It undergoes intracellular metabolism to form an active uridine analog triphosphate. Hepatitis C virus NS5B RNA polymerase incorporates this metabolite into the viral RNA, where it acts as a chain terminator. It does not inhibit human DNA or RNA polymerase, nor does it block mitochondrial RNA polymerase
Velpatasvir: Inhibits the HCV NS5A protein, which is required for viral replication

Therapeutic outcome: Decreased symptoms of chronic hepatitis C

USES: Treatment of chronic hepatitis C infection, including genotypes 1, 2, 3, 4, 5, and 6 in those without cirrhosis and in patients with compensated cirrhosis (Child-Pugh A); treatment of chronic hepatitis C infection in patients with decompensated cirrhosis (Child-Pugh B or C)

Pharmacokinetics

Absorption	Unknown
Distribution	Sofosbuvir: 61%-65% protein binding; velpatasvir 99.5% protein binding

Metabolism	Sofosbuvir: Converted in the liver from the nucleotide prodrug to active nucleoside analog triphosphate
	Velpatasvir: Metabolized by CYP2B6, CYP2C8, and CYP3A4
Excretion	Sofosbuvir: Elimination via kidneys 80%, feces 14%, expired air 2.5%
	Velpatasvir: Excretion in bile 77% of the parent drug, 95% feces, 0.4% urine
Half-life	Sofosbuvir: Half-life of 25 hr
	Velpatasvir: Terminal elimination half-life 15 hr

Pharmacodynamics

Onset	Unknown
Peak	Sofosbuvir: Peak 0.5-1 hr Velpatasvir: Peak 3 hr, increased by high-fat meal
Duration	Unknown

CONTRAINDICATIONS
Hypersensitivity

Precautions: Breastfeeding, hepatitis C and HIV coinfection, male-mediated teratogenicity, pregnancy, renal failure/impairment

> **BLACK BOX WARNING:** Hepatitis B exacerbation

DOSAGE AND ROUTES
Chronic hepatitis C infection in patients without cirrhosis and in patients with compensated cirrhosis (Child-Pugh A)
Adult: PO 1 tablet (400 mg sofosbuvir; 100 mg velpatasvir) qday × 12 wk

Chronic hepatitis C infection in patients with decompensated cirrhosis (Child-Pugh B or C)
Adult: PO 1 tablet (400 mg sofosbuvir; 100 mg velpatasvir) qday plus ribavirin × 12 wk. The dose of ribavirin is based on weight as follows: <75 kg give 500 mg bid; ≥75 kg 600 mg bid

Available forms: Tablet 400 sofosbuvir-100 mg velpatasvir

ADVERSE EFFECTS
CNS: *Fatigue, headache, insomnia,* depression, irritability, asthenia
GI: *Nausea, diarrhea*
HEMA: Anemia
INTEG: Rash
META: Hyperbilirubinemia

INTERACTIONS
Drug classifications
CYP3A4 inducers (armodafinil, barbiturates, bexarotene, bosentan, carbamazepine, dexamethasone, efavirenz, enzalutamide, eslicarbazepine, ethanol, etravirine, felbamate, flutamide, griseofulvin, lesinurad, modafinil, nafcillin, nevirapine, primidone, phenytoin, phenobarbital, pioglitazone, rifampin, rifapentine, rifabutin); antacids, PPIs: separate by 4 hr: decreased velpatasvir level

CYP3A4 inhibitors (aldesleukin, aliskiren, amlodipine, amprenavir, aprepitant, atazanavir, boceprevir, bromocriptine, chloramphenicol, ciprofloxacin, clarithromycin, cyclosporine, dalfopristin/quinupristin, danazol, darunavir, dasatinib, delavirdine, diltiazem, dronedarone, erythromycin, fluconazole, fluoxetine, fluvoxamine, fosaprepitant, idelalisib, imatinib, indinavir, isavuconazonium, isoniazid, itraconazole, ketoconazole, miconazole, ritonavir, tipranavir), P-gp inhibitors: increased velpatasvir level
P-glycoprotein (P-gp) inducers avoid concurrent use: decreased sofosbuvir level

Individual drugs
Amiodarone, avoid using together: increased bradycardia
Atorvastatin: increased myopathy, rhabdomyolysis
Azithromycin, boceprevir, canagliflozin, carvedilol, clarithromycin, crizotinib: increased effect of both products
Carvedilol, cobicistat: increased sofosbuvir level
Ritonavir: decreased levels of ritonavir

Drug/herb
St. John's wort, do not use together: decreased sofosbuvir level

NURSING CONSIDERATIONS
Assessment

> **BLACK BOX WARNING: Hepatitis B exacerbation:** Monitor serum HCV-RNC baseline and periodically, continue to monitor coinfected patients during and after treatment for clinical and laboratory signs of hepatitis B exacerbation (HBsAg, HBV DNA, hepatic enzymes, bilirubin), assess for signs of liver toxicity (yellow eyes or skin, fatigue, weakness, loss of appetite, nausea, vomiting, or light-colored stools); to decrease the risk of reactivating an HBV infection, screen all potential recipients for evidence of current or prior HBV infection by testing HBsAg and anti-HBc concentrations. For those patients whose screening reveals serologic evidence of HBV infection, a baseline HBV DNA concentration should be obtained before starting this product; monitor LFTs

S

• Severe renal disease/GFR <30 ml/min/1.73 m^2, monitor BUN, creatinine
• Geriatric patients more carefully, may develop renal, cardiac symptoms more rapidly
• **Pregnancy:** The use of sofosbuvir/velpatasvir in combination with ribavirin is contraindicated in pregnant women and in the male partners of women who are pregnant, birth defects and/or death of the fetus may occur. Ribavirin therapy also may cause male-mediated teratogenicity and is contraindicated for use during pregnancy, in females who may become pregnant, or in men whose female partners are pregnant. Patients and their partners are required to use 2 reliable forms of effective contraception during treatment and for 6 months after use of these combination therapies. Females must also undergo a pregnancy test immediately before initiation of therapy, monthly during therapy, and for 6 months post-therapy. Ribavirin Pregnancy Registry; telephone (800) 593-2214. For patients who are also infected with HIV and taking concomitant antiretrovirals, an Antiretroviral Pregnancy Registry is available at (800) 258-4263, not to breastfeed
• **Anemia:** Monitor Hgb/Hct if anemia is suspected

Patient problem
Infection (uses)

Implementation:
• Take without regard to food
• If given with ribavirin, take ribavirin with food

Patient/family education
• That optimal duration of treatment is unknown; that product is not a cure, that transmission to others may still occur
• To avoid use with other products unless approved by prescriber
• Not to stop abruptly unless directed, worsening of hepatitis may occur, keep in original container

> **BLACK BOX WARNING: Hepatitis exacerbation:** report to provider immediately signs of liver toxicity (yellow eyes or skin, fatigue, weakness, loss of appetite, nausea, vomiting, or light-colored stools)

• **Pregnancy:** Teach patients that they and their partners are required to use 2 reliable forms of effective contraception during treatment and for 6 months after use of these combination therapies, pregnancy tests are needed immediately before initiation of

therapy, monthly during therapy, and for 6 months post-therapy, not to breastfeed

Evaluation
• Decreased symptoms of chronic hepatitis C

RARELY USED

sofosbuvir/velpatasvir/voxilaprevir
(soe-fos′bue-vir/vel-pat′as-vir/vox-i-la′pre-vir)
Vosevi
Func. class.: Antiviral, antihepatitis Agent
Chem. class.: NS5A/NS5B inhibitor, protease inhibitor

USES: Treatment of chronic hepatitis C infection, including genotypes 1, 2, 3, 4, 5, and 6, in those without cirrhosis and in patients with compensated cirrhosis (Child-Pugh A) who have previously been treated with an NS5A inhibitor; treatment of chronic HCV genotype 1a, 3 in those without cirrhosis or compensated cirrhosis who were treated without an NS5A inhibitor

CONTRAINDICATIONS: Hypersensitivity

Precautions: Breastfeeding, hepatitis C and HIV coinfection, male-mediated teratogenicity, pregnancy, renal failure/impairment

> **BLACK BOX WARNING:** Hepatitis B exacerbation

DOSAGE AND ROUTES
Adult: PO 1 tablet q day × 12 wk

solifenacin (Rx)
(sol-i-fen′a-sin)
VESIcare
Func. class.: Urinary antispasmodic, anticholinergic
Chem. class.: Antimuscarinic receptor antagonist

Do not confuse: Vesicare/Vesanoid

ACTION: Relaxes smooth muscles in urinary tract by inhibiting acetylcholine at postganglionic sites

Therapeutic outcome: Decreased dysuria, frequency, nocturia, incontinence

USES: Overactive bladder (urinary frequency, urgency, incontinence)

Pharmacokinetics

Absorption	Rapid (90%)
Distribution	98% protein bound
Metabolism	Extensively metabolized by CYP3A4
Excretion	Excreted in urine (69%)/feces (22%)
Half-life	45-68 hr

Pharmacodynamics

Onset	Unknown
Peak	4-8 hr
Duration	Up to 24 hr

CONTRAINDICATIONS

Hypersensitivity, uncontrolled closed-angle glaucoma, urinary retention, gastric retention

Precautions: Pregnancy, breastfeeding, children, geriatric patients, renal/hepatic disease, controlled closed-angle glaucoma, bladder outflow obstruction, GI obstruction, decreased GI motility, history of QT prolongation

DOSAGE AND ROUTES
Adult: PO 5 mg/day, max 10 mg/day

Renal/hepatic dose
Adult: PO CCr <30 ml/min 5 mg/day; Child-Pugh B max 5 mg/day

Available forms: Tabs 5, 10 mg

ADVERSE EFFECTS
CNS: *Dizziness,* headache, confusion, depression, drowsiness
CV: Palpitations, tachycardia
EENT: *Vision abnormalities*
GI: *Nausea, anorexia,* abdominal pain, *constipation,* dry mouth
INTEG: Angioedema

INTERACTIONS
Drug classifications
Azoles, macrolides, fluoroquinolones, class IA, III antidysrhythmics: increased QT prolongation

Benzodiazepines, hypnotics, opioids, sedatives: increased CNS depression

CYP3A4 inducers (carBAMazepine, nevirapine, phenobarbital, phenytoin): decreased effects of solifenacin

CYP3A4 inhibitors (clarithromycin, diclofenac, doxycycline, erythromycin, isoniazid, ketoconazole, nefazodone, propofol, protease inhibitors, verapamil): increased action of solifenacin, max dose 5 mg

Drug/herb
St. John's wort: decreased effects

Drug/food
Grapefruit juice: increased effect

Drug/lab test
Increased: LFTs

NURSING CONSIDERATIONS
Assessment
• **Urinary patterns:** assess for distention, nocturia, frequency, urgency, incontinence
• **Allergic reactions:** assess for rash; if this occurs, product should be discontinued

Patient problem
Impaired urination (uses)

Implementation
PO route
• Without regard to meals
• Swallow product whole with water, liquid

Patient/family education
• Caution patient to avoid hazardous activities; dizziness may occur
• Advise patient that constipation, blurred vision may occur, to notify prescriber if abdominal pain with constipation occurs
• Instruct patient to call prescriber if severe abdominal pain or constipation lasts for 3 or more days
• Advise patient that heat prostration may occur if used in a hot environment, sweating is decreased
• Teach patient to take without regard to food
• Teach patient to swallow tab whole, do not crush, chew

Evaluation
Positive therapeutic outcome
• Urinary status: decreased dysuria, frequency, nocturia, incontinence

S

⚠ HIGH ALERT

sotalol (Rx)
(soe-ta'lole)
Betapace, Betapace AF, Rylosol ✽, Sorine, Sotylize
Func. class.: Antidysrhythmic, group III
Chem. class.: Nonselective β-blocker

Do not confuse: sotalol/Sudafed

ACTION: Blockade of β_1- and β_2-receptors leads to antidysrhythmic effect, prolongs action potential in myocardial fibers without affecting conduction, prolongs QT interval, no effect on QRS duration

---

Therapeutic outcome: Decreased B/P, heart rate, AV conduction

USES: Life-threatening ventricular dysrhythmias; Betapace AF: to maintain sinus rhythm in symptomatic atrial fibrillation/flutter

Pharmacokinetics

Absorption	Well
Distribution	Crosses placenta
Metabolism	Liver
Excretion	70% unchanged—kidneys
Half-life	10-24 hr, increased in renal disease

Pharmacodynamics

	PO	IV
Onset	Several hr	5-10 min
Peak	Unknown	Unknown
Duration	Unknown	Unknown

CONTRAINDICATIONS

Hypersensitivity to β-blockers, cardiogenic shock, heart block (2nd or 3rd degree), sinus bradycardia, HF, bronchial asthma, CCr <40 ml/min, hypokalemia

> **BLACK BOX WARNING:** Congenital or acquired long QT syndrome

Precautions: Pregnancy, breastfeeding, major surgery, diabetes mellitus, renal/thyroid disease, COPD, well-compensated heart failure, CAD, nonallergic bronchospasm, electrolyte disturbances, bradycardia, peripheral vascular disease

> **BLACK BOX WARNING:** Cardiac dysrhythmias, torsades de pointes, ventricular dysrhythmias, ventricular fibrillation, requires a specialized care setting

DOSAGE AND ROUTES

Ventricular dysrhythmias

Adult: PO 80 mg bid, increase gradually to 160-320 mg/day in divided doses; IV 75 mg bid, may increase by 75 mg q 3 days if QTc <500 sec

Renal dose

Adult: PO CCr 30-59 mL/min 80 mg initially, give doses after initial q24hr; CCr 10-29 mL/min 80 mg initially, then q 36-48 hr

Atrial fibrillation/flutter

Adult: PO 80 mg bid increase up to 120 m bid if needed

Renal dose

Adult: PO CCr 40-60 mL/min give dose q 24 hr

Available forms: Tabs 80, 120, 160, 240 mg; (Betapace AF) 80, 120, 160 mg; inj 150 mg/10 ml (15 mg/ml)

ADVERSE EFFECTS

CNS: Dizziness, mental changes, drowsiness, fatigue, headache, depression, anxiety, paresthesia, insomnia, decreased concentration
CV: Orthostatic hypotension, HF, dysrhythmias, palpitations, torsades de pointes; Betapace AF: life-threatening ventricular dysrhythmias
EENT: Tinnitus, visual changes
GI: Nausea, vomiting, diarrhea, dry mouth, constipation, anorexia
GU: Impotence, dysuria
INTEG: Rash, urticaria, pruritus, fever
MS: Arthralgia, muscle cramps, pain
RESP: Bronchospasm, wheezing

INTERACTIONS
Individual drugs

> **BLACK BOX WARNING:** Haloperidol, chloroquine, droperidol, pentamidine; arsenic trioxide, levomethadyl: increased QT prolongation

Insulin: increased hypoglycemia
Lidocaine: increased effects of lidocaine
Nitroglycerin: increased hypotension
Theophylline: decreased bronchodilating effects of theophylline

Drug classifications

Antihypertensives, diuretics: increased hypotension
β₂-Agonists: decreased bronchodilating effects
Class IA/III antidysrhythmics, some phenothiazines, β-agonists, local anesthetics, tricyclics, CYP3A4 inhibitors (amiodarone, clarithromycin, erythromycin, telithromycin, troleandomycin), CYP3A4 substrates (methadone, pimozide, QUEtiapine, quiNIDine, risperiDONE, ziprasidone): increased QT prolongation
Sulfonylureas: decreased hypoglycemic effects
Sympathomimetics: decreased β-blocker effects

Drug/herb
Hawthorn: do not use concurrently

Drug/lab test
False: increased urinary catecholamines
Interference: glucose, insulin tolerance tests

NURSING CONSIDERATIONS
Assessment

> **BLACK BOX WARNING: QT syndrome:**
> Monitor B/P during beginning treatment,
> periodically thereafter; pulse q4hr; note rate,
> rhythm, quality: apical/radial pulse before
> administration; notify prescriber of any signifi-
> cant changes (pulse ⌐60 bpm); monitor ECG
> continuously (Betapace AF); use QT interval to
> determine patient eligibility; baseline QT must
> be ≤450 msec, if ≥500 msec, frequency or
> dosage must be decreased or drug must be
> discontinued

> **BLACK BOX WARNING:** Requires a special-
> ized care setting: for a minimum of at least 3
> days on maintenance dose with continuous
> ECG monitoring, creatinine clearance, calcu-
> late before dosing

> **BLACK BOX WARNING:** Cardiogenic shock,
> acute pulmonary edema: do not use, as effect
> can further depress cardiac output

• Check for baselines in renal function tests,
before therapy begins
• Assess for edema in feet, legs daily, monitor
I&O ratio, daily weight; check for jugular vein
distention, crackles, bilaterally, dyspnea (HF)
• **Abrupt discontinuation:** do not discontinue abruptly; taper over 1-2 wk
• Dose should be adjusted slowly, with at least
3 days between changes; monitor ECG for QT
interval
• Monitor electrolytes (hypokalemia, hypomagnesemia); may increase dysrhythmias
• **Pregnancy/breastfeeding:** Use only if
benefits outweigh fetal risk, do not breastfeed,
excreted in breast milk

Patient problem
Impaired cardiac functioning (uses)
Impaired cardiac output (adverse reactions)
Nonadherence (teaching)

Implementation
PO route
• Given before meals, at bedtime, tab may be
crushed or swallowed whole; give with food
to prevent GI upset; reduce dosage in renal
dysfunction
• Betapace and Betapace AF are not interchangeable
• Store in dry area at room temp; do not freeze

IV route
• Dilute to a volume of either 120 ml or 300 ml
with D_5W, LR
• **75-mg dose:** withdraw 6 ml sotalol inj
(90 mg), add 114 ml diluent to make 120 ml
(0.75% mg/ml); or withdraw 6 ml sotalol inj
(90 mg), add 294 ml diluent to make 300 ml
(0.3 mg/ml)
• **112.5-mg dose:** withdraw 9 ml sotalol inj,
(135 ml), add 111 ml diluent to 120 ml (1.125
mg/ml); or withdraw 9 ml sotalol (135 mg) and
add 291 ml diluent to 300 ml (0.45 mg/ml)
• **150-mg dose:** withdraw 12 ml sotalol (180
mg), add 108 ml to 120 ml (1.5 mg/ml); or
withdraw 12 ml of sotalol (180 mg), add 288 ml
to 300 ml (0.6 mg/ml)
• Use inf pump and infuse 100 or 250 ml over
5 hr at a constant rate

Patient/family education
• Teach patient not to discontinue product
abruptly, taper over 2 wk; may cause precipitate
angina if stopped abruptly
• Teach patient not to use OTC products containing α-adrenergic stimulants (such as nasal
decongestants, cold preparations); to avoid
alcohol and smoking and to limit sodium intake
as prescribed
• Teach patient how to take pulse and B/P at
home, advise when to notify prescriber
• Instruct patient to comply with weight control,
dietary adjustments, modified exercise program
• Caution patient to carry/wear emergency ID to
identify product being taken, allergies
• Inform patient that product controls symptoms but does not cure
• Caution patient to avoid hazardous activities if
dizziness, drowsiness are present
• Teach patient to report symptoms of **HF:** difficulty breathing, especially on exertion or when
lying down; night cough; swelling of extremities;
bradycardia; dizziness; confusion; depression;
fever
• Teach patient to take product as prescribed,
not to double or skip doses; take any missed
doses as soon as remembered if at least 4 hr
until next dose
• Teach patient that hospitalization will be
required for ≥3 days

Evaluation
Positive therapeutic outcome
• Absence of dysrhythmias

spironolactone (Rx)

(speer′on-oh-lak′tone)

Aldactone

Func. class.: Potassium-sparing diuretic

Chem. class.: Aldosterone antagonist

Do not confuse: Aldactone/Aldactazide

ACTION: Competes with aldosterone at receptor sites in the distal tubule in the renal system, resulting in excretion of sodium chloride, water, retention of potassium, phosphate

Therapeutic outcome: Diuretic and antihypertensive effect while retaining potassium; lowered aldosterone levels

USES: Edema of HF, hypertension, diuretic-induced hypokalemia, primary hyperaldosteronism (diagnosis, short-term treatment, long-term treatment), edema of nephrotic syndrome, cirrhosis of the liver with ascites

Unlabeled uses: HF

Pharmacokinetics

Absorption	GI tract; well absorbed
Distribution	Crosses placenta
Metabolism	Liver to canrenone (active metabolite)
Excretion	Renal; breast milk
Half-life	12-24 hr (canrenone)

Pharmacodynamics

Onset	24-48 hr
Peak	48-72 hr
Duration	Unknown

CONTRAINDICATIONS

Pregnancy, hypersensitivity, anuria, severe renal disease, hyperkalemia

Precautions: Breastfeeding, dehydration, renal/hepatic disease, electrolyte imbalances, metabolic acidosis, gynecomastia

> **BLACK BOX WARNING:** Secondary malignancy

DOSAGE AND ROUTES

Edema/hypertension

Adult: PO 25-200 mg/day in 1-2 divided doses

HF (unlabeled)

Adult: PO 12.5-25 mg/day, max 50 mg/day

Edema

Child: PO 1.5-3.3 mg/kg/day in single or divided doses

Hypertension

Child (unlabeled): PO 1.5-3.3 mg/kg in divided doses

Hypokalemia

Adult: PO 25-100 mg/day; if PO, potassium supplements must not be used

Primary hyperaldosteronism diagnosis

Adult: PO 400 mg/day × 4 days or 4 wk depending on the test, then 100-400 mg/day maintenance

Edema (nephrotic syndrome, HF, hepatic disease)

Adult: PO 100 mg/day given as a single dose or in divided doses, titrate to response

Child: PO 1.5-3.3 mg/kg/day or 60 mg/m^2/day given once daily or in 2-4 divided doses

Renal dose

Adult: PO CCr 10-50 ml/min; give dose q12-24hr; CCr <10 ml/min, avoid use

Available forms: Tabs 25, 50, 100 mg

ADVERSE EFFECTS

CNS: Headache, confusion, drowsiness, lethargy, ataxia

ELECT: Hyperchloremic metabolic acidosis, hyperkalemia, hyponatremia

ENDO: Impotence, gynecomastia, irregular menses, amenorrhea, postmenopausal bleeding, hirsutism, deepening voice, breast pain

GI: Diarrhea, cramps, bleeding, gastritis, vomiting, anorexia, nausea, hepatocellular toxicity

HEMA: Agranulocytosis

INTEG: *Rash, pruritus,* urticaria

INTERACTIONS

Individual drugs

Aspirin: decreased action of spironolactone

Cholestyramine: increased hyperchloremic acidosis in cirrhosis

Digoxin: increased digoxin action

Lithium: increased action, toxicity

Drug classifications

ACE inhibitors, diuretics (potassium-sparing), angiotensin II receptor antagonists potassium products, salt substitute: increased hyperkalemia

Anticoagulants: decreased effects of anticoagulants, monitor INR/PT

Antihypertensives: increased action

NSAIDs: decreased effect of spironolactone

Drug/food

Potassium-rich foods, potassium salt substitutes: increased hyperkalemia

Drug/herb
Ephedra: decreased antihypertensive effect
Hawthorn, horse chestnut: increased hypotension
St. John's wort: severe photosensitivity

Drug/lab test
Increased: BUN, potassium
Decreased: sodium, magnesium
Interference: 17-OHCS, 17-KS, radioimmunoassay, digoxin assay

NURSING CONSIDERATIONS
Assessment
- **Hypokalemia:** assess for polyuria, polydipsia, dysrhythmias including a U wave on ECG
- **Hyperkalemia:** assess for weakness, fatigue, dyspnea, dysrhythmias, confusion
- **HF assessment daily:** Assess fluid volume status: I&O ratios and record, count or weigh diapers as appropriate, weight, distended red veins, crackles in lung, color, quality, and specific gravity of urine, skin turgor, adequacy of pulses, moist mucous membranes, bilateral lung sounds, peripheral pitting edema; dehydration symptoms of decreasing output, thirst, hypotension, dry mouth and mucous membranes should be reported, potassium must be checked within 3 days, 1 wk, 1 mo × 3, then q3mo, recheck after starting products that alter potassium
- Monitor electrolytes: potassium, sodium, calcium, magnesium; also include BUN, ABGs, uric acid, CBC, blood glucose

> **BLACK BOX WARNING:** Secondary malignancy: assess periodically

- **Beers:** Avoid in older adults with heart failure or CCr <30 ml/min

Patient problem
Fluid imbalance (uses)

Implementation
- Give in AM to avoid interference with sleep
- Give with food if nausea occurs; absorption may be increased; take at same time each day
- Effect may take 2 wk

Patient/family education
- Teach patient to take medication early in day to prevent nocturia
- Instruct patient to take with food or milk if GI symptoms of nausea and anorexia occur
- Teach patient to maintain a record of weight on a weekly basis and notify prescriber of weight loss of >5 lb
- Caution patient that this product causes an increase in potassium levels, that foods high in potassium should be avoided: oranges, bananas, salt substitutes, dried apricots, dates; avoid potassium salt substitutes; refer to dietitian for assistance planning

- Teach patient to take in AM, to prevent sleeplessness
- Teach patient to avoid hazardous activities until reaction is known
- Teach patient not to use alcohol or any OTC medications without prescriber's approval; serious product reactions may occur
- Emphasize the need to contact prescriber immediately if muscle cramps, weakness, nausea, dizziness, or numbness occur
- Teach patient to take own B/P and pulse and record
- Teach patient to notify prescriber of cramps, diarrhea, lethargy, thirst, headache, skin rash, menstrual abnormalities, deepening voice, breast enlargement
- Advise patient that dizziness and confusion may occur; avoid driving or other hazardous activities if alertness is decreased
- Teach patient to continue taking medication even if feeling better; this product controls symptoms but does not cure the condition
- Advise patient with hypertension to continue other treatment (exercise, weight loss, relaxation techniques, cessation of smoking)
- Teach patient to notify prescriber if pregnancy is planned or suspected; do not breastfeed

Evaluation
Positive therapeutic outcome
- Prevention of hypokalemia (diuretic use)
- Decreased edema
- Decreased B/P
- Decreased aldosterone levels
- Increased diuresis

TREATMENT OF OVERDOSE
- Lavage if taken orally, monitor electrolytes
- Administer sodium bicarbonate
- Monitor hydration, CV, renal status

streptomycin (Rx)
(strep-toe-mye'sin)
Func. class.: Antiinfective, antituberculosis
Chem. class.: Aminoglycoside

ACTION: Interferes with protein synthesis in bacterial cell by binding to ribosomal subunit, causing inaccurate peptide sequence to form in protein chain; bactericidal

Therapeutic outcome: Bactericidal effects for the following organisms: sensitive strains of *Mycobacterium tuberculosis*, nontuberculous infections caused by sensitive strains of *Yersinia pestis*, *Brucella*, *Haemophilus influenzae*, *Klebsiella pneumoniae*, *Escherichia coli*, *Enterobacter aerogenes*, *Streptococcus viridans*, *Francisella tularensis*, *Proteus*

USES: Active TB; used in combination for streptococcal and enterococcal infections; endocarditis, tularemia, plague

Pharmacokinetics

Absorption	Well absorbed
Distribution	Widely distributed in extracellular fluids, poorly distributed in CSF; crosses placenta
Metabolism	Minimal—liver
Excretion	Mostly unchanged (>90%) kidneys
Half-life	2–2 1/2 hr, increase in renal disease

Pharmacodynamics

Onset	Rapid
Peak	1-2 hr
Duration	Unknown

CONTRAINDICATIONS: Hypersensitivity

> **BLACK BOX WARNING:** Pregnancy, severe renal disease

Precautions: Breastfeeding, geriatric, neonates, mild renal disease, myasthenia gravis, Parkinson's disease, hepatic disease

> **BLACK BOX WARNING:** Hearing deficits, neuromuscular disease

DOSAGE AND ROUTES
General dosing
Adults: IM 1-2 g in divided doses q6-12hr
Child: IM 20-40 mg/kg/day in divided doses q6-12hr, max adult dose

Tuberculosis (HIV negative)
Adult: IM 15 mg/kg (max 1 g) daily 2-3 mo, then 1 g 2-3/wk given with other antitubercular products for up to 1 yr
Child: IM 20–40 mg/kg/day; max 1 g/day

Enterococcal endocarditis
Adult: IM, **IV** 15 mg/kg/day divided q12h
Child: IM/IV 20-30 mg/kg/day divided q12hr

Available forms: Inj 500 mg, 1 g/ml

ADVERSE EFFECTS
CNS: Confusion, dizziness, depression, numbness, tremors, seizures, muscle twitching, neurotoxicity, dizziness, headache
CV: Hypotension, myocarditis, palpitations
EENT: *Ototoxicity*, tinnitus, deafness, visual disturbances

GI: *Nausea, vomiting, anorexia,* increased ALT, AST, bilirubin, hepatomegaly, hepatic necrosis, splenomegaly
GU: Oliguria, hematuria, renal damage, azotemia, renal failure, nephrotoxicity
HEMA: Agranulocytosis, thrombocytopenia, leukopenia, eosinophilia, anemia
INTEG: *Rash*, burning, urticaria, dermatitis, alopecia
MS: Arthralgia, weakness

INTERACTIONS
Individual drugs
Amphotericin B, cidofovir, CISplatin, ethacrynic acid, furosemide, mannitol, methoxyflurane, polymyxin, tacrolimus, vancomycin: increased ototoxicity, neurotoxicity, nephrotoxicity
Succinylcholine, warfarin: increased effects of streptomycin

Drug classifications
Aminoglycosides, cephalosporins: increased ototoxicity, neurotoxicity, nephrotoxicity
Nondepolarizing neuromuscular blockers, NSAIDs: increased effects of streptomycin

NURSING CONSIDERATIONS
Assessment
• **Infection:** monitor urine, stool, sputum, wound characteristics, fever; monitor WBC for changes
• Assess patient for previous sensitivity reaction
• Complete C&S testing before and after product therapy to identify if correct treatment has been initiated
• **Assess for allergic reactions:** rash, urticaria, pruritus, chills, fever, joint pain; angioedema may occur a few days after therapy begins; epinephrine, resuscitation equipment should be available for anaphylactic reaction
• **Severe renal disease:** identify urine output; if decreasing, notify prescriber (may indicate nephrotoxicity); also increased BUN, creatinine, urine CCr 80 ml/min
• Monitor blood tests: AST, ALT, CBC, Hct, bilirubin, LDH, alkaline phosphatase, Coombs' test monthly if patient is on long-term therapy
• Monitor electrolytes: potassium, sodium, chloride, magnesium monthly if patient is on long-term therapy
• Monitor for bleeding: ecchymosis, bleeding gums, hematuria, stool guaiac daily if on long-term therapy
• Assess for overgrowth of infection: perineal itching, fever, malaise, redness, pain, swelling, drainage, rash, diarrhea, change in cough, sputum

---

• Obtain weight before treatment; calculation of dosage is usually based on ideal body weight but may be calculated on actual body weight
• Monitor I&O ratio; urinalysis daily for proteinuria, cells, casts; report sudden change in urine output
• Obtain serum peak 30-60 min after IM inj, trough level drawn 30-60 min before next dose; therapeutic peak 15-40 mg/L, therapeutic trough 5 mg/L.

BLACK BOX WARNING: Deafness: assess by audiometric testing, ringing, roaring in ears, vertigo; assess hearing before, during, after treatment
Dehydration: monitor for high specific gravity, decrease in skin turgor, dry mucous membranes, dark urine

Patient problems
• Diarrhea (adverse reactions)
• Infection (uses)
• Risk for injury (adverse reactions)
• Lack of knowledge of medication (teaching)
• Nonadherence (teaching)

Implementation
• Give deeply in large muscle mass
• Reconstitute with 4.2-4.5 ml of sterile water for inj or 0.9% NaCl/1 g (200 mg/ml), 3.2-3.5 ml/1 g (250 mg/ml), 17 ml/5 g (250 mg/ml); give at 500 mg/ml or less

Patient/family education
• Teach patient to report sore throat, bruising, bleeding, joint pain, may indicate blood dyscrasias (rare); ringing, roaring in the ears
• Advise patient to contact prescriber if vaginal itching; loose, foul-smelling stools; furry tongue occur; may indicate superinfection

Evaluation

Positive therapeutic outcome
• Absence of signs/symptoms of infection
• Reported improvement in symptoms of infection

TREATMENT OF OVERDOSE:
Withdraw product, hemodialysis, monitor serum levels of product, may give ticarcillin or carbenicillin

sucralfate (Rx)
(soo-kral'fate)
Carafate, Sulcrate ✹
Func. class.: Antiulcer
Chem. class.: Aluminum hydroxide/sulfated sucrose

ACTION: Forms a complex that adheres to ulcer site, adsorbs pepsin

Therapeutic outcome: Healing of ulcers

USES: Duodenal ulcer, oral mucositis, stomatitis after radiation of head and neck

Unlabeled uses: Gastric ulcers, gastroesophageal reflux

Pharmacokinetics
Absorption	Minimally absorbed
Distribution	Unknown
Metabolism	Not metabolized
Excretion	Feces (90%)
Half-life	6-20 hr

Pharmacodynamics
Onset	½ hr
Peak	Unknown
Duration	6 hr

CONTRAINDICATIONS
Hypersensitivity

Precautions: Pregnancy, breastfeeding, children, renal failure, hypoglycemia (diabetics)

DOSAGE AND ROUTES
Duodenal ulcers
Adult: PO 1 g qid 1 hr before meals and at bedtime
Child: PO 40-80 mg/kg/day divided

Available forms: Tabs 1 g; oral susp 1 g/10 ml

ADVERSE EFFECTS
GI: *Dry mouth, constipation,* bezoar (critically ill patients)

INTERACTIONS
Individual drugs
Cimetidine, ranitidine: decreased absorption of sucralfate
Digoxin, ketoconazole, phenytoin, tetracycline, theophylline: decreased action of each specific product

Drug classifications
Antacids: decreased absorption of sucralfate
Fat-soluble vitamins: decreased action of fat-soluble vitamins
Fluoroquinolones: decreased absorption

NURSING CONSIDERATIONS
Assessment
• **GI symptoms:** assess for abdominal pain, blood in stools
• **Hypoglycemia:** may occur in those with diabetes mellitus, monitor blood glucose carefully

Patient problem
Pain (uses)
Lack of knowledge of medication (teaching)

Implementation
• Do not break, crush, or chew tabs
• Give on empty stomach 1 hr before meals and at bedtime
• Avoid antacids ½ hr before or 1 hr after taking this product
• Store at room temperature

Patient/family education
• Instruct patient to take medication on empty stomach
• Caution patient to take full course of therapy, not to use >8 wk, to avoid smoking
• Caution patient to take 2 hr after product, to avoid antacids, milk alkalotics, water within 2 hr of the product
• Advise patient to increase fluids, bulk, exercise to lessen constipation

Evaluation

Positive therapeutic outcome
• Absence of pain or GI complaints

---

sulfamethoxazole/ trimethoprim (cotrimoxazole) (Rx)
(sul-fa-meth-ox′a-zole/trye-meth′oh-prim [ko-trye-mox′a-zole])
Bactrim, Bactrim DS, Nu-Cotrimox ❋, Septra, Protin DF ❋, Septra DS, SMZ/ TMP, Trisulfa DS ❋, Trisulfa S ❋
Func. class.: Antiinfective
Chem. class.: Sulfonamide— miscellaneous

ACTION: Sulfamethoxazole (SMZ) interferes with bacterial biosynthesis of proteins by competitive antagonism of PABA when adequate levels are maintained; trimethoprim (TMP) blocks synthesis of tetrahydrofolic acid; combination blocks two consecutive steps in bacterial synthesis of essential nucleic acids, protein

Therapeutic outcome: Absence of infection, based on C&S

USES: UTI, otitis media, acute and chronic prostatitis, shigellosis, chancroid, traveler's diarrhea, *Enterobacter, Escherichia coli, Haemophilus influenzae* (beta-lactamase negative), *Haemophilus influenzae* (beta-lactamase positive), *Klebsiella, Morganella morganii, Pneumocystis carinii, Pneumocystis jiroveci, Proteus mirabilis, Proteus, Shigella flexneri, Shigella sonnei, Streptococcus* pneumonia; **may also be effective for** *Acinetobacter baumannii, Actinomadura madurae, Actinomadura pelletieri, Bordetella pertussis, Burkholderia pseudomallei, Cyclospora cayetanensis, Haemophilus ducreyi, Isospora belli, Klebsiella granulomatis, Legionella micdadei, Legionella pneumophila, Listeria monocytogenes, Moraxella catarrhalis, Neisseria gonorrhoeae, Nocardia asteroides, Nocardia brasiliensis, Nocardia otitidiscaviarum, Pediculus capitis, Plasmodium falciparum, Providencia, Salmonella, Serratia, Shigella, Staphylococcus aureus* (MRSA), *Staphylococcus aureus* (MSSA), *Staphylococcus epidermidis, Stenotrophomonas maltophilia, Streptococcus pyogenes* (group A beta-hemolytic streptococci), *Streptomyces somaliensis, Toxoplasma gondii, Vibrio cholerae, Viridans* streptococci, *Yersinia enterocolitica*

Pharmacokinetics

Absorption	Rapid
Distribution	Breast milk, crosses placenta, 68% protein bound
Metabolism	Liver
Excretion	Kidneys
Half-life	8-13 hr

Pharmacodynamics

Onset	Unknown
Peak	1-4 hr
Duration	Unknown

CONTRAINDICATIONS
Pregnancy at term, breastfeeding, infants <2 mo, hypersensitivity to trimethoprim or sulfonamides, megaloblastic anemia, CCr <15 ml/min

Precautions: Pregnancy, infants, geriatric, renal disease, G6PD deficiency, impaired renal/ hepatic function, possible folate deficiency, severe allergy, bronchial asthma, UV exposure, porphyria, hyperkalemia, hypothyroidism

DOSAGE AND ROUTES
Based on TMP content

Most infections
Adult/child >2 mo: PO/IV 6-12 mg TMP/kg/day divided q12hr

UTI
Adult: PO 160 mg TMP q12hr × 10-14 days
Child: PO 8 mg/kg TMP daily in 2 divided doses q12hr (treatment); 2 mg/kg/day (prophylaxis)

Otitic media
Child: PO 8 mg/kg TMP daily in 2 divided doses q12hr × 10 days

Chronic bronchitis
Adult: PO 160 mg TMP q12hr × 10-14 days

Serious infections/Pneumocystis jiroveci pneumonitis
Adult and child: PO 15-20 mg/kg TMP daily in 4 divided doses q6hr × 14-21 days; IV 15-20 mg/kg/day (based on TMP) in 3-4 divided doses for up to 14 days

Renal dose
Dosage reduction necessary in moderate to severe renal impairment (CCr <30 ml/min)

Available forms: Tabs 20 mg TMP/100 SMX ✤, 80 mg TMP/400 mg SMZ, 160 mg TMP/800 mg SMZ; susp 200 mg-40 mg/5 ml, 800 mg-160 mg/20 ml; **IV** 16 mg/80 mg/ml

ADVERSE EFFECTS
CNS: Headache, insomnia, hallucinations, depression, vertigo, fatigue, anxiety, seizures, drug fever, chills, aseptic meningitis
CV: Allergic myocarditis
EENT: Tinnitus
GI: *Nausea, vomiting, abdominal pain,* stomatitis, hepatitis, glossitis, pancreatitis, diarrhea, enterocolitis, anorexia, pseudomembranous colitis
GU: Renal failure, toxic nephrosis; increased BUN, creatinine; crystalluria
HEMA: Leukopenia, neutropenia, thrombocytopenia, agranulocytosis, hemolytic anemia, hypoprothrombinemia, Henoch-Schölein purpura, methemoglobinemia, eosinophilia
INTEG: Rash, dermatitis, urticaria, erythema, photosensitivity, pain, inflammation at injection site, toxic epidermal necrolysis, erythema multiforme
RESP: Cough, shortness of breath
SYST: Anaphylaxis, systemic lupus erythematosus, Stevens-Johnson syndrome

INTERACTIONS
Individual drugs
CycloSPORINE: decreased response
Dofetilide: increased levels of dofetilide
Methenamine: increased crystalluria
Methotrexate: increased bone marrow depression
Phenytoin: decreased hepatic clearance of phenytoin

Drug classifications
Anticoagulants (oral): increased anticoagulant effect
CYP2C9, CYP3A4 inducers: decreased hepatic clearance
Diuretics (potassium-sparing), potassium supplements: increased potassium levels
Diuretics (thiazide): increased thrombocytopenia
Sulfonylureas: increased hypoglycemic response

Drug/lab test
Increased: creatinine, bilirubin
Decreased: Hgb, platelets

NURSING CONSIDERATIONS
Assessment
• Monitor I&O ratio; note color, character, pH of urine if product administered for UTI; output should be 800 ml less than intake; if urine is highly acidic, alkalization may be needed
• Monitor renal function tests: BUN, creatinine, urinalysis (long-term therapy)
• Assess type of infection; obtain C&S before starting therapy
• Assess blood dyscrasias, skin rash, fever, sore throat, bruising, bleeding, fatigue, joint pain
• Assess allergic reaction: rash, dermatitis, urticaria, pruritus, dyspnea, bronchospasm, AIDS patients are more susceptible, identify if patient has a sulfa allergy

Patient problem
Infection (uses)

Implementation
• Give with full glass of water to maintain adequate hydration; increase fluids to 2 L/day to decrease crystallization in kidneys
• Give medication after C&S; repeat C&S after full course of medication
• Store in airtight, light-resistant container at room temp
• Give without regard to meals

Intermittent IV infusion route
• Dilute 5 ml ampule/100-125 ml of D_5W, stable for 6 hr, give over ½ hr, do not refrigerate, if using Septra ADD-Vantage vials dilute each 10-ml vial in ADD-Vantage diluent containers containing 250 ml of D_5W, infuse over 60-90 min, change site q48-72hr

Y-site compatibilities: Acyclovir, aldesleukin, allopurinol, amifostine, atracurium, aztreonam, cefepime, cyclophosphamide, diltiazem, enalaprilat, esmolol, filgrastim, fludarabine,

S

gallium, granisetron, HYDROmorphone, labetalol, LORazepam, magnesium sulfate, melphalan, meperidine, morphine, pancuronium, perphenazine, piperacillin/tazobactam, sargramostim, tacrolimus, teniposide, thiotepa, vecuronium, zidovudine

Patient family education
• Teach patient to take each oral dose with full glass of water to prevent crystalluria; drink 8-10 glasses of water/day, not to treat diarrhea with OTC product, to call health care professional if diarrhea lasts more than 2 days
• Teach patient to complete full course of treatment to prevent superinfection
• Teach patient to avoid sunlight or use sunscreen to prevent burns
• Teach patient to avoid OTC medications (aspirin, vit C) unless directed by prescriber
• If diabetic, teach patient to use Clinistix or Tes-Tape
• Teach patient to notify prescriber if skin rash, sore throat, fever, mouth sores, unusual bruising, bleeding occur

Evaluation
Positive therapeutic outcome
• Absence of pain, fever, C&S negative

---

sulfaSALAzine (Rx)
(sul-fa-sal′a-zeen)
Azulfidine, Azulfidine EN-tabs, Salazopyrin ✤
Func. class.: GI Antiinflammatory, antirheumatic (DMARD)
Chem. class.: GI Sulfonamide

Do not confuse: sulfaSALAzine/sulfadiazine

ACTION: Proproduct to deliver sulfapyridine and 5-aminosalicylic acid to colon; antiinflammatory in connective tissue

Therapeutic outcome: Treatment of ulcerative colitis, rheumatoid arthritis

USES: Ulcerative colitis, rheumatoid arthritis, juvenile rheumatoid arthritis (Azulfidine EN-tabs)

Unlabeled uses: Crohn's disease

Pharmacokinetics

Absorption	Partially absorbed
Distribution	Crosses placenta
Metabolism	Liver
Excretion	Kidneys, breast milk
Half-life	6 hr

Pharmacodynamics

Onset	1 hr
Peak	1½-6 hr
Duration	6-12 hr

CONTRAINDICATIONS
Pregnancy at term, children <2 yr, hypersensitivity to sulfonamides or salicylates, intestinal, urinary obstruction, porphyria

Precautions: Pregnancy, breastfeeding, impaired renal/hepatic function, severe allergy, bronchial asthma, megaloblastic anemia

DOSAGE AND ROUTES
Ulcerative colitis
Adult: PO 3-4 g/day in divided doses; maintenance 2 g/day in divided doses q6hr
Child ≥2 yr: PO 40-60 mg/kg/day in 4-6 divided doses, then 30 mg/kg/day in 4 doses, max 2 g/day

Rheumatoid arthritis
Adult: PO 0.5-1 g/day, then increase daily dose by 500 mg qwk to 2 g/day in 2-3 divided doses

Juvenile rheumatoid arthritis
Child ≥6 yr: PO 30-50 mg/kg/24 hr, divided into 2 doses

Renal dose
Adult: PO CCr 10-30 ml/min give bid; CCr <10 ml/min give daily

Available forms: Tabs 500 mg; oral susp 250 mg/5 ml; del rel tabs 500 mg

ADVERSE EFFECTS
CNS: Headache, neuropathy
GI: *Nausea, vomiting, abdominal pain,* stomatitis, hepatitis, glossitis, pancreatitis, diarrhea
GU: Crystalluria, orange-colored urine
HEMA: Leukopenia, neutropenia, thrombocytopenia, agranulocytosis, hemolytic anemia
INTEG: Rash, dermatitis, urticaria, Stevens-Johnson syndrome, erythema, photosensitivity
SYST: Anaphylaxis

INTERACTIONS
Individual drugs
AzaTHIOprine, mercaptopurine: increased leucopenia risk
CycloSPORINE: decreased effect of cycloSPORINE
Digoxin: decreased digoxin effect
Folic acid: decreased folic acid effect
Methotrexate: decreased renal excretion

Drug classifications

Anticoagulants (oral): increased anticoagulant effect

Hypoglycemics (oral): increased hypoglycemic response

Drug/food

Iron, folic acid will be poorly absorbed

Drug/lab test

False positive: urinary glucose test

NURSING CONSIDERATIONS
Assessment

• **Ulcerative colitis, proctitis, other inflammatory bowel disease:** monitor character, amount, consistency of stools, abdominal pain, cramping, blood, mucus

• **Rheumatoid arthritis:** assess mobility, joint swelling, pain, activities of daily living

• Monitor I&O ratio; note color, amount, character, pH of urine if product administered for UTIs; output should be 800 ml less than intake; if urine is highly acidic, alkalization may be needed

• Monitor kidney function tests: BUN, creatinine, urinalysis if on long-term therapy

• **Blood dyscrasias:** assess for rash, fever, sore throat, bruising, bleeding, fatigue, joint pain; monitor CBC before and q3mo

• **Allergic reaction:** assess for rash, dermatitis, urticaria, pruritus, dyspnea, bronchospasm, identify sulfa, salicylate allergy

Patient problem

Pain (uses)

Diarrhea (uses)

Lack of knowledge of medication (teaching)

Implementation

• Give with full glass of water to maintain adequate hydration; increase fluids to 2 L/day to decrease crystallization in kidneys; contact lenses, urine, skin may be yellow-orange

• Give total daily dose in evenly spaced doses and after meals to help minimize GI intolerance

• Give at bedtime

• Store in airtight, light-resistant container at room temperature

Patient/family education

• Advise patient to take each oral dose with full glass of water to prevent crystalluria

• Teach patient to avoid sunlight or to use sunscreen to prevent burns

• Teach patient to avoid OTC medication (aspirin, vit C) unless directed by prescriber

• Advise patient to notify prescriber if skin rash, sore throat, fever, mouth sores, unusual bruising, bleeding occur

• Advise patient to use rectal susp at bedtime and retain all night

• Advise patient that decreased sperm production may occur and resolves after completion of product

• Notify prescriber if enteric-coated tablets are seen in the stool, discontinue if present

Evaluation

Positive therapeutic outcome

• Absence of fever, mucus in stools or pain in joints

SUMAtriptan (Rx)

(soo-ma-trip′tan)

ALSUMA Auto-injector, Imitrex, Imitrex DF ✦, Imitrex STAT-dose, Oneztra Xsuil, Zembrance, Symtouch, Sumavel Dose Pro

Func. class.: Antimigraine agent

Chem. class.: 5-HT₁ receptor agonist

Do not confuse: SUMAtriptan/ somatropin

ACTION: Binds selectively to the vascular 5-HT₁ receptor subtype and exerts antimigraine effect; causes vasoconstriction in cranial arteries

Therapeutic outcome: Absence of migraines

USES: Acute treatment of migraine with or without aura and cluster headache

Pharmacokinetics

Absorption	Well absorbed (SUBCUT)
Distribution	10%-20% plasma protein binding
Metabolism	Liver (metabolite)
Excretion	Urine, feces
Half-life	2 hr

Pharmacodynamics

	PO	Nasal	SUBCUT
Onset	30 min	60 min	10-20 min
Peak	2-4 hr	2 hr	10 min-2 hr
Duration	Up to 24 hr	Unknown	Up to 24 hr (pain relief)

CONTRAINDICATIONS

Angina pectoris, history of MI, documented silent ischemia, Prinzmetal's angina, ischemic heart

---

disease, **IV** use, concurrent ergotamine-containing preparations, uncontrolled hypertension, hypersensitivity, basilar or hemiplegic migraine

Precautions: Pregnancy, breastfeeding, children <18 yr, postmenopausal women, men >40 yr, geriatric, risk factors for CAD, hypercholesterolemia, obesity, diabetes, impaired renal/hepatic function, overuse

DOSAGE AND ROUTES
Adult: SUBCUT 6 mg or less, may repeat in 1 hr, max 12 mg/24 hr; **PO** 25 mg with fluids if no relief in 2 hr, give another dose, max 200 mg/day; **NASAL** 1 dose of 5, 10, or 20 mg in one nostril, may repeat in 2 hr, max 40 mg/24 hr, 1 puff each nostril q2hr; **nasal powder** 11 mg in each nostril; may repeat after 2 hr

Hepatic dose
Adult: PO 25 mg, if no response after 2 hr, give up to 50 mg

Available forms: Inj 4, 6 mg/0.5 ml; tabs 25, 50, 100 mg; nasal spray 5 mg/100 mcl-units dose spray device 20 mg/100 mcl-units

ADVERSE EFFECTS
CNS: *Tingling, hot sensation, burning, feeling of pressure, tightness, numbness, dizziness, sedation,* headache, anxiety, fatigue, cold sensation
CV: *Flushing,* MI, hypo/hypertension
EENT: Throat, mouth, nasal discomfort, vision changes
GI: Abdominal discomfort
INTEG: *Inj site reaction,* sweating
MS: *Weakness, neck stiffness,* myalgia
RESP: Chest tightness, pressure

INTERACTIONS
Individual drugs
Ergotamine: increased risk of vasospastic reaction

Drug classifications
Ergot derivatives: extended vasospastic effects
MAOIs, SSRIs, SNRIs, serotonin-receptor agonists: increased SUMAtriptan levels

Drug/herb
SAM-e, St. John's wort: increase: serotonin syndrome

NURSING CONSIDERATIONS
Assessment
• **Serotonin syndrome:** assess for delirium, coma, agitation, diaphoresis, hypertension, fever, tremors, may resemble neuroleptic malignant syndrome (in patients taking SSRIs, SNRIs)

• Assess for tingling, hot sensation, burning, feeling of pressure, numbness, flushing, inj site reaction
• Assess B/P; signs/symptoms of coronary vasospasm
• Monitor stress level, activity, reaction, coping mechanisms of patient
• Assess neurologic status: LOC, blurring vision, nausea, vomiting, tingling in extremities preceding headache
• Assess for ingestion of tyramine-containing foods (pickled products, beer, wine, aged cheese), food additives, preservatives, colorings, artificial sweeteners, chocolate, caffeine, which may precipitate these types of headaches

Patient problem
Pain (uses)
Diarrhea (uses)
Nonadherence (teaching)

Implementation
PO route
• Swallow tab whole; do not break, crush, or chew
• Take with fluids as soon as symptoms appear; may take a second dose >4 hr, max 200 mg/24 hr
SUBCUT route
• Give by SUBCUT route only, avoid IM or **IV** administration, use only for actual migraine attack
• Give 1st dose supervised by medical staff in those with CAD or those at risk for CAD
Nasal route
• Spray once in 1 nostril, may repeat if headache returns, do not repeat if pain continues after 1st dose
Nasal powder: fully press and release button, insert into nostril with tight seal, rotate mouthpiece to place in mouth, blow forcefully to deliver powder, discard nosepiece, repeat

Patient/family education
• Caution patient not to take more than 2 doses/day or 12 mg/day; allow at least 1 hr between doses
• Caution patient to avoid driving or hazardous activities if dizziness or drowsiness occurs
• Teach patient to report chest tightness, heat, flushing, drowsiness, dizziness, fatigue, sudden severe abdominal pain or any allergic reactions that occur to prescriber immediately
• Inform patient to report any side effects to prescriber
• Caution patient to use contraception when taking product, to notify prescriber if pregnancy is suspected or planned
• **Nasal spray:** one spray in one nostril, may repeat if headache returns, do not repeat if pain continues after 1st dose

- **Nasal powder:** use in each nostril using nosepiece and mouthpiece
- **Subcut:** provide pamphlet from manufacturer, review with patient

Evaluation
Positive therapeutic outcome
- Decrease in frequency, severity of headache

⚠ HIGH ALERT

SUNItinib (Rx)
(soo-nit'in-ib)
Sutent
Func. class.: Antineoplastic—miscellaneous
Chem. class.: Protein-tyrosine kinase inhibitor

ACTION: Inhibits multiple receptor tyrosine kinases (RTKs), some are responsible for tumor growth

Therapeutic outcome: Decrease in size of tumor

USES: Gastrointestinal stromal tumors (GIST) after disease progression or intolerance to imatinib; advanced renal carcinoma, pancreatic neuroendocrine tumors (pNET) in those with unresectable locally advanced/metastatic disease

Pharmacokinetics

Absorption	Well
Distribution	Protein binding 95%
Metabolism	By CYP3A4
Excretion	Feces, small amount in urine
Half-life	40-60 hr (SUNItinib); active metabolite 80-110 hr

Pharmacodynamics

Onset	Unknown
Peak	6-12 hr
Duration	Unknown

CONTRAINDICATIONS
Pregnancy, breastfeeding, hypersensitivity

Precautions: Children, geriatric, active infections, QT prolongation, torsades de pointes, stroke, heart failure

BLACK BOX WARNING: Hepatotoxicity

DOSAGE AND ROUTES
Gastrointestinal stromal tumors (GIST)/renal cell cancer
Adult: PO 50 mg/day × 4 wk, then 2 wk off; may increase or decrease dose by 12.5 mg; if adminis-

tered with CYP3A4 inducers, give 87.5 mg/day; if given with CYP3A4 inhibitors give 37.5 mg/day

Pancreatic neuroendocrine (pNET)
Adult: PO 37.5 mg/day continuously, increase or decrease by 12.5 mg based on tolerance, avoid potent CYP3A4 inhibitors/inducers, if used with CYP3A4 inhibitor decrease SUNItinib dose to a minimum of 25 mg/day; if used with CYP3A4 inducer increase SUNItinib to a max of 62.5 mg/day

Available forms: Caps 12.5, 25, 37.5, 50 mg

ADVERSE EFFECTS
CNS: Headache, dizziness, insomnia, fatigue, reversible posterior leukoencephalopathy syndrome (RPLS)
CV: Hypertension, QT prolongation, thrombotic microangiopathy, torsades de pointes
ENDO: Hyper/hypothyroidism
GI: *Nausea,* hepatotoxicity, vomiting, dyspepsia, *anorexia, abdominal pain,* altered taste, *constipation,* stomatitis, mucositis, pancreatitis, diarrhea, GI bleeding/perforation
GU: Nephrotic syndrome
HEMA: Neutropenia, thrombocytopenia, hemolytic anemia, leukopenia
INTEG: *Rash, yellow skin discoloration,* depigmentation of hair or skin, alopecia
MS: Pain, arthralgia, myalgia, myopathy, rhabdomyolysis
RESP: Cough, dyspnea, pulmonary embolism
SYST: Bleeding, electrolyte abnormalities, hand-foot syndrome, serious infection, tumor lysis syndrome

INTERACTIONS
Individual drugs
Acetaminophen: increased hepatotoxicity
Bevacizumab: microangiopathic hemolytic anemia; avoid concurrent use
Dexamethasone, carBAMazepine, PHENobarbital, phenytoin, rifampin: decreased SUNItinib concentrations
Haloperidol, chloroquine, droperidol, pentamidine, arsenic trioxide, levomethadyl: increased QT prolongation
Simvastatin: increased plasma concentrations
Warfarin: increased plasma concentration; avoid use with warfarin, use low-molecular-weight anticoagulants instead

Drug classifications
Calcium channel blockers: increased plasma concentrations
Class IA/III antidysrhythmics, some phenothiazines, β-agonists, local anesthetics, tricyclics, CYP3A4 inhibitors (amiodarone,

S

---

clarithromycin, erythromycin, telithromycin, troleandomycin), CYP3A4 substrates (methadone, pimozide, QUEtiapine, quiNIDine, risperiDONE, ziprasidone): increased QT prolongation

Drug/herb
St. John's wort: decreased SUNItinib concentration

Drug/food
Grapefruit juice: increased plasma concentrations

NURSING CONSIDERATIONS
Assessment
• Monitor ANC and platelets; if ANC <1 × 10⁹/L and/or platelets <50 × 10⁹/L, stop until ANC >1.5 × 10⁹/L and platelets >75 × 10⁹/L; if ANC <0.5 × 10⁹/L and/or platelets <10 × 10⁹/L, reduce dose by 200 mg; if cytopenia continues, reduce dose by another 100 mg; if cytopenia continues for 4 wk, stop product until ANC ≥1 × 10⁹/L
• Assess CV status: hypertension, QT prolongation can occur; monitor left ventricular ejection fraction (LVEF) MUGA baseline periodically, ECG, B/P
• **Assess for renal toxicity:** if bilirubin >3 × IULN, withhold SUNItinib until bilirubin levels return to <1.5 × IULN; electrolytes
• **Tumor lysis syndrome:** Usually in renal cell carcinoma or GI stromal tumor, may be fatal, monitor for hyperkalemia, severe muscle weakness, hypocalcemia, hyperphosphatemia, myopathy, hyperuricemia, monitor serum electrolytes before each dose
• **Osteonecrosis of the jaw:** Dental disease or use of bisphosphonates may increase risk, invasive dental procedures should be avoided
• **QT prolongation:** Those taking CYP3A4 inhibitors, those with bradycardia, cardiac disease, or electrolyte disturbances are at greater risk, monitor electrolytes, especially magnesium, potassium; ECG
• **Hand-foot syndrome:** Assess for redness, swelling, numbness, desquamation on palms and soles of the feet, may occur days after use; if these occur, product should be discontinued
• **Nephrotic syndrome:** Monitor urinalysis and proteinuria

> **BLACK BOX WARNING: Hepatotoxicity:** monitor liver function tests, before treatment and qmo; if liver transaminases >5 × IULN, withhold SUNItinib until transaminase levels return to <2.5 × IULN

• Assess for **HF, adrenal insufficiency** in those experiencing trauma
• Assess for bleeding: epistaxis rectal, gingival, upper GI, genital, wound bleeding; tumor-related hemorrhage may occur rapidly
• **Pregnancy/breastfeeding:** Do not use in pregnancy, breastfeeding

Patient problem
Nausea (adverse reactions)
Risk for injury (uses, adverse reactions)

Implementation
• Give with meal and large glass of water to decrease GI symptoms
• Give nutritious diet with iron, vitamin supplement, low fiber, few dairy products
• Store at 25°C (77°F)

Patient/family education
• Advise patient to report adverse reactions immediately: shortness of breath, bleeding
• Teach patient reason for treatment, expected result
• Teach patient that many adverse reactions may occur: high B/P, bleeding, mouth swelling, taste change, skin discoloration, depigmentation of hair/skin
• Teach patient to avoid persons with known upper respiratory infections; immunosuppression is common
• Teach to avoid grapefruit juice
• Teach patient to report if pregnancy is planned or suspected or if breastfeeding, not to be used in pregnancy

Evaluation
Positive therapeutic outcome
• Decrease in size of tumor

---

suvorexant
(soo'voe-rex'ant)
Belsomra
Func. class.: Psychotropic—sedative/hypnotic, anxiolytic
Chem. class.: Orexin receptor antagonist
Controlled Substance Schedule IV

ACTION: Alters the signaling of neurotransmitters called orexins, which are responsible for regulating the sleep–wake cycle

Therapeutic outcome: Normalized sleeping patterns

USES: The treatment of insomnia characterized by difficulties with sleep onset and/or sleep maintenance

---

Pharmacokinetics

Absorption	Unknown
Distribution	High-protein binding
Metabolism	Unknown
Excretion	Feces (66%), urine (23%)
Half-life	12 hr

Pharmacodynamics

Onset	Unknown
Peak	2 hr
Duration	Unknown

CONTRAINDICATIONS: Narcolepsy, hypersensitivity

Precautions: Preexisting respiratory disease, COPD, breastfeeding, pregnancy, labor, geriatrics, hepatic disease, sleep apnea, substance abuse, alcohol use, suicidal ideation, mental changes, depression

DOSAGE AND ROUTES

Adult: PO 10 mg every night within 30 min of going to bed, and with ≥7 hr remaining before the planned time of awakening, may increase to maximum 20 mg every night

Available forms: Tabs 5, 10, 15, 20 mg

ADVERSE EFFECTS

CNS: Amnesia, suicidal ideation, anxiety, dizziness, drowsiness, hallucinations, headache, memory impairment, sleep paralysis
GI: Diarrhea

INTERACTIONS
Drug classifications

CNS depressants: increased effects of both products
CYP3A inducers: decreased suvorexant effect
CYP3A inhibitors: avoid concurrent use

Drug/herb

Kava kava, melatonin, valerian: increased suvorexant effect

NURSING CONSIDERATIONS
Assessment

• **Sleeping patterns:** waking in the night, inability to fall asleep, stay asleep, amnesia
• **Beers:** Avoid in older adults with or at high risk for delirium

Patient problem

Impaired sleep (uses)
Risk for injury (adverse reactions)

Implementation

• Give 30 min before bedtime
• Effect may be delayed if taken with food, take on empty stomach for faster effect

Patient/family education

• Teach patient that daytime drowsiness or dizziness may occur, to avoid hazardous activities until response is known
• Teach patient to avoid grapefruit juice
• Advise patient to use on an empty stomach for faster effect
• Teach patient to report suicidal thoughts/ behaviors immediately or if depression worsens
• Teach patient to avoid use with other products unless approved by prescriber
• Pregnancy/breastfeeding: Teach patient to notify provider if pregnancy is planned or suspected, or if breastfeeding
• Teach patient that complex sleep behaviors may occur (sleep driving, sleep eating)
• Identify if pregnancy is planned or suspected or if breastfeeding

Evaluation
Therapeutic response

• Normalized sleeping patterns

tacrolimus (PO, IV) (Rx)
(tak-row'lim-us)
Advagraf ✲, **Astagraf XL,
Envarsus ER, Prograf**
tacrolimus (topical) (Rx)
Protopic
Func. class.: Immunosuppressant
Chem. class.: Macrolide

Do not confuse: Prograf/PROzac

ACTION: Produces immunosuppression by inhibiting lymphocytes (T)

Therapeutic outcome: Prevention of rejection in organ transplant

USES: Organ transplants, to prevent rejection; **topical:** atopic dermatitis

Pharmacokinetics

Absorption	Erratically absorbed (PO), completely absorbed **(IV)**
Distribution	Crosses placenta, 75% protein binding
Metabolism	Liver to metabolite
Excretion	Kidney—minimal; breast milk, bile
Half-life	10 hr

Pharmacodynamics

	PO	IV
Onset	Unknown	Unknown
Peak	1-4 hr	Unknown
Duration	12 hr	12 hr

CONTRAINDICATIONS
Hypersensitivity to this product or to some kinds of castor oil, long-term use (topical), child <2 yr (topical)

Precautions: Pregnancy, breastfeeding, children <12 yr, severe renal/hepatic disease, diabetes mellitus, hyperkalemia, hyperuricemia, lymphomas, hypertension, acute bronchospasm, African descent, heart failure, seizures, QT prolongation

> **BLACK BOX WARNING:** Children <12 yr, lymphomas, infection, neoplastic disease, neonates, infants; requires a specialized setting and an experienced clinician; liver transplant (ext rel)

DOSAGE AND ROUTES-NTI
Kidney transplant rejection prophylaxis
Adult: **IV** 0.03-0.05 mg/kg/day as cont INF, may begin with 24 hr of transplantation, delay until renal function has recovered; PO 0.2 mg/kg/day in 2 divided doses q12hr with azathioprine and corticosteroids; may give first dose within 24 hr of transplantation; delay until renal function has recovered; **ext rel caps** 0.1 mg/kg qday preoperatively on empty stomach, 1st dose 12 hr prior to reperfusion and 0.2 mg/kg once daily postoperatively 1st dose within 12 hr of reperfusion but ≥4 hr after preoperative dose in combination with mycophenolate and corticosteroids

Liver transplant rejection prophylaxis
Adult: PO 0.1-0.15 mg/kg/day in 2 divided doses q12h, give no sooner than 6 hr after transplantation; **IV** 0.03-0.05 mg/kg/day as a cont INF, give no sooner than 6 hr after transplantation

Heart transplant rejection prophylaxis
Adult: PO 0.075 mg/kg/day in 2 divided doses q12h, give no sooner than 6 hr after transplantation; **IV** 0.01 mg/kg/day as a cont INF, give no sooner than 6 hr after transplantation

Atopic dermatitis
Adult: TOP use 0.03% or 0.1% ointment, apply bid × 7 days after clearing of signs
Child 2-5 yr: TOP 0.03% ointment, apply bid × 7 days after clearing of signs

Available forms: Inj **IV** 5 mg/ml; caps 0.5, 1, 5 mg; ext rel cap (Astragraf XL) 0.5, 1, 3 ✲, 5 mg; ointment 0.03%, 0.1%; ext rel cap (Envarsus XR) 0.75, 1.4 mg

ADVERSE EFFECTS
CNS: *Tremors, headache,* insomnia, paresthesia, chills, fever, seizures, posterior reversible encephalopathy syndrome, BK-virus-associated nephropathy, coma, post-transplant lymphoproliferation time disorder (PTLD)
CV: Hypertension, myocardial hypertrophy, prolonged QTc, cardiomyopathy
EENT: Blurred vision, photophobia
GI: Nausea, vomiting, diarrhea, constipation, GI bleeding, GI preforation
GU: Urinary tract infections, albuminuria, hematuria, proteinuria, renal failure, hemolytic uremic syndrome
HEMA: Anemia, leukocytosis, thrombocytopenia, purpura
INTEG: Rash, flushing, itching, alopecia
META: Hyperglycemia, hyperuricemia, hypokalemia, hyperkalemia, hypomagnesemia

MS: Back pain, muscle spasms
RESP: Pleural effusion, atelectasis, dyspnea, interstitial lung disease
SYST: Anaphylaxis, infection, malignancy

INTERACTIONS
Individual drugs
CarBAMazepine, PHENobarbital, phenytoin, rifampycin: decreased blood levels

Cimetidine, danazol, erythromycin, mycophenolate, mofetil: increased blood levels

CISplatin, cycloSPORINE: increased toxicity

Haloperidol, chloroquine, droperidol, pentamidine, arsenic trioxide, CYP3A4 substrates (methadone, pimozide, QUEtiapine, quiNIDine, risperiDONE, ziprasidone): increased QT prolongation; do not use together

Ibuprofen: increased oliguria

Drug classifications
Aminoglycosides: increased toxicity

Antifungals, calcium channel blockers: increased blood levels

Class IA/III antidysrhythmics, some phenothiazines, β-agonists, local anesthetics, tricyclics, CYP3A4 inhibitors (amiodarone, clarithromycin, erythromycin, telithromycin, troleandomycin), CYP3A4 substrates (methadone, pimozide, QUEtiapine, quiNIDine, risperiDONE, ziprasidone): increased QT prolongation

Live virus vaccines: decreased effect of vaccines

Drug/herb
Astragalus, echinacea, melatonin: decreased immunosuppression, ginseng, St. John's wort

Drug/food
Decreased absorption of food
Grapefruit juice: increased effect of tacrolimus

Drug/lab test
Increased: glucose, BUN, creatinine
Decreased: magnesium, Hgb, platelets
Increased or decreased: LFTs, potassium

NURSING CONSIDERATIONS
Assessment
• Assess for caster oil allergy (HCO-60) do not use if present
• **Monitor blood studies:** Hgb, WBC, platelets during treatment monthly; if WBC is <3000/mm³ or platelet count <100,000/mm³, product should be discontinued or reduced; decreased Hgb level may indicate bone marrow suppression
• **PTLD:** Assess for malaise, fever, weight loss, night sweats, decreased appetite can be fatal, allogeneic hematopoietic stem cell transplant (HCST) may be required

• **Blood level monitoring:** maintain tacrolimus whole blood (7-20 mg/ml), then 5-15 mg/ml for 1 yr in kidney transplant; 1-3 month maintain whole blood at 8-20 mg/ml, then 6-18 ng/ml 3-18 months after transplant (heart transplant)
• **QT prolongation:** ECG for QT prolongation, ejection fraction; assess for chest pain, palpitations, dyspnea
• **Monitor liver function tests:** alkaline phosphatase, AST, ALT, amylase, bilirubin, and for hepatotoxicity: dark urine, jaundice, itching, light-colored stools; product should be discontinued
• Monitor serum creatinine/BUN, serum electrolytes, lipid profile, serum tacrolimus concentration
• **Atopic dermatitis:** check lesions baseline and during treatment
• **Assess for anaphylaxis:** assess for rash, pruritus, wheezing, laryngeal edema; stop inf, initiate emergency procedures

Patient problem
Immunologic impairment (uses)
Risk for infection (adverse reactions)

Implementation
Conventional immediate-release capsules
• Give consistently with or without food
Extended-release capsules (Astagraf XL)
• Take in the morning, preferably on an empty stomach, at least 1 hr before a meal or at least 2 hr after a meal
• Swallow whole; do not chew, divide, or crush capsules
• Do not administer with an alcoholic beverage
• If a dose is missed up to 14 hr from the scheduled time, take the dose. If a dose is missed at more than 14 hr from the scheduled time, skip the dose and take the next dose at the regularly scheduled time
Extended-release tablets (Envarsus XR)
• Take in the morning, preferably on an empty stomach, at least 1 hr before a meal or at least 2 hr after a meal
• Swallow whole; do not chew, divide, or crush capsules
• Do not administer with an alcoholic beverage
• If a dose is missed up to 15 hr from the scheduled time, take the dose. If a dose is missed at more than 15 hr from the scheduled time, skip the dose and take the next dose at the regularly scheduled time
• Topical ointment has risk of developing cancer; use only when other options have failed

IV route
• Visually inspect for particulate matter and discoloration before use

---

- Because of the risk of hypersensitivity reactions, IV use should be reserved for those who cannot take tacrolimus orally. Oral therapy should replace IV therapy as soon as possible
- Observe patients for 30 min after beginning the infusion and frequently thereafter for possible hypersensitivity reactions
- Due to chemical instability, tacrolimus should not be mixed or infused with solutions with a pH of 9 or more (acyclovir or ganciclovir)

Dilution

- The concentrate for injection must be diluted with NS or D5W injection to a final concentration between 0.004 mg/ml and 0.02 mg/ml
- Prepare solutions in polyethylene or glass containers to allow storage for 24 hr, do not use polyvinyl chloride (PVC) containers because stability is decreased and the polyoxyl 60 hydrogenated castor oil in the formulation may leach phthalates from PVC containers

Continuous IV infusion

- Give through non-PVC tubing to minimize the potential for drug adsorption onto the tubing
- Infuse the required daily dose of the diluted IV solution over 24 hr

Y-site compatibilities: Alemtuzumab, alfentanil, amifostine, amikacin, aminophylline, amiodarone, amphotericin B colloidal, amphotericin B liposome, anidulafungin, atracurium, aztreonam, benztropine, bivalirudin, bleomycin, bumetanide, buprenorphine, busulfan, butorphanol, calcium acetate/chloride/gluconate, CARBOplatin, carmustine, caspofungin, ceFAZolin, cefoperazone, cefotaxime, cefoTEtan, cefOXitin, cefTAZidime, ceftizoxime, cefTRIAXone, cefuroxime, chloramphenicol, chlorproMAZINE, cimetidine, ciprofloxacin, cisatracurium, CISplatin, clindamycin, cyclophosphamide, cycloSPORINE, cytarabine, DACTINomycin, DAPTOmycin, dexamethasone, dexmedetomidine, dexrazoxane, digoxin, diltiazem, diphenhydrAMINE, DOBUTamine, DOCEtaxel, dolasetron, DOPamine, doripenem, doxacurium, DOXOrubicin hydrochloride, doxycycline, droperidol, enalaprilat, ePHEDrine, EPINEPHrine, epirubicin, ertapenem, erythromycin, esmolol, etoposide, etoposide phosphate, famotidine, fenoldopam, fentaNYL, fluconazole, fludarabine, foscarnet, fosphenytoin, gemcitabine, gentamicin, glycopyrrolate, granisetron, haloperidol, heparin, hydrALAZINE, hydrocortisone, HYDROmorphone, IDArubicin, ifosfamide, imipenem/cilastatin, inamrinone, insulin, isoproterenol, ketorolac, labetalol, leucovorin, levofloxacin, levorphanol, lidocaine, linezolid, LORazepam, magnesium sulfate, mannitol, mechlorethamine, meperidine, meropenem, mesna, metaraminol, methotrexate, methyldopate,

methylPREDNISolone, metoclopramide, metoprolol, metroNIDAZOLE, micafungin, midazolam, milrinone, mitoMYcin, mitoXANtrone, mivacurium, morphine, multivitamins, nafcillin, nalbuphine, naloxone, nesiritide, niCARdipine, nitroglycerin, nitroprusside, norepinephrine, octreotide, ondansetron, oxacillin, oxaliplatin, oxytocin, PACLitaxel, palonosetron, pancuronium, PEMEtrexed, penicillin G, pentamidine, pentazocine, perphenazine, phentolamine, phenylephrine, piperacillin/tazobactam, potassium chloride/phosphates, procainamide, prochlorperazine, promethazine, propranolol, quinupristin/dalfopristin, ranitidine, remifentanil, rocuronium, sodium acetate/bicarbonate/phosphates, streptozocin, succinylcholine, SUFentanil, teniposide, theophylline, thiotepa, ticarcillin/clavulanate, tigecycline, tirofiban, tobramycin, tolazoline, trimethobenzamide, vancomycin, vasopressin, vecuronium, verapamil, vinCRIStine, vinorelbine, voriconazole, zidovudine, zoledronic acid

Patient/family education

> **BLACK BOX WARNING:** Advise patient to report if pregnancy is planned or suspected

> **BLACK BOX WARNING:** Advise patient to report symptoms of lymphoma, or skin cancer

- Instruct patient to report fever, rash, severe diarrhea, chills, sore throat, fatigue because serious infections may occur; clay-colored stools, cramping may indicate hepatotoxicity, signs of diabetes mellitus
- Caution patient to avoid crowds or persons with known infections to reduce risk of infection, to avoid eating raw shellfish
- **Organ rejection:** monitor B/P, provide treatment for hypertension

> **BLACK BOX WARNING: Liver transplant:** extended-release product should not be used due to increased female death rate

> **BLACK BOX WARNING: Specialized care setting, experienced clinician:** this product should only be used when equipped and staffed with adequate supportive medical services and by those experienced in immunosuppressive therapy and organ transplantation

> **BLACK BOX WARNING: Children, infants, neonates:** Not approved use of ointment in those <2 yr old, ext rel in those <16 yr not approved for pediatric kidney/heart transplant

- **Topical:** teach patient to stop using topical product when atopic dermatitis is resolved, not

---

to use over 6 wk if symptoms do not improve, not to shower or swim after applying
• Teach patient not to consume grapefruit juice
• **Pregnancy/breastfeeding:** Identify if pregnancy is planned or suspected or if breastfeeding

Evaluation

Positive therapeutic outcome
• Absence of graft rejection
• Immunosuppression in autoimmune disorders

tadalafil (Rx)
(tah-dal′a-fil)
Adcirca, Cialis
Func. class.: Impotence agent
Chem. class.: Phosphodiesterase type 5 inhibitor

ACTION: Inhibits phosphodiesterase type 5 (PDE5); enhances erectile function by increasing the amount of cyclic GMP, which causes smooth muscle relaxation and increased blood flow into the corpus cavernosum; improves erectile function for up to 36 hr

Therapeutic outcome: Erection

USES: Treatment of erectile dysfunction (Cialis); pulmonary arterial hypertension (PAH) (Adcirca only), benign prostatic hyperplasia (BPH) with or without erectile dysfunction

Pharmacokinetics

Absorption	Rapid; rate and extent of absorption of tadalafil are not influenced by food
Distribution	94% protein bound
Metabolism	Liver
Excretion	Excreted primarily as metabolites, feces, urine; plasma concentration 61% in feces, 36% in urine
Half-life	17.5 hr

Pharmacodynamics

Onset	Rapid
Peak	6 hr
Duration	Unknown

CONTRAINDICATIONS
Newborns, women, children, hypersensitivity, patients taking organic nitrates regularly or intermittently, patients taking any α-adrenergic antagonist other than 0.4 mg once-daily tamsulosin

Precautions: Pregnancy, anatomic penile deformities, sickle cell anemia, leukemia, multiple myeloma, CV/renal/hepatic disease, bleeding disorders, active peptic ulcer, prolonged erection

DOSAGE AND ROUTES
Erectile dysfunction
Adult: PO (Cialis) 10 mg, taken prior to sexual activity, dose may be reduced to 5 mg or increased to a max of 20 mg; usual max dosing frequency is once per day; once-daily dosing 2.5 mg/day at same time each day

For improvement in exercise ability in patients with WHO Group I pulmonary hypertension (Adcirca)
Adult: PO 40 mg (two 20-mg tablets) qday with or without food

BPH
Adult: PO 5 mg qday at the same time every day

Renal dose
Adult: PO CCr 31-50 ml/min 5 mg/day, max 10 mg q48hr; CCr <30 ml/min, max 5 mg q72hr

Hepatic dose
Adult: PO Child-Pugh class A, B, max 10 mg/day or 20 mg/day (pulmonary hypertension) max 40 mg/day; Child-Pugh class C, not recommended

Concomitant medications
Ketoconazole, itraconazole, ritonavir, max 10 mg q72hr

Available forms: Tabs (Cialis) 2.5, 5, 10, 20 mg; tab 20 mg (Adcirca)

ADVERSE EFFECTS
CNS: *Headache, flushing, dizziness,* seizures, transient global amnesia
CV: MI, hypotension, QT prolongation
INTEG: Stevens-Johnson syndrome, exfoliative dermatitis, urticaria
MISC: Back pain/myalgia, *dyspepsia, nasal congestion, UTI,* blurred vision, changes in color vision, *diarrhea,* pruritus, priapism, nonarteritic ischemic optic neuropathy (NAION), hearing loss

INTERACTIONS
Individual drugs
Alcohol, amlodipine, enalapril: decreased B/P
Bosentan: decreased effects of tadalafil
Itraconazole, ketoconazole, ritonavir: increased levels (although not studied, may also include other HIV protease inhibitors)

Drug classifications
• Do not use with nitrates because of unsafe drop in B/P that could result in heart attack or stroke

---

α-blockers, angiotensin II receptor blockers: decreased B/P

Antacids: decreased effects of tadalafil

Drug/food
Grapefruit: increased tadalafil effect

NURSING CONSIDERATIONS
Assessment
• **Cialis:** assess for underlying cause of erectile dysfunction prior to treatment; organic nitrates that should not be used with this product; assess for severe loss of vision; BPH: assess for urinary hesitancy, poor stream, dribbling baseline and periodically

• **Adcirca:** monitor hemodynamic parameters, exercise tolerance baseline and periodically

• **Beers:** Use with caution in older adults, may exacerbate syncope, monitor frequently for syncope

• Teach patient to notify provider immediately and to stop taking product if vision, hearing loss occurs

• **Pregnancy/breastfeeding:** Use only if clearly needed (Adcirca only). Cialis is not indicated for women, cautious use in breastfeeding

Patient problem
Impaired sexual functioning (uses)
Impaired urination (uses)

Implementation
• **Sexual dysfunction:** give before sexual activity; do not use more than once a day

• **Pulmonary hypertension:** give Adcirca without regard to meals

• Product should not be used with nitrates in any form

Patient/family education
• Teach patient to take 1 hr before sexual activity

• Teach patient not to drink large amounts of alcohol

• Advise that product does not protect against STDs, including HIV

• Instruct to tell physician if patient has a bleeding problem

• Advise that product should not be used with nitrates in any form

• Advise that product has no effect in the absence of sexual stimulation

• Instruct to seek medical help if an erection lasts more than 4 hr or if chest pain occurs

• Advise patient to discuss with health care professional all OTC, Rx, herbals, supplements taken

• Advise to notify physician of all medicines, vitamins, and herbs patient is taking, especially α-blockers, erythromycin, indinavir, itraconazole, ketoconazole, nitrates, ritonavir

• Advise that tadalafil is contraindicated for use with α-blockers except 0.4 mg/daily tamsulosin

Evaluation
Positive therapeutic outcome
• Sustainable erection
• Decrease BPH symptoms
• Improvement in exercise ability (pulmonary hypertension)

tafenoquine
(ta fen′ oh-kwin)
Krintafel, Arakoda
Func. class.: Antimalarial
Chem. class.: 8-aminoquinoline

ACTION: The activity against the pre-erythrocytic liver stages of the parasite prevents the development of the erythrocytic forms, which are responsible for malaria relapse; may inhibit hematin polymerization and induce apoptotic-like death of the parasite

Therapeutic outcome: Prevention of relapse or prevention of malaria

USES: Prevention of relapse of *Plasmodium vivax* malaria in those receiving antimalarial therapy for acute *P. vivax* infection (Krintafel); for malaria prophylaxis (Arakoda)

Pharmacokinetics

Absorption	Unknown
Distribution	Protein binding 99.5%
Metabolism	Affected cytochrome P450 isoenzymes and drug transporters: OCT2, MATE-1, MATE2-K
Excretion	Unknown
Half-life	12-15 days (Krintafel)

Pharmacodynamics

Onset	Unknown
Peak	12-15 hr
Duration	Unknown

CONTRAINDICATIONS: Hypersensitivity to this product or iodoquinol or primaquine, G6PD deficiency, psychosis

PRECAUTIONS: Breastfeeding, contraception requirements, hepatic disease, methemoglobin reductase deficiency, pregnancy, pregnancy testing, psychiatric events, renal disease, reproductive risk

DOSAGE AND ROUTES
Prevention of relapse of *Plasmodium vivax* malaria in those receiving antimalarial therapy for acute *P.* vivax infection (Krintafel)
Adult/adolescent ≥16 yr PO 300 mg as a single dose on the first or second day of the antimalarial therapy (chloroquine)

For malaria prophylaxis (Arakoda)
Adult: PO 200 mg PO daily for 3 days prior to travel as loading dose, then 200 mg weekly starting 7 days after the last loading dose, continuing during travel to malarious area as maintenance, then 200 mg once at 7 days after the last maintenance dose in the wk after exit from malarious area; may be given for ≤6 months of continuous dosing

Available forms: Tablets 100 mg (Arakoda); 150 mg (Krintafel)

ADVERSE EFFECTS
GI: Nausea, vomiting
Hema: Decreased Hgb
Integ: Angioedema, urticaria
EENT: Vortex keratopathy, photophobia

INTERACTIONS
Drug classifications
Avoid use with MATE (multidrug and toxin extrusion substrates) and OCT2 (organic cation transporter-2) (dofetilide, metformin); if these products must be given, monitor for toxicity

Drug/lab test
Increased: Methemoglobin, ALT, creatinine

NURSING CONSIDERATIONS
Assessment
• **Malaria symptoms:** Monitor for anemia, jaundice, diarrhea, sweating, vomiting, fast heart rate, low B/P; report symptoms to healthcare provider
• **Methemoglobinemia:** Monitor lab for increased methemoglobin; report immediately shortness of breath, cyanosis, mental status changes; O_2 and methylene blue may be given
• **Psychiatric effects:** Assess for serious psychiatric adverse reactions that have been observed in patients with a previous history of psychiatric conditions at doses higher than the approved dose; the effects may occur during or after treatment
• **Hypersensitivity reactions:** Assess for serious hypersensitivity reactions (angioedema); these reactions may occur during or after conclusion of therapy

• **Pregnancy/breastfeeding:** Avoid use in pregnancy; a pregnancy test is required in all females of reproductive potential; adequate contraception is required during and for 3 months after last dose; infant should be tested for G6PD deficiency before breastfeeding

Implementation
• Give with food
• Swallow tablets whole; do not break, crush, or chew
• If vomiting occurs within 1 hr after dosing, repeat; do not redose more than once (prevention of relapse single-dose therapy)
• **Storage:** At room temperature in original container; protect from moisture
CNS: *Dizziness, headache, anxiety,* abnormal dreams, insomnia, somnolence

Patient/family education
• **Pregnancy/breastfeeding:** Teach patient not to use during pregnancy; adequate contraception should be used during and for 3 months after last dose; infant should have a lab test performed before breastfeeding
• Advise patient to swallow tablets whole, not to split or cut, and to take with food
• Inform patient to report immediately dark urine or lips as these may be symptoms of hemolytic anemia
• Teach patient to use sunglasses in bright light to prevent photophobia

Evaluation
• Prevention of relapse or prevention of malaria

⚠ HIGH ALERT
tamoxifen (Rx)
(ta-mox′i-fen)
Nolvadex-D ♦, Tamofen ♦, Tamone ♦, Tamoplex ♦
Func. class.: Antineoplastic
Chem. class.: Antiestrogen

ACTION: Inhibits cell division by binding to cytoplasmic estrogen receptors; resembles normal cell complex but inhibits DNA synthesis and estrogen response of target tissue

Therapeutic outcome: Prevention of rapidly growing malignant cells

USES: Advanced breast carcinoma that has not responded to other therapy in estrogen receptor–positive patients (usually postmenopausal), prevention of breast cancer, after breast surgery/radiation in ductal carcinoma in situ (DCIS)

Pharmacokinetics

Absorption	Adequately absorbed
Distribution	Unknown
Metabolism	Liver—extensively
Excretion	Feces—slowly, small amounts (kidneys)
Half-life	1 wk

Pharmacodynamics

Onset	Unknown
Peak	4-7 hr
Duration	Unknown

CONTRAINDICATIONS
Pregnancy, breastfeeding, hypersensitivity

> **BLACK BOX WARNING:** Thromboembolic disease, endometrial cancer, stroke

Precautions: Leukopenia, thrombocytopenia, cataracts, women of childbearing age

> **BLACK BOX WARNING:** Uterine cancer

DOSAGE AND ROUTES
Breast cancer (men/women)
Adult: PO 20-40 mg/day × 5 yr, doses >20 mg/day divide AM/PM

High risk for breast cancer
Adult: PO 20 mg/day × 5 yr

Ductal carcinoma in situ
Adult: PO 20 mg/day × 5 yr

Available forms: Tabs 10, 20 mg; oral solution 10 mg/5 ml

ADVERSE EFFECTS
CNS: *Hot flashes, headache, light-headedness,* depression, mood changes, stroke
CV: Chest pain, stroke, fluid retention, flushing, thromboembolism
EENT: Blurred vision (high doses)
GI: *Nausea, vomiting,* altered taste
GU: Vaginal bleeding, uterine malignancies, *altered menses, amenorrhea*
HEMA: Thrombocytopenia, leukopenia, deep vein thrombosis
INTEG: *Rash,* alopecia
META: Hypercalcemia
RESP: Pulmonary embolism

INTERACTIONS
Individual drugs
Aminoglutethimide, rifamycin: decreased tamoxifen levels
Bromocriptine: increased tamoxifen level
Letrozole: decreased levels of letrozole

PARoxetine: increased risk for death from breast cancer
Radiation: increased myelosuppression

Drug classifications
Anticoagulants: increased risk of bleeding
Cytotoxics: increased thromboembolic action
CYP2D6 inhibitors (antidepressants): decreased tamoxifen effect
CYP3A4 inducers (barbiturates, bosentan, carBAMazepine, efavirenz, phenytoin, nevirapine, rifabutin, rifampin): decreased tamoxifen effect
CYP3A4 inhibitors (aprepitant, antiretroviral protease inhibitors, clarithromycin, danazol, delavirdine, diltiazem, erythromycin, fluconazole, FLUoxetine, fluvoxaMINE, imatinib, ketoconazole, mibefradil, nefazodone, telithromycin, voriconazole): increased toxicity

Drug/herb
Black cohosh, dong quai, St. John's wort: avoid use

Drug/lab test
Increased: serum calcium, T_4, AST, ALT, cholesterol, triglycerides, BUN

NURSING CONSIDERATIONS
Assessment
• Monitor CBC, differential, platelet count baseline and periodically notify prescriber of results; monitor calcium levels (hypercalcemia is common); breast exam, mammogram, pregnancy test, bone mineral density, LFTs, serum calcium, serum lipid profile, periodic eye exams (cataracts, retinopathy), Pap smear
• **Assess for tumor flare:** increase in bone, tumor pain during beginning treatment; give analgesics as ordered to decrease pain
• **Assess for bleeding:** hematuria, guaiac, bruising or petechiae, mucosa or orifices q8hr, no rectal temp
• **Severe allergic reactions:** Rash, pruritus, urticaria, purpuric skin lesions, itching, flushing
• Bone pain; may give analgesics; pain usually transient

> **BLACK BOX WARNING: Assess for uterine malignancies:** symptoms of stroke, PE that may occur in women with DCIS and women at high risk for breast cancer, monitor gynecologic exams periodically

• **Pregnancy/breastfeeding:** Do not use in pregnancy, breastfeeding

Patient problem
Risk for infection (adverse reactions)
Risk for injury (uses, adverse reactions)

Implementation
- Do not break, crush, or chew tabs
- Give with food or fluids for GI upset; repeat dose may be needed if vomiting occurs
- Store in light-resistant container at room temperature
- Oral solution: use calibrated container; dose >20 mg/day should be divided morning and evening; may be used with food for gastric irritation

Patient/family education
- **Teach patient to notify prescriber immediately of stroke:** blurred vision, headache, weakness on one side of the body; pulmonary embolism: chest pain, fainting, sweating, difficulty breathing; this is a medical emergency
- Instruct patient to report any complaints, side effects to prescriber; if dose is missed, do not double next dose; that use may be 5 yr
- Advise patient that vaginal bleeding, pruritus, hot flashes can occur and are reversible after discontinuing treatment
- Instruct patient to report immediately decreased visual acuity, which may be irreversible; stress need for routine eye exams
- Inform patient about who should be told about tamoxifen therapy
- Advise patient to report vaginal bleeding immediately; that tumor flare (increase in size or tumor, increased bone pain) may occur and will subside rapidly; may take analgesics for pain; that premenopausal women must use mechanical birth control method because ovulation may be induced (teratogenic product)
- **Tumor flare:** Advise patient that increase in size of tumor, increased bone pain may occur and will subside rapidly; may take analgesics for pain
- Teach patient that hair loss may occur during treatment; a wig or hairpiece may make patient feel better; new hair may be different in color, texture
- Advise patient to increase fluids to 2 L/day unless contraindicated
- Teach patient to use nonhormonal contraception during treatment and for 2 mo after discontinuing treatment

Evaluation

Positive therapeutic outcome
- Decreased spread of malignant cells in breast cancer

---

tamsulosin (Rx)
(tam-sue-lo′sen)
Flomax
Func. class.: Selective α-adrenergic blocker, BPH agent
Chem. class.: Sulfamoyl phenethylamine derivative

Do not confuse: Tamsulosin/tacrolimus

ACTION: Binds preferentially to α IA-adrenoceptor subtype located mainly in the prostate

Therapeutic outcome: Decreased symptoms of benign prostatic hyperplasia (BPH)

USES: Symptoms of BPH

Pharmacokinetics
Absorption	Well absorbed
Distribution	Not known; 98% plasma protein bound
Metabolism	Liver, extensively
Excretion	Kidneys
Half-life	9-15 hr

Pharmacodynamics
Unknown

CONTRAINDICATIONS
Hypersensitivity

Precautions: Pregnancy, breastfeeding, children, hepatic disease, CAD, severe renal disease, prostate cancer; cataract surgery (floppy iris syndrome)

DOSAGE AND ROUTES
Adult: PO 0.4 mg/day, increasing to 0.8 mg/day if required

Hepatic dose (moderate impairment)
Adult: PO reg rel 50 mg q8hr, titrate; ext rel 50 mg q24hr, titrate, max 100 mg q24hr; avoid use in severe impairment

Available forms: Caps 0.4 mg

ADVERSE EFFECTS
CNS: *Dizziness, headache,* asthenia, insomnia
CV: Chest pain, orthostatic hypotension
EENT: Amblyopia, floppy iris syndrome
GI: Nausea, diarrhea, dysgeusia
GU: Decreased libido, abnormal ejaculation, priapism
MS: Back pain
RESP: Rhinitis, pharyngitis, cough
SYST: Angioedema

T

INTERACTIONS
Individual drugs
Cimetidine: increased toxicity
Doxazosin, prazosin, terazosin, vardenafil: do not use together

Drug classifications
α-blockers: do not use together

Drug/food
Decreased: absorption with food

NURSING CONSIDERATIONS
Assessment
• **Assess for BPH:** change in urinary patterns, baseline, throughout treatment; monitor I&O ratios, weight daily, edema, report weight gain or edema
• Monitor CBC with differential and liver function tests; B/P and heart rate
• Monitor urodynamic studies/urinary flow rates, residual volume
• **Orthostatic hypotension:** monitor B/P standing, sitting
• **Pregnancy/breastfeeding:** Not to be used for women

Patient problem
Impaired urination (uses)
Impaired sexual functioning (adverse reactions)

Implementation
• Swallow caps whole; do not break, crush, or chew
• Store in airtight container at 86° F (30° C) or less
• Give without regard to food, but may be given with food to prevent GI symptoms; ½ hr after same meal each day
• If treatment is interrupted for several days, restart at lowest dose (0.4 mg/day)

Patient/family education
• Teach patient not to discontinue product abruptly; emphasize the importance of complying with dosage schedule, even if feeling better; if dose is missed, take as soon as remembered; take at same time each day
• Teach patient not to use OTC products (cough, cold, allergy) unless directed by prescriber; also to avoid large amounts of caffeine
• Caution patient that product may cause dizziness, may occur during 1st few days of therapy; to avoid hazardous activities
• Teach patient to take ½ hr after same meal each day
• Teach patient about priapism (rare)
• Advise patient not to crush, break, chew caps
• Teach patient that decreased ejaculate or absence may occur, resolves after discontinuing

Evaluation
Positive therapeutic outcome
• Decreased symptoms of BPH

> **⚠ HIGH ALERT**
>
> ## tapentadol (Rx)
> (ta-pen′ta-dol)
> **Nucynta, Nucynta IR ✽, Nucynta ER**
> *Func. class.:* Analgesic, miscellaneous
> *Chem. class.:* μ-Opioid receptor agonist
> **Controlled substance schedule II**

ACTION: Centrally acting synthetic analgesic; μ-opioid agonist activity is thought to result in analgesia; inhibits norepinephrine uptake

Therapeutic outcome: Relief of pain

USES: Moderate to severe pain

Pharmacokinetics
Absorption	32%
Distribution	Protein binding 20%, widely
Metabolism	Liver, extensively
Excretion	Urine 99%
Half-life	4 hr

Pharmacodynamics
Onset	Unknown
Peak	1 hr
Duration	4-6 hr

CONTRAINDICATIONS
Hypersensitivity, asthma, ileus

> **BLACK BOX WARNING:** Respiratory depression

Precautions: Pregnancy, breastfeeding, children <18 yr, increased intracranial pressure, MI (acute), severe heart disease, respiratory depression, renal/hepatic disease, GI obstruction, ulcerative colitis, sleep apnea, seizure disorder

> **BLACK BOX WARNING:** Accidental exposure, avoid ethanol, substance abuse, neonatal opioid withdrawal/syndrome, potential for overdose, poisoning, coadministration with other CNS depressants

DOSAGE AND ROUTES
Adult: PO 50-100 mg q4-6hr; may give second dose 1 hr or more after 1st dose; max 700 mg on day 1, 600 mg/day thereafter; **ext rel** 50 mg q12hr (opioid-naive), titrate 50 mg/dose bid q3 days; max 250 mg q12hr

---

Hepatic disease

Adult: PO immediate rel sol 50 mg q8hr; may titrate to response; ext rel 50 mg qday max 100 mg/day

Available forms: Tab 50, 75, 100 mg; tabs, ext rel 50, 100, 150, 200, 250 mg; oral solution 20 mg/ml

Oral solution: Measure using calibrated syringe

ADVERSE EFFECTS

CNS: *Drowsiness, dizziness, confusion, headache, euphoria,* hallucinations, restlessness, syncope, anxiety, flushing, psychological dependence, insomnia, lethargy, tremor, seizures
CV: Palpitations, bradycardia, hypo/hypertension, orthostatic hypotension, sinus tachycardia
GI: *Nausea, vomiting, anorexia, constipation, cramps,* gastritis, dyspepsia, biliary spasms
GU: Urinary retention/frequency
INTEG: *Rash,* urticaria, diaphoresis, pruritus
RESP: Respiratory depression, cough
SYST: Anaphylaxis, infection, serotonin syndrome

INTERACTIONS
Individual drugs

> **BLACK BOX WARNING:** Alcohol: increased effects with other CNS depressants

Drug classifications

Antipsychotics, opioids, sedatives/hypnotics, skeletal muscle relaxants: increased effects with other CNS depressants
MAOIs: increased toxicity
Serotonin-receptor agonists, SSRIs, SNRIs, tricyclics: increased serotonin syndrome

> **BLACK BOX WARNING:** Do not use with alcohol; fatal overdose may occur

Drug/herb

Kava, St. John's wort, valerian: increased sedative effect

NURSING CONSIDERATIONS
Assessment

• Monitor I&O ratio; check for decreasing output; may indicate urinary retention
• Assess CNS changes: dizziness, drowsiness, hallucinations, euphoria, LOC, pupil reaction
• Assess for allergic reactions: rash, urticaria, anaphylaxis
• **Seizures:** Assess for history of seizures, increased with SSRIs, SNRIs, tricyclic antidepressants
• **Serotonin syndrome:** Assess for increased heart rate, shivering, sweating, dilated pupils, tremors, high B/P, hyperthermia, headache,

confusion; if these occur, stop product, administer a serotonin antagonist if needed

> **BLACK BOX WARNING: Addiction risk, previous substance abuse** before using extended-release product, some may crush extended-release product and snort, inject product that is dissolved

> **BLACK BOX WARNING: Accidental exposure:** Identify if alcohol has been used before giving this product; may be fatal if used with tapentadol; keep from children, pets; avoid coadministration with other CNS depressants

> **BLACK BOX WARNING: Assess for respiratory dysfunction:** respiratory depression, character, rate, rhythm; notify prescriber if respirations are <10/min; also B/P, pulse

• **Assess for pain:** intensity, location, type, characteristics; need for pain medication by pain/sedation scoring; physical dependence

> **BLACK BOX WARNING: Neonatal opioid withdrawal syndrome:** May be fatal, monitor neonates for irritability, hyperactivity, abnormal sleep patterns, high-pitched cry, tremors, vomiting, diarrhea, failure to gain weight

> **BLACK BOX WARNING: Pregnancy/ breastfeeding:** Use only if benefits outweigh fetal risk, including neonatal opioid withdrawal syndrome, do not breastfeed, excretion unknown

Patient problem

Pain (uses)
Risk for injury (adverse reactions)

Implementation

• Give with antiemetic if nausea, vomiting occur
• Give when pain is beginning to return; determine dosing interval by response
• Store in light-resistant area at room temperature
• Provide assistance with ambulation
• Provide safety measures: night-light, call bell within easy reach
• Not to crush, chew, break ext rel product or use with alcohol
• This is the preferred analgesic in those with altered cytochrome P450 or mild hepatic disease, mild to moderate renal disease

> **BLACK BOX WARNING:** These products have high potential for overdose, poisoning; may be fatal due to respiratory depression

T

Patient/family education
• Teach patient to report any symptoms of CNS changes, allergic reactions
• Advise that physical dependency may result from extended use
• Inform that withdrawal symptoms may occur: nausea, vomiting, cramps, fever, faintness, anorexia
• Instruct patient to discuss with provider OTC, Rx, herbals, supplements taken; to avoid CNS depressants, alcohol
• Advise to avoid driving, operating machinery if drowsiness occurs

> **BLACK BOX WARNING:** Not to use with alcohol, may be fatal

• Teach patient to take as directed, not to double doses; if breakthrough pain occurs, notify provider; do not discontinue abruptly, gradually taper
• **Seizures:** Teach patient that if seizures occur, discontinue, notify provider
• Advise patient not to drive or perform other hazardous activities until response is known
• **Orthostatic hypertension:** Teach patient to rise slowly to prevent orthostatic hypertension
• **Serotonin syndrome:** Teach patient symptoms of serotonin syndrome and when to contact provider
• **Pregnancy/breastfeeding:** Identify if pregnancy is planned or suspected or if breastfeeding

Evaluation
Positive therapeutic outcome
• Decrease in pain

tavaborole topical
See Appendix B

tazobactam
See piperacillin/tazobactam

telavancin (Rx)
(tel-a-van'sin)
Vibativ
Func. class.: Antiinfective—miscellaneous
Chem. class.: Lipoglycopeptide

ACTION: Inhibits bacterial cell wall synthesis, disrupts cell membrane integrity, blocks glycopeptides

Therapeutic outcome: Negative culture

USES: Skin/skin structure infections caused by *Enterococcus faecalis, E. faecium, Staphylococcus aureus* (MSRA), *S. aureus* (MSSA), *S. epidermidis, S. haemolyticus, Streptococcus agalactiae* (group B), *S. dysgalactiae, S. pyogenes* (group A beta tremolytic), *S. anginosus, S. intermedius, S. constellatus,* nosocomial pneumonia caused by susceptible gram-positive bacteria

Pharmacokinetics
Absorption	Unknown
Distribution	Unknown, protein binding 90%
Metabolism	Unknown, hepatic metabolism
Excretion	Urine 76%
Half-life	8-9 hr

Pharmacodynamics
Onset	Rapid
Peak	Unknown
Duration	Unknown

CONTRAINDICATIONS
Hypersensitivity

Precautions: Breastfeeding, geriatric patients, renal disease, antimicrobial resistance, children, diabetes mellitus, diarrhea, GI disease, heart failure, hypertension, pseudomembranous colitis, QT prolongation, vancomycin hypersensitivity

> **BLACK BOX WARNING:** Pregnancy, females, renal disease

DOSAGE AND ROUTES
Complicated skin/skin structure infections
Adult: **IV** INF 10 mg/kg over 60 min q24hr × 7-14 days

Nosocomial pneumonia
Adult: **IV** INF 10 mg/kg q24hr × 7-21 days

Renal dose
Adult: IV CCr 30-50 ml/min 7.5 mg/kg q24hr; CCr 10-29 ml/min 10 mg/kg q48hr

Available forms: Lyophilized powder for inj 250, 750 mg

ADVERSE EFFECTS
CNS: Anxiety, chills, flushing, headache, insomnia, dizziness
CV: QT prolongation, irregular heartbeat
EENT: Hearing loss

GI: Nausea, vomiting, CDAD, abdominal pain, constipation, diarrhea, metallic/soapy taste

GU: Nephrotoxicity, *increased BUN, creatinine*, renal failure, foamy urine

HEMA: Leukopenia, eosinophilia, anemia, thrombocytopenia

INTEG: Chills, fever, rash, thrombophlebitis at inj site, urticaria, pruritus, necrosis (red man syndrome)

SYST: Anaphylaxis, superinfection

INTERACTIONS
Individual drugs
Adefovir, amphotericin B, bacitracin, cidofovir, CISplatin, colistin, cycloSPO-RINE, foscarnet, ganciclovir, IV pentamidine, acyclovir, pamidronate, polymyxin, streptozotocin, tacrolimus, zoledronic acid: increased toxicity, nephrotoxicity

Chloroquine, clarithromycin, dronedarone, droperidol, erythromycin, grepafloxacin, haloperidol, levomethadyl, methadone, pimozide, ziprasidone: increased QT prolongation

Drug classifications
Aminoglycosides, cephalosporins, nondepolarizing muscle relaxants: increased toxicity, nephrotoxicity

Class IA, III antidysrhythmics, some phenothiazines: increased QT prolongation

Drug/lab test
False increase: INR, PT, PTT

NURSING CONSIDERATIONS
Assessment
• **Nephrotoxicity:** Monitor I&O ratio; report hematuria, oliguria; avoid in those with CCr ≤50 mL/min; more common in those with diabetes, heart failure, hypertension, geriatrics, renal disease

• Monitor C&S throughout treatment

• Assess auditory function during, after treatment, hearing loss, ringing, roaring in ears; product should be discontinued

• **CDAD:** Monitor for diarrhea, fever, blood in stools, abdominal cramps; may be several weeks after therapy ends; report to prescriber immediately

> **BLACK BOX WARNING:** Pregnancy/breastfeeding: Obtain a pregnancy test before use; if a woman has taken this product during pregnancy, the national registry should be notified at 866-658-4228

• **Anaphylaxis:** Monitor for rash, itching, wheezing, laryngeal edema; discontinue and notify prescriber immediately; emergency equipment and EPINEPHrine should be nearby

• Monitor B/P during administration; sudden drop may indicate red man syndrome; also flushing, pruritus, rash, use slow IV infusion to prevent

• Assess respiratory status: rate, character, wheezing, tightness in chest

Patient problem
Infection (uses)
Nausea (adverse reactions)
Diarrhea (adverse reactions)

Implementation
• Use only for susceptible organisms to prevent drug-resistant bacteria

• Give antihistamine if red man syndrome occurs: decreased B/P, flushing of neck, face

• Store in refrigerator

• Have EPINEPHrine, suction, tracheostomy set, endotracheal intubation equipment on unit; anaphylaxis may occur

• Give adequate intake of fluids (2 L/day) to prevent nephrotoxicity

• Avoid IM, subcut use

Intermittent IV infusion route
• Administer after reconstituting with 15 ml D₅W sterile water for inj; 0.9% NaCl (15 mg/ml) 250 mg vial; add 45 ml to 750 mg vial (15 mg/ml) for dose of 150-800 mg; further dilute with 100-250 ml of compatible sol; for dose <150 mg or 800 mg, further dilute to a conc of 0.6-8 mg/ml with compatible sol; give over 60 min, avoid rapid IV, may cause red man syndrome; reconstituted or diluted solution is stable for 4 hr at room temperature, 7 hr refrigerated

Y-site compatibilities: Amphotericin B lipid complex (Abelcet), ampicillin-sulbactam, azithromycin, calcium gluconate, caspofungin, cefepime, cefTAZidime, cefTRIAXone, ciprofloxacin, dexamethasone, diltiazem, DOBUTamine, DOPamine, doripenem, doxycycline, ertapenem, famotidine, fluconazole, gentamicin, hydrocortisone, labetalol, magnesium sulfate, mannitol, meropenem, metoclopramide, milrinone, norepinephrine, ondansetron, pantoprazole, phenylephrine, piperacillin-tazobactam, potassium chloride/phosphates, ranitidine, sodium bicarbonate, sodium phosphates, tigecycline, tobramycin, vasopressin

Patient/family education
• Teach all aspects of product therapy; culture may be taken after completed course of medication

- Advise patient to notify prescriber if infection continues
- That bitter taste, nausea, vomiting, headache may occur
- Advise to report sore throat, fever, fatigue; could indicate superinfection; diarrhea; CDAD; hearing loss; rash, wheezing, tightness of chest, itching, tightening of throat (anaphylaxis)

> **BLACK BOX WARNING:** Teach patient to use contraception while taking this product; do not breastfeed; to notify prescriber if pregnancy is planned or suspected

Evaluation

Positive therapeutic outcome
- Negative culture

---

telmisartan (Rx)

(tel-mih-sar′tan)
Micardis
Func. class.: Antihypertensive
Chem. class.: Angiotensin II receptor (type AT₁)

ACTION: Blocks the vasoconstrictor and aldosterone-secreting effects of angiotensin II; selectively blocks the binding of angiotensin II to the AT_1 receptor found in tissues

Therapeutic outcome: Decreased B/P

USES: Hypertension, alone or in combination; stroke, MI prophylaxis (>55 yr) in those unable to take ACE inhibitors

Unlabeled uses: Heart failure, proteinuria in diabetic nephropathy

Pharmacokinetics

Absorption	Unknown
Distribution	Highly protein bound
Metabolism	Liver, extensively
Excretion	Urine/feces
Half-life	Terminal 24 hr

Pharmacodynamics

Onset	3-hr
Peak	0.5-1 hr
Duration	Unknown

CONTRAINDICATIONS

Hypersensitivity

> **BLACK BOX WARNING:** Pregnancy

Precautions: Pregnancy (1st trimester), breastfeeding, children, geriatric, hypersensitivity to angiotensin-converting enzyme (ACE) inhibitors, renal/hepatic disease, renal artery stenosis, dialysis, HF, hyperkalemia, hypotension, hypovolemia, African descent

DOSAGE AND ROUTES

Adult: PO 40 mg/day; range 20-80 mg/day

Stroke, MI prophylaxis
Adult >55 yr: PO 80 mg/day

Available forms: Tabs 20, 40, 80 mg

ADVERSE EFFECTS

CNS: Dizziness, insomnia, *anxiety,* headache, fatigue, syncope
GI: *Diarrhea,* dyspepsia, *anorexia, vomiting*
META: Hyperkalemia
MS: *Myalgia, pain*
RESP: *Cough, upper respiratory tract infection,* sinusitis, pharyngitis
SYST: Angioedema

INTERACTIONS
Individual drugs
Digoxin: increased digoxin peak, trough concentrations

Drug classifications
ACE inhibitors, potassium-sparing diuretics, potassium salt substitutes: increased hyperkalemia
Antihypertensives, diuretics, NSAIDs: increased antihypertensive action
NSAIDs, salicylates: decreased antihypertensive effect

Drug/lab test
Increased: LFTs

NURSING CONSIDERATIONS
Assessment

> **BLACK BOX WARNING:** Pregnancy test: if positive, stop treatment, can cause death to fetus, do not breastfeed

- Monitor B/P, pulse q4hr; note rate, rhythm, quality; if severe hypotension occurs, place in supine position **IV** NS, usually occurs during first few weeks of treatment
- Monitor baselines in renal, electrolytes, liver function tests before therapy begins
- Assess edema in feet, legs daily
- Assess skin turgor, dryness of mucous membranes for hydration status
- **Overdose:** dizziness, bradycardia or tachycardia

Patient problem
Risk for injury (uses, adverse reactions)
Nonadherence (teaching)

Implementation
• Give without regard to meals
• Give increased dose to African American, Hispanic patients; B/P response may be reduced
• Do not remove from blister pack until ready to use

Patient/family education
• Instruct patient to comply with dosage schedule, even if feeling better
• Advise patient to notify prescriber immediately of mouth sores, fever, swelling of hands or feet, face, lips irregular heartbeat, chest pain
• Teach patient that excessive perspiration, dehydration, vomiting, diarrhea may lead to fall in blood pressure; consult prescriber if these occur
• Teach patient not to stop medication abruptly, increased B/P will occur

> **BLACK BOX WARNING:** Teach patient that product may cause dizziness, fainting; lightheadedness may occur; to avoid hazardous activities until response is known; to rise slowly from sitting to prevent drop in B/P

> **BLACK BOX WARNING:** Advise patient to use contraception while taking this product, do not use in pregnancy, breastfeeding

• Teach patient to notify prescriber of all prescriptions, OTC preparations, and supplements taken

Evaluation

Positive therapeutic outcome
• Decreased B/P

telotristat
(tel-oh'tri-stat)
Xermelo
Func. class.: Antidiarrheal
Chem. class.: Tryptophan hydroxylase inhibitor

Do not confuse: Xermelo/Xarelto

ACTION: Reduces serotonin production; this decreases stools in carcinoid syndrome

Therapeutic outcome: Decreased diarrhea without abdominal pain or severe constipation

USES: Carcinoid syndrome diarrhea; used with somatostatin analogue (SSA), when an SSA alone does not control symptoms

Pharmacokinetics

Absorption	Unknown
Distribution	99% protein binding
Metabolism	CYP3A4, P-glycoprotein (P-gp) unknown
Excretion	Urine 93.2%
Half-life	0.6 hr

Pharmacodynamics

Onset	Unknown
Peak	1/2-2 hr
Duration	Unknown

CONTRAINDICATIONS: Hypersensitivity

PRECAUTIONS: Abdominal pain, breastfeeding, constipation, GI perforation/obstruction, pregnancy

DOSAGE AND ROUTES
Adult: PO 250 mg tid

Available forms: Tablets 250 mg

ADVERSE EFFECTS
CNS: *Headache*, depression, fever
CV: Peripheral edema
GI: *Nausea*, *constipation*, flatulence, anorexia, abdominal pain

INTERACTIONS
Drug classifications
CYP3A4 substrates: monitor for ineffective results
CYP3A4 inducers: decreased effect; may need to be increased
P-glycoprotein (P-gp) products: Increased telotristat effect

Individual drugs
Octreotide: Decreased effects of telotristat give short-acting octreotide 30-60 min after telotristat

Drug/lab test
Increase: ALT/AST, alkaline phosphatase

NURSING CONSIDERATIONS
Assessment
• **Stools:** Monitor volume, color, characteristics, frequency, bowel pattern before product, rebound constipation, abdominal pain; discontinue if abdominal pain or constipation is severe
• **Pregnancy/breastfeeding:** Use only if benefits outweigh fetal risk; not studied in pregnancy; breastfeeding is not recommended, effects unknown

Patient problem
Diarrhea (uses)

T

Implementation
- With food to increase effect
- Do not double dose; if a dose is missed, give next dose as usual
- Store at room temperature

Patient/family education
- Advise patient to take with food
- Teach patient if dose is missed, do not double; take regular dose at next scheduled time
- **Pregnancy/breastfeeding:** Teach patient to contact healthcare professional if pregnancy is suspected or planned or if breastfeeding
- Advise patient to discontinue if abdominal pain or severe constipation occurs; notify healthcare professional

Evaluation
- Decreased diarrhea without abdominal pain or severe constipation

---

⚠ HIGH ALERT

temazepam (Rx)
(tem-az′a-pam)
Restoril
Func. class.: Sedative-hypnotic
Chem. class.: Benzodiazepine, short-intermediate acting
Controlled substance schedule IV (USA), schedule F (Canada)

Do not confuse: Restoril/RisperDAL

ACTION: Produces CNS depression at limbic, thalamic, hypothalamic levels of the CNS; may be mediated by neurotransmitter γ-aminobutyric acid (GABA); results are sedation, hypnosis, skeletal muscle relaxation, anticonvulsant activity, anxiolytic action

Therapeutic outcome: Decreased insomnia

USES: Insomnia (short-term treatment, generally 7-10 days)

Pharmacokinetics

Absorption	Well absorbed
Distribution	Widely distributed, crosses placenta, crosses blood-brain barrier
Metabolism	Liver
Excretion	Kidneys, breast milk
Half-life	10-20 hr

Pharmacodynamics

Onset	½ hr
Peak	1-2 hr
Duration	6-8 hr

CONTRAINDICATIONS
Pregnancy, breastfeeding, hypersensitivity to benzodiazepines

Precautions: Children <15 yr, geriatric, anemia, pulmonary/renal/hepatic disease, suicidal patients, product abuse, psychosis, acute closed-angle glaucoma, seizure disorders, angioedema, sleep-related behavior (sleep walking), COPD, dementia, myasthenia gravis, intermittent porphyria

> **BLACK BOX WARNING:** Coadministration with other CNS depressants

DOSAGE AND ROUTES
Adult: PO 7.5-30 mg at bedtime
Geriatric: PO 7.5 mg at bedtime

Available forms: Caps 7.5, 15, 22.5, 30 mg

ADVERSE EFFECTS
CNS: *Lethargy, drowsiness, daytime sedation,* dizziness, confusion, light-headedness, headache, anxiety, irritability, complex sleep-related reactions (sleep driving, sleep eating), fatigue
CV: Chest pain, pulse changes, hypotension
EENT: Blurred vision
GI: Nausea, vomiting, diarrhea, heartburn, abdominal pain, constipation, anorexia
SYST: Severe allergic reactions

INTERACTIONS
Individual drugs

> **BLACK BOX WARNING:** Alcohol: increased actions of both products

Cimetidine, disulfiram: increased effect of each specific product
Probenecid: increased effect of temazepam
Rifampin: decreased action of rifampin
Theophylline: decreased effects of theophylline

Drug classifications
Antacids: decreased effect of antacids
Contraceptives (oral): increased effect
CNS depressants: increased action of both products

Drug/herb
Chamomile, skullcap, valerian: increased CNS depression

Drug/food
Caffeine: decreased temazepam effect

Drug/lab test
Increased: AST/ALT
Decreased: radioactive iodine uptake
False increase: 17-OHCS

NURSING CONSIDERATIONS
Assessment
- Assess mental status: mood, sensorium, anxiety, affect, (baseline, periodically),

drowsiness, dizziness, especially geriatric; physical dependency, withdrawal symptoms: anxiety, panic attacks, agitation, orientation, headache, nausea, vomiting, muscle pain, weakness; indications of increasing tolerance and abuse

• **Insomnia:** Assess for characteristics of sleep, length of insomnia, baseline and periodically

• **Beers:** Avoid in older adults, increased sensitivity to benzodiazepines and decreased metabolism, may cause delirium

Patient problem
Impaired sleep (uses)
Risk for injury (adverse reactions)

Implementation
• Without regard to food
• Give with food or milk to decrease GI symptoms; if patient is unable to swallow medication whole, tab may be crushed and mixed with foods or fluids
• Give sugarless gum, hard candy, frequent sips of water for dry mouth

> **BLACK BOX WARNING:** Avoid use with CNS depressants; serious CNS depression may result

• Store in tight container in cool environment
• 15-30 min before bedtime for sleeplessness

Patient/family education
• Inform patient that product may be taken with food, and that tab may be crushed or swallowed whole
• Advise patient not to use for everyday stress or longer than 3 mo unless directed by prescriber; not to take more than prescribed amount; may be habit forming; not to double or skip doses
• Caution patient to avoid OTC preparations unless approved by prescriber; alcohol and CNS depressants will increase CNS depression, may cause dizziness, drowsiness
• Advise patient to avoid driving, activities that require alertness, drowsiness may occur; to avoid alcohol ingestion or other psychotropic medications; to rise slowly or fainting may occur, especially in geriatric; that drowsiness may worsen at beginning of treatment
• Caution patient not to discontinue medication abruptly after long-term use; withdrawal symptoms include vomiting, cramping, tremors, seizures
• Advise patient that complex sleep-related behavior may occur (sleep driving/eating/walking)
• Teach patient to limit to 7-10 days continuous use, to take as directed, not to increase dose unless approved by prescriber
• Advise patient to use contraception while taking this product, to notify prescriber if pregnancy is planned or suspected, do not use in pregnancy, cautious use in breastfeeding, excretion unknown

Evaluation
Positive therapeutic outcome
• Decreased anxiety, restlessness, sleeplessness (short-term treatment only)

TREATMENT OF OVERDOSE:
Lavage, VS, supportive care

> **A HIGH ALERT**

tenecteplase (TNK-tPA) (Rx)
(ten-ek′ta-place)
TNKase
Func. class.: Thrombolytic
Chem. class.: Tissue plasminogen activator

Do not confuse: TNKase/Activase

ACTION: Activates conversion of plasminogen to plasmin (fibrinolysin): plasmin breaks down clots (fibrin), fibrinogen, factors V, VII; occlusion of venous access lines

Therapeutic outcome: Resolution of MI

USES: Acute MI, coronary artery thrombosis

Pharmacokinetics

Absorption	Complete
Distribution	Unknown
Metabolism	Liver
Excretion	Unknown
Half-life	20-24 min

Pharmacodynamics

Onset	Immediate
Peak	Unknown
Duration	Unknown

CONTRAINDICATIONS
Hypersensitivity, arteriovenous malformation, aneurysm, active bleeding, intracranial, intraspinal surgery or trauma within 2 mo, CNS neoplasms, severe hypertension, severe renal disease, hepatic disease, history of CVA, increased ICP, stroke

Precautions: Pregnancy, breastfeeding, children, geriatric, arterial emboli from left side of heart, hypocoagulation, subacute bacterial endocarditis, rheumatic valvular disease, cerebral embolism/thrombosis/hemorrhage, intraarterial diagnostic procedure or surgery (10 days), recent major surgery, dysrhythmias, hypertension

DOSAGE AND ROUTES
Total dose, max 50 mg, based on patient's weight
Adult <60 kg: IV BOL 30 mg, give over 5 sec
Adult 60-70 kg: IV BOL 35 mg, give over 5 sec

Adult 70-80 kg: IV BOL 40 mg, give over 5 sec
Adult 80-90 kg: IV BOL 45 mg, give over 5 sec
Adult ≥90 kg: IV BOL 50 mg, give over 5 sec, max 50 mg total dose

Available forms: Powder for inj, lyophilized 50 mg

ADVERSE EFFECTS
CV: Dysrhythmias, hypotension, pulmonary edema, pulmonary embolism, cardiogenic shock, cardiac arrest, heart failure, myocardial reinfarction, myocardial rupture, tamponade, pericarditis, pericardial effusion, thrombosis, CVA
HEMA: Decreased Hct, bleeding
INTEG: Rash, urticaria, phlebitis at IV inf site, itching, flushing
SYST: GI, GU, intracranial, retroperitoneal bleeding, surface bleeding, anaphylaxis

INTERACTIONS
Individual drugs
Aspirin, cefamandole, cefoperazone, cefoTEtan, clopidogrel, dipyridamole, indomethacin, phenylbutazone, ticlopidine: increased bleeding potential

Drug classifications
Anticoagulants, antithrombolytics, glycoprotein IIb, IIIa inhibitors, NSAIDs, SNRIs, SSRIs: increased bleeding

Drug/herb
Anise, basil, dong quai, fenugreek, feverfew, garlic, ginger, ginkgo, ginseng, green tea, horse chestnut: increased risk of bleeding

Drug/lab test
Increased: INR, PT, PTT

NURSING CONSIDERATIONS
Assessment
• **Assess for allergy:** fever, rash, itching, chills; mild reaction may be treated with antihistamines
• Assess for bleeding during 1st hr of treatment; hematuria, hematemesis, bleeding from mucous membranes, epistaxis, ecchymosis; may require transfusion (rare), continue to assess for bleeding for 24 hr
• **AVM, recent surgery, active bleeding:** Assess for contraindications before use
• Monitor blood tests (Hct, platelets, PTT, protime, TT, aPTT) before starting therapy; protime or aPTT must be less than 2 × control before starting therapy; PTT or pro-time q3-4hr during treatment
• **Cholesterol embolism:** assess for blue-toe syndrome, renal failure, MI, cerebral/spinal cord/bowel/retinal infarction, hypertension; can be fatal

• **Assess for hypersensitive reactions:** fever, rash, dyspnea; product should be discontinued
• Monitor VS, B/P, pulse, respirations, neurologic signs, temp at least q4hr; temp >104° F (40° C) indicates internal bleeding; systolic pressure increase >25 mm Hg should be reported to prescriber
• Assess for neurologic changes that may indicate intracranial bleeding
• **Assess for retroperitoneal bleeding:** back pain, leg weakness, diminished pulses
• **Pregnancy/breastfeeding:** Use only if benefits outweigh fetal risk, cautious use in breastfeeding, excretion unknown

Patient problem
Ineffective tissue perfusion (uses)
Risk for injury (uses, adverse reactions)

Implementation
Intermittent IV infusion route
• Give as soon as thrombi are identified; not useful for thrombi >1 wk old
• Administer cryoprecipitate or fresh frozen plasma if bleeding occurs
• Give heparin after fibrinogen level >100 mg/dl; heparin inf to increase PTT to 1.5-2 × baseline for 3-7 days; IV heparin with loading dose is recommended
• Aseptically withdraw 10 ml of sterile water for inj from diluent vial, use red cannula syringe-filling device, inject all contents of syringe into product vial, direct into powder, swirl, withdraw correct dose, discard any unused sol; stand the shield with dose vertically on flat surface and passively recap the red cannula; remove entire shield assembly by twisting counterclockwise; give by IV bol
• IV therapy: use upper extremity vessel that is accessible to manual compression
• Provide bed rest during entire course of treatment
• Avoid venous or arterial puncture, inj, rectal temp, any invasive treatment
• Treat fever with acetaminophen or aspirin
• Apply pressure for 30 sec to minor bleeding sites; inform prescriber if this does not attain hemostasis; apply pressure dressing

Patient/family education
• Teach patient to notify prescriber immediately of severe headache
• Advise patient to notify prescriber of bleeding, hypersensitivity, fast, slow, or uneven heart rate, feeling of fainting, blood in urine/stools, nose bleeds
• Teach patient about proper dental care to avoid bleeding

Evaluation

Positive therapeutic outcome
• Resolution of myocardial infarction

tenofovir (Rx)
(ten-oh-foh'veer)
Viread
Func. class.: Antiretroviral
Chem. class.: Nucleoside reverse transcriptase inhibitor (NRTI)

ACTION: Inhibits replication of HIV-1 virus by competing with the natural substrate and then incorporating into cellular DNA by viral reverse transcriptase, thereby terminating cellular DNA chain

Therapeutic outcome: Improved symptoms of HIV-1 infection

USES: HIV-1 infection with at least 2 other antiretrovirals, hepatitis B

Pharmacokinetics

Absorption	Rapidly absorbed
Distribution	Extravascular space; bound to serum plasma <0.7%, to serum proteins <7.2%
Metabolism	Unknown
Excretion	Urine, unchanged (70%-80%)
Half-life	Terminal 17 hr

Pharmacodynamics

Onset	Unknown
Peak	1-2 hr
Duration	Unknown

CONTRAINDICATIONS
Hypersensitivity

BLACK BOX WARNING: Lactic acidosis

Precautions: Pregnancy, breastfeeding, children, geriatric, renal disease, hepatic insufficiency, CCr <60 ml/min, osteoporosis, immune reconstitution syndrome

BLACK BOX WARNING: Hepatic disease, hepatitis

DOSAGE AND ROUTES
HIV infection in combination with other antiretroviral agents
Adult, adolescent, and child ≥ 35 kg: PO tablet: 300 mg PO once daily; PO oral powder 300 mg (7.5 scoops) qday with 2-4 oz of soft food
Child and adolescent weighing 28-34 kg: PO tablet: 250 mg qday
Child ≥ 2 yr and older and 22-27 kg: PO tablet 200 mg qday

Child ≥ 2 yr and 17-21 kg: PO tablet 150 mg qday
Child and adolescent ≥ 2 yr and < 35 kg: PO oral powder 8 mg/kg/dose qday with 2-4 oz of soft food. Round dose to the nearest 20-mg increment

Renal dose
Adult: PO CCr 30-49 ml/min 300 mg q48hr; CCr 10-29 ml/min 300 mg q72-96hr; CCr <10 ml/min not recommended
Child ≥2 yr: PO 8 mg/kg/day approximate; ≥35 kg 300 mg/day; 28-34 kg 250 mg/day; 22-27 kg 200 mg/day; 17-21 kg 150 mg/day

Available forms: Tabs 150, 200, 250, 300 mg; oral powder 40 mg/scoop

ADVERSE EFFECTS
CNS: *Headache,* asthenia
GI: *Nausea, vomiting, diarrhea,* anorexia, *flatulence, abdominal pain,* pancreatitis
GU: Renal failure, renal tubular acidosis/necrosis, Fanconi syndrome
HEMA: Neutropenia, osteopenia
INTEG: *Rash,* angioedema
META: Lactic acidosis, hypokalemia, hypophosphatemia
MS: Arthralgia, myalgia, decreased bone mineral density
SYST: Lipodystrophy

INTERACTIONS
Individual drugs
Acyclovir, cidofovir, ganciclovir, valacyclovir, valganciclovir: increased level of tenofovir
Didanosine: increased level of didanosine when coadministered with tenofovir

Drug classifications
Increased: levels of tenofovir with any product that decreases renal function

NURSING CONSIDERATIONS
Assessment
• Monitor viral load, CD4+ T cell count, plasma HIV RNA, serum creatinine/BUN/phosphate

BLACK BOX WARNING: Hepatitis exacerbations: Monitor resistance testing at start of therapy and at treatment failure, after treatment assess for exacerbations for 6 mo after last dose

• Assess liver function tests: AST, ALT, bilirubin; amylase, lipase, triglycerides baseline, periodically during treatment
• **Assess for bone, renal toxicity:** if bone abnormalities are suspected, obtain tests: serum phosphorus, creatinine, creatinine clearance, urine glucose

T

BLACK BOX WARNING: Lactic acidosis, severe hepatomegaly with steatosis: Obtain baseline LFTs, if elevated discontinue treatment; discontinue even if LFTs are normal but lactic acidosis, hepatomegaly are present, may be fatal

- **Pregnancy/breastfeeding:** Use only if clearly needed, register pregnant patient in the Antiretroviral Pregnancy Registry 800-258-4263, do not breastfeed

Patient problem
Infection (uses)
Risk for injury (adverse reactions)

Implementation
- Administer PO without regard to meals
- Store at 25° C (77° F)
- **Oral powder:** use scoop provided, mix powder into 2-4 oz (¼-½ cup) of applesauce or yogurt, do not mix with liquid, product will not mix; product is bitter; use immediately after mixing, clean scoop

Patient/family education
- Instruct patient to take product with meal
- Advise patients that GI complaints resolve after 3-4 wk of treatment
- Caution patient not to breastfeed while taking this product
- Teach patient to discuss wth provider OTC, Rx, herbals, supplements
- Inform patient that product must be taken daily even if patient feels better
- Advise patient to continue follow-up visits since serious toxicity may occur; blood counts must be done q2wk
- Inform patient that product controls symptoms but is not a cure for HIV; patient is still infectious, may pass HIV virus on to others
- Advise patient that other products may be necessary to prevent other infections
- Advise patient that changes in body fat distribution may occur usually breast, neck, back

BLACK BOX WARNING: Lactic acidosis: teach patient symptoms of lactic acidosis, to notify prescriber (nausea, vomiting, weakness, abdominal pain)

- **Hepatotoxicity:** Teach patient to notify provider of yellow skin, eyes, dark urine, clay-colored stools, nausea, abdominal pain

Evaluation

Positive therapeutic outcome
- Decrease in signs/symptoms of HIV

terazosin (Rx)
(ter-ay′zoe-sin)
Hytrin ✦
Func. class.: Antihypertensive
Chem. class.: α-Adrenergic blocker (peripherally acting)

ACTION: Peripheral blood vessels are dilated, peripheral resistance is lowered; reduction in blood pressure results from α-adrenergic receptors being blocked

Therapeutic outcome: Decreased B/P in hypertension, decreased symptoms of benign prostatic hyperplasia (BPH)

USES: Hypertension, as a single agent or in combination with diuretics or β-blockers, BPH

Pharmacokinetics
Absorption	Well absorbed
Distribution	Not known
Metabolism	Liver (50%)
Excretion	Kidneys unchanged (10%), feces unchanged (20%)
Half-life	9-12 hr

Pharmacodynamics
Onset	15 min
Peak	2-3 hr
Duration	24 hr

CONTRAINDICATIONS
Hypersensitivity

Precautions: Pregnancy, breastfeeding, children, prostate cancer, renal disease, syncope

DOSAGE AND ROUTES
Hypertension
Adult: PO 1 mg at bedtime, may increase dosage slowly to desired response; max 20 mg/day divided q12hr

Benign prostatic hyperplasia
Adult: PO 1 mg at bedtime, gradually increase up to 5-10 mg, max 20 mg divided q12hr

Available forms: Caps 1, 2, 5, 10 mg

ADVERSE EFFECTS
CNS: *Dizziness, headache, drowsiness,* anxiety, depression, vertigo, weakness, fatigue, syncope
CV: *Palpitations, orthostatic hypotension,* tachycardia, *edema,* rebound hypertension
EENT: Blurred vision, epistaxis, tinnitus, dry mouth, red sclera, nasal congestion, sinusitis
GI: *Nausea,* vomiting, diarrhea, constipation, abdominal pain

GU: Urinary frequency, incontinence, impotence, priapism
RESP: Dyspnea, cough, pharyngitis

INTERACTIONS
Individual drugs
Alcohol, nitroglycerin, verapamil: increased hypotensive effects, not to drink alcohol

Drug classifications
Antihypertensives (other): increased hypotension
β-Blockers: increased hypotensive effects
Estrogens, NSAIDs, salicylates, sympathomimetics: decreased antihypertensive effect

Drug/herb
Hawthorn: increased antihypertensive effect
Ephedra: decreased antihypertensive effect

NURSING CONSIDERATIONS
Assessment
• **Hypertension:** monitor B/P, orthostatic hypotension, syncope; check for edema in feet, legs daily; I&O ratio; weight daily; notify prescriber of changes
• **Benign prostatic hyperplasia (BPH):** assess urinary patterns (hesitancy, frequency, change in stream, dribbling, dysuria, urgency)
• **Pregnancy/breastfeeding:** Use only if benefits outweigh fetal risk, cautious use in breastfeeding, excretion unknown
• **Beers:** Avoid use in older adults as an antihypertensive, high risk of orthostatic hypotension

Patient problem
Risk for injury (uses, adverse reactions)
Nonadherence (teaching)

Implementation
• May be used in combination with other antihypertensives
• Give at same time each day
• May be given with food to prevent GI symptoms
• Store in airtight container at 86° F (30° C) or less
• If treatment is interrupted for several days, restart with initial dose
• Give without regard to food
• Feeding tube: place cap in 60 ml of warm tap water, stir until liquid spills from ruptured shell (5 min), stir until cap dissolves, draw solution into oral syringe, give through feeding tube, flush with water

Patient/family education
• Caution patient not to discontinue product abruptly; the importance of complying with dosage schedule, even if feeling better; if dose is missed take as soon as remembered; take medication at same time each day

• Teach patient not to use OTC products (cough, cold, allergy) unless directed by prescriber; to avoid large amounts of caffeine
• Emphasize the need to rise slowly to sitting or standing position to minimize orthostatic hypotension
• Teach patient to notify prescriber of mouth sores, sore throat, fever, swelling of hands or feet, irregular heartbeat, chest pain
• Caution patient to report excessive perspiration, dehydration, vomiting, diarrhea; may lead to fall in B/P
• Caution patient that product may cause dizziness, fainting, light-headedness; may occur during 1st few days of therapy; to avoid hazardous activities
• **Hypertension:** teach patient how to take B/P and normal readings for age group; to take B/P q7day; to continue with regimen including diet and exercise

Evaluation

Positive therapeutic outcome
• Decreased B/P in hypertension
• Decreased symptoms of BPH

TREATMENT OF OVERDOSE:
Administer volume expanders or vasopressors; discontinue product; place patient in supine position

terbinafine, oral (Rx)
(ter-bin′a-feen)
LamISIL, Lamisil AT
Func. class.: Antifungal, systemic
Chem. class.: Synthetic allylamine derivative

Do not confuse: LamISIL/LaMICtal/lamoTRIgine

ACTION: Interferes with cell membrane permeability in fungi such as *Trichophyton rubrum, Trichophyton mentagrophytes, Trichophyton tonsurans, Epidermophyton floccosum, Microsporum canis, Microsporum audouinii, Microsporum gypseum, Candida,* broad-spectrum antifungal

Therapeutic outcome: Resolution of fungal infection

USES: Onychomycosis of the toenail or fingernail due to dermatophytes, tinea capitis/corporis/cruris/pedis/versicolor

Pharmacokinetics

Pharmacokinetics	
Absorption	80%
Distribution	Extensive, most to hair, scalp, nails; excreted in breast milk; protein binding 99%
Metabolism	Liver, extensively
Excretion	Unknown
Half-life	22 days or longer

Pharmacodynamics	
Onset	Up to 1 wk
Peak	Several days-weeks
Duration	Several weeks

CONTRAINDICATIONS
Hypersensitivity

Precautions: Pregnancy, breastfeeding, children, chronic/active renal/hepatic disease GFR ≤50 mg/min, immunosuppression

DOSAGE AND ROUTES
Adult: PO 250 mg/day × 6 wk (fingernail); × 12 wk (toenail)

Available forms: Tabs 250 mg; oral granules 125, 187.5 mg

ADVERSE EFFECTS
CNS: Depression
EENT: Tinnitus, hearing impairment
GI: Diarrhea, dyspepsia, abdominal pain, nausea, hepatitis
HEMA: Neutropenia
INTEG: Rash, pruritus, urticaria, Stevens-Johnson syndrome, photosensitivity
MISC: Headache, hepatic enzyme changes, taste, visual/olfactory disturbance

INTERACTIONS
Individual drugs
Atomoxetine: decreased metabolism of atomoxetine
Cimetidine: increased effect
CycloSPORINE: increased cycloSPORINE clearance
Dextromethorphan: increased levels
Rifampin: increased terbinafine clearance

Drug/herb
Cola nut, guarana, yerba maté, tea (black, green), coffee: side effects

Drug/lab test
Increased: LFTs

NURSING CONSIDERATIONS
Assessment
• Assess hepatic studies (ALT, AST) before beginning treatment; do not use in presence of hepatic disease
• Monitor CBC in treatment >6 wk
• Assess for continuing infection
• **Pregnancy/breastfeeding:** Use only if benefits outweigh fetal risk, avoid during pregnancy, breastfeeding

Patient problem
Infection (uses)

Implementation
• **PO:** give without regard to food
• **Granules:** take with food, sprinkle packet contents on pudding or non-acidic soft food, swallow without chewing, do not use fruit-based foods
• Store at 25° C (77° F), protect from light

Patient/family education
• Teach patient to notify prescriber of nausea, vomiting, fatigue, jaundice, dark urine, clay-colored stool, RUQ pain, that may indicate hepatic dysfunction
• Teach patient to avoid using OTC medication unless approved by prescriber
• Teach patient that treatment may take 12 wk (toenail), 6 wk (fingernail)
• Teach patient to take without regard to meals, granules may be sprinkled on soft food but not chewed, do not mix with fruit-based products
• Advise patient to report vision changes immediately

Evaluation

Positive therapeutic outcome
• Decrease in size, number of lesions

terbinafine topical
See Appendix B

terbutaline (Rx)
(ter-byoo'ta-leen)
Func. class.: Selective β_2-agonist; bronchodilator
Chem. class.: Catecholamine

Do not confuse: Brethine/Methergine

ACTION: Relaxes bronchial smooth muscle by direct action on β_2-adrenergic receptors through accumulation of cyclic AMP at β-adrenergic receptor sites; results are bronchodilatation, diuresis, and CNS and cardiac stimulation; relaxes uterine smooth muscle

Therapeutic outcome: Bronchodilation with ease of breathing

USES: Bronchospasm

Unlabeled uses: Premature labor

Pharmacokinetics

Absorption	Well absorbed (SUBCUT), partially absorbed (PO)
Distribution	Unknown
Metabolism	Liver, partially
Excretion	Unknown
Half-life	PO 3-4 hr, subcut 5-7 hr

Pharmacodynamics

	PO	INH	SUB-CUT	IV
Onset	½ hr	5-15 min	10-15 min	Rapid
Peak	1-2 hr	1-2 hr	½-1 hr	Unknown
Duration	4-8 hr	4-6 hr	1½-4 hr	Unknown

CONTRAINDICATIONS

Hypersensitivity to sympathomimetics; closed-angle glaucoma, tachydysrhythmias

Precautions: Pregnancy, breastfeeding, geriatric, cardiac disorders, hyperthyroidism, diabetes mellitus, prostatic hypertension, hypertension, seizure disorder

> **BLACK BOX WARNING:** Labor

DOSAGE AND ROUTES
Bronchospasm

Adult and child >12 yr: PO 2.5-5 mg q8hr; SUBCUT 0.25 mg q15-30min, max 0.5 mg in 4 hr
Adolescent ≤15 yr and child ≥12 yr: PO 2.5 mg tid, max 7.5 mg/day

Renal dose
Adult: PO CCr 10-50 ml/min 50% of dose; CCr <10 ml/min avoid use

Severe renal failure
Adult: PO avoid if GFR <10 ml/min

Tocolytic (preterm labor) (unlabeled)
Adult: SUBCUT 0.25 mg q20min to 6 hr, hold if pulse >120 bpm

Available forms: Tabs 2.5, 5 mg; inj 1 mg/ml

ADVERSE EFFECTS
CNS: Tremors, anxiety, insomnia, headache, dizziness, stimulation

CV: Palpitations, tachycardia, hypertension, dysrhythmias, cardiac arrest, QT prolongation
GI: Nausea, vomiting
META: Hypokalemia, hyperglycemia
RESP: Paradoxical bronchospasm, dyspnea

INTERACTIONS
Individual drugs
Arsenic trioxide, chloroquine, droperidol, haloperidol, levomethadyl, pentamidine: increased QT prolongation

Drug classifications
Beta agonists, class IA/III antidysrhythmics, CYP3A4 inhibitors (amiodarone, clarithromycin, erythromycin, telithromycin, troleandomycin), CYP3A4 substrates (methadone, pimozide, QUEtiapine, quiNIDine, risperiDONE, ziprasidone), local anesthetics, some phenothiazines, tricyclics: increased QT prolongation
β-Adrenergic blockers: do not use together, block therapeutic effect
MAOIs: increased chance of hypertensive crisis
Sympathomimetics: increased effects of both products

Drug/herb
Green tea (large amounts), guarana: increased effect

NURSING CONSIDERATIONS
Assessment
• **Monitor respiratory function:** vital capacity, FEV, ABGs, lung sounds, heart rate, rhythm (baseline)
• Determine that patient has not received theophylline therapy before giving dose; assess client's ability to self-medicate
• Monitor for evidence of allergic reactions; withhold dose and notify prescriber
• **Assess for paradoxical bronchospasm:** dyspnea, wheezing; keep emergency resuscitative equipment nearby

> **BLACK BOX WARNING: Assess for labor:** maternal heart rate, B/P, contractions, fetal heart rate; can inhibit uterine contractions, labor; monitor for hypoglycemia, do not use injectable product for prevention or treatment over 72 hr in preterm labor; do not use oral product for preterm labor, avoid in breastfeeding

Patient problem
Ineffective airway clearance (uses)
Impaired breathing (uses)

Implementation
• Use this medication before other medications and allow 5 min between each to prevent overstimulation
PO route
• Give PO with meals to decrease gastric irritation; tab may be crushed and mixed with food or fluid
SUBCUT route
• May give by SUBCUT route; do not give by IM route
Aerosol route
• Give after shaking; ask patient to exhale, place mouthpiece in mouth, then inhale slowly; hold breath, remove, exhale slowly; allow at least 1 min between inhalations
• Store in light-resistant container, do not expose to temperatures over 86° F (30° C)

IV route
• Give at 5 mcg q10min until contractions are stopped; use inf pump for correct dose; after ½-1 hr with no contraction decrease dose by 5 mcg; switch to PO dose when possible

Y-site compatibilities: Regular insulin

Patient/family education
• Advise patient not to use OTC medications; extra stimulation may occur; to use this medication before other medications and allow at least 5 min between each to prevent overstimulation
• Teach patient how to use inhaler; to avoid getting aerosol in eyes because blurring may result; to wash inhaler in warm water daily and dry; to avoid smoking, smoke-filled rooms, persons with respiratory infections; review package insert with patient
• Teach patient that paradoxical bronchospasm may occur; to stop product immediately and notify prescriber; to limit caffeine products such as chocolate, coffee, tea, and colas
• Instruct patient on administration of dose, not to use more than prescribed; serious side effects may occur; if taking PO regularly and dose is missed, take when remembered; space other doses on new time schedule

Evaluation

Positive therapeutic outcome
• Absence of dyspnea, wheezing after 1 hr
• Improved airway exchange
• Improved ABGs

TREATMENT OF OVERDOSE:
Administer a β_2-adrenergic blocker

---

terconazole vaginal antifungal
See Appendix B

teriflunomide
(ter'i-floo'noe-mide)
Aubagio
Func. class.: Multiple sclerosis agent
Chem. class.: Pyrimidine synthesis inhibitor

ACTION: Antiproliferative effects including peripheral T- and B-lymphocytes, might reduce inflammatory demyelination

Therapeutic outcome: Decreased symptoms of MS

USES: Reduction of the frequency of relapses or remitting MS

Pharmacokinetics
Absorption	Unknown
Distribution	Protein binding >99%
Metabolism	Unknown
Excretion	Unknown
Half-life	Median 18–19 days

Pharmacodynamics
Onset	Unknown
Peak	1-4 hr
Duration	Unknown

CONTRAINDICATIONS
Hypersensitivity

BLACK BOX WARNING: Pregnancy

Precautions: Breastfeeding, alcoholism, diabetes mellitus, eosinophilic pneumonia, hepatitis, jaundice, male-mediated teratogenicity, pneumonitis, pulmonary disease/fibrosis, sarcoidosis, TB, vaccination

BLACK BOX WARNING: Hepatic disease, contraception requirements, male medicated teratogenicity

DOSAGE AND ROUTES
Adult: **PO** 7 or 14 mg/day

Available forms: Tabs 7, 14 mg

ADVERSE EFFECTS
CNS: Anxiety, headache
CV: Palpitations, hypertension, MI
EENT: Blurred vision, conjunctivitis, sinusitis

GI: Nausea, vomiting, diarrhea, cystitis, hepatotoxicity
HEMA: Leukopenia, lymphopenia, neutropenia
INTEG: Acne vulgaris, alopecia, pruritus
META: Weight loss
MISC: Infection, cystitis, Stevens-Johnson syndrome

INTERACTIONS
Individual drugs
Do not use with leflunomide
CycloSPORINE, eltrombopag, gefitinib: increased teriflunomide effect

> **BLACK BOX WARNING:** Methotrexate: increased hepatotoxicity

Zidovudine: increased hematologic toxicity
Repaglinide, pioglitazone, rosiglitazone, PACLitaxel, naproxen, topotecan, bosentan, furosemide: increased effect of each agent
Warfarin, alosetron, DULoxetine, theophylline, tiZANidine, quiNINE, tamoxifen, bendamustine, rasagiline, rOPINIRole, selegiline, propafenone, mexiletine, lidocaine, anagrelide, cloZAPine, cinacalcet, caffeine: decreased effect of each agent, monitor closely
Cholestyramine: decreased effect of teriflunomide

Drug classifications
Do not use with live virus vaccines
HMG-CoA reductase inhibitors: Increase: hepatotoxicity
Oral contraceptives: increased effect of oral contraceptives

NURSING CONSIDERATIONS
Assessment
• CNS symptoms: assess for anxiety, confusion, vertigo
• GI status: assess for diarrhea, vomiting, abdominal pain
• Cardiac status: assess for tachycardia, palpitations, vasodilation, chest pain
• **Stevens-Johnson syndrome, toxic epidermal necrolysis:** Assess for fever, blisters, aches, fatigue; if these occur, stop product immediately
• **Hepatotoxicity:** Monitor LFTs after 6 mo or less of treatment and q mo after start of treatment; do not use if ALT >2x ULN, discontinue if >3x ULN; monitor bilirubin
• **Blood dycriasis:** Monitor CBC, platelets 6 mo prior to use and periodically, monitor for infection, monitor INR

• Advise patient that hair may be lost, to use a hair piece or wig

> **BLACK BOX WARNING: Pregnancy/breastfeeding:** Do not start treatment until pregnancy is ruled out, this product should not be used during or for 2 yr after discontinuing this product, those wishing to become pregnant must discontinue this product and undergo an accelerated elimination procedure, with verification of teriflunomide plasma level <0.02 mg/L, do not use in pregnancy, breastfeeding

Patient problem
Impaired mobility (uses)
Risk for injury (adverse reactions)

Implementation
PO route
May be taken without regard to food

Patient/family education
• Teach patient that blurred vision can occur

> **BLACK BOX WARNING:** Advise patient to notify prescriber if pregnancy is planned or suspected

• Inform patient not to change dosing or stop taking without advice of prescriber
• Teach patient to take as directed, provide "Medication Guide"
• Teach patient to notify provider of nausea, vomiting, loss of appetite, dark urine, yellow eyes or skin
• Advise patient not to receive any live virus vaccines during treatment

Evaluation
Positive therapeutic outcome
• Decreased symptoms of MS

tesamorelin
(tes-a-moe-rel′in)
Egrifta
Func. class.: Pituitary hormone, growth hormone modifiers

ACTION: Binds to growth hormone releasing factor receptors on the pituitary somatotroph cells; binding stimulates the production, release of endogenous growth hormone (GH)

Therapeutic outcome: Decreasing lipodystrophy in HIV patients

USES: Treatment of excess abdominal fat in HIV-infected patients with lipodystrophy

Pharmacokinetics

Absorption	Unknown
Distribution	Unknown
Metabolism	Unknown
Excretion	Unknown
Half-life	26 and 38 mins in healthy and HIV-infected patients, respectively, peak 0.15 hrs

Pharmacodynamics

Onset	Unknown
Peak	0.15 hrs
Duration	Unknown

CONTRAINDICATIONS

Hypersensitivity to this product or mannitol, neoplastic disease, pregnancy, disruption of the hypothalamic-pituitary axis (hypothalamic-pituitary-adrenal [HPA] suppression) resulting from hypophysectomy, hypopituitarism, pituitary tumor/surgery, radiation therapy of the head, head trauma, IV/IM administration

Precautions: Breastfeeding, CABG, diabetes, diabetic retinopathy, edema, geriatrics, children, infants, adolescents

DOSAGE AND ROUTES

Adult: SUBCUT 2 mg/day

Available forms: Powder for injection 1 mg

ADVERSE EFFECTS

CNS: Depression, flushing, headache, hypoesthesia, insomnia, night sweats, peripheral neuropathy paresthesias
CV: Peripheral edema
GI: Diarrhea, dyspepsia, nausea, upper abdominal pain, vomiting, constipation
INTEG: Flushing, injection site reactions, pruritus, rash, urticaria
MS: Arthralgia, carpal tunnel syndrome, joint swelling, myalgias, stiffness
RESP: *Upper respiratory tract infection*
SYST: Secondary malignancy
META: Hypercalcemia, hyperuricemia

INTERACTIONS
Individual drugs

Cortisone, predniSONE, simvastatin, ritonavir: decreased effect of each specific product

NURSING CONSIDERATIONS
Assessment

• **Lipodystrophy:** Assess for sunken cheeks; thinning arms and legs; fat accumulation in the abdomen, jaws, and back of neck; after treatment these should lessen

• Monitor glycosylated hemoglobin A1C (HbA1C), serum IGF-1 concentrations, ophthalmologic exam
• Assess for edema, joint pains, carpal tunnel syndrome; therapy may need to be discontinued
• **Pregnancy/breastfeeding:** Do not use in pregnancy, breastfeeding
• Teach patient that lab exams will be needed
• **Beers:** Avoid in older adults except as hormone replacement after pituitary gland removal, may cause edema, arthralgia

Patient problem
Lack of knowledge of medication (teaching)

Implementation
SUBCUT route

• Visually inspect parenteral products for particulate matter and discoloration before use whenever solution and container permit
• To reconstitute use 2, 1-mg vials, inject 2.1 ml sterile water for injection into the first 1-mg vial; use the syringe with the needle already attached. To avoid foaming, push the plunger in slowly with the needle at a slight angle, keep the vial upright and gently roll the vial for 30 sec until mixed; do not shake; remove all contents and put in next 1-mg vial, roll; withdraw 2.1 ml of the reconstituted solution
• Take the syringe out of the vial, place the needle cap on its side against a clean, flat surface; do not touch needle; hold syringe and slide the needle into cap; push the cap all the way or until it snaps shut; do not touch cap until it covers the needle completely
• Remove needle and insert a ½″ 27-G safety injection needle onto the syringe; use immediately; throw away any unused product or used sterile water for injection
• Solution should be clear; do not use if discolored, cloudy, or has particles, but slight foaming is acceptable
• Inject subcut into abdomen; avoid scar tissues, bruises, or the navel; rotate injection sites in the abdomen; slowly push plunger down until all solution has been injected
• After removing the injection from the skin, flip back the needle shield until it snaps, covering the injection needle completely; keep pressing until you hear a click
• Use a piece of sterile gauze to rub the injection site clean; if there is bleeding, apply pressure to the injection site with gauze for 30 seconds
• Properly dispose of used equipment

Patient/family education
• Explain reason for product and expected result

- **Hypersensitivity:** Teach patient to report rash, swelling of face, trouble breathing immediately
- **Fluid retention:** Teach patient to report edema, joint pains
- Advise patient on correct use and how to prepare injection
- Teach patient to use contraception (pregnancy)

Evaluation

Positive therapeutic outcome
- Decreasing lipodystrophy in HIV patients

testosterone (Rx)
(tess-toss′te-rone)
testosterone enanthate (Rx)
Delatestryl
testosterone undecanoate
Aveed
testosterone cypionate (Rx)
Depo-Testosterone
testosterone pellets (Rx)
Testopel
testosterone transdermal (Rx)
Androderm
testosterone gel (Rx)
AndroGel, Fortesta, Testim, Vogel XO
testosterone buccal (Rx)
Striant
testosterone nasal gel (Rx)
Natesto

Func. class.: Androgenic anabolic steroid
Chem. class.: Halogenated testosterone derivative
Controlled substance schedule III

Do not confuse: Testoderm/Testoderm TTS

ACTION: Increases weight by building body tissue; increases potassium, phosphorus, chloride, nitrogen levels; increases bone development; responsible for maintenance of secondary sex characteristics (male)

Therapeutic outcome: Increased hormone levels in eunuchoidism, decreased tumor growth in female breast cancer, onset of male puberty

USES: Female breast cancer, hypogonadism, eunuchoidism, male climacteric, oligospermia, impotence, vulvar dystrophies, low testosterone levels, delayed male puberty (inj)

Pharmacokinetics

Absorption	Well but slowly absorbed
Distribution	Crosses placenta
Metabolism	Liver
Excretion	Kidneys, breast milk
Half-life	8 days (cypionate)
	10-100 min (base)

Pharmacodynamics

	IM (base)	IM (cypionate)	IM (enanthate)	IM (propionate)
Onset	Unknown	Unknown	Unknown	Unknown
Peak	Unknown	Unknown	Unknown	Unknown
Duration	1-3 days	2-4 wk	2-4 wk	1-3 days

CONTRAINDICATIONS
Pregnancy, breastfeeding, severe renal/cardiac/hepatic disease, hypersensitivity, genital bleeding (rare), male breast/prostate cancer

Precautions: Diabetes mellitus, CV disease, MI, urinary tract disorders, prostate cancer, hypercalcemia

> **BLACK BOX WARNING:** Children, accidental exposure, pulmonary oil microembolism, risk of serious hypersensitivity reactions or anaphylaxis

DOSAGE AND ROUTES
Replacement
Adult: IM (enanthate or cypionate) 50-400 mg q2-4wk; **TRANSDERMAL** (Testoderm) 4-6 mg applied q24hr; (Androderm, AndroGel) 5 mg applied q24hr; once daily (gel); **TOPICAL SOL** (Axiron) 60 mg (2 pump activations) each AM; **BUCCAL** 1 buccal system (30 mg) to the gum region q12hr before meals/PM
Adult (male) and child: SUBCUT (pellets) 150-450 mg (2-6 pellets) inserted q3-6mo

Breast cancer
Adult: IM 50-100 mg 3×/wk (propionate) or 200-400 mg q2-4wk (cypionate or enanthate)

Delayed male puberty
Child >12 yr: IM up to 100 mg/mo for up to 6 mo

Available forms: Enanthate: inj 200 mg/ml; **cypionate:** inj 100, 200 mg/ml; pellets 75 mg; **transdermal** 2, 4 mg/24 hr; **gel** 1%, 1.62%, 10 mg/actuation; **buccal system** 30 mg; **topical solution** 30 mg/actuation

ADVERSE EFFECTS

CNS: Dizziness, headache, fatigue, tremors, paresthesias, flushing, sweating, anxiety, lability, insomnia, carpal tunnel syndrome

CV: Increased B/P

EENT: Conjunctival edema, nasal congestion

ENDO: Abnormal GTT

GI: Nausea, vomiting, constipation, weight gain, cholestatic jaundice

GU: Hematuria, amenorrhea, vaginitis, decreased libido, decreased breast size, clitoral hypertrophy, testicular atrophy, gynecomastia, enlarged prostate

HEMA: Polycythemia

INTEG: Rash, acneiform lesions, oily hair and skin, flushing, sweating, acne vulgaris, alopecia, hirsutism

MS: Cramps, spasms

INTERACTIONS
Individual drugs
ACTH, buPROPion: increased edema

Insulin: decreased glucose levels may alter need for insulin

Oxyphenbutazone: increased effects of oxyphenbutazone

Drug classifications
Adrenal steroids: increased edema

Anticoagulants: increased pro-time

Antidiabetics, oral: decreased need for oral antidiabetics

Drug/lab test
Increased: serum cholesterol, blood glucose, urine glucose

Decreased: serum Ca, serum K, T_4, T_3, thyroid ^{131}I uptake test, urine 17-OHCS, 17-KS, PBI

NURSING CONSIDERATIONS
Assessment
• Monitor patient's weight daily; notify prescriber if weekly weight gain is >5 lb; assess I&O ratio; be alert for decreasing urinary output, increasing edema

• Monitor B/P q4hr, Hgb/Hct

• Assess growth rate, bone age in adolescent because growth rate may be uneven (linear/bone growth) if used for extended periods

• Monitor electrolytes: potassium, sodium, chloride, calcium; cholesterol

• Monitor liver function tests: ALT, AST, bilirubin

• Assess edema, hypertension, cardiac symptoms, jaundice

• Assess mental status: affect, mood, behavioral changes, aggression

• **Assess signs of masculinization** in female: increased libido, deepening of voice, decreased breast tissue, enlarged clitoris, menstrual irregularities; male: gynecomastia, impotence, testicular atrophy

• **Assess hypercalcemia:** lethargy, polyuria, polydipsia, nausea, vomiting, constipation; product may have to be decreased

• **Assess hypoglycemia** in diabetics because oral antidiabetic action is increased

---

BLACK BOX WARNING: Accidental exposure: In children have occurred with the topical product after contact with application site in adults, cover site in adult, cover site with clothing, wash hands with soap and water

---

BLACK BOX WARNING: Anaphylaxis: Usually with testosterone undecanoate (Aveed) oil for injection, may occur after any injection, observe for 30 min after each use, product is contraindicated in those with castor oil, benzyl/alcohol, benzoic acid hypersensitivity

---

BLACK BOX WARNING: Pulmonary embolism: Occurs immediately after 1000 mg IM of testosterone undecanoate, symptoms include cough, dyspnea, chest pain, dizziness, throat tightening and resolve after a few minutes or with supportive measure, some require emergency measures

---

• **Beers:** Avoid in older adults unless indicated for confirmed hypogonadism with clinical symptoms, potential for cardiac problems, do not use in prostate cancer

• **Pregnancy/breastfeeding:** Do not use in pregnancy, breastfeeding

Patient problem
Impaired sexual functioning (uses)

Risk for injury (adverse reactions)

Implementation
• Administer diet with increased calories, protein; decreased sodium if edema occurs

• Administer supportive product if anemia occurs

• Give titrated dose; use lowest effective dose

• Give IM inj deep into upper outer quadrant of gluteal muscle; route can be painful

Transdermal route

• Apply Testoderm to skin of scrotum, Androderm to skin of back, upper arms, thighs, abdomen; area must be clean and dry, free of hair

Gel route

• Products are not interchangeable, dosage and administration for AndroGel 1% differs from AndroGel 1.62%

• Apply daily to clean dry area on shoulders, upper arms, or abdomen; women, children should not touch gel or treated skin

---

Buccal system route
- Do not chew or swallow buccal system
- Rotate sites; place above incisor tooth on either side of mouth
- Open packet; place rounded side of surface against gum and hold firmly in place with finger over lip for 30 sec; if product falls off, replace with new system; discard in trash can away from children or pets

Topical solution
- Using the provided applicator, apply the solution to clean, dry, intact skin of the axilla, preferably at the same time each morning. Do not apply to any other part of the body. Allow the solution to dry completely before dressing. If an antiperspirant or deodorant is used, apply at least 2 min before applying the solution. The pump must be primed before the first use by fully depressing the pump mechanism 3 times and discarding any solution that is released during the priming. To dispense the solution, position the nozzle over the applicator cup and carefully depress the pump once fully; the cup should be filled with no more than 1 pump actuation (30 mg). With the applicator upright, place it up into the axilla and wipe steadily down and up into the axilla. Do not use fingers or hand to rub the solution. If multiple applications are necessary for the required dose, alternate application between the left and right axilla. When repeat application to the same axilla is necessary, allow the solution to dry completely before the next application. After use, rinse the applicator under running water and pat dry with tissue. Wash hands with soap and water
- Following application, allow the site to dry a few minutes before putting on clothing
- Direct contact of the medicated skin with the skin of another person can result in the transfer of residual testosterone and absorption by the other person. To reduce accidental transfer, the patient should cover the application site(s) with clothing after the solution has dried. The application site should be washed with soap and water prior to any skin-to-skin contact regardless of the length of time since application. In the case of direct contact, the other person should wash the area of contact with soap and water as soon as possible
- Do not use near fire, flame, and smoking; flammable
- Advise patients to avoid swimming or washing the application site until 2 hr following application

Patient/family education
- Inform patient that product needs to be combined with complete health plan: diet, rest, exercise

- Caution patient to notify prescriber if therapeutic response decreases; not to discontinue this medication abruptly
- Inform women patients to report menstrual irregularities; about changes in sex characteristics, if pregnancy is planned or suspected
- Discuss that 1-3 mo course is necessary for response in breast cancer
- Teach about changes in sex characteristics: priapism, gynecomastia, increased libido
- **Nasal:** Teach patient to report nasal bleeding, irritation, pain
- **Topical:** Teach patient to avoid contact with area that has been treated, to wash area before contact
- **Buccal:** Teach patient how to administer buccal tab to gum
- **Transdermal:** Advise patient to notify provider of viralization in females; inform patient about application of transdermal patches: Testoderm to skin of scrotum; Androderm to skin of back, upper arms, thighs, abdomen; area must be dry and free of hair; may be reapplied after bathing, swimming

Evaluation

Positive therapeutic outcome
- Decrease size of tumor in breast cancer
- Increased androgen levels

tetracaine ophthalmic
See Appendix B

tetracaine topical
See Appendix B

tetracycline (Rx)
(tet-ra-sye′kleen)
Func. class.: Antiinfective—broad-spectrum
Chem. class.: Tetracycline

ACTION: Inhibits protein synthesis and phosphorylation in microorganisms; bacteriostatic

Therapeutic outcome: Bactericidal action against susceptible organisms: gram-positive pathogens *Bacillus anthracis, Clostridium perfringens, Clostridium tetani, Listeria monocytogenes, Nocardia, Propionibacterium acnes, Actinomyces israelii;* gram-negative pathogens *Haemophilus influenzae, Legionella pneumophila, Yersinia enterocolitica, Yersinia pestis, Neisseria gonorrhoeae, Neisseria meningitidis*

USES: Syphilis, *Chlamydia trachomatis,* gonorrhea, lymphogranuloma venereum, uncommon gram-positive, gram-negative organisms, rickettsial infections

Absorption	60%-80% (PO), lower (IM)
Distribution	Widely distributed, some in CSF; crosses placenta
Metabolism	Not metabolized
Excretion	Unchanged—kidneys
Half-life	6-10 hr

Pharmacodynamics

Onset	1-2 hr
Peak	2-3 hr
Duration	Unknown

CONTRAINDICATIONS
Pregnancy, breastfeeding, children <8 yr, hypersensitivity to tetracyclines

Precautions: Renal/hepatic disease, UV exposure

DOSAGE AND ROUTES
Susceptible gram-positive/gram-negative infections
Adult: PO 250-500 mg q6hr
Child >8 yr: PO 25-50 mg/kg/day in divided doses q6hr

Chlamydia trachomatis
Adult: PO 500 mg qid × 7 days

Syphilis
Adult and adolescent: PO 500 mg qid × 2 wk; if syphilis duration >1 yr, must treat 30 days

Brucellosis
Adult: PO 500 mg qid × 3 wk with 1 g of streptomycin IM 2 ×/day × 1 wk, and 1 ×/day the 2nd wk

Urethral, endocervical, rectal infections (C. trachomatis)
Adult: PO 500 mg qid × 7 days

Acne
Adult and adolescent: PO 250 mg q6hr, then 125-500 mg/day or every other day

Renal dose
Adult: PO CCr 51-90 ml/min give dose q8-12hr, CCr 10-50 ml/min give dose q12-24hr, CCr <10 ml/min give dose q24hr

Available forms: Caps 250, 500 mg

ADVERSE EFFECTS
CNS: Fever, headache, paresthesia
CV: Pericarditis
EENT: Dysphagia, glossitis, decreased calcification (permanent discoloration) of deciduous teeth, oral candidiasis, oral ulcers
GI: *Nausea,* abdominal pain, *vomiting, diarrhea,* anorexia, enterocolitis, hepatotoxicity, flatulence, abdominal cramps, epigastric burning, stomatitis, hepatitis, CDAD
GU: *Increased BUN,* azotemia, acute renal failure
HEMA: Eosinophilia, neutropenia, thrombocytopenia, leukocytosis, hemolytic anemia
INTEG: *Rash, urticaria, photosensitivity, increased pigmentation,* exfoliative dermatitis, pruritus, angioedema, Stevens-Johnson syndrome
MISC: Increased intracranial pressure, candidiasis

INTERACTIONS
Individual drugs
Cimetidine, NaHCO$_3$: decreased tetracycline effect
Digoxin: increased digoxin effect
Iron: forms chelates, decreased absorption
Isotretinoin: Increase: Pseudotumor cerebi, avoid concurrent use
Methoxyflurane: fatal nephrotoxicity, do not use together
Warfarin: increased warfarin effect

Drug classifications
Alkali products, antacids: decreased tetracycline effect
Hormonal contraception: Decrease: possible, but unlikely, use additional contraception
Penicillins: decreased penicillin effect

Drug/herb
Dong quai: increased photosensitivity

Drug/food
Decreased: absorption with dairy products; forms insoluble chelate

Drug/lab test
Increased: BUN, LFTs

NURSING CONSIDERATIONS
Assessment
• **Serious skin reactions:** angioedema, Stevens-Johnson syndrome, exfoliative dermatitis, report immediately after stopping product
• Assess patient for previous sensitivity reaction
• Assess patient for signs and symptoms of infection including characteristics of wounds, sputum, urine, stool, WBC >10,000/mm^3, temp; obtain baseline information before, during treatment
• Complete C&S testing before beginning product therapy to identify if correct treatment has been initiated, therapy may start before results are received

• **Assess for allergic reactions:** rash, urticaria, pruritus, chills, fever, joint pain; angioedema may occur a few days after therapy begins; EPINEPHrine, resuscitation equipment should be available for anaphylactic reaction

• Identify urine output; if decreasing, notify prescriber (may indicate nephrotoxicity); increased BUN, creatinine

• **CDAD:** assess for diarrhea, abdominal pain, fever, fatigue, anorexia; possible anemia, elevated WBC and low serum albumin; stop product and usually give either vancomycin or IV metroNIDAZOLE

• **Assess for superinfection:** perineal itching, fever, malaise, redness, pain, swelling, drainage, rash, diarrhea, change in cough, sputum if on prolonged therapy

• **Pregnancy/breastfeeding:** Do not use in pregnancy, toxic to fetus, do not breastfeed, excreted in breast milk

Patient problem

Infection (uses)
Diarrhea (adverse reactions)

Implementation
PO route

• Give around the clock to maintain proper blood levels; give with food to increase absorption of product; do not give within 3 hr of other agents; product interactions may occur; take on an empty stomach (1 hr before or 2 hr after meals)

• Give with 8 oz of water

• Shake liquid preparation well before giving; use calibrated device for proper dosing

• Store in tight, light-resistant container at room temp

Patient/family education

• Teach patient to report sore throat, bruising, bleeding, joint pain; may indicate blood dyscrasias (rare)

• Advise patient to use sunscreen when outdoors to decrease photosensitivity reaction

• Advise patient to contact prescriber if vaginal itching, loose foul-smelling stools, furry tongue occur; may indicate superinfection; report itching, rash, pruritus, urticaria

• Teach patient to take 1 hr before bedtime to prevent esophageal ulceration

• Instruct patient to take all medication prescribed for the length of time ordered; product must be taken around the clock to maintain blood levels; do not give medication to others

• Teach patient to notify prescriber immediately of diarrhea with pus, mucus, fever, abdominal pain

• Teach patient not to use outdated products, as Fanconi syndrome (nephrotoxicity) may occur

• Teach patient that tooth discoloration may occur, especially in children, do not use in child <8 yr, may cause bone formation abnormalities

• Teach patient to notify prescriber if pregnancy is planned or suspected

Evaluation

Positive therapeutic outcome

• Absence of signs/symptoms of infection (WBC <10,000/mm³; temp WNL; absence of red, draining wounds)

• Reported improvement in symptoms of infection, resolution of infection, prevention of malaria

tetrahydrozoline nasal agent
See Appendix B

tetrahydrozoline ophthalmic
See Appendix B

thiamine (vitamin B₁) (PO, OTC; IV, IM, Rx)
Betaxin ✦, Betalin S, Biamine, Revitonus, Thiamilate
Func. class.: Vitamin B₁
Chem. class.: Water soluble

Do not confuse: thiamine/Tenormin

ACTION: Needed for pyruvate metabolism, carbohydrate metabolism

Therapeutic outcome: Prevention and treatment of thiamine deficiency

USES: Vit B₁ deficiency or polyneuritis, cheilosis adjunct with thiamine beriberi, Wernicke-Korsakoff syndrome, pellagra, metabolic disorders, alcoholism

Pharmacokinetics

Absorption	Well absorbed (PO, IM), completely absorbed (IV)
Distribution	Widely distributed
Metabolism	Liver
Excretion	Kidneys (unchanged—excess amounts)
Half-life	Unknown

Pharmacodynamics

Unknown

CONTRAINDICATIONS
Hypersensitivity

Precautions: Pregnancy

DOSAGE AND ROUTES
RDA
Adult: PO (Male) 1.2-1.5 mg; (female) 1.1 mg; (pregnancy) 1.4 mg; (breastfeeding) 1.4 mg
Child 9-13 yr: PO 0.9 mg
Child 4-8 yr: PO 0.6 mg
Child 1-3 yr: PO 0.5 mg
Infant 6 mo-1 yr: PO 0.3 mg
Neonate and infant to 6 mo: PO 0.3 mg

Beriberi
Adult: PO 5-30 mg qd or given in 3 divided doses × 1 month; IM/IV 5-30 mg qd or in 3 doses, then convert to PO
Child/infant: PO 10-50 mg qd × 2 wk, then 5-10 mg qd × 1 mo; IV/IM 10-25 mg/day × 2 wk, then 5-10 mg qd × 1 mo

Wernicke-Korsakoff syndrome
Adult: IV 100 mg, then 50-100 mg IM q day

Available forms: Tabs 50, 100, 250, 500 mg; inj 100 mg/ml; enteric-coated tabs 20 mg

ADVERSE EFFECTS
CNS: Weakness, restlessness
CV: Collapse, pulmonary edema, hypotension
EENT: Tightness of throat
GI: Hemorrhage, *nausea*, *diarrhea*
INTEG: Angioneurotic edema, cyanosis, sweating, warmth
SYST: Anaphylaxis

NURSING CONSIDERATIONS
Assessment
• **Anaphylaxis (IV only):** assess for swelling of face, eyes, lips, throat, wheezing
• **Thiamine deficiency:** assess for anorexia, weakness, pain, depression, confusion, blurred vision, tachycardia
• Assess nutritional status: yeast, beef, liver, whole or enriched grains, legumes
• Application of cold to help decrease pain at injection site
• **Pregnancy/breastfeeding:** Considered compatible with pregnancy, breastfeeding

Patient problem
Impaired nutritional intake (uses)

Implementation
IM route
• Give by IM inj; rotate sites if pain and inflammation occur; do not mix with alkaline sol; Z-track to minimize pain
• Application of cold compress may decrease pain
• Store in airtight, light-resistant container

Direct IV route
• **IV** undiluted given over 5 min
Continuous IV infusion route
• Dilute in compatible **IV** sol

Y-site compatibilities: Famotidine

Patient/family education
• Teach patient necessary foods to be included in diet: yeast, beef, liver, legumes, whole grains

Evaluation
Positive therapeutic outcome
• Absence of nausea, vomiting, anorexia, insomnia, tachycardia, paresthesias, depression, muscle weakness

tiaGABine (Rx)
(tie-ah-ga′been)
Gabitril
Func. class.: Anticonvulsant

Do not confuse: tiaGABine/tiZANidine

ACTION: Inhibits reuptake and metabolism of GABA; may increase seizure threshold, structurally similar to GABA; tiaGABine binding sites in neocortex, hippocampus

USES: Adjunct treatment of partial seizures in adults and children ≥12 yr

Pharmacokinetics
Absorption	>95%
Distribution	Protein binding 96%
Metabolism	Liver
Excretion	Kidneys
Half-life	7-9 hr

Pharmacodynamics
Onset	Unknown
Peak	45 min
Duration	Unknown

CONTRAINDICATIONS
Hypersensitivity

Precautions: Pregnancy, breastfeeding, child <12 yr, geriatric, renal/hepatic disease, suicidal ideation/behavior, status epilepticus, mania, bipolar disorder, abrupt discontinuation, depression

DOSAGE AND ROUTES
When not given with a CYP3A4 enzyme, effect of tiaGABine is doubled; lower dosages are indicated
Adult: PO (those on an enzyme-inducing antiepileptic) 4 mg/day in divided doses, may increase by 4-8 mg qwk until desired response, max 56 mg/day

Child 12-18 yr: PO 4 mg/day, may increase by 4 mg at beginning of wk 2, may increase by 4-8 mg qwk until desired response, max 32 mg/day

Hepatic dose
Adult: PO reduce dose or increase dosing interval

Available forms: Tabs 2, 4, 12, 16 mg

ADVERSE EFFECTS
CNS: *Dizziness, anxiety,* somnolence, ataxia, confusion, *asthenia,* unsteady gait, depression, suicidal ideation, seizures, tremor, hostility, EEG changes, insomnia
CV: Vasodilatation, tachycardia, hypertension
ENDO: Goiter, hypothyroidism
GI: Nausea, diarrhea, vomiting, increased appetite
INTEG: Pruritus, rash, Stevens-Johnson syndrome, alopecia, hyperhidrosis
MS: Myalgia
RESP: Pharyngitis, coughing

INTERACTIONS
Individual drugs
CarBAMazepine, PHENobarbital, phenytoin, primidone: decreased effect of these products
Sevelamer: decreased tiagabine effect
Valproate: lower dose of tiaGABine may be required

Drug classifications
Alcohol, CNS depressants: increased CNS depression

Drug/food
High-fat meal: decreased rate of absorption

NURSING CONSIDERATIONS
Assessment
• Assess description of seizures: location, duration, presence of aura; assess for weakness
• Monitor renal function tests: urinalysis, BUN, urine creatinine q3mo
• Monitor liver function tests: ALT, AST, bilirubin
• Withdraw gradually to prevent seizures
• May cause status epilepticus and unexplained death
• **Assess mental status:** mood, sensorium, affect, behavioral changes, suicidal thoughts; if mental status changes, notify prescriber, increased affect and hypomania may be present
• **Beers:** Avoid in older adults, unless safer alternatives are not available, may cause ataxia, impaired psychomotor function

Patient problem
Risk for injury (uses, adverse reactions)
Suicidal ideation (adverse reactions)

Implementation
• Store at room temperature away from heat and light
• Provide assistance with ambulation during early part of treatment; dizziness occurs
• Provide seizure precautions: padded side rails; move objects that may harm patient
• Use with food

Patient/family education
• Advise patient to carry/wear emergency ID stating patient's name, products taken, condition, prescriber's name and phone number
• Advise patient to avoid driving, other activities that require alertness, until response is known
• Teach patient not to discontinue medication quickly after long-term use
• Teach patient to report suicidal thoughts, behaviors immediately
• Teach patient to notify prescriber if pregnancy is planned or suspected; avoid breastfeeding

Evaluation
Positive therapeutic outcome
• Decreased seizure activity; document on patient's chart

⚠ HIGH ALERT
ticagrelor
(tye-ka′gre-lor)
Brilinta
Func. class.: Platelet inhibitor
Chem. class.: ADP receptor antagonist

Do not confuse: Brilinta/Brintellix

ACTION: Reversibly binds to the platelet receptor, preventing platelet activation

Therapeutic outcome: Prevention of thromboembolism

USES: Arterial thromboembolism prophylaxis in acute coronary syndrome (ACS) (unstable angina, acute MI), including in patients undergoing percutaneous coronary intervention (PCI)

Pharmacokinetics
Absorption	36%
Distribution	Protein binding >99%
Metabolism	By CYP3A4
Excretion	26% (urine)
Half-life	7 hr; 9 hr metabolite

Pharmacodynamics

Onset	Unknown
Peak	1.5 hr (product), 2.5 hr (metabolite)
Duration	≥8 hr

CONTRAINDICATIONS
Hypersensitivity, severe hepatic disease, bleeding

Precautions: Abrupt discontinuation, breast-feeding, children, infants, neonates, GI bleeding, hepatic disease, pregnancy

> **BLACK BOX WARNING:** Bleeding, intracranial bleeding

> **BLACK BOX WARNING:** Coronary artery bypass graft (CABG) surgery, abrupt discontinuation, aspirin coadministration

DOSAGE AND ROUTES
Adult: PO Loading dose 180 mg with aspirin (usually 325 mg PO); then, give 90 mg bid with aspirin 75-100 mg/day, do not give **maintenance doses** of aspirin >100 mg/day

Available forms: Tab 60, 90 mg

ADVERSE EFFECTS
CNS: Dizziness, fatigue, headache
CV: Atrial fibrillation, bradyarrhythmias, chest pain, hypertension, hypotension, syncope, ventricular pauses
GI: Diarrhea, nausea
HEMA: Fatal bleeding
MISC: Back pain, gynecomastia, hyperuricemia
RESP: Cough, dyspnea

INTERACTIONS
Individual drugs
Simvastatin, lovastatin: increased effect
Digoxin: change in effect

Drug classifications

> **BLACK BOX WARNING:** Anticoagulants, NSAIDs, platelet inhibitors: increased bleeding risk

CYP3A4 inducers (carBAMazepine, dexamethasone, PHENobarbital, phenytoin, rifampin): decreased ticagrelor action

> **BLACK BOX WARNING:** CYP3A4 inhibitors (atazanavir, clarithromycin, dalfopristin, delavirdine, indinavir, isoniazid, itraconazole, ketoconazole, lopinavir, nefazodone, nelfinavir, quinupristin, ritonavir, saquinavir, telithromycin, tipranavir, voriconazole): increased bleeding risk

Drug/lab
Serum creatinine: increased

NURSING CONSIDERATIONS
Assessment
• **Thromboembolism:** Monitor CBC differential with platelet count baseline and periodically during treatment

> **BLACK BOX WARNING:** Assess for **bleeding** that may occur when aspirin is combined with this product, some bleeding can be fatal, usually aspirin doses >100 mg/day; watch for frank bleeding, hypotension, avoid use with active bleeding, history of intracranial bleeding

> **BLACK BOX WARNING: CABG:** Do not use in those undergoing CABG; discontinue ≥5 days before surgery

> **BLACK BOX WARNING: Abrupt discontinuation:** Do not discontinue abruptly, may increase risk for MI, stent thrombosis, death

> **BLACK BOX WARNING: Aspirin coadministration:** Use with 75-100 mg of aspirin/day, avoid higher doses, ticagrelor efficiency is decreased with aspirin >100 mg/day

• **Pregnancy/breastfeeding:** Use only if benefits outweigh fetal risk, may be fetal toxic, do not breastfeed, excretion unknown

Patient problem
Risk for injury (uses, adverse reactions)

Implementation
PO route
• May be taken without regard to food
• Store at room temperature, in original container in dry place
• Discontinue 5-7 days before surgery
• May be crushed (90-mg tab) and mixed with purified water, 100 ml (PO), 50 ml (NG); ensure entire dose is given by flushing mortar, syringe, NG tube with 2 additional 50 ml of water

Patient/family education
• Teach patient to take only as prescribed, do not skip or double doses, if a dose is missed, take next dose at scheduled time

> **BLACK BOX WARNING:** Advise patient to notify prescriber of chills, fever, bruising, bleeding; not to use aspirin ≥100 mg/day

• Teach patient not to use any Rx, OTC products, herbs without approval of prescriber; products with aspirin, NSAIDs may cause bleeding
• Instruct patient to notify all health care providers of product use
• Advise patient that product can be taken without regard to meals

---

⚠ Nurse Alert   ✴ Key NCLEX® Drug   ≫ Drug Specifics

- Teach patient it may take longer for bleeding to stop

BLACK BOX WARNING: Advise patient to notify prescriber if pregnancy is planned or suspected; not to breastfeed

Evaluation
Positive therapeutic outcome
- Prevention of thromboembolism

tigecycline (Rx)
(tye-ge-sye′kleen)
Tygacil
Func. class.: Broad-spectrum antiinfective
Chem. class.: Glycylcyclines

ACTION: Inhibits protein synthesis and phosphorylation in microorganisms; bacteriostatic, structurally similar to the tetracyclines

Therapeutic outcome: Resolution of infection

USES: Complicated skin/skin structure infections: *Escherichia coli, Enterococcus faecalis* (vancomycin-susceptible only), *Staphylococcus aureus, Streptococcus agalactiae, S. anginosus* group, *S. pyogenes, Bacteroides fragilis;* complicated intraabdominal infections *(Citrobacter freundii), Enterobacter cloacae, Escherichia coli, Klebsiella oxytoca, K. pneumoniae, E. faecalis* (vancomycin-susceptible only), *S. aureus* (methicillin-susceptible only), *S. anginosus* group, *B. fragilis, Bacteroides thetaiotaomicron, B. uniformis, B. vulgatus, Clostridium perfringens, Peptostreptococcus micros,* community-acquired pneumonia

Pharmacokinetics

Absorption	Unknown
Distribution	Protein binding 71%-89%
Metabolism	Not extensively
Excretion	22% unchanged, urine; primarily biliarily excreted
Half-life	Terminal 42 hr

Pharmacodynamics
Unknown

CONTRAINDICATIONS
Pregnancy, breastfeeding, children <18 yr, hypersensitivity to tigecycline

Precautions: Renal/hepatic disease, hypersensitivity to tetracyclines, ventricular-associated hospital-acquired pneumonias

BLACK BOX WARNING: Infection

DOSAGE AND ROUTES
Adult: IV 100 mg, then 50 mg q12hr, IV INF is given over 30 min to 60 min q12hr; given for 5-14 days depending on infection

Hepatic dose (Child-Pugh C)
Adult: IV 100 mg, then 25 mg q12hr

Available forms: Powder for inj, lyophilized 50 mg

ADVERSE EFFECTS
CNS: Headache, dizziness, insomnia
CV: Hypo/hypertension, phlebitis
EENT: Tooth discoloration
GI: *Nausea, vomiting, diarrhea,* anorexia, constipation, dyspepsia, hepatotoxicity, hepatic failure, CDAD
HEMA: Anemia, leukocytosis, thrombocytopenia
INTEG: *Rash,* pruritus, sweating, photosensitivity
META: Increased ALT, AST, BUN, lactic acid, alkaline phosphatase, amylase, hyperglycemia, hypokalemia, hypoproteinemia, bilirubinemia
MISC: Back pain, fever, abnormal healing, abdominal pain, abscess, asthenia, infection, pain, peripheral edema, local reactions
RESP: Cough, dyspnea
SYST: Anaphylaxis

INTERACTIONS
Individual drugs
Warfarin: increased effect of tigecycline

Drug classifications
Oral contraceptives: decreased effect of tigecycline

Drug/lab test
Increased: amylase, LFTs, alk phos, BUN, creatinine, LDH, WBC, INR, PTT, PT
Decreased: potassium, calcium, sodium, Hgb/Hct, platelets

NURSING CONSIDERATIONS
Assessment

BLACK BOX WARNING: Increased mortality risk: Use only with confirmed or strongly suspected bacterial infection; do not use as a prophylactic

- **CDAD:** assess for diarrhea, abdominal pain, fever, fatigue, anorexia; possible anemia, elevated WBC, low serum albumin; stop product and usually give either vancomycin or IV metroNIDAZOLE
- Assess for signs of anemia: Hct, Hgb, fatigue
- Monitor blood tests: PT, CBC, AST, ALT, BUN creatinine
- **Assess for allergic reactions:** rash, itching, pruritus, angioedema, serious allergic skin

T

reactions: assess for Stevens-Johnson syndrome, anaphylaxis
• Assess for nausea, vomiting, diarrhea; administer antiemetic, antacids as ordered
• **Assess for overgrowth of infection:** fever, malaise, redness, pain, swelling, drainage, perineal itching, diarrhea, changes in cough or sputum
• **Toxicity:** assess for pseudotumor cerebri, photosensitivity, anti-anabolic actions (azotemia, BUN, hypophosphatemia, metabolic acidosis): tigecycline is structurally similar to tetracycline
• **Assess for pancreatitis, hyperamylasemia:** may be fatal; if these occur, discontinue; improvement usually occurs after product is discontinued
• **Pregnancy/breastfeeding:** Do not use in pregnancy, breastfeeding, may cause fetal harm

Patient problem
Infection (uses)
Diarrhea (adverse reactions)

Implementation
• Tigecycline allergy test before using, obtain C&S, do not begin treatment before results

Intermittent IV infusion route
• Reconstitute each vial with 5.3 ml of 0.9% NaCl, or D₅W (10 mg/ml); swirl to dissolve; immediately withdraw 5 ml of the reconstituted sol and add to a 100-ml **IV** bag for inf (1 mg/ml); may be yellow or orange, if not, sol should be discarded; do not give if particulate matter is present, use a dedicated IV line or Y-site, flush with NS before and after use, give over ½ hr
• Store in tight, light-resistant container at room temperature, diluted sol at room temp for up to 24 hr, 6 hr in vial, and remaining time in IV bag, 48 hr refrigerated

Y-site compatibilities: Acyclovir, alfentanil, allopurinol, amifostine, amikacin, aminocaproic acid, aminophylline, amphotericin B liposome, ampicillin, ampicillin/sulbactam, argatroban, azithromycin, aztreonam, bivalirudin, bumetanide, buprenorphine, butorphanol, calcium chloride/gluconate, CARBOplatin, carmustine, caspofungin, ceFAZolin, cefepime, cefotaxime, cefoTEtan, cefOXitin, cefTAZidime, ceftizoxime, cefTRIAXone, cefuroxime, cimetidine, ciprofloxacin, cisatracurium, CISplatin, clindamycin, cyclophosphamide, cycloSPORINE, cytarabine, dacarbazine, DACTINomycin, DAPTOmycin, DAUNOrubicin hydrochloride, dexamethasone, dexmedetomidine, dexrazoxane, digoxin, diltiazem, diphenhydrAMINE, DOBUTamine, DOCEtaxel, dolasetron, DOPamine, doripenem, DOXOrubicin hydrochloride, DOXOrubicin liposome, droperidol, enalaprilat, EPINEPHrine, eptifibatide, ertapenem, erythromycin, esmolol, etoposide, etoposide phosphate, famotidine, fenoldopam, fentaNYL, fluconazole, fludarabine, fluorouracil, foscarnet, fosphenytoin, furosemide, ganciclovir, gemcitabine, gentamicin, glycopyrrolate, granisetron, haloperidol, heparin, hydrocortisone, HYDROmorphone, ifosfamide, imipenem/cilastatin, insulin, irinotecan, isoproterenol, ketorolac, labetalol, lansoprazole, lepirudin, leucovorin, levofloxacin, lidocaine, linezolid, LORazepam, magnesium sulfate, mannitol, mechlorethamine, melphalan, meperidine, meropenem, mesna, methohexital, methotrexate, methyldopa, metoclopramide, metoprolol, metroNIDAZOLE, midazolam, milrinone, mitoMYcin, mitoXANtrone, morphine, moxifloxacin, mycophenolate, nafcillin, nalbuphine, naloxone, nesiritide, nitroglycerin, nitroprusside, norepinephrine, octreotide, ondansetron, oxaliplatin, oxytocin, PACLitaxel, palonosetron, pamidronate, pancuronium, pantoprazole, PEMEtrexed, pentamidine, pentazocine, PENTobarbital, PHENobarbital, phenylephrine, piperacillin/tazobactam, potassium acetate/chloride/phosphate, procainamide, prochlorperazine, promethazine, propofol, propranolol, ranitidine, remifentanil, rocuronium, sodium acetate/bicarbonate/phosphate, streptozocin, succinylcholine, SUFentanil, tacrolimus, teniposide, theophylline, thiopental, thiotepa, ticarcillin/clavulanate, tirofiban, tobramycin, topotecan, trimethoprim/sulfamethoxazole, vancomycin, vasopressin, vecuronium, vinBLAStine, vinCRIStine, vinorelbine, zidovudine, zoledronic acid

Patient/family education
• Teach patient to avoid sun exposure; sunscreen does not seem to decrease photosensitivity
• Teach patient to avoid pregnancy while taking this product; fetal harm may occur; to avoid breastfeeding
• Teach patient to report burning, pain at inj site
• Teach patient to report diarrhea, fatigue, abdominal pain, severe nausea, vomiting

Evaluation

Positive therapeutic outcome
• Decreased temp, absence of lesions, negative C&S

timolol ophthalmic
See Appendix B

tioconazole vaginal antifungal
See Appendix B

tiotropium (Rx)

(ty-oh′tro-pee-um)

Spiriva Handihaler Spiriva Respimat

Func. class.: Anticholinergic, bronchodilator

Chem. class.: Synthetic quaternary ammonium compound

Do not confuse: Spiriva/Inspra/Apidra

ACTION: Inhibits interaction of acetylcholine at receptor sites on the bronchial smooth muscle, resulting in decreased cGMP and bronchodilatation

Therapeutic outcome: Improved breathing

USES: COPD, for long-term treatment, once daily maintenance of bronchospasm, associated with COPD including chronic bronchitis and emphysema

Pharmacokinetics

Absorption	Unknown
Distribution	Does not cross blood-brain barrier
Metabolism	Very little metabolized in the liver
Excretion	Excreted in urine, 72% protein binding
Half-life	5-6 days in animals

Pharmacodynamics

Unknown

CONTRAINDICATIONS

Hypersensitivity to this product, atropine, or its derivatives

Precautions: Pregnancy, breastfeeding, children, geriatric, closed-angle glaucoma, prostatic hypertrophy, bladder neck obstruction, renal disease

DOSAGE AND ROUTES

Adult: INH content of 1 cap/day (18 mcg) using HandiHaler inhalation device or 2 inh (spray) (2.5 mcg each) qday

Available forms: Powder for inhalation 18 mcg in blister packs containing 6 caps with inhaler; 30 caps with inhaler; spray inhaler (Respimat) 2.5 mcg/spray

ADVERSE EFFECTS

CNS: Depression, paresthesia

CV: Chest pain, increased heart rate

EENT: Dry mouth, blurred vision, glaucoma

GI: *Vomiting,* abdominal pain, constipation, dyspepsia

GU: Urinary difficulty, urinary retention, UTI

INTEG: Rash, angioedema

MISC: Candidiasis, flulike syndrome, herpes zoster, infections, angina pectoris

MS: Arthritis, myalgic leg/skeletal pain

RESP: *Cough, worsening of symptoms,* sinusitis, URI, epistaxis, pharyngitis

INTERACTIONS

Drug classifications

Anticholinergics: avoid use with other anticholinergics

Drug/lab test

Increased: cholesterol, glucose

NURSING CONSIDERATIONS

Assessment

• **Respiratory status:** assess for dyspnea, rate, breath sounds before and during treatment; pulmonary function tests baseline and periodically; upper respiratory infection, cough, sinusitis

• Assess for tolerance over long-term therapy; dose may have to be increased or changed

• **Pregnancy/breastfeeding:** Use only if benefits outweigh fetal risk, cautious use in breastfeeding, unlikely to cause harm in the infant

Patient problem

Ineffective airway clearance (uses)

Impaired breathing (uses)

Implementation

Inhalation route

• Caps are for INH only; do not swallow

• Immediately before administration, peel back foil until cap is visible (until "stop" line); open dust cap of HandiHaler by pulling upward, then open mouthpiece

• Place cap in center chamber; firmly close mouthpiece until it clicks, leaving dust cap open

• Hold HandiHaler with mouthpiece upward; press button in once, completely, and release; this allows medication to be released

• Breathe out completely; do not breathe into mouthpiece at any time

• Raise device to mouth and close lips tightly around mouthpiece

• With head upright, breathe in slowly/deeply, but allowing the cap to vibrate; breathe until lungs fill; hold breath and remove mouthpiece; resume normal breathing

• Repeat

• Remove used capsule and discard; close the mouthpiece and dust cap; store

Inhalation route (spray)

• Insert cartridge into inhaler; prime inhaler; must reprime once if not used for >3 days; if

T

not used for >21 days, prime until aerosol is visible and 3 more times

Patient/family education
- Teach patient how to use HandiHaler
- Teach patient signs of closed-angle glaucoma (eye pain, blurred vision, visual halos)
- Advise patient that product is used for long-term maintenance, not for immediate relief of breathing problems
- Caution patient to avoid getting the powder in the eyes; may cause blurred vision and pupil dilatation
- Teach patient to hold hand/haler with mouthpiece upward; to press button in once, completely; and release; this allows for medication to be released
- Teach patient to breathe out completely; not to breathe into mouthpiece at any time
- Teach patient to raise device to mouth and close lips tightly around mouthpiece
- Teach patient to rinse mouth after use; to use hard candy or regular oral hygiene to reduce dry mouth
- With head upright, to breathe in slowly and deeply, but allow the cap to vibrate; to breathe until the lungs fill; to hold breath and remove mouthpiece; to resume normal breathing
- Teach patient to report immediately blurred vision, eye pain, halos
- Teach patient to keep caps in sealed blisters before use, store at room temperature

Evaluation

Positive therapeutic outcome
- Ability to breathe easier

⚠ HIGH ALERT

tirofiban (Rx)
(tie-roh-fee′ban)
Aggrastat
Func. class.: Antiplatelet
Chem. class.: Glycoprotein IIb/IIIa inhibitor

Do not confuse: Aggrastat/argatroban

ACTION: Antagonist of platelet glycoprotein (GP) IIb/IIIa receptor that leads to binding of fibrinogen and von Willebrand's factor, which inhibits platelet aggregation

Therapeutic outcome: Decreased platelet count

USES: Acute coronary syndrome in combination with heparin

Pharmacokinetics

Absorption	Unknown
Distribution	Plasma clearance 20%-25%
Metabolism	Liver
Excretion	Urine/feces
Half-life	2 hr

Pharmacodynamics
Unknown

CONTRAINDICATIONS
Hypersensitivity, active internal bleeding, stroke, major surgery, severe trauma within 30 days, intracranial neoplasm, aneurysm, hemorrhage, acute pericarditis, platelets <100,000/mm^3, history of thrombocytopenia, coagulopathy, systolic B/P >180 mm Hg or diastolic B/P >110 mm Hg

Precautions: Pregnancy, breastfeeding, children, geriatric, renal disease, bleeding tendencies, hypertension, platelets <150,000/mm^3

DOSAGE AND ROUTES
Adult: IV 25 mcg/kg within 5 min, then 0.15 mcg/kg/min for up to 18 hr

Renal dose
Adult: IV CCr <60 ml/min 25 mcg/kg, then 0.075 mcg/kg/min

Available forms: Inj 50-ml vials; inj premixed bag 50 mcg/ml in 100, 250 ml

ADVERSE EFFECTS
CNS: Dizziness, headache
CV: Bradycardia, hypotension
GI: Nausea, vomiting
HEMA: Bleeding, thrombocytopenia
INTEG: *Rash*
MISC: Dissection, edema, pain in legs/pelvis, sweating
SYST: Anaphylaxis

INTERACTIONS
Individual drugs
Abciximab, aspirin, cefamandole, cefoperazone, cefoTEtan, clopidogrel, dipyridamole, eptifibatide, heparin, ticlopidine, valproic acid: increased bleeding risk

Drug classifications
Heparins, NSAIDs, SNRIs, SSRIs, thrombin inhibitors: increased bleeding risk
Increase: Tirofiban clearance: levothyroxine, omeprazole

Drug/lab
Decrease: Platelets, Hct, Hgb

NURSING CONSIDERATIONS
Assessment
• **Bleeding:** Monitor platelet counts, Hct, Hgb before treatment, within 6 hr of loading dose and at least daily thereafter; watch for bleeding from puncture sites, catheters, or in stools, urine
• Assess for contraindications to therapy; recent major surgery, active bleeding trauma within 30 days
• **Pregnancy/breastfeeding:** Do not use unless clearly needed, do not breastfeed, excretion unknown

Patient problem
Ineffective tissue perfusion (uses)
Risk for injury (uses, adverse reactions)

Implementation
Intermittent IV infusion route
• Discontinue no less than 2-4 hrs before CABG
• Dilute inj: withdraw and discard 100 ml from a 500-ml bag of sterile 0.9% NaCl or D_5 and replace this vol with 100 ml of tirofiban inj from two vials
• Tirofiban inj for sol is premixed in containers of 500 ml 0.9% NaCl (50 mg/ml), give over 30 min
• Minimize other arterial/venous punctures, IM inj, catheter use, intubation to reduce bleeding risks
• Do not use if particulates are present
• Discard unused solution after 24 hr from start of infusion

Y-site compatibilities: Acyclovir, alfentanil, allopurinol, amifostine, amikacin, aminocaproic acid, aminophylline, amiodarone, ampicillin, ampicillin/sulbactam, anidulafungin, argatroban, arsenic trioxide, atracurium, atropine, azithromycin, aztreonam, bivalirudin, bleomycin, bumetanide, buprenorphine, butorphanol, calcium chloride/gluconate, capreomycin, CARBOplatin, carmustine, caspofungin, ceFAZolin, cefepime, cefotaxime, cefoTEtan, cefOXitin, cefTAZidime, ceftizoxime, cefTRIAXone, cefuroxime, chloramphenicol, chlorproMAZINE, cimetidine, ciprofloxacin, cisatracurium, CISplatin, clindamycin, cyclophosphamide, cycloSPORINE, cytarabine, DACTINomycin, DAPTOmycin, dexamethasone, dexmedetomidine, dexrazoxane, digoxin, diltiazem, diphenhydrAMINE, DOBUTamine, DOCEtaxel, dolasetron, DOPamine, doxacurium, DOXOrubicin, DOXOrubicin liposome, doxycycline, droperidol, enalaprilat, ePHEDrine, EPINEPHrine, epirubicin, eptifibatide, ertapenem, erythromycin, esmolol, etoposide, etoposide phosphate, famotidine, fenoldopam, fentaNYL, fluconazole, fludarabine, fluorouracil, foscarnet, fosphenytoin, furosemide, ganciclovir, gemcitabine, gentamicin, glycopyrrolate, granisetron, haloperidol, heparin, hydrALAZINE, hydrocortisone, HYDROmorphone, IDArubicin, ifosfamide, imipenem/cilastatin, insulin, irinotecan, isoproterenol, ketorolac, labetalol, leucovorin, lidocaine, linezolid, LORazepam, magnesium sulfate, mannitol, mechlorethamine, melphalan, meperidine, meropenem, mesna, methylhexital, methotrexate, methyldopate, methylPREDNISolone, metoclopramide, metoprolol, metroNIDAZOLE, midazolam, milrinone, mitoXANtrone, morphine, mycophenolate, nafcillin, nalbuphine, naloxone, nesiritide, niCARdipine, nitroglycerin, nitroprusside, norepinephrine, octreotide, ondansetron, oxaliplatin, oxytocin, PACLitaxel, palonosetron, pamidronate, pancuronium, pantoprazole, PEMEtrexed, PENTobarbital, PHENobarbital, phentolamine, phenylephrine, piperacillin/tazobactam, potassium acetate/chloride/phosphates, procainamide, prochlorperazine, promethazine, propranolol, quinupristin/dalfopristin, ranitidine, remifentanil, rocuronium, sodium acetate/bicarbonate, streptozocin, succinylcholine, SUFentanil, tacrolimus, teniposide, theophylline, thiopental, thiotepa, ticarcillin/clavulanate, tigecycline, tobramycin, topotecan, vancomycin, vasopressin, vecuronium, verapamil, vinBLAStine, vinCRIStine, vinorelbine, voriconazole, zidovudine, zoledronic acid

Patient/family education
• Advise patient that it is necessary to quit smoking to prevent excessive vasoconstriction
• Teach signs/symptoms of bleeding, low platelets
• Advise that there are many drug and herb interactions, do not use unless approved by prescriber

Evaluation
Positive therapeutic outcome
• Treatment of acute coronary syndrome

⚠ HIGH ALERT
RARELY USED

tisagenlecleucel
(tid'-suh-jen-lek'-loo-sel)
Kymriah
Func. class.: Antineoplastic

USES: For the treatment of refractory B-cell precursor acute lymphoblastic leukemia

Dosage and routes
Adult: ≤ 25 yr, **adolescent, child, infant, and neonate: IV** (> 50 kg), infuse a single dose of 0.1 to 2.5 × 10⁸ CAR-positive viable T-cells (non-weight based); (≤ 50 kg) infuse a single dose of 0.2 to 5 × 10⁶ CAR-positive viable T-cells per kg of body weight. Give at 2 to 14 days

after the completion of lymphocyte depletion with fludarabine and cyclophosphamide

---

tobramycin (Rx)
(toe-bra-mye′sin)
Aktob, Bethkis, Kitabis, TOBI, TOBI Podhaler
Func. class.: Antiinfective
Chem. class.: Aminoglycoside

ACTION: Interferes with protein synthesis in bacterial cell by binding to ribosomal subunit, causing inaccurate peptide sequence to form in protein chain, causing bacterial death

Therapeutic outcome: Bactericidal effects for the following organisms: *Pseudomonas aeruginosa, Enterobacter, Escherichia coli, Providencia, Citrobacter, Staphylococcus, Proteus, Klebsiella, Serratia*

USES: Severe systemic infections of CNS, respiratory, GI, urinary tract, bone, skin, soft tissues, cystic fibrosis (nebulizer), *Acinetobacter calcoaceticus, Citrobacter, Enterobacter, Enterococcus, Escherichia coli, Haemophilus aegyptius, Haemophilus influenzae* (beta-lactamase negative), *Haemophilus influenzae* (beta-lactamase positive), *Klebsiella, Moraxella lacunata, Morganella morganii, Neisseria, Proteus mirabilis, Proteus vulgaris, Providencia, Pseudomonas aeruginosa, Serratia, Staphylococcus aureus* (MSSA), *Staphylococcus epidermidis, Staphylococcus, Streptococcus;* **may also be used for the following:** *Acinetobacter, Aeromonas, Bacillus anthracis, Salmonella, Shigella*

Pharmacokinetics

Absorption	Well absorbed (IM), completely absorbed (**IV**)
Distribution	Widely distributed in extracellular fluids
Metabolism	Minimal liver
Excretion	Mostly unchanged (>90%) kidneys
Half-life	2-3 hr, increased in renal disease, neonates

Pharmacodynamics

	IM	IV	OPHTH
Onset	Rapid	Rapid	Rapid
Peak	1 hr	Inf end	Unknown
Duration	Unknown	Unknown	Unknown

CONTRAINDICATIONS
Hypersensitivity to aminoglycosides

BLACK BOX WARNING: Pregnancy, severe renal disease

Precautions: Breastfeeding, geriatric, neonates, mild renal disease, myasthenia gravis, Parkinson's disease

BLACK BOX WARNING: Hearing deficits, neuromuscular disease

DOSAGE AND ROUTES
Adult: IM/IV 3 mg/kg/day in divided doses q8hr; may give up to 6 mg/kg/day in divided doses q8-12hr; once-daily dosing (pulse dosing) (unlabeled) **IV** 5-7 mg/kg; dosing intervals are determined using a nomogram and are based on random levels drawn 8-12 hr after first dose
Child: IM/IV 6-7.5 mg/kg/day in 3-4 equal divided doses
Neonate <1 wk: IM/IV ≤4 mg/kg/day divided q12hr
Conventional dosing: Multiply the serum creatinine (mg/100 ml) by 6 to determine the dosing; to decrease the dose, divide the standard dose by the serum creatinine (mg/100 ml) to determine the lower recommended dose
Interval adjustment of extended-interval dosing of 5 or 7 mg/kg (unlabeled): Adjust doses based on serum concentrations and organism MIC; CCr 40-59 ml/min: 5 or 7 mg/kg IV q36hr; CCr 20-39 ml/min: 5 or 7 mg/kg IV q48hr; CCr <20 ml/min: 5 or 7 mg/kg IV once, then follow serial levels to determine time of next dose (serum concentration <1 mcg/ml)
Dose adjustment of extended dosing of 5 mg/kg (unlabeled): Adjust doses based on serum concentrations and organism MIC; CCr >80 ml/min: no dosage adjustment is needed; CCr 60-79 ml/min: 4 mg/kg **IV** q24hr; CCr 50 ml/min: 3.5 mg/kg **IV** q24hr CrCl 40 ml/min: 2.5 mg/kg **IV** q24hr; CrCl <30 ml/min: Use traditional dosing

Cystic fibrosis with *Pseudomonas aeruginosa*
Child 6 yr: NEB 300 mg bid in repeating cycles of 28 days on/28 days off; give inh over 10-15 min using a hand-held PARI LC PLUS reusable nebulizer with a DeVilbiss Pulmo-Aid compressor

Available forms: Inj 10, 40 mg/ml; powder for inj 1.2 g; neb sol 300 mg/5 ml; powder for inh 28 mg

ADVERSE EFFECTS
CNS: Confusion, depression, numbness, tremors, seizures, muscle twitching, neurotoxicity, dizziness, vertigo

---

CV: Hypo/hypertension, palpitations

EENT: *Ototoxicity*, deafness, visual disturbances, tinnitus

GI: *Nausea, vomiting, anorexia*, increased ALT, AST, bilirubin, hepatomegaly, hepatic necrosis, splenomegaly

GU: Oliguria, hematuria, renal damage, azotemia, renal failure, nephrotoxicity

HEMA: Agranulocytosis, thrombocytopenia, leukopenia, eosinophilia, anemia

INTEG: *Rash*, burning, urticaria, dermatitis, alopecia

INTERACTIONS
Individual drugs
Acyclovir, amphotericin B, bacitracin, cidofovir, CISplatin, ethacrynic acid, furosemide, mannitol, methoxyflurane, polymyxin, vancomycin: increased ototoxicity, neurotoxicity, nephrotoxicity

Drug classifications

> **BLACK BOX WARNING: Aminoglycosides,** cephalosporins, penicillins: increased otoxicity, neurotoxicity, nephrotoxicity

NURSING CONSIDERATIONS
Assessment
• Assess patient for previous sensitivity reaction
Systemic route
• Assess patient for signs and symptoms of infection including characteristics of wounds, sputum, urine, stool, WBC >10,000/mm³, temp baseline, during treatment
• Complete C&S testing before beginning product therapy to identify if correct treatment has been initiated
• Assess for allergic reactions: rash, urticaria, pruritus, chills, fever, joint pain

> **BLACK BOX WARNING: Renal disease:** Identify urine output; if decreasing, notify prescriber (may indicate nephrotoxicity); also, obtain BUN, creatinine, urine CCr (<80 ml/min) values; urinalysis daily for proteinuria, cells, casts; report sudden change in urine output

> **BLACK BOX WARNING: Pregnancy:** identify if pregnancy is planned or suspected; do not use in pregnancy, breastfeeding

> **BLACK BOX WARNING:** Serum aminoglycoside concentration: Serum peak drawn at 30-60 min after IV infusion or 60 min after IM inj; trough drawn just before next dose, peak 4-10 mcg/ml, trough 0.5-2 mcg/ml, increased level may lead to serious toxicity

> **BLACK BOX WARNING:** Deafness by audiometric testing; ringing, roaring in ears; vertigo; assess hearing before, during, after treatment

• Monitor blood studies: AST, ALT, CBC, Hct, bilirubin, LDH, alkaline phosphatase, Coombs' test monthly if patient is on long-term therapy
• Monitor electrolytes: potassium, sodium, chloride, magnesium monthly if patient is on long-term therapy
• Monitor for bleeding: ecchymosis, bleeding gums, hematuria, stool guaiac daily if patient is on long-term therapy
• **Assess for overgrowth of infection:** perineal itching, fever, malaise, redness, pain, swelling, drainage, rash, diarrhea, change in cough, sputum
• Obtain weight before treatment; calculation of dosage is usually based on ideal body weight but may be calculated on actual body weight
• Monitor VS during inf, watch for hypotension, change in pulse
• Assess IV site for thrombophlebitis including pain, redness, swelling q30min; change site if needed; apply warm compresses to discontinued site

> **BLACK BOX WARNING:** Obtain serum peak, drawn at 30-60 min after IV inf or 60 min after IM inj, trough level drawn just before next dose; peak 4-12 mcg/ml, trough 1-2 mcg/ml, increased level may lead to serious toxicity

> **BLACK BOX WARNING: Monitor for deafness by audiometric testing,** ringing, roaring in ears, vertigo; assess hearing before, during, after treatment, promptly

Patient problem
Infection (uses)

Implementation
IM route
• Give inj deeply in large muscle mass, aspirate
• Draw peak 1 hr after dose, trough right before next dose; absorption erratic
Nebulizer route
• The solution for nebulization is for inhalation only; use over 10-15 min
Inhalation route (TOBI Podhaler)
• Use with Podhaler device, do not swallow caps, use device for 7 days then discard
• Keep caps in blister pack until ready to use, administer other inhaled products or chest physiotherapy before
• While holding base of Podhaler device, unscrew lid, stand upright, unscrew mouthpiece; while holding body, tear blister card in half lengthwise along precut lines; peel back foil, place cap in

chamber at top of device, reattach mouthpiece, and tighten; with mouthpiece pointed down, press blue button down with thumb, release; exhale completely, place mouth over mouthpiece, close lips, inhale with single breath, hold 5 sec, and exhale normally away from device; after a few normal breaths, repeat, unscrew mouthpiece, and remove cap: cap should be empty; repeat process 3 more times (total 4 caps); after use reattach mouthpiece and wipe with clean, dry cloth

Intermittent IV infusion route
• Visually inspect solution; do not use if discolored or if particulate is present
• ADD-Vantage vials are for IV only and only for exactly 60 or 80 mg
• Give **IV** diluted in 50-100 ml of 0.9% NaCl, $D_{10}W$, D_5/0.9% NaCl, 0.9% NaCl, Ringer's, LR, D_5W (adult), inf over 20-60 min, volume for pediatric patients needs and should be sufficient to allow for 20-60 min infusion
• Flush after inf with D_5W, 0.9% NaCl
• Separate aminoglycosides and penicillins by ≥1 hr

Y-site compatibilities: Acyclovir, aldesleukin, alfentanil, alprostadil, amifostine, aminophylline, amiodarone, amsacrine, anidulafungin, ascorbic acid, atracurium, atropine, aztreonam, bivalirudin, bretylium, bumetanide, buprenorphine, butorphanol, calcium chloride/gluconate, CARBOplatin, caspofungin, chloramphenicol, cimetidine, ciprofloxacin, cisatracurium, CISplatin, clindamycin, cyanocobalamin, cyclophosphamide, cycloSPORINE, cytarabine, DACTINomycin, DAPTOmycin, dexmedetomidine, digoxin, diltiazem, diphenhydrAMINE, DOBUTamine, DOCEtaxel, DOPamine, doripenem, doxacurium, DOXOrubicin hydrochloride, DOXOrubicin liposome, doxycycline, enalaprilat, ePHEDrine, EPINEPHrine, epirubicin, epoetin alfa, ertapenem, esmolol, etoposide, etoposide phosphate, famotidine, fenoldopam, fentaNYL, filgrastim, fluconazole, fludarabine, fluorouracil, foscarnet, furosemide, gemcitabine, gentamicin, glycopyrrolate, granisetron, HYDROmorphone, ifosfamide, imipenem/cilastatin, isoproterenol, ketorolac, labetalol, levofloxacin, lidocaine, linezolid, LORazepam, magnesium sulfate, mannitol, mechlorethamine, melphalan, meperidine, metaraminol, methicillin, methotrexate, methoxamine, methyldopate, methylPREDNISolone, metoclopramide, metoprolol, metroNIDAZOLE, miconazole, midazolam, milrinone, minocycline, mitoXANtrone, morphine, moxalactam, multiple vitamins, nafcillin, nalbuphine, naloxone, niCARdipine, nitroglycerin, nitroprusside, norepinephrine, octreotide, ondansetron, oxaliplatin, oxytocin, PAClitaxel, palonosetron, pantoprazole, papaverine, penicillin G, pentazocine, perphenazine, PHENobarbital, phentolamine, phenylephrine, phytonadione, potassium chloride, procainamide, prochlorperazine, promethazine, propranolol, protamine, pyridoxine, quinupristin/dalfopristin, ranitidine, remifentanil, riTUXimab, rocuronium, sodium acetate/bicarbonate, succinylcholine, SUFentanil, tacrolimus, teniposide, theophylline, thiamine, thiotepa, ticarcillin/clavulanate, tigecycline, tirofiban, tolazoline, trastuzumab, trimetaphan, urokinase, vancomycin, vasopressin, vecuronium, verapamil, vinCRIStine, vinorelbine, voriconazole, zidovudine

Patient/family education
• Teach patient to report sore throat, bruising, bleeding, joint pain; may indicate blood dyscrasias (rare)
• Advise patient to contact prescriber if vaginal itching, loose foul-smelling stools, furry tongue occur; may indicate superinfection

> **BLACK BOX WARNING:** Advise patient to notify prescriber if pregnancy is planned or suspected, not to use in pregnancy, breastfeeding

• Advise patient to notify prescriber of diarrhea with blood or pus; may indicate pseudomembranous colitis
• Teach patient to avoid hazardous activities until response is known

Nebulizer route
• Advise patient to use multiple therapies first, then tobramycin, not to use if cloudy or contains particulates

Evaluation
Positive therapeutic outcome
• Absence of signs/symptoms of infection (WBC <10,000/mm³; temp WNL; absence of red, draining wounds)
• Reported improvement in symptoms of infection

TREATMENT OF OVERDOSE:
Withdraw product, hemodialysis, exchange transfusion in the newborn, monitor serum levels of product, may give ticarcillin or carbenicillin

tobramycin ophthalmic
See Appendix B

tocilizumab (Rx)
(toe′si-liz′oo-mab)
Actemra
Func. class.: DMARDs (Disease modifying anti-rheumatoid drugs)/tumor necrosis factor (TNF) modifier

ACTION: Interleukin- 6 (IL-6) receptor inhibiting monoclonal antibody

Therapeutic outcome: Ability to move more easily with less pain

USES: Rheumatoid arthritis, active systemic juvenile idiopathic arthritis

Pharmacokinetics

Absorption	Unknown
Distribution	Unknown
Metabolism	Unknown
Excretion	Unknown
Half-life	~6 days with a single dose and ~11 days with multiple (steady state) doses

Pharmacodynamics

Unknown

CONTRAINDICATIONS
Hypersensitivity

Precautions: Breastfeeding, pregnancy, risk for GI perforation, active hepatic disease, severe neutropenia/thrombocytopenia, demyelinating disorders

> **BLACK BOX WARNING:** Invasive fungal infection, active TB

DOSAGE AND ROUTES
Monotherapy with or without methotrexate or other DMARDs, moderate-severe rheumatoid arthritis

Adult: IV 4 mg/kg over 1 hr q4wk, may increase to 8 mg/kg q4wk based on clinical response, max dose 800 mg/inf; do not initiate if ANC is >2000 and platelets are <100,000/mm^3; subcut adult <100 kg 162 mg q other wk, increase to 162 mg q wk if no response; >100 kg 162 mg qwk

Juvenile idiopathic arthritis
Child ≥2 yr/adolescent ≥30 kg: IV 8 mg/kg over 1 hr q2wk
Child ≥2 yr/adolescent <30 kg: IV 10 mg/kg over 1 hr q2wk

Available forms: Sol for inj 20 mg/ml; prefilled syringes 162 mg/0.9 ml

ADVERSE EFFECTS
CNS: Headache, dizziness
CV: Hypertension
GI: Perforation, abdominal pain, gastritis, mouth ulcerations
HEMA: Neutropenia, thrombocytopenia
INTEG: Rash, infusion reactions
RESP: Upper respiratory infections, nasopharyngitis, bronchitis

SYST: Serious infections, anaphylaxis, infusion-related reactions, anti-tocilizumab antibody formation, secondary malignancy

INTERACTIONS
Individual drugs
CycloSPORINE, theophylline, warfarin: decreased product level

Drug classifications
CYP3A4 substrates (hormonal contraceptives, omeprazole, atorvastatin, simvastatin): decreased levels of these products
Live virus vaccines: Do not use together
TNF modifiers, DMARDs, immunosuppressives: avoid use due to increased risk of infection

NURSING CONSIDERATIONS
Assessment
• **Rheumatoid arthritis:** assess ROM, pain, stiffness baseline q1-2wk
• Monitor blood studies: CBC with differential, LFTs, platelet count, serum lipid profile, baseline and periodically; LFTs 1-3 × ULN, reduce dose, if 3-5 × ULN interrupt; platelets 50,000-100,000/mm^3 interrupt until platelets are >100,000/mm^3, then resume at lower dose

> **BLACK BOX WARNING: Infection:** Before treatment and periodically; obtain TB screening before beginning treatment, invasive fungal infections; discontinue if infection occurs during administration; may use antituberculosis therapy before tocilizumab in past history of latent or active TB when adequate course of treatment cannot be confirmed and those with a negative TB with risk factors for infections

• **Secondary malignancy:** Assess for malignancy periodically
• **Pregnancy/breastfeeding:** Use only if benefits outweigh fetal risk, pregnant patients should enroll in the Mother To Baby Autoimmune Disease Pregnancy Registry, do not breastfeed, excretion unknown
• **Anaphylaxis:** Assess for rash, facial swelling, dyspnea, antihistamine, corticosteroids, emergency equipment should be available
• **Fungal infections:** Assess for flu-like symptoms, dyspnea; may lead to shock; notify provider immediately

Patient problem
Pain (uses)
Risk for infection (adverse reactions)
Risk for injury (adverse reactions)

Implementation
SUBCUT route
• Remove syringe, allow to warm for 30 min at room temperature. Do not warm in any other way
• Use injection site such as the front of a thigh, outer area of an upper arm, or the abdomen except for the 2-inch area around the navel. Do not inject into moles, scars, or areas where the skin is tender, bruised, red, hard, or not intact. Rotate injection sites with each injection. Inject at >1 inch from the last area injected
• Remove the needle cap immediately before injection, and gently pinch a cleaned area of skin. Using a dartlike motion, insert the needle at a 45- or 90-degree angle to the skin. Release the pinched skin, and gently push the plunger all the way down to inject the full amount in the prefilled syringe (0.9 ml), which provides 162 mg of product
• The prefilled syringe is single-use only, as it does not have a preservative
• Remove the needle from the skin while continuing to depress the plunger. After the needle is completely removed, release the plunger, which will allow the needle-shield to protect the needle. Do not rub the site

Intermittent IV route
• Visually inspect for particulate matter and discoloration before administration should be colorless to pale yellow liquid
• From a 100-ml infusion bag or bottle, withdraw a volume of 0.9% NaCl for inj equal to the volume of the tocilizumab solution required for the patient's dose
• Slowly add tocilizumab from each vial into the infusion bag or bottle. Gently invert the bag to avoid foaming. Fully diluted solutions are compatible with polypropylene, polyethylene, and polyvinyl chloride infusion bags and polypropylene, polyethylene, and glass infusion bottles
• The fully diluted sol for inf may be stored refrigerated or at room temp for up to 24 hours and should be protected from light. Do not use unused product remaining in vials; no preservatives
• Allow the fully diluted solution to reach room temp before infusing
• Give over 60 min with an infusion set. Do not administer as an **IV** push or bolus
• Do not infuse concomitantly in the same intravenous line with other drugs

Patient/family education
• Teach patient that this treatment must continue unless safety or effectiveness is an issue; reason for use and expected result

> **BLACK BOX WARNING:** Advise patient to avoid use of live vaccines, bring immunizations up to date before treatment

> **BLACK BOX WARNING:** Instruct patient to report signs/symptoms of infection (including TB and Hepatitis B), invasive fungal infections, discontinue if infection occurs during administration; may use antituberculosis therapy prior to tocilizumab in past history of latent or active TB when adequate course of treatment cannot be confirmed and those with a negative TB with risk factors for infections, to avoid others with infections

• Teach patient to notify prescriber if pregnancy is planned or suspected, pregnancy; do not use if breastfeeding, consider using a nonhormonal contraceptive because contraception may be decreased
• **Secondary malignancy:** assess for malignancy periodically

Evaluation
Positive therapeutic outcome
• Ability to move more easily with less pain

tofacitinib
(toe'fa-sye'ti-nib)
Xeljanz, Xelganz XR
Func. class.: antirheumatic agent (disease modifying), immunomodulator/biologic DMARD
Chem. class.: Janus kinase inhibitor

ACTION: Affects the signaling pathway of Janus kinase

Therapeutic outcome: Decreased inflammation, pain in joints, decreased joint destruction

USES: Rheumatoid arthritis (moderately to severely active) in those who have taken methotrexate with inadequate response or intolerance

Pharmacokinetics

Absorption	Bioavailability 70%
Distribution	Protein binding 40% (albumin)
Metabolism	Mediated by CYP3A4
Excretion	Unknown
Half-life	3 hr

Pharmacodynamics

Onset	Unknown
Peak	0.5–1 hr
Duration	Unknown

CONTRAINDICATIONS
Hypersensitivity

Precautions: Pregnancy, breastfeeding, neonates, infants, children, geriatric patients, neoplastic disease, ulcerative colitis, neutropenia, peptic ulcer disease, active infections, risk of lymphomas/leukemias, TB, posttransplant lymphoproliferative disorder (PTLD), kidney disease, diabetes mellitus, HIV, hypercholesterolemia, herpes virus infection reactivation, patients of Asian descent

> **BLACK BOX WARNING: Infection, secondary malignancy**

DOSAGE AND ROUTES
RA
Adult: PO 5 mg/bid with or without methotrexate or other nonbiologic DMARDs; ext rel 11 mg q day

Ulcerative colitis
Adult: PO 10 mg bid x 8 wk or more, then 5-10 mg bid

Available forms: Tabs 5, 10 mg; ext rel tab 11 mg

ADVERSE EFFECTS
CNS: Headache, paresthesias, insomnia, fatigue
CV: Hypertension
GI: Abdominal pain, nausea, liver damage, dyspepsia, vomiting, diarrhea, gastritis, GI perforation, steatosis
HEMA: Anemia, lymphocytosis, lymphopenia, neutropenia
INTEG: Rash, pruritus
MISC: Increased cancer risk, risk of infection (TB, invasive fungal infections, other opportunistic infections), may be fatal, posttransplant lymphoproliferative disorder (PTLD)

INTERACTIONS
Drug classifications

> **BLACK BOX WARNING: Do not use with TNF modifiers, vaccines, potent immunosuppressants, other biologic DMARDS, serious infection may occur**

CYP3A4 inhibitors (amprenavir, boceprevir, delavirdine, ketoconazole, indinavir, itraconazole, dalfopristin/quinupristin, ritonavir, tipranavir, fluconazole, isoniazid, miconazole): increased tofacitinib effect
CYP3A4 inducers (rifampin, rifapentine, rifabutin, primidone, phenytoin, PHENobarbital, nevirapine, nafcillin, modafinil, griseofulvin, etravirine, efavirenz, barbiturates, bexarotene, bosentan, carBAMazepine, enzalutamide, dexamethasone): decreased tofacitinib effect

Drug/lab test
Increase: LFTs, cholesterol
Decrease: neutrophils, lymphocytes, Hct, Hgb

NURSING CONSIDERATIONS
Assessment
• Monitor lipid profile, Hct/Hgb WBC, LFTs
• **RA:** assess for pain, stiffness, ROM, swelling of joints before, during treatment

> **BLACK BOX WARNING: Active infection, including localized infection:** evaluate and test patients for latent or active TB before use; treat with antimycobacterials before use of product; this product increases the risk of serious illness including fatal infections (pulmonary or extrapulmonary TB; invasive fungal infections; and bacterial, viral, and opportunistic infections); during and after use, monitor for infection including TB in those who tested negative for latent TB before use; if a serious infection develops, interrupt receipt until the infection is controlled, reactivation or viral infections is higher in those of Asian descent

> **BLACK BOX WARNING: Secondary malignancy:** lymphoma and other malignancies have been noted with product use

• **Epstein–Barr virus–associated post transplant lymphoproliferative disorder (PTLD):** in kidney transplant patients when used with this product and immunosuppressives
• **Liver disease:** not recommended in severe liver disease, impairment; dose modification is needed with moderate liver impairment, monitor LFTs
• **GI perforation:** assess in those with diverticulitis, peptic ulcer disease, or ulcerative colitis

> **BLACK BOX WARNING: Immunosuppression:** obtain neutrophil and lymphocyte counts before use, do not start the product in lymphocyte count < 500 cells/mm^3 or < ANC 1000 cells/mm^3; for ANC >1000 cells/mm^3, monitor neutrophil counts after 4-8 wk and every 3 mo thereafter; lymphocyte count > 500 cells/ mm^3, monitor lymphocyte counts every 3 mo

• **Anemia:** determine Hgb, do not start in Hgb 9 g/dl; monitor Hgb after 4-8 wk and every 3 mo thereafter

T

> **BLACK BOX WARNING: Neoplastic disease** (lymphomas/leukemias)

• **Pregnancy/breastfeeding:** use during pregnancy only if the potential benefit justifies the potential risk to the fetus; if pregnancy occurs, enrollment in the pregnancy registry is encouraged by calling 877–311–8972; discontinue product or breastfeeding, serious adverse reactions can occur in nursing infants

Patient problem
Impaired mobility (uses)
Risk for infection (adverse reactions)

Implementation
PO route
Give without regard to food

Patient/family education
• Teach patient not to have vaccines while taking this product
• Advise patient not to take any live virus vaccines during treatment, vaccinations should be brought up to date before starting treatment
• Inform patient to report signs of infection, allergic reaction
• **Pregnancy:** teach patient to report if pregnancy is planned or suspected, do not breastfeed

Evaluation

Positive therapeutic outcome
• Decreased inflammation, pain in joints, decreased joint destruction

tolcapone (Rx)
(toll'cah-pone)
Tasmar
Func. class.: Antiparkinson agent
Chem. class.: Catecholamine inhibitor (COMT)

ACTION: Selective, reversible inhibitor of catecholamine; used as adjunct to levodopa/carbidopa therapy

Therapeutic outcome: Increased ability to move and speak

USES: Parkinsonism

Pharmacokinetics

Absorption	Rapidly absorbed
Distribution	Protein binding 99%
Metabolism	Liver, extensively
Excretion	Urine (60%), feces (40%)
Half-life	2-3 hr

Pharmacodynamics

Onset	Unknown
Peak	2 hr
Duration	Unknown

CONTRAINDICATIONS
Hypersensitivity, rhabdomyolysis

Precautions: Pregnancy, breastfeeding, cardiac/renal disease, hypertension, asthma, history of rhabdomyolysis, hepatic disease

DOSAGE AND ROUTES
Adult: PO 100-200 mg tid, with levodopa/carbidopa therapy; max 600 mg/day; discontinue if no benefit in 3 wk

Available forms: Tabs 100, 200 mg

ADVERSE EFFECTS
CNS: Dystonia, dyskinesia, dreaming, *fatigue, headache, confusion,* psychosis, hallucination, dizziness, sleep disorders
CV: *Orthostatic hypotension,* chest pain, hypotension
EENT: Cataract, eye inflammation
GI: *Nausea, vomiting, abdominal distress,* diarrhea, constipation, fatal liver failure, elevated liver function tests
GU: UTI, urine discoloration, uterine tumor, micturition disorder, hematuria
HEMA: Hemolytic anemia, leukopenia, agranulocytosis
INTEG: Sweating, alopecia
MS: Rhabdomyolysis

INTERACTIONS
Individual drugs
Apomorphine, DOBUTamine, isoproterenol, α-methyldopa: may influence pharmacokinetics

Drug classifications
CNS depressants: increased CNS depression
MAOIs: decreased normal catecholamine metabolism; MAO-B inhibitor may be used

NURSING CONSIDERATIONS
Assessment

> **BLACK BOX WARNING: Hepatic disease:** monitor liver function tests: AST, ALT, alkaline phosphatase, LDH, bilirubin, CBC; monitor ALT, AST q2wk x 1 yr, then q4wk x 6 mo, then q8wk thereafter; if LFTs are elevated product should not be used, if no improvement in 3 wk, discontinue, do not use in hepatic disease

• Assess involuntary movements in parkinsonism: akinesia, tremors, staggering gait, muscle rigidity, drooling

---

- Monitor B/P, respiration during initial treatment; hypo/hypertension should be reported
- Monitor mental status: affect, mood, behavioral changes, avoid use in those with dystonia

Patient problem
Impaired mobility (uses)
Risk for injury (uses, adverse reactions)

Implementation
- Administer tid with levodopa/carbidopa therapy
- Provide assistance with ambulation during beginning therapy
- Give without regard to food

Patient/family education
- Advise patient to change positions slowly to prevent orthostatic hypotension
- Advise patient that urine, sweat may change color
- Teach patient that CNS changes may occur, hallucinations, involuntary movement
- Teach patient to avoid hazardous activities until reaction is known, dizziness occurs
- Teach patient to report poor impulse control, urges to gamble, spend wildly (rare)

> **BLACK BOX WARNING:** Advise patient to report signs of **hepatic injury:** clay-colored stools, jaundice, fatigue, appetite loss, lethargy, fatigue, itching, right upper abdominal pain

- Teach patient to report nausea, vomiting, anorexia, diarrhea
- May be taken without regard to food
- Teach patient to notify prescriber if pregnancy is planned or suspected

Evaluation

Positive therapeutic outcome
- Decrease in akathisia, improved mood

tolnaftate topical
See Appendix B

tolterodine (Rx)
(tol-tehr′oh-deen)
Detrol, Detrol LA
Func. class.: Overactive bladder product
Chem. class.: Muscarinic receptor antagonist

ACTION: Relaxes smooth muscles in urinary tract by inhibiting acetylcholine at postganglionic sites

Therapeutic outcome: Decreased symptoms of overactive bladder

USES: Overactive bladder (frequency, urgency), urinary incontinence

Pharmacokinetics

Absorption	Rapidly absorbed
Distribution	Highly protein bound
Metabolism	Liver, extensively by CYP2D6, a portion of the population may be poor metabolizers
Excretion	Urine/feces
Half-life	2-3.7 hr

Pharmacodynamics
Unknown

CONTRAINDICATIONS
Hypersensitivity, uncontrolled closed-angle glaucoma, urinary retention, gastric retention ⚕

Precautions: Pregnancy, breastfeeding, children, renal/hepatic disease, controlled closed-angle glaucoma, bladder obstruction, QT prolongation, decreased GI motility

DOSAGE AND ROUTES
Overactive bladder
Adult and geriatric: PO 2 mg bid, may decrease to 1 mg bid; EXT REL 4 mg/day, may decrease to 2 mg if needed, max 4 mg/day

Hepatic disease
Adult: PO 1 mg bid (50% dose) or EXT REL 2 mg/day

Renal dose
Adult: PO CCr ≤30 ml/min reduce by 50%

CYP3A4 inhibitor dose
Adult: PO 1 mg bid; extended-release 2 mg qday if using with CYP3A4 inhibitor

Available forms: Tabs 1, 2 mg; ext rel caps 2, 4 mg

ADVERSE EFFECTS
CNS: *Anxiety,* paresthesia, fatigue, *dizziness,* headache, increasing dementia, memory impairment
CV: Chest pain, hypertension, QT prolongation
EENT: Vision abnormalities, xerophthalmia
GI: *Nausea, vomiting, anorexia,* abdominal pain, constipation, dry mouth, dyspepsia
GU: Dysuria, retention, frequency, UTI
INTEG: Rash, pruritus
RESP: Bronchitis, cough, pharyngitis, upper respiratory tract infection
SYST: Angioedema, Stevens-Johnson syndrome

INTERACTIONS
Individual drugs
Chloroquine, clarithromycin, droperidol, erythromycin, grepafloxacin, halofantrine,

---

haloperidol, methadone, pentamidine: increased QT prolongation

Fesoterodine: do not use in those with known hypersensitivity

Drug classifications

Antibiotics (macrolide), antifungal agents, antiretroviral protease inhibitors: increased action of tolterodine

Antimuscarinics: increased anticholinergic effect

β-agonists, class IA/III antidysrhythmics, local anesthetics, some phenothiazines, tricyclics: increased QT prolongation

Diuretics: increased urinary frequency

Drug/food

Increased: bioavailability of tolterodine

Drug/lab test

Increased: LFTs, bilirubin

NURSING CONSIDERATIONS
Assessment

• **Assess urinary patterns:** distention, nocturia, frequency, urgency, incontinence, residual urine

• **Serious skin disorders:** assess for angioedema, Stevens-Johnson syndrome; assess allergic reactions: rash; if this occurs, product should be discontinued

• **QT prolongation:** ECG for QT prolongation, ejection fraction; assess for chest pain, palpitations, dyspnea, may be compounded in those taking Class IA/III dysrythmics

> **BLACK BOX WARNING: Fatal hepatic injury:** increased LFTs, bilirubin during first 18 mo of therapy in those with autosomal dominant polycystic kidney disease; assess for fatigue, anorexia, right upper abdominal pain, dark urine, jaundice; if these occur, discontinue product and do not restart if cause is liver injury

• **Beers:** Avoid in older adults with or at high risk for delirium; monitor for confusion, delirium frequency

• **Pregnancy/breastfeeding:** Use only if benefits outweigh fetal risk, no well-controlled studies, do not breastfeed, excretion unknown

Patient problem

Impaired urination (uses)

Implementation

• Swallow whole; give with liquids

Patient/family education

• Advise patient to avoid hazardous activities; dizziness may occur, shortness of breath, urinary retention

• Advise patient not to drink liquids before bedtime, to swallow extended-release product whole

• Teach patient importance of bladder maintenance

• Teach patient to take with liquids; swallow whole

• Notify prescriber if pregnancy is planned or suspected

Evaluation

Positive therapeutic outcome

• Decreased urinary frequency, urgency

---

tolvaptan (Rx)

(tole-vap′tan)

Jinarc ✦, **Samsca**

Func. class.: Antihypertensive

Chem. class.: Vasopressin receptor antagonist, V2

ACTION: Arginine vasopressin (AVP) antagonist with affinity for V_2 receptors; level of circulating AVP in circulating blood is critical for regulation of water, electrolyte balance and is usually elevated in euvolemic/hypervolemic hyponatremia

Therapeutic outcome: Normal serum sodium level

USES: Hypervolemic/euvolemic hyponatremia in heart failure, cirrhosis, SIADH

Pharmacokinetics

Absorption	Unknown
Distribution	Protein binding 99%
Metabolism	CYP3A4
Excretion	Unknown
Half-life	12 hr

Pharmacodynamics

Onset	Unknown
Peak	2-4 hr
Duration	Unknown

CONTRAINDICATIONS

Hypersensitivity, hypovolemia, anuria

Precautions: Pregnancy, breastfeeding, children, dehydration, geriatric patients, hyperkalemia, autosomal dominant PKD, malnutrition, alcoholism, hepatic disease

> **BLACK BOX WARNING:** Osmotic demyelination syndrome, requires a specialized care setting

DOSAGE AND ROUTES

Adult: PO 15 mg qd; after 24 hr, may increase to 30 mg qd; max 60 mg/day max 30 days

Available forms: Tab 15, 30 mg

ADVERSE EFFECTS

CNS: Fever, dizziness
CV: Ventricular fibrillation, DIC, stroke, thrombosis
GI: *Nausea*, vomiting, *constipation*, colitis, hepatic injury
GU: Polyuria
HEMA: Bleeding
META: *Dehydration, hyperglycemia,* hyperkalemia, hypernatremia
MS: Rhabdomyolysis
RESP: Respiratory depression, pulmonary embolism

INTERACTIONS

Drug classifications

CYP3A4 inducers (carBAMazepine, dexamethasone, etravirine, flutamide, griseofulvin, metyrapone, modafinil, nafcillin, nevirapine, OXcarbazepine, phenytoin, rifampin, rifabutin, rifapentine, topiramate): decreased concentrations of tolvaptan

CYP3A4 inhibitors (efavirenz, fosamprenavir, quiNINE), P-gp inhibitors (azithromycin, cycloSPORINE, mefloquine, paliperidone, propafenone, quiNIDine, testosterone): increased concentrations of tolvaptan

Drug/herb

St. John's wort: decreased tolvaptan effect

Drug/food

Grapefruit/grapefruit juice: do not use together

NURSING CONSIDERATIONS

Assessment

• Assess renal, hepatic function

BLACK BOX WARNING: Osmotic demyelination syndrome, frequent sodium volume status; overly rapid correction of sodium concentration (>12 mEq/L per 24 hr) may occur in alcoholism, severe malnutrition, advanced liver disease, SIADH, correct sodium levels slowly, may result in dysarthria, mutism, dysphagia, coma, seizures, death

• **Liver injury:** monitor for fatigue, abdominal pain, dark urine, clay-colored stool, jaundice
• Assess CV status: ventricular fibrillation, hypertension, monitor B/P, pulse
• Monitor electrolytes (sodium, potassium)

BLACK BOX WARNING: Specialized care setting needed so neurologic status, sodium levels can be monitored

• **Pregnancy/breastfeeding:** Use only if benefits outweigh fetal risk, do not breastfeed

Patient problem

Fluid imbalance (uses)

Implementation

• Give PO with or without food
• Avoid fluid restriction the first 24 hr
• Initiate in hospital setting
• Do not use with grapefruit or grapefruit juice

Patient/family education

• Advise of administration procedure and expected result
• Teach patient to report difficulty swallowing or speaking, seizures, dizziness, drowsiness: embolism may be the cause
• Teach patient to drink fluid in response to thirst
• Teach patient to not use grapefruit juice
• Teach patient to notify prescriber before using other products
• Teach patient to report upper-right abdominal pain, nausea, vomiting, anorexia, dark urine, yellowing of skin/eyes (hepatic injury)
• Teach patient to avoid pregnancy, breastfeeding while taking this product

Evaluation

Positive therapeutic outcome

• Correction of serum sodium levels

---

topiramate (Rx)

(toh-pire'a-mate)
Topamax, Topamax Sprinkle, Trokendi XR, Qudexy XR
Func. class.: Anticonvulsant—miscellaneous
Chem. class.: Monosaccharide derivative

Do not confuse: Topamax/Toprol XL

ACTION: Increased GABA activity; may prevent seizure spread as opposed to an elevation of seizure threshold

Therapeutic outcome: Absence of seizures

USES: Partial seizures in adults and children 2-16 yr old; tonic-clonic seizures; seizures in Lennox-Gastaut syndrome, migraine prophylaxis

Unlabeled uses: Infantile spasms, bulimia nervosa

Pharmacokinetics

Absorption	Well absorbed
Distribution	Crosses placenta, plasma protein binding (9%-17%), steady state 4 days
Metabolism	Unknown
Excretion	Kidneys unchanged 55%-97%
Half-life	19-25 hr

Pharmacodynamics

Onset	Unknown
Peak	2-4 hr
Duration	Unknown

CONTRAINDICATIONS

Hypersensitivity, metabolic acidosis, pregnancy

Precautions: Breastfeeding, children, renal/hepatic disease, acute myopia, secondary closed-angle glaucoma, behavioral disorders, COPD, dialysis, encephalopathy, status asthmaticus, status epilepticus, surgery, paresthesias, maculopathy, nephrolithiasis

DOSAGE AND ROUTES
Adjunctive therapy

Adult/adolescent/child ≥10 yr: PO 25-50 mg/day initially, titrate by 25-50 mg/wk, up to 200-400 mg/day in 2 divided doses

Adult/adolescent/child ≥10 yr: PO (Qudexy XR, Trokendi XR) 50 mg qday; increase by 50 mg qwk during wk 2, 3, 4; increase by 100 mg qwk, wk 5, 6; final dose 400 mg qday

Child 2-9 yr: PO week 1 25 mg q PM, then 25 mg bid if tolerated (week 2), then increase by 25-50 mg/day each week as tolerated over 5-7 wk titration period, maintenance given in 2 divided doses; <11 kg minimum 150 mg/day, max 250 mg/day; 12-22 kg minimum 200 mg/day, max 300 mg/day; 23-31 kg minimum 200 mg, max 350 mg/day, 32-38 kg minimum 250 mg/kg, max 350 mg/day; >38 kg minimum 250 mg/day, max 400 mg/day; Qudexy XR 25 mg qday at night; may increase to 50 mg wk 2, if tolerated; increase by 25-50 mg each wk over 5-7 wk titration period; max dose based on weight

Migraine prophylaxis

Child ≤11 kg: PO Qudexy XR minimum 150 mg daily, max 250 mg daily; 12-22 kg minimum 200 mg daily, max 300 mg daily; 23-31 kg minimum 200 mg daily, max 350 mg daily; 32-38 kg minimum 250 mg daily, max 350 mg daily; >38 kg minimum 250 mg daily, max 400 mg daily

Adult: PO 25 mg/day initially, increase by 25 mg/day qwk up to 100 mg/day in 2 divided doses

Renal dose

Adult: PO CCr <70 ml/min ½ dose

Available forms: Tabs 25, 50, 100, 200 mg; sprinkle caps 15, 25 mg; ext rel caps 25, 50, 100, 200 mg; ext rel cap (sprinkles 24 hr) 25, 50, 100, 150, 200 mg

ADVERSE EFFECTS

CNS: Dizziness, fatigue, cognitive disorder, *insomnia,* anxiety, depression, paresthesia, motor retardation, suicidal ideation, memory loss, tremor, poor balance, ataxia

CV: Flushing, chest pain

EENT: Diplopia, vision abnormality

GI: *Diarrhea, anorexia,* nausea, dyspepsia, abdominal pain, constipation, dry mouth, pancreatitis

GU: Breast pain, dysmenorrhea, menstrual disorder

INTEG: Rash, alopecia

MISC: Weight loss, leukopenia, metabolic acidosis, increased body temperature, unexplained death (epilepsy)

RESP: Upper respiratory tract infection, pharyngitis, sinusitis

INTERACTIONS
Individual drugs

Alcohol: increased CNS depression

Amitriptyline: increased effect of amitriptyline

CarBAMazepine, phenytoin, probenecid: decreased levels of topiramate

Digoxin: decreased levels of digoxin

Estrogen: decreased levels of estrogen

Hydrochlorothiazide, lamoTRIgine, metformin: increased topiramate levels

Lithium: decreased levels of lithium

RisperiDONE: decreased levels of risperidone

Valproic acid: decreased levels of both products

Drug classifications

Carbonic anhydrase inhibitors: increased kidney stone formation

CNS depressants: increased CNS depression

hormonal contraceptives: decreased level of oral contraceptives

NURSING CONSIDERATIONS
Assessment

• **Bipolar disorder:** assess mood, behavior, activity

• **Assess mental status:** mood, sensorium, affect, memory (long, short), especially in geriatric; suicidal thoughts/behavior

• Assess for blood dyscrasias: fever, sore throat, bruising, rash, jaundice, epistaxis (long-term treatment only)

• **Assess seizure activity** including type, location, duration, and character; provide seizure precaution

• Monitor CBC during long-term therapy; serum bicarbonate

• Assess body weight, perception of body image, eating disorders may occur or be exacerbated especially in adolescents; and evidence of cognitive disorder

• **Beers:** Avoid in older adults unless safer alternative is not available, may cause ataxia, impaired psychomotor function

- **Pregnancy/breastfeeding:** Use only if benefits outweigh fetal risk, birth defects have occurred, pregnant patients should register with the Antiepileptic Drug Pregnancy Registry 888-233-2334, may decrease hormonal contraceptives, caution use in breastfeeding, excretion unknown

Patient problem
Pain (uses)
Distorted thinking process (uses)
Risk for injury (uses, adverse reactions)

Implementation
- Do not break, crush, or chew tabs; very bitter
- May take without regard to meals
- Sprinkle cap can be given whole or opened and sprinkled on soft food; do not chew, drink water after sprinkle
- Store at room temp away from heat, light
Trokendi XR: swallow whole; do not sprinkle on food, crush, chew; not recommended for child <6 yr
Qudexy XR: may swallow whole or sprinkle on food (teaspoon); swallow immediately; do not crush, chew

Patient/family education
- Teach patient to carry/wear emergency ID stating name, products taken, condition, prescriber's name and phone number
- Advise patient to avoid driving, other activities that require alertness, until response is known
- Teach patient not to discontinue medication abruptly after long-term use, do not restart if several doses are missed without close supervision, to follow prescriber's directions closely
- Advise patient to use nonhormonal contraceptive; effect of oral contraceptives is decreased, pregnancy
- Teach patient to drink plenty of fluids to prevent kidney stones, vision loss may occur
- Teach patient that increased dietary intake might be necessary, weight loss may occur
- Teach patient to swallow extended-release product whole
- Teach patient minor hair loss may occur, report to provider if severe

Evaluation

Positive therapeutic outcome
- Decreased seizure activity

TREATMENT OF OVERDOSE:
Lavage, VS

⚠ HIGH ALERT

topotecan (Rx)
(to-poe'ti-kan)
Hycamtin
Func. class: Antineoplastic natural;
topoisomerase inhibitor
Chem. class: Camptothecin analog

ACTION: Antitumor product with topoisomerase I–inhibitory activity; topoisomerase I relieves torsional strain in DNA by causing single-strand breaks; causes double-strand DNA damage

Therapeutic outcome: Decreased tumor size

USES: Metastatic ovarian cancer after failure of traditional chemotherapy, relapsed small cell lung cancer, cervical cancer

Pharmacokinetics

Absorption	Rapidly, completely absorbed
Distribution	7%-35% protein binding
Metabolism	Liver
Excretion	Urine, feces to metabolites
Half-life	2.8 hr

Pharmacodynamics

	IV	PO
Onset	Unknown	Unknown
Peak	Unknown	1-2 hr
Duration	Unknown	Unknown

CONTRAINDICATIONS
Pregnancy, breastfeeding, hypersensitivity, severe bone marrow depression

BLACK BOX WARNING: Neutropenia, bone marrow supression

Precautions: Children, renal disease, gelatin hypersensitivity, anemia, contraceptive requirements, dehydration, diarrhea, extravasation, herpes, infertility, neutropenia, pulmonary fibrosis, varicella

DOSAGE AND ROUTES
Metastatic carcinoma of the ovary
Adult: IV INF 1.5 mg/m^2 over 30 min/day × 5 days starting on day 1 of a 21-day course × 4 courses; may be reduced to 0.25 mg/m^2 for subsequent courses if severe neutropenia occurs

---

Cervical cancer unresponsive to surgery or radiation
Adult: IV infusion 0.75 mg/m^2 on days 1, 2, 3 then 50 mg/m^2 CISplatin IV on day 1 then repeat q21day, adjust for toxicity

Relapsed small-cell lung cancer (SCLC)
Adult: PO 2.3 mg/m^2/day on days 1-5 of a 21-day course

Therapeutic drug monitoring
Dosage adjustments for treatment-related toxicities:
Hematologic toxicity: Do not administer subsequent courses until neutrophils recover to >1000 cells/mm^3, platelets to >100,000 cells/mm^3, and hemoglobin to >9 g/dl
Neutropenia:
• *Single agent (IV) (ANC <500 cells/mm^3):* Reduce the dose of topotecan to 1.25 mg/m^2. Alternatively, granulocyte-colony stimulating factor (G-CSF) may be administered, starting at least 24 hr after the last dose of topotecan
• *Single agent (oral) (ANC <500 cells/mm^3 for ≥7 days, or ANC 500-1000 cells/mm^3 lasting beyond day 21):* Reduce the dose of topotecan to 1.9 mg/m^2/day, with subsequent dose reductions by 0.4 mg/m^2/day if necessary
Thrombocytopenia:
• *Single agent (IV) (platelets <25,000 cells/mm^3 in the previous cycle):* Reduce dose to 1.25 mg/m^2
• *Single agent (oral) (platelets <25,000 cells/mm^3):* Reduce dose to 1.9 mg/m^2/day, with subsequent dose reductions by 0.4 mg/m^2/day if necessary
• *In combination with cisplatin (IV) (platelets <25,000 cells/mm^3 in the previous cycle):* Reduce dose to 0.6 mg/m^2 and further to 0.45 mg/m^2 if necessary
Neutropenic fever:
• *Single agent (oral) (ANC <500 cells/mm^3 associated with fever or infection):* Reduce to 1.9 mg/m^2/day, with subsequent dose reductions by 0.4 mg/m^2/day if necessary
• *In combination with cisplatin (IV) (ANC <1000 cells/mm^3 with temperature ≥ 38° C or 100.4° F):* Reduce dose to 0.6 mg/m^2 and further to 0.45 mg/m^2 if necessary. Alternatively, G-CSF may be given, starting at least 24 hr after the last dose
Diarrhea (grade 3 or 4):
• *Single agent (oral):* Hold, when diarrhea resolves to grade ≤1, resume at 1.9 mg/m^2/day, with subsequent dose reductions by 0.4 mg/m^2/day if necessary

Renal dose
Adult: PO: CCr: 50-80ml/min No change; **CCr 30-49 ml/min:** Reduce dose to 1.5 mg/m^2/day; dose may be increased by 0.4 mg/m^2/day after the first course if no severe hematologic or gastrointestinal toxicities occur; **CCr <30 ml/min:** Reduce dose to 0.6 mg/m^2/day; dose may be increased by 0.4 mg/m^2/day after the first course if no severe hematologic or gastrointestinal toxicities occur

Adult: IV: CCr 40-60 ml/min: No change; **CCr 20-39 ml/min:** Reduce dose to 0.75 mg/m^2; **CCr <20 ml/min:** unknown

Available forms: Lyophilized powder for inj 4 mg; cap 0.25, 1 mg

ADVERSE EFFECTS
CNS: Arthralgia, *asthenia, headache,* myalgia, *pain,* weakness
GI: *Abdominal pain, constipation,* diarrhea, obstruction, *nausea,* stomatitis, *vomiting,* increased ALT, AST, anorexia
HEMA: Neutropenia, leukopenia, thrombocytopenia, anemia, sepsis
INTEG: *Total alopecia*
RESP: Dyspnea, cough, interstitial lung disease

INTERACTIONS
Individual drugs
CISplatin: increased myelosuppression
Itraconazole, mefloquine, niCARdipine, quiNIDine, RU-486, tamoxifen, testosterone, verapamil: avoid giving together

Drug classifications
Anticoagulants, NSAIDs, platelet inhibitors, thrombolytics: increased bleeding risk
P-glycoprotein, breast cancer resistance protein inhibitors (amiodarone, clarithromycin, diltiazem, erythromycin, indinavir vaccines, toxoids: avoid using together

Drug/food
Grapefruit juice: avoid use

NURSING CONSIDERATIONS
Assessment
• Monitor liver function tests: AST, ALT, alkaline phosphatase, which may be elevated; creatinine, BUN

BLACK BOX WARNING: Bone marrow suppression: Monitor CBC, differential, platelet count weekly; withhold product if WBC is <3500/mm^3 or platelet count is <100,000/mm^3; notify prescriber of these results; product should be discontinued

---

• Assess buccal cavity for dryness, sores or ulceration, white patches, oral pain, bleeding, dysphagia

• **Interstitial lung disease (ILD):** assess for fever, cough, dyspnea, hypoxia, may be fatal
• **Pregnancy/breastfeeding:** Do not use in pregnancy or breastfeeding, can cause fetal harm, use contraception during and for $\geq$ 1 mo after final dose (female), during and for 3 mo after final dose (males), may cause infertility in both males/females

Patient problem

Risk for infection (adverse reactions)
Risk for injury (uses, adverse reactions)

Implementation

• Provide increased fluid intake to 2-3 L/day to prevent dehydration, unless contraindicated
• Change **IV** site q48hr
• Store caps in refrigerator; IV INF unopened at room temperature; protect both from light

Intermittent IV infusion route

• Visually inspect for particulate matter and discoloration prior to use
• Reconstitute each 4-mg vial with 4 ml sterile water for injection; use immediately, no preservative
• Withdraw the appropriate volume of the reconstituted solution; dilute further in 0.9% NaCl or D_5W prior to administration
• The reconstituted solution is yellow or yellow-green
• Topotecan injection diluted for infusion is stable at room temperature with normal light for 24 hr
• Infuse over 30 min

Patient/family education

• Advise patient to avoid foods with citric acid or hot flavor or rough texture if stomatitis is present; to drink adequate fluids
• Advise patient that total alopecia may occur; hair grows back but may be different in color and texture
• Advise patient to report stomatitis; any bleeding, white spots, ulcerations in mouth; tell patient to examine mouth daily; report symptoms

BLACK BOX WARNING: Teach patient to report signs of anemia; fatigue, headache, faintness, shortness of breath, irritability

• Teach patient to rinse mouth tid-qid with water, club soda; brush teeth bid-tid with soft brush or cotton-tipped applicator for stomatitis; use unwaxed dental floss
• Advise patient to avoid OTC products without approval of prescriber
• Advise to avoid driving or other activities requiring alertness
• Advise to avoid vaccines, toxoids
• Teach patient not to crush or chew capsules

• Advise patient not to retake dose if vomiting occurs, notify provider
• Teach patient to use effective contraception during treatment and at least 1 mo after; males should use contraception during and for 3 mo after final dose; not to breastfeed

Evaluation

Positive therapeutic outcome

• Decreased tumor size, spread of malignancy

---

torsemide (Rx)
(tor' suh-mide)
Demadex
Func. class.: Loop diuretic
Chem. class.: Sulfonamide derivative

ACTION: Acts on loop of Henle by inhibiting absorption of chloride, sodium, water

USES: Treatment of hypertension and edema with HF, ascites

Pharmacokinetics

Absorption	Rapidly absorbed; duration 6 hr
Distribution	Excreted in breast milk; crosses placenta; protein binding 97%-98%
Metabolism	Liver
Excretion	Urine 20%
Half-life	3.5 hr

Pharmacodynamics

Onset	1 hr
Peak	1-2 hr
Duration	6-8 hr

CONTRAINDICATIONS: Infants, hypersensitivity to sulfonamides, anuria

Precautions: Pregnancy, breastfeeding, diabetes mellitus, dehydration, severe renal disease, electrolyte depletion, hypovolemia, syncope, ventricular dysrhythmias

DOSAGE AND ROUTES
HF diuresis
Adult: PO 10-20 mg/day, may increase as needed, max 200 mg/day

Diuresis in chronic renal failure
Adult: PO 20 mg/day, may increase to 200 mg/day

Hepatic cirrhosis
Adult: PO 5-10 mg/day, may increase as needed, max 40 mg/day

Hypertension

Adult: **PO** 5 mg/day, may increase to 10 mg/day

Available forms: Tabs 5, 10, 20, 100 mg

SIDE EFFECTS

CNS: Headache, dizziness, asthenia, insomnia, nervousness

CV: Orthostatic hypotension, chest pain, ECG changes, circulatory collapse, ventricular tachycardia, edema

EENT: *Loss of hearing*, ear pain, tinnitus, blurred vision

ELECT: *Hypokalemia, hypochloremic alkalosis, hyponatremia*, metabolic alkalosis

ENDO: *Hyperglycemia, hyperuricemia*

GI: *Nausea*, diarrhea, dyspepsia, cramps, constipation

GU: *Polyuria*, renal failure, glycosuria

INTEG: *Rash*, photosensitivity, pruritus

MS: Cramps, stiffness

RESP: Rhinitis, cough increase

INTERACTIONS
Individual drugs

CISplatin, vancomycin; cautious use— **increase:** ototoxicity

Lithium, digoxin— **increase:** toxicity

Indomethacin, carBAMazepine, PHENobarbital, phenytoin, rifAMPin— **decrease:** antihypertensive effect of torsemide

Drug classifications

Nondepolarizing skeletal muscle relaxants— **increase:** toxicity

Antihypertensives, oral anticoagulants, nitrates; cautious use— **increase:** action of each

Aminoglycosides cautious use— **increase:** ototoxicity antidiabetics; monitor blood glucose levels often— **decrease:** hypoglycemic effect

NSAIDs— **decrease:** antihypertensive effect of torsemide

Drug/herb

• Severe photosensitivity: St. John's wort

Drug/lab test

Increase: BUN, creatinine, uric acid, blood glucose, cholesterol

Decrease: potassium, magnesium, chloride sodium

NURSING CONSIDERATIONS
Assessment:

• **Heart failure**: Monitor B/P lying, standing; postural hypotension may occur; weight, I&O daily to determine fluid loss; effect of product may be decreased if used daily

• Monitor hearing when giving high doses

• **Sulfa allergy:** determine before using product

• Electrolytes: monitor potassium, sodium, chlorine; include blood glucose, CBC, blood pH, ABGs, uric acid; calcium, magnesium, potassium supplements may be required

• Monitor blood glucose of diabetic patients, glycosuria

• Renal failure: monitor urinalysis, BUN, CCr

• **Hyperuricemia:** Monitor for exacerbation of gout

• **Metabolic alkalosis:** Assess for drowsiness, restlessness

• **Hypokalemia:** Monitor for postural hypotension, malaise, fatigue, tachycardia, leg cramps, weakness

• Assess for rashes, temperature elevation daily

• Assess for confusion, especially in geriatric patients; take safety precautions if needed

• **Beers:** use with caution in older adults; may exacerbate or cause SIADH or hyponatremia; monitor sodium levels frequently

Patient problem

Fluid imbalance (uses)

Implementation
PO route

• Give in AM to avoid interference with sleep if using product as diuretic

• Give with food or milk if nausea occurs; absorption may be decreased slightly

Patient/family education:

• Teach patient to rise slowly from lying, sitting position

• Teach patient to recognize adverse reactions: muscle cramps, weakness, nausea, dizziness, tinnitus

• Advise patient to take with food or milk for GI symptoms; to limit alcohol use

• Advise patient to take early during the day to prevent nocturia

• Inform patient to use sunscreen, protective clothing to prevent sunburn

• Teach patient to notify prescriber if pregnancy is planned or suspected or if breastfeeding

• Advise patient to report tinnitus immediately; may indicate toxicity

• Teach patient not to use any OTC medications, herbal products before approved by prescriber

Evaluation:

Therapeutic response: Improvement in edema of feet, legs, sacral area daily if medication is being used with HF

TREATMENT OF OVERDOSE:

Lavage if taken orally; monitor electrolytes; administer dextrose in saline; monitor hydration, CV, renal status

---

A HIGH ALERT

traMADol (Rx)

(trah'mah-dol)

ConZip, Durela ✦, Raliva ✦, Tridural ✦, Ultram, Ultram ER, Zytram ✦

Func. class.: Analgesic, miscellaneous

Controlled Substance IV

Do not confuse: traMADol/traZODone Ultram/lithium

ACTION: Binds to μ-opioid receptors and inhibits reuptake of norepinephrine, serotonin

Therapeutic outcome: Relief of pain

USES: Management of moderate to severe pain, chronic pain, headache, osteoarthritis

Pharmacokinetics

Absorption	Rapidly, almost completely absorbed
Distribution	Steady state 2 days
Metabolism	Extensively in liver, may cross blood-brain barrier
Excretion	Unchanged product 30% in urine, protein binding 20%
Half-life	6-7 hr; ext rel 8-10 hr

Pharmacodynamics

	PO	Ext rel
Onset	1 hr	Unknown
Peak	2 hr	10-12 hr
Duration	Unknown	Unknown

CONTRAINDICATIONS

Hypersensitivity, acute intoxication with any CNS depressant, alcohol, asthma, children, adenoidectomy, GI obstruction, ileus, MAOIs

BLACK BOX WARNING: Respiratory depression

Precautions: Pregnancy, breastfeeding, children, geriatric, seizure disorder, renal/hepatic disease, head trauma, increased ICP, acute abdominal condition, product abuse, depression, suicidal ideation, abrupt discontinuation, constipation

BLACK BOX WARNING: Coadministration with other CNS depressants, neonatal opioid withdrawal syndrome

DOSAGE AND ROUTES
Mild to moderate pain

Adult: PO 25 mg qd, titrate by 25 mg ≥3 days to 100 mg/day (25 mg qid), then may increase by 50 mg ≥3 days to 200 mg (50 mg qid), then 50-100 mg q4-6hr, max 400 mg/day; use caution in elderly

Geriatric >75 yr: PO <300 mg/day in divided dose

Hepatic dose
Adult: PO 50 mg q12hr

Renal dose
Adult (Child-Pugh C): PO CCr <30 ml/min q12hr, max 200 mg/day; do not use ext rel tabs

Moderate to severe chronic pain
Adult: PO-ER (Ultram ER) 100 mg daily, titrate upward q5day by 100 mg, max 300 mg/day; (Ryzolt) 100 mg, titrate upward q2-3day in 100 mg increments; max 300 mg/day; products are not interchangeable

Available forms: Tabs 50 mg; ext rel tab 100, 200, 300 mg; orally disintegrating tab 50 mg

ADVERSE EFFECTS

CNS: Dizziness, CNS stimulation, somnolence, headache, anxiety, confusion, euphoria, seizures, hallucinations, sedation, neuroleptic malignant syndrome–like reactions

CV: Vasodilatation, orthostatic hypotension, tachycardia, hypertension, abnormal ECG

EENT: Visual disturbances

GI: Nausea, constipation, vomiting, dry mouth, diarrhea, abdominal pain, anorexia, flatulence, GI bleeding

GU: Urinary retention/frequency, menopausal symptoms, dysuria, menstrual disorder

INTEG: Pruritus, rash, urticaria, vesicles, flushing

SYST: Anaphylaxis, Stevens-Johnson syndrome, toxic epidermal necrolysis, serotonin syndrome

INTERACTIONS
Individual drugs

BLACK BOX WARNING: Alcohol: increased CNS depression

CarBAMazepine: decreased tramadol level

Drug classifications

CYP3A4 inducers (barbiturates, bosentan, carBAMazepine, efavirenz, nevirapine, phenytoin, rifabutin, rifampin): decreased tramadol effect

CYP3A4 inhibitors (aprepitant, antiretroviral protease inhibitors, clarithromycin, danazol, delavirdine, diltiazem, erythromycin, fluconazole, FLUoxetine, fluvoxaMINE, imatinib, ketoconazole, mibefradil, nefazodone, telithromycin, voriconazole): increased traMADol levels

T

MAOIs: inhibition of norepinephrine and serotonin reuptake; use together with caution

Opiates, sedative/hypnotics: increased CNS depression

SSRIs, SNRIs, serotonin-receptor agonists: increased serotonin syndrome

Drug/herb

Chamomile, hops, kava, skullcap, valerian: increased CNS depression

St. John's wort: avoid use

Drug/lab test

Increased: creatinine, liver enzymes

Decreased: Hgb

NURSING CONSIDERATIONS

Assessment

• **Pain:** assess location, type, character; give before pain becomes extreme

• Assess for increased side effects in renal/hepatic disease

> **BLACK BOX WARNING: Respiratory depression:** withhold if respirations ,12/min, may be compounded with use of other CNS depressants

• Monitor I&O ratio: check for decreasing output; may indicate urinary retention

• Assess need for product

• Assess for constipation and bowel pattern; increase fluids, bulk in diet

• **Hypersensitivity:** usually after beginning treatment

• **Beers:** Avoid in older adults, lowers seizure threshold, monitor for seizures frequently in those with a seizure disorder

> **BLACK BOX WARNING:** Monitor CNS changes: dizziness, drowsiness, hallucinations, euphoria, LOC, pupil reaction

• Determine allergic reactions: rash, urticaria

• **Serotonin syndrome, neuroleptic malignant syndrome:** assess for increased heart rate, shivering, sweating, dilated pupils, tremors, high B/P, hyperthermia, headache, confusion; if these occur, stop product, administer a serotonin antagonist if needed

> **BLACK BOX WARNING: Neonatal opioid withdrawal syndrome:** Prolonged use of opioids in the mother may result in withdrawal effects in the neonate, can be fatal, assess for irritability, hyperactivity, abnormal sleep pattern, high-pitched cry, tremor, vomiting, diarrhea, failure to gain weight in the neonate

• **Pregnancy/breastfeeding:** Use only if benefits outweigh fetal risk, no well-controlled studies, do not use in labor/delivery, do not breastfeed

Patient problem

Pain (uses)

Risk of injury (adverse reactions)

Impaired breathing (adverse reactions)

Implementation

• Do not break, crush, or chew ext rel product

• Give with antiemetic for nausea, vomiting

• Administer when pain is beginning to return; determine dosage interval by patient response

• Store in cool environment, protect from sunlight

• Give with or without food; ext rel: always give with food, or always give on empty stomach

Patient/family education

• Before taking, to tell health care provider if history of head injury, seizures, liver, kidney, thyroid problems, problems urinating, pancreas or gallbladder problems, abuse of street or prescription drugs, alcohol addiction, or mental health problems

• To tell health care provider if pregnant or planning to become pregnant. Prolonged use during pregnancy can cause withdrawal symptoms in the newborn baby that could be life-threatening if not recognized and treated. Do not breastfeed

• Not to take prescription, OTC products, vitamins, or herbal supplements without health care provider's approval

• Do not change dose, take exactly as prescribed by health care provider. Do not take more than prescribed dose and do not take more than 8 tablets per day. If a dose is missed, take next dose at usual time

• Notify health care provider if the dose does not control pain

• Do not stop taking product abruptly if taking regularly without talking to health care provider

• Do not drive or operate heavy machinery until affect is known, product may cause dizziness or lightheadedness

• Do not drink alcohol or use prescription or OTC products that contain alcohol

• Notify health care provider of severe constipation, nausea, sleepiness, vomiting, tiredness, headache, dizziness, abdominal pain

• Get emergency medical help if there is trouble breathing, shortness of breath, fast heartbeat, chest pain, swelling of face, tongue, or throat, extreme drowsiness, lightheadedness when changing positions, feeling faint, agitation, high body temperature, trouble walking, stiff muscles, or mental changes such as confusion

Evaluation

Positive therapeutic outcome

• Decreased pain

trandolapril (Rx)

(tran-doe′la-prill)
Mavik
Func. class.: Antihypertensive
Chem. class.: Angiotensin-converting
enzyme (ACE) inhibitor

ACTION: Selectively suppresses renin-
angiotensin-aldosterone system; inhibits ACE;
prevents conversion of angiotensin I to angiotensin II, resulting in dilatation of arterial and
venous vessels and lowered B/P

Therapeutic outcome: Decreased B/P in
hypertension

USES: Hypertension alone or in combination,
heart failure, after MI, LV dysfunction after MI

Pharmacokinetics

Absorption	40%-60%
Distribution	Unknown
Metabolism	Liver
Excretion	Kidneys (33%), feces (66%)
Half-life	0.6-1.1 hr, 16-24 hr

Pharmacodynamics

Onset	½ hr
Peak	4-10 hr
Duration	>8 days

CONTRAINDICATIONS

Breastfeeding, hypersensitivity, history of angioedema

> **BLACK BOX WARNING:** Pregnancy

Precautions: Geriatric, hyperkalemia, hepatic disease, bilateral renal stenosis, after
kidney transplant, aortal/mitral valve stenosis,
cirrhosis, severe renal disease, untreated HF,
autoimmune diseases, cough

DOSAGE AND ROUTES
Hypertension

Adult: PO 1 mg/day, 2 mg/day in African
Americans, make dosage adjustment ≥1 wk; up
to 8 mg/day

Heart failure (after MI/left ventricular dysfunction)

Adult: PO 1 mg/day, titrate upward to 4 mg/day
if tolerated, for 2-4 yr

Renal dose/hepatic dose

Adult: PO CCr <30 ml/min or hepatic disease 0.5 mg/day

Available forms: Tabs 1, 2, 4 mg

ADVERSE EFFECTS

CNS: *Dizziness,* paresthesias, headache, *syn-
cope,* fatigue, drowsiness, depression, sleep dis-
turbances, anxiety, syncope
CV: *Hypotension,* MI, palpitations, angina,
TIAs, stroke, bradycardia, dysrhythmias
GI: Nausea, vomiting, cramps, diarrhea, consti-
pation, pancreatitis, *dyspepsia*
GU: Proteinuria, renal failure
HEMA: Agranulocytosis, neutropenia, leu-
kopenia, anemia
INTEG: Rash, purpura, pruritus, angioedema
MISC: Hyperkalemia, hyponatremia, impo-
tence, *myalgia,* angioedema, muscle cramps,
asthenia, hypocalcemia, gout
RESP: Dyspnea, cough

INTERACTIONS
Individual drugs

Levodopa, lithium, reserpine: increased effect of
each specific product

Drug classifications

Antacids, NSAIDs, salicylates: decreased effect of
trandolapril
Antihypertensives, diuretics: increased severe
hypotension
Barbiturates, ergots, hypoglycemics, neuromuscular blocking agents: increased effects of
each specific product
Diuretics (potassium-sparing): increased potassium levels
Phenothiazines: increased antihypertensive
effects
Potassium supplements: increased potassium
levels
Salt substitutes: increased potassium levels

Drug/lab test

Increased: potassium, LFTs, BUN, creatinine
Decreased: sodium, WBC

NURSING CONSIDERATIONS
Assessment

• Monitor blood tests: neutrophils, decreased
platelets
• Monitor B/P, orthostatic hypotension,
syncope; if changes occur dosage change may
be required
• Monitor renal studies: protein, BUN, creatinine; increased levels may indicate nephrotic
syndrome and renal failure
• Monitor renal symptoms: polyuria, oliguria,
frequency, dysuria
• Establish baselines in renal, liver function
tests before therapy begins
• Check potassium levels throughout treatment,
although hyperkalemia rarely occurs
• Check for edema in feet, legs daily

T

• Assess for allergic reactions: rash, fever, pruritus, urticaria; product should be discontinued if antihistamines fail to help

> **BLACK BOX WARNING:** Pregnancy: Identify if pregnancy is planned or suspected; pregnancy

• **Hepatotoxicity (rare):** assess for increased LFTs, jaundice, fulminating hepatic necrosis; if jaundice occurs, discontinue product
• **Angioedema:** of the face, edema of the extremities, mucus membranes, may need to discontinue
• **Hyperkalemia:** monitor electrolytes, check potassium

Patient problem
Risk for injury (uses, adverse reactions)
Nonadherence (teaching)

Implementation
• Store in airtight container at ≤77° F (≤25° C) or less
• Give without regard to food
• Space antacids by 2 hr after dose

Patient/family education
• Advise patient not to discontinue product abruptly; advise patient to tell all persons associated with health care
• Teach patient not to use OTC products (cough, cold, allergy) unless directed by physician; serious side effects can occur; xanthines, such as coffee, tea, chocolate, cola, can prevent action of product
• Instruct patient on the importance of complying with dosage schedule, even if feeling better; to continue with medical regimen to decrease B/P: exercise, cessation of smoking, decreasing stress, diet modifications
• Emphasize the need to rise slowly to sitting or standing position to minimize orthostatic hypotension; not to exercise in hot weather, which can cause increased hypotension
• Advise patient to notify prescriber of mouth sores, sore throat, fever, swelling of hands or feet, irregular heartbeat, chest pain, coughing, shortness of breath
• Caution patient to report excessive perspiration, dehydration, vomiting, diarrhea; may lead to fall in B/P
• Caution patient that product may cause dizziness, fainting, light-headedness; may occur during 1st few days of therapy; to avoid activities that may be hazardous
• Teach patient how to take B/P and normal readings for age group

> **BLACK BOX WARNING:** Teach patient to notify prescriber if pregnancy is suspected or planned, pregnancy

Evaluation
Positive therapeutic outcome
• Decreased B/P in hypertension

TREATMENT OF OVERDOSE:
Lavage, **IV** atropine for bradycardia, **IV** theophylline for bronchospasm, digoxin, O₂, diuretic for cardiac failure, hemodialysis

---

> **⚠ HIGH ALERT**
>
> ### trastuzumab (Rx)
> (tras-tuz′uh-mab)
> **Herceptin**
> *Func. class.:* Antineoplastic—miscellaneous
> *Chem. class.:* Humanized monoclonal antibody

ACTION: DNA-derived monoclonal antibody selectively binds to extracellular portion of human epidermal growth factor receptor 2 (HER2); it inhibits proliferation of cancer cells

Therapeutic outcome: Decreasing symptoms of breast cancer

USES: Metastatic breast cancer with overexpression of ⟐ HER2, early breast cancer (adjuvant, neoadjuvant), gastric cancer; previously untreated HER2 overexpressing metastatic gastric or gastroesophageal junction adenocarcinoma with CISplatin, 5-fluorouracil or capecitabine

Pharmacokinetics

Absorption	Unknown
Distribution	Unknown
Metabolism	Unknown
Excretion	Unknown
Half-life	1-32 days, 97% of washout by 7 mo after end of treatment

Pharmacodynamics
Unknown

CONTRAINDICATIONS
Hypersensitivity to this product, Chinese hamster ovary cell protein

Precautions: Breastfeeding, children, geriatric, pulmonary disease, anemia, leukopenia

---

BLACK BOX WARNING: Cardiac disease, respiratory distress syndrome, respiratory insufficiency, infusion-related reactions, cardiomyopathy, pregnancy, pulmonary toxicity, contraception requirement

DOSAGE AND ROUTES
For adjuvant treatment of breast cancer
Adult: IV 4 mg/kg over 90 min on day 1, then 2 mg/kg over 30 min qwk for a total of 12 wk, with PACLitaxel (either 80 mg/m² IV wk or 175 mg/m² q3wk) beginning on day 1 for a total of 4 cycles (12 wk). On week 13, begin trastuzumab 6 mg/kg over 30 to 90 min q3wk as monotherapy for a total of 52 wk of trastuzumab therapy; begin PACLitaxel plus trastuzumab after the completion of 4 cycles of AC chemotherapy (DOXOrubicin 60 mg/m² IV and cyclophosphamide 600 mg/m² IV q21days)

Metastatic breast cancer
Adult: IV 4 mg/kg IV over 90 min on day 1, then 2 mg/kg over 30 min qwk (total of 12 wk), with docetaxel 100 mg/m² IV q21days beginning on day 1 for a total of 4 cycles (12 wk). On week 13, begin trastuzumab 6 mg/kg IV over 30 to 90 min q3wk as monotherapy for a total of 52 wk of trastuzumab therapy. Begin docetaxel plus trastuzumab after the completion of 4 cycles of AC chemotherapy (DOXOrubicin 60 mg/m² IV and cyclophosphamide 600 mg/m² IV q21days)

Metastatic gastric cancer
Adult: IV 8 mg/kg, then 6 mg/kg q 3 wk until disease progression

Therapeutic drug monitoring
Dosage adjustments for cardiotoxicity
• *First, second, or third occurrence, ≥16% absolute decrease in left ventricular ejection fraction (LVEF) from baseline, or LVEF below institutional limit of normal with ≥10% absolute decrease in LVEF from baseline:* Hold for 4 to 8 wk and monitor ejection fraction with a MUGA scan or echocardiogram q4wk. If LVEF returns to normal limits with an absolute decrease from baseline of ≤15% within 4-8 weeks, resume, if decrease in LVEF persists >8 wk, permanently discontinue
• *Fourth occurrence, ≥16% absolute decrease in left ventricular ejection fraction (LVEF) from baseline, or LVEF below institutional limit of normal with ≥10% absolute decrease in LVEF from baseline:* Permanently discontinue

Available forms: Lyophilized powder 150, 440 mg

ADVERSE EFFECTS
CNS: *Dizziness, numbness, paresthesias,* depression, *insomnia,* neuropathy, peripheral neuritis
CV: Tachycardia, HF
GI: Nausea, vomiting, *anorexia, diarrhea,* abdominal pain, hepatotoxicity, dysgeusia
HEMA: *Anemia,* leukopenia
INTEG: *Rash,* acne, herpes simplex
META: Edema, peripheral edema
MISC: *Flulike symptoms; fever, headache, chills*
MS: Arthralgia, *bone pain*
RESP: *Cough, dyspnea, pharyngitis, rhinitis,* sinusitis, pneumonia, pulmonary edema/fibrosis, acute respiratory distress syndrome (ARDS)
SYST: Anaphylaxis, angioedema

INTERACTIONS
Individual drugs
Cyclophosphamide: increased cardiomyopathy risk; avoid use
Warfarin: increased bleeding risk

Drug classifications
Anthracyclines: increased cardiomyopathy risk
Vaccines/toxoids: decreased immune response

Drug/lab
Decrease: WBC, RBC

NURSING CONSIDERATIONS
Assessment
• Monitor CBC, HER2 overexpression
• Assess for symptoms of infection; may be masked by product
• Assess CNS reaction: LOC, mental status, dizziness, confusion

BLACK BOX WARNING: HF and other cardiac symptoms: assess for dyspnea, coughing, gallop; obtain a full cardiac workup including before and q3mo during treatment and q6mo for ≥ 2 yr after adjuvant treatment (LVEF, MUGA, or ECHO, monitor for clinical deterioration in those with decreased LEVF)

• Hypersensitivity reactions, anaphylaxis

BLACK BOX WARNING: Potentially fatal infusion reactions: assess for fever, chills, nausea, vomiting, pain, headache, dizziness, hypotension; discontinue product

• **Pulmonary toxicity:** assess for dyspnea, interstitial pneumonitis, pulmonary hypertension, ARDS; can occur after infusion reaction, those with lung disease may have more severe toxicity
• **Benzyl alcohol hypersensitivity:** reconstitute with sterile water for injection, USP. Discard any unused portion

• **Hamster protein hypersensitivity (Chinese hamster ovary cell hypersensitivity):** Assess for hypersensitivity due to increased risk of severe allergic reactions

BLACK BOX WARNING: Pregnancy/breast-feeding: Fetal harm may occur if given during pregnancy or within 7 mo of conception; monitoring for oligohydramnios is recommended. If oligohydramnios occurs, fetal testing should be done that is appropriate for gestational age. Encourage these women to enroll in the MotHER Pregnancy Registry by contacting 800-690-6720 or visiting http://www.motherpregnancyregistry.com. Counsel patients about the reproductive risk and contraception requirements during trastuzumab treatment. Trastuzumab can be teratogenic if taken by the mother during pregnancy or within 7 mo before conception. Effective contraception should be used during and for at least 7 mo after treatment. Females of reproductive potential should undergo pregnancy testing before use. Women who become pregnant while receiving or within 7 mo of the last dose should be apprised of the potential hazard to the fetus. It is not known whether the product is excreted into human milk, advise women to discontinue breastfeeding during treatment and for 7 mo after the last dose

Patient problem
Risk for infection (adverse reactions)
Diarrhea (adverse reactions)
Risk for injury (uses, adverse reactions)

Implementation
• Give acetaminophen as ordered to alleviate fever and headache
• Increase fluid intake to 2-3 L/day

Intermittent IV infusion route
• Use cytotoxic handling procedures, avoid treatment over 1 yr
• Administer after reconstituting vial with 20 ml of bacteriostatic water for inj, 1.1% benzyl alcohol preserved (supplied) to yield 21 mg/ml, mark date on vial 28 days from reconstitution date; if patient is allergic to benzyl alcohol, reconstitute with sterile water for inj; use immediately; inf over 90 min; q3wk give 8 mg/kg loading dose over 90 min; subsequent doses 6 mg/kg may be given over 30-60 min
• Do not mix or dilute with other products or dextrose sol

Patient/family education
• Advise patient to take acetaminophen for fever
• Teach patient to avoid hazardous tasks, since confusion, dizziness may occur

• Teach patient to report signs of infection: sore throat, fever, diarrhea, vomiting
• Inform patient that emotional lability is common; instruct patient to notify prescriber if severe or incapacitating

BLACK BOX WARNING: Teach patient to report pain at infusion site, usually with first dose

BLACK BOX WARNING: Cardiomyopathy: Teach patient to report cough, swelling in extremities, shortness of breath, may occur during or after completion of treatment

BLACK BOX WARNING: Advise patient to use contraception while taking this product or within 7 mo of pregnancy; not to breastfeed

Evaluation
Positive therapeutic outcome
• Decrease in size of tumors

travoprost ophthalmic
See Appendix B

traZODone (Rx)
(tray'zoe-done)
Oleptro ✦, **Trazorel** ✦
Func. class.: Antidepressant—miscellaneous
Chem. class.: Triazolopyridine

ACTION: Selectively inhibits serotonin, norepinephrine uptake by brain, potentiates behavioral changes

Therapeutic outcome: Decreased symptoms of depression after 2-3 wk

USES: Depression

Unlabeled uses: Insomnia, chronic pain, anxiety

Pharmacokinetics
Absorption	Well absorbed
Distribution	Widely distributed
Metabolism	Liver, extensively
Excretion	Kidneys, minimally unchanged
Half-life	4½-7½ hr

Pharmacodynamics
Onset	Unknown
Peak	1 hr without food, 2 hr with food
Duration	Unknown

CONTRAINDICATIONS
Hypersensitivity to tricyclics

Precautions: Pregnancy, suicidal patients, severe depression, increased intraocular pressure, closed-angle glaucoma, urinary retention, cardiac/hepatic disease, hyperthyroidism, electroshock therapy, elective surgery, bleeding, abrupt discontinuation, bipolar disorder, breastfeeding, dehydration, hyponatremia, hypovolemia, recovery phase of MI, seizure disorders, prostatic hypertrophy, family history of long QT

> **BLACK BOX WARNING:** Suicidal ideation in children/adolescents

DOSAGE AND ROUTES
Depression
Adult: PO 150 mg/day in divided doses; may increase by 50 mg/day q3-4day, max 400 mg/day (outpatient), 600 mg/day (inpatient); EXT REL 150 mg/day in the evening, may increase gradually by 75 mg/day at 3 day intervals, max 375 mg/day
Geriatric: PO 25-50 at bedtime, increase by 25-50 mg q3-7day to desired dose, usual 75-150 mg/day
Child 6-18 yr (unlabeled): PO 1.5-2 mg/kg/day in divided doses, may increase q3-4day up to 6 mg/kg/day or 400 mg/day in divided doses, whichever is less

Available forms: Tabs 50, 100, 150, 300 mg; ext rel tabs 150, 300 mg

ADVERSE EFFECTS
CNS: *Dizziness, drowsiness,* confusion, headache, anxiety, tremors, stimulation, weakness, insomnia, nightmares, EPS (geriatric), increase in psychiatric symptoms, suicide in children/adolescents
CV: *Orthostatic hypotension, ECG changes, tachycardia,* hypertension, palpitations
EENT: *Blurred vision,* tinnitus, mydriasis
GI: *Diarrhea, dry mouth,* nausea, vomiting, paralytic ileus, increased appetite, cramps, epigastric distress, jaundice, hepatitis, stomatitis, constipation
GU: *Retention,* acute renal failure, priapism
HEMA: Agranulocytosis, thrombocytopenia, eosinophilia, leukopenia
INTEG: Rash, urticaria, sweating, pruritus, photosensitivity

INTERACTIONS
Individual drugs
Alcohol, carBAMazepine, digoxin, phenytoin: increased effect of each product
FLUoxetine, nefazodone: increased levels, increased toxicity, serotonin syndrome
Guanethidine, cloNIDine: decreased effects of each product

Warfarin: increased or decreased effects of warfarin

Drug classifications
Barbiturates, benzodiazepines, CNS depressants: increased effects
CYP3A4, 2D6 inhibitors (phenothiazines, protease inhibitors, azole antifungals): increased effects of trazodone
MAOIs: increased hyperpyretic crisis, seizures, hypertensive episode, do not use within 14 days
SNRIs, SSRIs: increased toxicity, serotonin syndrome
Sympathomimetics (direct-acting): increased sympathomimetic effects
Sympathomimetics (indirect-acting): decreased effects

Drug/herb
Hops, kava, lavender, valerian: increased CNS depression
SAM-e, St. John's wort: increased serotonin syndrome

Drug/lab test
Increased: LFTs
Decreased: Hgb

NURSING CONSIDERATIONS
Assessment
• Monitor B/P (lying, standing), pulse q4hr; if systolic B/P drops 20 mm Hg hold product, notify prescriber; take vital signs q4hr in patients with CV disease
• Monitor blood tests: CBC, leukocytes, differential
• Monitor liver function tests: AST, ALT, bilirubin
• Check weight qwk; appetite may increase with product
• Assess ECG for flattening of T wave, bundle branch block, AV block, dysrhythmias in cardiac patients
• Assess for EPS primarily in geriatric: rigidity, dystonia, akathisia

> **BLACK BOX WARNING:** Assess mental status: mood, sensorium, affect, suicidal tendencies in children/adolescents; increase in psychiatric symptoms: depression, panic, not approved for children, if worsening depression occurs, product may need to be tapered as rapidly as possible without abrupt discontinuation

• Monitor urinary retention, constipation; constipation is more likely to occur in children or geriatric
• **Withdrawal symptoms:** assess for headache, nausea, vomiting, muscle pain, weakness;

do not usually occur unless product was discontinued abruptly
• Identify alcohol consumption; if alcohol is consumed, hold dose until AM
• **Serotonin syndrome, neuroleptic malignant syndrome:** assess for increased heart rate, shivering, sweating, dilated pupils, tremors, high B/P, hyperthermia, headache, confusion; if these occur, stop product, administer a serotonin antagonist if needed
• **Pregnancy/breastfeeding:** Use only if benefits outweigh fetal risk, no well-controlled studies, cautious use in breastfeeding, excreted in breast milk

Patient problem
Depression (uses)
Impaired sexual functioning (adverse reactions)

Implementation
• Give with food or milk for GI symptoms; crush if patient is unable to swallow medication whole
• Give dose at bedtime if oversedation occurs during day; may take entire dose at bedtime; geriatric may not tolerate once/day dosing
• Store in tight, light-resistant container at room temp; do not freeze

Patient/family education
• Teach patient that therapeutic effects may take 2-3 wk
• Teach patient to use caution in driving or other activities requiring alertness because of drowsiness, dizziness, blurred vision; to avoid rising quickly from sitting to standing, especially geriatric
• Teach patient not to crush, chew ext rel product
• Caution patient to avoid alcohol ingestion, other CNS depressants
• Teach patient not to discontinue medication quickly after long-term use: may cause nausea, headache, malaise
• Advise patient to wear sunscreen or large hat because photosensitivity occurs
• Teach patient to increase fluids, bulk in diet if constipation, urinary retention occur, especially geriatric
• Advise patient to take gum, hard sugarless candy, or frequent sips of water for dry mouth
• Advise patient to rise slowly to prevent dizziness

> **BLACK BOX WARNING:** Teach family to watch for suicidal ideation or tendencies, usually in children/adolescents, to notify provider if there is an increase in depression, agitation

• Teach patient to notify prescriber if pregnancy is planned or suspected, pregnancy, avoid breastfeeding

Evaluation
Positive therapeutic outcome
• Decrease in depression
• Absence of suicidal thoughts

TREATMENT OF OVERDOSE:
ECG monitoring, induce emesis, lavage, administer anticonvulsant

---

tretinoin (vitamin A acid, retinoic acid) (Rx)
(tret′i-noyn)
Avita, Renova, Retin-A, Retin-A Micro, Stieva-A ✤
Func. class.: Vitamin A acid/acne product, antineoplastic—miscellaneous
Chem. class.: Tretinoin derivative

ACTION: (Topical) Decreases cohesiveness of follicular epithelium, decreases microcomedone formation; (PO) induces maturation of acute promyelocytic leukemia, exact action is unknown

Therapeutic outcome: Decreased signs/symptoms of leukemia

USES: (Topical) Acne vulgaris (grades 1-3); (PO) acute promyelocytic leukemia, facial wrinkles, photoaging

Pharmacokinetics
Absorption	Small amounts
Distribution	Unknown
Metabolism	Unknown
Excretion	Kidneys
Half-life	Unknown

Pharmacodynamics
Unknown

CONTRAINDICATIONS
Hypersensitivity to retinoids or sensitivity to parabens

> **BLACK BOX WARNING:** Pregnancy

Precautions: Pregnancy (topical), breastfeeding, eczema, sunburn, sun exposure

> **BLACK BOX WARNING:** Rapid-evolving leukocytosis, respiratory compromise, acute promyelocytic leukemia differentiation syndrome, requires a specialized care setting, experienced clinician

DOSAGE AND ROUTES

Adult and child: TOP cleanse area, apply 0.025%-0.1% cream or 0.05% liquid at bedtime; cover lightly

Promyelocytic leukemia

Adult: PO 45 mg/m²/day given as 2 evenly divided doses until remission; discontinue treatment 30 days after remission or after 90 days of treatment, whichever is first

Available forms: Topical cream 0.01%, 0.02%, 0.025%, 0.05%, 0.1%; topical gel 0.025%, 0.04%, 0.05%, 0.1%; topical liquid 0.05%; caps 10 mg

ADVERSE EFFECTS

PO route

CNS: Headache, fever, sweating, fatigue
CV: Cardiac dysrhythmias, pericardial effusion
GI: Nausea, vomiting, *hemorrhage*, abdominal pain, diarrhea, constipation, dyspepsia, distention, *hepatitis*
META: Hypercholesterolemia, hypertriglyceridemia
RESP: Pneumonia, upper respiratory tract disease

Topical route

INTEG: Rash, stinging, warmth, redness, erythema, blistering, crusting, peeling, contact dermatitis, hypo/hyperpigmentation, dry skin, pruritus, scaly skin, retinoic acid syndrome (RAS)

INTERACTIONS

Individual drugs

Aminocaproic acid, aprotinin, tranexamic acid: increased thrombotic complications
Benzoyl peroxide, resorcinol, salicylic acid (topical), sulfur: increased peeling
Ketoconazole: increased plasma concentrations of tretinoin (oral)

Drug classifications

Alcohol, astringents, cleansers with drying effect, medicated, abrasive soaps: use with caution (topical)
Diuretics (thiazide), phenothiazines, quinolones, retinoids, sulfonamides, sulfonylureas: increased photosensitivity
Tetracyclines: increased ICP, risk of pseudotumor cerebri; do not use together

Drug/lab test

Increased: AST, ALT

NURSING CONSIDERATIONS

Assessment

Topical route
• Assess part of body involved, including time involved, what helps or aggravates condition, cysts, dryness, itching; lesions may become worse at beginning of treatment
PO route
• Monitor hepatic function, coagulation, hematologic parameters, also cholesterol, triglycerides
• **Pregnancy/breastfeeding:** Do not use in pregnancy/breastfeeding (PO)

Patient problem

Impaired skin integrity (uses)

Implementation

Topical route
• Apply using gloves or cotton, once daily before bedtime; cover area lightly using gauze
• Store at room temperature
• Wash hands after application
• Apply only to affected areas

Patient/family education

Topical route
• Instruct patient to avoid application on normal skin; to avoid getting cream in eyes, nose, other mucous membranes
• Advise patient to avoid sunlight, sunlamps or to use protective clothing or sunscreen to prevent burns
• Advise patient that treatment may cause warmth, stinging; dryness, peeling will occur
• Inform patient that cosmetics may be used over product; not to use shaving lotions
• Inform patient that rash may occur during first 1-3 wk of therapy
• Caution patient that product does not cure condition, only relieves symptoms; that therapeutic results may be seen in 2-3 wk but may not be optimal until after 6 wk
PO route

> **BLACK BOX WARNING:** Advise patient to report to prescriber if pregnancy is planned or suspected, pregnancy (PO)

Evaluation

Positive therapeutic outcome
• Decrease in size and number of lesions

T

tretinoin topical
See Appendix B

triamcinolone (Rx)
(trye-am-sin'oh-lone)
Aristospan, Kenalog-10, Kenalog-40, Tac-3, Tac-40, Triesence
Func. class.: Corticosteroid, synthetic; antiinflammatory
Chem. class.: Glucocorticoid, intermediate-acting

ACTION: Decreases inflammation by suppressing migration of polymorphonuclear leukocytes, fibroblasts, reversal of increased capillary permeability and lysosomal stabilization

Therapeutic outcome: Decreased inflammation, normal immune response

USES: Severe inflammation, immunosuppression, neoplasms, asthma (steroid dependent), collagen, respiratory, dermatologic disorders, rheumatic disorders

Pharmacokinetics

Absorption	Well absorbed (PO, IM)
Distribution	Crosses placenta, widely distributed
Metabolism	Liver, extensively
Excretion	Kidney, breast milk
Half-life	2-5 hr, adrenal suppression 3-4 days

Pharmacodynamics

	PO	IM	TOPICAL	INH	INTRANASAL
Onset	Unknown	Unknown	Min to hr	1-2 wk	Unknown
Peak	1-2 hr	1-2 hr	Hr to days	Unknown	2-3 wk
Duration	3 days	Unknown	Hr to days	Unknown	Unknown

CONTRAINDICATIONS
Hypersensitivity, neonatal prematurity, epidural/intrathecal administration (triamcinolone acetonide injections [Kenalog]), systemic fungal infections

Precautions: Pregnancy, breastfeeding, diabetes mellitus, glaucoma, osteoporosis, seizure disorders, ulcerative colitis, HF, myasthenia gravis, renal disease, esophagitis, peptic ulcer, acne, cataracts, coagulopathy, head trauma, children <2 yr, psychosis, idiopathic thrombocytopenia, acute glomerulonephritis, amebiasis, fungal infections, nonasthmatic bronchial disease, AIDS, TB, adrenal insufficiency, acute bronchospasm, acne rosacea, Cushing's syndrome, acute MI, thromboembolism

DOSAGE AND ROUTES
Adult: IM (acetonide) 40-80 mg q 4 wk; intraarticular (hexacetonide) 2-20 mg q 3-4 wk
Child: IM acetonide 40 mg q 4 wk or 30-200 mcg/kg (1-6.25 mg/m2) q 1-7 days

Available forms: Inj 10, 40 mg/ml acetonide; inj 5, 20 mg/ml hexacetonide
Inhalation route
• Use spacer device for geriatric
• Give inh with water to decrease possibility of fungal infections; titrated dose, use lowest effective dose

• Give after cleaning aerosol top daily with warm water, dry thoroughly
• Store in cool environment; do not puncture or incinerate container
Topical route
• Apply only to affected areas; do not get in eyes
• Apply medication, then cover with occlusive dressing (only if prescribed), seal to normal skin, change q12hr; systemic absorption may occur
• Apply only to dermatoses; do not use on weeping, denuded, or infected areas
• Cleanse skin before applying product
• Continue treatment for a few days after area has cleared
• Store at room temperature
Nasal route
• Have patient clear nasal passages before administration; use decongestant if needed; shake inhaler, invert, tilt head backward, insert nozzle into nostril, away from septum; hold other nostril closed and depress activator, inhale through nose, exhale through mouth

ADVERSE EFFECTS
CNS: *Depression,* headache, mood changes
CV: *Hypertension,* circulatory collapse, embolism, tachycardia, edema

EENT: Fungal infections, increased intraocular pressure, blurred vision
GI: *Diarrhea, nausea, abdominal distention,* GI hemorrhage, *increased appetite,* pancreatitis
HEMA: Thrombocytopenia
INTEG: Acne, poor wound healing, ecchymosis, petechiae
MS: Fractures, osteoporosis, weakness

INTERACTIONS
Individual drugs
Alcohol, amphotericin B, cycloSPORINE, digoxin, indomethacin, quinolones: increased side effects
Ambenonium, isoniazid, neostigmine, somatrem: decreased effects of each specific product
Cholestyramine, colestipol, ePHEDrine, phenytoin, rifampin, theophylline: decreased action of triamcinolone
Indomethacin, ketoconazole: increased action of triamcinolone

Drug classifications
Anticholinesterases, anticoagulants, anticonvulsants, antidiabetics, salicylates: decreased effects of each specific product
Antidiabetic agents: increased need for antidiabetic agents
Antiinfectives (macrolide), carBAMazepine, contraceptives (oral), estrogens, salicylates: increased action of triamcinolone
Barbiturates: decreased action of triamcinolone
Diuretics, salicylates: increased side effects
Toxoids, vaccines: decreased effects of toxoids, vaccines

Drug/herb
Aloe, cascara sagrada, senna: increased hypokalemia

Drug/lab test
Increased: cholesterol, sodium, blood glucose, uric acid, calcium, urine glucose
Decreased: calcium, potassium, T_4, T_3, thyroid ^{131}I uptake test, urine 17-OHCS, 17-KS
False negative: skin allergy tests

NURSING CONSIDERATIONS
Assessment
• Monitor potassium, blood glucose, urine glucose while on long-term therapy; hypokalemia and hyperglycemia
• Monitor weight daily; notify prescriber of weekly gain >5 lb; I&O ratio; be alert for decreasing urinary output and increasing edema
• Monitor B/P q4hr, pulse; notify prescriber if chest pain occurs
• Monitor plasma cortisol levels during long-term therapy (normal level 138-635 nmol/L

[SI units] when measured at 8 AM); adrenal function periodically for hypothalamic-pituitary-adrenal axis suppression
• Assess for infection: increased temp, WBC even after withdrawal of medication; product masks infection symptoms
• Assess for potassium depletion: paresthesias, fatigue, nausea, vomiting, depression, polyuria, dysrhythmias, weakness
• Assess mental status: affect, mood, behavioral changes, aggression
• Assess nasal passages during long-term treatment for changes in mucus (nasal)
• Monitor temp; if fever develops, product should be discontinued
• Assess for systemic absorption: increased temp, inflammation, irritation (topical)
• **Beers:** Avoid in older adults with or at high risk of delirium, monitor for confusion, delirium
• **Pregnancy/breastfeeding:** Use only if benefits outweigh fetal risk; cleft lip/palate has occurred (1st trimester); cautious use in breastfeeding, excreted in breast milk

Patient problem
Risk for infection (adverse reactions)
Risk for injury (uses, adverse reactions)

Implementation
PO route
• Give with food or milk to decrease GI symptoms; tablet may be crushed
IM route
• Give IM inj deeply in large muscle mass; rotate sites; avoid deltoid; use 21-G needle
• Avoid SUBCUT administration, may damage tissue

Patient/family education
• Advise patient that emergency ID as corticosteroid user should be carried/worn; not to discontinue abruptly, taper dose
• Instruct patient to notify prescriber if therapeutic response decreases; dosage adjustment may be needed
• Caution patient to avoid OTC products: salicylates, alcohol in cough products, cold preparations unless directed by prescriber; to avoid live vaccines
• Advise patient on all aspects of product use including cushingoid symptoms
• Teach patient symptoms of adrenal insufficiency: nausea, anorexia, fatigue, dizziness, dyspnea, weakness, joint pain
• Teach patient that long-term therapy may be needed to clear infection (1-2 mo depending on type of infection)

T

🍁 Canada only   👁‍🗨 Genetic Warning   Adverse effects: *italics* = common; red = life-threatening

Inhalation route
• Teach patient proper administration technique; to wash inhaler with warm water and dry after each use
• Teach patient all aspects of product use including cushingoid symptoms

Topical route
• Instruct patient to avoid sunlight on affected area; burns may occur

Nasal route
• Instruct patient to clear nasal passages if sneezing attack occurs, repeat dose
• Advise patient to continue using product even if mild nasal bleeding occurs; is usually transient
• Teach patient method of instillation after providing written instruction from manufacturer

Evaluation

Positive therapeutic outcome
• Decrease in runny nose (nasal)
• Decreased dyspnea, wheezing, dry crackles on auscultation (inh)
• Ease of respirations, decreased inflammation
• Absence of severe itching, patches on skin, flaking (topical)

---

triamcinolone nasal agent
See Appendix B

---

triamcinolone topical
See Appendix B

⚠ HIGH ALERT

triazolam (Rx)
(trye-az′oh-lam)
Halcion
Func. class.: Sedative-hypnotic, antianxiety
Chem. class.: Benzodiazepine, short acting
Controlled substance schedule IV (USA), targeted (CDSA IV) (Canada)

Do not confuse: Halcion/Haldol/halcinonide

ACTION: Produces CNS depression at limbic, thalamic, hypothalamic levels of CNS; may be mediated by neurotransmitter; γ-aminobutyric acid (GABA); results are sedation, hypnosis, skeletal muscle relaxation, anticonvulsant activity, anxiolytic action

Therapeutic outcome: Decreased anxiety, insomnia

USES: Insomnia (short-term), sedative/hypnotic

Pharmacokinetics

Absorption	Well absorbed
Distribution	Widely distributed, crosses placenta, crosses blood-brain barrier
Metabolism	Liver
Excretion	Kidneys, breast milk
Half-life	1.5-5.5 hr

Pharmacodynamics

Onset	15-30 min
Peak	Unknown
Duration	6-8 hr

CONTRAINDICATIONS
Pregnancy, breastfeeding, hypersensitivity to benzodiazepines

Precautions: Children <15 yr, geriatric, anemia, renal/hepatic disease, suicidal individuals, product abuse, psychosis, acute closed-angle glaucoma, seizure disorders, angioedema, respiratory disease, depression, sleep-related behaviors (sleep walking), intermittent porphyria, myasthenia gravis, Parkinson's disease

> **BLACK BOX WARNING:** Coadministration with other CNS depressants, respiratory depression

DOSAGE AND ROUTES
Adult: PO 0.125-0.5 mg at bedtime, max 0.5 mg/day
Geriatric: PO 0.0625-0.125 mg at bedtime, max 0.25 mg/day

Available forms: Tabs 0.125, 0.25 mg

ADVERSE EFFECTS
CNS: *Headache, lethargy, drowsiness, daytime sedation,* dizziness, confusion, light-headedness, anxiety, irritability, amnesia, poor coordination, complex sleep-related reactions (sleep driving, sleep eating)
CV: Chest pain, pulse changes, ECG changes
GI: Nausea, vomiting, diarrhea, heartburn, abdominal pain, constipation, hepatic injury
SYST: Severe allergic reactions

INTERACTIONS
Individual drugs

> **BLACK BOX WARNING:** Alcohol: increased action of both products

Cimetidine, clarithromycin, disulfiram, erythromycin, isoniazid, probenecid: increased effects; do not use concurrently

Rifampin: decreased action of rifampin
Theophylline: decreased effects of theophylline

Drug classifications
Antacids: decreased effects of antacids
Antiinfectives (clarithromycin): increased effects
CNS depressants: increased effects of both products
Contraceptives (oral): increased effects; do not use concurrently
CYP3A4 inhibitors, protease inhibitors: increased triazolam levels
Smoking: decreased hypnotic effects

Drug/food
Grapefruit may increase action, avoid concurrent use

Drug/herb
Chamomile, hops, kava, lavender, valerian: increased CNS depression

Drug/lab test
Increased: AST, ALT, serum bilirubin
Decreased: radioactive iodine uptake
False increase: 17-OHCS

NURSING CONSIDERATIONS
Assessment
• Assess patient's mental status: mood, sensorium, anxiety, affect, sleeping pattern, drowsiness, dizziness, especially geriatric; physical dependency, withdrawal symptoms: anxiety, panic attacks, agitation, seizures, headache, nausea, vomiting, muscle pain, weakness; suicidal tendencies; for indications of increasing tolerance and abuse
• Monitor patient's B/P (lying, standing), pulse; if systolic B/P drops 20 mm Hg, hold product, notify prescriber
• Monitor blood tests: CBC during long-term therapy; blood dyscrasias have occurred rarely; decreased hematocrit, neutropenia may occur
• Monitor liver function tests: AST, ALT, bilirubin, creatinine LDH, alkaline phosphatase
• Monitor I&O ratio; indicate renal dysfunction
• Severe allergic reactions: May occur any time during use

BLACK BOX WARNING: Respiratory depression: May occur more frequently with coadministration of other CNS depressants, monitor respirations often

• **Beers:** Avoid use in older adults; increased sensitivity to benzodiazepine and decreased metabolism; may cause or worsen delirium

• **Pregnancy/breastfeeding:** Do not use in pregnancy, not recommended in breastfeeding

Patient problem
Impaired sleeping (uses)
Risk for injury (adverse reactions)

Implementation
• Give with food or milk to decrease GI symptoms; if patient is unable to swallow medication whole, tab may be crushed and mixed with food or fluid
• Give sugarless gum, hard candy, frequent sips of water for dry mouth

Patient/family education
• Advise patient that product may be taken with food or fluids, and tab may be crushed or swallowed whole
• Caution patient not to use for everyday stress or longer than 3 mo unless directed by prescriber; not to take more than prescribed amount; may be habit forming; not to double doses or skip doses

BLACK BOX WARNING: Instruct patient to avoid OTC preparations unless approved by prescriber; alcohol and CNS, sedatives, hypnotics depressants will increase CNS depression

• Caution patient to avoid driving, activities that require alertness because drowsiness may occur; to avoid alcohol ingestion or other psychotropic medications; to rise slowly or fainting may occur, especially geriatric; that drowsiness may worsen at beginning of treatment
• Teach patient that complex sleep-related behaviors (sleep eating/driving) may occur
• Advise patient not to discontinue medication abruptly after long-term use; withdrawal symptoms include vomiting, cramping, tremors, seizures; decrease dosage by 50% q2nights until 0.125 mg for 2 nights, then stop
• Teach patient to use reliable contraception

Evaluation
Positive therapeutic outcome
• Decreased anxiety, restlessness, sleeplessness (short-term treatment only)

TREATMENT OF OVERDOSE:
Lavage, VS, supportive care

trifluridine ophthalmic
See Appendix B

ulipristal (Rx)

(ue′li-pris′tal)

Ella

Func. class.: Progesterone agonist/antagonist-abortifacient

ACTION: Binds to the progesterone receptor and prevents progesterone from occupying the receptor, postpones follicular rupture when taken immediately prior to ovulation

Therapeutic outcome: Absence of pregnancy

USES: Emergency contraception

Pharmacokinetics

Absorption	Unknown
Distribution	Protein binding >94%
Metabolism	Metabolized by CYP3A4
Excretion	Unknown
Half-life	27-38 hrs

Pharmacodynamics

Onset	Unknown
Peak	1 hr
Duration	Unknown

CONTRAINDICATIONS

Pregnancy, children/infants/neonates, postmenopausal females

Precautions: History of ectopic pregnancy, HIV

DOSAGE AND ROUTES

Adult/adolescent females: PO 30 mg (1 tab) as soon as possible within 120 hr (5 days) of unprotected intercourse or a known or suspected contraceptive failure

Available forms: Tab 30 mg

ADVERSE EFFECTS

CNS: Dizziness, headache, fatigue
GI: Nausea, vomiting, abdominal pain
GU: Dysmenorrhea, breakthrough bleeding
INTEG: Acne vulgaris

INTERACTIONS

Individual drugs

Bosentan, carBAMazepine, felbamate, griseofulvin, OXcarbazepine, phenytoin, rifampin, St. John's wort, topiramate, bexarotene, dexamethasone, etravirine, flutamide, metyrapone, modafinil, nafcillin, nevirapine, pioglitazone, rifabutin, itraconazole, ketoconazole: decreased effect of ulipristal

Aldesleukin, IL-2, amiodarone, atazanavir, basiliximab, chloramphenicol, cimetidine, clarithromycin, dalfopristin, danazol, darunavir, delavirdine, diltiazem, dronedarone, erythromycin, fluconazole, FLUoxetine, fluvoxaMINE, imatinib, isoniazid, lapatinib, nefazodone, nelfinavir, niCARdipine, octreotide, pantoprazole, quinupristin, ranolazine, saquinavir, tamoxifen, telithromycin, tipranavir, verapamil, voriconazole, zafirlukast: increased ulipristal effect and adverse reactions

Aprepitant, fosaprepitant, efavirenz, fosamprenavir, quiNINE, ritonavir: increased or decreased ulipristal effect

Drug classifications

Regular hormonal contraceptive methods: decreased contraceptive action

CYP3A4 inducers, barbiturates: decreased effect of ulipristal

CYP3A4 inhibitors: increased ulipristal effect and adverse reactions

Drug/herb

St. John's wort: decreased effect of ulipristal

NURSING CONSIDERATIONS

Assessment

• **Assess need for emergency contraception,** pregnancy planned or suspected, obtain pregnancy test before use (pregnancy)
• Assess medications taken, many drug interactions may occur

Patient problem

Risk of injury (adverse reactions)

Implementation

• Administer without regard to food
• Store at room temperature, protect from light

Patient/family education

• Instruct patient that if vomiting occurs within 3 hours of taking the tablet, consider repeating the dose
• Advise patient to report to provider any side effects
• Explain reason for medication and expected results
• Advise patient to avoid use in breastfeeding

Evaluation

Positive therapeutic outcome

• Absence of pregnancy

undecylenic acid topical

See Appendix B

unoprostone ophthalmic

See Appendix B

valACYclovir (Rx)
(val-a-sye′kloh-vir)
Valtrex
Func. class.: Antiviral
Chem. class.: Synthetic acyclic purine nucleoside analog

Do not confuse: valACYclovir/ valGANciclovir, **Valtrex**/Valcyte

ACTION: Interferes with DNA synthesis by conversion to acyclovir, causing decreased viral replication, time of lesional healing

Therapeutic outcome: Absence of itching, painful lesions; crusting and healing of lesions

USES: Treatment or suppression of herpes zoster (shingles), recurrent genital herpes, herpes labialis (cold sores), varicella, varicella-zoster

Pharmacokinetics

Absorption	50%
Distribution	Crosses placenta, enters breast milk, protein binding 13.5%-17.9%
Metabolism	Converts to acyclovir in intestine, liver
Excretion	Urine, as acyclovir
Half-life	2½-3½ hr

Pharmacodynamics

Onset	Unknown
Peak	1.5-2.5 hr
Duration	Up to 24 hr

CONTRAINDICATIONS
Hypersensitivity to this product, acyclovir, valGANciclovir

Precautions: Pregnancy, breastfeeding, geriatric, renal/hepatic disease, electrolyte imbalance, dehydration, hypersensitivity to penciclovir, famciclovir, ganciclovir, varicella

DOSAGE AND ROUTES
Herpes Zoster (shingles)
Adult: PO 1 g tid × 1 wk

Herpes labialis
Adult: PO 2 g bid × 1 day at first sign of lesions

Genital herpes (suppressive initial)
Adult: PO 1 g bid × 10 days initially

Genital herpes (recurrent episodes)
Adult: PO 500 mg bid × 3 days

Genital herpes (suppressive therapy)
Adult: PO 1 g/day with normal immune function; 500 mg/day for those with ≤9 recurrences/ yr; 500 mg bid in HIV-infected patients with CD4 ≥100

Reduction of transmission
Adult: PO 500 mg/day for source partner

Varicella (chickenpox)
Adolescent and child ≥2 yr: PO 20 mg/kg/ dose tid × 5 days, max 3 g/day; start at first sign, preferably within 24 hr of rash

Renal dose
Adult: PO CCr 30-49 ml/min 1g q12hr (herpes zoster); 1 g q12hr × 1 day (herpes labialis); CCr 10-29 ml/min 1 g q24hr (genital herpes/ herpes zoster); 500 mg q24hr (recurrent genital herpes); CCr <10 ml/min 500 mg q24hr (genital herpes/herpes zoster), 500 mg q24hr (recurrent genital herpes)

Available forms: Tabs 500, 1000 mg

ADVERSE EFFECTS
CNS: Tremors, lethargy, *dizziness, headache, weakness,* depression, hallucinations, seizures, encephalopathy
ENDO: *Dysmenorrhea*
GI: *Nausea, vomiting, diarrhea, abdominal pain, constipation*
HEMA: Thrombocytopenic purpura, hemolytic uremic syndrome
INTEG: *Rash*
GU: Crystalluria, renal failure

INTERACTIONS
Individual drugs
Cimetidine, probenecid: increased blood levels of valACYclovir (only if renal disease is significant)

Drug/lab test
Increased: LFTs, creatinine
Decreased: WBC, platelets

NURSING CONSIDERATIONS
Assessment
• **Assess for signs of infection;** characteristics of lesions; therapy should be started at first sign of herpes and is most effective within 72 hr of outbreak
• Assess C&S before product therapy; product may be given as soon as culture is performed, lesion must be unroofed to obtain specimen; repeat C&S after treatment; determine the presence of other STDs
• Assess allergies before treatment, reaction of each medication

• Assess for thrombocytopenic purpura, hemolytic uremic syndrome, may be fatal

Patient problem

Infection (uses)

Implementation

• Give without regard to meals
• Give within 72 hr of outbreak (herpes zoster); as soon as possible (herpes labialis, genital herpes), within 24 hr (chicken pox)
• Give orally before infection occurs
• Store at room temp; protect from light, moisture

Patient/family education

• Advise patient to take as prescribed; if dose is missed, take as soon as remembered up to 2 hr before next dose; do not double dose, without regard to meals
• Instruct patient to take product orally before infection occurs; product should be taken when itching or pain occurs, usually before eruptions
• Inform patient that partners need to be told that patient has herpes; they can become infected; condoms must be worn to prevent reinfections
• Tell patient that product does not cure infection, just controls symptoms and does not prevent infection to others; to use safe sex techniques in genital herpes, herpes labialis
• Teach patient to discuss all Rx, OTC, herbals, supplements taken with health care professional
• Advise patient that adequate hydration is needed to prevent crystalluria
• **Pregnancy/breastfeeding:** Identify if pregnancy is planned or suspected or if breastfeeding
• Teach patient to report CNS changes (tremors, weakness, lethargy, hallucinations) immediately

Evaluation

Positive therapeutic outcome

• Absence of itching, painful lesions; crusting and healed lesions

---

RARELY USED

valbenazine

(val-ben´-a-zeen)

Ingrezza

Func. class.: CNS agent; monoamine depletor

USES: For the treatment of tardive dyskinesia

DOSAGE AND ROUTES

Adult: **PO** Initially, 40 mg qday, after 1 wk, increase to 80 mg qday. Continuation of 40 mg qday may be considered for some patients

CONTRAINDICATIONS

Hypersensitivity

---

valGANciclovir (Rx)

(val-gan-sy´kloh-veer)

Valcyte

Func. class.: Antiviral

Chem. class.: Synthetic nucleoside

Do not confuse: valGANciclovir/ valACYclovir, **Valcyte/**Valtrex

ACTION: valGANciclovir is metabolized to ganciclovir; inhibits replication of human CMV in vivo and in vitro by selectively inhibiting viral DNA synthesis

Therapeutic outcome: Decreased proliferation of virus responsible for CMV retinitis

USES: Cytomegalovirus (CMV) retinitis in immunocompromised persons, including those with AIDS, after indirect ophthalmoscopy confirms diagnosis; prevention of CMV in transplantation; prevention of CMV in patients at risk going through transplant (kidney, heart, pancreas)

Pharmacokinetics

Absorption	60% absorbed from GI tract
Distribution	Plasma protein binding unknown; crosses blood-brain barrier, CSF
Metabolism	Rapidly metabolized in intestinal wall and liver to ganciclovir
Excretion	Kidneys (ganciclovir)
Half-life	3-4½ hr

Pharmacodynamics

Onset	Unknown
Peak	1-3 hr
Duration	up to 24 hr

CONTRAINDICATIONS

Breastfeeding, hypersensitivity to ganciclovir or valACYclovir, absolute neutrophil count $<500/mm^3$, platelet count $<25,000/mm^3$, hemodialysis, liver transplant

Precautions: Children, geriatric, renal function impairment, hypersensitivity to acyclovir, penciclovir, famciclovir

BLACK BOX WARNING: Preexisting cytopenias, secondary malignancy, infertility, anemia, pregnancy

DOSAGE AND ROUTES

Treatment of CMV

Adult: **PO** induction 900 mg bid × 21 days with food; maintenance 900 mg/day with food

---

Transplant (CMV prophylaxis)

Adult/adolescent >16 yr: PO 900 mg/day with food starting within 10 days before transplantation until 100 days after transplantation (kidney/pancreas, heart); continue for 200 days (kidney)

Infant ≥4 mo/child/adolescent ≤16 yr: PO give within 10 days of heart/kidney transplant; calculate dose as 7 × BSA × CCr and give a single daily dose

Renal dose

Adult: PO CCr ≥60 ml/min same dosage as above; CCr 40-59 ml/min 450 mg bid × 21 days, then 450 mg/day; CCr 25-39 ml/min 450 mg/day × 21 days, then 450 mg q2day; CCr 10-24 ml/min 450 mg q2day, then 450 mg 2 ×/ week

Available forms: Tabs 450 mg; powder for oral sol 50 mg/ml

ADVERSE EFFECTS

CNS: *Fever*, chills, *confusion*, dizziness, *headache*, psychosis, tremors, *paresthesia*, *weakness*, seizures, insomnia

GI: *Nausea, vomiting, anorexia, diarrhea, abdominal pain*

GU: Renal dysfunction

HEMA: Thrombocytopenia, irreversible neutropenia, anemia, pancytopenia

INTEG: *Rash*, alopecia, *pruritus*, urticaria, pain at inj site, phlebitis, Stevens-Johnson syndrome

MISC: Local and systemic infections and sepsis

INTERACTIONS

Individual drugs

Adriamycin, amphotericin B, cycloSPORINE, dapsone, DOXOrubicin, flucytosine, pentamidine, trimethoprim/sulfamethoxazole, vinBLAStine, vinCRIStine: increased toxicity

Didanosine: increased effect; monitor for adverse effects, toxicity

Imipenem/cilastatin: increased seizures

Mycophenolate: increased effect of both drugs

Probenecid: decreased renal clearance of valGANciclovir

Radiation, zidovudine: severe granulocytopenia; do not coadminister

Drug classifications

Antineoplastics, immunosuppressants: increased severe granulocytopenia; do not coadminister

Nucleoside analogs, other: increased toxicity

Drug/food

Absorption: increased with high-fat meal

Drug/lab test

Increased: creatinine, BUN

Decreased: RBC/WBC, Hct/Hgb

NURSING CONSIDERATIONS

Assessment

• **CMV retinitis:** Determine diagnosis by opthalmoscopy before use; culture may be used, negative results do not confirm that CMV retinitis is not present, use ophthalmoscopy q 2 wk during treatment

> **BLACK BOX WARNING: Assess for leukopenia/ neutropenia/thrombocytopenia:** monitor WBCs, platelets q2day during 2 ×/day dosing and then qwk, do not use if ANC <500/mm³, platelets <25,000/mm³, hgb <8 g/dl

> **BLACK BOX WARNING: Malignancy:** monitor for malignancy; avoid accidental exposure of broken, crushed tabs, powder for solution; if these were in contact with skin, wash well with soap and water

• Assess serum creatinine or CCr, BUN ≥q2wk

Patient problem

Infection (uses)

Implementation

PO tab

• Give with food for better absorption, avoid getting on skin, do not break, crush, or chew tab; wash hands if contact with skin

Oral SOL

• Give with food

• Measure 9 ml of purified water in graduated cylinder, shake bottle to loosen powder, add ½ liquid, shake well, add remaining water, shake, remove child-resistant cap and push bottle adapter into neck of bottle, close with cap, give using the dispenser provided

• Store liquid in refrigerator; do not freeze; throw away any unused portion after 49 days

Patient/family education

• Inform patient that product does not cure condition, that regular ophthalmologic exams will be needed q 1 month and blood tests are necessary

• Caution patient that major toxicities may necessitate discontinuing product

• Instruct patient to take with food, avoid high-fat meals

• Instruct patient to report seizures, dizziness; to avoid hazardous activities

• Caution patient to use sunscreen to prevent burns

Evaluation

Positive therapeutic outcome
• Decreased symptoms of CMV

TREATMENT OF OVERDOSE:
Maintain adequate hydration; dialysis may help reduce serum concentrations; consider use of hematopoietic growth factors

valproate (Rx)
(val-proh'ate)
Depacon
valproic acid (Rx)
Depakene
divalproex sodium (Rx)
Depakote, Depakote ER, Depakote Sprinkle, Epival ✿

Func. class.: Anticonvulsant, vascular headache suppressant
Chem. class.: Carboxylic acid derivative

ACTION: Increases levels of γ-aminobutyric acid (GABA) in the brain, which decreases seizure activity

Therapeutic outcome: Decreased symptoms of epilepsy, bipolar disorder

USES: Simple (petit mal), complex (petit mal), absence, mixed seizures, manic episode associated with bipolar disorder, prophylaxis of migraine, adjunct in schizophrenia, tardive dyskinesia, aggression in children with ADHD, organic brain syndrome, tonic-clonic (grand mal)/ myoclonic seizures

Unlabeled uses: Rectal for seizures (valproic acid)

Pharmacokinetics

Absorption	Well (PO), complete (IV)
Distribution	Breast milk, crosses placenta, blood, brain barrier, widely distributed, protein binding 90%
Metabolism	Liver
Excretion	Kidneys
Half-life	6-16 hr

Pharmacodynamics

Onset	15-30 min
Peak	1-4 hr
Duration	4-6 hr

CONTRAINDICATIONS
Hypersensitivity, urea cycle disorders, mitochondrial disease, hepatic disease

Precautions: Breastfeeding, geriatric abrupt discontinuation, carnitine deficiency, coagulopathy, head trauma, organic brain syndrome, HIV, renal disease, suicidal ideation, surgery, thrombocytopenia

DOSAGE AND ROUTES
Seizures
Adult, adolescent, and child 10 yr and older: PO/IV: Initially, 10-15 mg/kg/day in 1-4 divided doses (≥250 mg should be given in divided doses), increase by 5-10 mg/kg/day qwk, max 60 mg/kg/day; **rectal enema** 17-20 mg/kg, then 10-15 mg/kg/dose q8h, dilute 1:1 (water)

Acute mania
Adult: PO (delayed-release divalproex [Depakote]): Initially, 750 mg/day in divided doses, then increase as rapidly as possible to the lowest effective dose, max 60 mg/kg/day; **PO (extended-release divalproex; Depakote ER):** Initially, 25 mg/kg/day, increase as rapidly as possible to achieve the desired clinical effect. Max 60 mg/kg/day

Migraine prophylaxis
Adult ≤ 65 yr: PO (delayed-release divalproex [Depakote]): Initially, 250 mg bid, titrate as needed up to a max 500 mg bid; (extended-release divalproex; Depakote ER): Initially, 500 mg qday × 1 wk, then increasing to 1000 mg qday, max 1000 mg/day

Available: Valproic acid: caps 250, 500 ✿ mg; syr 250 mg/5 ml; **divalproex:** del rel tabs 125, 250, 500 mg; ext rel tabs 250, 500 mg; sprinkle caps 125 mg; **valproate:** inj 100 mg/ml

ADVERSE EFFECTS
CNS: *Sedation, drowsiness,* dizziness, headache, depression, behavioral changes, tremors, aggression, weakness, suicidal ideation
CV: Peripheral edema
EENT: Visual disturbances, taste perversion
GI: *Nausea, vomiting, constipation, diarrhea, dyspepsia,* anorexia, pancreatitis, stomatitis, weight gain, dry mouth, hepatotoxicity

HEMA: Thrombocytopenia, leukopenia
INTEG: *Rash,* alopecia, photosensitivity, dry skin, DRESS
META: Hyperammonemia, SIADH

INTERACTIONS
Individual drugs
Abciximab, cefoperazone, cefoTEtan, eptifibatide, heparin, tirofiban: increased bleeding risk
Alcohol: increased CNS depression
Aspirin, carbamazepine, cimetidine, chlorpromazine, erythromycin, felbamate: increased valproic acid level, toxicity
Warfarin: increased bleeding

Drug classifications
Antidepressants (tricyclics), barbiturates: increased action
Antihistamines, barbiturates, MAOIs, opioids, sedative/hypnotics: increased CNS depression
Carbamazepine, cholestyramin, estrogens, hormonal contraceptives, neropenem, phenobarbital, phenytoins, rifampin: Decreased valproate levels
Tricyclics: decreased seizure threshold

Drug/lab test
Increased: LFTs, bleeding time, ammonia
Decreased: sodium
False positive: ketones, urine
Interference: thyroid function tests

NURSING CONSIDERATIONS
Assessment
• **Assess seizure disorder:** location, aura, activity, duration; seizure precautions should be in place
• **Assess bipolar disorder:** mood, activity, sleeping, eating, behavior; suicidal thoughts/behaviors
• **Assess migraines:** frequency, intensity
• Monitor blood tests: Hct, Hgb, RBC, serum folate, ammonia, platelets, pro-time, PTT, vit D if on long-term therapy
• Monitor liver function tests: AST, ALT, bilirubin, creatinine, failure; monitor for fever, anorexia, vomiting, lethargy, jaundice of skin, eyes that may occur during treatment, those with organic brain disorders, mental retardation, child <2 yr
• Monitor blood levels: therapeutic level 50-125 mcg/ml
• **Hyperammonemic encephalopathy:** can be fatal in those with urea cycle disorders (UCD); assess for lethargy, confusion, coma, CV, respiratory changes; discontinue

> **BLACK BOX WARNING:** Assess for **pancreatitis**, may be fatal; may occur anytime during treatment or several months/years after discontinuing treatment

• **Beers:** Avoid in older adults unless safer alternative is not available, ataxia, impaired psychomotor function may occur
• **Suicidal thoughts/behaviors:** Usually occurs during beginning therapy, limited amount of product should be given to patient
• **DRESS:** Assess for eosinophilia, changes in lab work, fever, rashes, lymphodenopathy, if present and condition confirmed discontinue immediately, do not restart
• **Trough/peak:** Monitor serum levels for peak, trough, toxicity
• **Hepatotoxicity:** Monitor AST/ALT, bilirubin, LDH, ammonia baseline and periodically during 6 mo or more; discontinue if hyperammonemia occurs

> **BLACK BOX WARNING:** Do not use in pregnancy (migraine prophylaxis), use only in pregnancy (epilepsy, manic episodes) if other alternatives are not available; major malformation may occur, enroll pregnant patients in the North American Antiepileptic Drug Pregnancy Registry (888-233-2334), cautious use in breastfeeding, excreted in breast milk

Patient problem
Distorted thinking process (uses) divalproex
Risk for injury (uses)
Lack of knowledge of medication (teaching)

Implementation
• Do not confuse different forms
• Swallow tabs and caps whole; do not break, crush, or chew
• Sprinkle cap contents on food
• Give syrup; do not dilute with carbonated beverage; do not give syrup to patients on sodium restriction, shake before use; may mix with foods or other liquids as taste is unpleasant
• May open sprinkle caps and use with food; should not chew
• Give with food or milk to decrease GI symptoms

Intermittent IV infusion route
• Dilute dose with ≥50 ml D$_5$W, NS, LR
• Run over 60 min (20 mg/min)

Y-site compatibilities: cefepime, ceftazidime, cloxacillin, naloxone, temocillin

Patient/family education
• Teach patient that physical dependency may result from extended use
• Instruct patient to report immediately suicidal thoughts/behaviors
• Instruct patient to avoid driving, other activities that require alertness, dizziness may occur

---

BLACK BOX WARNING: Advise patient not to discontinue medication quickly after long-term use; seizures may result

---

BLACK BOX WARNING: Advise patient to report visual disturbances, rash, diarrhea, light-colored stools, jaundice, protracted vomiting to prescriber

---

• Advise patient to use contraception while taking this product, to notify provider if pregnancy is planned or suspected
• Instruct patient to drink plenty of fluids
• Teach patient that continuing follow-up exams and blood work will be needed
• Advise patient to carry emergency ID with condition, medications
• **Hepatotoxicity/pancreatitis:** Teach patient to report immediately nausea, vomiting, abdominal pain, fever
• **DRESS:** Teach patient to report fever, swelling of lymph glands, rash
• Advise patient to discuss with health care professional all Rx, OTC, herbals, supplements taken
• Advise patient to take as directed; not to skip, double doses; not to discontinue abruptly

Evaluation

Positive therapeutic outcome
• Decreased seizures

---

valsartan (Rx)

(val-zar'tan)
Diovan
Func. class.: Antihypertensive
Chem. class.: Angiotensin II receptor antagonist (type AT_1)

Do not confuse: Diovan/Zyban

ACTION: Blocks the vasoconstrictor and aldosterone-secreting effects of angiotensin II; selectively blocks the binding of angiotensin II to the AT_1 receptor found in tissues

Therapeutic outcome: Decreased B/P

USES: Hypertension, alone or in combination, in patients >6 yr; HF, after MI with left ventricular dysfunction/failure in stable patients

Pharmacokinetics

Absorption	Well absorbed
Distribution	Bound to plasma proteins
Metabolism	Extensive
Excretion	Feces, urine, breast milk
Half-life	9 hr

Pharmacodynamics

Onset	Up to 2 hr
Peak	2-4 hr
Duration	24 hr

CONTRAINDICATIONS

Hypersensitivity, severe hepatic disease, bilateral renal artery stenosis

---

BLACK BOX WARNING: Pregnancy

Precautions: Breastfeeding, children, geriatric, HF, hypertrophic cardiomyopathy, aortic/mitral valve stenosis, CAD, angioedema, renal/hepatic disease, hypersensitivity to ACE inhibitors, hyperkalemia, hypovolemia, African descent

DOSAGE AND ROUTES
Hypertension (alone or in combination)

Adult: PO 80 or 160 mg/day alone or in combination with other antihypertensives, may increase to 320 mg HF Class II to IV
Geriatric: PO Adjust based on clinical response; may start with lower dose
Child/adolescent 6-16 yr: PO 1.3 mg/kg/dose, q day max 40 mg/day, initially, adjust dose on clinical response max 2.7 mg/kg/day

HF
Adult: PO 40 mg bid, up to 60 mg bid

Post MI
Adult: PO 20 mg bid as early as 12 hr after MI, may be titrated within 7 days to 40 mg bid, then titrate to maintenance of 160 mg bid

Available forms: Tabs 80, 160, 320 mg

ADVERSE EFFECTS
CNS: *Dizziness, insomnia,* drowsiness, vertigo, headache, fatigue
CV: Angina pectoris, 2nd-degree AV block, cerebrovascular accident, hypotension, MI, dysrhythmias
EENT: Conjunctivitis
GI: Diarrhea, abdominal pain, nausea, hepatotoxicity
GU: Impotence, nephrotoxicity, renal failure
HEMA: *Anemia,* neutropenia
META: Hyperkalemia
MISC: Vasculitis, angioedema
MS: Cramps, myalgia, pain, stiffness
RESP: *Cough*

INTERACTIONS
Individual drugs

Aliskiren: do not use concurrently
Gemfibrozil, rifampin, ritonavir, telithromycin: increased valsartan levels
Lithium: increased effects of lithium

Drug classifications

Diuretics (potassium-sparing, potassium supplements, ACE inhibitors): increased hyperkalemia

NSAIDs, salicylates: decreased antihypertensive effects

Drug/herb

Ephedra, ma huang: decreased antihypertensive effect

Garlic, Hawthorn. increased antihypertensive effect

Drug/food

Decreased AUC by 40%

Salt substitutes with potassium: increased hyperkalemia

NURSING CONSIDERATIONS
Assessment

• Assess B/P (lying, sitting, standing), pulse q4hr; note rate, rhythm, quality periodically

• Monitor electrolytes: potassium, sodium, chloride; total CO_2

• **Assess for angioedema:** facial swelling, shortness of breath, edema in feet, legs daily

• Obtain baselines in renal, liver function tests before therapy begins

• Assess blood tests: BUN, creatinine, before treatment

• Monitor for edema in feet, legs daily

• Assess for skin turgor, dryness of mucous membranes for hydration status; correct volume depletion before initiating therapy

• **Overdose symptoms:** bradycardia or tachycardia, circulatory collapse

> **BLACK BOX WARNING: Pregnancy/breastfeeding:** Do not use in pregnancy, may cause fetal death, do not breastfeed

Patient problem

Risk for injury (uses, adverse reactions)

Nonadherence (teaching)

Implementation

• Administer without regard to meals

Patient/family education

• Teach patient not to take this product if breastfeeding or pregnant, or have had an allergic reaction to this product

• If a dose is missed, instruct patient to take as soon as possible, unless it is within an hour before next dose

• Advise patient to comply with dosage schedule, even if feeling better

• Teach patient to notify prescriber of fever, swelling of hands or feet, irregular heartbeat, chest pain, persistent cough

• Advise patient excessive perspiration, dehydration, diarrhea may lead to fall in blood pressure; consult prescriber if these occur

• Inform patient that product may cause dizziness, fainting; light-headedness may occur, maintain hydration

• Instruct patient to avoid potassium supplements and foods, salt substitutes

• Caution patient to rise slowly to sitting or standing position to minimize orthostatic hypotension; how to take B/P

> **BLACK BOX WARNING:** Teach patient not to take this medication if pregnant or breastfeeding

Evaluation

Positive therapeutic outcome
• Decreased B/P

vancomycin
(van-koe-mye′sin)

Vancocin

Func. class.: Antiinfective—miscellaneous

Chem. class.: Tricyclic glycopeptide

ACTION: Inhibits bacterial cell wall synthesis, blocks glycopeptides

Therapeutic outcome: Bactericidal for the following organisms: staphylococci, streptococci, *Corynebacterium*, *Clostridium*

USES: *Actinomyces* sp., *Bacillus* sp., *Clostridium difficile*, *Clostridium* sp., *Enterococcus faecalis*, *Enterococcus faecium*, *Enterococcus* sp., *Lactobacillus* sp., *Listeria monocytogenes*, *Staphylococcus aureus* (MRSA), *Staphylococcus aureus* (MSSA), *Staphylococcus epidermidis*, *Staphylococcus* sp., *Streptococcus agalactiae* (group B streptococci), *Streptococcus bovis*, *Streptococcus pneumoniae*, *Streptococcus pyogenes* (group A beta-hemolytic streptococci), *Viridans streptococci*; may be effective against *Corynebacterium jeikeium*, *Corynebacterium* sp.; pseudomembranous colitis, staphylococcal enterocolitis, group A β-hemolytic streptococci, endocarditis prophylaxis for dental procedures, bacteremia, joint/bone infections, osteomyelitis, pneumonia, septicemia

Pharmacokinetics

Absorption	Poorly absorbed (PO), completely absorbed (**IV**)
Distribution	Widely distributed, crosses placenta, penetration in CSF (20%-30%)
Metabolism	Liver
Excretion	PO, feces; **IV**, kidneys
Half-life	4-8 hr (adult), 2-2.5 (child >3 yr)

	IV
Onset	Immediate
Peak	Inf end
Duration	Up to 24 hr

CONTRAINDICATIONS
Hypersensitivity, previous hearing loss

Precautions: Pregnancy, breastfeeding, neonates, geriatric, renal disease

DOSAGE AND ROUTES
Serious systemic infections
Adult: **IV** 500 mg (7.5 mg/kg) q6-8hr or 1 g (15 mg/kg) q12hr or 15-20 mg/kg q12hr
Child: **IV** 40-60 mg/kg/day divided q6-8hr
Neonate: **IV** 15 mg/kg initially followed by 10 mg/kg q8-24hr

CDAD
Adult: PO 125 mg qid × 10-14 days
Child: PO (unlabeled) 40 mg/kg/day divided q6hr × 7-10 days, max 2 g/day

Staphylococcal endocarditis
Adult: **IV** 2 g divided (500 mg q6hr or 1 g q12hr)
Child: **IV** 20 mg/kg over 1 hr; 1 hr before procedure

Staphylococcal enterocolitis
Adult: **PO** 500-2000 mg/day in 3-4 divided doses × 7-10 days
Child: **PO** 40 mg/kg/day in 3-4 divided doses × 7-10 days, max 2000 mg/day

Renal dose
Adult: IV 15-20 mg/kg loading dose in seriously ill; individualize all other doses

Available forms: Cap 125, 250 mg; powder for inj **IV** 500, 750 mg; vials 1, 5, 10 g; dextrose sol for inj 500 mg/100 ml, 750 mg/150 ml, 1 g/200 ml

ADVERSE EFFECTS
CNS: Headache
CV: Hypotension, peripheral edema
EENT: *Ototoxicity*
GI: Nausea, CDAD
GU: Nephrotoxicity
HEMA: Leukopenia, eosinophilia, neutropenia
INTEG: Chills, fever, rash, thrombophlebitis at inj site, (red man syndrome), skin/subcutaneous tissue disorders
MS: Back pain
SYST: Anaphylaxis, superinfection

INTERACTIONS
Individual drugs
Acyclovir, adefovir, amphotericin B, capreomycin, CISplatin, colistin, cycloSPORINE, foscarnet, ganciclovir, methotrexate, pamidronate, IV pentamidine, polymyxin B, streptozocin, tacrolimus, zoledronic acid: increased ototoxicity or nephrotoxicity

Drug classifications
Aminoglycosides, cephalosporins, NSAIDs: increased ototoxicity or nephrotoxicity
Nondepolarizing muscle relaxants: increased neuromuscular effects

Drug/lab test
Increased: BUN/creatinine, eosinophils
Decreased: WBC

NURSING CONSIDERATIONS
Assessment
• **Assess for infection:** WBC, urine, stools, sputum, wound characteristics, throughout treatment, obtain C&S before starting treatment, may start treatment before results are received
• **Nephrotoxicity** Monitor I&O ratio, BUN, creatinine; report hematuria, oliguria because nephrotoxicity may occur
• Monitor blood tests: WBC; serum levels; peak 1 hr after 1-hr inf 25-40 mg/L; trough before next dose 5-10 mg/L, especially in renal disease, no trough levels are needed for PO form
• **CDAD:** Assess for watery or bloody diarrhea, abdominal cramps, fever, pus, mucus, nausea, dehydration, discontinue immediately
• Assess auditory function during, after treatment; hearing loss, ringing, roaring in ears; product should be discontinued
• Monitor B/P during administration; sudden drop may indicate red man syndrome
• Assess for signs of infection
• **Red man syndrome:** Assess for flushing of neck, face, upper body, arms, back; may lead to anaphylaxis, slow IV infusion to >1 hr

Patient problem
Infection (uses)
Diarrhea (adverse reactions)

Implementation
• Give antihistamine if red man syndrome occurs: decreased B/P, flushing of neck, face; stop or slow infusion
• Give dose based on serum conc
• Give in equal intervals around the clock to maintain blood levels
• Store at room temp for up to 2 wk after reconstitution
• Have adrenaline, suction, tracheostomy set, endotracheal intubation equipment on unit; anaphylaxis may occur

---

- Provide adequate intake of fluids (2 L) to prevent nephrotoxicity

PO route

- Give without regard to food, swallow whole (only used for *Clostridium difficile*, staphylococcus enterocolitis)
- Use calibrated measuring for liquid
- IV form may be used NG after diluting in 30 mL water

IT route

- Dilute with preservative-free normal saline (1-5 mg/mL) given into ventricular cerebrospinal fluid, dose based on CSF concentration

Intermittent IV INF route

- Give after reconstitution with 10 ml of sterile water for inj (500 mg/10 ml); further dilution is needed for **IV**, 500 mg/100 ml of 0.9% NaCl, D₅W given as intermittent inf over 1 hr; decrease rate of inf if red man syndrome occurs

Continuous IV INF route (unlabeled)

- Reconstitute, then may inf 1-2 g in volume to give over 24 hr if intermittent **IV** route cannot be used
- A central line may be considered for long-term therapy; assess peripheral lines for phlebitis

Y-site compatibilities: Acetylcysteine, acyclovir, alatrofloxacin, aldesleukin, alemtuzumab, alfentanil, allopurinol, alprostadil, amifostine, amikacin, amino acids injection, aminocaproic acid, amiodarone, amoxicillin-clavulanate, amsacrine, anidulafungin, argatroban, ascorbic acid injection, atenolol, atracurium, atropine, azithromycin, benztropine, bleomycin, bretylium, bumetanide, buprenorphine, butorphanol, calcium chloride/gluconate, CARBOplatin, carmustine, caspofungin, cefpirome, chlorproMAZINE, cimetidine, ciprofloxacin, cisatracurium, CISplatin, clarithromycin, clindamycin, codeine, cyanocobalamin, cyclophosphamide, cycloSPORINE, cytarabine, DACTINomycin, DAUNOrubicin liposome, dexamethasone, dexmedetomidine, dexrazoxane, digoxin, diltiazem, diphenhydrAMINE, DOBUTamine, DOCEtaxel, dolasetron, DOPamine, doripenem, doxacurium, doxapram, DOXOrubicin, DOXOrubicin liposomal, doxycycline, enalaprilat, ePHEDrine, EPINEPHrine, epirubicin, eptifibatide, ertapenem, erythromycin, esmolol, etoposide, etoposide phosphate, famotidine, fenoldopam, fentaNYL, filgrastim, fluconazole, fludarabine, folic acid (as sodium salt), gallium, gemcitabine, gentamicin, glycopyrrolate, granisetron, HYDROmorphone, hydrOXYzine, ifosfamide, insulin regular, irinotecan, isoproterenol, isosorbide, ketamine, labetalol, lactated Ringer's injection, lepirudin, levofloxacin, lidocaine, linezolid, LORazepam, magnesium sulfate, mannitol, mechlorethamine, melphalan, meperidine, meropenem, metaraminol, methyldopate,

metoclopramide, metoprolol, metroNIDAZOLE, midazolam, milrinone, minocycline, mitoXANtrone, morphine, multiple vitamins injection, mycophenolate, nalbuphine, naloxone, nesiritide, netilmicin, niCARdipine, nitroglycerin, nitroprusside, norepinephrine, octreotide, ofloxacin, ondansetron, oxacillin, oxaliplatin, oxytocin, PACLitaxel (solvent/surfactant), palonosetron, pamidronate, pancuronium, papaverine, PEMEtrexed, penicillin G potassium/sodium, pentamidine, pentazocine, PENTobarbital, perphenazine, PHENobarbital, phentolamine, phenylephrine, phytonadione, piritramide, polymyxin B, potassium acetate/chloride, procainamide, prochlorperazine, promethazine, propranolol, protamine, pyridoxine, quiNIDine, ranitidine, remifentanil, rifampin, Ringer's injection, riTUXimab, sodium acetate/bicarbonate/citrate, succinylcholine, SUFentanil, tacrolimus, teniposide, thiamine, thiotepa, tigecycline, tirofiban, TNA (3-in-1), tobramycin, tolazoline, TPN (2-in-1), trastuzumab, urapidil, vasopressin, vecuronium, verapamil, vinBLAStine, vinCRIStine, vinorelbine, voriconazole, zidovudine, zoledronic acid

Patient/family education

- Teach patient aspects of product therapy: need to complete entire course of medication to ensure organism death (7-10 days); culture may be performed after completed course of medication
- Advise patient to report sore throat, fever, fatigue; could indicate superinfection
- Instruct patient that product must be taken in equal intervals around the clock to maintain blood levels
- **Pregnancy/breastfeeding:** Identify if pregnancy is planned or suspected or if breastfeeding
- Advise patient to take PO as directed, not to double or skip doses
- Teach patient to notify prescriber if there are no changes in 72-96 hr
- Teach patient that antiinfectives must be taken before dental/medical invasive procedures in rheumatic heart disease

Evaluation

Positive therapeutic outcome

- Absence of fever, sore throat
- Negative culture after treatment

vardenafil (Rx)

(var-den′a-fil)

Levitra, Staxyn

Func. class.: Impotence agent

Chem. class.: Phosphodiesterase type 5 inhibitor

ACTION: Inhibits phosphodiesterase type 5 (PDE5); enhances erectile function by increasing the amount of cyclic GMP, which causes smooth muscle relaxation and increased blood flow into the corpus cavernosum

Therapeutic outcome: Erection

USES: Treatment of erectile dysfunction

Pharmacokinetics

Absorption	Rapid; reduced absorption with high-fat meal, Bioavailability 15%
Distribution	Protein binding 95%, semen
Metabolism	Liver (CYP3A4)
Excretion	Primarily in feces (91%-95%)
Half-life	4-5 hr

Pharmacodynamics

Onset	20 min
Peak	½-1½ hr
Duration	<5 hr

CONTRAINDICATIONS

Hypersensitivity, coadministration of α-blockers or nitrates, renal failure, congenital or acquired QT prolongation

Precautions: Pregnancy; not indicated for women, children, or newborns; hepatic impairment; retinitis pigmentosa; cardiovascular disease; anatomic penile deformities; sickle cell anemia; leukemia; multiple myeloma; bleeding disorders; active peptic ulceration; renal disease

DOSAGE AND ROUTES

Levitra

Adult: PO 10 mg, taken 1 hr before sexual activity, dose may be reduced to 5 mg or increased to a max of 20 mg; max dosing frequency is once/day; orally disintegrating tab 10 mg 60 min before sexual activity; do not use with potent CYP3A4 inhibitors

Geriatric >65 yr: PO 5 mg initially, titrate as needed/tolerated

Hepatic dose (Child-Pugh B)

Adult: PO 5 mg, max 10 mg

Staxyn

Adult PO 10 mg 1 hr prior to sexual activity, max 10 mg/24 hr

Available forms: Levitra tabs 2.5, 5, 10, 20 mg; **Staxyn orally disintegrating tab** 10 mg

ADVERSE EFFECTS

CNS: *Headache, flushing, dizziness, insomnia*
EENT: Diminished vision, hearing loss
GU: Abnormal ejaculation, priapism
GI: Nausea

MISC: Flu-like symptoms

INTERACTIONS
Individual drugs

Alcohol, amLODIPine, metoprolol, NIFEdipine: increased hypotension, do not use concurrently

Cimetidine, erythromycin, itraconazole, ketoconazole: increased levels

Clarithromycin, droperidol, procainamide, quiNIDine: serious dysrhythmias; do not use concurrently

Drug classifications

Do not use with nitrates because of unsafe decrease in B/P that could result in heart attack or stroke

α-Blockers, protease inhibitors, angiotensin II receptor blockers, antidysrhythmics class Ia, III, quinolones: serious dysrhythmias; do not use together

Drug/food

High-fat meal: decreased absorption

Drug/lab test

Increase: CK

NURSING CONSIDERATIONS
Assessment

• **Erectile dysfunction:** Determine the presence of ED before use
• Assess for use of organic nitrates that should not be used with this product
• Assess for severe loss of vision while taking this or any similar products; these products should not be used if vision loss has occurred

Patient problem

Impaired sexual functioning (uses)

Implementation

• Take approximately 1 hr before sexual activity; do not use more than once a day
• Orally disintegrating tabs are not interchangeable with film-coated tabs
• **Orally disintegrating tab:** place on tongue immediately after opening blister pack, allow to dissolve, do not use water

Patient/family education

• Advise that product does not protect against STDs, including HIV
• Teach that product absorption is reduced with a high-fat meal
• Instruct that product should not be used with nitrates in any form
• Inform that product has no effect in the absence of sexual stimulation
• Teach that patient should seek immediate medical attention if erection lasts for more than 4 hr

• Advise to inform physician of all medications being taken
• Teach patient to notify prescriber immediately and stop taking product if vision loss occurs

Evaluation

Positive therapeutic outcome
• Sustainable erection

---

varenicline (Rx)
(var-e-ni'kleen)
Champix ✦, Chantix
Func. class.: Smoking cessation agent
Chem. class.: Nicotine agonist

ACTION: Partial agonist for nicotine receptors; partially activates receptors to help curb cravings; occupies receptors to prevent nicotine binding

Therapeutic outcome: Smoking cessation

USES: Smoking deterrent

Pharmacokinetics

Absorption	100%
Distribution	Steady state 4 days
Metabolism	Minimal
Excretion	Urine 92%, unchanged
Half-life	24 hr

Pharmacodynamics

Onset	Unknown
Peak	3-4 hr
Duration	24 hr

CONTRAINDICATIONS
Hypersensitivity, eating disorders

Precautions: Pregnancy, breastfeeding, children <18 yr, geriatric, renal disease, recent MI, angioedema
• Bipolar disorder, depression, schizophrenia, suicidal ideation

DOSAGE AND ROUTES
Adult: PO therapy should begin 1 week prior to smoking stop date (i.e., take product plus tobacco for 7 days); titrate for 1 wk, days 1 through 3, 0.5 mg/day; days 4 through 7, 0.5 mg bid; day 8 through end of treatment 1 mg bid; treatment is 12 wk and may repeat for another 12 wk

Renal dose
Adult: PO CCr ≤50 ml/min, titrate to max 0.5 mg bid

Available forms: Tabs 0.5, 1 mg

ADVERSE EFFECTS
CNS: Headache, agitation, dizziness, insomnia, abnormal dreams, fatigue, malaise, behavior changes, depression, homicidal/suicidal ideation, amnesia, hallucinations, hostility, mania, psychosis, tremor, seizures, stroke
CV: Dysrhythmias, MI
EENT: *Blurred vision*
GI: *Nausea, vomiting,* anorexia, *dry mouth,* increased/decreased appetite, *constipation,* flatulence, GERD, diarrhea, gingivitis, dyspepsia, enterocolitis
GU: Erectile dysfunction, urinary frequency, menstrual irregularities
INTEG: Rash, pruritus, angioedema, Stevens-Johnson syndrome, flushing dermatitis
MS: Back pain, myalgia, *arthralgia*
HEMA: Anemia

NURSING CONSIDERATIONS
Assessment
• **Assess smoking history:** motivation for smoking cessation, years used, amount each day, assess for smoking cessation after 12 wk; if progress has not been made, product may be used for an additional 12 wk
• **Neuropsychiatric symptoms:** assess for mood, sensorium, affect, behavioral changes, agitation, suicidal ideation; suicide has occurred; possible worsening of depression, schizophrenia, bipolar disorder; risk is increased in adolescents
• **Angioedema/Stevens-Johnson syndrome:** Assess for rash during treatment, discontinue if rash, fever, fatigue, joint pain, lesions occur
• **Pregnancy/breastfeeding:** Not used in women

Patient problem
Risk for injury (uses, adverse reactions)

Implementation
• Do not break, crush, or chew tabs
• Give increased fluids, bulk in diet if constipation occurs
• Give with a full glass of water after eating
• Give sugarless gum, hard candy, or frequent sips of water for dry mouth

Patient/family education
• Teach patient that treatment for smoking cessation lasts 12 wk and another 12 wk may be required
• Teach patient to use caution in driving, other activities requiring alertness; blurred vision may occur
• Advise patient to set a date to quit smoking and initiate treatment 1 wk prior to that date
• Teach patient how to titrate product

V

- Advise patient not to use with nicotine patches unless directed by prescriber; may increase B/P
- Advise patient to notify prescriber if pregnancy is suspected or planned
- Teach patient that vivid dreams, insomnia may occur during beginning of treatment, but usually subside
- To notify all prescribers of all OTC/Rx/herbs used
- Instruct patient to notify prescriber immediately of change in thought/behavior (suicidal ideation, hostility, depression); stop product
- Advise patient to notify prescriber if pregnancy is planned or suspected

Evaluation
Positive therapeutic outcome
- Smoking cessation

⚠ HIGH ALERT

vasopressin (Rx)
(vay-soe-press′in)
Vasostrict
Func. class.: Pituitary hormone
Chem. class.: Lysine vasopressin

ACTION: Promotes reabsorption of water by action on renal tubular epithelium; causes vasoconstriction on muscles in the GI system

Therapeutic outcome: Increased osmolality, decreased urine output in diabetes insipidus

USES: Diabetes insipidus (nonnephrogenic/nonpsychogenic), hypotension, postcardiotomy shock, septic shock

Unlabeled uses: GI hemorrhage, cardiac arrest, CPR

Pharmacokinetics

Absorption	Erratically absorbed (IM)
Distribution	Widely distributed extracellular fluid
Metabolism	Liver, rapidly
Excretion	Kidneys, unchanged
Half-life	10 min

Pharmacodynamics

	IM	IV
Onset	1 hr	Unknown
Peak	Unknown	Unknown
Duration	3-8 hr	60 min

CONTRAINDICATIONS
Hypersensitivity, chronic nephritis

Precautions: Pregnancy, breastfeeding, CAD, asthma, renal/vascular disease, migraines, seizures

DOSAGE AND ROUTES
Diabetes insipidus
Adult: IM/SUBCUT 5-10 units bid-qid prn; CONT **IV** INF 0.0005 units/kg/hr, (0.5 milliunit/kg/hr), double dose q30min as needed
Child: IM/SUBCUT 2.5-10 units bid-qid prn

Hypotension in septic shock
Adult: IV 0.01 units/min, titrate by 0.005 units/min q10-15min until target B/P is achieved, to max 0.07 units/min after target B/P of 8 hr without use of catecholamines; taper 0.005 units/min qhr to maintain B/P

GI hemorrhage (unlabeled)
Adults IV 0.2-0.4 units/min titrate, max 0.8 units/min

Available forms: Sol for inj 20 units/ml

ADVERSE EFFECTS
CNS: Headache, lethargy, flushing
CV: Chest pain, MI
GI: Nausea, heartburn, cramps, vomiting, flatus
MISC: Urticaria

INTERACTIONS
Individual drugs
Clozapine, foscaret, lithium: decreased antidiuretic effect
Demeclocycline, lithium, chlorpropamide, cyclophosphamide, enalapril, felbamate, haloperidol, pentamine: increased antidiuretic effect

Drug classifications
Tricyclics: increased antidiuretic effect

NURSING CONSIDERATIONS
Assessment
- Monitor pulse, B/P, ECG periodically during treatment, if using for CPR monitor continuously
- Monitor for **Diabetes insipidus:** I&O ratio, weight daily, fluid/electrolyte balance, urine specific gravity, check for extreme thirst, poor skin turgor, dilute urine, large urine volume; check for water intoxication: lethargy, behavioral changes, disorientation, neuromuscular excitability
- Small doses may precipitate coronary adverse effects; keep emergency equipment nearby
- **Pregnancy/breastfeeding:** Use only if benefits outweigh fetal risk, breastfeeding women should pump and discard milk for 1.5 hr after receiving product

Patient problem
Fluid imbalance (uses)

Implementation
IM/SUBCUT route
• May be given IM/SUBCUT for diagnosis of diabetes insipidus (aqeous vassopressin)
• Give patient 16 oz water at administration to prevent nausea, vomiting, cramping
Continuous IV infusion
• Dilute in 0.9% NaCl or D5W (0.1 units/mL or 1 units/mL); store refrigerated for 24 hr, room temperature 18 hr

Patient/family education
• Caution patient to avoid OTC products for cough, hay fever because these preparations may contain EPINEPHrine, decrease product response; do not use with alcohol
• Advise patient to carry/wear emergency ID specifying therapy, disease process (diabetes insipidus)
• Teach patient to measure/record I&O
• Teach patient to avoid all OTC, herbals, supplements, medications unless approved by prescriber

Evaluation
Positive therapeutic outcome
• Absence of severe thirst
• Decreased urine output, osmolality

vedolizumab
(ve'-doe-liz'ue-mab)
Entyvio
Func. class.: GI antiinflammatory
Chem. class.: Integrin receptor antagonist

ACTION: A specific integrin receptor antagonist that inhibits the migration of specific memory T lymphocytes across the endothelium into inflamed gastrointestinal parenchymal tissue. The action reduces the chronic inflammatory process present in both ulcerative colitis and Crohn's disease

Therapeutic outcome: Lessening of ulcerative colitis and Crohn's disease

USES: For moderately to severely active ulcerative colitis/Crohn's disease; to reduce signs and symptoms, and to induce and maintain clinical remission in patients who have an inadequate response to conventional therapy

Pharmacokinetics

Absorption	Complete
Distribution	Unknown
Metabolism	Unknown
Excretion	Unknown
Half-life	25 days

Pharmacodynamics

Onset	Up to 6 wk
Peak	Unknown
Duration	Up to 8 wk

CONTRAINDICATIONS: Hypersensitivity

Precautions: Hepatic disease, infections, progressive multifocal leukoencephalopathy (PML), pregnancy, breastfeeding, live vaccines, TB, human antichimeric antibody (HACA)

DOSAGE AND ROUTES
Adult: IV INF 300 mg; give over 30 min at weeks 0, 2, and 6 as induction therapy, then 300 mg q8wk continue if response occurs by wk 14

Available forms: Powder for injection 300 mg/20 mL vial

ADVERSE EFFECTS
CNS: *Headache*, fatigue, dizziness
GI: Nausea, vomiting
MISC: Rash, pruritus, infusion-related reactions
MS: *Arthralgia*, back pain
RESP: Cough
SYST: Anaphylaxis, progressive multifocal leukoencephalopathy (PML), increased infection risk

INTERACTIONS
Drug classifications
Antineoplastics, immunosuppressives: increased infection risk
Do not use with tumor necrosis factor (TNF) modifiers
Toxoids, vaccines: decreased immune response

NURSING CONSIDERATIONS
Assessment
• **Ulcerative colitis/Crohn's disease:** Monitor symptoms before and after treatment
• **Hypersensitivity:** Swelling of lips, tongue, throat, face, rash, wheezing, hypertension; if serious reactions occur discontinue product
• **Liver dysfunction:** Monitor for elevated hepatic enzymes, jaundice, malaise, nausea, vomiting, abdominal pain, and anorexia; these signs are predictive of severe liver injury that may be fatal or may require a liver transplant in some patients; if hepatic dysfunction is suspected, discontinue
• **Tuberculosis (TB) latent/active:** Obtain TB skin test both before and during treatment. Do not give in active infection such as influenza or sepsis

V

- **Progressive multifocal leukoencephalopathy (PML):** Assess for increased weakness on one side of the body or clumsiness of limbs, visual disturbance, and changes in thinking, memory, and orientation leading to confusion and personality changes; severe disability or death can come over weeks or months

Patient problem
Pain (uses)
Risk for infection (adverse reactions)

Implementation
- Full response is usually observed by 6 wk; those who do not respond by week 14 are unlikely to respond
- Give as IV infusion only, do not use as an IV push or bolus
- Make sure all immunizations are up to date
- Reconstitute with 4.8 ml of sterile water for injection, using a syringe with a 21- to 25-gauge needle
- Insert the syringe needle into the vial and direct the stream of sterile water for injection to the glass wall of the vial; gently swirl the solution for 15 sec; do not shake
- Allow the solution to stand for up to 20 min at room temperature to allow for reconstitution and for any foam to settle
- Once dissolved, product should be clear or opalescent, colorless to light brownish yellow, and free of visible particulates. Discard if discolored or if foreign particles are present.
- Before withdrawing solution from vial, gently invert vial 3 times. Withdraw 5 ml (300 mg) of reconstituted product using a 21- to 25-gauge needle. Discard remaining product.
- Add the 5 ml (300 mg) of reconstituted product to 250 ml of sterile 0.9% sodium chloride and gently mix infusion bag. Do not mix with other medications. Administer solution as soon as possible; if necessary, solution may be stored for up to 4 hr refrigerated; do not freeze. Infuse over 30 min; after infusion, flush line with 30 ml of sterile 0.9% sodium chloride injection. Discard any unused infusion solution.

Patient/family education
- Teach patient about the symptoms of infection and to report to health care provider immediately
- Advise patient to report planned or suspected pregnancy, or if breastfeeding, if pregnant, to call 1-877-825-3327 to enroll in the Entyvia Pregnancy Registry
- Teach patient not to use live virus vaccines while taking this product, bring vaccinations up to date before starting product
- Teach patient to report allergic reactions, hepatotoxicity, PML, teach symptoms
- Inform patient reason for product, expected result
- Teach patient that risk of infection is increased; to notify health care professional of fever, chills, trouble breathing, sore throat
- Teach patient to discuss with health care professional all Rx, OTC, herbals, supplements taken

Evaluation
Positive therapeutic response
- Lessening of ulcerative colitis and Crohn's disease

⚠ HIGH ALERT
vemurafenib
(vem-ue-raf′e-nib)
Zelboraf
Func. class.: Antineoplastic
Chem. class.: Kinase inhibitor

ACTION: Inhibitor of some mutated forms of ▶◀ BRAF serine threonine kinase, thereby blocking cellular proliferation in melanoma cells with the mutation. It also inhibits other kinases including ▶◀ CRAF, ARAF, wild-type BRAF, SRMA, ACK1, MAP4H5, and FGR. It is a potent adenosine triphosphate-competitive inhibitor of RAFs with a modest preference for mutant BRAF and CRAF as compared with wild-type BRAF.

Therapeutic outcome: Decreased spread of malignancy

USES: Unresectable or metastatic malignant melanoma with V600E mutation of the BRAF gene

Pharmacokinetics
Absorption	Minimal
Distribution	Protein binding 99%
Metabolism	Liver by CYP3A4
Excretion	94% feces
Half-life	30-120 hr

Pharmacodynamics
Onset	Unknown
Peak	3 hr
Duration	Up to 12 hr

CONTRAINDICATIONS
Hypersensitivity

Precautions: Pregnancy, breastfeeding, children, infants, neonates, hepatic disease, QT prolongation, secondary malignancy, torsades de pointes, hypokalemia, hypomagnesium, sunlight exposure

---

DOSAGE AND ROUTES
Adult: PO 960 mg (4 tabs) bid about q12h, continue until unacceptable toxicity or disease progression; if strong CYP3A4 inducers are used increase dose to 1200 mg (5 tablets) bid

Available forms: Tab 240 mg

ADVERSE EFFECTS
CNS: *Fatigue*, fever, dizziness, headache, muscle paralysis, peripheral neuropathy, weakness
CV: Atrial fibrillation, hypotension, QT prolongation
EENT: Blurred vision, iritis, photophobia, uveitis
GI: Dysgeusia, nausea, hepatotoxicity
INTEG: Actinic keratosis, *alopecia*, hyperkeratosis, *maculopapular rash*, palmar-plantar erythrodysesthesia (hand and foot syndrome), papular rash, *photosensitivity, pruritus, xerosis/dry skin*
MS: *Arthralgia*, arthritis, back pain, extremity pain, musculoskeletal pain, *myalgias*
GU: Acute tubular necrosis, interstitial nephritis
SYST: Anaphylaxis, secondary malignancy, Stevens-Johnson syndrome, toxic epidermal necrolysis, drug reaction with eosinophilia/anaphylaxis

INTERACTIONS
Individual drugs
Abarelix, alfuzosin, amoxapine, apomorphine, arsenic trioxide, asenapine, chloroquine, ciprofloxacin, citalopram, clarithromycin, cloZAPine, cyclobenzaprine, dasatinib, dolasetron, dronedarone, droperidol, eribulin, erythromycin, ezogabine, flecainide, fluconazole, gatifloxacin, gemifloxacin, grepafloxacin, halofantrine, haloperidol, iloperidone, indacaterol, lapatinib, levofloxacin, levomethadyl, lopinavir/ritonavir, magnesium sulfate, maprotiline, mefloquine, methadone, moxifloxacin, nilotinib, norfloxacin, octreotide, ofloxacin, OLANZapine, ondansetron, paliperidone, palonosetron, pentamidine, pimozide, posaconazole, potassium sulfate, probucol, propafenone, QUEtiapine, quiNIDine, ranolazine, rilpivirine, risperiDONE, saquinavir, sodium, sparfloxacin, SUNItinib, tacrolimus, telavancin, telithromycin, tetrabenazine, troleandomycin, vardenafil, vemurafenib, venlafaxine, vorinostat, ziprasidone: increased QT prolongation, torsades de pointes

Drug classifications
β-agonists, Class IA antiarrhythmics (disopyramide, procainamide, quiNIDine), Class III antiarrhythmics (amiodarone, dofetilide, ibutilide, sotalol), halogenated anesthetics, local anesthetics, certain phenothiazines (chlorproMAZINE, fluPHENAZine, mesoridazine, perphenazine, prochlorperazine, thioridazine and trifluoperazine), tricyclic antidepressants: increased QT prolongation, torsades de pointes
CYP3A4 inducers (alcohol, barbiturates, bexarotono, carBAMazepine, erythromycin, etravirine, fluvoxaMINE, ketoconazole, metyrapone, modafinil, nevirapine, OXcarbazepine, phenytoin, rifabutin, rifampin, ritonavir): decreased vemurafenib effect
CYP3A4/CYP1A2 inhibitors (cimetidine, dalfopristin, delavirdine, enoxacin, indinavir, isoniazid, itraconazole, quinupristin, tipranavir): increased vemurafenib effect

Drug/lab test
Alkaline phosphatase, bilirubin, LFTs, serum creatinine: increase

NURSING CONSIDERATIONS
Assessment
• **Hepatotoxicity:** Monitor LFTs and bilirubin levels prior to treatment, then monthly; more frequent testing is needed in those presenting with grade 2 or greater toxicities; Laboratory alterations should be managed with dose reduction, treatment interruption, or discontinuation
• **QT prolongation:** Avoid in patients with QT prolongation; Monitor ECG and electrolytes in those with congestive heart failure, bradycardia, electrolyte imbalance (hypokalemia, hypomagnesemia), or in those who are taking concomitant medications known to prolong the QT interval; treatment interruption, dosage adjustment, treatment discontinuation may be needed in those who develop QT prolongation
• Serum electrolytes, CCR, bilirubin, ECG
• **BRAF testing:** Obtain testing before use, do not use in wild-type *BRAF*, confirm *BRAF* V600E mutation
• **Skin reactions:** Assess for cuSCC skin reactions

Patient problem
Risk for injury (uses, adverse reactions)

Implementation
• Continue until disease progresses or unacceptable toxicity occurs
• Missed doses can be taken up to 4 hr before the next dose is due; take about 12 hr apart; take without regard to meals
• Swallow whole with a full glass of water; do not crush or chew
• Store at room temperature in original container

V

Patient/family education
• Teach patient/family that missed doses can be taken up to 4 hr before the next dose is due to maintain the twice-daily regimen; if vomiting occurs, do not retake dose, take next scheduled dose
• Teach patient to notify provider of new skin lesions
• Advise patient to notify health care professional of hepatotoxicity, yellow skin, eyes, dark urine, clay-colored stool, nausea/vomiting, pain in right side of abdomen; allergic reactions: rash, trouble breathing, swelling of face, lips, blisters
• Advise patient to discuss with health care professional all Rx, OTC, herbals, supplements taken
• Advise patient to avoid sun exposure, wear sunscreen, protective clothing
• **Pregnancy/breastfeeding:** Identify if pregnancy is planned or suspected; do not use in pregnancy, avoid breastfeeding. Teach patient to use reliable contraception; both women and men of childbearing age should use adequate contraceptive methods during therapy and for at least 90 days after completing treatment

Evaluation
Positive therapeutic outcome
• Decreased spread of malignancy

⚠ HIGH ALERT
RARELY USED

venetoclax
(veh-neh′toh-klax)
Venclexta
Func. class.: Antineoplastic, signal transduction inhibitor

USES: Treatment of CLL in patients with a 17p deletion who have received at least one prior therapy

CONTRAINDICATIONS
Hypersensitivity, pregnancy

DOSAGE AND ROUTES
Adult: PO initially 20 mg qday × 7 days, increase dose qwk × 5 wk: wk 2, 50 mg/day; wk 3, 100 mg/day; wk 4, 200 mg/day; wk 5 and beyond, 400 mg/day. Continue therapy until disease progression. A dose reduction and/or therapy interruption may be necessary in patients who develop toxicity

venlafaxine (Rx)
(ven-la-fax′een)
Effexor XR
Func. class.: Second-generation SNRI antidepressant—miscellaneous

ACTION: Potent inhibitor of neuronal serotonin and norepinephrine uptake, weak inhibitor of dopamine; no muscarinic, histaminergic, or α-adrenergic receptors in vitro

Therapeutic outcome: Relief of depression

USES: Prevention/treatment of major depression, to treat depression at end of life; long-term treatment of generalized anxiety disorder, panic disorder, social anxiety disorder (Effexor XR only)

Pharmacokinetics
Absorption	Well absorbed
Distribution	Widely distributed, 27% protein binding
Metabolism	Liver, extensively (CYP2D6), some are poor metabolizers ⚕
Excretion	Kidneys, 87%
Half-life	5 hr, 11 hr (active metabolite)

Pharmacodynamics
Onset	Up to 14 day
Peak	Up to 4 wks
Duration	Unknown

CONTRAINDICATIONS
Hypersensitivity, MAOIs

Precautions: Pregnancy, breastfeeding, geriatric, mania, recent MI, cardiac/renal/hepatic disease, seizure disorder, hypertension, eosinophilic pneumonia, desvenlafaxine hypersensitivity

BLACK BOX WARNING: Children, suicidal ideation

DOSAGE AND ROUTES
Major depression
Adult: PO 75 mg/day in 2 or 3 divided doses; taken with food, may be increased to 150 mg/day; if needed may be further increased to 225 mg/day; increments of 75 mg/day should be made at intervals of no less than 4 days; some hospitalized patients may require up to 375 mg/day in 3 divided doses; EXT REL 37.5-75 mg PO daily, max 225 mg/day; give Effexor XR daily

Anxiety disorders
Adult: PO 75 mg/day or 37.5 mg/day × 4-7 days initially, max 225 mg/day

---

Hepatic dose
Adult: PO moderate impairment 50% of dose

Renal dose
Adult: PO CCr 10-70 ml/min reduce dose by 25%-50%; CCr <10 ml/min reduce by 50%

Available forms: Tabs scored (Effexor) 25, 37.5, 50, 75, 100 mg; ext rel caps (Effexor XR) 37.5, 75, 150, 225 mg

ADVERSE EFFECTS
CNS: *Emotional lability, dizziness, weakness,* headache, hallucinations, insomnia, anxiety, suicidal ideation in children/adolescents, seizures, neuroleptic malignant syndrome–like reaction, anxiety, abnormal dreams, paresthesia
CV: Chest pain, postural hypotension, syncope, hypertension, tachycardia
EENT: *Abnormal vision,* taste, *ear pain*
GI: *Dysphagia, eructation,* colitis, gastritis, gingivitis, *constipation,* stomatitis, stomach and mouth ulceration, nausea, anorexia, dry mouth, *abdominal pain, vomiting, weight loss*
GU: *Anorgasmia,* abnormal ejaculation, urinary frequency, decreased libido, impotence, menstrual changes
INTEG: Ecchymosis, acne, alopecia, brittle nails, dry skin, photosensitivity, sweating, angioedema (ext rel), Stevens-Johnson syndrome
META: *Peripheral edema, weight loss*

INTERACTIONS
Individual drugs
Alcohol: increased CNS depression
Cimetidine: increased venlafaxine effect
CloZAPine, desipramine, haloperidol, warfarin: increased levels of these products
Cyproheptadine: decreased venlafaxine effect
Indinavir: decreased effect of indinavir
Linezolid, methylene blue, sibutramine, SUMAtriptan, traMADol, traZODone, tryptophan: increased serotonin syndrome

Drug classifications
Antihistamines, opioids, sedative-hypnotics: increased CNS depression
MAOIs: hyperthermia, rigidity, rapid fluctuations of vital signs, mental status changes, neuroleptic malignant syndrome
Salicylates, NSAIDs, platelet inhibitors, anticoagulants: increased bleeding risk
SSRIs, SNRIs, serotonin-receptor agonists: increased serotonin syndrome

Drug/herb
Chamomile, hops, Kava, valerian: increased CNS depression
St. John's wort: serotonin syndrome

Drug/lab test
Increased: alkaline phosphatase, bilirubin, AST, ALT, BUN, creatinine, serum cholesterol, CPK, LDH
False positive: amphetamines, phencyclidine

NURSING CONSIDERATIONS
Assessment

BLACK BOX WARNING: Assess mental status: mood, sensorium, affect; increase in psychiatric symptoms: depression, panic; for suicidal ideation in children/adolescents, discuss with family members and in early treatment

• Monitor B/P (lying, standing), pulse q4hr; if systolic B/P drops 20 mm Hg hold product, notify prescriber; take vital signs q4hr in patients with CV disease
• Monitor blood tests: CBC, leukocytes, differential, cardiac enzymes if patient is receiving long-term therapy
• Monitor liver function tests: AST, ALT, bilirubin
• Check weight qwk; weight loss or gain; appetite may increase, peripheral edema may occur
• Monitor urinary retention, constipation; constipation is more likely to occur in children or geriatrics
• **Assess for withdrawal symptoms:** headache, nausea, vomiting, muscle pain, weakness; do not usually occur unless product was discontinued abruptly, taper over 14 days
• Identify alcohol consumption; if alcohol is consumed, hold dose
• **Serotonin syndrome, neuroleptic malignant syndrome:** assess for increased heart rate, shivering, sweating, dilated pupils, tremors, high B/P, hyperthermia, headache, confusion; if these occur, stop product, administer a serotonin antagonist if needed; usually worse if given with linezolid, methylene blue, tryptophan
• **Beers:** Use with caution in older adults, may exacerbate or cause syndrome of inappropriate antidiuretic hormone secretion
• **Pregnancy/breastfeeding:** Use only if benefits outweigh fetal risk, use in late 3rd trimester has resulted in neonatal complications, do not breastfeed, excreted in breast milk

Patient problem
Risk for depression (uses)
Suicidal ideation (adverse reactions)

Implementation
• Give with food or milk for GI symptoms
• Swallow ext rel whole; do not break, crush, chew
• May open cap and sprinkle on soft food, use immediately
• Store at room temperature; do not freeze

Patient/family education
• Advise patient to notify prescriber of rash, hives, or allergic reactions
• Teach patient that therapeutic effects may take 2-3 wk
• Teach patient to use caution in driving or other activities requiring alertness because of drowsiness, dizziness, blurred vision; to avoid rising quickly from sitting to standing, especially geriatric
• Teach patient to avoid alcohol ingestion, other CNS depressants
Serotonin syndrome, neuroleptic malignant syndrome: advise patient to report immediately shivering, sweating, tremors, fever, dilated pupils
• Advise patient to avoid pregnancy, breast-feeding while taking this product, birth defects have occurred when used in the 3rd trimester
• Teach patient that worsening of symptoms, suicidal thoughts/behavior may occur in children, young adults
• Advise patient to take as prescribed, contents of capsule may be sprinkled on applesauce if unable to swallow whole

Evaluation

Positive therapeutic outcome
• Decreased depression, anxiety; sense of well-being
• Absence of suicidal thoughts

TREATMENT OF OVERDOSE:
ECG monitoring, induce emesis, lavage, administer anticonvulsant

---

⚠ HIGH ALERT

verapamil (Rx)
(ver-ap′a-mil)
Calan, Calan SR, Covera ✦, Isoptin, Isoptin SR, Verelan, Verelan PM
Func. class.: Calcium-channel blocker; antihypertensive; antianginal, antidysrhythmic (Class IV)
Chem. class.: Diphenylalkylamine

ACTION: Inhibits calcium ion influx across cell membrane during cardiac depolarization; produces relaxation of coronary vascular smooth muscle, peripheral vascular smooth muscle; dilates coronary vascular arteries; decreases SA/AV node conduction; dilates peripheral arteries

Therapeutic outcome: Decreased angina pectoris, dysrhythmias, B/P

USES: Chronic stable vasospastic, unstable angina; dysrhythmias, hypertension, supraventricular tachycardia, atrial flutter or fibrillation

Pharmacokinetics
Absorption	Well absorbed (PO)
Distribution	Protein binding 90%
Metabolism	Liver, extensively, by CYP3A4
Excretion	Kidneys (70%)
Half-life	3-12 hr

Pharmacodynamics
	PO	PO-EXT REL	IV
Onset	1-2 hr	Unknown	1-5 min
Peak	½-1½ hr	5-7 hr	3-5 min
Duration	3-7 hr	24 hr	2 hr

CONTRAINDICATIONS
Sick sinus syndrome, 2nd- or 3rd-degree heart block, hypotension <90 mm Hg systolic, cardiogenic shock, severe HF, Lown-Ganong-Levine syndrome, Wolff-Parkinson-White syndrome

Precautions: Pregnancy, breastfeeding, children, geriatric, HF, hypotension, hepatic injury, renal disease, concomitant β-blocker therapy

DOSAGE AND ROUTES
Angina
Adult: PO 80-120 mg tid, increase qwk, max 480 mg/day

Dysrhythmias
Adult: PO 240-320 mg/day in 3-4 divided doses in digitalized patients
Adult: IV BOL 5-10 mg (0.075-0.15 mg/kg) over 2 min, may repeat 10 mg (0.15 mg/kg) ½ hr after first dose
Child 1-15 yr: IV BOL 0.1-0.3 mg/kg over >2 min, repeat in 30 min, max 5 mg in a single dose
Child 0-1 yr: IV BOL 0.1-0.2 mg/kg over ≥2 min, may repeat after 30 min

Hypertension
Adult: PO 80 mg tid, may titrate upward; EXT REL 120-240 mg/day as a single dose, may increase to 240-480 mg/day

Hepatic dose/geriatric/compromised ventricular function
Adult: PO 40 mg tid initially, increase as tolerated

Available forms: Tabs 40, 80, 120 mg; ext rel tabs 120, 180, 240 mg; inj 2.5 mg/ml in ampules, syringes, vials; ext rel caps 100, 200, 240, 300 mg

---

ADVERSE EFFECTS
CNS: *Headache, drowsiness,* dizziness, anxiety, depression, weakness, asthenia, fatigue, insomnia, confusion, light-headedness
CV: *Edema,* HF, bradycardia, hypotension, palpitations, AV block, dysrhythmias
EENT: Blurred vision, tinnitus, equilibrium change, epistaxis
GI: *Nausea,* diarrhea, gastric upset, *constipation,* elevated liver function tests
GU: Impotence, nocturia, polyuria, gynecomastia
HEMA: Bruising, petechiae, bleeding
INTEG: Rash, bruising
MISC: Gingival hyperplasia
RESP: Cough, dyspnea
SYST: Stevens-Johnson syndrome

INTERACTIONS
Individual drugs
CarBAMazepine, cycloSPORINE, digoxin, theophylline: increased levels of each specific product
Cimetidine, clarithromycin, erythromycin: increased effect of verapamil
FentaNYL, prazosin, quiNIDine: increased hypotension
Lithium: decreased lithium levels

Drug classifications
Antihypertensive, β-adrenergic blockers, nitrates: increased effects of verapamil, monitor for CV effects
Nondepolarizing muscle relaxants: increased effect
NSAIDs: decreased antihypertensive effect

Drug/herb
Ephedra (ma huang): increased hypertension
Ginseng, ginkgo: increased verapamil effect
St. John's wort: decreased verapamil effect

Drug/food
Grapefruit juice: increased hypotension

Drug/lab test
Increased: alkaline phosphatase, AST, ALT, BUN, creatinine, serum cholesterol

NURSING CONSIDERATIONS
Assessment
• **HF:** Assess fluid volume status: I&O ratio and record; weight; distended red veins; crackles in lung; color; quality, specific gravity of urine; skin turgor; adequacy of pulses; moist mucous membranes; bilateral lung sounds; peripheral pitting edema; dehydration symptoms of decreasing output, thirst, hypotension, dry mouth, and mucous membranes should be reported
• Monitor B/P and pulse, pulmonary capillary wedge pressure (PCWP), central venous pressure,

index, often during inf; notify prescriber if <50 bpm, systolic B/P <90 mm Hg
• Monitor ALT, AST, bilirubin daily; if these are elevated, hepatotoxicity is suspected
• Monitor platelets; if <150,000/mm³, product is usually discontinued and another product started
• Assess for extravasation; change site q48hr
• **Monitor cardiac status:** B/P, pulse, respiration, ECG
• Monitor renal/hepatic function tests during long-term treatment, serum potassium, periodically
• **Beers:** Avoid use in older adults, may cause fluid retention or exacerbate heart failure

Patient problem
Impaired cardiac output (uses)
Pain (uses)

Implementation
PO route
• **Regular release:** give without regard to food, give with meals or milk to prevent gastric upset
• **Extended release:** do not crush or chew ext rel products
• **Verelan PM:** cap may be opened and contents sprinkled on food; do not dissolve, chew cap
• Give once a day before meals at bedtime; sus rel give with food to decrease GI symptoms

Direct IV route
• Give by direct **IV** undiluted (Y-site, 3-way stopcock) over at least 2 min, or 3 min geriatric; discard unused sol; to prevent serious hypotension, patient should be recumbent for 1 hr or more, with continuous ECG and B/P monitoring
• Do not use IV with IV β-blockers, may cause AV nodal blockade

Y-site compatibilities: Alfentanil, amikacin, argatroban, ascorbic acid, atracurium, atropine, aztreonam, bivalirudin, bumetanide, buprenorphine, butorphanol, calcium chloride/gluconate, CARBOplatin, caspofungin, ceFAZolin, cefonicid, cefotaxime, cefoTEtan, cefOXitin, ceftizoxime, cefTRIAXone, cefuroxime, chlorproMAZINE, cimetidine, ciprofloxacin, clindamycin, cyanocobalamin, cyclophosphamide, cycloSPORINE, cytarabine, DACTINomycin, DAPTOmycin, dexamethasone, dexmedetomidine, digoxin, diltiazem, diphenhydrAMINE, DOBUTamine, DOCEtaxel, DOPamine, doxacurium, DOXOrubicin hydrochloride, doxycycline, enalaprilat, ePHEDrine, EPINEPHrine, epirubicin, epoetin alfa, eptifibatide, erythromycin, esmolol, etoposide, etoposide phosphate, famotidine, fenoldopam, fentaNYL, fluconazole, fludarabine, gemcitabine, gentamicin, glycopyrrolate, granisetron, heparin, hydrALAZINE, hydrocortisone, HYDRO-morphone, ifosfamide, imipenem/cilastatin, in-amrinone, insulin, isoproterenol, ketorolac, la-betalol, levofloxacin, lidocaine, linezolid, LORazepam, magnesium sulfate, mannitol, mechlorethamine, meperidine, metaraminol, methotrexate, methoxamine, methyldopate, methylPREDNISolone, metoclopramide, meto-prolol, metroNIDAZOLE, miconazole, mid-azolam, milrinone, mitoXANtrone, morphine, multivitamins, nalbuphine, naloxone, nesiritide, nitroglycerin, nitroprusside, norepinephrine, octreotide, ondansetron, oxaliplatin, oxytocin, PACLitaxel, palonosetron, papaverine, PEME-trexed, penicillin G, pentamidine, pentazocine, phentolamine, phenylephrine, phytonadione, piperacillin/tazobactam, potassium chloride, procainamide, prochlorperazine, promethazine, propranolol, protamine, pyridoxine, quinupris-tin/dalfopristin, ranitidine, rocuronium, sodium acetate, succinylcholine, SUFentanil, tacrolimus, teniposide, theophylline, thiamine, ticarcillin/clavulanate, tirofiban, tobramycin, tolazoline, trimethaphan, urokinase, vancomycin, vasopres-sin, vecuronium, vinCRIStine, vinorelbine, vori-conazole

Patient/family education
• Advise patient to increase fluids/fiber to counteract constipation
• Caution patient to avoid hazardous activities until stabilized on product and dizziness is no longer a problem
• Teach patient how to take pulse, B/P before taking product; to keep record or graph
• Instruct patient to limit caffeine consumption; to avoid alcohol, grapefruit, and OTC products unless directed by prescriber
• Advise patient to comply with medical regimen: diet, exercise, stress reduction, product therapy; to notify prescriber of irregular heartbeat, shortness of breath, swelling of feet and hands, pronounced dizziness, constipation, nausea, hypotension, **IV** calcium
• Teach patient to use as directed even if feeling better; may be taken with other CV products (nitrates, β-blockers)
• Caution patient not to discontinue abruptly; chest pain may occur
• **Stevens-Johnson syndrome:** Rash, fever, fatigue, joint pain, lesions, discontinue immediately
• Advise to report chest pain, palpitations, irregular heartbeats, swelling of extremities, skin irritation, rash, tremors, weakness
• Instruct patient to notify prescriber if preg-nancy is planned; avoid breastfeeding

Evaluation
Positive therapeutic outcome
• Decreased anginal pain
• Decreased dysrhythmias
• Decreased B/P

TREATMENT OF OVERDOSE:
Defibrillation, atropine for AV block, vasopressor for hypotension, **IV** calcium

---

vilazodone (Rx)
(vil-az'oh-done)
Viibryd
Func. class.: Antidepressant
Chem. class.: SSRI, benzofuran

ACTION: A novel antidepressant unrelated to other antidepressants, enhances serotoniner-gic action by a dual mechanism

Therapeutic outcome: Remission of de-pressive symptoms

USES: Major depression

Pharmacokinetics

Absorption	Unknown
Distribution	Protein binding 96-99%
Metabolism	Metabolized by the liver by CYP 3A4 (major) and CY-P2C19 and CYP2D (minor) and non-CYP pathways
Excretion	Unknown
Half-life	25 hr

Pharmacodynamics

Onset	Unknown
Peak	4-5 hr
Duration	Unknown

CONTRAINDICATIONS
Concomitant use of MAOIs or within 14 days af-ter discontinuing an MAOI or within 14 days after discontinuing vilazodone

Precautions: Abrupt discontinuation, bipo-lar disorder, bleeding, operating machinery, ECT, geriatrics, hepatic disease, hyponatremia, hypo-volemia, infants, labor, pregnancy, substance abuse, history of seizures, serotonin syndrome, neuroleptic malignant syndrome, use with sero-tonin precursors, serotonergic drugs, suicidal ideation and worsening depression or behavior

BLACK BOX WARNING: Child, suicidal ideation

DOSAGE AND ROUTES
Major depressive disorder
Adult: PO 10 mg ×7 days, then 20 mg ×7 days, then 40 mg/day; with a potent CYP3A4 inhibitor, max 20 mg/day; with a potent CYP3A4 inducer-increased dose up to double may be needed, max 80 mg/day

Available forms: Tabs 10, 20, 40 mg

ADVERSE EFFECTS
CNS: Restlessness, dizziness, drowsiness, fatigue, mania, insomnia, migraine, neuroleptic malignant-like syndrome, paresthesias, seizures, suicidal ideation, tremor, night sweats, dream disorders
CV: Palpitations, ventricular extrasystole
EENT: Cataracts, blurred vision
GI: *Nausea*, vomiting, flatulence, *diarrhea*, *xerostomia*, altered taste, gastroenteritis, increased appetite
GU: Decreased libido, ejaculation disorder, increased frequency of urination, sexual dysfunction
HEMA: Bleeding, decreased platelets
INTEG: Sweating
MS: Arthralgia
SYST: Neonatal abstinence syndrome, withdrawal, serotonin syndrome

INTERACTIONS
Individual drugs
Selegiline, busPIRone, dextromethorphan, fenfluramine, dexfluramine, linezolid, methylene blue lithium, meperidine, fentaNYL, methylphenidate, dexmethylphenidate, metoclopramide, mirtazapine, nefazodone, pentazocine, phenothiazines, haloperidol, loxapine, thiothixene, molindone: increased serotonin syndrome

Drug classifications
MAO inhibitors: do not use within 2 wk of this product
SSRIs, SNRIs, serotonin receptor agonists, ergots, amphetamines: increased serotonin syndrome
Anticoagulants, NSAIDs, platelet inhibitors, salicylates, thrombolytics: increased bleeding
CYP3A4 inducers (carbamazepine): decreased vilazodone effect
CYP3A4 inhibitors (clarithromycin, dronedarone, efavirenz, erythromycin, ketoconazole and others): increased vilazodone levels

Drug/herb
St. John's wort: increased serotonin syndrome

Drug/food
Grapefruit juice: avoid use

Drug/lab test
Decreased: sodium

NURSING CONSIDERATIONS
Assessment
• Assess mental status: orientation, mood behavior initially and periodically report significant changes; bipolar disorder should be determined before use; if used in bipolar disorder use cautiously.

> **BLACK BOX WARNING:** Initiate suicide precautions if indicated, suicide more likely at beginning therapy; risk is increased in children, young adults

• Assess for history of seizures, mania
• Monitor renal, hepatic status: hyponatremia (confusion, weakness, headache); monitor serum sodium
• **Abrupt discontinuation:** do not discontinue abruptly; taper, monitor for symptoms of withdrawal; if intolerable, resume previous dose and decrease more slowly
• **Neuroleptic malignant syndrome:** Assess for fever, hyper/hypotension, dyspnea, change in mental status, rigidity, tachycardia, discontinue and notify health care professional
• **Serotonin syndrome,** nausea, vomiting, sedation, sweating, facial flushing, high B/P: discontinue product, notify prescriber; higher incidence in those taking other products cause serotonin syndrome

Patient problem
Depression (uses)
Risk for injury (adverse reactions)

Implementation
• Administer with food to increase absorption
• Store at room temperature, away from moisture, heat
• Do not use within 2 wk of MAOIs

Patient/family education
• Teach patient to take as directed, with food, do not double doses, that follow-up will be needed
• Advise patient to avoid abrupt discontinuation unless approved by prescriber
• Instruct patient not to drive or operate machinery until effects are known
• Instruct patient not to use other products unless approved by prescriber, do not use alcohol
• Advise patient to contact prescriber if allergic reactions, personality changes (aggression, anxiety, anger, hostility), extreme sleepiness or drowsiness, confusion, nervousness, restlessness, clumsiness, numbness, tingling or burning pain

V

in hands, arms, legs, or feet, tremors, or having unusual behavior or thoughts about self-harm
• **Pregnancy/breastfeeding:** Use only if benefits outweigh fetal risk; if used in 3rd trimester, fetal complications may occur; avoid breastfeeding, excreted in breast milk; instruct patient to notify prescriber if pregnancy is planned or suspected

> **BLACK BOX WARNING: Suicidal thoughts/ behaviors:** discuss with family the possibility of suicidal thoughts/behaviors, to notify prescriber immediately if these occur

• **Neuroleptic malignant syndrome:** Teach patient symptoms, fever, change in mental status, seizures, rigidity, discontinue product, notify health care professional immediately

Evaluation

Positive therapeutic outcome
• Remission of depressive symptoms
• Decreased anxiety

> **⚠ HIGH ALERT**
>
> ## vinBLAStine (VLB) (Rx)
> (vin-blast'een)
> *Func. class.:* Antineoplastic
> *Chem. class.:* Vinca rosea alkaloid

Do not confuse: vinBLAStine/vinCRIStine/ vinorelbine

ACTION: Inhibits mitotic activity, arrests cell cycle at metaphase; inhibits RNA synthesis, blocks cellular use of glutamic acid needed for purine synthesis; a vesicant

Therapeutic outcome: Prevention of rapid growth of malignant cells; immunosuppression

USES: Breast, testicular cancer; lymphomas; neuroblastoma; Hodgkin's, non-Hodgkin's lymphomas; mycosis fungoides; histiocytosis; Kaposi's sarcoma, Langerhans' cell histiocytosis

Pharmacokinetics

Absorption	Complete bioavailability
Distribution	Crosses blood-brain barrier slightly
Metabolism	Liver—active antineoplastic
Excretion	Biliary, kidneys
Half-life	Triphasic <5 min, 50-155 min, 23-85 hr

Pharmacodynamics
Unknown

CONTRAINDICATIONS
Pregnancy, breastfeeding, infants, hypersensitivity, leukopenia, granulocytopenia, bone marrow suppression, infection

Precautions: Renal/hepatic disease, tumor lysis syndrome

> **BLACK BOX WARNING:** Extravasation, intrathecal use

DOSAGE AND ROUTES
Doses vary greatly
Breast cancer
Adult: **IV** 4.5 mg/m² on day 1 of every 21 days in combination with DOXOrubicin and thiotepa

Hodgkin's disease
Adult: **IV** 6 mg/m² on days 1 and 15 q28 days with DOXOrubicin (ABVD)
Child: **IV** 2.5-6 mg/m²/day once q 1-2 wk × 3-6 wks; max weekly dose 12.5 mg/m²

Available forms: Inj powder 10 mg for 10 ml **IV** inj; sol for inj 1 mg/ml

ADVERSE EFFECTS
CNS: Paresthesias, peripheral neuropathy, depression, headache, seizures, malaise
CV: Tachycardia, orthostatic hypotension, hypertension
GI: *Nausea, vomiting,* ileus, *anorexia, stomatitis, constipation,* abdominal pain, GI and rectal bleeding, hepatotoxicity, pharyngitis
GU: Urinary retention, renal failure, hyperuricemia
HEMA: Thrombocytopenia, leukopenia, myelosuppression, agranulocytosis, granulocytosis, aplastic anemia, neutropenia, pancytopenia
INTEG: *Rash, alopecia,* photosensitivity, extravasation, tissue necrosis
META: SIADH
SYST: Tumor lysis syndrome (TLS)
RESP: Fibrosis, pulmonary infiltrate, bronchospasm

INTERACTIONS
Individual drugs
Bleomycin: increased synergism
Methotrexate: increased methotrexate action
MitoMYcin: increased bronchospasm
Phenytoin: decreased phenytoin level
Radiation: increased toxicity, bone marrow suppression; do not use together

Drug classifications

Anticoagulants, antiplatelets, NSAIDs, thrombolytics: increased bleeding risk

Antineoplastics: increased toxicity, bone marrow suppression

CYP3A4 inducers (barbiturates, bosentan, carBAMazepine, efavirenz, phenytoin, nevirapine, rifabutin, rifampin): decreased vinBLAStine effect

CYP3A4 inhibitors (aprepitant, antiretroviral protease inhibitors, clarithromycin, danazol, delavirdine, diltiazem, erythromycin, fluconazole, FLUoxetine, fluvoxaMINE, imatinib, ketoconazole, mibefradil, nefazodone, telithromycin, voriconazole): increased toxicity

Live virus vaccines: increased adverse reactions

Drug/herb

St. John's wort: avoid use

Drug/lab test

Increased: uric acid, bilirubin
Decreased: Hgb, platelets, WBC

NURSING CONSIDERATIONS
Assessment

• Monitor B/P baseline and during administration
• Monitor CBC, differential, platelet count weekly; withhold product if WBC is <2000/mm³ or platelet count is <75,000/mm³; notify prescriber of results; recovery will take 3 wk; RBC, Hct, Hgb may be decreased; nadir occurs on days 4-10 (leukopenia), and continues for another 1-2 wk
• **Tumor lysis syndrome:** monitor for hyperkalemia, hyperphosphatemia, hyperuricemia; usually occurs with leukemia, lymphoma; alkalinization of the urine; allopurinol should be used to prevent urate nephropathy; monitor electrolytes and renal function (BUN, uric acid, urine CCR)
• Monitor renal function tests: BUN, serum uric acid, urine CCr before, during therapy; I&O ratio; report fall in urine output of 30 ml/hr; for decreased hyperuricemia
• **Bronchospasm:** can be life threatening; usually occurs when giving mitoMYcin
• Monitor for cold, fever, sore throat (may indicate beginning of infection); notify prescriber if these occur
• Assess for bleeding: hematuria, guaiac, bruising or petechiae, mucosa or orifices q8hr, no rectal temp; avoid IM inj; use pressure to venipuncture sites
• Identify nutritional status: an antiemetic may need to be prescribed

• Assess for gout, joint pain, swelling, increased uric acid; allopurinol or other treatment may be used
• **Assess for symptoms indicating severe allergic reactions:** rash, pruritus, urticaria, itching, flushing, bronchospasm, hypotension; EPINEPHrine and resuscitative equipment should be nearby
• **Hepatitis:** transient hepatitis may occur with continuous IV

Patient problem

Risk for infection (adverse reactions, teaching)
Impaired nutritional intake (adverse reactions)

Implementation

IV inj route
• Administer **IV** after diluting 10 mg/10 ml NaCl; give through Y-tube or 3-way stopcock or directly over 1 min
Intermittent IV INF route
• Further dilute in 50-100 ml of NS, inf over 15-30 min
• Give by intermittent inf
• Sol should be prepared by qualified personnel only under controlled conditions
• Use Luer-Lok tubing to prevent leakage; do not let sol come in contact with skin; if contact occurs, wash well with soap and water

> **BLACK BOX WARNING:** Give hyaluronidase 150 units/ml in 1 ml of NaCl, through IV catheter or SUBCUT in circular pattern around extravasated site warm compress for extravasation for vesicant activity treatment

> **BLACK BOX WARNING:** Do not administer intrathecally: fatal

Y-site compatibilities: Acyclovir, alemtuzumab, alfentanil, allopurinol, amifostine, amikacin, aminocaproic acid, aminophylline, amiodarone, amphotericin B cholesteryl, amphotericin B lipid complex, amphotericin B liposome, ampicillin, ampicillin-sulbactam, anidulafungin, argatroban, arsenic trioxide, asparaginase, atenolol, atracurium, azithromycin, aztreonam, bivalirudin, bleomycin, bumetanide, buprenorphine, butorphanol, calcium chloride/gluconate, capreomycin, CARBOplatin, carmustine, caspofungin, ceFAZolin, cefoperazone, cefoTEtan, cefOXitin, cefTAZidime, ceftizoxime, cefTRIAXone, cefuroxime, chlorproMAZINE, cimetidine, ciprofloxacin, cisatracurium, CISplatin, cladribine, clindamycin, codeine, cyclophosphamide, cycloSPORINE, cytarabine, D₅W-dextrose 5%, dacarbazine, DACTINomycin, DAPTOmycin, DAUNOrubicin, DAUNOrubicin citrate liposome, dexamethasone, dexmedetomidine, dexrazoxane, digoxin, diltiazem, diphenhydrAMINE, DOBUTamine, DOCEtaxel, dolasetron, DOPamine, doxacurium, doxapram, DOXOrubicin, DOXOrubicin liposomal, doxycycline, droperidol, enalaprilat, ePHEDrine, EPINEPHrine, epirubicin, ertapenem, erythromycin, esmolol, etoposide, famotidine, fenoldopam, fentaNYL, filgrastim, fluconazole, fludarabine, fluorouracil, foscarnet, fosphenytoin, gallium, ganciclovir, garenoxacin, gatifloxacin, gemcitabine, gentamicin, granisetron, haloperidol, heparin, hydrocortisone sodium phosphate/succinate, HYDROmorphone, hydrOXYzine, ifosfamide, imipenem-cilastatin, inamrinone, insulin regular, isoproterenol, ketorolac, labetalol, lepirudin, leucovorin, levofloxacin, levorphanol, lidocaine, linezolid, LORazepam, magnesium sulfate, mannitol, mechlorethamine, melphalan, meperidine, meropenem, mesna, methadone, methohexital, methotrexate, methylPREDNISolone, metoclopramide, metoprolol, metroNIDAZOLE, midazolam, milrinone, minocycline, mitoMYcin, mitoXANtrone, mivacurium, morphine, moxifloxacin, nalbuphine, naloxone, nesiritide, niCARdipine, nitroglycerin, nitroprusside, norepinephrine, octreotide, ondansetron, oxaliplatin, PACLitaxel (solvent/surfactant), palonosetron, pamidronate, pancuronium, PEMEtrexed, pentamidine, pentazocine, PENTobarbital, PHENobarbital, phenylephrine, piperacillin, piperacillin–tazobactam, potassium acetate/chloride/phosphates, procainamide, prochlorperazine, promethazine, propranolol, quinupristin-dalfopristin, ranitidine, remifentanil, riTUXimab, rocuronium, sargramostim, sodium acetate/phosphates, succinylcholine, SUFentanil, sulfamethoxazole-trimethoprim, tacrolimus, teniposide, theophylline, thiopental, thiotepa, ticarcillin, ticarcillin-clavulanate, tigecycline, tirofiban, tobramycin, topotecan, trastuzumab, trimethobenzamide, vancomycin, vasopressin, vecuronium, verapamil, vinBLAStine, vinorelbine, voriconazole, zidovudine, zoledronic acid

Y-site incompatibilities: Amphotericin B conventional colloidal, cefepime, diazepam, gemtuzumab, IDArubicin, lansoprazole, nafcillin, pantoprazole, phenytoin

Patient/family education
• Teach patient to avoid use of products containing aspirin or NSAIDs, razors, commercial mouthwash because bleeding may occur; to report symptoms of bleeding (hematuria, tarry stools)
• Instruct patient to report signs of anemia, (fatigue, headache, irritability, faintness, shortness of breath)

• Caution patient to report any changes in breathing or coughing even several mo after treatment; avoid breastfeeding; may cause male infertility
• Advise patient to use sunscreen, wear protective clothing and sunglasses
• Inform patient that hair may be lost during treatment; a wig or hairpiece may make patient feel better; new hair will be different in color, texture
• Advise patient to avoid vaccinations during treatment; serious reactions may occur

BLACK BOX WARNING: Teach patient to report irritation, pain, burning, discoloration at IV site extravasation

• Teach patient to report signs/symptoms of infection: fever, chills, sore throat; patient should avoid crowds and persons with known infections
• Instruct patient to avoid persons with known infections
• **Infection:** instruct patient to report sore throat, flulike symptoms
• **Pregnancy:** teach patient to notify prescriber if pregnancy is planned or suspected, not to breastfeed; may cause male infertility; advise patient that contraception will be necessary during treatment; teratogenesis may occur

Evaluation

Positive therapeutic outcome
• Decreased spread of malignant cells

⚠ HIGH ALERT

vinCRIStine (VCR) (Rx)
(vin-kris'teen)
Func. class.: Antineoplastic—miscellaneous
Chem. class.: Vinca alkaloid

Do not confuse: vinCRIStine/vinBLAStine/vinorelbine

ACTION: Inhibits mitotic activity, arrests cell cycle at metaphase; inhibits RNA synthesis, blocks cellular use of glutamic acid needed for purine synthesis; a vesicant

Therapeutic outcome: Prevention of rapid growth of malignant cells, immunosuppression

USES: Lymphomas, neuroblastomas, Hodgkin's disease, acute lymphoblastic and other leukemias, rhabdomyosarcoma, Wilms' tumor, non-Hodgkin's lymphoma, malignant glioma, soft-tissue sarcoma; **liposomal:** Philadelphia chromosome-negative ALL in second or greater relapse or that has progressed after 2 or more antileukemia therapies

Pharmacokinetics

Absorption	Complete bioavailability
Distribution	Rapidly, widely distributed; crosses blood-brain barrier
Metabolism	Liver
Excretion	Biliary, in feces, crosses placenta
Half-life	Triphasic <5 min, 50-155 min, 23-85 hr

Pharmacodynamics

Onset	Unknown
Peak	Unknown
Duration	1 wk

CONTRAINDICATIONS

Pregnancy, breastfeeding, infants, hypersensitivity, radiation therapy

> **BLACK BOX WARNING:** Intrathecal use

Precautions: Renal/hepatic disease, hypertension, neuromuscular disease

> **BLACK BOX WARNING:** Extravasation

DOSAGE AND ROUTES

Adult: IV 0.4-1.4 mg/m²/wk, max 2 mg
Child >10 kg: IV 1-2 mg/m²/wk, max 2 mg

Available forms: Inj 1 mg/ml; liposomal 5 mg/31 ml injection kit

ADVERSE EFFECTS

CNS: *Decreased reflexes, numbness, weakness, motor difficulties,* CNS depression, cranial nerve paralysis, seizures, peripheral neuropathy
CV: Orthostatic hypotension
EENT: *Diplopia*
GI: *Nausea, vomiting, anorexia, stomatitis, constipation,* paralytic ileus, abdominal pain, hepatotoxicity
GU: Renal tubular obstruction
HEMA: Thrombocytopenia, leukopenia, myelosuppression, anemia
INTEG: *Alopecia,* extravasation
SYST: Tumor lysis syndrome (TLS)

INTERACTIONS
Individual drugs

Digoxin: decreased digoxin level
MitoMYcin-C: increased acute pulmonary reactions
Radiation: increased toxicity, bone marrow suppression; do not use together

Drug classifications

CYP3A4 inducers (barbiturates, bosentan, carBAMazepine, efavirenz, phenytoins, nevirapine, rifabutin, rifampin): decreased vinCRIStine effect
CYP3A4 inhibitors (aprepitant, antiretroviral protease inhibitors, clarithromycin, danazol, delavirdine, diltiazem, erythromycin, fluconazole, FLUoxetine, fluvoxaMINE, imatinib, ketoconazole, mibefradil, nefazodone, telithromycin, voriconazole): increased toxicity
Peripheral nervous system products: increased neurotoxicity
Vaccines/toxoids: decreased immune response

Drug/herb
St. John's wort: avoid use

Drug/lab test
Increased: uric acid
Decreased: Hgb, WBC, platelets, sodium

NURSING CONSIDERATIONS
Assessment

• Monitor CBC, differential, platelet count weekly; withhold product if WBC is <4000/mm³ or platelet count is <75,000/mm³; notify prescriber of results; platelets may increase or decrease, nadir occurs on days 4-10 (leukopenia) and continuous for another 1-2 wk
• Assess neurologic status: paresthesia, weakness, cranial nerve palsies, orthostatic hypotension, lethargy, agitation, psychosis; notify prescriber
• **Bronchospasm:** more common with mitoMYcin
• Identify for increased uric acid levels, joint pain in extremities; increase fluid intake to 2-3 L/day unless contraindicated
• **Tumor lysis syndrome:** hyperkalemia, hyperphosphatemia, hyperuricemia, hypocalcemia; more common in leukemia, lymphoma, use alkalinization of urine with allopurinol, monitor electrolytes, renal function (BUN, urine, CCR, uric acid)

> **BLACK BOX WARNING:** Extravasation: Assess for pain, swelling, poor blood return; if extravasation occurs, local injection of hyaluronidase and moderate heat to area may help disperse product

• **Pregnancy/breastfeeding:** Do not use in pregnancy, breastfeeding

Patient problem
Impaired nutritional intake (adverse reactions)
Nausea (adverse reactions)
Risk for injury (adverse reactions)

Implementation
IV route

> **BLACK BOX WARNING:** Do not give intrathecally: fatal

- Administer **IV** after diluting with diluent provided or 1 mg/10 ml of sterile water or 0.9% NaCl; give through Y-tube or 3-way stopcock or directly over 1 min; do not use 5-mg vial for single doses

> **BLACK BOX WARNING:** Hyaluronidase 150 units/ml in 1 ml of NaCl; apply warm compress for extravasation

Y-site compatibilities: Acyclovir, alemtuzumab, alfentanil, allopurinol, amifostine, amikacin, aminocaproic acid, aminophylline, amiodarone, amphotericin B cholesteryl, amphotericin B lipid complex, amphotericin B liposome, ampicillin, ampicillin-sulbactam, anidulafungin, argatroban, arsenic trioxide, asparaginase, atenolol, atracurium, azithromycin, aztreonam, bivalirudin, bleomycin, bumetanide, buprenorphine, butorphanol, calcium chloride/gluconate, capreomycin, CARBOplatin, carmustine, caspofungin, ceFAZolin, cefoperazone, cefoTEtan, cefOXitin, cefTAZidime, ceftizoxime, cefTRIAXone, cefuroxime, chlorproMAZINE, cimetidine, ciprofloxacin, cisatracurium, CISplatin, cladribine, clindamycin, codeine, cyclophosphamide, cycloSPORINE, cytarabine, D₅W-dextrose 5%, dacarbazine, DACTINomycin, DAPTOmycin, DAUNOrubicin, DAUNOrubicin citrate liposome, dexamethasone, dexmedetomidine, dexrazoxane, digoxin, diltiazem, diphenhydrAMINE, DOBUTamine, DOCEtaxel, dolasetron, DOPamine, doxacurium, doxapram, DOXOrubicin, DOXOrubicin liposomal, doxycycline, droperidol, enalaprilat, ePHEDrine, EPINEPHrine, epirubicin, ertapenem, erythromycin, esmolol, etoposide, famotidine, fenoldopam, fentaNYL, filgrastim, fluconazole, fludarabine, fluorouracil, foscarnet, fosphenytoin, gallium, ganciclovir, garenoxacin, gatifloxacin, gemcitabine, gentamicin, granisetron, haloperidol, heparin, hydrocortisone sodium phosphate/succinate, HYDROmorphone, hydrOXYzine, ifosfamide, imipenem-cilastatin, inamrinone, insulin regular, isoproterenol, ketorolac, labetalol, lepirudin, leucovorin, levofloxacin, levorphanol, lidocaine, linezolid, LORazepam, magnesium sulfate, mannitol, mechlorethamine, melphalan, meperidine, meropenem, mesna, methadone, methohexital, methotrexate, methylPREDNISolone, metoclopramide, metoprolol, metroNIDAZOLE, midazolam, milrinone, minocycline, mitoMYcin, mitoXANtrone, mivacurium, morphine, moxifloxacin, nalbuphine, naloxone, nesiritide, niCARdipine, nitroglycerin, nitroprusside, norepinephrine, octreotide, ondansetron, oxaliplatin, PACLitaxel (solvent/surfactant), palonosetron, pamidronate, pancuronium, PEMEtrexed, pentamidine, pentazocine, PENTobarbital, PHENobarbital, phenylephrine, piperacillin, piperacillin–tazobactam, potassium acetate/chloride/phosphates, procainamide, prochlorperazine, promethazine, propranolol, quinupristin-dalfopristin, ranitidine, remifentanil, riTUXimab, rocuronium, sargramostim, sodium acetate/phosphates, succinylcholine, SUFentanil, sulfamethoxazole-trimethoprim, tacrolimus, teniposide, theophylline, thiopental, thiotepa, ticarcillin, ticarcillin–clavulanate, tigecycline, tirofiban, tobramycin, topotecan, trastuzumab, trimethobenzamide, vancomycin, vasopressin, vecuronium, verapamil, vinBLAStine, vinorelbine, voriconazole, zidovudine, zoledronic acid

Patient/family education

- Teach patient to avoid use of products containing aspirin or NSAIDs, razors, commercial mouthwash because bleeding may occur; to report symptoms of bleeding (hematuria, tarry stools)
- Instruct patient to report signs of anemia (fatigue, headache, irritability, faintness, shortness of breath)
- Caution patient to report any changes in breathing or coughing, even several mo after treatment
- Inform patient that hair may be lost during treatment; a wig or hairpiece may make patient feel better; new hair will be different in color, texture
- Advise patient to avoid vaccinations during treatment; serious reactions may occur
- Teach patient to report signs/symptoms of infection: fever, chills, sore throat; patient should avoid crowds or persons with known infections
- Advise patient to increase fluids, bulk in diet, exercise to prevent constipation
- **Infection:** instruct patient to report sore throat, fever, flulike symptoms; avoid persons with known infection
- **Pregnancy:** instruct patient to notify prescriber if pregnancy is planned or suspected; advise patient that contraception will be necessary during and 2 mo after treatment; may be teratogenic, not to breastfeed

Evaluation

Positive therapeutic outcome

- Decreased spread of malignancies

⚠ HIGH ALERT

vinorelbine (Rx)
(vi-nor'el-bine)
Navelbine
Func. class.: Antineoplastic—miscellaneous
Chem. class.: Semisynthetic vinca alkaloid

ACTION: Inhibits mitotic spindle activity, arrests cell cycle at metaphase; inhibits RNA synthesis, blocks cellular use of glutamic acid needed for purine synthesis; a vesicant

Therapeutic outcome: Decreased spread of malignancy

USES: Unresectable, advanced non–small-cell lung cancer (NSCLC) stage IV; may be used alone or in combination with cisplatin for stage III or IV NSCLC

Pharmacokinetics

Absorption	Poor bioavailability (<50%)
Distribution	Highly bound to platelets, lymphocytes
Metabolism	Liver, to metabolite
Excretion	Bile
Half-life	43 hr

Pharmacodynamics

Onset	Unknown
Peak	1-2 hr
Duration	Unknown

CONTRAINDICATIONS
Pregnancy, breastfeeding, hypersensitivity, infants, granulocyte count <1000 cells/mm³ pretreatment

Precautions: Children, geriatric, hepatic/pulmonary/neurologic/renal disease, bone marrow suppression

BLACK BOX WARNING: Extravasation severe neutropenia, intrathecal use

DOSAGE AND ROUTES
Adult: IV 30 mg/m² qwk

ANC: 1000-1499/mm³, give 50% dose; <1000 hold dose; <1000/mm³ × 3 wk, discontinue

Hepatic dose
Adult: IV total bilirubin 2.1-3 mg/dl 15 mg/m² qwk; total bilirubin ≥3 mg/dl 7.5 mg/m²/day

Available forms: Inj 10 mg/ml

ADVERSE EFFECTS
CNS: Paresthesias, peripheral neuropathy, depression, headache, seizures, weakness, jaw pain, asthenia
CV: Chest pain
GI: *Nausea, vomiting,* ileus, *anorexia, stomatitis,* constipation, abdominal pain, *diarrhea,* hepatotoxicity, GI obstruction/perforation
HEMA: Neutropenia, anemia, thrombocytopenia, granulocytopenia
INTEG: *Rash, alopecia,* photosensitivity, inj site reaction, necrosis
META: Syndrome of inappropriate diuretic hormone
MS: Myalgia
RESP: Shortness of breath, dyspnea, pulmonary edema, acute bronchospasm, acute respiratory distress syndrome (ARDS)

INTERACTIONS
Drug classifications
NSAIDs, anticoagulants: increased bleeding risk
CYP3A4 inhibitors (antiretroviral protease inhibitors, aprepitant, clarithromycin, danazol, delavirdine, diltiazem, erythromycin, fluconazole, FLUoxetine, fluvoxaMINE, imatinib, ketoconazole, mibefradil, nefazodone, telithromycin, voriconazole): increased toxicity
CYP3A4 inducers (barbiturates, bosentan, carBAMazepine, efavirenz, nevirapine, phenytoins, rifabutin, rifampin): decreased vinorelbine effect

Drug/herb
St. John's wort: avoid use

Drug/lab test
Increased: LFTs, bilirubin
Decreased: Hgb, WBC, platelets

NURSING CONSIDERATIONS
Assessment
• Monitor B/P baseline during administration

BLACK BOX WARNING: Bone marrow suppression: Monitor CBC, differential, platelet count before each dose; withhold product if WBC is <4000/mm³ or platelet count is <75,000/mm³; notify prescriber of results; recovery will take 3 wk; liver function tests: AST, ALT, bilirubin, LDH

• **Bronchospasm:** more common with mitoMYcin; also dyspnea, wheezing; may be treated with oxygen, bronchodilators, corticosteroids, especially if there is underlying pulmonary disease
• **Neurological status:** Paresthesia, peripheral neuropathy, weakness, these may occur even after termination of treatment

V

• Monitor renal function tests: BUN, serum uric acid, urine CCr before, during therapy, I&O ratio; report fall in urine output of 30 ml/hr; for decreased hyperuricemia
• Monitor for cold, fever, sore throat (may indicate beginning **infection**); notify prescriber if these occur; effects of alopecia on body image
• **Assess for bleeding:** hematuria, guaiac, bruising or petechiae, mucosa or orifices q8hr: no rectal temp; avoid IM inj; use pressure on venipuncture sites
• **Assess for symptoms indicating severe allergic reactions:** rash, pruritus, urticaria, itching, flushing, bronchospasm, hypotension; EPINEPHrine and resuscitative equipment should be nearby
• Assess neurologic status: numbness, pain, tingling, loss of Achilles reflex, weakness, palsies

Patient problem
Risk for infection (adverse reactions)
Risk for injury (adverse reactions)
Nausea (adverse reactions)

Implementation

> **BLACK BOX WARNING:** Do not give intrathecally: fatal, syringes with this product should be labeled "Warning: For IV use only, fatal if given intrathecally"

• **Extravasation:** Stop infusion, aspirate, then hyaluronidase 150 units/ml in 1 ml of 0.9% NaCl, thorough IV catheter or SUBCUT in circular pattern around site; warm compress for extravasation, for vesicant activity treatment

Intermittent IV infusion route
• Dilute to 0.5-2 mg/ml with 0.9% NaCl, 0.45% NaCl, D₅W, D₅/0.45% NaCl, LR, Ringer's; give over 6-10 min into Y-site or central line; flush line
Continuous IV infusion route
• Give 40 mg/m² q3wk after **IV** bol of 8 mg/m²; may be given in combination with DOXOrubicin, fluorouracil, cisplatin

Y-site compatibilities: Amikacin, aztreonam, bleomycin, buprenorphine, butorphanol, calcium gluconate, CARBOplatin, cefotaxime, cimetidine, CISplatin, clindamycin, dexamethasone, enalaprilat, etoposide, famotidine, filgrastim, fluconazole, fludarabine, gentamicin, hydrocortisone, LORazepam, meperidine, morphine, netilmicin, ondansetron, plicamycin, streptozocin, teniposide, ticarcillin, tobramycin, vancomycin, vinBLAStine, vinCRIStine, zidovudine

Patient/family education
• Teach patient to use liquid diet: cola, gelatin; dry toast or crackers may be added if patient is not nauseated or vomiting

• Advise patient to rinse mouth 3-4 ×/day with water and brush teeth 2-3 ×/day with soft brush or cotton-tipped applicators for stomatitis; use unwaxed dental floss
• Advise patient to avoid crowds, people with infections, vaccinations
• Teach patient hair may be lost but will grow back; new hair may be different texture, color
• **Infection:** report sore throat, fever, flulike symptoms
• **Pregnancy:** notify prescriber if pregnancy is planned or suspected; advise patient to use effective contraception during and for ≥2 mo after product is discontinued; do not use in pregnancy, breastfeeding

Evaluation

Positive therapeutic outcome
• Decreased spread of malignant cells

vitamin A (PO, OTC; IM, Rx)
Aquasol A, Del-Vi-A, Vitamin A
Func. class.: Vitamin, fat-soluble
Chem. class.: Retinol

ACTION: Needed for normal bone and tooth development, visual dark adaptation, skin disease, mucosa tissue repair; assists in production of adrenal steroids, cholesterol, RNA

Therapeutic outcome: Prevention, absence of vit A deficiency

USES: Vit A deficiency

Pharmacokinetics

Absorption	Rapidly absorbed
Distribution	Stored in liver, kidneys, lungs
Metabolism	Liver
Excretion	Breast milk
Half-life	Unknown

Pharmacodynamics
Unknown

CONTRAINDICATIONS
Pregnancy (parenteral), hypersensitivity to vit A, malabsorption syndrome (PO), hypervitaminosis A, parenteral, **IV** administration

Precautions: Pregnancy (PO), breastfeeding, impaired renal function, children, hepatic disease, infants, alcoholism, hepatitis

DOSAGE AND ROUTES
Adult and child >8 yr: PO 100,000-500,000 international units/day × 3 days, then 50,000 international units/day × 2 wk; dose based on

severity of deficiency; maintenance 10,000-20,000 international units for 2 mo

Child 1-8 yr: IM 5000-15,000 international units/day × 10 days

Infant <1 yr: IM 5000-15,000 international units × 10 days

Maintenance

Child 4-8 yr: IM 15,000 international units/day × 2 mo

Child <4 yr: IM 10,000 international units/ day × 2 mo

Available forms: Caps 10,000, 25,000, 50,000 international units; drops 5000 international units/ml; inj 50,000 international units/ml; tabs 10,000, 25,000, 50,000 international units

ADVERSE EFFECTS

CNS: Headache, increased ICP, intracranial hypertension, lethargy, malaise

EENT: Gingivitis, papilledema, exophthalmos, inflammation of tongue and lips

GI: Nausea, vomiting, anorexia, abdominal pain, *jaundice*

INTEG: Drying of skin, pruritus, increased pigmentation, night sweats, alopecia

META: Hypomenorrhea, hypercalcemia

MS: Arthralgia, retarded growth, hard areas on bone

INTERACTIONS
Individual drugs
Cholestyramine, colestipol, mineral oil: decreased absorption of vit A

Drug classifications
Contraceptives (oral), corticosteroids: increased levels of vit A

Drug/lab test
False increase: bilirubin, serum cholesterol

NURSING CONSIDERATIONS
Assessment
• Assess nutritional status: increase intake of yellow and dark green vegetables, yellow/orange fruits, vit A–fortified foods, liver, egg yolks

• Assess vit A deficiency: decreased growth; night blindness; dry, brittle nails; hair loss; urinary stones; increased infection; hyperkeratosis of skin; drying of cornea

• Identify vit A deficiency by plasma vit A, carotene level

• Assess for chronic vit A toxicity: increased calcium, BUN, glucose, cholesterol, triglyceride level

• **Pregnancy/breastfeeding:** Do not use IM in pregnancy, fetal complications may occur; breastfeeding is considered safe at recommended dietary levels

Patient problem
Impaired nutritional intake (uses)

Implementation
PO route
• Give with food (PO) for better absorption; do not give **IV** because anaphylaxis may occur, IM only

• Oral preparations are not indicated for vit A deficiency in those with malabsorption syndrome

• Store in airtight, light-resistant container

IM route
• Give deep in large muscle mass; do not use deltoid muscle for administration of >1 ml

Patient/family education
• Instruct patient that if dose is missed, it should be omitted

• Inform patient that ophth exams may be required periodically throughout therapy

• Instruct patient not to use mineral oil while taking this product because absorption will be decreased

• Advise patient to notify prescriber of nausea, vomiting, lip cracking, loss of hair, headache

• Caution patient not to take more than the prescribed amount

Evaluation
Positive therapeutic outcome
• Increase in growth rate, weight

• Absence of dry skin and mucous membranes, night blindness

TREATMENT OF OVERDOSE:
Discontinue product

vitamin A acid
See tretinoin

vitamin B₁
See thiamine

vitamin B₁₂ (cyanocobalamin) (PO, OTC; IM/SUBCUT, Rx)
(sye-an-oh-koe-bal′a-min)
Func. class.: Vitamin B₁₂, water-soluble vitamin

vitamin B₁₂a (hydroxocobalamin) (vit B₁₂) (Rx)
(hye-drox′o-ko-bal′a-min)
CyanoKit

ACTION: Needed for adequate nerve functioning, protein and carbohydrate metabolism, normal growth, RBC development and cell reproduction

Therapeutic outcome: Prevention, correction of vit B$_{12}$ deficiency

USES: Vit B$_{12}$ deficiency; pernicious anemia; vit B$_{12}$ malabsorption syndrome; Schilling test; increased requirements with pregnancy, thyrotoxicosis, hemolytic anemia, hemorrhage, renal and hepatic disease

Pharmacokinetics

Absorption	Well absorbed (IM, SUBCUT)
Distribution	Crosses placenta
Metabolism	Stored in liver, kidney, stomach
Excretion	50%-90% (urine), breast milk
Half-life	Unknown

Pharmacodynamics

Unknown

CONTRAINDICATIONS

Hypersensitivity, optic nerve atrophy

Precautions: Pregnancy, breastfeeding, children

DOSAGE AND ROUTES
Cyanocobalamin
Adult: PO up to 1000 mcg/day; SUBCUT/IM 30-100 mcg/day × 1 wk, then 100-200 mcg/mo

Schilling test
Adult and child: IM 1000 mcg in 1 dose
Child: PO up to 1000 mcg/day; SUBCUT/IM 30-50 mcg/day × 2 wk, then 100 mcg/mo; NASAL 500 mcg qwk

Hydroxocobalamin
Adult: SUBCUT/IM 30-50 mcg/day × 5-10 days, then 100-200 mcg/mo
Child: SUBCUT/IM 30-50 mcg/day × 5-10 days, then 30-50 mcg/mo

Available forms: Cyanocobalamin: tabs 25, 50, 100, 250, 500, 1000, 5000 mcg; ext rel tabs 100, 200, 500, 1000 mcg; lozenges: 100, 250, 500 mcg; nasal gel 500 mcg/spray; inj 100, 1000 mcg/ml; hydroxocobalamin: inj 1000 mcg/ml

ADVERSE EFFECTS
CNS: Flushing, optic nerve atrophy
CV: HF, peripheral vascular thrombosis, pulmonary edema
GI: *Diarrhea*
INTEG: Itching, rash, pain at inj site
META: Hypokalemia
SYST: Anaphylactic shock

INTERACTIONS
Individual drugs
Aminosalicylic acid, chloramphenicol, cimetidine, colchicine: decreased absorption
PredniSONE: increased absorption

Drug classifications
Aminoglycosides, anticonvulsants, potassium products: decreased absorption

Drug/herb
Goldenseal: decreased vit B$_{12}$ absorption

Drug/lab test
False positive: intrinsic factor

NURSING CONSIDERATIONS
Assessment
• Assess for deficiency: anorexia, dyspepsia on exertion, palpitations, paresthesias, psychosis, visual disturbances, pallor, red inflamed tongue, neuropathy, edema of legs
• Monitor potassium levels during beginning treatment in patients with megaloblastic anemia
• Monitor CBC for increase in reticulocyte count during 1st wk of therapy, then increase in RBC and hemoglobin; folic acid levels, vit B$_{12}$ levels
• Assess nutritional status: egg yolks, fish, organ meats, dairy products, clams, oysters, which are good sources of vit B$_{12}$
• Monitor for pulmonary edema or worsening of HF in cardiac patients

Patient problem
Impaired nutritional intake (uses)

Implementation
PO route
• Give with fruit juice to disguise taste; administer immediately after mixing
• Give with meals if possible for better absorption; large doses should not be used because most is excreted
IM route
• Give by IM inj for pernicious anemia for life unless contraindicated

IV route
• May be mixed with TPN sol, but **IV** route is not recommended

Y-site compatibilities: Heparin, hydrocortisone sodium succinate, potassium chloride

Solution compatibilities: Dextrose/Ringer's or LR's combinations, dextrose/saline combinations, D$_5$W, D$_{10}$W, 0.45% NaCl, Ringer's or LR's sol, ascorbic acid

Patient/family education
• Instruct patient that treatment must continue for life if diagnosed as having pernicious anemia

---

• Advise patient to eat well-balanced diet from the food pyramid and comply with dietary recommendation

• Caution patient not to exceed the RDA of vit B_{12} because adverse reactions may occur

Evaluation

Positive therapeutic outcome
• Decreased anorexia, dyspnea on exertion, palpitations, paresthesias, psychosis, visual disturbances, edema of legs
• Prevention or correction of vit B_{12} deficiency

TREATMENT OF OVERDOSE:
Discontinue products

---

vitamin C (ascorbic acid) (OTC, Rx)
(as-kor′bic)
Func. class.: Vitamin C, water-soluble vitamin

ACTION: Needed for wound healing, collagen synthesis, antioxidant, carbohydrate metabolism

Therapeutic outcome: Replacement and supplementation of vit C

USES: Vit C deficiency, scurvy, delayed wound and bone healing, chronic disease, before gastrectomy, dietary supplement

Unlabeled uses: Common cold prevention

Pharmacokinetics

Absorption	Readily absorbed (PO)
Distribution	Widely distributed; crosses placenta
Metabolism	Oxidation
Excretion	Kidneys, inactive; breast milk
Half-life	Unknown

Pharmacodynamics

Unknown

CONTRAINDICATIONS
Tartrazine, sulfite sensitivity; G6PD deficiency

Precautions: Pregnancy, gout, diabetes, renal calculi (large doses)

DOSAGE AND ROUTES
RDA
Neonate and up to 6 mo: PO 30 mg/day
Infant: PO 40-50 mg/day
Child 1-3 yr: PO 15 mg/day
Child 4-8 yr: PO 25 mg/day
Child 9-13 yr: PO 45 mg/day
Child 14-18 yr: PO 65 mg/day (females), 75 mg/day (males)

Adult: PO 50-500 mg/day

Scurvy
Adult: PO/SUBCUT/IM/IV 100 mg-250 mg daily × 2 wk, then 50 mg or more daily
Child: PO/SUBCUT/IM/IV 100-300 mg daily × 2 wk, then 35 mg or more daily

Wound healing/chronic disease/fracture
May be given with zinc
Adult: SUBCUT/IM/IV/PO 200-500 mg daily for 1-2 mo
Child: SUBCUT/IM/IV/PO 100-200 mg added doses for 1-2 mo

Urine acidification
Adult: 4-12 g daily in divided doses
Child: 500 mg q6-8hr

Available forms: Tabs 25, 50, 100, 250, 500, 1000, 1500 mg; effervescent tabs 1000 mg; chewable tabs 100, 250, 500 mg; time-release tabs 500, 750, 1000, 1500 mg; time-release caps 500 mg; crystals 4 g/tsp; powder 4 g/tsp; liquid 35 mg/0.6 ml; sol 100 mg/ml; syr 20 mg/ml, 500 mg/5 ml; inj SUBCUT, IM, **IV** 100, 250, 500 mg/ml

ADVERSE EFFECTS

CNS: Headache, insomnia, dizziness, fatigue, flushing
GI: Nausea, vomiting, diarrhea, anorexia, heartburn, cramps
GU: Polyuria, urine acidification, oxalate or urate renal stones, dysuria
HEMA: Hemolytic anemia in patients with G6PD
INTEG: Inflammation at inj site

INTERACTIONS
Drug/lab test
False positive: negative in glucose tests (Clinitest, Tes-Tape)
False negative: occult blood (large dose), urine bilirubin, leukocyte determination

NURSING CONSIDERATIONS
Assessment
• Assess nutritional status for inclusion of foods high in vit C: citrus fruits, cantaloupe, tomatoes
• Assess for vit C deficiency before, during, and after treatment; scurvy (gingivitis, bleeding gums, loose teeth); poor bone development
• Monitor I&O ratio, polyuria; in patients receiving large doses, renal stones may occur; urine pH (acidification)
• Monitor ascorbic acid levels throughout treatment if continued deficiency is suspected
• Assess inj sites for inflammation, pain, redness, thrombophlebitis if in large doses

---

• **Pregnancy/breastfeeding:** Use only recommended dietary allowances in pregnancy, breastfeeding

Patient problem
Impaired nutritional intake (uses)

Implementation
PO route
• Swallow time rel tabs or caps whole; do not break, crush, or chew
• Mix oral sol with foods or fluids
IM route
• Not to be diluted; give deep in large muscle mass

IV, direct route
• Give undiluted by *direct* IV 100 mg over at least 1 min, rapid inf may cause fainting
Intermittent IV infusion route
• Give by intermittent inf after diluting with D₅W, D₁₀W, 0.9% NaCl, 0.45% NaCl, LR, Ringer's sol, dextrose/saline, dextrose/Ringer's combinations; temp will increase pressure in ampules; wrap with gauze before breaking

Syringe compatibilities: Metoclopramide, aminophylline, theophylline

Syringe incompatibilities: CeFAZolin, doxapram

Y-site compatibilities: Warfarin

Patient/family education
• Teach patient necessary foods to be included in diet that are rich in vit C: citrus fruits, cantaloupe, tomatoes, chili peppers (red)
• Teach patient that smoking decreases vit C levels; not to exceed prescribed dose; increases will be excreted in urine, except time release
• Teach patient not to exceed RDA recommended dose, urinary stones may occur
• Teach patient using ascorbic acid for acidification of urine to test urine pH periodically

Evaluation
Positive therapeutic outcome
• Absence of anorexia, irritability, pallor, joint pain, hyperkeratosis, petechiae, poor wound healing
• Reversal of scurvy: bleeding gums, gingivitis, loose teeth

vitamin D (cholecalciferol, vitamin D₃ or ergocalciferol, vitamin D₂) (Rx, OTC)
Delta-D, Drisdol, vitamin D, vitamin D₃
Func. class.: Vitamin D
Chem. class.: Fat-soluble vitamin

Do not confuse: Calciferol/calcitriol

ACTION: Needed for regulation of calcium, phosphate levels; normal bone development; parathyroid activity; neuromuscular functioning

Therapeutic outcome: Prevention of rickets, osteomalacia, normal calcium/phosphate levels

USES: Vit D deficiency, rickets, renal osteodystrophy, hypoparathyroidism, hypophosphatemia, psoriasis, rheumatoid arthritis

Pharmacokinetics
Absorption	Well absorbed
Distribution	Stored in liver
Metabolism	Liver, sun
Excretion	Bile, kidney
Half-life	12-22 hr

Pharmacodynamics
	PO	IM
Onset	Unknown	Unknown
Peak	4 hr	Unknown
Duration	15-20 days	Unknown

CONTRAINDICATIONS
Hypersensitivity, hypercalcemia, renal dysfunction, hyperphosphatemia

Precautions: Pregnancy, CV disease, renal calculi

DOSAGE AND ROUTES
Deficiency
Adult: PO/IM 12,000 international units/day, then increased to 500,000 international units/day
Child: PO/IM 1500-5000 international units/day × 2-4 wk, may repeat after 2 wk or 600,000 international units as single dose

Hypoparathyroidism
Adult and child: PO/IM 200,000 international units given with 4 g calcium tab

Available forms: Tabs 400, 1000, 50,000 international units; caps 25,000, 50,000 international units; oral sol 8000 international units/ml; inj 500,000 international units/ml, 500,000 international units/5 ml

ADVERSE EFFECTS
CNS: Fatigue, weakness, drowsiness, seizures, headache, psychosis
CV: Hypertension, dysrhythmias
GI: Nausea, vomiting, anorexia, cramps, diarrhea, constipation, metallic taste, dry mouth
GU: Polyuria, nocturia, hematuria, albuminuria, renal failure, decreased libido
INTEG: Pruritus, photophobia

MS: Decreased bone growth, early joint pain, early muscle pain

INTERACTIONS
Individual drugs
Cholestyramine, colestipol, PHENobarbital, phenytoin: decreased effects of vit D
Verapamil: increased toxicity

Drug classifications
Antacids, diuretics (thiazide): increased toxicity

NURSING CONSIDERATIONS
Assessment
• Monitor BUN, urinary calcium, AST, ALT, cholesterol, creatinine, uric acid, chloride, magnesium, electrolytes, urine pH, phosphate—may increase; calcium should be kept at 9-10 mg/dl; vit D at 50-135 international units/dl, phosphate at 70 mg/dl; alkaline phosphatase may be decreased
• Monitor for increased blood level; toxic reactions may occur rapidly
• Assess for dry mouth, metallic taste, polyuria, bone pain, muscle weakness, headache, fatigue, tinnitus, change in LOC, irregular pulse, dysrhythmias, increased respirations, anorexia, nausea, vomiting, cramps, diarrhea, constipation; may indicate hypercalcemia
• Assess renal status: decreased urinary output (oliguria, anuria), edema in extremities, weight gain ≥5 lb, periorbital edema
• Assess nutritional status, diet for sources of vit D (milk, cod, halibut, salmon, sardines, egg yolk), calcium (dairy products, dark green vegetables), phosphates (dairy products)
• **Pregnancy/breastfeeding:** Use only recommended dietary allowances in pregnancy, breastfeeding

Patient problem
Impaired nutritional intake (uses)

Implementation
PO route
• PO may be increased q4wk depending on blood level
• Store in airtight, light-resistant container at room temperature
IM route
• Give inj deeply in large muscle mass, administer slowly, aspirate to avoid **IV** administration, rotate inj site

Patient/family education
• Advise patient to omit dose if missed; to avoid vitamin supplements unless directed by prescriber
• Inform patient of necessary foods to be included in diet

• Advise patient to keep appointments for evaluation because therapeutic and toxic levels are narrow
• Instruct patient to report weakness, lethargy, headache, anorexia, loss of weight; to report nausea, vomiting, abdominal cramps, diarrhea, constipation, excessive thirst, polyuria, muscle and bone pain
• Caution patient to decrease intake of antacids and laxatives containing magnesium

Evaluation

Positive therapeutic outcome
• Calcium levels 9-10 ml/dl
• Decreasing symptoms of bone disease

vitamin E (OTC)
Aquasol E
Func. class.: Vitamin E
Chem. class.: Fat-soluble vitamin

ACTION: Needed for digestion and metabolism of polyunsaturated fats, decreases platelet aggregation, decreases blood clot formation, promotes normal growth and development of muscle tissue, prostaglandin synthesis

Therapeutic outcome: Prevention and treatment of vit E deficiency

USES: Vit E deficiency, impaired fat absorption, hemolytic anemia in premature neonates, prevention of retrolental fibroplasia, sickle cell anemia, supplement in malabsorption syndrome

Pharmacokinetics

Absorption	20%-80% (PO)
Distribution	Widely distributed, stored in fat
Metabolism	Liver
Excretion	Bile
Half-life	Unknown

Pharmacodynamics
Unknown

CONTRAINDICATIONS
IV use in infants

Precautions: Pregnancy, anemia, breastfeeding, hypothrombinemia

DOSAGE AND ROUTES
Deficiency
Adult: PO 60-75 international units/day
Child: PO 1 international unit/kg (malabsorption)

Prevention of deficiency
Adult: PO 30 international units/day
Infant: PO 5 international units/day

Topical route
Adult and child: TOP apply to affected areas as needed

Available forms: Caps 100, 200, 400, 500, 600, 1000 international units; tabs 100, 200, 400 international units; drops 15 mg/0.3 ml; chew tabs 400 units; ointment, cream, lotion, oil

ADVERSE EFFECTS
CNS: Headache, fatigue
CV: Increased risk of thrombophlebitis
EENT: Blurred vision
GI: Nausea, cramps, diarrhea
GU: Gonadal dysfunction
INTEG: Sterile abscess, contact dermatitis
META: Altered metabolism of hormones (thyroid, pituitary, adrenal), altered immunity
MS: Weakness

INTERACTIONS
Individual drugs

Cholestyramine, colestipol, mineral oil, sucralfate: decreased absorption

Drug classification

Anticoagulants (oral): increased action of anticoagulants

NURSING CONSIDERATIONS
Assessment
• Assess nutritional status: intake of wheat germ, dark green leafy vegetables, nuts, eggs, liver, vegetable oils, dairy products, cereals
• Assess for vit E deficiency (usually in neonates): irritability, restlessness, hemolytic anemia
• **Pregnancy/breastfeeding:** Use only recommended dietary allowances in pregnancy, breastfeeding

Patient problem
Impaired nutritional intake (uses)

Implementation
PO route
• Chew chewable tabs well
• Sol may be dropped in mouth or mixed with food
• Store in airtight, light-resistant container
Topical route
• Apply topical to moisturize dry skin

Patient/family education
• Inform patient necessary foods to be included in diet high in vit E
• Instruct patient to omit if dose is missed
• Instruct patient to avoid vit supplements unless directed by prescriber because overdose may occur

Evaluation
Positive therapeutic outcome
• Absence of hemolytic anemia
• Adequate vit E levels
• Improvement in skin lesions
• Decrease in edema

⚠ HIGH ALERT

voriconazole (Rx)
(vohr-i-kahn′a-zol)
Vfend
Func. class.: Antifungal

Do not confuse: Vfend/Venofer

ACTION: Inhibits fungal CYP 450-mediation demethylation, needed for biosynthesis, causing leakage from cell membrane

Therapeutic outcome: Decreasing signs, symptoms of infection

USES: Invasive aspergillosis, serious fungal infections (*Candida* sp., *Scedosporium apiospermum, Fusarium* sp.), *Monosporium, apiospermum*

Pharmacokinetics

Absorption	Unknown
Distribution	Unknown
Metabolism	✿ CYP3A4/CYP2C9
Excretion	Via hepatic metabolism
Half-life	Elimination 6 hr (dose dependent)

Pharmacodynamics

Onset	Unknown
Peak	1-2 hr
Duration	Unknown

CONTRAINDICATIONS
Pregnancy, breastfeeding, children, hypersensitivity, severe bone marrow depression, severe hepatic disease

Precautions: Renal disease (**IV**); Asian/African descent, cardiomyopathy, cholestasis, chemotherapy, lactase deficiency, visual disturbances, renal failure, pancreatitis, QT prolongation, hypokalemia, ventricular dysrhythmias, torsades de pointes

DOSAGE AND ROUTES
Esophageal candidiasis
Adult/geriatric/child ≥12 yr: PO IV ≥**40 kg** 200 mg q12hr; <**40 kg** 100 mg q12hr

---

Candidemia

Adult/child ≥12 yr: **IV** loading dose 6 mg/kg q12hr × 24 hr, then 3-4 mg/kg q12hr × ≥14 days and ≥7 days after resolution of symptoms; **PO** after loading dose >**40 kg** 200 mg q12hr × ≥14 days and ≥7 days after resolution of symptoms; <**40 kg** 100 mg q12hr × ≥14 days and ≥7 days after resolution of symptoms

Invasive aspergillosis

Adult/adolescent: **IV** 6 mg/kg q12hr (loading dose) then 4 mg/kg q12hr, may reduce to 3 mg/kg q12hr if intolerable
Child ≥12 yr: **IV** 6 mg/kg q12hr, then 4 mg/kg q12hr

Renal dose

Adult: PO CCr <50 ml/min, use only orally

Hepatic dose

Adult: PO/IV (Child-Pugh Class A or B): Standard loading dose, then 50% of maintenance dose; (Child-Pugh Class C): Avoid use

Available forms: Tabs 50, 200 mg; powder for inj, lyophilized 200 mg, powder for oral susp 45 g (40 mg/ml after reconstitution)

ADVERSE EFFECTS

CNS: *Headache*, paresthesias, peripheral neuropathy, *hallucinations*, psychosis, EPS, depression, Guillain-Barré syndrome, insomnia, suicidal ideation, dizziness, fever
CV: Tachycardia, hyper/hypotension, vasodilatation, atrial dysrhythmias, atrial fibrillation, AV block, bradycardia, HF, MI, QT prolongation, torsades de pointes, peripheral edema
EENT: *Blurred vision*, eye hemorrhage, *visual disturbances*
GI: *Nausea, vomiting, anorexia, diarrhea*, cramps, hemorrhagic gastroenteritis, acute liver failure, hepatitis, intestinal perforation, pancreatitis
GU: *Hypokalemia*, azotemia, renal tubular necrosis, permanent renal impairment, anuria, oliguria
HEMA: Anemia, eosinophilia, hypomagnesemia, thrombocytopenia, leukopenia, pancytopenia
INTEG: *Burning, irritation*, pain, necrosis at inj site with extravasation, dermatitis, *rash*, photosensitivity
MISC: Respiratory disorder
SYST: Stevens-Johnson syndrome, toxic epidermal necrolysis, sepsis, melanoma (photosensitivity reaction)

INTERACTIONS
Individual drugs
CISplatin, cycloSPORINE, polymyxin B, vancomycin: increased nephrotoxicity

CycloSPORINE, phenytoin, pimozide, predniso-LONE, quiNIDine, rifabutin, sirolimus, tacrolimus, warfarin: increased effects of each specific product
Digoxin: increased hypokalemia
Haloperidol, chloroquine, droperidol, pentamidine; arsenic trioxide, levomethadyl: increased QT prolongation

Drug classifications
Aminoglycosides: increased nephrotoxicity
Benzodiazepines, calcium channel blockers, ergots, HMG-CoA reductase inhibitors, nonnucleoside reverse transcriptase inhibitors, protease inhibitors, proton pump inhibitors, sulfonylureas, vinca alkaloids: increased effects of each specific product
Class IA/III antidysrhythmics, some phenothiazines, beta agonists, local anesthetics, tricyclics, CYP3A4 inhibitors (amiodarone, clarithromycin, erythromycin, telithromycin, troleandomycin); CYP3A4 substrates (methadone, pimozide, QUEtiapine, quiNIDine, risperiDONE, ziprasidone): increased QT prolongation
Corticosteroids, diuretics (thiazide), skeletal muscle relaxants: increased hypokalemia

Drug/herb
St. John's wort: do not use together

Drug/food
High-fat foods: avoid use with high-fat meals, take 1 hr before or after a meal

Drug/lab test
Increased: AST/ALT, alkaline phosphatase, creatinine, bilirubin
Decreased: Hgb/Hct, platelets, WBC

NURSING CONSIDERATIONS
Assessment
• Monitor VS q15-30min during first inf; note changes in pulse, B/P
• Monitor I&O ratio; watch for decreasing urinary output, change in specific gravity; discontinue product to prevent permanent damage to renal tubules
• Monitor blood tests: CBC, K, Na, Ca, Mg q2wk; BUN, creatinine weekly
• Monitor weight weekly; if weight increases >2 lb/wk, edema is present; renal damage should be considered
• **Assess for renal toxicity:** increasing BUN, serum creatinine; if BUN is >40 mg/dl or if serum creatinine >3 mg/dl, product may be discontinued or dosage reduced
• **Assess for hepatotoxicity:** increasing AST, ALT, alkaline phosphatase, bilirubin, baseline and periodically

- **Assess for allergic reaction:** dermatitis, rash; product should be discontinued, antihistamines (mild reaction) or EPINEPHrine (severe reaction) administered
- **Assess for hypokalemia:** anorexia, drowsiness, weakness, decreased reflexes, dizziness, increased urinary output, increased thirst, paresthesias
- **Assess for ototoxicity:** tinnitus (ringing, roaring in ears), vertigo, loss of hearing (rare)
- **QT prolongation:** ECG for QT prolongation, ejection fraction; assess for chest pain, palpitations, dyspnea
- **Pregnancy/breastfeeding:** Do not use in pregnancy, may cause fetal harm, do not breastfeed

Patient problem
Impaired nutritional intake (uses)

Implementation
- Give 1 hr before or after meals
- Store at room temperature (powder, tabs)

Intermittent IV infusion route
- Give product only after C&S confirms organism, and product needed to treat condition; make sure product only is used in life-threatening infections
- Reconstitute powder with 19 ml water for inj to 10 mg/ml, shake until dissolved; infuse over 1-2 hr at a conc of 5 mg/ml or less; do not admix with other products, 4.2% sodium bicarbonate inf

Y-site compatibilities: Acyclovir, alfentanil, allopurinol, amifostine, amikacin, aminocaproic acid, aminophylline, amiodarone, amphotericin B liposome, ampicillin, ampicillin/sulbactam, anidulafungin, azithromycin, aztreonam, bivalirudin, bleomycin, bumetanide, buprenorphine, butorphanol, calcium acetate/chloride/gluconate, CARBOplatin, carmustine, caspofungin, ceFAZolin, cefotaxime, cefoTEtan, cefOXitin, cefTAZidime, ceftizoxime, cefTRIAXone, chloramphenicol, chlorproMAZINE, cimetidine, ciprofloxacin, cisatracurium, CISplatin, clindamycin, cyclophosphamide, cytarabine, dacarbazine, DACTINomycin, DAPTOmycin, DAUNOrubicin, dexamethasone, dexmedetomidine, dexrazoxane, digoxin, diltiazem, diphenhydrAMINE, DOBUTamine, DOCEtaxel, dolasetron, DOPamine, doripenem, doxacurium, doxycycline, droperidol, enalaprilat, ePHEDrine, EPINEPHrine, epirubicin, ertapenem, erythromycin, esmolol, etoposide, etoposide phosphate, famotidine, fenoldopam, fentaNYL, fluconazole, fludarabine, fluorouracil, foscarnet, fosphenytoin, furosemide, ganciclovir, gemcitabine, gentamicin, glycopyrrolate, granisetron, haloperidol, heparin, hydrALAZINE, hydrocortisone, ifosfamide, imipenem/cilastatin, inamrinone, insulin, irinotecan, isoproterenol, ketorolac, labetalol, leucovorin, levofloxacin, lidocaine, linezolid, LORazepam, magnesium sulfate, mannitol, mechlorethamine, melphalan, meperidine, meropenem, mesna, metaraminol, methohexital, methotrexate, methyldopate, methylPREDNISolone, metoclopramide, metoprolol, metroNIDAZOLE, midazolam, milrinone, mitoMYcin, morphine, nafcillin, nalbuphine, naloxone, niCARdipine, nitroglycerin, norepinephrine, octreotide, ondansetron, oxaliplatin, oxytocin, PACLitaxel, palonosetron, pancuronium, pentamidine, pentazocine, PENTobarbital, PHENobarbital, phentolamine, phenylephrine, piperacillin/tazobactam, potassium chloride/phosphates, procainamide, promethazine, propranolol, quinupristin/dalfopristin, remifentanil, rocuronium, sodium acetate/bicarbonate/phosphates, streptozocin, succinylcholine, SUFentanil, tacrolimus, teniposide, theophylline, thiotepa, ticarcillin/clavulanate, tirofiban, tobramycin, topotecan, trimethobenzamide, trimethoprim/sulfamethoxazole, vancomycin, vasopressin, vecuronium, verapamil, vinBLAStine, vinCRIStine, vinorelbine, zidovudine

Patient/family education
- Teach that long-term therapy may be needed to clear infection (2 wk-3 mo depending on type of infection)
- Advise patient to notify prescriber of bleeding, bruising, or soft tissue swelling
- Teach to take 1 hr before or after meal (PO)
- Advise patient not to drive at night because of vision changes
- Advise to avoid strong, direct sunlight
- Advise women of childbearing age to use effective contraceptive

Evaluation

Positive therapeutic outcome
- Decreased fever, malaise, rash, negative C&S for infecting organism

---

> ⚠ **HIGH ALERT**

warfarin (Rx)
(war'far-in)
Coumadin, Jantoven
Func. class.: Anticoagulant
Chem. class: Coumarins

Do not confuse: Coumadin/Cardura/
Avandia Jantoven/Janumet/Januvia

ACTION: Interferes with blood clotting by
indirect means; depresses hepatic synthesis of vit
K–dependent coagulation factors (II, VII, IX, X)

Therapeutic outcome: Prevention of
clotting or pulmonary embolism

USES: Antiphospholipid antibody syndrome,
arterial thromboembolism prophylaxis, deep
vein thrombosis, MI prophylaxis, post MI, stroke
prophylaxis, thrombosis prophylaxis, pulmonary
embolism

Pharmacokinetics

Absorption	Well absorbed (PO), completely absorbed
Distribution	Crosses placenta, 99% plasma protein binding
Metabolism	Liver
Excretion	Kidney, feces (active, inactive metabolites)
Half-life	Effective ½-2½ days

Pharmacodynamics

	PO
Onset	12-24 hr
Peak	½-4 days
Duration	3-5 days

CONTRAINDICATIONS
Pregnancy, breastfeeding, hypersensitivity, hemophilia, leukemia with bleeding, peptic ulcer disease, thrombocytopenic purpura, hepatic disease
(severe), malignant hypertension, subacute bacterial endocarditis, acute nephritis, blood dyscrasias, preeclampsia, eclampsia, hemorrhagic
tendencies, surgery of CNS, eye, traumatic surgery
with large open surface, bleeding tendencies of
GI/GU/respiratory, stroke, aneurysms, pericardial
effusion, spinal puncture, major regional/lumbar
block anesthesia

> **BLACK BOX WARNING:** Bleeding

Precautions: Alcoholism, geriatric, HF, debilitated patients, trauma, indwelling catheters,
severe hypertension, active infections, protein C
deficiency, polycythemia vera, vasculitis, severe
diabetes, ⟡ Asian patients (CYP2C9, protein C,S
deficiency or VKORC1)

DOSAGE AND ROUTES
Adult: PO 2-5 mg/day × 3 days, then titrated to
INR/pro-time
Adolescent/child/infant: PO 0.2 mg/kg/day
titrated to INR, max 10 mg

Available forms: Tabs 1, 2, 2.5, 3, 4, 5, 6,
7.5, 10 mg

ADVERSE EFFECTS
GI: nausea, cramps
GU: Hematuria, calciphylaxis
HEMA: Hemorrhage
INTEG: *Rash,* dermal necrosis
MISC: Fever
MS: Bone fractures
SYST: Anaphylaxis, coma, cholesterol, mi-
croembolisms, exfoliative dermatitis, purple
toe syndrome

INTERACTIONS
Individual drugs
Allopurinol, amiodarone, azithromycin, chloral
hydrate, chloramphenicol, cimetidine, clofibrate, clotrimazole, dextrothyroxine, diflunisal, disulfiram, erythromycin, furosemide,
glucagon, heparin, indomethacin, isoniazid,
levofloxacin, mefenamic acid, metroNIDAZOLE,
mifepristone, phenylbutazone, quiNIDine,
RU-486, sulfinpyrazone, sulindac, thyroid:
increased warfarin action

Aprepitant, azoTHIOprine, bosentan, carBAM-
azepine, dicloxicillin, ethchlorvynol, factor
IX/VIIa, griseofulvin, nafcillin, phenytoin,
rifampin, sucralfate, sulfaSALAzine, thyroid,
vitamin K: decreased warfarin action
Phenytoin: increased toxicity

Drug classifications
Antidepressants (tricyclic), ethacrynic acids,
HMG-CoA reductase inhibitors, NSAIDs,
oxyphenbutazones, COX-2 selective inhibitors,
penicillins, quinolones, salicylates, selective
serotonin reuptake inhibitors, steroids,
sulfonamides, thrombolytics: increased
warfarin action
Barbiturates, bile acid sequestrants, contraceptives (oral), estrogens: decreased warfarin
action
Sulfonylureas (oral): increased toxicity

Drug/herb
Anise, chamomile, dong quai, evening primrose,
feverfew, garlic, ginger, ginkgo, ginseng,
horse chestnut, kava, licorice, melatonin,

W

---

red yeast rice, saw palmetto: increased risk of bleeding

Coenzyme Q10, St. John's wort: decreased anticoagulant effect

Drug/food

Vit K foods: decreased warfarin action

Drug/lab test

Increased: T_3 uptake, liver function tests
Decreased: uric acid

NURSING CONSIDERATIONS
Assessment

> **BLACK BOX WARNING:** Monitor blood studies (Hct, PT, platelets, occult blood in stools) q3mo; INR: in hospital daily after 2nd or 3rd dose; once in therapeutic range for 2 consecutive days, monitor 2-3× wk for 1-2 wk, then less frequently depending on stability of INR results; *Outpatient:* monitor every few days until stable dose, then periodically thereafter depending on stability of INR results, usually at least monthly

> **BLACK BOX WARNING:** Assess for bleeding gums, petechiae, ecchymosis, black tarry stools, hematuria, occult, cerebral, (intra abdominal); fatal hemorrhage can occur

- Monitor B/P, watch for increasing signs of hypertension
- Assess for fever, skin rash, urticaria
- Assess for needed dosage change q1-2wk

Patient problem

Risk for injury (uses, adverse reactions)
Ineffective tissue perfusion (uses)

Implementation
PO route

- Warfarin is usually given with **IV** heparin for 3 or more days, warfarin blood level may take several days

Patient/family education

- Caution patient to avoid OTC preparations unless directed by prescriber; may cause serious product interactions; avoid alcohol
- Advise patient that product may be withheld during active bleeding (menstruation), depending on condition
- Advise patient to use soft-bristle toothbrush to avoid bleeding gums, avoid contact sports, use electric razor, avoid IM inj
- Instruct patient to carry/wear emergency ID identifying product taken

> **BLACK BOX WARNING:** Advise patient to report any signs of bleeding: nosebleed, gums, under skin, urine, stools

- Teach patient to read food labels; limited intake of vit K foods (green leafy vegetables) is necessary to maintain consistent prothrombin levels
- Teach patient to take as prescribed, not to skip or double doses, take missed dose as soon as remembered
- Advise patient to report if pregnancy is planned or suspected or if breastfeeding
- Advise patient that continuing follow-up exams and lab work will be needed

Evaluation

Positive therapeutic outcome

- Decrease of deep vein thrombosis
- Pro-time (1.3-2.0 × control)
- Absence of pulmonary embolism

⚠ HIGH ALERT

zaleplon (Rx)

(zal'eh-plon)

Sonata

Func. class.: Hypnotic, nonbarbiturate

Chem. class.: Pyrazolopyrimidine

Controlled substance schedule IV

Do not confuse: Sonata/Soriatane

ACTION: Binds selectively to ω-1 receptor of the γ-aminobutyric acid type A (GABA_A) receptor complex; results are sedation, hypnosis, skeletal muscle relaxation, anticonvulsant activity, anxiolytic action

Therapeutic outcome: Ability to sleep

USES: Insomnia (short-term treatment)

Pharmacokinetics

Absorption	Rapidly absorbed
Distribution	Extravascular tissues, crosses blood-brain barrier; crosses placenta
Metabolism	Extensively, liver to inactive metabolites
Excretion	Kidneys
Half-life	1 hr

Pharmacodynamics

Onset	Rapid
Peak	1 hr
Duration	3-4 hr

CONTRAINDICATIONS

Hypersensitivity, severe hepatic disease

Precautions: Pregnancy, breastfeeding, children <15 yr, geriatric, renal/hepatic disease, psychosis, angioedema, respiratory disease, depression, sleep-related behavior (sleep walking), Asian descent, CNS depression

DOSAGE AND ROUTES

Adult: PO 10 mg at bedtime; may increase dosage to 20 mg at bedtime if needed; 5 mg may be used in low-weight persons

Geriatric: PO 5 mg at bedtime; may increase if needed

Hepatic dose: Adult PO 5 mg at bedtime, max 10 mg

Available forms: Caps 5, 10 mg

ADVERSE EFFECTS

CNS: *Drowsiness,* amnesia, depersonalization, hallucinations, hyperesthesia, paresthesia, somnolence, tremor, vertigo, dizziness, anxiety, *lethargy, daytime sedation,* confusion, complex sleep-related reactions (sleep driving, sleep eating)

CV: Chest pain, peripheral edema

EENT: Vision changes, ear/eye pain, hyperacusis, parosmia

GI: Nausea, anorexia, colitis, dyspepsia, dry mouth, constipation, abdominal pain

MISC: Asthenia, fever, headache, myalgia, dysmenorrhea

MS: Myalgia, back pain, arthritis

RESP: Bronchitis

SYST: Severe allergic reactions

INTERACTIONS

Individual drugs

Cimetidine: increased action of zaleplon

Drug classifications

CYP3A4 inhibitors/inducers: increased or decreased zaleplon levels

Drug/herb

Chamomile, hops, kava, valerian: increased CNS depression

Drug/food

High-fat/heavy meal: prolonged absorption, sleep onset reduced

NURSING CONSIDERATIONS

Assessment

• **Sleep disorders:** assess for type of sleep problem, falling asleep, staying asleep; monitor for complex sleep disorders

• Assess for previous product dependence or tolerance; if product dependent or tolerant, amount of medication should be restricted

• Monitor patient's mental status: mood, sensorium, affect, sleeping patterns, drowsiness, dizziness, suicidal tendencies, excessive sedation, impaired coordination

• **Beers:** Avoid in older adults with or at high risk for delirium, potential for worsening or inducing delirium

Patient problem

Impaired sleep (uses)

Implementation

• Give ½-1 hr before bedtime for sleeplessness; give on empty stomach

• Store in tight container in cool environment

Patient/family education

• Inform patient that product is for short-term use only

• Teach patient to take immediately before going to bed

• Advise patient that product may cause memory problems, dependence (if used for

Z

---

longer periods of time), changes in behavior/thinking, complex sleep-related behavior (sleep eating/driving)
• Advise patient not to ingest a high-fat/heavy meal before taking
• Advise patient to avoid OTC preparations unless approved by a physician, to avoid alcohol ingestion or other psychotropic medications unless prescribed by a health care provider, that 1-2 wk of therapy may be required before therapeutic effects occur
• Caution patient to avoid driving, activities requiring alertness; drowsiness may occur; until medication response is known, tell patient that drowsiness may worsen at beginning of treatment
• Instruct patient not to discontinue medication abruptly after long-term use
• **Pregnancy/breastfeeding:** Identify if pregnancy is planned or suspected or if breastfeeding

Evaluation
Positive therapeutic outcome
• Decreased sleeplessness

zidovudine (Rx)
(zye-doe′vue-deen)
Retrovir
Func. class.: Antiretroviral
Chem. class.: Nucleoside reverse transcriptase inhibitor (NRTI)

Do not confuse: Retrovir/ritonavir

ACTION: Inhibits replication of HIV-1 by incorporating into cellular DNA by viral reverse transcriptase, thereby terminating the cellular DNA chain

Therapeutic outcome: Decreased symptoms of HIV-1 infection

USES: Used in combination with at least 2 other antiretrovirals for HIV-1 infection

Pharmacokinetics
Absorption	Well absorbed (PO), completely absorbed (**IV**)
Distribution	Widely distributed—crosses placenta, CSF, protein binding 38%
Metabolism	Liver, mostly
Excretion	Kidneys
Half-life	Terminal ½-3 hr

Pharmacodynamics
	PO	IV
Onset	Unknown	Rapid
Peak	½-1½ hr	Inf end
Duration	4 hr	4 hr

CONTRAINDICATIONS
Hypersensitivity

Precautions: Pregnancy, breastfeeding, children, granulocyte count $<1000/mm^3$ or Hgb <9.5 g/dl, severe renal disease, obesity

> **BLACK BOX WARNING:** Hepatotoxicity, anemia, lactic acidosis, myopathy, neutropenia

DOSAGE AND ROUTES
Human immunodeficiency virus (HIV) infection in combination with other antiretroviral agents
Adults: PO 300 mg BID or 200 mg TID; **IV Infusion** 1 mg/kg over 1 h q4hr around the clock (total daily dose: 6 mg/kg/day). Initiate oral therapy as soon as possible. Monotherapy with zidovudine is not recommended for treatment of HIV
Children and Adolescents: ≥ 30 kg PO 300 mg BID (preferred) or 200 mg TID
Infants and Children: 9 to 29 kg PO 9 mg/kg/dose BID (preferred) or 6 mg/kg/dose tid
• **Infants and Children 4 to 8 kg PO** 12 mg/kg/dose BID (preferred) or 8 mg/kg/dose TID
• **Neonates 35 wks gestational age and older (unlabeled)** PO 4 mg/kg/dose BID initially; increase to 12 mg/kg/dose BID after 4 wks of age.
• **Premature Neonates 30 to 34 wks gestational age (unlabeled)** PO 2 mg/kg/dose BID initially increase to 3 mg/kg/dose BID at 2 wks of age, and then increase to 12 mg/kg/dose BID after 6 to 8 wks of age
• **Premature Neonates less than 30 weeks gestational age** 2 mg/kg/dose **PO** twice daily initially. Increase to 3 mg/kg/dose PO twice daily at 4 weeks of age, and then increase to 12 mg/kg/dose PO twice daily after 8 to 10 weeks of age

For perinatal human immunodeficiency virus (HIV) prophylaxis
Pregnant Females (intrapartum) IV Infusion 2 mg/kg over 1 h, followed by 1 mg/kg/h IV continuous infusion until clamping of the umbilical cord
Neonates ≥ 35 wks gestational age IV 3 mg/kg/dose q12hr beginning as soon as possible

---

after birth (preferably within 6 to 12 hours). Increase to 9 mg/kg/dose q12 hr after 4 wks of age

Renal dose
Adult: PO CCr 15 ml/min or more: No change; CCr <15 ml/min: 100 mg q8hr or 300 mg qday
Pediatric patients: PO GFR 10 ml/min/1.73 m2 or more: No change; GFR < 10 ml/min/1.73 m2: Reduce dose by 50%

Available forms: Caps 100 mg; tabs 300 mg; inj 10 mg/ml; oral syr 50 mg/5 ml

ADVERSE EFFECTS
CNS: *Fever, headache, malaise,* diaphoresis, *dizziness, insomnia,* paresthesia, somnolence, chills, tremor, twitching, anxiety, confusion, depression, lability, vertigo, loss of mental acuity, seizures, malaise
EENT: Taste change, hearing loss, photophobia
GI: *Nausea, vomiting, diarrhea,* anorexia, cramps, *dyspepsia, constipation,* dysphagia, *flatulence,* rectal bleeding, mouth ulcer, abdominal pain, hepatomegaly
GU: Dysuria, polyuria, frequency, hesitancy
HEMA: Granulocytopenia, anemia
INTEG: *Rash,* acne, pruritus, urticaria
MS: Myalgia, arthralgia, muscle spasm
RESP: Dyspnea, cough, wheezing
SYST: Lactic acidosis

INTERACTIONS
Individual drugs
Clarithromycin: decreased effects of zidovudine
DOXOrubicin, ribavirin, staduvine: avoid concurrent use
Fluconazole, probenecid: increased toxicity
Ganciclovir, radiation, SMZ/TMP, valganciclovir: increased bone marrow suppression
Methadone: increased zidovudine level

Drug classifications
Antineoplastics: increased bone marrow suppression
Interferons, NRTIs: decreased zidovudine levels

Drug/lab test
Increased: LFTs, granulocytes
Decreased: platelets, amylase, CPK

NURSING CONSIDERATIONS
Assessment
• **HIV:** Monitor symptoms of HIV baseline and throughout treatment
• **Assess for peripheral neuropathy:** tingling or pain in hands and feet, distal numbness; if these occur, product may be decreased or discontinued

• **Assess for pancreatitis:** abdominal pain, nausea, vomiting, elevated liver enzymes; product should be discontinued because condition can be fatal
• Assess children by dilated retinal examination q6mo to rule out retinal depigmentation

> **BLACK BOX WARNING: Bone marrow suppression:** Monitor blood counts q2wk; watch for decreasing granulocytes, Hgb; if low, therapy may have to be discontinued and restarted after hematologic recovery; blood transfusions may be required; monitor viral load, CD4 counts, LFTs, plasma HIV RNA, serum creatinine/BUN baseline and throughout treatment

• Monitor lipid profile, blood glucose, hepatitis B serology, plasma hepatitis C RNA, more common in females

> **BLACK BOX WARNING: Lactic acidosis, severe hepatomegaly with steatosis:** obtain baseline LFTs; if elevated, discontinue treatment; discontinue even if LFTs are normal but lactic acidosis, hepatomegaly are present; may be fatal

• **Pregnancy/breastfeeding:** Register pregnant patients at the Antiretroviral Pregnancy Registry 800-258-4263, do not breastfeed, excreted in breast milk

Patient problem
Infection (uses)

Implementation
PO route
• Latex is the vial stopper
• Give on empty stomach
• Do not take dapsone at same time as didanosine
• Store in cool environment; protect from light

> **Intermittent IV infusion route**
> • Give after diluting with D₅W; give over 1 hr (<4 mg/ml), do not give by direct **IV**
> • Protect unopened product from light; use diluted solutions within 8 hr if stored at room temperature, 48 hr if refrigerated, do not use discolored solutions

Y-site compatibilities: Acyclovir, alemtuzumab, allopurinol, amikacin, amphotericin B, anidulafungin, argatroban, aztreonam, ceftazidime, cefTRIAXone, cimetidine, clindamycin, dexamethasone, DOBUTamine, DOPamine, erythromycin, fluconazole, fludarabine, gentamicin, heparin, imipenem/cilastatin, LORazepam, metoclopramide, morphine, nafcillin, ondansetron, oxacillin, pentamidine, phenylephrine, piperacillin, potassium chloride, ranitidine, sargramostim, tacrolimus, tobramycin, trimethoprim/sulfamethoxazole, vancomycin, zoledronic acid

Additive incompatibilities: Blood products or protein solutions

Patient/family education

• Caution patient to take on empty stomach; to use exactly as prescribed

• Advise patient to report signs of infection: increased temp, sore throat, shortness of breath flulike symptoms; to avoid crowds and those with known infections; to avoid crowds or people with known infections

• Advise that fainting, dizziness may occur, to avoid driving or other hazardous activities until response is known

• Instruct patient to report signs of anemia: fatigue, headache, faintness, shortness of breath, irritability

• Advise patient to report bleeding; avoid use of razors or commercial mouthwash

• Inform patient that hair may be lost during therapy (rare); a wig or hairpiece may make patient feel better

• Caution patient to avoid OTC products or other medications without approval of prescriber serious drug interactions may occur

• Caution patient not to have any sexual contact without use of a condom; needles should not be shared; blood from infected individual should not come in contact with another's mucous membranes, compliance with treatment is required

• Teach patient that redistribution of body fat may occur

• **Pregnancy/breastfeeding:** Identify if pregnancy is planned or suspected or if breastfeeding

Evaluation

Positive therapeutic outcome

• Decreased infection; decreased symptoms of HIV infection, decreased viral load, increased CD4 counts

---

zinc (PO, OTC; IV, Rx)
(zink sul′fate)
Orazinc, PMS Egozinc ✦, Verazinc, Zinca-Pak, Zincate, Zinc 15, Zinc-220
Func. class.: Trace element; nutritional supplement

ACTION: Needed for adequate healing, bone and joint development, (23% zinc)

Therapeutic outcome: Replacement of zinc

USES: Prevention of zinc deficiency, adjunct to vit A therapy

Unlabeled uses: Wound healing

Precautions: Pregnancy (parenteral), breastfeeding, hypocupremia, neonatal prematurity, neonates, renal disease

Pharmacokinetics

Absorption	Poorly absorbed (**PO**), completely absorbed (**IV**)
Distribution	Widely distributed
Metabolism	Liver
Excretion	90% (feces), 10% (kidneys)
Half-life	Unknown

Pharmacodynamics
Unknown

DOSAGE AND ROUTES
Dietary supplement (elemental zinc)
Adult/adolescent pregnant females: PO 11-13 mg/day

Nutritional supplement (IV)
Adult: IV 2.5-4 mg/day, may increase by 2 mg/day if needed
Child 1-5 yr: IV 50 mcg/kg/day
Adult and lactating female: PO 12-14 mg/day × 12 mo
Adult and adolescent male ≥14 yr: PO 11 mg/day
Adult female ≥19 yr: PO 8 mg/day
Adolescent female ≥14 yr: PO 9 mg/day
Child 9-13 yr: PO 8 mg/day
Child 4-8 yr: PO 5 mg/day
Child 1-3 yr: PO 3 mg/day
Infant 7-12 mo: PO 3 mg/day
Infant birth to 6 mo: PO 2 mg/day (adequate intake)

Wound healing (unlabeled)
Adult: PO 50 mg tid until healed (elemental iron)

Available forms: Tabs 66, 110, 220 mg; inj 1, 5 mg/ml, Caps 25, 50 mg

ADVERSE EFFECTS
GI: Nausea, vomiting, cramps, heartburn, ulcer formation

INTERACTIONS
Drug classifications
Fluoroquinolones, tetracyclines: decreased absorption

Drug/food
Caffeine, dairy products: decreased absorption of PO zinc

NURSING CONSIDERATIONS
Assessment
- Zinc deficiency: poor wound healing, absence of taste, smell, slowing growth
- Alkaline phosphatase, HDL monthly in long-term therapy
- Monitor zinc levels during treatment, CBC
- **Pregnancy/breastfeeding:** Use only if benefits outweigh fetal risk (IV), considered safe in breastfeeding

Patient problem
Impaired nutritional intake (uses)

Implementation
PO route
- Give with meals to decrease gastric upset; restrict dairy products, caffeine, which decrease absorption

IV route
- Part of TPN

Patient/family education
- Inform patient that element must be taken for 3 mo to be effective
- Advise patient to report immediately nausea, diarrhea, rash, severe vomiting, restlessness, abdominal pain, tarry stools

Evaluation
Positive therapeutic outcome
- Absence of zinc deficiency
- Improved wound healing

OVERDOSE: Diarrhea, rash, dehydration, restlessness

ziprasidone (Rx)
(zi-praz'ih-dohn)
Geodon, Zeldox ✿
Func. class.: Antipsychotic/neuroleptic
Chem. class.: Benzisoxazole derivative

ACTION: Unknown; may be mediated through both dopamine type 2 (D_2) and serotonin type 2 ($5-HT_2$) antagonism

Therapeutic outcome: Decreased signs/symptoms of psychosis

USES: Schizophrenia, acute agitation, acute psychosis, bipolar disorder, mania, psychotic depression, agitation

Pharmacokinetics

Absorption	Unknown
Distribution	Protein binding 99%
Metabolism	Liver, extensively to metabolite
Excretion	Unknown
Half-life	7 hr (IM), 2-5 hr (PO)

Pharmacodynamics

Onset	Unknown
Peak	PO 6-8 hr; IM 60 min
Duration	PO 12 hr

CONTRAINDICATIONS
Hypersensitivity, breastfeeding

Precautions: Pregnancy, children, geriatric, renal/cardiac/hepatic disease, breast cancer, diabetes, AV block, CNS depression, seizure disorders, abrupt discontinuation, agranulocytosis, ambient temperature increase, suicidal ideation, torsades de pointes, strenuous exercise

> **BLACK BOX WARNING:** Increased mortality in elderly patients with dementia-related psychosis

DOSAGE AND ROUTES
Schizophrenia
Adult: PO 20 mg bid with food, adjust dosage every 2 days upward to max of 80 mg bid; **IM** 10-20 mg per dose; may give 10 mg q2hr, doses of 20 mg may be given q4hr, max 40 mg/day

Bipolar disorder
Adult: PO 40 mg bid with food, on day 2 increase to 60 or 80 mg bid, then adjust to response; maintenance as adjunct to lithium/valproate 40-80 mg bid

Available forms: Tabs 20, 40, 60, 80 mg; inj 20 mg/ml single-dose vials

ADVERSE EFFECTS
CNS: *EPS (pseudoparkinsonism, akathisia, dystonia, tardive dyskinesia), drowsiness, insomnia, agitation, anxiety, headache,* seizures, neuroleptic malignant syndrome, dizziness, tremor, facial droop
CV: Orthostatic hypotension, tachycardia, prolonged QT/QTc, sudden death, heart failure (geriatric), torsades de pointes
HEMA: Agranulocytosis
EENT: Blurred vision, diplopia
ENDO: Hyperglycemia
GI: *Nausea,* vomiting, *anorexia, constipation,* jaundice, weight gain, diarrhea, dry mouth, abdominal pain
GU: Priapism
RESP: Infection, cough
INTEG: Rash, inj site pain, sweating, drug reaction with eosinophilia and systemic symptoms (DRESS), Stevens-Johnson syndrome

INTERACTIONS
Individual drugs
Alcohol: increased sedation

Chloroquine, clarithromycin, droperidol, erythromycin, grepafloxacin, haloperidol, methadone, moxifloxacin, pentamidine: increased QT prolongation

CarBAMazepine, phenytoin, rifampin: increased excretion of ziprasidone

Lithium: increased EPS, possible neurotoxicity

Drug classifications

Antihypertensives: increased hypotension, monitor B/P

Antipsychotics: increased EPS

β-agonists, class IA/III antidysrhythmics, local anesthetics, phenothiazines (some), tricyclics: increased QT prolongation

Barbiturates: increased excretion of ziprasidone

CNS depressants: increased sedation

CYP3A4 inhibitors (ketoconazole, itraconazole): increased ziprasidone level, dose may need to be reduced

Opioids: increased respiratory depression, avoid concurrent use

SSRIs, SNRIs: increased serotonin syndrome, increased neuroleptic malignant syndrome

NURSING CONSIDERATIONS
Assessment

> **BLACK BOX WARNING:** Assess geriatric with dementia closely; heart failure, sudden death have occurred

• Assess mental status before initial administration, AIMS assessment

• Monitor bilirubin, CBC, liver function tests, fasting blood glucose, cholesterol profile; potassium, magnesium when taken with loop/thiazide diuretics qmo

• Monitor B/P standing and lying; also pulse, respirations; take these q4hr during initial treatment; establish baseline before starting treatment; report drops of 30 mm Hg; watch for ECG changes; QT prolongation may occur, QTc >500 msec should have products discontinued

• Assess dizziness, faintness, palpitations, tachycardia on rising

• Assess EPS, including akathisia (inability to sit still, no pattern to movements), tardive dyskinesia (bizarre movements of the jaw, mouth, tongue, extremities), pseudoparkinsonism (rigidity, tremors, pill rolling, shuffling gait)

• **DRESS:** monitor for rash, fever, swollen lymph nodes, product should be discontinued

• **Assess for neuroleptic malignant syndrome:** hyperthermia, increased CPK, altered mental status, muscle rigidity

• **Stevens-Johnson syndrome:** Assess for rash, with fever aches, blisters, swelling of face, discontinue product immediately

• **Seizures:** Assess for seizures in those with seizure disorders, provide seizure precautions seizure threshold is lowered

• Assess constipation, urinary retention daily; if these occur, increase bulk and water in diet

• **Pregnancy/breastfeeding:** May cause EPS in the neonate, enroll in the Atypical Antipsychotic Pregnancy Registry 866-961-2388, avoid breastfeeding, excretion unknown

• **Beers:** Avoid use in older adults except for schizophrenia, bipolar disorder, or short-term as an antiemetic during chemotherapy, increased risk of stroke and cognitive decline

Patient problem

Distorted thinking process (uses)
Excess food intake (adverse reactions)

Implementation

• Give reduced dosage in geriatric patient

• Give antiparkinsonian agent to be used for EPS

• Store in tight, light-resistant container

• Provide supervised ambulation until patient is stabilized on medication; do not involve in strenuous exercise program because fainting is possible; patient should not stand still for a long time

PO route

• Take cap whole and with food, with plenty of fluid at same time of day

• Food increases absorption

• Store in airtight, light-resistant container

IM route

• Add 1.2 ml sterile water for inj to vial, shake vigorously until product is dissolved; give deeply in large muscle; do not mix with other products; do not use if particulates are present, keep patient recumbent for 30 min after injection

• Do not give over 3 consecutive days

• Store injection at room temperature; protect from light; after reconstituting may be stored at room temperature × 24 hr, 7 days refrigerated

Patient/family education

• Advise patient that orthostatic hypotension may occur and to rise from sitting or lying position gradually; avoid hot tubs, hot showers, tub baths because hypotension may occur

• Advise patient to avoid abrupt withdrawal of this product; EPS may result; product should be withdrawn slowly

• Advise patient to avoid OTC preparations (cough, hay fever, cold), herbals, supplements

---

⚠ Nurse Alert   ✴ Key NCLEX® Drug   >> Drug Specifics

unless approved by prescriber, since serious product interactions may occur; avoid use with alcohol, CNS depressants; increased drowsiness may occur

• Teach patient to avoid hazardous activities if drowsy or dizzy

• Advise patient to increase fluids, bulk in diet to prevent constipation

• Teach patient to use sips of water, candy, gum for dry mouth

• Teach patient to report impaired vision, tremors, muscle twitching

• Teach patient that in hot weather, heat stroke may occur; take extra precautions to stay cool, take adequate liquids

• Advise patient that continuing follow-up exams will be needed

• **Pregnancy/breastfeeding:** Identify if pregnancy is planned or suspected, or if breastfeeding

Evaluation

Positive therapeutic outcome

• Decrease in emotional excitement, hallucinations, delusions, paranoia; reorganization of patterns of thought, speech

TREATMENT OF OVERDOSE:
Lavage if orally ingested; provide airway; *do not induce vomiting*

⚠ HIGH ALERT

ziv-aflibercept
(ziv-a-flih′ber-sept)

Zaltrap

Func. class.: Antineoplastic

Chem. class.: Signal transduction inhibitor (STI), fusion protein

ACTION: An angiogenesis inhibitor, a fusion protein that binds to vascular endothelial growth factors (🗝 VEGF-A, VEGF-B) and placental growth factor 1 and 2

Therapeutic outcome: Decrease in spread or size of tumor

USES: Metastatic colorectal cancer that is resistant or has progressed after an oxaliplatin-containing regimen in combination with 5-fluorouracil, leucovorin, irinotecan (FOLFIRI)

Pharmacokinetics

Absorption	Complete
Distribution	Unknown
Metabolism	Unknown
Excretion	Unknown
Half-life	6 days

Pharmacodynamics

Onset	Unknown
Peak	Unknown
Duration	Unknown

CONTRAINDICATIONS
Hypersensitivity

Precautions: Infertility, male-mediated teratogenicity, encephalopathy, hypertension, dental work, breastfeeding, children, neonates, geriatric patients, infection, neutropenia, pregnancy

> **BLACK BOX WARNING:** Bleeding, GI bleeding/perforation, intracranial bleeding, surgery

DOSAGE AND ROUTES
Adult: IV 4 mg/kg over 1 hr on day 1 every 2 wk in combination with the FOLFIRI regimen (irinotecan 180 mg/m² over 90 min on day 1 with dl-racemic leucovorin 400 mg/m² over 2 hr) (infused at the same time, in same Y-line; then on day 1 by 5-fluorouracil 400 mg/m² as a bolus, then 2400 mg/m² as a 46-hr cont IV inf)

Available forms: Solution for injection 100 mg/4 ml; 200 mg/8 ml

ADVERSE EFFECTS
CNS: Intracranial bleeding, *headache, dizziness,* reversible posterior leukoencephalopathy

CV: Hypertensive crisis, *hypertension,* stroke

GI: Nausea, hepatotoxicity, dyspepsia, GI hemorrhage, *abdominal pain,* GI perforation

GU: Proteinuria, hematuria

HEMA: Neutropenia, leukopenia

INTEG: Rash, pruritus, alopecia, hypersensitivity, palmar plantar erythrodysesthesia

MISC: Fatigue, epistaxis, night sweats, decreased weight, flulike symptoms, infection

RESP: Dyspnea, pulmonary embolism

NURSING CONSIDERATIONS
Assessment

> **BLACK BOX WARNING: Severe bleeding:** Assess for GI bleeding, intracranial bleeding, and pulmonary hemorrhage/hemoptysis; may be fatal; monitor patients for signs and symptoms of bleeding

> **BLACK BOX WARNING: GI perforation:** some cases are fatal; monitor patients for signs and symptoms of GI perforation; discontinue therapy if GI perforation develops

• **Poor wound healing:** hold ≥4 wk before elective surgery; after major surgery, do not

Z

---

restart for ≥4 wk and until the surgical wound is entirely healed
- **Severe hypertension/hypertensive crisis:** usually occurs within the first 2 cycles (grade 3 or 4 hypertension); monitor B/P every 2 wk or more often if needed; treatment with antihypertensives may be needed; product may need to be discontinued
- **Severe proteinuria/nephrotic syndrome/ thrombotic microangiopathy (TMA):** monitor urine protein by dipstick analysis and urinary protein–to–creatinine ratio (UPCR); obtain a 24-hr urine collection for a UPCR >1; for proteinuria of <2 g/24 hr, temporarily hold doses until proteinuria is <2 g/24 hr; if proteinuria recurs, hold doses until proteinuria is <2 g/24 hr, then permanently reduce; discontinue in nephrotic syndrome or TMA
- **Febrile neutropenia, neutropenic infection/sepsis:** monitor CBC with differential at baseline and before each cycle, hold FOLFIRI until the neutrophil count is ≥1.5 × 10^9/L
- **Geriatric toxicity:** assess for diarrhea, dizziness, asthenia, weight loss, and dehydration that can indicate toxicity

Patient problem
Risk for injury (uses, adverse reactions)
Diarrhea (adverse reactions)

Implementation
- Give before FOLFIRI chemotherapy; visually inspect for particulate matter and discoloration before use

Dilution and preparation
- Withdraw the calculated dose, add to 0.9% sodium chloride or dextrose 5% solution to 0.6–8 mg/ml; use polyvinyl chloride (PVC) infusion bags containing bis (2-ethylhexyl) phthalate (DHEP) or polyolefin infusion bags; do not re-enter the vial after first puncture; discard any unused portion; do not mix or combine with other drugs in the same infusion bag; the diluted solution may be stored refrigerated for ≤4 hr; discard any unused portion in the infusion bag

IV infusion
- Give diluted solution over 1 hr using a 0.2 micrometer polyethersulfone filter; do not use nylon or polyvinylidene fluoride (PVDF) filters; do not give IV push or bolus; do not mix or combine with other drugs in the same IV line; give using an infusion set made of one of the following: PVC containing DEHP, DEHP-free PVC containing trioctyl-trimellitate (TOTM), polypropylene, polyethylene-lined PVC, or polyurethane

Dosage adjustments for recurrent or severe hypertension

Hold until B/P is controlled and then permanently reduce dose to 2 mg/kg; discontinue in hypertensive crisis or hypertensive encephalopathy

Dosage adjustments for proteinuria (2 g/24 hr)

Hold until proteinuria is <2 g/24 hr; if proteinuria recurs, hold therapy until proteinuria is <2 g/24 hr, then reduce to 2 mg/kg; discontinue in nephrotic syndrome or thrombotic microangiopathy

Patient/family education
- **Pregnancy/breastfeeding:** Teach that highly effective contraception should be used during treatment and up to 3 mo after the last dose in all patients of reproductive potential, infertility and male-mediated teratogenicity can occur; infertility is reversible within 18 wk after stopping product; do not breastfeed
- Teach patient about reason for treatment, expected results

BLACK BOX WARNING: Notify prescriber immediately of bleeding, severe abdominal pain, poor wound healing

Evaluation

Positive therapeutic outcome
- Decrease in spread of size of tumor

zoledronic acid (Rx)
(zoh'leh-drah'nick ass'id)
Aclasta ✢, Reclast, Zometa
Func. class.: Bone-resorption inhibitor
Chem. class.: Bisphosphonate

Do not confuse: Zometa/Zofran/Zoladex

ACTION: Inhibits normal and abnormal bone resorption; potent inhibitor of osteoclastic bone resorption; inhibits osteoclastic activity, reduces bone resorption and inhibits skeletal calcium release caused by stimulating factors released by tumors; reduction of abnormal bone resorption is responsible for therapeutic effect in hypercalcemia; may directly block dissolution of hydroxyapatite bone crystals

Therapeutic outcome: Serum calcium at normal level

USES: Moderate to severe hypercalcemia associated with malignancy; multiple myeloma; bone metastases from solid tumors (used with antineoplastics), active Paget's disease, osteoporosis, glucocorticoid-induced osteoporosis, osteoporosis prophylaxis in postmenopausal women

---

Pharmacokinetics

Absorption	Rapidly cleared from circulation, complete
Distribution	Taken up mainly by bones; plasma protein binding ~22%
Metabolism	Not metabolized
Excretion	Kidneys (~50% eliminated in urine within 24 hr)
Half-life	167 hr

Pharmacodynamics

Onset	Unknown
Peak	15 min
Duration	Max effect 7 days

CONTRAINDICATIONS

Pregnancy, breastfeeding, hypocalcemia, hypersensitivity to this product or bisphosphonates

Precautions: Children, geriatric, renal dysfunction, asthmatic patients, asthma, acute bronchospasm, anemia, chemotherapy, coagulopathy, dehydration, dental disease, diabetes mellitus, renal disease, electrolyte imbalance, hypertension, hypovolemia, phosphate hypersensitivity, infection, multiple myeloma

DOSAGE AND ROUTES
Hypercalcemia of malignancy
Adult: IV INF 4 mg, given as a single INF over ≥15 min, may re-treat with 4 mg if serum calcium does not return to normal within 1 wk

Multiple myeloma/metastatic bone lesions
Adult: IV INF 4 mg, given over 15 min q3-4wk

Osteoporosis
Adult: IV 5 mg over 15 min or more q12mo

Active Paget's disease
Adult: IV INF 5 mg over ≥15 min

Osteoporosis prophylaxis (Reclast), postmenopausal women
Adult: IV INF 5 mg every other yr

Osteoporosis prophylaxis (Reclast) taking systemic glucocorticoids
Adult: IV 5 mg qyr

Renal dose
Adult: IV INF CCr 50-60 ml/min 3.5 mg; CCr 40-49 ml/min 3.3 mg; CCR 30-39 ml/min 3 mg; CCr <30 ml/min don't use

Early breast cancer (unlabeled)
Adult: IV 4 mg q6mo with goserelin 3.6 mg subcut qmo and tamoxifen 20 mg/day or anastrozole 1 mg/day for 3 yr

Available forms: Sol for inj 4 mg/5 ml (Zometa); inj 5 mg/100 ml (Reclast)

ADVERSE EFFECTS
CNS: Dizziness, headache, anxiety, confusion, insomnia, agitation
CV: Hypotension, leg edema, chest pain
GI: Abdominal pain, anorexia, constipation, nausea, diarrhea, vomiting, taste change
GU: UTI, possible reduced renal function, renal damage
INTEG: Stevens-Johnson syndrome, toxic epidermal necrolysis
META: Anemia, hypokalemia, hypomagnesemia, hypophosphatemia, hypocalcemia, increased serum creatinine
MISC: *Fever, chills, flulike symptoms*
MS: Severe bone pain, *arthralgias, myalgias,* osteonecrosis of the jaw

INTERACTIONS
Individual drugs
Calcium, vitamin D: decreased zoledronic acid effect
Digoxin: hypomagnesemia, hypokalemia

Drug classifications
Aminoglycosides, NSAIDs, radiopaque contrast agents: increased neurotoxicity
Aminoglycosides, loop diuretics: decreased serum calcium
Infusion solutions (calcium-containing): do not mix with calcium-containing inf sol such as lactated Ringer's sol

Drug/lab test
Increased: creatinine
Decreased: calcium, phosphorus, magnesium, potassium, Hct/Hgb, RBC, platelets, WBC

NURSING CONSIDERATIONS
Assessment
• Assess renal function tests and calcium, phosphate, magnesium, potassium, creatinine; if creatinine is elevated hold treatment
• **Assess for hypocalcemia:** paresthesia, twitching, laryngospasm; Chvostek's/Trousseau's signs
• **Assess dental status;** dental health may be required before starting this product, assess mouth for sores, dental cavities, gingivitis, a dental professional exam should be done; cover with antiinfectives for dental extraction
• Assess for atrial fibrillation
• **Fluid volume status:** Encourage additional fluid intake or give bolus before use, monitor I&O ratio, renal status screening before use in renal disease
• **Skeletal survey:** Bone fractures may occur, prevent falls and injury

Z

Patient problem
Risk for injury (uses, adverse reactins)

Implementation
• Give acetaminophen before and for 72 hr after to decrease pain
• Sol reconstituted with sterile water may be stored under refrigeration for up to 24 hr **IV**
• Administer in separate **IV** line from all other products

Zometa
• Administer after reconstituting by adding 5 ml of sterile water for inj to each vial, then add up to ≥100 ml of sterile 0.9% NaCl, D₅W, run over ≥15 min

Reclast
• No further dilution required; inf over ≥15 min at constant rate; max 5 mg

Patient/family education
• Instruct patient to report hypercalcemic relapse: nausea, vomiting, bone pain, thirst
• Advise patient to continue with dietary recommendations including calcium and vit D; take a multiple vitamin daily, 500 mg of calcium, 400 international units vit D in multiple myeloma
• Teach patient if nausea/vomiting occur, eat small meals, use lozenges or chewing gum
• Advise patient if bone pain occurs, notify prescriber to obtain analgesic
• Instruct patient to continue good oral hygiene
• Teach patient that oral health may be required before starting product in high-risk patients, repair of dental cavities, treatment of gingivitis
• Advise patient to report ocular infection or eye pain immediately
• Teach patient to use, expected results of product
• Teach patient that musculoskeletal pain and weakness may occur
• Advise patient to have regular checkups, report mouth sores or jaw pain (osteoporosis of the jaw)
• Advise patient not to use during pregnancy, breastfeeding

Evaluation

Positive therapeutic outcome
• Calcium levels decreased to normal

TREATMENT OF OVERDOSE:
Correct reductions in serum calcium by administering **IV** calcium gluconate; in serum phosphorus, with potassium or sodium phosphate; in serum magnesium, with magnesium sulfate

ZOLMitriptan (Rx)
(zole-mih-trip'tan)
Zomig, Zomig-ZMT
Func. class.: Migraine agent, abortive
Chem. class.: 5HT₁ᴮ/5HT₁ᴰ receptor agonist (triptan)

ACTION: Binds selectively to the vascular serotonin type 1 (5HT₁ᴮ/5HT₁ᴰ) receptor subtype, exerts antimigraine effect; causes vasoconstriction in cranial arteries

Therapeutic outcome: Decreased severity, frequency of headache

USES: Acute treatment of migraine with or without aura

Pharmacokinetics
Absorption	Unknown
Distribution	25% plasma protein binding
Metabolism	Liver
Excretion	Urine, feces
Half-life	3-3½ hr

Pharmacodynamics
Onset	Unknown
Peak	Unknown
Duration	2-3½ hr

CONTRAINDICATIONS
Angina pectoris, history of MI, documented silent ischemia, ischemic heart disease, uncontrolled hypertension, hypersensitivity, basilar or hemiplegic migraine, risk of CV events

Precautions: Pregnancy, breastfeeding, children, postmenopausal women, men >40 yr, geriatric, risk factors for CAD, hypercholesterolemia, obesity, diabetes, impaired renal/hepatic function

DOSAGE AND ROUTES
Adult: PO start at 2.5 mg or lower (tab may be broken), may repeat after 2 hr, max single dose 5 mg, max 10 mg/24 hr; NASAL 1 spray in 1 nostril at onset of migraine, repeat in 2 hr if no relief

Available forms: Tabs 2.5, 5 mg; orally disintegrating tabs 2.5, 5 mg; nasal spray 2.5, 5 mg

ADVERSE EFFECTS
CNS: *Tingling, hot sensation, burning, feeling of pressure, tightness, numbness, dizziness, sedation*

CV: Palpitations, chest pain
GI: Abdominal discomfort, nausea, dry mouth, dyspepsia, dysphagia
MISC: Odd taste (spray)
MS: *Weakness, neck stiffness,* myalgia
RESP: Chest tightness, pressure

INTERACTIONS
Individual drugs
Cimetidine: increased half-life of ZOLMitriptan
Ergot: increased vasospastic effects
FLUoxetine, fluvoxaMINE, PARoxetine, sertraline: increased weakness, hyperreflexia, incoordination
Sibutramine: increased ZOLMitriptan levels

Drug classifications
Contraceptives (oral): increased half-life of ZOLMitriptan
Ergot derivatives: increased vasospastic effects
MAOIs: do not use within 2 wk
Selective serotonin reuptake inhibitors: increased weakness, hyperreflexia, incoordination

Drug/herb
SAM-e, St. John's wort: serotonin syndrome

Drug/lab test
Increased: alkaline phosphatase

NURSING CONSIDERATIONS
Assessment
• Assess for tingling, hot sensation, burning; feeling of pressure, numbness, flushing
• Assess neurologic status: LOC, blurring vision, nausea, vomiting, tingling in extremities preceding headache
• Monitor ingestion of tyramine foods (pickled products, beer, wine, aged cheese), food additives, preservatives, colorings, artificial sweeteners, chocolate, caffeine, which may precipitate these types of headaches
• Assess for serotonin syndrome if also taking an SSRI
• **Pregnancy/breastfeeding:** May cause fetal harm and death, do not breastfeed, excreted in breast milk
• **Beers:** Avoid use in older adults, may cause CNS effects

Patient problem
Pain (uses)

Implementation
PO route
• Give with fluids as soon as symptoms of migraine occur
• Provide quiet, calm environment with decreased stimulation for noise, bright light, excessive talking

Orally disintegrating tablet
• Give orally disintegrating tablet immediately after opening; do not crush or chew, allow to dissolve on tongue
Nasal route
• Blow nose before use
• Remove top, insert in nostril, hold other nostril shut
• Press on plunger while breathing
• Discard, for single use only

Patient/family education
• Teach patient to report any side effects to prescriber
• Advise patient to use contraception while taking product
• Teach patient to report pain, rash, swelling of face
• Instruct patient not to double doses; if second dose is needed, wait at least 2 hr; disintegrating dosage form: do not split, break, alter, to remove from blister pack immediately before use
• Teach patient that product does not reduce or prevent number of migraines and not to use for other headaches, use over 10 days per month, may lead to exacerbation of headache

Evaluation

Positive therapeutic outcome
• Decrease in frequency, severity of headache

⚠ HIGH ALERT

zolpidem (Rx)
(zole-pi′dem)
Ambien, Ambien CR, Edluar, Intermezzo, Sublinox ✦, Zolpimist
Func. class.: Sedative-hypnotic
Chem. class.: Nonbenzodiazepine of imidazopyridine class
Controlled substance schedule IV

Do not confuse: Ambien/Abilify/Ativan/Coumadin/zolpidem/lorazepam/zaleplon/zolmitriptan

ACTION: Produces CNS depression at limbic, thalamic, hypothalamic levels of CNS; may be mediated by neurotransmitter γ-aminobutyric acid (GABA); results are sedation, hypnosis, skeletal muscle relaxation, anticonvulsant activity, anxiolytic action

Therapeutic outcome: Ability to sleep, sedation

USES: Insomnia, short-term treatment; insomnia with difficulty of sleep onset/maintenance (ext rel)

Pharmacokinetics

Absorption	Rapidly absorbed
Distribution	Unknown
Metabolism	Liver—inactive metabolite
Excretion	Kidneys, breast milk
Half-life	2½ hr, increased in geriatric, hepatic disease

Pharmacodynamics

	PO	EXT	REL SL	Spray
Onset	Unknown	Unknown	Unknown	Unknown
Peak	1-2 hr	2-4 hr	Unknown	Unknown
Duration	6-8 hr	Unknown	Unknown	Unknown

CONTRAINDICATIONS
Hypersensitivity to benzodiazepines

Precautions: Pregnancy, breastfeeding, children <18 yr, geriatric, anemia, hepatic disease, suicidal individuals, product abuse, seizure disorders, angioedema, depression, respiratory disease, sleep apnea, sleep-related behavior (sleep walking), myasthenia gravis, pulmonary disease, next-morning impairments; females (lower dose needed)

DOSAGE AND ROUTES
Adult: PO 10 mg at bedtime × 7-10 days only; total dose max 10 mg; **EXT REL** 12.5 mg immediately before bedtime, may be useful for up to 24 wk in people 18-64 yr with primary insomnia; **oral spray (Zolpimist)** 10 mg (2 sprays) immediately before bedtime, max 10 mg/day; **SL (Edluar)** 10 mg just before bedtime
Geriatric: PO 5 mg at bedtime; EXT REL 6.25 mg

Available forms: Tabs 5, 10 mg; **ext rel tabs** 6.25, 12.5 mg; **SL** 1.75, 3.5, 5, 10 mg; **oral spray** 5 mg/spray

ADVERSE EFFECTS
CNS: Headache, lethargy, drowsiness, daytime sedation, dizziness, confusion, light-headedness, anxiety, irritability, amnesia, poor coordination, complex sleep-related reactions (sleep driving, sleep eating), depression, somnolence, suicidal ideation, abnormal thinking/behavioral changes
CV: Chest pain, palpitation
GI: Nausea, vomiting, diarrhea, heartburn, abdominal pain, constipation
HEMA: Leukopenia, granulocytopenia (rare)
MISC: Myalgia
SYST: Severe allergic reactions, angioedema, anaphylaxis

INTERACTIONS
Individual drugs
Alcohol: increased action of both products

Drug classifications
CNS depressants: increased action of both products
CYP3A4 inhibitors/inducers: increased or decreased zolpidem levels

Drug/herb
Chamomile, kava, valerian: increased CNS depression
St. John's wort: decreased action

NURSING CONSIDERATIONS
Assessment
• Assess mental status: mood, sensorium, anxiety, affect, sleeping pattern, drowsiness, dizziness, especially geriatric; physical dependency, withdrawal symptoms: anxiety, panic attacks, agitation, seizures, headache, nausea, vomiting, muscle pain, weakness; suicidal tendencies; for indications of increasing tolerance and abuse
• Monitor B/P (lying, standing), pulse; if systolic B/P drops 20 mm Hg, hold product, notify prescriber
• Monitor I&O ratio for renal dysfunction
• **Beers:** Avoid in older adults, CNS effects occur

Patient problem
Impaired sleep (uses)
Risk for injury (adverse reactions)

Implementation
PO route
• Do not break, crush, or chew ext rel product or orally disintegrating tab
• Give ½-1 hr before bedtime for sleeplessness; give several hr before patient is to rise (to avoid hangover)
• Give with food or fluids; tab may be crushed or swallowed whole
• Do not use spray with or after a meal
• Store in airtight container in cool environment

Patient/family education
• Advise patient that complex sleep-related behavior may occur (sleep driving/eating)
• Instruct patient that product may be taken with food or fluids, next-morning impairment may occur
• Caution patient not to use for everyday stress or longer than 3 mo unless directed by prescriber; not to take more than prescribed amount; may be habit forming; not to double or skip doses
• Caution patient to avoid OTC preparations unless approved by prescriber; alcohol and CNS depressants will increase CNS depression

• Advise patient to avoid driving, activities that require alertness, because drowsiness may occur; to avoid alcohol ingestion or other psychotropic medications; to rise slowly or fainting may occur, especially geriatric; that drowsiness may worsen at beginning of treatment

• Instruct patient not to discontinue medication abruptly after long-term use; withdrawal symptoms include vomiting, cramping, tremors, seizures may occur

• Teach patient use of orally disintegrating tabs: place on tongue, allow to dissolve before swallowing

• Teach patient not to crush, chew, break ext rel tabs

• Teach patient to prime spray pump before using

• **Pregnancy/breastfeeding:** Identify if pregnancy is planned or suspected or if breastfeeding

Evaluation

Positive therapeutic outcome

• Ability to sleep at night

• Decreased amount of early-morning awakening if taking product for insomnia

TREATMENT OF OVERDOSE:

Lavage, VS, supportive care

Alpha-adrenergic Blockers

ACTION: α-Adrenergic blockers bind to α-adrenergic receptors, causing dilatation of peripheral blood vessels and lower peripheral resistance resulting in decreased blood pressure.

USES: α-Adrenergic blockers are used for benign prostatic hyperplasia, pheochromocytoma, prevention of tissue necrosis, and sloughing associated with extravasation of IV vasopressors.

CONTRAINDICATIONS
Hypersensitive reactions may occur, and allergies should be identified before these products are given. Patients with myocardial infarction, coronary insufficiency, angina, or other evidence of coronary artery disease should not use these products.

IMPLEMENTATION
PO route
• Start with low dose, gradually increasing to prevent side effects
• Give with food or milk for GI symptoms

ADVERSE EFFECTS: The most common side effects are hypotension, tachycardia, nasal stuffiness, nausea, vomiting, and diarrhea.

PHARMACOKINETICS: Onset, peak, and duration vary among products.

INTERACTIONS: Vasoconstrictive and hypertensive effects of EPINEPHrine are antagonized by α-adrenergic blockers.

NURSING CONSIDERATIONS
Assessment
• Monitor electrolytes: potassium, sodium chloride, carbon dioxide
• Monitor weight daily, I&O
• Monitor B/P with patient lying, standing before starting treatment, q4hr thereafter
• Assess for nausea, vomiting, diarrhea
• Assess for skin turgor, dryness of mucous membranes for hydration status

Patient/family education
• Caution patient to avoid alcoholic beverages
• Advise patient to report dizziness, palpitations, fainting
• Instruct patient to change position slowly or fainting may occur
• Teach patient to take product exactly as prescribed; to avoid all OTC products (cough, cold, allergy) unless directed by prescriber

Evaluation
Positive therapeutic outcome
• Decreased B/P
• Increased peripheral pulses

Generic Names
α 1 blockers:
silodosin

Anesthetics—general/local

ACTION: Anesthetics (general) act on the CNS to produce tranquilization and sleep before invasive procedures. Anesthetics (local) inhibit conduction of nerve impulses from sensory nerves.

USES: General anesthetics are used to premedicate for surgery, and for induction and maintenance in general anesthesia. For local anesthetics, refer to individual product listing for indications.

CONTRAINDICATIONS
Persons with CVA, increased ICP, severe hypertension, and cardiac decompensation should not use these products since severe adverse reactions can occur.

Precautions: Anesthetics (general) should be used with caution in the geriatric, children <2 yr, and those with cardiovascular disease (hypotension, bradydysrhythmias), renal/hepatic disease, and Parkinson's disease. The precaution for anesthetics (local) is pregnancy.

IMPLEMENTATION
• Give anticholinergic preoperatively to decrease secretions
• Administer only with resuscitative equipment nearby
• Provide quiet environment for recovery to decrease psychotic symptoms

ADVERSE EFFECTS: The most common side effects are dystonia, akathisia, flexion of arms, fine tremors, drowsiness, restlessness, and hypotension. Also common are chills, respiratory depression, and laryngospasm.

PHARMACOKINETICS: Onset, peak, and duration vary widely among products. Most products are metabolized in the liver and excreted in urine.

INTERACTIONS: AOIs, tricyclics, and phenothiazines may cause severe hypo/hypertension when used with local anesthetics. CNS depressants will potentiate general and local anesthetics.

NURSING CONSIDERATIONS
Assessment
• Monitor VS q10min during **IV** administration, q30min after IM dose

Evaluation

Positive therapeutic outcome
• Maintenance of anesthesia
• Decreased pain

Generic Names

General anesthetics:
droperidol (high alert), **fentaNYL** (high alert), fentaNYL/droperidol, fentaNYL transdermal, fospropofol, midazolam, **propofol** (high alert)

Local anesthetics:
lidocaine, parenteral (high alert), penicillin G procaine, ropivacaine

Antacids

ACTION: Antacids are basic compounds that neutralize gastric acidity and decrease the rate of gastric emptying. Products are divided into those containing aluminum, magnesium, calcium, or a combination of these.

USES: Antacids decrease hyperacidity in conditions such as peptic ulcer disease, reflux esophagitis, gastritis, or hiatal hernia.

CONTRAINDICATIONS
Sensitivity to aluminum or magnesium products may cause hypersensitive reactions. Aluminum products should not be used by persons sensitive to aluminum. Magnesium products should not be used by persons sensitive to magnesium. Check for sensitivity before administering.

Precautions: Magnesium products should be given cautiously to patients with renal insufficiency, and during pregnancy and breastfeeding. Sodium content of antacids may be significant. Use with caution for patients with hypertension, or HF or those on a low-sodium diet.

IMPLEMENTATION
• Advise patient not to take other products within 1-2 hr of antacid administration, since antacids may impair absorption of other products
• Give all products with an 8-oz glass of water to ensure absorption in the stomach
• Give another antacid if constipation occurs with aluminum products

ADVERSE EFFECTS: The most common side effect caused by aluminum-containing antacids is constipation, which may lead to fecal impaction and bowel obstruction. Diarrhea occurs often when magnesium products are given. Alkalosis may occur when systemic products are used. Constipation occurs more frequently than laxation with calcium carbonate. The release of CO_2 from carbonate-containing antacids causes belching, abdominal distention, and flatulence. Sodium bicarbonate may act as a systemic antacid and produce systemic electrolyte disturbances and alkalosis. Calcium carbonate and sodium bicarbonate may cause rebound hyperacidity and milk-alkali syndrome. Alkaluria may occur when products are used on a long-term basis, particularly in persons with abnormal renal function.

PHARMACOKINETICS: Duration is 20-40 min. If ingested 1 hr after meals, acidity is reduced for at least 3hr.

INTERACTIONS: Products whose effects may be increased by some antacids include quiNIDine, amphetamines, pseudoephedrine, levodopa, valproic acid, and dicumarol. Products whose effects may be decreased by some antacids include cimetidine, corticosteroids, ranitidine, iron salts, phenothiazines, phenytoin, digoxin, tetracyclines, ketoconazole, salicylates, and isoniazid.

NURSING CONSIDERATIONS
Assessment
• Assess for aggravating and alleviating factors of epigastric pain or hyperacidity; identify the location, duration, and characteristics of epigastric pain
• Assess GI symptoms, including constipation, diarrhea, abdominal pain; if severe abdominal pain with fever occurs, these products should not be given
• Assess renal symptoms, including increasing urinary pH, electrolytes

Evaluation

Positive therapeutic outcome
• Absence of epigastric pain
• Decreased acidity

Generic Names
aluminum hydroxide, bismuth subsalicylate, calcium carbonate, magaldrate, magnesium oxide, sodium bicarbonate

Anti-Alzheimer Agents

ACTION: Anti-Alzheimer agents improve cognitive functioning by increasing acetylcholine and inhibiting cholinesterase in the CNS. They do not cure the condition, but improve symptoms.

USES: Anti-Alzheimer agents are used for the treatment of Alzheimer's symptoms.

CONTRAINDICATIONS
Persons with hypersensitivity reactions should not use these products.

Precautions: Anti-Alzheimer agents should be used cautiously in pregnancy, breastfeeding, sick sinus syndrome, GI bleeding, bladder obstruction, and seizures.

IMPLEMENTATION
• Give lowest possible dose for therapeutic result; adjust dose to response
• Provide assistance with ambulation during beginning therapy if dizziness, ataxia occur

ADVERSE EFFECTS: The most common side effects are nausea, vomiting, diarrhea, dry mouth, insomnia, dizziness, urinary frequency, incontinence, and rash. The most serious side effects are seizures and dysrhythmias.

PHARMACOKINETICS: Onset, peak, and duration vary widely among products. Most products are metabolized in the liver and excreted by the kidneys.

INTERACTIONS: Increased synergistic reactions may occur with succinylcholine, cholinesterase inhibitors, and cholinergic agonists. There may be a decrease in the action of anticholinergics, and there may be additive effects when used with cholinergic agents.

NURSING CONSIDERATIONS
Assessment
• B/P, hypo/hypertension
• Mental status: affect, mood, behavioral changes, depression, confusion
• GI status: nausea, vomiting, anorexia, diarrhea
• GU status: urinary frequency, incontinence

Patient/family education
• Instruct patient to report side effects, adverse reactions to healthcare provider
• Advise patient to use exactly as prescribed, at regular intervals
• Caution patient not to increase or abruptly decrease dose; serious consequences may result
• Inform patient that product is not a cure, but relieves symptoms

Evaluation

Positive therapeutic outcome
• Decrease in confusion
• Improved mood

Generic Names
donepezil, memantine, rivastigmine

Antianginals

ACTION: Antianginals are divided into the nitrates, calcium channel blockers, and β-adrenergic blockers. The nitrates dilate coronary arteries, causing decreased preload, and dilate systemic arteries, causing decreased afterload. Calcium channel blockers dilate coronary arteries and decrease SA/AV node conduction. β-adrenergic blockers decrease heart rate so that myocardial O_2 use is decreased. Dipyridamole selectively dilates coronary arteries to increase coronary blood flow.

USES: Antianginals are used in chronic stable angina pectoris, unstable angina, and vasospastic angina. Some (i.e., calcium channel blockers and β-blockers) may be used as dysrhythmics and in hypertension.

CONTRAINDICATIONS
Persons with known hypersensitivity, increased ICP, or cerebral hemorrhage should not use some of these products.

Precautions: Antianginals should be used with caution in pregnancy, breastfeeding, children, postural hypotension, renal disease, and hepatic injury.

IMPLEMENTATION
• Store protected from light, moisture; place in cool environment

ADVERSE EFFECTS: The most common side effects are postural hypotension, headache, flushing, dizziness, nausea, edema, and drowsiness. Also common are rash, dysrhythmias, and fatigue.

PHARMACOKINETICS: Onset, peak, and duration vary widely among coronary products. Most products are metabolized in the liver and excreted in urine.

INTERACTIONS: Interactions vary widely among products. Check individual monographs for specific information.

NURSING CONSIDERATIONS
Assessment
• Monitor orthostatic B/P, pulse
• Assess for pain: duration, time started, activity being performed, character
• Assess for tolerance if taken over long period
• Assess for headache, light-headedness, decreased B/P; may indicate a need for decreased dosage

Patient/family education

• Instruct patient to keep tabs in original container
• Instruct patient not to use OTC products unless directed by prescriber
• Advise patient to report bradycardia, dizziness, confusion, depression, fever
• Teach patient to take pulse at home; advise when to notify prescriber
• Advise patient to avoid alcohol, smoking, sodium intake
• Advise patient to comply with weight control, dietary adjustments, modified exercise program
• Teach patient to carry/wear emergency ID to identify product being taken, allergies
• Caution patient to make position changes slowly to prevent fainting

Evaluation

Positive therapeutic outcome
• Decrease, prevention of anginal pain

Generic Names

Nitrates:
isosorbide, nitroglycerin

β-adrenergic blockers:
atenolol, dipyridamole, metoprolol, nadolol, propranolol

Calcium channel blockers:
amLODIPine, **diltiazem** (high alert), niCARdipine, NIFEdipine, verapamil

Miscellaneous:
ranolazine

Antianxiety Agents

ACTION: Benzodiazepines potentiate the action of GABA, including any other inhibitory transmitters in the CNS, resulting in decreased anxiety. Most agents cause a decrease in CNS excitability.

USES: Anxiety is relieved in conditions such as generalized anxiety disorder and phobic disorders. Benzodiazepines are also used for acute alcohol withdrawal to prevent delirium tremens, and some products are used for relaxation before surgery.

CONTRAINDICATIONS

These products are contraindicated in hypersensitivity, acute closed-angle glaucoma, breastfeeding (diazepam), children <6 mo, and hepatic disease (clonazePAM).

Precautions: Antianxiety agents should be used cautiously in geriatric or debilitated patients.

Usually smaller doses are needed since metabolism is slowed. Persons with renal/hepatic disease may show delayed excretion. ClonazePAM may increase the incidence of seizures.

IMPLEMENTATION

• Give with food or milk for GI symptoms; may give crushed if patient is unable to swallow whole (tabs only, no controlled or sustained-release products)

ADVERSE EFFECTS: The most common side effects are dizziness, drowsiness, blurred vision, and orthostatic hypotension. Most adverse reactions are mediated through the CNS. There is potential for abuse and physical dependence with some products.

PHARMACOKINETICS: Most of these agents are metabolized by the liver and excreted via the kidneys.

INTERACTIONS: Increased CNS depression may occur when given with other CNS depressants. These products should be used together cautiously. Alcohol should not be used, as fatal reactions have occurred. The serum concentration and toxicity may be increased when used with benzodiazepines.

NURSING CONSIDERATIONS
Assessment

• Assess B/P (lying and standing), pulse; if systolic B/P drops 20 mm Hg, hold product and notify prescriber; orthostatic hypotension can be severe
• Monitor renal/hepatic function tests: AST, ALT, bilirubin, creatinine, LDH, alkaline phosphatase
• Monitor physical dependency and withdrawal with some products, including headache, nausea, vomiting, muscle pain, and weakness after long-term use

Patient/family education

• Inform patient that product should not be used for everyday stress or long-term use; not to take more than prescribed amount since product is habit forming
• Caution patient to avoid driving and activities that require alertness since drowsiness and dizziness may occur
• Instruct patient to abstain from alcohol, other psychotropic medications unless directed by prescriber
• Caution patient not to discontinue abruptly; after extended periods, withdrawal symptoms may occur

Evaluation

Positive therapeutic outcome
• Decreased anxiety
• Increased relaxation

Generic Names

Benzodiazepines:
ALPRAZolam, chlordiazePOXIDE, clonazePAM, diazepam, LORazepam, midazolam, triazolam

Miscellaneous:
busPIRone, doxepin, hydrOXYzine, PARoxetine, venlafaxine

Antiasthmatics

ACTION: Bronchodilators are divided into anticholinergics, α/β-adrenergic agonists, β-adrenergic agonists, and phosphodiesterase inhibitors. Also included in antiasthmatic agents are corticosteroids, leukotriene antagonists, mast cell stabilizers, and monoclonal antibodies. Anticholinergics act by inhibiting interaction of acetylcholine at receptor sites on bronchial smooth muscle. α/β-adrenergic agonists act by relaxing bronchial smooth muscle and increasing diameter of nasal passages. β-adrenergic agonists act by action on β_2-receptors, which relaxes bronchial smooth muscle. Phosphodiesterase inhibitors act by blocking phosphodiesterase and increasing cAMP, which mediates smooth muscle relaxation in the respiratory system. Corticosteroids act by decreasing inflammation in the bronchial system. Leukotriene receptor antagonists decrease leukotrienes, and mast cell stabilizers decrease histamine; both act to decrease bronchospasm.

USES: Antiasthmatics are used for bronchial asthma; bronchospasm associated with bronchitis, emphysema, or other obstructive pulmonary diseases; Cheyne-Stokes respirations; and prevention of exercise-induced asthma. Some products are used for rhinitis and other allergic reactions.

CONTRAINDICATIONS

Persons with hypersensitivity, closed-angle glaucoma, tachydysrhythmias, and severe cardiac disease should not use some of these products.

Precautions: Antiasthmatics should be used with caution in pregnancy, breastfeeding, hyperthyroidism, hypertension, prostatic hypertrophy, and seizure disorders.

IMPLEMENTATION

• Give inhaled product after shaking; exhale, place mouthpiece in mouth, inhale slowly, hold breath, remove, exhale slowly
• Give PO product with meals to decrease gastric irritation

• Store inhaled product in light-resistant container; do not expose to temperatures >86° F (30° C)
• Give gum, small sips of water for dry mouth

ADVERSE EFFECTS: The most common side effects are tremors, anxiety, nausea, vomiting and irritation in the throat. The most serious adverse reactions are bronchospasm and dyspnea.

PHARMACOKINETICS: Onset, peak, and duration vary widely among products. Most products are metabolized by the liver and excreted in urine.

INTERACTIONS: Interactions vary widely among products. Check individual monographs for specific information.

NURSING CONSIDERATIONS
Assessment

• Monitor respiratory function: vital capacity, forced expiratory volume, ABGs, lung sounds, heart rate and rhythm, aggravating and alleviating factors

Patient/family education

• Caution patient to avoid hazardous activities; drowsiness or dizziness may occur with some products
• Instruct patient to obtain bloodwork as required; some products require blood levels to be drawn
• Advise patient to avoid all OTC medications unless approved by provider
• Instruct patient to report side effects, including insomnia, heart palpitations, light-headedness; these side effects may occur with some products

Evaluation

Positive therapeutic outcome
• Decreased severity and number of asthma attacks
• Absence of dyspnea, wheezing

Generic Names

Bronchodilators:
albuterol, arformoterol, **atropine** (high alert), formoterol, ipratropium, levalbuterol, terbutaline, theophylline, tiotropium

Adrenergics:
EPINEPHrine (high alert)

Corticosteroids:
beclomethasone, betamethasone, budesonide, cortisone, dexamethasone, flunisolide, fluticasone, hydrocortisone, methylPREDNISolone, predniSONE, triamcinolone

Leukotriene antagonists:
zafirlukast

Monoclonal antibodies:
omalizumab

Anticholinergics

ACTION: Anticholinergics inhibit the muscarinic actions of acetylcholine at receptor sites in the autonomic nervous system. Anticholinergics are also known as antimuscarinic products.

USES: Anticholinergics are used for a variety of conditions: decreasing involuntary movements in parkinsonism (benztropine, trihexyphenidyl); bradydysrhythmias (atropine); nausea and vomiting (scopolamine); and as cycloplegic mydriatics (atropine, homatropine, scopalamine, cyclopentolate, tropicamide). Gastrointestinal anticholinergics are used to decrease motility (smooth muscle tone) in the GI, biliary, and urinary tracts and for their ability to decrease gastric secretions (propantheline, glycopyrrolate).

CONTRAINDICATIONS
Persons with closed-angle glaucoma, myasthenia gravis, or GI/GU obstruction should not use some of these products.

Precautions: Anticholinergics should be used with caution in pregnant, breastfeeding, or geriatric patients, or in those with prostatic hypertrophy, HF, or hypertension. Use with caution in the presence of high environmental temperature.

IMPLEMENTATION
PO route
• Give with or after meals to prevent GI upset; may give with fluids other than water
• Store at room temperature
• Give hard candy, frequent drinks, sugarless gum to relieve dry mouth

IM/IV route
• Give parenteral dose with patient recumbent to prevent postural hypotension
• Give parenteral dose slowly; keep in bed for at least 1 hr after dose; monitor VS
• Give after checking dose carefully; even slight overdose could lead to toxicity

ADVERSE EFFECTS: The most common side effects are dry mouth, constipation, urinary retention, urinary hesitancy, headache, and dizziness. Also common is paralytic ileus.

PHARMACOKINETICS: Onset, peak, and duration vary widely among products. Most products are metabolized in the liver and excreted in urine.

INTERACTIONS: Increased anticholinergic effects may occur when used with MAOIs, tricyclics, and amantadine. Anticholinergics may cause a decreased effect of phenothiazines and levodopa.

NURSING CONSIDERATIONS
Assessment
• Assess I&O ratio; retention commonly causes decreased urinary output
• Assess for urinary hesitancy, retention; palpate bladder if retention occurs
• Assess for constipation; increase fluids, bulk, exercise if this occurs
• Identify tolerance over long-term therapy; dosage may need to be increased or changed
• Assess mental status: affect, mood, CNS depression, worsening of mental symptoms during early therapy

Patient/family education
• Caution patient to avoid driving and other hazardous activities; drowsiness may occur
• Advise patient to avoid OTC medication: cough, cold preparations with alcohol, antihistamines unless directed by prescriber

Evaluation

Positive therapeutic outcome
• Decreased secretions
• Absence of nausea and vomiting

Generic Names
atropine (high alert), benztropine, glycopyrrolate, hyoscyamine, scopolamine (transdermal), solifenacin

Anticoagulants

ACTION: Anticoagulants interfere with blood clotting by preventing clot formation.

USES: Anticoagulants are used for DVT, pulmonary emboli, myocardial infarction, open heart surgery, disseminated intravascular clotting syndrome, atrial fibrillation with embolization, and in transfusion and dialysis.

CONTRAINDICATIONS
Persons with hemophilia and related disorders, leukemia with bleeding, peptic ulcer disease, thrombocytopenic purpura, blood dyscrasias, acute nephritis, and subacute bacterial endocarditis should not use these products.

Precautions: Anticoagulants should be used with caution in pregnancy, geriatric, and alcoholism.

IMPLEMENTATION
• Store in tight container (PO dose)

SUBCUT route
- Give at same time each day to maintain steady blood levels
- Do not massage area or aspirate when giving SUBCUT inj; give in abdomen between pelvic bones; rotate sites; do not pull back on plunger, leave in for 10 sec; apply gentle pressure for 1 min
- Do not change needles
- Avoid all IM inj that may cause bleeding

ADVERSE EFFECTS: The most serious adverse reactions are hemorrhage, agranulocytosis, leukopenia, eosinophilia, and thrombocytopenia, depending on the specific product. The most common side effects are diarrhea, rash, and fever.

PHARMACOKINETICS: Onset, peak, and duration vary widely among products. Most products are metabolized in the liver and excreted in urine.

INTERACTIONS: Salicylates, steroids, and nonsteroidal antiinflammatories will potentiate the action of anticoagulants. Anticoagulants may cause serious effects. Check individual monographs for specific information.

NURSING CONSIDERATIONS
Assessment
- Monitor blood tests (Hct, platelets, occult blood in stools) q3mo
- Monitor PTT, which should be 1½-2 × control, PPT; daily, APTT, ACT, INR
- Monitor B/P; watch for increasing signs of hypertension
- Monitor for bleeding gums, petechiae, ecchymosis, black tarry stools, hematuria
- Monitor for fever, skin rash, urticaria
- Monitor for needed dosage change q1-2wk

Patient/family education
- Advise patient to avoid OTC preparations that may cause serious product interactions unless directed by prescriber
- Inform patient that product may be held during active bleeding (menstruation), depending on condition
- Caution patient to use soft-bristle toothbrush to prevent bleeding gums; avoid contact sports; use electric razor
- Instruct patient to carry/wear emergency ID identifying product taken
- Instruct patient to report any signs of bleeding: gums, under skin, urine, stools

Evaluation

Positive therapeutic outcome
- Decrease of DVT

Generic Names
argatroban, dabigatran, **dalteparin** (high alert), **enoxaparin** (high alert), fondaparinux, **heparin** (high alert), **lepirudin** (high alert), **tinzaparin** (high alert), **warfarin** (high alert)

Anticonvulsants

ACTION: Anticonvulsants are divided into the barbiturates, benzodiazepines, hydantoins, succinimides, and miscellaneous products. Barbiturates and benzodiazepines are discussed in separate sections. Hydantoins act by inhibiting the spread of seizure activity in the motor cortex. Succinimides act by inhibiting spike and wave formation; they also decrease amplitude, frequency, duration, and spread of discharge in seizures.

USES: Hydantoins are used in generalized tonic-clonic seizures, status epilepticus, and psychomotor seizures. Succinimides are used for absence (or petit mal) seizures. Barbiturates are used in generalized tonic-clonic and cortical focal seizures.

CONTRAINDICATIONS
Hypersensitive reactions may occur, and allergies should be identified before these products are given.

Precautions: Persons with renal/hepatic disease should be watched closely.

IMPLEMENTATION
PO route
- Give with food, milk to decrease GI symptoms
- Provide good oral hygiene as it is important for patients taking hydantoins

ADVERSE EFFECTS: Bone marrow depression is the most life-threatening adverse reaction associated with hydantoins or succinimides. The most common side effects are GI symptoms. Other common side effects for hydantoins are gingival hyperplasia and CNS effects such as nystagmus, ataxia, slurred speech, and confusion.

PHARMACOKINETICS: Onset, peak, and duration vary widely among products. Most products are metabolized in the liver and excreted in urine, bile, and feces.

INTERACTIONS: Hydantoins cause decreased effects of estrogens, and oral contraceptives.

NURSING CONSIDERATIONS
Assessment
- Monitor renal function tests, including BUN, creatinine, serum uric acid, urine CCr before, during therapy

• Monitor blood tests: RBC, Hct, Hgb, reticulocyte counts weekly for 4 wk then monthly
• Monitor hepatic function tests: AST, ALT, bilirubin, creatinine
• Assess mental status, including mood, sensorium, affect, behavioral changes; if mental status changes, notify prescriber
• Assess for eye problems, including need for ophth examinations before, during, and after treatment (slit lamp, fundoscopy, tonometry)
• Assess for allergic reaction, including red, raised rash; if this occurs, product should be discontinued
• Assess for blood dyscrasias, including fever, sore throat, bruising, rash, jaundice
• Monitor toxicity, including bone marrow depression, nausea, vomiting, ataxia, diplopia, cardiovascular collapse, Stevens-Johnson syndrome

Patient/family education
• Advise patient to carry/wear emergency ID stating products taken, condition, prescriber's name, phone number
• Advise patient to avoid driving, other activities that require alertness

Evaluation

Positive therapeutic outcome
• Decreased seizure activity; document on patient's chart

Generic Names
Succinimides:
ethosuximide

Hydantoins:
fosphenytoin, phenytoin

Miscellaneous:
acetaZOLAMIDE, cannabidiol, carBAMazepine, clonazePAM, diazepam, eslicarbazepine, ezogabine, fenfluramine, gabapentin, lacosamide, lamoTRIgine, **magnesium sulfate** (high alert), rufinamide, tiaGABine, topiramate, valproate/valproic acid/divalproex sodium, vigabatrin, zonisamide

Barbiturates:
PHENobarbital (high alert), primidone, **thiopental** (high alert)

Antidepressants

ACTION: Antidepressants are divided into the tricyclics, MAOIs, and miscellaneous antidepressants (SSRIs). The tricyclics work by blocking reuptake of norepinephrine and serotonin into nerve endings and increasing action of norepinephrine and serotonin in nerve cells. MAOIs act by increasing concentrations of endogenous EPINEPHrine, norepinephrine, serotonin, and dopamine in storage sites in the CNS by inhibition of MAO; increased concentration reduces depression.

USES: Antidepressants are used for depression and, in some cases, enuresis in children.

CONTRAINDICATIONS
The contraindications for antidepressants are seizure disorders, prostatic hypertrophy, and severe renal/hepatic/cardiac disease depending on the type of medication.

Precautions: Antidepressants should be used cautiously in pregnant, geriatric, and suicidal patients; severe depression; schizophrenia; hyperactivity; and diabetes mellitus.

IMPLEMENTATION
PO route
• Give increased fluids, bulk in diet if constipation, urinary retention occur
• Give with food or milk for GI symptoms
• Give gum, hard candy, or frequent sips of water for dry mouth
• Store in airtight container at room temperature; do not refreeze
• Provide assistance with ambulation during beginning therapy since drowsiness/dizziness occurs

ADVERSE EFFECTS: The most serious adverse reactions are paralytic ileus, acute renal failure, hypertension, and hypertensive crisis, depending on the specific product. Common side effects are dizziness, drowsiness, diarrhea, dry mouth, urinary retention, and orthostatic hypotension.

PHARMACOKINETICS: Onset, peak, and duration vary widely among products. Most products are metabolized in the liver and excreted in urine.

INTERACTIONS: Interactions vary widely among products. Check individual monographs for specific information.

NURSING CONSIDERATIONS
Assessment
• Monitor B/P (lying, standing), pulse q4hr; if systolic B/P drops 20 mm Hg, hold product, notify prescriber; take VS q4hr in patients with CV disease
• Monitor blood tests: CBC, leukocytes, differential, cardiac enzymes if patient is receiving long-term therapy
• Monitor hepatic function tests: AST, ALT, bilirubin, creatinine
• Monitor weight weekly; appetite may increase with product

• Monitor for EPS primarily in geriatric: rigidity, dystonia, akathisia
• Assess mental status: mood, sensorium, affect, suicidal tendencies, increase in psychiatric symptoms (depression, panic)
• Check for urinary retention, constipation; constipation is more likely to occur in children, geriatric patients
• Assess for withdrawal symptoms: headache, nausea, vomiting, muscle pain, weakness; do not usually occur unless product was discontinued abruptly
• Identify alcohol consumption; if alcohol is consumed, hold dose until AM

Patient/family education
• Teach patient that therapeutic effects may take 2-3 wk
• Advise patient to use caution in driving or other activities requiring alertness because of drowsiness, dizziness, blurred vision
• Caution patient to avoid alcohol ingestion, other CNS depressants
• Instruct patient not to discontinue medication quickly after long-term use; may cause nausea, headache, malaise
• Instruct patient to wear sunscreen or large hat, since photosensitivity may occur

Evaluation

Positive therapeutic outcome
• Decreased depression

Generic Names

Tetracyclics:
mirtazapine

Tricyclics:
amitriptyline, clomiPRAMINE, desipramine, doxepin, imipramine, nortriptyline

Miscellaneous:
brexanolone, buPROPion, DULoxetine, esketamine, levomilnacipran, traZODone, venlafaxine, vortioxetine

SSRIs:
citalopram, escitalopram, FLUoxetine, PARoxetine, sertraline

Antidiabetics

ACTION: Antidiabetics are divided into the insulins that decrease blood glucose, phosphate, and potassium and increase blood pyruvate and lactate and oral antidiabetics that cause functioning β-cells in the pancreas to release insulin and improve the effect of endogenous and exogenous insulin.

USES: Insulins are used for ketoacidosis and diabetes mellitus types 1 and 2; oral antidiabetics are used for diabetes mellitus type 2.

CONTRAINDICATIONS
Hypersensitive reactions may occur, and allergies should be identified before these products are given. Oral antidiabetics should not be used in juvenile or brittle diabetes, diabetic ketoacidosis, or severe renal/hepatic disease.

Precautions: Oral antidiabetics should be used with caution in pregnancy, breastfeeding, geriatric, cardiac disease, and in the presence of alcohol.

IMPLEMENTATION
PO route
• Give oral antidiabetic 30 min before meals
SUBCUT route
• Give insulin after warming to room temperature by rotating in palms to prevent lipodystrophy from injecting cold insulin
• Give human insulin to those allergic to beef or pork
• Rotate inj sites when giving insulin; use abdomen, upper back, thighs, upper arm, buttocks; keep a record of sites

ADVERSE EFFECTS: The most common side effect of insulin and oral antidiabetics is hypoglycemia. Other adverse reactions for oral antidiabetics include blood dyscrasias, hepatotoxicity, and, rarely, cholestatic jaundice. Adverse reactions for insulin products include allergic responses and, more rarely, anaphylaxis.

PHARMACOKINETICS: Onset, peak, and duration vary widely among products. Oral antidiabetics are metabolized in the liver, with metabolites excreted in urine, bile, and feces.

INTERACTIONS: Interactions vary widely among products. Check individual monographs for specific information.

NURSING CONSIDERATIONS
Assessment
• Monitor blood, urine glucose levels during treatment to determine diabetes control (oral products)
• Monitor fasting blood glucose, 2 hr PP (60-100 mg/dl normal fasting level) (70-130 mg/dl—normal 2-hr level)
• Assess for hypoglycemic reaction that can occur during peak time

Patient/family education
• Advise patient to avoid alcohol and salicylates except on advice of prescriber

---

- Teach patient symptoms of ketoacidosis: nausea, thirst, polyuria, dry mouth, decreased B/P, dry, flushed skin, acetone breath, drowsiness, Kussmaul respirations
- Teach patient symptoms of hypoglycemia: headache, tremors, fatigue, weakness; that candy or sugar should be carried to treat hypoglycemia
- Advise patient to test urine for glucose/ketones tid if this product is replacing insulin
- Advise patient to continue weight control, dietary restrictions, exercise, hygiene

Evaluation

Positive therapeutic outcome
- Decrease in polyuria, polydipsia, polyphagia
- Clear sensorium
- Absence of dizziness
- Stable gait

Generic Names
albiglutide, canagliflozin, dapagliflozin, **dulaglutide** (high alert), empagliflozin, ertugliflozin, glipiZIDE, glyBURIDE, **insulin aspart** (high alert), **insulin detemir** (high alert), **insulin glargine** (high alert), **insulin glulisine** (high alert), **insulin lispro** (high alert), **insulin, regular** (high alert), **insulin, regular concentrated** (high alert), insulin, zinc suspension (Lente), insulin, zinc suspension extended (Ultralente), liraglutide, linagliptin, metFORMIN, miglitol, pioglitazone, repaglinide, rosiglitazone, saxagliptin, semaglutide, sitaGLIPtin

Antidiarrheals

ACTION: Antidiarrheals work by various actions including direct action on intestinal muscles to decrease GI peristalsis or by inhibiting prostaglandin synthesis responsible for GI hypermotility, acting on mucosal receptors responsible for peristalsis, or decreasing water content of stools.

USES: Antidiarrheals are used for diarrhea of undetermined causes.

CONTRAINDICATIONS
The contraindications are persons with severe ulcerative colitis, and pseudomembranous colitis with some products.

Precautions: Antidiarrheals should be used with caution in pregnancy, breastfeeding, children, geriatric patients, dehydration.

IMPLEMENTATION
PO route
- Give for 48 hr only

ADVERSE EFFECTS: The most serious adverse reactions of some products are paralytic ileus, toxic megacolon, and angioneurotic edema. The most common side effects are constipation, nausea, dry mouth, and abdominal pain.

PHARMACOKINETICS: Onset, peak, and duration vary widely among products. Most products are metabolized in the liver and excreted in urine.

INTERACTIONS: Interactions vary widely among products. Check individual monographs for specific information.

NURSING CONSIDERATIONS
Assessment
- Monitor electrolytes (potassium, sodium, chloride) if on long-term therapy
- Monitor bowel pattern before; for rebound constipation after termination of medication
- Assess response after 48 hr; if no response, product should be discontinued
- Identify dehydration in children

Patient/family education
- Advise patient to avoid OTC products
- Caution patient not to exceed recommended dose

Evaluation

Positive therapeutic outcome
- Decreased diarrhea

Generic Names
bismuth subsalicylate, kaolin/pectin, loperamide, telotristat

Antidysrhythmics

ACTION: Antidysrhythmics are divided into four classes and miscellaneous antidysrhythmics:
- Class I increases the duration of action potential and the effective refractory period and reduces disparity in the refractory period between a normal and infarcted myocardium; further subclasses include Ia, Ib, Ic
- Class II decreases the rate of SA node discharge, increases recovery time, slows conduction through the AV node, and decreases heart rate, which decreases O_2 consumption in the myocardium
- Class III increases the duration of action potential and the effective refractory period
- Class IV inhibits calcium ion influx across the cell membrane during cardiac depolarization; decreases SA node discharge, decreases conduction velocity through the AV node

• Miscellaneous antidysrhythmics include those such as adenosine, which slows conduction through the AV node, and digoxin, which decreases conduction velocity and prolongs the effective refractory period in the AV node

USES: Antidysrhythmics are used for PVCs, tachycardia, hypertension, atrial fibrillation, and angina pectoris.

CONTRAINDICATIONS
Contraindications vary widely among products.

Precautions: Precautions vary widely among products.

ADVERSE EFFECTS: Side effects and adverse reactions vary widely among products.

PHARMACOKINETICS: Onset, peak, and duration vary widely among products.

INTERACTIONS: Interactions vary widely among products. Check individual monographs for specific information.

NURSING CONSIDERATIONS
Assessment
• Monitor ECG continuously to determine product effectiveness, PVCs, or other dysrhythmias
• Assess for dehydration or hypovolemia
• Monitor B/P continuously for hypo/hypertension
• Monitor I&O ratio
• Monitor serum potassium
• Assess for edema in feet and legs daily

Patient/family education
• Advise patient to comply with dosage schedule, even if patient is feeling better
• Instruct patient to report bradycardia, dizziness, confusion, depression, fever

Evaluation

Positive therapeutic outcome
• Decrease in B/P in hypertension
• Decreased B/P, edema, moist crackles in HF

Generic Names
Class Ia:
disopyramide, procainamide, quiNIDine

Class Ib:
lidocaine, parenteral (high alert), phenytoin

Class Ic:
flecainide, propafenone

Class II:
acebutolol, esmolol, propranolol, sotalol

Class III:
amiodarone (high alert), **dronedarone** (high alert), **ibutilide** (high alert)

Class IV:
verapamil

Miscellaneous:
adenosine (high alert), **atropine** (high alert), **digoxin** (high alert)

Antiemetics

ACTION: The antiemetics are divided into the 5-HT$_3$ receptor antagonists, the phenothiazines, and the miscellaneous products. The 5-HT$_3$ receptor antagonists work by blocking serotonin peripherally, centrally, and in the small intestine. The phenothiazines act by blocking the chemoreceptor trigger zone in the brain. The miscellaneous products work by either decreasing motion sickness or delaying gastric emptying.

USES: Antiemetics are used to prevent nausea and vomiting due to cancer chemotherapy, radiotherapy, and surgery (5-HT$_3$ receptor antagonists); some of the miscellaneous products (antihistamines) work by decreasing motion sickness. Most other products are used for many types of nausea and vomiting.

CONTRAINDICATIONS
Persons developing hypersensitive reactions should not use these products.

Precautions: Antiemetics should be used cautiously in pregnancy, breastfeeding, hepatic disease, and some GI disorders.

IMPLEMENTATION
• Give prophylactically, before nausea and vomiting occur, in cancer chemotherapy
• Store at room temperature vial/ampules, oral products

ADVERSE EFFECTS: The most common side effects are headache, dizziness, fatigue, and diarrhea.

PHARMACOKINETICS: Onset, peak, and duration vary widely among products. Most products are metabolized by the liver and excreted by the kidneys.

INTERACTIONS: Interactions vary widely among products. Check individual monographs for specific information. Other CNS depressants increase CNS depression.

NURSING CONSIDERATIONS
Assessment
• Assess reason for nausea, vomiting; absence of nausea and vomiting after giving product
• Monitor hypersensitivity reactions: rash, bronchospasm with some products

Patient/family education

• Caution patient to avoid hazardous activities if dizziness occurs; ask for assistance if hospitalized
• Instruct patient to rise slowly to prevent orthostatic hypotension
• Teach patient all aspects of product usage
• Teach patient conservative methods to control nausea and vomiting such as sips of water or other fluids and dry crackers

Evaluation

Positive therapeutic outcome
• Absence or decreasing nausea and vomiting after use

Generic Names

5-HT₃ antagonists:
dolasetron, granisetron, ondansetron, palonosetron

Phenothiazines:
chlorproMAZINE, prochlorperazine, promethazine

Miscellaneous:
amisulpride, aprepitant, meclizine, metoclopramide, scopolamine, trimethobenzamide

Antifungals (systemic)

ACTION: Antifungals act by increasing cell membrane permeability in susceptible organisms by binding sterols and decreasing potassium, sodium, and nutrients in the cell.

USES: Antifungals are used for infections of histoplasmosis, blastomycosis, coccidioidomycosis, cryptococcosis, aspergillosis, phycomycosis, candidiasis, sporotrichosis causing severe meningitis, septicemia, and skin infections.

CONTRAINDICATIONS

Persons with severe bone marrow depression or hypersensitivity should not use these products.

Precautions: Antifungals should be used with caution in renal/hepatic disease and pregnancy.

IMPLEMENTATION

IV route
• Give by **IV** using in-line filter (mean pore diameter >1 μm) using distal veins; check for extravasation, necrosis q8hr
• Give product only after C&S confirms organism, make sure product is used in life-threatening infections
• Provide protection from light during infusion; cover with foil
• Give symptomatic treatment as ordered for adverse reactions: aspirin, antihistamines, antiemetics, antispasmodics
• Store protected from moisture and light; diluted sol is stable for 24 hr

ADVERSE EFFECTS: The most serious adverse reactions include renal tubular acidosis, permanent renal impairment, anuria, oliguria, hemorrhagic gastroenteritis, acute liver failure, and blood dyscrasias. Some common side effects include hypokalemia, nausea, vomiting, anorexia, headache, fever, and chills.

PHARMACOKINETICS: Onset, peak, and duration vary widely among products. Most products are metabolized in the liver and excreted in urine.

INTERACTIONS: Interactions vary widely among products. Check individual monographs for specific information.

NURSING CONSIDERATIONS
Assessment
• Monitor VS q15-30min during first infusion; note changes in pulse, B/P
• Monitor I&O ratio; watch for decreasing urinary output, change in specific gravity; discontinue product to prevent permanent damage to renal tubules
• Monitor blood tests; CBC, potassium, sodium, calcium, magnesium q2wk
• Monitor weight weekly; if weight increases over 2 lb/wk, edema is present; renal damage should be considered
• Assess for renal toxicity: increasing BUN, if >40 mg/dl or if serum creatinine >3 mg/dl; product may be discontinued or dosage reduced
• Assess for hepatotoxicity: increasing AST, ALT, alkaline phosphatase, bilirubin
• Assess for allergic reaction: dermatitis, rash; product should be discontinued; antihistamines (mild reaction) or EPINEPHrine (severe reaction) administered
• Assess for hypokalemia: anorexia, drowsiness, weakness, decreased reflexes, dizziness, increased urinary output, increased thirst, paresthesias
• Assess for ototoxicity: tinnitus (ringing, roaring in ears), vertigo, loss of hearing (rare)

Patient/family education
• Teach patient that long-term therapy may be needed to clear infection (2 wk-3 mo depending on type of infection)

Evaluation
Positive therapeutic outcome
• Decreased fever, malaise, rash
• Negative C&S for infecting organism

Generic Names
amphotericin B, anidulafungin, fluconazole, isavuconazonium, itraconazole, ketoconazole, micafungin, nystatin, posaconazole, voriconazole

Antihistamines

ACTION: Antihistamines compete with histamines for H_1 receptor sites. They antagonize in varying degrees most of the pharmacologic effects of histamines.

USES: Antihistamines are used to control the symptoms of allergies, rhinitis, and pruritus.

CONTRAINDICATIONS
Hypersensitivity to H_1-receptor antagonists occurs rarely. Patients with acute asthma and lower respiratory tract disease should not use these products since thick secretions may result. Other contraindications include closed-angle glaucoma, bladder neck obstruction, stenosing peptic ulcer, symptomatic prostatic hypertrophy, breastfeeding, and in the newborn.

Precautions: Antihistamines must be used cautiously in conjunction with intraocular pressure since they increase intraocular pressure. Caution should also be used in pregnancy, breastfeeding, and geriatric patients and patients with renal/cardiac disease, hypertension, and seizure disorders.

ADVERSE EFFECTS: Most products cause drowsiness; however, loratadine and fexofenadine produce little, if any, drowsiness. Other common side effects are headache and thickening of bronchial secretions. Serious blood dyscrasias may occur, but are rare. Urinary retention, GI effects occur with many of these products.

PHARMACOKINETICS: Onset varies from 20-60 min, with duration lasting 4-24 hr. In general, pharmacokinetics vary widely among products.

INTERACTIONS: Barbiturates, opioids, hypnotics, tricyclics, and alcohol can increase CNS depression when taken with antihistamines.

NURSING CONSIDERATIONS
Assessment
• Check I&O ratio; be alert for urinary retention, frequency, dysuria; product should be discontinued if these occur
• Assess for blood dyscrasias: thrombocytopenia, agranulocytosis (rare)
• Assess for respiratory status, including rate, rhythm, increase in bronchial secretions, wheezing, chest tightness
• Assess for cardiac status, including palpitations, increased pulse, hypotension
• Assess CBC during long-term therapy, since hemolytic anemia, although rare, may occur
• Administer with food or milk to decrease GI symptoms; absorption may be decreased slightly

• Administer whole (sus rel tab)
• Provide hard candy, gum, frequent rinsing of mouth for dryness

Patient/family education
• Advise patient to notify prescriber if confusion, sedation, hypotension occur
• Caution patient to avoid driving and other hazardous activity if drowsiness occurs
• Instruct patient to avoid concurrent use of alcohol and other CNS depressants
• Inform patient to discontinue a few days before skin testing

Evaluation

Positive therapeutic outcome
• Absence of allergy symptoms, itching

Generic Names
brompheniramine, budesonide, cetirizine, chlorpheniramine, cyproheptadine, desloratadine, diphenhydrAMINE, fexofenadine, levocetirizine, loratadine, promethazine

Antihypertensives

ACTION: Antihypertensives are divided into angiotensin converting enzyme (ACE) inhibitors, β-adrenergic blockers, calcium channel blockers, centrally acting adrenergics, diuretics, peripherally acting antiadrenergics, and vasodilators. β-blockers, calcium channel blockers, and diuretics are discussed in separate sections. ACE inhibitors selectively suppress conversion of renin-angiotensin I to angiotensin II; dilation of arterial and venous vessels occurs. Centrally acting adrenergics act by inhibiting the sympathetic vasomotor center in the CNS, which reduces impulses in the sympathetic nervous system; blood pressure, pulse rate, and cardiac output decrease. Peripherally acting antiadrenergics inhibit sympathetic vasoconstriction by inhibiting release of norepinephrine and/or depleting norepinephrine stores in adrenergic nerve endings. Vasodilators act on arteriolar smooth muscle by producing direct relaxation or vasodilatation; a reduction in blood pressure, with concomitant increases in heart rate and cardiac output, occurs.

USES: Antihypertensives are used for hypertension and for heart failure not responsive to conventional therapy. Some products are used in hypertensive crisis, angina, and for some cardiac dysrhythmias.

CONTRAINDICATIONS
Hypersensitive reactions may occur, and allergies should be identified before these products are

given. Antihypertensives should not be used in children or in patients with heart block.

Precautions: Antihypertensives should be used with caution in geriatric and dialysis patients, and in the presence of hypovolemia, leukemia, and electrolyte imbalances.

IMPLEMENTATION
• Place patient in supine or Trendelenburg position for severe hypotension

ADVERSE EFFECTS: The most common side effects are marked hypotension, bradycardia, tachycardia, headache, nausea, and vomiting. Side effects and adverse reactions may vary widely between classes and specific products.

PHARMACOKINETICS: Onset, peak, and duration vary widely among products. Most products are metabolized in the liver, with metabolites excreted in urine, bile, and feces.

INTERACTIONS: Interactions vary widely among products. Check individual monographs for specific information.

NURSING CONSIDERATIONS
Assessment
• Monitor blood tests: neutrophil; decreased platelets occur with many of the products
• Monitor renal function tests: protein, BUN, creatinine; watch for increased levels, which may indicate nephrotic syndrome; obtain baselines in renal/hepatic function tests before beginning treatment
• Assess for edema in feet and legs daily
• Identify allergic reaction, including rash, fever, pruritus, urticaria: product should be discontinued if antihistamines fail to help
• Identify symptoms of HF: edema, dyspnea, wet crackles, B/P
• Assess for renal symptoms: polyuria, oliguria, frequency

Patient/family education
• Instruct patient to comply with dosage schedule, even if feeling better
• Advise patient to rise slowly to sitting or standing position to minimize orthostatic hypotension

Evaluation
Positive therapeutic outcome
• Decrease in B/P in hypertension
• Decreased B/P, edema, moist crackles in HF

Generic Names

Angiotensin-converting enzyme inhibitors:
benazepril, enalapril, fosinopril, lisinopril, quinapril, ramipril, trandolapril

Angiotensin II receptor blockers:
azilsartan, candesartan, eprosartan, irbesartan, losartan, olmesartan, telmisartan, valsartan

Centrally acting adrenergics:
cloNIDine, guanFACINE, methyldopa

Peripherally acting antiadrenergics:
doxazosin, prazosin, reserpine

Vasodilators:
ambrisentan, fenoldopam, hydrALAZINE, macitentan, minoxidil, **nitroprusside** (high alert)

Antiadrenergic: Combined α/β-blocker:
labetalol

Direct renin inhibitors:
aliskiren

Antiinfectives

ACTION: Antiinfectives are divided into several groups, which include but are not limited to penicillins, cephalosporins, aminoglycosides, sulfonamides, tetracyclines, monobactam, erythromycins, and quinolones. These products inhibit the growth and replication of susceptible bacterial organisms.

USES: Antiinfectives are used for infections of susceptible organisms. These products are effective against bacterial, rickettsial, and spirochete infections.

CONTRAINDICATIONS
Hypersensitive reactions may occur, and allergies should be identified before these products are given. Cross-sensitivity can occur between products of different classes (penicillins or cephalosporins). Often persons allergic to penicillins are also allergic to cephalosporins.

Precautions: Antiinfectives should be used with caution in persons with renal/hepatic disease.

IMPLEMENTATION
• Give for 10-14 days to ensure organism death, prevention of superinfection
• Give after C&S completed; product may be taken as soon as culture is obtained

ADVERSE EFFECTS: The most common side effects are nausea, vomiting, and diarrhea. Adverse reactions include bone marrow depression and anaphylaxis.

PHARMACOKINETICS: Onset, peak, and duration vary widely among products. Most products are metabolized in the liver. Metabolites are excreted in urine, bile, and feces.

INTERACTIONS: Interactions vary widely among products. Check individual monographs for specific information.

NURSING CONSIDERATIONS
Assessment
• Assess for nephrotoxicity: increased BUN, creatinine
• Monitor blood tests: AST, ALT, CBC, Hct, bilirubin; test monthly if patient is on long-term therapy
• Monitor bowel pattern daily; if severe diarrhea occurs, product should be discontinued
• Monitor urine output; if decreasing, notify prescriber; may indicate nephrotoxicity
• Assess for allergic reaction: rash, fever, pruritus, urticaria; product should be discontinued
• Assess for bleeding: ecchymosis, bleeding gums, hematuria, stool guaiac daily
• Assess for overgrowth of infection: perineal itching, fever, malaise, redness, pain, swelling, drainage, rash, diarrhea, change in cough, sputum

Patient/family education
• Teach patient to comply with dosage schedule, even if feeling better
• Advise patient to report sore throat, bruising, bleeding, joint pain; may indicate blood dyscrasias (rare)

Evaluation
Positive therapeutic outcome
• Absence of fever, fatigue, malaise, draining wounds

Generic Names
Aminoglycosides:
amikacin, azithromycin, clarithromycin, gentamicin, neomycin, plazomicin, streptomycin, tobramycin

Cephalosporins:
cefaclor, cefadroxil, ceFAZolin, cefdinir, cefditoren, cefepime, cefixime, cefotaxime, cefprozil, ceftibuten, cefuroxime, cephalexin, cephradine

Fluoroquinolones:
ciprofloxacin, gemifloxacin, levofloxacin, norfloxacin, ofloxacin

Ketolides:
telithromycin

Miscellaneous:
adefovir, atoltivimab/maftivimab/odesivimab, dalbavancin, DAPTOmycin, delafloxacin, doripenem, ertapenem, fidaxomicin, lefamulin, meropenem, meropenem/vaborbactam, oritavancin, peginterferon alfa-2a, telavancin, vancomycin

Penicillins:
amoxicillin/clavulanate, ampicillin/sulbactam, imipenem/cilastatin, nafcillin, penicillin G

benzathine, penicillin G, penicillin G procaine, penicillin V, piperacillin/tazobactam, ticarcillin, ticarcillin/clavulanate

Sulfonamides:
sulfaSALAzine

Tetracyclines:
doxycycline, eravacycline, minocycline, tetracycline

Antilipidemics

ACTION: Antilipidemics are divided into three categories or subclassifications; HMG-CoA reductase inhibitors (statins), bile acid sequestrants, and miscellaneous products. The HMG-CoA reductase inhibitors work by reduction of an enzyme that is responsible for the beginning step in cholesterol production. Bile acid sequestrants work by binding cholesterol in the GI system. The miscellaneous products work by various actions.

USES: Primary hypercholesterolemia in individuals as an adjunct with other lifestyle changes.

CONTRAINDICATIONS
Persons breastfeeding (some products) or those with hypersensitivity to any product or severe hepatic disease should not take these products. Antilipidemics are identified as pregnancy on some products.

Precautions: Some products are identified as pregnancy.

IMPLEMENTATION
• Give as directed by health care provider; times will vary with medication used
• Provide protection from sunlight and heat

ADVERSE EFFECTS: The most common side effects are headache, dizziness, fatigue, insomnia, peripheral edema, dysrhythmias, sinusitis, pharyngitis, abdominal pain, diarrhea, constipation, flatulence, and back pain.

PHARMACOKINETICS: Pharmacokinetics and pharmacodynamics vary with each product.

INTERACTIONS: Interactions vary widely among products. Check individual monographs for specific information.

NURSING CONSIDERATIONS
Assessment
• Obtain a diet and lifestyle history, including exercise, smoking, alcohol, and stress-related activities

Patient/family education
• Teach patient all aspects of medication use

- Instruct patient to combine medication with lifestyle changes, including low-cholesterol diet, decreasing LDL in diet; avoid smoking, alcohol, and sedentary daily routine

Evaluation

Positive therapeutic outcome
- Decrease in triglycerides and LDL cholesterol levels

Generic Names

HMG-CoA reductase inhibitors:
atorvastatin, fluvastatin, lovastatin, pitavastatin, pravastatin, simvastatin

Bile acid sequestrants:
cholestyramine, colesevelam

Miscellaneous:
alirocumab, avapritinib, bempedoic acid/ezetimibe, capmatinib, daratumumab/hyaluronidase-fihj evolocumab, ezetimibe, fenofibrate, fenofibric acid, gemfibrozil, mipomersen, niacin, niacinamide

Antineoplastics

ACTION: Antineoplastics are divided into alkylating agents, antimetabolites, antibiotic agents, hormonal agents, and miscellaneous agents. Alkylating agents act by cross-linking strands of DNA. Antimetabolites act by inhibiting DNA synthesis. Antibiotic agents act by inhibiting RNA synthesis and by delaying or inhibiting mitosis. Hormones alter the effect of androgens, luteinizing hormone, follicle-stimulating hormone, or estrogen by changing the hormonal environment.

USES: Antineoplastics vary widely among products and classes of products. They are used to treat leukemia, Hodgkin's disease, lymphomas, and other tumors throughout the body.

CONTRAINDICATIONS
Hypersensitive reactions may occur, and allergies should be identified before these products are given. Also, persons with severe renal/hepatic disease should not use these products unless the benefits outweigh the risks.

Precautions: Persons with bleeding, severe bone marrow depression, or renal/hepatic disease should be watched closely.

IMPLEMENTATION
- Check IV site for irritation; phlebitis
- Have EPINEPHrine available for hypersensitivity reaction
- Give antibiotics for prophylaxis of infection

- Provide strict medical asepsis, protective isolation if WBC levels are low
- Provide comprehensive oral hygiene, using careful technique and soft-bristle brush

ADVERSE EFFECTS: Most products cause thrombocytopenia, leukopenia, and anemia. If these reactions occur, the product may need to be stopped until the problem is corrected. Other side effects include nausea, vomiting, glossitis, and hair loss. Some products also cause hepatotoxicity, nephrotoxicity, and cardiotoxicity.

PHARMACOKINETICS: Onset, peak, and duration vary widely among products. Most products cross the placenta and are excreted in breast milk and in urine.

INTERACTIONS: Toxicity may occur when used with other antineoplastics or radiation.

NURSING CONSIDERATIONS
Assessment
- Monitor CBC, differential, platelet count weekly; withhold product if WBC is <4000 or platelet count is <75,000; notify prescriber of results
- Monitor renal function tests: BUN, creatinine, serum uric acid, and urine creatinine clearance before, during therapy
- Monitor I&O ratio; report fall in urine output of 30 ml/hr
- Monitor temp q4hr (may indicate beginning infection)
- Monitor hepatic function tests before, during therapy (bilirubin, AST, ALT, LDH) monthly or as needed
- Assess for bleeding, including hematuria, guaiac, bruising or petechiae, mucosa, or orifices q8hr; obtain prescription for viscous lidocaine (Xylocaine)
- Identify jaundice of skin, sclera, dark urine, clay-colored stools, itchy skin, abdominal pain, fever, diarrhea
- Assess for edema in feet, joint pain, stomach pain, shaking
- Assess for inflammation of mucosa, breaks in skin

Patient/family education
- Advise patient to report signs of infection, including increased temp, sore throat, malaise
- Instruct patient to report signs of anemia, including fatigue, headache, faintness, shortness of breath, irritability
- Instruct patient to report bleeding and to avoid use of razors and commercial mouthwash

Evaluation

Positive therapeutic outcome
- Decreased tumor size

Generic Names

Alkylating agents:
bendamustine, **busulfan** (high alert), **CARBO-platin** (high alert), **carmustine** (high alert), chlorambucil, **CISplatin** (high alert), **cyclophosphamide** (high alert), **dacarbazine** (high alert), lurbinectedin **melphalan** (high alert), oxaliplatin

Antimetabolites:
capecitabine, **cytarabine** (high alert), decitabine, decitabine/cedazuridine, **etoposide** (high alert), **fluorouracil** (high alert), mercaptopurine, **methotrexate** (high alert), PEMEtrexed

Antibiotic agents:
bleomycin (high alert), **DACTINomycin** (high alert), **DAUNOrubicin** (high alert), **DOXO-rubicin** (high alert), **mitoMYcin** (high alert), **mitoXANtrone** (high alert)

Hormonal agents:
apalutamide, darolutamide, flutamide, fulvestrant, goserelin, **irinotecan** (high alert), **leuprolide** (high alert), megestrol, tamoxifen, **topotecan** (high alert)

Miscellaneous agents:
abemaciclib, acalabrutinib, ado-trastuzumab, afatinib, alemtuzumab, alpelisib, anastrozole, avapritinib, axicabtegene, azaCITIDine, belantamab mafodotin-blmf, belinostat, bortezomib, brentuximab, cabazitaxel, capmatinib, cemiplimab, **ceritinib** (high alert), cetuximab, crizotinib, dabrafenib, daratumumab/hyaluronidase-fihj, dasatinib, decitabine/cedazuridine, durvalumab, enasidenib, entrectinib, erdafitinib, eribulin, erlotinib, fam-trastuzumab, gemcitabine, ibritumomab, ibrutinib, idelalisib, imatinib, interferon alfa-2a, interferon alfa-2b, ipilimumab, irinotecan, ixabepilone, lapatinib, midostaurin, nilotinib, niraparib, olaparib, palbociclib, panitumumab, pembrolizumab, pemigatinib, pertuzumab trastuzumab hyaluronidase, pexidertinib, pomalidomide, pralsetinib, procarbazine, ramucirumab, ranibizumab, ripretinib, riTUXimab, sacituzumab govitecan, selinexor, selumetinib, sipuleucel-T, sonidegib, tazemetostat, tisagenlecleucel, trametinib, tucatinib, vemurafenib, **vinBLAStine** (high alert), **vinCRIStine** (high alert), **vinorelbine** (high alert)

PARP inhibitor:
rucaparib

Antiparkinsonian Agents

ACTION: Antiparkinsonian agents are divided into cholinergics, dopamine agonists, and monoamine oxidase type B inhibitors. Cholinergics work by blocking or competing at central acetylcholine receptors. Dopamine agonists work by decarboxylation to dopamine or by activation of dopamine receptors. Monoamine oxidase type B inhibitors increase dopamine activity by inhibiting MAO type B activity.

USES: Antiparkinson agents are used alone or in combination for patients with Parkinson's disease.

CONTRAINDICATIONS

Persons with hypersensitivity, closed-angle glaucoma, and undiagnosed skin lesions should not use these products.

Precautions: Antiparkinsonian agents should be used with caution in pregnancy, breastfeeding, children, renal/cardiac/hepatic disease, and affective disorder.

IMPLEMENTATION

- Give product up until NPO before surgery
- Adjust dosage depending on patient response
- Give with meals; limit protein taken with product
- Give only after MAOIs have been discontinued for 2 wk
- Assist with ambulation during beginning therapy if needed
- Test for diabetes mellitus and acromegaly if on long-term therapy

ADVERSE EFFECTS: Side effects and adverse reactions vary widely among products. The most common side effects include involuntary movements, headache, numbness, insomnia, nightmares, nausea, vomiting, dry mouth, and orthostatic hypotension.

PHARMACOKINETICS: Onset, peak, and duration vary widely among products. Most products are metabolized in the liver and excreted in urine.

INTERACTIONS: Interactions vary widely among products. Check individual monographs for specific information.

NURSING CONSIDERATIONS
Assessment
- Monitor B/P, respiration
- Assess mental status: affect, behavioral changes, depression, complete suicide assessment

Patient/family education
- Advise patient to change positions slowly to prevent orthostatic hypotension
- Instruct patient to report side effects: twitching, eye spasm; indicate overdose
- Advise patient to use product exactly as prescribed; if product is discontinued abruptly, parkinsonian crisis may occur

Evaluation

Positive therapeutic outcome
- Decrease in akathisia
- Improvement in mood

Generic Names
amantadine, benztropine, bromocriptine, carbidopa-levodopa, istradefylline, opicapone, pramipexole, rasagiline, selegiline, tolcapone

Antiplatelets

ACTION: The antiplatelets are divided into the platelet aggregation inhibitors, platelet adhesion inhibitors, and the glycoprotein IIb, IIIa inhibitors. The platelet aggregation inhibitors work by action on thrombin; the platelet adhesion inhibitors work by inhibition of phosphodiesterase; and the glycoprotein IIb, IIIa inhibitors work by preventing fibrin from binding to glycoprotein IIb, IIIa receptors.

USES: Antiplatelets are used to prevent myocardial infarction and stroke; other products are used for coronary syndromes.

CONTRAINDICATIONS
Persons developing hypersensitive reactions should not use these products.

Precautions: Antiplatelets should be used cautiously in pregnancy, breastfeeding, and bleeding disorders.

IMPLEMENTATION
- Give with heparin or other aspirin (some products)
- Store at room temperature vial/ampules, oral products

ADVERSE EFFECTS: The most common side effects are headache, dizziness, bleeding, and diarrhea.

PHARMACOKINETICS: Onset, peak, and duration vary widely among products. Most products are metabolized by the liver and excreted by the kidneys.

INTERACTIONS: Interactions vary widely among products. Check individual monographs for specific information.

NURSING CONSIDERATIONS
Assessment
- Assess reason for use of these products
- Monitor hypersensitivity reactions with some products
- Monitor bleeding from orifices, stool urine
- Monitor blood tests: platelets, Hgb, Hct, PT/APTT, and INR

Patient/family education
- Caution patient to avoid hazardous activities if drowsiness, dizziness occurs; ask for assistance if hospitalized
- Teach patient all aspects of product usage

Evaluation

Positive therapeutic outcome
- Absence of MI, stroke, or other coronary syndromes

Generic Names
Platelet aggregation inhibitors:
cilostazol, clopidogrel, ticagrelor, ticlopidine

Platelet adhesion inhibitors:
dipyridamole

Glycoprotein IIb, IIIa inhibitors:
eptifibatide (high alert), **tirofiban** (high alert)

Antipsychotics

ACTION: Antipsychotics/neuroleptics are divided into several subgroups: phenothiazines, thioxanthenes, butyrophenones, dibenzoxazepines, dibenzodiazepines, and indolones and other heterocyclic compounds. Although chemically different, these subgroups share many pharmacologic and clinical properties. All antipsychotics work to block postsynaptic DOPamine receptors in the brain that are responsible for psychotic behavior, including hallucinations, delusions, and paranoia.

USES: Antipsychotic behavior is decreased in conditions such as schizophrenia, paranoia, and mania. These agents are also effective for severe anxiety, intractable hiccups, nausea, vomiting, behavioral problems in children, and for relaxation before surgery.

CONTRAINDICATIONS
Persons with liver damage, severe hypertension or coronary disease, cerebral arteriosclerosis, blood dyscrasias, bone marrow depression, parkinsonism, severe depression, or closed-angle glaucoma; children <12 yr; persons withdrawing from alcohol or barbiturates should not use antipsychotics until these conditions are corrected.

Precautions: Caution must be used when antipsychotics are given to geriatric patients, since metabolism is slowed and adverse reactions can occur rapidly. Renal/hepatic disease may cause poor metabolism and excretion of the product. Seizure threshold is decreased with these products; increases in the dose of anticonvulsants may be required. Persons with diabetes mellitus, prostatic hypertrophy, chronic respiratory disease, and peptic ulcer disease should be monitored closely.

IMPLEMENTATION

• Give antiparkinsonian agent if extrapyramidal symptoms occur
• Administer liquid conc mixed in glass of juice or cola since taste is unpleasant; avoid contact with skin when preparing liquid conc or parenteral medications
• Supervise ambulation until stabilized on medication; do not involve in strenuous exercise program, since fainting is possible; patient should not stand still for long periods
• Increase fluids to prevent constipation
• Give sips of water, candy, gum for dry mouth
• Patient should remain lying down for at least 30 min after IM inj

ADVERSE EFFECTS: The most common side effects include extrapyramidal symptoms such as pseudoparkinsonism, akathisia, dystonia, and tardive dyskinesia, which may be controlled by use of antiparkinsonian agents. Serious adverse reactions such as hypotension, agranulocytosis, cardiac arrest, and laryngospasm have occurred. Other common side effects include dry mouth and photosensitivity.

PHARMACOKINETICS: Onset, peak, and duration vary widely with different products and routes. Products are metabolized by the liver, are excreted in urine as metabolites, are highly bound to plasma proteins, cross the placenta, and enter breast milk. Half-life can be extended over 3 days.

INTERACTIONS: Because other CNS depressants can cause oversedation, these combinations should be used carefully. Anticholinergics may decrease the therapeutic actions of phenothiazines and also cause increased anticholinergic effects.

NURSING CONSIDERATIONS
Assessment

• Monitor bilirubin, CBC, hepatic function tests monthly, since these products are metabolized in the liver and excreted in urine
• Monitor I&O ratio: palpate bladder if low urinary output occurs, since urinary retention occurs with many of these products
• Assess affect, orientation, LOC, reflexes, gait, coordination, sleep pattern disturbances
• Assess dizziness, faintness, palpitations, tachycardia on rising
• Check B/P with patient lying and standing; wide fluctuations between lying and standing B/P

may require dosage or product change, since orthostatic hypotension is occurring
• Assess for EPS, including akathisia, tardive dyskinesia, pseudoparkinsonism

Patient/family education

• Advise patient to rise from sitting or lying position gradually, since fainting may occur
• Caution patient to avoid hot tubs, hot showers, or tub baths, since hypotension may occur
• Advise patient to wear sunscreen or protective clothing to prevent burns
• Advise patient to take extra precautions during hot weather to stay cool; heat stroke can occur
• Caution patient to avoid driving and other activities requiring alertness until response to medication is known
• Inform patient that drowsiness or impaired mental/motor activity is evident the first 2 wk, but tends to decrease over time

Evaluation

Positive therapeutic outcome

• Decrease in excitement, hallucinations, delusions, paranoia
• Reorganization of thought patterns, speech

Generic Names
Phenothiazines:
chlorproMAZINE, fluPHENAZine

Butyrophenone:
haloperidol

Miscellaneous:
amisulpride, ARIPiprazole, asenapine, iloperidone, loxapine, OLANZapine, paliperidone, QUEtiapine, risperiDONE, ziprasidone

Antipyretics

ACTION: The antipyretics act on the CNS to control fever and also inhibit prostaglandin production.

USES: Antipyretics are used to decrease fever.

CONTRAINDICATIONS
Persons developing hypersensitive reactions should not use these products.

Precautions: Antipyretics should be used cautiously in pregnancy, breastfeeding, geriatric patients, hepatic disease, and those with certain GI disorders.

IMPLEMENTATION
• Give around the clock to keep fever reduced
• Store at room temperature

ADVERSE EFFECTS: The most common side effects are nausea, vomiting, and rash.

PHARMACOKINETICS: Onset, peak, and duration vary widely among products. Most products are metabolized by the liver and excreted by the kidneys.

INTERACTIONS: Interactions vary widely among products. Check individual monographs for specific information.

NURSING CONSIDERATIONS
Assessment
• Monitor temp frequently
• Assess reason for use and expected outcome
• Monitor hypersensitivity reactions: rash, bronchospasm with some products

Patient/family education
• Teach patient all aspects of product usage

Evaluation

Positive therapeutic outcome
• Absence or decreasing fever after use

Generic Names
acetaminophen, aspirin, choline/magnesium salicylates, ibuprofen, ketoprofen, magnesium salicylate, naproxen, salsalate

Antiretrovirals

ACTION: Antiretrovirals act by blocking DNA synthesis.

USES: Antiretrovirals are used in HIV infections, chronic hepatitis C to slow the progression of the disease.

CONTRAINDICATIONS
Persons with hypersensitivity should not use these products.

Precautions: Antiretrovirals should be used cautiously in pregnancy, breastfeeding, and renal/hepatic disease. Protease inhibitors should be used cautiously in diabetes.

IMPLEMENTATION
• Give in equal intervals around the clock
• Store at room temperature

ADVERSE EFFECTS: The most common side effects are nausea, vomiting, anorexia, headache, and diarrhea. The most serious adverse reactions are nephrotoxicity and blood dyscrasias.

PHARMACOKINETICS: Onset, peak, and duration vary widely among products. Most products are metabolized by the liver and excreted by the kidneys.

INTERACTIONS: Interactions vary widely among products. Check individual monographs for specific information.

NURSING CONSIDERATIONS
Assessment
• Monitor for signs of HIV infection: increased CD4 counts, decreased viral load; signs of chronic hepatitis C
• Monitor patients with compromised renal system; since product is excreted slowly in poor renal system function, toxicity may occur rapidly

Patient/family education
• Instruct patient to report sore throat, fever, fatigue; may indicate superinfection
• Caution patient that product does not cure condition or prevent infecting others, but controls symptoms
• Instruct patient that product must be taken around the clock, in equal intervals to maintain blood levels for duration of therapy
• Instruct patient to notify prescriber of side effects such as bruising, bleeding, fatigue, malaise; may indicate blood dyscrasias

Evaluation

Positive therapeutic outcome
• Decreased viral load
• Increased CD4 count
• Improvement in the symptoms of HIV/AIDS

Generic Names
Nonnucleoside reverse transcriptase inhibitors:
delavirdine, efavirenz, etravirine, nevirapine, rilpivirine

Nucleoside reverse transcriptase inhibitors:
abacavir, didanosine, emtricitabine, lamiVUDine, stavudine d4t, tenofovir, zidovudine

Protease inhibitors:
atazanavir, **atazanavir/cobistat** (high alert), boceprevir, fosamprenavir, indinavir, nelfinavir, ritonavir, saquinavir, telaprevir, tipranavir

Fusion inhibitors:
enfuvirtide

Miscellaneous:
daclatasvir, dolutegravir, dolutegravir/lamivudine, dolutegravir/rilpivirine, fostemsavir, raltegravir

Antituberculars

ACTION: Antituberculars act by inhibiting RNA or DNA, or interfering with lipid and protein synthesis, thereby decreasing tubercle bacilli replication.

USES: Antituberculars are used for pulmonary tuberculosis.

CONTRAINDICATIONS
Persons with severe renal disease or hypersensitivity should not use these products.

Precautions: Antituberculars should be used with caution in pregnancy, breastfeeding, and hepatic disease.

IMPLEMENTATION
• Give some of these agents on empty stomach, 1 hr before meals (only for isoniazid and rifampin) or 2 hr after meals
• Give antiemetic if vomiting occurs
• Give after C&S is completed; monthly to detect resistance

ADVERSE EFFECTS: Adverse effects vary widely among products. Most products can cause nausea, vomiting, anorexia, and rash. Serious adverse reactions include renal failure, nephrotoxicity, ototoxicity, and hepatic necrosis.

PHARMACOKINETICS: Onset, peak, and duration vary widely among products. Most products are metabolized in the liver and excreted in urine.

INTERACTIONS: Interactions vary widely among products. Check individual monographs for specific information.

NURSING CONSIDERATIONS
Assessment
• Assess for signs of anemia: Hct, Hgb, fatigue
• Monitor hepatic function tests weekly: ALT, AST, bilirubin
• Monitor renal status before treatment and monthly thereafter: BUN, creatinine, output, specific gravity, urinalysis
• Monitor hepatic status: decreased appetite, jaundice, dark urine, fatigue

Patient/family education
• Teach patient that compliance with dosage schedule, duration is necessary
• Teach patient that scheduled appointments must be kept; relapse may occur
• Advise patient to avoid alcohol while taking product
• Advise patient to report flulike symptoms: excessive fatigue, anorexia, vomiting, sore throat; unusual bleeding, yellowish discoloration of skin/eyes

Evaluation

Positive therapeutic outcome
• Decreased symptoms of TB
• Negative culture

Generic Names
ethambutol, isoniazid, pyrazinamide, rifabutin, rifampin, streptomycin

Antitussives/Expectorants

ACTION: Antitussives suppress the cough reflex by direct action on the cough center in the medulla. Expectorants act by liquefying and reducing the viscosity of thick, tenacious secretions.

USES: Antitussives/expectorants are used to treat cough occurring in pneumonia, bronchitis, TB, cystic fibrosis, and emphysema; as an adjunct in atelectasis (expectorants); and for nonproductive cough (antitussives).

CONTRAINDICATIONS
Some products are contraindicated in pregnancy, breastfeeding, and hypothyroidism

Precautions: Some products should be used cautiously with asthma and in geriatric and debilitated patients.

IMPLEMENTATION
• Give decreased dosage to geriatric patients; their metabolism may be slowed
• Increase fluids to liquefy secretions
• Humidify patient's room

ADVERSE EFFECTS: The most common side effects are drowsiness, dizziness, and nausea.

PHARMACOKINETICS: Onset, peak, and duration vary widely among products. Some products are metabolized in the liver and excreted in urine.

INTERACTIONS: Interactions vary widely among products. Check individual monographs for specific information.

NURSING CONSIDERATIONS
Assessment
• Assess cough: type, frequency, character including sputum

Patient/family education
• Advise patient to avoid driving and other hazardous activities until stabilized on this medication
• Caution patient to avoid smoking, smoke-filled rooms, perfumes, dust, environmental pollutants, cleaners that increase cough

Evaluation

Positive therapeutic outcome
• Absence of cough

Generic Names

acetylcysteine, codeine, dextromethorphan, diphenhydrAMINE, guaiFENesin, HYDROcodone

Antivirals

ACTION: Antivirals act by interfering with DNA synthesis that is needed for viral replication.

USES: Antivirals are used for mucocutaneous herpes simplex virus, herpes genitalis (HSV-1, HSV-2), varicella infections, herpes zoster, and herpes simplex encephalitis.

CONTRAINDICATIONS

Persons with hypersensitivity or immunosuppressed individuals should not use these products.

Precautions: Antivirals should be used cautiously in pregnancy, breastfeeding, and renal/hepatic disease.

IMPLEMENTATION

• Give increased fluids to 3 L/day to decrease crystalluria when given **IV**
• Store at room temperature for up to 12 hr after reconstitution

ADVERSE EFFECTS: The most common side effects are nausea, vomiting, anorexia, headache, and diarrhea. The most serious adverse reactions are nephrotoxicity and blood dyscrasias.

PHARMACOKINETICS: Onset, peak, and duration vary widely among products. Most products are metabolized by the liver and excreted by the kidneys.

INTERACTIONS: Interactions vary widely among products. Check individual monographs for specific information.

NURSING CONSIDERATIONS
Assessment

• Monitor for signs of infection, anemia
• Monitor patients with a compromised renal system; since product is excreted slowly in poor renal system function, toxicity may occur rapidly
• Monitor renal function tests: urinalysis, BUN, serum creatinine or decreased CCr may indicate nephrotoxicity; I&O ratio; report hematuria, oliguria, fatigue, weakness; check for protein in the urine during treatment
• Assess C&S before treatment; agent may be given as soon as culture is taken; repeat C&S after treatment
• Monitor bowel pattern before, during treatment; if severe abdominal pain with bleeding occurs, agent should be discontinued
• Monitor skin reactions: rash, urticaria, itching

• Monitor hepatic function tests: AST, ALT
• Monitor blood tests: WBC, RBC, Hct, Hgb, bleeding time; blood dyscrasias

Patient/family education

• Instruct patient to report sore throat, fever, fatigue; may indicate superinfection
• Caution patient that product does not prevent infecting others or cure condition but controls symptoms
• Instruct patient that product must be taken around the clock in equal intervals to maintain blood levels for duration of therapy
• Instruct patient to notify prescriber of side effects such as bruising, bleeding, fatigue, malaise; may indicate blood dyscrasias

Evaluation

Positive therapeutic outcome

• Absence or control of infection

Generic Names

acyclovir, atoltivimab/maftivimab/odesivimab-ebgn, amantadine, baloxavir, cidofovir, daclatasvir, docosanol, entecavir, famciclovir, foscarnet, ganciclovir, glecaprevir/pibrentasvir, lamiVUDine, maraviroc, oseltamivir, penciclovir, rapivab, remdesivir, ribavirin, simeprevir, sofosbuvir, valACYclovir, valGANciclovir, zanamivir

β-adrenergic Blockers

ACTION: β-blockers are divided into selective and nonselective blockers. Selective β-blockers competitively block stimulation of β_1-receptors in cardiac smooth muscle; these products produce chronotropic and inotropic effects. Nonselective blockers produce a fall in blood pressure without reflex tachycardia or reduction in heart rate through a mixture of β-blocking effects; elevated plasma renins are reduced.

USES: β-blockers are used for hypertension, ventricular dysrhythmias, and prophylaxis of angina pectoris.

CONTRAINDICATIONS

Hypersensitive reactions may occur, and allergies should be identified before these products are given. β-adrenergic blockers should not be used in heart block, HF, or cardiogenic shock.

Precautions: β-blockers should be used with caution in pregnant and geriatric patients or in renal/thyroid disease, COPD, CAD, diabetes mellitus, and asthma.

IMPLEMENTATION

• Give PO before meals and at bedtime; tab may be crushed or swallowed whole
• Give reduced dosage in renal dysfunction

ADVERSE EFFECTS: The most common side effects are orthostatic hypotension, bradycardia, diarrhea, nausea, and vomiting. Serious adverse reactions include blood dyscrasias, bronchospasm, and HF.

PHARMACOKINETICS: Onset, peak, and duration vary widely among products. Most products are metabolized in the liver, with metabolites excreted in urine, bile, and feces.

INTERACTIONS: Interactions vary widely among products. Check individual monographs for specific information.

NURSING CONSIDERATIONS
Assessment
• Monitor renal function tests: protein, BUN, creatinine; watch for increased levels that may indicate nephrotic syndrome; obtain baselines in renal/hepatic function tests before beginning treatment
• Monitor I&O ratio, weight daily
• Monitor B/P during beginning of treatment and periodically thereafter, pulse q4hr; note rate, rhythm, quality
• Monitor apical/radial pulse before administration; notify prescriber of significant changes
• Check for edema in feet and legs daily

Patient/family education
• Instruct patient to comply with dosage schedule, even if feeling better
• Caution patient to rise slowly to sitting or standing position to minimize orthostatic hypotension
• Advise patient to report bradycardia, dizziness, confusion, depression, fever
• Teach patient to take pulse at home; advise when to notify prescriber
• Instruct patient to comply with weight control, dietary adjustment, modified exercise program
• Advise patient to wear support hose to minimize effects of orthostatic hypotension
• Advise patient not to discontinue product abruptly; taper over 2 wk; may precipitate angina

Evaluation

Positive therapeutic outcome
• Decrease in B/P in hypertension
• Decreased B/P, edema, moist crackles in HF

Generic Names
Selective β₁-receptor blockers:
acebutolol, atenolol, esmolol, metoprolol, nebibolol

β₂-receptor blocker:
indacaterol

Nonselective β₁ and β₂-blockers:
carteolol, nadolol, propranolol, timolol

Combined α₁, β₁, and β₂-receptor blocker:
labetalol

Bone Resorption Inhibitors

ACTION: Bone resorption inhibitors are divided into the bisphosphonates and the selective estrogen receptor modulators. The bisphosphonates act by absorbing calcium phosphate crystals in bone and may directly block dissolution of hydroxyapatite crystals of bone, inhibiting normal and abnormal bone resorption and mineralization. Selective estrogen receptor modulators act by reducing resorption of bone and decreasing bone turnover, mediated through estrogen receptor binding.

USES: Bone resorption inhibitors are used for prevention and treatment of osteoporosis in postmenopausal women, treatment of Paget's disease, and treatment of osteoporosis in men.

CONTRAINDICATIONS
Persons developing hypersensitive reactions or those with hypocalcemia should not use these products.

Precautions: Bone resorption inhibitors should be used cautiously in pregnancy, breastfeeding, the geriatric patient, renal/hepatic disease, and some GI disorders.

IMPLEMENTATION
• Give for 6 months or more in Paget's disease
• Store at room temperature

ADVERSE EFFECTS: The most common side effects are nausea, vomiting, headache, bone pain, and rash.

PHARMACOKINETICS: Onset, peak, and duration vary widely among products. Most products are taken up by the bones and excreted by the kidneys.

INTERACTIONS: Interactions vary widely among products. Check individual monographs for specific information.

NURSING CONSIDERATIONS
Assessment
• Assess reason for use and expected outcome
• Monitor bone density test; hormonal status (women) before starting treatment and thereafter
• Monitor hypercalcemia: paresthesia, twitching, laryngospasm; Chvostek's, Trousseau's signs

Patient/family education
- Instruct patient to remain upright for at least 30 min after taking to prevent esophageal irritation
- Teach patient all aspects of product usage
- Instruct patient to use weight-bearing exercise to increase bone density

Evaluation

Positive therapeutic outcome
- Increase in bone mass
- Absence of fractures

Generic Names
Bisphosphonates:
alendronate, etidronate, ibandronate, pamidronate, risedronate

Selective estrogen receptor modulator:
raloxifene

Monoclonal antibody:
denosumab

Calcium Channel Blockers

ACTION: Calcium channel blockers inhibit calcium ion influx across the cell membrane in cardiac and vascular smooth muscle. This action produces relaxation of coronary vascular smooth muscle, dilates coronary arteries, slows SA/AV node conduction, and dilates peripheral arteries.

USES: Calcium channel blockers are used for chronic stable angina pectoris, vasospastic angina, dysrhythmias, hypertension, and unstable angina.

CONTRAINDICATIONS
Persons with 2nd- or 3rd-degree heart block, sick sinus syndrome, hypotension of <90 mm Hg systolic, Wolff-Parkinson-White syndrome, or cardiogenic shock should not use these products, since worsening of those conditions may occur.

Precautions: HF may worsen since edema may be increased. Hypotension may worsen, since B/P is decreased. Patients with renal/hepatic disease should use these products cautiously since they are metabolized in the liver and excreted by the kidneys.

IMPLEMENTATION
- Give PO before meals and at bedtime

ADVERSE EFFECTS: The most common side effects are dysrhythmias and edema. Also common are headache, fatigue, drowsiness, and flushing.

PHARMACOKINETICS: Onset, peak, and duration vary widely with route of administration. Products are metabolized by the liver and excreted in the urine primarily as metabolites.

INTERACTIONS: Increased levels of digoxin and theophylline may occur when used with these products. Increased effects of β-blockers and antihypertensives may occur with calcium channel blockers.

NURSING CONSIDERATIONS
Assessment
- Monitor cardiac system: B/P, pulse, respirations, ECG intervals (PR, QRS, QT)

Patient/family education
- Teach patient how to take pulse before taking product; patient should record or graph pulses to identify changes
- Advise patient to avoid hazardous activities until stabilized on this product since dizziness occurs frequently
- Inform patient of the need for compliance to all areas of medical regimen, including diet, exercise, stress reduction, and product therapy

Evaluation

Positive therapeutic outcome
- Decreased anginal pain
- Decreased B/P, dysrhythmias

Generic Names
amLODIPine, clevidipine, **diltiazem** (high alert), felodipine, isradipine, niCARdipine, NIFEdipine, verapamil

Cardiac Glycosides

ACTION: Cardiac glycosides act by inhibiting sodium and potassium ATPase and then making more calcium available to activate contracted proteins. Cardiac contractility and cardiac output are increased.

USES: Cardiac glycosides are used for HF, atrial fibrillation, atrial flutter, atrial tachycardia, and rapid digitalization in these disorders.

CONTRAINDICATIONS
Hypersensitive reactions may occur, and allergies should be identified before these products are given. Also, persons with ventricular tachycardia, ventricular fibrillation, and carotid sinus syndrome should not use these products.

Precautions: Persons with acute MI and those who have or may develop serum potassium, calcium, or magnesium imbalances should use these products cautiously. Also, geriatric patients and those with AV block, severe respiratory disease, hypothyroidism, or renal/hepatic disease should exercise caution when these products are prescribed.

IMPLEMENTATION
• Give potassium supplements if ordered for potassium levels <3

ADVERSE EFFECTS:
The most common side effects are cardiac disturbances, headache, hypotension, and GI symptoms. Also common are blurred vision and yellow-green halos.

PHARMACOKINETICS:
Onset, peak, and duration vary widely with the route of administration. Digitoxin is inactivated by the liver, and inactive metabolites are excreted in urine. Digoxin is excreted in urine mainly as the parent product and metabolites.

INTERACTIONS:
Toxicity may occur when used with diuretics, succinylcholine, quiNIDine, and thioamines. Increased blood levels may occur with propantheline bromide, spironolactone, quiNIDine, verapamil, aminoglycosides (PO), amiodarone, anticholinergics, and quiNINE. Diuretics may increase toxicity.

NURSING CONSIDERATIONS
Assessment
• Monitor cardiac system: B/P, pulse, respirations, and increased urine output
• Monitor apical pulse for 1 min before giving product; if pulse <60, take again in 1 hr; if <60 notify prescriber
• Monitor electrolytes: potassium, sodium, chloride, calcium, magnesium; renal function tests, including BUN and creatinine; and blood tests, including AST, ALT, bilirubin
• Monitor I&O ratio, daily weights
• Monitor therapeutic product levels

Patient/family education
• Teach patient how to take pulse before taking product; patient should record or graph pulse to identify changes
• Advise patient to avoid hazardous activities until stabilized on this product since dizziness occurs frequently
• Inform patient of the need for compliance to all areas of medical regimen, including diet, exercise, stress reduction, product therapy

Evaluation
Positive therapeutic outcome
• Decreased weight, edema, pulse, respiration
• Increased urine output

Generic Names
digoxin (high alert)

Cholinergics

ACTION:
Cholinergics act by preventing destruction of acetylcholine, which increases concentration at sites where acetylcholine is released. This exaggerates the effects of acetylcholine and facilitates transmission of impulses across the myoneural junction. Cholinergics may also act by stimulating receptors for acetylcholine.

USES:
Cholinergics are used for myasthenia gravis, as antagonists of nondepolarizing neuromuscular blockade, postoperative bladder distention and urinary distention, postoperative ileus.

CONTRAINDICATIONS
Persons with obstruction of the intestine or renal system should not use these products.

Precautions: Caution should be used in patients with bradycardia, hypotension, seizure disorders, bronchial asthma, coronary occlusion, and hyperthyroidism, and in breastfeeding and children.

IMPLEMENTATION
• Give only with atropine sulfate available for cholinergic crisis
• Give only after all other cholinergics have been discontinued
• Give increased dosages if tolerance occurs
• Give larger doses after exercise or fatigue
• Give on empty stomach for better absorption
• Store at room temperature

ADVERSE EFFECTS:
The most serious adverse reactions are respiratory depression, bronchospasm, constriction, laryngospasm, respiratory arrest, convulsions, and paralysis. The most common side effects are nausea, diarrhea, and vomiting.

PHARMACOKINETICS:
Onset, peak, and duration vary widely among products. Most products are metabolized in the liver and excreted in urine.

INTERACTIONS:
Interactions vary widely among products. Check individual monographs for specific information.

NURSING CONSIDERATIONS
Assessment
• Monitor VS, respiration q8hr
• Monitor I&O ratio; check for urinary retention or incontinence

• Assess for bradycardia, hypotension, bronchospasm, headache, dizziness, seizures, respiratory depression; product should be discontinued if toxicity occurs

Patient/family education
• Inform patient that product is not a cure; it only relieves symptoms (myasthenia gravis)
• Advise patient to carry/wear emergency ID specifying myasthenia gravis, products taken

Evaluation

Positive therapeutic outcome
• Increased muscle strength, hand grasp
• Improved muscle gait
• Absence of labored breathing (if severe)

Generic Names
bethanechol, physostigmine, pyridostigmine

Cholinergic Blockers

ACTION: Cholinergic blockers inhibit or block acetylcholine at receptor sites in the autonomic nervous system.

USES: Many cholinergic blockers are used to decrease secretions before surgery, to reverse neuromuscular blockade, and to decrease motility of the GI, biliary, and urinary tracts. Other products are used for parkinsonian symptoms, including dystonia associated with neuroleptic products.

CONTRAINDICATIONS
Hypersensitivity can occur, and allergies should be identified before administering these products. Persons with GI and GU obstruction should not use these products, since constipation and urinary retention may occur. They are also contraindicated in closed-angle glaucoma and myasthenia gravis.

Precautions: Caution must be used when these products are given to the geriatric patient, since metabolism is slowed. Also, persons with tachycardia or prostatic hypertrophy should use these products with caution.

IMPLEMENTATION
• Give with food or milk to decrease GI symptoms
• Give parenteral dose with patient recumbent to prevent postural hypotension; give dose slowly, monitoring VS
• Give hard candy, gum, frequent rinsing of mouth for dryness

ADVERSE EFFECTS: The most common side effects are dryness of the mouth and constipation, which can be prevented by frequent rinsing of the mouth and increasing water and bulk in the diet.

PHARMACOKINETICS: Onset, peak, and duration vary with route.

INTERACTIONS: Increase in anticholinergic effect occurs when used with opioids, barbiturates, antihistamines, MAOIs, phenothiazines, amantadine.

NURSING CONSIDERATIONS
Assessment
• Assess I&O ratio; be alert for urinary retention, frequency, dysuria; product should be discontinued if these occur
• Assess urinary hesitancy, retention; palpate bladder if retention occurs
• Assess constipation; increase fluids, bulk, exercise
• Assess for tolerance over long-term therapy; dosage may need to be changed
• Assess mental status: affect, mood, CNS depression, worsening of mental symptoms during early therapy

Patient/family education
• Caution patient to avoid driving and other hazardous activities if drowsiness occurs
• Advise patient to avoid concurrent use of cough, cold preparations with alcohol, antihistamines unless directed by prescriber
• Caution patient to use with caution in hot weather, since medication may increase susceptibility to heat stroke

Evaluation

Positive therapeutic outcome
• Absence of cramps
• Absence of EPS

Generic Names
atropine (high alert), benztropine, glycopyrrolate, scopolamine

Corticosteroids

ACTION: Corticosteroids are divided into glucocorticoids and mineralocorticoids. Glucocorticoids decrease inflammation by the suppression of migration of polymorphonuclear leukocytes, fibroblasts, increased capillary permeability, and lysosomal stabilization. They also have varied metabolic effects and modify the body's immune responses to many different stimuli. Mineralocorticoids act by increasing resorption of sodium by increasing hydrogen and potassium excretion in the distal tubule.

USES: Glucocorticoids are used to decrease inflammation and for immunosuppression. In addition, some products may be given for allergy, adrenal insufficiency, or cerebral edema. Mineralocorticoids are given for adrenal insufficiency or adrenogenital syndrome.

CONTRAINDICATIONS
Hypersensitivity may occur and should be identified before administering. Since these products mask infection, they should not be used in systemic fungal infections or amebiasis. Mothers taking pharmacologic doses of corticosteroids should not breastfeed.

Precautions: Caution must be used when these products are prescribed for diabetic patients since hyperglycemia may occur. Also, patients with glaucoma, seizure disorders, peptic ulcer, impaired renal function, HF, hypertension, ulcerative colitis, or myasthenia gravis should be monitored closely if corticosteroids are given. Use with caution during pregnancy, in children, and in the geriatric patient.

IMPLEMENTATION
• Give with food or milk to decrease GI symptoms
• Give single daily or alternate-day doses in the morning before 9 AM (for replacement therapy)

ADVERSE EFFECTS: The most common side effects include change in behavior, including insomnia and euphoria; GI irritation, including peptic ulcer; metabolic reactions, including hypokalemia, hyperglycemia, and carbohydrate intolerance; and sodium and fluid retention. Most adverse reactions are dose dependent.

PHARMACOKINETICS: For oral preparations the onset of action occurs between 1-2 hr, and duration can be up to 2 days, with a half-life of 2-4 days. Pharmacokinetics vary widely among products. These products cross the placenta and appear in breast milk.

INTERACTIONS: Decreased corticosteroid effect may occur with barbiturates, rifampin, and phenytoin; corticosteroid dosage may need to be increased. There is a possibility of GI bleeding when used with salicylates and indomethacin. Steroids may reduce salicylate levels. When using with digoxin, glycosides, potassium-depleting diuretics, and amphotericin, serum potassium levels should be monitored.

NURSING CONSIDERATIONS
Assessment
• Monitor potassium, blood glucose, urine glucose while on long-term therapy; hypokalemia and hyperglycemia are common

• Monitor weight daily; notify prescriber if weekly gain of >5 lb since these products alter fluid and electrolyte balance
• Assess for potassium depletion: paresthesias, fatigue, nausea, vomiting, depression, polyuria, dysrhythmias, weakness
• Assess for mental status: affect, mood, behavioral changes, aggression; if severe personality changes occur, including depression, product may need to be tapered and then discontinued
• Monitor I&O ratio; be alert for decreasing urinary output and increasing edema
• Monitor plasma cortisol levels during long-term therapy (normal level is 138-635 nmol/L when drawn at 8 AM)
• Assess for infection: increased temp, WBC, even after withdrawal of medication; product masks symptoms of infection
• Assess for adrenal insufficiency: nausea, anorexia, fatigue, dizziness, dyspnea, weakness, joint pain

Patient/family education
• Advise patient that emergency ID as steroid user should be carried/worn
• Advise patient not to discontinue this medication abruptly; adrenal crisis can result
• Teach patient all aspects of product use, including cushingoid symptoms
• Instruct patient to take with meals or a snack
• Teach patient to avoid exposure to chickenpox or measles if taking immunosuppressives

Evaluation
Positive therapeutic outcome
• Decreased inflammation

Generic Names
Glucocorticoids:
beclomethasone, betamethasone, cortisone, dexamethasone, hydrocortisone, hydrocortisone sodium succinate, methylPREDNISolone, predniSOLONE, predniSONE, triamcinolone

Diuretics

ACTION: Diuretics are divided into subgroups: thiazides and thiazidelike diuretics, loop diuretics, carbonic anhydrase inhibitors, osmotic diuretics, and potassium-sparing diuretics. Each one of these subgroups differs in its mechanism of action. Thiazides and thiazide-like diuretics increase excretion of water and sodium by inhibiting resorption in the early distal tubule. Loop diuretics inhibit resorption of sodium and chloride in the thick ascending limb of the loop of Henle. Carbonic anhydrase inhibitors increase sodium excretion by decreasing sodium-hydrogen ion exchange throughout the renal tubule. Carbonic anhydrase inhibitors also decrease secretion of aqueous humor in the eye and thus decrease intraocular pressure. Osmotic diuretics increase the osmotic pressure of glomerular filtrate, thus decreasing net absorption of sodium. The potassium-sparing diuretics interfere with sodium resorption at the distal tubule, thus decreasing potassium excretion.

USES: Blood pressure is reduced in hypertension; edema is reduced in HF; intraocular pressure is decreased in glaucoma.

CONTRAINDICATIONS
Persons with electrolyte imbalances (sodium, chloride, potassium), dehydration, or anuria should not be given these products until the problem is corrected.

Precautions: Caution must be used when diuretics are given to the geriatric patient, since electrolyte disturbances and dehydration can occur rapidly. Renal/hepatic disorders may cause poor metabolism and excretion of the product.

IMPLEMENTATION
- Give in AM to avoid interference with sleep if using product as a diuretic
- Give potassium replacement if potassium is less than 3 mg/dl

ADVERSE EFFECTS: Hypokalemia, hyperuricemia, and hyperglycemia occur most frequently with thiazide diuretics. Aplastic anemia, blood dyscrasias, volume depletion, and dehydration may occur when thiazide-like diuretics, loop diuretics, or carbonic anhydrase inhibitors are given. Side effects and adverse reactions vary widely for the miscellaneous products.

PHARMACOKINETICS: Onset, peak, and duration vary widely among the different subgroups of these products.

INTERACTIONS: Cholestyramine and colestipol decrease the absorption of thiazide diuretics. Concurrent use of thiazides with diazoxide may increase hyperuricemia, hyperglycemia, and antihypertensive effects of thiazides. Ototoxicity may occur when loop diuretics are used with aminoglycosides. Thiazide and loop diuretics may increase therapeutic and toxic effects of lithium.

NURSING CONSIDERATIONS
Assessment
- Monitor weight, I&O ratio daily to determine fluid loss; check skin turgor for dehydration
- Monitor electrolytes: potassium, sodium, chloride: include BUN, blood glucose, CBC, serum creatinine, blood pH, ABGs, uric acid, calcium; electrolyte imbalances may occur quickly
- Monitor B/P with patient lying, standing; postural hypotension may occur since fluid loss occurs from intravascular spaces first
- Assess for signs of metabolic alkalosis, including drowsiness and restlessness
- Assess for signs of hypokalemia with some products: postural hypotension, malaise, fatigue, tachycardia, leg cramps, weakness

Patient/family education
- Teach patient to take product early in the day (diuretic) to prevent nocturia

Evaluation
Positive therapeutic outcome
- Improvement in edema of feet, legs, sacral area daily if medication is being used in HF
- Improvement in B/P if medication is being used as a diuretic
- Improvement in intraocular pressure if medication is being used to decrease aqueous humor in the eye

Generic Names
Thiazides:
chlorothiazide, hydrochlorothiazide

Thiazidelike:
chlorthalidone, indapamide, metolazone

Loop:
bumetanide, furosemide

Carbonic anhydrase inhibitors:
acetaZOLAMIDE

Potassium-sparing:
aMILoride, spironolactone

Osmotic:
mannitol, urea

Histamine H$_2$ Antagonists

ACTION: Histamine H$_2$ antagonists act by inhibiting histamine at H$_2$ receptor site in parietal cells, which inhibits gastric acid secretion.

USES: Histamine H$_2$ antagonists are used for short-term treatment of duodenal and gastric ulcers and maintenance therapy for duodenal ulcer and for gastroesophageal reflux disease.

CONTRAINDICATIONS
Persons with hypersensitivity should not use these products.

Precautions: Caution should be used in pregnancy, breastfeeding, children <16 yr, organic brain syndrome, and renal/hepatic disease.

IMPLEMENTATION
- Give with meals for prolonged product effect
- Give antacids 1 hr before or 1 hr after cimetidine
- Give IV slowly; bradycardia may occur; give over 30 min
- Store diluted sol at room temperature for up to 48 hr

ADVERSE EFFECTS: The most serious adverse reactions are agranulocytosis, thrombocytopenia, neutropenia, aplastic anemia, and exfoliative dermatitis. The most common side effects are confusion (not with ranitidine), headache, and diarrhea.

PHARMACOKINETICS: Onset, peak, and duration vary widely among products. Most products are metabolized in the liver and excreted in urine.

INTERACTIONS: Antacids interfere with absorption of histamine H_2 antagonists. Check individual monographs for specific information.

NURSING CONSIDERATIONS
Assessment
- Monitor gastric pH (>5 should be maintained)
- Monitor I&O ratio, BUN, creatinine

Patient/family education
- Advise patient that gynecomastia, impotence may occur but is reversible
- Caution patient to avoid driving and other hazardous activities until patient is stabilized on this medication
- Caution patient to avoid black pepper, caffeine, alcohol, harsh spices, extremes in temperature of food
- Caution patient to avoid OTC preparations: aspirin, cough, cold preparations
- Inform patient that product must be continued for prescribed time to be effective
- Advise patient to report bruising, fatigue, malaise; blood dyscrasias may occur

Evaluation

Positive therapeutic outcome
- Decreased pain in abdomen

Generic Names
cimetidine, famotidine, ranitidine

Immunosuppressants

ACTION: Immunosuppressants produce immunosuppression by inhibiting T lymphocytes.

USES: Most immunosuppressants are used for organ transplants to prevent rejection.

CONTRAINDICATIONS
Products are contraindicated in hypersensitivity.

Precautions: Caution should be used in pregnancy and severe renal/hepatic disease.

IMPLEMENTATION
- Give for several days before transplant surgery
- Give with meals for GI upset or place product in chocolate milk
- Give with oral antifungal for *Candida* infections

ADVERSE EFFECTS: The most serious adverse reactions are albuminuria, hematuria, proteinuria, renal failure, and hepatotoxicity. The most common side effects are oral *Candida* infection, gum hyperplasia, tremors, and headache. The most serious adverse reactions for azaTHIOprine are hematologic (leukopenia and thrombocytopenia) and GI (nausea and vomiting). There is a risk of secondary infection.

PHARMACOKINETICS: Onset, peak, and duration vary widely among products. Most products are metabolized in the liver and excreted in urine.

INTERACTIONS: Interactions vary widely among products. Check individual monographs for specific information.

NURSING CONSIDERATIONS
Assessment
- Monitor renal function tests: BUN, creatinine at least monthly during treatment, 3 mo after treatment
- Monitor hepatic function tests: alkaline phosphatase, AST, ALT, bilirubin
- Monitor product blood levels during treatment
- Assess for hepatotoxicity: dark urine, jaundice, itching, light-colored stools; product should be discontinued

Patient/family education
- Advise patient to report fever, chills, sore throat, fatigue since serious infections may occur
- Caution patient to use contraceptive measures during treatment and for 12 wk after ending therapy

Evaluation

Positive therapeutic outcome
- Absence of rejection

Generic Names

azaTHIOprine, **basiliximab** (high alert), cycloSPORINE, everolimus, muromonab-CD3, secukinumab, sirolimus, tacrolimus, vedolizumab

Laxatives

ACTION: Laxatives are divided into bulk products, lubricants, osmotics, saline laxative stimulants, and stool softeners. Bulks work by absorbing water and expanding to increase moisture content and bulk in the stool. Lubricants increase water retention in the stool, causing reabsorption of water in the bowel. Saline draws water into the intestinal lumen. Osmotics increase distention and promote peristalsis. Stimulants act by increasing peristalsis by direct effect on the intestine. Stool softeners reduce surface tension of liquid in the bowel.

USES: Laxatives are used as a preparation for bowel or rectal examination, for constipation, or as stool softeners.

CONTRAINDICATIONS

Persons with GI obstruction, perforation, gastric retention, toxic colitis, megacolon, abdominal pain, nausea, vomiting, and fecal impaction should not use these products.

Precautions: Caution should be used in rectal bleeding, large hemorrhoids, and anal excoriation.

IMPLEMENTATION

• Give alone only with water for better absorption; do not take within 1 hr of antacids, milk, or cimetidine
• Swallow tab whole; do not break, crush, or chew

ADVERSE EFFECTS: The most common side effects are nausea, abdominal cramps, and diarrhea.

PHARMACOKINETICS: Onset, peak, and duration vary among products.

INTERACTIONS: Interactions vary widely among products. Check individual monographs for specific information.

NURSING CONSIDERATIONS
Assessment

• Monitor blood, urine electrolytes if product is used often by patient
• Monitor I&O ratio to identify fluid loss
• Determine cause of constipation; identify whether fluids, bulk, or exercise is missing from lifestyle

• Assess for cramping, rectal bleeding, nausea, vomiting; if these symptoms occur, product should be discontinued

Patient/family education

• Caution patient not to use laxatives for long-term therapy; bowel tone will be lost; that normal bowel movements do not always occur daily
• Caution patient not to use in presence of abdominal pain, nausea, vomiting
• Advise patient to notify prescriber of abdominal pain, nausea, vomiting
• Advise patient to notify prescriber if constipation is unrelieved or if symptoms of electrolyte imbalance occur: muscle cramps, pain, weakness, dizziness

Evaluation

Positive therapeutic outcome
• Decrease in constipation

Generic Names

Bulk laxative:
psyllium

Osmotic agent:
lactulose

Saline laxatives:
magnesium salts, sodium biphosphate/sodium phosphate

Stimulants:
bisacodyl, senna

Stool softener:
docusate

Neuromuscular Blocking Agents

ACTION: Neuromuscular blocking agents are divided into depolarizing and nondepolarizing blockers. They act by inhibiting transmission of nerve impulses by binding with cholinergic receptor sites.

USES: Neuromuscular blocking agents are used to facilitate endotracheal intubation and skeletal muscle relaxation during mechanical ventilation, surgery, or general anesthesia.

CONTRAINDICATIONS

Persons who are hypersensitive should not be given this product.

Precautions: Caution should be used in pregnancy, breastfeeding, children <2 yr, thyroid disease, collagen disease, cardiac disease, electrolyte imbalances, dehydration, neuromuscular disease (myasthenia gravis), and respiratory disease.

IMPLEMENTATION

- Administer using nerve stimulator by anesthesiologist to determine neuromuscular blockade
- Administer anticholinesterase to reverse neuromuscular blockade
- Give **IV** undiluted over 1-2 min (only by qualified person, usually an anesthesiologist)
- Store in light-resistant, cool area
- Reassure patient if communication is difficult during recovery from neuromuscular blockade

ADVERSE EFFECTS: The most serious adverse reactions are prolonged apnea, bronchospasm, cyanosis, respiratory depression, and malignant hyperthermia. The most common side effects are bradycardia and decreased motility.

PHARMACOKINETICS: Onset, peak, and duration vary widely among products. Most products are metabolized in the liver and excreted in urine.

INTERACTIONS: Aminoglycosides potentiate neuromuscular blockade. Check individual monographs for specific information.

NURSING CONSIDERATIONS
Assessment

- Monitor for electrolyte imbalances (potassium, magnesium); may lead to increased action of this product
- Monitor VS (B/P, pulse, respirations, airway) q15min until fully recovered; rate, depth, pattern of respirations, strength of hand grip
- Monitor I&O ratio; check for urinary retention, frequency, hesitancy
- Assess for recovery: decreased paralysis of face, diaphragm, leg, arm, rest of body
- Assess for allergic reactions: rash, fever, respiratory distress, pruritus; product should be discontinued

Evaluation

Positive therapeutic outcome
- Paralysis of jaw, eyelid, head, neck, rest of body

Generic Names
pancuronium (high alert), succinylcholine (high alert), vecuronium (high alert)

Nonsteroidal Antiinflammatories

ACTION: Nonsteroidal antiinflammatories decrease prostaglandin synthesis by inhibiting an enzyme needed for biosynthesis.

USES: Nonsteroidal antiinflammatories are used to treat mild to moderate pain, osteoarthritis, rheumatoid arthritis, and dysmenorrhea.

CONTRAINDICATIONS
Persons with hypersensitivity, asthma, or severe renal/hepatic disease should not use these products.

Precautions: Caution should be used in pregnancy, breastfeeding, children, geriatric patients, bleeding/GI/cardiac disorders, and hypersensitivity to other antiinflammatory agents.

IMPLEMENTATION
- Give with food to decrease GI symptoms; however, best to take on empty stomach to facilitate absorption
- Store at room temperature

ADVERSE EFFECTS: The most serious adverse reactions are nephrotoxicity (dysuria, hematuria, oliguria, azotemia), blood dyscrasias, and cholestatic hepatitis. The most common side effects are nausea, abdominal pain, anorexia, dizziness, and drowsiness.

PHARMACOKINETICS: Onset, peak, and duration vary widely among products. Most products are metabolized in the liver and excreted in urine.

INTERACTIONS: Interactions vary widely among products. Check individual monographs for specific information.

NURSING CONSIDERATIONS
Assessment
- Monitor renal, hepatic, blood tests: BUN, creatinine, AST, ALT, Hgb, before treatment, periodically thereafter
- Monitor audiometric, ophth examination before, during, and after treatment.
- Check for eye, ear problems: blurred vision, tinnitus; may indicate toxicity

Patient/family education
- Advise patient to report blurred vision, ringing, roaring in ears; may indicate toxicity
- Caution patient to avoid driving, other hazardous activities if dizziness, drowsiness occurs, especially in geriatric patients
- Advise patient to report change in urine pattern, increased weight, edema, increased pain in

joints, fever, blood in urine; indicate nephrotoxicity
• Inform patient that therapeutic effects may take up to 1 mo to occur

Evaluation

Positive therapeutic outcome
• Decreased pain, stiffness in joints
• Decreased swelling in joints
• Ability to move more easily

Generic Names
celecoxib, diclofenac, etodolac, ibuprofen, indomethacin, ketoprofen, ketorolac, nabumetone, naproxen, piroxicam, sulindac

Opioid Analgesics

ACTION: These agents depress pain impulse transmission at the spinal cord level by interacting with opioid receptors. Products are divided into opiates and nonopiates.

USES: Most opioid analgesics are used to control moderate to severe pain and are used before and after surgery.

CONTRAINDICATIONS
Hypersensitive reactions occur frequently. Check for sensitivity before administering. These products should not be used if opioid addiction is suspected.

Precautions: Caution must be used when these products are given to persons with an addictive personality, since the possibility of addiction is so great. Also, persons with increased ICP may experience an even greater increase in ICP. Persons with severe heart disease, renal/hepatic disease, respiratory conditions, and seizure disorders should be monitored closely for worsening condition.

IMPLEMENTATION
• Give with antiemetic if nausea or vomiting occurs
• Give when pain is beginning to return; determine dosage interval by patient response
• Provide assistance with ambulation; patient should not be ambulating during product peak

ADVERSE EFFECTS: GI symptoms, including nausea, vomiting, anorexia, constipation, and cramps are the most common side effects. Other common side effects include lightheadedness, dizziness, and sedation. Serious adverse reactions such as respiratory depression, respiratory arrest, circulatory depression, and increased ICP may result but are less common and usually dose dependent.

PHARMACOKINETICS: Onset of action is immediate by **IV** route and rapid by IM and PO routes. Peak occurs from 1-2 hr, depending on route, with a duration of 2-8 hr. These agents cross the placenta and appear in breast milk.

INTERACTIONS: Barbiturates, other opioids, hypnotics, antipsychotics, or alcohol can increase CNS depression when taken with opioids.

NURSING CONSIDERATIONS
Assessment
• Monitor I&O ratio; be alert for urinary retention, frequency, dysuria; product should be discontinued if these occur
• Assess for respiratory dysfunction: respiratory depression, rate, rhythm, character; notify prescriber if respirations are <12/min
• Assess for CNS changes: dizziness, drowsiness, hallucinations, euphoria, LOC, pupil reaction
• Assess for allergic reactions: rash, urticaria
• Assess for need for pain medication, use pain scoring

Patient/family education
• Advise patient to report any symptoms of CNS changes, allergic reactions, or shortness of breath
• Caution patient that physical dependency may result when used for extended periods
• Teach patient that withdrawal symptoms may occur, including nausea, vomiting, cramps, fever, faintness, anorexia
• Advise patient to avoid alcohol and other CNS depressants

Evaluation

Positive therapeutic outcome
• Decrease in pain

Generic Names
buprenorphine, butorphanol, codeine, **fentaNYL** (high alert), fentaNYL transdermal, **HYDROmorphone** (high alert), **meperidine** (high alert), **methadone** (high alert), **morphine** (high alert), nalbuphine, oxyCODONE (high alert), **oxymorphone** (high alert), **pentazocine** (high alert), **remifentanil** (high alert)

Salicylates

ACTION: Salicylates have analgesic, antipyretic, and antiinflammatory effects. The analgesic and antiinflammatory activities may be mediated through the inhibition of prostaglandin

---

synthesis. Antipyretic action results from inhibition of the hypothalamic heat-regulating center.

USES: The primary uses of salicylates are relief of mild to moderate pain and fever and in inflammatory conditions such as arthritis, thromboembolic disorders, and rheumatic fever.

CONTRAINDICATIONS
Hypersensitivity to salicylates is common. Check for sensitivity before administering. Persons with bleeding disorders, GI bleeding, and vit K deficiency should not use these products since salicylates increase pro-time. Children should not use these products since salicylates have been associated with Reye's syndrome.

Precautions: Caution is needed when salicylates are given to patients with anemia, renal/hepatic disease, and Hodgkin's disease. Caution should also be exercised in pregnancy and breastfeeding.

IMPLEMENTATION
• Give with food or milk to decrease gastric irritation; give 30 min before or 1 hr after meals with a full glass of water

ADVERSE EFFECTS: The most common side effects are GI symptoms and rash. Serious blood dyscrasias and hepatotoxicity may result when used for long periods at high doses. Tinnitus or impaired hearing may indicate that blood salicylate levels are reaching or exceeding the upper limit of the therapeutic range.

PHARMACOKINETICS: Onset of action occurs in 15-30 min, with a peak of 1-2 hr and a duration up to 6 hr. These products are metabolized by the liver and excreted by the kidneys.

INTERACTIONS: Increased effects of anticoagulants, insulin, methotrexate, heparin, valproic acid, and oral sulfonylureas may occur when used with salicylates. Aspirin may decrease serum concentrations of nonsteroidal antiinflammatory agents.

NURSING CONSIDERATIONS
Assessment
• Monitor renal/hepatic function tests: AST, ALT, bilirubin, creatinine, LDH, alkaline phosphatase, BUN if patient is on long-term therapy since these products are metabolized and excreted by the liver and kidney
• Monitor blood tests: CBC, Hct, Hgb, and pro-time if patient is on long-term therapy, since these products increase the possibility of bleeding and blood dyscrasias

• Assess for hepatotoxicity: dark urine, clay-colored stools, jaundiced skin and sclera, itching, abdominal pain, fever, diarrhea, which may occur with long-term use
• Assess for ototoxicity: tinnitus, ringing, roaring in ears; audiometric testing is needed before and after long-term therapy

Patient/family education
• Advise patient that blood sugar levels should be monitored closely if patient is diabetic
• Caution patient not to exceed recommended dosage; acute poisoning may result
• Inform patient that therapeutic response takes 2 wk in arthritis
• Caution patient to avoid use of alcohol since GI bleeding may result
• Advise patient to notify prescriber if ringing in the ears or persistent GI pain occurs
• Advise patient to take with full glass of water to reduce risk of lodging in esophagus

Evaluation
Positive therapeutic outcome
• Decreased pain, fever

Generic Names
aspirin, magnesium salicylate, salsalate

Sedatives/Hypnotics

ACTION: The sedatives/hypnotics depress the CNS; some products at the cerebral cortex, others inhibit transmitters in the CNS.

USES: Sedatives/hypnotics are used for the treatment of sleep disorders, seizures, muscle spasms, and alcohol withdrawal.

CONTRAINDICATIONS
Persons with hypersensitivity reactions should not use these products.

Precautions: Sedatives/hypnotics should be used cautiously in pregnancy and breastfeeding.

IMPLEMENTATION
• Give lowest possible dose for therapeutic result; adjust dose to response
• Provide assistance with ambulation during beginning therapy if dizziness, ataxia occur

ADVERSE EFFECTS: The most common side effects are nausea and drowsiness. The most serious side effects are Stevens-Johnson syndrome, blood dyscrasias, and risk of dependency.

PHARMACOKINETICS: Onset, peak, and duration vary widely among products. Most products are metabolized in the liver and excreted by the kidneys.

INTERACTIONS: Increased CNS depression may occur with other CNS depressants such as alcohol, opiates, antipsychotics, and antidepressants.

NURSING CONSIDERATIONS
Assessment
• Monitor mental status: affect, mood, behavioral changes, depression, confusion; seizure activity

Patient/family education
• Inform patient that these products should only be used for short-term insomnia
• Caution patient not to drive or engage in other hazardous activities while taking these products
• Instruct patient to avoid breastfeeding while taking these products
• Instruct patient to avoid alcohol or other CNS depressants as drowsiness will increase
• Teach patient that some of the products take two nights to be effective
• Advise patient to report side effects, adverse reactions to health care provider
• Instruct patient to use exactly as prescribed, at regular intervals

Evaluation
Positive therapeutic outcome
• Ability to sleep throughout the night
• Absence or decreasing seizure activity

Generic Names
Barbiturates:
PHENobarbital (high alert)

Benzodiazepines:
chlordiazePOXIDE, clorazepate, diazepam, flurazepam, LORazepam, midazolam, oxazepam, temazepam, triazolam

Miscellaneous products:
chloral hydrate, dexmedetomidine, **droperidol** (high alert), eszopiclone, hydrOXYzine, promethazine, ramelteon, suvorexant, tasimelton, zaleplon, zolpidem

Skeletal Muscle Relaxants

ACTION: Most skeletal muscle relaxants inhibit synaptic responses in the CNS by stimulating receptors and decreasing neurotransmission, decreasing pain and spasticity.

USES: Skeletal muscle relaxants are used for musculoskeletal disorders with pain or spasticity related to spinal cord injuries.

CONTRAINDICATIONS
Persons with hypersensitivity should not use these products.

Precautions: Skeletal muscle relaxants should be used cautiously in pregnancy, breastfeeding, the geriatric patient, peptic ulcer, renal/hepatic disease, stroke, seizure disorder, and diabetes.

IMPLEMENTATION
• Give when pain is beginning to return, not after pain is severe
• Store in dry area, away from heat and sunlight

ADVERSE EFFECTS: The most common side effects are dizziness, weakness, fatigue, drowsiness, and headache. Some products can cause seizures, cardiovascular collapse, and severe CNS depression.

PHARMACOKINETICS: Pharmacokinetics vary widely among products. Check individual monographs for specific information.

INTERACTIONS: CNS depressants used with skeletal muscle relaxants may lead to increased CNS depression.

NURSING CONSIDERATIONS
Assessment
• Monitor pain: character, location, duration, alleviating/aggravating factors

Patient/family education
• Advise patient not to use with other CNS depressant unless prescriber approved
• Inform patient that many products require 1-2 mo of treatment for full effect
• Caution patient to avoid hazardous activities until response to medication is known
• Caution patient that most products should not be discontinued quickly, but tapered over 1-2 wk

Evaluation
Positive therapeutic outcome
• Decrease in pain or spasticity

Generic Names
Centrally acting:
baclofen, carisoprodol, cyclobenzaprine, diazepam, methocarbamol

Direct-acting:
dantrolene

Thrombolytics

ACTION: Thrombolytics activate conversion of plasminogen to plasmin (fibrinolysin). Plasmin is able to break down clots (fibrin).

USES: Thrombolytics are used to treat DVT, PE, arterial thrombosis, arterial embolism, arteriovenous cannula occlusion, lysis of coronary artery thrombi after MI, and acute evolving transmural MI.

CONTRAINDICATIONS

Persons with hypersensitivity, active bleeding, intraspinal surgery, neoplasms of the CNS, ulcerative colitis/enteritis, severe hypertension, renal/hepatic disease, hypocoagulation, COPD, subacute bacterial endocarditis, rheumatic valvular disease, cerebral embolism/thrombosis/hemorrhage, intra-arterial diagnostic procedure or surgery (10 days), and recent major surgery should not use these products.

Precautions: Caution should be used in arterial emboli from left side of heart and pregnancy.

IMPLEMENTATION

• Administer as soon as thrombi identified; not useful for thrombi over 1wk old
• Administer cryoprecipitate or fresh, frozen plasma if bleeding occurs
• Give loading dose at beginning of therapy; may require increased loading doses
• Give heparin after fibrinogen level is over 100 mg/dl; heparin INF to increase PTT to 1.5-2 × baseline for 3-7 days
• About 10% of patients have high streptococcal antibody titers requiring increased loading doses
• Give **IV** therapy using 0.8-μm filter
• Store reconstituted sol in refrigerator; discard after 24 hr
• Provide bed rest during entire course of treatment

ADVERSE EFFECTS: Serious adverse reactions include GI, GU, intracranial, and retroperitoneal bleeding and anaphylaxis. The most common side effects are decreased Hct, urticaria, headache, and nausea.

PHARMACOKINETICS: Onset, peak, and duration vary widely among products. Most products are metabolized in the liver and excreted in urine.

INTERACTIONS: Interactions vary widely among products. Check individual monographs for specific information.

NURSING CONSIDERATIONS
Assessment
• Monitor VS, B/P, pulse, respirations, neurologic signs, temp at least q4hr (increased temp is an indicator of internal bleeding), cardiac rhythm following intracoronary administration; systolic pressure increase of >25 mm Hg should be reported to prescriber
• Assess for neurologic changes that may indicate intracranial bleeding
• Assess retroperitoneal bleeding: back pain, leg weakness, diminished pulses
• Assess for allergy: fever, rash, itching, chills; mild reaction may be treated with antihistamines
• Assess for bleeding during 1st hr of treatment: hematuria, hematemesis, bleeding from mucous membranes, epistaxis, ecchymosis
• Monitor blood tests (Hct, platelets, PTT, PT, TT, APTT) before starting therapy; PT or APTT must be less than 2 times control before starting therapy; TT or PT q3-4hr during treatment

Patient/family education
• Teach patient to avoid venous or arterial puncture, injection, rectal temp
• Teach patient to treat fever with acetaminophen or aspirin
• Teach patient to apply pressure for 30 sec to minor bleeding sites; inform prescriber if this does not attain hemostasis; apply pressure dressing

Evaluation
Positive therapeutic outcome
• Resolution of thrombosis, embolism

Generic Names
alteplase (high alert), drotrecogin alfa, tenecteplase (high alert), urokinase (high alert)

Thyroid Hormones

ACTION: Thyroid hormones increase metabolic rates, resulting in increased cardiac output, O_2 consumption, body temp, blood volume, growth, development at cellular level, respiratory rate, and enzyme system activity.

USES: Thyroid hormones are used for thyroid replacement.

CONTRAINDICATIONS

Persons with adrenal insufficiency, myocardial infarction, or thyrotoxicosis should not use these products.

Precautions: Caution should be used in pregnancy and breastfeeding. Geriatric patients and those with angina pectoris, hypertension, ischemia, cardiac disease, or diabetes mellitus or insipidus should be watched closely when using these products.

IMPLEMENTATION

• Give at same time each day to maintain product level
• Give only for hormone imbalances; not to be used for obesity, male infertility, menstrual conditions, lethargy
• Remove medication 4 wk before RAIU test

ADVERSE EFFECTS: The most common side effects include insomnia, tremors, tachycardia, palpitations, angina, dysrhythmias, weight loss, and changes in appetite. Serious adverse reactions include thyroid storm.

PHARMACOKINETICS: Pharmacokinetics vary widely among products. Check individual monographs for specific information.

INTERACTIONS
• Impaired absorption of thyroid products may occur when administered with cholestyramine, iron products (separate by 4-5 hr).
• Increased effects of anticoagulants, sympathomimetics, tricyclics, catecholamines may occur.
• Decreased effects of digoxin, glycosides, insulin, hypoglycemics may occur.
• Decreased effects of thyroid products may occur with estrogens.

NURSING CONSIDERATIONS
Assessment
• Monitor B/P, pulse before each dose
• Monitor I&O ratio
• Monitor weight daily in same clothing, using same scale, at same time of day
• Monitor height, growth rate if given to a child
• Monitor T_3, T_4, which are decreased; radioimmunoassay of TSH, which is increased; ratio uptake, which is decreased if patient is on too low a dosage of medication
• Assess for increased nervousness, excitability, irritability; may indicate too high a dosage of medication, usually after 1-3 wk of treatment
• Assess for cardiac status: angina, palpitation, chest pain, change in VS

Patient/family education
• Advise patient/family that hair loss will occur in children and is temporary
• Advise patient to report excitability, irritability, anxiety; indicates overdose
• Caution patient not to switch brands unless directed by prescriber
• Caution family that hypothyroid children will show almost immediate behavior/personality change
• Advise patient that treatment product is not to be taken to reduce weight
• Advise patient to avoid OTC preparations with iodine; read labels; to avoid iodine-containing foods: iodized salt, soybeans, tofu, turnips, some seafood, some bread

Evaluation

Positive therapeutic outcome
• Absence of depression

• Increased weight loss, diuresis, pulse, appetite
• Absence of constipation, peripheral edema, cold intolerance, pale, cool, dry skin, brittle nails, alopecia, coarse hair, menorrhagia, night blindness, paresthesias, syncope, stupor, coma, rosy cheeks

Generic Names
levothyroxine, liothyronine (T_3), liotrix, thyroid USP

Vasodilators

ACTION: Vasodilators act in various ways. Check individual monographs for specific action.

USES: Vasodilators are used to treat intermittent claudication, arteriosclerosis obliterans, vasospasm and muscular ischemia, ischemic cerebral vascular disease, hypertension, and angina.

CONTRAINDICATIONS
Some products are contraindicated in acute MI, paroxysmal tachycardia, and thyrotoxicosis.

Precautions: Caution should be used in uncompensated heart disease or peptic ulcer disease.

IMPLEMENTATION
• Give with meals to reduce GI symptoms
• Store in tight container at room temperature

ADVERSE EFFECTS: The most common side effects are headache, nausea, hypotension, hypertension, and ECG changes.

PHARMACOKINETICS: Onset, peak, and duration vary widely among products. Most products are metabolized in the liver and excreted in urine.

INTERACTIONS: Interactions vary widely among products. Check individual monographs for specific information.

NURSING CONSIDERATIONS
Assessment
• Assess bleeding time in individuals with bleeding disorders
• Assess cardiac status: B/P, pulse, rate, rhythm, character; watch for increasing pulse

Patient/family education
• Inform patient that medication is not cure, may need to be taken continuously
• Advise patient that it is necessary to quit smoking to prevent excessive vasoconstriction
• Advise patient that improvement may be sudden, but usually occurs gradually over several weeks

• Instruct patient to report headache, weakness, increased pulse, since product may need to be decreased or discontinued
• Instruct patient to avoid hazardous activities until stabilized on medication; dizziness may occur

Evaluation

Positive therapeutic outcome
• Ability to walk without pain
• Increased temp in extremities
• Increased pulse volume

Generic Names
amyl nitrite, bosentan, dipyridamole, hydrALA-ZINE, minoxidil, nesiritide

Vitamins

ACTION: The action of vitamins varies widely among products and classes. Check individual monographs for specific action.

USES: Vitamins are used to correct and prevent vitamin deficiencies.

CONTRAINDICATIONS
Hypersensitive reactions may occur, and allergies should be identified before these products are given.

IMPLEMENTATION
• Give PO with food for better absorption
• Store in tight, light-resistant container

ADVERSE EFFECTS: There is an absence of side effects or adverse reactions with the water-soluble vitamins (C, B). However, fat-soluble vitamins (A, D, E, K) may accumulate in the body and cause adverse reactions (refer to individual monographs).

PHARMACOKINETICS: Onset, peak, and duration vary widely among products. Check individual monographs for specific information.

NURSING CONSIDERATIONS
Patient/family education
• Advise patient not to take more than prescribed amount

Evaluation

Positive therapeutic outcome
• Absence of vitamin deficiency

Generic Names
Fat-soluble:
phytonadione (vitamin K_1), vitamin A, vitamin D, vitamin E

Water-soluble:
ascorbic acid (C), cyanocobalamin (B_{12}), pyridoxine (B_6), riboflavin (B_2), thiamine (B_1)

Miscellaneous:
multivitamins

Appendix A

Selected New Drugs

aclidinium/formoterol (Rx)
Duaklir Pressair
Func. class: Respiratory agent
Chem. class: Respiratory corticosteroid; long-acting β_2 agonist; respiratory long-acting muscarinic antagonist

USES: Maintenance treatment of chronic obstructive pulmonary disease (COPD)

CONTRAINDICATIONS
Hypersensitivity.

DOSAGE AND ROUTES
• **Adult: INH** 1 inhalation (400 mcg aclidinium and 12 mcg formoterol per actuation) inhaled bid (morning and evening). Max: 1 INH bid.

⚠ HIGH ALERT

alpelisib
(al-peh-lih′-sib)
Pigray
Func. class.: Antineoplastic
Chem. class.: Small molecule antineoplastic phosphatidylinositol-3-kinase (PI3K) inhibitors

ACTION: In breast cancer cell lines, inhibits the phosphorylation of PI3K downstream targets, including Akt, and shows activity in cell lines harboring a PI3KCA mutation

USES: Hormone receptor (HR)-positive, HER2-negative, PIK3CA-mutated, advanced, or metastatic breast cancer in men and postmenopausal women following progression of or after an endocrine-based regimen, in combination with fulvestrant

CONTRAINDICATIONS
Hypersensitivity, pregnancy

Precautions: Breast feeding, chronic lung disorders, contraceptive requirement, diabetes mellitus, diarrhea, hyperglycemia, infertility, interstitial lung disease, male-mediated teratogenicity

DOSAGE AND ROUTES
• **Males and postmenopausal females**
PO: 300 mg per os (PO) daily with food, in combination with fulvestrant (500 mg intramuscular [IM] on days 1, 15, 29, and monthly thereafter) until disease progression or unacceptable toxicity

Available forms: Tabs 200, 250, 300 mg

SIDE EFFECTS
CNS: *Fever, headache*
ENDO: Hypoglycemia, hyperglycemia
INTEG: *Rash, pruritus*
GU: Renal dysfunction
GI: *Nausea, vomiting, diarrhea, anorexia, abdominal pain, anorexia, weight loss*
SYST: Infection, anaphylaxis, Stevens-Johnson syndrome

Pharmacokinetics

Absorption	Unknown
Distribution	89% protein binding
Metabolism	Affected by CYP2C9, CYP3A4, BCRP
Excretion	81% excreted in feces
	(36% unchanged, 32% as metabolite, 14% excreted in urine)
	(2% unchanged, 7.1% metabolite)
Half-life	8–9 hr

Pharmacodynamics

Onset	Unknown
Peak	2–4 hr
Duration	Unknown

INTERACTIONS
Drug classifications: Avoid use with CYP3A4 inhibitors, inducers, substrates

Drug/Lab Test
Increase: LFTs

NURSING CONSIDERATIONS
Assess:
• **Diabetes mellitus:** Fasting blood glucose and hemoglobin A1c (HbA1c) should be monitored before starting treatment and before any antidiabetic treatment change; continue to monitor blood glucose weekly for the first 2 weeks, then q4wk; monitor HbA1c q3mo

• **Severe diarrhea:** May use with antidiarrheal medication (loperamide). An interruption of therapy, dose reduction, or discontinuation of therapy may be necessary

• **Severe hypersensitivity reactions (anaphylaxis and anaphylactic shock):** Monitor for severe hypersensitivity reactions (dyspnea, flushing, rash, fever, or tachycardia), permanently discontinue if this occurs

• **Pregnancy/breastfeeding:** Do not use in pregnancy/breastfeeding, obtain pregnancy testing before use

Patient problem:
• Risk for injury (adverse reactions)

Implementation:
• Give with food at approximately the same time each day

• Do not crush, chew, or split, do not use any tablet that is broken, cracked, or otherwise not intact

• If a dose is missed, it can be taken with food within 9 hr after the time it is usually taken. After more than 9 hr, skip the dose for that day and resume dosing on the following day at the usual time

• If vomiting occurs, do not administer an additional dose on that day. Resume dosing the following day at the usual time

Patient/family education:
• **Pregnancy/breastfeeding:** Teach patient to report planned or suspected pregnancy; to use effective contraception during treatment and for at least 1 month after the last dose; to avoid breastfeeding

• Advise patient to report new or worsening side effects

• Inform patient to take tabs whole, not to crush or chew, to take with food

• **Pre-existing chronic lung disease (CLD), severe pneumonitis/interstitial lung disease:** Advise patient to immediately report any new or worsening respiratory symptoms (hypoxia, cough, dyspnea)

• **Diarrhea:** Teach patients to begin antidiarrheal treatment, increase oral fluids, and notify their healthcare provider if diarrhea occurs

Evaluation
Positive therapeutic outcome
• Decreased disease progression in breast cancer

---

brexanolone (Rx) (REMS)
(brek-san' oh-lone)
Zulresso
Func. class.: Antidepressants
Chem. class.: Gamma-aminobutyric acid (GABA) modulator

ACTION: Not fully known but thought to be related to its positive modulation of GABA-A receptors. GABA is a major inhibitory neurotransmitter in the brain

USES: Postpartum depression

THERAPEUTIC OUTCOME
Resolution of postpartum depression

CONTRAINDICATIONS
Hypersensitivity

Precautions: Abrupt discontinuation, driving or hazardous activities, breastfeeding, coadministration with other central nervous system (CNS) depressants, alcohol use, hypoxia, pregnancy, renal failure, suicidal ideation

> **BLACK BOX WARNING:** CNS depression, loss of consciousness, requires a specialized setting

DOSAGE AND ROUTES
• **Adult females continuous IV:** Give over a total of 60 hrs (2.5 days) as follows: 0 to 4 hrs: initiate with a dosage of 30 mcg/kg/hr; 4 to 24 hrs: increase dose to 60 mcg/kg/hr; 24 to 52 hrs: increase dosage to 90 mcg/kg/hr; 52 to 56 hrs: decrease dosage to 60 mcg/kg/hr; 56 to 60 hrs: decrease dosage to 30 mcg/kg/hr

Available forms: Solution for injection 100 mg/20 mL

SIDE EFFECTS
CNS: Sedation, drowsiness, loss of consciousness, suicidal ideation
CV: Tachycardia
RESP: Hypoxia
INTEG: Injection site reaction

Pharmacokinetics

Absorption	Unknown
Distribution	Extensive into tissues, protein binding >99%
Metabolism	Extensively metabolized by non-CYP pathways (keto-reduction, glucuronidation, sulfation)
Excretion	Metabolites in feces (47%) and urine (42%), less than 1% of the drug is excreted as unchanged
Half-life	9 hr

Pharmacodynamics

Onset	Unknown
Peak	Unknown
Duration	Unknown

INTERACTIONS
None known

NURSING CONSIDERATIONS
Assess:
• Monitor for hypoxia using continuous pulse oximetry with an alarm. If hypoxia occurs, discontinue and do not reinitiate

BLACK BOX WARNING: Assess for excessive sedation q2hr during planned, nonsleep periods, and stop the infusion if excessive sedation occurs until the symptom resolves. Thereafter, the infusion may be resumed at the same or lower dose

• Available only through the Zulresso Risk Evaluation and Mitigation Strategy (Zulresso REMS) program, risks of serious adverse outcomes (excessive sedation or sudden loss/alteration of consciousness)

BLACK BOX WARNING: Requires a specialized care setting: Healthcare settings must be certified in the REMS program. For further information, including a list of certified healthcare facilities, visit www.zulressorems.com or call 1-844-472-4379

• **Suicidal ideation:** Assess for suicidal thoughts or behavior, which are more common in young adults

Patient problem:
• Suicidal ideation (uses)

Implementation:
• The vials require dilution

• Visually inspect product. Vial will be clear and colorless without particulate matter and discoloration. Do not use discolored vials or vials with particulate matter
• Five infusion bags will be required for the 60-hr infusion; additional bags will be needed for those ≥90 kg
• Prepare and store in a polyolefin, non-DEHP, nonlatex bag only. Do not use in-line filter
• Dilute in the infusion bag immediately after the initial puncture of the vial
• Withdraw 20 mL of product from the vial and place in the infusion bag. Dilute with 40 mL of sterile water for injection, and further dilute with 40 mL of 0.9% sodium chloride injection (total volume of 100 mL) to achieve a target concentration of 1 mg/mL.
• Immediately place the infusion bag in a refrigerator until use
• Give as a continuous intravenous (IV) infusion over a total of 60 hrs (2.5 days) via a dedicated line. Do not inject other medications into the infusion bag or admix
• Use a programmable peristaltic infusion pump, and prime infusion sets with admixture before inserting into the pump and connecting to the venous catheter
• A healthcare provider must be available on site to continuously monitor
• Initiate treatment early enough during the day to allow for recognition of excessive sedation.
• After the product is diluted, it can be stored in infusion bags under refrigerated conditions for up to 96 hr
• Each diluted product can be used for up to 12 hr of infusion time at room temperature. Discard any unused product after 12 hr of infusion

Patient/family education:
• Teach patient reason for product and expected result
• Advise patient to discuss all prescriptions, over-the-counter (OTC) medicines, herbals, and supplements with healthcare provider
• Inform patient to report pain, inflammation at injection site
• **Excessive sedation and sudden loss of consciousness.** Teach patient about excessive sedation or loss of consciousness, and that checking q2hr for these symptoms will be required. If these occur she should tell the healthcare provider
• Advise the patient that a family member or caregiver needs to help care for her and her children during the infusion

• Inform the patient not to drive or engage in hazardous tasks while sleepiness occurs
• Advise the patient not to use alcohol or other CNS depressants
• **Pregnancy/breastfeeding:** Identify if pregnancy is planned or suspected or if breastfeeding; if pregnant register with the National Pregnancy Registry for Antidepressants at 1-844-405-6185 or visit https://womensmentalhealth.org/clinical-and-research-programs/pregnancyregistry/antidepressants/

Evaluation
Positive therapeutic outcome
• Decrease in postpartum depression, improved mood

caplacizumab (Rx)
(kap′ luh-sih′-zoo-mab)
Cablivi
Func. class: Hematologic agent

USES: Acquired thrombotic thrombocytopenia purpura (aTTP), in combination with plasma exchange and immunosuppressive therapy

CONTRAINDICATIONS
Hypersensitivity

DOSAGE AND ROUTES
Adults: IV 11 mg once at least 15 min before plasma exchange on the first day of treatment (initial dose); subcut 11 mg daily starting after the completion of plasma exchange on day 1 and continuing for 30 days after the last daily plasma exchange; treatment may be extended for a maximum of 28 days after the initial treatment (maintenance dose)

▲ HIGH ALERT

cladribine (Rx)
(klad′ dri-been)
Leustatin, Mavenclad
Func. class.: Multiple sclerosis agent/antineoplastic
Chem. class.: Purine nucleoside antimetabolite

ACTION: May be lymphocyte depletion through cytotoxic effects on B and T lymphocytes through impairment of deoxyribonucleic acid (DNA) synthesis

THERAPEUTIC OUTCOME: Decreasing symptoms of multiple sclerosis, prevention of spread of cancer

USES: Relapsing multiple sclerosis, active hairy-cell leukemia

CONTRAINDICATIONS
Breastfeeding, human immunodeficiency virus (HIV), TB

BLACK BOX WARNING: Pregnancy

Precautions: Contraceptive requirements, hepatic disease, infection, renal disease, progressive multifocal leukoencephalopathy (PML), neonates, premature

BLACK BOX WARNING: Bone marrow suppression, neurotoxicity, nephrotoxicity, new primary malignancy, reproductive risk, requires an experienced clinician

DOSAGE AND ROUTES
Relapsing forms of multiple sclerosis
• **Adults:** Per os (PO) 1.75 mg/kg per treatment course divided into 2 cycles and given as divided doses of 1 or 2 tablets daily over 4 or 5 days for each cycle with second cycle starting 23 to 27 days after the last dose of the first cycle. Give a second course at least 43 wks after the last dose of the first course, second cycle for a cumulative dosage of 3.5 mg/kg. Max: 20 mg (2 tablets)/cycle day.

Active hairy-cell leukemia (orphan drug)
• **Adults:** Continuous infusion 0.09 mg/kg/day × 7 days.

Available forms: Tablet 10 mg, solution for injection 1 mg/mL

SIDE EFFECTS
CNS: Fatigue, fever, headache, neurotoxicity
HEMA: Anemia, neutropenia, thrombocytopenia, lymphopenia
GI: Nausea
GU: Nephrotoxicity
INTEG: Rash

Pharmacokinetics

Absorption	Inhibition of breast cancer resistance protein (BCRP) in the GI tract may increase oral bioavailability and systemic exposure
Distribution	Protein binding is 20%, crosses the blood-brain barrier

Metabolism	A substrate of BCRP, P-glycoprotein (P-gp), equilibrative nucleoside transporter 1 (ENT1), and concentrative nucleoside transporter 3 (CNT3, PO product is decreased by a high-fat meal excretion)
	Potent ENT1 or CNT3 inhibition may alter renal elimination
Half-life	1 day

Pharmacodynamics

Onset	Unknown
Peak	Unknown
Duration	Unknown

INTERACTIONS
Drug classifications:
• Do not use with live virus vaccines
• Immunosupressives: Duplicate effects, avoid using together
• Antiviral and antiretroviral drugs: Avoid concomitant use
• BCRP or ENT/CNT inhibitors: May alter bioavailability, avoid using together

NURSING CONSIDERATIONS
Assess:
• **PML:** Assess for new or worsening neurological, cognitive, or behavioral signs or symptoms, irreversible paraparesis and quadraparesis, may be more common in those who received continuous infusion at high doses (4 to 9 times the recommended dose for hairy-cell leukemia)

> **BLACK BOX WARNING: Bone marrow suppression:** Assess for neutropenia, anemia, thrombocytopenia; usually reversible and appears to be dose dependent. During the first 2 weeks after treatment initiation, mean platelet count, absolute neutrophil count (ANC), and HGB declines and then increases with normalization of mean counts by day 15, week 5 and week 8. Monitor hematologic parameters especially during the first 4 to 8 weeks after treatment

> **BLACK BOX WARNING: Secondary malignancies:** Monitor for secondary malignancies

> **BLACK BOX WARNING: Pregnancy/breastfeeding:** Assess if pregnancy is planned or suspected or if breastfeeding

Patient problem:
• Risk for injury (adverse reactions)

Implementation:
• Follow cytotoxic handling and disposal procedures
• Separate all other products by ≥3 hrs during the 4- or 5-day treatment cycles.
PO Route
• Use dry hands. Wash hands after use. Avoid prolonged contact with skin
• If a tablet is left on a surface, broken, or fragmented, wash the area with water
• Take without regard to meals, swallow whole with water immediately after removal from blister. Do not chew
IV Route
• Visually inspect for particulate matter and discoloration before use. A precipitate may occur during the exposure of injection to low temperatures; it may be resolubilized by allowing the solution to warm naturally to room temperature and by shaking vigorously. Do not heat or microwave the solution
• Use aseptic technique, does not contain preservative
• The concentrate for injection must be diluted before use, do not use dextrose 5% injection or benzyl alcohol in neonates, do not admix
Daily IV Infusion:
• Add the calculated single daily dose of the concentrate through a sterile 0.22-micrometer disposable hydrophilic syringe filter to a polyvinyl chloride infusion bag containing 500 mL of 0.9% sodium chloride injection. Prepare each solution daily. Discard any unused portion; vials are for single-use only. Once solutions are diluted, promptly administer or store at 2°C to 8°C for no more than 8 hrs before the start of administration
• Infuse continuously over 24 hrs
• Admixtures are stable for at least 24 hrs at room temperature under normal room fluorescent light in Baxter Viaflex PVC infusion containers.
Seven (7) Day IV Infusion:
• Calculate the dose for a 7-day period and withdraw from the concentrate for injection. Dilute in bacteriostatic 0.9% sodium chloride injection containing benzyl alcohol as a preservative. To minimize the risk of microbial contamination, first the calculated 7-day dose and then the amount of diluent needed to bring the total volume to 100 mL should be passed through a sterile 0.22-micrometer disposable hydrophilic syringe filter as each solution is being added to the infusion reservoir. After completing solution preparation, clamp off the

line, disconnect, and discard the filter. Aseptically aspirate air bubbles from the reservoir as necessary using the syringe and a dry second sterile filter or a sterile vent filter assembly. Reclamp the line, and discard the syringe and filter assembly.

• Discard any unused portion of injection; vials are for single-use only. Once solutions are diluted, promptly administer or store at 2°C to 8°C for no more than 8 hr before the start of administration

• Solutions prepared for individuals weighing more than 85 kg may have reduced preservative effectiveness due to greater dilution of the benzyl alcohol. Admixtures for the 7-day infusion have demonstrated acceptable chemical and physical stability for at least 7 days in the SIMS DELTEC MEDICATION CASSETTE RESERVOIR, Infuse continuously over 7 days

Patient/family education:
• Teach patient if a dose is missed, take the missed dose on the following day and extend the number of days in that treatment cycle. If 2 consecutive doses are missed, extend the treatment cycle by 2 days

---

BLACK BOX WARNING: Pregnancy/breastfeeding: Advise females of reproductive potential to use effective contraception during treatment with PO product and for at least 6 months after the last dose in each treatment course. Instruct women who are using systemic hormonal contraceptives to add a barrier method during PO product and for at least 4 wk after the last treatment. Advise male patients of reproductive potential to take precautions to prevent pregnancy of their partner during PO treatment and for at least 6 months after the last dose in each treatment course. Highly effective contraception is recommended during treatment with IV product

---

Evaluation
Therapeutic response
• Decrease in spread of malignancy, decreasing symptoms of multiple sclerosis

---

⚠ HIGH ALERT

darolutamide (Rx)
(dar'oh-loo'-tuh-mide)
Nubeqa
Func. class.: Antineoplastic, hormone

ACTION: Competitively inhibits androgen binding, AR nuclear translocation, and AR-mediated transcription

USES: Nonmetastatic castration-resistant prostate cancer

CONTRAINDICATIONS
Hypersensitivity

Precautions: Breastfeeding, pregnancy, hepatic disease, contraception requirements, renal disease

DOSAGE AND ROUTES
• **Adults per os (PO):** 600 mg bid until disease progression or unacceptable toxicity

Available forms: Tablets 300 mg

SIDE EFFECTS
CNS: Fatigue
GI: Elevated LFTs, hyperbilirubinemia, diarrhea, nausea
GU: Hot flashes
HEMA: Neutropenia, anemia
MS: MS pain
CV: Hyper-hypotension, heart failure
INTEG: Rash

Pharmacokinetics

Absorption	Food increases the bioavailability by 2- to 2.5-fold
Distribution	Protein binding (albumin) is 92% for darolutamide, 99.8% for the active metabolite, keto-darolutamide
Metabolism	CYP3A4, UGT1A9, and UGT1A1, a BCRP inhibitor, inhibits OATP1B1 and OATP1B3
Excretion	63.4% urine, 32.4% feces (30% unchanged)
Half-life	20 hrs

Pharmacodynamics

Onset	Unknown
Peak	Unknown
Duration	Unknown

INTERACTIONS
Avoid use with CYP3A4 , UGT1A9, UGT1A1

NURSING CONSIDERATIONS
Assess:
• **Prostate cancer:** Assess for decreasing signs/symptoms of prostate cancer
• **Hepatic/renal disease:** Monitor for hepatic and renal involvement
• **Pregnancy:** Males with female partners of reproductive potential should avoid

---

pregnancy and use effective contraception during and for at least 1 wk after treatment

Patient problem:
• Risk for injury (adverse reactions)

Implementation:
• Patient should be receiving a GnRH analog or should have had a bilateral orchiectomy
• Give with food
• Have the patient swallow the tablet whole. Do not crush or chew
• If a dose is missed, it should be taken as soon as the patient remembers before the next scheduled dose. Do not take 2 doses at the same time if a dose is missed

Patient/family education:
• **Pregnancy:** Teach patients with female partners of reproductive potential that they should avoid pregnancy and use effective contraception during and for at least 1 wk after treatment. There is a possibility of infertility

Evaluation
Positive therapeutic outcome
• Decreased progression of prostate cancer

diroximel
(dye-rox' i-mel)
Vumerity
Func. class: MS agent

USES
Relapsing multiple sclerosis

CONTRAINDICATIONS
Hypersensitivity

DOSAGE AND ROUTES
Adults: PO 231 mg bid for 7 days, then increase to 462 mg bid

dolutegravir/lamivudine
(doe-loo-leg' ra-vir la-mi' vyoo-deen)
Dovato
Func. class.: Antiretroviral/antiviral
Chem. class.: INST/NRTI

ACTION: Dolutegravir/lamivudine is active against infections caused by human immunodeficiency virus type 1 (HIV-1). Lamivudine is a nucleoside analog that works by inhibiting HIV reverse transcriptase, while dolutegravir works by inhibiting HIV integrase

USES: HIV-1 infection in adults

CONTRAINDICATIONS
Hypersensitivity

Precautions: Alcoholism, autoimmune disease, bone fractures, breastfeeding, children, depression, females, Graves' disease, Guillain-Barré syndrome, hepatic disease, hepatitis, hepatitis B and HIV coinfection, hepatitis C and HIV coinfection, hepatomegaly, HIV resistance, hypercholesterolemia, hyperlipidemia, hypertriglyceridemia, hypophosphatemia, immune reconstitution syndrome, lactic acidosis, obesity, osteomalacia, osteoporosis, pregnancy, renal failure, renal impairment, serious rash, suicidal ideation, torsades de pointes

> **BLACK BOX WARNING:** Hepatitis B exacerbation, hepatotoxicity

DOSAGE AND ROUTES
• **Adults who are treatment-naïve per os (PO):** One tablet (50 mg dolutegravir; 300 mg lamivudine) daily

Available forms: Tablet 50 mg – 300 mg

SIDE EFFECTS
CNS: Headache, abnormal dreams, depression, dizziness, *insomnia,* neuropathy, paresthesia, asthenia, fatigue, drowsiness
GI: *Nausea, vomiting, anorexia, diarrhea, abdominal pain, dyspepsia,* hepatomegaly with stenosis (may be fatal), hyperbilirubinemia, hypercholesterolemia, pancreatitis
GU: Glomerulonephritis membranous/mesangial proliferative
INTEG: *Rash,* skin discoloration
MS: Arthralgia, myalgia, rhabdomyolysis
RESP: *Cough*
SYST: Change in body fat distribution, lactic acidosis

THERAPEUTIC OUTCOME
Improvement in CD4, HIV RNC counts, decreasing signs and symptoms of HIV

PHARMACOKINETICS
Lamivudine:

Absorption	Unknown
Distribution	36% bound to plasma protein
Metabolism	Parent drug is not metabolized
Excretion	70% unchanged urine by active organic cationic secretion
Half-life	13-19 hrs

Dolutegravir:

Absorption	Unknown
Distribution	99% protein binding
Metabolism	Via UDP-glucuronosyltransferase (UGT)1A1 (major), CYP3A (minor)
Excretion	53% unchanged feces, urine 31%
Half-life	14 hrs

INTERACTIONS
Drug classifications: CYP3A4 inhibitors (aldesleukin IL-2, amiodarone, aprepitant, atazanavir, basiliximab, boceprevir, bromocriptine, chloramphenicol, clarithromycin, conivaptan, danazol, dalfopristin, darunavir, dasatinib, delavirdine, diltiazem, dronedarone, efavirenz, erythromycin, ethinyl estradiol, fluconazole, fluoxetine, fluvoxamine, fosamprenavir, fosaprepitant, imatinib, indinavir, isoniazid, itraconazole, ketoconazole, lanreotide, lapatinib, miconazole, nefazodone, nelfinavir, nicardipine, octreotide, posaconazole, quinine, ranolazine, rifaximin, tamoxifen, telaprevir, telithromycin, tipranavir, troleandomycin, verapamil, voriconazole, zafirlukast): Increased dolutegravir level

Metformin: Increased level

Dofetilide: Increased level, coadministration is contraindicated

Dolutegravir-carbamazepine, rifampin: Decreased level, an additional dolutegravir 50-mg dose should be taken

Dolutegravir-oxcarbazepine, phenytoin, phenobarbital: Avoid coadministration

Drug/Herb St. John's Wort: Decrease dolutegravir, avoid concurrent use

Drug/Lab Test
Increase: AST/ALT, amylase, bilirubin, CK, glucose, lipase

Decrease: Neutrophils

NURSING CONSIDERATIONS
Assess:
• **HIV infection:** Assess symptoms of HIV, including opportunistic infections, before and during treatment, some may be life threatening; monitor plasma CD4, CD8 cell counts, serum beta-2 microglobulin, and serum ICD 24 antigen levels, because treatment failures occur more often in those with baseline HIV-1 RNA concentrations (>100,000 copies/mL) than in those (<100,000 copies/mL); monitor blood glucose, CBC with differential, serum cholesterol, lipid panel

> **BLACK BOX WARNING**
> • Hepatotoxicity/lactic acidosis: Monitor hepatitis B serology, LFTs, plasma hepatitis C RNA, lactic acidosis levels. If lab reports confirm these conditions, discontinue product. More common in females or those who are overweight. Avoid use in alcoholism

> **BLACK BOX WARNING**
> • **Pregnancy:** Obtain pregnancy testing before use. Hepatitis B exacerbation: Those with coexisting HBV and HIV infections who discontinue this product may experience severe acute hepatitis B exacerbation, with some cases resulting in hepatic decompensation and hepatic failure. Patients coinfected with HBV and HIV who discontinue this product should have transaminase concentrations monitored q6wk for the first 3 months, and q3-6 months thereafter.

> **BLACK BOX WARNING**
> • Resumption of antihepatitis B treatment may be required. For patients who refuse a fully suppressive antiretroviral regimen but still require treatment for HBV, consider 48 wk of peginterferon alfa; do not administer HIV-active medications in the absence.

> **BLACK BOX WARNING**
> • Periodically monitor serum bilirubin (total and direct), serum creatinine, urinalysis, LFTs, amylase, lipase

Patient problem:
• Infection (uses)

Implementation:
• Give without regard to food
• During coadministration with carbamazepine or rifampin, the dolutegravir dose needs to be increased to 50 mg bid; add 50 mg/day of dolutegravir (separated by 12 hrs from dolutegravir/lamivudine)
• Avoid use in treatment-experienced patients and in patients with known substitutions associated with resistance to dolutegravir or lamivudine
• Do not use within 2 hrs before or 6 hrs after iron or calcium supplement. If coadministration is unavoidable, give the supplement and dolutegravir/lamivudine with food
• Do not use within 2 hrs before or 6 hrs after antacids, laxatives, or other medicines that contain aluminum, magnesium, sucralfate, or buffered medicines

Patient/family education:
- Teach patient that hepatitis and HIV coinfected patients should avoid consuming alcohol; offer vaccinations against hepatitis A/hepatitis B as appropriate
- Advise patient that GI complaints resolve after 2-3 wks of treatment
- Inform patient to report suspected or planned pregnancy, not to breastfeed. Instruct mothers with HIV-1 infection not to breastfeed because HIV-1 can be passed to the baby in the breast milk, inform patients that there is an antiretroviral pregnancy registry to monitor fetal outcomes
- Advise patient to take at the same time of day to maintain blood level, not to crush, break, or chew
- Inform patient that product controls the symptoms of HIV but does not cure, that patient is still able to infect others, that other products may be necessary to prevent other infections
- Lactic acidosis: Teach patient to notify prescriber of fatigue, muscle aches/pains, abdominal pain, difficulty breathing, nausea, vomiting, change in heart rhythm

BLACK BOX WARNING:
- **Hepatotoxicity:** Teach patient to notify prescriber of dark urine, yellowing skin or eyes, clay-colored stools, anorexia, nausea, vomiting

BLACK BOX WARNING:
- Teach patient to discuss with provider all Rx, over-the-counter (OTC), herbs, and supplements taken as there are many drug interactions

BLACK BOX WARNING:
- **Immune Reconstitution Syndrome:** Advise patients to inform their healthcare provider immediately of any signs and symptoms of infection as inflammation from previous infection may occur

BLACK BOX WARNING:
- Instruct patients that if they miss a dose to take it as soon as they remember, not to double their next dose or take more than the prescribed dose

Evaluation
Positive therapeutic outcome
- Improvement in CD4, HIV RNC counts, decreasing signs and symptoms of HIV

entrectinib (Rx)
(en-trex' tih-nib)
Rozlytrek
Func. class: Antineoplastic orphan drug
Chem. class: tyrosine kinase ROS1 inhibitor, tropomyosin receptor kinase (TRK) inhibitor

USES
ROS1-positive non–small cell lung cancer and *NTRK* gene fusion–positive solid tumors

CONTRAINDICATIONS
Hypersensitivity, pregnancy, breastfeeding

DOSAGE AND ROUTES
Adults: PO 600 mg daily until disease progression or unacceptable toxicity

⚠ HIGH ALERT
erdafitinib (Rx)
(er'-duh-fih'-tih-nib)
Balversa
Func. class.: Antineoplastic-kinase inhibitor
Chem. class.: Fibroblast growth factor receptor (FGFR) inhibitors

ACTION: Inhibits the enzymatic activity of FGFR1, FGFR2, FGFR3, and FGFR4

USES: Locally advanced or metastatic urothelial carcinoma

DOSAGE AND ROUTES
- **Adults per os (PO):** 8 mg daily initially, then after 14 to 21 days of treatment, increase the dose to 9 mg daily if the serum phosphate level is < 5.5 mg/dL and there are no ocular disorders or grade 2 or higher adverse reactions. Continue treatment until disease progression or unacceptable toxicity

Available forms: Tabs 3, 4, 5 mg

SIDE EFFECTS
GI: Abdominal pain, nausea, vomiting, anorexia, constipation, diarrhea
CNS: Fatigue, fever
EENT: Stomatitis, blurred vision, retinal detachment
INTEG: Rash, nail discoloration
META: Hyperglycemia, hyper-hypophosphatemia, hypomagnesemia, hyponatremia, hypoalbuminemia
HEMA: Leukopenia, anemia, thrombocytopenia
SYST: Infection

THERAPEUTIC OUTCOME
Decreased spread of cancer

PHARMACOKINETICS

Absorption	Unknown
Distribution	99.8% protein bound to alpha-1-acid glycoprotein
Metabolism	CYP2C9 (39%) and CYP3A4 (20%); an inhibitor of OCT2
Excretion	69% feces (19% unchanged), 19% urine (13% unchanged)
Half-life	59 hrs

Pharmacodynamics

Onset	Unknown
Peak	2.5 hrs
Duration	Unknown

INTERACTIONS
Avoid use with CYP3A4 inducers, inhibitors

NURSING CONSIDERATIONS
Assess:
• **Ocular disease:** Provide dry eye prophylaxis with ocular demulcents as needed. Perform monthly ophthalmological examinations during the first 4 months of treatment and every 3 months thereafter, and urgently at any time for visual disturbance; examinations should include an assessment of visual acuity, slit lamp examination, fundoscopy, and optical coherence tomography. An interruption of therapy, discontinuation of therapy, or dose reduction may be necessary for ocular adverse reactions
• **Infection:** Assess for infection (fever, flu-like symptoms)
• Avoid coadministration with agents that alter serum phosphate levels before the initial dose increase period (days 14 to 21), monitor phosphate levels monthly for hyperphosphatemia and follow dose modification guidelines when required. In patients with hyperphosphatemia, restrict phosphate intake to 600 mg to 800 mg daily. If serum phosphate is above 7 mg/dL, consider adding an oral phosphate binder until the serum phosphate level returns to less than 5.5 mg/dL.
• **Pregnancy/breastfeeding:** Pregnancy should be avoided during and for at least 1 month after the last dose, obtain pregnancy testing before use

Patient problem:
• Risk for injury (uses)

Implementation:
• Swallow tablets whole, with or without food
• If vomiting occurs, do not replace the dose; the next dose should be taken the next day

• If a dose is missed, it can be taken as soon as possible on the same day; do not take extra tablets to make up for the missed dose. Resume the regular daily schedule the next day

Patient/family education:
• Counsel patients about the reproductive risk and contraception requirements during treatment. Men with female partners of reproductive potential should also use effective contraception during treatment and for 1 month after the last dose. Teach patient not to breastfeed during and for 1 month after last dose
• Teach patient that ophthalmic exams will be needed periodically

Evaluation
Positive therapeutic outcome
• Decreased progression of cancer

---

esketamine (Rx)
(es- ket′ a- meen)
Spravato nasal spray
Func. class.: Antidepressant
Chem. class.: Augmentation agent
Controlled substance III

ACTION: Noncompetitively blocks the NMDA receptor, which is an ionotropic glutamate receptor. The mechanism of action for antidepressant effect is unknown; however, the activity on NMDA receptors may be responsible for both the therapeutic and the adverse psychiatric effects

USES: Treatment-resistant depression in adults with an oral antidepressant

CONTRAINDICATIONS
Aneurysm, arteriovenous malformation, intracranial bleeding, ketamine hypersensitivity

Precautions: Alcoholism, breastfeeding, cardiac disease, cerebrovascular disease, coadministration with other central nervous system (CNS) depressants, driving or operating machinery, encephalopathy, geriatrics, hepatic disease, hypertension, hypertensive crisis, loss of consciousness, pregnancy, psychosis, schizophrenia

> **BLACK BOX WARNING:** Children, CNS depression, dissociation, requires a specialized care setting, substance abuse, suicidal ideation

DOSAGE AND ROUTES
• **Adults NASAL: INDUCTION PHASE:** On day 1, give 56 mg. For subsequent doses during wks 1 through 4, give 56 mg or 84 mg twice per wk. Use 2 devices for the 56 mg dose and 3 devices for the 84 mg dose with a 5-min rest between use of each device. **MAINTENANCE PHASE:** During

---

weeks 5 through 8, give 56 mg or 84 mg weekly. During week 9 and thereafter, give 56 mg or 84 mg q2wk or weekly.

Available forms: Nasal spray 56, 84 dose kit

SIDE EFFECTS

CNS: Anxiety, dissociation, drowsiness, dizziness, headache, vertigo, dependence, impaired cognition, hallucinations, confusion, lethargy, suicidal ideation
CV: Hypertension, hypertensive crisis
GI: Nausea

THERAPEUTIC OUTCOME

Decreased depression, increased sense of well-being

Pharmacokinetics

Absorption	48%
Distribution	Unknown
Metabolism	Metabolized to noresketamine, the active metabolite, by CYP2B6 and CYP3A4, lesser extent by CYP2C9 and CYP2C19 through glucuronidation
Excretion	Metabolites are excreted in urine (78%) and feces (2%)
Half-life	7-12 hrs

Pharmacodynamics

Onset	Unknown
Peak	20-40 mins
Duration	Unknown

INTERACTIONS

> **BLACK BOX WARNING:** CNS depression- other CNS depressants: Increased-CNS depression, do not use together

MAOIs, psychostimulants: Increased-sedation, B/P, do not use together

NURSING CONSIDERATIONS
Assess:

> **BLACK BOX WARNING: Dissociation:**
> Monitor patient for at least 2 hrs after each treatment session, then provide an assessment to determine when the patient is stable and ready to leave the healthcare setting. Special care is needed with those with schizophrenia

> **BLACK BOX WARNING: Substance abuse:**
> Monitor for signs of abuse or dependence. Physical dependence has been reported with prolonged use of ketamine. Withdrawal symptoms of ketamine include cravings, fatigue, poor appetite, and anxiety

> **BLACK BOX WARNING: Suicidal ideation:**
> Behavior should be closely monitored during treatment. Consider that the therapeutic regimen may need changing, including discontinuing esketamine and/or the concurrent oral antidepressant in patients with worsening of depression or emergent suicidality

Patient problem:
• Suicidal ideation (uses, adverse reactions)

Implementation:
Nasal route
• Must be given under the direct supervision of a healthcare provider and include supervised postadministration observation
• Each device contains 28 mg; use 2 devices for a 56 mg dose and 3 devices for an 84 mg dose with a 5-min rest between use of each device
• To prevent loss of medication, do not prime the device before use
• During and after use at each treatment session, observe the patient for at least 2 hrs until the patient is safe to leave
• Assess B/P before use. If baseline B/P is systolic greater than 140 mm Hg or diastolic greater than 90 mm Hg, do not use if an increase in B/P or intracranial pressure poses a serious risk
• Reassess B/P about 40 min after dosing and subsequently as clinically indicated. If B/P is decreasing and the patient appears clinically stable for at least 2 hrs, the patient may be discharged at the end of the postdose monitoring period; if not, continue to monitor
• Due to the potential for drug-induced nausea and vomiting, advise patients to avoid food for at least 2 hrs before use and avoid liquids at least 30 min before administration
• Patients requiring a nasal corticosteroid or nasal decongestant on dosing day should use these at least 1 hr before receiving this product
• If treatment sessions are missed and there is a worsening of depression symptoms, consider returning to the previous dosing schedule

Patient/family education:

> **BLACK BOX WARNING: Suicidal ideation:**
> Teach family members or caregivers to monitor for changes in behavior and to alert the healthcare provider if such behaviors occur

> **BLACK BOX WARNING: CNS depression:** Tell healthcare provider about all the Rx, over-the-counter (OTC), vitamins, and herbal supplements used, and don't use with other CNS depressants unless discussed with healthcare provider

- Before use instruct patients not to engage in potentially hazardous activities (driving, operating heavy machinery) until the next day after a restful sleep
- How to use:
  - Step 1: Instruct patient to blow nose before the first device use only. Confirm the required number of devices (56 mg = 2 devices; 84 mg = 3 devices)
  - Step 2: Check expiration date. Peel blister and remove device. Do not prime the device - this will cause loss of medication. Ensure that the indicator on the device shows 2 green dots. Give device to patient
  - Step 3: Instruct patient to hold device with thumb gently supporting but not pressing the plunger as shown in the product labeling. The patient should recline head at about 45 degrees during administration to keep medication in nose
  - Step 4: Instruct patient as follows: insert tip straight into the first nostril (the nose rest should touch the skin between the nostrils); close the opposite nostril; breathe in through nose while pushing plunger all the way up until it stops; sniff gently after spraying to keep medication inside nose; switch hands to insert tip into the second nostril; repeat steps to deliver second spray
  - Step 5: After administration is complete, take the device from the patient. Check that indicator on device shows no green dots. If green dot remains, have patient spray again into the second nostril. Instruct patient to rest comfortably (preferably semireclined) for 5 min after each device is used. If liquid drips out, dab nose with a tissue. DO NOT blow nose. If a second device is required, ensure a 5-min waiting period before use to allow medication from first device to be absorbed.
- **Pregnancy/breastfeeding:** Identify if pregnancy is planned or suspected or if breastfeeding; if patient is pregnant she should register with the National Pregnancy Registry for Antidepressants online at https://womensmentalhealth.org/clinical-and-research-programs/pregnancyregistry/antidepressants/ or by calling 1-844-405-6185

Evaluation
Positive therapeutic outcome
- Decreasing depression

fam-trastuzumab deruxtecan-nxki
Enhertu
Func. class.: Antineoplastic, *HER2*-directed antibody

USES: *HER2* breast cancer

DOSAGE AND ROUTES
Adult: Intermittent IV Infusion 5.4 mg/kg once q3wk (21-day cycle) until disease progression or unacceptable toxicity

CONTRAINDICATIONS
Hypersensitivity

fedratinib (Rx)
(fed-ra' ti-nib)
Inrebic
Func. class.: Antineoplastic

USES: Intermediate-2 or high-risk primary or secondary (post-polycythemia vera or post-essential thrombocythemia) myelofibrosis, orphan drug

CONTRAINDICATIONS
Hypersensitivity, encephalopathy, thiamine deficiency

DOSAGE AND ROUTES
Adults PO 400 mg q day in patients with a baseline platelet count of 50×10^9 cells/L or greater

istradefylline (Rx)
(iz-tra' de-fye' leen)
Nourianz
Func. class.: Anti-Parkinson Agent
Chem. class.: Adenosine receptor antagonist

ACTION: An adenosine A_{2A} receptor antagonist that acts through a nondopaminergic mechanism to improve motor function

USES: Adjuvant treatment for patients with Parkinson disease experiencing "off" episodes

CONTRAINDICATIONS
Hypersensitivity

Precautions: Behavioral changes, breastfeeding, children, contraception requirements, dyskinesia, geriatric, hepatic disease, impulse control symptoms, infants, pregnancy, psychosis, reproductive risk, tobacco smoking

DOSAGE AND ROUTES
• **Adults per os (PO):** 20 mg daily. Adjust the dose based on response and tolerability. Max: 40 mg daily; if patient smokes 20 or more cigarettes per day, use 40 mg daily

Available forms: Tabs 20, 40 mg

SIDE EFFECTS
CNS: *Dyskinesia,* psychosis, dizziness, hallucinations, insomnia
GI: Nausea, constipation

THERAPEUTIC OUTCOME
Decreasing symptoms of Parkinson disease

PHARMACOKINETICS

Absorption	Unknown
Distribution	Protein binding 98%
Metabolism	CYP1A1,CYP3A4, with a minor contribution from CYP1A2, CYP2B6, CYP2C8, CYP2C9, CYP2C18, and CYP2D6 to metabolites
Excretion	Urine (39%), feces (48%)
Half-life	83 hrs

Pharmacodynamics

Onset	Unknown
Peak	4 hrs (fasting), increased with high fat meal
Duration	Unknown

INTERACTIONS
Drug classifications:
• Strong CYP3A4 inhibitors (ketoconazole, itraconazole, clarithromycin): Increased -istradefylline effect, max 20 mg daily
• Strong CYP3A4 inducers (carbamazepine, rifampin, phenytoin, rifampin): Decreased-istradefylline effect, avoid using together

Drug/Herb
• St. John's Wort, avoid using together

NURSING CONSIDERATIONS
Assess:
• Parkinson disease: Assess for decreasing "off episodes," tremors usually first appearing in hands/feet while at rest, slow movement, rigidity, postural instability, problems with speech and voice, incontinence, difficulty swallowing, inability to start movements or continue repeated movement, excessive sweating, constipation, dry skin, or mood changes
• Dyskinesia: Assess for grimacing, eye blinking, lip smacking, repetitive movements,. These should lessen with treatment

• Hallucinations/psychosis/impulse control/compulsive behaviors: Assess for these effects, and if present decreasing dose or discontinuing treatment may be necessary
• Monitor LFTs in hepatic disease

Patient problem:
• Impaired mobility (uses)

Implementation:
• May give without regard to meals

Patient/family education:
• Identify if tobacco is used and if so, how much per day. Dosage change may be needed
• Identify all Rx, over-the-counter (OTC), herbals, supplements that are used and discuss with healthcare provider
• Pregnancy/breastfeeding: Identify if pregnancy is planned or suspected or if breastfeeding. Use in pregnancy is not recommended; adequate contraception should be used in women of child-bearing age

Evaluation
Positive therapeutic outcome
• Decreasing symptoms of Parkinson disease

lasmiditan
(las-mid' i- tan)
Reyvow
Func. class.: Antimigraine

USES
Migraine with or without aura in adults

CONTRAINDICATIONS
Hypersensitivity

DOSAGE AND ROUTES
Adults PO 50, 100, or 200 mg as a single dose; max: 1 dose in 24 hr

Lumateperone
(Luma-tep'-erone)
Caplyta

USES: Schizophrenia

DOSAGE AND ROUTES
Adult: PO 42 mg/day

CONTRAINDICATIONS
Hypersensitivity

BLACK BOX WARNING: Dementia-related psychosis

meropenem/vaborbactam (Rx)

(mer-oh-pen'em/va bor bak' tam)
Vabomere
Func. class.: Antiinfective—miscellaneous
Chem. class.: Carbapenem

ACTION: Bactericidal; interferes with cell wall replication of susceptible organisms

USES: For the treatment of complicated urinary tract infections caused by *Citrobacter* freundii, *Citrobacter koseri*, *Enterobacter aerogenes*, *Enterobacter cloacae*, *Escherichia coli*, *Klebsiella oxytoca*, *Klebsiella pneumoniae*, *Morganella morganii*, *Proteus mirabilis*, *Providencia* spp., *Pseudomonas aeruginosa*, *Serratia marcescens*

Pharmacokinetics

Distribution	Protein binding 2% (meropenem), 33% (vaborbactam)
Metabolism	Meropenem is a substrate of OAT1 and OAT3 transporters, use after hemodialysis
Excretion	Kidneys
Half-life	1.22 hr (meropenem), 1.68 hr (vaborbactam)

Pharmacodynamics

Onset, peak, duration   Unknown

CONTRAINDICATIONS

Hypersensitivity to this product, carbapenems

Precautions: Pregnancy, breastfeeding, geriatric patients, renal disease, seizure disorder, gram-negative infection, pneumonia, hypersensitivity to cephalosporins, penicillins

DOSAGE AND ROUTES
Complicated urinary tract infection (UTI), including pyelonephritis
Adult: **IV:** 4 g (2 g meropenem and 2 g vaborbactam) q8hr for up to 14 days

Renal dose
Adult: IV; eGFR 50 ml/min/1.73 m^2 or more: No change; eGFR 30 to 49 ml/min/1.73 m^2: 2 g (1 g meropenem and 1 g vaborbactam) q8hr; eGFR 15 to 29 ml/min/1.73 m^2: 2 g (1 g meropenem and 1 g vaborbactam) q12hr; eGFR less than 15 ml/min/1.73 m^2: 1 g (0.5 g meropenem and 0.5 g vaborbactam) q12hr

Intermittent hemodialysis: Meropenem and vaborbactam are removed by hemodialysis, give appropriate renal dose of meropenem; vaborbactam after hemodialysis

Available forms: Powder for injection 2 g
ADVERSE EFFECTS
CNS: Seizures, dizziness, weakness, headache, insomnia, agitation, confusion, drowsiness

CV: Hypotension, tachycardia

ENDO: Hypoglycemia

GI: Diarrhea, nausea, vomiting, pseudomembranous colitis, hepatitis, glossitis, jaundice

INTEG: Rash, urticaria, pruritus, pain at inj site, phlebitis, erythema at inj site

RESP: Dyspnea, hyperventilation, cough, sputum

SYST: Anaphylaxis, Stevens-Johnson syndrome, angioedema

INTERACTIONS
Individual drugs
Probenecid: Increased meropenem levels
Valproic acid: Increased effect of this agent

Drug/lab test
Increase: AST, ALT, LDH, BUN, alk phos, bilirubin, creatinine
Decrease: Prothrombin time
False positive: Direct Coomb's test

NURSING CONSIDERATIONS
Assessment
• Assess for sensitivity to carbapenem antibiotics, penicillins, cephalosporins
• **Renal disease:** Lower dose may be required; monitor serum creatinine/BUN sodium, before, during therapy
• **CDAD:** Assess bowel pattern daily; if severe diarrhea, abdominal pain, fatigue occurs, product should be discontinued
• **Infection:** Assess temperature, sputum, characteristics of wound before, during, and after treatment
• **Allergic reactions, anaphylaxis:** Assess for rash, laryngeal edema, wheezing, urticaria, pruritus; may occur immediately or several days after therapy begins; identify if there has been hypersensitivity to penicillins, cephalosporins, beta-lactams, cross-sensitivity may occur
• **Seizures:** May occur in those with brain lesions, seizure disorder, bacterial meningitis, or renal disease; stop product and notify prescriber if seizures occur
• **Overgrowth of infection:** Assess for perineal itching, fever, malaise, redness, pain, swelling, drainage, rash, diarrhea, change in cough, sputum

Patient problems
Infection (uses)

Implementation
IV route
• Visually inspect for particulate matter and discoloration before use
Reconstitution
• Constitute the appropriate number of vials as needed for the dose
• 2 vials are used for 4 g (2 g meropenem and 2 g vaborbactam) dose
• 1 vial is used for 2 g (1 g meropenem and 1 g vaborbactam) or 1 g (0.5 g meropenem and 0.5 g vaborbactam) doses
• Withdraw 20 ml of 0.9% sodium chloride Injection from an infusion bag and constitute each vial
• For 4 g (2 g meropenem and 2 g vaborbactam) dose/250 to 1000 ml
• For 2 g (1 g meropenem and 1 g vaborbactam) dose/125 to 500 ml
• For 1 g (0.5 g meropenem and 0.5 g vaborbactam) dose 70 to 250 ml
• Mix gently to dissolve. The constituted solution is concentrations of 0.05 g/ml meropenem and 0.05 g/ml vaborbactam; the final volume is 21.3 ml
• Further dilute before use; do not use by direct injection
Dilution
• Withdraw the full or partial constituted vial contents from each vial and add back into the 0.9% sodium chloride Injection infusion bag
• The final concentration of meropenem and vaborbactam will be between 2 and 8 mg/ml
• *Storage:* Complete infusion within 4 hr if stored at room temperature or 22 hr if refrigerated at 2 to 8° C (36 to 46° F)

Intermittent IV infusion
• Give over 3 hr

Patient/family education
• **CDAD:** Teach patient to report severe diarrhea
• Advise patient to report sore throat, bruising, bleeding, joint pain, may indicate blood dyscrasias (rare)
• Teach patient to report overgrowth of infection: Black furry tongue, vaginal itching, foul-smelling stools

Evaluation
Positive therapeutic outcome
• Negative C&S; absence of symptoms and signs of infection

pexidartinib (Rx)
(pex'-i-dar'-ti-nib)
Turalio
Func. class.: Antineoplastic-orphan drug
Chem. class.: Colony stimulating factor-1 receptor (CSF-1R) inhibitor

USES: Symptomatic tenosynovial giant cell tumor

CONTRAINDICATIONS
Hypersensitivity, pregnancy, breastfeeding

> **BLACK BOX WARNING:** Hepatotoxicity

DOSAGE AND ROUTE
Adults PO 400 mg bid on an empty stomach until disease progression

polatuzumab vedotin (Rx)
(poh'lah-too'zoo-mab veh-doh'-tin)
Polivy
Func. class.: Antineoplastic

USES: Relapsed or refractory diffuse large B-cell lymphoma (DLBCL) following at least 2 prior therapies, in combination with bendamustine and rituximab, orphan drug

CONTRAINDICATIONS
Hypersensitivity, pregnancy, breastfeeding

DOSAGE AND ROUTES
• Adults: Intravenous (IV) 1.8 mg/kg on day 1 in combination with bendamustine 90 mg/m^2 IV on days 1 and 2 and rituximab 375 mg/m^2 IV on day 1 repeated q21 days for 6 cycles; premedicate with an antihistamine and antipyretic 30 to 60 min before use

ramucirumab
(ra-mue-sir' ue-mab)
Cyramza
Func. class.: Antineoplastic
Chem. class.: Vascular endothelial growth factor antagonist

ACTION: Binds to vascular endothelial growth factor receptor 2 (VEGFR2; kinase insert domain-containing receptor [KDR]), preventing the binding of ligands. As a result, ramucirumab inhibits ligand-induced proliferation, and migration of human endothelial cells.

Therapeutic outcome: Decreased progression of cancer

USES: Advanced or metastatic gastric or gastro-esophageal cancer after fluoropyrimidine- or platinum-containing chemotherapy; non-small cell lung cancer (NSCLC) with disease progression on or after platinum-based chemotherapy, in combination with docetaxel; metastatic colorectal cancer after prior therapy with bevacizumab, oxaliplatin, and a fluoropyrimidine, in combination with irinotecan, folinic acid (leucovorin), and fluorouracil (FOLFIRI); advanced hepatocellular cancer in patients with an alpha-fetoprotein (AFP) of 400 ng/mL or more and who have previously been treated with sorafenib

Pharmacokinetics

Absorption	Unknown
Distribution	Unknown
Metabolism	Unknown
Excretion	Unknown
Half-life	14 days

Pharmacodynamics

Onset	Unknown
Peak	Unknown
Duration	Unknown

CONTRAINDICATIONS

Hypersensitivity, pregnancy, breastfeeding

Precautions: Anticoagulant therapy, bleeding, cirrhosis, MI, contraception requirements, GI perforation, hepatic disease, human anti-human antibody (HAHA), hypertension, hypothyroidism, infusion-related reactions, renal disease, stroke, surgery

DOSAGE AND ROUTES

For the treatment of gastric cancer or gastro-esophageal junction adenocarcinoma

Adults IV Infusion 8 mg/kg over 60 min q 2 wk until disease progression or unacceptable toxicity. If the first infusion is tolerated, all subsequent infusions may be administered over 30 min.

For the treatment of non-small cell lung cancer (NSCLC)

Adult IV Infusion: 10 mg/kg over 60 min with docetaxel (75 mg/m^2 IV) on day 1, q 21 days until disease progression or unacceptable toxicity.

For the treatment of metastatic colorectal cancer (mCRC)

Adult IV 8 mg/kg IV over 60 min on day 1 prior to FOLFIRI use, q 2 wk until disease progression

or unacceptable toxicity. FOLFIRI consists of irinotecan 180 mg/m^2 IV over 90 min and folinic acid (leucovorin) 400 mg/m^2 given with over 120 min on day 1, followed by fluorouracil 400 mg/m^2 IV bolus over 2 to 4 min on day 1, followed by fluorouracil 2,400 mg/m^2 by continuous IV infusion over 46 to 48 hr. If the first infusion is tolerated, all subsequent infusions may be given over 30 min.

For the treatment of hepatocellular cancer

Adult IV Infusion 8 mg/kg over 60 min q 2 wk until disease progression or unacceptable toxicity. If the first infusion is tolerated, all subsequent infusions may be administered over 30 min.

Hepatic dose

Adult IV mild to moderate hepatic impairment (Child-Pugh A; total bilirubin 1.1 to 3 times the upper limit of normal [ULN] and any AST, OR, or total bilirubin within ULN and AST greater than ULN): no change; severe hepatic impairment (Child-Pugh B or C): use only if the potential benefits outweigh the risks

Available forms: Injection 10 mg/mL single dose vial

SIDE EFFECTS

CNS: Headache, fatigue RPLS
CV: Hypertension, arterial thromboembolic events, hemorrhage
EENT: Epistaxis
GI: Intestinal obstruction, diarrhea
GU: Proteinuria
HEMA: Neutropenia, anemia
INTEG: Rash
MISC: Hypothyroidism, hyponatremia, IRR, antibody formation, infusion site reactions, poor wound healing

INTERACTIONS:
Drug classifications

Anticoagulants, NSAIDs, antiplatelets: Increased bleeding risk

Drug/lab test
Increase: Urine protein
Decrease: RBCs, serum sodium

NURSING CONSIDERATIONS
Assess

• **Bleeding/hemorrhage:** Assess for GI bleeding, perforation (severe abdominal pain, nausea, vomiting, fever) may be fatal; discontinue and do not restarts if this occurs.
• **Poor wound healing**: Assess all wounds for changes, avoid use if present.

• **Hypertension:** Monitor B/P frequently at least q 2 wk; if hypertension occurs, withhold until controlled
• **RPLS:** Assess for hypertension, blurred vision, impaired consciousness, seizures, headache; may be confirmed with MRI; discontinue and do not restart if confirmed
• **ATE:** Assess for serious cardiac events including MI and stroke, and discontinue permanently if these occur.
• **Pregnancy/breastfeeding:** Do not use in pregnancy; women should use adequate contraception during and for $\geq$ 3 months after last dose; if childbearing potential, do not breastfeed

Patient problem
Risk for injury (adverse reactions)

Implementation:
Intermittent IV infusion route
• Use cytotoxic handling precautions.
• Premedicate with an IV histamine-1 (H1) receptor antagonist (diphenhydramine); for patients who have had a prior grade 1 or 2 infusion-related reaction, premedicate with an H1-receptor antagonist, dexamethasone (or equivalent), and acetaminophen prior to each infusion.
• Dilute with normal saline to a final volume of 250 mL, invert to mix, do not shake; stable for 4 hr at room temperature.
• Inspect for particles and discoloration before using.
• Use a protein-sparing 0.22 micron filter, use separate line, flush with normal saline after use.
• Do not admix with other solutions or medications.
• Store vials in refrigerator, protect from light, do not freeze.

Patient/family education
• **Bleeding:** Teach patient that bleeding may occur, to contact provider for bleeding.
• **Poor wound healing**: Teach patient to report wound changes, to discuss with all providers use of product.
• **Hypertension:** Teach patient to monitor B/P frequently at least q 2 wk; if high or if headache is present, notify provider.
• **RPLS:** Assess for hypertension, blurred vision, impaired consciousness, seizures, headache; may be confirmed with MRI; discontinue and do not restart if confirmed
• **Pregnancy/breastfeeding:** Identify if pregnancy is planned or suspected; do not use in pregnancy; use adequate contraception during and for $\geq$ 3 months after last dose, if childbearing potential; do not breastfeed; product may impair fertility

Evaluation
Positive therapeutic outcome
• Decreased progression of cancer

ravulizumab
(rav'-yoo-liz'-yoo-mab)
Ultomiris
Func. class.:

USES: Atypical hemolytic uremic syndrome in adults and pediatrics

CONTRAINDICATIONS
Hypersensitivity

DOSAGE AND ROUTES
Treat for at least 6 months
Adults $\geq$ 100 kg: **IV** 3,000 mg load, then 3,600 mg q8wk starting 2 wk after loading dose
Adults 60 to 99 kg: **IV** 2,700 mg load, then 3,300 mg q8wk starting 2 wk after loading dose
Adults 40 to 59 kg: **IV** 2,400 mg load, then 3,000 mg q8wk starting 2 wk after loading dose
Adolescents $\geq$ 100 kg: **IV** 3,000 mg load, then 3,600 mg q8wk starting 2 wk after the loading dose
Children and adolescents 60 to 99 kg: **IV** 2,700 mg load, then 3,300 mg q8wk starting 2 wk after loading dose
Children and adolescents 40 to 59 kg: **IV** 2,400 mg load, then 3,000 mg q8wk starting 2 wk after loading dose
Children and adolescents 30 to 39 kg: **IV** 1,200 mg load, then 2,700 mg qy 8 wk starting 2 wk after loading dose
Children 20 to 29 kg: **IV** 900 mg load, then 2,100 mg q8wk starting 2 wk after the loading dose
Infants and children 10 to 19 kg: **IV** 600 mg load, then 600 mg q4wk starting 2 wk after loading dose
Infants and children 5 to 9 kg: **IV** 600 mg load, then 300 mg q4wk starting 2 wk after loading dose.

risankizumab (Rx)
(ris' an- kiz' ue- mab)
Skyrizi
Func. class: Systemic Antipsoriasis Agents

ACTION: A humanized immunoglobulin G1 (IgG1) monoclonal antibody that selectively binds to the p19 subunit of human interleukin-23 (IL-23), thereby inhibiting its interaction with the IL-23 receptor. Human IL-23 is a naturally occurring cytokine involved in inflammatory and immune responses. By blocking IL-23 from binding to its receptor, it prevents the release of proinflammatory cytokines and chemokines.

USES
Moderate to severe plaque psoriasis

Pharmacokinetics

Absorption	89%
Distribution	Unknown
Metabolism	Unknown
Excretion	Unknown
Half-life	Unknown

Pharmacodynamics

Onset	Unknown
Peak	3 to 14 days
Duration	Unknown

CONTRAINDICATIONS
Hypersensitivity

Precautions
Pregnancy, breastfeeding, TB, infection, immunosuppression

DOSAGE AND ROUTES
Adults subcut 150 mg (two 75 mg injections) at wk 0 and 4, and q 12 wk thereafter

Available forms: Prefilled syringe solution for injection 75 mg/0.83 mL 2-pack

INTERACTIONS
Avoid use with live virus vaccines.

NURSING CONSIDERATIONS
Assessment:
• **Plaque psoriasis:** Assess for red, raised, inflamed patches of skin; whitish-silver scales or plaques on the red patches; dry skin that may crack and bleed; soreness around patches; itching and burning sensations around patches; thick, pitted nails; painful, swollen joints.
• Assess for inj site pain, swelling, redness, usually occur after 2 inj (4-5 days); use cold compress to relieve pain/swelling.
• **Infections:** Assess for fever, flulike symptoms, dyspnea, change in urination, redness/swelling around any wounds; stop treatment if present; some serious infections, including sepsis, may occur; patients with active infections should not be started on this product.
• Latent TB before therapy; treat before starting this product.

Patient problem
Impaired skin integrity (uses)

Implementation
Subcut route
• Keep in the original carton to protect from light until time of use.
• Do not shake the carton or prefilled syringe.
• Prior to use, allow to reach room temperature out of direct sunlight (15 to 30 min). Do not use other methods to speed the warming process.
• Visually inspect parenteral products for particulate matter and discoloration. The solution should be clear to slightly opalescent, colorless to slightly yellow. The solution may contain a few translucent white particles.
• Do not use if: solution contains large particles or is cloudy or discolored; solution has been frozen; syringe has been dropped or damaged; syringe tray seal is broken or missing.
• Only an individual trained in subcutaneous drug delivery should administer the injection. An adult who is properly trained in injection technique may self-inject; the first injection needs to be under the supervision of a qualified health care professional.
• Wash and dry hands.
• Select an injection site, right or left thigh or abdomen (at least 2 inches from the navel) and wipe with an alcohol swab. Do not inject into skin that is tender, bruised, red, hard, or affected by psoriasis. Do not inject into a scar or stretch mark. Administer the injections at different sites at least 1 inch apart.
• Remove the needle cover from the first prefilled syringe.
• With one hand, gently pinch the cleaned injection site. Use the other hand to insert the needle at a 45-degree angle using a quick short movement.
• Slowly push the plunger until all the solution is injected.
• Pull the needle out of the skin. Release the plunger and allow the prefilled syringe to move up until the entire needle is covered by the needle guard.
• Apply a cotton ball or gauze pad over the injection site for 10 seconds. Do not rub the injection site.
• To obtain the full dose, repeat the injection process using the second prefilled syringe. Select and cleanse an alternative injection site that is at least 1 inch away from the first site; do not inject into the same site as the first syringe.
• If a dose is missed, administer the dose as soon as possible, then resume dosing at the regular schedule.

Patient/family education
• Teach patient about self-administration if appropriate: inj should be made in thigh,

abdomen, upper arm; rotate sites at least 1 inch from old site; do not inject in areas that are bruised, red, hard.

• Inform patient to refrigerate in the container in which the product was received and to dispose of needles and equipment as instructed.

• Teach patient that if medication is not taken when due, inject dose as soon as remembered and inject next dose as scheduled.

• Advise patient not to take any live virus vaccines during treatment.

Teach patient to report signs of infection, allergic reaction, or TB immediately.

Evaluation
Positive therapeutic outcome
• Decreasing plaques and painful, swollen joints

romosozumab-aqqg (Rx)
(roe′ moe-soz′ ue-mab)
Evenity
Func. class.: Monoclonal antibody

USES
Osteoporosis in postmenopausal women at high risk for fracture

CONTRAINDICATIONS:
Hypersensitivity, hypocalcemia, pregnancy

DOSAGE AND ROUTES
Adult females Subcut 210 mg q monthly x 12 months

selinexor
(sel-ih-nex′-or)
Xpovio
Func. class.: Antineoplastic
Chem class.: Small molecule antineoplastic nuclear export inhibitor

USES
Multiple myeloma in those who have received at least 4 prior therapies and who are refractory to at least 2 proteasome inhibitors, at least 2 immunomodulatory agents, and an anti-CD38 monoclonal antibody, in combination with dexamethasone

CONTRAINDICATIONS
Hypersensitivity, pregnancy, breastfeeding

DOSAGE AND ROUTES
Adults PO 80 mg in combination with dexamethasone 20 mg orally on days 1 and 3 of each week; repeat weekly until disease progression or unacceptable toxicity

solriamfetol (Rx)
(sol′ ri- am′ fe-tol)
Sunosi
Func. class.: Narcolepsy agents
Chem. class: Dopamine norepinephrine reuptake inhibitor
Controlled substance IV

ACTION: Unknown; action may be due to its inhibitor of a dopamine and norepinephrine reuptake

Therapeutic outcome: Ability to stay awake

USES: Excessive daytime sleepiness due to narcolepsy or obstructive sleep apnea

Pharmacokinetics

Absorption	
Distribution	Protein binding <20%
Metabolism	Minimal
Excretion	95% unchanged, urine
Half-life	7.1 hr

Pharmacodynamics

Onset	Unknown
Peak	1.2-3 hr
Duration	Unknown

CONTRAINDICATIONS
Hypersensitivity, MAOIs

Precautions
Alcoholism, bipolar disorder, cardiac disease, breastfeeding, diabetes mellitus, geriatrics, heart failure, hepatic disease, hypertension, MI, pregnancy, renal disease, schizophrenia, stroke, substance abuse, valvular heart disease, ventricular dysfunction

DOSAGE AND ROUTES
Narcolepsy
Adults PO Initially, 75 mg q day upon awakening; may increase to 150 mg after ≥3 days, max 150 mg q day

Obstructive sleep apnea
Adults PO Initially, 37.5 mg q day upon awakening; double the dose at intervals of at least 3 days if needed, max 150 mg q day

Renal dose
Adult: PO 37.5 mg q day; may increase to 75 mg q day after ≥7 days

Available forms
Tablet 75, 150 mg

ADVERSE REACTIONS

CNS: *Insomnia, anxiety, headache,* dizziness
CV: Palpitations, chest discomfort
GI: *Anorexia, nausea, dry mouth, constipation,* abdominal pain
INTEG: Hyperhidrosis

INTERACTIONS
Drug classifications

MAOIs: Increased hypertensive reaction, do not use within 14 days

Use caution with dopaminergic agents or drugs that increase B/P or heart rate

NURSING CONSIDERATIONS
Assess

• **Narcolepsy:** Assess for trouble staying awake at baseline and after 1 week, 2 weeks.
• Monitor B/P and heart rate baseline and periodically; hypertension should be treated before starting this product.
• Psychiatric symptoms: Assess for symptoms baseline and periodically; those with renal disease may be at higher risk.
• Abuse: Assess for those with a recent history of drug abuse, especially alcohol, amphetamines, cocaine, methylphenidate; watch for drug-seeking behaviors.

Patient problem
Sleep disturbance (uses)

Implementation
• Give without regard to food
• Take upon awakening; avoid within 9 hr of bedtime

Patient/family education
• Teach patient to discuss all Rx, OTC, herbs, and supplements taken, and if they are taking an MAOI.
• If a dose is missed, skip the missed dose and administer the next dose the following day in the morning upon wakening.
• Report to health care provider if inability to stay awake continues or if you develop anxiety, agitation, irritability, problems sleeping.
• **Pregnancy/breastfeeding:** Identify if pregnancy is planned or suspected; encourage enrolling in the pregnancy registry if patient becomes pregnant. To enroll or obtain information from the registry, go online at www.SunosiPregnancyRegistry.com or call 1-877-283-6220; present in breast milk.

Evaluation
Positive therapeutic outcome
• Ability to stay awake

---

tenapanor
(ten-a′ pa- nor)
Ibsrela
Func. class.: IBS agent

USES: Irritable bowel syndrome with constipation in adults

CONTRAINDICATIONS
Hypersensitivity, GI obstruction

DOSAGE AND ROUTES
Adult: PO 50 mg bid immediately before breakfast or the first meal of the day and immediately before dinner

---

ubrogepant
Ubrelvy
Func. class.: Calcitonin gene–related peptide (CGRP) receptor antagonist

USES: Acute migraine

DOSAGE AND ROUTES
Adult PO 50 or 100 mg; If needed, may take second dose at least 2 hr after initial dose; max: 200 mg/24 hr

CONTRAINIDCATIONS
Hypersensitivity, strong CYP3A4 inhibitors

---

upadacitinib (Rx)
(ue-pad′ a-sye′ ti-nib)
Rinvoq
Func. class.: Immunomodulating agent
Chem. class.: Janus-associated kinase (JAK) inhibitor

ACTION: An oral Janus kinase (JAK) inhibitor. Janus kinases are a tyrosine kinase enzyme that transmit signals arising from cytokine or growth factor-receptor interactions on the cellular membrane to influence cellular processes of immune cell function and hematopoiesis.

Therapeutic outcome: Decreasing pain, inflammation of joints

USES:
Treatment of rheumatoid arthritis

Pharmacokinetics

Absorption	Unknown
Distribution	Protein binding 52%, equally between RBCs and plasma
Metabolism	Hepatic by CYP3A4, minor CYP2D6
Excretion	Unchanged 38% urine, 24% feces
Half-life	8-14 hr

Pharmacodynamics

Onset	Unknown
Peak	2-4 hr
Duration	Unknown

CONTRAINDICATIONS
Hypersensitivity

Precautions:
AIDS, anemia, breastfeeding, children, contraception requirements, corticosteroid use, diverticulitis, geriatrics, GI perforation, hepatic disease, hepatitis B exacerbation, herpes, HIV, neutropenia, pregnancy, pregnancy testing, vaccination

> **BLACK BOX WARNING:** Infection, new primary malignancy, thrombosis

DOSAGE AND ROUTES
Adults PO 15 mg q day with or without methotrexate or other nonbiologic disease-modifying antirheumatic drugs (DMARDs)

Available forms: Extended release tablet 15 mg

ADVERSE REACTIONS
SYST: Infection

INTERACTIONS
Drug classifications
Live virus vaccines, avoid use
Strong CYP3A4 inhibitors (ketoconazole), use cautiously
Strong CYP3A4 inducers (rifampin), not recommended

NURSING CONSIDERATIONS
Assessment:
• **RA:** Assess for pain, stiffness, ROM, swelling of joints before, during treatment

> **BLACK BOX WARNING: Infections:** Assess for fever, flulike symptoms, dyspnea, change in urination, redness/swelling around any wounds—stop treatment if present; some serious infections, including sepsis, may occur, may be fatal; patients with active infections should not be started on this product

> **BLACK BOX WARNING:** Thrombosis (DVT, PE, arterial thrombosis): Assess for symptoms and treat immediately; some have been fatal

• May reactivate hepatitis B in chronic carriers; may be fatal

> **BLACK BOX WARNING:** Latent TB before therapy; treat before starting this product

• Blood dyscrasias: monitor CBC, differential periodically

> **BLACK BOX WARNING:** Neoplastic disease (lymphomas/leukemia): monitor for these and skin cancer

• Pregnancy/breastfeeding: use only if clearly needed; no well-controlled studies; do not breastfeed, excreted in breast milk

Patient problem
Infection (adverse reactions)

Implementation
• Give with or without food.
• Swallow whole, do not split, crush, or chew.

Patient/family education:
• Teach patient not to take any live virus vaccines during treatment.
• Advise patient to report signs of infection, TB, immediately.

Evaluation
Positive therapeutic outcome
• Decreased inflammation, pain in joints, decreased joint destruction

Appendix B

Ophthalmic, Nasal, Topical, and Otic Products

OPHTHALMIC PRODUCTS

ANESTHETICS
lidocaine (Rx)
(lye'doe-kane)
Akten
proparacaine (Rx)
(proe-par'a-kane)
Alcaine, Diocaine ✿, Parcaine
tetracaine (Rx)
(tet'ra-kane)
Minims Tetracaine ✿, Tetracaine,
TetraVisc

ANTIHISTAMINES
alcaftadine
(al-caf'tah-deen)
Lastacaft
azelastine (Rx)
(ay-zell'ah-steen)
cetirizine (Rx)
(se-teer'-i-zeen)
Zerviate
emedastine (Rx)
(ee-med'a-steen)
Emadine
epinastine (Rx)
(ep-een-as'teen)
Elestat
ketotifen (Rx, OTC)
(kee-toh-tif'en)
Alaway, Claritin Eye, Zaditor, ZyrTEC
Itchy Eye
levocabastine (Rx)
(lee-voh-cab'ah-steen)
Livostin
olopatadine (Rx)
(oh-loh-pat'ah-deen)
Pataday, Patanase, Pazeo

ANTIINFECTIVES
azithromycin (Rx)
(ay-zi-thro-my'sin)
AzaSite
besifloxacin (Rx)
(be'si-flox'a-sin)
Besivance
ciprofloxacin (Rx)
(sip-ro-floks'a-sin)
Ciloxan
erythromycin (Rx)
(er-ith-roe-mye'sin)
Ilotycin, Romycin
ganciclovir (Rx)
(gan-sye'kloe-vir)
Zirgan
gatifloxacin (Rx)
(gat-ih-floks'ah-sin)
Zymaxid
gentamicin (Rx)
(jen-ta-mye'sin)
Garamycin Ophthalmic, Gentak,
Gentasol
levofloxacin (Rx)
(lee-voh-flock'sah-sin)
moxifloxacin (Rx)
(mox-i-flox'a-sin)
Moxeza, Vigamox
natamycin (Rx)
(nat-a-mye'sin)
Natacyn
ofloxacin (Rx)
(oh-floks'a-sin)
Ocuflox
silver nitrate 1% (Rx)
silver nitrate
sulfacetamide sodium (Rx)
(sul-fa-seet'a-mide)
Bleph-10
tobramycin (Rx)
(toe-bra-mye'sin)
Tobrasol, Tobrex

trifluridine (Rx)
(trye-floor'i-deen)
Viroptic

β-ADRENERGIC BLOCKERS
betaxolol (Rx)
(beh-tax'oh-lole)
Botoptic
carteolol (Rx)
(kar-tee'oh-lole)
levobetaxolol (Rx)
(lee-voh-beh-tax'oh-lohl)
Betaxon
levobunolol (Rx)
(lee-voe-byoo'no-lole)
Betagen
metipranolol (Rx)
(met-ee-pran'oh-lole)
OptiPranolol
timolol (Rx)
(tym'moe-lole)
Betimol

CARBONIC ANHYDRASE INHIBITORS
brinzolamide (Rx)
(brin-zoh'la-mide)
Azopt
dorzolamide (Rx)
(dor-zol'a-mide)
Trusopt

CHOLINERGICS
(Direct-acting)
acetylcholine (Rx)
(ah-see-til-koe'leen)
Miochol-E
carbachol (Rx)
(kar'ba-kole)
Isopto Carbachol
pilocarpine (Rx)
(pye-loe-kar'peen)
Isopto Carpine

CHOLINESTERASE INHIBITORS
physostigmine (Rx)
(fi-zoe-stig'meen)

CORTICOSTEROIDS
dexamethasone (Rx)
(dex-a-meth'a-sone)
Maxidex

fluorometholone (Rx)
(flure-oh-meth'oh-lone)
Flarex, FML, FML Forte, FML S.O.P.
loteprednol (Rx)
(loe-tee-pred-nole)
Alrex, Lotemax
prednisoLONE (Rx)
(pred-niss'oh-lone)
Econopred Plus, Omnipred,
Pred-Forte, Pred Mild
rimexolone (Rx)
(ri-mex'a-lone)
Vexol

MYDRIATICS
atropine (Rx)
(a'troe-peen)
cyclopentolate (Rx)
(sye-kloe-pen'toe-late)
Cyclogyl, Cylate
homatropine (Rx)
(home-a'troe-peen)
Isopto Homatropine
phenylephrine (OTC)
(fen-ill-ef'rin)
Neofrin

NONSTEROIDAL
ANTIINFLAMMATORIES
bromfenac (Rx)
(brome'fen-ak)
Prolensa
diclofenac (Rx)
(dye-kloe'fen-ak)
flurbiprofen (Rx)
(flure-bi'pro-fen)
Ocufen
ketorolac (Rx)
(kee-toe'role-ak)
Acular, Acuvail
nepafenac (Rx)
(ne-pa-fen'ak)
Ilevro, Nevanac

SYMPATHOMIMETICS
apraclonidine (Rx)
(a-pra-klon'i-deen)
Iopidine
brimonidine (Rx)
(brem-on'i-dine)
Alphagan P

latanoprostene bunod (Rx)
(la-tan-oh-pros'-teen bu'-nod)
Vyzulta

OPHTHALMIC DECONGESTANTS/ VASOCONSTRICTORS
lodoxamide
(loe-dox'ah-mide)
Alomide
naphazoline (Rx, OTC)
(naf-az'oh-leen)
AK-Con, All Clear AR Maximum Strength Ophthalmic Solution, All Clear Eye Drops, CVS Maximum Redness Relief Eye Drops, CVS Redness Relief Lubricant Eye Drops
oxymetazoline (Rx)
(ox-i-met-ah-zoh'leen)
Visine L.R.
tetrahydrozoline (OTC)
(tet-ra-hye-dro'zoe-leen)
Visine Original

MISCELLANEOUS OPHTHALMICS
bimatoprost (Rx)
(bih-mat'o-prost)
Latisse, Lumigan
latanoprost (Rx)
(la-tan'oh-prost)
Xalatan
travoprost (Rx)
(tra'voe-prost)
Travatan
unoprostone (Rx)
(yoo-noe-pros'tone)
Rescula

β-ADRENERGIC BLOCKERS

ACTION: Reduces production of aqueous humor by unknown mechanism

USES: Ocular hypertension, chronic open angle glaucoma

ANESTHETICS

ACTION: Decreases ion permeability by stabilizing neuronal membrane

USES: Cataract extraction, tonometry, gonioscopy, removal of foreign objects, corneal suture removal, glaucoma surgery (ophthalmic); pruritus, sunburn, toothache, sore throat, cold sores, oral pain, rectal pain and irritation, control of gagging (topical)

ANTIINFECTIVES

ACTION: Inhibits folic acid synthesis by preventing PABA use, which is necessary for bacterial growth

USES: Conjunctivitis, superficial eye infections, corneal ulcers, prophylaxis against infection after removal of foreign matter from the eye

ANTIINFLAMMATORIES

ACTION: Decreases inflammation, resulting in decreased pain, photophobia, hyperemia, cellular infiltration

USES: Inflammation of eye, eyelids, conjunctiva, cornea; uveitis, iridocyclitis, allergic conditions, burns, foreign bodies, postoperatively in cataract

CARBONIC ANHYDRASE INHIBITOR

ACTION: Converted to EPINEPHrine, which decreases aqueous production and increases outflow

USES: Open angle glaucoma, ocular hypertension

DIRECT-ACTING MIOTIC

ACTION: Acts directly on cholinergic receptor sites; induces miosis, spasm of accommodation, fall in intraocular pressure, caused by stimulation of ciliary, pupillary sphincter muscles, which leads to pulling away of iris from filtration angle, resulting in increased outflow of aqueous humor

USES: Primary glaucoma, early stages of wide angle glaucoma (less useful in advanced stages), chronic open angle glaucoma, acute closed angle glaucoma before emergency surgery; also neutralizes mydriatics used during eye exam; may be used alternately with mydriatics to break adhesions between iris and lens

CONTRAINDICATIONS
Hypersensitivity

Precautions: Pregnancy, breastfeeding, children, aphakia, hypersensitivity to carbonic anhydrase inhibitors, sulfonamides, thiazide diuretics, ocular inhibitors, renal/hepatic insufficiency

ADVERSE EFFECTS
CNS: Headache

CV: Hypertension, tachycardia, dysrhythmias
EENT: Burning, stinging
GI: Bitter taste

NURSING CONSIDERATIONS
Assessment
• Monitor ophthalmic exams and intraocular pressure readings
• Monitor blood counts, renal/hepatic function tests and serum electrolytes during long-term treatment

Implementation
• Storage at room temperature away from light

Patient/family education
• Teach how to instill drops
• Advise patient that product may cause burning, itching, blurring, dryness of eye area

Evaluation

Positive therapeutic outcome
• Absence of increased intraocular pressure

NASAL AGENTS

NASAL ANTIHISTAMINES
olopatadine (Rx)
(oh-low-pat'uh-deen)
Patanase

NASAL DECONGESTANTS
azelastine (Rx)
(ay-zell'ah-steen)
Astepro
EPINEPHrine (OTC)
(ep-i-neff'rin)
Adrenalin Nasal Solution
oxymetazoline (OTC)
(ox-i-met-az'oh-leen)
Afrin No Drip, Dristan 12-HR Nasal Spray, Mucinex Moisture, Mucinex Sinus-Max, Vicks Sinex, Vicks QlearQuil
phenylephrine (OTC)
(fen-ill-eff'rin)
4-Way Nasal Spray, Neo-Synephrine
tetrahydrozoline (OTC)
(tet-ra-hye-dro'zoe-leen)
Tyzine, Tyzine Pediatric

NASAL STEROIDS
beclomethasone (Rx)
(be-kloe-meth'a-sone)
Beconase AQ Nasal, Qnasl

budesonide (Rx)
(byoo-des'oh-nide)
Rhinocort Aqua
flunisolide (Rx)
(floo-niss'oh-lide)
fluticasone (Rx)
(floo-tic'a-son)
Veramyst
triamcinolone (Rx)
(trye-am-sin'oh-lone)
Allergy 24 HR Nasal Spray, Nasacort

NONSTEROIDAL ANTIINFLAMMATORY
ketorolac (Rx)
(kee'toe-role-ak)
Sprix

ACTION: Produces vasoconstriction (rapid, long acting) of arterioles, thereby decreasing fluid exudation, mucosal engorgement by stimulation of α-adrenergic receptors in vascular smooth muscle

Therapeutic outcome: Absence of nasal congestion

USES: Nasal congestion

CONTRAINDICATIONS
Hypersensitivity to sympathomimetic amines

Precautions: Pregnancy, children <6 yr, geriatric, diabetes, CV disease, hypertension, hyperthyroidism, increased ICP, prostatic hypertrophy, glaucoma

ADVERSE EFFECTS
CNS: Anxiety, restlessness, tremors, weakness, insomnia, dizziness, fever, headache
EENT: Irritation, burning, sneezing, stinging, dryness, rebound congestion
GI: Nausea, vomiting, anorexia
INTEG: Contact dermatitis

NURSING CONSIDERATIONS
Assessment
• Assess for redness, swelling, pain in nasal passages before, during treatment
• Assess for systemic absorption; hypertension, tachycardia; notify prescriber; systemic absorption occurs at high doses or after prolonged use

Implementation
• Have patient tilt head back, squeeze bulb to create a vacuum, and draw correct amount of sol into dropper; insert 2 gtt of sol into nostril; repeat in other nostril
• Store in light-resistant container; do not expose to high temperature or let sol come into contact with aluminum

- Give for <4 consecutive days
- Provide environmental humidification to decrease nasal congestion, dryness

Patient/family education
- Advise patient that stinging may occur for several applications; drying of mucosa may be decreased by environmental humidification
- Caution patient to notify prescriber if irregular pulse, insomnia, dizziness, or tremors occur
- Teach patient proper administration to avoid systemic absorption
- Advise patient to rinse dropper with very hot water to prevent contamination

Evaluation
Positive therapeutic outcome
- Decreased nasal congestion

TOPICAL GLUCOCORTICOIDS

betamethasone (Rx)
(bay-ta-meth′a-sone)
Beben ✹, Betacort ✹, Betanate, Betnovate ✹, Celestoderm ✹, Del-Beta, Ectosone ✹, Metaderm ✹
betamethasone (augmented) (Rx)
(bay-ta-meth′a-sone)
Diprolene AF
clobetasol (Rx)
(kloe-bay′ta-sol)
Clobex, Cormax, Dermovate ✹, Olux Topical Foam, Temovate
desonide (Rx)
(dess′oh-nide)
Desonate, DesOwen, LoKara, Verdeso Foam
desoximetasone (Rx)
(dess-ox-i-met′a-sone)
Topicort
fluocinolone (Rx)
(floo-oh-sin′oh-lone)
Derma-Smoothe/FS oil, Lidemol ✹, Lyderm ✹, Synalar, Topsyn ✹
flurandrenolide (Rx)
(flure-an-dren′oh-lide)
Cordran, Drenison 1/4 ✹, Drenison Tape ✹
fluticasone (Rx)
(floo-tik′a-sone)
Cutivate

halcinonide (Rx)
(hal-sin′oh-nide)
Halog
hydrocortisone (Rx)
(hye-droe-kor′ti-sone)
Barriere-HC ✹, CaldeCORT Cortacet ✹, Cortalo, Cortate ✹, Cortef ✹, Corticreme ✹, Cortifoam, Cortoderm ✹, Hyderm ✹, Instacort, Neosporin Eczema Anti-Itch, Novo Hydrocort ✹, Nutracort , Nuzon, Sarna HC ✹, Unicort ✹
triamcinolone (Rx)
(trye-am-sin′oh-lone)
Dermasorb TA, Kenalog, Pediaderm TA, Trianide ✹, Triderm

ACTION: Antipruritic, antiinflammatory

Therapeutic outcome: Decreased itching, inflammation

USES: Psoriasis, eczema, contact dermatitis, pruritus; usually reserved for severe dermatoses that have not responded to less potent formulation

CONTRAINDICATIONS
Hypersensitivity, viral infections, fungal infections

Precautions: Pregnancy

DOSAGE AND ROUTES
Adult and child: Apply to affected area

ADVERSE EFFECTS
INTEG: *Acne, atrophy, epidermal thinning, purpura, striae*

NURSING CONSIDERATIONS
Assessment
- Monitor temp; if fever develops, product should be discontinued
- Monitor for systemic absorption, increased temp, inflammation, irritation

Implementation
- Apply only to affected areas; do not get in eyes
- Apply and leave site uncovered or lightly covered; occlusive dressing is not recommended—systemic absorption may occur
- Use only on dermatoses; do not use on weeping, denuded, or infected area
- Cleanse area before application of product
- Continue treatment for a few days after area has cleared
- Store at room temperature

Patient/family education
- Teach patient to avoid sunlight on affected area; burns may occur
- Teach patient to limit treatment to 14 days

Evaluation
Positive therapeutic outcome
- Absence of severe itching, patches on skin, flaking

TOPICAL ANTIFUNGALS

clotrimazole (OTC)
(kloe-trye'ma-zole)
Canesten ✽, Clotrimaderm ✽, Cruex, Crux, Desenex, Lotrimin AF, Myclo ✽, Neo-Zol ✽

econazole (OTC)
(ee-kon'a-zole)
Ecoza
efinaconazole
(ef'in-a-kon'a-zole)
Jublia
ketoconazole (OTC)
(kee-toe-kon'a-zole)
Extina, Ketodan, Kuric, Xolegel
luliconazole
(loo'li-kon'a-zole)
Luzu
miconazole (OTC)
(mye-kon'a-zole)
Antifungal, Azolen, Baza, Cruex, Lotrimin AF, Micaderm, Novana, Triple Paste AF, Zeasorb-AF
nystatin (OTC)
(nye-stat'in)
Nodostine ✽, Nyamyc, Nyaderm ✽, Nystop, Pediaderm AF
selenium (OTC)
(see-leen'ee-um)
tavaborole
(ta'va-bor'ole)
Kerydin
terbinafine (OTC)
(ter-bin'a-feen)
LamISIL
tolnaftate (OTC)
(tole-naf'tate)
Absorbine Athlete's Foot Cream, Lamasil AF Topical Spray, Ting
undecylenic acid (OTC)
(un-deh-sih-len'ik)

ACTION: Interferes with fungal cell membrane permeability

Therapeutic outcome: Absence of itching and white patches of the skin

USES: Tinea cruris, tinea pedis, diaper rash, minor skin irritations; amphotericin B is used for *Candida* infections

CONTRAINDICATIONS
Hypersensitivity

Precautions: Pregnancy, breastfeeding, children

DOSAGE AND ROUTES
Massage into affected area, surrounding area daily or bid, continue for 7-14 days, max 4 wk

ADVERSE EFFECTS
INTEG: Burning, stinging, dryness, itching, local irritation

NURSING CONSIDERATIONS
Assessment
- Assess skin for fungal infections: peeling, dryness, itching before, throughout treatment
- Assess for continuing infection; increased size, number of lesions

Implementation
- Apply to affected area, surrounding area; do not cover with occlusive dressings
- Store below 30° C (86° F)

Patient/family education
- Instruct to apply with glove to prevent further infection; not to cover with occlusive dressings
- Teach patient that long-term therapy may be needed to clear infection (2 wk-6 mo depending on organism); compliance is needed even after feeling better
- Teach patient proper hygiene: hand-washing technique, nail care, use of concomitant top agents if prescribed
- Caution patient to avoid use of OTC creams, ointments, lotions unless directed by prescriber
- Instruct patient to use medical asepsis (hand washing) before, after each application; to change socks and shoes once a day during treatment of tinea pedis
- Advise patient to report to health care prescriber if infection persists or recurs; if blisters, burning, oozing, swelling occur
- Caution patient to avoid alcohol because nausea, vomiting, hypertension may occur
- Caution patient to use sunscreen or avoid direct sunlight to prevent photosensitivity
- Advise patient to notify prescriber of sore throat, fever, skin rash, which may indicate overgrowth of organisms

---

Evaluation

Positive therapeutic outcome
• Decrease in size, number of lesions

TOPICAL ANTIINFECTIVES

azelaic acid (Rx)
(a-zuh-lay'ic)
Azelex, Finacea
bacitracin (OTC)
(bass-i-tray'sin)
Bacitin ✿
clindamycin (Rx)
(klin-da-my'sin)
Cleocin T, Clindacin ETZ, Clindacin PAC, Evocin
erythromycin (Rx, OTC)
(er-ith-roe-mye'sin)
Emgel, Emcin Clear, Ery, Erygel
gentamicin (Rx)
(jen-ta-mye'sin)
mafenide (Rx)
(ma'fe-nide)
Sulfamylon
metroNIDAZOLE (Rx)
(met-roh-nye'da-zole)
MetroGel, MetroCream, Noritate, Rosadan
mupirocin (Rx)
(myoo-peer'oh-sin)
Bactroban, Centany
retapamulin (Rx)
(re-tap'a-mue'lin)
Altabax
salicylic acid (Rx)
(sal'i-sil'ik)
Bensal HP, Demarest, Keralyt, Salacyn, Salvax, UltraSal-ER
silver sulfADIAZINE (Rx)
(sul-fa-dye'a-zeen)
Flamazine ✿**, Silvadene, SSD, Thermazene**
tretinoin (Rx)
(treh'tih-noyn)
Atralin, Avita, Refissa, Retin-A, Rrnova, Tretin-X

ACTION: Interferes with bacterial protein synthesis

Therapeutic outcome: Resolution of infection

USES: Skin infections, minor burns, wounds, skin grafts, primary pyodermas, otitis externa

CONTRAINDICATIONS
Hypersensitivity, large areas, burns, ulcerations

Precautions: Pregnancy, breastfeeding, impaired renal function, external ear or perforated eardrum

ADVERSE EFFECTS
INTEG: Rash, urticaria, scaling, redness

NURSING CONSIDERATIONS
Assessment
• Assess for allergic reaction: burning, stinging, swelling, redness
• Assess for signs of nephrotoxicity or ototoxicity

Implementation
• Apply enough medication to cover lesions completely
• Apply after cleansing with soap, water before each application; dry well
• Apply to less than 20% of body surface area when patient has impaired renal function
• Store at room temperature in dry place

Evaluation

Positive therapeutic outcome
• Decrease in size, number of lesions

TOPICAL ANTIVIRALS

acyclovir (Rx)
(ay-sye'kloe-ver)
Zovirax Topical
penciclovir (Rx)
(pen-sye'kloe-ver)
Denavir

ACTION: Interferes with viral DNA replication

Therapeutic outcome: Resolution of infection

USES: Simple mucocutaneous herpes simplex, in immunocompromised clients with initial herpes genitalis

CONTRAINDICATIONS
Hypersensitivity

Precautions: Pregnancy, breastfeeding

ADVERSE EFFECTS
INTEG: Rash, urticaria, stinging, burning, pruritus, vulvitis

NURSING CONSIDERATIONS
Assessment
- Assess for allergic reaction: burning, stinging, swelling, redness, rash, vulvitis, pruritus
- Assess for signs of nephrotoxicity or ototoxicity

Implementation
- Apply with finger cot or rubber glove to prevent further infection
- Apply enough medication to cover lesions completely
- Apply after cleansing with soap, water before each application; dry well
- Store at room temperature in dry place

Patient/family education
- Teach patient not to use in eyes or when there is no evidence of infection
- Advise patient to apply with glove to prevent further infection
- Advise patient to avoid use of OTC creams, ointments, lotions unless directed by prescriber
- Advise patient to use medical asepsis (hand washing) before, after each application and avoid contact with eyes
- Advise patient to adhere strictly to prescribed regimen to maximize successful treatment outcome
- Advise patient to begin using product when symptoms arise

Evaluation
Positive therapeutic outcome
- Decrease in size, number of lesions

TOPICAL ANESTHETICS

benzocaine (OTC)
(ben′zoe-kane)
Americaine Anesthetic, Anbesol Maximum Strength, Boil-Ease, Orajel
dibucaine (OTC)
(dye′byoo-kane)
Nupercainal
lidocaine (Rx, OTC)
(lye′doe-kane)
EnovaRx, Glydo, Lidomar, LidoRx, LTA, Solarcaine, Zilactin-L
pramoxine (OTC)
(pra-mox′een)
Prax, Proctofoam
tetracaine (OTC, Rx)
(tet′ra-cane)
Pontocaine, Viractin

ACTION: Inhibits conduction of nerve impulses from sensory nerves

Therapeutic outcome: Decreasing inflammation, itching, pain

USES: Oral irritation, sore throat, toothache, cold sore, canker sore, sunburn, minor cuts, insect bites, pain, itching

CONTRAINDICATIONS
Hypersensitivity, infants <1 yr, application to large areas

Precautions: Pregnancy, children <6 yr, sepsis, denuded skin

DOSAGE AND ROUTES
Adult and child: TOP apply qid as needed; RECT insert tid and after each BM

ADVERSE EFFECTS
INTEG: Rash, irritation, sensitization

NURSING CONSIDERATIONS
Assessment
- Assess pain: location, duration, characteristics before, after administration
- Assess for infection: redness, drainage, inflammation; this product should not be used until infection is treated

Implementation
- Store in tight, light-resistant container; do not freeze, puncture, or incinerate aerosol container

Patient/family education
- Teach patient to avoid contact with eyes
- Teach patient not to use for prolonged periods: use for <1 wk; if condition remains, prescriber should be contacted

Evaluation
Positive therapeutic outcome
- Decreased redness, swelling, pain

TOPICAL MISCELLANEOUS

docosanol (OTC)
(doh-koh′sah-nohl)
Abreva
pimecrolimus (Rx)
(pim-eh-kroh-ly′mus)
Elidel
oxymetazoline hydrochloride (Rx)
(ox-EE-meh-taz-oh-lin)
Rhofade

ACTION: Docosanol unknown; pimecrolimus may bind with macrophilin and inhibit calcium-dependent phosphatase

---

Therapeutic outcome: Decreased redness, swelling, pain

USES: Docosanol applied to fever blisters to promote more rapid healing; pimecrolimus used to treat mild to moderate atopic dermatitis in nonimmunocompromised patients ≥2 yr who are unresponsive to other treatment

CONTRAINDICATIONS
Hypersensitivity

Precautions: Pregnancy, breastfeeding, dermal infections

DOSAGE AND ROUTES
Docosanol
Adult: TOP rub into blisters 5 ×/day until healing occurs

Pimecrolimus
Adult and child ≥2 yr: TOP apply thin layer 2 ×/day and rub in; use as long as needed

ADVERSE EFFECTS
Docosanol
NONE known

Pimecrolimus
INTEG: Burning

NURSING CONSIDERATIONS
Assessment
• Assess skin condition (color, pain, inflammation) before, after administration
• Assess for signs and symptoms of skin infections (redness, draining lesions); if present, avoid use of product (pimecrolimus)

Implementation
• Apply to skin, rub in gently

Patient/family education
• Advise patient to avoid contact between medication and eyes
• Instruct patient to discontinue use of product when condition clears

Evaluation

Positive therapeutic outcome
• Decreased inflammation, redness

VAGINAL ANTIFUNGALS

butoconazole (OTC)
(byoo-toh-kone′ah-zole)
Gynazol-1
clotrimazole (OTC)
(kloe-trye′ma-zole)
Canesten ✦, Gyne-Lotrimin 3, Gyne-Lotrimin 7, Myclo ✦

---

miconazole (OTC)
(mye-kon′a-zole)
Monistat 3, Monistat 7
terconazole (OTC)
(ter-kone′ah-zole)
Terazol 7, Tetrazol 3, Zazole
tioconazole (OTC)
(tye-oh-kone′ah-zole)
Gyne-Trosyd ✦, Monistat 1, Vagistat-1

ACTION: Interferes with fungal DNA replication; binds sterols in fungal cell membranes, which increases permeability, leaking of nutrients

Therapeutic outcome: Fungistatic/fungicidal against susceptible organisms: *Candida* only

USES: Vaginal, vulval, vulvovaginal candidiasis (moniliasis)

CONTRAINDICATIONS
Hypersensitivity

Precautions: Pregnancy, breastfeeding, children <2 yr

ADVERSE EFFECTS
GU: Vulvovaginal burning, itching, pelvic cramps
INTEG: Rash, urticaria, stinging, burning
MISC: *Headache,* body pain

NURSING CONSIDERATIONS
Assessment
• Assess for allergic reaction: burning, stinging, itching, discharge, soreness

Implementation
Topical route
• Administer one full applicator every night high into the vagina
• Store at room temperature in dry place

Patient/family education
• Instruct patient in asepsis (hand washing) before, after each application
• Teach patient to apply with applicator only; to avoid use of any other vaginal product unless directed by prescriber; sanitary napkin may prevent soiling of undergarments
• Instruct patient to abstain from sexual intercourse until treatment is completed; reinfection and irritation may occur
• Advise patient to notify prescriber if symptoms persist

Evaluation

Positive therapeutic outcome
• Decrease in itching or white discharge (vaginal)

OTIC ANTIINFECTIVES

ciprofloxacin (Rx)
(sip′roe-flox′a-sin)
Cetraxal, Ofloxacin, Otiprio

ACTION: Inhibits protein synthesis in susceptible microorganisms

USES: Ear infection (external), short-term use

CONTRAINDICATIONS
Hypersensitivity, perforated eardrum

Precautions: Pregnancy

ADVERSE EFFECTS
EENT: Itching, irritation in ear
INTEG: Rash, urticaria

NURSING CONSIDERATIONS
Assessment
• Assess for redness, swelling, fever, pain in ear, which indicates superinfection

Implementation
• After removing impacted cerumen by irrigation
• After cleaning stopper with alcohol
• After restraining child if necessary
• After warming sol to body temp

Patient/family education
• Teach patient correct method of instillation using aseptic technique, including not touching dropper to ear
• Inform patient that dizziness may occur after instillation

Evaluation

Positive therapeutic outcome
• Decreased ear pain

Appendix C   Vaccines and toxoids

GENERIC NAME	TRADE NAME	USES	DOSAGE AND ROUTES	CONTRAINDICATIONS
anthrax vaccine	BioThrax	Pre-/postexposure prophylaxis	**Preexposure** Adult: SUBCUT 0.5 ml at 0, 2, 4 wk, then 0.5 ml at 6, 12, 18 mo **Postexposure** Adult: SUBCUT 0.5 ml 0, 2, 4 wk, with antibiotics	Hypersensitivity
BCG vaccine	TICE BCG	TB exposure	Adult and child >1 mo: 0.2-0.3 ml Child <1 mo: Reduce dose by 50% using 2 ml of sterile water after re-constituting	Hypersensitivity, hypogamma-globulinemia, pos-itive TB test, burns
dengue tatravalent vaccine, live	Dengvaxia	Prevention of dengue disease	Child 9-16 yrs SUBCUT 0.5 mL × 3 doses, 6 mon apart at mon 1, 6, 12	Hypersensitivity
diphtheria and tetanus tox-oids, adsorbed	Tenivac	Induces antitoxins to provide immu-nity to diphtheria and tetanus	Adult and child ≥7 yr: IM (adult strength) 0.5 ml q4-8wk × 2 doses, then 3rd dose 6-12 mo after 2nd dose, booster IM 0.5 ml q10yr Child 1-6 yr: IM (pediatric strength) 0.5 ml q4wk × 2 doses, booster 6-12 mo after 2nd dose Infant 6 wk-1 yr: IM (pediatric strength) 0.5 ml q4wk × 3 doses, booster 6-12 mo after 3rd dose	Hypersensitivity to mercury, thimerosal; immu-nocompromised patients; radiation; cortico-steroids; acute illness
diphtheria and tetanus tox-oids and whole-cell per-tussis vaccine (DPT, DTP)	DTwP, Tr-Immunol	Prevention of diphtheria, tetanus, pertussis	Doses vary Check product information	Hypersensitivity, active infection, poliomyelitis outbreak, immunosuppression, febrile illness
diphtheria and tetanus tox-oids and acellular pertus-sis vaccine	Adacel, Boostrix, Daptacel, Infranrix	Prevention of diphtheria, tetanus, pertussis		
diphtheria, tetanus, pertus-sis, haemophilus, polio IPV	Pentacel	Immunity to diphtheria, tetanus, per-tussis, haemophilus, polio IPV	Infant >6 wk and child ≤5 yr: IM 0.5 ml at 2, 4, 6, and 15-18 mo	Hypersensitivity, polio outbreak, acute infection, immunosuppression
diphtheria, tetanus, pertus-sis, polio vaccine IPV	Kinrix, Quadracel	Immunity to diphtheria, tetanus, per-tussis, polio vaccine IPV	Child: IM 0.5 ml	Hypersensitivity, polio outbreak, acute infection, immunosuppression

H1N1 influenza A (swine flu) virus vaccine	Influenza A (H1N1)	Immunity to H1N1	Adult <50 yr, adolescent, child ≥2 yr: Intranasal 1 dose (roughly 0.1 ml) into each nostril; child 2-9 repeat dose ≥4 wk later Adult, adolescent, child ≥3 yr: IM 0.5 ml as a single dose; child 3-9 yr repeat dose ≥4 wk later (Sanofi) (CSL); child 4-9 yr repeat dose ≥4 wk later (Novartis); infants ≥6 mo, child <36 mo: IM 0.25 ml, repeat in 4 wk (Sanofi) Adult: IM 0.5 ml as a single dose (GSK)	Hypersensitivity; febrile illness, active infection
haemophilus b conjugate vaccine, diphtheria CRM$_{197}$ protein conjugate (HbOC)	HibTITER	Polysaccharide immunization of children 2-6 yr against *H. influenzae* b, conjugate	**HibTITER (IM only)** Child: IM 0.5 ml Child 2-6 mo: 0.5 ml q2mo × 3 inj	
haemophilus b conjugate vaccine, meningococcal protein conjugate (PRP-OMP)	PedvaxHIB	Immunization of child 2, 4, 6 mo	Child 7-11 mo: Previously unvaccinated 0.5 ml q2mo inj Child 12-14 mo: Previously unvaccinated 0.5 ml × 1 inj **PedvaxHIB (IM only)** Child 2-14 mo: 0.5 ml × 2 inj at 2, 4 mo of age (6 mo dose not needed), then booster at 12-18 mo against invasive disease Child ≥15 mo: Previously unvaccinated 0.5 ml inj	
hepatitis A vaccine, inactivated	Havrix, VAQTA	Active immunization against hepatitis A virus	Adult: IM 1440 EL units (Havrix) or 50 units (VAQTA) as a single dose; booster dose is the same given at 6, 12 mo Child 2-18 yr: IM 720 EL units (Havrix) or 25 units (VAQTA) as a single dose, booster dose is the same given at 6, 12 mo	Hypersensitivity
hepatitis B vaccine, recombinant	Engerix-B, Recombivax HB	Immunization against all subtypes of hepatitis B virus	Varies widely	Hypersensitivity to this vaccine or yeast
human papillomavirus recombinant vaccine, quadrivalent	Gardasil	Prevention of HPV types 6, 11, 16, 18, cervical cancer, genital warts, precancerous dysplastic lesions, anal cancer/anal intraepithelial neoplasia	Adult up to 26 yr and child >9 yr to 26 yr: IM give as 3 separate doses; 1st dose as elected; 2nd dose 2 mo after 1st dose; 3rd dose 6 mo after 1st dose	Child <9 yr, pregnancy, breastfeeding, geriatric, active disease, hypersensitivity

Continued

Appendix C Vaccines and toxoids—cont'd

GENERIC NAME	TRADE NAME	USES	DOSAGE AND ROUTES	CONTRAINDICATIONS
influenza virus vaccine	Afluria, FluMist, Fluvirin, Fluzone	Prevention of seasonal influenza	Adult and child >12 yr: IM 0.5 ml in 1 dose Adult 18-64 yr: ID 0.1 ml as a single dose Child 3-12 yr: IM 0.5 ml, repeat in 1 mo (split) unless 1978-1985 vaccine was given; also given nasal Child 6 mo to 3 yr: IM 0.25 ml, repeat in 1 mo (split) unless 1978-1985 vaccine was given; also given nasal child ≤2 yr	Hypersensitivity, active infection, chicken egg allergy, Guillain-Barré syndrome, active neurologic disorders
Japanese encephalitis virus vaccine, inactivated	Ixiaro	Active immunity against Japanese encephalitis (JE)	Adult/child >3 yr: IM 0.5 ml (deltoid), then 0.5 ml 28 days later. Give the second dose ≥1 wk before potential exposure Child ≥2 mo to <3 yr: IM 0.25 ml (anterolateral aspect of the thigh or deltoid for children 1-2 yr with adequate muscle mass), then 0.25 ml 28 days later	Hypersensitivity to murine, thimerosal; allergic reactions to previous dose
measles, mumps, and rubella vaccine, live	M-R-II	Prevention of measles, mumps, rubella	Adult: SUBCUT 1 vial; 2 vials separated by 1 mo, in person born after 1957 Child >15 mo and adult: SUBCUT 0.5 ml	Hypersensitivity, blood dyscrasias, anemia, active infection, immunosuppression; egg, chicken allergy; pregnancy, febrile illness, neomycin allergy, neoplasms
measles, mumps, rubella, varicella	ProQuad	Immunity to measles, mumps, rubella, varicella	Child: SUBCUT 0.5 ml	Hypersensitivity to eggs, neomycin, cancer, radiation, corticosteroids, blood dyscrasias, active untreated TB
meningococcal polysaccharide vaccine	Menomune-A/C	Prophylaxis to meningococcal meningitis	Adult and child >2 yr: SUBCUT 0.5 ml	Hypersensitivity to thimerosal, pregnancy; acute illness
pneumococcal 7-valent conjugate vaccine	Prevnar	Immunity against *Streptococcus pneumoniae*	Child: IM 0.5 ml × 3 doses (7-11 mo); × 2 doses (12-23 mo); × 1 dose >2-9 yr	Hypersensitivity to diphtheria toxoid or this product
pneumococcal vaccine, polyvalent	Pneumovax 23	Pneumococcal immunization	Adult and child >2 yr: IM/SUBCUT 0.5 ml	Hypersensitivity, Hodgkin's disease, ARDS
poliovirus vaccine (IPV)	IPOL	Prevention of polio	Adult and child >2 yr: PO 0.5 ml, given q8wk × 2 doses, then 0.5 ml ½-1 yr after dose 2 Infant: PO 0.5 ml at 2, 4, 18 mo; booster at 4-6 yr; may also be given: IPV at 2, 4 mo, then TOPV at 12-18 mo, booster at 4-6 yr	Hypersensitivity, active infection, allergy to neomycin/streptomycin, immunosuppression, vomiting, diarrhea
rabies vaccine, human diploid cell (HDCV)	Imovax, RabAvert	Active immunity to rabies	**Preexposure** Adult and child: IM 1 ml on day 0, 7, 21, or 28 (total 4 doses) **Postexposure** Adult and child: IM 1 ml on day 0, 3, 7, 14, 28 (total 5 doses)	No contraindications

Drug	Trade Name	Uses	Dosage and Routes	Contraindications
rotavirus	RotaTeq, Rotarix	Prevents rotavirus	Infant: PO 3 doses given between 6 and 32 wk of age; 1st dose between 6-12 wk of age; 2nd and 3rd doses q4-10wk	Hypersensitivity to this product or latex, immunocompromised, blood products given within 6 wk, lymphatic disorders
smallpox and monkeypox vaccine, live, nonreplicating	Jynneos	Prevention of smallpox and monkeypox disease	Adult: SUBCUT 0.5 mL × 2 doses, 4 wks apart	Hypersensitivity
tetanus toxoid, adsorbed	No trade name	Tetanus toxoid: Used for prophylactic treatment of wounds	Adult and child: IM 0.5 ml q4-6wk × 2 doses, then 0.5 ml 1 yr after dose 2 (adsorbed); SUBCUT/IM 0.5 ml q4-8wk × 3 doses, then 0.5 ml ½-1 yr after dose 3, booster dose 0.5 ml q10yr	Hypersensitivity, active infection, poliomyelitis outbreak, immunosuppression
typhoid vaccine, parenteral typhoid vaccine, oral	Typhim Vi Vivotif Berna Vaccine	Active immunity to typhoid fever	Adult: PO 1 cap 1 hr before meals × 4 doses, booster q5yr; Adult and child >10 yr: SUBCUT 0.5 ml, repeat in 4 wk, booster q3yr; Child 6 mo-10 yr: SUBCUT 0.25 ml, repeat in 4 wk, booster q3yr	Parenteral: Systemic or allergic reaction, acute respiratory or other acute infection, intensive physical exercise in high temperatures; Oral: Hypersensitivity, acute febrile illness, suppressive or antibiotic products
typhoid Vi polysaccharide vaccine	Typhim Vi	Active immunity to typhoid fever	Adult and child ≥2 yr: IM 0.5 ml as a single dose, reimmunize q2yr 0.5 ml IM, if needed	Hypersensitivity chronic typhoid carriers
Varicella-Zoster Virus Vaccine	Varivax, Zostavax	Prevention of varicella-zoster (chickenpox)	Adult and child ≥13 yr: SUBCUT 0.5 ml, 2nd dose SUBCUT 0.5 ml 4-8 wk later	Hypersensitivity to neomycin; blood dyscrasias, immunosuppression, active untreated TB, acute illness, pregnancy, diseases of lymphatic system
yellow fever vaccine	YF-Vax	Active immunity to yellow fever	Adult and child ≥9 mo: SUBCUT 0.5 ml deeply, booster q10yr; Child 6-9 mo: same as above if exposed	Hypersensitivity to egg or chicken embryo protein, pregnancy, child <6 mo, immunodeficiency
Zoster vaccine recombinant, adjuvanted	Shingrix	For the prevention of herpes zoster (shingles)	Adult: IM 2 doses (0.5 mL each) at 0 and 2 to 6 months	History of severe allergic reaction (e.g., anaphylaxis) to any component of the vaccine or after a previous dose

Appendix D

Abbreviations

abd	abdomen	GPC	giant papillary conjunctivitis
ABG	arterial blood gas	gr	grain
ac	before meals	GTT	glucose tolerance test
ACE	angiotensin-converting enzyme	gtt	drops
ACT	activated clotting time	GU	genitourinary
ADA	American Diabetes Association	GVHD	graft-versus-host disease
ADH	antidiuretic hormone	H_2	histamine$_2$
ALT	alanine aminotransferase	hCG	human chorionic gonadotropin
ANA	antinuclear antibody	Hct	hematocrit
AP	anteroposterior	HDCV	human diploid cell rabies vaccine
APLA	antiphospholipid antibody syndrome	Hgb	hemoglobin
APTT	activated partial thromboplastin time	H&H	hematocrit and hemoglobin
ASA	acetylsalicylic acid, aspirin	5-HIAA	5-hydroxyindoleacetic acid
ASHD	arteriosclerotic heart disease	HIV	human immunodeficiency virus (AIDS)
AST	aspartate aminotransferase (SGOT)	H_2O	water
AV	atrioventricular	HOB	head of bed
bid	twice a day	HR	heart rate
BM	bowel movement	hr	hour
BMR	basal metabolic rate	IBD	inflammatory bowel disease
B/P	blood pressure	IC	intracardiac
BPH	benign prostatic hypertrophy	ICP	intracranial pressure
BPM	beats per minute	ID	intradermal
BS	blood sugar	IgG	immunoglobulin G
BUN	blood urea nitrogen	IM	intramuscular
C	Celsius (centigrade)	inf	infusion
CAD	coronary artery disease	INH	inhalation
cap	capsule	inj	injection
Cath	catheterization or catheterize	I&O	intake and output
CBC	complete blood cell count	IPPB	intermittent positive-pressure breathing
HF	heart failure	IT	intrathecal
CHo	carbohydrates	ITP	idiopathic thrombocytopenic purpura
cm	centimeter	IUD	intrauterine device
CNS	central nervous system	IV	intravenous
CO_2	carbon dioxide	IVP	intravenous pyelogram
cont	continuous	K	potassium
COPD	chronic obstructive pulmonary disease	kg	kilogram
CPAP	continuous positive airway pressure	L	liter
CPK	creatinine phosphokinase	lb	pound
CPR	cardiopulmonary resuscitation	LDH	lactic dehydrogenase
CCr	creatinine clearance	LE	lupus erythematosus
C&S	culture and sensitivity	LH	luteinizing hormone
C sect	cesarean section	LLQ	left lower quadrant
CSF	cerebrospinal fluid	LMP	last menstrual period
CTCL	cutaneous T-cell lymphoma	LOC	level of consciousness
CV	cardiovascular	LR	lactated Ringer's solution
CVA	cerebrovascular accident	LUQ	left upper quadrant
CVP	central venous pressure	M	meter
D&C	dilatation and curettage	m	minim
dir inf	direct infusion	m^2	square meter
dr	dram	MAOI	monoamine oxidase inhibitor
D_5W	5% glucose in distilled water	mcg	microgram
DVT	deep vein thrombosis	mEq	milliequivalent
ECG	electrocardiogram (EKG)	mg	milligram
EDTA	ethylenediamine tetraacetic acid	MI	myocardial infarction
EEG	electroencephalogram	min	minute
EENT	ear, eye, nose, and throat	ml	milliliter
EPS	extrapyramidal symptoms	mm	millimeter
ESR	erythrocyte sedimentation rate	mo	month
ext rel	extended release	Na	sodium
FBS	fasting blood sugar	neg	negative
FHT	fetal heart tones	NGU	nongonococcal urethritis
FSH	follicle-stimulating hormone	NHL	non-Hodgkin's lymphoma
g	gram	NPO	nothing by mouth (Lat. *nulla per os*)
GABA	γ-aminobutyric acid	NS	normal saline
GI	gastrointestinal	O_2	oxygen

🅰 Nurse Alert   ✴ Key NCLEX® Drug   ≫ Drug Specifics

OBS	organic brain syndrome
OD	right eye
OR	operating room
OS	left eye
OTC	over-the-counter
OU	each eye
oz	ounce
p̄	after
P56	Plasma-Lyte 56
PaCO₂	arterial carbon dioxide tension (pressure)
PaO₂	arterial oxygen tension (pressure)
PAT	paroxysmal atrial tachycardia
PBI	protein-bound iodine
pc	after meals
PCI	percutaneous coronary intervention
PCWP	pulmonary capillary wedge pressure
PEEP	positive end-expiratory pressure
PERRLA	pupils equal, round, react to light and accommodation
pH	hydrogen ion concentration
PO	by mouth
postop	postoperative
PP	postprandial
PPHN	persistent pulmonary hypertension of the newborn
preop	preoperative
prn	as required
PT	prothrombin time
PTT	partial thromboplastin time
PVC	premature ventricular contraction
q	every
qAM	every morning
qhr	every hour
q2hr	every 2 hours
q3hr	every 3 hours
q4hr	every 4 hours
q6hr	every 6 hours
q12hr	every 12 hours
qid	four times daily
qmo	every month
qPM	every night
qs	sufficient quantity
qt	quart
qwk	every week
R	right
RAIU	radioactive iodine uptake
RBC	red blood count or cell
RLQ	right lower quadrant
ROM	range of motion

RUQ	right upper quadrant
Rx	prescription
SARS	severe acute respiratory syndrome
SCr	serum creatinine
SIMV	synchronous intermittent mandatory ventilation
SL	sublingual
SLE	systemic lupus erythematosus
SOB	shortness of breath
sol	solution
sp gr	specific gravity
ss	one half
STD	sexually transmitted disease
SUBCUT	subcutaneous
supp	suppository
sus rel	sustained release
syr	syrup
T&A	tonsillectomy and adenoidectomy
tab	tablet
tbsp	tablespoon
TD	transdermal
temp	temperature
tid	three times daily
tinc	tincture
TPN	total parenteral nutrition
TOP	topical
TSH	thyroid-stimulating hormone
tsp	teaspoon
TT	thrombin time
UA	urinalysis
UTI	urinary tract infection
UV	ultraviolet
vag	vaginal
VMA	vanillylmandelic acid
vol	volume
VS	vital sign
WBC	white blood cell count
wk	week
wt	weight
yr	year
>	greater than
<	less than
=	equal
°	degree
%	percent
α	alpha
γ	gamma
β	beta

- For a list of the Institute for Safe Medicine Practices (ISMP) error-prone abbreviations, symbols, and dose designations, please see http://www.ismp.org/tools/errorproneabbreviations.pdf.
- For frequently asked questions regarding the 2018 National Patient Safety Goals, please visit The Joint Commission website at http://www.jointcommission.org/PatientSafety/NationalPatientSafetyGoals.

Appendix E

Immunization Schedules

Recommended Child and Adolescent Immunization Schedule for ages 18 years or younger, United States, 2020

These recommendations must be read with the notes that follow[1]. For those who fall behind or start late, provide catch-up vaccination at the earliest opportunity as indicated by the green bars. To determine minimum intervals between doses, see the catch-up schedule[1]. School entry and adolescent vaccine age groups are shaded in gray.

Vaccine	Birth	1 mo	2 mos	4 mos	6 mos	9 mos	12 mos	15 mos	18 mos	19-23 mos	2-3 yrs	4-6 yrs	7-10 yrs	11-12 yrs	13-15 yrs	16 yrs	17-18 yrs
Hepatitis B (HepB)	1st dose	2nd dose			◄------- 3rd dose -------►												
Rotavirus (RV): RV1 (2-dose series), RV5 (3-dose series)			1st dose	2nd dose	See Notes[1]												
Diphtheria, tetanus, acellular pertussis (DTaP <7 yrs)			1st dose	2nd dose	3rd dose			◄---- 4th dose ----►				5th dose					
Haemophilus influenzae type b (Hib)			1st dose	2nd dose	See Notes[1]		◄-- 3rd or 4th dose --► See Notes[1]										
Pneumococcal conjugate (PCV13)			1st dose	2nd dose	3rd dose		◄---- 4th dose ----►										
Inactivated poliovirus (IPV <18 yrs)			1st dose	2nd dose	◄-------- 3rd dose --------►							4th dose					
Influenza (IIV) or **Influenza (LAIV)**						Annual vaccination 1 or 2 doses						Annual vaccination 1 or 2 doses		Annual vaccination 1 dose only			
Measles, mumps, rubella (MMR)					See Notes[1]		◄-- 1st dose --►					2nd dose					

Vaccine									
Varicella (VAR)	1st dose			2nd dose					
Hepatitis A (HepA)	See Notes[1]	2nd dose series, See Notes[1]							
Tetanus, diphtheria, acellular pertussis (Tdap ≥7 yrs)							Tdap		
Human papillomavirus (HPV)						See Notes[1]			
Meningococcal (MenACWY-D ≥9 mos, MenACWY-CRM ≥2 mos)		See Notes[1]					1st dose		2nd dose
Meningococcal B							*		See Notes[1]
Pneumococcal polysaccharide (PPSV23)							See Notes[1]		

Legend:

- ☐ Range of recommended ages for all children
- ☐ Range of recommended ages for catch-up immunization
- ☐ Range of recommended ages for certain high-risk groups
- ☐ Recommended based on shared clinical decision-making or *can be used in this age group
- ☐ No recommendation/ not applicable

Consult relevant ACIP statements for detailed recommendations at www.cdc.gov/vaccines/hcp/acip-recs/index.html. For information on contraindications and precautions for the use of a vaccine, consult the General Best Practice Guidelines for Immunization at www.cdc.gov/vaccines/hcp/acip-recs/general-recs/contraindications.html and relevant ACIP statements at www.cdc.gov/vaccines/hcp/acip-recs/index.html. For calculating intervals between doses, 4 weeks = 28 days. Intervals of ≥4 months are determined by calendar months. Within a number range (e.g., 12–18), a dash (–) should be read as "through." Vaccine doses administered ≤4 days before the minimum age or interval are considered valid. Doses of any vaccine administered ≥5 days earlier than the minimum age or minimum interval should not be counted as valid and should be repeated as age appropriate. The repeat dose should be spaced after the invalid dose by the recommended minimum interval. For further details, see Table 3-1, Recommended and minimum ages and intervals between vaccine doses, in General Best Practice Guidelines for Immunization at www.cdc.gov/vaccines/hcp/acip-recs/general-recs/timing.html. yInformation on travel vaccine requirements and recommendations is available at www.cdc.gov/travel/. yFor vaccination of persons with immunodeficiencies, see Table 8-1, Vaccination of persons with primary and secondary immunodeficiencies, in General Best Practice Guidelines for Immunization at www.cdc.gov/vaccines/hcp/acip-recs/general-recs/immunocompetence.html, and Immunization in Special Clinical Circumstances (In: Kimberlin DW, Brady MT, Jackson MA, Long SS, eds. Red Book: 2018 Report of the Committee on Infectious Diseases. 31st ed. Itasca, IL: American Academy of Pediatrics; 2018:67–111). For information regarding vaccination in the setting of a vaccine preventable disease outbreak, contact your state or local health department. The National Vaccine Injury Compensation Program (VICP) is a no-fault alternative to the traditional legal system for resolving vaccine injury claims. All routine child and adolescent vaccines are covered by VICP except for pneumococcal polysaccharide vaccine (PPSV23). For more information, see www.hrsa.gov/vaccinecompensation/index.html.

[1]For complete information and notes, refer to https://www.cdc.gov/vaccines/schedules/hcp/imz/child-adolescent.html
Table adapted from: https://www.cdc.gov/vaccines/schedules/hcp/imz/child-adolescent.html

Appendix F

Standard Precautions

The following precautions are used in the care of all patients regardless of their diagnosis or disease. They are also applied when handling or cleaning equipment or supplies that are potentially contaminated.

1. Wear gloves any time that you may contact blood, any moist body fluid (except sweat), secretions, excretions, nonintact skin, or mucous membranes.
2. Remove your gloves, wash your hands, and reapply clean gloves if your gloves become soiled with infective material.
3. Even if you are wearing gloves, remove them, wash your hands, and apply clean gloves *immediately before* contact with mucous membranes or nonintact skin.
4. Wear a protective cover gown of waterproof material if your clothing is likely to have substantial contact with infective material or if splashing of body fluids is likely.
5. Wear a face shield or goggles to protect your eyes if splashing of secretions is likely.
6. Any time a face shield or goggles are worn, wear a surgical mask to protect the mucous membranes of your nose and mouth. A surgical mask may be worn during certain sterile procedures without protective eyewear. However, protective eyewear is *never* worn without a surgical mask.
7. Handle needles, razors, broken glass, and other sharp objects with care. Needles should never be recapped. All sharps should be disposed of in a puncture-resistant sharps container.
8. Wash your hands before and after each patient contact.
9. Wash your hands before you apply and after you remove gloves. Do not assume that hand washing is unnecessary because gloves were worn. Do not wash your hands with gloves on them.
10. Gloves are used for the care of one patient only, then discarded.
11. Follow your facility policy for disposal of gloves and other contaminated items. These items are generally not disposed of in open trash containers. Facilities have designated disposal sites for these biohazardous waste materials.
12. Use resuscitation barrier devices as an alternative to mouth-to-mouth resuscitation.
13. Linen should be handled in a manner that prevents contamination of the outside of the container. Linen from isolation rooms was previously double bagged. Double bagging is no longer recommended since all linen is handled as potentially infectious. Double bag linen only if the outside of the bag becomes contaminated during the bagging process.

Appendix G

Illustrated Mechanisms and Sites of Action

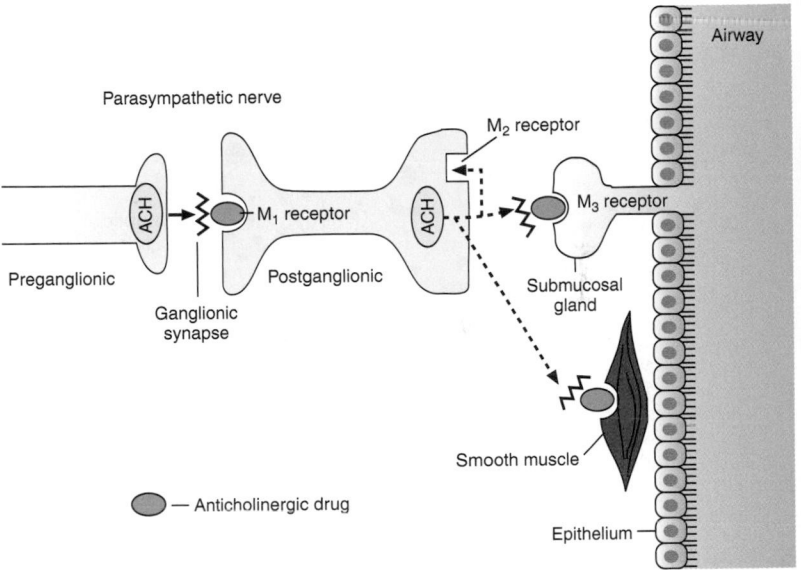

Fig. G-1 Sites and Mechanisms of Action: Anticholinergic Bronchodilators: Anticholinergic bronchodilators, such as ipratropium, work by blocking muscarinic-1 (M_1) receptors on postganglionic parasympathetic nerve endings and muscarinic-3 (M_3) receptors on the cell membranes of bronchial smooth muscles and submucosal glands. Normally, stimulation of the M_1 and M_3 receptors by acetylcholine (ACH) causes bronchoconstriction and mucus secretion from submucosal glands. Anticholinergic bronchodilators block these specific muscarinic receptors from the effects of acetylcholine, causing bronchial smooth muscle relaxation, bronchodilatation, and decreased mucus production. (From Gardenhire OS: *Rau's Respiratory Care Pharmacology,* ed 8, St. Louis, 2012, Mosby.)

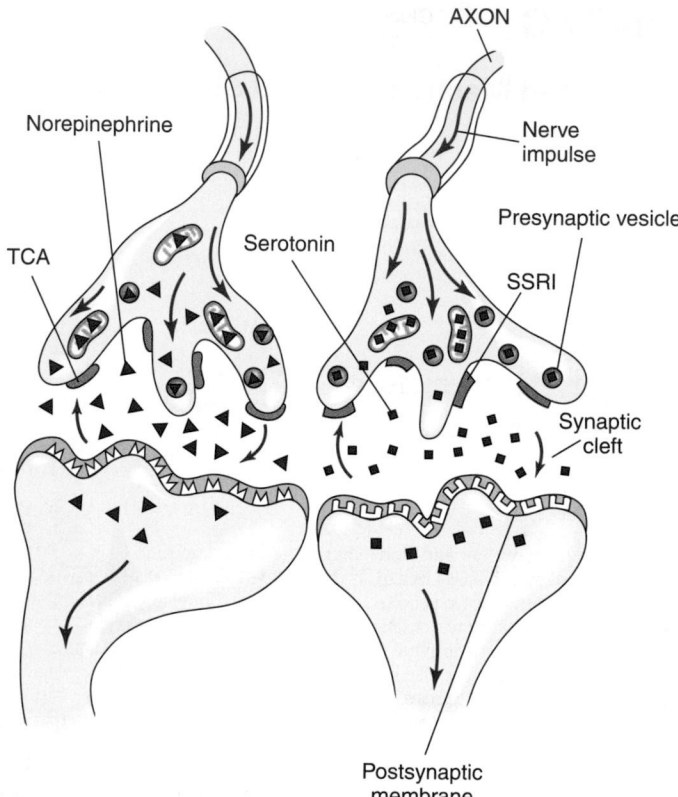

Fig. G-2 Mechanisms of Action: Antidepressants. Depression is thought to occur when levels of neurotransmitters, such as norepinephrine and serotonin, are reduced at postsynaptic receptor sites. These neurotransmitters affect a wide array of functions, including mood, obsessions, appetite, and anxiety. Antidepressants work by increasing the availability of these neurotransmitters at postsynaptic membranes and by enhancing and prolonging their effects. As a result, these agents improve mood, reduce anxiety, and minimize obsessions.

Antidepressants typically are classified as tricyclic antidepressants (TCAs), monoamine oxidase inhibitors (not shown), selective serotonin reuptake inhibitors (SSRIs), and atypical antidepressants (not shown). TCAs, such as amitriptyline and desipramine, primarily block norepinephrine reuptake at presynaptic membranes, thereby increasing the norepinephrine concentration at synapses and making more available at postsynaptic receptors.

SSRIs, such as FLUoxetine and PARoxetine, selectively inhibit serotonin uptake at presynaptic membranes. This action leads to increased serotonin availability at postsynaptic receptors. (From Gutierrez K: *Pharmacotherapeutics: Clinical Reasoning in Primary Care,* ed 2, Philadelphia, 2008, Saunders.)

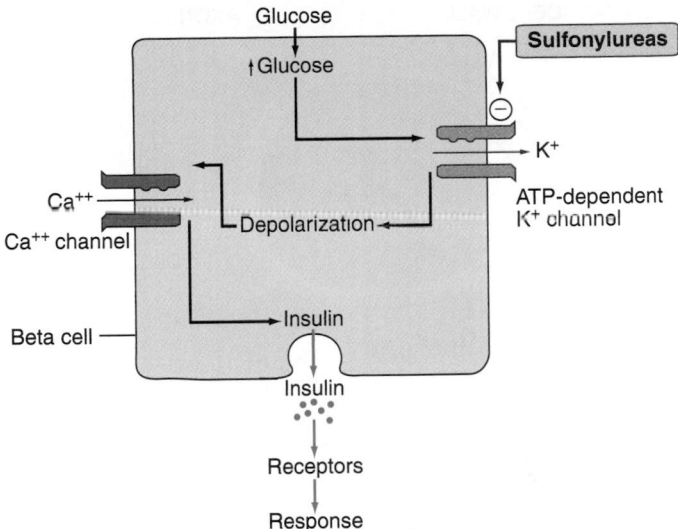

Fig. G-3 Mechanisms of Action: Antidiabetic Agents. Diabetes mellitus takes two forms: type 1 diabetes characterized by a complete lack of insulin and type 2 diabetes marked by insufficient insulin secretion, insulin resistance in peripheral tissues, or both. Normally, the beta cells in the pancreatic islets of Langerhans are responsible for secreting insulin. The rise of glucose levels in the beta cell triggers adenosine triphosphate (ATP)-dependent potassium (K^+) channels in the membranes of beta cells to close. Then the beta cells depolarize and calcium (Ca^{++}) enters the cell through Ca^{++} channel, and insulin is released from the cell. When circulating insulin engages with insulin receptors on cell membranes, it facilitates the movement of glucose into the cell, among other actions.

Type 1 diabetes is treated with the use of exogenous insulin, which mimics natural insulin in the body. Insulin takes many forms with varying degrees of onset, peak, and duration, including rapid, regular, intermediate, and long acting.

Type 2 diabetes is usually treated with oral agents. Sulfonylureas, such as glyBURIDE, block ATP-dependent K^+ channels in the cell membranes of beta cells, ultimately resulting in the release of insulin. (From Taylor: *Mosby's Crash Course Pharmacology*, St. Louis, 1998, Mosby.)

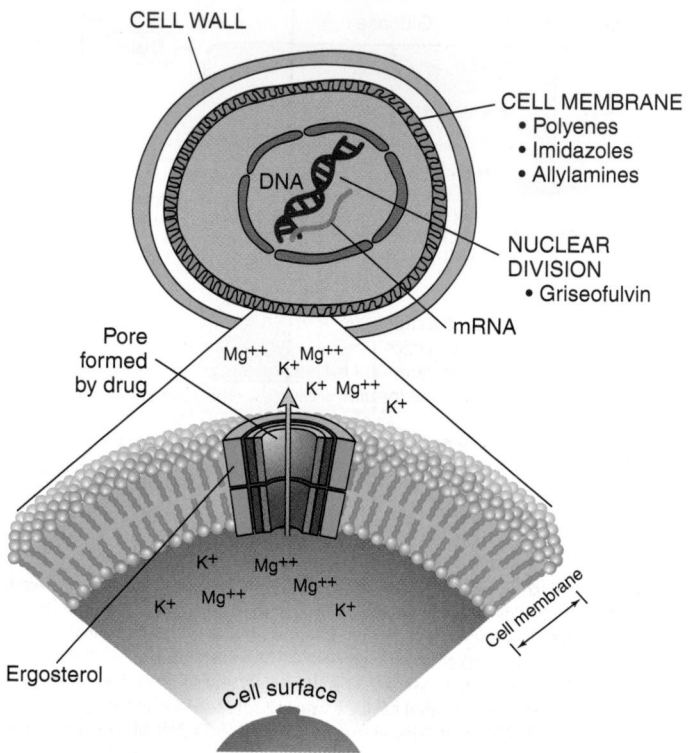

Fig. G-4 Sites and Mechanisms of Action: Antifungal Agents. Antifungal agents primarily affect fungi at one of two sites: the cell membrane or the cell nucleus. Most of these agents, such as polyene, imidazole, and allylamine antifungals, act on the fungal cell membrane. Polyene antifungals, such as amphotericin B, bind to ergosterol and increase cell membrane permeability. Imidazole antifungals, such as fluconazole and ketoconazole, interfere with ergosterol synthesis by inhibiting the cytochrome P_{450} enzyme system, altering the cell membrane, and inhibiting fungal growth. Allylamine antifungals, such as terbinafine, inhibit the enzyme squalene epoxidase, which disrupts ergosterol production—and cell membrane integrity. When cell membrane permeability increases, cellular components, including potassium (K^+) and magnesium (Mg^{++}), leak out. Loss of these cellular components leads to cell death.

Another antifungal agent, griseofulvin, directly affects the fungal nucleus, interfering with mitosis. By binding to structures in the mitotic spindle, it prevents cells from dividing, which eventually leads to their death. (From Gutierrez K: *Pharmacotherapeutics: Clinical Reasoning in Primary Care,* ed 2, Philadelphia, 2008, Saunders.)

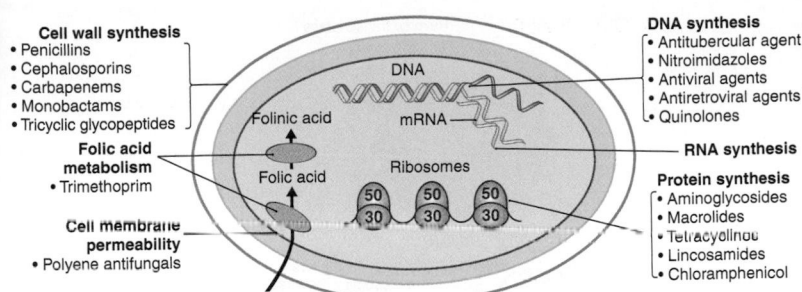

Fig. G-5 Sites and Mechanisms of Action: Antiinfective Agents. The goal of antiinfective therapy is to kill or inhibit the growth of microorganisms such as bacteria, viruses, and fungi. To achieve this goal, antiinfective agents must reach their targets, which usually occurs through absorption and distribution by the circulatory system. When the target is reached, a drug can kill or suppress microorganisms by:

• Inhibiting cell wall synthesis or activating enzymes that disrupt the cell wall, which leads to cellular weakening, lysis, and death. Penicillins (ampicillin), cephalosporins (ceFAZolin), carbapenems (imipenem), monobactams (aztreonam), and tricyclic glycopeptides (vancomycin) act in this way.

• Altering cell membrane permeability through direct action on the cell wall, which allows intracellular substances to leak out and destabilizes the cell. Polyene antifungals (amphotericin) work by this mechanism.

• Altering protein synthesis by binding to bacterial ribosomes (50/30) or affecting ribosomal function, which leads to cell death or slowed growth respectively. Aminoglycosides (gentamicin), macrolides (erythromycin), tetracyclines (doxycycline), lincosamides (clindamycin), and the miscellaneous antiinfective chloramphenicol use this action.

• Inhibiting DNA or RNA, including messenger RNA (mRNA), synthesis by binding to nucleic acids or interacting with enzymes required for their synthesis. Antitubercular agents (rifampin), nitroimidazoles (metroNIDAZOLE), antiviral agents (acyclovir), antiretroviral agents (stavudine), and quinolones (ciprofloxacin) act like this.

• Inhibiting the metabolism of folic acid and folinic acid or other cellular components that are essential for bacterial cell growth. The miscellaneous antiinfective trimethoprim employs this mechanism of action. (From Page C et al: *Integrated Pharmacology,* ed 3, St. Louis, 2006, Mosby.)

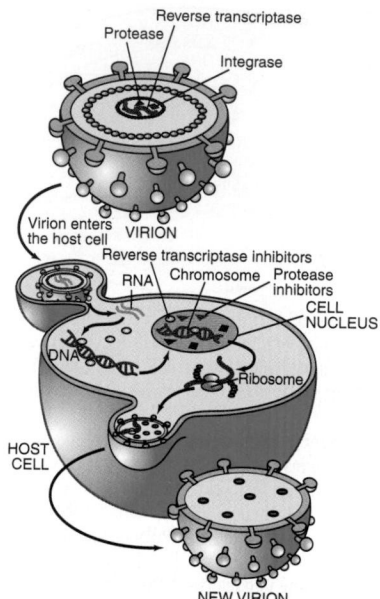

Fig. G-6 Mechanisms and Sites of Action: Antiretroviral Agents. When viruses reproduce, the infectious viral particle, or virion (**A**), enters the host cell. The virion attaches to the cell's surface and then inserts itself into the host cell (**B**). Once inside, the virion uncoats, and the enzyme reverse transcriptase makes two copies of the viral RNA: one copy is identical; the other is a mirror image. These two copies form double-stranded viral DNA that enters the host cell's nucleus, where it inserts itself into the host cell's DNA with the help of the enzyme integrase. Then viral DNA reprograms the host cell to produce additional viral RNA, which begins the process of forming new viruses. Specifically, messenger RNA (mRNA) instructs ribosomal RNA (rRNA) to produce a new chain of proteins and enzymes that are used to form new viruses. Protease cuts the chains, creating individual proteins. These combine with new RNA to create new virions, which bud and are released from the host cell (**C**).

Antiretroviral agents target specific enzymes during viral reproduction. Nucleoside reverse transcriptase inhibitors, such as stavudine, interfere with the action of reverse transcriptase by mimicking naturally occurring nucleosides. Nucleotide reverse transcriptase inhibitors, such as tenofovir, block reverse transcriptase by competing with the natural substrate deoxyadenosine triphosphate and by causing DNA chain termination. Nonnucleoside reverse transcriptase inhibitors, such as delavirdine, work by directly binding to reverse transcriptase. As a result, no viral DNA is available to insert itself into the host cell's DNA. Protease inhibitors, such as indinavir, bind to and interfere with the action of protease; thus, the new chain of proteins formed by rRNA cannot be cut into individual proteins to make new viruses. (From Gutierrez K: *Pharmacotherapeutics: Clinical Reasoning in Primary Care,* ed 2, Philadelphia, 2008, Saunders.)

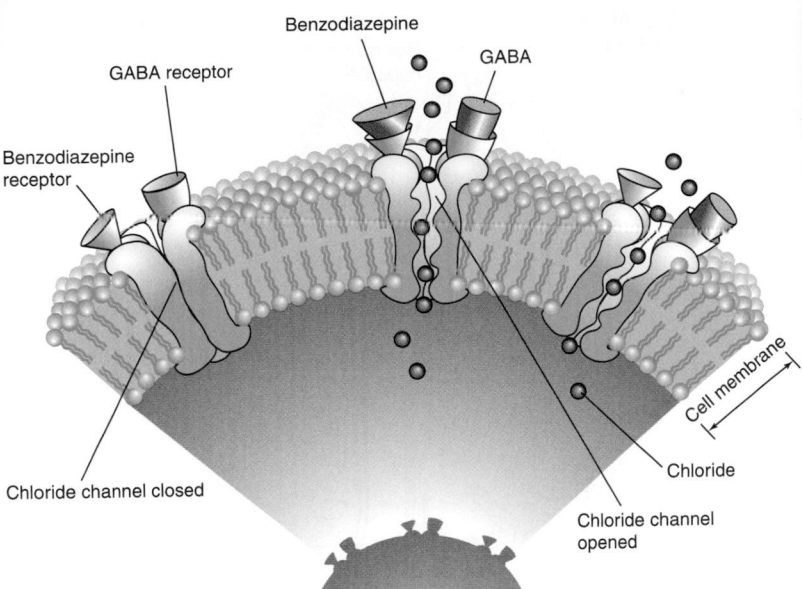

Fig. G-7 Mechanisms of Action: Benzodiazepines. Benzodiazepines reduce anxiety by stimulating the action of the inhibitory neurotransmitter, gamma-aminobutyric acid (GABA), in the limbic system. The limbic system plays an important role in the regulation of human behavior. Dysfunction of GABA neurotransmission in the limbic system may be linked to the development of certain anxiety disorders.

The limbic system contains a highly dense area of benzodiazepine receptors that may be linked to the antianxiety effects of benzodiazepines. These benzodiazepine receptors are located on the surface of neuronal cell membranes and are adjacent to GABA receptors. The binding of a benzodiazepine to its receptor enhances the affinity of a GABA receptor for GABA. In the absence of a benzodiazepine, the binding of GABA to its receptor causes the chloride channel in the cell membrane to open, which increases the influx of chloride into the cell. This influx of chloride results in hyperpolarization of the neuronal cell membrane and reduces the neuron's ability to fire, which is why GABA is considered an inhibitory neurotransmitter.

A benzodiazepine acts only in the presence of GABA. When it binds to a benzodiazepine receptor, it prolongs the time that the chloride channel remains open. This results in greater depression of neuronal function and a reduction in anxiety. (From Gutierrez K: *Pharmacotherapeutics: Clinical Reasoning in Primary Care,* ed 2, Philadelphia, 2008, Saunders.)

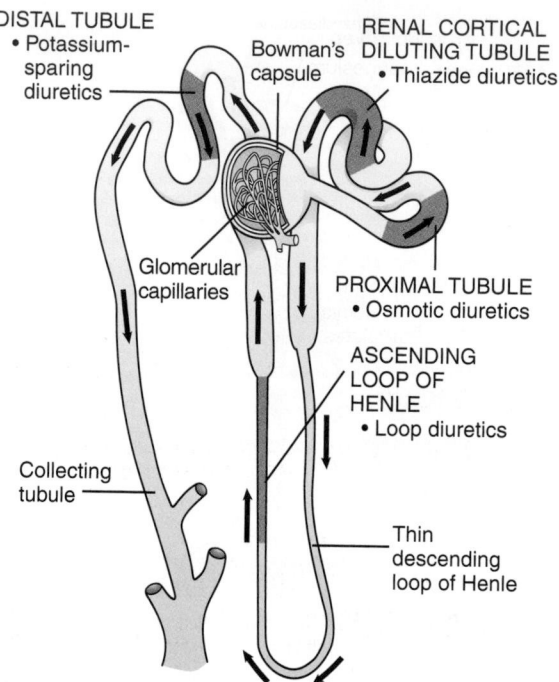

Fig. G-8 Sites of Action: Diuretics. Diuretics act primarily to increase water and sodium excretion by the kidneys, thereby increasing urine output. In the process, chloride, potassium, and other electrolytes may also be excreted. Most diuretics act by blocking sodium, water, and chloride reabsorption by peritubular capillaries in the nephrons. As a result, water and electrolytes remain in the convoluted tubules to be excreted as urine. The increased water and electrolyte excretion reduces blood volume—and ultimately blood pressure.

Diuretics belong to four major subclasses:

1. Thiazide diuretics, such as hydrochlorothiazide, act in the early portion of the distal convoluted tubule, called the cortical diluting segment. These drugs block sodium, chloride, and water reabsorption and promote their excretion along with potassium.

2. Loop diuretics, such as furosemide, act primarily in the thick ascending limb of the loop of Henle, blocking sodium, water, and chloride reabsorption. Then these substances are excreted along with potassium.

3. Potassium-sparing diuretics, such as spironolactone, act in the late portion of the distal convoluted tubule and collecting tubule. Here, they inhibit the action of aldosterone, leading to sodium excretion and potassium retention. Although triamterene and amiloride, two other potassium-sparing diuretics, act at the same site, they do not affect aldosterone. Instead, these drugs directly block the exchange of sodium and potassium, leading to decreased sodium reabsorption and decreased potassium excretion.

4. Osmotic diuretics, such as mannitol, work in the proximal convoluted tubule. As their name implies, these diuretics increase the osmotic pressure of the glomerular filtrate, inhibiting the passive reabsorption of water, sodium, and chloride. (From Gutierrez K: *Pharmacotherapeutics: Clinical Reasoning in Primary Care,* ed 2, Philadelphia, 2008, Saunders.)

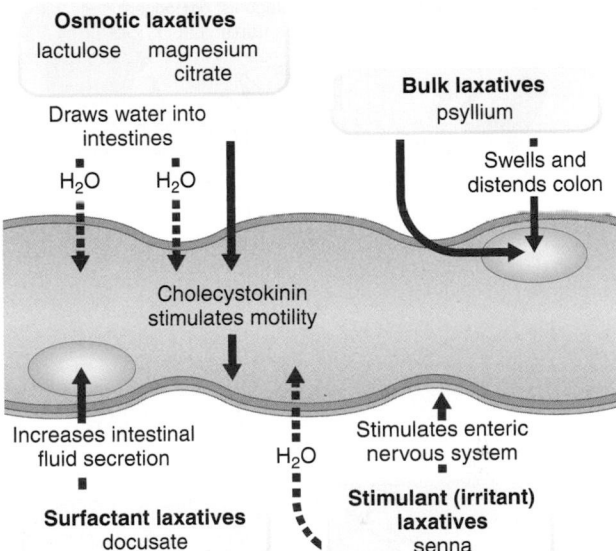

Fig. G-9 Mechanisms of Action: Laxatives. Laxatives ease or stimulate defecation. Typically, they are classified by their mechanism of action as bulk-forming, osmotic, stimulant, or surfactant laxatives.

Bulk-forming laxatives, such as psyllium, act in the small and large bowel. Because ingredients in these laxatives are undigestible, they remain within the stool and increase the fecal mass by drawing in water. These agents also enhance bacterial growth in the colon, further adding to the fecal mass.

Osmotic laxatives, such as lactulose, draw water into the intestinal lumen, causing the fecal mass to soften and swell. This osmotic action may be enhanced by the metabolism of colonic bacteria to lactate and other organic acids. These acids decrease colonic pH and increase colonic motility.

Stimulant (or irritant) laxatives, such as senna, act on the intestinal wall to increase water and electrolytes in the intestinal lumen. In addition, they directly irritate the colon, increasing motility.

Surfactant laxatives (or fecal softeners), such as docusate, reduce the surface tension of the stool, allowing water to enter it. These laxatives may also help to increase water and electrolyte excretion into the intestinal lumen, softening and increasing the fecal mass. (From Page C et al: *Integrated Pharmacology,* ed 3, St. Louis, 2006, Mosby.)

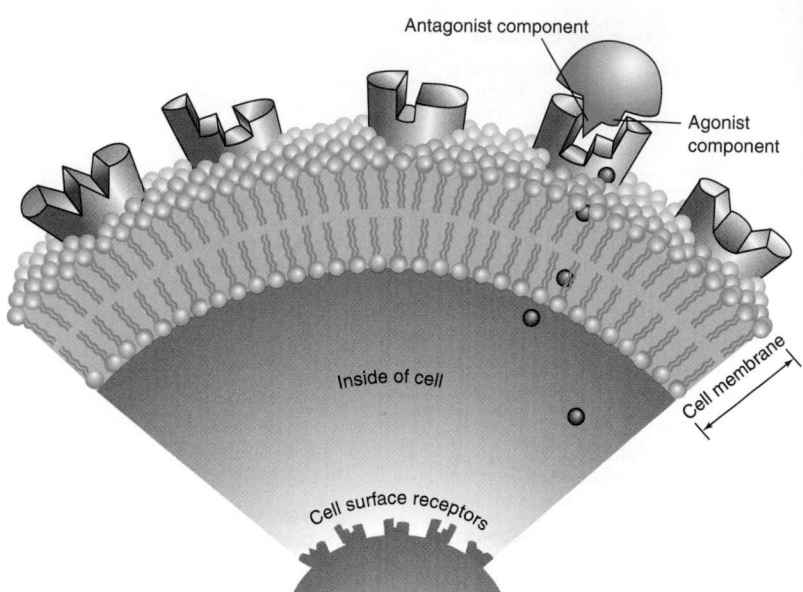

Fig. G-10 Mechanisms of Action: Narcotic Agonist-Antagonist Analgesics. Cell membranes have different types of opioid receptors, such as mu, kappa, and delta receptors. Opioid agonist-antagonists work by stimulating one type of receptor, while simultaneously blocking another type. As agonists, they work primarily by activating kappa receptors to produce analgesia and such other effects as CNS and respiratory depression, decreased GI motility, and euphoria. As antagonists, they compete with opioids at mu receptors, helping to reverse or block some of the other effects of agonists. (From Gutierrez K: *Pharmacotherapeutics: Clinical Reasoning in Primary Care,* ed 2, Philadelphia, 2008, Saunders.)

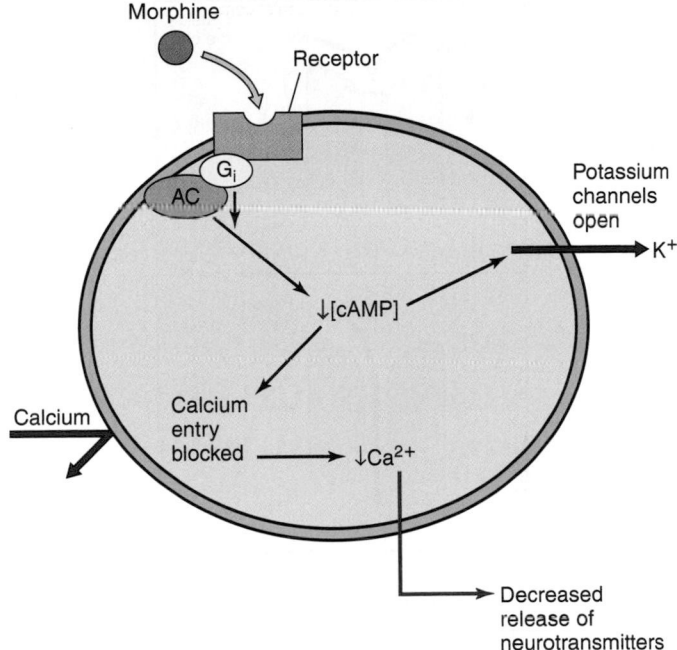

Fig. G-11 Mechanisms of Action: Narcotic Analgesics. Narcotic analgesics bind to three types of opioid receptors: mu, kappa, and delta receptors. They produce analgesia primarily by activating mu receptors. However, they also engage with and activate kappa and delta receptors, producing other effects, such as sedation and vasomotor stimulation.

When morphine or another narcotic analgesic binds to opioid receptors, activation occurs. The receptors send signals to the enzyme adenyl cyclase (AC) to slow activity by way of G proteins (G_i). Decreased adenyl cyclase activity causes reduced production of cyclic adenosine monophosphate (cAMP). A secondary messenger substance, cAMP is important for regulating cell membrane channels. A reduced cAMP level allows fewer potassium ions to leave the cell and blocks calcium ions from entering the cell. This ion imbalance—especially the reduced intracellular calcium level—ultimately decreases the release of neurotransmitters from the cell, thereby blocking or reducing pain impulse transmission. (From Minneman KP, Wecker L: *Brody's Human Pharmacology: Molecular to Clinical,* ed 4, St. Louis, 2005, Mosby.)

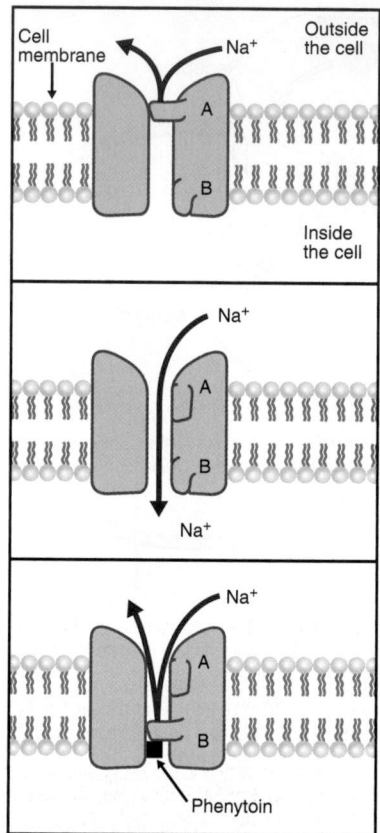

Fig. G-12 Mechanisms of Action: Phenytoin. Phenytoin, which is used to treat tonic-clonic seizures, acts in the motor cortex and brain stem, where the tonic phase of tonic-clonic seizures originates. By altering sodium transport across neuronal cell membranes, phenytoin stabilizes the cell membrane, reduces repetitive firing of the neurons, and halts or limits the spread of seizures. The first illustration shows a neuronal cell membrane in its resting state. The activation gate (**A**) of the sodium channel in the cell membrane is closed and blocks sodium (Na^+) from entering the cell. In the second illustration, a nerve impulse has caused depolarization and opening of the activation gate, allowing Na^+ to move into the cell. In the third illustration, depolarization continues and an inactivation gate (**B**) moves into the channel. This prevents Na^+ from moving into the cell. Phenytoin prolongs the inactivated state of the sodium channel by preventing reopening of the inactivation gate. By further preventing Na^+ from entering the cell, phenytoin slows impulse transmission, and thus slows the rate at which neurons fire. (From Minneman KP, Wecker L: *Brody's Human Pharmacology: Molecular to Clinical,* ed 4, St. Louis, 2005, Mosby.)

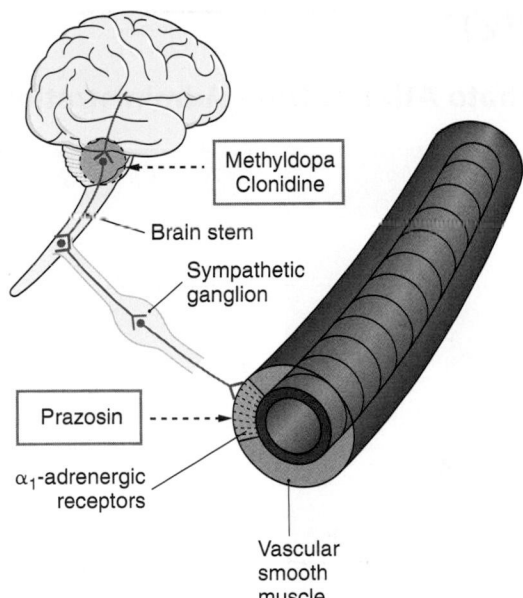

Fig. G-13 Sites of Action: Sympatholytics. Sympatholytics inhibit sympathetic nervous system (SNS) activity, which plays a major role in regulating B/P. Normally when the SNS is stimulated, nerve impulses travel from the cardiovascular center of the CNS to the sympathetic ganglia. From there, the impulses travel along postganglionic fibers to specific effector organs, such as the heart and blood vessels. SNS stimulation also triggers the release of norepinephrine, which acts primarily at alpha-adrenergic receptors.

Sympatholytics fall into two subclasses: central-acting α_2 agonists and peripheral-acting α_1-adrenergic antagonists. Central-acting α_2 agonists, such as methyldopa and cloNIDine, stimulate α_2-adrenergic receptors in the cardiovascular center of the CNS and reduce activity in the vasomotor center of the brain, interfering with sympathetic stimulation of the heart and blood vessels. This causes blood vessel dilatation and decreased cardiac output, which leads to reduced B/P.

Peripheral-acting α_1-adrenergic antagonists, such as prazosin, inhibit the stimulation of α_1-adrenergic receptors by norepinephrine in vascular smooth muscle, interfering with SNS-induced vasoconstriction. As a result, the blood vessels dilate, reducing peripheral vascular resistance and venous return to the heart. These effects, in turn, lead to decreased B/P. (From Prosser S, Worster B, Dewar K: *Applied Pharmacology for Nurses and Other Health Care Professionals,* St. Louis, 2000, Mosby.)

Appendix H

Photo Atlas of Drug Administration

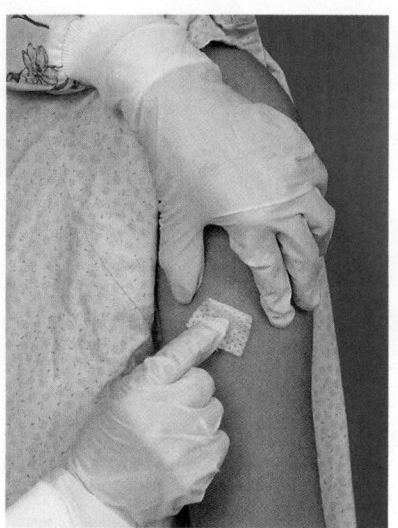

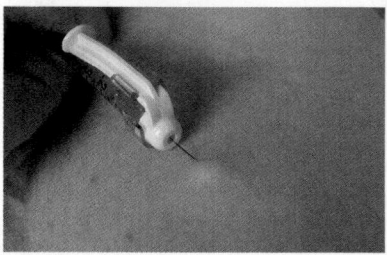

Fig. H-2 Intradermal Injection. For an intradermal injection, note formation of small bleb approximately 6 mm (¼ in) in diameter at injection site. (From Perry AG, Potter PA, and Elkin MK: *Nursing Interventions & Clinical Skills,* ed 5, St. Louis, 2012, Mosby.)

Fig. H-1 Administering an Injection. Cleanse site with antiseptic swab. Apply swab at center of site and rotate outward in circular direction for about 5 cm (2 in). (From Perry AG, Potter PA, and Elkin MK: *Nursing Interventions & Clinical Skills,* ed 5, St. Louis, 2012, Mosby.)

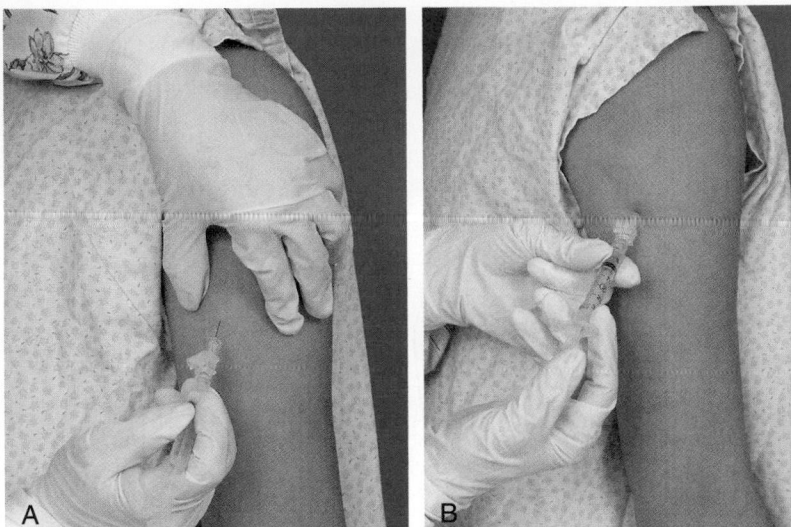

Fig. H-3 Subcutaneous Injection. **A,** For a subcutaneous injection, hold the syringe between the thumb and forefinger of the dominant hand as a dart, with the palm down. **B,** After injecting the needle at a 45- to 90-degree angle, grasp lower end of syringe barrel with nondominant hand to end of plunger. Avoid moving syringe while slowly pulling back on plunger to aspirate drug. If blood appears in syringe, remove needle, discard medication and syringe, and repeat procedure. *Exception:* Do not aspirate when giving heparin. (From Perry AG, Potter PA, and Elkin MK: *Nursing Interventions & Clinical Skills,* ed 5, St. Louis, 2012, Mosby.)

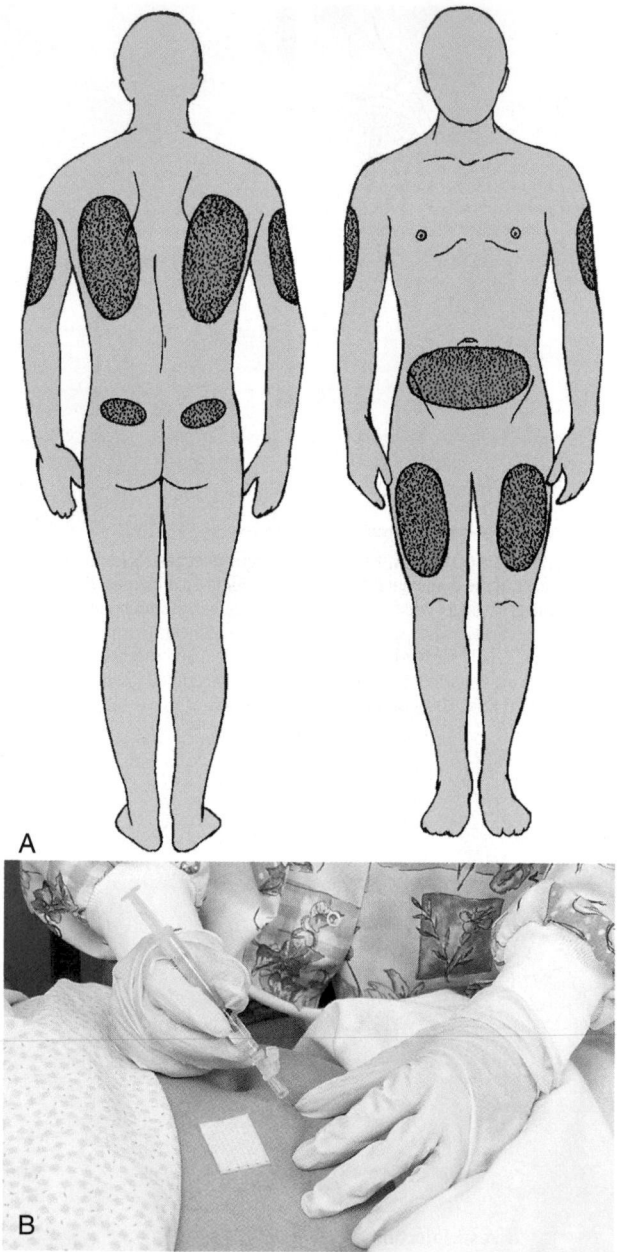

Fig. H-4 Subcutaneous Injection. A, Sites recommended for subcutaneous injections. **B,** Giving subcutaneous injection in the abdomen. (From Perry AG, Potter PA, and Elkin MK: *Nursing Interventions & Clinical Skills,* ed 5, St. Louis, 2012, Mosby.)

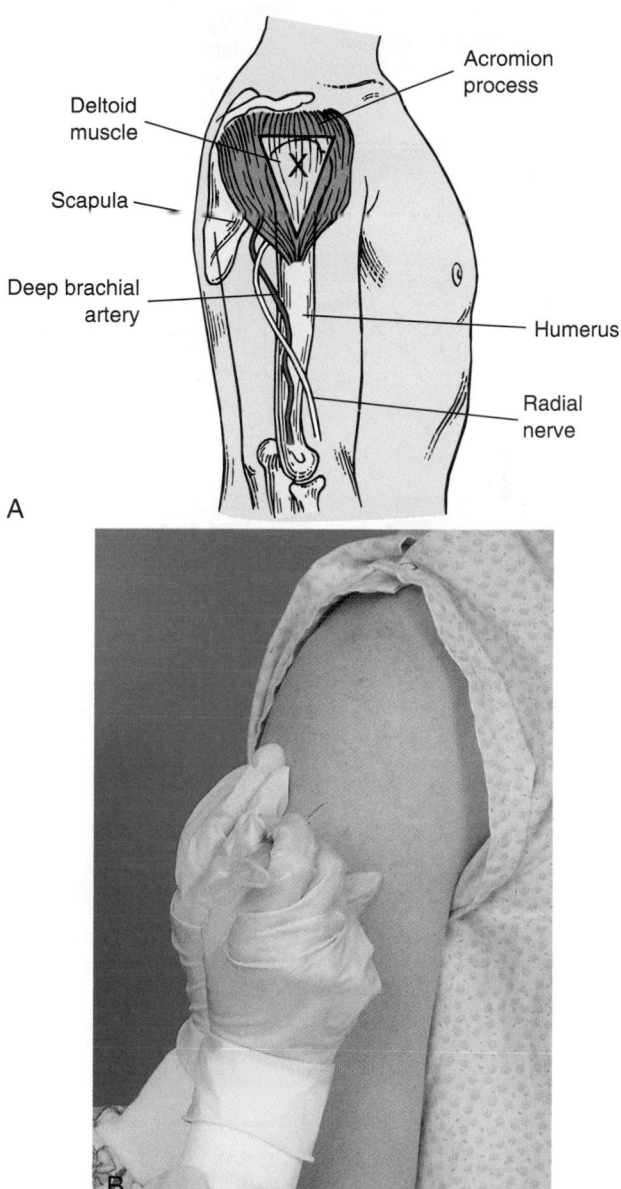

Fig. H-5 Deltoid Intradermal Injection. A, Landmarks for IM injection into the deltoid muscle. **B,** Giving IM injection in deltoid muscle. (From Perry AG, Potter PA, and Elkin MK: *Nursing Interventions & Clinical Skills,* ed 5, St. Louis, 2012, Mosby.)

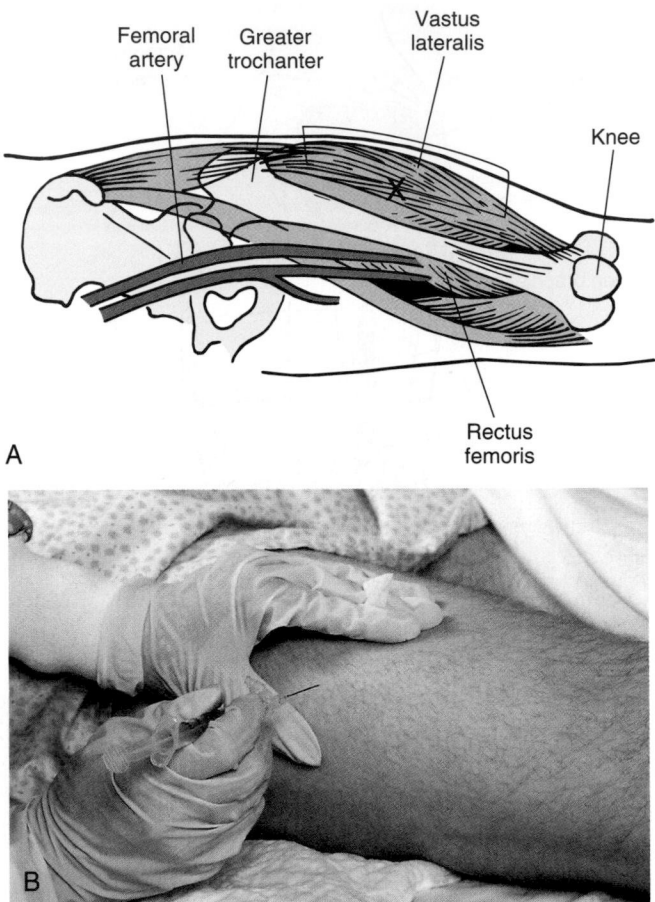

Femoral
artery

Greater
trochanter

Vastus
lateralis

Knee

A

Rectus
femoris

B

Fig. H-6 Vastus Lateralis Intramuscular Injection. A, Landmarks for IM injection in vastus lateralis. **B,** Giving IM injection in vastus lateralis site. (From Perry AG, Potter PA, and Elkin MK: *Nursing Interventions & Clinical Skills,* ed 5, St. Louis, 2012, Mosby.)

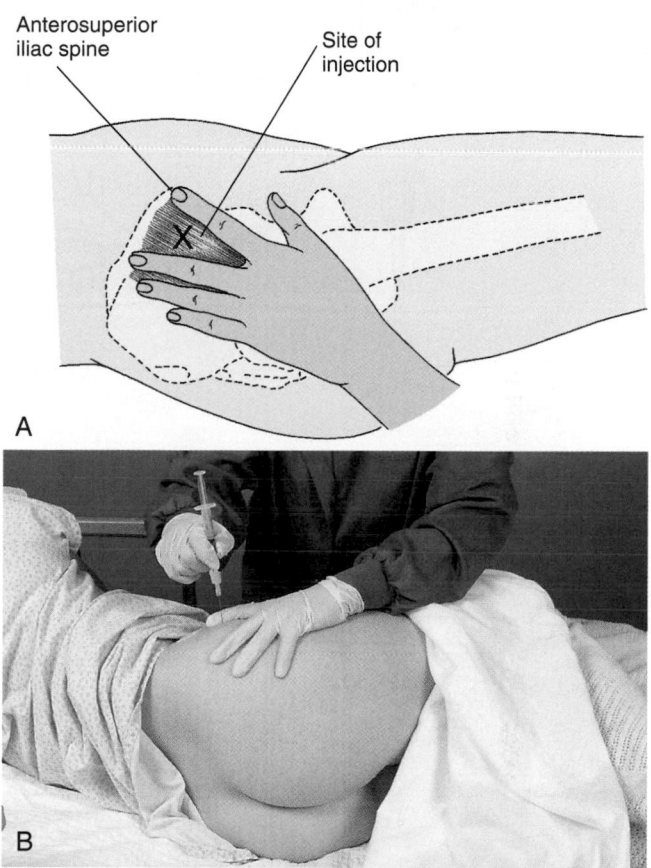

Fig. H-7 Ventrogluteal Intramuscular Injection. A, Anatomical view of ventrogluteal site.
B, Giving IM injection into ventrogluteal muscle to avoid major nerves and blood vessels. (From
Perry AG, Potter PA, and Elkin MK: *Nursing Interventions & Clinical Skills,* ed 5, St. Louis, 2012,
Mosby.)

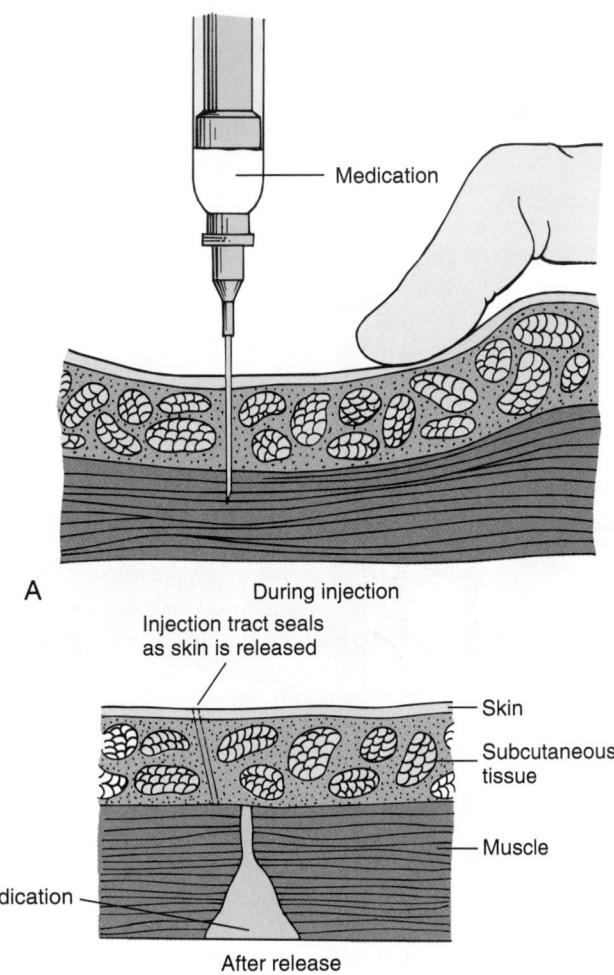

Fig. H-8 Z-Track Method of Injection. A, Pulling on overlying skin during IM injection moves tissues to prevent later tracking. **B,** The Z-track left after injection prevents the deposit of medication through sensitive tissue. (From Perry AG, Potter PA, and Elkin MK: *Nursing Interventions & Clinical Skills,* ed 5, St. Louis, 2012, Mosby.)

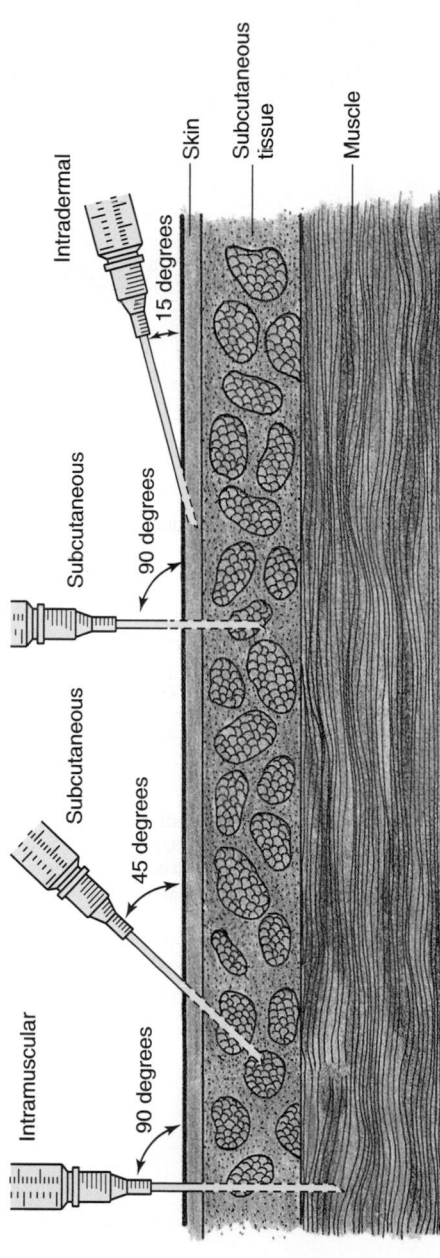

Fig. H-9 Comparison of Needle Angles. Comparison of angles of insertion for IM (90 degrees), SUBCUT (45 degrees and 90 degrees), and ID (15 degrees) injections. (From Potter PA, Perry AG: *Fundamentals of Nursing*, ed 7, St. Louis, 2009, Mosby.)

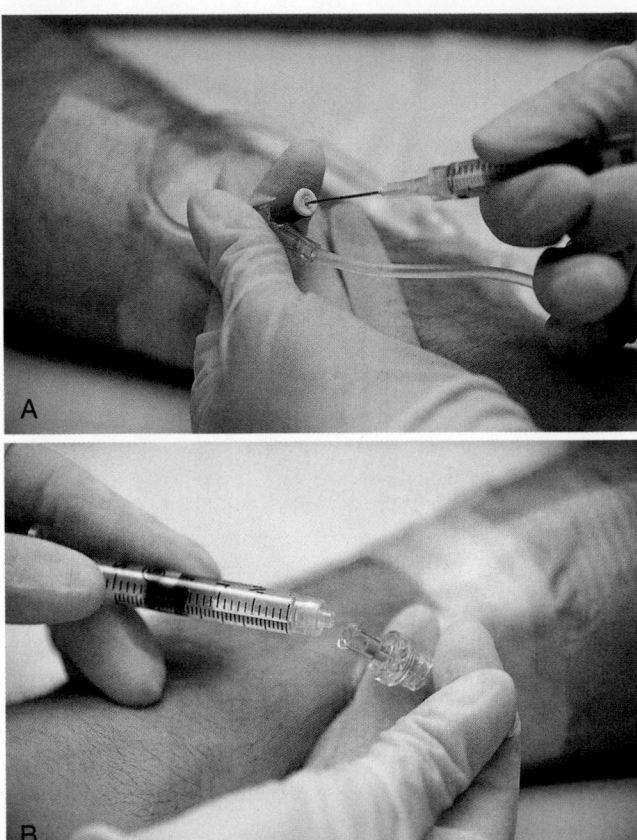

Fig. H-10 Administering Medication by IV Bolus (push). **A,** Needle system: Insert small-gauge needle of syringe containing prepared drug through center of injection port. **B,** Needleless system: Remove cap of needleless injection port. Connect tip of syringe directly. (From Potter PA, Perry AG: *Fundamentals of Nursing,* ed 6, St. Louis, 2005, Mosby.)

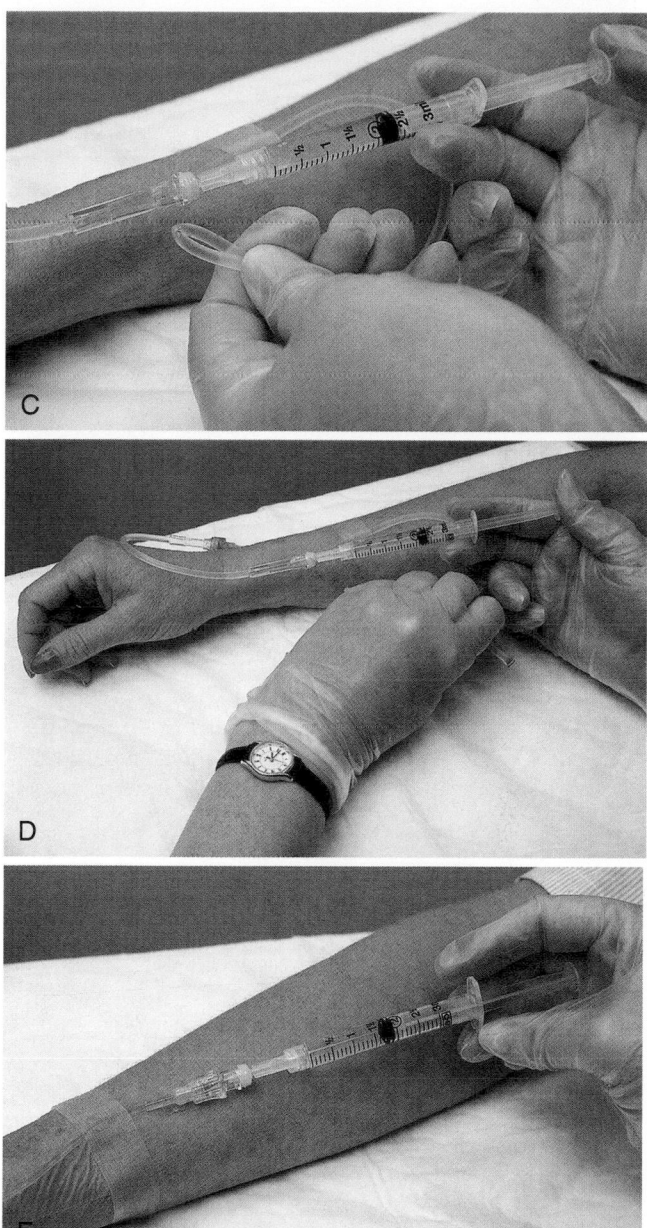

Fig. H-10, cont'd C, Occlude **IV** line by pinching tubing just above injection port. Pull back gently on syringe's plunger to aspirate blood return. **D,** After noting blood return, continue to occlude tubing and inject medication slowly over several minutes (read directions on drug package). Use watch to time administration. **E, IV** lock: Insert needle of syringe containing prepared drug through center of diaphragm. (From Potter PA, Perry AG: *Fundamentals of Nursing,* ed 6, St. Louis, 2005, Mosby.)

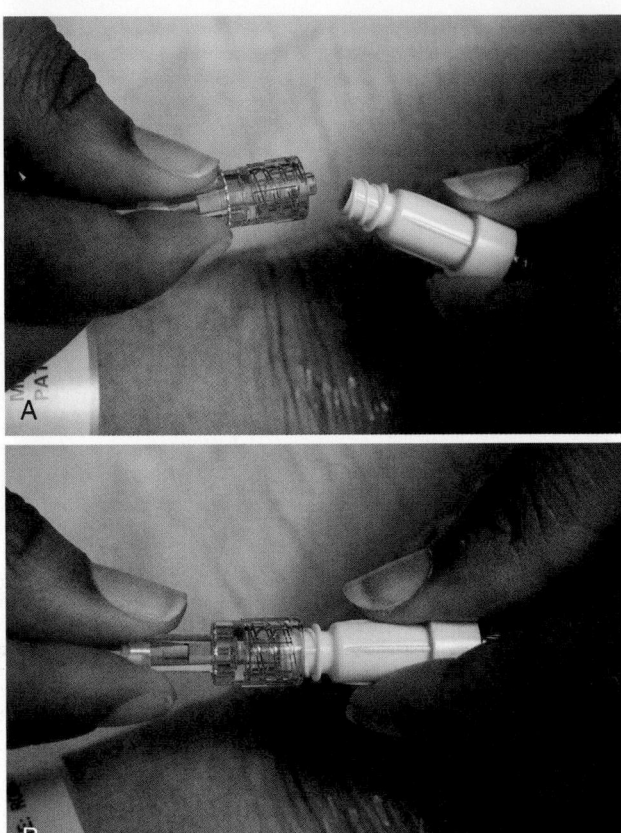

Fig. H-11 Administering IV Medication by Piggyback, Volume Administration Sets of Miniinfusors (Syringe Pump). Use needle-lock device to secure needle of secondary piggyback line through injection port of main line. (From Perry AG, Potter PA, and Elkin MK: *Nursing Interventions & Clinical Skills,* ed 5, St. Louis, 2012, Mosby.)

Appendix I

Common Herbs

aloe
(a'low)

Scientific names: Aloe vera L., *Aloe perryi,*
Aloe barbadensis, Aloe ferox, Aloe spicata
Other common names: Aloe, aloe barbadensis, aloe vera, Barbados, bitter al-
oes, burn plant, Cape aloe, Curacao aloe,
elephant's gall, hsiang-dan, lily of the
desert, lu-hui, socotrine aloe, Venezuela
aloe, Zanzibar aloe

ORIGIN: Aloe is a succulent found throughout the world. It is native to Africa.

USES: Aloe is used topically to treat minor
burns, sunburn, cuts, abrasions, bedsores, diabetic ulcers, acne, and stomatitis. It is used internally as a stimulant laxative. Aloe may also be
used to relieve radiation burns suffered by cancer patients and may help slow the development
of wrinkles.

ACTIONS
Aloe products have been used for centuries for a
variety of purposes.

Antiinflammatory and wound-
healing actions
The actions of topical aloe products are well
documented. Numerous studies have demonstrated their antiinflammatory, wound-healing
properties. Aloe products have been used to reduce inflammation by inactivation of bradykinin,
to inhibit prostaglandin A2, to oxidize arachidonic acids, and to block thromboxane A. The
wound-healing action of aloe may result from it
causing increased blood flow in the affected
area. There is demonstrated the antiinflammatory activity of aloe vera gel extract when used to
treat induced edema of the rat paw. The extract
reduced edema and the number of neutrophils
migrating into the rat's peritoneal cavity. In addition, aloe has been shown to be an effective
treatment for aphthous stomatitis.

Laxative action
The laxative effects of aloe result from its ability to inhibit absorption without stimulating
peristalsis.

PRODUCT AVAILABILITY
Available forms: Capsules: 75, 100, 200
mg extract or powder; cream; gel: 98%, 99.5%,
99.6%; jelly; juice: 99.6%, 99.7%; tincture
(1:10, 50% alcohol) shampoo and conditioner

Plant parts used: Large, blade-like leaf;
secretory cells below leaf epidermis; roots
(rarely)

DOSAGES
Laxative
Adult PO dried juice: 50-300 mg at bedtime
Adult PO aloe latex extract: 100-200 mg
aloe or 50 mg aloe extract at bedtime

Skin irritation/wounds
Adult and child: PO capsules: 100-200 mg
at bedtime
Adult and child: PO extract: 50-100 mg at
bedtime
Adult and child topical leaf gel: apply prn;
do not use on deep wounds

CONTRAINDICATIONS
Aloe should not be given to children younger
than 12 years of age. It should not be used by
persons with kidney disease, cardiac disease, or
bowel obstruction. Aloe gel should be used cautiously in intestinal obstruction, Crohn's disease,
ulcerative colitis, appendicitis, and other bowel
disorders because aloe gel could be contaminated with aloe latex. Aloe should not be used
topically by persons who are hypersensitive to
this plant or to garlic, onions, tulips, or other
plants of the Liliaceae family. It should not be
used topically on deep wounds. Dried aloe juice
is not for long-term use.

SIDE EFFECTS/ADVERSE
REACTIONS
GI: Spasms, intestinal mucosa damage (irreversible), hemorrhagic, *diarrhea* (internal use
of dried juice)
GU: Red-colored urine, *nephrotoxicity* (internal use of dried juice)
INTEG: Contact dermatitis, delayed healing of
deep wounds (topical use)

META: Hypokalemia (frequent internal use)
Reproductive: Uterine contractions causing spontaneous abortion, premature labor (internal use of dried juice)

INTERACTIONS
Drug
Antiarrhythmics, antidiabetics, cardiac glycosides, loop diuretics, potassium-wasting drugs, systemic steroids, thiazides: aloe products taken internally may increase the effects of antiarrhythmics, cardiac glycosides, antidiabetics, loop diuretics, potassium-wasting drugs, systemic steroids, and thiazides.

Herb
Jimsonweed: The action of jimsonweed is increased in cases of chronic use or abuse of aloe.
Licorice/horsetail: Licorice/horsetail may cause hypokalemia when used with aloe taken internally; avoid concurrent use.

Lab test
Serum potassium: Aloe may lower test values with long-term aloe use.

NURSING CONSIDERATIONS
Assess
General Use
• Assess the reason the client is using this product.
• Assess whether the client is taking cardiac or renal medications (antidysrhythmics, cardiac glycosides, loop diuretics, antidiabetes agents, thiazide diuretics).
• Assess whether systemic steroids or potassium-wasting drugs are being used. Inform the client that aloe products taken internally may increase the effects of these drugs.
• Assess for the use of licorice, jimsonweed, or other herbs that contain cardiac glycosides (see Interactions).
• Assess for internal use. Caution client that dried juice aloe products taken internally can be dangerous.
Laxative use of dried juice products
• Assess for repeated laxative use of aloe or traditional products.
• Assess blood and urine electrolytes if herb is used often.
• Assess for cramping, gastrointestinal spasms, and hemorrhagic diarrhea.
• Assess for cause of constipation: identify whether fluids, bulk, or exercise is lacking from lifestyle.
Skin disorders
• Assess area to be treated with topical aloe products. Identify characteristics of burns, rashes, inflammation, and color.

• Aloe products should not be used on deep wounds; healing can be delayed.
• Assess for route of use.
• Refrigerate 100% aloe vera gel after opening.

Patient problems
Impaired skin integrity (uses)
Constipation (uses)

Teach client/family
• Caution the client not to use aloe in children younger than 12 years of age.
• Caution the client not to use aloe topically if hypersensitive to this plant or to garlic, onions, or tulips.
• Caution the client not to use aloe topically on deep wounds.
• Caution the client that dried aloe juice is not for long-term use.

arnica
(ahr'ni-kuh)
Scientific name: Arnica montana L.; may also include *A. chamissonis less., A. cordifolia hook, A. fulgens Pursh, A. sororia Greene*
Other common names: Leopard's bane, common arnica, sneezewort, mountain snuff, mountain tobacco, wolf's bane

ORIGIN: Arnica grows wild in the mountains of Europe and Russia. Some species can be found in the western United States.

USES: Arnica is used topically to decrease inflammation in bruises, sprains, wounds, acne, boils, and rashes. Arnica should not be used internally. It is used in small quantities as a flavor in beverages and desserts.

ACTIONS
Antiinflammatory action
Antiinflammatory properties of arnica, possibly due to a decrease in interleukin-6. Antiinflammatory effect of helenalin, one of the chemical components of arnica. Clients who took homeopathic arnica had much less postoperative swelling after arthroscopy.

Cytotoxic action
Low cytotoxicity when compared with other antineoplastics. Helenalin showed the greatest cytotoxic effect.

Other actions
Arnica montana decreased mild postpartum bleeding.

PRODUCT AVAILABILITY
Topical: spray, cream, salve, ointment; oral: tablets, tea, tincture, sublingual

Plant parts used: Dried flower heads, rhizome

DOSAGES
Adult topical: apply to affected area as needed. Very little information is available on dosages.

CONTRAINDICATIONS
Pregnancy, breastfeeding.

Because arnica is considered poisonous, injection is contraindicated. Death can occur. Internal use is contraindicated unless supervised by an expert; serious renal and hepatic damage can occur. Arnica should not be used in children.

Do not use full-strength tincture on broken skin as contact dermatitis can occur. Do not use for prolonged periods.

SIDE EFFECTS/ADVERSE REACTIONS
INTEG: Rash, contact dermatitis
Taken internally (contraindicated)
CNS: Nervousness, restlessness, *coma*, *death*
CV: Cardiac arrest, cardiotoxicity, hypertension
GI: Abdominal pain, diarrhea, vomiting, anorexia, *hepatic failure*
HEMA: Bleeding
INTEG: Contact dermatitis (topical), *Sweet syndrome*
MS: Weakness
RESP: Dyspnea

INTERACTIONS
Drug
Antihypertensives: May decrease the antihypertensive effect if arnica is taken internally.

Lab test
APTT, PT, INR: Arnica increases these lab tests.
Primary

NURSING CONSIDERATIONS
Assess
• Assess the reason the client is using this product.
• Assess the condition of the skin: broken, bruised, rashes. Arnica should not be used for prolonged periods on this type of skin.
• Assess for Sweet syndrome, psoriasis.

Patient problem
Impaired skin integrity

Implementation
• Use only topically, unless under the supervision of a qualified expert.
• Do not use for prolonged periods; allergic reactions may occur.
• Do not use full-strength on broken, hypersensitive skin. Do not use on open wounds or abrasions.

Patient/family education
• Teach the patient not to use internally unless supervised by a competent herbalist.
• Arnica is considered poisonous and can be cardiotoxic. Serious hepatic and renal toxicity can occur.
• Inform the patient not to use in pregnancy and breastfeeding.
• Instruct the patient not to use for extended periods on broken or bruised skin; contact dermatitis can occur.
• Keep out of reach of children; ingestion of flowers or roots can lead to death.

bilberry
(bil'beh-ree)
Scientific name: Vaccinium myrtillus
Other common names: Airelle, bilberry, black whortle, bleaberry, bog bilberry, European blueberry, huckleberry, trackleberry, whinberry, whortleberry

ORIGIN: Bilberry is found in the central, northern, and southeastern regions of Europe.

USES: Bilberry has been used to improve night vision; to prevent cataracts, macular degeneration, and glaucoma; to treat varicose veins and hemorrhoids; to prevent hemorrhage after surgery; and to prevent and treat diabetic retinopathy and myopia. Other uses for bilberry include decreasing diarrhea and dyspepsia in adults or children, controlling insulin levels, and using as a diuretic and/or a urinary antiseptic.

ACTIONS
Research is more extensive for bilberry than for many other commonly used herbs. Areas of research include the use of bilberry for treating circulatory disorders, glaucoma, cataracts, macular degeneration, poor night vision, and diabetic/hypertensive retinopathy. Studies have also focused on its use as an antilipemic.

Ophthalmologic action
Studies indicate that night vision improved significantly when individuals were given bilberry. Participants experienced improved night visual acuity, improved adjustment to darkness, and restoration of acuity after glare. These actions may be due to the affinity of bilberry for the retina. In addition, bilberry may be useful for the prevention and treatment of glaucoma, cataracts, and macular degeneration of the eye. Chemical components in bilberry may alter the collagen structure of the eye and decrease intraocular pressure. The collagen-stabilizing effects of Vaccinium may offer protection against glaucoma

and the development of cataracts and macular degeneration of the eye.

Antidiabetic action
The anthocyanoside components of bilberry have been shown to decrease hyperglycemia. Their effect is somewhat weaker than that of insulin. However, a single dose has an extended duration of up to several weeks.

Other actions
Some of the other proposed actions of bilberry include its lipid-lowering effect and its ability to treat inflammatory joint disease, microscopic hematuria, and varicose veins. Studies in rats have shown that the anthocyanosides promote collagen synthesis and inhibit collagen loss. Bilberry also has been studied for its antioxidant effect.

PRODUCT AVAILABILITY
Capsules: 60, 80, 120, 450 mg; fluid extract; fresh berries, dried berries; liquid; tincture; dried roots, dried leaves.

Plant parts used: Berries, roots, leaves

DOSAGES
Cataracts
Adult PO extract: 40-80 mg standardized to 25% anthocyanosides (anthocyanadin) tid

Diabetes mellitus
Adult PO extract: 80-160 mg standardized to 25% anthocyanosides tid

Glaucoma
Adult PO extract: 80 mg standardized to 25% anthocyanosides tid

Other
Adult PO fresh berries: 55-115 g tid
Adult topical decoction: ⅛-¼ ounce (5-8 g) of crushed, dried fruit in 150 ml of water; boil 10 min; strain; use warm
Adult gargle/mouthwash: prepare decoction 10%, rinse or gargle

CONTRAINDICATIONS
Bilberry has been used traditionally to help stop breastfeeding.
Avoid large doses in those with clotting/bleeding disorders.

SIDE EFFECTS/ADVERSE REACTIONS
GI: Constipation (large consumption of dried fruits)

INTERACTIONS
Drug
Anticoagulants (heparin, warfarin), **NSAIDs:** Bilberry may increase the action of anticoagulants, NSAIDs; use caution if taking concurrently!

Antidiabetics: Bilberry may increase hypoglycemia; use caution if taking concurrently.

Antiplatelet agents: Bilberry may cause anti-aggregation of platelets; use caution if taking concurrently.

Aspirin: Bilberry may increase the anticoagulation action of aspirin; use caution if taking concurrently.

Insulin: Bilberry leaves may significantly decrease blood glucose levels; monitor carefully.

Iron: Bilberry interferes with iron absorption; avoid concurrent use.

Herb
Hypoglycemic herbs (devil's claw, fenugreek, garlic, horse chestnut, ginseng [Panax, Siberian]): Bilberry may increase hypoglycemic effect when used with hypoglycemic herbs.

Lab test
Blood glucose: Bilberry may decrease blood glucose.

NURSING CONSIDERATIONS
Assess
• Assess whether the client is taking anticoagulants, antidiabetic agents, or antiplatelet agents. Bilberry is known to induce hypoglycemia, anticoagulation, and antiplatelet aggregation (see Interactions).

Pharmacology
Pharmacokinetics
Peak 15 minutes; eliminated via bile. Therapeutic properties vary by harvest area.

NURSING CONSIDERATIONS
Assess
• Assess whether the client is taking anticoagulants, antidiabetic agents, or antiplatelet agents. Bilberry is known to induce hypoglycemia, anticoagulation, and antiplatelet aggregation (see Interactions).
• Monitor for improvement in vision if using to treat cataracts or glaucoma.
• Monitor blood glucose if using to treat diabetes mellitus.

Patient problems
Risk for injury (uses)
Diarrhea (uses)

Implementation
• Instruct the client to take bilberry PO in the form of tincture, capsules, fluid extract, or fresh berries.

Patient/family education
• Advise the client to notify the health care provider if diarrhea persists for more than 4 days.
• Advise the client that use of higher-than-recommended doses or use of this herb for extended periods will result in toxicity and may result in death (leaves).

black cohosh
(blak koe'hahsh)
Scientific names: Actaea racemosa, Cimicifuga racemosa
Other common names: Black snakeroot, bugbane, bugwort, cimicifuga, rattleroot, rattleweed, squaw root

ORIGIN: Black cohosh is a perennial that grows in the eastern region of the United States and in parts of Canada.

USES: Black cohosh is used as a smooth-muscle relaxant, an antispasmodic, an antitussive, an astringent, a diuretic, an antidiarrheal, an antiarthritic, and a hormone balancer in perimenopausal women. It is also used to decrease uterine spasms in the first trimester of pregnancy, as an antiabortion agent, and as a treatment for dysmenorrhea.

Investigational uses
Investigation is ongoing into the use of black cohosh to treat menopausal symptoms.

ACTIONS
Black cohosh has been researched extensively in the past few years, primarily for its effects when used to treat menopausal symptoms. The triterpene glycosides may be responsible for black cohosh's antiinflammatory and hormonal effects.

Estrogenic action
There is adequate evidence to support the use of black cohosh as an alternative to estrogen therapy in menopausal women. When cimicifuga extract is given, both physical and psychologic menopausal symptoms improve significantly within 6 to 8 weeks. Most improve within 4 weeks. Unlike estrogens, black cohosh does not affect the secretion of prolactin, follicle-stimulating hormone, and luteinizing hormone. Some information is contradictory. Antiestrogen results occur when estradiol activities are antagonized. LH levels may be altered.
Black cohosh was studied for safety and efficacy in breast/prostate cancer patients. A critical assessment of clinical and preclinical studies of black cohosh and cancer (breast, prostate) was presented. It appears that black cohosh is safe in breast cancer without risk for liver disease.

PRODUCT AVAILABILITY
Caplets: 40, 400, 420 mg; capsules: 25, 525 mg; fluid extract; powdered rhizome; solid (dry) powdered extract; tincture

Plant parts used: Rhizome (dried and fresh); roots

DOSAGES
Adult PO caplets/capsules: 40-80 mg bid standardized to 1 mg triterpenes (27-deoxyactein) (20 mg) per caplet/capsule (total of 4-8 mg triterpene glycosides/day)
Adult PO liquid extract: 0.9-6 ml/day (1:1)
Adult PO powdered rhizome: 1-2 g
Adult PO solid dry powdered extract: 250-500 mg (4:1)
Adult PO tincture: 6-12 ml/day (1:10)
Adult PO decoction 1.5-9 g daily

CONTRAINDICATIONS
Do not use in pregnancy or breastfeeding.
Black cohosh should not be given to children except under the supervision of a qualified expert. Black cohosh should not be used in patients with a history of estrogen receptor-positive breast cancer, cholestasis, or celiac disease.

SIDE EFFECTS/ADVERSE REACTIONS
CV: Hypotension, slow heart rate
ENDO: Uterine stimulation, miscarriage
GI: Nausea, vomiting, anorexia

INTERACTIONS
Drug
Antihypertensives: Black cohosh increases the action of antihypertensives; avoid concurrent use.
Docetaxel, doxorubicin: Black cohosh may increase the toxicity of docetaxel and doxorubicin; avoid concurrent use.
Hormonal contraceptives: Black cohosh may increase the effects; avoid concurrent use.
Hormone replacement therapy: Black cohosh may alter the effects of other hormone replacement therapies; use together cautiously.
Sedatives/hypnotics: Black cohosh may increase the hypotension; avoid concurrent use.
Tamoxifen: Black cohosh may augment the antiproliferative properties of tamoxifen.

Lab test
Luteinizing hormone (LH): Black cohosh

NURSING CONSIDERATIONS
Assess
• Assess for menopausal and menstrual irregularities: length of cycle, amount of flow, spotting, pain, and hot flashes.

- Assess for the presence of ovarian cysts or fibroids.
- Assess for the use of other hormonal products: estrogen, progesterone, contraceptives, thyroid products, steroids, and androgens. Concurrent use requires caution (see Interactions).
- Assess for breast cancer or other cancers; avoid concurrent use.

Patient problems
Risk for injury (uses)

Implementation
- Instruct the client to take black cohosh PO using standardized products.
- Advise the client that effects are usually not seen until black cohosh is taken for at least 4 weeks.

Patient/family education
- Inform the client not to use in pregnancy and breastfeeding.
- Caution the client not to give black cohosh to children.

chondroitin
(kahn-droe'uh-tuhn)
Scientific names: Chondroitin sulfate, chondroitin sulfuric acid, chonsurid
Other common names: CAS, chondroitin sulfate, chondroitin C

ORIGIN: Chondroitin is obtained from bovine tracheal cartilage.

USES: Chondroitin is used alone or in combination with glucosamine to treat joint conditions such as arthritis. It is also used as an antithrombotic, an extravasation therapy agent, and as a treatment for ischemic heart disease and hyperlipidemia.

ACTIONS
Antiarthritic action
Chondroitin attracts essential fluid into the joints, which acts as a shock absorber. It also attracts needed nutrients into cartilage. It may protect cartilage from degradation.

Extravasation action
Chondroitin has been used to treat extravasation after ifosfamide therapy.

Antithrombolytic action
Because of its ability to inhibit thrombi, chondroitin is used as an anticoagulant in hemodialysis.

PRODUCT AVAILABILITY
Capsules: 200, 400 mg; source: cartilage of the bovine trachea

DOSAGES
Adult PO weight <120 pounds: 1000 mg glucosamine and 800 mg chondroitin
Adult PO weight 120-200 pounds: 1500 mg glucosamine and 1200 mg chondroitin
Adult PO weight >200 pounds: 2000 mg glucosamine and 1600 mg chondroitin

CONTRAINDICATIONS
Until more research is available, chondroitin should not be used during pregnancy and breastfeeding. It should not be given to children. Chondroitin should not be used by persons with bleeding disorders, asthma, prostate cancer, or renal failure.

SIDE EFFECTS/ADVERSE REACTIONS
CNS: Headache, restlessness, euphoria
GI: Nausea, vomiting, anorexia
SYST: Bleeding

INTERACTIONS
Drug
Anticoagulants, NSAIDs, salicylates: Chondroitin used with anticoagulants, NSAIDs, or salicylates can cause increased bleeding; do not use chondroitin at high doses.

Lab test
Anti-factor Xa: May be increased when used with chondroitin.
Prothrombin time: May be increased when used with high dose of chondroitin and glucosamine.

Pharmacology
Pharmacokinetics
Very little is known about the pharmacokinetics. The half-life of this herb is extended when used by persons with renal failure.

NURSING CONSIDERATIONS
Assessment
- Assess the reason the client is using chondroitin.
- Assess for joint conditions: joints involved; aggravating and ameliorating factors; and pain location, intensity, and duration.
- Assess for other medications used; chondroitin should not be used concurrently with anticoagulants, NSAIDs, or salicylates because of the risk of increased bleeding.

Patient problems
Impaired mobility (uses)

Implementation
- Instruct the patient to store chondroitin in a cool, dry place, away from heat and moisture.

Teach client/family
• Caution the patient not to use chondroitin in children or in those who are pregnant or breastfeeding until more research is available.

dong quai
Scientific name: Angelica polymorpha var. sinensis
Other common names: Chinese angelica, danggui, dry-kuei, tanggwi, tang-kuei, toki, women's ginseng

ORIGIN: Dong quai is a perennial found in Japan, China, and Korea.

USES: Dong quai has been used extensively to treat the symptoms of menopause.

It is also used to treat menstrual irregularities such as dysmenorrhea, premenstrual syndrome, and menorrhagia. Other uses include treatment for headaches, neuralgia, herpes infections, and malaria. In traditional Chinese medicine, dong quai is used to treat vitiligo and anemia. Dong quai should not be confused with other *Angelica* spp.

ACTIONS
Dong quai has been used since the sixth century as a blood and liver tonic. In Chinese medicine, it has been used to treat hormonal irregularities and anemia.

Hormonal action
Research on the hormonal actions of dong quai shows conflicting results.

Other actions
Angelica sinensis root on melanocyte proliferation showed no stimulation of melanocyte division. Instead, cell cytotoxicity resulted at higher doses. Other cell actions include decreased intraocular pressure, decreased blood pressure, decreased premature ventricular contractions, inhibition of platelet aggregation, increased tumor necrosis factor (TNF), and decreased atherosclerosis. Antiinflammatory and mild analgesic properties have also been reported.

PRODUCT AVAILABILITY
Capsules, fluid extract, raw roots (powdered), tablets, tea, tincture; available in many combination products; not available as a standardized extract

Plant part used: Roots

DOSAGES
Symptoms of menopause and premenstrual syndrome
Adult PO fluid extract: 1 ml (¼ tsp) tid
Adult PO powdered root: 1-2 g tid
Adult PO tea: 1-2 g tid
Adult PO tincture: 4 ml (1 tsp) (1:5 dilution) tid

>> Other
Adult PO capsules/tablets: 500 mg ≤6 times/day
Adult PO raw root: 1 g/day
Adult PO tea: 1 cup bid-tid
Adult PO tincture: 5-20 drops (1:5 concentration) ≤tid

CONTRAINDICATIONS
Do not use in pregnancy or breastfeeding. Until more research is available, dong quai should not be given to children. In Chinese medicine, dong quai has been used during pregnancy, but its use must be monitored by a qualified expert. This herb should not be used by persons who are hypersensitive to it or by those with bleeding disorders, excessive menstrual flow, or acute illness.

SIDE EFFECTS/ADVERSE REACTIONS
GI: Nausea, vomiting, diarrhea, anorexia
GU: Increased menstrual flow
INTEG: Hypersensitivity reactions, photosensitivity
SYST: Fever, *bleeding*, cancer

INTERACTIONS
Drug
Anticoagulants (anisindione, dicumarol, warfarin), **antiplatelets, estrogens, hormonal contraceptives:** Dong quai may increase the effects of anticoagulants, antiplatelets, estrogens, hormonal contraceptives.

Herb
Chamomile, dandelion, horse chestnut, red clover: Dong quai may potentiate anticoagulant activity.
St. John's wort: Dong quai may increase photosensitivity (theoretical).

Lab test
APTT, prothrombin time (PT), international normalized ratio (INR): Dong quai may increase levels of APTT, PT, INR.

NURSING CONSIDERATIONS
Assess
- Assess the reason the patient is using dong quai.
- Assess for hypersensitivity reactions. If present, discontinue use of dong quai and administer an antihistamine or other appropriate therapy.
- Determine whether the patient is using anticoagulants; dong quai may increase bleeding tendencies (see Interactions).

Patient problems
Impaired sexual functioning (uses)

Implementation
- Instruct the patient to store dong quai products in a sealed container away from moisture and heat.

Patient/family education
- Inform the patient not to use in pregnancy or breastfeeding. Caution the patient not to use dong quai in children until more research is available.
- Advise the patient that photosensitivity may occur. Sunscreen or protective clothing should be worn in sunlight.

echinacea
Scientific names: Echinacea angustifolia, Echinacea pallida, Echinacea purpurea
Other common names: American cone flower, black sampson, black susans, cock-up-hat, comb flower, coneflower, hedgehog, Indian head, Kansas snakeroot, Missouri snakeroot, purple coneflower, red sunflower, rudbeckia, sampson root, scurvy root, snakeroot

ORIGIN: Echinacea is a perennial found in only three states: Missouri, Nebraska, and Kansas. It is cultivated in much of the world. Echinacea is a Native American remedy.

USES: Echinacea is used internally, primarily as an immune stimulant and for immune support, and as prophylaxis for colds, influenza, and other viral, fungal, and bacterial infections. It may be used topically to promote wound healing and to treat wounds, bruises, burns, scratches, and leg ulcers. Echinacea is more effective when taken at the onset or first signs of an illness, not after the illness is well established.

Investigational uses
Researchers are experimenting with the use of echinacea to stimulate the immune system of HIV/AIDS patients. It may also be used as a prophylaxis for colds or urinary tract infections.

ACTIONS
Echinacea has been studied extensively and found to be effective in both the prevention and treatment of acute colds and upper respiratory tract infections. Native Americans have used this herb to treat various illnesses. For the past several years echinacea has been among a group of herbs accepted by practitioners of mainstream medicine.

Immunostimulant action
Echinacea stimulates the nonspecific immune response via phagocytosis, which plays a major role in the immune response. It also stimulates T-lymphocytes. It may significantly increase the phagocytosis of red blood cells, enhanced interleukin-6 (IL-6) production in response to strenuous exercise.

Antiinfective action
Echinacea has been shown to inhibit streptococcal growth and tissue hyaluronidase and to stabilize hyaluronic acid. Hyaluronidase is found in pathogenic organisms. In recent years there has been a lot of controversy about echinacea's use in the common cold. Preparations vary widely, and this could account for the differences in studies.

PRODUCT AVAILABILITY
Capsules, fluid extract, juice, solid (dry powdered) extract, sublingual tablets, tablets, tea, tincture
  NOTE: Some extracts may be standardized to 4% to 5% echinacoside; others are standardized to phenolics.

Plant parts used: Rhizome, roots; depending on developmental stage of growth: flowers, juice from the stem, leaves, whole plant

DOSAGES
Adult parenteral: Dose individualized to age of patient and condition. (NOTE: parenteral route not used in the United States; herb used parenterally in Germany.)
Adult PO capsules: 500 mg-1 g tid
Adult PO dried root: 0.5-1 g tid; can use as tea
Adult PO fluid extract: 1-2 ml tid (1:1 dilution) mixed in a little water
Adult PO freeze-dried plant: 325-650 mg tid
Adult PO pressed juice: 6-9 ml daily in divided doses (25:1 dilution in 22% alcohol)

Adult PO solid (dry powdered) extract: 150-300 mg tid (6.5:1 dilution or 3.5% echinacoside)

Adult PO tea: 2 tsp (4 g) powdered herb simmered 15 min in hot water

Adult PO tincture: 15-30 drops bid-qid or 30-60 drops bid

Acute infections
Child PO root tincture: ½-1 tsp up to q2hr

Skin infections
Child topical tincture: 1 tbsp root/¼ cup water, use as topical rinse

To prevent colds and infections
Child: PO root tincture: ½ tsp bid

CONTRAINDICATIONS
Pregnancy category is 1; breastfeeding category is 2A.

Echinacea should not be given to children younger than 2 years of age. It should not be used by persons who have autoimmune diseases such as lupus erythematosus, multiple sclerosis, HIV/AIDS, or collagen disease, or by those with tuberculosis or hypersensitivity to *Bellis* sp. or composite family herbs. Immunosuppression may occur after extended therapy with this herb; do not use for longer than 8 weeks without a 3-week rest period.

SIDE EFFECTS/ADVERSE REACTIONS
GI: Hepatotoxicity
INTEG: Hypersensitivity reactions
RESP: Acute asthma attack
SYST: Anaphylaxis, angioedema

INTERACTIONS
Drug
Cytochrome P4503A4 substrates: Echinacea may inhibit cytochrome P4503A4 enzymes
Econazole vaginal cream: The action of this cream may be decreased by echinacea; avoid concurrent use.
Immunomodulators (*azathioprine, basiliximab, cyclosporine, daclizumab, muromonab, mycophenolate, tacrolimus, protease inhibitors, corticosteroids*): Echinacea may decrease the effects of immunosuppressants, protease inhibitors, and corticosteroids and should not be used immediately before, during, or after transplant surgery.

Lab test
ALT, AST, lymphocyte counts (*Echinacea purpurea*), serum immunoglobulin E (IgE), blood erythrocyte sedimentation rate (ESR): Echinacea may increase these tests.
Sperm enzyme activity: High doses of echinacea interfere with sperm enzyme activity.

NURSING CONSIDERATIONS
Assess
• Assess for hypersensitivity reactions to this herb, members of the daisy family (genus *Bellis*), or composite family herbs. If hypersensitivity is present, discontinue the use of this herb and administer an antihistamine or other appropriate therapy.
• Assess for use of econazole vaginal cream, immunomodulators, cytochrome.
• P4503A4 substrates, protease inhibitors, and corticosteroids (see Interactions).

Patient problems
Infection (uses)

Implementation
• Instruct the patient to store echinacea products in sealed container away from heat and moisture.
• Instruct the patient not to use this herb for longer than 8 weeks without a 3-week rest period.

Patient/family education
• Inform the patient it is considered safe in pregnancy and breastfeeding.
• Caution the patient not to give echinacea to children younger than 2 years of age.
• Caution the patient to be careful not to confuse this herb with other *Echinacea* spp. that have different uses.

garlic
(gahr'lik)
Scientific name: Allium sativum
Other common names: Ail, allium, camphor of the poor, da-suan, knoblauch, la-suan, nectar of the gods, poor-man's treacle, rustic treacle, stinking rose

ORIGIN: Garlic is a perennial bulb found throughout the world.

USES: Garlic is used as an antilipidemic, antimicrobial, antiasthmatic, and antiinflammatory. It is a possible antihypertensive agent and is used to treat some types of heavy metal poisoning.

Investigational uses
Studies are underway to determine the role of garlic as an anticancer, antioxidant, antiplatelet, and antidiabetic treatment.

ACTIONS

The main actions attributed to garlic are antimicrobial, antilipidemic, antitriglyceride, antiplatelet, antioxidant, and cancer preventive.

Antimicrobial action

Garlic inhibits both gram-positive and gram-negative organisms, and various studies identified the antifungal, antiviral, and antiparasitic actions of garlic.

Cardiovascular action

Garlic has been shown to exert cholesterol-lowering, triglyceride-lowering, and antiplatelet actions.

Cholesterol-lowering and triglyceride-lowering actions

The chemical component believed to be responsible for the anticholesterol action is allicin, which is believed to reduce cholesterol production by preventing gastric lipase fat digestion and fecal excretion of sterols and bile acids.

Antiplatelet action

The antiplatelet effect of garlic has been demonstrated, with ajoene apparently functioning as the chemical component responsible. Several investigations have demonstrated the ability of garlic to reduce platelet aggregation and cyclooxygenase.

Cancer prevention

A large amount of evidence is available to support the beneficial effects of garlic in the prevention of cancer and the slowing of its progression. There may be a decrease in the development of gastric cancer when garlic is added to the diet. The protective effects may be due to the antioxidant properties of these vegetables and their ability to inhibit cancer cell proliferation.

Other actions

Garlic has been shown to inhibit free radicals, which may be responsible for cancer proliferation, and to decrease lipid peroxidation.

PRODUCT AVAILABILITY

Bulbs, capsules, extract, fresh garlic, oil, powder, syrup, tablets, tea

Plant part used: Bulb (root)

DOSAGES

Garlic may be standardized to its allicin (active ingredient) content.

Chronic candidiasis
Adult PO fresh garlic: 4 g daily

General use
Adult PO extract, aged: 4 ml daily
Adult PO fresh garlic: 4 g daily
Adult PO oil, perles: 10 mg daily

Hypercholesteremia/hypertension
Adult PO: 40,000 mcg daily (allicin)
Adult PO capsules/powder/tablets: 600-900 mg daily in divided doses to decrease lipids

General use
Child PO fresh garlic: ½-3 cloves daily
Child PO syrup: ½-1 tsp/day
Child PO tea: 1 cup daily; may give up to 4 cups daily to treat colds

CONTRAINDICATIONS

May be used in pregnancy and breastfeeding.

Because garlic may reduce iodine uptake, it should not be used by persons with hypothyroidism. Because garlic may cause clotting time to be increased, it should not be used by persons who recently have had or are about to have surgery. Garlic should not be used by persons with stomach inflammation, gastritis, or hypersensitivity to this herb.

SIDE EFFECTS/ADVERSE REACTIONS

CNS: Dizziness, headache, irritability, fatigue, insomnia
CV: Tachycardia, orthostatic hypotension
GI: Nausea, vomiting, anorexia
GU: Hypothyroidism
INTEG: Hypersensitivity reactions, contact dermatitis
RESP: Asthma, shortness of breath
SYST: Diaphoresis, garlic odor, irritation of the oral cavity, decreased red blood cells, hypothyroidism

INTERACTIONS
Drug

Anticoagulants (anisindione, dicumerol, heparin, warfarin), **antiplatelets, NSAIDs, salicylates:** Garlic may increase bleeding when used with these products; do not use concurrently.

Antidiabetics (acetohexamide, chlorpropamide, glipizide, metformin, tolazamide, tolbutamide, troglitazone): Because of the hypoglycemic effects of garlic, oral antidiabetic dosages may need to be adjusted.

Cytochrome P4503A4 substrates: Garlic containing allicin may increase the action of cytochrome P4503A4.

Hormonal contraceptives, nonnucleoside reverse transcriptase inhibitors: Garlic with allicin may decrease the action of hormonal contraceptives, nonnucleoside reverse transcriptase inhibitors.

Insulin: Because of the hypoglycemic effects of garlic, insulin dosages may need to be adjusted.

Herb

Acidophilus: Acidophilus may decrease the absorption of garlic. If taken concurrently, separate the dosages by 3 hours.

Anticoagulant/antiplatelet, fish oils herbs: Garlic used with herbs having anticoagulant/antiplatelet properties may increase risk of bleeding.

Lab test

LDL, platelet aggregation, triglycerides, blood lipid profile: Garlic may decrease LDL cholesterol (aged extract taken continuously), platelet aggregation (aged extract of garlic taken over extended period of time), triglycerides (aged extract of garlic taken over extended period of time), blood lipid profile.

Prothrombin time INR, APTT, serum IgE: Garlic may increase prothrombin time, INR, APTT, and serum immunoglobulin E (IgE).

NURSING CONSIDERATIONS
Assessment

• Assess the reason the patient is using garlic.
• Because garlic is a common allergen, assess for hypersensitivity reactions and contact dermatitis. If such reactions are present, discontinue the use of garlic and administer an antihistamine or other appropriate therapy.
• Assess lipid levels if the patient is using garlic to decrease lipids.
• Monitor CBC and coagulation studies if the patient is using garlic at high doses or with anticoagulants. Identify anticoagulants the patient is using, including salicylates (see Interactions).
• Determine whether the patient is diabetic and is using insulin or antidiabetics; dosages may need to be adjusted (see Interactions).

Patient problems

Infection (uses)

Implementation

• Instruct the patient to avoid the daily use of medicinal garlic, unless under the supervision of a qualified expert. Blood clotting may be affected.
• Instruct the patient to store garlic products in a sealed container away from heat and moisture.

Patient/family education

• Inform the patient that garlic is considered safe in small amounts in pregnancy and breastfeeding
• Inform the patient that some studies have indicated that garlic may be helpful in treating children with hypercholesterolemia.
• Advise the patient to inform all health care providers of garlic use.

• Caution the patient to discontinue the use of garlic before undergoing any invasive procedure in which bleeding may occur.

ginger

(jin'juhr)

Scientific name: Zingiber officinale
Other common names: Black ginger, race ginger, zinyibor

ORIGIN: Ginger is found in the tropics of Asia and is now cultivated in the tropics of South America, China, India, Africa, the Caribbean, and parts of the United States.

USES: Ginger is used to prevent and relieve motion and morning sickness; to relieve sore throat, nausea, and vomiting; to treat migraine headaches; and as an antioxidant.

Investigational uses

Preliminary research is available that documents the efficacy of ginger in decreasing the pain and inflammation associated with arthritis and other joint disorders. Some evidence indicates that it may also reduce platelet aggregation. Ginger may decrease hyperglycemia, ulcers, and fever.

ACTIONS
Antiemetic and antinausea actions

Several studies have documented the antiemetic and antinausea actions of ginger. When dried ginger powder was evaluated against dimenhydrinate and a placebo, ginger was found to reduce nausea and vomiting more effectively than dimenhydrinate. This effect is postulated to result from action on the digestive tract instead of the central nervous system. Ginger lacks any anticholinergic effects.

Antiinflammatory action

Its ability to inhibit arachidonic acid metabolism is believed to be responsible for antiinflammatory action. Ginger has been used in traditional medicine to treat rheumatic disorders.

Other actions

Other actions for ginger include antiulcer, antiplatelet, antipyretic, antiinfective, antioxidant, and antidiabetic action; improved digestive function and positive inotropic action.

Improved digestive functioning

Improved digestive functioning may occur as a result of increased amylase and salivary production. Ginger has been shown to increase the absorption of other drugs and to prevent degradation during the first hepatic pass.

Antiulcer action
The antiulcer effects of ginger may be due to two of its chemical components, gingerol and ginge-sulphonic acid. Improvements in ulcer patients occurred with the use of ginger decocted in water. However, relapse was common and complete cure did not occur.

Antiplatelet action
The antiplatelet action of ginger may be a result of the inhibition of thromboxane formation. Increases occurred in ADP, collagen, arachidonic acid, and epinephrine when ginger was used.

Antipyretic action
The antipyretic effect of ginger is due to its prostaglandin inhibition. Ginger is as effective as aspirin in reducing fever.

Antiinfective action
Ginger exerts antiinfective action against both gram-positive and gram-negative bacteria. Its antiinfective action was very weak when tested; however, one class of chemical components, the sesquiterpenes, did exert significant action against antirhinoviral infections.

Antioxidant action
The antioxidant effects of ginger may be the result of the actions of gingerol and zingerone, two of its chemical components. These components inhibit lipoxygenase and eliminate the radicals superoxide and hydroxyl.

Antidiabetes action
Ginger may be useful in the treatment of hyperglycemia.

PRODUCT AVAILABILITY
Capsules, dried root, extract, fresh root, powder, tablets, tea, tincture

Plant part used: Rhizome

DOSAGES
Ginger may be standardized to its volatile oil (4%) or essential oil (8%).

General use
Adult PO dried ginger capsules: 1 g/day
Adult PO dried root equivalent: 500 mg bid-qid
Adult PO fluid extract: 0.7-2 ml/day (1:2 dilution)
Adult PO fresh root equivalent: 500-1000 mg tid
Adult PO tablets/caps: 500 mg bid-qid
Adult PO tincture: 1.7-5 ml/day (1:5 dilution)
Migraine
Adult PO dried ginger: 500 mg qid

Adult PO extract: 100-200 mg, standardized to 20% gingerol and shogaol
Adult PO fresh ginger: 10 g/day (¼-inch slice)

Motion sickness and morning sickness prevention
Adult PO extract: 100-200 mg, standardized to 20% gingerol and shogaol
Adult PO powder: 1-2 g ½-1 hr before traveling or upon arising
Adult PO tea, dried root: 1½ tsp ground dried root in 1 cup water, boil 5-10 min, drink prn
Adult PO tea, fresh root: 1 tsp fresh root in 1 cup water, infuse 5 min, drink prn

Rheumatoid arthritis
Adult PO extract: 100-200 mg, standardized to 20% gingerol and shogaol
Adult PO fresh ginger: 8-10 g/day

Sore throat
Adult PO fresh root tea: 1 tsp fresh root in 1 cup water, infuse 5 min, gargle prn

General use
Child PO ginger root tea: ¼-1 cup prn
Child PO tincture: 5-25 drops in water prn

CONTRAINDICATIONS
Avoid use in pregnancy and breastfeeding. Ginger should not be used by persons with hypersensitivity to it. Unless directed by a physician, ginger should not be used by persons with cholelithiasis.

SIDE EFFECTS/ADVERSE REACTIONS
CV: Arrhythmias
GI: Nausea, vomiting, anorexia
INTEG: Hypersensitivity reactions

INTERACTIONS
Drug
All oral medications: Ginger may increase absorption of all medications taken orally.
Antacids, antidiabetics, antihypertensives, H2-blockers, proton pump inhibitors: Ginger may decrease the action of these agents (theoretical).
Anticoagulants *(ardeparin, anisindione, aspirin, dicumerol, dalteparin, heparin, warfarin),* ***antiplatelets*** *(abciximab):* Ginger may increase the risk for bleeding when used concurrently with anticoagulants, antiplatelets (theoretical).

Herb
Anticoagulant/antiplatelet herbs: When used with anticoagulant/antiplatelet herbs, ginger may increase the risk for bleeding (theoretical).

Lab test
Plasma partial prothrombin time, prothrombin time: Ginger may increase plasma partial prothrombin time in clients taking warfarin concurrently and may increase prothrombin time.

Pharmacokinetics
Information on the pharmacokinetics and pharmacodynamics of ginger is limited. Its metabolites are known to be eliminated via urinary excretion within 24 hours, and it is 90% bound to plasma proteins.

NURSING CONSIDERATIONS
Assessment
- Assess the reason the patient is taking ginger.
- Assess for hypersensitivity reactions. If present, discontinue use of this herb and administer an antihistamine or other appropriate therapy.
- Assess all medications used (see Interactions).

Patient problems
Implementation
- Instruct the patient to store ginger products in a cool, dry place away from heat and moisture.

Patient/family education
- Inform the patient that ginger should be avoided in pregnancy and breastfeeding.

ginkgo
(ging'koe)

Scientific name: *Ginkgo* biloba
Other common names: Maidenhair tree, rokan, sophium, tanakan, tebofortan, tebonin

ORIGIN: Ginkgo is a tree native to China and Japan. It is now also found in the United States and Europe.

USES: Ginkgo is used to decrease disturbances of cerebral functioning and peripheral vascular insufficiency in persons with Alzheimer's disease or other types of age-related dementia. It is also used as an antioxidant, to improve peripheral artery disease, and to enhance circulation throughout the body. Other reported uses include the treatment of depressive mood disorders, sexual dysfunction, asthma, glaucoma, menopausal symptoms, multiple sclerosis, headaches, tinnitus, dizziness, arthritis, altitude sickness, and intermittent claudication.

ACTIONS
Much research is available documenting the uses and actions of *Ginkgo biloba* L. Ginkgo has been used in China since ancient times. Initial research began in Europe in the 1960s.

Cognitive enhancement action
The cognitive enhancement action of ginkgo is a result of the flavonoids present in the extract. The pharmacologic actions involve increased release of neurotransmitters, including catecholamines, and inhibition of monoamine oxidase.

Vasoprotective and tissue-protective actions
The vasoprotective and tissue-protective actions of ginkgo result from several factors: its ability to relax blood vessels, to protect against capillary permeability, to inhibit platelet aggregation, and to decrease ischemia and edema.

Other actions
Ginkgo has been studied for its antioxidant effects, its relief of altitude sickness, its antiarthritic and analgesic effects, and its relief of ischemia in intermittent claudication.

Antioxidant action
Ginkgo has been studied for its antioxidant effects. It has been found to eliminate free radicals and is able to inhibit polymorphonuclear neutrophils.

Altitude sickness relief
Ginkgo can relieve altitude sickness.

Antiarthritic and analgesic actions
Ginkgetin, a chemical component of ginkgo, has been studied for its antiarthritic and analgesic effects.

PRODUCT AVAILABILITY
Capsules, fluid extract, tablets, tincture

Plant part used: Leaves

DOSAGES
Ginkgo may be standardized to 24% ginkgo flavonglycosides and 6% terpene trilactones.

Alzheimer's disease
Adult PO capsules/extract/tablets: 80 mg tid standardized to 24% flavonglycosides

Asthma
Adult PO extract: 80 mg tid

Cerebral vascular insufficiency
Adult PO extract: 80 mg tid standardized to 24% flavonglycosides

General use
Adult PO standardized extract: 40 mg tid

Glaucoma
Extract: 40-80 mg tid standardized to 24% flavonglycosides

Impotence from arterial insufficiency
Adult PO extract: 80 mg tid standardized to 24% flavonglycosides

Menopause
Adult PO extract: 40 mg tid standardized to 24% flavonglycosides

Multiple sclerosis
Adult PO extract: 40-80 mg tid standardized to 24% flavonglycosides

CONTRAINDICATIONS
Avoid use in pregnancy and breastfeeding. Ginkgo should not be given to children. It should not be used by persons with coagulation or platelet disorders, hemophilia, seizures, or hypersensitivity to this herb.

SIDE EFFECTS/ADVERSE REACTIONS
CNS: Transient headache, anxiety, restlessness
GI: Nausea, vomiting, anorexia, diarrhea, flatulence
INTEG: Hypersensitivity reactions, rash

INTERACTIONS
Drug
Anticoagulants (anisindione, dalteparin, dicumerol, heparin, salicylates, warfarin), **platelet inhibitor** (abciximab), **salicylates:** Because of the increased risk of bleeding, ginkgo should not be taken concurrently with these products.
Anticonvulsants (carbamazepine, gabapentin, phenobarbital, phenytoin): Ginkgo components may decrease the anticonvulsant effect; avoid concurrent use.
Buspirone, fluoxetine: Ginkgo given with these agents may cause hypomania (Jellin et al., 2008).
Cytochrome P450IA2/P4502D6/P4503A4 substrates: Ginkgo may affect drugs metabolized by these agents; use caution if giving concurrently.
MAOIs: MAOI action may be increased if taken with ginkgo; do not use concurrently (theoretical).
SSRIs: Ginkgo is often used to reverse the sexual side effects of SSRIs.
Trazodone: Ginkgo with trazodone may cause coma.

Herb
Anticoagulant/antiplatelet herbs: Ginkgo may increase the risk of bleeding when used with these herbs.
St. John's wort: Ginkgo with St. John's wort can lead to hypomania.

Lab test
Partial thromboplastin time, ASA tolerance test: Ginkgo may cause increased bleeding (partial thromboplastin time, ASA tolerance test).
Platelet activity: Ginkgo may decrease platelet activity.
Prothrombin time, blood salicylate: Ginkgo may increase prothrombin time and blood salicylate.

NURSING CONSIDERATIONS
Assessment
• Assess the reason the patient is using ginkgo.
• Assess for hypersensitivity reactions. If present, discontinue the use of this herb and administer an antihistamine or other appropriate therapy.
• Assess for the use of anticoagulants, platelet inhibitors, or MAOIs (see Interactions).

Implementation
• Inform the patient that ginkgo takes 1 to 6 months before it becomes effective.

Patient/family education
• Inform the patient to avoid in pregnancy and breastfeeding.
• Caution the patient not to give ginkgo to children.
• Caution the client not to use ginkgo with anticoagulants, platelet inhibitors, trazodone, or MAOIs.

ginseng
(jin'sing)
Scientific names: Panax quinquefolius, Panax ginseng
Other common names: American ginseng, Asiatic ginseng, Chinese ginseng, five-fingers, Japanese ginseng, jintsam, Korean ginseng, ninjin, Oriental ginseng, schinsent, seng and sang, tartar root, Western ginseng

ORIGIN: Ginseng is now found throughout the world. *Panax quinquefolius* is native to North America; *Panax ginseng* is native to the Far East.

USES: Ginseng has been used for a variety of purposes for about 5000 years. It has been used to increase physical endurance and lessen fatigue, to improve the ability to cope with stress, and to improve concentration. It also may improve overall well-being. Many herbalists consider it a tonic.

Investigational uses
Initial research is exploring the use of ginseng to improve cognitive functioning and to treat diabetes mellitus, hyperlipidemia, seizure disorders,

cancer, male infertility, male erectile dysfunction, emphysema, and rheumatoid arthritis and to enhance immunity.

ACTIONS

Most of the available research on ginseng comes from Asia, where this herb has been studied extensively. Investigators have completed research on the abilities of ginseng. It has been shown to decrease fatigue, increase physical performance, and improve mental functioning. Studies have also been done on its anticancer and antidiabetes effects.

Decreased fatigue, increased physical performance, *and improved mental function*
Decreased fatigue
There may be significant improvement in fatigue with the use of ginseng as compared with the use of a placebo.
Increased physical performance
Studies using both human subjects and laboratory animals indicate that ginseng increases physical performance.
Improved mental function
In both animal and human studies, ginseng has been shown to improve mental functioning.

Anticonvulsant action
Panax ginseng may show promise as an anticonvulsant.

Antidiabetic action
Ginseng has been used for centuries to treat diabetes mellitus. Its antidiabetic action results from the chemical components from adenosine, known as panaxans, and others. Ginseng has shown glucoregulating properties even when administered with glucose.

PRODUCT AVAILABILITY
Capsules, dried root used for decoction, extract, powder, standardized extract, tea, tincture; may be found in creams and lotions used to treat wrinkles.

Plant part used: Roots
DOSAGES
Standardized extracts contain 5% ginsenosides (an aglycone chemical component believed to act as a stimulant).

General use
Adult PO capsules: 200-500 mg extract daily
Adult PO infusion: pour boiling water over 3 g herb, let stand 10 min, strain; may be taken tid for 3-4 weeks
Adult PO powdered root: 1-4 g daily

Adult PO standardized extract: 200-500 mg daily
Adult PO tincture: 1-2 ml extract daily (1:1 dilution)

Male infertility
Adult PO crude herb (root, high quality): 1.5-2 g tid
Adult PO extract: 100-200 mg tid standardized to 5% ginsenosides

Rheumatoid arthritis
Adult PO crude herb: 4.5-6 g/day in divided doses
Adult PO extract: 500 mg daily tid

CONTRAINDICATIONS
Avoid use in pregnancy and breastfeeding
Ginseng should not be given to children. It should not be used by persons with hypertension, cardiac disorders, or hypersensitivity to it. If breast cancer or other estrogen-dependent conditions are present, ginseng should not be used.

SIDE EFFECTS/ADVERSE REACTIONS
CNS: Anxiety, insomnia, restlessness (high doses), headache
CV: Hypertension, chest pain, palpitations, decreased diastolic blood pressure, increased QTc interval.
GI: Nausea, vomiting, anorexia, diarrhea (high doses)
Ginseng abuse syndrome: Edema, insomnia, hypertonia
INTEG: Hypersensitivity reactions, rash

INTERACTIONS
Drug
Anticoagulants (anisindione, dicumarol, heparin, warfarin), **antiplatelets, salicylates:** Ginseng may decrease the action of these products.
Anticonvulsants: Ginseng may provide an additive anticonvulsant action (theoretical).
Antidiabetics (acetohexamide, chlorpropamide, glipizide, metformin, tolazamide, tolbutamide, troglitazone): Because ginseng is known to decrease blood glucose levels, it may increase the hypoglycemic effect of antidiabetics; avoid concurrent use.
Immunosuppressants (azathioprine, basiliximab, cyclosporine, daclizumab, muromonab, mycophenolate, tacrolimus): Ginseng may diminish the effect of immunosuppressants; do not use immediately before, during, or after transplant surgery.
Insulin: Because ginseng is known to decrease blood glucose levels, it may increase the

hypoglycemic effect of insulin; avoid concurrent use.

MAOIs (isocarboxazid, phenelzine, tranylcypromine): Concurrent use of MAOIs with ginseng may result in manic-like syndrome.

Stimulants: Use of stimulants (e.g., xanthines) concurrently with ginseng is not recommended; overstimulation may occur.

Herb
Caffeine, guarana, yerba maté, tea: Ginseng with these agents may lead to added stimulation (Jellin et al., 2008).

Ephedra: Concurrent use of ephedra and ginseng may increase hypertension and central nervous system stimulation; avoid concurrent use.

Food
Caffeinated coffee, cola, tea: Overstimulation may occur when ginseng is used with caffeinated coffee, cola, and tea; avoid concurrent use.

Lab test
Blood glucose: Ginseng may decrease blood glucose (decoctions, infusions).

Plasma partial thromboplastin time, INR: Ginseng may increase plasma partial thromboplastin time and INR.

Serum, urine estrogens: Ginseng may have an additive effect on serum and 24-hour urine estrogens.

Serum digoxin: Ginseng may falsely increase serum digoxin.

NURSING CONSIDERATIONS
Assessment
• Assess the reason the patient is using ginseng.
• Assess for hypersensitivity reactions and rash. If these are present, discontinue the use of this herb and administer an antihistamine or other appropriate therapy.
• Assess for ginseng abuse syndrome: insomnia, edema, and hypertonia.
• Assess for the use of stimulants, anticoagulants, MAOIs, and antidiabetics (see Interactions).

Patient problems
Fatigue (uses)

Implementation
• Instruct the patient to store ginseng products in a cool, dry place away from heat and moisture.
• Instruct the patient to avoid the continuous use of ginseng. The recommendation is to use this herb for no more than 3 continuous months, taking a break between courses.

Patient/family education
• Inform the patient to avoid use in pregnancy and breastfeeding. Caution the patient not to give ginseng to children.
• Advise the patient to use other stimulants and antidiabetics carefully if taking concurrently with ginseng (see Interactions).
• Warn the patient of the life-threatening side effects of ginseng abuse syndrome.
• Instruct the patient that *Siberian ginseng* and *Panax ginseng* are not the same.

glucosamine
(glew-koe'suh-meen)
Scientific name: 2-amino-2-deoxyglucose
Other common names: Chitosamine, GS

ORIGIN: Glucosamine is found in mucopolysaccharides, chitin, and mucoproteins. Glucosamine is a naturally occurring substance; glucosamine sulfate is manufactured synthetically.

USES: Glucosamine typically is used in conjunction with chondroitin to treat joint conditions such as those associated with arthritis.

Investigational uses
Researchers are working to determine whether glucosamine may be effective in the treatment of diabetes mellitus.

ACTIONS
Antiarthritic action
The primary action of glucosamine is to protect against and prevent osteoarthritis. Several studies have focused on the results of glucosamine use as compared with that of nonsteroidal antiinflammatories and placebos.

PRODUCT AVAILABILITY
Capsules, tablets

Dosages
General use
Adult PO capsules/tablets: 1500 mg glucosamine and 1200 mg chondroitin for average-weight individuals; lower doses for underweight individuals; higher doses for overweight individuals
Osteoarthritis
Adult PO capsules/tablets: 1500 mg/day

CONTRAINDICATIONS
Until more research is available, glucosamine should not be used during pregnancy or breastfeeding. It should not be given to children because its effects on them are unknown. Glucosamine should not be used by persons with hypersensitivity to it.

SIDE EFFECTS/ADVERSE REACTIONS
CNS: Drowsiness, headache
GI: Nausea, vomiting, anorexia, constipation or diarrhea, heartburn, epigastric pain and cramps, indigestion
INTEG: Hypersensitivity reactions, rash (rare)

INTERACTIONS
Drug
Anticoagulants, antiplatelets: Glucosamine and chondroitin at high levels can lead to bleeding risk
Antidiabetics: Glucosamine may increase the effects of antidiabetics (theoretical).

Lab test
International normalized ratio (INR): Glucosamine and chondroitin in high doses may lead to increased INR.

Pharmacology
Chemical properties
Glucosamine sulfate is a synthetically manufactured product or derived from chitin (marine exoskeletons). Glucosamine is required for synthesis of certain proteins needed for tendons, ligaments, and cartilage.

NURSING CONSIDERATIONS
Assessment
• Assess the reason the patient is using glucosamine.
• Assess for hypersensitivity reactions, rash (rare). If these are present, discontinue use of glucosamine and administer an antihistamine or other appropriate therapy.
• Assess for joint pain, stiffness, and aggravating or ameliorating factors.
• Monitor blood glucose in diabetic patients (see Interactions).

Patient problems
Impaired mobility (uses)

Implementation
• Instruct the patient to take glucosamine PO with food to reduce gastric upset.
• Instruct the patient to store glucosamine products in a cool, dry place away from heat and moisture.

Teach client/family
• Caution the patient not to use glucosamine in children or those who are pregnant or breastfeeding until more research is available.
• Inform the diabetic patient that glucosamine may lower blood glucose levels.

grapeseed
(grayp'seed)
Scientific name: Vitis vinifera
Other common name: Muskat

ORIGIN: Grapeseed is found throughout the world.

USES: Grapeseed may be used as an antioxidant and an anticancer treatment. It may also be used to treat varicose veins, circulatory problems, and vision problems such as cataracts as well as to improve vision by lessening eye strain.

Investigational uses
Researchers are experimenting with the use of grapeseed to treat diabetes mellitus and inflammatory, degenerative, diverticular, and heart diseases.

ACTIONS
Vision improvement
Grapeseed has produced beneficial effects in people with vision problems.

Other actions
Grapeseed has shown protective effects against carbon tetrachloride hepatic poisoning in mice, as well as photoprotective properties of melanins. A significant antioxidant, grapeseed is stronger than the antioxidant properties of vitamin C or E for the skin.

PRODUCT AVAILABILITY
Capsules, tablets, drops, liquid concentrate, cream

Plant part used: Seeds

DOSAGES
Dosages are standardized to 85%-95% procyanidins.

Supplementation
Adult PO capsules/tablets: 50-100 daily

Therapeutic use
Adult PO capsules/tablets: 150-300 mg daily for 21 days, then 50-80 mg daily maintenance

CONTRAINDICATIONS
Until more research is available, grapeseed should not be used during pregnancy and breastfeeding. It should not be given to children.

SIDE EFFECTS/ADVERSE REACTIONS
CNS: Dizziness
GI: Nausea, anorexia, hepatotoxicity (theoretical)
INTEG: Rash

INTERACTIONS
Drug
Anticoagulants, antiplatelets: Grapeseed given with these agents may increase the risk of bleeding (theoretical).

NURSING CONSIDERATIONS
Assessment
- Assess the reason the patient is using grapeseed.
- If the patient is using grapeseed to improve cardiovascular disorders, assess cardiovascular status: edema in legs, improvement in atherosclerosis, and improvement in varicose veins. Monitor blood pressure and pulse.
- Identify other cardiovascular medications taken by the patient.
- Assess for hepatotoxicity.

Patient problems
Risk of injury (uses)

Implementation
- Instruct the patient to take grapeseed PO only once per day.
- Instruct the patient to store grapeseed products in a cool, dry place away from heat and moisture.

Patient/family education
- Caution the patient not to use grapeseed in children or those who are pregnant or breastfeeding until more research is available.

---

green tea
(green tee)
Scientific name: Camellia sinensis
Other common name: Matsu-cha

ORIGIN: Green tea is a shrub found in Asia.

USES: Green tea is used as a general antioxidant, anticancer agent, diuretic, stimulant, antibacterial, antilipidemic, and antiatherosclerotic.

Investigational uses
Research is underway to confirm the use of green tea in treating HIV, increasing muscle health, reducing total cholesterol, and supporting vascular protection. Green tea is shown to be effective in reducing the risk of bladder, ovarian, esophageal, gastric, and pancreatic cancer. Green tea may reduce the risk of breast cancer reoccurring (Jellin et al., 2008). It increases cognitive function and delays Parkinson's disease.

ACTIONS
Green tea and black tea come from the same plant, *Camellia sinensis*. Black tea is produced by allowing the leaves to oxidize, while green tea is cut and steamed. The major actions of green tea result from its antioxidant, anticancer, and antilipidemic properties.

Antioxidant and anticancer actions
Green tea exerts protective effects against gastrointestinal cancers of the stomach, intestine, colon, rectum, and pancreas. Green tea also has been shown to decrease the incidence of breast cancer in vitro by inhibiting the interaction with estrogen receptors.

Antilipidemic action
Green tea can produce a significant increase in HDL and a decrease in LDL lipoproteins. These reactions occurred in direct proportion to the amount of green tea consumed.

Other actions
Green tea was able to improve muscle health by reducing or delaying necrosis in mice by an antioxidant mechanism. Green tea can prevent cold and flu symptoms and enhance gamma delta T-cell function.

PRODUCT AVAILABILITY
Tablets, capsules, dried/liquid extract, tea

Plant part used: Dried leaves

DOSAGES
Green tea is standardized to 60% polyphenols.
Adult PO extract: 250-400 mg/day of standardized to 90% polyphenols
Adult PO tea: 1 tsp tea leaves in 8 oz hot water, drink 2-5 cups/day

CONTRAINDICATIONS
Green tea should not be used by persons with hypersensitivity to this product or by those with kidney inflammation, gastrointestinal ulcers, insomnia, cardiovascular disease, or increased intraocular pressure. This herb contains caffeine. Decaffeinated tea is available, although some caffeine may remain.

SIDE EFFECTS/ADVERSE REACTIONS
CNS: Anxiety, nervousness, insomnia (high doses)
CV: Increased blood pressure, palpitations, irregular heartbeat (high doses)
GI: Nausea, heartburn, increased stomach acid (high doses)
INTEG: Hypersensitivity reactions

INTERACTIONS
Drug
Antacids: Antacids may decrease the therapeutic effects of green tea (theoretical).
Anticoagulants, antiplatelets: Green tea with anticoagulants, antiplatelets may increase risk of bleeding (theoretical).

Beta-adrenergic blockers: Green tea used with these agents can lead to increased inotropic effects.

Benzodiazepines: Green tea with these agents increases sedation (theoretical).

Bronchodilators, xanthines (theophylline): Large amounts of green tea increase the action of xanthines and some bronchodilators.

MAOIs (isocarboxazid, phenelzine, tranylcypromine): Green tea used in large amounts taken with MAOIs can lead to hypertensive crisis; do not use together.

Herb
Ephedra: Concurrent use of ephedra and caffeinated green tea may increase hypertension and CNS stimulation; avoid concurrent use with caffeinated green tea products.

Food
Dairy products: Dairy products may decrease the therapeutic effects of green tea.

Iron: Green tea may decrease iron absorption.

Lab test
Glucose, VMA, urine creatine, urine catecholamine: green tea may increase these levels.

NURSING CONSIDERATIONS
Assessment
- Assess the reason the patient is using green tea.
- Assess for hypersensitivity reactions. If present, discontinue the use of this herb and administer an antihistamine or other appropriate therapy.
- Assess for other conditions that are contraindications to green tea use, including cardiovascular and renal disease, and increased intraocular pressure.
- Assess for use of antacids, dairy products, and ephedra (see Interactions).

Patient problems
Infection (uses)

Implementation
- Instruct the patient to store green tea in a cool, dry place, protected from heat and moisture.

Patient/family education
- Caution the patient with renal or cardiovascular disease, or increased intraocular pressure, not to use green tea products that contain caffeine.
- Teach the patient not to use green tea with antacids or milk because its effect is decreased.

hawthorn
(haw'thawrn)

Scientific name: Crataegus spp.

Other common names: Li 132, may, maybush, quickset, thorn-apple tree, whitethorn

ORIGIN: Hawthorn is a bush or tree found throughout the United States, Canada, Europe, and Asia.

USES: Hawthorn is one of the most commonly used herbs. It is used to treat cardiovascular disorders such as hypertension, arrhythmias, arteriosclerosis, congestive heart failure, Buerger's disease, and stable angina pectoris.

ACTIONS
Cardiovascular action
Hawthorn exerts both antihypertensive and antihyperlipidemic effects. It increases blood supply to the heart, increases the force of contractions, and indirectly inhibits angiotensin-converting enzyme (ACE). The proanthocyanidins, among the chemical components of hawthorn, have been shown to inhibit ACE in a manner similar to that of the drug captopril. Hawthorn also stabilizes collagen, reduces atherosclerosis, and decreases cholesterol. The collagen-stabilizing action of hawthorn helps to keep the artery strong and free of plaque development. Hawthorn can be used with cardiac glycosides in the treatment of congestive heart failure. Hawthorn has been shown to reduce hypertension in laboratory animals.

Other actions
The hawthorn extract is a scavenger, increases intracellular GSH levels, and is not cytotoxic. Therefore, it is considered an adequate antioxidant.

Product availability
Capsules of berries, extended release capsules, fluid extract, leaves, solid extract, tea, tincture, topical cream

Plant parts used: Flowers, fruit, leaves

DOSAGES
Angina
Adult PO berries of flowers, dried: 3-5 g tid or as a tea

Adult PO fluid extract: 1-2 ml (¼-½ tsp) tid (1:1 dilution)

Adult PO solid extract: 100-250 mg tid (10% procyanidin or 1.8% vitexin-4´-rhamnoside)

Adult PO tincture: 4-6 ml (1-1½ tsp) tid (1:5 dilution)

Coronary artery disease
Adult PO solid extract: 100-250 mg tid (10% procyanidin content or 1.8% vitexin-4´-rhamnoside)

Adult PO solid extract: 120-240 mg tid of a standardized product (18.75% procyanidins or 2.2% flavonoids)

Adult PO tea: 1-2 tsp berries, steep in 8 oz water for 15 min, strain, drink tid

Adult PO tincture: 5 ml tid (1:5 dilution)

Moderate hypertension
Adult PO solid extract: 100-250 mg tid (10% procyanidin content or 1.8% vitexin-4´-rhamnoside)

General use
Child PO tea: 1 cup several times/wk
Child PO tincture: ¼-1 tsp up to tid
Child topical cream: apply prn

CONTRAINDICATIONS
Considered safe in breastfeeding. Hawthorn may be given to children. It should not be used by persons with hypersensitivity to this herb or *Rosaceae* spp.

SIDE EFFECTS/ADVERSE REACTIONS
CNS: Fatigue, sedation
CV: Hypotension, *arrhythmias*
GI: Nausea, vomiting, anorexia
INTEG: Hypersensitivity reactions

INTERACTIONS
Drug
Antihypertensives (beta-blockers): Hawthorn may increase hypotension when used with antihypertensives; avoid concurrent use.
Cardiac glycosides: Hawthorn may increase the effects of cardiac glycosides; monitor concurrent use carefully.
CNS depressants: Hawthorn may increase the sedative effects of CNS depressants such as alcohol, barbiturates, and psychotropics; avoid concurrent use.
Iron salts: Hawthorn tea may decrease the absorption of iron salts; separate by at least 2 hours.

>> Herb
Adonis, lily of the valley, squill: Hawthorn increases the action of *Adonis vernalis*, *Convallaria majalis*, and *Scillae bulbus* when taken concurrently.
Fenugreek, ginger: Hawthorn may increase cardiac events when used with these products.

Lab test
Serum digoxin: Hawthorn may cause false increase of serum digoxin.

NURSING CONSIDERATIONS
Assessment
• Assess the reason the patient is using hawthorn.
• Assess for hypersensitivity reactions. If present, discontinue the use of hawthorn and administer an antihistamine or other appropriate therapy.
• Assess cardiovascular status if the patient is taking hawthorn to treat congestive heart failure.
• Assess for other cardiovascular drugs the patient may be taking, including beta blockers, cardiac glycosides, central nervous system depressants, and antihypertensives; assess for use of the herbs (see Interactions).

Patient problems
Impaired cardiac function (uses)

Implementation
• Instruct the patient to take hawthorn PO as an extract, tincture, or tea.
• Instruct the patient to store hawthorn products in a cool, dry place away from heat and moisture.

Patient/family education
• Inform the patient it is considered safe in breastfeeding.
• Inform the patient that hawthorn may be given to children.
• Caution the patient to check with the prescriber before giving hawthorn to a child who is taking cardiovascular medications.
• Advise the patient not to use this herb if allergic to *Rosaceae* spp.

horse chestnut
(hoers chehs´nuht)
Scientific names: Aesculus hippocastanum, Aesculus california, Aesculus glabra
Other common names: Aescin, buckeye, California buckeye, chestnut, escine, Ohio buckeye

ORIGIN: Horse chestnut is a tree or shrub found worldwide.

USES: Traditional uses of horse chestnut include treatment of fever, phlebitis, hemorrhoids, prostate enlargement, edema, inflammation, and diarrhea. It is commonly used in Germany to treat varicose veins.

Investigational uses
Researchers are investigating the use of horse chestnut for treatment of venous insufficiency and varicose veins.

ACTIONS
Antiinflammatory action
The chemical component aescin, a saponin present in horse chestnut, is responsible for its antiinflammatory properties.

PRODUCT AVAILABILITY

Standardized extract, tincture

Plant parts used: Seeds, young bark

DOSAGES

Adult PO standardized extract: 100-150 mg daily in two divided doses

Adult PO tincture: 1-2 ml in ½ cup water, bid-qid

CONTRAINDICATIONS

Do not use in pregnancy or breastfeeding. Horse chestnut should not be given to children.

SIDE EFFECTS/ADVERSE REACTIONS

GI: Nausea, vomiting, anorexia, *hepatotoxicity*

GU: Nephropathy, nephrotoxicity

INTEG: Pruritus, hypersensitivity, rash, urticaria

MS: Spasms

SYST: Bruising, severe bleeding, shock; seeds are toxic

INTERACTIONS

Drug

Anticoagulants (anisindione, dicumarol, heparin, warfarin), **aspirin, and other salicylates:** Because of the presence of hydroxycoumarin, a chemical component of the herb that possesses anticoagulant activity, concurrent use of horse chestnut and anticoagulants, aspirin, and other salicylates increases the risk of severe bleeding. Do not use concurrently.

Antidiabetics: May increase the hypoglycemic effects of diabetes medications.

Iron salts: Horse chestnut tea may decrease the absorption of iron salts; separate by 2 hours.

Herb

Anticoagulant, antiplatelet herbs: Horse chestnut given with anticoagulant, antiplatelet herbs increases risk of bleeding.

Hypoglycemic herbs: Horse chestnut given with hypoglycemic herbs increases hypoglycemia.

NURSING CONSIDERATIONS

Assess

• Assess the reason the patient is using horse chestnut.

• Assess for symptoms of hepatotoxicity (increased AST, ALT, and bilirubin levels; clay-colored stools; jaundice; right upper-quadrant pain). If any of these symptoms are present, discontinue the use of this herb.

• Assess for bleeding, bruising, and allergic reactions such as a rash or itching. If present, discontinue the use of this herb.

• Assess renal function if high dosage is suspected. Obtain blood urea nitrogen (BUN) and creatinine levels. Monitor for nephrotoxicity.

• Assess for medications used (see Interactions).

• Assess for toxicity (see Side Effects).

Patient problems

Risk of injury (adverse reactions)

Implementation

• Instruct the client to store horse chestnut in a cool, dry place away from heat and moisture.

Teach client/family

• Inform the patient not to use in pregnancy and breastfeeding.

• Caution the patient not to give horse chestnut to children.

• Warn the patient of the life-threatening side effects of horse chestnut. Do not use older bark as it is poisonous.

kava
(kah'vah)

Scientific name: Piper methysticum

Other common names: Ava, awa, kava-kava, kawa, kew, sakau, tonga, yagona

ORIGIN: Kava is a shrub found on the South Sea Islands.

USES: Kava is used as an anxiolytic, antiepileptic, antidepressant, and antipsychotic, as well as for antianxiety, attention deficit-hyperactivity disorder, insomnia, restlessness, and headaches.

It is also used as a muscle relaxant and to promote wound healing.

Investigational use

Research is underway for use in cancer.

ACTIONS

Kava acts as a sedative, an analgesic, and an anxiolytic. It has been used for ceremonial purposes in Micronesia and Polynesia for thousands of years in the place of alcoholic beverages, which have not always been available.

Sedative action

The sedative action of kava is unlike any other. It appears to act directly on the limbic system. Kava lactones may actually modify receptor areas rather than bind to receptor-binding sites.

Analgesic, antiinflammatory action

The analgesic effect of kava appears to be unrelated to that of other pain relievers. Kava does not bind to opiate receptors and does not block pain impulses in the central nervous system. Its mechanism of action is unknown at present.

PRODUCT AVAILABILITY
Capsules, beverage, extract, tablets, tincture

Plant parts used: Dried rhizome, dried roots

DOSAGES
Anxiolytic
Adult PO extract, standardized: 45-70 mg kava lactones tid

Depression
Adult PO extract, standardized: 45-70 mg kava lactones tid

General use
Adult PO extract, standardized: 70 mg kava lactones tid
Adult PO capsules/tablets: 400-500 mg up to 6 times/day
Adult PO tincture: 15-30 drops (dilution 1:2) taken tid in water

Sedative
Adult PO extract, standardized: 190-200 mg kava lactones 60 min at bedtime

CONTRAINDICATIONS
Avoid use in pregnancy and breastfeeding. Kava should not be given to children younger than 12 years of age. This herb should not be used by persons with major depressive disorder or Parkinson's disease, or by those with hypersensitivity to it.

SIDE EFFECTS/ADVERSE REACTIONS
Most side effects and adverse reactions occur when high doses are taken for a long period.
CNS: Increased reflexes, drowsiness
EENT: Blurred vision, red eyes
GI: Nausea, vomiting, anorexia, weight loss, *hepatic damage*
GU: Hematuria
HEMA: Decreased platelets, lymphocytes, bilirubin, protein, and albumin; increased red blood cell volume
INTEG: Hypersensitivity reactions; skin yellowing and scaling (high doses)
RESP: Shortness of breath, pulmonary hypertension

INTERACTIONS
Drug
Antiparkinsonians (carbidopa, levodopa): Antiparkinsonian drugs may increase symptoms of parkinsonism when used with kava; do not use concurrently.

Antipsychotics (chlorpromazine, fluphenazine, loxapine, mesoridazine, molindone, perphenazine, prochlorperazine, promazine, thioridazine, thiothixene, trifluoperazine, triflupromazine): Antipsychotics taken with kava may result in neuroleptic movement disorders.

Barbiturates (amobarbital, aprobarbital, butabarbital, phenobarbital, secobarbital): Barbiturates taken with kava may result in increased sedation.

Benzodiazepines: Increased sedation and coma (theoretical) may result when kava is used with benzodiazepines, including alprazolam; do not use concurrently.

CNS depressants: CNS depressants such as alcohol, benzodiazepines, and barbiturates may cause increased sedation when used with kava; avoid concurrent use.

Cytochrome P450 1A2, 2C9, 2C19, 2D6, 3A4 substrates: Kava significantly decreases these substrates; use cautiously in patients taking these agents.

Food
Increased absorption of kava occurs when taken with food.

Lab test
AST, ALT, LDH, bilirubin: Kava may increase hepatic function tests.

Pharmacology
Pharmacokinetics
Most pharmacokinetics and pharmacodynamics are unknown. Kava lactones are more readily absorbed orally when taken as an extract of the root than as kava lactones alone. Kava may cross the placenta and enter breast milk.

NURSING CONSIDERATIONS
Assess
• Assess the reason the patient is using kava.
• Assess for hypersensitivity reactions. If present, discontinue the use of kava and administer an antihistamine or other appropriate therapy.
• Assess for use of other central nervous system depressants, including alcohol, barbiturates, benzodiazepines, antianxiety medications, and sedatives/hypnotics (see Interactions).

Patient problems
Anxiety (Uses)

Implementation
• Instruct the patient to store kava products in a cool, dry place away from heat and moisture.
• Instruct the patient not to use kava for longer than 3 months unless under the direction of an herbalist. This herb may be habit forming.

• Inform the patient that kava absorption is increased when kava is taken with food.

Patient/family education
• Inform the patient that pregnancy category is 2 and breastfeeding category is 3A.
• Caution the patient not to give kava to children younger than 12 years of age.
• Inform the patient that excessive doses may result in daytime drowsiness. Advise the client not to operate heavy machinery or engage in hazardous activities if drowsiness occurs.
• Caution the patient not to use kava with other central nervous system depressants (see Interactions).

melatonin
(meh-luh-toe'nuhn)
Scientific name: N-Acetyl-5-methoxytryptamine
Other common name: MEL, MLT, Pineal hormone

ORIGIN: Melatonin is a naturally occurring hormone in the body.

USES: Melatonin is used to treat insomnia and inhibit cataract formation. It is also used to increase longevity and treat epilepsy, hypertension, various cancers, and jet lag, as well as prevent weight loss in cancer patients. Because it lowers luteinizing hormone (LH), estradiol, and progesterone levels, melatonin could possibly be useful as a contraceptive.

ACTIONS
Melatonin is a hormone produced in the body by the pineal gland. It is an antioxidant and a free-radical scavenger. When tryptophan is converted to serotonin, melatonin results from enzymatic processes in the pineal gland. Melatonin production increases during sleep and decreases during waking hours; melatonin supplementation has been found to induce and maintain sleep in adults who have low melatonin levels. The most promising use is for the geriatric client, who typically has low melatonin levels. Melatonin treatment in vivo caused a significant increase in blood glucose and a decreased level of free fatty acids. Parkinson's disease may be treated with melatonin, which lacks any serious side effects.

PRODUCT AVAILABILITY
Extended release capsules: 3 mg; injectable; liquid: 500 mcg/ml; tablets: 500 mcg, 1 mg, 1.5 mg, 3 mg

DOSAGES
Cancer (as a single agent)
Adult PO: 20 mg daily <2 mo IM (injectable form), then 10 mg PO daily

Cancer (in combination with interleukin-2)
Adult PO: 40-50 mg at bedtime for 1 wk before interleukin-2

Chronic insomnia
Adult PO tablets: 75 mg at bedtime

Delayed sleep-phase syndrome
Adult PO: 5 mg at bedtime

Jet lag
Adult PO: 5 mg daily 2-3 days before and 3 days after travel

Chronic insomnia
Geriatric PO tablets: extended release 1-2 mg 2 hr before meals

CONTRAINDICATIONS
Until more research is available, melatonin should not be used during pregnancy and breastfeeding. It should not be given to children. Persons with hypersensitivity to melatonin and those with hepatic or cardiovascular disease, central nervous system disorders, or depression should not use it. Persons with renal disease should use melatonin with caution. Use only synthetic forms due to contamination of animal products.

SIDE EFFECTS/ADVERSE REACTIONS
CNS: Headache, change in sleep patterns, confusion, hypothermia, sedation
CV: Tachycardia
GI: Nausea, vomiting, anorexia
INTEG: Hypersensitivity reactions (rash, pruritus)
Reproductive: Decreased progesterone, estradiol, LH levels

INTERACTIONS
Drug
Anticoagulants, antiplatelets: Melatonin with anticoagulants, antiplatelets may increase the risk of bleeding (theoretical).
Antidiabetics: Melatonin with antidiabetics may decrease hypoglycemia (theoretical).
Benzodiazepines: Melatonin may increase the anxiolytic effects of benzodiazepines; use together cautiously.
Beta-blockers: Melatonin is able to reverse the negative action of beta-blockers on sleep.
CNS depressants: Melatonin with central nervous system depressants may increase sedation (theoretical).

Cerebral stimulants: Cerebral stimulants used with melatonin may have a synergistic effect and exacerbate insomnia; avoid concurrent use.

DHEA: DHEA (dehydroepiandrosterone) used with melatonin may decrease cytokine production; avoid concurrent use.

Immunosuppressants: Melatonin with immunosuppressants concurrently may decrease response to immunosuppressants.

Magnesium: Magnesium used with melatonin increases inhibition of *N*-methyl-D-aspartate (NMDA) receptors; avoid concurrent use.

Succinylcholine: Melatonin increases the blocking properties of succinylcholine; avoid concurrent use.

Zinc: Zinc used with melatonin increases inhibition of NMDA receptors; avoid concurrent use.

Herb

Anticoagulant/antiplatelet herbs: Melatonin with anticoagulant/antiplatelet herbs may increase the risk of bleeding (theoretical).

Sedative herbs: Melatonin with sedative herbs may increase sedation (theoretical)

NURSING CONSIDERATIONS
Assess

• Assess for hypersensitivity reactions. If present, discontinue the use of melatonin and administer an antihistamine or other appropriate therapy.

• Assess sleep patterns: ability to fall asleep, stay asleep, hours slept, and napping, if using for insomnia.

• Assess for CNS effects: confusion, headache, sedation, and changes in sleeping patterns.

• Assess for medications used (see Interactions).

Patient problems
Impaired sleep (uses)

Implementation

• Instruct the patient to take melatonin PO to treat insomnia or jet lag. Melatonin is administered both PO and IM to cancer patients.

• Instruct the patient to store melatonin products in a sealed container away from heat and moisture.

Patient/family education

• Caution the patient not to use melatonin in children or those who are pregnant or breastfeeding.

• Advise the patient to avoid use with magnesium, zinc, and DHEA.

• Advise the patient to notify their health care provider of all supplements taken.

milk thistle
(milk thi'suhl)

Scientific name: *Silybum marianum*
Other common names: Holy thistle, lady's thistle, Marian thistle, Mary thistle, St. Mary thistle

ORIGIN: Milk thistle is found in Kashmir, Mexico, Canada, and the United States.

USES: Milk thistle has been used to treat hepatotoxicity caused by poisonous mushrooms, cirrhosis of the liver, chronic candidiasis, hepatitis C, exposure to toxic chemicals, and liver transplantation.

ACTIONS
Hepatoprotective action

Several studies have demonstrated the hepatoprotective action of silymarin, a chemical component of milk thistle; silymarin has been used for centuries to treat hepatic and gallbladder conditions. Silymarin has been found to act as an antioxidant, decreasing free radicals and increasing hepatocyte synthesis as well as exerting other hepatoprotective effects. It has been used to treat acute and chronic hepatic disease and has been found to inhibit cytochrome P450 enzymes in liver microsomes. It is possible that drugs metabolized by CYP3A4 or CYP2C9 may interact with this herb.

Nephroprotective action

There may be nephroprotective effects of silibinin and silicristin, two of milk thistle's chemical components. Kidney cells that had been damaged by cisplatin, vincristine, and paracetamol showed lessened or no nephrotoxic effects.

PRODUCT AVAILABILITY
Tincture, capsule

Plant parts used: Seeds, above-ground parts

DOSAGES
Alcoholism
Adult PO tincture: 70-210 mg tid (70%-80% silymarin)

General dosages
Adult PO tincture: 200-400 mg daily (dosage standardized to silymarin content)

Hepatitis
Adult PO tincture: 140-210 mg tid (70%-80% silymarin)

CONTRAINDICATIONS
Until more research is available, milk thistle should not be used during pregnancy and

---

breastfeeding. It should not be given to children. Milk thistle should not be used by persons with hypersensitivity to this herb or other plants in the Asteraceae family (ragweed, daisy, marigolds, chrysanthemums). Do not use in those with hormone-sensitive cancers.

SIDE EFFECTS/ADVERSE REACTIONS

CNS: Headache
GI: Nausea, vomiting, anorexia, diarrhea
GU: Menstrual changes
INTEG: Hypersensitivity reactions

INTERACTIONS
Drug
Antineoplastics (platinum): Milk thistle may prevent nephrotoxicity from platinum antineoplastics.
Cytochrome P450 2C9, 3A4 substrates: Milk thistle may inhibit these substrates.
Estrogens: Milk thistle may inhibit the clearance of estrogen (theoretical).

Lab test
AST, ALT, alkaline phosphatase, blood glucose: Milk thistle may decrease AST, ALT, alkaline phosphatase, blood glucose levels.

NURSING CONSIDERATIONS
Assessment
- Assess the reason the patient is using milk thistle.
- Assess for hypersensitivity reactions. If present, discontinue the use of milk thistle and administer an antihistamine or other appropriate therapy.
- Monitor hepatic function tests (ALT, AST, bilirubin) if the client is using milk thistle to treat hepatic disease.
- Assess all medications used (see Interactions).

Patient problems
Risk for injury (uses)

Implementation
- Instruct the patient to store milk thistle products in a cool, dry place away from heat and moisture.

Patient/family education
- Caution the patient not to use milk thistle in children or those who are pregnant or breast-feeding until more research is available.

SAM-e
Scientific name: S-Adenosylmethionine
Origin: SAM-e is found in all living cells and is a precursor in some amino acids.

USES: SAM-e is used to treat depression, Alzheimer's disease, migraine headaches, attention deficit-hyperactivity disorder, chronic hepatic disease, and pain in fibromyalgia. It is also used as an antiinflammatory in osteoarthritis.

ACTIONS
SAM-e plays an important role in normal cell function and survival and is present naturally in the human body. It is necessary for adequate functioning of the central nervous system. SAM-e is considered to be hepatoprotective, as well as an antioxidant and antidepressant. It may also play a role in decreasing *Pneumocystis jiroveci,* improving cognition in Alzheimer's disease, and protecting against coronary artery disease (CAD).

Antidepressant and central nervous system actions
SAM-e has been shown to be effective in the treatment of depressive disorders by acting on the methylation process in the brain. It also has been shown to be effective in the treatment of Alzheimer's disease, HIV-associated neuropathies, and spinal cord degeneration. Deficiencies of certain vitamins, such as folate and B12, decrease levels of SAM-e. Lowered levels of SAM-e are accompanied by a decrease in serotonin levels, which can lead to depression. It is thought to increase dopamine and serotonin, as well as other neurotransmitters.

Antiinflammatory action
The antiinflammatory and analgesic effects of SAM-e have been found to be equal to those of NSAIDs, with far fewer side effects than NSAIDs. SAM-e is thought to protect cartilage and to assist in the repair of cartilage.

Hepatoprotective action
Studies have found that SAM-e decreases hepatic injury associated with alcoholic cirrhosis. The addition of SAM-e allowed liver transplantation to be delayed in alcoholic cirrhosis.

Other actions
SAM-e has been found to decrease the intensity of migraine headaches at dosages of 200 to 400 mg twice daily.

PRODUCT AVAILABILITY
Capsules, tablets

Dosages
Migraine
Adult PO capsules/tablets: 200-400 mg bid

CONTRAINDICATIONS
Until more research is available, SAM-e supplements should not be used during pregnancy and breastfeeding. They should not be given to children. Persons with bipolar disorder or Parkinson's disease should not use SAM-e supplements.

SIDE EFFECTS/ADVERSE REACTIONS
CNS: Headache, dizziness, insomnia, sweating
GI: Nausea, vomiting, anorexia, diarrhea, flatulence

INTERACTIONS
Drug
Antidepressants (amitriptyline, amoxapine, citalopram, desipramine, doxepin, fluoxetine, fluvoxamine, imipramine, naratriptan, nefazodone, nortriptyline, paroxetine, phenelzine, sertraline, sumatriptan, tramadol, tranylcypromine, venlafaxine, zolmitriptan): Combining SAM-e with antidepressants may lead to serotonin syndrome; do not use concurrently.
MAOIs: SAM-e may lead to hypertensive crisis when used with MAOIs; do not use concurrently.

NURSING CONSIDERATIONS
Assessment
• Assess the reason the client is taking SAM-e.
• Assess for depression or bipolar disorder; SAM-e should not be used with these patients as it may precipitate manic episode.

Patient problems
Depression (uses)

Implementation
• Instruct the patient to store SAM-e in a cool, dry place away from heat and moisture.

Patient/family education
• Caution the patient not to use SAM-e supplements in children or those who are pregnant or breastfeeding until more research is available.

saw palmetto
(saw pal-meh'toe)
Scientific names: Serenoa repens, Sabul serrulata
Other common names: American dwarf palm tree, cabbage palm, fan palm, IDS 89, LSESR, sabal, scrub palm

ORIGIN: Saw palmetto is a palm found in the United States.

USES: Saw palmetto is primarily used to treat mild to moderate benign prostatic hypertrophy (BPH), stages I and II. It is also used to treat chronic and subacute cystitis; to increase breast size, sperm count, and sexual potency; and as a mild diuretic.

Investigational uses
Research is underway to confirm the use in prostate cancer.

ACTIONS
Benign prostatic hypertrophy action
Saw palmetto has been studied extensively for its use in the treatment of BPH. The herb has been found to decrease both the symptoms of BPH and the swelling of the prostate. A study of a saw palmetto herbal blend versus a placebo noted a decrease in the symptoms and swelling in moderately symptomatic clients with BPH in the experimental group.

Cytotoxicity in prostate cancer
Serenoa repens may be cytotoxic to prostate cancer cells. The chemical component responsible for the cytotoxic action is myristoleic acid.

PRODUCT AVAILABILITY
Berries, capsules, fluid extract, tablets, tea

Plant part used: Fruit

DOSAGES
Saw palmetto is standardized to 85% to 95% fatty acids and sterols.

Benign prostatic hypertrophy
Adult PO capsules/tablets: 585 mg up to tid for 4-6 months (Foster, 1998)
Adult PO fluid extract, standardized: 160 mg bid, or 320 mg daily
Adult PO tincture: 20-30 drops up to qid (1:2 dilution)

Other
Adult PO decoction: 0.5-1 g dried berries tid
Adult PO decoction: 1-2 g fresh berries tid

CONTRAINDICATIONS
Avoid use in pregnancy and breastfeeding. Saw palmetto is an antiandrogen herb that is usually given to men. It should not be given to children. Persons with hypersensitivity to saw palmetto should not use it.

SIDE EFFECTS/ADVERSE REACTIONS
CNS: Headache
GI: Nausea, vomiting, anorexia, constipation, diarrhea, abdominal pain, and cramping
GU: Dysuria, urine retention, impotence
INTEG: Hypersensitivity reactions
MS: Back pain

INTERACTIONS
Drug
Anticoagulants (anisindione, ardeparin, dalteparin, dicumarol, heparin, warfarin): Saw palmetto may potentiate the anticoagulant effects of salicylates; avoid concurrent use.
Antiplatelets: Saw palmetto may lead to increased bleeding; avoid concurrent use.

Hormones (estrogens, hormonal contraceptives, and androgens): Saw palmetto may antagonize hormone therapy; avoid concurrent use (theoretical).

Immunostimulants: Saw palmetto may increase or decrease the effect of immunostimulants; avoid concurrent use (theoretical).

NSAIDs (bromfenac, diclofenac, etodolac, fenoprofen, flurbiprofen, ibuprofen, indomethacin, ketoprofen, ketorolac, meclofenamate, mefenamic acid, nabumetone, naproxen, oxaprozin, piroxicam, sulindac, tolmetin): Saw palmetto may lead to increased bleeding time; avoid concurrent use.

Lab test
Bleeding time: Saw palmetto can increase bleeding time.

Semen analysis: Saw palmetto may cause metabolic changes in specimen semen analysis.

NURSING CONSIDERATIONS
Assessment
• Assess for hypersensitivity reactions. If present, discontinue the use of saw palmetto and administer an antihistamine or other appropriate therapy.
• Assess the client's urinary patterns, including retention, frequency, pain, urge, residual urine, and nocturia.
• Assess for the use of antiinflammatories, hormones, and immunostimulants (see Interactions).

Patient problems
Impaired urination (uses)

Implementation
• Instruct the patient to store saw palmetto products in a cool, dry place away from heat and moisture.
• Saw palmetto should be taken with meals to minimize gastrointestinal symptoms.

Patient/family education
• Inform the patient not to use in pregnancy and breastfeeding.
• Caution the patient not to give saw palmetto to children.
• Advise the patient who is taking saw palmetto for BPH to consult a qualified expert for supervision.
• Advise the patient to obtain a prostate-specific antigen (PSA) test before using this herb.

St. John's wort
(saynt jahnz wawrt)
Scientific name: Hypericum perforatum L
Other common names: Amber, goatweed, hardhay, John's wort, Klamath weed, millepertuis, rosin rose, witches' herb

ORIGIN: St. John's wort is found in Europe, Asia, and the United States.

USES: St. John's wort is used to treat mild to moderate depression and anxiety. It may be used topically as an antiinflammatory to relieve hemorrhoids, as well as to treat vitiligo and burns.

Investigational uses
St. John's wort is used experimentally to treat warts, Kaposi's sarcoma, cutaneous T-cell lymphoma, and other viruses such as influenzae. It is also used experimentally as an antiretroviral in the treatment of HIV, as an antiinfective against methicillin-resistant strains of *Staphylococcus aureus,* and for phytotherapy in the treatment of psoriasis. Studies are underway to confirm the use of St. John's wort in menopausal symptoms and seasonal affective disorder. It may be effective for nicotine withdrawal symptoms.

ACTIONS
Several different possible actions have been researched in the United States and abroad, primarily in the 1980s and 1990s.

Antidepressant action
The inhibition of MAO (monoamine oxidase) and COMT (catechol *O*-methyltransferase) by *Hypericum* extracts and hypericin was researched (Bladt, Wagner, 1994; Suzuki et al., 1984; Thiede et al., 1994). Hypericin was found to inhibit in vitro type A and B MAOs. In rats, MAO-A inhibition was greater than MAO-B inhibition. The inhibition of MAO was determined to be the result of flavonoids in the hypericin. Much of the antidepressant action may be attributed to hyperforin and adhyperforin. These two constituents are found in the reproductive parts of the plant.

Antiretroviral/antimicrobial action
Investigation is underway into the possible antiretroviral action of St. John's wort and its use in the treatment of HIV infections. Antiretroviral action may be due to protein kinase-C-mediated phosphorylation.

PRODUCT AVAILABILITY
Cream; sublingual capsules; solid forms: 100, 300, 500 (0.3% hypericin), 250 (0.14% hypericin) mg; tincture

Plant part used: Flowers

DOSAGES
Adult PO: 300 mg hypericum extract, standardized to 0.3% hypericin, tid
Adult topical: apply prn

CONTRAINDICATIONS
Avoid use in pregnancy and breastfeeding. St. John's wort should not be given to children.

Persons who are hypersensitive to this herb should not use it.

SIDE EFFECTS/ADVERSE REACTIONS

CNS: Dizziness, insomnia, restlessness, fatigue (PO)

GI: Constipation, abdominal cramps (PO)

INTEG: Photosensitivity, rash, hypersensitivity

INTERACTIONS
Drug

ACE inhibitors, hormonal contraceptives, loop diuretics, NSAIDs, sulfonamides, sulfonylureas, tetracyclines, thiazide diuretics: St. John's wort combined with these products may lead to severe photosensitivity; avoid concurrent use.

Alcohol, MAOIs: St. John's wort may increase MAO inhibition (suggested by early studies); do not use alcohol, MAOIs, and St. John's wort concurrently until research is available.

Amphetamines, antidepressants, trazodone, tricyclics: St. John's wort used with these products may cause serotonin syndrome.

Antiretrovirals, nonnucleoside reverse transcriptase inhibitors (NNRTIs), protease inhibitors: Studies indicate that St. John's wort taken PO in combination with indinavir may decrease the antiretroviral action of this drug; do not use together.

Cytodrome P450 1A2, 2C9, 3A4: St. John's wort induces these enzyme systems.

Immunosuppressants: Rejection of transplanted hearts has occurred when St. John's wort was taken PO with cyclosporine, an immunosuppressant. Other immunosuppressants may have the same drug interaction in heart transplants, as well as other transplants.

Paroxetine: Increased sedation may result when paroxetine is combined with St. John's wort.

SSRIs: Serotonin syndrome and an additive effect may occur when SSRIs are combined with St. John's wort. Concurrent use may lead to coma. Do not use concurrently.

Food

Catecholamines, tyramine: Limit foods high in tyramine or catecholamines until further research confirms or denies the MAOI action of St. John's wort taken PO.

Lab test

Growth hormone: St. John's wort may cause increased growth hormone (somatotropin, GH).

Digoxin, serum iron, serum prolactin, theophylline: St. John's wort may cause decreased serum prolactin, theophylline (aminophylline), serum iron, and digoxin (peak and trough concentrations).

Pharmacology
Pharmacokinetics

Very little is known about the pharmacokinetics in humans. St. John's wort is thought to cross the blood-brain and placental barriers and possibly enter breast milk.

NURSING CONSIDERATIONS
Assess
Antidepressant use

• Assess the client's mental status: mood, sensorium, affect, memory (long, short), change in depression, or anxiety levels.

• Assess for the use of MAOIs and SSRIs, which should not be used with St. John's wort (taken PO) until further research is available.

• Assess for other drugs, foods, and herbs the client uses on a regular basis (see Interactions).

Antiretroviral use

• Assess for signs of infection.

• Assess CBC, blood chemistry, plasma HIV, RNA, absolute CD4/CD8+ cell counts, serum b-2 microglobulin, and serum ICD+ 24 antigen levels.

Patient problems

Depression (uses)

Implementation

• PO: use 2 tsp herb in 150 ml boiling water. Steep 15 minutes to create infusion.

• Topical: use oily hypericum preparations to treat inflammation or burns. Apply as needed.

Patient/family education

• Inform the patient to avoid in pregnancy and breastfeeding.

• Caution the patient not to give St. John's wort to children.

• Advise the patient to avoid high-tyramine foods such as aged cheese, sour cream, beer, wine, pickled products, liver, raisins, bananas, figs, avocados, meat tenderizers, chocolate, and yogurt, and to avoid increased caffeine intake when using this herb PO.

• Inform the patient that the therapeutic effect may take 4 to 6 weeks for the treatment of depression. If no improvement occurs in that time, another therapy should be considered.

• Advise the patient to avoid the use of alcohol or over-the-counter products that contain alcohol when using this herb PO.

• Advise the patient to avoid the sun or use sunscreen or protective clothing to prevent photosensitivity when using this herb.

turmeric
(tuhr'muh-rik)
Scientific name: Curcuma longa
Other common names: Curcuma, Indian saffron, Indian valerian, jiang huang, kyoo, radix, red valerian, tumeric, ukon

ORIGIN: Turmeric is found in the Far East and tropical regions.

USES: Turmeric traditionally has been used in both Chinese and Ayurvedic medicine to treat menstrual disorders, colic, inflammation, bruising, dyspepsia, hematuria, and flatulence. It is also used to improve stomach and liver function.

Investigational uses
Research has begun to focus on the use of turmeric for the treatment of lung, gastrointestinal, oral, and breast cancers; viruses such as HIV/AIDS; cholecystitis; and joint pain associated with arthritis and other joint disorders.

ACTIONS
The three chemical components of turmeric, curcumins I, II, and III, may have anticancer and antioxidant actions on leukemia, central nervous system disorders, renal cancer, breast cancer, colon cancer, and melanoma. Turmeric is also known to inhibit tissue necrosis factor (TNF)-alpha. The chemical component diferuloylmethane has been shown to cause the most significant inhibition. Turmeric may also exert hepatoprotective, antiinflammatory, antispasmodic, and hypolipidemic effects.

PRODUCT AVAILABILITY
Capsules, dried rhizome, fluid extract, oil, spice, tincture

Plant part used: Rhizome

DOSAGES
Adult PO: 400-600 mg tid (standardized to curcumin content)
Adult PO cut root: 1.5-3 g/day
Adult PO fluid extract: 1.5-3 ml (1:1 dilution)
Adult PO tincture: 10 ml (1:5 dilution)

CONTRAINDICATIONS
Considered safe in pregnancy and breastfeeding. Turmeric should not be used therapeutically by persons with bile duct obstruction, peptic ulcer, hyperacidity, gallstones, bleeding disorders, or hypersensitivity to this herb.

SIDE EFFECTS/ADVERSE REACTIONS
GI: Nausea, vomiting, anorexia, gastrointestinal ulceration (high doses)

INTEG: Hypersensitivity reactions

INTERACTIONS
Drug
Anticoagulants (heparin, salicylates, warfarin), **antiplatelets, NSAIDs** (bromfenac, diclofenac, etodolac, fenoprofen, flurbiprofen, ibuprofen, indomethacin, ketoprofen, ketorolac, meclofenamate, mefenamic acid, nabumetone, naproxen, oxaprozin, piroxicam, sulindac, tolmetin): Use of turmeric with anticoagulants, antiplatelets, NSAIDs may result in an increased risk of bleeding; avoid concurrent use.
Immunosuppressants (cyclosporine): Turmeric may decrease the effectiveness of immunosuppressants; avoid concurrent use.

Herb
Anticoagulant/antiplatelet herbs: Turmeric with anticoagulant/antiplatelet herbs increase the risk of bleeding.

NURSING CONSIDERATIONS
Assess
• Assess for hypersensitivity reactions, including contact dermatitis. If present, discontinue the use of turmeric and administer an antihistamine or other appropriate therapy.
• Assess for the use of anticoagulants, NSAIDs, and immunosuppressants (see Interactions).
• Monitor coagulation studies if the client is using turmeric for long-term treatment.

Patient problems
Risk of injury (uses)

Implementation
• Instruct the patient to store turmeric in a cool, dry place away from heat and moisture.
• Instruct the patient to take turmeric on an empty stomach.

Teach client/family
• Inform the patient turmeric is considered safe in pregnancy and breastfeeding.
• Advise the patient to report bleeding gums, blood in the urine or stool, and bruising.

valerian
(vuh-lir'ee-uhn)
Scientific name: Valeriana officinalis
Other common names: All heal, amantilla, baldrianwurzel, capon's tail, great wild valerian, herba benedicta, katzenwurzel, phu germanicum, phu parvum, setewale, setwell, theriacaria, valeriana

ORIGIN: Valerian is a perennial that is now cultivated throughout the world.

USES: Valerian is used to treat nervous disorders such as anxiety, restlessness, and insomnia.

ACTIONS
Antianxiety Action
Valerian has been studied almost as extensively as St. John's wort. Its effects are primarily neurochemical, acting on gamma-aminobutyric acid A (GABA) receptors and possibly also with other presynaptic components.

Antiinsomnia action
Valerian is most effective in long-term treatment.

Other actions
Valerian has shown positive results in the treatment of angina, decreasing the frequency and shortening the duration of anginal attacks.

PRODUCT AVAILABILITY
Capsules, crude herb, extract, tablets, tea, tincture; combination products containing other herbs

Plant parts used: Rhizomes, roots

DOSAGES
Insomnia
Adult PO extract: 400-900 mg ½-1 hr before bedtime (standardized)
Adult PO tea (crude herb): 1 tsp crude herb qid
Adult PO tincture: 3-5 ml qid (standardized)

CONTRAINDICATIONS
Avoid use in pregnancy and breastfeeding. Caution should be used when giving valerian to children. Persons with hepatic disease and those with hypersensitivity to valerian should not use it.

SIDE EFFECTS/ADVERSE REACTIONS
CNS: Insomnia, headache, restlessness
GI: Nausea, vomiting, anorexia, *hepatotoxicity (overdose)*
INTEG: Hypersensitivity reactions
MISC: Vision changes, palpitations

INTERACTIONS
Drug
CNS depressants (alcohol, barbiturates, benzodiazepines, opiates, sedatives/hypnotics): Valerian may increase the effects of central nervous system depressants; avoid concurrent use.

Cytochrome P4503A4 substrates: Valerian may inhibit these enzyme systems.
Iron salts: Valerian may interfere with the absorption of iron salts; separate by 2 hours.
MAOIs, phenytoin, warfarin: Valerian may negate the therapeutic effects of MAOIs, warfarin, and products containing phenytoin; do not use concurrently.

Lab test
ALT, AST, total bilirubin, urine bilirubin: Valerian may cause increased ALT, AST, total bilirubin, and urine bilirubin.

NURSING CONSIDERATIONS
Assess
• Assess for hypersensitivity reactions. If present, discontinue the use of valerian and administer an antihistamine or other appropriate therapy.
• Assess liver function studies (AST, ALT, bilirubin) if the client is using valerian for long-term treatment. If results are elevated, discontinue use of the herb.
• Assess medications used (see Interactions).

Patient problems
Impaired sleep

Implementation
• Instruct the client that valerian products should be kept away from heat and moisture.

Patient/family education
• Inform the patient to avoid in pregnancy and breastfeeding.
• Advise the patient to use caution when giving valerian to children.
• Advise the patient not to perform hazardous activities such as driving or operating heavy machinery until physical response to the herb can be evaluated. Valerian causes sedation and dizziness.
• Advise the patient to discontinue the use of valerian if symptoms worsen.

Entries can be identified as follows: generic name, Trade Name, DRUG CATEGORY

Entries can be identified as follows: generic name, Trade Name, DRUG CATEGORY

Entries can be identified as follows: generic name, Trade Name, DRUG CATEGORY

NEW DRUGS FOR 2022

atoltivimab/maftivimab/odesivimab-ebgn (Rx)
Inmazeb
Func. class.: Antiinfective

USES: Treatment of *Zaire ebolavirus* infection

CONTRAINDICATIONS
Hypersensitivity

DOSAGE AND ROUTES
Adult/child: IV 50-mg atoltivimab, 50-mg maftivimab, 50-mg odesivimab per kg diluted and administered as a single IV infusion

amisulpride (Rx)
(a' mi-sul' pride)
Barhemsys
Func. class.: Antiemetic
Chem. class.: Dopamine receptor

ACTION: Blocks dopamine receptors. D_2 receptors are in the chemoreceptor trigger zone (CTZ) and respond to the dopamine released from the nerve endings. CTZ activation is responsible for stimulating the vomiting center, which causes emesis

USES: Prevention/treatment of postoperative nausea/vomiting

Pharmacokinetics

Absorption	Complete
Distribution	Protein binding 25%-30%, to erythrocytes
Metabolism	Unknown
Excretion	Urine 74%, feces 23%; breast milk
Half-life	4-5 hr

Pharmacodynamics

Onset	Rapid
Peak	End of dose
Duration	Unknown

CONTRAINDICATIONS
Hypersensitivity

Precautions: QT prolongation, pregnancy, child, renal disease, infertility, preexisting arrhythmias/cardiac conduction disorders, hypokalemia, hypomagnesemia, congestive heart failure

DOSAGE AND ROUTES
Prevention of postoperative nausea/vomiting
Adult: IV 5 mg as a single dose given over 1-2 min at the time of induction of anesthesia

Treatment of postoperative nausea/vomiting
Adult: IV 10 mg as a single dose given over 1-2 min for nausea/vomiting after surgery

Available forms: Injection 5 mg/2 mL (2.5 mg/mL), 10 mg/4 mL (2.5 mg/mL) single-dose vial

ADVERSE EFFECTS
CNS: Chills, agitation, seizures, confusion, insomnia, somnolence, EPS, confusion, psychiatric symptoms
CV: Postural hypotension bradycardia, torsades de pointes, ventricular tachycardia, prolonged QT
META: Hypokalemia, hypomagnesemia
GI: Abdominal distention, increased LFTs
HEMA: Agranulocytosis
SYST: Neuroleptic malignant syndrome, angioedema, hypersensitivity

INTERACTIONS
CNS depressants: Increased—CNS depression
Dopamine agonists (levodopa): Increase—antagonism, avoid using together
Drugs that increase QT prolongation (ondansetron): Increase—QT prolongation, monitor ECG

NURSING CONSIDERATIONS
Assessment
• Nausea/vomiting: Monitor baseline and after using product
• QT prolongation: Monitor ECG if other QT prolongation medications are used or history of QT prolongation
• Pregnancy/breastfeeding: Identify if pregnant or breastfeeding

Patient problems
Nausea (uses)

Implementation
• Visually inspect for particulate matter and discoloration, discard if present
• Dilution is not needed
• Protect from light, give within 12 hr of removing from carton

Solution compatibilities: Water for Injection, D_5W, 0.9% NaCl

Patient/family education
• **QT prolongation:** Instruct patients to contact their health care provider immediately about change in their heart rate, lightheadedness, syncope
• Teach patients to report to their health care provider if they are taking drugs that prolong the QT interval
• **Pregnancy/breastfeeding:** Suggest pumping and discarding breast milk for 48 hours after product

Evaluation
Positive therapeutic outcome: Absence of nausea/vomiting

avapritinib (Rx)
(a′va-pri′ti-nib)
Ayvakit
Func. class.: Antineoplastic

USES: PDGFRA exon 18 mutation–positive unresectable/metastatic GI stromal tumor (GIST)

CONTRAINDICATIONS
Hypersensitivity

DOSAGE AND ROUTES
Adult: PO 300 mg daily on an empty stomach, continue until disease progression or unacceptable toxicity

belantamab mafodotin-blmf (Rx)
(bel-an′ta-mab ma-foe-doe′tin)
Blenrep
Func. class.: Antineoplastic agent
Chem. class.: Anti-BCMA

ACTION: A humanized antibody targeted against B-cell maturation antigen (BCMA) that is expressed on multiple myeloma cells

USES: Treatment of relapsed/refractory multiple myeloma in those who have received ≥4 prior therapies

Pharmacokinetics
Absorption	Complete
Distribution	Unknown
Metabolism	To small peptides/amino acids by catabolism
Excretion	Unknown
Half-life	14 days

Pharmacodynamics
Onset	Of response 1-4 mo
Peak	End of infusion
Duration	Of response ≥ 6 mo

CONTRAINDICATIONS
Hypersensitivity

BLACK BOX WARNING: Ocular toxicity, restricted access

Precautions: Bleeding, breastfeeding, driving/operating machinery, geriatric, pregnancy, infusion-related reactions, requires a specialized care setting, requires an experienced clinician, thrombocytopenia, visual impairment

DOSAGE AND ROUTES
Multiple myeloma
Adult: IV: 2.5 mg/kg q3wk until disease progression/unacceptable toxicity

Available forms: IV solution (preservative free) 100 mg/vial

ADVERSE EFFECTS
CNS: Fatigue, fever, asthenia
GI: Constipation, anorexia, diarrhea, nausea, vomiting, increased LFTs
GU: Increased serum creatinine, renal insufficiency, albuminuria
META: Decreased serum albumin (43%), hypokalemia, hyponatremia, increased gamma-glutamyl transferase, hyperglycemia, hypercalcemia
HEMA: Decreased hgb, decreased neutrophils, lymphocytopenia, thrombocytopenia
MS: Arthralgia, back pain, increased CPK
EENT: Blurred vision, decreased visual acuity, dry eye syndrome, epithelial keratopathy, eye irritation, photophobia
RESP: URI, pneumonia
MISC: Infusion related reaction, sepsis

INTERACTIONS: BCG (intravesical), chloramphenicol (ophthalmic), cladribine, clozapine, deferiprone, promazine, salicylates: Increased-myelosuppression

NURSING CONSIDERATIONS
Assessment
• Monitor CBC at baseline and as needed
• Obtain hepatitis B virus screening with hepatitis B surface antigen (HBsAg), hepatitis B core antibody (anti-HBc), total Ig or IgG, and antibody to hepatitis B surface antigen (anti-HBs) before use, may start treatment before results are received
• Monitor for bleeding, infusion site reactions

BLACK BOX WARNING: REMS: Ocular toxicity: available only through a restricted program under a Risk Evaluation and Mitigation Strategy (REMS) called the BLENREP REMS; obtain ophthalmic examinations (visual acuity/slit lamp) baseline within 3 wk of first dose, before each dose, and for worsening ocular symptoms

• **Pregnancy/breastfeeding:** Obtain pregnancy testing before use in females of reproductive potential; contraception is needed during and for 4 mo after the last dose, males with female partners of reproductive potential should use contraception during and for 6 mo after the last dose

Patient problems
Risk for injury (adverse reactions)
Risk for infection (adverse reactions)

Implementation
• Allow to warm to room temperature for 10 min
• Reconstitute 100 mg/2 mL 0.9% NaCl (50 mg/mL); gently swirl
• Solution should be clear to opalescent, colorless-yellow-brown liquid; discard if particulates are observed
• Withdraw needed amount and dilute in a 250 mL 0.9% NaCl infusion bag (0.2-2 mg/mL) use only infusion bag of PVC or polyolefin
• Mix by gentle inversion; do not shake
• Solutions diluted for infusion should be clear and colorless; discard if particulate matter is observed
• Do not admix
• Give over ≥30 min using PVC or polyolefin infusion set, may use a polyethersulfone-based filter (0.2 micron)
• Do not give with other medications
• If refrigerated, allow to warm to room temperature before use; use within 6 hr, including time to warm and infusion time
• Assess for infusion-related reactions
• Store vials refrigerated, reconstituted solution may be stored refrigerated or room temperature for ≤4 hr; discard if not diluted within 4 hr; solutions diluted for infusion may be stored refrigerated ≤24 hr

Patient/family education
• Teach patient to use preservative-free lubricant eye drops and avoid contact lenses, that ophthalmic testing will be needed during treatment
• Identify if pregnancy is planned or suspected, or if breastfeeding; discuss contraception

Evaluation
Positive therapeutic outcome: Decreasing spread of multiple myeloma

bempedoic acid/ezetimibe (Rx)
(bem'pe-doe'ik as'id)
Nexlizet
Func. class.: Antilipemic

USES: Atherosclerotic CV disease, heterozygous familial hypercholesterolemia as an adjunct to diet/statin therapy

CONTRAINDICATIONS
Hypersensitivity

DOSAGE AND ROUTES
Adult: PO 1 tablet (180 mg bempedoic acid/10 mg ezetimibe) daily with statins

capmatinib (Rx)
(kap-ma'ti-nib)
Tabrecta
Func. class.: Antineoplastic

USES: Treatment of metastatic non-small cell lung cancer with a mutation of mesenchymal-epithelial transition (MET) exon 14 skipping

CONTRAINDICATIONS
Hypersensitivity, pregnancy, breastfeeding

DOSAGE AND ROUTES
Adult: PO 400 mg bid, continue until disease progression or unacceptable toxicity

collagenase clostridium histolyticum-aaes (Rx)
(kol'la-je-nase)
Xiaflex
Func. class.: Enzyme

USES: Treatment of adults with Dupuytren contracture with a palpable cord; treatment of adult men with Peyronie disease with a palpable plaque/curvature deformity of at least 30 degrees

CONTRAINDICATIONS
Treatment of Peyronie plaques that involve the penile urethra; hypersensitivity to collagenase

DOSAGE AND ROUTES
Dupuytren contracture
Adult: Intralesional: Inject 0.58 mg per cord affecting a metacarpophalangeal (MP) joint or a proximal interphalangeal (PIP) joint. If contracture persists, finger extension procedure should be performed 24 to 72 hr after injection

Peyronie disease
Adult male: Intralesional: Inject 0.58 mg into a Peyronie plaque; repeat 1-3 days later. Perform

a penile modeling procedure 1-3 days after 2nd injection. Use a 2nd treatment cycle (two 0.58-mg injections and a penile modeling procedure) in 6 wk if needed (max 4 cycles)

daratumumab/ hyaluronidase-fihj (Rx)
(dar′a-toom′ue-mab/hye′al-ureon′i-dase)
Darzalex
Func. class.: Antineoplastic

USES: Multiple myeloma

CONTRAINDICATIONS
Hypersensitivity, pregnancy, breastfeeding

DOSAGE AND ROUTES
Multiple myeloma (newly diagnosed)
Adult: SUBCUT with *lenalidomide and dexamethasone in those ineligible for autologous stem cell transplant:* Weeks 1-8: Daratumumab 1800 mg/hyaluronidase 30,000 units weekly × 8 doses; weeks 9-24: Daratumumab 1800 mg/hyaluronidase 30,000 units q2wk × 8 doses; weeks 25 and thereafter: Daratumumab 1800 mg/hyaluronidase 30,000 units q4wk until disease progression or unacceptable toxicity
Adult: SUBCUT with **bortezomib, melphalan, prednisone; in those ineligible for autologous stem cell transplant:** Weeks 1-6: Daratumumab 1800 mg/hyaluronidase 30,000 units weekly × 6 doses; weeks 7-54: Daratumumab 1800 mg/hyaluronidase 30,000 units q3wk × 16 doses; weeks 55 and thereafter: Daratumumab 1800 mg/hyaluronidase 30,000 units q4wk until disease progression or unacceptable toxicity

decitabine/cedazuridine (Rx)
(de-sye′ta-been/sed′az-ure′i-deen)
Inqovi
Func. class.: Antineoplastic, antimetabolite

USES: Treatment of myelodysplastic syndromes (MDSs)

CONTRAINDICATIONS
Hypersensitivity

DOSAGE AND ROUTES
Adult: PO 35 mg decitabine/100 mg cedazuridine daily × 5 days of each 28-day cycle, complete at least 4 cycles

eptinezumab-jjmr (Rx)
(ep′ti-nez′ue-mab)
Vyepti
Func. class.: Antimigraine agent
Chem. class.: Calcitonin gene–related peptide receptor antagonist

ACTION: A humanized monoclonal antibody, binds to calcitonin gene–related peptide ligand and blocks binding to the receptor

USES: Prevention of migraine

Pharmacokinetics

Absorption	Complete
Distribution	Unknown
Metabolism	Amino acids, small peptides by proteolysis
Excretion	Unknown
Half-life	27 days

Pharmacokinetics

Onset	1 day
Peak	Infusion's end
Duration	Unknown

CONTRAINDICATIONS
Serious hypersensitivity

Precautions: Pregnancy, breastfeeding

DOSAGE AND ROUTES
Migraine prophylaxis
Adult: IV: 100 mg q3mo; may use 300 mg q3mo

Available forms: IV solution, preservative free, 100 mg/mL (1 mL)

ADVERSE EFFECTS
MISC: Antibody development
RESP: Nasopharyngitis
CNS: Fatigue
GI: Nausea
INTEG: Hypersensitivity, angioedema

INTERACTIONS: None known

NURSING CONSIDERATIONS
Assessment
• **Migraine:** Baseline and periodically, presence of aura, nausea/vomiting
• Assess for hypersensitivity, dyspnea; reaction may be delayed, discontinue if these occur

Patient problems
Pain (uses)

Implementation
Intermittent IV infusion
- Contains polysorbate 80
- Dilute in 100 mL NS; infusion bags must be made of polyvinyl chloride, polyethylene, polyolefin; mix by gentle inverting; do not shake; discard unused portion; **100-mg dose:** Withdraw 1 mL eptinezumab/100 mL NS (1 mg/mL); **300-mg dose:** Withdraw 1 mL eptinezumab from 3 vials/100 mL NS (3 mg/mL)
- Run over 30 min using an infusion set with a 0.2 micron or 0.22 micron in-line or add-on sterile filter; do not give IV push/bolus
- Do not admix or infuse other medications in same infusion set
- After infusion, flush line with 20 mL NS
- Store intact vial at 2°C to 8°C (36°F to 46°F), protect from light, do not freeze; diluted solution may be stored at room temperature, infuse within 8 hr

Patient/family education
- Reason for product and expected result
- Identify if pregnancy is planned or suspected

Evaluation
Positive therapeutic response: Prevention of migraine

---

fenfluramine (Rx)
(fen-flur′a-meen)
Fintepla
Func. class.: Anticonvulsant

USES: Dravet syndrome

CONTRAINDICATIONS
Hypersensitivity, MAOIs

DOSAGE AND ROUTES
Child ≥ 2 yr: PO 0.1 mg/kg BID; titrate q wk, increase to 0.2 mg/kg BID on day 7 and to 0.35 mg/kg BID on day 14; dose may be increased q 4 days; max 0.35 mg/ kg BID, up to 26 mg/day

---

fostemsavir (Rx)
(fos-tem′sa-vir)
Rukobia
Func. class.: Antiretroviral
Chem. class.: gp120 attachment inhibitor

ACTION: Binds to the HIV-1 protein glycoprotein 120 subunit, inhibits the interaction between the virus and cellular CD4 receptors, prevents attachment

USES: Treatment of HIV-1 infection with other antiretrovirals in multidrug-resistant HIV-1 infection

Pharmacokinetics

Absorption	Increased with high-fat meal
Distribution	Protein binding 88.4%
Metabolism	Hydrolysis, oxidation
Excretion	Urine 51%, feces 33%
Half-life	11 hr

Pharmacodynamics

Onset	Unknown
Peak	2 hr
Duration	Unknown

CONTRAINDICATIONS
Breastfeeding, hypersensitivity, use of strong CYP3A inducers (enzalutamide, carbamazepine, phenytoin, rifampin, St. John's wort)

Precautions: Pregnancy, infants, liver disease, myelosuppression, infections

DOSAGE AND ROUTES
HIV-1 infection
Adult: PO 600 mg bid with other antiretrovirals

Available forms: Ext Rel tablets 600 mg

ADVERSE EFFECTS
CNS: Fatigue, headache, dizziness, drowsiness, insomnia, abnormal dreams, peripheral neuropathy
CV: QT prolongation
GI: Nausea, vomiting, abdominal pain, diarrhea, dyspepsia, increased LFTs
META: Hyperbilirubinemia, hypercholesterolemia, hyperglycemia, hypertriglyceridemia
HEMA: Anemia, neutropenia
INTEG: Rash, pruritus

INTERACTIONS: Many drug interactions, refer to manufacturer's information

NURSING CONSIDERATIONS
Assessment
- HIV: Monitor CBC, with differential, blood chemistry, blood glucose, plasma HIV RNA, absolute CD4+/CD8+ cell counts, serum ICD+24 antigen levels, cholesterol, serum bilirubin (total and direct), serum lipid profile, urinalysis baseline and periodically
- **Hepatotoxicity:** Monitor LFTs, signs of hepatotoxicity in HBV and/or HCV coinfection; continue with or start anti-HBV therapy in those coinfected with HBV
- Monitor for QT prolongation in those with a history of prolonged QT interval, preexisting cardiac disease, or those taking drugs known to cause torsades de pointes

---

• **Hepatitis B virus coinfection:** Use with caution; elevations in liver function tests may occur more often with HBV coinfection, which may be related to HBV reactivation, monitor hepatitis B serology, plasma hepatitis C RNA

• **Peripheral neuropathy:** May occur and last for several months, where nerves are close to the skin, monitor for peripheral neuropathy

• Assess bowel pattern before, during treatment; if severe abdominal pain or constipation occurs, notify prescriber; monitor hydration

• **Hypersensitivity:** Assess for skin eruptions, rash, urticaria, itching; assess allergies before treatment, reaction to each medication; may occur quickly or later after continued use

• **Immune reconstitution syndrome:** With combination therapy, patients may develop immune reconstitution syndrome with an inflammatory response to opportunistic infection during initial HIV treatment or activation of autoimmune disorders (Graves disease, polymyositis, Guillain-Barre syndrome, autoimmune hepatitis)

• **Pregnancy/breastfeeding:** Identify if pregnancy is planned or suspected, or if breastfeeding; if pregnant, register with the Antiretroviral Pregnancy Registry, 800-258-4263, obtain a pregnancy test

Patient problems
Infection (uses)
Risk for injury (adverse reactions)

Implementation
PO route
Give without regard to food; swallow whole; do not chew, crush, split

Patient/family education
• Teach patient that hypersensitive reactions may occur; rash, pruritus; to stop product, contact provider

• Advise patient that product is not a cure for HIV-1 infection but controls symptoms; HIV-1 can still be transmitted to others; that product is to be used in combination only with other antiretrovirals

• Inform patient to notify provider if pregnancy is suspected; not to breastfeed

Evaluation
Positive therapeutic outcome: Increased CD4 cell counts; decreased viral load; slowing progression of HIV-1 infection

lumasiran (Rx)
(loo′ma-sir′an)
Oxlumo
Func. class.: Metabolic disorder agent

USES: Primary hyperoxaluria type 1

CONTRAINDICATIONS
Hypersensitivity, breastfeeding, pregnancy

DOSAGE AND ROUTES
Adults: SUBCUT 3 mg/kg/dose monthly × 3 doses, then 3 mg/kg/dose q3mo
Child/adolescent ≥20 kg: SUBCUT 3 mg/kg/dose monthly × 3 doses, then 3 mg/kg/dose q3mo
Infant/child 10-19 kg: SUBCUT 6 mg/kg/dose monthly × 3 doses, then 6 mg/kg/dose q3mo
Infant/child <10 kg: SUBCUT 6 mg/kg/dose monthly × 3 doses, then 3 mg/kg/dose monthly
Neonates: SUBCUT 6 mg/kg/dose monthly × 3 doses, then 3 mg/kg/dose monthly

lurbinectedin (Rx)
(loor bin-ek′te-din)
Zepzelca
Func. class.: Antineoplastic, alkylating agent

USES: Treatment of metastatic small cell lung cancer with disease progression after platinum-type chemotherapy

CONTRAINDICATIONS
Hypersensitivity

DOSAGE AND ROUTES
Small cell lung cancer, metastatic
Adult: IV: 3.2 mg/m^2 q21 days until disease progression/unacceptable toxicity

moderna COVID-19 Vaccine (Rx)
Func. class.: Vaccine for COVID-19

ACTION: Formulated in lipid particles, delivers RNA into cells to allow for the SARS-CoV-2 immune response to the S antigen, which protects against COVID-19

USES: Emergency use authorization (EUA) for active immunization to prevent coronavirus disease 2019 (COVID-19) caused by severe acute respiratory syndrome coronavirus 2 (SARS-CoV-2) in those ≥18 yr. Vaccination providers enrolled in the federal COVID-19 vaccination program must report all vaccine administration errors, all serious adverse events, cases of multisystem inflammatory syndrome (MIS) in adults, and cases of COVID-19 that result in hospitalization or death following administration of the Moderna COVID-19 vaccine.

CONTRAINDICATIONS
History of a severe allergic reaction (anaphylaxis) to any component

Precautions: Immunocompromised, immunosuppressant treatment, may not protect all patients, emergency equipment nearby

DOSAGE AND ROUTES
Adult/adolescent ≥18 yr: IM single dose of 0.5 mL, then another dose in 1 mo

Available forms: Multiple-dose vial, frozen suspension, without preservative

ADVERSE EFFECTS
CNS: Fatigue, headache, chills, fever, malaise
GI: Nausea, vomiting
MS: Joint/muscle pain
SYST: Allergic reactions, anaphylaxis, lymphadenopathy
INTEG: Pain/swelling/redness at the injection site

INTERACTIONS: Several drug interactions, check specific products

NURSING CONSIDERATIONS
Assessment:
• Allergic reactions: Assess for serious allergic reactions after use
• Report to the Vaccine Adverse Event Reporting System (VAERS) all administration errors, all serious adverse events, cases of MIS, and hospitalized or fatal cases of COVID-19 following vaccination

Patient problems
• Risk of infection (uses)
• Risk of injury (adverse reactions)

Implementation
IM route
• Multiple-dose vials are stored frozen between −25° and −15°C (−13° and 5°F)
• Store in the original carton to protect from light
• Do not store on dry ice or below −40°C (−40°F)
• Vials can be stored refrigerated between 2° and 8°C (36° and 46°F) ≤30 days before first use
• Unpunctured vials may be stored between 8° and 25°C (46° and 77°F) ≤12 hr, do not dilute
• Do not refreeze once thawed
• After the first dose has been withdrawn, the vial should be held between 2° and 25°C (36° and 77°F)
• Discard vial after 6 hr, do not refreeze

Evaluation
Positive therapeutic outcome: Absence of COVID-19 infection

Patient/family education
• FDA has authorized the emergency use of the Moderna COVID-19 vaccine, which is not an FDA-approved vaccine
• You or your caregiver can accept or refuse the vaccine
• Known risks and benefits are unknown
• Give patient information about other vaccines and risks/benefits of alternatives
• Teach patient to report serious adverse reactions immediately
• Identify if pregnancy is suspected, or if breastfeeding
• Provide a vaccination card to the recipient or caregiver with the date when the second dose should be given
• Provide the v-safe information sheet to patient/caregiver and encourage to participate in v-safe
• V-safe is a new voluntary smartphone-based tool that uses text messaging and web surveys to check in with people who have been vaccinated to identify potential side effects after vaccination. V-safe asks questions that help the CDC monitor the safety of COVID-19 vaccines
• V-safe also provides second-dose reminders if needed and live telephone follow-up by CDC if participants report a significant health impact following COVID-19 vaccination, visit: www.cdc.gov/vsafe

nifurtimox (Rx)
(nye-fure′ ti-mox)
Lampit
Func. class.: Antiprotozoal

USES: Treatment of Chagas disease in children

CONTRAINDICATIONS
Hypersensitivity, alcohol use

DOSAGE AND ROUTES
Birth (term neonate to ≤18 yr and 2.5 to <40 kg: PO 10-20 mg/kg/day in divided doses tid; **≥40 kg:** 8-10 mg/kg/day in divided doses tid

oliceridine (Rx)
(oh′li-ser′i-deen)
Olinvyk
Func. class.: Opioid analgesic
Controlled substance II

ACTION: Binds to the opioid *mu* receptor to produce analgesia

USES: Acute pain

Pharmacokinetics

Absorption	Complete
Distribution	Protein binding 77%
Metabolism	Hepatic by CYP3A4, 2D6 (major); 2C9, 2C19 (minor)
Excretion	Urine 70%, feces 30%
Half-life	1.3-3 hr, metabolite 44 hr

Pharmacodynamics

Onset	<5 min
Peak	Unknown
Duration	Unknown

CONTRAINDICATIONS

Hypersensitivity, severe respiratory depression; GI obstruction, asthma

Precautions: Pregnancy, breastfeeding, abuse, neonatal opioid withdrawal syndrome, use with benzodiazepine or other CNS depressants, QT prolongation, chronic pulmonary disease, adrenal insufficiency, hypotension, GI disease, seizures

DOSAGE AND ROUTES
Acute pain

Adult: IV bolus: 1.5 mg; may give another dose of 0.75 mg after 1 hr; subsequent supplemental doses may be repeated no more frequently than hourly and titrated based on tolerability and response; max single supplemental dose: 3 mg; max total daily dose: 27 mg

Adult: PCA: 1.5 mg (given by provider); demand dose: Range: 0.35-0.5 mg; lockout interval: 6 min; supplemental dose (administered by health care provider): 0.75 mg; may be administered beginning 1 hr after the initial dose and repeated hourly as needed; may be used in addition to the demand dose if needed for adequate analgesia

Max cumulative daily dose: 27 mg; an initial dose of oliceridine 1 mg = morphine 5 mg

Available forms: IV solution (preservative free): 1 mg/mL (1 mL); 2 mg/2 mL (2 mL); 30 mg/30 mL (30 mL)

ADVERSE EFFECTS

CNS: Dizziness, somnolence, sedation, headache, flushing
GI: Nausea, vomiting, constipation
INTEG: Pruritus
RESP: Respiratory depression, decreased O_2 saturation
MS: Back pain

INTERACTIONS: Moderate-strong inhibitors of CYP3A4 (macrolides, azoles, protease inhibitors); moderate-strong CYP2D6 inhibitors

(fluoxetine, quinidine, bupropion); benzodiazepines, other CNS depressant—Increase: oliceridine effect; monitor for respiratory depression/sedation

SSRIs, SNRIs tricyclic antidepressants, triptans, 5-HT3 receptor antagonists, mirtazapine, trazodone, tramadol, cyclobenzaprine, metaxalone, MAOIs, linezolid, IV methylene blue: Increase—Serotonin effects, observe for serotonin symptoms

Muscle relaxants; monitor for respiratory depression: Increase—respiratory depression

Anticholinergics; monitor for urinary retention, paralytic ileus: Increase—urinary retention, paralytic ileus

CYP3A4 inducers (rifampin, carbamazepine, phenytoin), mixed agonist/antagonists, partial agonist opioids: Decrease: oliceridine effect—monitor for signs of opioid withdrawal

Diuretics: Decrease: diuretic effect—monitor B/P, urinary output

NURSING CONSIDERATIONS
Assessment

• **Pain:** Assess location, intensity, type, character; check for pain relief 20 min following IV, to relieve pain; give dose before pain becomes severe

• Bowel status; assess for constipation is common, use stimulant laxative if needed; provide increased bulk, fluids in diet

• Monitor B/P, pulse, respirations (character, depth, rate)

• CNS changes: Assess for dizziness, drowsiness, euphoria, LOC, pupil reaction

• **Abrupt discontinuation:** Gradually taper to prevent withdrawal symptoms

• **Respiratory dysfunction:** Assess for depression, character, rate, rhythm; notify prescriber if respirations are <12/min

• **Pregnancy/breastfeeding:** Use only if benefits outweigh risk to fetus; longer use can result in neonatal opioid withdrawal syndrome; do not breastfeed, identify if pregnancy is planned or suspected, or if breastfeeding

Patient problems

Pain (uses)
Risk for injury (adverse reactions)

Implementation
IV direct route

• No dilution needed

• Use the 1 mg/mL and 2 mg/2 mL single-dose vials for direct use only

• **PCA:** Withdraw directly into a PCA syringe or IV bag; no dilution needed; 30 mg/30 mL vial is for PCA only

• Store at room temperature, do not freeze, protect from light

Patient/family education
- Advise patient to report change in pain control
- Teach patient to report constipation, as other products will need to be used
- Teach patient to change position slowly; orthostatic hypotension may occur
- Advise patient to report any symptoms of CNS changes, allergic reactions
- Inform patient that physical dependency may result from long-term use
- Teach patient that withdrawal symptoms may occur: nausea, vomiting, cramps, fever, faintness, anorexia
- Teach patient to report serotonin syndrome: shivering, sweating, dilated pupils, increased B/P, increased heart rate, twitching

Evaluation
Positive therapeutic outcome: Control of pain without adverse reactions

TREATMENT OF OVERDOSE:
Naloxone (Narcan) O_2, IV fluids, vasopressors

opicapone (Rx)
(oh-pik′a-pone)
Ongentys
Func. class.: Anti-parkinson agent, COMT inhibitor

USES: Adjunct with levodopa/carbidopa in Parkinson disease "off" episodes

CONTRAINDICATIONS
Hypersensitivity, MAOIs, pheochromocytoma, paraganglioma

DOSAGE AND ROUTES
Adult: PO 50 mg daily at bedtime

peanut (*Arachis hypogaea*) allergen powder-dnfp
Palforzia

USES
Mitigation of allergic reactions to peanuts

CONTRAINDICATIONS
Hypersensitivity, uncontrolled asthma, eosinophilic esophagitis

DOSAGE AND ROUTES
See manufacturer's information

pemigatinib
(pem′i-ga′ti-nib)
Penazyre
Func. class.: Antineoplastic agent, fibroblast growth factor receptor (FGFR) inhibitor

USES: Treatment of previously treated, unresectable, locally advanced/metastatic cholangiocarcinoma with an FGFR 2 fusion or other rearrangement

CONTRAINDICATIONS
Hypersensitivity, pregnancy, breastfeeding

DOSAGE AND ROUTES
Adult: PO: 13.5 mg daily on days 1-14 of a 21-day cycle; continue until disease progression or unacceptable toxicity

pertuzumab/trastuzumab/hyaluronidase-zzxf (Rx)
(per-tu′zoo-mab/tras-tu′zoo-mab/hye-al-yoor-on′i-dase)
Phesgo
Func. class.: Antineoplastic

USES: Neoadjuvant treatment of HER2-positive, locally advanced, inflammatory, or early stage breast cancer (either >2 cm in diameter or node positive); treatment of HER2-positive metastatic breast cancer (in combination with docetaxel) in those who have not received prior anti-HER2 therapy/chemotherapy for metastatic disease

CONTRAINDICATIONS
Hypersensitivity to pertuzumab, trastuzumab, hyaluronidase, or any component

BLACK BOX WARNING: Cardiomyopathy, embryo-fetal toxicity, pulmonary toxicity

DOSAGE AND ROUTES
Adult: **SUBCUT Initial loading dose:** Pertuzumab 1200 mg/trastuzumab 600 mg/hyaluronidase 30,000 units, then after 3 wk, **maintenance:** Pertuzumab 600 mg/trastuzumab 600 mg/hyaluronidase 20,000 units q3wk; after surgery, continue to complete 1 yr

Pfizer-BioNTech COVID-19 Vaccine (Rx)
Func. class.: Vaccine for COVID-19

ACTION: Formulated in lipid particles, delivers RNA into cells to allow for the SARS-CoV-2 immune response to the S antigen, which protects against COVID-19

USES: Emergency use authorization (EUA) for active immunization to prevent coronavirus disease 2019 (COVID-19) caused by severe acute respiratory syndrome coronavirus 2 (SARS-CoV-2) in those ≥16 yr

CONTRAINDICATIONS

History of a severe allergic reaction (anaphylaxis) to any component

Precautions: Immunocompromised, immunosuppressant treatment, may not protect all patients, emergency equipment nearby

DOSAGE AND ROUTES

Adult/adolescent ≥16 yr: IM Single dose of 0.3 mL, then another dose in 21 days

Available forms: Multiple-dose vial (volume of 0.45 mL), frozen suspension, without preservative

ADVERSE EFFECTS

CNS: Fatigue, headache, chills, fever, malaise
GI: Nausea, vomiting
MS: Joint/muscle pain
SYST: Allergic reactions, anaphylaxis, lymphadenopathy
INTEG: Pain/swelling/redness at the injection site

INTERACTIONS: None known

NURSING CONSIDERATIONS
Assessment

• Allergic reactions: Assess for serious allergic reactions after use
• Report to the Vaccine Adverse Event Reporting System (VAERS) all administration errors, all serious adverse events, cases of multisystem inflammatory syndrome (MIS), and hospitalized or fatal cases of COVID-19 following vaccination

Patient problems

Infection (uses)
Risk for injury (adverse reactions)

Implementation
IM route

• Thaw the vial in refrigerator or at room temperature
• Inspect the liquid in the vial before dilution; it is a white to off-white suspension and contains white to off-white opaque particles
• Do not use if liquid is discolored or if other particles are present
• Before dilution invert 10 times, do not shake
• Dilute the vial contents using 1.8 mL of 0.9% NaCl Injection, do not use bacteriostatic 0.9% NaCl
• After dilution, one vial contains up to 6 doses of 0.3 mL

• Record the date/time of dilution on vial label
• Store between 2°C and 25°C (35°F and 77°F).
• Discard any unused vaccine 6 hr after dilution
• Minimize exposure to light
• Do not refreeze thawed vials

Patient/family education

• Teach patient to report serious adverse reactions immediately
• Identify if pregnancy is suspected or if breastfeeding

Evaluation

Positive therapeutic outcome: Absence of COVID-19 infection

---

pralsetinib (Rx)
(pral'se'ti'nib)
Gavreto
Func. class.: Antineoplastic
Chem. class.: RET kinase inhibitor

ACTION: Inhibits wild-type RET, oncogenic RET fusions, and RET mutations; antitumor activity occurs in cells harboring oncogenic RET fusions or mutations

USES: Treatment of non-small cell lung cancer (NSCLC)

Pharmacokinetics

Absorption	Unknown
Distribution	Protein binding 97%
Metabolism	Unknown
Excretion	Unknown
Half-life	22 hr

Pharmacodynamics

Onset	Unknown
Peak	2-4 hr
Duration	Unknown

CONTRAINDICATIONS

Hypersensitivity

Precautions: Breastfeeding, children, chronic lung disease, contraception requirements, growth inhibition, hepatic disease, hypertension, impaired wound healing, infertility, interstitial lung disease, male-mediated teratogenicity, pneumonitis, pregnancy, renal impairment, surgery, tumor lysis syndrome

DOSAGE AND ROUTES
Metastatic non-small cell lung cancer RET fusion-positive

Adult: PO 400 mg daily until disease progression/unacceptable toxicity

---

Available forms: Capsule 100 mg

Administer
- On empty stomach ≥1 hr before or ≥2 hr after food
- Store at room temperature

ADVERSE EFFECTS
CNS: Fatigue
GI: Constipation, diarrhea, xerostomia, increased LFTs, hepatotoxicity
CV: Edema, hypertension
META: Hypocalcaemia, hyponatremia, hyper/hypophosphatemia
HEMA: Decreased Hgb, neutropenia, lymphocytopenia, thrombocytopenia, hemorrhage
MS: MS pain
GU: Increased serum creatinine, UTI
RESP: Cough, pneumonia, pneumonitis
MISC: Fever, sepsis

INTERACTIONS
Decrease: Pralsetinib effect—CYP3A4 inducers, depending on if moderate or strong monitor or alter dose
Increase: Pralsetinib effect—Strong CYP3A4 inhibitors, avoid using together

NURSING CONSIDERATIONS
Assessment
- **Lung cancer:** Obtain RET gene fusion status, hepatitis B surface antigen (HBsAg), hepatitis B core antibody (anti-HBc), total Ig or IgG before starting treatment, treatment may start before results
- **Bone marrow suppression:** Monitor CBC with differential, platelets; anemia, lymphocytopenia, neutropenia, thrombocytopenia may occur
- **Bleeding/hemorrhage:** Monitor for bleeding/hemorrhage, including ≥3; permanently discontinue if severe
- **Hepatotoxicity:** Monitor LFTs baseline, q2wk × 3 months, then monthly; if elevated, dosage modification or discontinuation may be needed, evaluate RET gene status
- **Hypertension:** Monitor B/P baseline, after 1 wk and ≤ monthly thereafter; do not use in uncontrolled hypertension
- **Interstitial lung disease/pulmonary toxicity:** Monitor for dyspnea, cough, fever, fatigue; withhold pralsetinib, evaluate for interstitial lung disease
- **Poor wound healing:** Withhold ≥5 days before elective surgery; do not use ≥2 wk after major surgery and until after adequate wound healing. The safety of resuming pralsetinib treatment after resolution of wound healing complications has not been established
- Identify if propylene glycol is present in product used: Monitor for toxicity if large amounts are present in the product (lactic acidosis, respiratory changes, seizures)
- **Pregnancy/breastfeeding:** Obtain pregnancy testing before use in females of reproductive potential, do not use in pregnancy or breastfeeding; nonhormonal contraceptive should be used during and for ≥2 wk after last dose; males should use contraception during and for ≥1 wk after last dose in those with partners of reproductive potential

Patient problems
Ineffective breathing (uses)
Risk of injury (adverse reactions)

Patient/family education
- Advise patient to report immediately poor wound healing after surgery, increased trouble breathing, bloody sputum, other bleeding, cough, fever
- Advise patient to take 1 hr before or 2 hr after food; do not crush, chew, open capsule; take whole
- Liver dysfunction: Teach patient to report yellow skin/sclera, clay-colored stools, dark urine
- Teach patient if a dose is missed, take on the same day; resume the regular dosing next day, do not take another dose if vomiting occurs
- Teach patient to identify if pregnancy is planned or suspected, not to breastfeed, discuss needed contraception

Evaluation:
Positive therapeutic outcome: Decreasing spread of lung cancer

remdesivir (Rx)
(rem-de′si-vir)
Veklury
Func. class.: Antiviral
Chem. class.: RNA polymerase inhibitor

ACTION: Inhibits SARS-CoV-2 RNA-dependent RNA polymerase needed for viral replication

USES: COVID-19

Pharmacokinetics

Absorption	Unknown
Distribution	Protein binding 88%-93%
Metabolism	Extensively
Excretion	Urine 10%
Half-life	1 hr, up to 27 hr metabolites

Pharmacodynamics

Onset	1 hr
Peak	Unknown
Duration	Unknown

DOSAGE AND ROUTES

Adult/child ≥12 yr and 40 kg: IV: Patients requiring low-flow/high-flow supplemental O₂ or noninvasive ventilation: 200 mg (single dose) on day 1, then 100 mg daily × 4 days or until hospital discharge, whichever is first; may continue up to 10 days in those without improvement at day 5; may use monotherapy or with dexamethasone; **patients requiring invasive mechanical ventilation/extracorporeal membrane oxygenation:** 200 mg (single dose) on day 1, then 100 mg daily, duration varies; total duration is 5 days or hospital discharge, whichever is first; may continue up to 10 days in those without improvement at day 5

Child ≥12 yr/adolescent <40 kg: Lyophilized powder only: IV: Loading dose: 5 mg/kg/dose on day 1, then 2.5 mg/kg/dose daily; **≥40 kg: Injection solution/lyophilized powder: IV:** Loading dose: 200 mg on day 1, then 100 mg daily; **in those not requiring mechanical ventilation/extracorporeal membrane oxygenation** use for 5 days or until hospital discharge, whichever is first; may continue up to 10 days in those without improvement at day 5; **in those requiring mechanical ventilation/ECMO use** for 10 days or start with a 5-day course and extend to 10 days on a case-by-case basis

Infant/child <12 yr: Lyophilized powder only 3.5 kg to <40 kg: IV: Loading dose: 5 mg/kg/dose on day 1, then 2.5 mg/kg/dose daily; **≥40 kg: IV:** Loading dose: 200 mg on day 1, then 100 mg daily; **in those not requiring mechanical ventilation/extracorporeal membrane oxygenation** use for 5 days or until hospital discharge, whichever is first; may continue up to 10 days in those without improvement at day 5; **in those requiring mechanical ventilation/ECMO** use for 10 days or start with a 5-day course and extend to 10 days on a case-by-case basis

Available forms: IV solution (preservative free) 100 mg/20 mL, 100 mg; IV solution reconstituted 150 mg

CONTRAINDICATIONS

Hypersensitivity

Precautions: Breastfeeding, child <12 yr, dialysis, hepatic disease, infusion-related reactions, pregnancy, renal disease

> **BLACK BOX WARNING:** Remdesivir is not an approved treatment for COVID-19 caused by SARS-CoV-2, but is investigational and is available under an FDA emergency use authorization (EUA) for the treatment of COVID-19 in hospitalized patients only

ADVERSE EFFECTS

GI: Diarrhea, constipation, increased LFTs, nausea
RESP: Dyspnea, hypoxia, respiratory arrest, wheezing
CNS: Fever, headache, delirium, seizures, shivering
INTEG: Anaphylaxis, angioedema, infusion-related reactions, phlebitis, rash, ecchymosis
HEMA: Anemia
CV: Atrial fibrillation, bradycardia, hypo/hypertension, sinus tachycardia
ENDO: Hyperbilirubinemia, hyperglycemia, hypernatremia, hypokalemia
GU: Hematuria

INTERACTIONS: Hydroxychloroquine, chloroquine, strong CYP3A4 inducers: Decrease—remdesivir effect, avoid using together

NURSING CONSIDERATIONS
Assessment

• **COVID-19:** Confirm presence of COVID-19 before starting treatment; obtain CBC with differential, PT, and serum electrolytes before and during treatment
• **Hepatic effects:** Obtain LFTs before and during treatment; discontinue in ALT >10 × upper normal limit; discontinue if ALT elevation with signs/symptoms of liver inflammation occur
• **Hypersensitivity:** Monitor for infusion-related reactions, anaphylaxis, angioedema, diaphoresis, dyspnea, hypo/hypertension, hypoxia, fever, rash, shivering, tachycardia, wheezing; slow infusion rate to max infusion time: 120 min; discontinue and provide treatment if severe
• **Renal disease:** Obtain BUN/creatinine baseline and during treatment; monitor for hematuria; avoid use in eGFR <30 mL/min, significant toxicity with a short duration of therapy 5-10 days is unlikely
• **CV reactions:** Monitor for atrial fibrillation, hyper/hypotension, sinus tachycardia, bradycardia
• **Pregnancy/breastfeeding:** Identify if pregnant or if breastfeeding

Patient problems
Infection (uses)
Risk for injury (adverse reactions)

Implementation
Intermittent IV infusion route
• **Injection solution:** Warm to room temperature before dilution, further dilute in 250 mL NS; withdraw and discard the required volume of NS from the infusion bag (40 mL/200 mg ; 20 mL/100 mg) before addition of remdesivir,

transfer required volume of remdesivir to the infusion bag and invert to mix; do not shake. Discard unused portion of the injection solution vial
• **Lyophilized powder:** Reconstitute vial/19 mL SWFI; shake for 30 sec, allow to sit for 2-3 min, repeat until contents are dissolved (5 mg/mL); further dilute in 100-250 mL NS; withdraw and discard the required volume of NS from the infusion bag (40 mL/200 mg; 20 mL/100 mg) before adding remdesivir; transfer needed volume of remdesivir to the infusion bag and invert to mix. Discard unused portion
• Give over 30-120 min

Teach patient/family
• Teach patient reason for product and expected results
• Teach patient to report immediately to provider rash, itching, injection-site reactions, trouble breathing, shivering, wheezing, rapid heartbeat
• Provide "fact sheet" to patient/caregiver and review
• Advise patient that this product has not been approved by the FDA and has been granted for emergency use only

Evaluation
Positive therapeutic outcome: Resolution of COVID-19 without serious adverse reactions

remimazolam (Rx)
Byfavo
Func. class.: Sedative/anesthetic
Chem. class.: Benzodiazepine
Controlled substance: Schedule IV

ACTION: Binds to benzodiazepine sites in the brain

USES: Ultra-short-acting IV sedation for procedures lasting ≤30 min

CONTRAINDICATIONS
Hypersensitivity to this product, dextran 40; child <18 yr

Precautions: Pregnancy, lactation, elderly, severe hepatic disease, breastfeeding, dementia, labor, sleep apnea

> **BLACK BOX WARNING:** Requires a specialized care setting, requires an experienced clinician, respiratory depression

Pharmacokinetics

Absorption	Unknown
Distribution	Unknown
Metabolism	Unknown
Excretion	Unknown
Half-life	37-53 min

Pharmacodynamics

Onset	Immediate
Peak	3-3.5 min
Duration	Unknown

DOSAGE AND ROUTES
Adult: IV direct 5 mg over 1 min, maintenance doses of 2.5 mg over a 15-sec time period, ≥2 min before additional dose

Available forms: Lyophilized powder single use 20 mg (2.5 mg/mL)

ADVERSE EFFECTS
CV: Hypo/hypertension, bradycardia, tachycardia, hypoxia
RESP: Increased respiratory rate, respiratory depression
GI: Nausea
CNS: Fever, headache

INTERACTIONS: Other CNS depressants (opioid analgesics, other benzodiazepines, sedatives/hypnotics): Increased CNS depression

NURSING CONSIDERATIONS
Assessment

> **BLACK BOX WARNING:** Continuously monitor for hypotension, airway obstruction, hypoventilation, apnea, O_2 desaturation, hypoxia, bradycardia; adverse reactions are more common in sleep apnea, the elderly, ASA-PS III/IV patients; provide O_2 during recovery period, have flumazenil available during use; have emergency equipment, including resuscitative drugs, appropriate equipment for assisted ventilation available

• Continuously monitor vital signs during sedation and through the recovery period. Titrate the dose when giving with opioids, sedative/hypnotics, other CNS depressants

> **BLACK BOX WARNING:** Only those trained in the use of procedural sedation should give this product

> **BLACK BOX WARNING: CNS depressants:** Increased sedation and respiratory depression may occur with opioids, other sedative/hypnotics

• **Pregnancy/breastfeeding:** Avoid use in pregnancy and breastfeeding, if breastfeeding, consider pumping and discarding during treatment and for 5 hr after use

• **Hypersensitivity:** Assess for hypersensitivity (rash, urticaria, pruritus), do not use in those allergic to dextran 40
• **Hepatic disease:** Titrate carefully in hepatic disease

Patient problems
Risk for injury (adverse reactions)

Implementation
IV direct route
• Use strict aseptic technique
• This product does not contain preservative
• Protect vials from light after removed from packaging
• Each single-patient-use vial contains 20 mg lyophilized powder for reconstitution. The product must be prepared immediately before use
• To reconstitute, add 8.2 mL sterile 0.9% NaCl Injection, directing the stream of solution toward the wall of the vial. Swirl the vial (do not shake) until dissolved (final concentration of 2.5 mg/mL)
• Check for particulate matter and discoloration before use. The solution should be a clear, colorless-pale yellow, discard if particulate matter or discoloration is present
• If not used immediately, reconstituted solution may be stored up to 8 hr at room temperature at 20°C to 25°C (68°F to 77°F), after 8 hr, discard
• Do not admix

Solution compatibilities
• 0.9% NaCl, D5 Injection, D20 Injection, D5/0.45% NaCl, Ringer's

Patient/family education
• Reason for use and expected result
• **Pregnancy/breastfeeding:** To notify provider if pregnancy is suspected or if breastfeeding
• **Hypersensitivity:** To notify provider if allergic to dextran 40
• **CNS depressants:** To notify provider if taking other CNS depressants, alcohol
• To notify provider of sleep apnea, respiratory conditions

Evaluation
Positive therapeutic outcome: Sedation without adverse effects

---

rimegepant (Rx)
(ri-me′je-pant)
Nurtec ODT
Func. class.: Antimigraine agent
Chem. class.: Calcitonin gene–related peptide receptor antagonist

---

ACTION: Involved in transmission through second- and third-order neurons and pain modulation in the brainstem

USES: Acute treatment of migraine with or without aura

Absorption	Unknown
Distribution	Protein binding 96%
Metabolism	Unknown
Excretion	Unknown
Half-life	11 hr

Pharmacodynamics

Onset	≤2 hr
Peak	1.5 hr
Duration	48 hr

CONTRAINDICATIONS
Hypersensitivity

Precautions: Pregnancy, breastfeeding, hepatic/renal disease

DOSAGE AND ROUTES
Migraine
Adult: PO 75 mg as a single dose; max 75 mg/24 hr

Available forms: Tablet ODT 75 mg

ADVERSE EFFECTS
GI: Nausea
INTEG: Rash, hypersensitivity
RESP: Dyspnea

INTERACTIONS
CYP3A4 substrates: Increase—effect of these substrates
CYP3A4 inhibitors: Increase—rimegepant effect
CY3A4 inducers: Decrease—rimegepant effect

NURSING CONSIDERATIONS
Assessment
• **Migraine:** Baseline and periodically, presence of aura, nausea/vomiting
• Assess for hypersensitivity, rash, dyspnea; reaction may be delayed, discontinue if these occur
• Avoid use in hepatic/renal disease

Patient problem
Pain (uses)

Implementation
• Peel foil covering blister to remove tablet with dry hands. Do not push tablet through the foil
• Place tablet on or under tongue, allow to dissolve
• Can be swallowed without additional fluids
• Store at 20°C to 25°C (68°F to 77°F)

Patient/family education
• Teach patient reason for product and expected result
• Identify if pregnancy is planned or suspected

Evaluation
Positive therapeutic outcome: Resolution of migraine

ripretinib (Rx)
(rip-re'ti-nib)
Qinlock
Func. class.: Antineoplastic, tyrosine kinase inhibitor

USES: Treatment of advanced gastrointestinal stromal tumor (GIST) in those who have received ≥3 kinase inhibitors, including imatinib

CONTRAINDICATIONS
Hypersensitivity, pregnancy, breastfeeding

DOSAGE AND ROUTES
Adult: PO 150 mg daily until disease progression or unacceptable toxicity

risdiplam (Rx)
(ris-dip'lam)
Evrysdi
Func. class.: Spinal muscular atrophy agent

USES: Treatment of spinal muscular atrophy in children ≥2 mo

CONTRAINDICATIONS
Hypersensitivity

DOSAGE AND ROUTES
Spinal muscular atrophy
Child ≥2 mo: PO 5 mg daily

sacituzumab govitecan-hziy (Rx)
(sak'i-tooz'ue-mab goe'vi-tee'kan)
Trodelvy
Func. class.: Antineoplastic-anti-trop-2

USES: Treatment of metastatic triple-negative breast cancer in those who have received ≥2 other therapies

CONTRAINDICATIONS
Hypersensitivity, pregnancy, breastfeeding

DOSAGE AND ROUTES
Adult: IV: 10 mg/kg on days 1 and 8 of a 21-day cycle; continue until disease progression or unacceptable toxicity

selumetinib (Rx)
(sel'ue-me'ti-nib)
Koselugo
Func. class.: Antineoplastic

USES: Treatment of neurofibromatosis type 1 in children ≥2 yr

CONTRAINDICATIONS
Hypersensitivity, pregnancy, breastfeeding

DOSAGE AND ROUTES
See manufacturer's information. Dose based on BSA

somapacitin-beco (Rx)
(soe'ma-pas'i-tan)
Sogroya
Func. class.: Growth hormone

USES: Growth hormone deficiency

CONTRAINDICATIONS
Hypersensitivity, open heart/abdominal surgery, trauma; respiratory failure; malignancy; diabetic retinopathy

DOSAGE AND ROUTES
Growth hormone deficiency
Adult: SUBCUT 1.5 mg weekly; may increase by 0.5-1.5 mg/wk q2-4wk based on response, max 8 mg/wk

tazemetostat (Rx)
(taz'e-met'oh-stat)
Tazverik
Func. class.: Antineoplastic

USES: Epithelioid sarcoma, metastatic/locally advanced, follicular lymphoma, relapsed/refractory

CONTRAINDICATIONS
Hypersensitivity

DOSAGE AND ROUTES
Adult: PO 800 mg bid until disease progression or unacceptable toxicity

teprotumumab-trbw (Rx)
(tep'roe-toom'ue-mab)
Tepezza
Func. class.: Insulin-like growth factor-1 antagonist

USES: Treatment of thyroid eye disease

CONTRAINDICATIONS
Hypersensitivity

DOSAGE AND ROUTES
Thyroid eye disease
Adult: IV: 10 mg/kg as a single dose, then 20 mg/kg q3wk × 7 more doses

tucatinib (Rx)

(too-ka'ti-nib)
Tukysa
Func. class.: Antineoplastic

USES: Breast cancer, human epidermal growth factor receptor 2 positive, advanced unresectable/metastatic

CONTRAINDICATIONS

Hypersensitivity, pregnancy, breastfeeding

DOSAGE AND ROUTES

Adult: PO 300 mg bid with trastuzumab and capecitabine until disease progression or unacceptable toxicity

vibegron (Rx)

(vye-beg'-ron)
Gemtesa
Func. class.: Beta-3 adrenergic agonist

USES: Overactive bladder

CONTRAINDICATIONS

Hypersensitivity

DOSAGE AND ROUTES

Adult: PO 75 mg tablet daily

viltolarsen (Rx)

(vil'toe-lar'sen)
Viltepso
Func. class.: Muscular dystrophy agent, antisense oligonucleotide

USES: Treatment of Duchenne muscular dystrophy with a mutation of the DMD gene with exon 53 skipping

CONTRAINDICATIONS

Hypersensitivity

DOSAGE AND ROUTES

Duchenne muscular dystrophy
Child/adolescent: IV: 80 mg/kg/dose weekly

- Does the patient have any allergies?
- Is the patient NPO?
- Is the patient taking any other medication and/or herbal supplements that may interact with this drug?
- Are there any vital signs that I need to check before administering the drug?
- Do I need to check any lab values (i.e., glucose)?
- Are there any other assessments that I need to make before giving this drug?

The 5 rights of medication administration

Always adhere to the 5 rights of medication administration when transcribing, preparing, administering, and documenting medications:

1. **Right patient:** Compare the patient's armband with the medication administration record. Compare the patient's name on the medication administration record (MAR) with that on the medication drawer or computerized equipment.
2. **Right drug:** Verify the correct medication by comparing the name on the label on the drug container with that written on the MAR.
3. **Right route:** Check the ordered route by reading the medication order, and verify the appropriateness of the route based on knowledge of the patient's condition.
4. **Right dose:** Always independently double-check dosages of medications with the pharmacy's calculations or with a second nurse. The nurse must also be aware of therapeutic dosages for each medication and question an order that is not within that range.
5. **Right time:** All medications should be administered within 30 minutes of the scheduled time. The medications must also be prepared to correlate appropriately with meal times and to avoid drug interactions.

Following appropriate drug administration, assess the patient for the expected therapeutic outcome and/or potential side effects.

Nomogram for Calculation of Body Surface Area

Place a straight edge from the patient's height in the left column to his or her weight in the right column. The point of intersection on the body surface area column indicates the body surface area (BSA). (Reproduced in Behrman RE, Kliegman RM, Jenson HB: *Nelson Textbook of Pediatrics,* ed 18, Philadelphia, 2007, WB Saunders; nomogram modified from data of E. Boyd by CD West.)

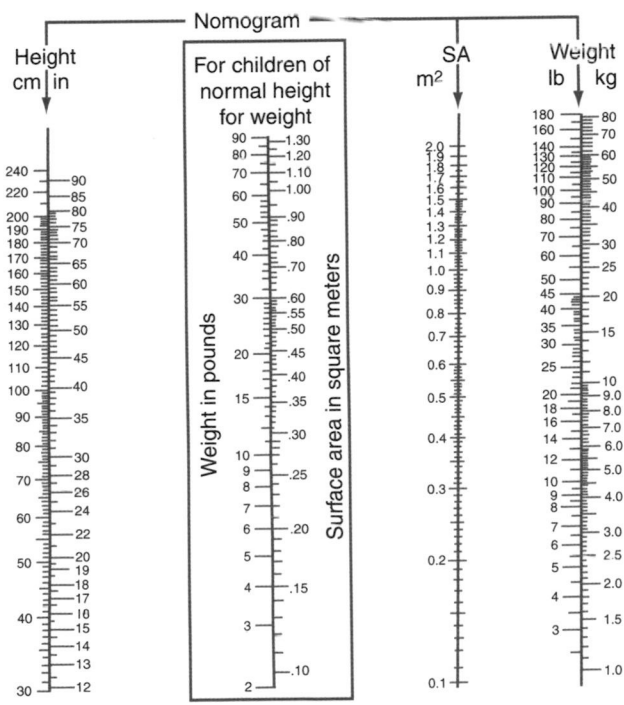

Alternative (Mosteller's formula):

$$\text{Surface area (m}^2) = \sqrt{\frac{\text{Height (cm)} \times \text{Weight (kg)}}{3600}}$$

Surface area rule:

$$\text{Child dose} = \frac{\text{Surface area (m}^2) \times \text{Adult dose}}{1.73 \text{ m}^2}$$

BMI formula:

$$\text{BMI} = \frac{\text{Weight (kg)}}{\text{Height (m}^2)}$$

Syringe Compatibility

	Atropine	Buprenorphine	Butorphanol	ChlorproMAZINE	Codeine	Diazepam	DimenhyDRINATE	DiphenhydrAMINE	Droperidol	Fentanyl	Glycopyrrolate	Heparin
Atropine	■		C	C		I	C	C	C	C	C	
Buprenorphine		■										
Butorphanol	C		■	C		I	I	C	C	C		
ChlorproMAZINE	C		C	■		I	I	C	C	C	C	C
Codeine					■	I						
Diazepam	I		I	I	I	■	I	I	I	I	I	
DimenhyDRINATE	C		I	I		I	■	C	C	C	I	
DiphenhydrAMINE	C		C	C		I	C	■	C	C	C	
Droperidol	C		C	C		I	C	C	■	C	C	I
Fentanyl	C		C	C		I	C	C	C	■	C	
Glycopyrrolate	C			C		I	I	C	C	C	■	
Heparin			I	C		I		I				■
HydrOXYzine	C		C	C		I	I	C	C	C		
Meperidine	C		C	C		I	C	C	C	C	C	I
Metoclopramide	C		C	C		I	C	C	C	C		
Midazolam	C		C	C		I	C	C	C	C		
Morphine	C		C	C		I	C	C	C	C	C	I
Nalbuphine	C					I		C				
Pentazocine	C		C	C		I	C	C	C	C	I	I
Pentobarbital	C		I	I	I	I	I	I	I	I	I	
Perphenazine	C		C	C		I	C	C	C	C		
Prochlorperazine	C		C	C		I	I	C	C	C	C	
Promazine	C			C		I	I	C	C	C	C	
Promethazine	C		C	C		I	I	C	C	C	C	
Ranitidine	C			C			C	C		C	C	
Scopolamine Hbr	C		C	C		I	C	C	C	C	C	
Secobarbital	I		I	I	I	I	I	I	I	I	I	
Thiethylperazine			C			I						

Developed by Providence Memorial Hospital, El Paso, Texas.
NOTE: Give within 15 minutes of mixing.
C = compatible; I = incompatible; ☐ = no documented information.
* = compatibility depends on manufacturer, Wyeth and DuPont forms are incompatible.